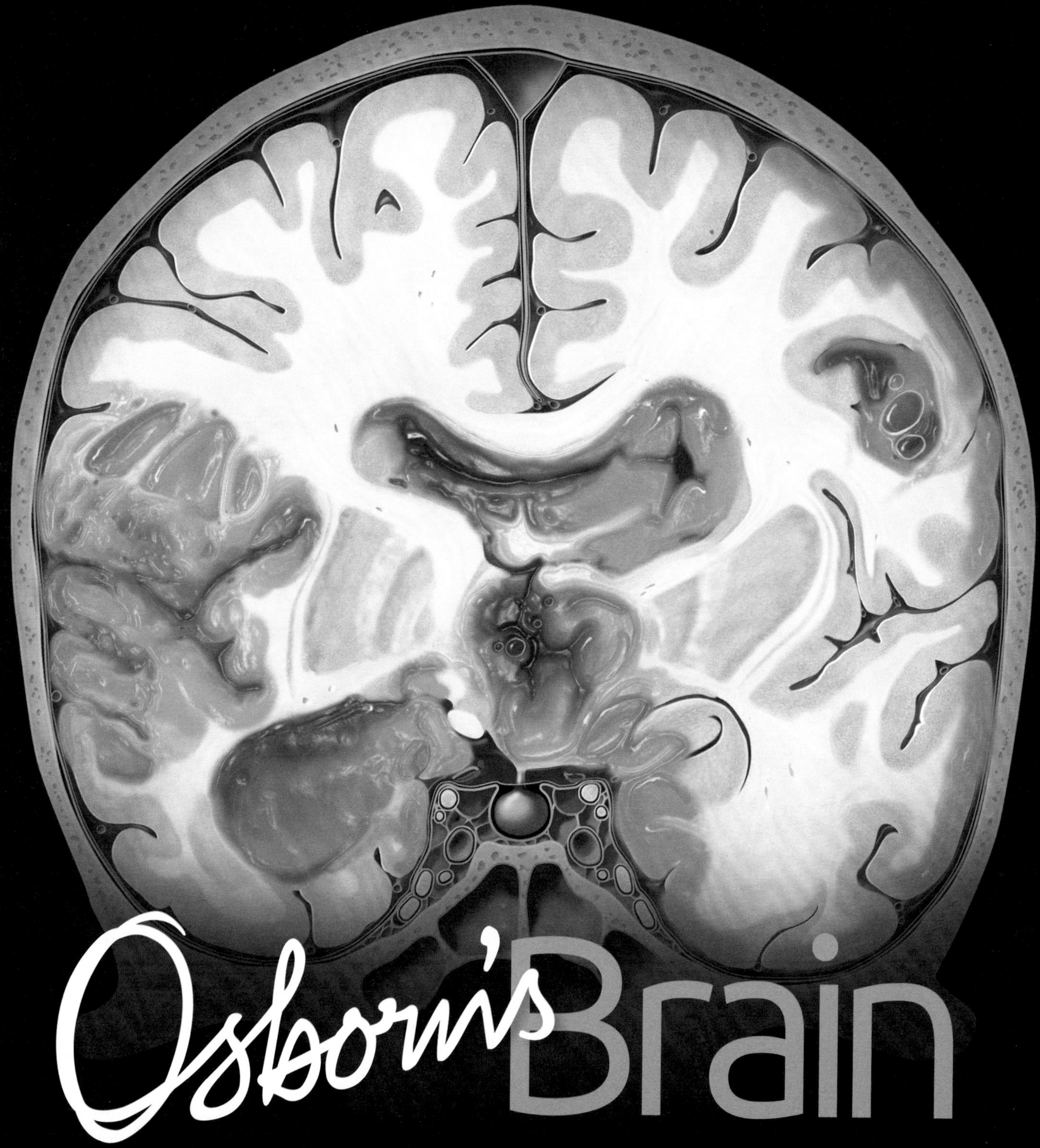

# Osborn's Brain

## IMAGING, PATHOLOGY, AND ANATOMY

THIRD EDITION

Anne G. Osborn

Salzman | Linscott

ELSEVIER

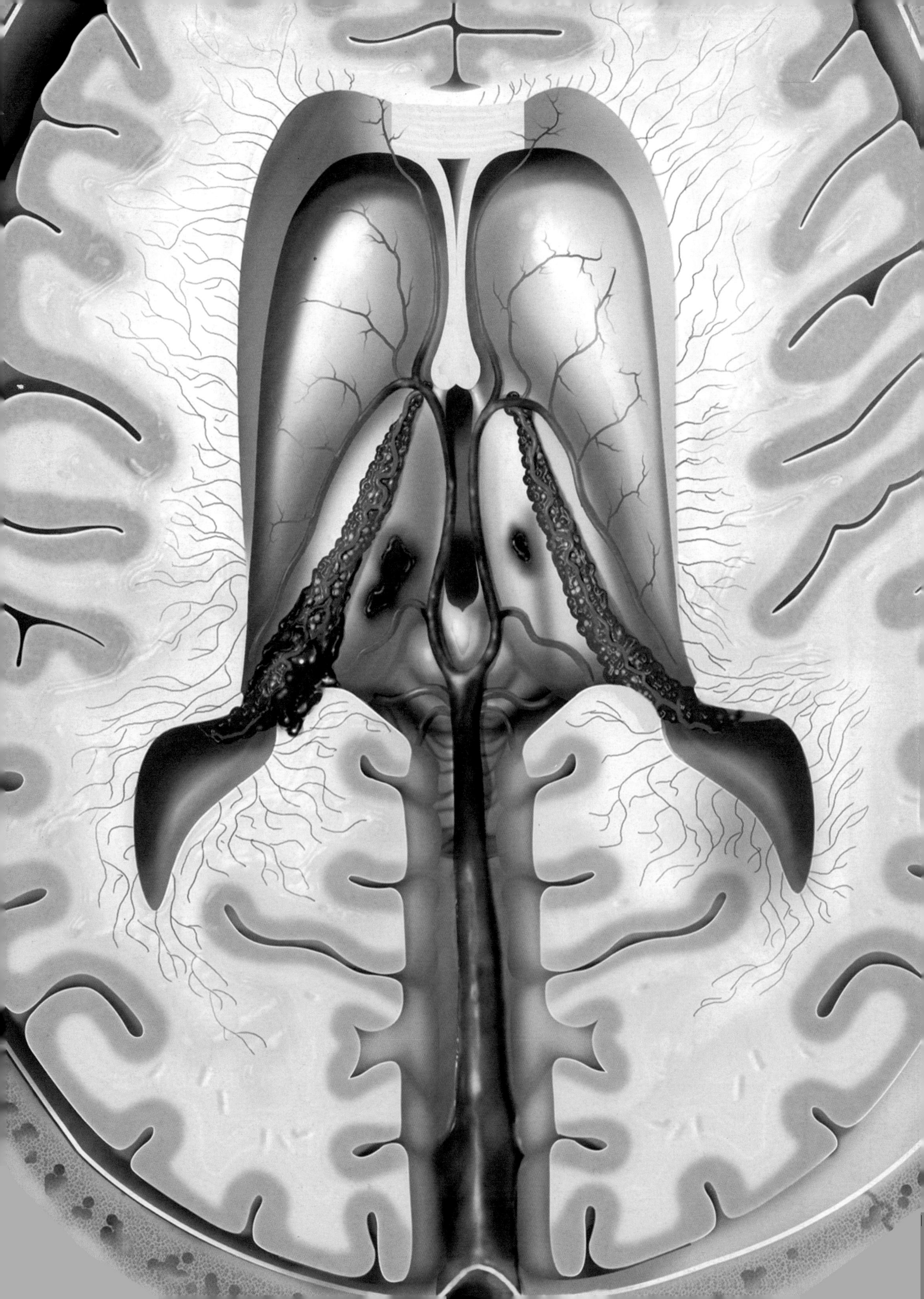

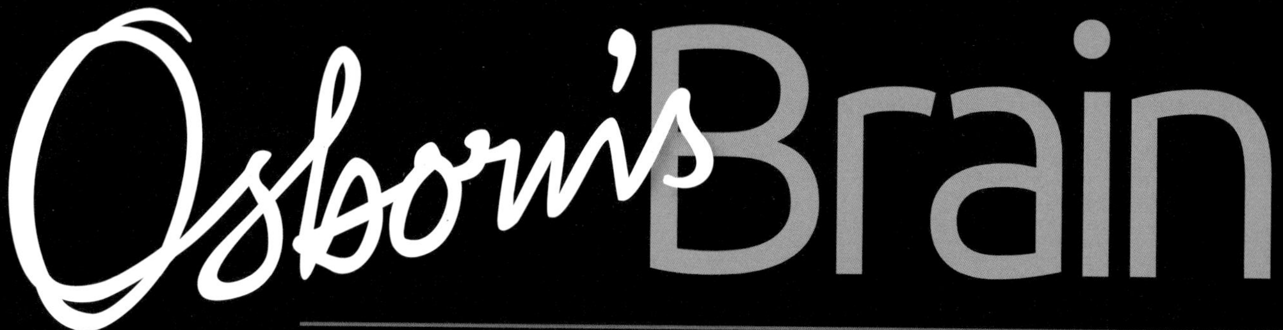


IMAGING, PATHOLOGY, AND ANATOMY

THIRD EDITION

**Anne G. Osborn, MD, FACR**
University Distinguished Professor and Professor of Radiology and Imaging Sciences
William H. and Patricia W. Child Presidential Endowed Chair in Radiology
University of Utah School of Medicine
Salt Lake City, Utah

**Karen L. Salzman, MD, FACR**
Professor of Radiology and Imaging Sciences
Neuroradiology Section Chief and Associate Fellowship Director
Leslie W. Davis Endowed Chair in Neuroradiology
University of Utah School of Medicine
Salt Lake City, Utah

**Luke L. Linscott, MD**
Pediatric Neuroradiologist
Vice Chair, Department of Medical Imaging
Primary Children's Hospital
Salt Lake City, Utah

Elsevier
1600 John F. Kennedy Blvd.
Ste 1800
Philadelphia, PA 19103-2899

OSBORN'S BRAIN, THIRD EDITION

ISBN: 978-0-443-10937-9



**Notices**

Practitioners and researchers must always rely on their own experience and knowledge in evaluating and using any information, methods, compounds or experiments described herein. Because of rapid advances in the medical sciences, in particular, independent verification of diagnoses and drug dosages should be made. To the fullest extent of the law, no responsibility is assumed by Elsevier, authors, editors or contributors for any injury and/or damage to persons or property as a matter of products liability, negligence or otherwise, or from any use or operation of any methods, products, instructions, or ideas contained in the material herein.

Previous edition copyrighted 2018.

**Library of Congress Control Number: 2023945203**

*Printed in Canada by Friesens, Altona, Manitoba, Canada*

**Last digit is the print number:** 9 8 7 6 5 4 3 2 1

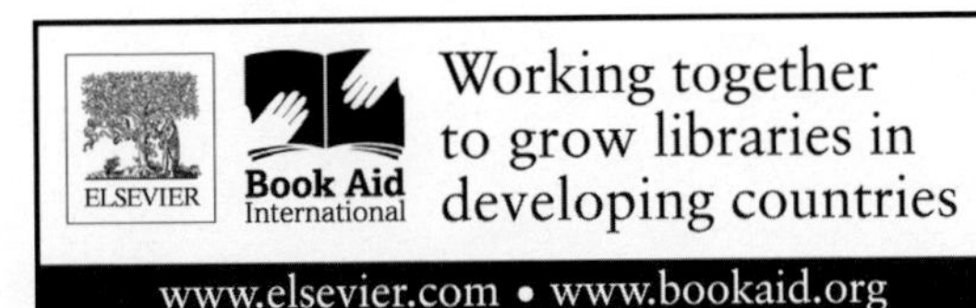

# DEDICATIONS

*FOR THE LATE DR. RICHARD HEWLETT*
*Neuropathologist and neuroradiologist extraordinaire…you are no longer with us, but you taught me the importance of really understanding pathology as the essential foundation of imaging. Thank you.*

**AGO**

*To the loves and lights of my life: Sophia, Aubrey, Ian, and Craig.*

**KLS**

*Enormous thanks to Anne Osborn, who has mentored me throughout my career ever since I was a young medical student. It is an honor and privilege for me to be a part of this impressive text!*

*So many thanks to my wife, Carrie, for her unfailing love and support, especially in the midst of the craziness of writing and editing! Thanks to my children, Abby, Katie, Alex, and Sarah, who sacrificed some fun time with Dad so I could help make this book happen.*

*Thanks to my parents for their love and support. My late father showed me how to find great satisfaction in the world of medicine and in sharing all that we've discovered with our friends and colleagues.*

**LLL**

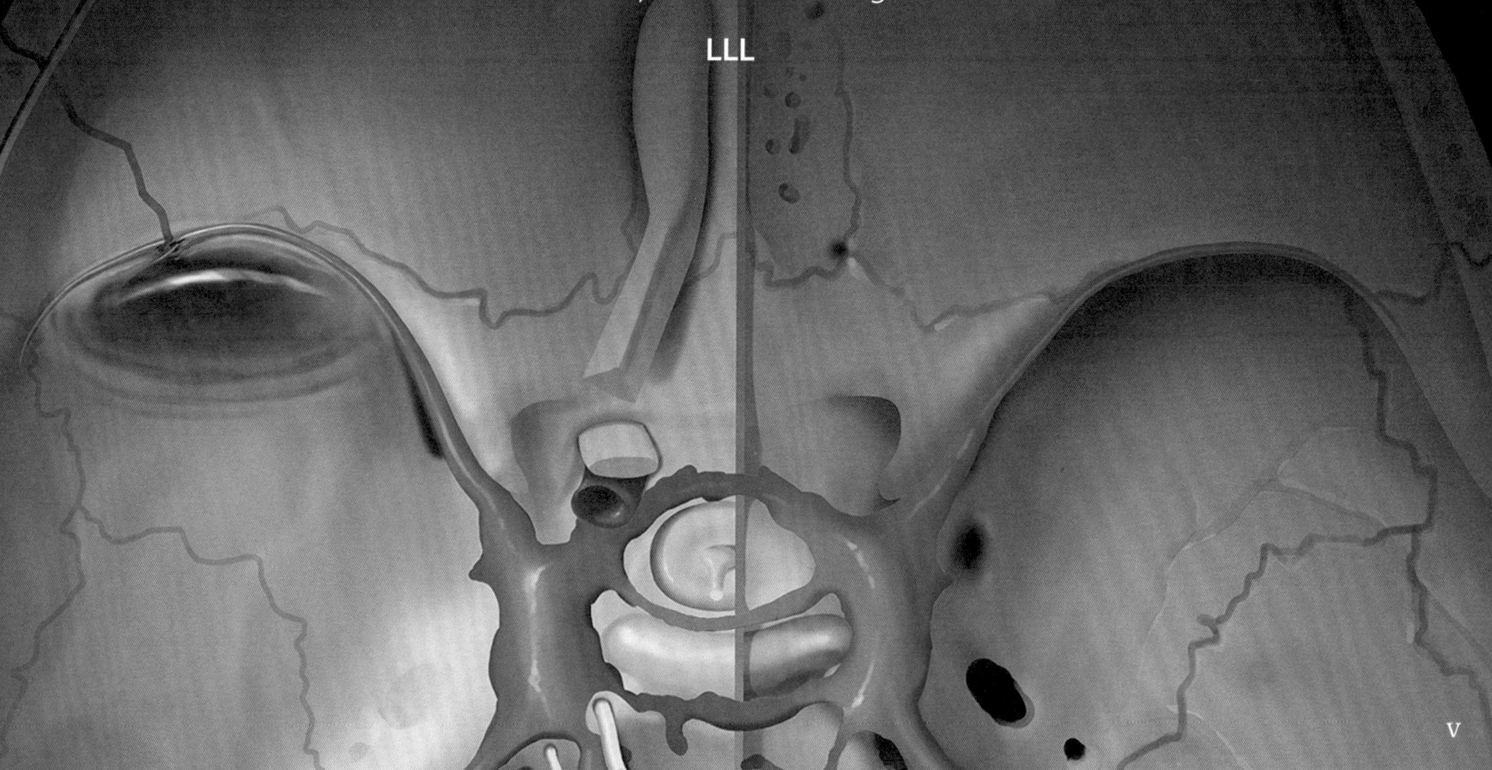

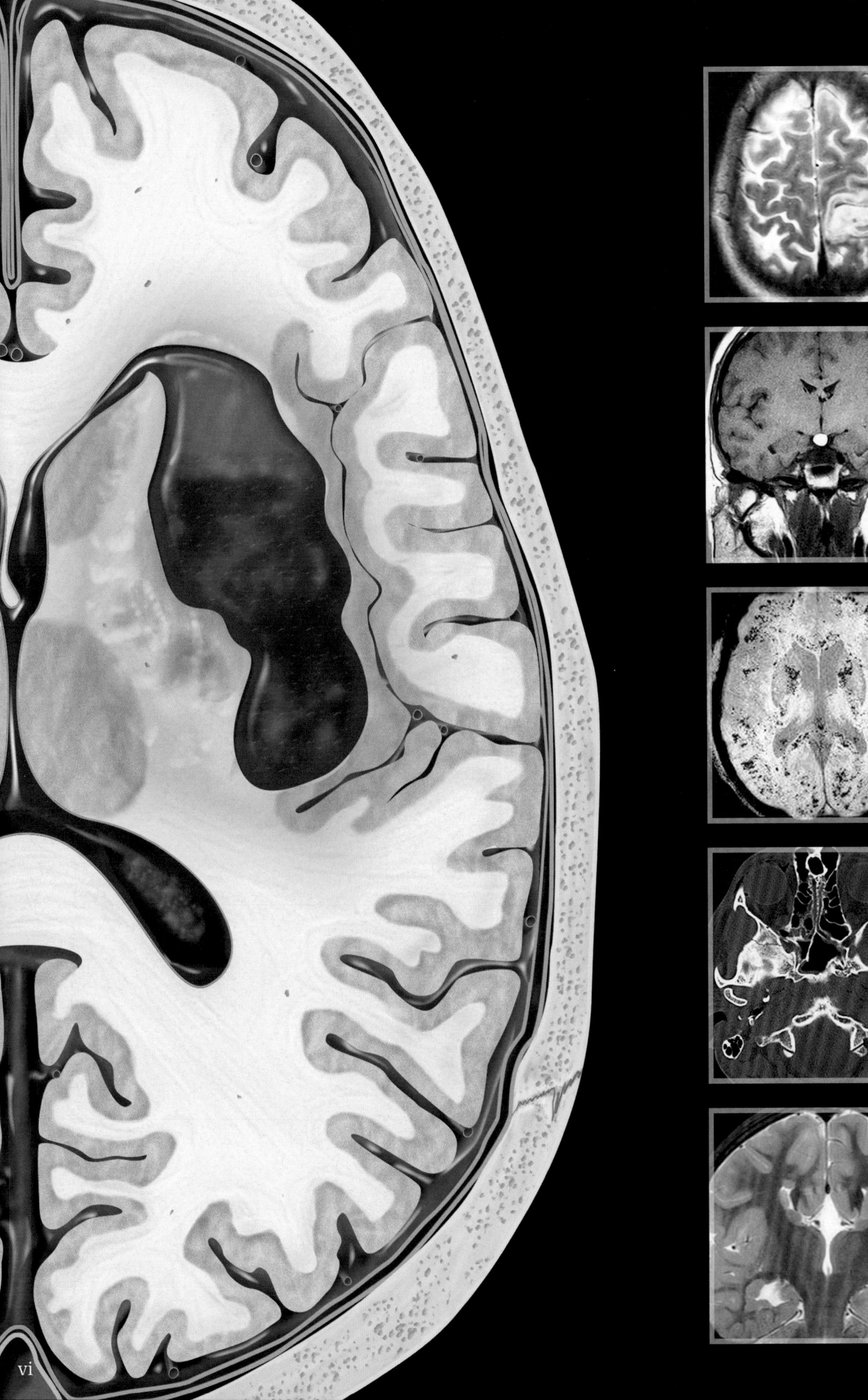

# PREFACE

It's hard to believe five years have passed by so quickly since the second edition of *Osborn's Brain* came off the press. With each passing edition, we mark some really significant changes in neuroradiology. We've made major changes in the new third edition to reflect publication of the *WHO Classification of Tumours: Central Nervous System Tumours*, fifth edition, in late 2021. Make no mistake about it—this is a landmark publication that enshrines molecular pathology as *the* essential information for diagnosis and treatment of CNS neoplasms. Accordingly, we've almost entirely reorganized, rewritten, and greatly expanded the tumors section of *Osborn's Brain* to reflect the updated WHO classification. I think you'll find it fascinating...knowing this stuff is absolutely required reading for neuroradiologists. I also highly recommend getting your own copy of the WHO "Blue Book" by going to https://publications.iarc.fr and buying the print book or subscribing online.

For those of you who are new to *Osborn's Brain*, the "must know—now!" topics, such as brain trauma, stroke, and brain bleeds, are always covered in the first few chapters. As with the first two editions, this book is image rich with hundreds of color graphics and gross pathology examples that inform the thousands of new, up-to-date images we've included. New in the third edition is the addition of a digital image gallery at the end of most chapters. We've included lots of additional images that will enrich your chapter reading.

Lastly, a comment about AI. As of this writing, we're just beginning to see its impact in our lives and in our beloved profession. I personally believe it won't replace us but will make our lives easier, intellectually richer, and even more fascinating than they already are. Will it make authoring texts like this obsolete? It might. But it also will likely make it a lot more fun. Personally, I plan to stick around and watch stuff unfold. See you in a few years for the fourth edition. Or, then again, maybe not...

**Anne G. Osborn, MD, FACR**
University Distinguished Professor and Professor of Radiology and Imaging Sciences
William H. and Patricia W. Child Presidential Endowed Chair in Radiology
University of Utah School of Medicine
Salt Lake City, Utah

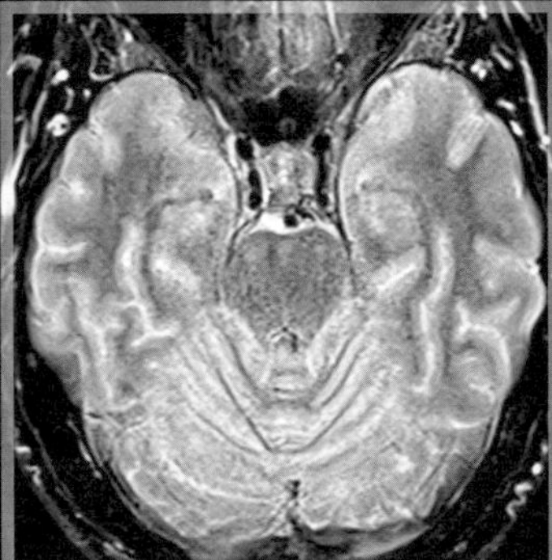

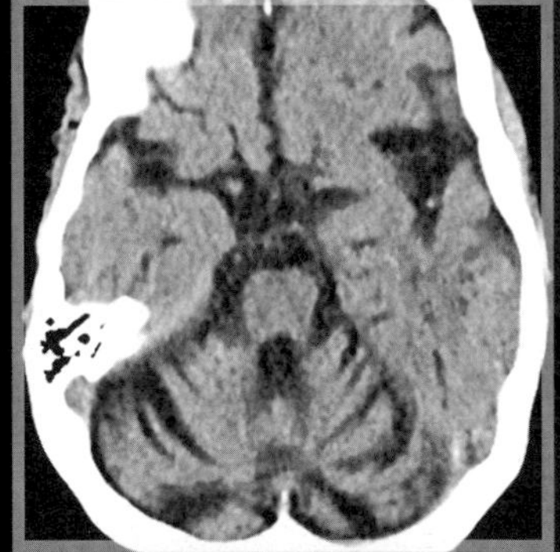

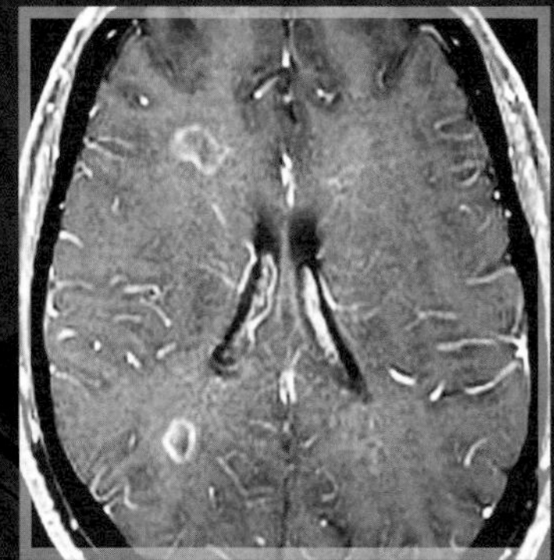

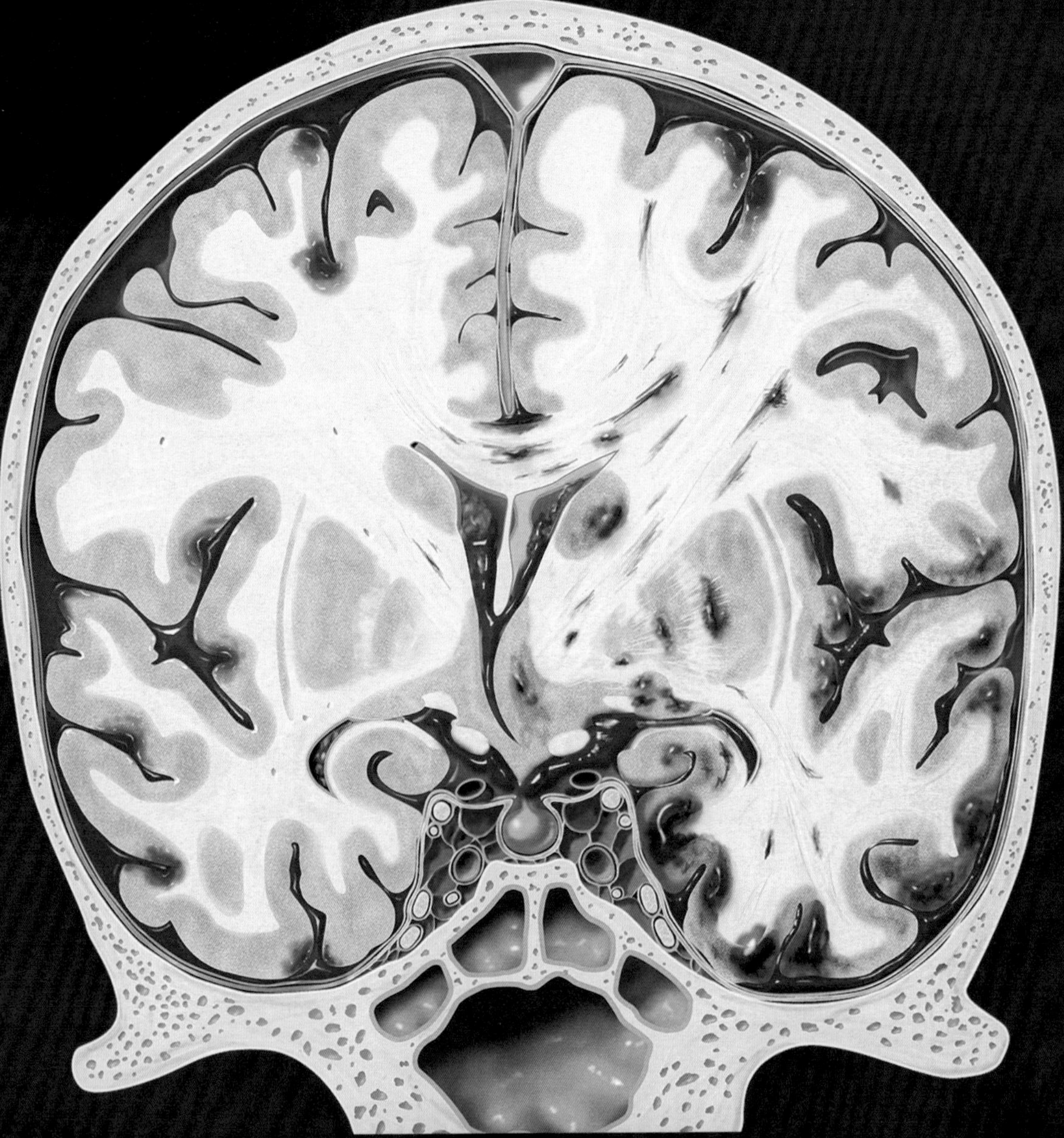

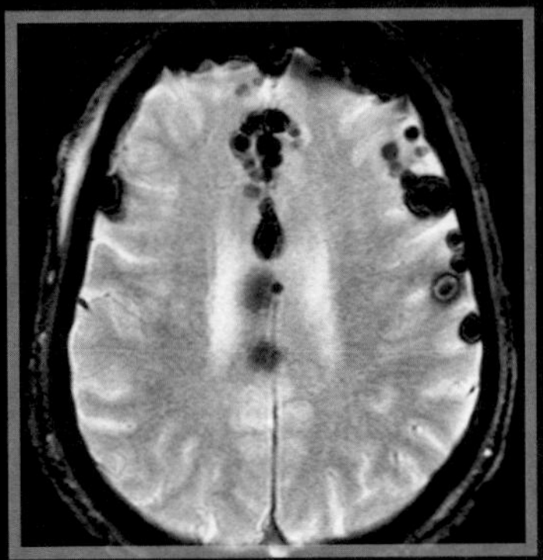
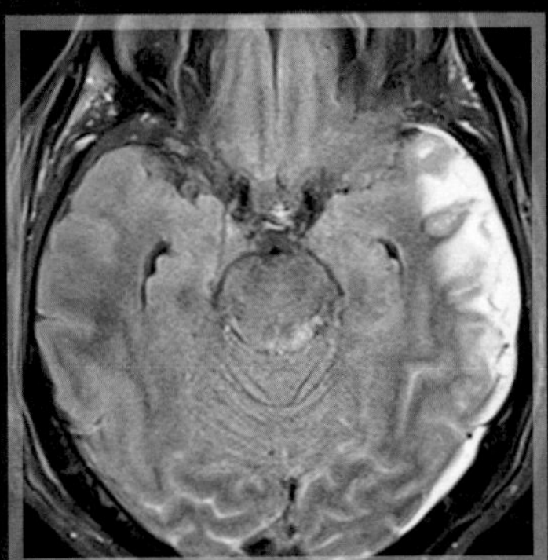
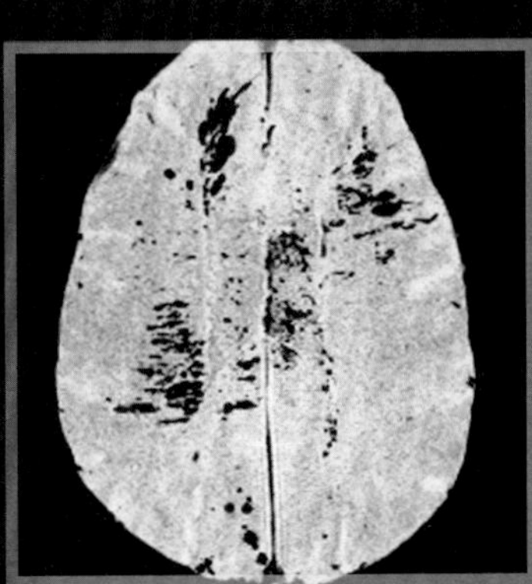

# IMAGE CONTRIBUTORS

AFIP Archives
D. P. Agamanolis, MD
N. Agarwal, MD
J. Ardyn, MD
M. Ayadi, MD
S. Aydin, MD
D. Bertholdo, MD
S. Blaser, MD
J. Boxerman, MD
M. Brant-Zawadski, MD
P. Burger, MD
S. Candy, MD
M. Castillo, MD
P. Chapman, MD
L. Chimelli, MD
S. Chung, MD
M. Colombo, MD
J. Comstock, MD
J. Curé, MD
B. Czerniak, MD
A. Datir, MD
B. N. Delman, MD
B. K. DeMasters, MD
K. Digre, MD
H. D. Dorfman, MD
M. Edwards-Brown, MD
D. Ellison, MD
H. Els, MD
A. Ersen, MD
W. Fang, MD
N. Foster, MD
C. E. Fuller, MD
S. Galetta, MD
C. Glastonbury, MBBS
S. Harder, MD
H. R. Harnsberger, MD
B. Hart, MD
E. T. Hedley-Whyte, MD
G. Hedlund, DO
R. Hewlett, MD
P. Hildenbrand, MD
C. Y. Ho, MD
B. Horten, MD
C. Hsu, MD
M. Huckman, MD
P. Hudgins, MD
A. Illner, MD
B. Jones, MD
J. A. Junker, MD
E. C. Klatt, MD
D. Kremens, MD
W. Kucharczyk, MD
P. Lasjaunias, MD
S. Lincoff, MD
T. Markel, MD
M. Martin, MD
A. Maydell, MD
S. McNally, MD
T. Mentzel, MD
C. Merrow, MD
M. Michel, MD
K. Moore, MD
S. Nagi, MD
T. P. Naidich, MD
N. Nakase, MD
S. Narendra, MD
K. Nelson, MD
R. Nguyen, MD
G. P. Nielsen, MD
M. Nielsen, MS
K. K. Oguz, MD
J. P. O'Malley, MD
N. Omar, MD
J. Paltan, MD
G. Parker, MD
T. Poussaint, MD
R. Ramakantan, MD
C. Rambaud, MD
M. L. Rivera-Zengotita, MD
C. Robson, MBChB
F. J. Rodriguez, MD
P. Rodriguez, MD
A. Rosenberg, MD
E. Ross, MD
A. Rossi, MD
L. Rourke, MD
Rubinstein Collection, AFIP Archives
E. Rushing, MD
M. Sage, MD
B. Scheithauer, MD
P. Shannon, MD
A. Sillag, MD
E. T. Tali, MD
M. Thurnher, MD
T. Tihan, MD
K. Tong, MD
J. Townsend, MD
University of Utah Dept. of Dermatology
S. van der Westhuizen, MD
M. Warmuth-Metz, MD
T. Winters, MD
A. T. Yachnis, MD
S. Yashar, MD

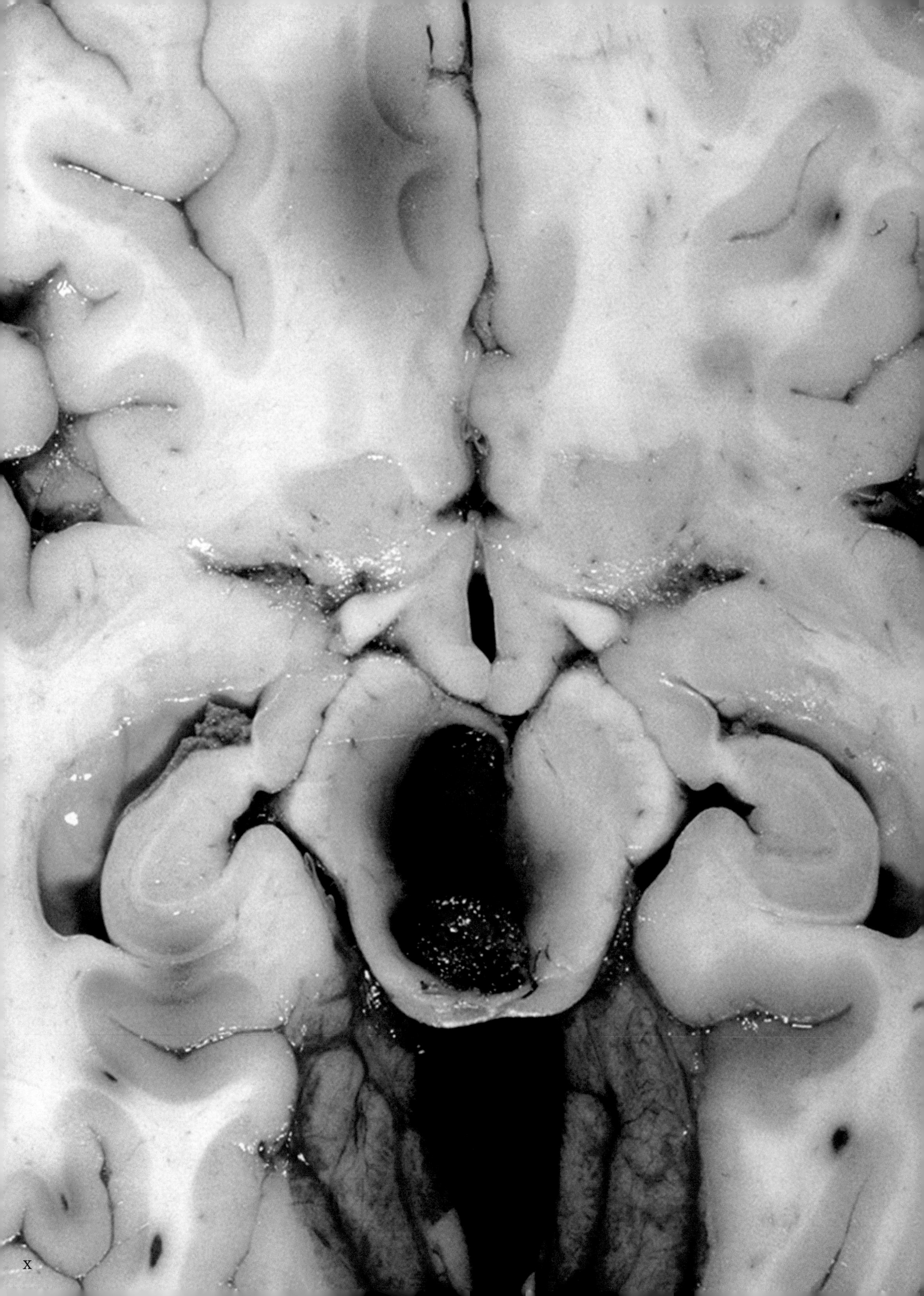

# ACKNOWLEDGMENTS


LEAD EDITORS
**Rebecca L. Bluth, BA**
**Kathryn Watkins, BA**

LEAD ILLUSTRATOR
**Lane R. Bennion, MS**

TEXT EDITORS
**Arthur G. Gelsinger, MA**
**Nina Themann, BA**
**Terry W. Ferrell, MS**
**Megg Morin, BA**
**Shannon Kelly, MA**

ILLUSTRATIONS
**James A. Cooper, MD**
**Richard Coombs, MS**
**Laura C. Wissler, MA**

IMAGE EDITORS
**Jeffrey J. Marmorstone, BS**
**Lisa A. M. Steadman, BS**

ART DIRECTION AND DESIGN
**Cindy Lin, BFA**

PRODUCTION EDITORS
**Emily C. Fassett, BA**
**John Pecorelli, BS**


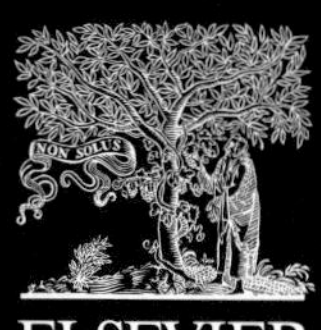

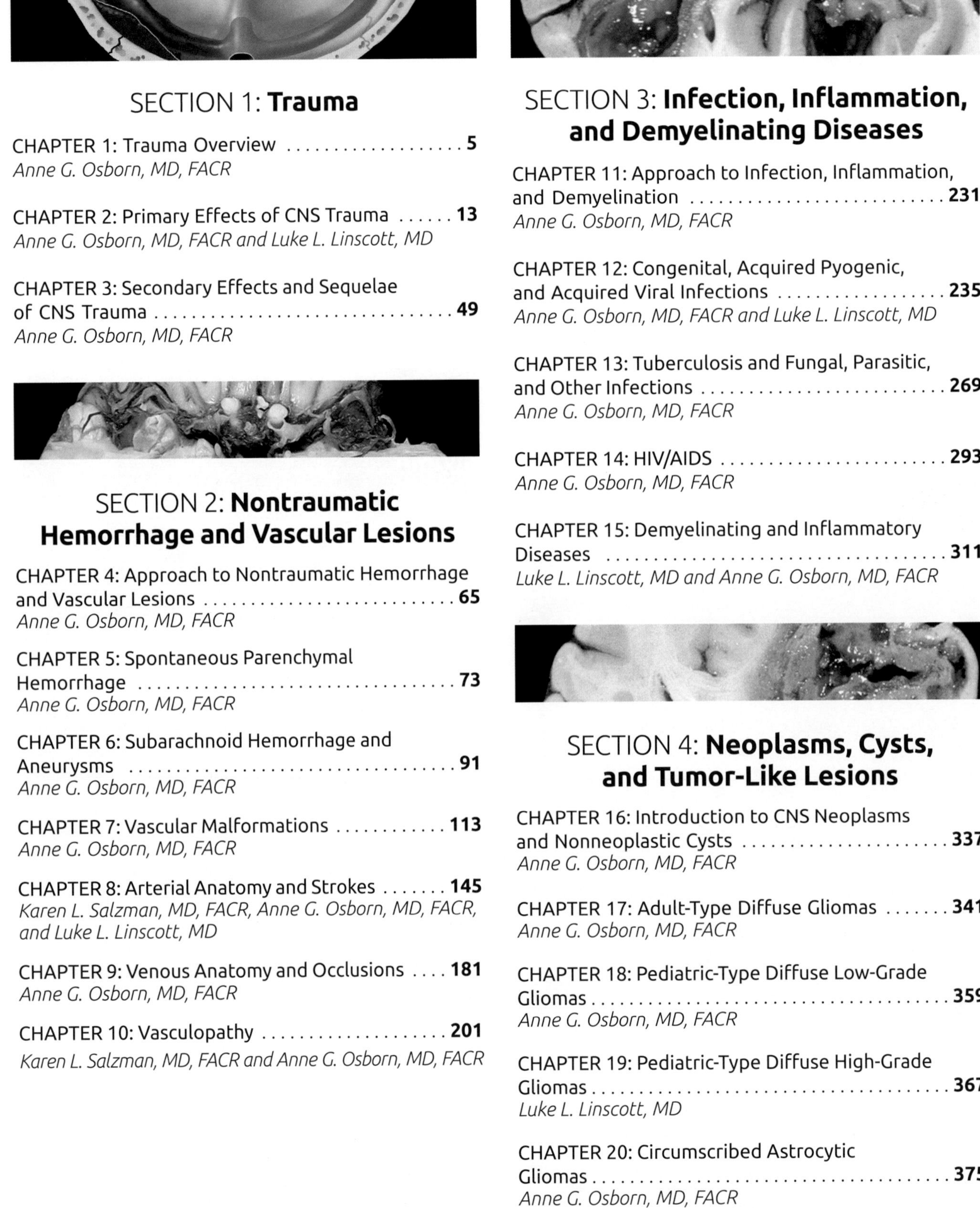

## SECTION 1: **Trauma**



## SECTION 2: **Nontraumatic Hemorrhage and Vascular Lesions**



## SECTION 3: **Infection, Inflammation, and Demyelinating Diseases**



## SECTION 4: **Neoplasms, Cysts, and Tumor-Like Lesions**

## SECTION 5: **Toxic, Metabolic, Degenerative, and CSF Disorders**



## SECTION 6: **Congenital Malformations and Genetic Tumor Syndromes**

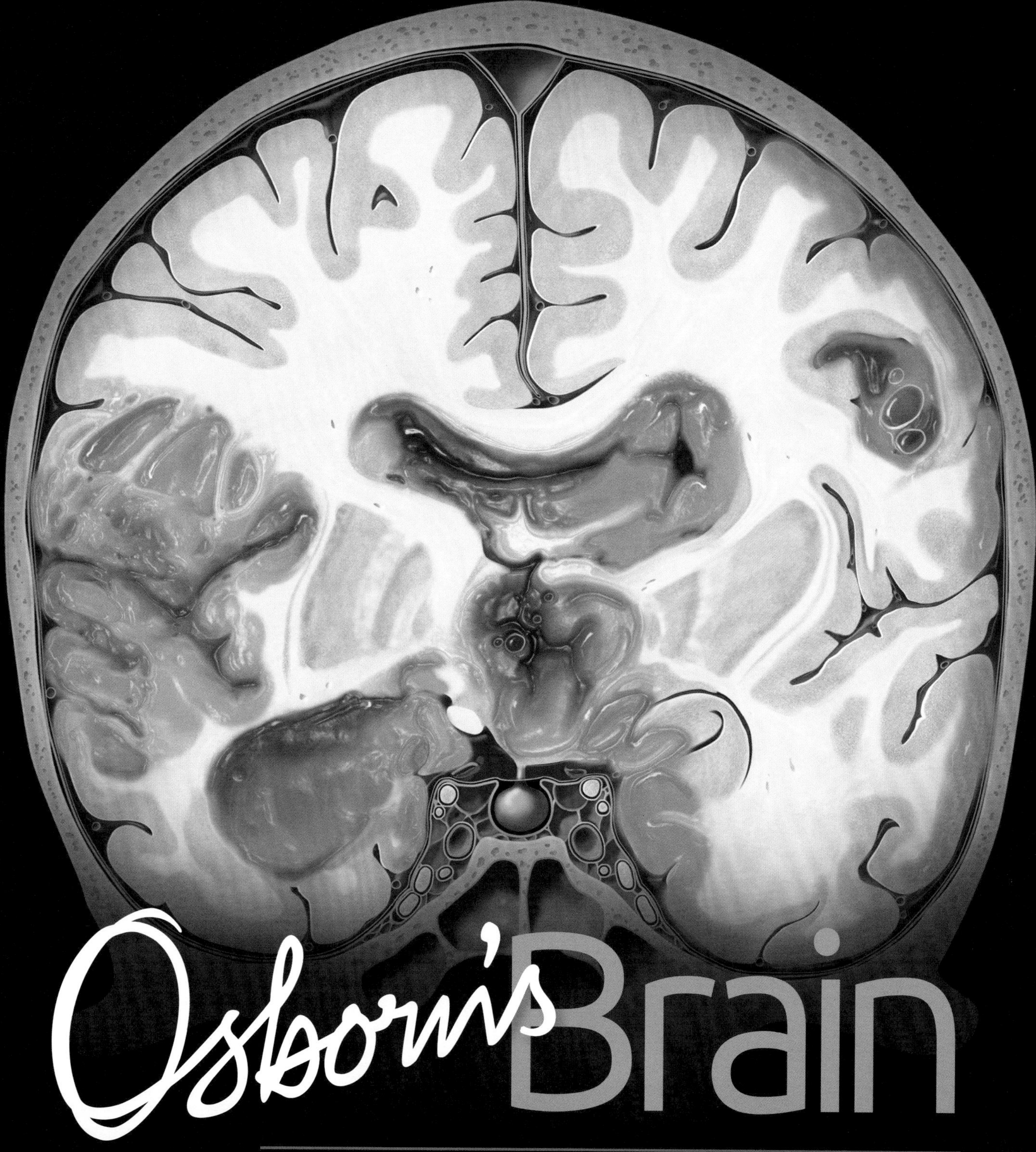

# Osborn's Brain

IMAGING, PATHOLOGY, AND ANATOMY

THIRD EDITION

Anne G. Osborn

Salzman | Linscott

ELSEVIER

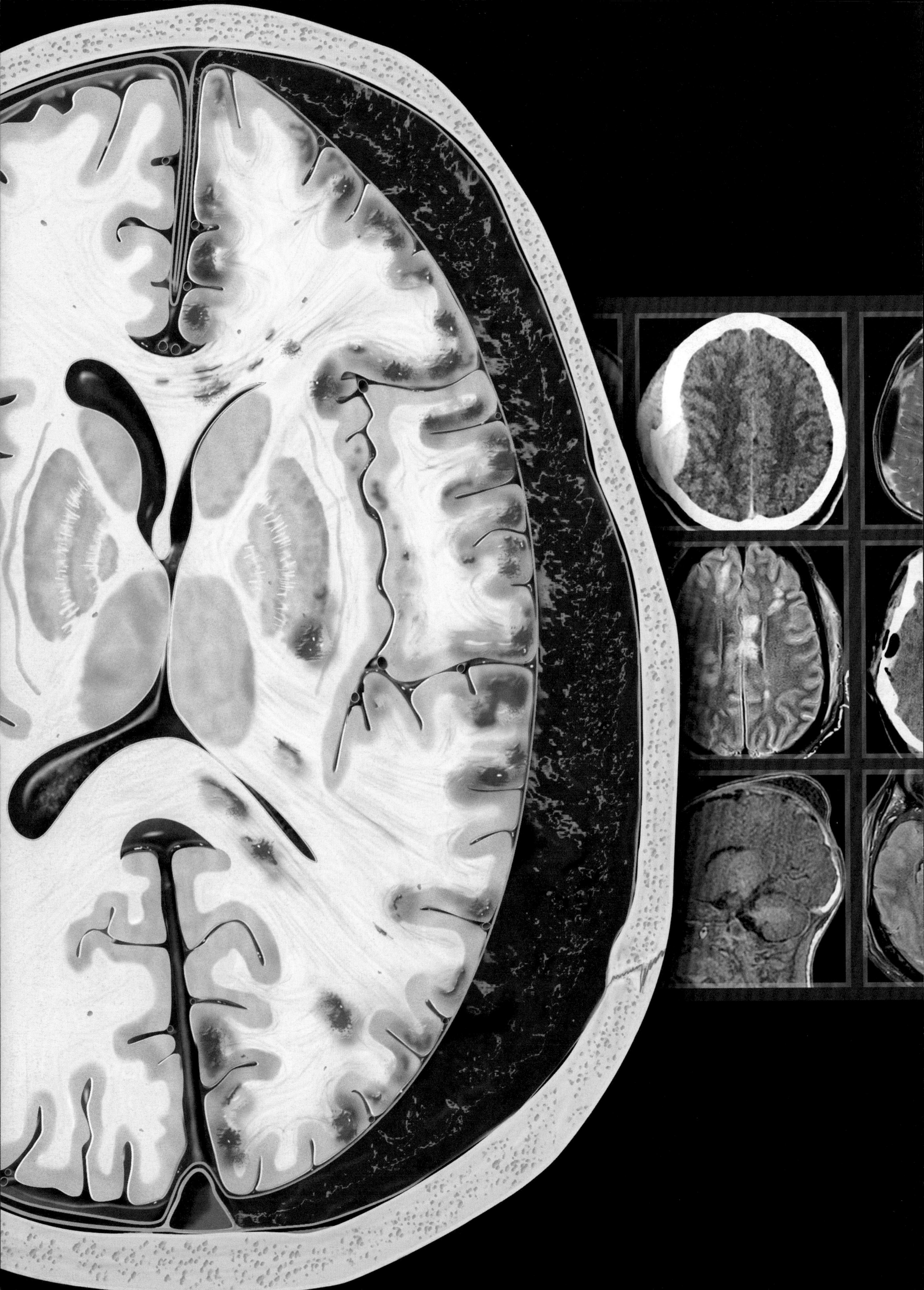

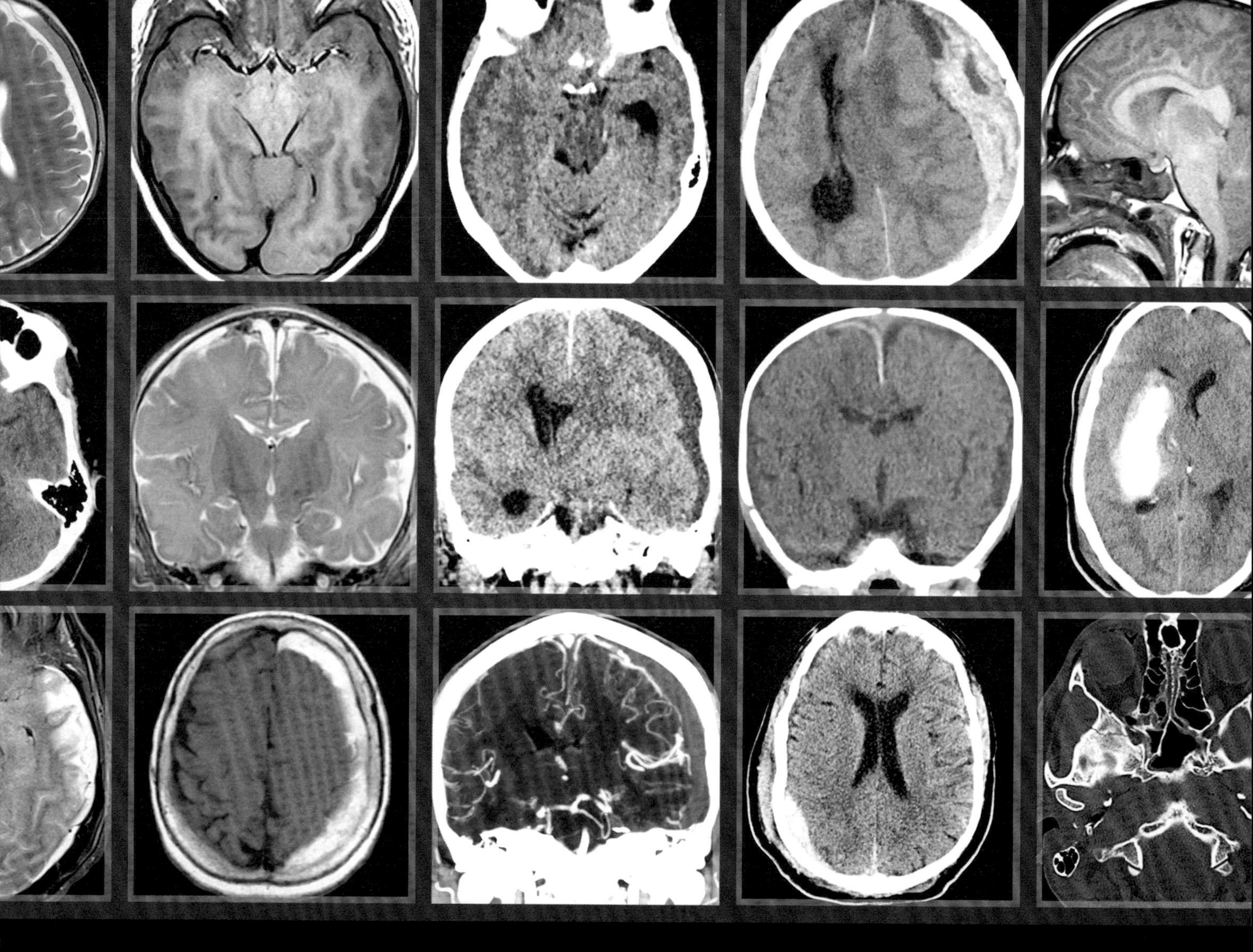

SECTION 1

# Trauma

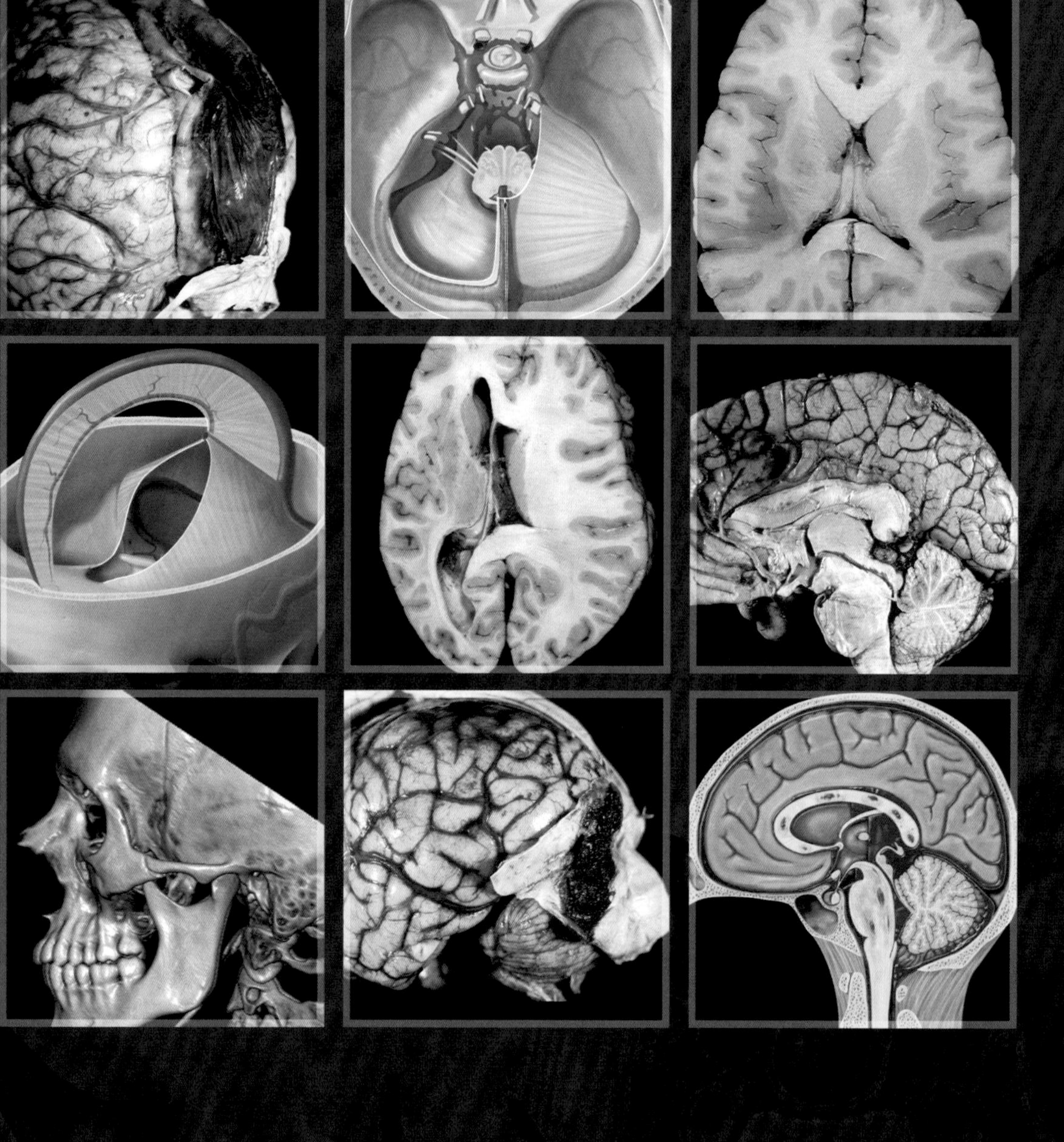

# Trauma Overview

*Trauma is one of the most frequent indications for emergent neuroimaging. Because imaging plays such a key role in patient triage and management, we begin this book by discussing skull and brain trauma.*

We start with a brief consideration of epidemiology. Traumatic brain injury (TBI) is a critical public health and socioeconomic problem throughout the world. The direct medical costs of caring for acutely traumatized patients are huge. The indirect costs of lost productivity and long-term care for TBI survivors are even larger than the short-term direct costs.

We then briefly discuss the etiology and mechanisms of head trauma. Understanding the different ways in which the skull and brain can be injured provides the context for understanding the spectrum of findings that can be identified on imaging studies.



## Introduction

### Epidemiology of Head Trauma

Trauma—sometimes called the silent epidemic—is the most common worldwide cause of death in children and young adults. Neurotrauma is responsible for the vast majority of these cases.

At least 10 million people worldwide sustain TBI each year. Approximately 10% sustain fatal brain injury. Lifelong disability is common in those who survive. Between 5-10% of TBI survivors have serious permanent neurologic deficits, and an additional 20-40% have moderate disability. Even more have subtle deficits ("minimal brain trauma").

### Etiology and Mechanisms of Injury

Trauma can be caused by missile or nonmissile injury. Missile injury results from penetration of the skull, meninges, &/or brain by an external object, such as a bullet. Gunshot wounds are most common in adolescent and young adult males but are relatively rare in other groups.

Nonmissile closed head injury (CHI) is a much more common cause of neurotrauma than missile injury. Falls have now surpassed road traffic incidents as the leading cause of TBI.

So-called ground-level falls (GLFs) are a common indication for neuroimaging in young children and older adults. In such cases, brain injury can be significant. With a GLF, a six-foot-tall adult's head impacts the ground at 20 MPH. Anticoagulated older adults are especially at risk for intracranial hemorrhages, even with minor head trauma.

Motor vehicle collisions occurring at high speed exert significant acceleration/deceleration forces, causing the brain to move suddenly within the skull. Forcible impaction of the brain against the unyielding calvarium and hard, knife-like dura results in gyral contusion. Rotation and sudden changes in angular momentum may deform, stretch, and damage long vulnerable axons, resulting in axonal injury.

## Classification of Head Trauma

The most widely used *clinical* classification of brain trauma, the Glasgow Coma Scale (GCS), depends on the assessment of three features: Best eye, verbal, and motor responses. With the use of the GCS, TBI can be designated as a mild, moderate, or severe injury.

TBI can also be divided chronologically and *pathoetiologically* into primary and secondary injury, the system used in this text. **Primary injuries** occur at the time of initial trauma. Skull fractures, epi- and subdural (SDH) hematomas, contusions, axonal injury, and brain lacerations are examples of primary injuries.

**Secondary injuries** occur later and include cerebral edema, perfusion alterations, brain herniations, and CSF leaks. Although vascular injury can be immediate (blunt impact) or secondary (vessel laceration from fractures, occlusion secondary to brain herniation), for purposes of discussion, it is included in the chapter on secondary injuries.

**CLASSIFICATION OF HEAD TRAUMA**

**Primary Effects**
- Scalp and skull injuries
- Extraaxial hemorrhage/hematomas
- Parenchymal injuries
- Miscellaneous injuries

**Secondary Effects**
- Herniation syndromes
- Cerebral edema
- Cerebral ischemia
- Vascular injury (can be primary or secondary)

# Imaging Acute Head Trauma

Imaging is absolutely critical to the diagnosis and management of the patient with acute TBI. The goal of emergent neuroimaging is twofold: (1) Identify treatable injuries, especially emergent ones, and (2) detect and delineate the presence of secondary injuries, such as herniation syndromes and vascular injury.

## How to Image

Injuries to the head and brain are often separated into acute (0-7 days), subacute (< 3 months), and chronic (> 3 months) phases. NECT is typically the first-line imaging modality for suspected acute head injury. CTA is helpful in cases with suspected injury to the cervical or intracranial vasculature. MR is rarely used in the acute trauma setting but can be useful for evaluating persistent subacute or chronic neurologic deficits.

### Skull Radiography

Skull radiography (whether "plain film" or "digital radiography") is no longer indicated in the initial evaluation of head injury. While it detects calvarial fractures reasonably well, skull radiography does not depict the far more important presence of extraaxial hemorrhages and parenchymal injuries and therefore has no appropriate role in the current management of the head-injured patient. *Keep in mind: Between 1/4 to 1/3 of autopsied patients with fatal brain injuries have no identifiable skull fracture!*

### NECT

CT is now accepted as the "workhorse" screening tool for imaging acute head trauma. The reasons are simple: CT depicts both bone and soft tissue injuries. It is also widely accessible, fast, effective, and comparatively inexpensive.

Nonenhanced CT (NECT) scans (4 or 5 mm thick) from just below the foramen magnum through the vertex should be performed. Two sets of images should be obtained: One using brain and one with bone reconstruction algorithms. In addition, viewing the brain images with a wider window width (150-200 HU, the so-called subdural window) should be performed on PACS. The scout view should **always** be displayed and examined as part of the study **(1-1)**.

Multidetector row CT (MDCT) is now routine in trauma triage. Coronal and sagittal reformatted images using the axial source data improve the detection rate of acute traumatic SDHs.

Three-dimensional shaded surface displays (3D SSDs) are helpful in depicting skull and facial fractures. If facial bone CT is also requested, a single MDCT acquisition can be obtained without overlapping radiation exposure to the eye and lower 1/2 of the brain.

Head trauma patients with acute intracranial lesions on CT have a higher risk for cervical spine fractures compared with patients with a CT-negative head injury. Because up to 1/3 of patients with moderate to severe head injury, as determined by the GCS, have concomitant spine injury, MDCT of the cervical spine is often obtained together with brain imaging. Soft tissue and bone algorithm reconstructions with multiplanar reformatted images of the cervical spine should be obtained.

### CTA

While there is no relevant literature to support the use of CT angiography (CTA) in the initial imaging evaluation of acute head trauma without suspected vascular injury, it is often obtained as part of a whole-body trauma CT protocol. Craniocervical CTA should also be specifically considered (1) in the setting of penetrating neck injury, (2) if a fractured foramen transversarium or facet subluxation is identified on cervical spine CT, or (3) if a skull base fracture traverses the

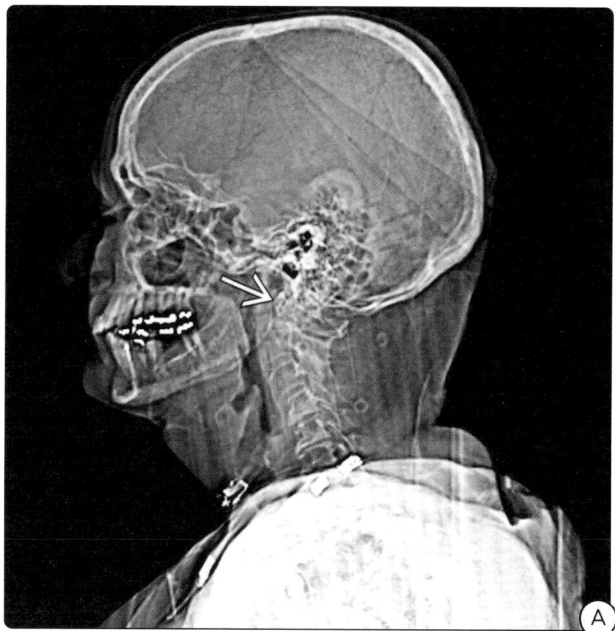


***(1-1A)** Scout view in a 66-year-old woman with a head CT requested to evaluate a ground-level fall shows a posteriorly angulated C1-odontoid complex ➡.*

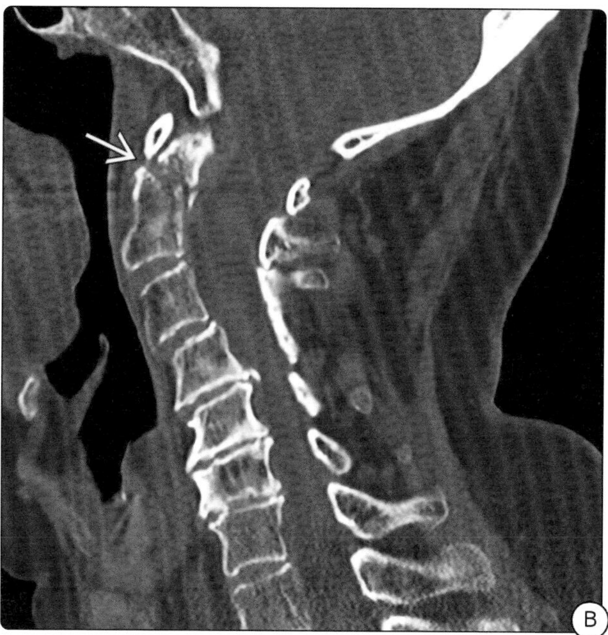


***(1-1B)** Head CT (not shown) in the same case was normal. Cervical spine CT was then performed. The sagittal image reformatted from the axial scan data shows a comminuted, posteriorly angulated dens fracture ➡.*

carotid canal or a dural venous sinus. Arterial laceration or dissection, traumatic pseudoaneurysm, carotid-cavernous fistula, or dural venous sinus injury are nicely depicted on high-resolution CTA.

### MR

Although MR can detect traumatic complications without radiation and is more sensitive for abnormalities, such as contusions and axonal injuries, there is general agreement that NECT is the procedure of choice in the initial evaluation of brain trauma. Limitations of MR include acquisition time, access, patient monitoring and instability, motion degradation of images, and cost.

With one important exception—suspected child abuse—using MR as a routine screening procedure in the setting of *acute* brain trauma is not appropriate. Standard MR together with susceptibility-weighted imaging and diffusion tensor imaging (DTI) is most useful in the subacute and chronic stages of TBI. Other modalities, such as fMRI, are playing an increasingly important role in detecting subtle abnormalities, especially in patients with mild cognitive deficits following minor TBI but are not utilized in the acute setting.

## Who and When to Image

Who to image and when to do it are paradoxically both well established and controversial. Patients with a GCS score indicating moderate (GCS = 9-12) or severe (GCS ≤ 8) neurologic impairment are invariably imaged. The real debate is about how best to manage patients with GCS scores of 13-15. Keep in mind that there is a **big** difference between a GCS of 15 (normal) and one of 13 or 14, as confusion, motor response localizing to pain, and eyes open only to verbal command do indicate some degree of neurologic impairment. Some investigators also distinguish between mild and minimal head trauma (i.e., GCS of 15 without loss of consciousness or posttraumatic amnesia).

### GLASGOW COMA SCALE

**Best Eye Response (Maximum = 4)**
- 1 = no eye opening
- 2 = eyes opening to pain
- 3 = eyes open to verbal command
- 4 = eyes open spontaneously

**Best Verbal Response (Maximum = 5)**
- 1 = none
- 2 = incomprehensible sounds
- 3 = inappropriate words
- 4 = confused
- 5 = oriented

**Best Motor Response (Maximum = 6)**
- 1 = none
- 2 = extension to pain
- 3 = flexion to pain
- 4 = withdrawal to pain
- 5 = localizing to pain
- 6 = obedience to commands

**Sum = "Coma Score" and Clinical Grading**
- 13-15 = mild brain injury (note: GCS of 13 is sometimes classified as moderate rather than mild)
- 9-12 = moderate brain injury
- ≤ 8 = severe brain injury

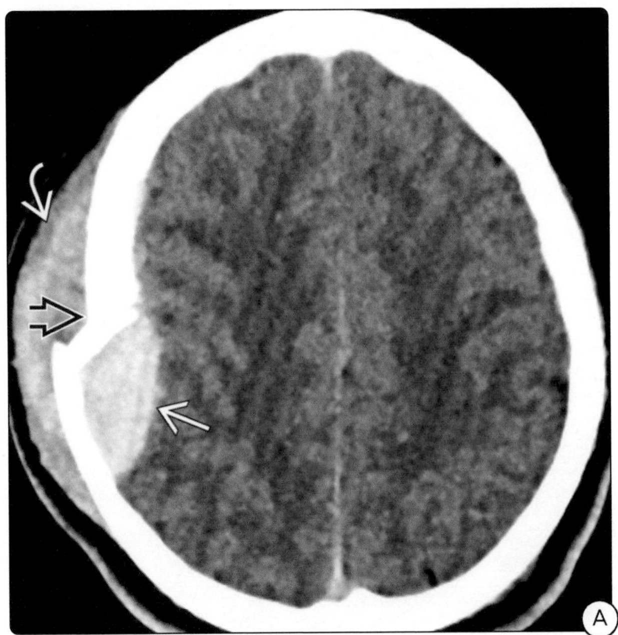


(1-2A) *NECT in a patient hit in the head with a baseball bat shows a large scalp hematoma ➡, a depressed skull fracture ⇨, and an epidural hematoma ➡ underlying the skull fracture.*

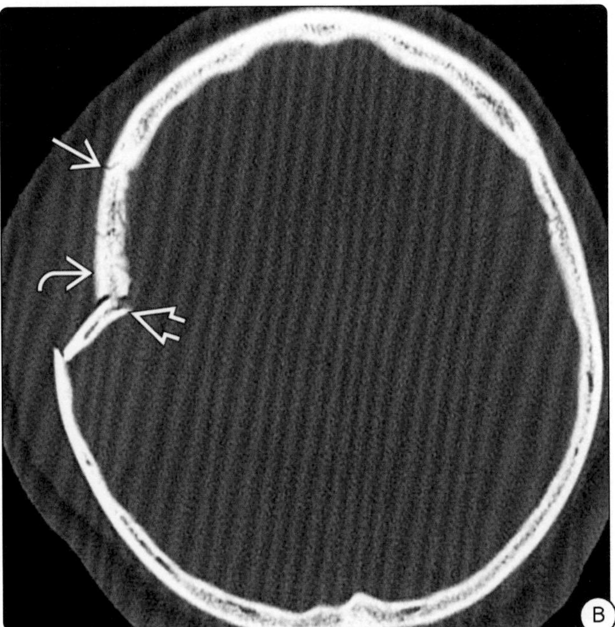


(1-2B) *Bone CT in the same case shows the comminuted, depressed skull fracture ⇨. Note fracture of the posterior frontal bone ➡ with subtle depression and angulation of the anterior fragment ➡.*

## Appropriateness Criteria

Head CT is useful for the evaluation of even mild acute head trauma when imaging is indicated by a validated clinical decision rule, such as the American College of Emergency Physicians (ACEP). However, many emergency physicians routinely order NECT scans on every patient with head trauma, regardless of GCS score or clinical findings.

In an attempt to reduce CT overutilization in emergency departments, several organizations have developed evidence-based clinical criteria that help separate "high-risk" from "low-risk" patients. Three major and widely used appropriateness criteria have been published: The American College of Radiology (ACR) Appropriateness Criteria, the New Orleans Criteria (NOC), and the Canadian Head CT Rule (CHCR).

**ACR Criteria**. The ACR Appropriateness Criteria are evidence-based guidelines for specific clinical conditions that are reviewed annually by a multidisciplinary expert panel and were most recently updated in 2021. Imaging in *adults* with mild acute head trauma (GCS of 13-15) "not indicated by clinical decision rule" (e.g., such as the ACEP) exposes patients to the negative impact of ionizing radiation and is considered "usually not appropriate." In contrast, emergent NECT in mild/minor CHI with the presence of a focal neurologic deficit &/or other risk factors is deemed "usually appropriate."

Imaging head trauma in *children* is considered separately and based on the Pediatric Emergency Care Network (PECARN) clinical criteria. PECARN is an age-based rule that can be implemented for children younger and older than two years of age to identify those at low risk for clinically important TBI so that CT scans can be safely avoided. A recent study demonstrated the safety and validity of the PECARN rule, concluding that for children < 18 years of age classified in the low-risk category, "it is a duty not to expose the child to ionizing radiation."

The ACR criteria recommends well-validated, pediatric-specific clinical decision guidelines, such as PECARN, should be used to identify very low-risk children who can safely forgo imaging. Of note, this specifically excludes cases of suspected abusive head trauma.

**NOC and CHCR**. Both the NOC and CHCR attempt to triage patients with minimal/mild head injuries in a cost-effective manner. A GCS score of 15 without any of the NOC indicators (e.g., headache, vomiting, patient > 60 years old, intoxication, loss of consciousness, anterograde amnesia, seizure, or visible trauma above the clavicles) is a highly sensitive negative predictor of clinically important brain injury or need for surgical intervention.

Between 6-7% of patients with minor head injury have positive findings on head CT scans. Most of these patients also have headache, vomiting, drug or alcohol intoxication, seizure, short-term memory deficits, or physical evidence of trauma above the clavicles. CT should be used liberally in these cases and in any patient with loss of consciousness or focal neurologic deficit.

CT should also be used liberally in patients over 65 years of age. Older adults are at higher risk of traumatic intracranial hemorrhage due to comorbidities, such as polypharmacy (including anticoagulation), brain atrophy, and loss of elastic integrity in the cerebral bridging veins. Note that falling on ground level is now the most common cause of traumatic intracranial bleeding worldwide! The mortality rate for fall-associated intracranial bleeding is 15%.

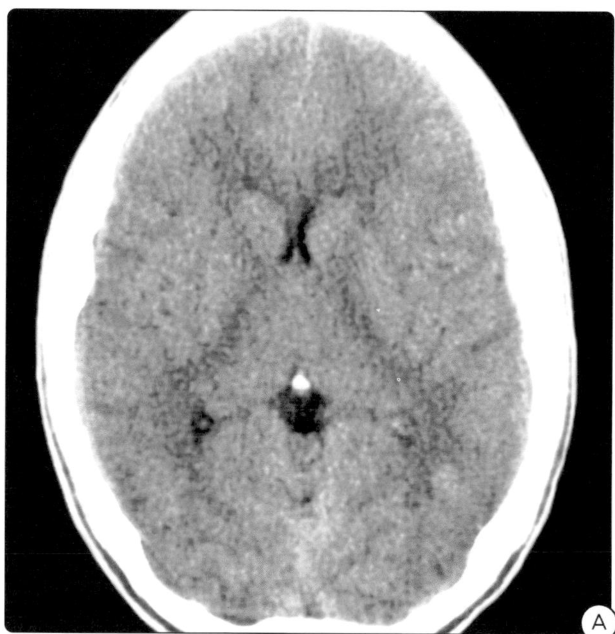

*(1-3A) Axial NECT in a patient with transient loss of consciousness after minor head injury appears relatively unremarkable.*

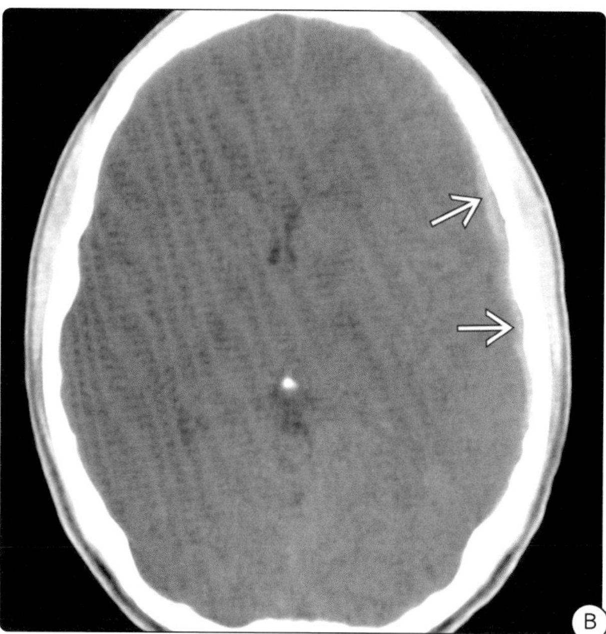

*(1-3B) Intermediate window ("subdural") width shows a 4-mm curvilinear hyperdensity ➡ under the intact skull. This is a small subdural hematoma. No surgery was required, and the patient was discharged after a 24-hour observation in the ED.*

# Trauma Imaging: Keys to Analysis

Four components are essential to the accurate interpretation of CT scans in patients with head injury: The scout image + brain, bone, and intermediate ("subdural") views of the NECT dataset. Critical information may be present on just one of these four components.

Suggestions on how to analyze NECT images in patients with acute head injury are delineated in this section.

## Scout Image

Before you look at the NECT scan, examine the digital scout image. Look for cervical spine abnormalities, such as fractures or dislocations, jaw &/or facial trauma, and the presence of foreign objects. If there is a suggestion of cervical spine fracture or malalignment on the scout image **(1-1A)**, MDCT of the cervical spine should be performed before the patient is removed from the scanner **(1-1B)**.

## Brain Windows

Methodically and meticulously work your way from the outside in. First, evaluate the soft tissue images, beginning with the scalp. Look for scalp swelling, which usually indicates the impact point. Carefully examine the periorbital soft tissues.

Next, look for extraaxial blood. The most common extraaxial hemorrhage is traumatic subarachnoid hemorrhage (tSAH) followed by sub- and epidural hematomas. The prevalence of tSAH in moderate to severe TBI approaches 100%. tSAH is usually found in the sulci adjacent to cortical contusions, along the sylvian fissures, and around the anteroinferior frontal and temporal lobes. The best place to look for subtle tSAH is the interpeduncular cistern, where blood collects when the patient is supine.

Any hypodensity within an extraaxial collection should raise suspicion of rapid hemorrhage with accumulation of unclotted blood or (especially in patients with alcohol abuse disorder or older patients) an underlying coagulopathy. This is an urgent finding that mandates immediate notification of the responsible clinician.

Look for intracranial air ("pneumocephalus"). Intracranial air is always abnormal and indicates the presence of a fracture that traverses either the paranasal sinuses or mastoid.

Now, move on to the brain itself. Carefully examine the cortex, especially the "high-yield" areas for cortical contusions (anteroinferior frontal and temporal lobes). If there is a scalp hematoma due to impact (a coup injury), look 180° in the opposite direction for a classic contrecoup injury. Hypodense areas around the hyperdense hemorrhagic foci indicate early edema and severe contusion.

Move inward from the cortex to the subcortical white and deep gray matter. Petechial hemorrhages often accompany axonal injury. If you see subcortical hemorrhages on the initial NECT scan, this is merely the "tip of the iceberg." There is usually *a lot* more damage than what is apparent on the first scan. A general rule: The deeper the lesion, the more severe the injury.

Finally, look inside the ventricles for blood-CSF levels and hemorrhage due to choroid plexus shearing injury.

## Subdural Windows

Look at the soft tissue image with both narrow ("brain") and intermediate ("subdural") windows. Small, subtle SDHs can sometimes be overlooked on standard narrow window widths (75-100 HU) yet are readily apparent when wider windows (150-200 HU) are used **(1-3)**.

## Bone CT

Bone CT refers to bone algorithm reconstruction viewed with wide (bone) windows. If you cannot do bone algorithm reconstruction from your dataset, widen the windows and use an edge-enhancement feature to sharpen the image. 3D SSDs are especially helpful in depicting complex or subtle fractures **(1-4)**.

Even though standard head scans are 4-5 mm thick, it is often possible to detect fractures on bone CT. Look for basisphenoid fractures with involvement of the carotid canal, temporal bone fractures (with or without ossicular dislocation), mandibular dislocation ("empty" condylar fossa), and calvarial fractures. Remember: Nondisplaced linear skull fractures that do not cross vascular structures (such as a dural venous sinus or middle meningeal artery) are in and of themselves basically meaningless. The brain and blood vessels are what matter!

The most difficult dilemma is deciding whether an observed lucency is a fracture or a normal structure (e.g., suture line or vascular channel). Keep in mind: It is virtually unheard of for a calvarial fracture to occur in the absence of overlying soft tissue injury. If there is no scalp "bump," it is unlikely that the lucency represents a nondisplaced linear fracture.

Bone CT images are also very helpful in distinguishing low density from air vs. fat. Although most PACS stations have a region of interest (ROI) function that can measure attenuation, fat fades away on bone CT images, and air remains very hypodense.

*__(1-4A)__ Axial NECT in an 18-year-old man who fell off his skateboard shows a small right epidural hematoma ➡ that also contains air ➡. __(1-4B)__ This 2-mm bone algorithm reconstruction in the same case shows a nondisplaced linear fracture ➡ of the squamous temporal bone adjacent to the epidural blood and air ➡.*

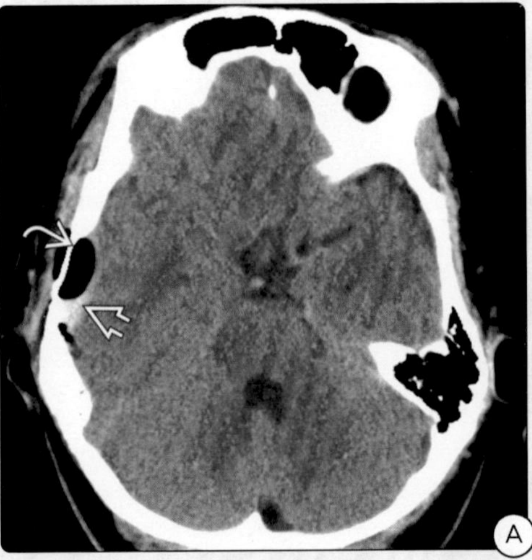


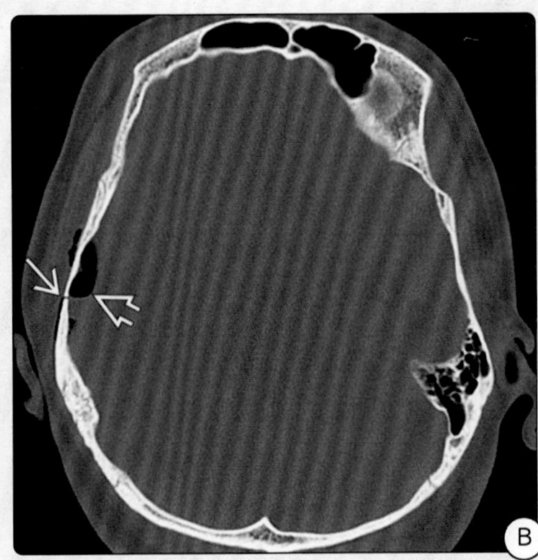


*__(1-4C)__ Coronal (left) and sagittal (right) bone CTs reconstructed from the axial source data show that the temporal bone fracture ➡ is comminuted and crosses the mastoid ➡ and middle ear ➡. __(1-4D)__ Bone CT with shaded surface display in the same case nicely shows the squamous ➡ and mastoid ➡ aspects of the nondisplaced but comminuted fracture.*

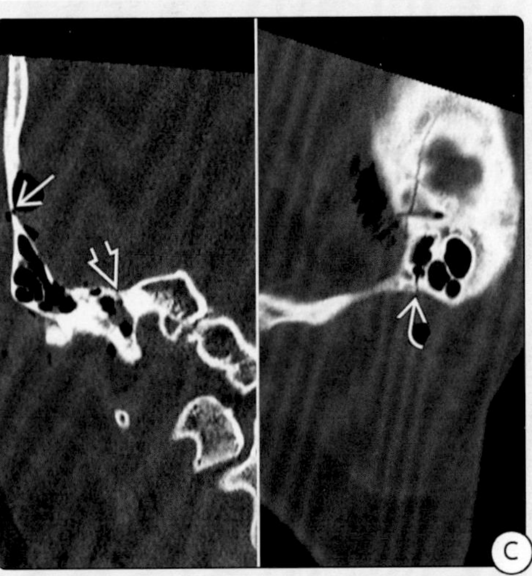


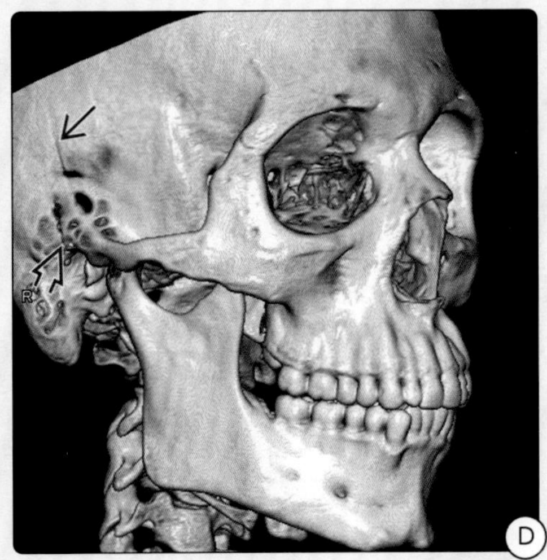

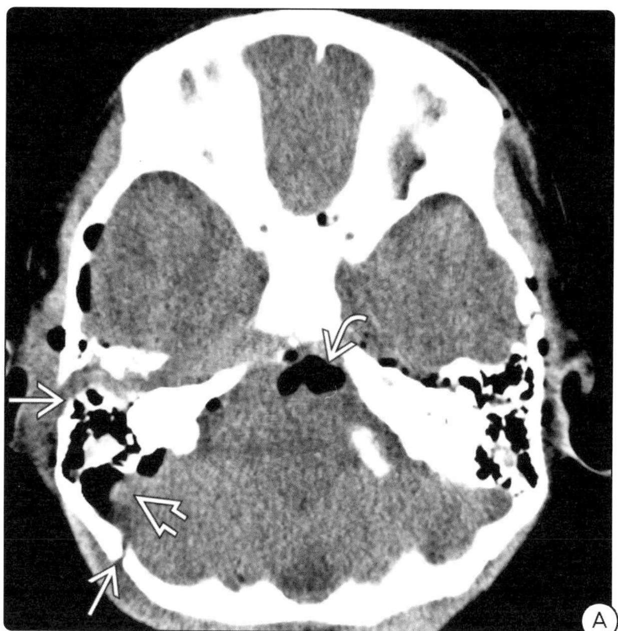

*(1-5A) NECT shows pneumocephalus ➡ and base of skull fractures ➡ adjacent to air, which seems to outline a displaced sigmoid sinus ➡.*

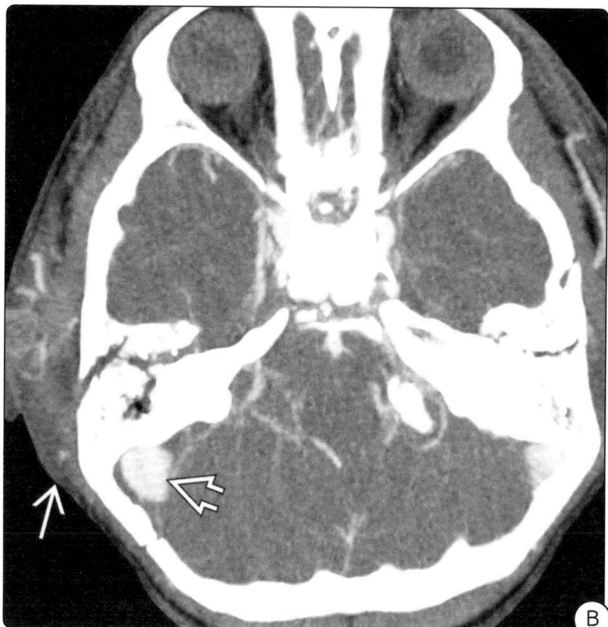

*(1-5B) MIP view of axial CTA in the same case obtained several minutes later shows that the sigmoid sinus ➡ is intact but displaced medially. Note a rapidly enlarging subgaleal hematoma ➡.*

## CTA

CTA is generally indicated if (1) basilar skull fractures cross the carotid canal or a dural venous sinus **(1-5)**, (2) if a cervical spine fracture dislocation is present, especially if the transverse foramina are involved, or (3) if the patient has stroke-like symptoms or unexplained clinical deterioration. Both the cervical and intracranial vasculature should be visualized.

Although it is important to scrutinize both the arterial and venous sides of the circulation, a CTA is generally sufficient. Standard CTAs typically show both the arteries and the dural venous sinuses well, whereas a CT venogram (CTV) often misses the arterial phase.

Examine the source images as well as the multiplanar reconstructions and maximum-intensity projection (MIP) reformatted scans. Traumatic dissection, vessel lacerations, intimal flaps, pseudoaneurysms, carotid-cavernous fistulas, and dural sinus occlusions can generally be identified on CTA.

### HEAD TRAUMA: CT CHECKLIST

**Scout Image**

- Evaluate for
    - Cervical spine fracture dislocation
    - Jaw dislocation, facial fractures
    - Foreign object

**Brain Windows**

- Scalp swelling (impact point)
- Extraaxial blood (focal hypodensity in clot suggests rapid bleeding)
    - Epidural hematoma
    - SDH
    - tSAH
- Pneumocephalus
- Cortical contusion
    - Anteroinferior frontal, temporal lobes
    - Opposite scalp laceration/skull fracture
- Hemorrhagic axonal injury
- Intraventricular hemorrhage

**Subdural Windows**

- 150-200 HU (for thin SDHs under skull)

**Bone CT**

- Bone algorithm reconstruction > bone windows
- Do any fractures cross a vascular channel?

*Selected References: The complete reference list is available on the eBooks+ version included with purchase.*

# Primary Effects of CNS Trauma

*Primary head injuries are defined as those that occur at the time of initial trauma, even though they may not be immediately apparent on initial evaluation.*



Head injury can be caused by direct or indirect trauma. **Direct trauma** involves a blow to the head and is usually caused by automobile collisions, falls, or injury inflicted by an object, such as a hammer or baseball bat. Scalp lacerations, hematomas, and skull fractures are common. Associated intracranial damage ranges from none to severe.

Significant forces of acceleration/deceleration, linear translation, and rotational loading can be applied to the brain **without** direct head blows. Such **indirect trauma** is caused by angular kinematics and typically occurs in high-speed motor vehicle collisions (MVCs). Here, the brain undergoes rapid deformation and distortion. Depending on the site and direction of the force applied, significant injury to the cortex, axons, penetrating blood vessels, and deep gray nuclei may occur. Severe brain injury can occur in the absence of skull fractures or visible scalp lesions.

We begin our discussion with a consideration of scalp and skull lesions as we work our way from the outside to the inside of the skull. We then delineate the spectrum of intracranial trauma, starting with extraaxial hemorrhages. We conclude this chapter with a detailed discussion of injuries to the brain parenchyma [e.g., cortical contusion, diffuse axonal injury (DAI), and the serious deep subcortical injuries (SCIs)].

## Scalp and Skull Injuries

Scalp and skull injuries are common manifestations of cranial trauma. Although brain injury is usually the most immediate concern in managing traumatized patients, superficial lesions, such as scalp swelling and focal hematoma, can be helpful in identifying the location of direct head trauma. On occasion, these initially innocent-appearing "lumps and bumps" can become life threatening. Before turning our attention to intracranial traumatic lesions, we therefore briefly review scalp and skull injuries, delineating their typical imaging findings and clinical significance.

### Scalp Injuries

Scalp injuries include lacerations and hematomas. Scalp **lacerations** can occur in both penetrating and closed head (CHIs) injuries. Lacerations may extend partially or entirely through all five layers of the scalp (skin, subcutaneous fibrofatty tissue, galea aponeurotica, loose areolar connective tissue, and periosteum) to the skull **(2-1)**.

Focal discontinuity, soft tissue swelling, and subcutaneous air are commonly identified in scalp lacerations. Scalp lacerations should be carefully evaluated for the presence of any foreign bodies. If not removed during wound debridement, foreign bodies can be a potential source of substantial morbidity and are very important to identify on initial imaging studies. Wood fragments are often hypodense, whereas leaded glass, gravel, and metallic shards are variably hyperdense **(2-2)**.

Scalp lacerations may or may not be associated with scalp **hematomas**. There are two distinctly different types of scalp hematomas: Cephalohematomas and subgaleal hematomas. The former are usually of no clinical significance, whereas the latter can cause hypovolemia and hypotension.

**Cephalohematomas** are **subperiosteal** blood collections that lie in the potential space between the outer surface of the calvarium and the pericranium, which serves as the periosteum of the skull **(2-3)**. The pericranium continues medially into cranial sutures and is anatomically contiguous with the outer (periosteal) layer of the dura.

Cephalohematomas are the extracranial equivalent of an intracranial epidural hematoma (EDH). Cephalohematomas do not cross suture lines and are typically unilateral. Because they are anatomically constrained by the tough fibrous periosteum and its insertions, cephalohematomas rarely attain a large size.

Cephalohematomas occur in 1% of newborns and are more common following instrumented delivery. They are often diagnosed clinically but imaged only if they are unusually prominent or if intracranial injuries are suspected. NECT scans show a somewhat lens-shaped soft tissue mass that overlies a single bone (usually the parietal or occipital bone) **(2-4)**. If more than one bone is affected, the two collections are separated by the intervening suture lines.

**Subgaleal hematomas** are **subaponeurotic** collections and are common findings in traumatized patients of all ages. Here, blood collects under the aponeurosis (the "galea") of the occipitofrontalis muscle **(2-5)**. Because a subgaleal hematoma lies deep to the scalp muscles and galea aponeurotica but

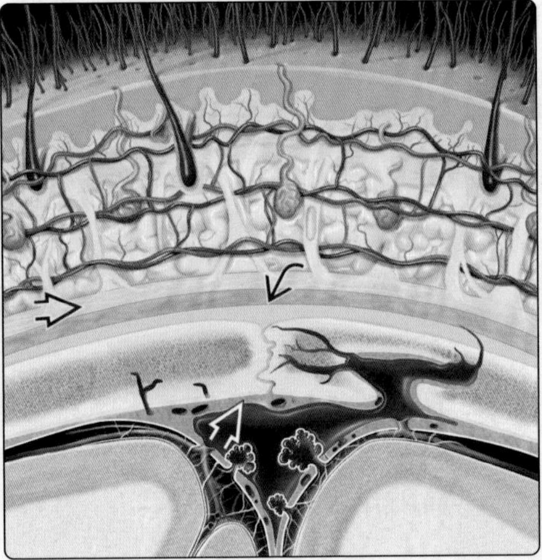

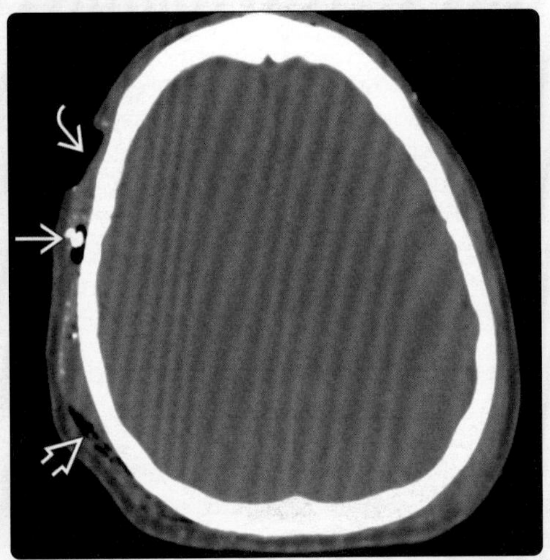

***(2-1)** Coronal graphic depicts normal layers of the scalp. Skin, subcutaneous fibrofatty tissue overlie the galea aponeurotica ⇨, loose areolar connective tissue. The pericranium ⇨ is the periosteum of the skull and continues into and through sutures to merge with the periosteal layer of the dura ➡. **(2-2)** NECT shows a scalp laceration ➡, hyperdense foreign bodies ➡, and subgaleal air ➡.*

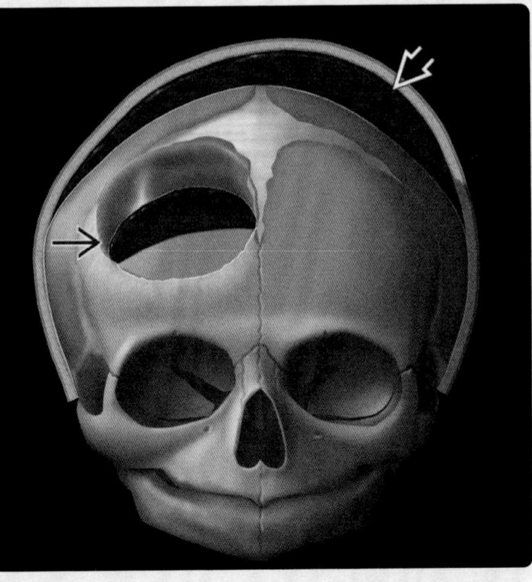

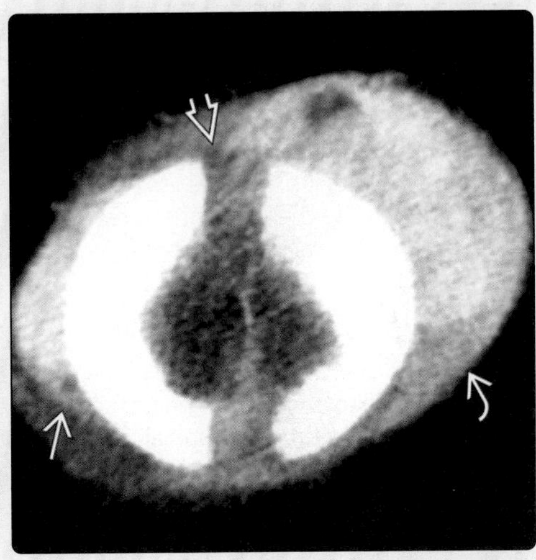

***(2-3)** Graphic shows the skull of a newborn, including the anterior fontanelle, coronal, metopic, sagittal sutures. Cephalohematoma ⇨ is subperiosteal, limited by sutures. Subgaleal hematoma ➡ is under the scalp aponeurosis, not bounded by sutures. **(2-4)** NECT in a newborn shows a small right ➡ and a large left ➡ parietal cephalohematoma. Neither crosses the sagittal suture ➡.*

external to the periosteum, it is not anatomically limited by suture lines.

Bleeding into the subgaleal space can be very extensive. Subgaleal hematomas are usually bilateral lesions that often spread diffusely around the entire calvarium. NECT scans show a heterogeneously hyperdense crescentic scalp mass that crosses one or more suture lines **(2-6)**. In contrast to benign self-limited cephalohematomas, expanding subgaleal hematomas in infants and small children can cause significant blood loss.

## Skull Fractures

Noticing a scalp "bump" or hematoma on initial imaging in head trauma is important, as calvarial fractures rarely—if ever—occur in the absence of overlying soft tissue swelling or scalp laceration. Skull fractures are present on initial CT scans in ~ 2/3 of patients with moderate head injury, although 25-35% of severely injured patients have no identifiable fracture, even with thin-section bone reconstructions.

Several types of acute skull fracture can be identified on imaging studies: Linear, depressed, and diastatic fractures **(2-7)**. Fractures can involve the calvarium, skull base, or both.

### Linear Skull Fractures

A **linear skull fracture** is a sharply marginated linear defect that typically involves both the inner and outer tables of the calvarium **(2-8)**.

Most linear skull fractures are caused by relatively low-energy blunt trauma that is delivered over a relatively wide surface area. Linear skull fractures that extend into and widen a suture become diastatic fractures. When multiple complex fractures are present, 3D shaded surface display (SSD) can be very helpful in depicting their anatomy and relationships to cranial sutures **(2-9)**.

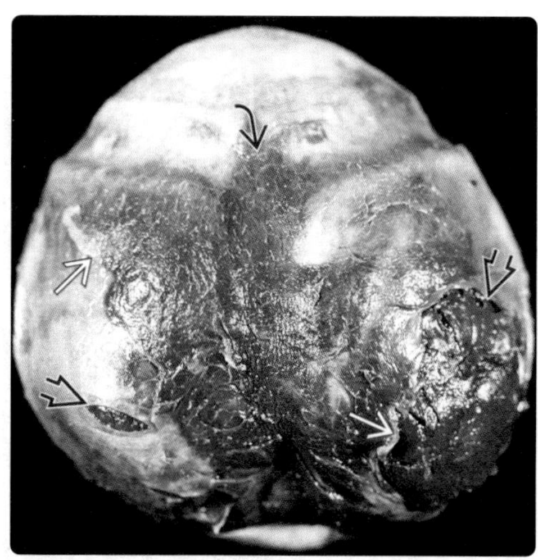

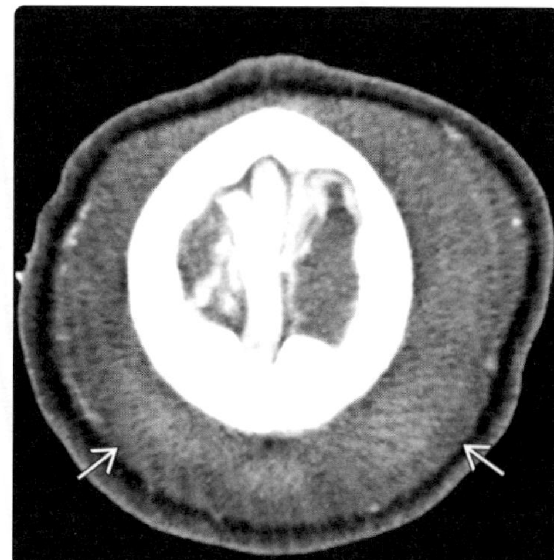

***(2-5)** Autopsy from a traumatized infant shows a massive biparietal subgaleal hematoma ➡. The galea aponeurotica has been partially opened ➡ to show large biparietal hematoma that crosses the sagittal suture ➡. **(2-6)** Axial CECT in a 3-yo shows massive subgaleal hematoma ➡ surrounding entire calvarium. Subgaleal hematomas cross sutures and can become life threatening, while cephalohematomas are anatomically limited.*

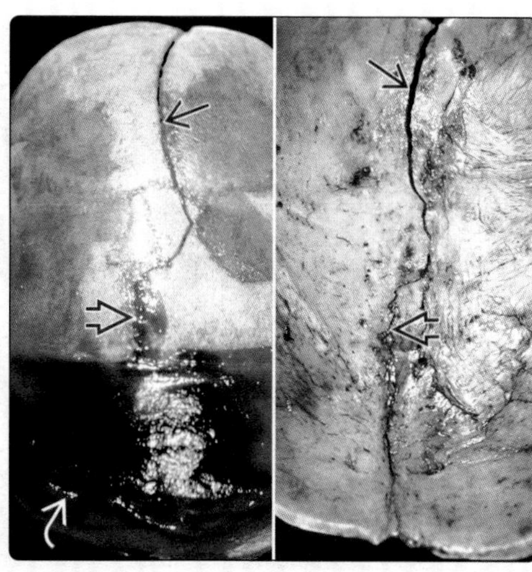

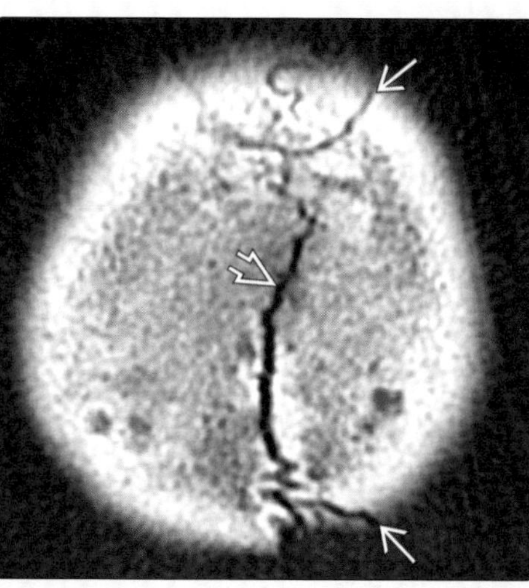

***(2-7)** Autopsied skull shows fatal trauma with exo- (L) and endocranial (R) views. A linear fracture ➡ extends into the superior sagittal suture ➡, causing diastasis and a subgaleal hematoma ➡. **(2-8)** Bone CT through the top of the calvarium shows linear skull fractures ➡ extending into and widening the sagittal suture, causing a diastatic fracture ➡.*

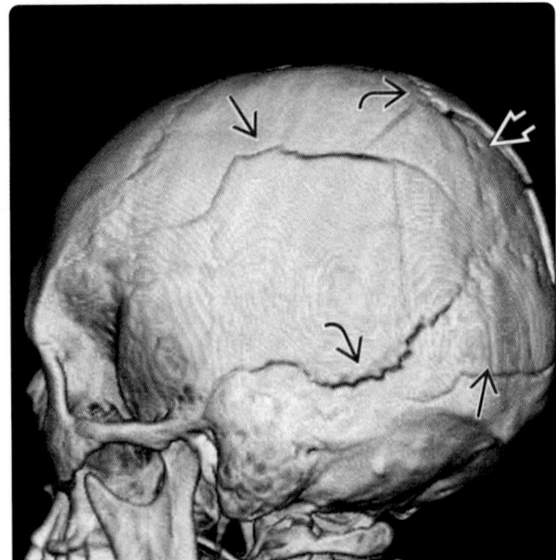

*(2-9) SSD nicely depicts linear ➔, diastatic fracture ➔ anatomy. Note slight depression ➔ of the fractured parietooccipital calvarium.*

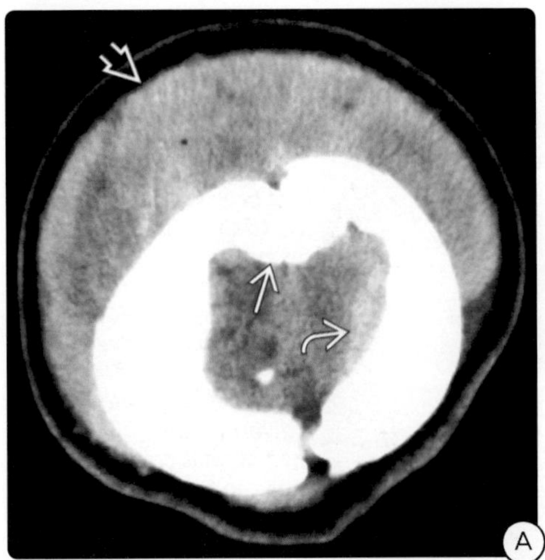


*(2-10A) NECT shows a massive subgaleal hematoma ➔ crossing the sagittal suture ➔. A small extraaxial hematoma ➔ is present.*

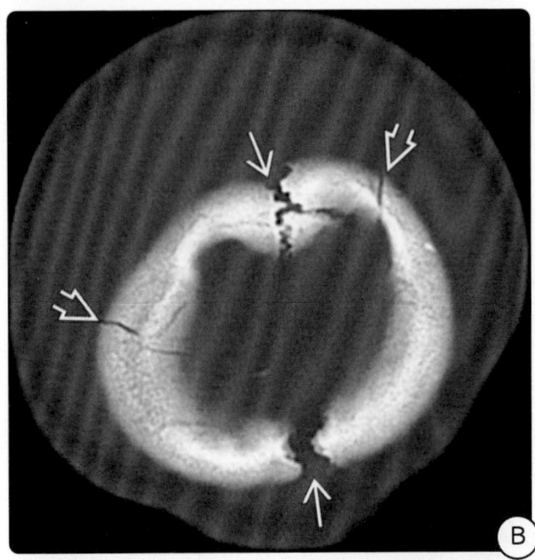


*(2-10B) Bone CT shows a diastatic fracture of the sagittal suture ➔. Nondisplaced linear fractures ➔ are also present.*

Patients with an isolated linear nondisplaced skull fracture (NDSF), no intracranial hemorrhage or pneumocephalus, normal neurologic examination, and absence of other injuries are at a very low risk for delayed hemorrhage or other life-threatening complication. Hospitalization is not necessary for many children with NDSFs.

## Depressed Skull Fractures

A **depressed skull fracture** is a fracture in which the fragments are displaced inward **(2-9)**. Comminution of the fracture fragments starts at the point of maximum impact and spreads centrifugally. Depressed fractures are most often caused by high-energy direct blows to a small surface with a blunt object (e.g., hammer, baseball bat, or metal pipe).

Depressed skull fractures typically tear the underlying dura and arachnoid and are often associated with cortical contusions and potential leakage of CSF into the subdural space. Fractures extending to a dural sinus or the jugular bulb are associated with venous sinus thrombosis in 40% of cases **(2-12A)**.

## Diastatic Skull Fractures

A **diastatic skull fracture** is a fracture that widens ("diastases" or "splits open") a suture or synchondrosis. Diastatic skull fractures usually occur in association with a linear skull fracture that extends into an adjacent suture **(2-10)**.

## Imaging

**General Features.** Both bone and soft tissue reconstruction algorithms should be used when evaluating patients with head injuries. Soft tissue reconstructions should be viewed with both narrow ("brain") and intermediate ("subdural") windows. Coronal and sagittal reformatted images obtained using the MDCT axial source data are helpful additions. SSDs can be useful in depicting complex and depressed fractures.

**CT Findings.** NECT scans demonstrate **linear** skull fractures as sharply marginated lucent lines. **Depressed** fractures are typically comminuted and show inward implosion of fracture fragments. Diastatic fractures appear as widened sutures or synchondroses **(2-10)** **(2-8)** and are usually associated with linear skull fractures.

**MR Findings.** MR is rarely used in the setting of acute head trauma because of the high cost, limited availability, and lengthy time required. Compared with CT, bone detail is poor, although parenchymal injuries are better seen. Adding T2* sequences, particularly SWI, is especially helpful in identifying hemorrhagic lesions.

**Angiography.** If a fracture crosses the site of a major vascular structure, such as the carotid canal or a dural venous sinus **(2-11)**, CTA is recommended. Sagittal, coronal, and MIP reconstructions help delineate the site and extent of vascular injuries.

Clival and skull base fractures are strongly associated with neurovascular trauma, and CTA/CTV should always be obtained in these cases **(2-12)**. Cervical fracture dislocations, distraction injuries, and penetrating neck trauma also merit further investigation. Uncomplicated asymptomatic soft tissue injuries of the neck rarely result in significant vascular injury.

SCALP AND SKULL INJURIES

**Scalp Injuries**
- Lacerations ± foreign bodies
- Cephalohematoma
  - Usually infants
  - Subperiosteal
  - Small, unilateral (limited by sutures)
- Subgaleal hematoma
  - Between galea, periosteum of skull
  - Circumferential, not limited by sutures
  - Can be very large, life threatening

**Skull Fractures**
- Linear
  - Sharp lucent line
  - Can be extensive and widespread
- Depressed
  - Focal
  - Inwardly displaced fragments
  - Often lacerates dura-arachnoid
- Diastatic
  - Typically associated with severe trauma
  - Usually caused by linear fracture that extends into suture
  - Widens, spreads apart suture or synchondrosis

# Extraaxial Hemorrhages

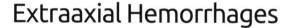

Extraaxial hemorrhages and hematomas are common manifestations of head trauma. They can occur in any intracranial compartment, within any space (potential or actual), and between any layers of the cranial meninges. Only the subarachnoid spaces exist normally; all the other spaces are potential spaces and occur only under pathologic conditions.

**Epidural hematomas (EDHs)** arise between the inner table of the skull and outer (periosteal) layer of the dura. **Subdural hematomas (SDHs)** are located between the inner (meningeal) layer of the dura and the arachnoid. **Traumatic subarachnoid hemorrhage (tSAH)** is found within the sulci and subarachnoid cisterns, between the arachnoid and the pia.

To discuss extraaxial hemorrhages, we work our way from the outside to the inside. We therefore begin this section with a discussion of EDHs (classic arterial as well as venous variants), then move deeper inside the cranium to the more common SDHs. We conclude with a consideration of tSAH.

## Arterial Epidural Hematoma

EDHs are uncommon but potentially lethal complications of head trauma. If an EDH is promptly recognized and appropriately treated, mortality and morbidity can be minimized.

### Terminology

An EDH is a collection of blood between the calvarium and outer (periosteal) layer of the dura.

### Etiology

Most EDHs arise from direct trauma to the skull that lacerates an adjacent blood vessel **(2-13)**. The vast majority (90%) are caused by arterial injury, most commonly to the middle meningeal artery. Approximately 10% of

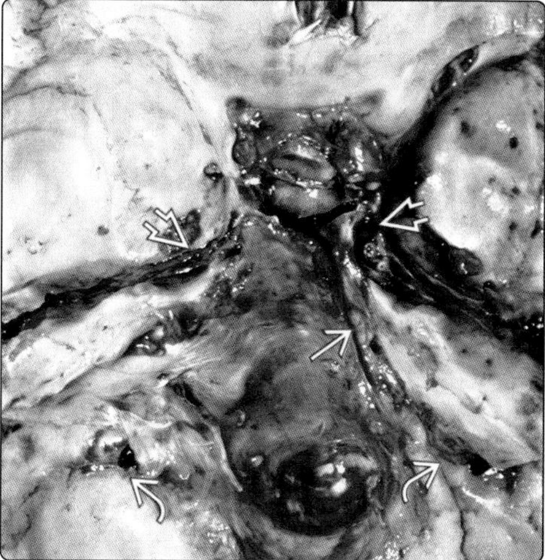

*(2-11) Multiple skull base fractures involving clivus ➡, carotid canals ➡, jugular foramina ➡ are shown. (Courtesy E. T. Hedley-Whyte, MD.)*

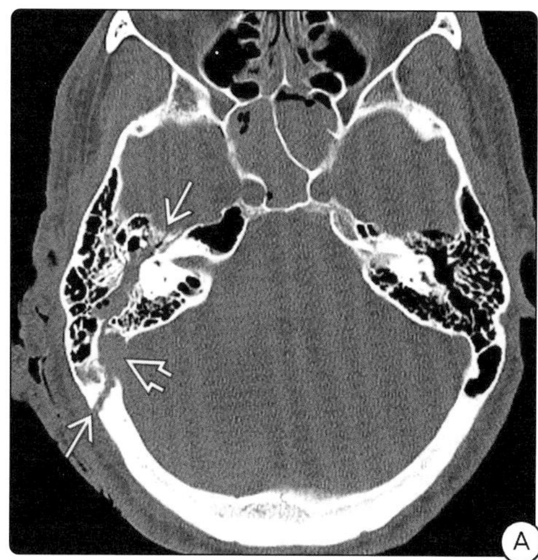

*(2-12A) Bone CT shows a slightly diastatic linear skull fracture ➡ crossing the temporal bone through the middle ear and jugular fossa ➡.*

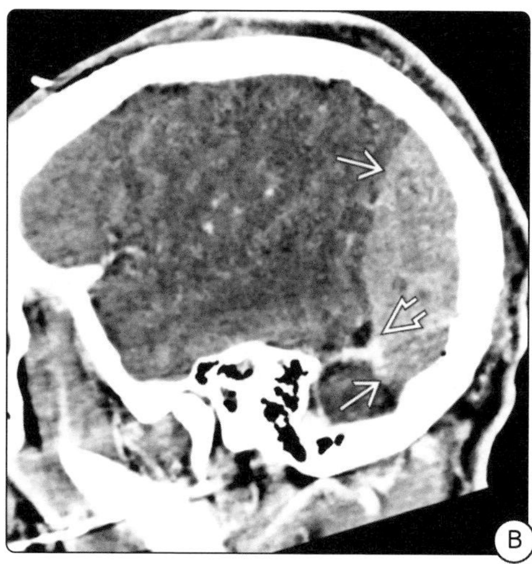

*(2-12B) Sagittal CT venogram (same case) shows an EDH ➡ crossing the tentorium. The right transverse sinus ➡ is displaced, occluded.*

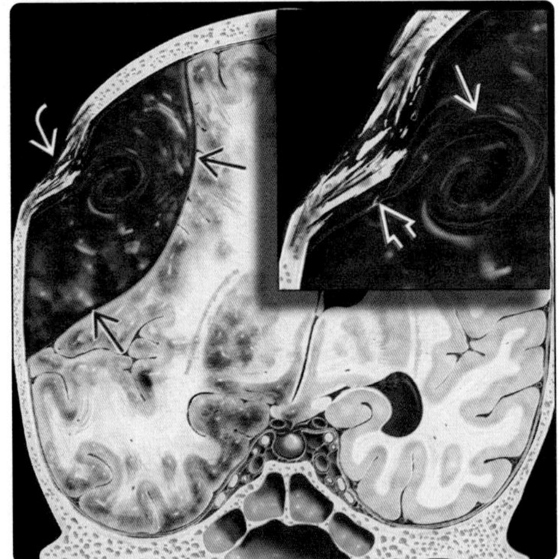

***(2-13)** EDH ⇒, depressed skull fracture ➡ are shown. Inset shows lacerated middle meningeal artery ➡, rapid bleeding, causing swirl sign ➡.*

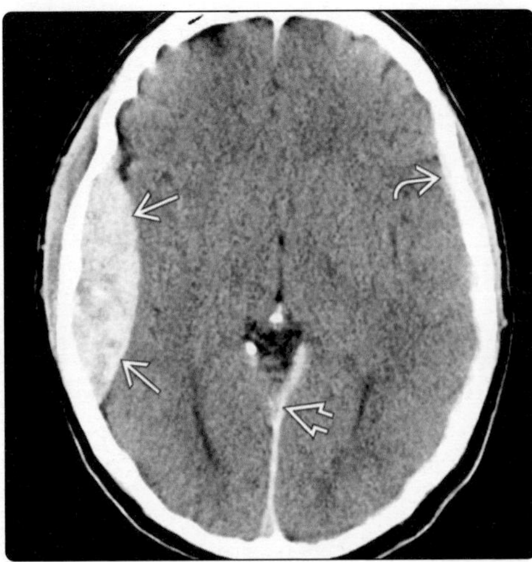

***(2-14)** Classic biconvex aEDH ➡ is shown with a thin subdural blood collection along the tentorium, falx ➡, and left hemisphere ➡.*

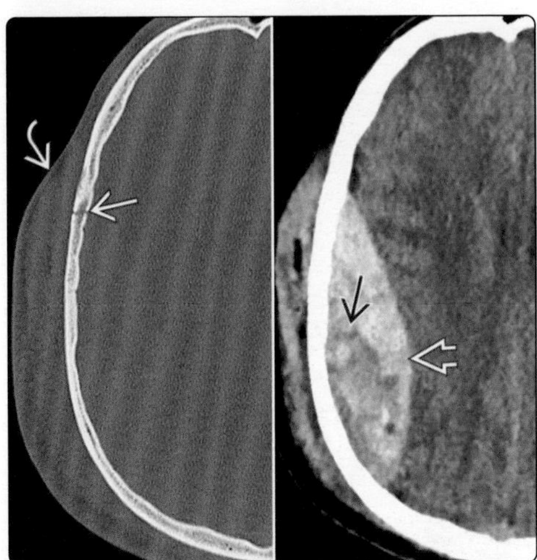

***(2-15)** Bone CT (L) shows skull fracture ➡ and scalp hematoma ➡. NECT (R) shows mixed-density, rapidly bleeding EDH ➡, swirl sign ⇒.*

EDHs are venous, usually secondary to a fracture that crosses a dural venous sinus.

## Pathology

**Location.** Over 90% of EDHs are unilateral and supratentorial. Between 90-95% are found directly adjacent to a skull fracture. The squamous portion of the temporal bone is the most common site.

**Gross Pathology.** EDHs are biconvex in shape. Adherence of the periosteal dura to the inner calvarium explains this typical configuration. As EDHs expand, they strip the dura away from the inner table of the skull, forming the classic lens-shaped hematoma **(2-13)**. Because the dura is especially tightly attached to sutures, EDHs in adults rarely cross suture lines (10% of EDHs in children *do* cross sutures, especially if a fracture traverses the suture or sutural diastasis is present).

The typical gross or intraoperative appearance of an acute EDH is a dark purple ("currant jelly") lentiform clot.

## Clinical Issues

**Epidemiology.** EDHs are much less common than either tSAH or SDH. Although EDHs represent up to 10% of fatal injuries in autopsy series, they are found in only 1-4% of patients imaged for craniocerebral trauma.

**Demographics.** EDHs are uncommon in infants and older adults. Most are found in older children and young adults. The M:F ratio is 4:1.

**Presentation.** The prototypical "lucid interval," during which a traumatized patient has an initial brief loss of consciousness followed by an asymptomatic period of various length prior to the onset of coma &/or neurologic deficit, occurs in only 50% of EDH cases. Headache, nausea, vomiting, symptoms of intracranial mass effect (e.g., pupil-involving third cranial nerve palsy) followed by somnolence and coma are common.

**Natural History.** Outcome depends on size and location of the hematoma, whether the EDH is arterial or venous, and whether there is active bleeding. In the absence of other associated traumatic brain injuries (TBIs), overall mortality rate with prompt recognition and appropriate treatment is < 5%.

Delayed development or enlargement of an EDH occurs in 10-15% of cases, usually within 24-36 hours following trauma.

**Treatment Options.** Many EDHs are now treated conservatively. Most traumatic EDHs are not surgical lesions at initial presentation, and the rate of conversion to surgery is low. Most venous and small classic hyperdense EDHs that do not exhibit a swirl sign and have minimal or no mass effect are managed conservatively with close clinical observation and follow-up imaging **(2-16)**. Significant clinical predictors of EDH progression requiring conversion to surgical therapy are coagulopathy and younger age.

## Imaging

**General Features.** EDHs, especially in adults, typically do not cross sutures unless a fracture with sutural diastasis is present. In children, 10% of EDHs cross suture lines, usually the coronal or sphenosquamous suture.

Look for other comorbid lesions, such as contrecoup injuries, tSAH, and secondary brain herniations, all of which are common findings in patients with EDHs.

**CT Findings.** NECT scan is the procedure of choice for initial imaging in patients with head injury. Both soft tissue and bone reconstruction algorithms should be obtained. Multiplanar reconstructions are especially useful in identifying vertex EDHs, which may be difficult to detect if only axial images are obtained.

The classic imaging appearance of **arterial EDHs** is a hyperdense (60-90 HU) biconvex extraaxial collection **(2-14)**. Presence of a hypodense component (swirl sign) is seen in ~ 1/3 of cases and indicates active, rapid bleeding with unretracted clot **(2-15)**.

EDHs compress the underlying subarachnoid space and displace the cortex medially, "buckling" the gray matter-white matter interface inward.

Air in an EDH occurs in ~ 20% of cases and is usually—but not invariably—associated with a sinus or mastoid fracture.

Patients with mixed-density EDHs tend to present earlier than patients with hyperdense hematomas and have lower Glasgow Coma Scale (GCS) scores, larger hematoma volumes, and poorer prognosis.

Imaging findings associated with adverse clinical outcome are thickness > 1.5 cm, volume > 30 mL, pterional (lateral aspect of the middle cranial fossa) location, midline shift > 5 mm, and the presence of a swirl sign within the hematoma on imaging.

Small, unoperated EDHs reduce in size and density with time and eventually resolve completely **(2-16)**.

**MR Findings.** Acute EDHs are typically isointense with underlying brain, especially on T1WI. The displaced dura can be identified as a displaced "black line" between the hematoma and the brain.

**Angiography.** DSA may show a lacerated middle meningeal artery with "tram-track" fistulization of contrast from the middle meningeal artery into the paired middle meningeal veins. Mass effect with displaced cortical arteries and veins is seen.

## ACUTE ARTERIAL EPIDURAL HEMATOMA

**Terminology**
- EDH = blood between skull, dura

**Etiology**
- Associated skull fracture in 90-95%
- Arterial in 90%
  - Most often middle meningeal artery
- Venous in 10%

**Pathology**
- Unilateral, supratentorial (> 90%)
- Dura stripped away from skull → biconvex hematoma
- Usually does not cross sutures (exception = children, 10%)
- Does cross sites of dural attachment

**Clinical**
- Rare (1-4% of head trauma)
- Older children, young adults most common
- M:F = 4:1
- Classic "lucid interval" in only 50%
- Delayed deterioration common
- Low mortality if recognized, treated
- Small EDHs
  - If minimal mass, no swirl sign often managed conservatively

**Imaging**
- Acute EDH = hyperdense, lens-shaped
- Swirl sign (hypodensity) = rapid bleeding
- Small EDHs ↓ in density with time, resolve

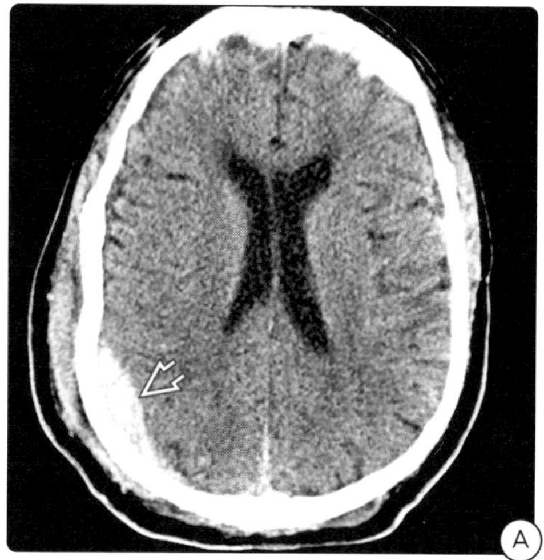


***(2-16A)** Serial imaging demonstrates temporal evolution of a small nonoperated EDH. Initial NECT scan shows a hyperdense biconvex EDH ➡.*

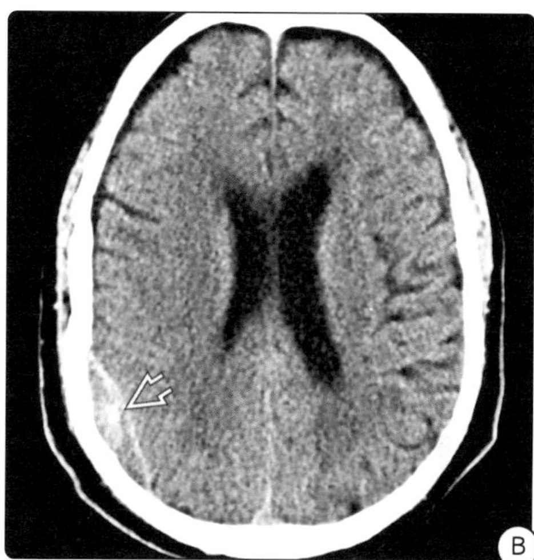


***(2-16B)** Repeat scan 10 days later reveals that density of the EDH ➡ has ↓ significantly.*

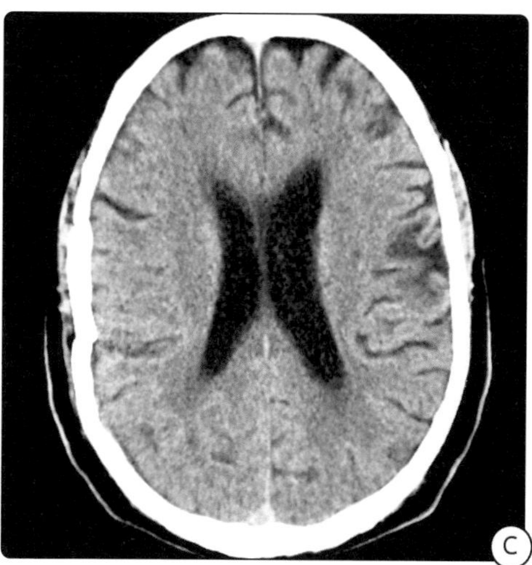


***(2-16C)** Repeat study 6 weeks after trauma reveals that the EDH has resolved completely.*

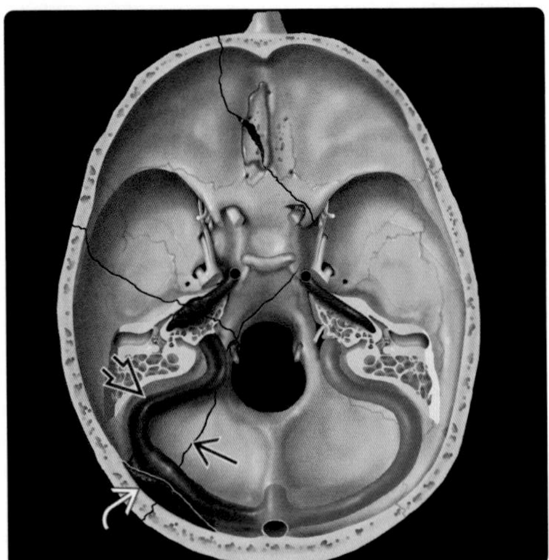

*(2-17) Graphic shows basilar skull fracture ➡ with transverse sinus occlusion ➡ and posterior fossa venous EDH ➡.*

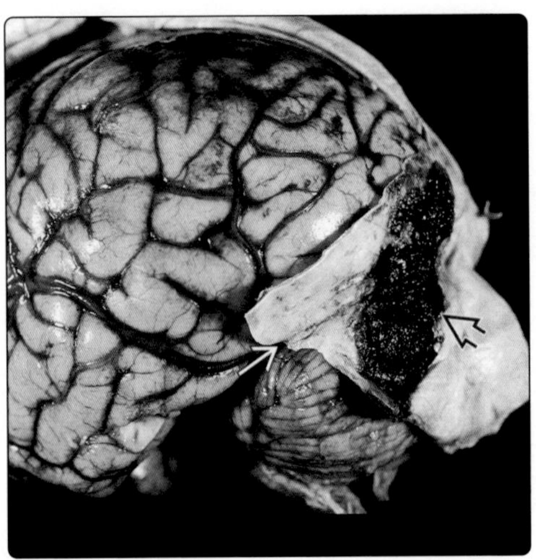

*(2-18) Autopsy shows that venous EDH ➡ caused by transverse sinus injury "straddles" the tentorium ➡. (Courtesy R. Hewlett, MD.)*

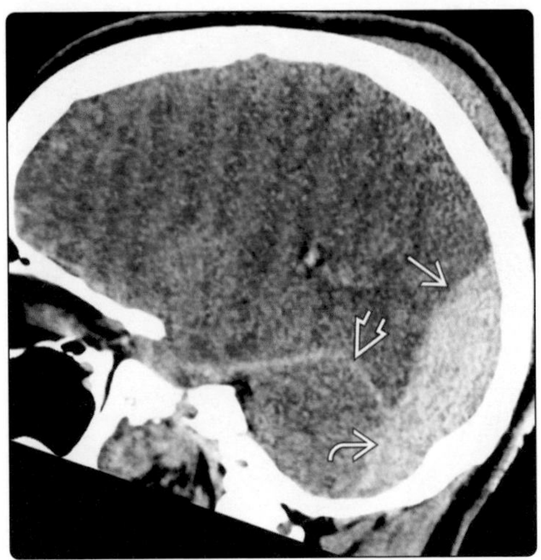

*(2-19) Sagittal NECT shows aEDH with supra- ➡ and infratentorial components ➡. Note subdural blood along displaced tentorium ➡.*

## Venous Epidural Hematomas

Not all EDHs are the same! **Venous EDHs** are often smaller, under lower pressure, and develop more slowly than their arterial counterparts. Most venous EDHs are caused by a skull fracture that crosses a dural venous sinus and therefore occur in the posterior fossa near the skull base (transverse/sigmoid sinus) **(2-17)** or the vertex of the brain [superior sagittal sinus (SSS)]. In contrast to their arterial counterparts, venous EDHs can "straddle" intracranial compartments, crossing both sutures and lines of dural attachment **(2-18)** and compressing or occluding the adjacent venous sinuses.

Venous EDHs can be subtle and easily overlooked. Coronal and sagittal reformatted images are key to the diagnosis and delineation of these variant EDHs. Several anatomic subtypes of venous EDHs, each with different treatment implications and prognosis, are recognized.

### Vertex EDH

"Vertex" EDHs are rare. Usually caused by a linear or diastatic fracture that crosses the SSS, they often accumulate over hours or even days with slow, subtle onset of symptoms. "Vertex" hematomas can be subtle and are easily overlooked unless coronal and sagittal reformatted images are obtained **(2-20)**.

### Anterior Temporal EDH

Anterior temporal EDHs are a unique subgroup of hematomas that occur in the anterior tip of the middle cranial fossa **(2-21)**. Anterior temporal EDHs are caused either by an isolated fracture of the adjacent greater sphenoid wing or by an isolated zygomaticomaxillary complex ("tripod") facial fracture. The sphenoparietal dural venous sinus is injured as it curves medially along the undersurface of the lesser sphenoid wing, extravasating blood into the epidural space. Limited anatomically by the sphenotemporal suture laterally and the orbital fissure medially, anterior temporal EDHs remain stable in size and do not require surgical evacuation **(2-22)**.

### Clival EDH

Clival EDHs usually develop after a hyperflexion or hyperextension injury to the neck and are possibly caused by stripping of the tectorial membrane from attachments to the clivus. Less commonly, they have been associated with basilar skull fractures that lacerate the clival dural venous plexus.

Clival EDHs most often occur in children and present with multiple cranial neuropathies. The abducens nerve is the most commonly affected followed by the glossopharyngeal and hypoglossal nerves. They are typically limited in size by the tight attachment of the dura to the basisphenoid and tectorial membrane.

Management of a clival EDH is dictated by the severity and progression of the neurologic deficits and stability of the atlantoaxial joint. In patients with minor cranial nerve involvement, the clinical course is usually benign, and treatment with a cervical collar is typical.

NECT scans show a hyperdense collection between the clivus and tectorial membrane. Sagittal MR of the craniocervical junction shows the hematoma elevating the clival dura and extending inferiorly between the basisphenoid and tectorial membrane anterior to the medulla **(2-23)**.

## VENOUS EPIDURAL HEMATOMA

**Not All Epidural Hematomas Are the Same!**
- Different etiologies in different anatomic locations
- Prognosis, treatment vary

**Venous Epidural Hematomas = 10% of All Epidural Hematomas**
- Skull fracture crosses dural venous sinus
  - Can cross sutures, dural attachments
- Often subtle, easily overlooked
  - Coronal, sagittal reformatted images are key to diagnosis
- Usually accumulate slowly
- Can be limited in size
- Often treated conservatively

**Subtypes**
- Vertex EDH
  - Skull fracture crosses SSS
  - SSS can be lacerated, compressed, thrombosed
  - Midline/paramidline EDH
  - Hematoma under low pressure, develops gradually
  - Delayed symptoms are common
  - May become large, cause significant mass effect
  - CTV shows displaced SSS, cortical veins
- Anterior temporal EDH
  - Sphenoid wing or zygomaticomaxillary fracture
  - Injures sphenoparietal venous sinus
  - Hematoma accumulates at anterior tip of middle cranial fossa
  - Limited anatomically
  - Extent constrained laterally by sphenotemporal suture, medially by orbital fissure
  - Benign clinical course
- Clival EDH
  - Most common = child with neck injury
  - May cause multiple cranial neuropathies (CNVI most common)
  - Hyperdense collection under clival dura
  - Limited by tight attachment of dura to basisphenoid, tectorial membrane
  - Usually benign course, resolves spontaneously

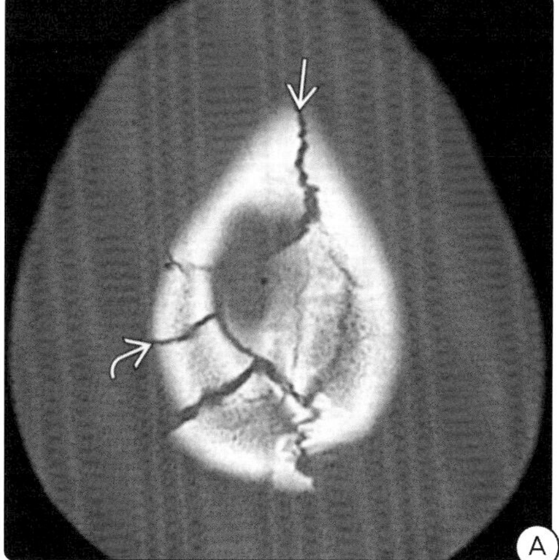

***(2-20A)** NECT shows multiple linear ➡, diastatic ➡ vertex skull fractures crossing the midline.*

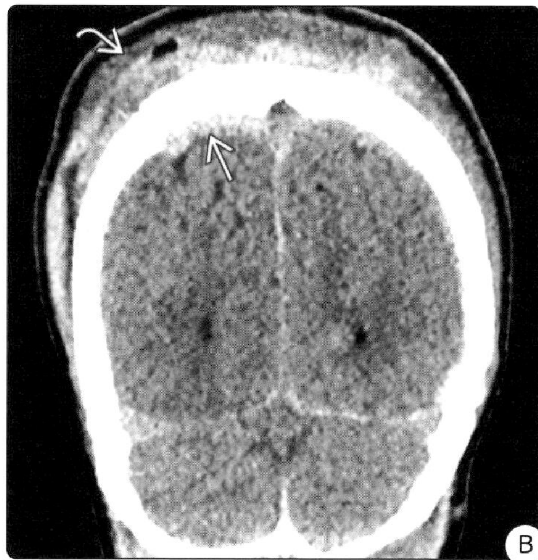

***(2-20B)** Coronal NECT shows a large cephalohematoma ➡ crossing the midline and a small extraaxial hematoma ➡.*

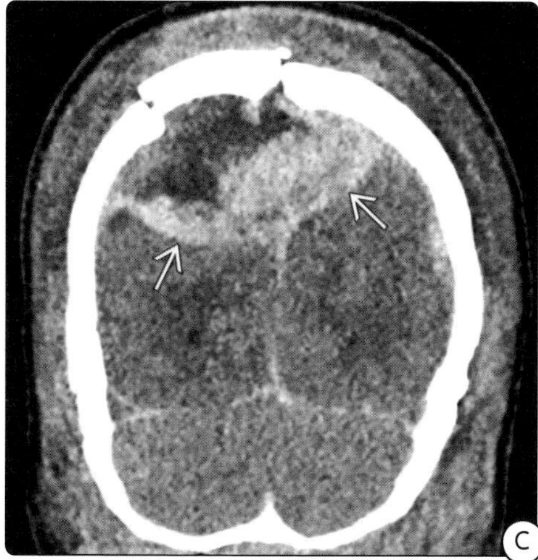

***(2-20C)** 24 hours later, the patient rapidly deteriorated. Repeat coronal NECT shows large, rapidly bleeding venous vertex EDH ➡.*

# Acute Subdural Hematoma

Acute SDHs (aSDHs) are one of the leading causes of death and disability in patients with severe TBI. Older adult patients with ground-level falls (GLFs) are especially prone to developing SDHs. Anticoagulation may lead to especially rapid expansion of an aSDH.

SDHs are much more common than EDHs. Most do not occur as isolated injuries; the vast majority of SDHs are associated with tSAH as well as significant parenchymal injuries, such as cortical contusions, brain lacerations, and DAIs.

## Terminology

An aSDH is a collection of acute blood products that lies in or between or within the inner border cell layer of the dura and the arachnoid **(2-24)**.

## Etiology

Trauma is the most common cause of aSDH. Both direct blows to the head and nonimpact injuries may result in formation of an aSDH. Tearing of bridging cortical veins as they cross the arachnoid and dural border cell layer to enter a dural venous sinus (usually the SSS) is the most common etiology.

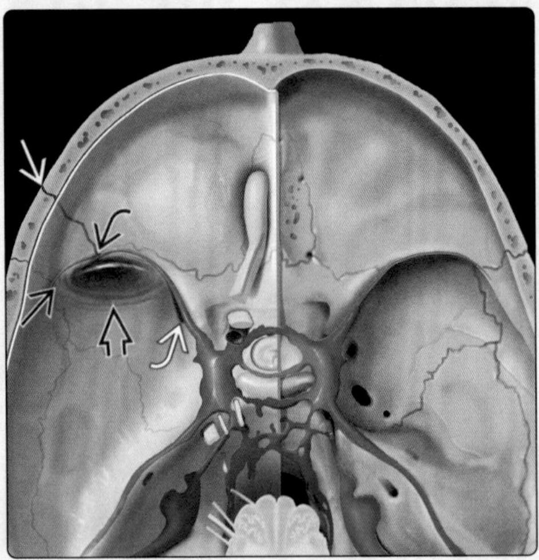

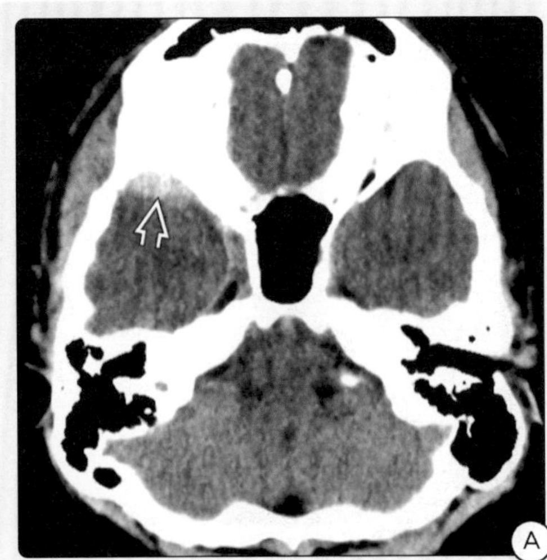

***(2-21)** Graphic depicts benign anterior temporal EDH. Fracture ➡ disrupts the sphenoparietal sinus ➡. Low-pressure venous EDH ➡ is anatomically limited, medially by the orbital fissure ➡ and laterally by the sphenotemporal suture ➡. **(2-22A)** NECT shows a small biconvex right anterior middle cranial fossa EDH ➡.*

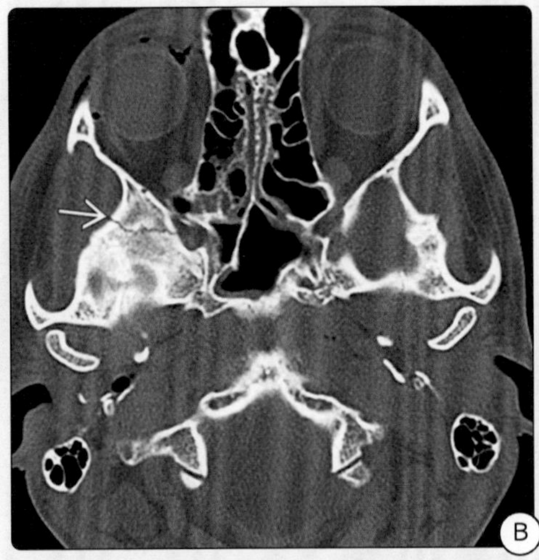

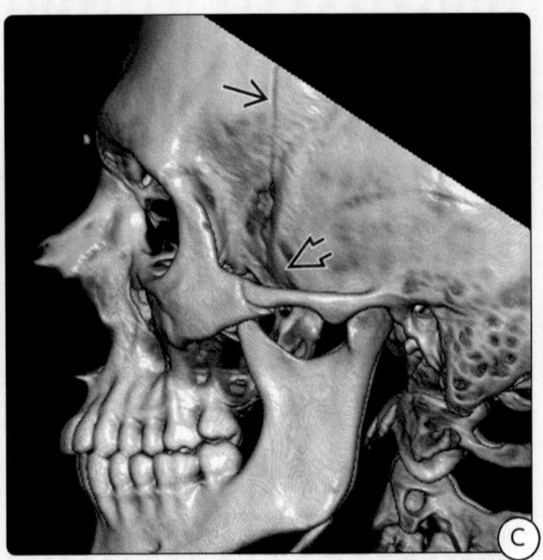

***(2-22B)** Bone CT in the same case shows a linear fracture ➡ extending across the floor of the right middle cranial fossa to the inferior orbital fissure. **(2-22C)** 3D SSD shows that the fracture ➡ extends across the sphenotemporal suture ➡. Middle fossa venous EDHs are anatomically limited by the orbital fissure medially and the sphenotemporal suture laterally.*

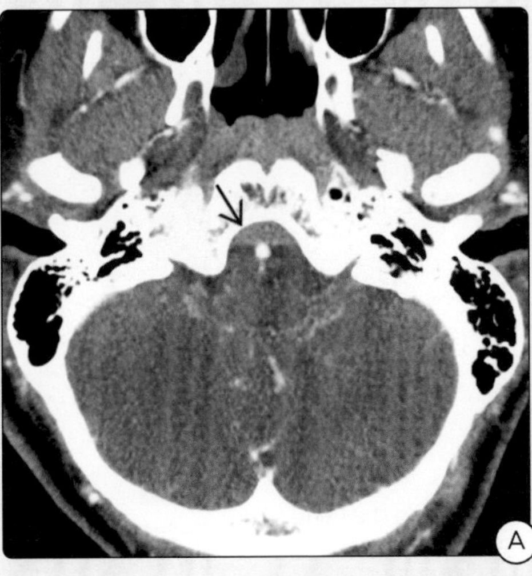

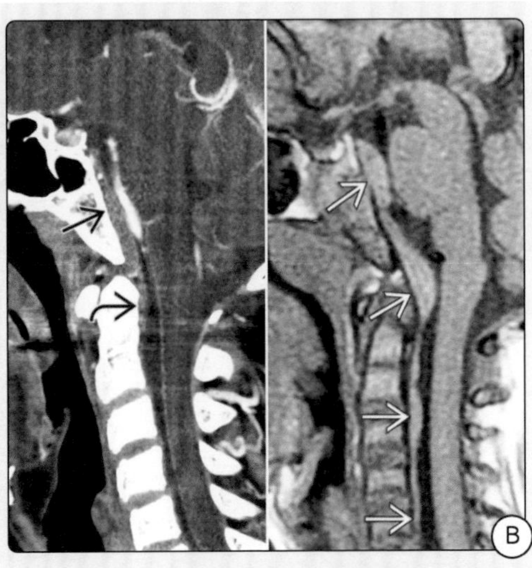

***(2-23A)** Axial CTA in a child with craniovertebral junction trauma shows a small clival EDH ➡. There was no evidence for vascular injury. **(2-23B)** (L) Sagittal CTA reformatted from the axial source data nicely demonstrates the clival EDH ➡. Note extension inferiorly ➡ to the middle of C2. (R) MR was obtained several hours later. The sagittal T1WI best shows the clival EDH ➡ now extends from the level of the dorsum sellae inferiorly to C5.*

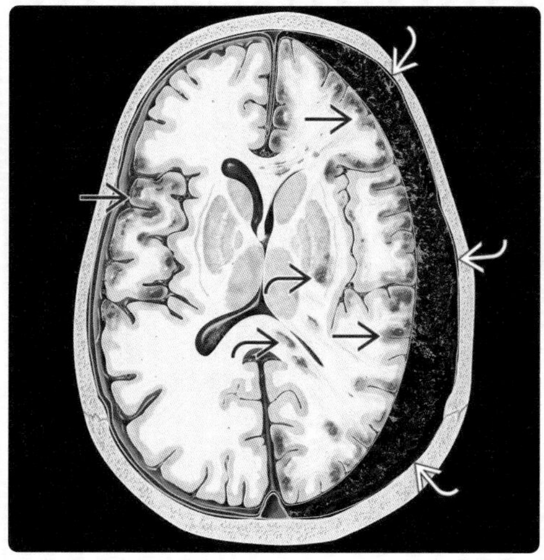

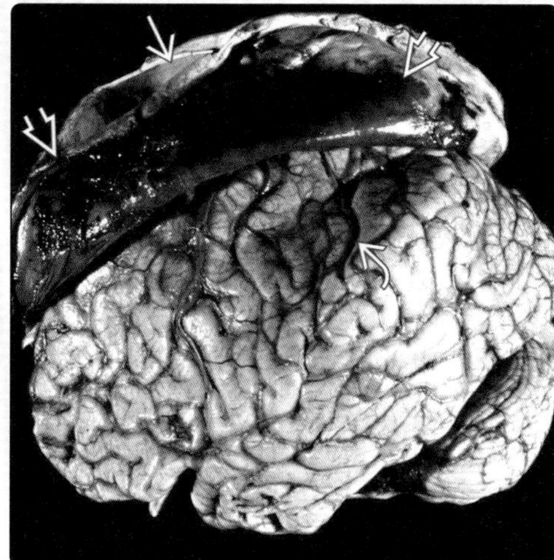

***(2-24)** Graphic depicts a crescent-shaped acute subdural hematoma (aSDH) ➡ with contusions and contrecoup injuries ➡ and diffuse axonal injuries ➡. **(2-25)** Autopsied brain shows a large subacute SDH (sSDH) ➡ that accumulated between the thickened, bulging dura ➡ and the arachnoid-covered brain. Note that the SDH extends over almost the entire hemisphere, displacing superficial cortical veins ➡ inward.*

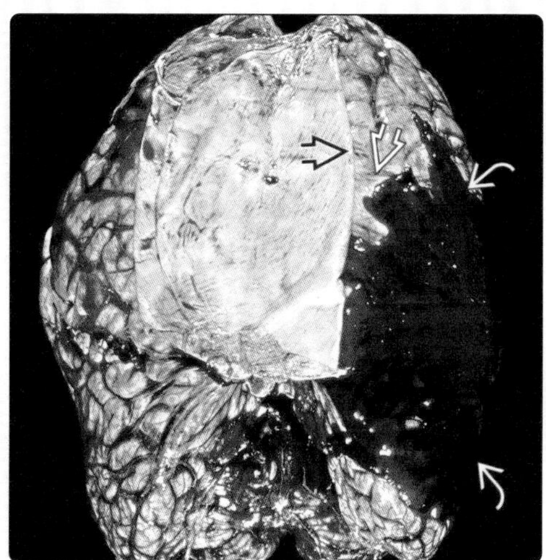

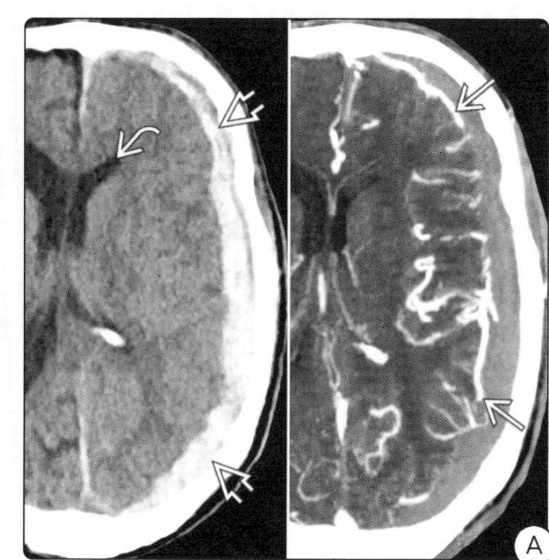

***(2-26)** Autopsy shows aSDH under dura ➡ but external to the arachnoid (seen here as glistening semitransparent membrane) ➡. The aSDH spreads diffusely over the brain, easily forming a crescent of blood ➡. **(2-27A)** (L) NECT shows hyperdense aSDH ➡ causing mass effect on the left lateral ventricle ➡. (R) Axial MIP CTA shows medially displaced cortical veins ➡ do not cross the SDH.*

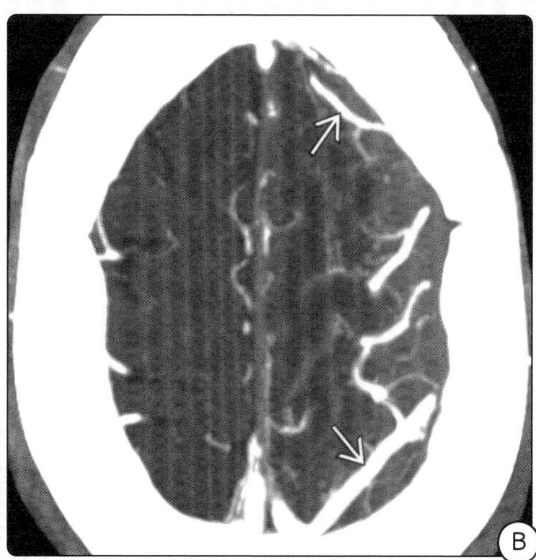

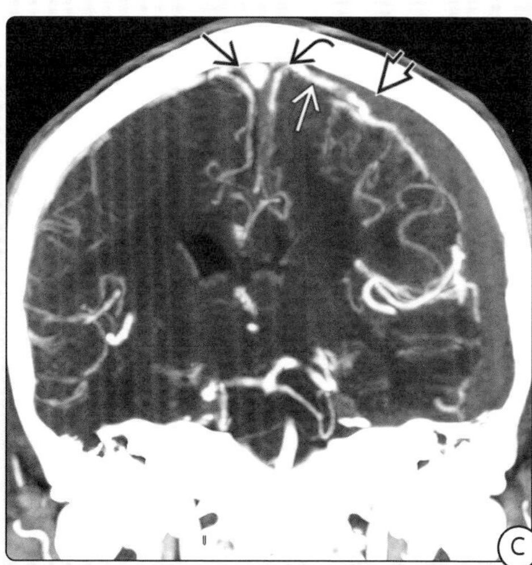

***(2-27B)** More cephalad MIP CTA shows stretched cortical veins ➡ crossing the aSDH toward the superior sagittal sinus (SSS). **(2-27C)** Coronal MIP CTA shows displaced cortical vein ➡ under the SDH ➡ crossing toward the SSS ➡. Vein appears narrowed ➡ as it crosses the dural border into the SSS.*

Cortical vein lacerations can occur with either a skull fracture or the sudden changes in velocity and brain rotation that occur during nonimpact CHI.

Blood from ruptured vessels spreads quickly through the potential space between the dura and the arachnoid. Large SDHs may spread over an entire hemisphere, also extending into the interhemispheric fissure and along the tentorium.

Tearing of cortical arteries or a venous sinus from a skull fracture may also give rise to an aSDH. The arachnoid itself may also rupture, creating a pathway for leakage of CSF into the subdural space that results in a subdural hygroma (SDHy) (pure CSF) or an admixture of both blood and CSF.

Less common causes of aSDH include aneurysm rupture, skull/dura-arachnoid metastases from vascular extracranial primary neoplasms, and spontaneous hemorrhage in patients with severe coagulopathy.

## Pathology

**Gross Pathology.** The gross appearance of an aSDH is that of a soft, purplish, "currant jelly" clot beneath a tense, bulging dura **(2-25)**. More than 95% are supratentorial. Most aSDHs spread diffusely over the affected hemisphere and are therefore typically crescent-shaped **(2-26)**.

## Clinical Issues

**Epidemiology.** An aSDH is the second most common extraaxial hematoma, exceeded only by tSAH. An aSDH is found in 10-20% of all patients with head injury and is observed in 30% of autopsied fatal injuries.

An aSDH may occur at any age from infancy to older adulthood. There is no sex predilection.

**Presentation.** Even relatively minor head trauma, especially in older adult patients who are often anticoagulated, may result

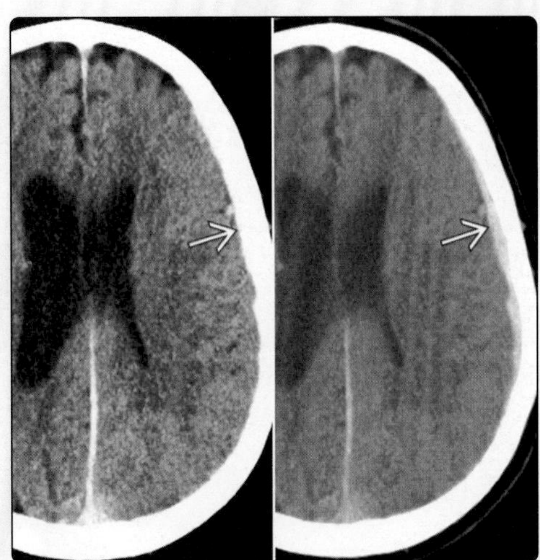

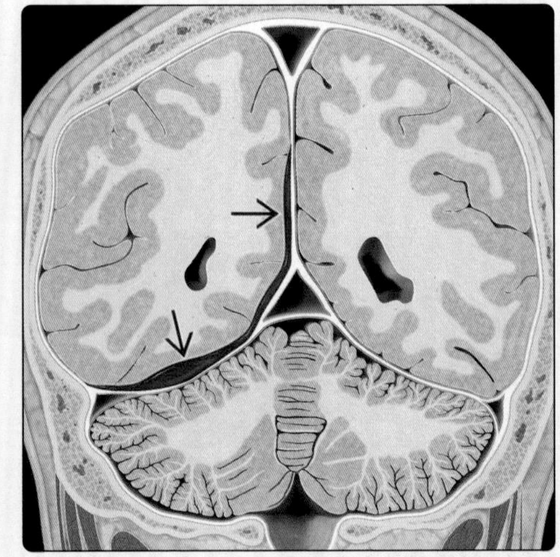

***(2-28)** NECT shows that a small SDH ➡ is easier to see with wider (R) compared with standard (L) windows. **(2-29)** Coronal graphic depicts thin aSDH layering along the tentorium and inferior falx cerebri ➡.*

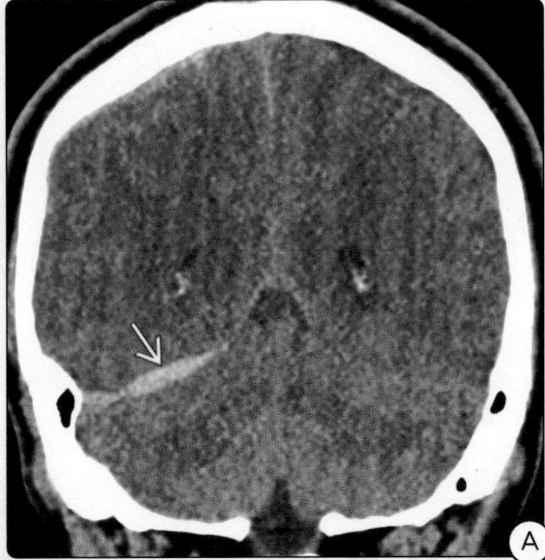



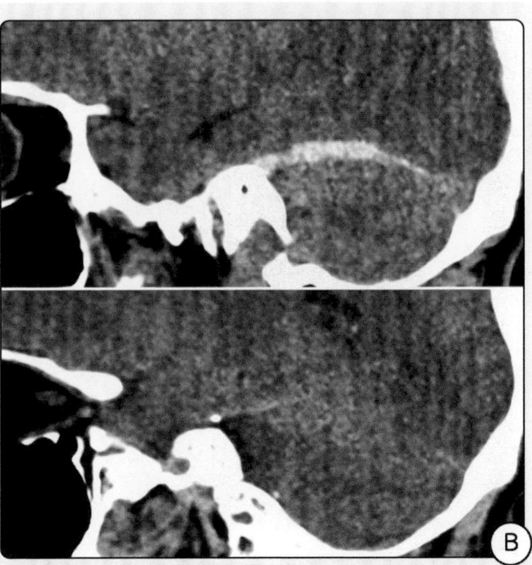



***(2-30A)** Reformatted coronal NECT using the axial source data shows a small right peritentorial aSDH ➡. **(2-30B)** Sagittal scans in the same case show the right peritentorial aSDH (top) with normal left sagittal dura (bottom) for comparison.*

in an aSDH. In such patients, a definite history of trauma may be lacking.

Clinical findings vary from none to loss of consciousness and coma. Most patients with aSDHs have low GCS scores on admission. Delayed deterioration, especially in older anticoagulated patients, is common.

**Natural History.** An aSDH may remain stable, grow slowly, or rapidly increase in size, causing mass effect and secondary brain herniations. Prognosis varies with hematoma thickness, midline shift, and the presence of associated parenchymal injuries. An aSDH that is thicker than 2 cm correlates with poor outcome (35-90% mortality). An aSDH that occupies more than 10% of the total available intracranial volume is usually lethal.

**Treatment Options.** The majority of patients with small SDHs are initially treated conservatively with close clinical observation and follow-up imaging. Small isolated falcine or tentorial SDHs typically do not increase in size and usually do not require short-term follow-up imaging.

Patients with larger SDHs, a lesion located at the convexity, alcohol abuse disorder, and repetitive falls are at the greatest risk for deterioration. Surveillance with follow-up CT scans is recommended until the SDH resolves or at least up to five weeks following the initial trauma.

## Imaging

**General Features.** The classic finding of an aSDH is a supratentorial crescent-shaped extraaxial collection that displaces the gray matter-white matter interface and cortical veins medially **(2-27)**. SDHs are typically more extensive than EDHs, easily spreading along the falx, tentorium, and around the anterior and middle fossa floors. SDHs may cross suture lines but generally do not cross dural attachments. Bilateral SDHs occur in 15% of cases. Contrecoup injuries, such as contusion of the contralateral hemisphere, are common.

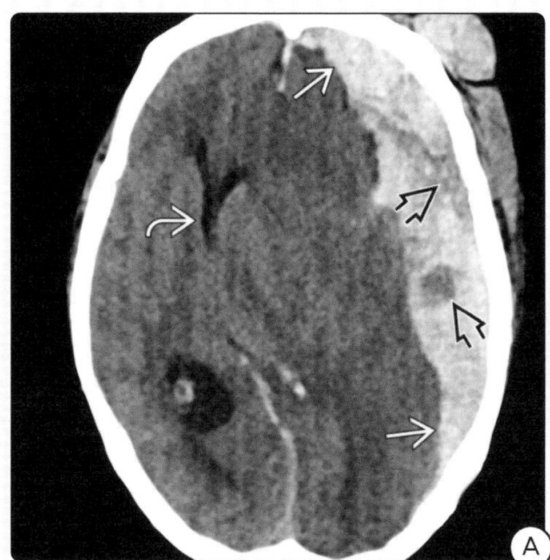


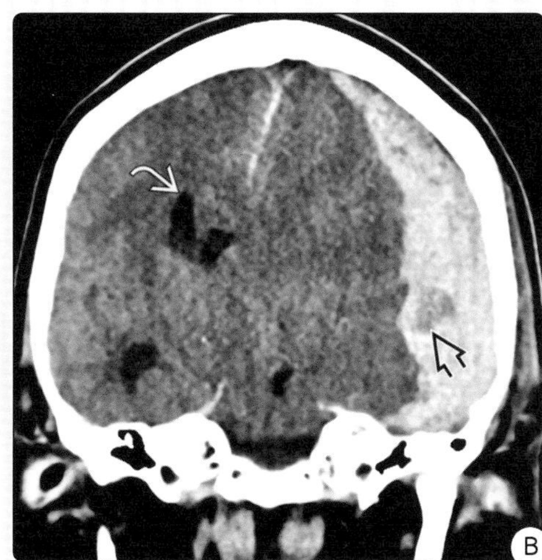


***(2-31A)** Axial NECT in a 74-yo anticoagulated patient with a ground-level fall shows a huge, mixed-density aSDH ➡ with severe subfalcine herniation of the lateral ventricles ➡. Low-density foci ⇨ within the aSDH indicate rapid bleeding with unclotted blood. **(2-31B)** Coronal NECT shows the subfalcine herniation ➡ and mixed-density aSDH with hypodense foci ⇨. The patient expired shortly after the scan.*

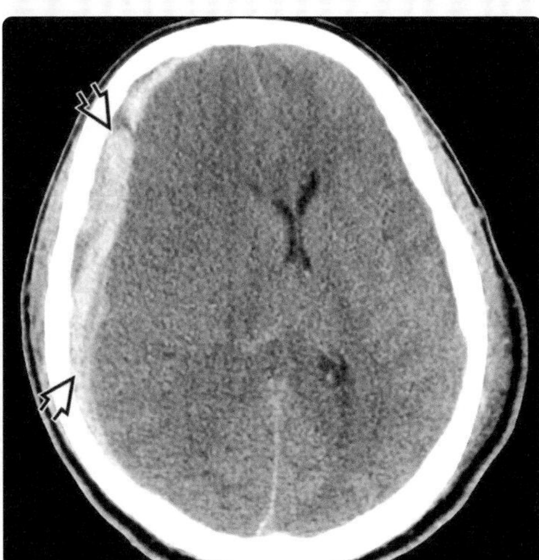

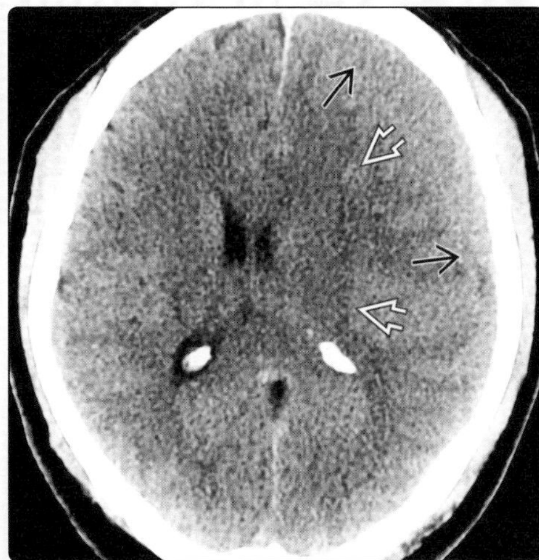

***(2-32)** NECT shows a mixed-density 12-mm aSDH ⇨ with a disproportionately large subfalcine herniation of the lateral ventricles (17 mm), indicating that diffuse holohemispheric brain swelling is present. Subfalcine herniation ≥ 3 mm portends a poor prognosis. **(2-33)** NECT in a very anemic patient shows an isodense aSDH ⇨. The aSDH is almost exactly the same density as the underlying cortex. The GM-WM interface is displaced inward ➡.*

Both standard soft tissue and intermediate ("subdural") windows as well as bone algorithm reconstructions should be used in all trauma patients, as small, subtle aSDHs can be obscured by the density of the overlying calvarium **(2-28)**. Coronal and sagittal reformatted images using the axial source data are especially helpful in visualizing small ("smear") peritentorial and parafalcine aSDHs **(2-29)** **(2-30)**.

### CT Findings

***NECT.*** Approximately 60% of aSDHs are hyperdense on NECT scans **(2-27A)**. Mixed-attenuation lesions are found in 40% of cases. Pockets of hypodensity within a larger hyperdense aSDH usually indicate rapid bleeding **(2-31)**. "Dots" or "lines" of CSF trapped within compressed, displaced sulci are often seen underlying an SDH **(2-33)**.

Mass effect with an aSDH is common and expected. Subfalcine herniation should be proportionate to the size of the subdural collection. However, **if the difference between the midline shift and thickness of the hematoma is 3 mm or more, then mortality is very high**. This discrepancy occurs when underlying cerebral edema is triggered by the traumatic event. Early recognition and aggressive treatment for potentially catastrophic brain swelling are essential **(2-32)**.

In other cases, especially in patients with repeated head injury, severe brain swelling with unilateral hemisphere vascular engorgement occurs very quickly. Here, the mass effect is greatly disproportionate to the size of the SDH, which may be relatively small.

Occasionally, an aSDH is nearly isodense with the underlying cortex. This unusual appearance is found in extremely anemic patients (Hgb < 8-10 g/dL) **(2-33)** and sometimes occurs in patients with coagulopathy. In rare cases, CSF leakage through a torn arachnoid may mix with—and dilute—the acute blood that collects in the subdural space.

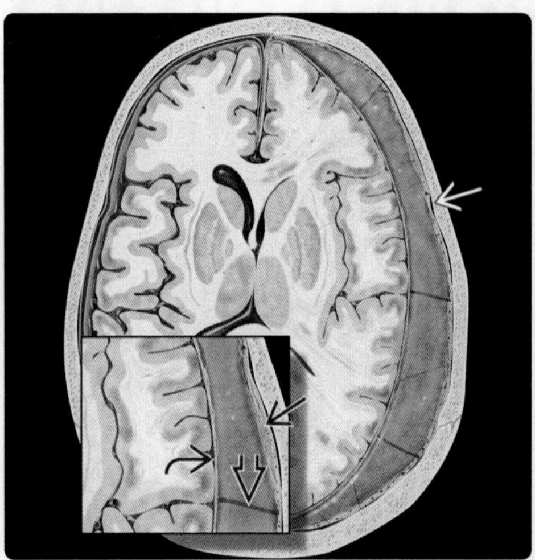

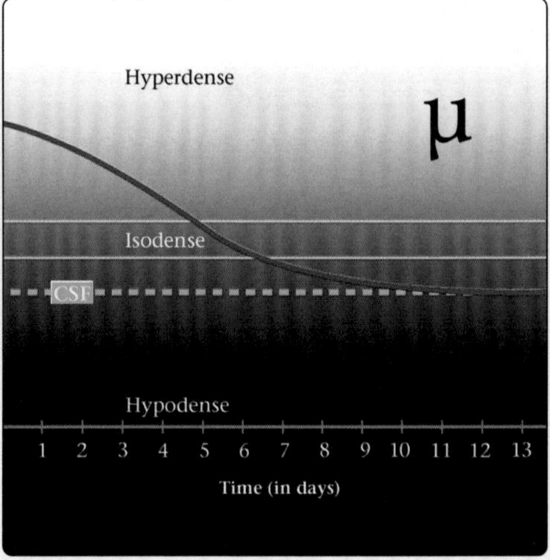


***(2-34)** Graphic depicts sSDH ➡. Inset shows bridging vein (BV) ➡ and thin inner ➡ and thick outer ➡ membranes. **(2-35)** SDHs ↓ ~ 1.5 HU/day. By 7-10 days, blood in hematoma is isodense with cortex. By 10 days, it is hypodense.*

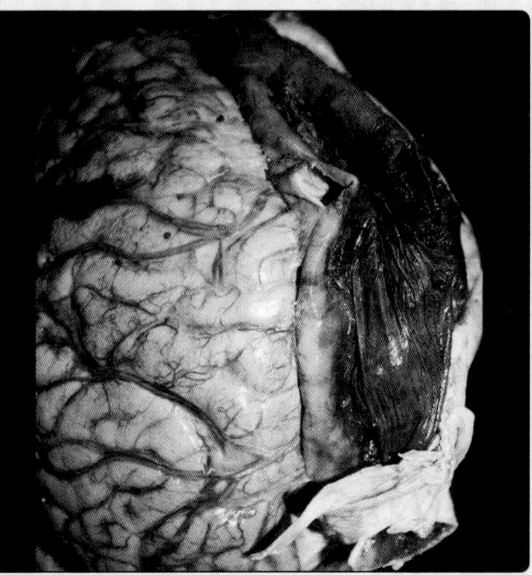

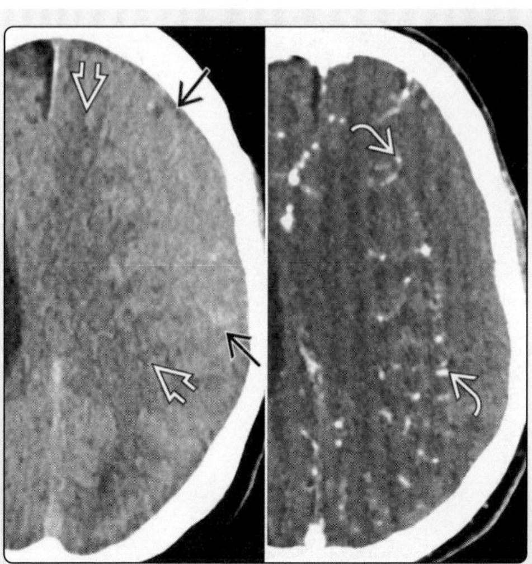

***(2-36)** Gross pathology of sSDH shows organized SDH slowing crescentic organized clot under dura. **(2-37)** (L) NECT of an sSDH shows the hematoma ➡ is isodense with the underlying cortex. Note the medial displacement ➡ of the GM-WM interface. (R) CTA shows cortical arteries and veins displaced medially ➡ by the avascular fluid collection.*

***CECT/CTA.*** CECT scans are helpful in detecting small isodense aSDHs. The normally enhancing cortical veins are displaced inward by the extraaxial fluid collection **(2-27)**. CTA may be useful in visualizing a cortical vessel that is actively bleeding into the subdural space.

**MR Findings.** MR scans are rarely obtained in acutely brain-injured patients. In such cases, aSDHs appear isointense on T1WI and hypointense on T2WI. Signal intensity on FLAIR scans is usually iso- to hyperintense compared with CSF but hypointense compared with the adjacent brain. aSDHs are hypointense on T2* scans.

DWI shows heterogeneous signal within the hematoma but may show patchy foci of restricted diffusion in the cortex underlying the aSDH.

## Differential Diagnosis

In the setting of acute trauma, the major differential diagnosis is EDH. Shape is a helpful feature, as most aSDHs are crescentic, whereas EDHs are biconvex. EDHs are almost always associated with skull fracture; SDHs frequently occur in the absence of skull fracture. EDHs may cross sites of dural attachment; SDHs do not cross the falx or tentorium.

# Subacute Subdural Hematoma

With time, SDHs undergo organization, lysis, and neomembrane formation. Within 2-3 days, the initial soft, loosely organized clot of an aSDH becomes organized. Breakdown of blood products and the formation of organizing granulation tissue change the imaging appearance of subacute (sSDH) and chronic (cSDH) SDHs.

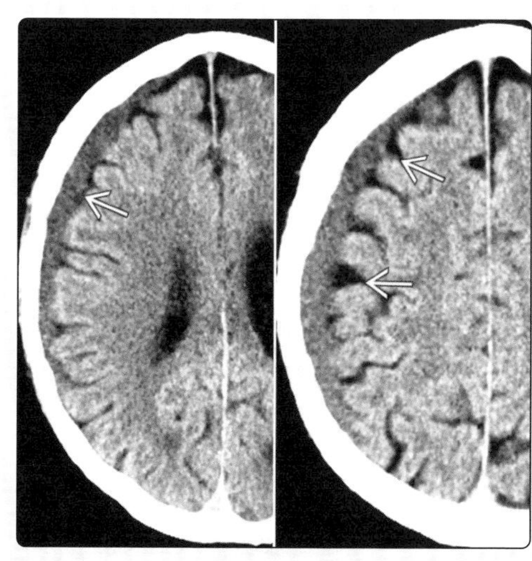

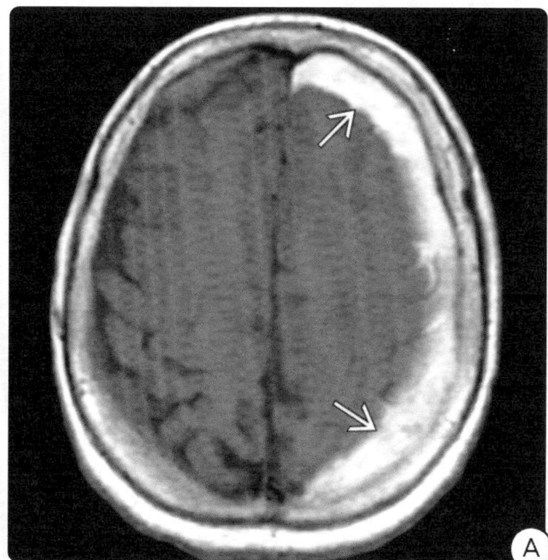


***(2-38) NECT in an older patient with sSDH and moderate cortical atrophy shows the difference between nearly isodense SDH and CSF in an underlying compressed subarachnoid space, sulci ➡. (2-39A) Axial T1WI MR in patient with a late-stage aSDH shows crescent-shaped hyperintense collection ➡ extending over entire surface of left hemisphere and gyral compression with almost obliterated sulci compared with normal right hemisphere.***

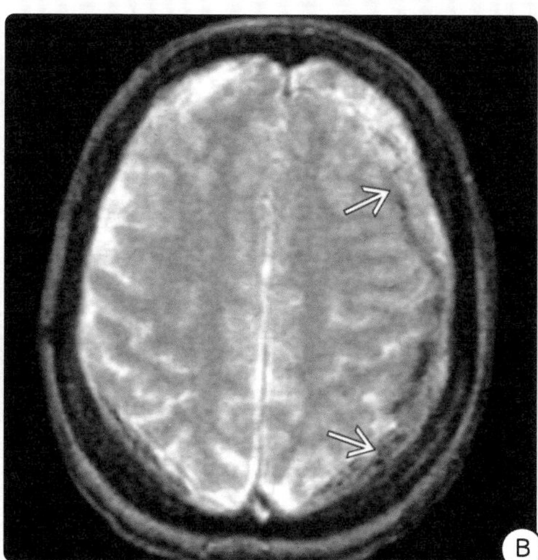


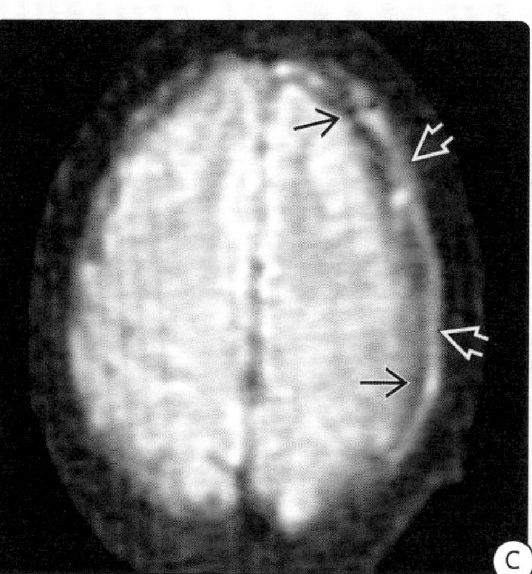


***(2-39B) T2* GRE MR shows some "blooming" ➡ in the sSDH. (2-39C) DWI MR shows the classic double-layer appearance of an sSDH with hypointense rim on the inside ➡ and mildly hyperintense rim on the outside ➡ of the clot.***

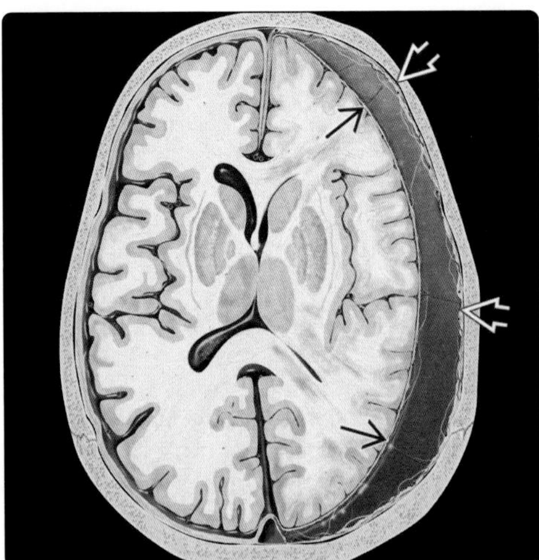

*(2-40) Simple cSDHs contain serosanguineous fluid with hematocrit effect and thin inner ⇨ and thick outer ➡ encapsulating membranes.*

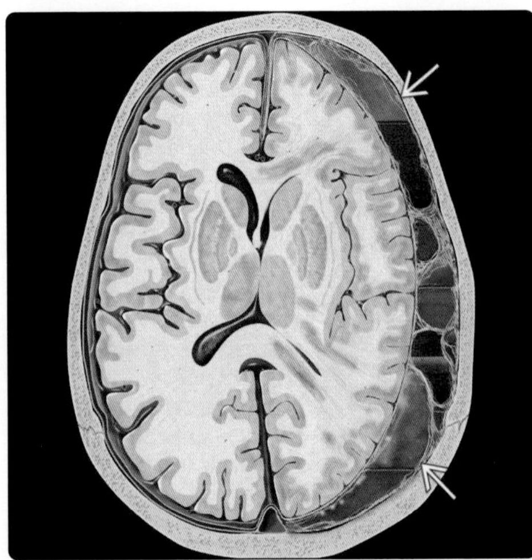

*(2-41) Complicated cSDHs contain loculated pockets of old and new blood seen as fluid-fluid levels ➡ within septated cavities.*

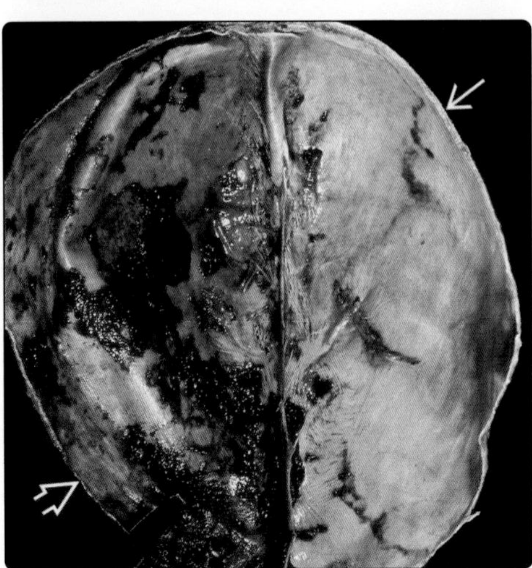

*(2-42) cSDH autopsy: 1 side has thickened dura ➡, the other has mixed acute, subacute, chronic hemorrhages ➡. (From DP: Hospital Autopsy.)*

## Terminology

An sSDH is between several days and several weeks old.

## Pathology

A collection of partially liquified clot with resorbing blood products is surrounded on both sides by a "membrane" of organizing granulation tissue **(2-34)**. The outermost membrane adheres to the dura and is typically thicker than the inner membrane, which abuts the thin, delicate arachnoid **(2-36)**.

In some cases, repetitive hemorrhages of different ages arising from the friable granulation tissue may be present. In others, liquefaction of the hematoma over time produces serous blood-tinged fluid.

## Clinical Issues

**Epidemiology and Demographics.** SDHs are common findings at imaging and autopsy. In contrast to aSDHs, sSDHs show a distinct bimodal distribution with children and older adults as the most commonly affected age groups.

**Presentation.** Clinical symptoms vary from asymptomatic to loss of consciousness and hemiparesis caused by sudden rehemorrhage into an sSDH. Headache and seizure are other common presentations.

**Natural History and Treatment Options.** Many sSDHs resolve spontaneously. In some cases, repeated hemorrhages may cause sudden enlargement and mass effect. Surgical drainage may be indicated if the sSDH is enlarging or becomes symptomatic.

## Imaging

**General Features.** Imaging findings are related to hematoma age and the presence of encasing membranes. Evolution of an untreated, uncomplicated SDH follows a very predictable pattern on CT. Density of an extraaxial hematoma decreases ~ 1-2 HU each day **(2-35)**. Therefore, an SDH will become nearly isodense with the underlying cerebral cortex within a few days following trauma.

**CT Findings.** sSDHs are typically crescent-shaped fluid collections that are iso- to slightly hypodense compared with the underlying cortex on NECT **(2-37)**. Medial displacement of the gray matter-white matter interface ("buckling") is often present, along with "dot-like" foci of CSF in the trapped, partially effaced sulci underlying the sSDH **(2-38)**. Mixed-density hemorrhages are common.

Bilateral sSDHs may be difficult to detect because of their "balanced" mass effect. Sulcal effacement with displaced gray matter-white matter interfaces is the typical appearance.

CECT/CTV shows that the enhanced cortical veins are displaced medially **(2-37)**. The encasing membranes, especially the thicker superficial layer, may enhance.

**MR Findings.** MR can be very helpful in identifying sSDHs, especially small lesions that are virtually isodense with underlying brain on CT scans.

Signal intensity varies with hematoma age but is less predictable than on CT, making precise "aging" of subdural collections more problematic. In general, early sSDHs are isointense with cortex on T1WI **(2-39A)** and hypointense on T2WI but gradually become more hyperintense as extracellular methemoglobin increases. Most late-stage sSDHs are T1/T2 "bright-bright." A linear T2 hypointensity representing the encasing membranes that surround the SDH is sometimes present.

FLAIR is the most sensitive standard sequence for detecting sSDH, as the collection is typically hyperintense. Because FLAIR signal intensity varies depending on the relative contribution of T1 and T2 effects, early sSDHs may initially appear hypointense due to their intrinsic T2 shortening.

T2* scans are also very sensitive, as sSDHs show distinct "blooming" **(2-39B)**.

Signal intensity on DWI also varies with hematoma age. DWI commonly shows a crescentic high-intensity area with a low-intensity rim closer to the brain surface (double-layer appearance) **(2-39C)**. The low-intensity area corresponds to a mixture of resolved clot and CSF, whereas the high-intensity area correlates with solid clot.

T1 C+ scans demonstrate enhancing, thickened, encasing membranes. The membrane surrounding an sSDH is usually thicker on the dural side of the collection. Delayed scans may show gradual "filling in" and increasing hyperintensity of the sSDH.

### Differential Diagnosis

The major differential diagnosis of an sSDH is an **isodense aSDH**. These are typically seen only in an extremely anemic or anticoagulated patient. A **subdural effusion** that follows surgery or meningitis or that occurs as a component of intracranial hypotension can also mimic an sSDH. An **SDHy** is typically isodense/isointense with CSF and does not demonstrate enhancing, encapsulating membranes.

## Chronic/Mixed Subdural Hematoma

### Terminology

A cSDH is an encapsulated collection of sanguineous or serosanguineous fluid confined within the subdural space. Recurrent hemorrhage(s) into a preexisting cSDH are common and produce a mixed-age (mSDH) or "acute-on-chronic" SDH.

### Etiology

With continued degradation of blood products, an SDH becomes progressively more liquified until it is largely serous fluid tinged with blood products **(2-40)**. Rehemorrhage from vascularized encapsulating membranes **(2-42)** or rupture of stretched cortical veins as they pass over the cSDH to enter the SSS **(2-27)** occurs in 5-10% of cSDHs and is considered "acute-on-chronic" SDH.

### Pathology

**Gross Pathology.** Blood within the subdural space incites tissue reaction around its margins. Organization and resorption of the hematoma contained within the "membranes" of surrounding granulation tissue continue. These neomembranes have fragile, easily disrupted capillaries and easily rebleed, creating an mSDH. Multiple hemorrhages of different ages are common in mSDHs **(2-41)** **(2-42)**.

Eventually, most of the liquified clot in a cSDH is resorbed. Only a thickened dura-arachnoid layer remains with a few scattered pockets of old blood trapped between the inner and outer membranes.

### Clinical Issues

**Epidemiology.** Unoperated, uncomplicated sSDHs eventually evolve into cSDHs. Approximately 5-10% will rehemorrhage, causing multiloculated mSDHs **(2-41)**.

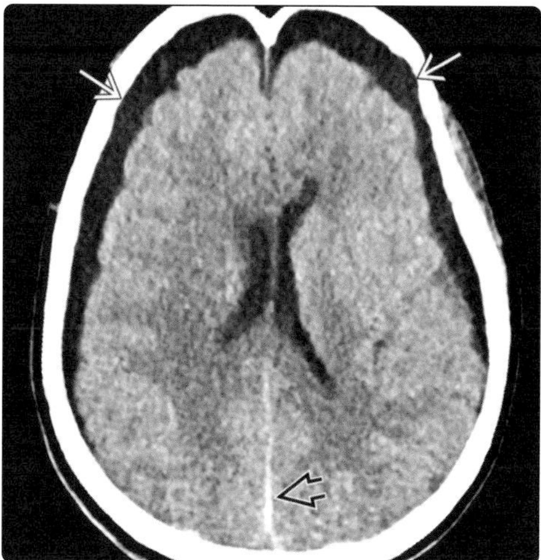

***(2-43)** NECT shows bilateral cSDHs ➡ causing mass effect on the underlying brain. A small left parafalcine aSDH is present ⇨.*

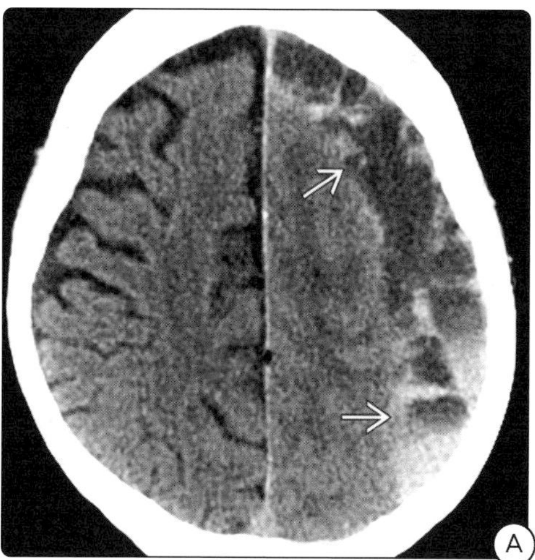


***(2-44A)** NECT shows mixed cSDH ➡ that features multiple loculated pockets of blood with old blood layered on top of recent hemorrhages.*

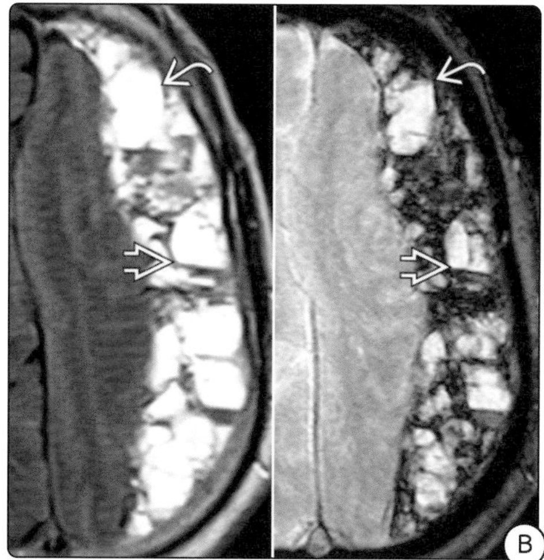


***(2-44B)** (L) FLAIR and (R) T2* in the same case show multiple pockets of loculated blood ➡ with varying signal intensities and fluid-fluid levels ➡.*

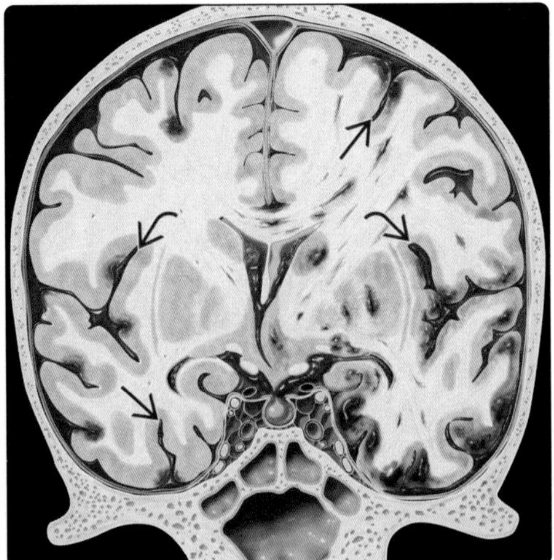

*(2-45) Graphic depicts traumatic subarachnoid hemorrhage (tSAH) around the sylvian fissures ➲ and in sulci ➲ adjacent to contused gyri.*

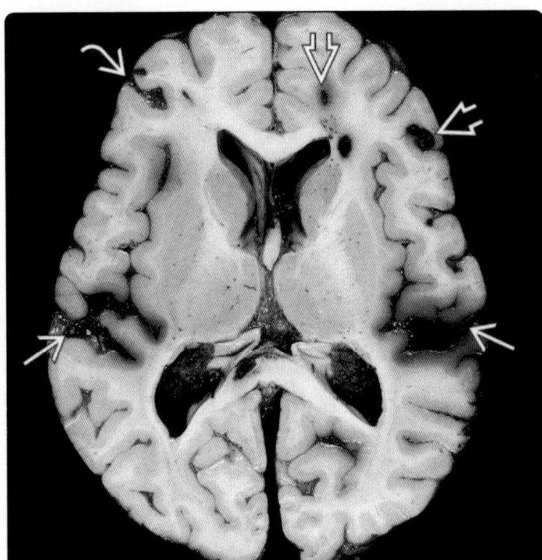

*(2-46) Autopsy of severe head trauma shows tSAH in sylvian fissures ➲, superficial sulci ➲, hemorrhagic axonal stretching/"shearing" ➲.*

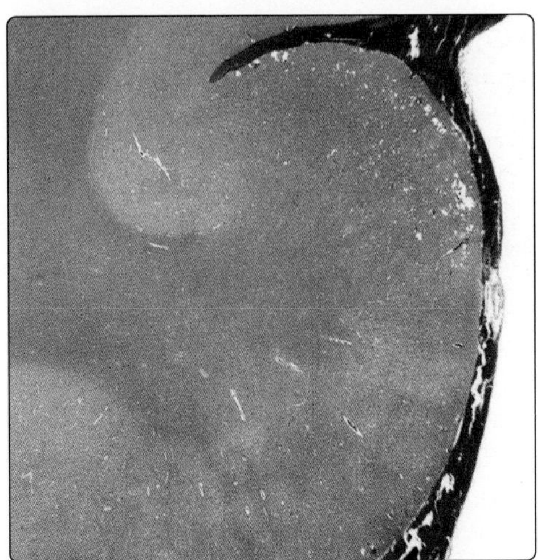

*(2-47) Photomicrograph of an autopsied boxer shows a typical tSAH covering the gyri and extending into the sulci. (Courtesy J. Paltan, MD.)*

**Demographics.** cSDHs may occur at any age. mSDHs are much more common in older adult patients.

**Presentation.** Presentation varies from no/mild symptoms (e.g., headache) to sudden neurologic deterioration if a preexisting cSDH rehemorrhages.

**Natural History.** In the absence of repeated hemorrhages, cSDHs gradually resorb and largely resolve, leaving a residue of thickened dura-arachnoid that may persist for months or even years. Older patients, especially those with brain atrophy, are subject to repeated hemorrhages.

**Treatment Options.** If follow-up imaging of an sSDH shows expected resorption and regression of the cSDH, no surgery may be required. Surgical drainage with evacuation of the cSDH and resection of its encapsulating membranes is performed if significant mass effect or repeated hemorrhages cause neurologic complications.

## Imaging

**General Features.** cSDHs have a spectrum of imaging appearances. **Uncomplicated cSDHs** show relatively homogeneous density/signal intensity **(2-43)** with slight gravity-dependent gradation of their contents ("hematocrit effect").

**mSDHs** with acute hemorrhage into a preexisting cSDH show a hematocrit level with distinct layering of the old (top) and new (bottom) hemorrhages. Sometimes, septated pockets that contain hemorrhages of different ages form **(2-44A)**. Dependent layering of blood within the loculated collections may appear quite bizarre.

Extremely old, **longstanding cSDHs** with virtually complete resorption of all liquid contents are seen as pachymeningopathies with diffuse dura-arachnoid thickening.

### CT Findings

***NECT.*** A hypodense crescentic fluid collection extending over the surface of one or both cerebral hemispheres is the classic finding in cSDH. Uncomplicated cSDHs approach CSF in density **(2-43)**. The hematocrit effect creates a slight gradation in density that increases from top to bottom.

Trabecular or loculated cSDHs show internal septations, often with evidence of repeated hemorrhages **(2-44A)**. With age, the encapsulating membranes surrounding the cSDH become thickened and may appear moderately hyperdense. Eventually, some cSDHs show peripheral calcifications that persist for many years. In rare cases, a cSDH may densely calcify or even ossify, a condition aptly termed "armored brain."

***CECT.*** The encapsulating membranes around a cSDH contain fragile neocapillaries that lack endothelial tight junctions. Therefore, the membranes show strong enhancement following contrast administration.

**MR Findings.** As with all intracranial hematomas, signal intensity of a cSDH or mSDH is quite variable and depends on the age of the blood products. On T1 scans, uncomplicated cSDHs are typically iso- to slightly hyperintense compared with CSF. Depending on the stage of evolution, cSDHs are iso- to hypointense compared with CSF on T2 scans.

Most cSDHs are hyperintense on FLAIR and may show "blooming" on T2* scans if subacute-chronic blood clots are still present **(2-39B)**. In ~ 1/4 of all cases, superficial siderosis can be identified over the gyri underlying a cSDH.

The encapsulating membranes of a cSDH enhance following contrast administration. Typically, the outer layer is thicker than the inner layer.

Uncomplicated cSDHs do not restrict on DWI. With cSDHs, a "double layer" effect—a crescent of hyperintensity medial to a nonrestricting fluid collection—indicates acute rehemorrhage **(2-39C)**.

### Differential Diagnosis

An mSDH is difficult to mistake for anything else. In older patients, a small uncomplicated cSDH may be difficult to distinguish from simple **brain atrophy** with enlarged bifrontal CSF spaces. However, cSDHs exhibit mass effect; they flatten the underlying gyri, often extending around the entire hemisphere and into the interhemispheric fissure. The increased extraaxial spaces in patients with cerebral atrophy are predominantly frontal and temporal.

A traumatic **SDHy** is an accumulation of CSF in the subdural space after head injury, probably secondary to an arachnoid tear. SDHys are sometimes detected within the first 24 hours after trauma; however, the mean time for appearance is nine days after injury. An SDHy or a hematohygroma in an infant or young child should be considered highly suspicious for abusive head trauma (AHT) (child abuse; see later discussion).

A classic uncomplicated SDHy is a hypodense, CSF-like, crescentic extraaxial collection that consists purely of CSF, has no blood products, lacks encapsulating membranes, and shows no enhancement following contrast administration. CSF leakage into the subdural space is also present in the vast majority of patients with cSDH. Therefore, many—if not most—cSDHs contain a mixture of *both* CSF and blood products.

A **subdural effusion** is an accumulation of clear fluid over the cerebral convexities or in the interhemispheric fissure. Subdural effusions are generally complications of meningitis; a history of prior infection, not trauma, is typical.

A **subdural empyema** (SDE) is a hypodense extraaxial fluid collection that contains pus. Most SDEs are secondary to sinusitis or mastoiditis, have strongly enhancing membranes, and often coexist with findings of meningitis. A typical SDE restricts strongly and uniformly on DWI. Look for underlying sulcal/cisternal hyperintensity on FLAIR and enhancement on T1 C+.

## Traumatic Subarachnoid Hemorrhage

tSAH is found in virtually all cases of moderate to severe head trauma. Indeed, trauma—**not** ruptured saccular aneurysm—is the most common cause of intracranial subarachnoid hemorrhage (SAH).

### Etiology

tSAH can occur with both direct trauma to the skull and nonimpact CHI. Tearing of cortical arteries and veins, rupture of contusions and lacerations into the contiguous subarachnoid space, and choroid plexus bleeds with intraventricular hemorrhage may all result in blood collecting within the subarachnoid cisterns.

Although tSAH occasionally occurs in isolation, it is usually accompanied by other manifestations of brain injury. Subtle tSAH *may be the only clue* on initial imaging studies that *more serious injuries lurk beneath the surface.*

### Pathology

**Location.** tSAHs are predominantly found in the anteroinferior frontal and temporal sulci, perisylvian regions, and over the hemispheric convexities **(2-45)**. In very severe cases, tSAH spreads over most of the brain. In mild cases,

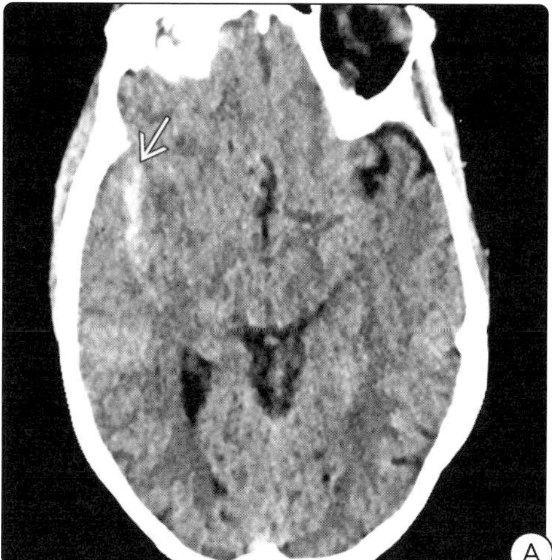


***(2-48A)** Axial NECT in a helmeted rider who fell off his bicycle shows tSAH in the right sylvian fissure ➡.*

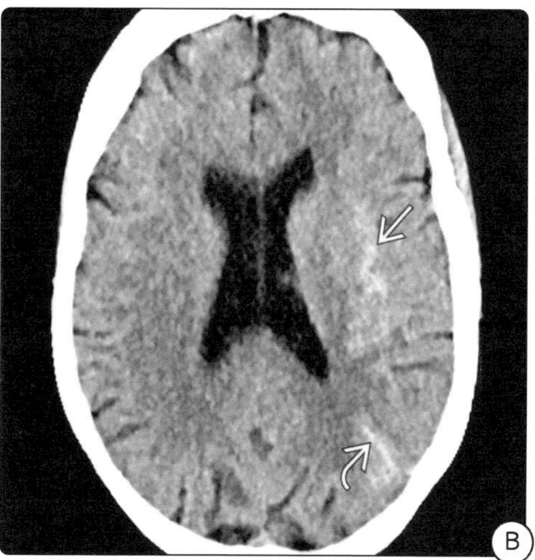


***(2-48B)** More cephalad NECT shows tSAH in the left sylvian fissure ➡ and parietal sulci ➡.*

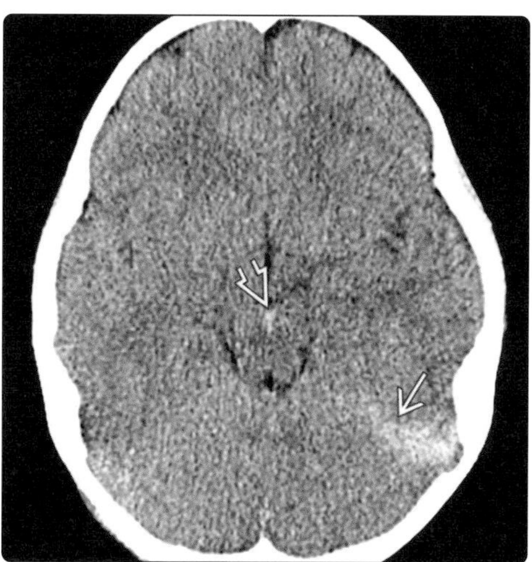

***(2-49)** Axial NECT shows a small peritentorial aSDH ➡ and a small amount of subarachnoid blood in the interpeduncular cistern ➡.*

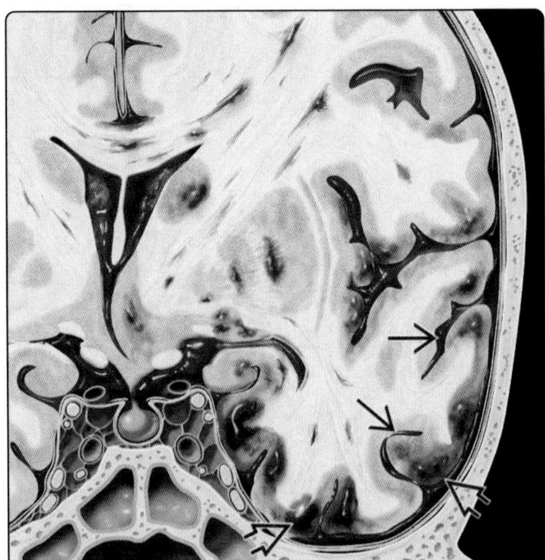

*(2-50) Cortical contusions are located primarily along gyral crests ⇒, around a sylvian fissure. tSAH is common in adjacent sulci ⇒.*

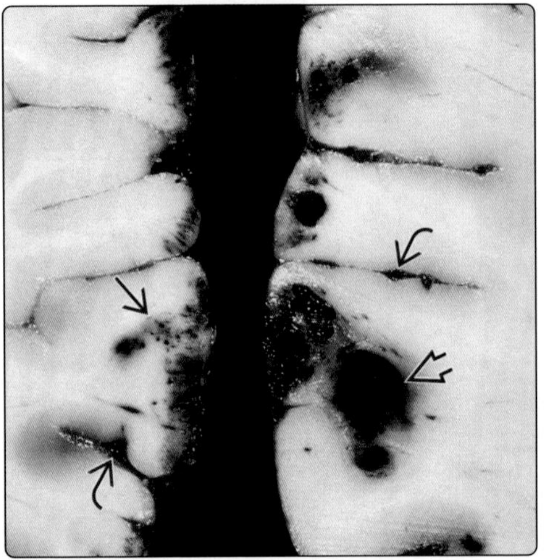

*(2-51) Autopsy shows petechial ⇒ and larger confluent cortical contusions ⇒ and tSAH in adjacent sulci ⇒. (Courtesy R. Hewlett, MD.)*

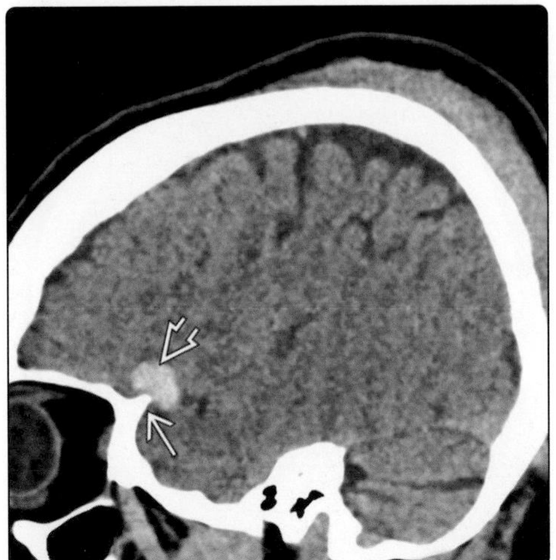

*(2-52) Sagittal NECT in CHI shows cortical contusion ⇒ immediately adjacent to bony ridge of greater sphenoid wing ⇒.*

blood collects in a single sulcus or the dependent portion of the interpeduncular fossa.

**Gross Pathology.** With the exception of location and associated parenchymal injuries, the gross appearance of tSAH is similar to that of aneurysmal SAH (aSAH). Curvilinear foci of bright red blood collect in cisterns and surface sulci **(2-46)** **(2-47)**.

tSAH typically occurs adjacent to cortical contusions. tSAH is also commonly identified under acute EDH and SDH.

## Clinical Issues

**Epidemiology.** tSAH is found in most cases of moderate trauma and is identified in virtually 100% of fatal brain injuries at autopsy.

**Natural History.** Breakdown and resorption of tSAH occurs gradually. Patients with isolated tSAH have very low rates of clinical or radiographic deterioration and typically do well.

## Imaging

**General Features.** With the exception of location, the general imaging appearance of tSAH is similar to that of aSAH, i.e., sulcal-cisternal hyperdensity/hyperintensity **(2-48)**. tSAH is typically more focal or patchy than the diffuse subarachnoid blood indicative of aneurysmal hemorrhage.

**CT Findings.** Acute tSAH is typically peripheral, appearing as linear hyperdensities in sulci adjacent to cortical contusions or under EDHs or SDHs. Occasionally, isolated tSAH is identified within the interpeduncular fossa **(2-49)**.

**MR Findings.** As acute blood is isointense with brain, it may be difficult to detect on T1WI. "Dirty" sulci with "smudging" of the perisylvian cisterns is typical. Subarachnoid blood is hyperintense to brain on T2WI and appears similar in signal intensity to cisternal CSF. FLAIR scans show hyperintensity in the affected sulci.

"Blooming" with hypointensity can be identified on T2* scans, typically adjacent to areas of cortical contusion. tSAH is recognized on GRE or SWI sequences as hypointense signal intensity surrounded by hyperintense CSF.

**Angiography.** Emergent CTA is usually unnecessary in cases with typical peripheral tSAH on NECT. Patients with suprasellar ("central") SAH may harbor a ruptured aneurysm and should be screened with CTA regardless of mechanism of injury.

## Differential Diagnosis

The major differential diagnosis of tSAH is **nontraumatic SAH** (ntSAH). Aneurysmal rupture causes 80-90% of all ntSAHs. In contrast to tSAH, aSAH is concentrated in the basal cisterns.

**Sulcal-cisternal hyperintensity** on FLAIR is nonspecific and can be caused by **meningitis, neoplasm, artifact** (incomplete CSF suppression), **contrast** leakage into the subarachnoid space (e.g., with renal failure), and **high inspired oxygen** during general anesthesia.

The term **pseudo-SAH** has been used to describe the CT appearance of a brain with severe cerebral edema. Hypodense brain makes circulating blood in arteries and veins look relatively hyperdense. The hyperdensity seen here is smooth and conforms to the expected shape of the vessels, not the subarachnoid spaces, and should not be mistaken for either tSAH or ntSAH.

**SUBDURAL AND SUBARACHNOID HEMORRHAGE**

**Acute Subdural Hemorrhage**
- 2nd most common traumatic extraaxial hemorrhage
  - aSDH > > EDH
- Crescentic collection of blood between dura, arachnoid
  - Supratentorial (95%), bilateral (15%)
  - SDHs cross sutures
  - SDHs do not cross dural attachments
- CT
  - Hyperdense (60%)
  - Mixed (40%)
  - Isodense aSDH rare (anemia, coagulopathy, CSF mixture)

**Subacute Subdural Hemorrhage**
- Clot organizes, lyses, forms "neomembranes"
- CT
  - Density ↓ 1-2 HU/day
  - Isodense with cortex in 7-10 days
  - Look for displaced "dots" of CSF under SDH
  - Gray matter-white matter interface "buckled" inward
  - Displaced cortical veins seen on CECT
- MR
  - Signal varies with clot age
  - T2* (GRE, SWI) shows "blooming"
  - T1 C+ shows clot inside enhancing membranes

**Chronic/Mixed Subdural Hemorrhage**
- Serosanguineous fluid
  - Hypodense on NECT
  - Rehemorrhage (5-10%)
  - Loculated blood "pockets" with fluid-fluid levels common
- Differential diagnosis of uncomplicated cSDH
  - Subdural **hygroma** (arachnoid tear → subdural CSF)
  - Subdural **effusion** (clear fluid accumulates after meningitis)
  - Subdural **empyema** (pus)

**Traumatic Subarachnoid Hemorrhage**
- Most common traumatic extraaxial hemorrhage
- tSAH > > aneurysmal SAH
- Adjacent to cortical contusions
- Superficial sulci > basilar cisterns

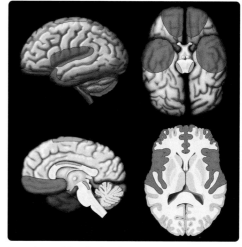

*(2-53) Graphics depict the most common sites of cerebral contusions in red. Less common sites are shown in green.*

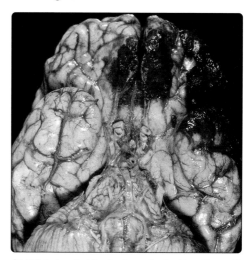

*(2-54) Autopsied brain shows typical locations of contusions, i.e., the anteroinferior frontal and temporal lobes. (Courtesy R. Hewlett, MD.)*

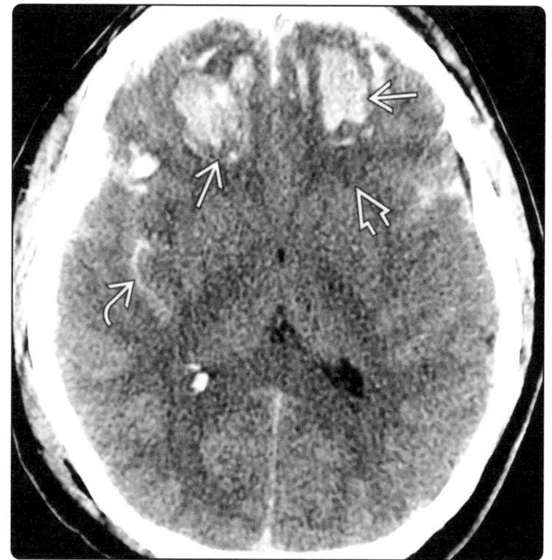

*(2-55) NECT shows bilateral inferior frontal confluent contusions ⇒, perilesional edema ⇒, and tSAH ⇒.*

# Parenchymal Injuries

Intraaxial traumatic injuries include cortical contusions and lacerations, diffuse axonal injury (DAI), subcortical injuries (SCIs), and intraventricular hemorrhages. In this section, we again begin with the most peripheral injuries—cortical contusions—and work our way inward, ending with the deepest (subcortical) injuries. **In general, the deeper the abnormalities, the more serious the injury**.

## Cerebral Contusions and Lacerations

Cerebral contusions are the most common of the intraaxial injuries. True brain lacerations are rare and typically occur only with severe (often fatal) head injury.

### Terminology

Cerebral contusions are basically "brain bruises." They evolve with time and are often more apparent on delayed scans than at the time of initial imaging.

*(2-56A) Contusions are a common contrecoup injury. In this case, the initial trauma was to the left parietooccipital region at the site of the scalp hematoma ➡. A large right frontal contusion ➡ is seen directly opposite the impact site. Note small ➡ peritentorial aSDH. (2-56B) Lower scan in the same case shows the scalp hematoma ➡ and tSAH ➡, also opposite the impact site.*

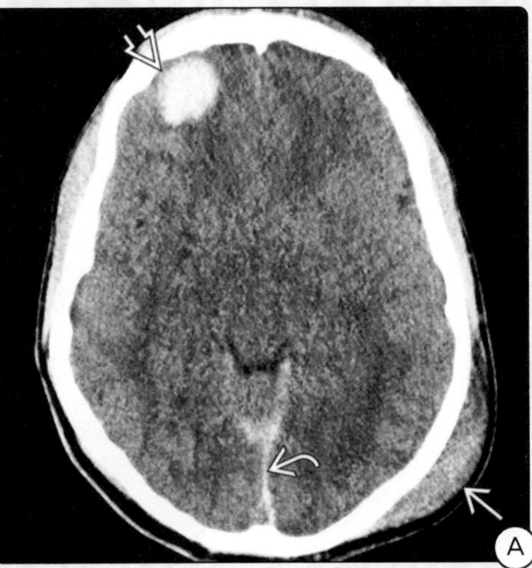


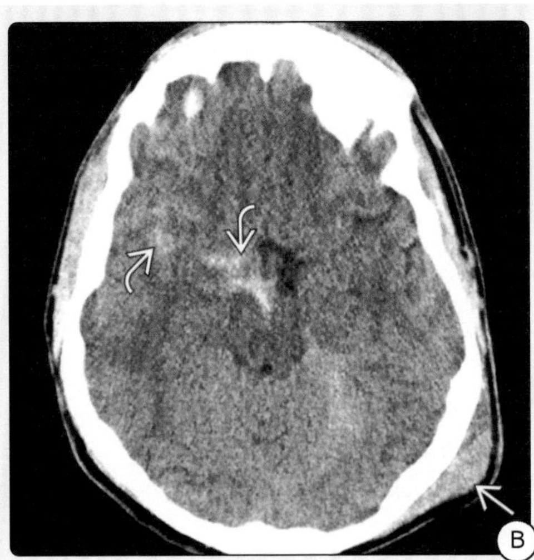


*(2-57A) Series of NECT scans demonstrates expected interval evolution of cortical contusions. Admission imaging shows bilateral inferior frontal contusions ➡, some tSAH ➡. (2-57B) Follow-up NECT 6 hours later shows that the contusions have enlarged ➡, and bifrontal hypodensities around the contusions have become apparent ➡. Note small peritentorial aSDH ➡.*

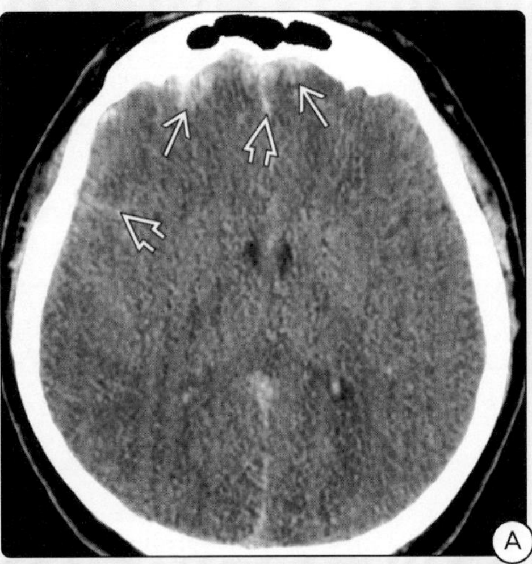


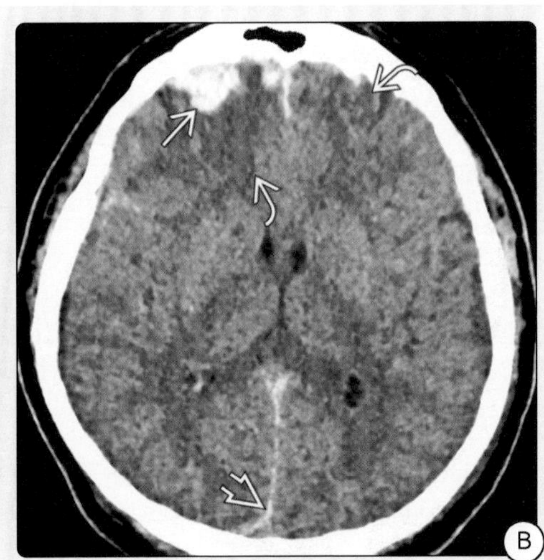


*(2-57C) Repeat NECT at 48 hours shows that the bifrontal hypodensities ➡ have consolidated around the hemorrhages. The tSAH and peritentorial aSDH have largely resolved. (2-57D) NECT at 2 months shows bifrontal encephalomalacia ➡, enlarged sylvian fissures ➡, and prominent 3rd ventricle ➡. These changes are common following moderately severe head trauma.*

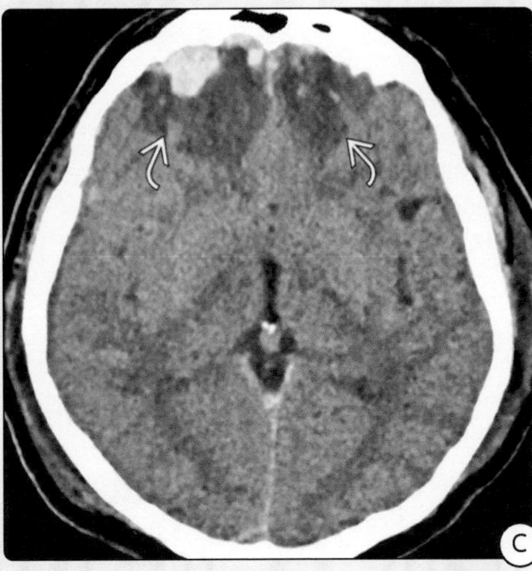


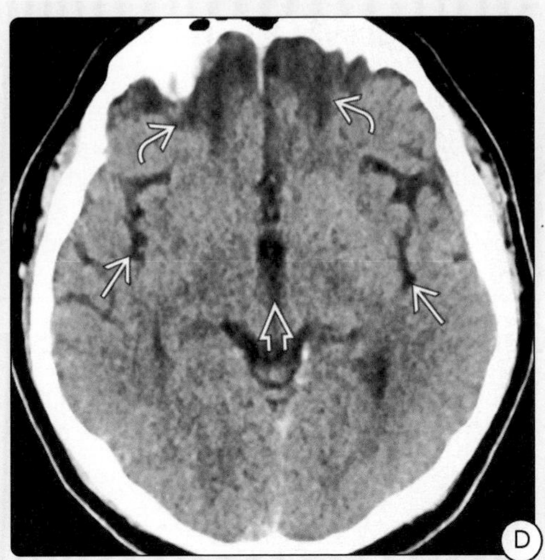

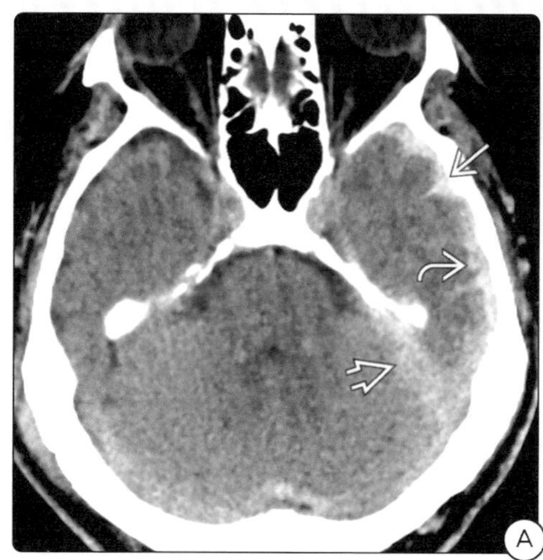

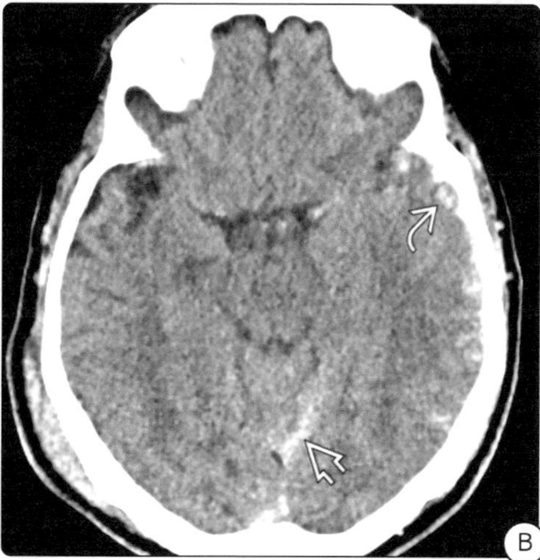

*(2-58A) NECT in severe CHI shows tSAH ➡, cortical contusions ➡, and small peritentorial aSDH ➡. (2-58B) More cephalad NECT shows extensive left temporal lobe cortical contusions ➡, small peritentorial SDH ➡.*

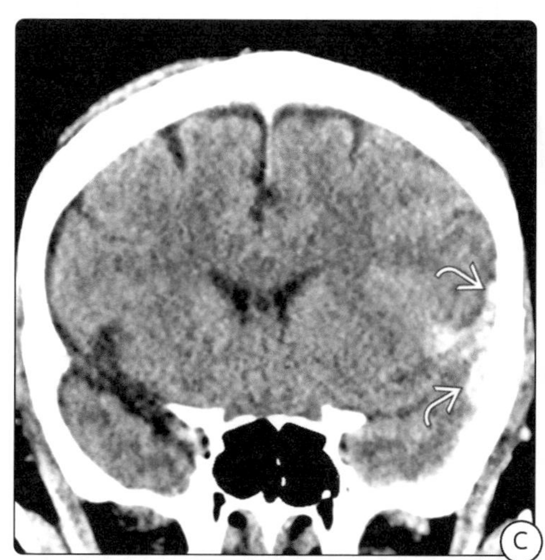

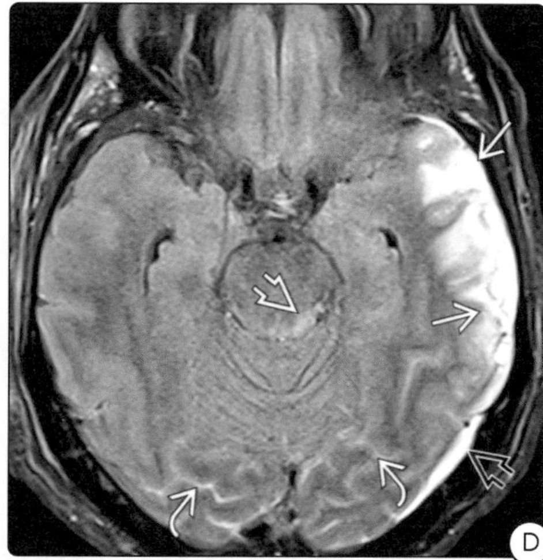

*(2-58C) Coronal reformatted NECT in the same case shows the extensive left temporal lobe cortical contusions ➡. (2-58D) Axial FLAIR MR in the same case 10 days later shows left temporal lobe contusions ➡, left dorsolateral midbrain contusion ➡, small sSDH ➡, and residual tSAH ➡.*

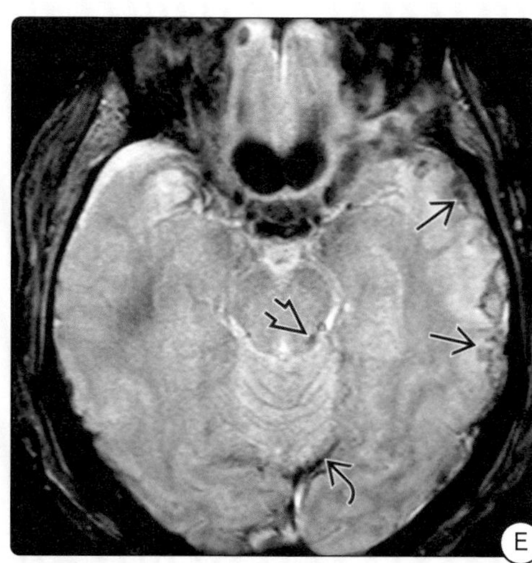

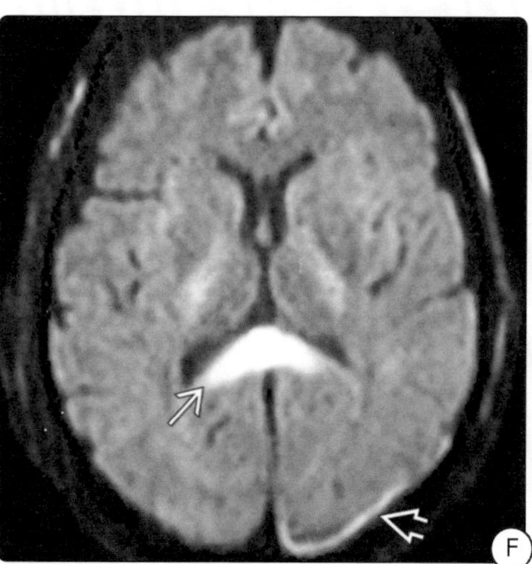

*(2-58E) T2* GRE MR shows "blooming" hemorrhagic cortical contusions ➡, dorsolateral midbrain contusion ➡, peritentorial SDH ➡. (2-58F) DWI MR shows excitotoxic injury of the corpus callosum ➡ and small residual left SDH ➡.*

Cerebral contusions are also called gyral "crest" injuries. The term "gliding" contusion is sometimes used to describe parasagittal contusions.

## Etiology

Most cerebral contusions result from nonmissile or blunt head injury. CHI induces abrupt changes in angular momentum and deceleration. The brain is suddenly and forcibly impacted against an osseous ridge or the hard, knife-like edge of the falx cerebri and tentorium cerebelli. Less commonly, a depressed skull fracture directly damages the underlying brain.

## Pathology

**Location.** Contusions are injuries of the brain surface that involve the gray matter and contiguous subcortical white matter **(2-50)** **(2-51)**. They occur in very characteristic, highly predictable locations. Nearly 1/2 involve the temporal lobes. The temporal tips, as well as the lateral and inferior surfaces and the perisylvian gyri, are most commonly affected **(2-53)**. The inferior (orbital) surfaces of the frontal lobes are also frequently affected **(2-54)**.

Convexity gyri, the dorsal corpus callosum body, dorsolateral midbrain, and cerebellum are less common sites of cerebral contusions. The occipital poles are rarely involved, even with relatively severe CHI.

**Size and Number.** Cerebral contusions vary in size from tiny lesions to large confluent hematomas. They are almost always multiple and often bilateral **(2-54)** **(2-55)**. Contusions that occur at 180° opposite the site of direct impact (the "coup") are common and called contrecoup lesions **(2-56)**.

## Clinical Issues

**Epidemiology and Demographics.** Cerebral contusions account for ~ 1/2 of all traumatic parenchymal lesions. They

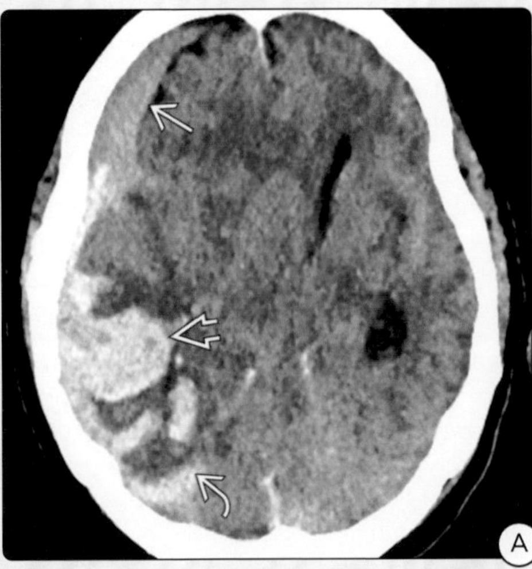
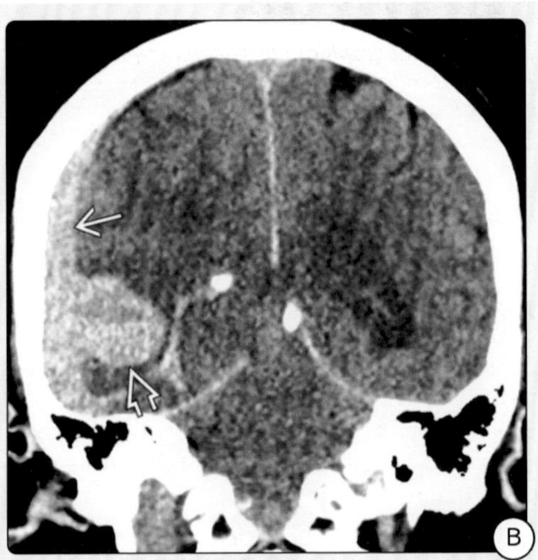

***(2-59A)** Axial NECT shows rapidly accumulating aSDH ➡, tSAH ➡, and parenchymal hematoma from a brain laceration ➡. **(2-59B)** Coronal NECT in the same case shows the aSDH ➡ communicates directly with the hematoma ➡ from the temporal lobe laceration. Small peritentorial and parafalcine subdural blood is also present.*

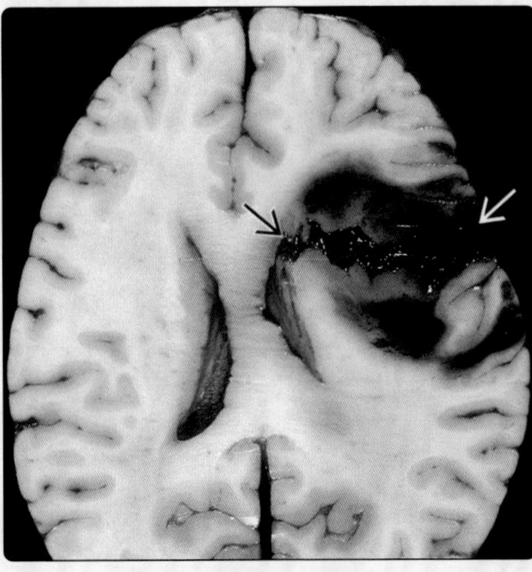
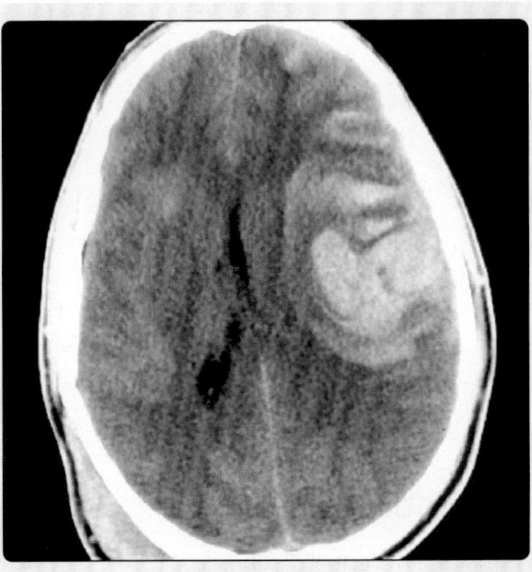

***(2-60)** Autopsy shows a "burst" lobe with a "full-thickness" laceration extending from the pial surface ➡ to the ventricle ➡. (Courtesy R. Hewlett, MD.) **(2-61)** NECT shows a "burst" lobe with rapid parenchymal hemorrhage extending deep into the brain. The patient died shortly after this scan was obtained.*

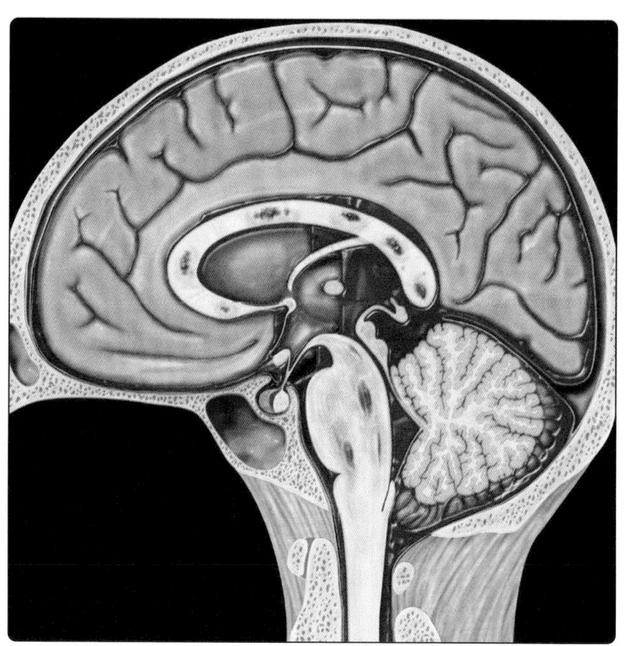

*(2-62) Sagittal graphic depicts common sites of axonal injury in the corpus callosum and midbrain. Traumatic intraventricular and subarachnoid hemorrhage are present.*

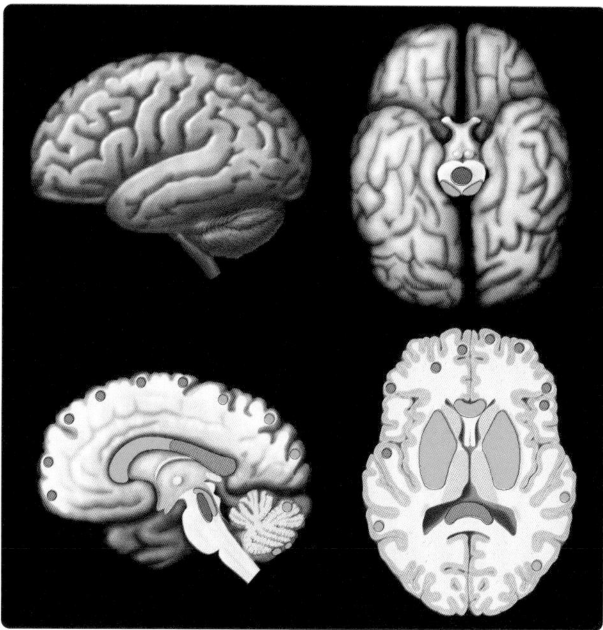

*(2-63) Graphics depict the most common sites of axonal injury in red. Frequent but relatively less common locations are shown in green. Injury to the midbrain/upper pons (purple) is uncommon but often lethal.*

occur at all ages, from infants to older adults. The peak age is 15-24 years, and the M:F ratio is 3:1.

## Imaging

**CT Findings.** Initial scans obtained soon after a CHI may be normal. The most frequent abnormality is the presence of focal or petechial hemorrhages along gyral crests immediately adjacent to the calvarium **(2-58B)**. A mixture of petechial hemorrhages surrounded by patchy ill-defined hypodense areas of edema is common **(2-55)** **(2-56)**.

A lesion "blooming" over time is frequent and seen with progressive increase in hemorrhage, edema, and mass effect **(2-57)**. Small lesions may coalesce, forming larger focal hematomas. Development of new lesions that were not present on initial imaging is also common.

**MR Findings.** MR is much more sensitive than CT in detecting cerebral contusions but is rarely obtained in the acute stage of TBI. T2 scans show patchy hyperintense areas (edema) surrounding hypointense foci of hemorrhage.

FLAIR scans are most sensitive for detecting cortical edema and associated tSAH, both of which appear as hyperintense foci on FLAIR **(2-58D)**. T2* (GRE, SWI) is the most sensitive sequence for imaging parenchymal hemorrhages **(2-58E)**. Significant "blooming" is typical in acute lesions. Complications, such as excitotoxic injury of the corpus callosum, may occur **(2-58F)**.

## Differential Diagnosis

The major differential diagnosis of cortical contusion is **DAI**. Both cerebral contusions and DAI are often present in patients who have sustained moderate to severe head injury.

Contusions tend to be superficial, located along gyral crests. DAI is most commonly found in the corona radiata and along compact white matter tracts, such as the internal capsule and corpus callosum.

Severe cortical contusion with confluent hematomas may be difficult to distinguish from brain laceration on imaging studies. **Brain laceration** occurs when severe trauma disrupts the pia and literally tears the underlying brain apart **(2-59)**. Parenchymal brain laceration (PBL) in infants and young children is typically associated with AHT.

A "burst lobe" is the most severe manifestation of frank brain laceration **(2-60)** **(2-61)**. Here, the affected lobe is grossly disrupted with large hematoma formation and adjacent tSAH. In some cases, especially those with depressed skull fracture, the arachnoid is also lacerated, and hemorrhage from the burst lobe extends to communicate directly with the subdural space, forming a coexisting SDH.

# Diffuse Axonal Injury

DAI is the second most common parenchymal lesion seen in TBI, exceeded only by cortical contusions. Patients with DAI often exhibit an apparent discrepancy between clinical status (often moderately to severely impaired) and initial imaging findings (often normal or minimally abnormal).

## Etiology

Most DAIs are caused by high-velocity MVCs and are dynamic, deformative, nonimpact injuries resulting from the inertial forces of rotation generated by sudden changes in acceleration/deceleration. The cortex moves at a different speed relative to underlying deep brain structures (white matter, deep gray nuclei). This results in axonal stretching, especially where brain tissues of different density intersect, i.e., the gray matter-white matter interface.

## Pathology

**Location.** DAI occurs in highly predictable locations. The cortex is typically spared; it is the subcortical and deep white matter that is most commonly affected. Lesions in compact white matter tracts, such as the corpus callosum, especially the genu and splenium, fornix, and internal capsule, are frequent. The midbrain and pons are less common sites of DAI **(2-62)** **(2-63)**.

**Gross Pathology.** The vast majority of DAIs are microscopic and nonhemorrhagic. Tears of penetrating vessels (diffuse vascular injury) may cause small round to ovoid or linear hemorrhages that sometimes are the only gross indications of underlying axonal injury **(2-64)**. These visible lesions are truly just the "tip of the iceberg."

## Clinical Issues

**Epidemiology and Demographics.** DAI is present in virtually all fatal TBIs and is found in almost 3/4 of patients with moderate or severe injury who survive the acute stage.

DAI may occur at any age, but peak incidence is in young adults (15-24 years old). Male patients are at least twice as often afflicted with TBI as female patients.

**Presentation.** DAI typically causes much more significant impairment compared with extracerebral hematomas and cortical contusions. DAI often causes immediate loss of consciousness, which may be transient (in the case of mild TBI) or progress to coma (with moderate to severe injury). In severe DAI, immediate coma from the moment of impact is typical. A very low GCS score, often < 6-8, is typical in patients who survive the initial impact.

***(2-64)** Autopsied brain from severe closed head trauma shows hemorrhagic deep axonal injuries in basal ganglia ➡ and subcortical WM ➡. **(2-65A)** NECT in severe head injury, GCS = 6, shows hemorrhagic deep axonal injuries ➡ and cortical contusion ➡.*

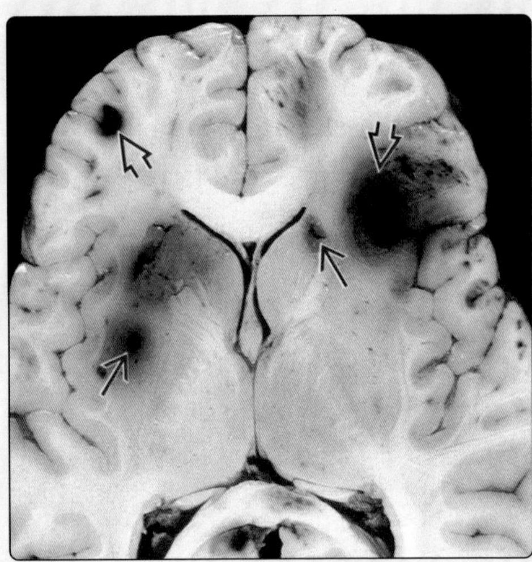

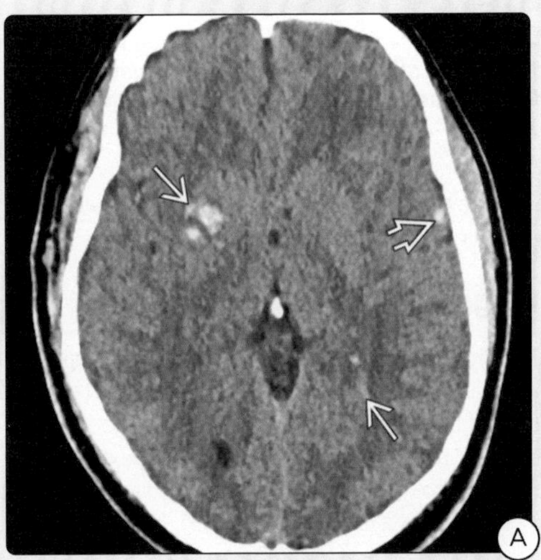


***(2-65B)** More cephalad NECT in the same case shows hemorrhagic axonal injuries in the deep corona radiata ➡. **(2-65C)** Coronal NECT in the same case shows the deep axonal injuries ➡.*

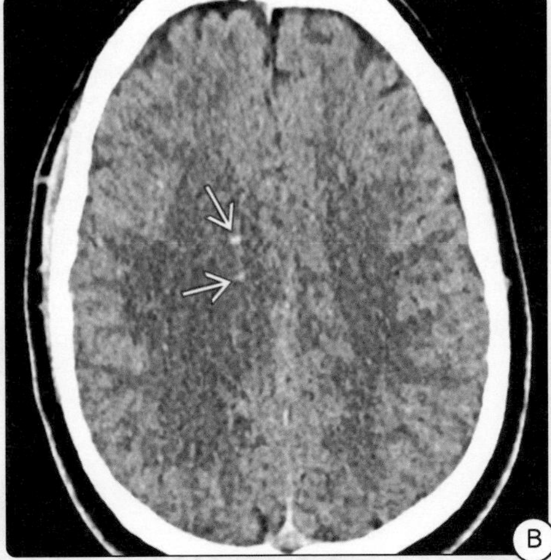


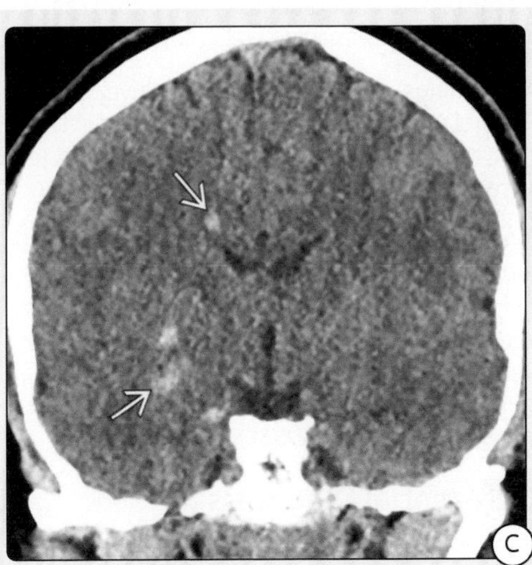

## Imaging

**CT Findings.** Initial NECT is often normal or minimally abnormal. Mild diffuse brain swelling with sulcal effacement may be present. A few small round or ovoid subcortical hemorrhages may be visible **(2-65)**, but the underlying damage is typically much more diffuse and much more severe than these relatively modest abnormalities would indicate.

**MR Findings.** MR is much more sensitive in detecting changes of DAI. T2WI and FLAIR may show hyperintense foci in the subcortical white matter and corpus callosum **(2-66A)**. Multiple lesions are the rule, and a combination of DAI and contusions or hematomas is very common.

T2* (GRE, SWI) scans are very sensitive to the microbleeds of DAI and typically show multifocal ovoid and linear hypointensities **(2-66B)** **(2-66C)**. DWI may show multiple foci of restricted diffusion **(2-66D)**.

## Differential Diagnosis

**Cortical contusions** often coexist with DAI in moderate to severe TBI. Cortical contusions are typically superficial lesions, usually located along gyral crests.

Multifocal hemorrhages with "blooming" on T2* (GRE, SWI) scans can be seen in numerous pathologies, including DAI. **Diffuse vascular injury** appears as multifocal parenchymal black dots. Pneumocephalus may cause multifocal "blooming" lesions in the subarachnoid spaces. Parenchymal lesions are rare.

# Subcortical (Deep Brain) Injury

## Terminology

SCIs are traumatic lesions of deep brain structures, such as the brainstem, basal ganglia, thalami, and ventricles. Most represent severe shear-strain injuries that disrupt axons, tear

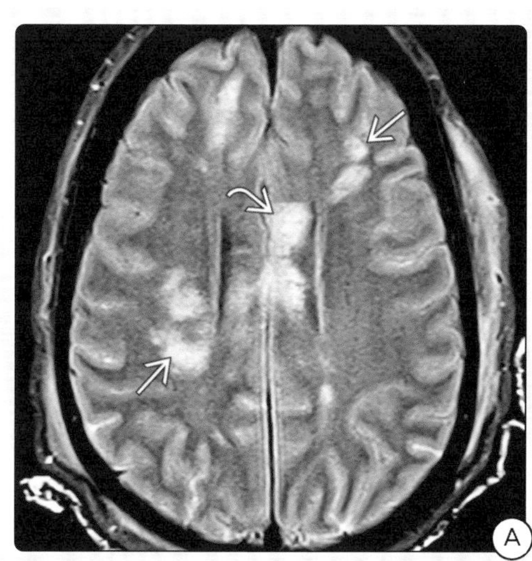


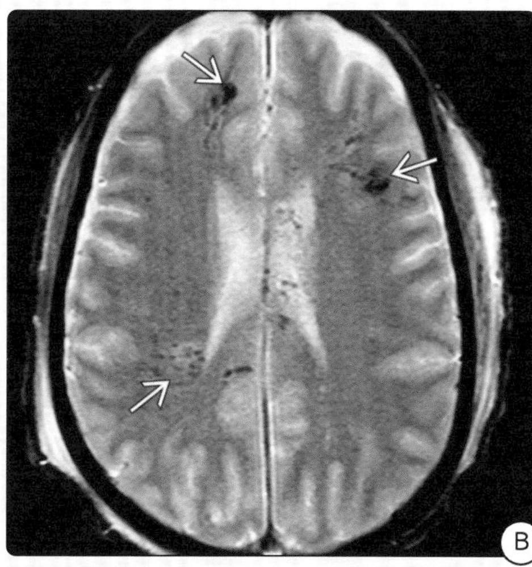


***(2-66A)** MR 2 days after a minimally abnormal initial NECT in a patient with severe CHI (GCS = 6) shows hyperintensities in subcortical/deep WM ➡ and corpus callosum ➡. **(2-66B)** T2* GRE MR shows multiple punctate and linear foci of gradient susceptibility ➡ in the subcortical, deep periventricular WM.*

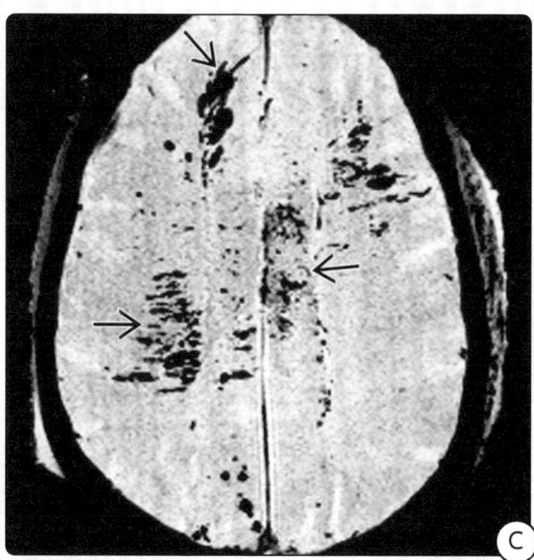


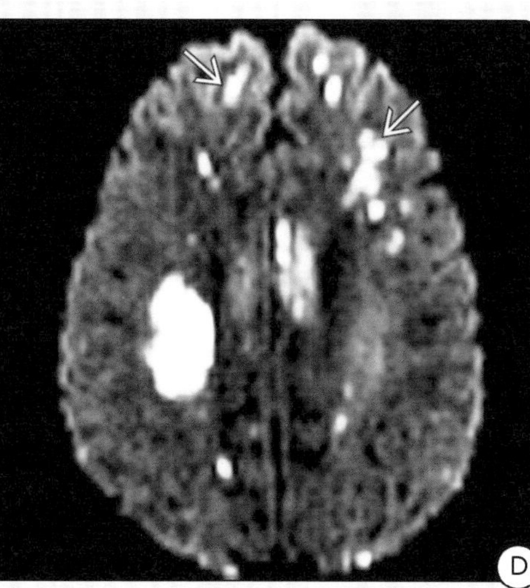


***(2-66C)** SWI MIP in the same case shows innumerable punctate and linear "blooming" hypointensities ➡, consistent with diffuse axonal injury/diffuse vascular injury. SWI sequences are much more sensitive to susceptibility artifacts than T2* GRE scans. **(2-66D)** DWI MR in the same case shows multiple foci of restricted diffusion ➡.*

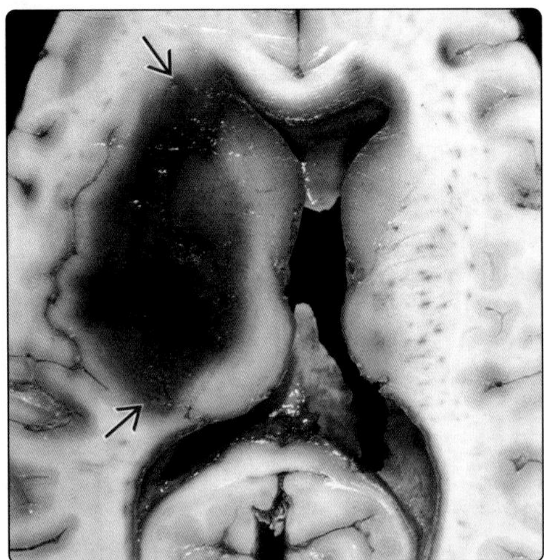

*(2-67) High-speed MVC case shows a large hemorrhage ⇒ characteristic of severe subcortical injury. (Courtesy R. Hewlett, MD.)*

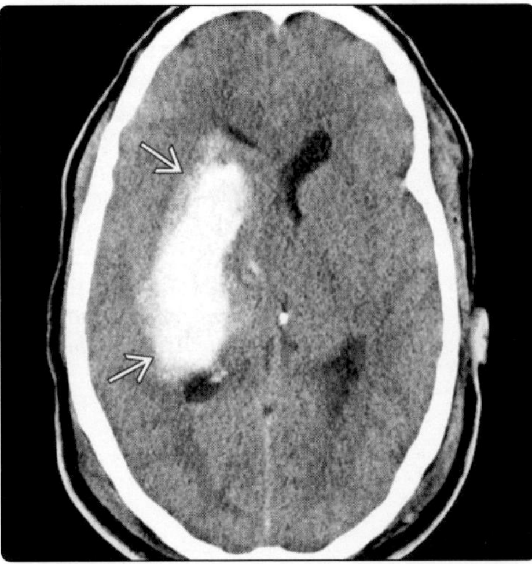

*(2-68) NECT in a 38-yo man in a severe MVA shows a large expanding basal ganglia hematoma ⇒. He expired 2 days later.*

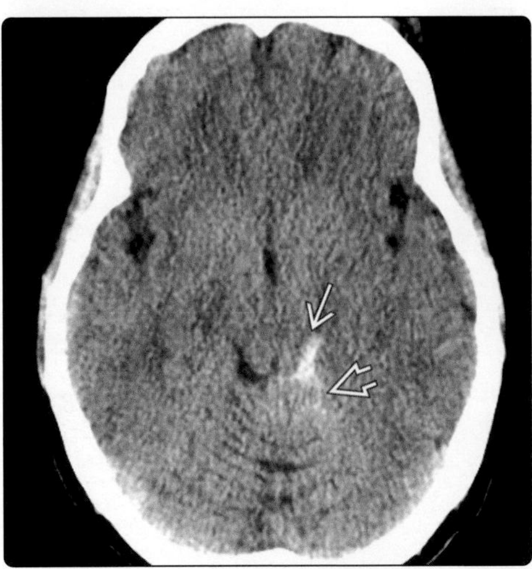

*(2-69) NECT of midbrain contusion shows hyperdensity in the left posterolateral midbrain ⇒ associated with focal tSAH ⇒.*

penetrating blood vessels, and damage the choroid plexus of the lateral ventricles.

## Pathology

**Gross Pathology.** Manifestations of SCI include deep hemorrhagic contusions, nonhemorrhagic lacerations, intraventricular bleeds, and tSAH **(2-67)**. SCIs usually occur with other traumatic lesions, such as cortical contusions and DAI.

## Clinical Issues

**Epidemiology.** Between 5-10% of patients with moderate to severe brain trauma sustain SCIs. SCIs are the third most common parenchymal brain injury after cortical contusions and DAI. As with most TBIs, SCIs are most common in male patients between 15-24 years of age.

**Natural History.** Prognosis is poor in these severely injured patients. Many do not survive; those who do typically have profound neurologic impairment with severe long-term disability.

### PARENCHYMAL BRAIN INJURIES

**Cerebral Contusions**
- Most common intraaxial injury
  - Brain impacts skull &/or dura
  - Causes "brain bruises" in gyral crests
  - Usually multiple, often bilateral
  - Anteroinferior frontal, temporal lobes most common sites
- Imaging
  - Superficial petechial, focal hemorrhage
  - Edema, hemorrhage more apparent with time
  - T2* (GRE, SWI) most sensitive imaging

**Diffuse Axonal Injury**
- 2nd most common intraaxial injury
  - Spares cortex, involves subcortical/deep white matter
- Imaging
  - GCS low; initial imaging often minimally abnormal
  - Subcortical, deep petechial hemorrhages ("tip of iceberg")
  - T2* (GRE, SWI) most sensitive technique

**Diffuse Vascular Injury**
- Rare, usually fatal
- High-speed, high-impact MVCs
- May represent extreme end of DAI spectrum
- Imaging
  - CT shows diffuse brain swelling
  - T2 and FLAIR show few scattered hyperintensities
  - SWI shows innumerable linear hypointensities

**Subcortical Injury**
- "The deeper the injury, the worse it is"
- Basal ganglia, thalami, midbrain, pons
  - Hemorrhages, axonal injury, brain tears

## Imaging

**General Features.** Minimal abnormalities may be present on initial imaging but show dramatic increase on follow-up scans.

SCI typically exists with numerous comorbid injuries. Lesions ranging from subtle tSAH to gross parenchymal hemorrhage are common **(2-68) (2-69)**.

Mass effect with cerebral herniation and gross disturbances in regional blood flow may develop.

**CT Findings.** NECT scans often show diffuse brain swelling with punctate &/or gross hemorrhage in the deep gray nuclei and midbrain. Intraventricular and choroid plexus hemorrhages are common and may form a "cast" of the lateral ventricles. Blood-fluid levels are common.

**MR Findings.** MR is much more sensitive than CT, even though acute hemorrhage is isointense with brain on T1 scans. FLAIR and T2* are the most sensitive sequences. DWI may show foci of restricted diffusion. DTI mapping delineates the pattern of white matter tract disruption.

### Differential Diagnosis

**Secondary midbrain ("Duret") hemorrhage** may occur with severe descending transtentorial herniation. These hemorrhages are typically centrally located within the midbrain, whereas contusional SCIs are dorsolateral.

# Miscellaneous Injuries

## Pneumocephalus

### Differential Diagnosis

Air is air and should not be mistaken for anything else. If wide windows are not used, a ruptured dermoid cyst with fat droplets in the CSF cisterns can mimic subarachnoid air.

### Terminology

Intracranial air does not exist under normal conditions. In **pneumocephalus**, air can be found anywhere within the cranium, including blood vessels, and within any compartment. While intracranial air is never normal, it can be an expected and therefore routine finding (e.g., after surgery).

**Tension pneumocephalus** is a collection of intracranial air under pressure that causes mass effect on the brain and results in neurologic deterioration. Intracerebral **pneumatocele** or "aerocele" is a less commonly used term and refers specifically to a focal gas collection within the brain parenchyma.

### Clinical Issues

**Epidemiology.** Pneumocephalus is present in 3% of all patients with skull fractures and 8% of those with paranasal sinus fractures. Virtually all patients who have supratentorial surgery have some degree of pneumocephalus on imaging studies obtained within the first 24-28 hours.

**Natural History and Treatment Options.** Unless it is under tension, most intracranial air resolves spontaneously within a few days after trauma or surgery. Occasionally, air collections increase and may require evacuation with duraplasty.

### Imaging

**General Features.** Intracranial air can exist in any compartment (epidural, subdural, subarachnoid, intraventricular, or intraparenchymal) and conforms to the shape of that compartment or potential compartment. The subdural space is the most frequent, and the most common site is frontal.

**Epidural air** is typically solitary, biconvex in configuration, may cross midline, and does not move with changes in head position **(2-70)**.

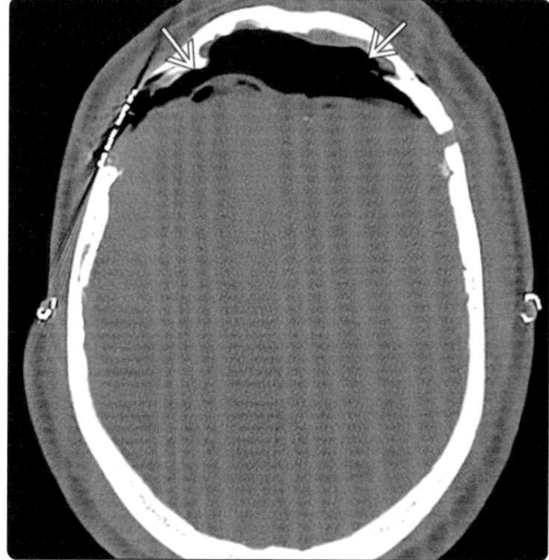

***(2-70)** Postbifrontal craniectomy NECT shows that the epidural air collection ➡ is continuous across the midline.*

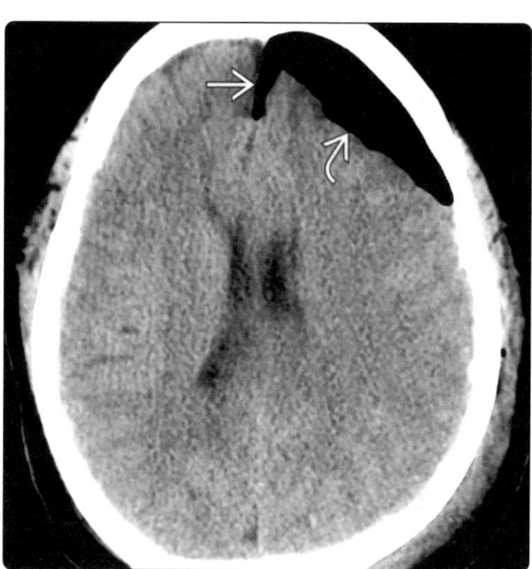

***(2-71)** Postoperative subdural air ➡ forms a crescent-shaped collection over the hemisphere and does not cross the midline ➡.*

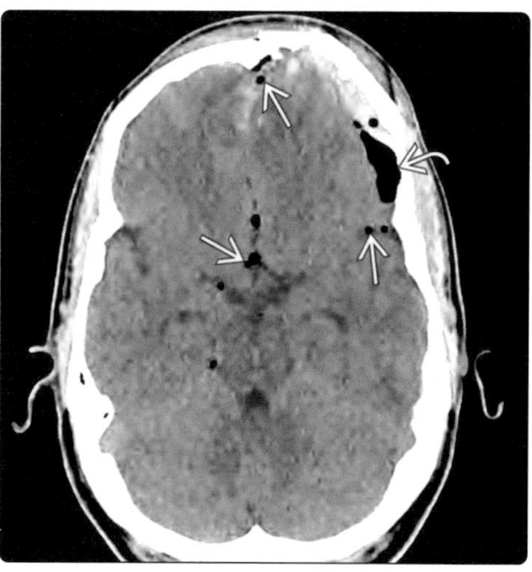

***(2-72)** NECT of frontal sinus fractures shows multiple "dots" of subarachnoid air ➡. A subdural air collection ➡ is also present.*

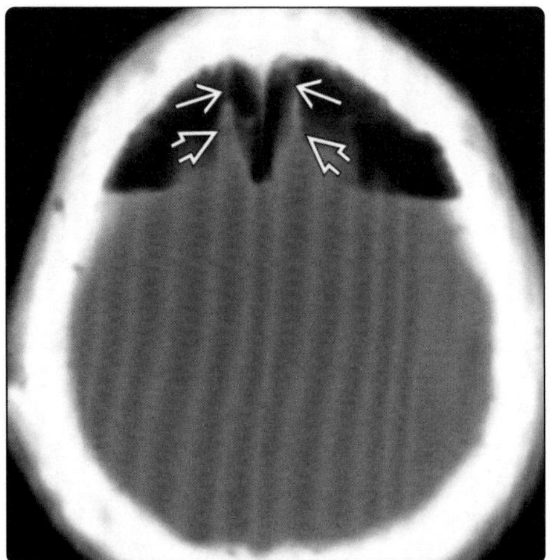

*(2-73) NECT shows tension pneumocephalus, Mount Fuji sign caused by cortical veins ➡ tethering frontal lobes ➡.*

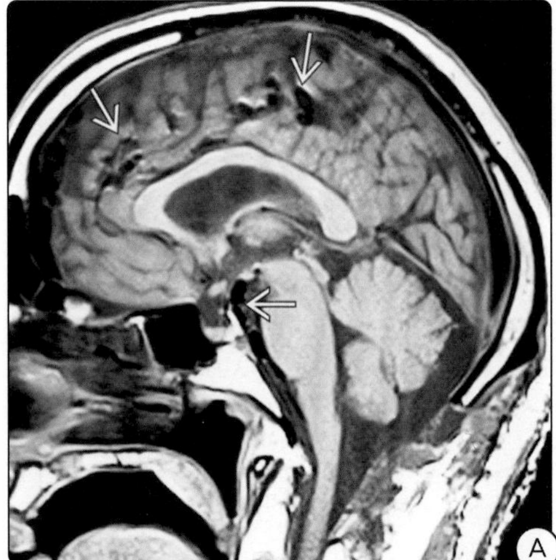

*(2-74A) Sagittal T1WI MR shows postoperative pneumocephalus with "spots" and "dots" of air ➡ in the subarachnoid spaces.*

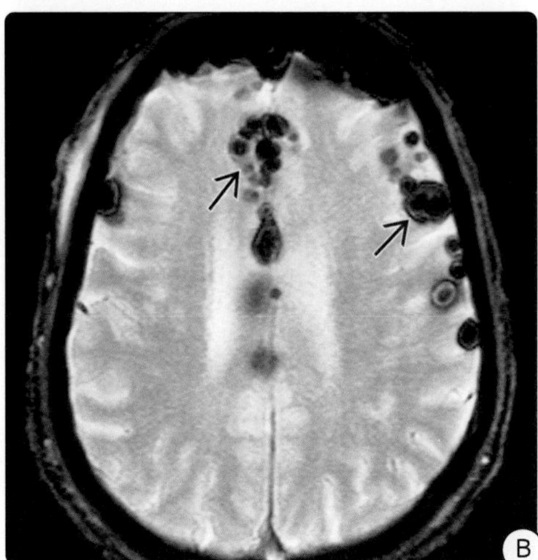

*(2-74B) T2* GRE MR in the same case shows multifocal "blooming" black dots ➡, representing air in the subarachnoid spaces.*

**Subdural air** is confluent, crescentic **(2-71)**, and often bilateral, frequently contains air-fluid levels, moves with changes in head position, and surrounds cortical veins as they cross the subdural space to enter the SSS.

**Subarachnoid air** is typically seen as multifocal small "dots" or "droplets" of air within and around cerebral sulci **(2-72)**. **Intraventricular air** forms air-fluid levels, most often in the frontal horns of the lateral ventricles. Intraparenchymal air is uncommon, and such a collection is termed a **pneumatocele**. **Intravascular air** conforms to the vascular structure(s) within which it resides. Air within venous sinuses is common; intraarterial air (air embolism) is rare and often fatal **(2-75)**.

**CT Findings.** Air is extremely hypodense on CT, measuring approximately -1,000 HU. The Mount Fuji sign of **tension pneumocephalus** is seen as bilateral subdural air collections that separate and compress the frontal lobes, widening the interhemispheric fissure **(2-73)**. The frontal lobes are displaced posteriorly by air under pressure and are typically pointed where they are tethered to the dura-arachnoid by cortical veins, mimicking the silhouette of Mount Fuji.

Distinguishing air from fat on CT is extremely important. With typical narrow soft tissue windows, both appear similarly hypodense. Increasing window width or simply looking at bone CT algorithms (on which air is clearly distinct from the less hypodense fat) helps differentiate fat from air.

**MR Findings.** Air is seen as areas of completely absent signal intensity on all sequences **(2-74A)**. On T2* GRE, intracranial air "blooms" and appears as multifocal "black dots" **(2-74B)**.

## PNEUMOCEPHALUS

**Etiology**

- Surgery (most common; expected after craniotomy)
- Trauma (8-10% of cases)
- "Spontaneous" (defect in temporal bone, sinus)

**Location**

- Epidural
  - Unilateral, biconvex
  - May cross midline
  - Does not move with change in position
- Subdural
  - Confluent, crescentic
  - Does not cross midline
  - Often bilateral ± air-fluid level
  - Changes with head position
- Subarachnoid
  - Discrete "spots" and "dots" in sulci, cisterns
- Miscellaneous
  - Intraventricular (air-fluid levels, usually frontal horns)
  - Intraparenchymal (confluent, well delineated)

**General Imaging Features**

- CT
  - Extremely hypodense (-1,000 HU)
  - Fat vs. air? Use wide windows!
- MR
  - Signal void
  - Prominent "blooming" on GRE
  - Alternating dark "holes" ± concentric bright rings
  - Chemical shift artifact in phase-encoding direction

## Abusive Head Trauma (Child Abuse)

Radiologists play a key role in the diagnosis of suspected child abuse. Imaging must be performed with care, interpreted with rigor, and precisely described. The final diagnosis of child abuse is typically made by a child abuse pediatrician, who leads a multidisciplinary team (in which the radiologist plays an important role). There is no rush to judgment. Detailed consideration of imaging and medicolegal issues in AHT is beyond the scope of *Osborn's Brain*.

### Terminology

The term nonaccidental trauma (NAT), a.k.a. nonaccidental injury (NAI) or shaken-baby syndrome (SBS), refers to intentionally inflicted injury. The American Academy of Pediatrics endorses the term **abusive head trauma (AHT)**, which encompasses a spectrum of potential mechanisms of intracranial injury acting independently or in concert, including shaking with or without impact, impact alone, strangulation/suffocation, and hypoxic-ischemic insult **(2-77)**.

### Etiology

Direct injuries are inflicted by blows to the head, impact of the cranium on an object, such as a wall, or the brain impacting a rigid internal structure, such as the pterion, rough floors of the anterior or middle cranial fossa, falx cerebri, or tentorium cerebelli. Direct impact may result in skull fractures **(2-76)**, acute subdural hemorrhage (aSDH), SAH, contusions in the subjacent brain, parenchymal brain lacerations (PBLs) of the subcortical white matter in the young infant, and contrecoup injuries. **Importantly, victims of AHT commonly exhibit no skin, scalp, or calvarial evidence of trauma**, thus supporting shaking alone as the underpinning of intracranial hemorrhage and brain injury in AHT.

AHT may involve linear translational forces with shaking and impact (impactive forces) or complex angular forces without impact (impulsive forces); AHT impulsive forces are commonly rapid acceleration and deceleration forces without impact. Resultant SDH and SAH, cerebral edema, infarction, and brainstem or cervical cord injury may predispose the patient to respiratory arrest. Irreversible hypoxic-ischemic injury may result. Death may follow.

Indirect injuries of AHT lead to death and significant neurologic morbidity. The head of an infant or young child is relatively large compared with its body, cervical musculature is comparatively weak, and the incompletely myelinated cerebral white matter is relatively fragile. Shaking motion alone and potential for whiplash injury of the brainstem and upper cervical cord may lead to death. The most common result of shaking is diffusely distributed aSDH. SAH is a common accompaniment of aSDH. These extraaxial hemorrhages often represent proxies for underlying cerebral edema, early herniation, infarction, parenchymal contusions, subcortical laceration, and axonal shear injuries.

### Pathology

SDH and subdural hygroma (SDHy) detected in a child under two years of age are strongly associated with trauma. SDH in a preambulatory infant (under one year of age) or young child is highly suspicious for AHT. SDHs of differing ages support multiple traumatic insults and are common in AHT. SDH is the most common intracranial imaging finding in confirmed cases of AHT **(2-81)**.

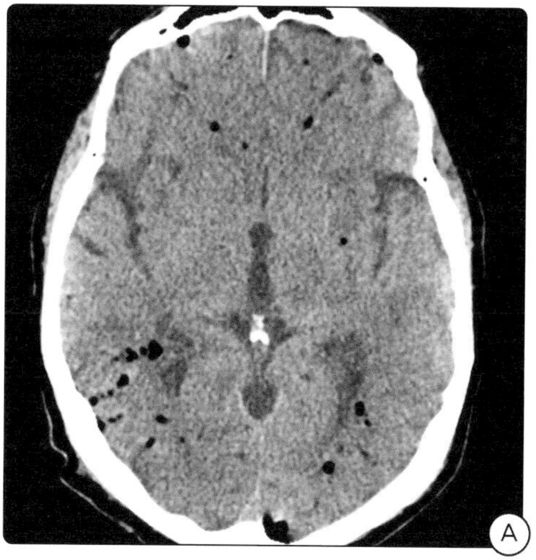


***(2-75A)** Axial NECT of an air embolism shows multifocal linear and punctate foci of intravascular air.*

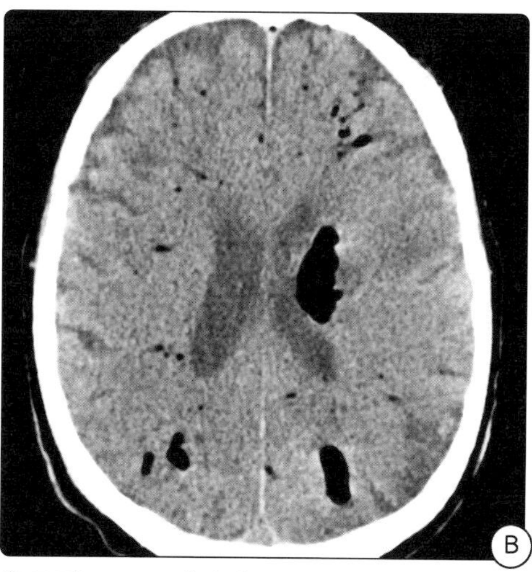


***(2-75B)** More cephalad NECT shows multiple small, round, and linear air foci with some large collections along the watershed zone.*

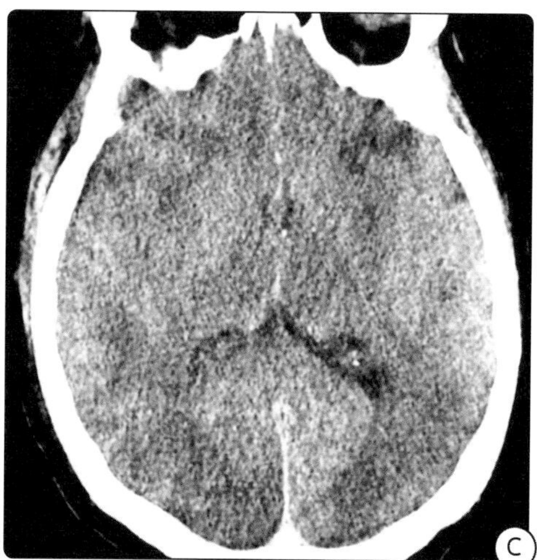


***(2-75C)** NECT 12 hours later, just before death, shows complete resorption of intravascular air, small ventricles, and hypodense brain.*

## Imaging

**General Features.** Initial imaging in cases of suspected child abuse should include a complete skeletal survey and NECT of the brain in the neurologically symptomatic infant or young child. MR is recommended for children two years old or younger. Brain MR obtained 3-5 days after admission optimizes identification of characteristic parenchymal injuries and helps to determine the acuity of the injury. Serial imaging (NECT and MR) plays an important role in dating AHT, extraaxial hemorrhage, and characterizing injury patterns.

Radiologists should refrain from using definitive timing language (e.g., "acute on chronic") when reporting hemorrhage on initial NECT findings in AHT. More precision in estimating hemorrhage age and magnitude of injury is achieved from serial imaging (NECT and MR).

Subdural collections discovered in the setting of benign enlargement of the subarachnoid spaces (BESS) (a benign transient communicating form of hydrocephalus) in normally developing infants and young children are a known association but often warrant a thoughtful investigation by the child protective services team, especially when the subdural collections contain frank hemorrhage or are moderate to large in size.

**CT Findings.** Identification and characterization of intracranial hemorrhage and detecting cerebral injury and herniation are critical. SDHs are shown in nearly 80% of all AHT cases **(2-80)**. These are often thin, parafalcine, and convexal in location. SAH frequently accompanies SDH.

Mixed-attenuation SDH is common in the acutely symptomatic AHT patient **(2-80A)** and is usually due to layering of blood and various mixtures of blood and CSF. Dependent SDH (hematohygroma and hematocrit effect) most commonly reflects a single event, not multiple bleeds or bleeds of varying ages **(2-85)**. SDHy (CSF-like on NECT) in children under two years old should be considered of

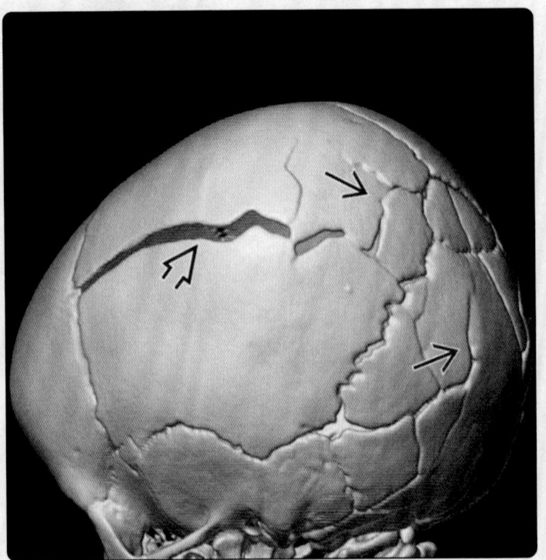

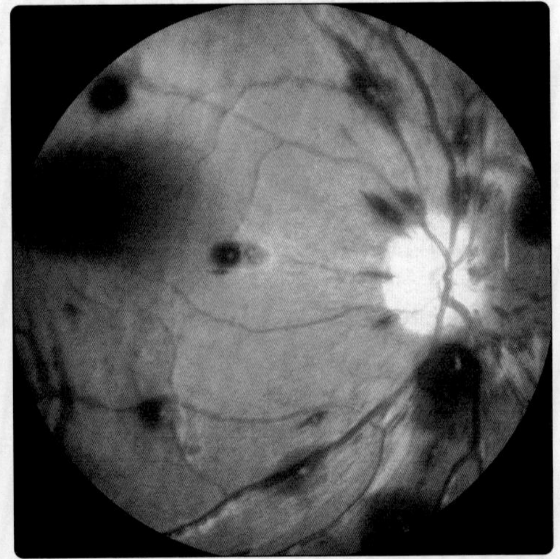

***(2-76)** 3D NECT in a 6-month-old boy with scalp swelling is shown. There was no history of prior head trauma. Note the diastatic right parietal fracture ➲ and innumerable occipital and parietal fractures ➲. Skull fractures are often absent in the setting of abusive head trauma (AHT). **(2-77)** Funduscopic exam in an infant victim of AHT (shaking) shows multiple retinal hemorrhages (RHs). RHs often accompany SDHs. (Courtesy K. Digre, MD.)*

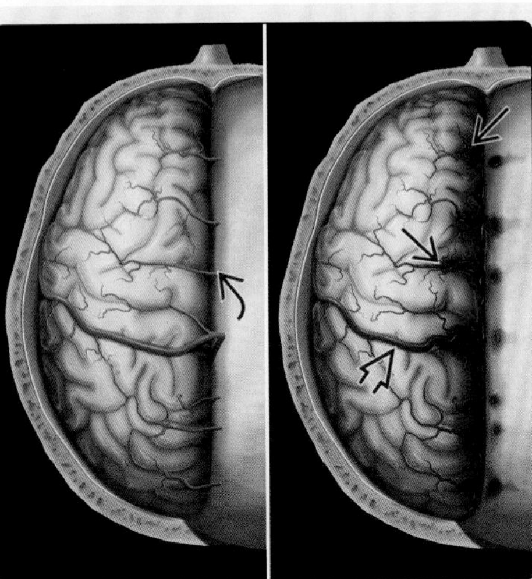

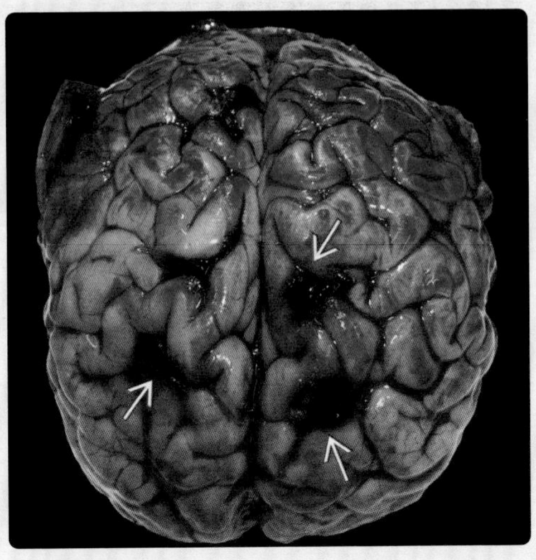

***(2-78)** (L) Cortical veins bridge subarachnoid space, enter dura ➲. In AHT (R), numerous torn BVs ➲ are present with thrombosis of the vein of Trolard ➲. BVs tear at the dural cuff where the veins penetrate the dura of the SSS. **(2-79)** Autopsy photograph in an infant victim of fatal AHT shows numerous traumatically torn and thrombosed convexity BVs ➲. (Courtesy C. Rambaud, MD.)*

traumatic etiology. SDHy can enlarge rapidly. EDH is rare in AHT. The presence of SDH and retinal hemorrhages increases the specificity of SDH as a proxy for AHT.

Causes of mixed-attenuation SDHs include the following: (1) aSDH, (2) hyperacute + acute hemorrhage, (3) hematohygroma (SDH + CSF), and (4) old and new SDH. When there is associated underlying cerebral edema and herniation, the subdural collection is one of the first three considerations. Innocent rebleeding into a cSDH rarely leads to shift and cerebral edema.

The common origin of SDH and SAH in AHT are torn bridging veins (BVs) **(2-78)**. On NECT, these appear as tubular or comma-shaped high-attenuation extraaxial collections over the parafalcine cerebral convexities **(2-82A)**. In the literature, these findings have been described as lollipop and tadpole signs. MR shows similarly shaped hypointensities on T2WI, GRE, and SWI **(2-82B)**. Underlying cerebral ischemia may be detected. These torn and thrombosed BVs represent a sign of trauma **(2-79)** and are more commonly encountered in AHT compared to accidental head trauma.

Careful evaluation and windowing of CT images may allow for detection of brain parenchymal injuries in AHT. Parenchymal injuries primarily affect the cerebral hemispheres and may be unilateral or bilateral. Looking for geographic areas of low attenuation and loss of gray matter-white matter differentiation allows for detection of these parenchymal injuries **(2-91)**.

**MR Findings.** Conventional T1, T2, and FLAIR sequences may show mixed hyper-, hypo-, and isointense components within subdural fluid collections. The heterogeneity of signal on these sequences may reflect various mixtures of blood and CSF or may reflect blood products of varying ages **(2-85)**. The interaction of SDH with the extraaxial space, and potentially CSF, confounds our ability to use MR signal intensity as a reliable estimate of the age of the subdural blood.

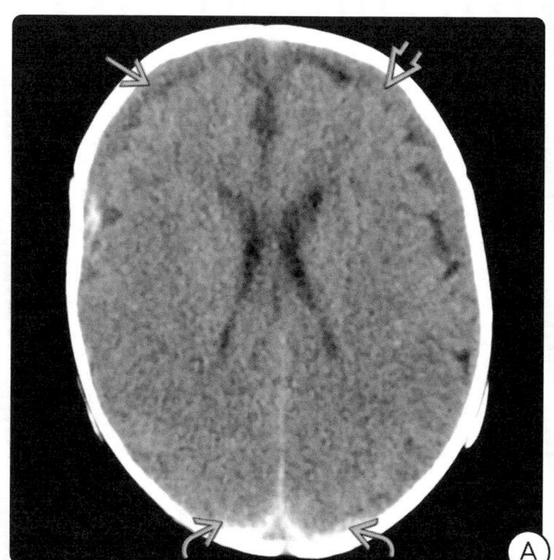

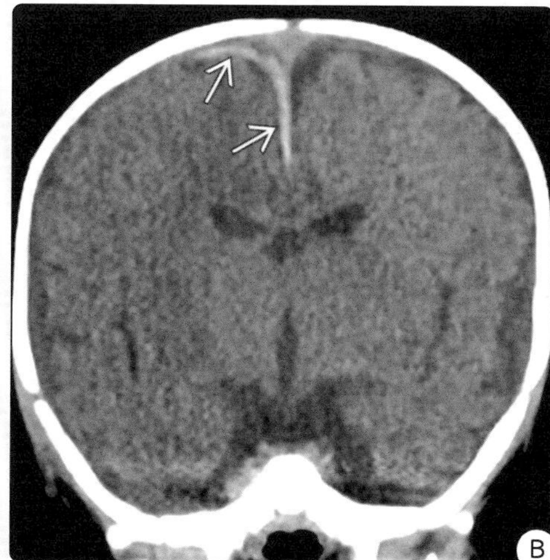

***(2-80A)** Axial NECT in a 2-month-old shows bilateral SDHs with hypodense ➔, isodense ➔, and hyperdense ➔ components. These various densities are likely the result of a single injury with varying mixtures of blood and hemorrhage as well as hematocrit effect. **(2-80B)** Coronal NECT shows an acute parafalcine and convexity SDH ➔. The falx cerebri limits the medial migration of the SDH.*

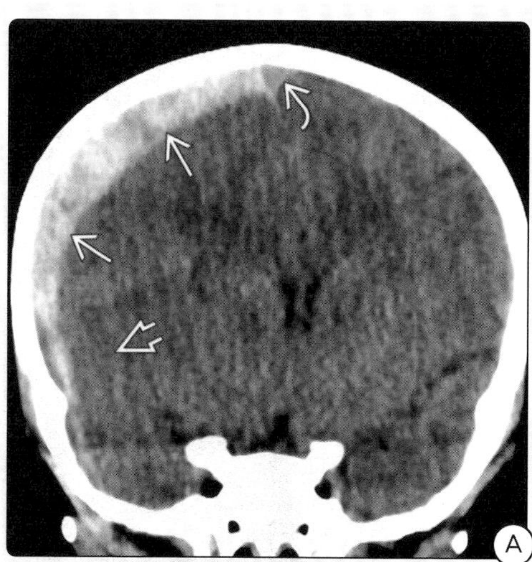

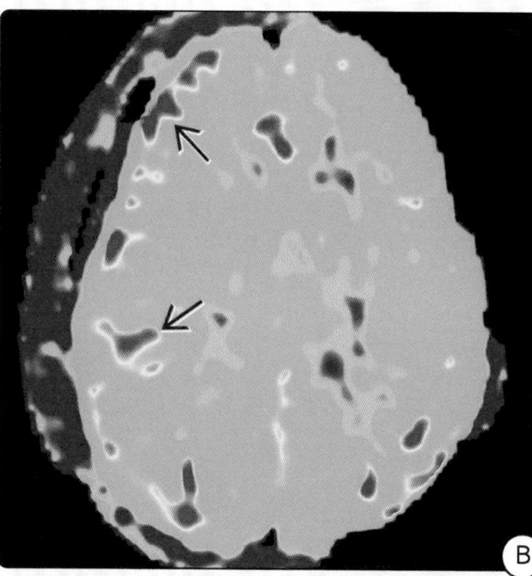

***(2-81A)** Coronal NECT in AHT shows mixed-attenuation SDH ➔ and subfalcine herniation ➔. An acute hematoma was evacuated. Note the loss of GM-WM differentiation ➔, representing cerebral edema. Extensive right hemispheric encephalomalacia followed. **(2-81B)** Arterial spin labeling (ASL) MR after SDH evacuation shows ↑ right cerebral hemispheric blood flow ➔, reflecting disordered autoregulation.*

Traumatic SDHy follows CSF on all MR pulse sequences (as in hematohygroma) **(2-87)** or proteinaceous content (as can be seen in cSDH). Trauma, both accidental and inflicted, represents a significant cause of SDHy and subdural hematohygroma in a child under two years of age.

T2* (GRE, SWI) scans are useful techniques for detecting blood products, particularly acute and subacute extraaxial and intraaxial hemorrhage, subtle petechial cortical contusions, PBLs, torn BVs, parenchymal lacerations, and hemorrhagic axonal injuries. Subcortical parenchymal lacerations, when present, are strongly suggestive of AHT **(2-90)**. Chronic convexity SDHs often lack susceptibility effect on T2* imaging (appearing deceptively as "simple fluid"); therefore, evaluation for presence of internal membrane structure within the SDH is important. T2* may show retinal hemorrhages, and their identification increases the imaging specificity for a diagnosis of AHT **(2-77)** **(2-84)**. MR can detect ~ 1/2 of those retinal hemorrhages that are identifiable by funduscopic examination.

FLAIR, FSE T2, T2*, and post-IV contrast 3D T1WI can detect membrane architecture within the SDH. Enhancing membranes that cause compartmentalization of the subdural collection are the most reliable imaging finding of a cSDH **(2-89)**. Macroscopic subdural membrane formation within the SDH requires ~ 4-6 weeks to form. 3D post-IV contrast T1 imaging may display the traumatic disruption of BVs and the presence of traumatic cerebral sinovenous thrombosis.

DWI and ADC are essential for evaluating foci of traumatic and ischemic injury in AHT. Patterns of cytotoxic edema in AHT vary from focal areas to large geographic areas (most common) **(2-92)**. In the setting of coexistent hypoxia and ischemia, a symmetric injury pattern may be present. Diffuse hemispheric patterns of cytotoxic edema are much more common in AHT compared to accidental injury. DWI is also helpful in establishing timing of injury, as acute injuries will

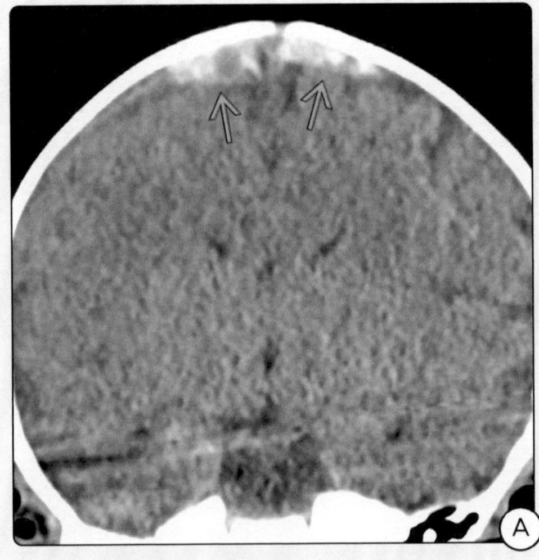

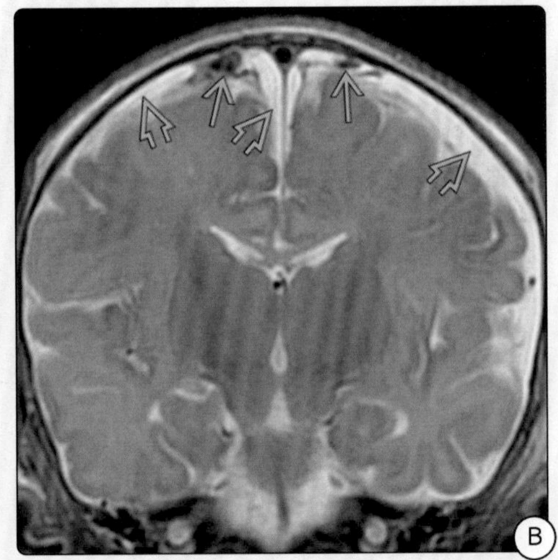

***(2-82A)** Coronal NECT in a 2-month-old shows globular areas of parafalcine hemorrhage ➩, typical of BV avulsion injuries. **(2-82B)** Coronal T2 in the same patient shows globular areas of hypointensity ➩ at the sites of BV avulsion injuries with adjacent CSF signal subdural collections ➩. While not pathognomonic for AHT, BV avulsion injuries are much more common in AHT vs. accidental injury.*

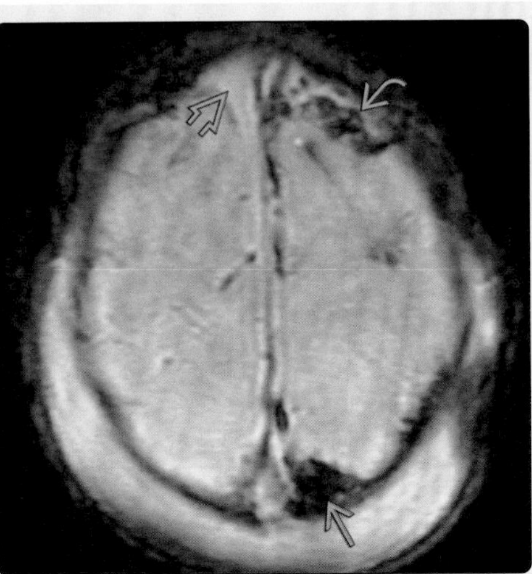

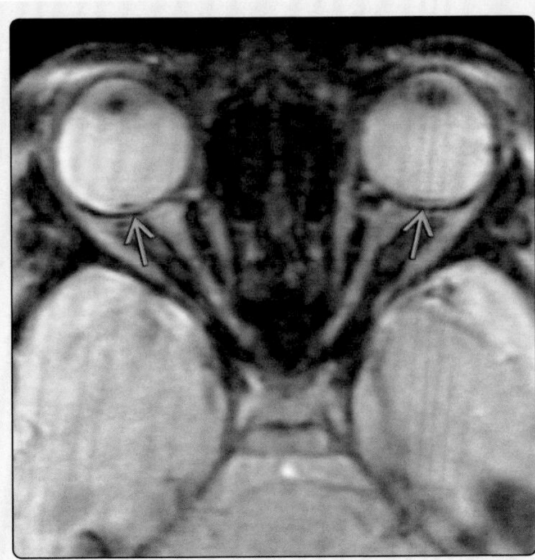

***(2-83)** Axial SWI shows parafalcine hemorrhage ➩ and injured/thrombosed BV ➩. Note the associated subdural collection ➩ on the right. SWI is a sensitive sequence for detection of BV avulsion injuries. **(2-84)** Axial SWI shows bilateral RHs ➩. It is important to look closely for RHs. MR has ~ 50% sensitivity for detection of RHs but is highly specific.*

show diffusion restriction. Chronic injuries demonstrate volume loss and encephalomalacia.

Arterial spin labeling (ASL) pre- and postoperatively reflects alterations in cerebral blood flow following trauma **(2-81B)**. Altered cerebral vascular regulation is a pathophysiologic underpinning of the potentially catastrophic **second impact syndrome**.

Spine and spinal cord injuries are common in infants and children with shaking injuries. MR is the procedure of choice, as significant injuries can occur in the absence of fractures or subluxations. MR of the cervical and thoracic spine is also often performed in conjunction with brain MR in the setting of suspected AHT.

## Differential Diagnosis

**Accidental TBI** is the most common differential diagnosis. Accidents are typically witnessed and more common after the child begins to ambulate. Household falls < 3 feet do not result in imaging findings that mimic AHT. Accidental head trauma is more commonly impactive as opposed to the more common impulsive forces of AHT.

Other uncommon diagnoses, such as **inborn error of metabolism** (e.g., glutaric aciduria and Menkes kinky hair syndrome), can cause retinal hemorrhages and bilateral SDHs.

*Selected References: The complete reference list is available on the eBooks+ version included with purchase.*

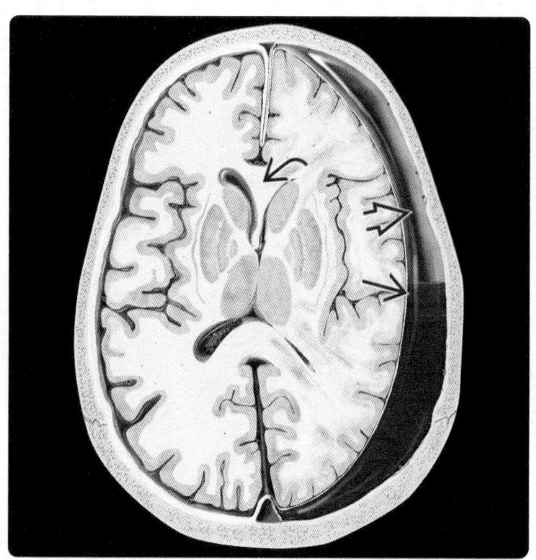

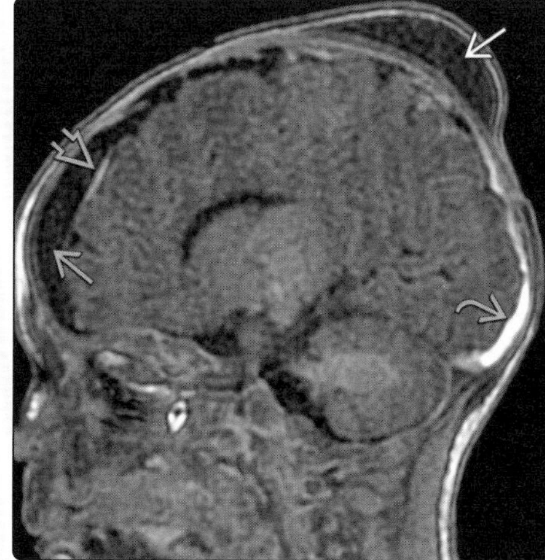

***(2-85)** Graphic demonstrates hematohygroma and subfalcine shift ➡. Dependent blood ➡ forms an interface with serum and CSF ➡. **(2-86)** Sagittal T1 MR shows a hematohygroma with CSF signal anteriorly ➡ and bright hemorrhage layering posteriorly ➡ and, to a lesser extent, anteriorly ➡. Nonhemorrhagic subgaleal fluid collection ➡ is also present.*

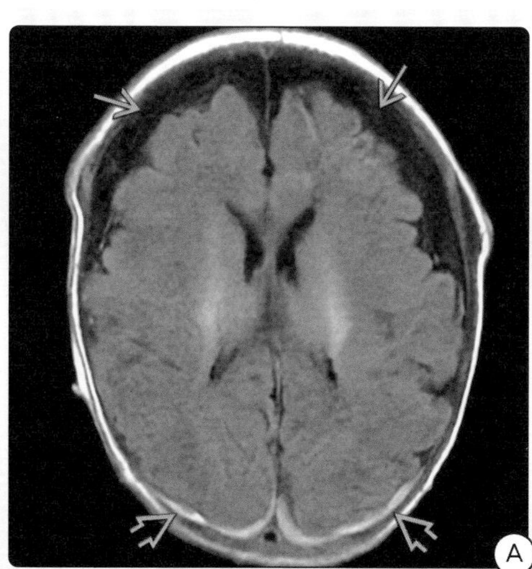

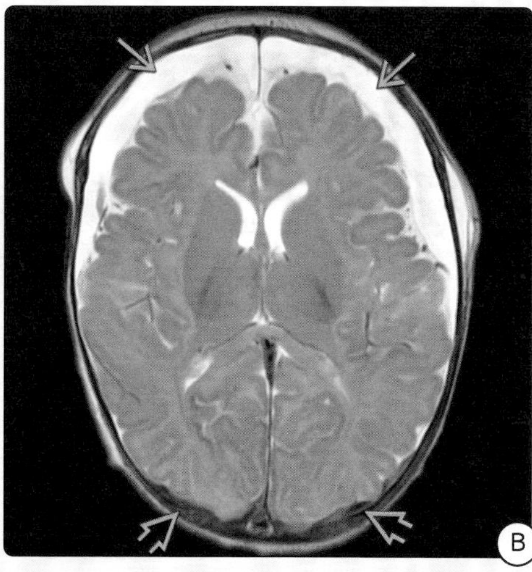

***(2-87A)** Axial T1 MR shows bilateral acute subdural hematohygromas. The dark subdural CSF ➡ is present anteriorly, and the bright blood ➡ is present posteriorly. **(2-87B)** Axial T2 MR in the same patient shows bright CSF fluid ➡ anteriorly and dark hemorrhage ➡ posteriorly. While mixed-signal subdural collections can be seen in cSDH, in the absence of membranes and compartmentalization, they are most likely due to a single acute injury.*

*__(2-88)__ Graphic shows aSDH ➡, subfalcine herniation, and cSDH ➡ with rebleed ➡. Note SAH ➡, cortical contusions ➡, and fracture ➡. __(2-89A)__ Axial T1 C+ MR in a 13-month-old with history of AHT shows bilateral cSDHs. Note the enhancing membranes ➡ and the compartmentalization of the subdural collections with collections of relatively high signal ➡ and relatively low signal ➡ intensity immediately adjacent to one another.*

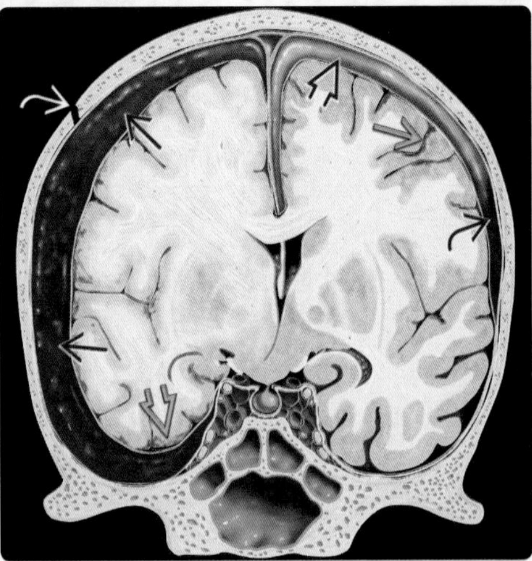

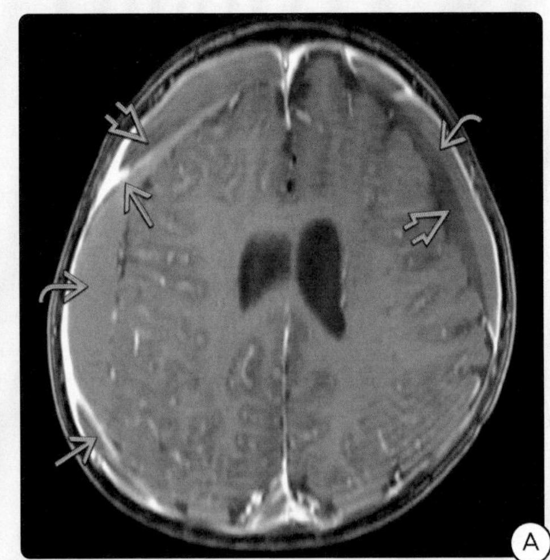

*__(2-89B)__ Axial T2 MR shows multiple compartments of SDH. The dark hemorrhage ➡ is separate from the CSF-like subdural fluid ➡ by a septation. The right SDH ➡ appears compartmentalized. __(2-90)__ Axial T2 MR in 1-month-old shows bifrontal subcortical lacerations ➡, bilateral subdural hematohygromas ➡, and parenchymal injury ➡ manifested as ↑ signal with loss of GM-WM differentiation in the parietal lobes.*

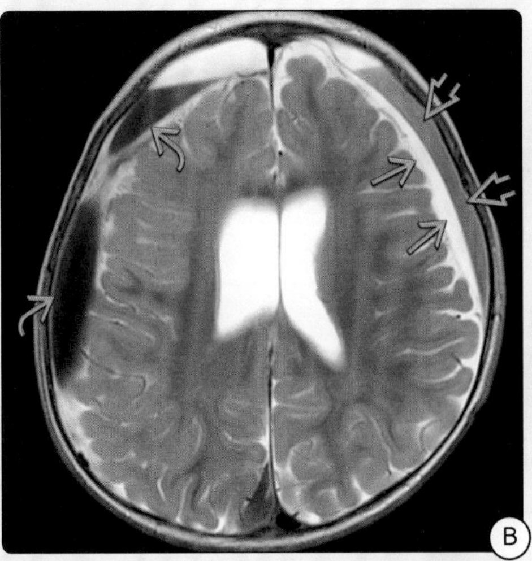

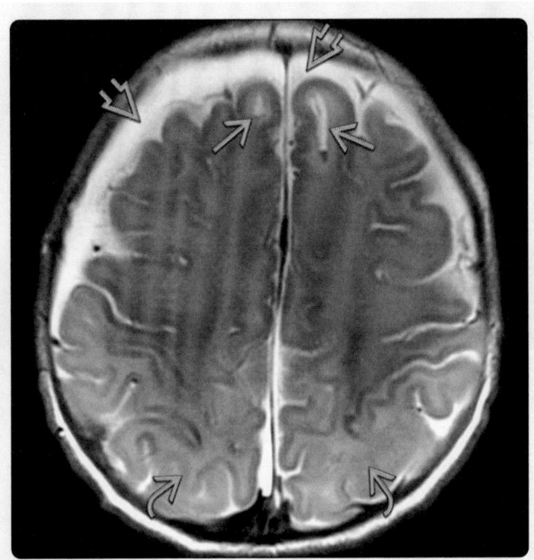

*__(2-91)__ Axial NECT in a toddler shows a hyperdense left subdural hematoma ➡. Associated parenchymal injury is also present with ↓ attenuation and loss of GM-WM differentiation ➡ in the left parietooccipital region. __(2-92)__ Axial DWI in a 2-month-old shows extensive bilateral cytotoxic edema, a common pattern of brain injury in AHT. Large geographic areas of cytotoxic edema are more common in AHT vs. accidental injury.*

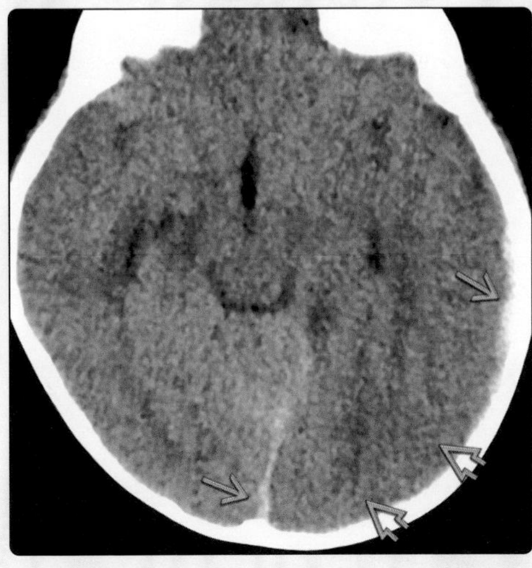

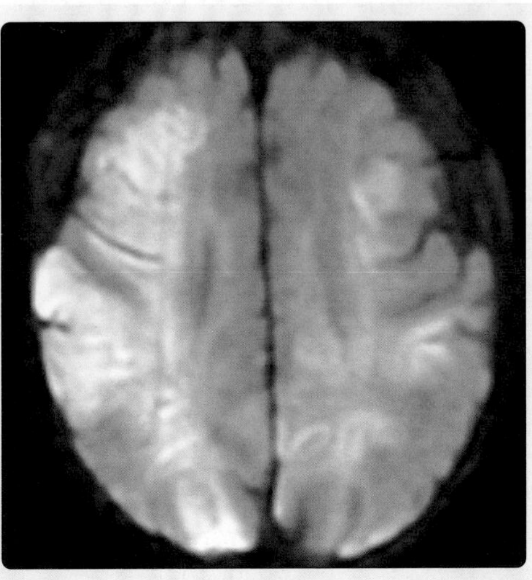

# Secondary Effects and Sequelae of CNS Trauma

*Traumatic brain injury is not a single "one and done" event. A veritable "cascade" of adverse pathophysiologic events continues to develop after the initial injury. Some—such as progressive hemorrhagic injury—occur within the first 24 hours after trauma. Others (e.g., brain swelling and herniation syndromes) may take a day or two to develop.*



Secondary effects of CNS trauma are defined as those that occur after the initial injury. These secondary effects are often more devastating than the initial injury itself and can become life threatening. Whereas many of the primary effects of CNS trauma (e.g., cortical contusions and axonal injuries) are permanent injuries, some secondary effects are either preventable or treatable.

Many potentially serious secondary effects are at least partially reversible if recognized early and treated promptly. Emergent imaging assessment, together with aggressive management of elevated intracranial pressure (ICP), perfusion alterations, and oxygenation deficits, may help mitigate both the immediate and long-term effects of brain trauma.

Chapter 2 focused on the primary effects of traumatic brain injury (TBI). In this chapter, we consider a broad spectrum of secondary effects that follow brain trauma, beginning with herniation syndromes.

## Herniation Syndromes

Brain herniations occur when one or more structures is displaced from its normal or "native" compartment into an adjacent space. They are the most common secondary manifestation of *any* expanding intracranial mass, regardless of etiology.

### Relevant Anatomy

Bony ridges and dural folds divide the intracranial cavity into three compartments: Two supratentorial hemicrania (the right and left halves) and the posterior fossa **(3-1)**.

The **falx cerebri** is a broad, sickle-shaped dural fold that attaches superiorly to the inside of the skull on either side of the midline, where it contains the superior sagittal sinus (SSS).

The concave inferior "free" margin of the falx contains the inferior sagittal sinus. As it courses posteriorly, the inferior margin of the falx forms a large open space above the corpus callosum and cingulate gyrus. This open space

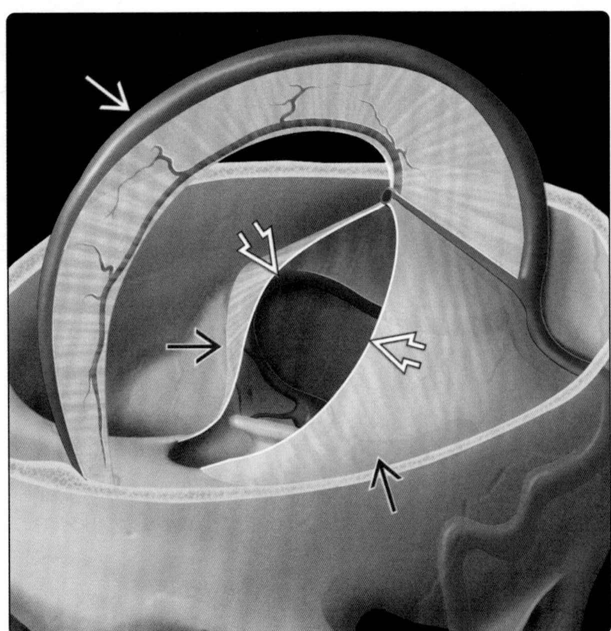

*(3-1) Falx ➡ divides the supratentorial compartment into 2 halves. Tentorium ➡ forms a U-shaped opening ➡, the tentorial incisura.*

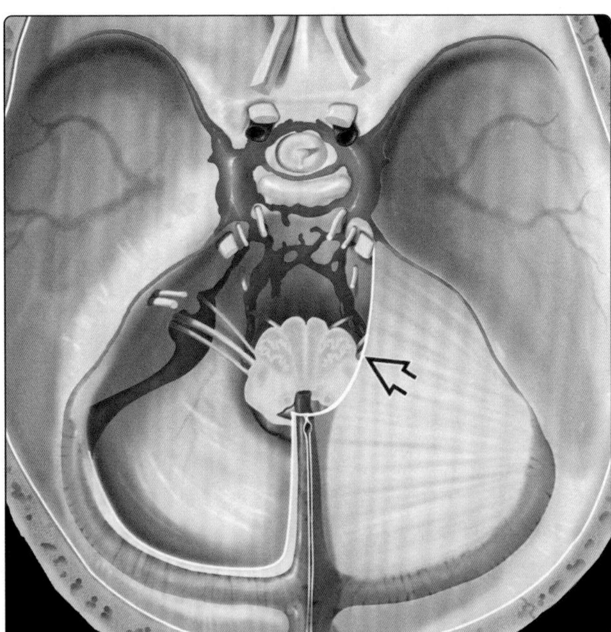

*(3-2) The right 1/2 of the tentorium has been removed to show the posterior fossa. The left 1/2 is shown forming the edge of the tentorial incisura ➡.*

allows potential displacement of brain and blood vessels from one side toward the other [subfalcine herniation (SFH)].

The **tentorium cerebelli** extends inferolaterally from its confluence with the falx, where their two merging dural folds contain the straight sinus. The straight sinus courses posteroinferiorly toward the sinus confluence with the SSS and transverse sinuses **(3-2)**.

The tentorium has two concave medial edges that contain a large U-shaped opening called the **tentorial incisura**. "Transtentorial" displacement of brain structures and accompanying blood vessels from the supratentorial compartment or posterior fossa can occur in either direction—up or down—through the tentorial incisura.

## Relevant Physiology

Once the sutures fuse and the fontanelles close, brain, CSF, and blood all coexist in a rigid, unyielding "bone box." The cerebral blood volume (CBV), perfusion, and CSF volume exist in a delicate balance within this closed box. Under normal conditions, pressures within the brain parenchyma and intracranial CSF spaces are equal.

When extra volume (blood, edema, tumor, etc.) is added to a cranial compartment, CSF in the sulci and subarachnoid cisterns is initially squeezed out. The ipsilateral ventricle becomes compressed and decreases in size. As intracranial volume continues to increase, the mass effect eventually exceeds the brain's compensatory capacity, and ICP begins to rise.

If a mass becomes sufficiently large, brain, CSF spaces, and blood vessels are displaced from one intracranial compartment into an adjacent one, resulting in one or more cerebral herniations.

In turn, cerebral herniations may cause their own cascade of secondary effects. Parenchyma, cranial nerves, &/or blood vessels can become compressed against the adjacent unyielding bone and dura. Secondary ischemic changes, frank brain infarcts, cranial neuropathies, and focal neurologic deficits may develop.

# Subfalcine Herniation

## Terminology and Etiology

SFH is the most common brain herniation and the easiest to understand. Here, an enlarging supratentorial mass in one hemicranium causes the brain to begin shifting toward the opposite side. Herniation occurs as the affected hemisphere pushes across the midline under the inferior "free" margin of the falx, extending into the contralateral hemicranium **(3-3)**. The cingulate gyrus and accompanying anterior cerebral artery (ACA) herniate under the falx anteriorly, but posterosuperiorly, the falx is wider and more rigid, anatomically limiting their displacement **(3-5)**.

## Imaging

Mass effect displaces the brain from one side toward the other ("midline shift"). The ipsilateral ventricle appears compressed and displaced across the midline, while the contralateral ventricle enlarges **(3-4)**. The cingulate gyrus and accompanying ACAs also herniate under the falx **(3-6)**.

## Complications

Early complications of SFH include unilateral hydrocephalus, seen on axial NECT as enlargement of the contralateral ventricle. As the mass effect increases, the lateral ventricles become progressively more displaced across the midline. This displacement initially just deforms, then kinks, and eventually occludes the foramen of Monro.

As herniation progresses, the choroid plexus in the contralateral ventricle continues to secrete CSF. Because the foramen of Monro is obstructed, CSF has no egress, and the contralateral ventricle enlarges while the ipsilateral ventricle is compressed by the mass effect.

If SFH becomes severe, the herniating ACA can become pinned against the inferior "free" margin of the falx cerebri and then occluded, causing secondary infarction of the cingulate gyrus.

### SUBFALCINE HERNIATION

**Etiology and Pathology**
- Unilateral hemispheric mass effect
- Brain shifts across midline under falx cerebri

**Epidemiology**
- Most common cerebral herniation

**Imaging**
- Cingulate gyrus, ACA, internal cerebral veins displaced across midline
- Foramen of Monro kinked, obstructed
- Ipsilateral ventricle small, contralateral enlarged

**Complications**
- Obstructive hydrocephalus
- Secondary ACA infarction (severe cases)

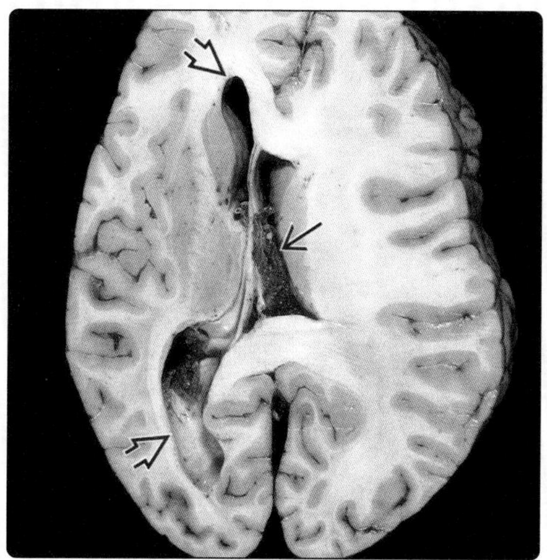

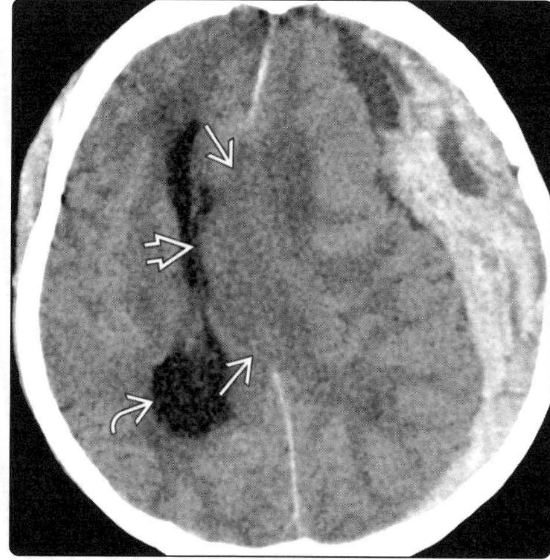

*(3-3) Subfalcine herniation (SFH): L lateral ventricle ⇨ is compressed, shifted across midline. Obstructed foramen of Monro causes enlarged R lateral ventricle ⇨. (Courtesy R. Hewlett, MD.) (3-4) NECT shows SFH of the cingulate gyrus ➡ caused by a rapidly bleeding subdural hematoma (SDH). The ipsilateral lateral ventricle is so severely compressed that it is almost inapparent ➡, while the contralateral ventricle is enlarged ➡.*

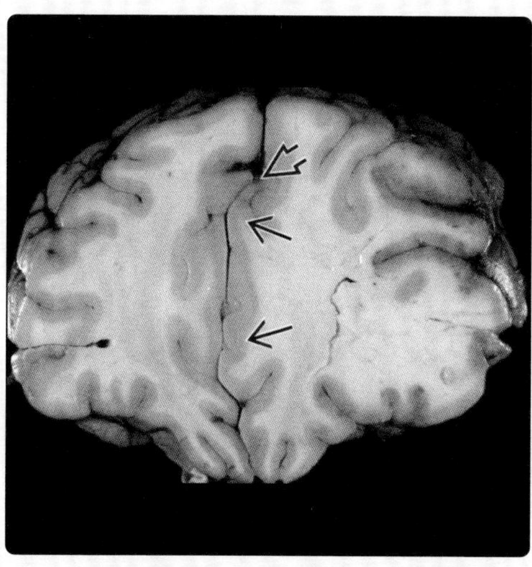

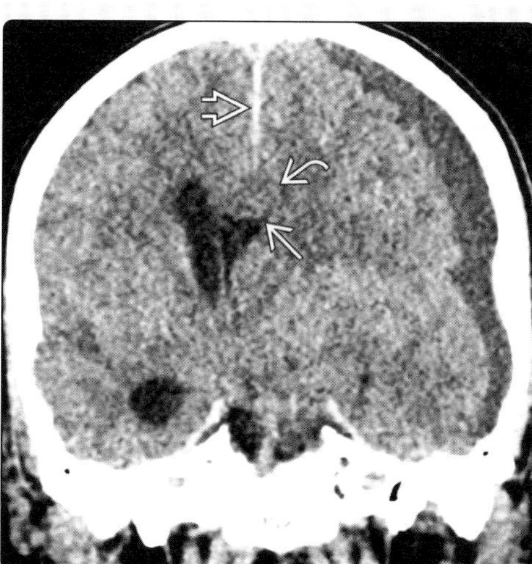

*(3-5) Coronal autopsy shows SFH. The brain is displaced across the midline ⇨ below the level of the falx cerebri ⇨. (3-6) Coronal NECT of a late subacute/early chronic SDH shows SFH of the lateral ventricles ➡ and cingulate gyrus ➡ under the falx cerebri ➡.*

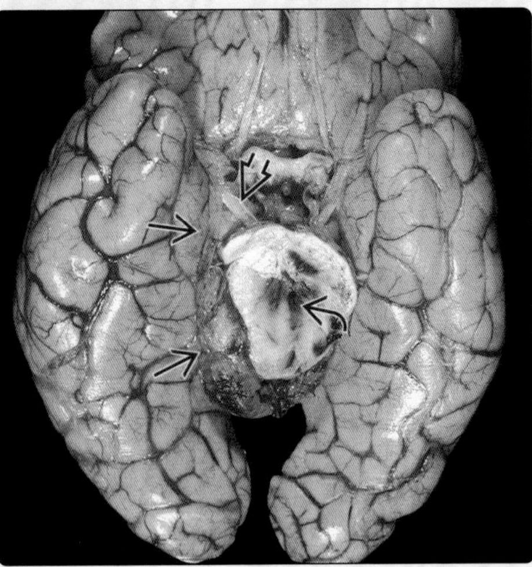

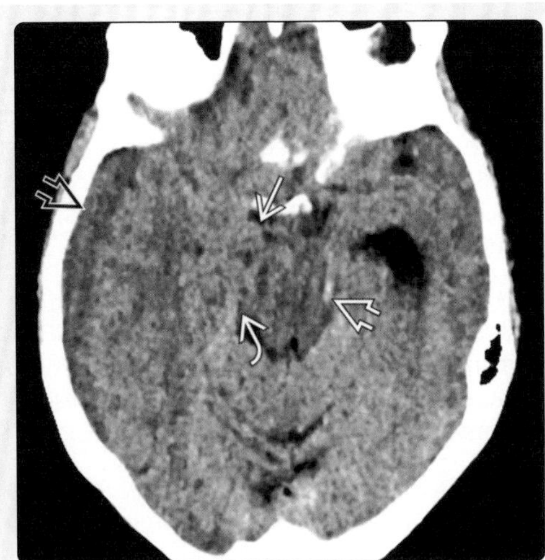

***(3-7)** Autopsy shows descending transtentorial herniation (DTH). Right uncus and hippocampus are displaced medially and demonstrate "grooving" → caused by impaction against tentorial incisura. CNIII is compressed → by herniating temporal lobe. Midbrain (Duret) hemorrhage is present →. **(3-8)** Subacute SDH →, DTH of uncus →, hippocampus →, and Kernohan notch → are shown.*

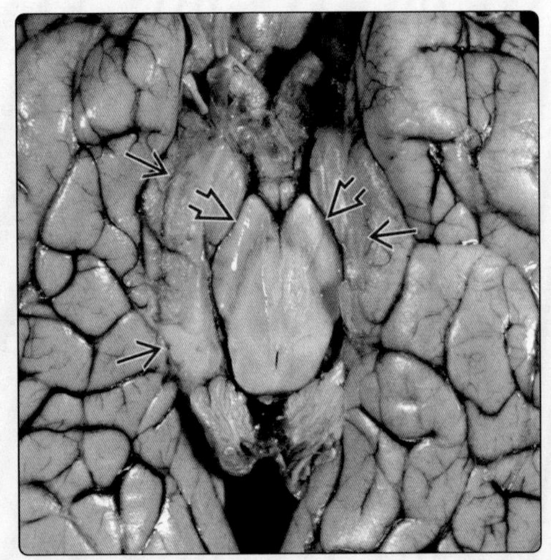

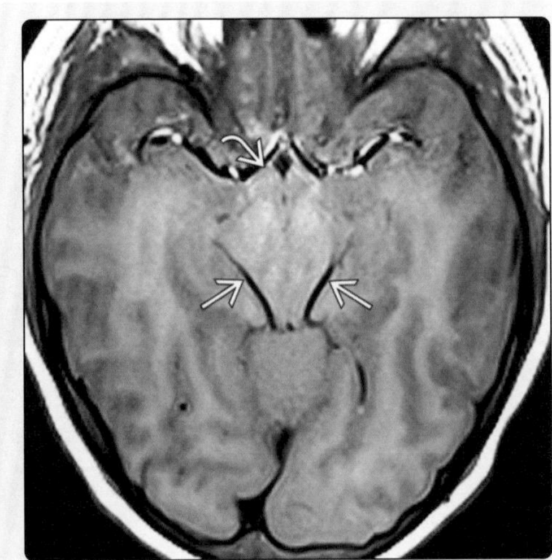

***(3-9)** Autopsy shows complete bilateral (central) DTH with "grooving" of the undersurface of the medial temporal lobes → caused by impaction against the tentorial incisura. The midbrain → is squeezed medially by the herniating temporal lobes. **(3-10)** Axial T1 MR shows bilateral DTH obliterating the suprasellar cistern →, herniating hippocampi, causing midbrain compression →.*

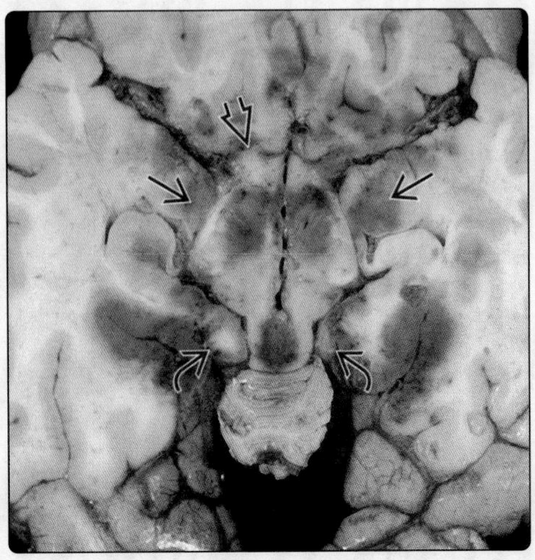

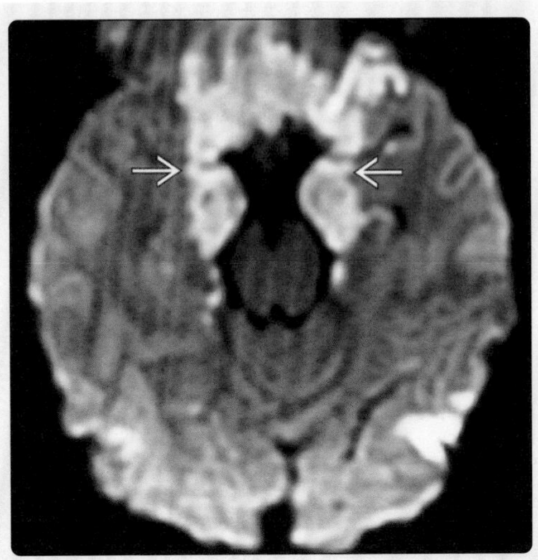

***(3-11)** Autopsy of complete bilateral ("central") herniation shows the suprasellar cistern obliterated by the inferiorly displaced hypothalamus →. The uncus → and hippocampi → are herniated medially and inferiorly into the tentorial incisura. **(3-12)** DWI MR after central DTH shows restricted diffusion in the same areas → as the autopsied brain in Fig. 3-11.*

## Descending Transtentorial Herniation

Transtentorial herniations are brain displacements that occur through the tentorial incisura. Although these displacements can occur in both directions (from top down or bottom up), descending herniations from supratentorial masses are far more common than ascending herniations.

### Terminology and Etiology

Descending transtentorial herniation (DTH) is the second most common type of intracranial herniation syndrome. DTH is caused by a hemispheric mass that initially produces side-to-side brain displacement (i.e., SFH). As the mass effect increases, the uncus of the temporal lobe is pushed medially and begins to encroach on the suprasellar cistern. With progressively increasing mass effect, both the uncus and hippocampus herniate inferiorly through the tentorial incisura.

DTH can be unilateral or bilateral. **Unilateral DTH** occurs when a hemispheric mass effect pushes the uncus and hippocampus of the ipsilateral temporal lobe over the edge of the tentorial incisura **(3-7)**. In **bilateral DTH**, both temporal lobes are displaced medially **(3-9)**.

"Complete" or **"central" descending herniation** occurs when the supratentorial mass effect becomes so severe that the hypothalamus and optic chiasm are flattened against the skull base, *both* temporal lobes are herniated, and the whole tentorial incisura is completely plugged with displaced tissue **(3-11)** **(3-12)**.

### Imaging

Axial CT scans in early **unilateral DTH** show that the uncus is displaced medially and the ipsilateral aspect of the suprasellar cistern is effaced **(3-8)**. As DTH increases, the hippocampus also herniates medially over the edge of the tentorium, compressing the quadrigeminal cistern and pushing the midbrain toward the opposite side of the incisura. In severe cases, the temporal horn can even be displaced almost into the midline.

With **bilateral DTH**, both temporal lobes herniate medially into the tentorial hiatus **(3-10)**. With **central descending herniation**, both hemispheres are so swollen that the whole central brain is flattened against the skull base **(3-13)**. All the basal cisterns are obliterated as the hypothalamus and optic chiasm are crushed against the sella turcica, and the suprasellar and quadrigeminal cisterns are completely effaced **(3-14)**.

In complete (central) bilateral DTH, the midbrain is compressed and squeezed medially from both sides. Sagittal images show that the midbrain is also pushed inferiorly through the tentorial incisura, displacing the pons downward. The angle between the midbrain and pons is progressively reduced from nearly 90° to almost 0° **(3-14)**. In terminal central herniation, the pons eventually pushes the cerebellar tonsils inferiorly through the foramen magnum **(3-15)**.

### Complications

Even mild DTH can compress the third cranial (oculomotor) nerve as it exits from the interpeduncular fossa and courses anterolaterally toward the cavernous sinus. This may produce a **pupil-involving third nerve palsy**.

Other, more severe complications may occur with DTH. As the temporal lobe is displaced inferomedially, it pushes the posterior cerebral artery (PCA) below the tentorial incisura. The PCA can become kinked and eventually even occluded as it passes back up over the medial edge of the tentorium, causing a **secondary PCA (occipital) infarct** **(3-28)** **(3-29)**.

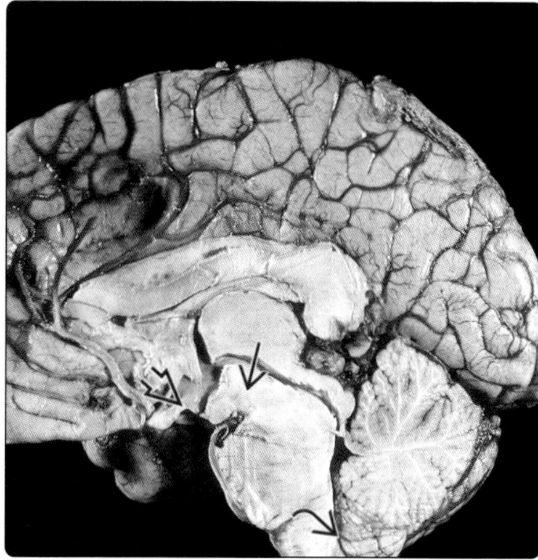

***(3-13)*** *DTH: Midbrain is kinked inferiorly ➙, hypothalamus is smashed over dorsum sellae ➙, tonsil is herniated ➙. (Courtesy R. Hewlett, MD.)*

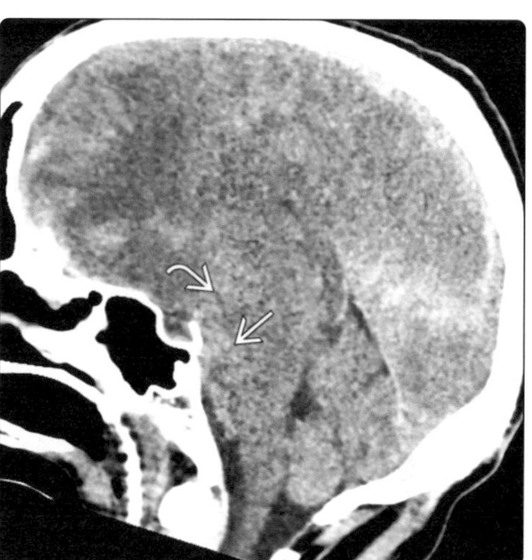

***(3-14)*** *Sagittal NECT of DTH shows midbrain displaced inferiorly ➙, and the midbrain-pons angle ➙ is obliterated.*

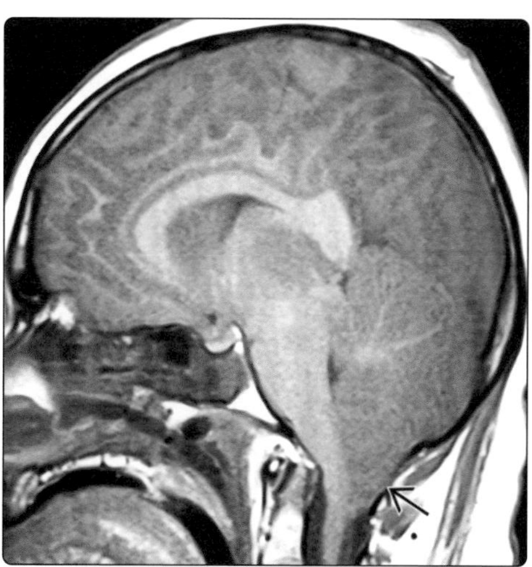

***(3-15)*** *Sagittal T1 MR shows diffuse brain swelling and DTH, similar to autopsy case shown in Fig. 3-13. Note severe tonsillar herniation ➙.*

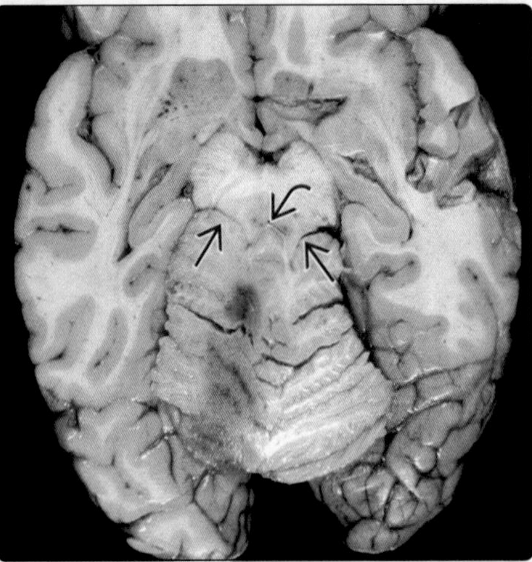

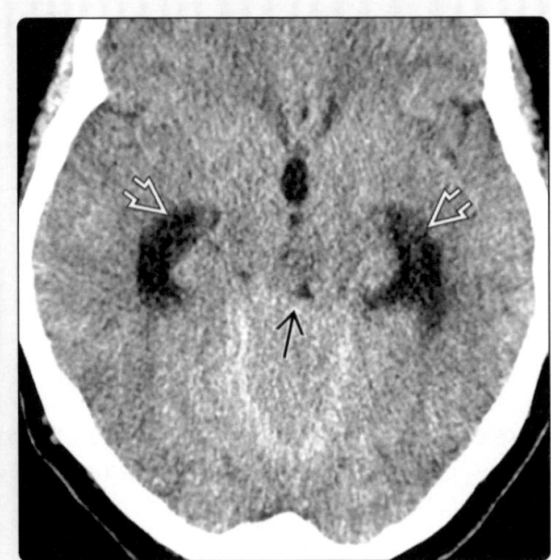

***(3-16)*** *Axial gross pathology of ascending transtentorial herniation (ATH) shows the cerebellum/vermis pushed upward, flattening the dorsal midbrain and obstructing the aqueduct.* ***(3-17)*** *NECT shows ATH with obliterated quadrigeminal cistern and compressed tectum. Note severe obstructive hydrocephalus.*

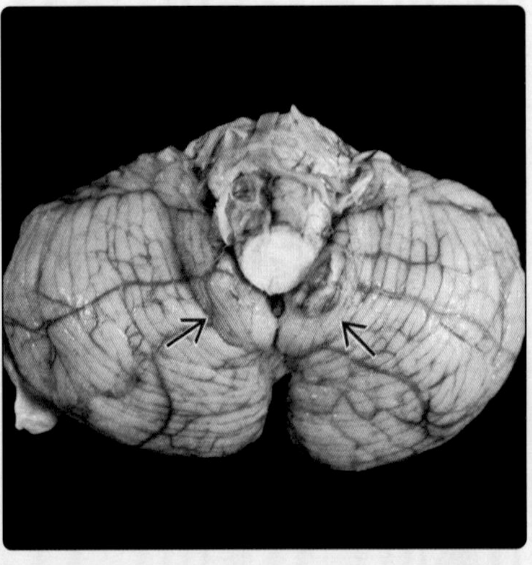

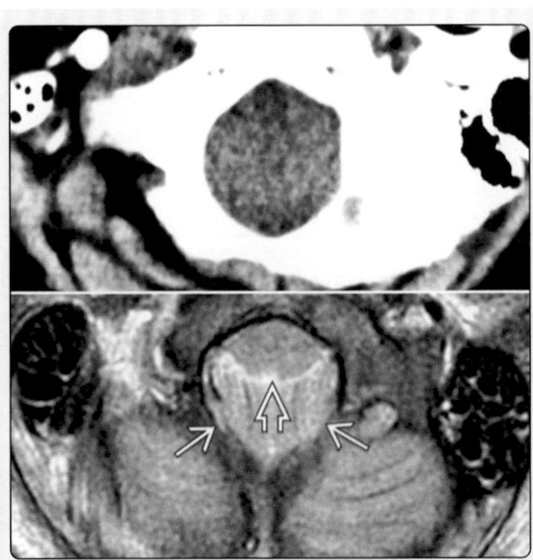

***(3-18)*** *Herniation shows tonsils displaced inferiorly, "grooved" by bony margins of foramen magnum. (Courtesy R. Hewlett, MD.)* ***(3-19)*** *(Top) NECT of tonsillar herniation only shows effacement of all CSF spaces within the foramen magnum. (Bottom) Axial T2 MR shows much more anatomic detail. The inferiorly displaced tonsils fill the foramen magnum and compress/displace the medulla anteriorly.*

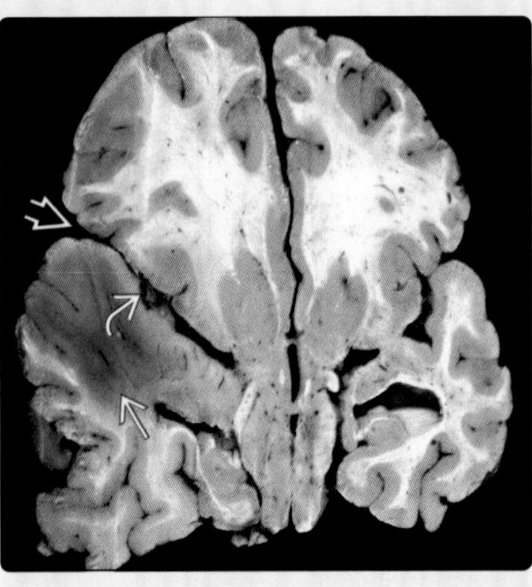

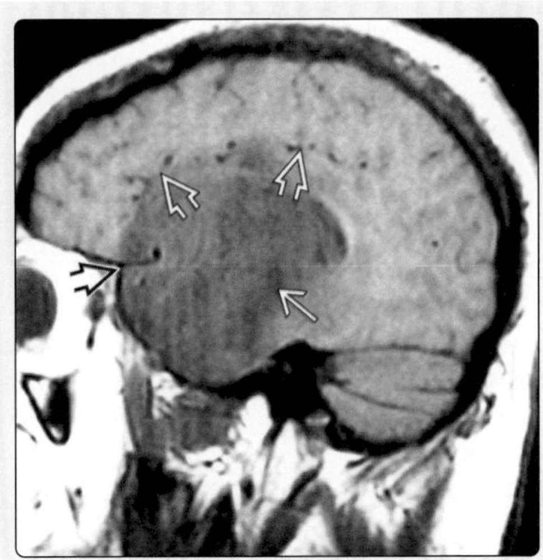

***(3-20)*** *Ascending transalar herniation shows a temporal lobe mass pushing the sylvian fissure and middle cerebral artery (MCA) up/over the site of the greater sphenoid wing. (Courtesy E. T. Hedley-Whyte, MD.)* ***(3-21)*** *Ascending transalar herniation shows the mass elevating the sylvian fissure and MCA, pushing the temporal lobe up/over the sphenoid wing.*

Severe bilateral DTH may cause pressure necrosis of the uncus and hippocampus **(3-11)**, causing a secondary hemorrhagic infarct in the midbrain or pons **(Duret hemorrhage)** **(3-7)**.

With complete central DTH, perforating arteries that arise from the circle of Willis are compressed against the central skull base and also occlude, causing multiple **hypothalamic and basal ganglia infarcts**.

In a vicious cycle, the hemispheres become more edematous, and ICP soars. If the rising pressure exceeds intraarterial pressure, perfusion is drastically reduced and eventually ceases, causing **brain death (BD)**.

**DESCENDING TRANSTENTORIAL HERNIATION**

**Terminology and Pathology**
- Unilateral DTH
  - Temporal lobe (uncus, hippocampus) pushed over tentorial incisura
- Severe bilateral DTH: "Complete" or "central" herniation
  - Hypothalamus, chiasm flattened against sella

**Epidemiology**
- 2nd most common cerebral herniation

**Imaging**
- Unilateral DTH
  - Suprasellar cistern initially encroached
  - Progressive effacement as herniation worsens
  - Herniating temporal lobe pushes midbrain to opposite side (may cause Kernohan "notch")
- Bilateral DTH
  - Basal cisterns completely effaced
  - Midbrain pushed down behind clivus, compressed on both sides
  - Midbrain-pons angle becomes more acute

**Complications**
- CNIII compression
  - May cause pupil-involving 3rd nerve palsy
- PCA occlusion
  - Becomes kinked against edge of tentorium
  - Secondary occipital (PCA) infarct may ensue
- Complete "central" DTH
  - If severe ± hypothalamus, basal infarcts
- Compression of contralateral cerebral peduncle (Kernohan "notch")
- Midbrain (Duret) hemorrhage

## Ascending Transtentorial Herniation

Two types of herniations occur with posterior fossa masses: Ascending transtentorial herniation (ATH) and tonsillar herniation.

### Terminology and Etiology

In ATH, the cerebellar vermis and hemispheres are pushed upward ("ascend") through the tentorial incisura into the supratentorial compartment. The superiorly herniating cerebellum first flattens and displaces, then effaces the quadrigeminal cistern and compresses the midbrain **(3-16)**.

### Imaging

Axial NECT scans show that CSF in the superior vermian cistern and cerebellar sulci is effaced. The quadrigeminal cistern is first compressed and then obliterated by the upwardly herniating cerebellum. As the herniation progresses, the tectal plate becomes compressed and flattened **(3-17)**. In severe cases, the dorsal midbrain may actually appear concave instead of convex. The most common complication of ATH is acute intraventricular obstructive hydrocephalus caused by compression of the cerebral aqueduct **(3-17)**.

**ASCENDING TRANSTENTORIAL HERNIATION**

**Relatively Rare**
- Caused by expanding posterior fossa mass
- Neoplasm > trauma
- Cerebellum pushed upward through incisura
- Compresses, deforms midbrain

**Imaging Findings**
- Incisura filled with tissue, CSF spaces obliterated
- Quadrigeminal cistern, tectal plate compressed/flattened
  - Eventually appear obliterated

**Complications**
- Hydrocephalus (secondary to aqueduct obstruction)

## Tonsillar Herniation

### Terminology and Etiology

In tonsillar herniation, the cerebellar tonsils are displaced inferiorly and become impacted into the foramen magnum **(3-18)**. Tonsillar herniation can be congenital (e.g., Chiari 1 malformation) or acquired.

Acquired tonsillar herniation occurs in two different circumstances. The most common cause is an expanding posterior fossa mass *pushing* the tonsils downward into the foramen magnum.

Inferior tonsillar displacement also occurs with intracranial hypotension. Here, the tonsils are *pulled* downward by abnormally low intraspinal CSF pressure (see Chapter 38).

### Imaging

Diagnosing tonsillar herniation on NECT scans may be problematic. The foramen magnum usually contains CSF that surrounds the medulla and cerebellar tonsils. Herniation of one or both tonsils into the foramen magnum obliterates most or all of the CSF in the cisterna magna **(3-19)**.

Tonsillar herniation is much more easily diagnosed on MR. In the sagittal plane, the normally horizontal tonsillar folia become vertically oriented, and the inferior aspect of the tonsils becomes pointed. Tonsils > 5 mm below the foramen magnum are generally abnormal, especially if they are peg-like or pointed (rather than rounded) **(3-15)**.

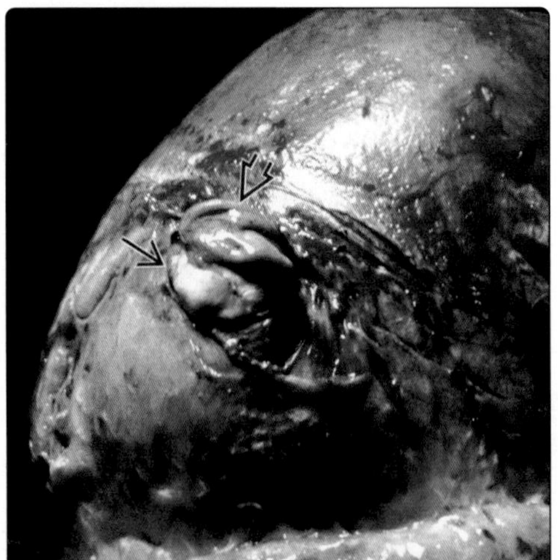

*(3-22) Autopsy of transdural/transcranial herniation with ↑ intracranial pressure shows the brain herniating → through a burr hole →.*

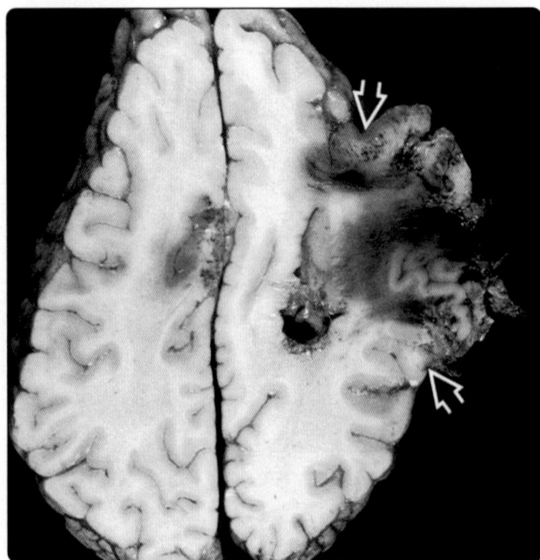

*(3-23) Transdural/transcranial herniation with brain extrusion through a large craniectomy defect →. (Courtesy E. T. Hedley-Whyte, MD.)*

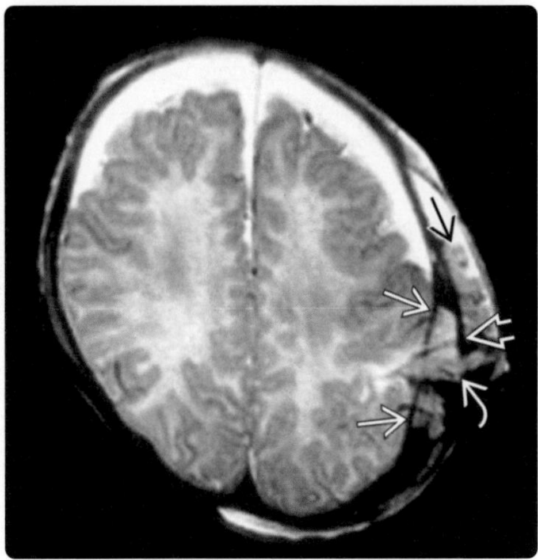

*(3-24) T2 MR in a case of abusive head trauma shows a fracture → and torn dura → with epidural brain → extruding under the scalp →.*

In the axial plane, T2 scans show that the tonsils are impacted into the foramen magnum, obliterating CSF in the cisterna magna and displacing the medulla anteriorly **(3-19)**.

## Complications

Complications of tonsillar herniation include obstructive hydrocephalus and tonsillar necrosis.

### TONSILLAR HERNIATION

**Etiology and Pathology**

- Most common posterior fossa herniation
- Can be congenital (Chiari 1) or acquired
- Acquired
  - Most common: Secondary to posterior fossa mass effect
  - Less common: Intracranial hypotension
  - Rare: Severe central DTH, BD

**Imaging Findings**

- 1 or both tonsils > 5 mm below foramen magnum
- CSF in foramen magnum effaced
- Foramen magnum appears tissue-filled on axial NECT, T2WI
- Inferior "pointing" or peg-like configuration of tonsils on sagittal T1WI

**Complications**

- Obstructive hydrocephalus
- Tonsillar necrosis

# Other Herniations

The vast majority of cerebral herniations are subfalcine, descending/ascending transtentorial, and tonsillar herniations. Other, less common herniation syndromes are transalar and transdural/transcranial herniations.

## Transalar Herniation

Transalar herniation occurs when the brain herniates across the greater sphenoid wing (GSW) or "ala" and can be either ascending (the most common) or descending.

**Ascending transalar herniation** is caused by a large *middle cranial fossa mass* **(3-20)**. The middle cerebral artery (MCA) branches and sylvian fissure are elevated, and the superior temporal gyrus is pushed above the GSW **(3-21)**.

**Descending transalar herniation** is caused by a large *anterior cranial fossa mass.* Here, the gyrus rectus is forced posteroinferiorly over the GSW, displacing the sylvian fissure and shifting the MCA backward.

## Transdural/Transcranial Herniation

This rare type of cerebral herniation, sometimes called a "brain fungus" by neurosurgeons, can be life threatening. For transdural/transcranial herniation to occur, the dura must be lacerated, a skull defect (fracture or craniotomy) must be present **(3-22)**, and ICP must be elevated **(3-23)**.

Traumatic transdural/transcranial herniations typically occur in infants or young children with a comminuted skull fracture that deforms inward with impact, lacerating the dura-arachnoid. When ICP increases, the brain can herniate through the torn dura and across the skull fracture into the subgaleal space **(3-24)**.

OTHER HERNIATIONS

**Ascending Transalar Herniation**
- Most common transalar herniation
- Caused by middle fossa mass
- Sagittal imaging (best appreciated on off-midline images)
  - Sylvian fissure, MCA displaced up/over greater sphenoid ala
- Axial imaging
  - Sylvian fissure/MCA bowed forward
  - Temporal lobe bulges into anterior fossa

**Descending Transalar Herniation**
- Caused by anterior fossa mass
- Sagittal imaging
  - Sylvian fissure, MCA displaced posteroinferiorly
  - Frontal lobe pushed backward over greater sphenoid ala
- Axial imaging
  - Gyrus rectus pushed posteriorly
  - MCA curved backward

**Transcranial/Transdural Herniation**
- Increased ICP + skull defect + dura-arachnoid tear
- Caused by
  - Comminuted, often depressed skull fracture
  - Craniectomy
- Brain extruded through skull, under scalp aponeurosis
- Best appreciated on axial T2WI

# Edema, Ischemia, and Vascular Injury

TBI can unleash a cascade of physiologic responses that may adversely affect the brain more than the initial trauma. These responses include diffuse brain swelling, excitotoxic responses elicited by glutamatergic pathway activation, perfusion alterations, and a variety of ischemic events, including territorial infarcts.

## Posttraumatic Brain Swelling

Cerebral edema is a major contributor to TBI morbidity. Massive brain swelling with severe intracranial hypertension is among the most serious of all secondary traumatic lesions. Mortality approaches 50%, so early recognition and aggressive treatment of this complication are imperative.

### Etiology and Epidemiology

Focal, regional, or diffuse brain swelling develops in 10-20% of patients with TBI. Whether this is caused by increased tissue fluid (cerebral edema) or elevated blood volume (cerebral hyperemia) secondary to vascular dysautoregulation is unclear. In some cases, the trigeminal system may mediate brain swelling associated with subdural bleeding, providing the link between small-volume, thin subdural bleeds and swelling of the underlying brain.

### Clinical Issues

Children, young adults, and individuals with repetitive concussive or subconcussive injuries are especially prone to developing posttraumatic brain swelling and are almost twice as likely as older adults to develop this complication. Although gross enlargement of one or both hemispheres

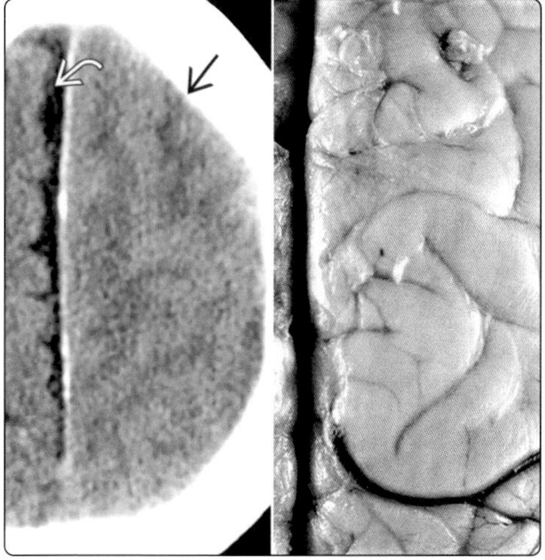

*(3-25) (L) NECT shows left hemisphere edema, obliterated sulci ➡, and normal right sulci ➡. (R) Autopsy shows unilateral hemispheric swelling.*

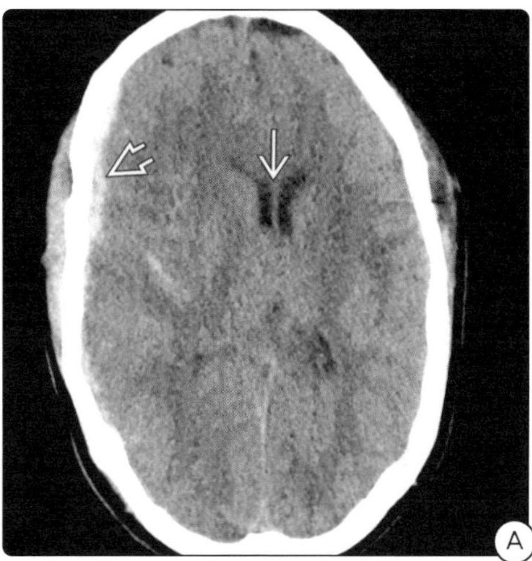


*(3-26A) NECT shows a 6-mm acute SDH ➡. Disproportionate 15-mm midline shift ➡ indicates imminent cerebral edema.*

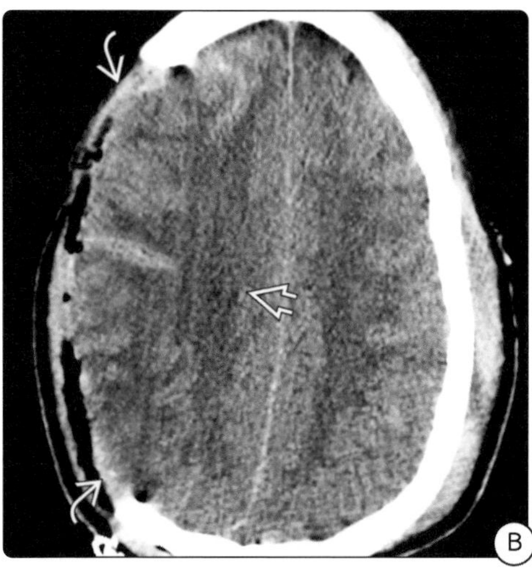


*(3-26B) Emergent decompressive craniectomy ➡ was performed due to an impending herniation. Note the right hemisphere edema ➡.*

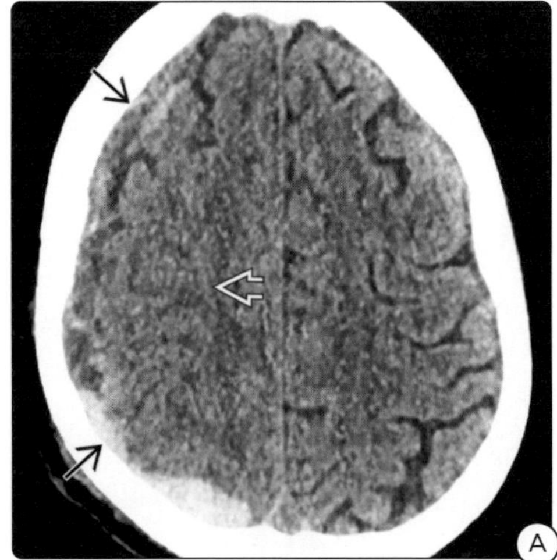


***(3-27A) NECT in a patient with left hemiparesis shows a mixed-age right SDH ⇨ and cortical swelling ➡ under the SDH.***

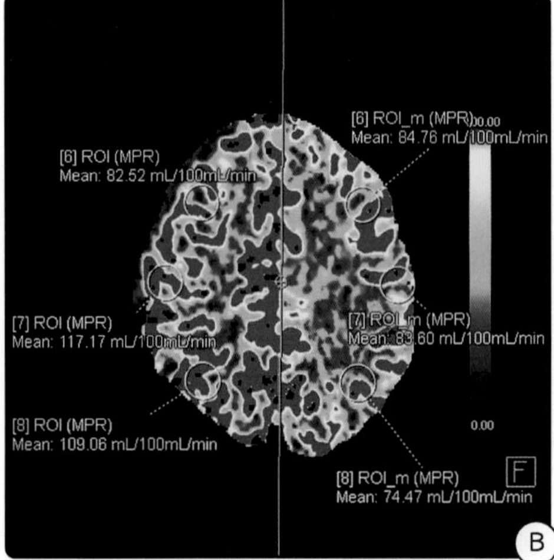


***(3-27B) Annotated CTP in the same case shows ↑ CBF in the right posterior frontal and anterior parietal lobes under the SDH.***

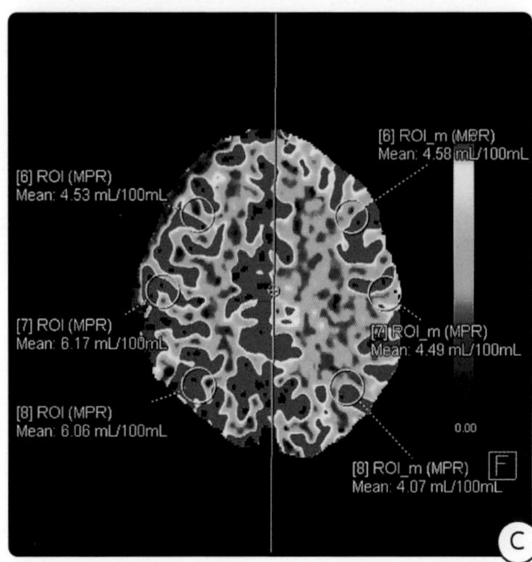


***(3-27C) CTP in the same case shows ↑ CBV in the same areas. This is posttraumatic hyperperfusion syndrome. (Courtesy C. Hsu, MD.)***

occasionally develops rapidly after the initial event, delayed onset is more typical. Severe cerebral edema generally takes between 24-48 hours to develop.

In some cases, aggressive measures for control of ICP fail to restore cerebral metabolism and improve neurologic outcome. Decompressive craniectomy as a last resort is often performed, but evidence for reduced risk of death or dependence in severe TBI is lacking.

## Imaging

The appearance of posttraumatic brain swelling evolves over time. Initially, mild hemispheric mass effect with sulcal/cisternal compression is seen on NECT scans **(3-25)**.

During the early stages of brain swelling, gray matter-white matter differentiation is relatively preserved. Although the ipsilateral ventricle may be slightly compressed, subfalcine displacement is generally minimal. **However, if the mass effect is disproportionately greater than the maximum width of an extraaxial collection, such as a subdural hematoma (SDH), early and potentially catastrophic swelling of the underlying brain parenchyma should be suspected and treated emergently (3-26)**.

MR shows swollen gyri that are hypointense on T1WI and hyperintense on T2WI. Diffusion-weighted scans show restricted diffusion with low apparent diffusion coefficient (ADC) values.

As brain swelling progresses, the demarcation between the cortex and underlying white matter becomes indistinct and eventually disappears **(3-31)**. The lateral ventricles appear smaller than normal, and the superficial sulci are no longer visible **(3-32)**.

### POSTTRAUMATIC BRAIN SWELLING

**Epidemiology**
- 10-20% of TBI
- Can be focal, regional, or diffuse
- Most common in children, young adults
- Potentially catastrophic

**Imaging**
- Earliest sign
  - SFH ≥ 3 mm than width of epidural or SDH
- Next
  - Sulcal effacement
- Later
  - Indistinct gray-white interfaces
- End stage
  - 1 or both hemispheres uniformly low density
  - All sulci, cisterns obliterated
  - Small ventricles

# Traumatic Cerebral Ischemia, Infarction, and Perfusion Abnormalities

Traumatic ischemia and infarction are uncommon but important complications of TBI. They have a variety of causes, including direct vascular compression, systemic hypoperfusion, vascular injury, vasospasm, and venous congestion. The most common cause of posttraumatic cerebral ischemia is mechanical vascular compression secondary to a brain herniation syndrome.

## Posttraumatic Infarcts

The most common brain herniation that causes secondary cerebral infarction is DTH. Severe unilateral DTH displaces the temporal lobe and accompanying PCA inferiorly into the tentorial incisura. As the herniating PCA passes posterior to the midbrain, it courses superiorly and is forced against the hard, knife-like edge of the tentorial incisura. The P3 PCA segment occludes, resulting in occipital lobe infarction **(3-28)** **(3-29)**.

Less commonly, SFH presses the callosomarginal branch of the ACA against the undersurface of the falx cerebri and causes cingulate gyrus infarction **(3-30)**.

With complete bilateral ("central") DTH, penetrating arteries that arise from the circle of Willis are crushed against the skull base, resulting in multiple scattered basal ganglia and hypothalamus infarcts. Pressure necrosis of the uncus and hippocampus can also occur as the herniated temporal lobes impact the free edge of the tentorial incisura **(3-12)**.

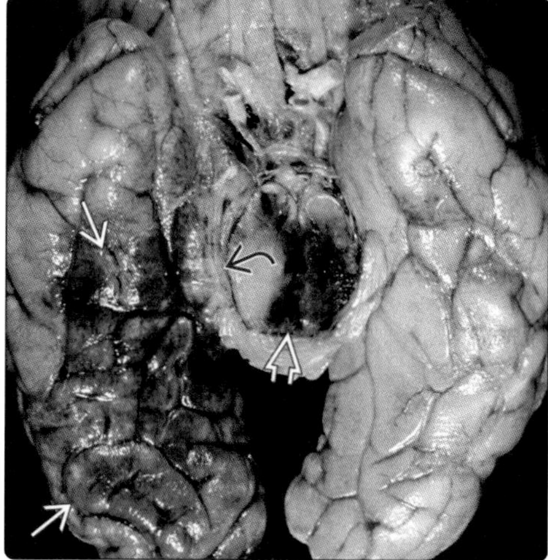

***(3-28)** DTH caused PCA occlusion against tentorium ➙, infarction ➙. Duret hemorrhage ➙ in midbrain. (Courtesy R. Hewlett, MD.)*

## Traumatic Cerebral Ischemia

Focal, regional, and generalized perfusion alterations also occur with TBI. Extraaxial hematomas that exert significant focal mass effect on the underlying brain may cause reduced arterial perfusion and cortical ischemia. They may also compress the underlying cortical veins, causing venous ischemia.

Global or generalized **cerebral ischemia** may result from hypoperfusion, hypoxia, membrane depolarization, or loss of cellular membrane integrity and ion homeostasis. Cellular energy failure may induce glutamate-mediated **acute excitotoxic brain injury**.

NECT scans show hypodensity with loss of gray-white differentiation in the affected parenchyma. CT perfusion (CTP) may show decreased cerebral blood flow (CBF) with prolonged time to drain. In cases of excitotoxic brain injury, MR shows swollen, hyperintense gyri on T2/FLAIR that do not correspond to defined vascular territories.

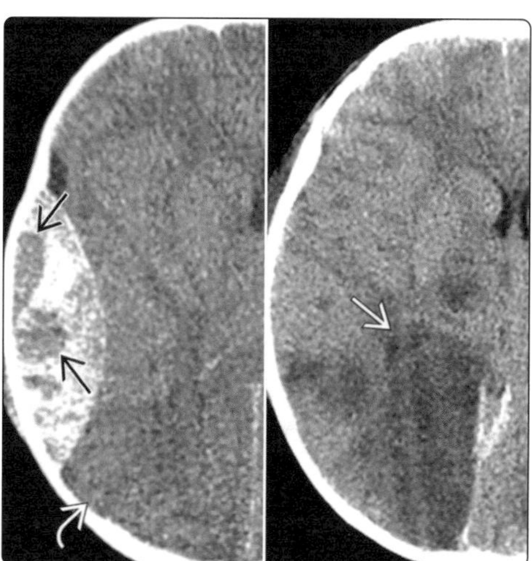

***(3-29)** (L) Acute EDH with rapid bleeding ➙, subtle occipital hypodensity ➙. (R) Postop scan shows infarct ➙ secondary to PCA herniation.*

## Traumatic Cerebral Perfusion Alterations

In patients with acute SDHs, raised ICP typically leads to reduced cerebral perfusion pressure and impaired CBF. In contrast, patients with mixed or chronic SDHs may have significantly upregulated CBV and CBF in the cortex underlying the chronic SDH **(3-27)**. Mean transit times (MTTs) are often elevated.

# Brain Death

## Terminology

The legal definition of BD varies from country to country. In the United States, the Uniform Determination of Death Act (UDDA) has served as a model statute for 40 years, embraced in whole or in part throughout the country. There is growing recognition that the UDDA needs to be revised and updated. A committee has been constituted that will be submitting its recommendations by July 2023.

## Clinical Issues

BD is primarily a clinical diagnosis. Three neurorespiratory findings are necessary to confirm irreversible cessation of all functions of the entire brain, *including the brainstem*: (1) Coma (with a known cause), (2) absence of brainstem reflexes, and (3) apnea.

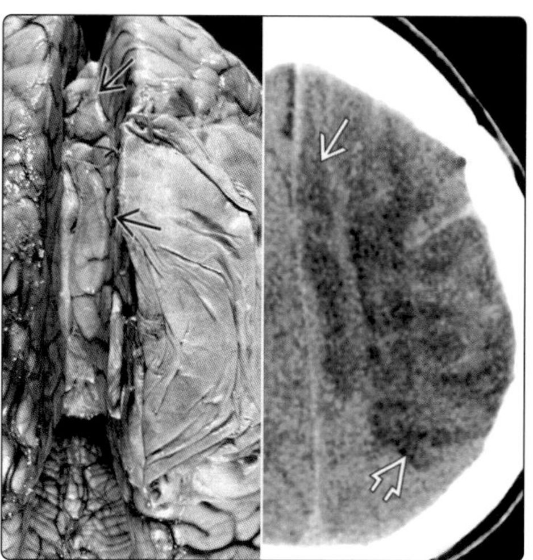

***(3-30)** (L) Cingulate herniation ➙ is shown. (R) Malignant MCA infarct ➙ caused ACA occlusion with cingulate gyrus infarct ➙.*

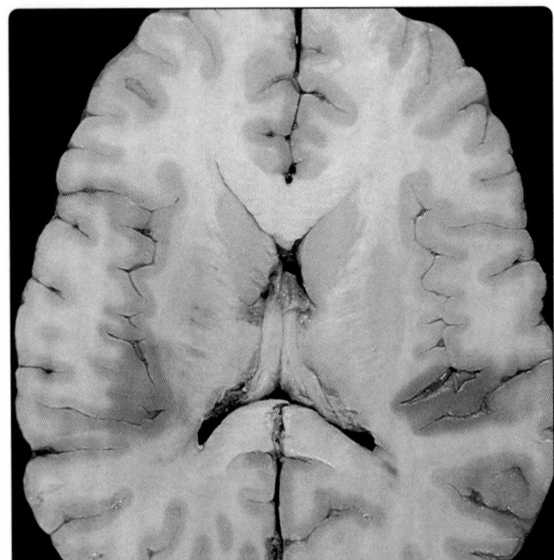

*(3-31) Brain death shows diffuse swelling, poor GM-WM discrimination, small ventricles, and effaced surface sulci. (Courtesy R. Hewlett, MD.)*

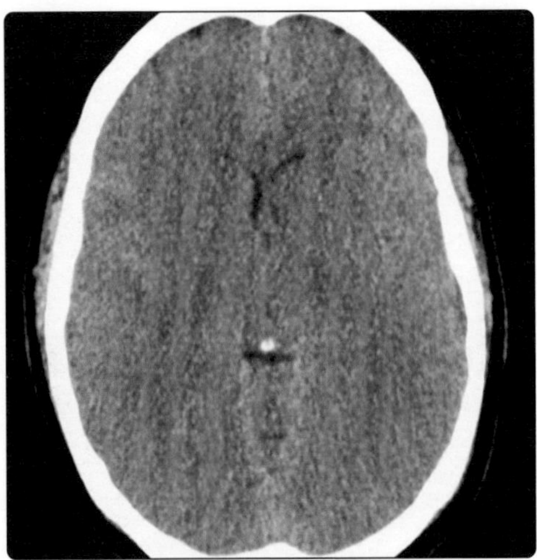

*(3-32) NECT shows severe cerebral edema with diffuse low-density brain, small ventricles, effaced sulci, and no GM-WM differentiation.*

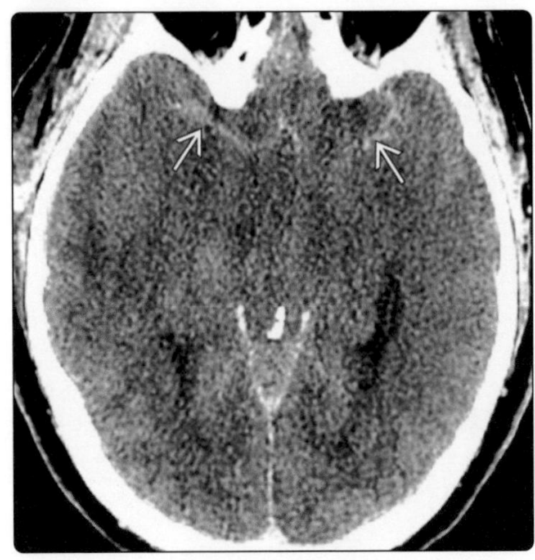

*(3-33) NECT in severe brain swelling shows diffuse hypodense brain. Attenuated MCAs appear hyperdense ➡, mimicking aSAH.*

Complex spontaneous motor movements and false-positive ventilator triggering may occur in patients who are brain dead, so expert assessment is crucial. Once reversible causes of coma (e.g., drug overdose, status epilepticus) are excluded, the clinical diagnosis of BD is highly reliable *if* the determination is made by experienced examiners using established, accepted criteria.

## Imaging

Although BD is a clinical diagnosis, ancillary and confirmatory tests, including imaging, are widely used. **While imaging studies may be helpful in confirming BD, they neither replace nor substitute for clinical diagnosis**.

To date, cerebral angiography, transcranial Doppler (TCD), and cerebral scintigraphy are the only imaging studies to have been validated by the American Academy of Neurology (AAN) for the diagnosis of BD. However, characteristic findings on CT, CTP, CTA, MR, and MRA may suggest the diagnosis.

**CT Findings.** NECT scans in BD show diffuse, severe cerebral edema **(3-32)**. The lateral ventricles appear small. The superficial sulci, sylvian fissures, and basilar cisterns of both hemispheres are completely effaced **(3-14)**. The normal gray matter-white matter differentiation is absent. Sometimes, the cortex becomes iso- or even hypodense relative to adjacent white matter **(reversal sign)**. Severely edematous, abnormally low-density brain accentuates the prominence of the cerebral vessels and may mimic subarachnoid hemorrhage (SAH) **(3-33)**.

Density of the deep gray nuclei and brainstem may be initially maintained; however, all supratentorial structures eventually assume a featureless, uniform hypodensity **(3-33)**. Density of the cerebellum initially appears relatively normal, but it too eventually becomes severely edematous.

**MR Findings.** Sagittal T1WI shows complete descending central brain herniation with the optic chiasm and hypothalamus compressed against the skull base and the midbrain "buckled" inferiorly through the tentorial incisura **(3-15)**. The hemispheres appear swollen and hypointense with indistinct gray matter-white matter differentiation.

T2 scans show swollen gyri with hyperintense cortex. DWI in patients with BD typically shows restricted diffusion with decreased ADC in both the cerebral cortex and white matter **(3-34)**.

**Angiography.** Conventional digital subtraction angiography (DSA) shows severe, prolonged contrast stasis in the internal carotid artery. Although most BD patients show no intracranial flow, almost 30% have some proximal opacification of intracranial arteries. The deep venous drainage remains unopacified throughout the examination.

CT angiography (CTA) is emerging as an acceptable, noninvasive alternative to DSA in many jurisdictions. Demonstrating lack of opacification in the MCA cortical segments and internal veins in CTA is an efficient and reliable method for confirming BD **(3-35)**.

**Nuclear Medicine.** Tc-99m scintigraphy shows scalp uptake but absent brain activity (light bulb sign). With increased extracranial activity (hot nose sign), these findings are both highly sensitive and specific for BD **(3-36)**.

## Differential Diagnosis

Potentially reversible causes of BD, such as deep coma due to **drug overdose** or **status epilepticus**, must be excluded. **Technical difficulties** that may mimic BD include a "missed bolus" on either CTA or nuclear medicine flow studies.

**End-stage brain swelling** from any cause (e.g., prolonged cardiopulmonary arrest) makes the cranial arteries, dura, and dural venous sinuses all seem relatively hyperdense compared with the diffusely edematous low-density brain.

With very low-density brain, comparatively high-density areas are seen along the basal cisterns, sylvian fissures, tentorium cerebelli, and sometimes even within the cortical sulci. This appearance is sometimes termed **pseudo-SAH** and should not be mistaken for "real" SAH **(3-33)**. The density of pseudo-SAH is significantly lower (between 30-40 HU) than the attenuation of "real" SAH (between 50-60 HU).

## BRAIN DEATH

### Terminology and Definition

- BD: Irreversible cessation of brain function
- Legal definition(s) vary with country, jurisdictions

### Clinical Issues

- AAN 2010 checklist (BD in adults)
  - Coma (irreversible, known cause)
  - Neuroimaging explains coma
  - Neurologic examination, apnea testing performed

### Ancillary Testing

- Only 1 needs to be performed
- Only if
  - Clinical examination cannot be fully performed, **or**
  - Apnea testing inconclusive/aborted
- Options
  - Cerebral angiogram (many jurisdictions accept DSA)
  - HMPAO SPECT
  - EEG
  - TCD

### Imaging Findings

- DSA
  - Severe, prolonged contrast stasis in ICA
  - Most show no intracranial flow
  - 30% have some proximal opacification of intracranial arteries
- CTA, CTP
  - **No** opacification of cortical MCAs and internal cerebral veins on CTA
  - Stasis filling on CTP
- HMPAO SPECT
  - No intracranial opacification of flow studies
  - Scalp uptake but no brain activity (light bulb sign)
  - Extracranial uptake (hot nose sign)

### Differential Diagnosis

- Reversible causes of coma (clinical, laboratory)
  - Drug overdose
  - Status epilepticus
  - Severe hypoglycemia
- Technical issues
  - "Missed" contrast bolus
- Severe brain swelling (other causes)
  - "Malignant" MCA infarct
  - Metabolic (e.g., hyperammonemia)
  - Hypoxic-ischemic encephalopathy

*Selected References: The complete reference list is available on the eBooks+ version included with purchase.*

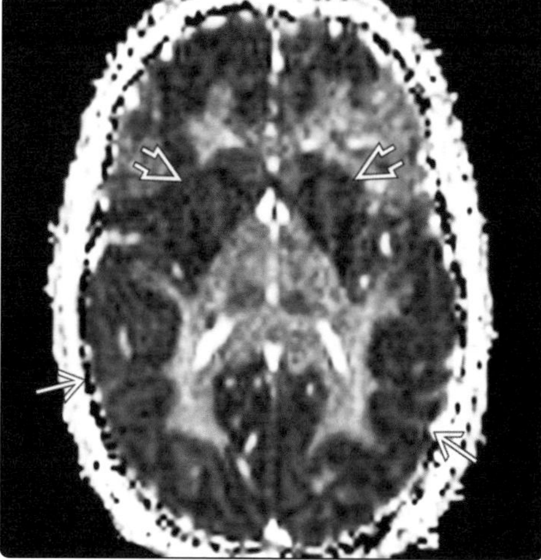

***(3-34)** ADC in documented brain death shows severely restricted diffusion in the cortex ➡ and basal ganglia ⇨.*

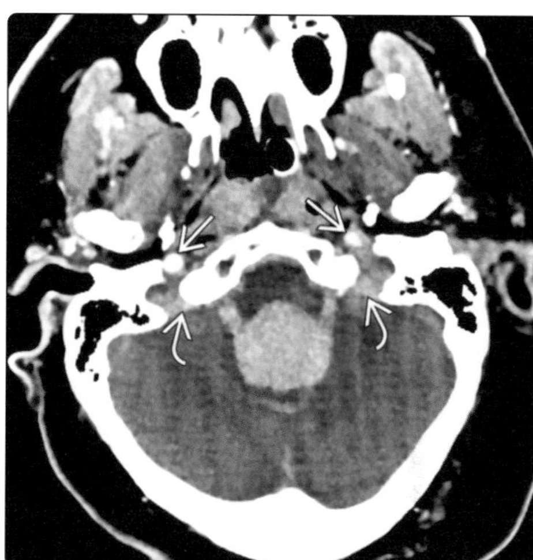

***(3-35)** CTA in brain death shows contrast in extracranial ICAs ➡ but none in the intracranial vertebral arteries or jugular veins ⇨.*

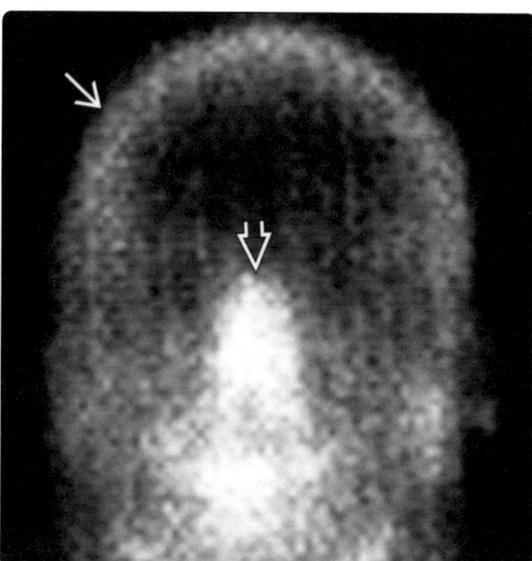

***(3-36)** Tc-99m Neurolite shows tracer accumulation in scalp ➡ (light bulb sign), nose ⇨ (hot nose sign), consistent with brain death.*

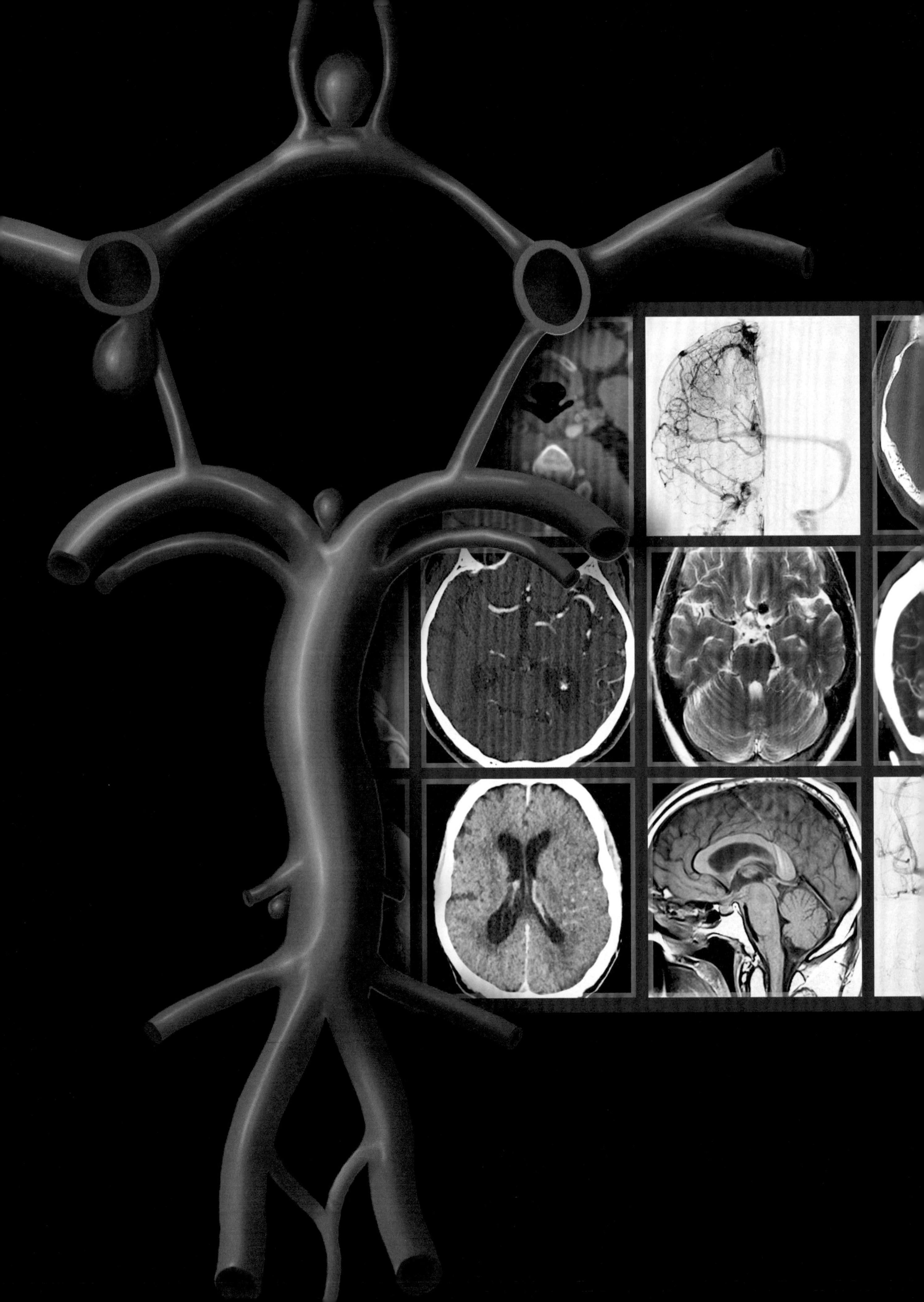

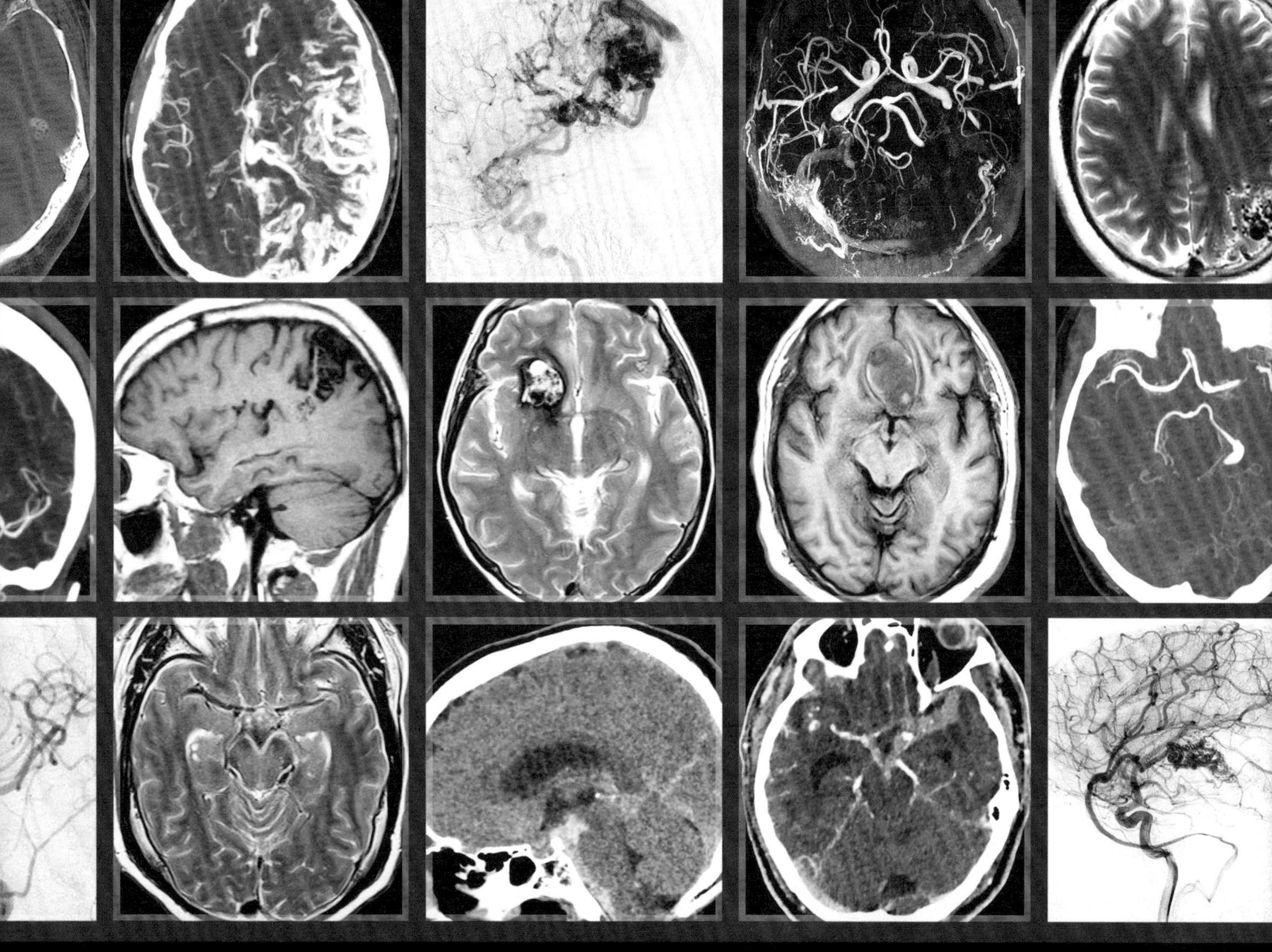

SECTION 2

# Nontraumatic Hemorrhage and Vascular Lesions

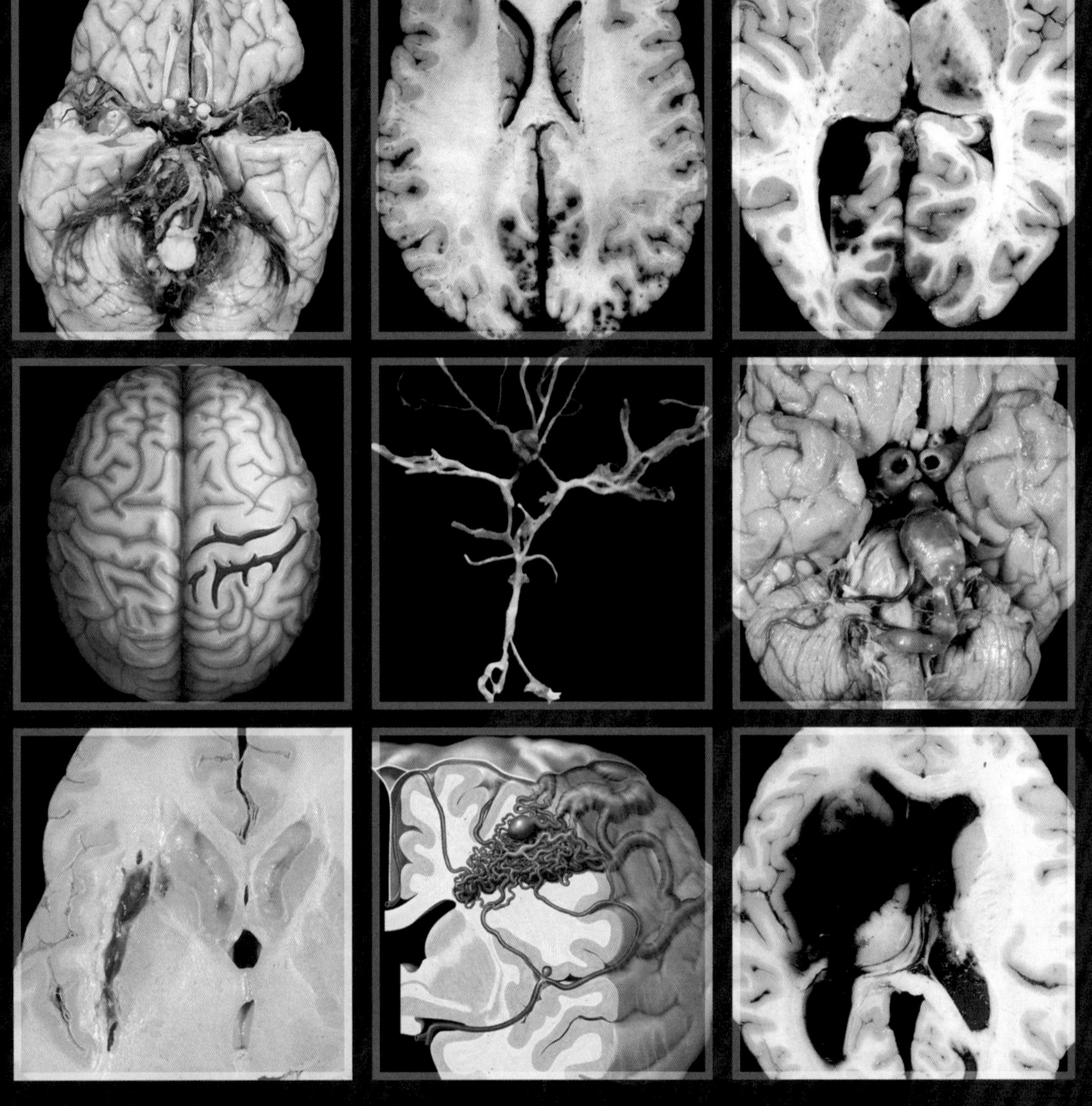

SECTION 2

# Nontraumatic Hemorrhage and Vascular Lesions

# Approach to Nontraumatic Hemorrhage and Vascular Lesions

*This part devoted to "spontaneous" (i.e., nontraumatic) hemorrhage and vascular lesions begins with a general discussion of brain bleeds. Subsequent chapters delineate a broad spectrum of vascular pathologies, ranging from aneurysms/subarachnoid hemorrhage and vascular malformations to cerebral vasculopathy and strokes. Where appropriate, anatomic considerations and the pathophysiology of specific disorders are included.*



Spontaneous (i.e., nontraumatic) intracranial hemorrhage (sICH) and vascular brain disorders are second only to trauma as neurologic causes of death and disability. Stroke or "brain attack"—defined as sudden onset of a neurologic event—is the third leading *overall* cause of death in industrialized countries. Imaging plays a crucial role in the management of stroke patients, both in establishing the diagnosis and stratifying patients for subsequent treatment.

We start this chapter with a brief overview of nontraumatic ICH and vascular diseases of the CNS, beginning with a short discussion of who, why, when, and how to image these patients. We then develop an anatomy-based approach to evaluating nontraumatic ICH. We close the discussion with a pathology-based introduction to the broad spectrum of congenital and acquired vascular lesions that affect the brain.

## Imaging Hemorrhage and Vascular Lesions

### Who, Why, and How to Image?

Because of its widespread availability and speed, an emergent NECT scan is generally the first-line imaging procedure of choice in patients with sudden onset of an unexplained neurologic deficit.

If the initial NECT scan is negative and no neurologic deficit is apparent, further imaging is often unnecessary. However, if the history and clinical findings suggest a thromboembolic stroke or transient ischemic attack (TIA), additional imaging is indicated, typically on an emergent basis.

Imaging studies are also frequently obtained in patients with headache of any kind, often with little or no initial evaluation. The first step in the evaluation of any headache patient should be a detailed clinical history and relevant clinical examinations. The American Academy of Neurology (AAN) and the American College of Radiology (ACR) do not recommend neuroimaging for patients with primary headache in the absence of so-called

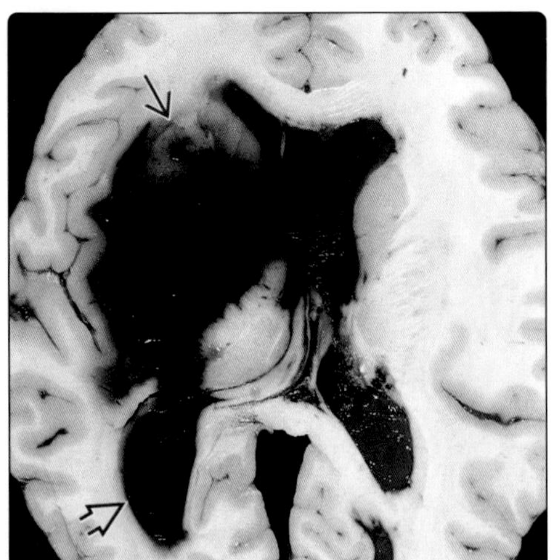

***(4-1)** Striatocapsular location is classic for hypertensive hemorrhage ⇨. Hematoma has ruptured into the lateral ventricle ⇨.*

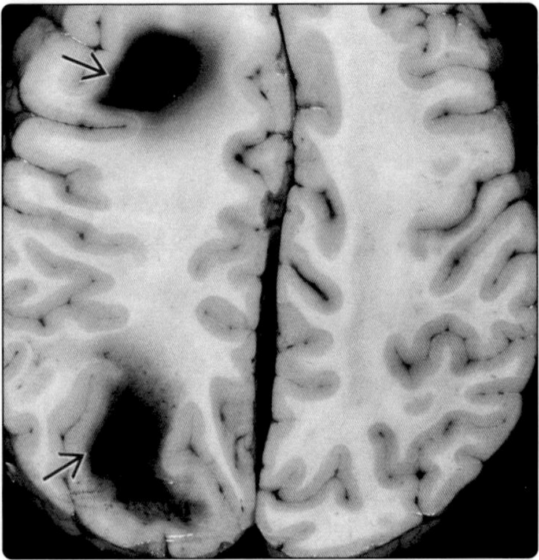

***(4-2)** Metastatic renal cell carcinoma shows 2 hemorrhagic lesions ⇨ at the gray matter-white matter interface, a typical location.*

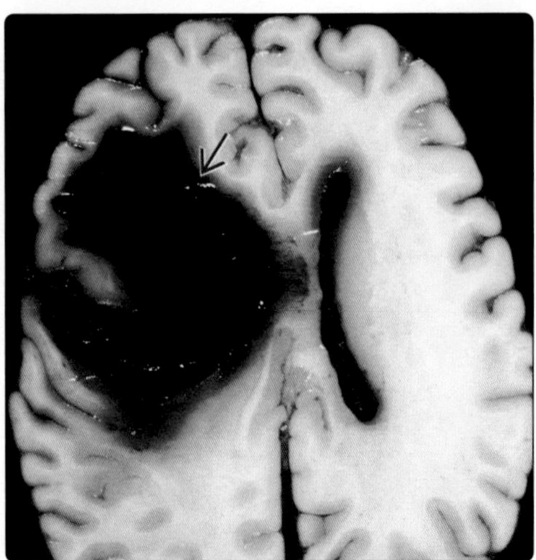

***(4-3)** Arteriovenous malformation (AVM) was the cause of this fatal intracranial hemorrhage (ICH) ⇨ in an adolescent patient.*

red flags [i.e., subacute head trauma, related activity (sexual activity, exertion, position), neurologic deficit, known or suspected cancer, immunosuppressed or immunocompromised state, pregnancy, age ≥ 50 years].

The ACR has established consensus Appropriateness Criteria for *initial* imaging in patients with different clinical types of headache, including those in which neuroimaging is mandatory. A variety of conditions are considered and given one of three appropriateness categories ("Usually Appropriate," "May Be Appropriate," and "Usually Not Appropriate"). These are briefly summarized in the following "ACR Appropriateness Criteria: Headache" table.

If ICH is identified, or if there is also a new neurologic deficit, further imaging should be considered using consensus studies, such as the ACR Appropriateness Criteria, summarized in the following table.

### ACR APPROPRIATENESS CRITERIA: HEADACHE

**Variant 1: Sudden Severe Headache ("Worst Headache of Life")**
- NECT usually appropriate
- CTA may be appropriate
- CECT, MR, MRA usually not appropriate

**Variant 2: New Headache With Optic Disc Edema**
- NECT, MR ± contrast usually appropriate
- CTV, MRV may be appropriate
- CECT, DSA usually not appropriate

**Variant 3: New/Worsening Headache With Clinical Red Flags**
- NECT, MR ± contrast usually appropriate
- CECT, MRA, DSA usually not appropriate

**Variant 4: New Headache (Classic Migraine/Tension-Type, Normal Neurologic Examination)**
- Imaging (CT, MR, etc.) usually not appropriate

**Variant 5: New Primary Headache, Suspected Trigeminal Autonomic Origin**
- MR ± contrast usually appropriate

**Variant 6: Chronic Headache, No New Features, No Neurologic Deficit**
- Imaging (CT, MR, etc.)

**Variant 7: Chronic Headache With New Features or Increasing Frequency**
- MR ± contrast usually appropriate
- CT ± contrast may be appropriate
- MRA, CTA, DSA usually not appropriate

## When and How to Image?

In sudden, severe headache, the negative predictive value of NECT performed with a modern scanner and obtained within the first six hours of symptoms is virtually 100% (sensitivity of 0.987 and specificity of 0.999).

Some of the most challenging questions arise when screening NECT discloses parenchymal hemorrhage. What are the potential causes? Should further emergent imaging be performed?

Spontaneous nontraumatic "brain bleeds" carry high mortality and morbidity **(4-1)**. The risk of rapid neurologic deterioration is high **(4-2)**. Rapid hematoma expansion and growth is common in the first few hours after onset **(4-3)**. High-quality, emergent imaging is crucial in further evaluating and managing these patients.

CTA is indicated in patients with sudden clinical deterioration *or* a mixed-density hematoma (indicating rapid bleeding or coagulopathy). A spot sign with active contrast extravasation caused by rupture of a lenticulostriate microaneurysm (Charcot-Bouchard aneurysm) can sometimes be identified. Contrast extravasation in sICH predicts hematoma expansion and poor clinical outcome.

CTA is also an appropriate next step in children and young/middle-aged adults with spontaneous (nontraumatic) ICH detected on screening NECT **(4-4)** **(4-5)**. In contrast to older adult patients—in whom hypertensive hemorrhage and amyloid angiopathy are the two most common etiologies of unexplained sICH—vascular malformation is the most common underlying etiology in younger age groups **(4-6)**.

Emergency MR is rarely necessary if CTA is negative. However, follow-up MR ± contrast enhancement can be very useful in patients with unexplained ICH. In addition to the standard sequences (i.e., T1WI, T2WI, FLAIR, DWI, and T1 C+), a T2* sequence—either (or both) GRE or susceptibility-weighted imaging (SWI)—should be obtained.

MR evidence for prior hemorrhage(s) and cerebral "microbleeds" can be very helpful in narrowing the differential diagnosis. Benign ICH typically follows an orderly, predictable evolution on MR scans. MR evidence of disordered or bizarre-looking hemorrhage should raise the possibility of neoplasm, underlying arteriovenous malformation (AVM), or coagulopathy.

If MR demonstrates multiple parenchymal hemorrhages of different ages, the underlying etiology varies with patient age. Multiple microbleeds in older adult patients are typically associated with chronic hypertension or amyloid angiopathy. Cavernous malformations or hematologic disorders **(4-16)** are the most common causes in children and young adults.

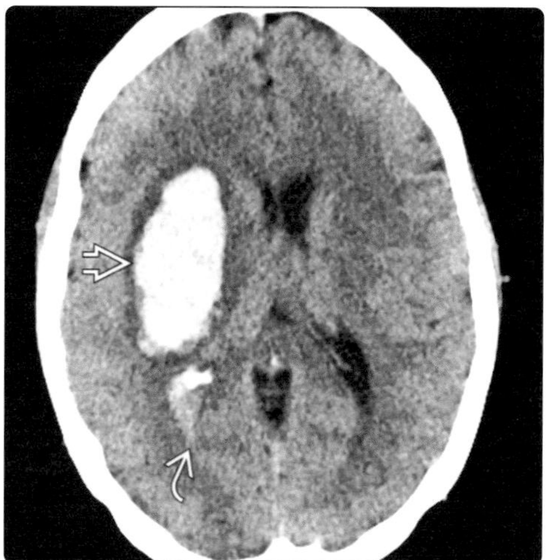

***(4-4)*** *NECT in a 60-yo hypertensive woman shows putamen-external capsule hemorrhage ➡. Note small amount of IVH ➡.*

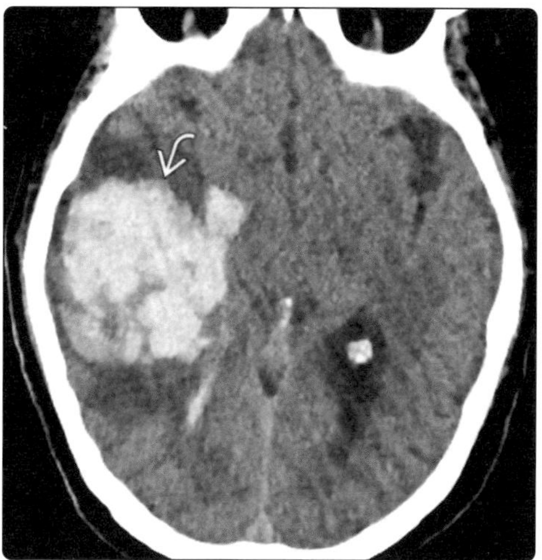

***(4-5)*** *NECT in 59-yo normotensive man shows a right temporal lobar hemorrhage ➡. CTA was negative. Surgery disclosed glioblastoma.*

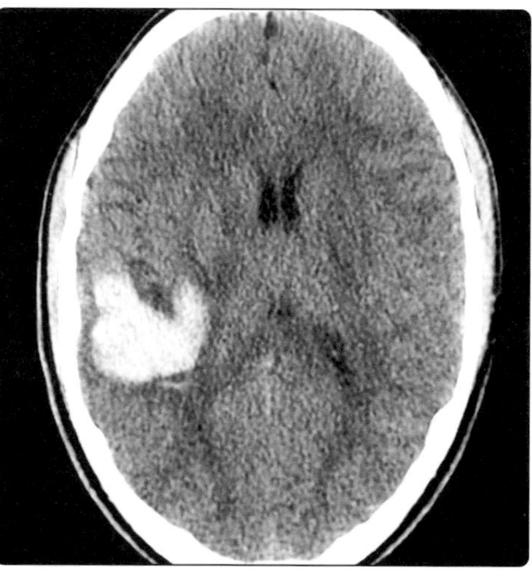

***(4-6)*** *NECT in a 15-yo with headache shows a right posterior temporal hematoma. DSA (not shown) disclosed a partially thrombosed AVM.*

# Approach to Nontraumatic Hemorrhage

Hematoma location, age, and number (solitary or multiple) should be noted.

The differential diagnosis of nontraumatic sICH varies widely with anatomic location and patient age. Because the brain itself is the most common site, we begin our discussion with intraaxial hematomas, then turn our attention to extraaxial bleeds.

## Intraaxial Hemorrhage

### Clinical Issues

Parenchymal hemorrhage is the most devastating type of stroke. Although recent advances have improved the treatment of ischemic strokes, few evidence-based treatments exist for ICH. Strategies are largely supportive, aimed at limiting further injury and preventing associated complications, such as hematoma expansion, elevated intracranial pressure, and intraventricular rupture with hydrocephalus.

### Imaging

Parenchymal hematomas are easily recognized on NECT scans by their hyperdensity or, in the case of rapid bleeding or coagulopathy, mixed iso-/hyperdense appearance. Expansion of a parenchymal hematoma into the ventricular system is commonly encountered on initial imaging in patients with sICH and associated with poor long-term outcome.

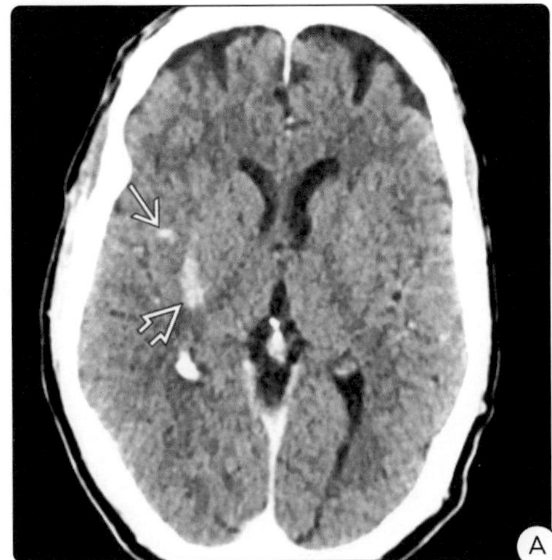

*(4-7A) 80-kV NECT performed immediately after thrombectomy shows 2 hyperdense foci ➡ ➡. Hemorrhage vs. contrast extravasation.*

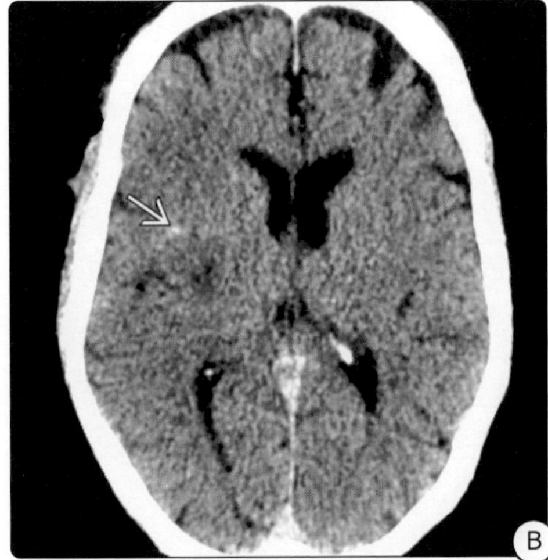

*(4-7B) Virtual noncontrast (VNC) image from dual-energy CT shows small focus ➡ is mostly blood; the larger (no longer visible) was contrast.*

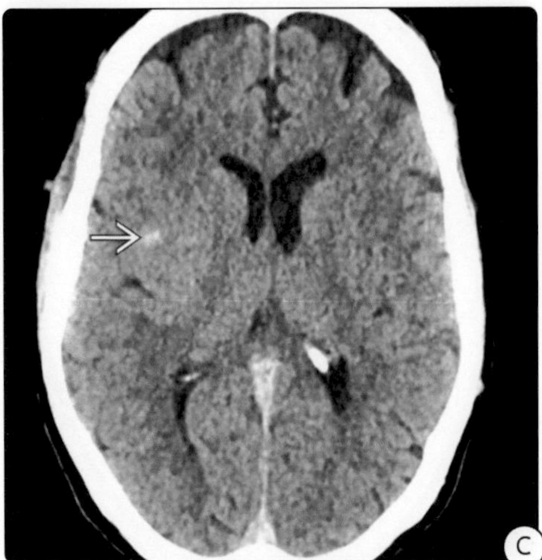

*(4-7C) Follow-up standard single-energy NECT 7 h later confirms small hyperdense focus on VNC ➡ was hemorrhage. Contrast has washed out.*

Hematomas typically expand the brain, displacing the cortex outward and producing mass effect on underlying structures, such as the cerebral ventricles. The sulci are often compressed, and the overlying gyri appear expanded and flattened. The surrounding brain may appear grossly edematous.

When immediate follow-up imaging after thrombolysis for acute stroke is obtained, it is important to differentiate parenchymal hemorrhage from contrast extravasation. Both are hyperdense on NECT on standard sequences. Dual-energy CT (DECT) acquires two datasets with different x-ray energy levels from the same anatomic region. Blended images are generated through a combination of the acquired low-energy (80-kilovoltage peak [kVp]) and high-energy (150-kVp) datasets to simulate a standard 120-kVp dataset. Virtual nonenhanced images can be generated using this dual-energy technique and may help differentiate contrast staining from true ICH **(4-7)**.

MR is often used to further evaluate unexplained nontraumatic ("spontaneous") parenchymal bleeds. Hematoma signal intensity on standard sequences varies with clot age and imaging sequence. T2* (GRE, SWI) scans are especially important in evaluating patients with brain hemorrhage. SWI is particularly useful in identifying the presence and location of cerebral microbleeds.

## Differential Diagnosis

The differential diagnosis of sICH varies widely with both anatomic location and patient age.

If a classic **striatocapsular** or **thalamic** hematoma is found in a *middle-aged or older adult patient*, hypertensive hemorrhage is, by far, the most common etiology **(4-1)** **(4-4)**. Drug abuse should be suspected in a *young adult* with a similar-appearing lesion. Ruptured aneurysms rarely cause lateral basal ganglionic hemorrhage, and neoplasms with hemorrhagic necrosis are far less common than hypertensive bleeds in this location.

**Lobar** hemorrhages present a different challenge, as the differential diagnosis is much broader. In older patients, amyloid angiopathy, hypertension, and underlying neoplasm (primary or metastatic) are the most common causes **(4-2)** **(4-5)**. Vascular malformations, especially AVMs **(4-3)** **(4-6)**, are more common in *children or young adults*. Chronic vascular diseases, especially moyamoya angiopathy and sickle cell disease-associated angiopathy, are rare but important causes of ICH in children, while neoplasm-associated hemorrhage is rare.

Dural sinus &/or cortical vein thrombosis are uncommon but occur in patients of all ages and should not be overlooked.

Hemorrhages at the **gray matter-white matter interface** are typical of metastases **(4-2)**, septic emboli, and fungal infection.

Multifocal hemorrhages confined to the white matter are rare **(4-10)**. **"Critical illness-associated" brain microbleeds** occur in intubated patients with acute respiratory distress syndrome (ARDS), especially those who are on extracorporeal membrane oxygenation (ECMO). These may be hypoxia related, similar to the microbleeds seen in high-altitude cerebral edema.

When microbleeds are identified in a patient with SARS-CoV-2 or a history of a febrile illness followed by sudden neurologic deterioration, they are most likely secondary to a hemorrhagic form of acute disseminated encephalomyelitis called acute hemorrhagic leukoencephalopathy **(AHLE, a.k.a. Weston-Hurst disease)**.

Clot age can likewise be helpful in suggesting the etiology of an ICH. A hemosiderin-laden encephalomalacic cavity in the basal ganglia or thalamus of an older patient is typically due to an old hypertensive hemorrhage. Cortical/subcortical microbleeds can be seen in cerebral amyloid angiopathy, particularly if siderosis is present.

Spontaneous (i.e., nontraumatic) primary intraventricular hemorrhage is rare. The most common causes are hypertension and occult vascular malformation in/around the ventricular wall.

**"UNEXPLAINED" (NONTRAUMATIC) PARENCHYMAL BRAIN BLEEDS**

**Key Clinical Information**
- Patient age, sex
- History (i.e., hypertension)
- Medications

**Initial Imaging Survey**
- NECT ± CTA
- Consider MR ± contrast if ≤ 55 years old

**Key Imaging Features for Report**
- Size
- Location
- Hematoma density (uniform vs. heterogeneous)
- Extent of edema, mass effect
- Hydrocephalus, intraventricular blood present?
- Spot sign on CTA?

**Age and Differential Diagnosis**
- Child/young adult (< 45 years old)
  - Vascular malformation
  - Drug abuse
  - Vasculitis/vasculopathy (Moyamoya, sickle cell)
  - Venous occlusion/infarct
- Middle aged, older adults
  - Hypertension (40-60%)
  - Amyloid angiopathy (2nd most common; 50% of sICH patients > 70 years old)
  - Primary neoplasm (up to 15% of primary tumors have associated hemorrhage; glioblastoma multiforme most common)
  - Metastasis
  - Venous occlusion/infarct
  - Vasculitis (including tumefactive)
  - Coagulopathy
  - Vascular malformation
  - Hemorrhagic transformation of ischemic infarct
  - Remote cerebellar hemorrhage (following craniotomy)

## Extraaxial Hemorrhage

Spontaneous extraaxial hemorrhages can occur in any of the three major anatomic compartments, i.e., the epidural space, subdural space, and the subarachnoid space. By far, the most common are subarachnoid hemorrhages (SAHs) **(4-8)** **(4-11)**. In contrast to traumatic hemorrhages, spontaneous bleeding into the epi- and subdural spaces is rare.

### Subarachnoid Hemorrhage

**Clinical Issues.** Patients with nontraumatic SAH (ntSAH) usually present with sudden onset of severe headache ("worst headache of my life"). A "thunderclap" headache is very common.

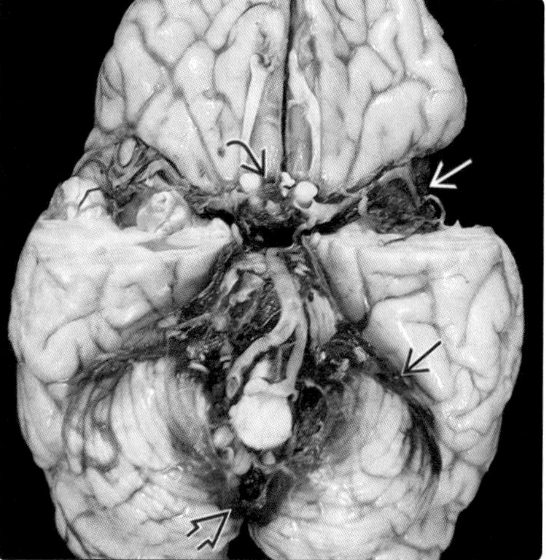

***(4-8)** In this acute SAH, blood fills sylvian fissures ➡, suprasellar cistern ⮕, and cisterna magna ⮕ and extends into the CPA cisterns ⮕.*

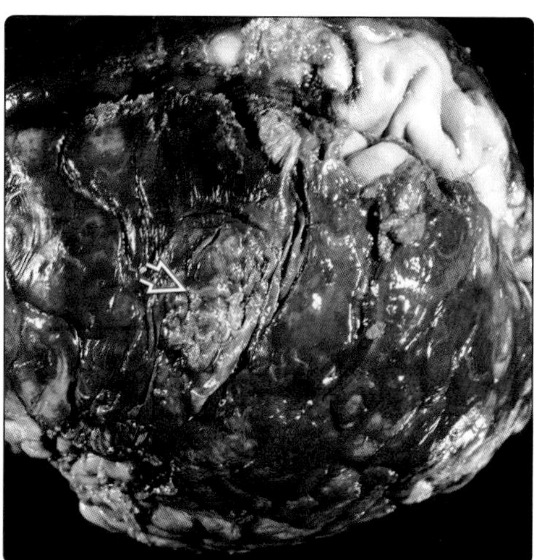

***(4-9)** Autopsy case shows an AVM ➡ causing massive ICH. (Courtesy R. Hewlett, MD.)*

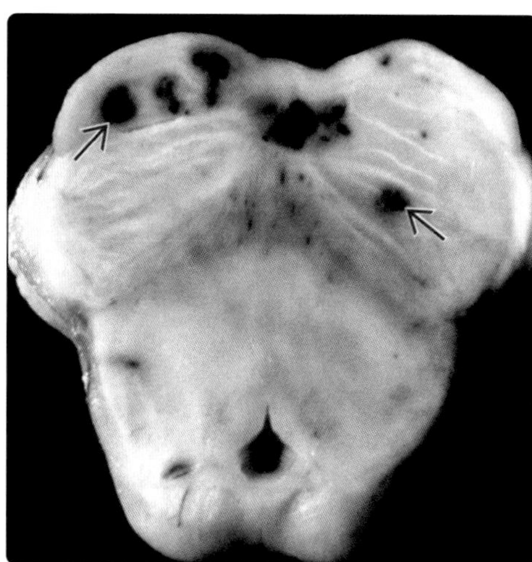

***(4-10)** Pathology shows hemorrhages ⮕ in upper pons from capillary telangiectasias. T2* SWI is most sensitive for microbleeds.*

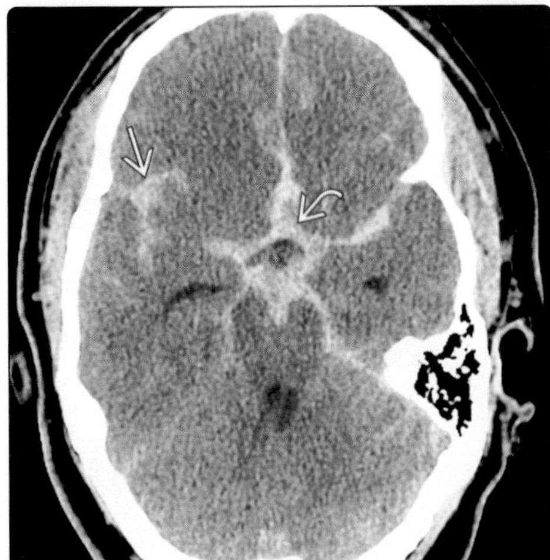

*(4-11) NECT shows a patient with aneurysmal SAH. Diffuse hemorrhage fills the suprasellar cistern ➡ and sylvian fissures ➡.*

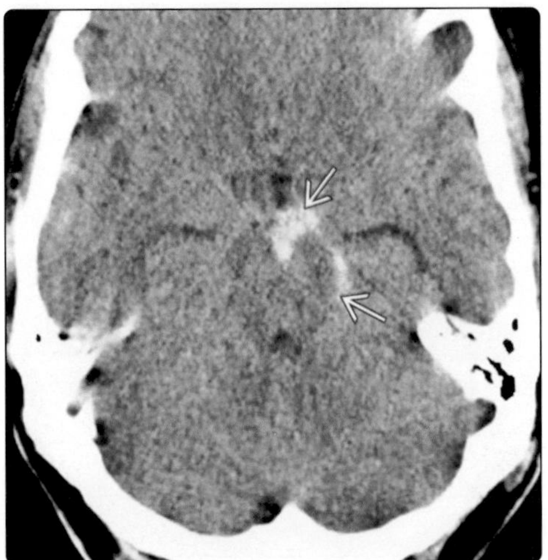

*(4-12) NECT shows classic perimesencephalic nonaneurysmal SAH ➡ with subarachnoid blood localized around the midbrain. CTA was negative.*

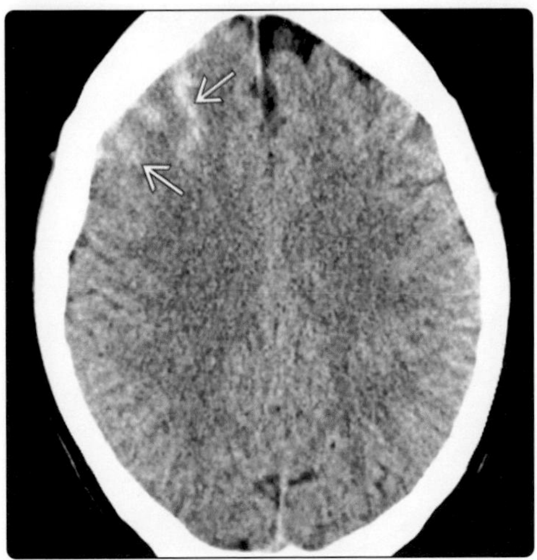

*(4-13) NECT shows focal subarachnoid blood in convexity sulci ➡. Basal cisterns were normal. Reversible cerebral vasoconstriction syndrome.*

**Imaging.** ntSAH is easily distinguished from a parenchymal hematoma by its location and configuration. Blood in the subarachnoid spaces has a feathery, curvilinear, or serpentine appearance as it fills the cisterns and surface sulci **(4-13)**. It follows brain surfaces and rarely causes a focal mass effect.

SAH is hyperdense on NECT scans. Bloody sulcal-cisternal CSF appears dirty on T1WI, hyperintense on FLAIR, and "blooms" on T2* sequences.

**Differential Diagnosis.** As with parenchymal bleeds, ntSAH sublocation is helpful in establishing an appropriate differential diagnosis. By far, the most common cause of ntSAH is **aneurysmal SAH** (aSAH). As most intracranial aneurysms arise from the circle of Willis and the middle cerebral bifurcation, aSAH tends to spread throughout the basal cisterns and extend into the sylvian fissures **(4-11)**.

Two special, easily recognizable subtypes of SAH are *not* associated with ruptured intracranial aneurysm. Blood localized to the subarachnoid spaces around the midbrain and anterior to the pons is called **perimesencephalic nonaneurysmal SAH** (pnSAH) **(4-12)**. This type of SAH is self-limited, rarely results in vasospasm, and is probably secondary to venous hemorrhage. CTA is a reliable technique to rule out a basilar tip aneurysm. DSA and noninvasive follow-up imaging have had no demonstrable increased diagnostic yield in such cases.

Blood in one or more sulci over the upper cerebral hemispheres is called **convexal SAH (4-13)**. This special subtype of SAH is associated with a number of diverse etiologies, including cortical vein thrombosis (all ages) and amyloid angiopathy in older patients, as well as reversible cerebral vasoconstriction syndrome in younger and middle-aged individuals.

Despite extensive imaging evaluation, the origin of spontaneous ntSAH remains unidentified in 10-20% of patients. Hydrocephalus and delayed cerebral ischemia in these patients are infrequent, and long-term neurologic outcomes are generally good.

## Epidural Hemorrhage

The pathogenesis of extradural hematomas is almost always traumatic and arises from lacerated meningeal arteries, fractures, or torn dural venous sinuses.

Most spontaneous epidural bleeds are found in the spinal—not the cranial—epidural space and are an emergent condition that may result in paraplegia, quadriplegia, and even death. Older adult anticoagulated patients are most at risk.

Intracranial spontaneous epidural hemorrhages are very rare. Most reported cases are associated with bleeding disorders, craniofacial infection (usually mastoiditis or sphenoid sinusitis), dural sinus thrombosis, bone infarction (e.g., in patients with sickle cell disease), or a vascular lesion of the calvarium (e.g., hemangioma, metastasis, or intradiploic epidermoid cyst).

## Subdural Hemorrhage

Trauma also causes the vast majority of subdural hematomas (SDHs). Nontraumatic SDHs represent < 5% of all cases and are more common in older adult &/or anticoagulated patients.

Many nontraumatic SDHs occur with CSF volume depletion and are strongly associated with intracranial hypotension. CSF hypovolemia can become life threatening if sufficiently severe.

Intracranial hypotension can be traumatic, iatrogenic, or spontaneous (see Chapter 34). Most cases of traumatic intracranial hypotension are secondary to CSF leak associated with spinal or dural injury. Iatrogenic intracranial hypotension occurs with dural tear following lumbar puncture, myelography, spinal anesthesia, or cranial surgery. Regardless of etiology, SDH is a common (but not invariable) association.

Nontraumatic SDHs have been reported in association with a number of other conditions, including hyponatremic dehydration, inherited or acquired coagulation disorders, dural venous sinus thrombosis, and meningitis.

A few cases of spontaneous SDH occur directly adjacent to a lobar peripheral hemorrhage and are associated with an underlying vasculopathy (such as cerebral amyloid disease with pseudoaneurysm formation) or vascular malformation. Others occur without an identifiable antecedent or predisposing condition.

Occasionally, a ruptured cortical artery or saccular aneurysm may result in a nontraumatic intracranial SDH. Dural hemangiomas have also been reported as causes of acute nontraumatic SDH. Older adult patients with intrinsic or iatrogenic coagulopathy can present with an SDH and either minor or no definite evidence for head trauma.

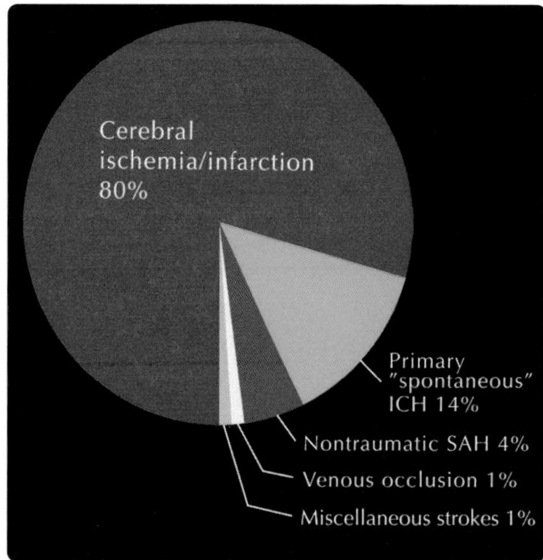


***(4-14)*** *Cerebral ischemia/infarction represents a vast majority of strokes. The 2nd most common is primary ICH followed by nontraumatic SAH.*

# Approach to Vascular Disorders of CNS

Here, we discuss a general approach to vascular disorders in the brain, briefly introducing the major chapters in this part. Details regarding pathoetiology, clinical features, imaging findings, and differential diagnosis are delineated in each individual chapter.

## Subarachnoid Hemorrhage and Aneurysms

Trauma is—by far—the most common cause of SAH. Traumatic SAH (tSAH) is found in 100% of patients with fatal severe head injuries and is common in those with moderate to severe nonfatal closed head trauma.

Chapter 6 focuses on *nontraumatic* "spontaneous" SAH, which causes 3-5% of all acute strokes. Of these, nearly 80% are caused by rupture of a saccular aneurysm. aSAH can generally be distinguished from nonaneurysmal SAH by its distribution on NECT scans.

Classic saccular ("berry") aneurysms as well as the less common dissecting aneurysms, pseudoaneurysms, fusiform aneurysms, and blood blister-like aneurysms, are discussed in this chapter.

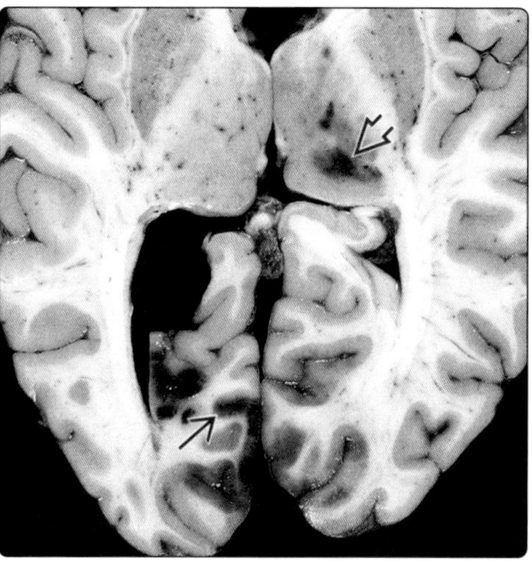

***(4-15)*** *Autopsy shows subacute cerebral infarct, hemorrhagic transformation in occipital cortex ⇒, and contralateral thalamus ⇒.*

## Vascular Malformations

Cerebrovascular malformations (CVMs) are a fascinating, remarkably heterogeneous group of disorders with unique pathophysiology and imaging features. Chapter 7 discusses the four major types of vascular malformations, grouping them according to whether they shunt blood directly from the arterial to the venous side of the circulation without passing through a capillary bed.

CVMs that display arteriovenous (AV) shunting include AVMs **(4-9)** and fistulas. Included in this discussion is the newly described entity called cerebral proliferative angiopathy. Cerebral proliferative angiopathy can mimic AVM on imaging studies but has unique features that may influence treatment decisions.

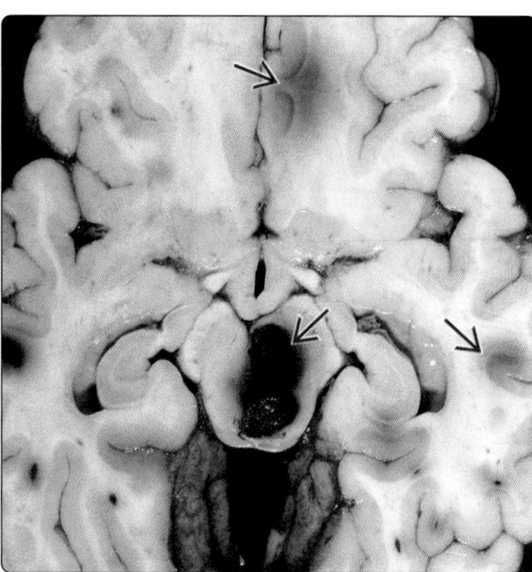

***(4-16)*** *Autopsy case is from a child with multifocal parenchymal hemorrhages ⇒ caused by leukemia.*

With few exceptions, most CVMs that lack AV shunting, i.e., developmental venous anomalies (venous "angiomas") along with cavernous malformations and capillary telangiectasias, rarely hemorrhage and are "leave me alone" lesions that are identified on imaging studies but generally do not require treatment.

Lastly, note that the topic of "occult" vascular malformation is not discussed. This is an outdated concept that originated in an era when angiography was the only available technique to diagnose brain vascular malformations prior to surgical exploration. Some vascular malformations, such as cavernous angiomas and capillary telangiectasias **(4-10)**, are invisible (and therefore "occult") at angiography but are easily identified on MR.

## Arterial Anatomy and Strokes

Chapter 8 begins with a discussion of normal intracranial arterial anatomy and vascular distributions, an essential foundation for understanding the imaging appearance of cerebral ischemia/infarction.

The major focus of the chapter is thromboembolic infarcts in major arterial territories, as they are, by far, the most common cause of acute strokes **(4-14)** **(4-15)**. The pros and cons of the increasing use of commercially available artificial intelligence software in acute stroke diagnosis are considered. The pathology and imaging of subacute and chronic infarcts are briefly discussed. Although typically not amenable to intravascular treatment, they are nevertheless seen on imaging studies and should be recognized as residua from a prior infarct.

The discussion of embolic infarcts includes cardiac and atheromatous emboli as well as lacunar infarcts and the distinct syndrome of fat emboli. The importance of recognizing calcified cerebral emboli on NECT scans is emphasized, as the risk of repeated stroke in these patients is very high.

The pathophysiology and imaging of watershed ("border zone") infarcts and global hypoxic-ischemic brain injury are also included. Miscellaneous strokes, such as cerebral hyperperfusion syndrome, are discussed.

The chapter concludes by illustrating strokes in unusual vascular distributions, including artery of Percheron and "top of the basilar" infarcts.

## Venous Anatomy and Occlusions

The venous side of the cerebral circulation is, quite literally, "terra incognita" (an unknown land) to many physicians who deal with brain disorders. Although many could sketch the major arterial territories with relative ease, few could diagram the intracranial venous drainage territories.

The brain veins and sinuses are unlike those of the body. Systemic veins typically travel parallel to arteries and mirror their vascular territories; not so in the brain. Systemic veins have valves, and flow is generally in one direction.

The cerebral veins and dural sinuses lack valves and may thus exhibit bidirectional flow. Systemic veins have numerous collateral pathways that can develop in the case of occlusion. Few such collaterals exist inside the calvarium.

Chapter 9 begins with a brief discussion of normal venous anatomy and drainage patterns before we consider the various manifestations of venous occlusion. Venous thrombosis causes just 1% of all strokes, and its clinical presentation is much less distinctive than that of major arterial occlusion. It is perhaps the type of stroke most frequently missed on imaging studies. Venous stroke can also mimic other diseases (e.g., neoplasm), and, in turn, a number of disorders can mimic venous thrombosis.

## Vasculopathy

Chapter 10, the final chapter in this part, is devoted to cerebral vasculopathy. This chapter begins with a review of normal extracranial arterial anatomy with special focus on the carotid arteries and their variants.

The bulk of the chapter is devoted to cerebral vasculopathy and is organized into two parts: Atherosclerosis and nonatherosclerotic disease. The concept of the "vulnerable" or "at-risk" atherosclerotic plaque is underscored. Indeed, although measuring the percentage of internal carotid artery stenosis has been emphasized since the 1990s as a major predictor of stroke risk and the basis for treatment-related decisions, identifying a rupture-prone plaque is at least as important as determining stenosis.

The relatively new but extremely important topic of high-resolution vessel wall imaging is introduced, and its role in distinguishing between different types of vasculopathy is emphasized.

The much-neglected but important topic of *intracranial* atherosclerosis is also discussed. Whereas major vessel and cardiac thromboemboli cause most arterial strokes, between 5-10% can be attributed to intracranial stenoocclusive disease. The topic of arteriolosclerosis (i.e., small vessel vascular disease) is also considered here and again in the subsequent section on metabolic disease.

Nonatheromatous diseases of the cerebral vasculature are much less common than atherosclerosis and its sequelae. However, a number of vasculopathies can have serious consequences and should be recognized on imaging studies. This heterogeneous group of disorders includes fibromuscular dysplasia, dissection, vasospasm, the unusual but important cerebral vasoconstriction syndromes, and the often-confusing topic of vasculitis.

The vasculopathy chapter concludes with the intriguing topic of nonatheromatous microvascular diseases, such as systemic lupus erythematosus, antiphospholipid syndrome, and amyloid angiopathy.

*Selected References: The complete reference list is available on the eBooks+ version included with purchase.*

# Spontaneous Parenchymal Hemorrhage

*Intracranial hemorrhage is not a single entity but results from a range of vascular pathologies that differ in implications for prognosis and treatment. In the absence of trauma, abrupt onset of focal neurologic symptoms is presumed to be vascular in origin until proven otherwise. Rapid neuroimaging to distinguish ischemic stroke from intracranial hemorrhage is crucial to patient management.*



## Primary (Spontaneous) Intracranial Hemorrhage

### Epidemiology

Cerebral ischemia/infarction is responsible for almost 80% of all "strokes." Spontaneous (nontraumatic) primary intracranial hemorrhage (pICH) causes 10-15% of first-time strokes and is a devastating subtype with unusually high mortality and morbidity. Death or dependent state is the outcome in > 70% of all patients.

### Clinical Considerations

The American Heart Association (AHA) is emphasizing the use of a baseline severity score as part of evaluating and managing patients with pICH. A widely used system is the intracerebral hemorrhage (ICH) score that combines Glasgow Coma Scale (GCS), patient age (≥ 80 years), ICH volume ≥ 30 mL, presence or absence of intraventricular hemorrhage, and whether the hemorrhage is infratentorial or supratentorial.

Early deterioration with spontaneous ICH (sICH) is common. More than 20% of patients experience a decrease in a GCS score of two or more points between initial assessment by paramedics and presentation in the ED.

Active bleeding with hematoma expansion (HE) occurs in 25-40% of patients and is common in the first 1-2 hours. Patients with large hematomas, history of anticoagulation, or hypertension (HTN) are at particular risk for HE, which may occur several hours after symptom onset. HE is predictive of clinical deterioration and carries significantly increased morbidity and mortality. Therefore, swift diagnosis is needed to direct treatment.

The prognosis is grave, even with prompt intervention. 20-30% of all patients die within 48 hours after the initial hemorrhage. The one-year mortality rate approaches 60%. Only 20% of patients who survive regain functional independence and recover without significant residual neurologic deficits.

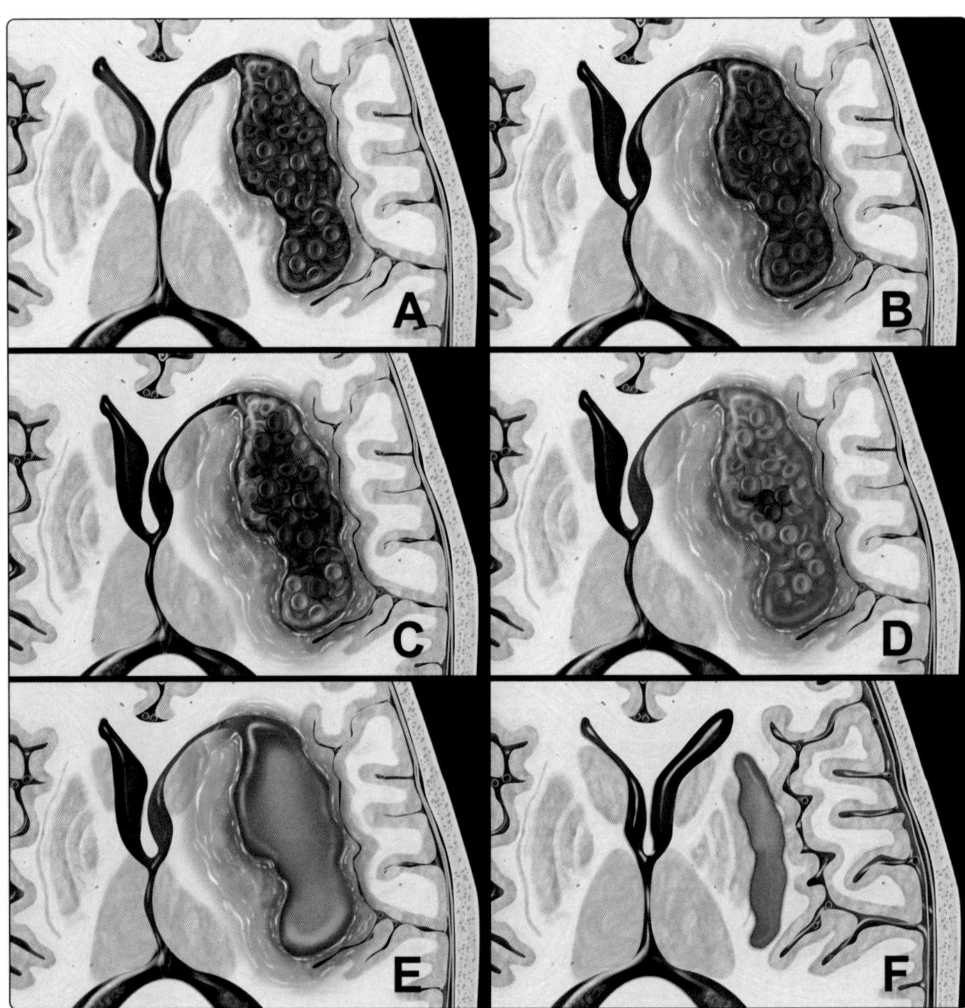


***(5-1)** Brain parenchymal hematomas have a fairly wide range of appearance, depending on age of the clot, size of the hematoma, and oxygen tension in the environment. (A) Hyperacute hemorrhage is defined as < 24 hours old. It consists of a water-rich clot that is 95-98% intracellular oxygenated hemoglobin (oxy-Hgb) (indicated by the intact RBCs colored red). (B) Acute clots are between 1-3 days old. Here, the hematoma consists mostly of RBCs (blue) containing intracellular deoxy-Hgb with the conversion first appearing in the intensely hypoxic clot center. Early subacute clots between 3 (C) and 7 (D) days contain mostly RBCs with intracellular met-Hgb (yellow). (E) Late subacute clots (between 1-2 weeks) consist primarily of lysed RBCs with a liquid pool of extracellular met-Hgb. The mostly liquidized clot gradually shrinks with time until only a thin, slit-like, yellowish residual fluid collection of extracellular met-Hgb surrounded by a hemosiderin rim remains (F).*

## Imaging Recommendations

The 2022 AHA/American Stroke Association (ASA) guidelines recommend emergent CT as the initial screening procedure to distinguish ICH from acute ischemic stroke (AIS), as the prognosis and management are strikingly different. The vast majority of strokes in high-income countries (~ 90%) are of ischemic origin (see Chapter 8).

If a parenchymal hematoma is identified on NECT, determining its size and etiology becomes critically important in patient triage. AI programs, such as RAPID ICH (SchemaView), can identify and quantitate hematomas on NECT studies. CTA is easily obtained at the time of initial imaging and is now included in many institutions as an integral part of acute stroke protocols. If contrast or extravasation within the clot (spot sign) is present, these patients are at risk of HE.

The management of unexplained brain bleeds also varies with patient age. If the patient is older than 45 years and has preexisting systemic HTN, a putaminal, thalamic, or posterior fossa ICH is almost always hypertensive in origin. Vascular imaging may or may not be requested.

In contrast, lobar or deep brain bleeds in younger patients or normotensive adults—regardless of age—almost always require further investigation. Contrast-enhanced CT/MR with angiography &/or venography may be helpful in detecting underlying abnormalities, such as arteriovenous malformation, neoplasm, and cerebral sinovenous thrombosis.

In older patients with pICH, MR with T2* (GRE, SWI) is also helpful in detecting the presence of "surrogate markers" of small vessel disease, such as brain microbleeds, white matter hyperintensities, and lacunar infarcts.

# Evolution of Intracranial Hemorrhage

## Overview

We begin with a discussion of the pathophysiology of ICH. This provides the basis for considering how pICH looks on imaging studies and why its appearance changes over time. We then consider some major causes of sICH, such as HTN and amyloid angiopathy.

Solitary lesions comprise the vast majority of pICHs. The presence of more than one simultaneous *macroscopic* brain bleed is actually quite uncommon, accounting for just 2-3% of all pICHs. Multifocal brain *microbleeds* are much more common. We therefore conclude this chapter with a discussion of multifocal brain microbleeds, their etiology, pathology, imaging appearance, and differential diagnosis.

## Pathophysiology of Intracranial Hemorrhage

### Clot Formation

Clot formation is a complex physiologic event that involves both cellular (mainly platelet) and soluble protein components. Platelets are activated by vascular injury and aggregate at the injured site. Soluble proteins are activated by both intrinsic and extrinsic arms that merge into a common coagulation pathway, resulting in a fibrin clot.

### Hemoglobin Degradation

Hemoglobin (Hgb) is composed of four protein (globin) subunits. Each subunit contains a heme molecule with an iron atom surrounded by a porphyrin ring.

Hgb within RBCs that are extravasating into a pICH rapidly desaturates. Fully oxygenated Hgb (oxy-Hgb) contains nonparamagnetic ferrous iron. In a hematoma, oxy-Hgb is initially converted to deoxyhemoglobin (deoxy-Hgb).

With time, deoxy-Hgb is metabolized to methemoglobin (met-Hgb), which contains ferric iron. As RBCs lyse, met-Hgb is released and eventually degraded and resorbed. Macrophages convert the ferric iron into hemosiderin and ferritin.

Ferritin is the major source of nonheme iron deposition in the human brain. Although iron is essential for normal brain function, iron overload may have devastating effects. Lipid peroxidation and free radical formation promote oxidative brain injury after ICH that may continue for weeks or months.

### Stages of Intraparenchymal Hemorrhage

Five general stages in temporal evolution of hematomas are recognized: Hyperacute, acute, early subacute, late subacute, and chronic. Each has its own features that depend on three key factors: (1) Clot structure, (2) RBC integrity, and (3) Hgb oxygenation status. In turn, imaging findings depend on hematoma stage **(5-1)**.

Hematomas consist of two distinct regions: A central core and a peripheral rim or boundary. In general, Hgb degradation begins in the clot periphery and progresses centrally toward the core.

**Hyperacute Hemorrhage.** Hyperacute hemorrhage is minutes (or even seconds) to under 24 hours old. Most imaged hyperacute hemorrhages are generally between 4-6, but < 24, hours old. Initially, a loose fibrin clot that contains plasma, platelets, and intact RBCs is formed. At this stage, diamagnetic intracellular oxyhemoglobin predominates in the hematoma.

In early clots, intact erythrocytes interdigitate with surrounding brain at the hematoma-tissue interface. Edema forms around the hematoma within hours after onset and is associated with mass effect, elevated intracranial pressure, and secondary brain injury.

**Acute Hemorrhage.** Acute ICH is defined as between 1-3 days old. Profound hypoxia within the center of the clot induces the transformation of oxy-Hgb to deoxy-Hgb. Iron in deoxy-Hgb is paramagnetic because it has four unpaired electrons.

Deoxy-Hgb is paramagnetic, but, as long as it remains within intact RBCs, it is shielded from direct dipole-dipole interactions with water protons in the extracellular plasma. At this stage, magnetic susceptibility is induced primarily because of differences between the microenvironments inside and outside of the RBCs.

**Early Subacute Hemorrhage.** Early subacute hemorrhage is defined as a clot that is from three days to one week old. Hgb remains contained within intact RBCs. Hgb at the hypoxic center of the clot persists as deoxy-Hgb. The periphery of the clot ages more rapidly and therefore contains intracellular

### Imaging Intraparenchymal Hemorrhage Stages

| Stage | Time (Range) | Blood Products | CT | T1 | T2 | T2* | DWI | ADC |
|---|---|---|---|---|---|---|---|---|
| Hyperacute | < 24 hours | Oxy-Hgb | Hyperdense | Isointense | Bright | Rim "blooms" | Bright | Dark |
| Acute | 1-3 days | Deoxy-Hgb | Hyperdense | Isointense | Dark | ↑ "blooming" | Dark | Dark |
| Early subacute | > 3 days to 1 week | Intracellular met-Hgb | Isodense | Bright | Dark | Very dark | Dark | Dark |
| Late subacute | 1 week to months | Extracellular met-Hgb | Hypodense | Bright | Bright | Dark rim, variable center | Bright | Dark |
| Chronic | > 14 days (≥ months) | Hemosiderin | Hypodense | Dark | Dark | Dark | Dark | Dark |

***(Table 5-1)*** *Deoxy-Hgb = deoxyhemoglobin; met-Hgb = methemoglobin; oxy-Hgb = oxygenated hemoglobin.*

met-Hgb. Intracellular met-Hgb is highly paramagnetic, but the intact RBC membrane prevents direct dipole-dipole interactions.

A cellular perihematomal inflammatory response develops. Microglial activation occurs as immune cells infiltrate the parenchyma surrounding the clot.

**Late Subacute Hemorrhage.** Late subacute hemorrhage lasts from one to several weeks. As RBCs lyse, met-Hgb becomes extracellular. Met-Hgb is now exposed directly to plasma water, reducing T1 relaxation time and prolonging the T2 relaxation time.

**Chronic Hemorrhage.** Parenchymal hemorrhagic residua persist for months to years. Heme proteins are phagocytized and stored as ferritin in macrophages. If the capacity to store ferritin is exceeded, excess iron is stored as hemosiderin. Intracellular ferritin and hemosiderin induce strong magnetic susceptibility.

Chronic hemorrhage in the subarachnoid space typically coats the pial surface of the brain, a condition termed "superficial siderosis" (see Chapter 6). Superficial siderosis is sometimes seen adjacent to intraparenchymal hematomas, especially those associated with amyloid angiopathy (see Chapter 10).

## Imaging of Intracranial Parenchymal Hemorrhage

The role of imaging in sICH is first to identify the presence and location of a clot (the easy part), to "age" the clot (harder), and then to detect other findings that may be clues to its etiology (the more difficult, demanding part).

The appearance of pICH on CT depends on just one factor: Electron density. In turn, the electron density of a clot depends almost entirely on its protein concentration, primarily the globin moiety of Hgb. Iron and other metals contribute <

*(5-3A) NECT in a hypertensive patient shows a large heterogeneous hematoma in the left cerebellar hemisphere ➡ and a smaller, much less hyperdense clot in the right cerebellum ➡. Findings are consistent with a hyperacute (loose, largely unretracted) clot. (5-3B) The patient suddenly deteriorated while still in the scanner. Repeat NECT scan now shows additional hemorrhage ➡. The patient died shortly after this scan was performed.*

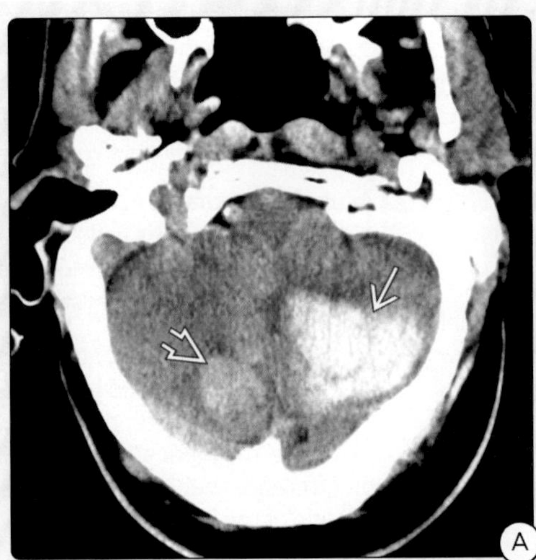

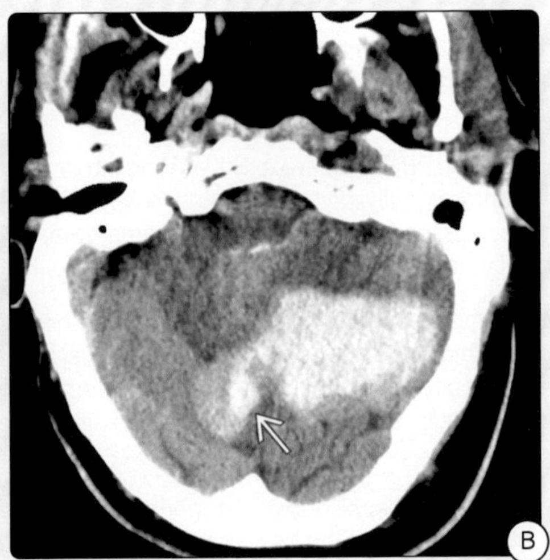

*(5-4A) NECT in 42-yo man with spontaneous onset of left-sided weakness shows right intraparenchymal hematoma ➡, moderate surrounding edema ➡. Faint subarachnoid hemorrhage (SAH) is also present along interhemispheric fissure ➡. CTA (not shown) was negative. (5-4B) (L) NECT 3 weeks later shows hematoma is now hypodense with mildly hyperdense rim ➡. (R) CECT shows some rim enhancement ➡.*

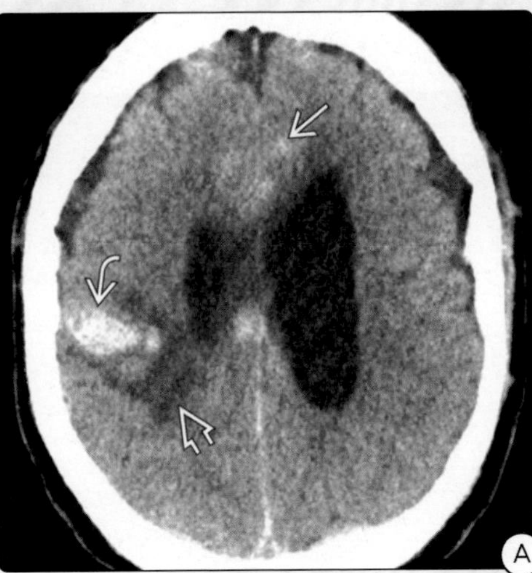

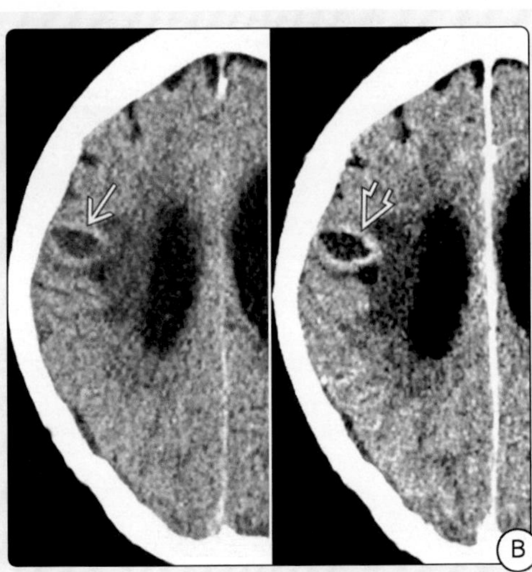

0.5% to total clot attenuation and so have no visible effect on hematoma density.

In contrast, the imaging appearance of ICH on MR is more complex and depends on a number of factors. Both intrinsic and extrinsic factors contribute to imaging appearance.

**Intrinsic biologic factors** that influence hematoma signal intensity are primarily related to macroscopic clot structure, RBC integrity, and Hgb oxygenation status. RBC concentration, tissue pH, arterial vs. venous source of the bleed, intracellular protein concentration, and the presence and integrity of the blood-brain barrier also contribute to the imaging appearance of an ICH.

**Extrinsic factors** include pulse sequence, sequence parameters, receiver bandwidth, and field strength of the magnet. Of these, pulse sequence and field strength are the most important determinants. T1- and T2-weighted images are the most helpful in estimating lesion age. T2* (GRE, SWI) is the most sensitive sequence in detecting parenchymal hemorrhages (especially microhemorrhages).

Field strength also affects imaging appearance of ICH. The MR findings delineated below and in the table **(Table 5-1)** are calculated for 1.5T scanners. At 3.0T, all parts of acute and early subacute clots have significantly increased hypointensity on FLAIR and T2WI.

## Hyperacute Hemorrhage

**CT.** If ICH is imaged within a few minutes of the ictus, the clot is loose, poorly organized, and largely unretracted **(5-3)**. Water content is still high, so a hyperacute hematoma may appear isodense or occasionally even hypodense relative to adjacent brain. If active hemorrhage is present, the presence of both clotted and unclotted blood results in a mixed-density hematoma with hypodense and mildly hyperdense components. Rapid bleeding and coagulopathy may result in fluid-fluid levels.

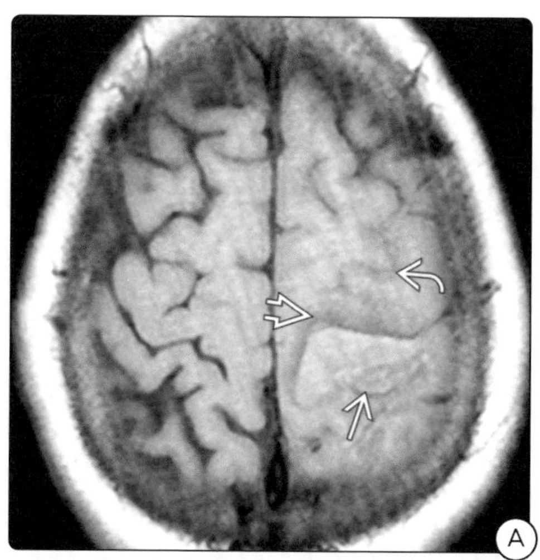


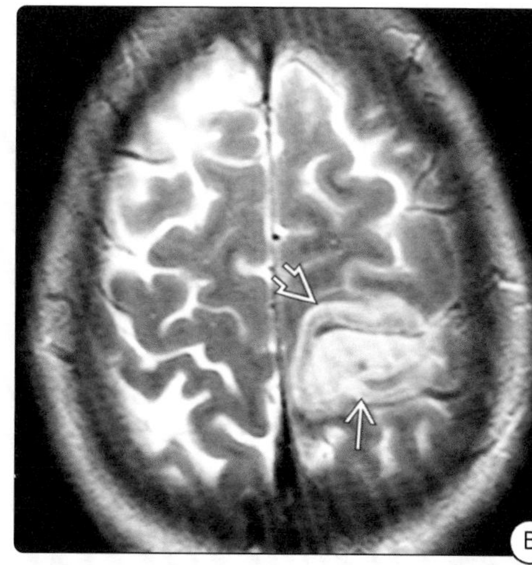


***(5-6A)** MR in a normotensive patient with acute spontaneous intracranial hemorrhage (sICH) on NECT is shown. T1WI shows acute hematoma is intermediate in SI ➡, surrounded by a rim of hypointense vasogenic edema ➡. Adjacent sulcal effacement ➡ may be from SAH. **(5-6B)** Clot is heterogeneously hyperintense on T2 MR ➡. Note vasogenic edema ➡. "Dirty" CSF probably represents SAH.*

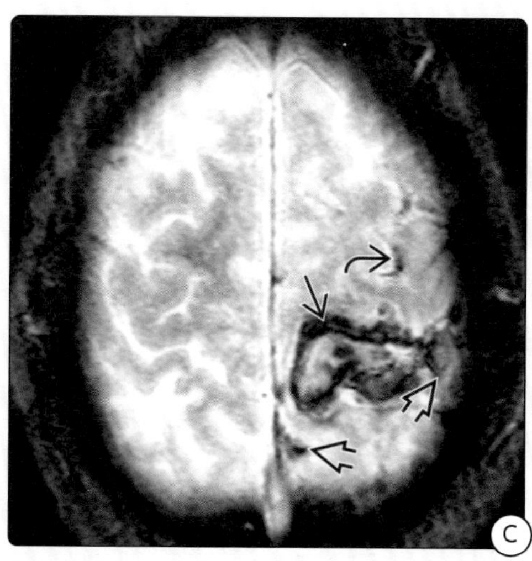


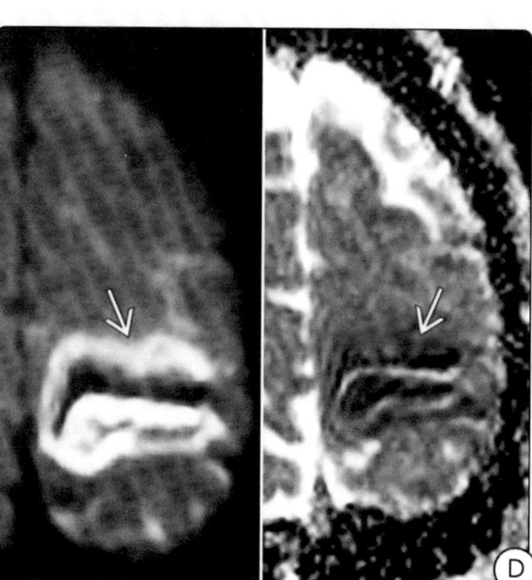


***(5-6C)** T2* GRE MR shows "blooming" around the periphery of the clot ➡ and in the sulci ➡. Tubular hypointensity in adjacent cortical veins ➡ suggests venous thrombosis. **(5-6D)** DWI (L) and ADC map (R) in the same case show restricted diffusion in the layered, heterogeneous acute hematoma ➡.*

**MR.** Oxy-Hgb has no unpaired electrons and is diamagnetic. Therefore, signal intensity of a hyperacute clot depends mostly on its water content. Hyperacute clots are isointense to slightly hypointense to gray matter on T1WI. A hyperacute clot is generally hyperintense on T2 scans, although they can appear quite heterogeneous.

Because the macroscopic structure of a hyperacute clot is so inhomogeneous, spin dephasing results in heterogeneous hypointensity ("blooming") on T2* sequences.

## Acute Hemorrhage

**CT.** The hematocrit of a retracted clot approaches 90%. Therefore, an acute hematoma is usually hyperdense on NECT, typically measuring 60-80 HU. Exceptions to this general rule are found if hemorrhage occurs in extremely anemic patients with very low hematocrits or in patients with coagulopathies.

**MR.** Acute hematomas are low/intermediate signal intensity on T1WI **(5-6A)**. Significant vasogenic edema develops around the clot and is T1 hypointense and T2/FLAIR hyperintense **(5-6B)**. As the clot retracts, water content diminishes. Intracellular deoxy-Hgb predominates. Deoxy-Hgb is paramagnetic with four unpaired electrons, and the hematoma becomes more profoundly hypointense on T2WI. Acute hematomas "bloom" on T2* (GRE, SWI) **(5-6C)**. Diffusion restriction is present on diffusion-weighted imaging (DWI) and ADC, although the presence of T2 and susceptibility effects can combine to produce a complex appearance in and around acute hematomas **(5-6D)**.

## Early Subacute Hemorrhage

**CT.** Hematoma density gradually decreases with time, beginning with the periphery of the clot. Clot attenuation diminishes by an average of 1.5 HU per day **(5-9)**. At around 7-10 days, the outside of a pICH becomes isodense with the

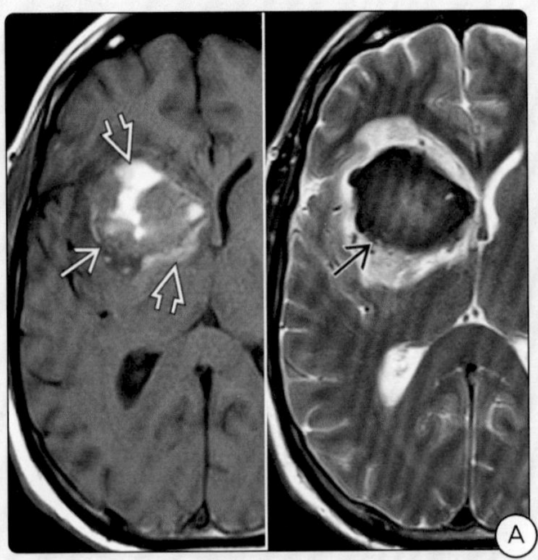

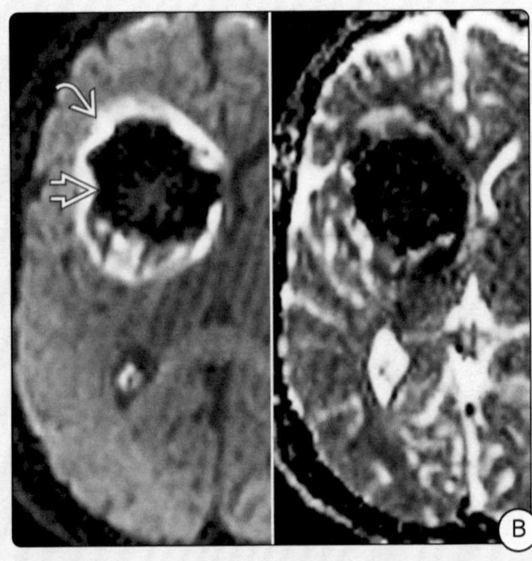

***(5-8A)** Axial T1 (L) and T2 (R) MR scans in a patient with a 3-day-old left basal ganglionic hematoma are shown. The clot is largely isointense with brain on T1WI and profoundly hypointense on T2WI. Some T1 shortening is beginning to appear in this late acute/early subacute hematoma. **(5-8B)** DTI DWI (L) and ADC (R) in the same case show "T2 blackout", which is surrounded by a hyperintense rim of "T2 shine-through".*

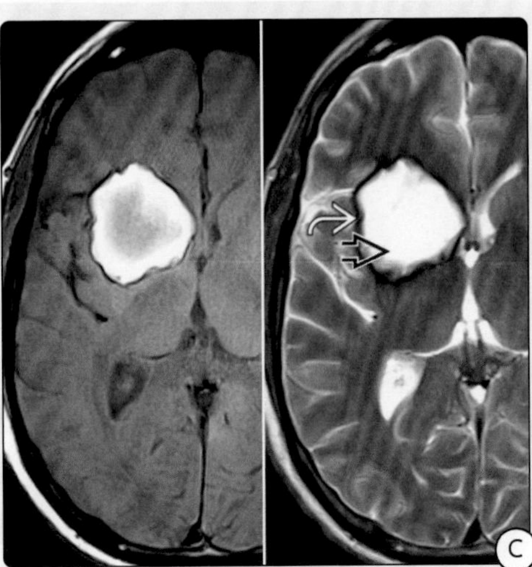

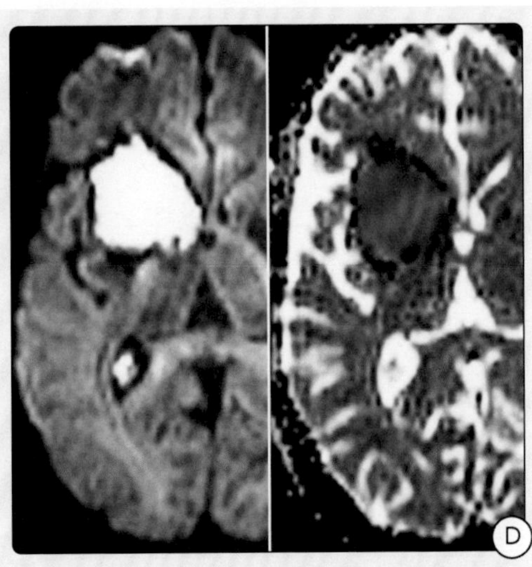

***(5-8C)** Axial T1 (L) and T2 (R) 3 months later in the same case shows the hematoma is composed mostly of "bright" extracellular dilute-free met-Hgb. Note hypointense rim (hemosiderin/ferritin) and some isointense clot remaining in the center of the hematoma. **(5-8D)** DWI (L) and ADC map (R) show that the T2 effect dominates in the DWI while the ADC is dark, indicating true diffusion restriction in the chronic hematoma.*

adjacent brain **(5-10B)**. The hyperdense center gradually shrinks, becoming less and less dense until the entire clot becomes hypodense. A subacute hematoma shows ring enhancement on CECT **(5-4)**.

**MR.** Intracellular met-Hgb predominates around the clot periphery, whereas deoxy-Hgb persists within the hematoma core. A rim of T1 shortening (hyperintensity) surrounding an isointense to slightly hypointense core is the typical appearance on T1WI **(5-10C)**. Paramagnetic met-Hgb is not very mobile and causes pronounced T2 shortening, so early subacute clots are hypointense on T2WI. Profound hypointensity on T2* persists.

Clot appearance on DWI varies. For many forms of hemorrhage, the T2/T2* effect comprises the dominant contribution to signal intensity and therefore appears markedly hypointense (T2 "blackout effect"). In acute and subacute hemorrhage, true restricted diffusion occurs with the intrinsically long T2 of these hematomas **(5-8D)**. The diffusion signal of hemorrhage at each stage of evolution is summarized in the table **(Table 5-1)**.

## Late Subacute Hemorrhage

**CT.** With progressive aging, a pICH gradually becomes hypodense relative to adjacent brain on NECT scans. Ring enhancement may persist for weeks or up to two or three months.

**MR.** Once cell lysis occurs, mobile free dilute extracellular met-Hgb predominates in determining signal intensity. Clots develop hyperintensity around their rim on both T1WI and T2WI **(5-8C)**. Eventually, the clot appears very hyperintense on both sequences. A rim of T2* "blooming" generally persists. With the exception of minor susceptibility artifacts, late subacute clots appear similar on both 1.5T and 3.0T.

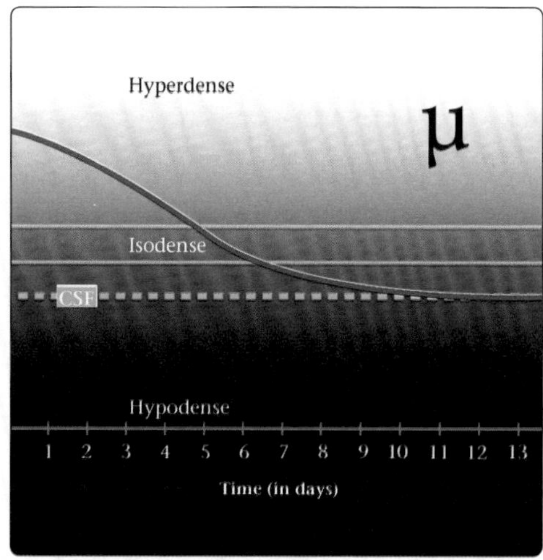


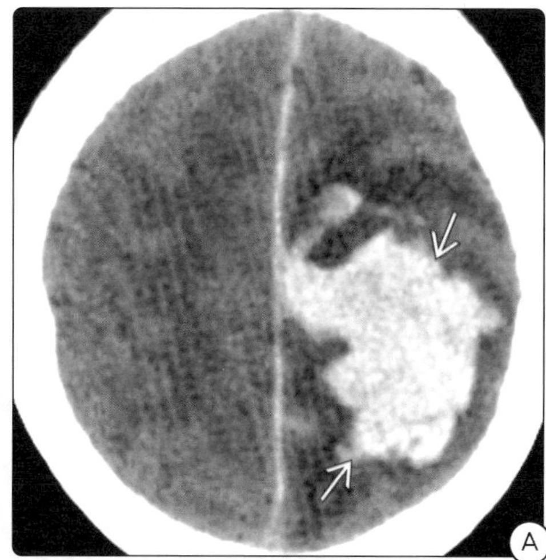


***(5-9)** Graphic depicts time-related progressive decrease in density of brain hematoma relative to parenchyma. Clots are initially hyperdense, become isodense between a few days to a week or so, and then are hypodense. Eventually, a resolving clot becomes nearly isodense with CSF. **(5-11A)** Axial NECT in a patient with an acute lobar hypertensive hemorrhage shows relatively uniform hyperdense clot in the left parietal lobe ➡.*

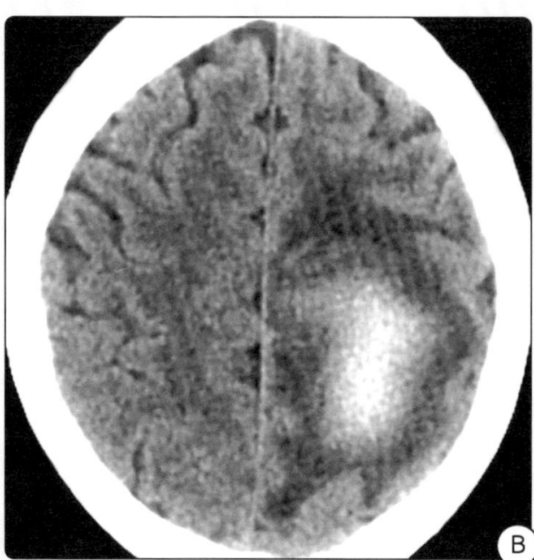


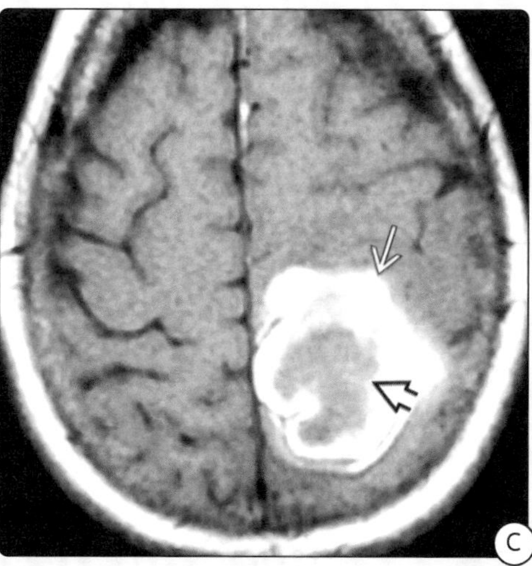


***(5-10B)** Follow-up NECT was obtained 1 week later. Clot density has decreased with a gradation from hyperdense in the center to isodense to hypodense at the periphery. **(5-10C)** MR was obtained immediately after the follow-up CT. T1WI shows that the subacute hematoma is hyperintense around the rim ➡ and nearly isointense in the center ⇨.*

## Chronic Hemorrhage

**CT.** A few very small healed hemorrhages may become invisible on NECT scan. Between 35-40% of chronic hematomas appear as a round or ovoid hypodense focus. Another 25% of patients develop slit-like hypodensities. Between 10-15% of healed hematomas calcify.

**MR.** Intracellular ferritin and hemosiderin are hypointense on both T1WI and T2WI. A hyperintense cavity surrounded by a "blooming" rim on T2* may persist for months or even years **(5-14)**. Eventually, only a slit-like scar remains as evidence of a prior parenchymal hemorrhage **(5-12)**.

# Etiology of Nontraumatic Parenchymal Hemorrhages

There are many causes of nontraumatic ("spontaneous") or unexplained ICH. The role of imaging in such cases is to localize the hematoma, estimate its age from its imaging features, and attempt to identify possible underlying causes.

The effect of age on the pathoetiology of sICH is profound. Knowing the patient's age is extremely important in establishing an appropriately narrowed differential diagnosis.

It can be difficult to discern enhancement within an already hyperdense acute hematoma on CECT scans. Dual-energy CT (DECT) can display the presence of contrast enhancement, potentially helping distinguish between tumor bleeding and nonneoplastic ("pure") hemorrhage. DECT can also help differentiate ICH from extravasated contrast material staining.

MR imaging with standard sequences as well as fat-saturated contrast-enhanced scans can be very helpful. A T2* sequence (GRE &/or SWI) should always be included, as the identification of other prior "silent" microhemorrhages affects both diagnosis and treatment decisions.

*(5-12) Gross autopsy case shows residua of remote striatocapsular hemorrhage. A slit-like cavity with a small amount of yellowish fluid is surrounded by dark hemosiderin staining ➙. Note volume loss with enlarged right frontal horn ➙ and gliotic brain ➙ surrounding old hematoma. (Courtesy R. Hewlett, MD.) (5-14A) Sagittal T1 MR in a patient 2 years following hypertensive hemorrhage shows ovoid hyperintense cavity ➙.*

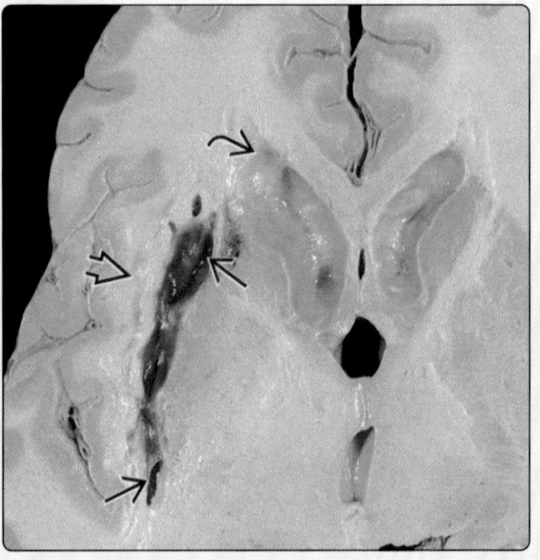

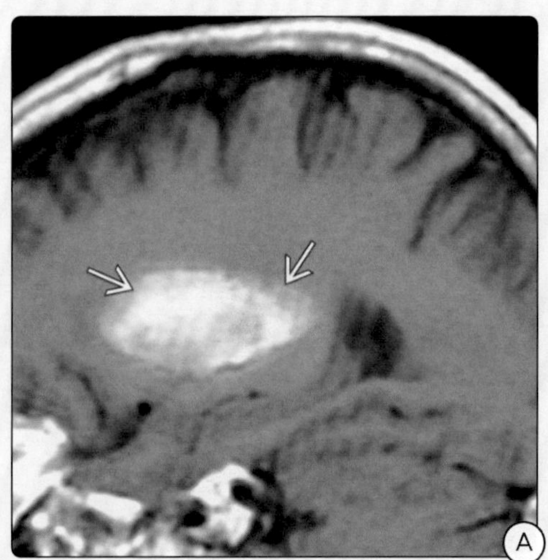

*(5-14B) Axial standard (not FSE) T2 MR shows that the cavity ➙ contains hyperintense fluid (dilute-free extracellular met-Hgb) and is surrounded by a hypointense rim of hemosiderin/ferritin ➙. (5-14C) T2* GRE MR shows "blooming" ➙ around the rim of the residual cavity. Findings are classic for chronic parenchymal hematoma.*

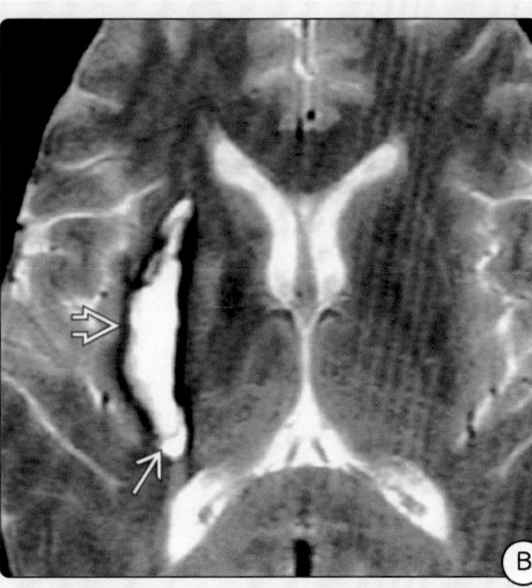

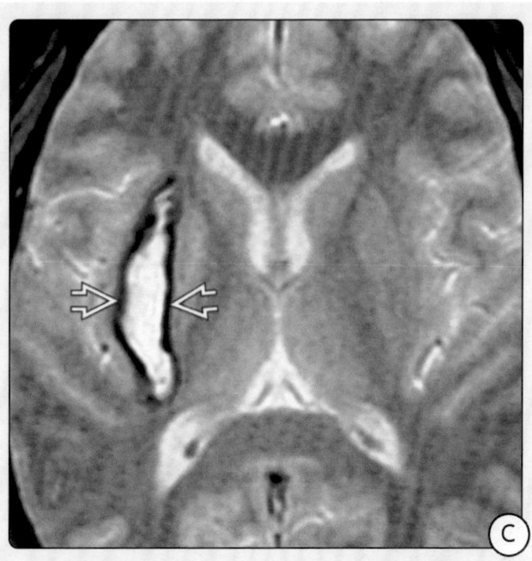

## Newborns and Infants With sICH

ICH in the term newborn is most frequently associated with prolonged or precipitous delivery, traumatic instrumented delivery (e.g., forceps assistance or vacuum extraction), and primiparity. The most common cause of ICH in infants < 34 gestational weeks is **germinal matrix hemorrhage** **(5-15)** **(5-16)**.

The germinal matrix is a highly vascular, developmentally dynamic structure in the brain subventricular zone. The germinal matrix contains multiple cell types, including premigratory/migratory neurons, glia, and neural stem cells. Rupture of the relatively fragile germinal matrix capillaries may occur in response to altered cerebral blood flow, increased venous pressure (e.g., with delivery), coagulopathy, or hypoxic-ischemic injury. Germinal matrix hemorrhage is discussed in greater detail in Chapter 8.

**Isolated choroid plexus** and **isolated intraventricular hemorrhage (IVH)** do not involve the germinal matrix. **White matter injury of prematurity** generally does not show evidence of hemorrhage ("blooming") on T2* imaging.

The most common nontraumatic cause of spontaneous IVH in *neonates beyond 34 gestational weeks* is **dural venous sinus thrombosis** (DVST) **(5-18)**. In contrast to older children and adults in whom the transverse sinus is most commonly affected, the straight sinus (85%) and superior sagittal sinus (65%) are the most frequent locations in infants. Multisinus involvement is seen in 80% of cases. Thalamic and punctate white matter lesions are common in infants with DVST.

## Children With sICH

The most common cause of sICH in children ages 1-18 years is an underlying **vascular malformation**. Vascular malformations are responsible for nearly 1/2 of spontaneous parenchymal hemorrhages in this age group **(5-20)**.

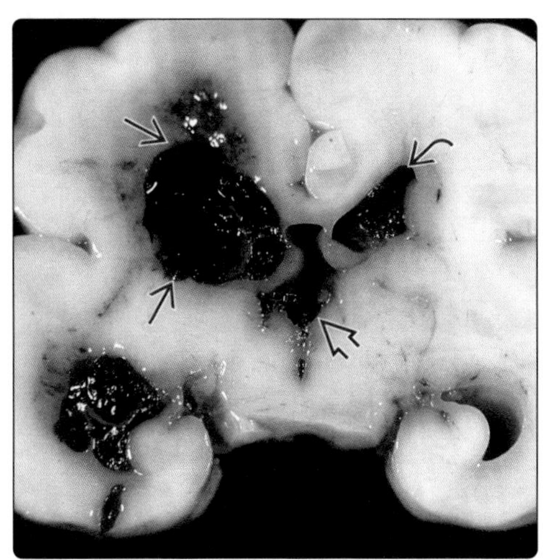

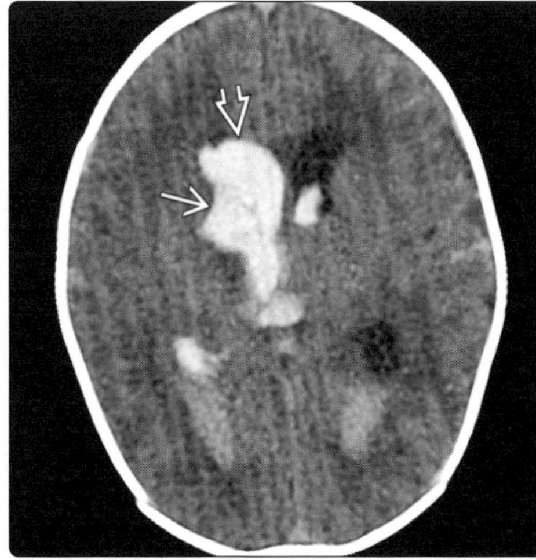

***(5-15)** Autopsied brain of a premature infant shows hemorrhage into the germinal matrix and the adjacent deep periventricular white matter (WM) ➡. Blood is also present in both lateral ↗ and 3rd ➡ ventricles. **(5-16)** NECT in a premature infant shows typical germinal matrix hemorrhage ➡ with dissection into the adjacent ventricles ➡.*

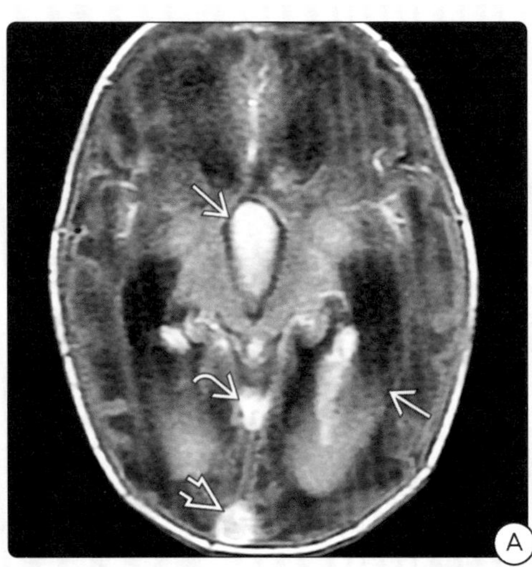


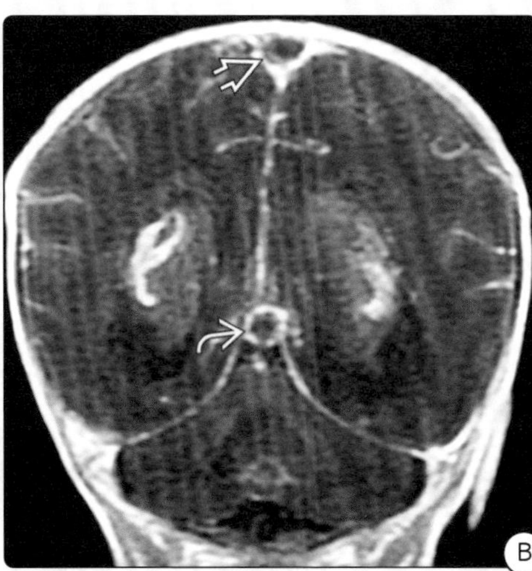


***(5-18A)** T1 MR in a septic newborn infant shows blood in the 3rd/lateral ventricles ➡, thrombus in straight sinus ➡, and torcular Herophili ➡. **(5-18B)** Coronal T1 C+ MR in the same case shows thrombosis of superior sagittal ➡ and straight sinuses ➡ seen here as enhancing dura around a nonenhancing clot (empty delta sign).*

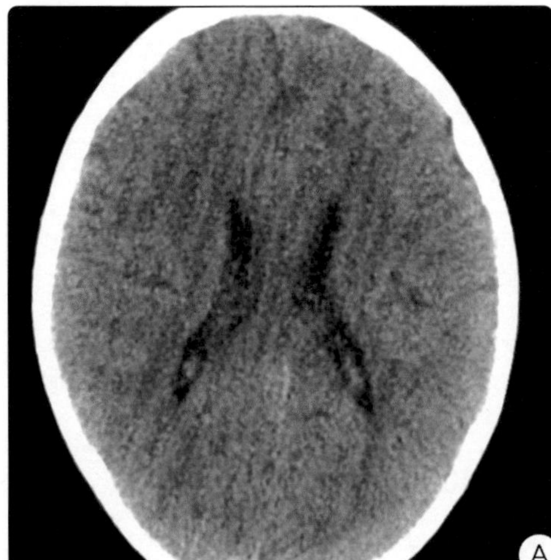

***(5-20A)** NECT in a child with headaches and family history of multiple cavernous malformations shows no abnormalities.*

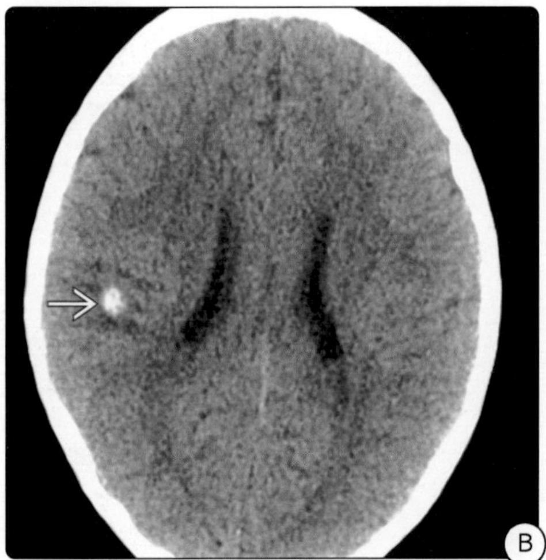

***(5-20B)** Follow-up scan 1 year later shows a small, solitary, calcified lesion in the right cerebral hemisphere ➡.*

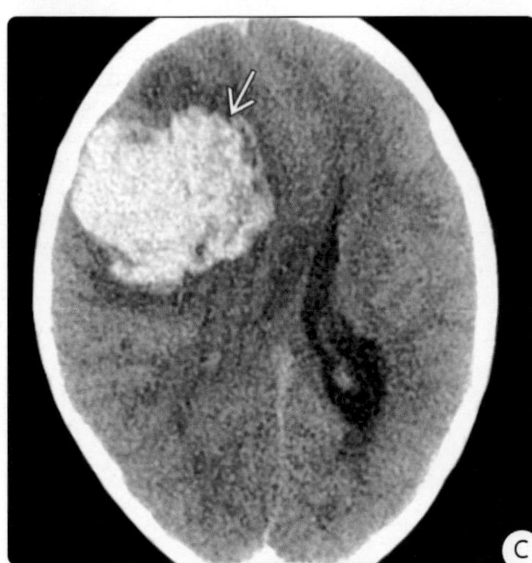

***(5-19C)** Several weeks later, the child had a severe headache, left-sided weakness, and bleeding into the cavernous malformation ➡.*

At least 25% of all arteriovenous malformations hemorrhage by the age of 15 years. Cavernous malformations, especially familial cavernous malformations ("cavernomas"), are a less common but important cause of sICH in children.

Other less common but important causes of pediatric sICH include **hematologic disorders** and **malignancies**, **vasculopathy**, and **venous occlusion/infarction**.

**Primary neoplasms** are a relatively rare cause of sICH in children **(5-22)**. Infratentorial tumors are more common than supratentorial neoplasms.

Posterior fossa neoplasms that frequently hemorrhage include ependymoma and rosette-forming glioneuronal tumor. Patchy or petechial hemorrhage is more common than large intratumoral bleeds.

Supratentorial tumors with a propensity to bleed include ependymoma and the spectrum of primitive neuroectodermal tumors. Malignant astrocytomas with hemorrhage occur but are rare. In contrast to middle-aged and older adults, hemorrhagic metastases from extracranial primary cancers are *very* rare in children.

### sICH IN INFANTS AND CHILDREN

**Newborns and Infants**

- Common
  - Germinal matrix hemorrhage (< 34 gestational weeks)
  - DVST (≥ 34 gestational weeks)
- Rare
  - Congenital prothrombotic disorder
  - Thrombocytopenia
  - Hemophilia
  - Vitamin K deficiency bleeding
  - Neoplasm

**Children**

- Common
  - Vascular malformation: ~ 50%
- Less common
  - Hematologic disorder
  - Vasculopathy
  - DVST or cortical vein thrombosis
- Rare but important
  - Neoplasm (primary)
  - Drug abuse

## Young Adults With sICH

An underlying **vascular malformation** is the most common cause of sICH in young adults as well **(5-25)**. **Drug abuse** is the second most common cause of unexplained hemorrhage **(5-23)**. Cocaine and methamphetamine may induce extreme systemic HTN, resulting in a putaminal-external capsule bleed that looks identical to those seen in older hypertensive adults.

**Vasculitis** and **reversible cerebral vasoconstriction syndrome** (RCVS) occasionally cause pICH in young adults **(5-29)**.

**Venous occlusion/infarction** with or without **dural sinus occlusion** is also relatively common in this age group, especially in young women taking oral contraceptives. Severe **eclampsia/preeclampsia** with posterior reversible encephalopathy syndrome (PRES) may cause multifocal posterior cortical and subcortical hemorrhages **(5-30)**. Hemorrhagic neoplasms (both primary and metastatic) are rare.

**sICH IN YOUNG AND MIDDLE-AGED ADULTS**

**Young Adults**
- Common
  - Vascular malformation
  - Drug abuse
- Less common
  - Venous occlusion
  - PRES
- Rare but important
  - Vasculitis
  - RCVS
  - Neoplasm

**Middle-Aged Adults**
- Common
  - HTN
  - Neoplasm (primary or metastatic)
- Less common
  - Dural sinus or cortical vein occlusion
  - Drug abuse
- Rare but important
  - Vascular malformation
  - Vasculitis
  - RCVS
  - Acute hemorrhagic leukoencephalopathy

## Middle-Aged and Older Adults With sICH

The two most common causes of sICH in middle-aged and older adult patients are **HTN** and **amyloid angiopathy**, both of which are discussed in detail. Approximately 10% of spontaneous parenchymal hemorrhages are caused by bleeding into a brain **neoplasm**, generally either a high-grade primary tumor, such as glioblastoma multiforme, or hemorrhagic metastasis from an extracranial primary, such as renal cell carcinoma **(5-32)**.

A less common but important cause of sICH in this age group is **venous infarct**. Venous infarcts are caused by cortical vein thrombosis with or without dural sinus occlusion. Iatrogenic **coagulopathy** is also common in older adult patients, as many take maintenance doses of warfarin for atrial fibrillation **(5-31)**.

Occasionally, a ruptured **saccular aneurysm** presents with a focal lobar hemorrhage rather than a subarachnoid hemorrhage. The most common source is an anterior communicating artery aneurysm that projects superolaterally and ruptures into the frontal lobe.

Underlying **vascular malformation** is a relatively rare cause of sICH in older patients. With a 2-4% per year cumulative rupture risk, a first-time arteriovenous malformation bleed at this age can occur but is unusual (as is hemorrhage from a cavernous malformation) **(5-26)**. However, **dural arteriovenous fistulas (dAVFs)** *do* occur in middle-aged and older adult patients. Although dAVFs rarely hemorrhage unless they have cortical venous (not just dural sinus) drainage, spontaneous thrombosis of the outlet veins may result in sudden ICH.

Rare but important causes of sICH in this age group include **vasculitis** (more common in younger patients) and **acute hemorrhagic leukoencephalopathy**.

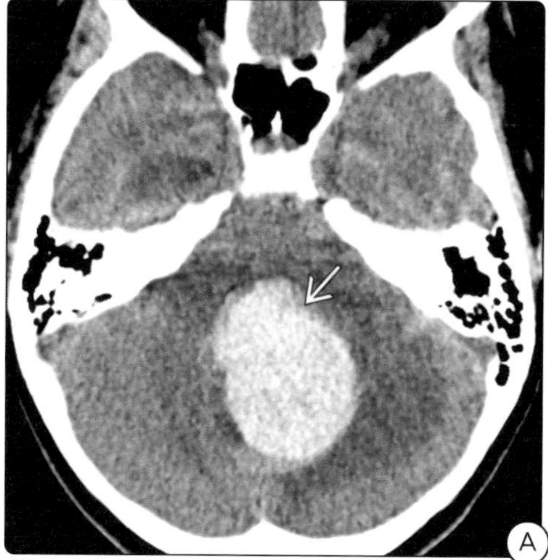

***(5-22A)** NECT in a 10-yo child shows large posterior fossa hemorrhage ➡ that involves the 4th ventricle/vermis.*

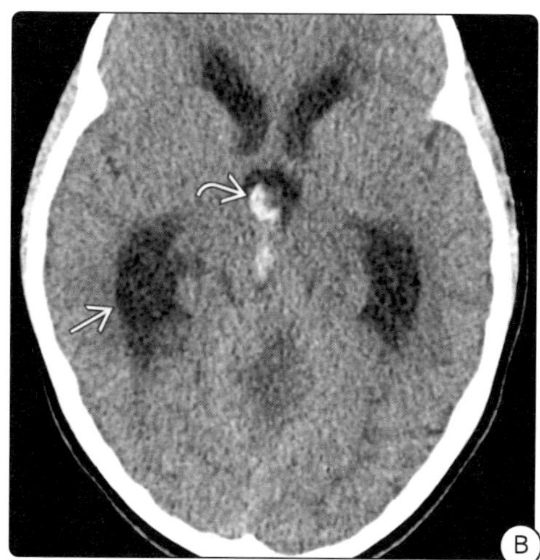

***(5-22B)** Hydrocephalus ➡ and intraventricular hemorrhage ➡ are present. Hemorrhagic pilocytic astrocytoma was found at surgery.*

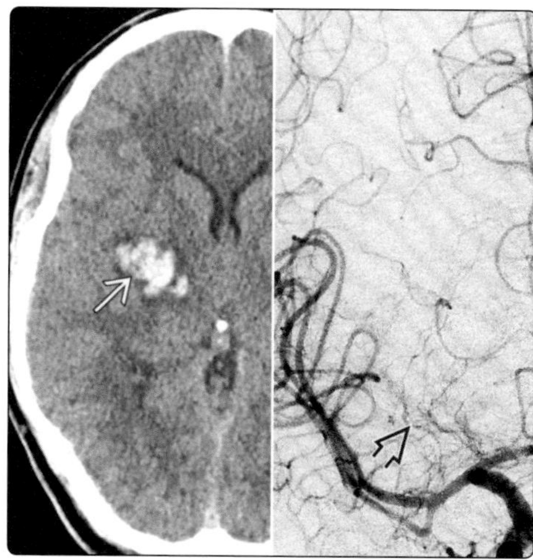

***(5-23)** (L) CT of basal ganglion hemorrhage ➡ and (R) DSA of irregular, beaded lenticulostriate arteries ➡ are shown in amphetamine vasculitis.*

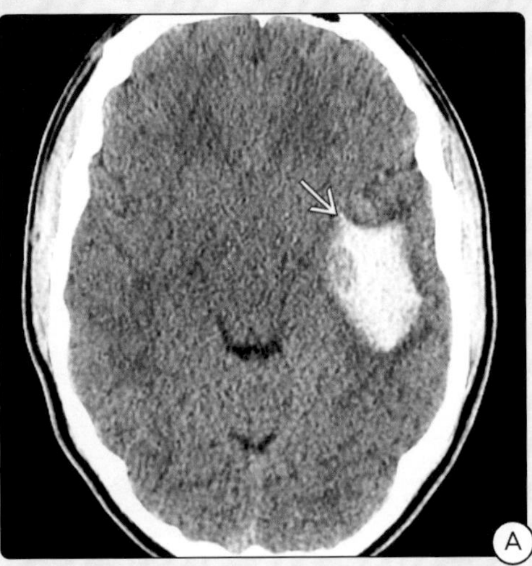

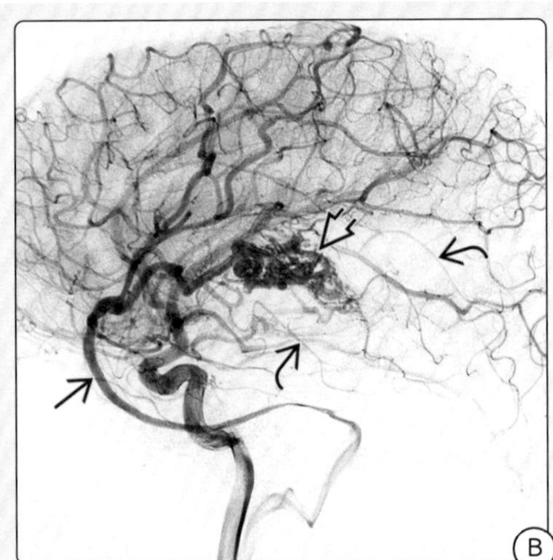

*(5-25A) NECT in a 15-yo boy with sudden-onset severe headache and right-sided weakness shows an acute left anterior temporal hematoma ➡. (5-25B) Lateral view of the internal carotid angiogram in the same case shows a partially thrombosed arteriovenous malformation (AVM) ⇨ with early draining superficial middle cerebral vein ➡. Most of the avascular mass effect ↗ is from the hematoma.*

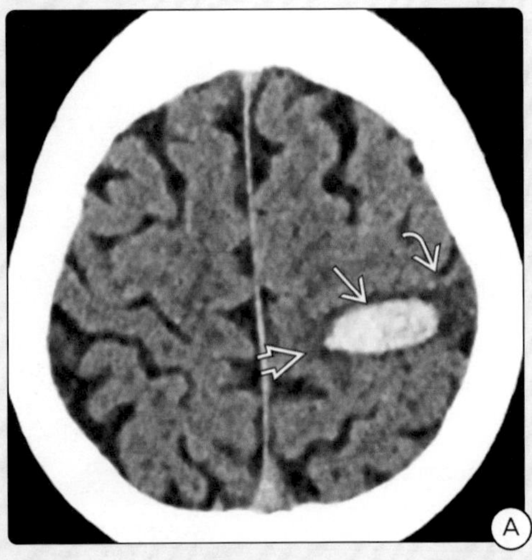

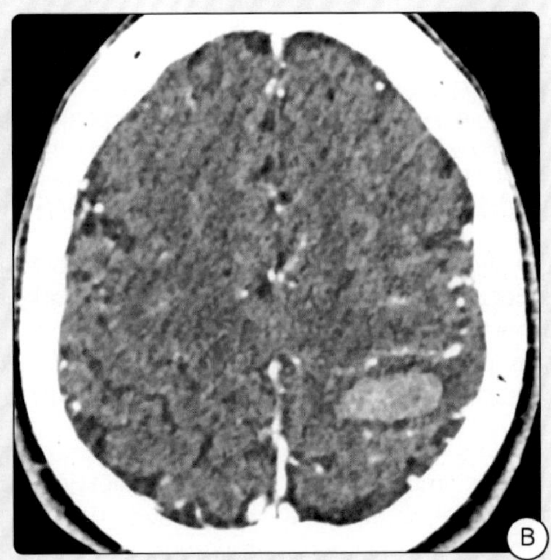

*(5-27A) NECT in a 60-yo man with sudden onset of right hemiparesis shows a well-delineated ovoid acute hematoma ➡ surrounded by parenchymal edema ➡. Mild mass effect on the adjacent cortical sulci ➡ is present. (5-27B) CTA shows no evidence for spot sign or abnormal vascularity. Superficial cortical veins were normal.*

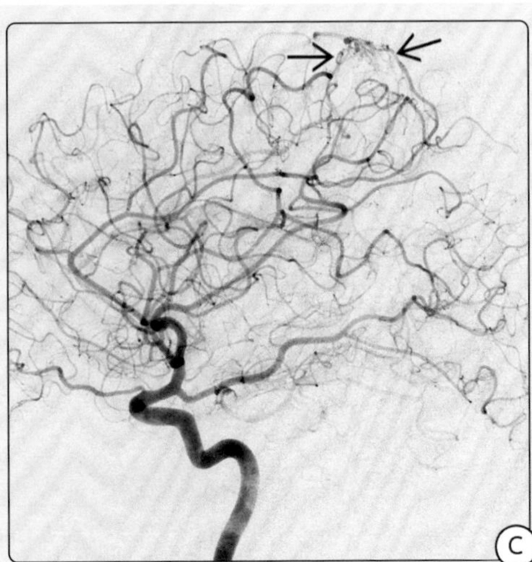

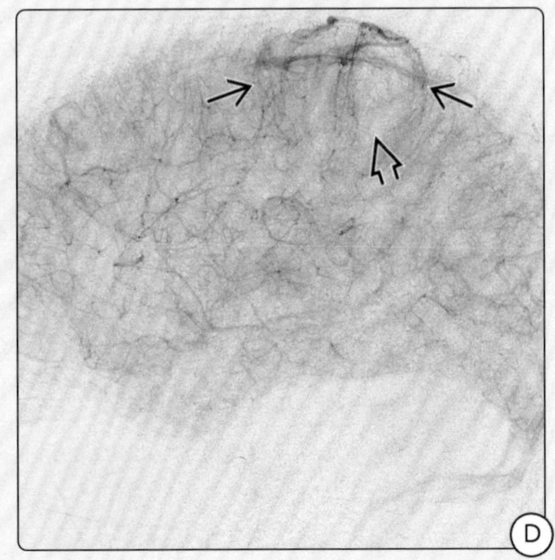

*(5-27C) Lateral view of left internal carotid DSA shows a small tangle of abnormal vessels ➡. (5-27D) Late capillary/early venous phase of the DSA in the same case shows an avascular mass effect ⇨ surrounded by a rim of stagnating contrast in early draining veins ➡. Mostly thrombosed AVM was found at surgery.*

**sICH IN OLDER ADULTS**

**Older Adults**
- Common
  - HTN
  - Amyloid angiopathy
  - Neoplasm (primary or metastatic)
- Less common
  - Dural sinus or cortical vein occlusion
  - Coagulopathy
- Rare but important
  - Vascular malformation (usually dAVF)

## Multiple sICHs

Solitary spontaneous parenchymal hemorrhages are much more common than multifocal bleeds. Etiology varies with patient age.

Multifocal brain bleeds that occur at all ages include venous thrombosis, PRES **(5-30)**, vasculitis (especially fungal), septic emboli, thrombotic microangiopathy, and acute hemorrhagic leukoencephalopathy.

Multiple *nontraumatic* brain bleeds in children and young adults are most often caused by multiple cavernous malformations and hematologic disorders (e.g., leukemia, thrombocytopenia).

The most common causes of multiple ICHs in middle-aged and older adults are HTN, amyloid angiopathy, hemorrhagic metastases, and impaired coagulation (either coagulopathy or anticoagulation).

**MULTIPLE sICHs**

**Children and Young Adults**
- Multiple cavernous malformations
- Hematologic disorder/malignancy

**Middle-Aged and Older Adults**
- Common
  - Chronic HTN
  - Amyloid angiopathy
- Less common
  - Hemorrhagic metastases
  - Coagulopathy, anticoagulation

**All Ages**
- Common
  - Dural sinus thrombosis
  - Cortical vein occlusion
- Less common
  - PRES
  - Vasculitis
  - Septic emboli
- Rare but important
  - Thrombotic microangiopathy
  - Acute hemorrhagic leukoencephalopathy

# Macrohemorrhages

HTN and amyloid angiopathy account for 78-88% of all nontraumatic ICHs. Although both can cause extensive nonhemorrhagic "microvascular" disease,

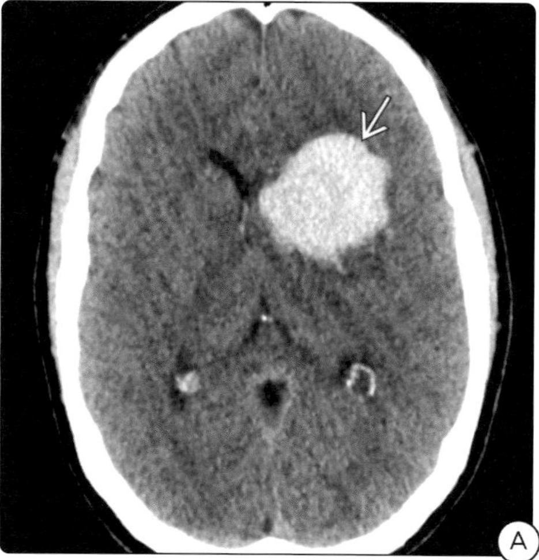


***(5-29A)** NECT in a 37-yo normotensive man with right-sided weakness shows left basal ganglionic hemorrhage ➡. Drug screen was negative.*

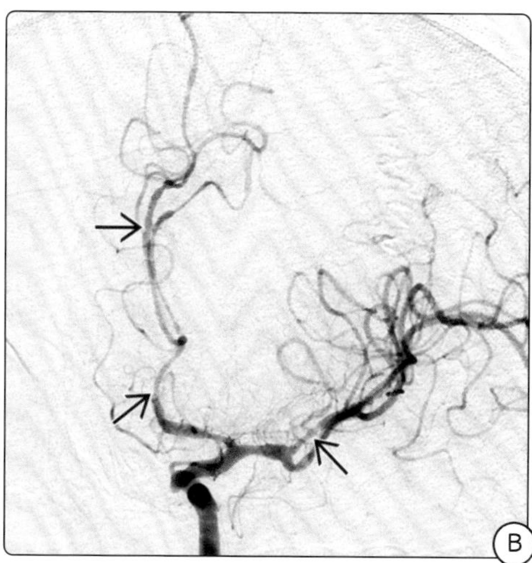


***(5-29B)** Oblique coronal DSA shows multiple areas of arterial dilatations, constrictions in the left ACA, MCA ➡. Initial diagnosis was vasculitis.*

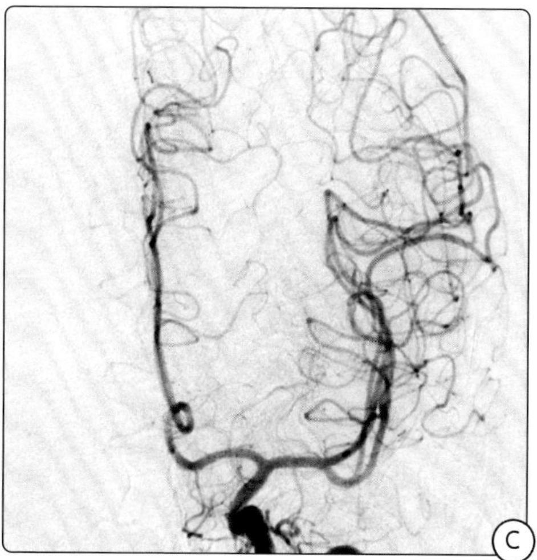


***(5-29C)** Repeat DSA 3 months later is normal. Final diagnosis was reversible cerebral vasoconstriction syndrome (RCVS).*

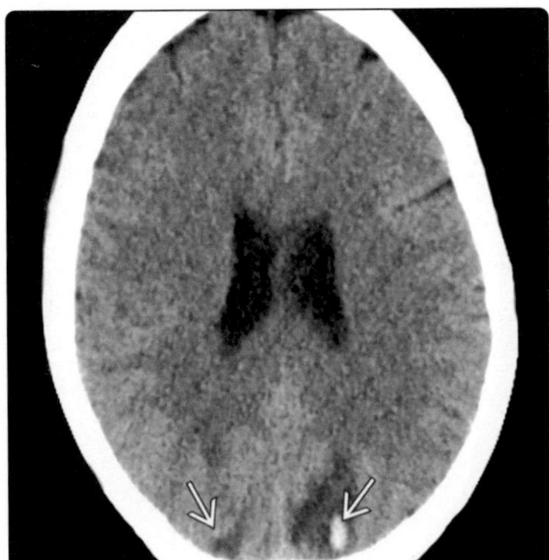

*(5-30) A 22-yo eclamptic woman has occipital lesions ➡ with edema, hemorrhage: Posterior reversible encephalopathy syndrome (PRES).*

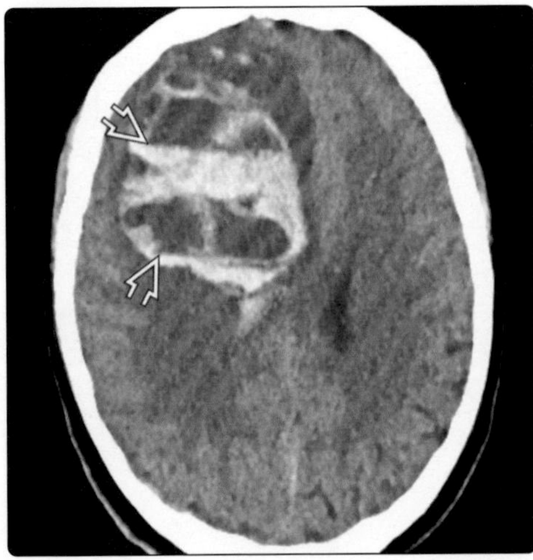

*(5-31) NECT in an anticoagulated 72-yo woman shows sICH with multiple blood-fluid levels ➡.*

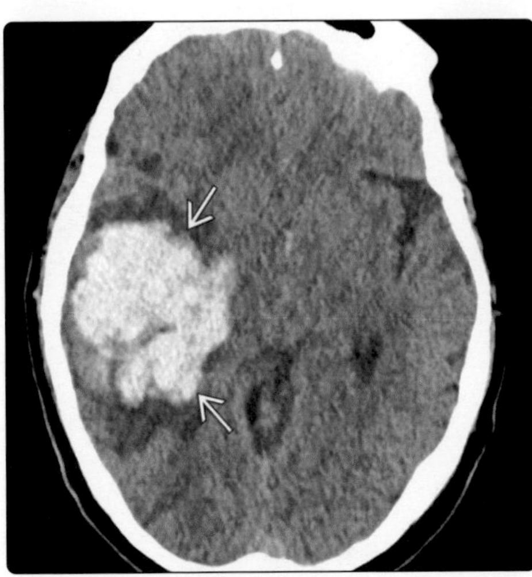

*(5-32) NECT in a normotensive 59-yo man with severe headaches shows right temporal lobe sICH ➡. Glioblastoma was found at surgery.*

their most common manifestations are gross lobar and multifocal microbleeds. We therefore discuss them here.

## Hypertensive Intracranial Hemorrhage

### Terminology

Hypertensive ICH (hICH) is the *acute* manifestation of nontraumatic ICH secondary to systemic HTN. *Chronic* hypertensive encephalopathy refers to the effects of longstanding HTN on the brain parenchyma and is mostly seen as subcortical white matter disease &/or multifocal microbleeds.

### Etiology

Atherosclerosis with lipohyalinosis and fibrinoid necrosis most severely affects the lenticulostriate arteries (LSAs). Progressive weakening and accelerated degeneration of the LSA wall forms small pseudoaneurysms (Charcot-Bouchard aneurysms or bleeding globes). Ruptured LSA pseudoaneurysm is thought to be the genesis of most striatocapsular hypertensive hemorrhages.

### Pathology

**Location.** The putamen/external capsule is the most common location **(5-33)**. These so-called striatocapsular hemorrhages account for nearly 2/3 of all hICHs. The thalamus is the next most common site, responsible for 15-25%. The pons and cerebellum are the third most common location and cause 10% of all hICHs. Lobar hemorrhages account for another 5-10%.

Multiple microbleeds are also common in patients with chronic HTN. These tend to cluster in the basal ganglia and cerebellum with fewer lesions in the cortex and subcortical white matter.

**Size and Number.** Size varies from tiny submillimeter microbleeds to large macroscopic lesions that measure several centimeters in diameter. When T2* sequences are used, the majority of patients with hICH have multiple lesions.

**Gross Pathology.** The most common gross finding in hICH is a large ganglionic hematoma that often extends medially into the ventricles. Hydrocephalus and mass effect with subfalcine herniation are common complications.

**Microscopic Features.** Generalized arteriosclerosis with lipohyalinosis and fibrinoid necrosis is common in patients with hICH. In some cases, small fibrosed pseudoaneurysms in the basal ganglia can be identified.

### Clinical Issues

**Epidemiology.** Although the prevalence of hICH has declined significantly, HTN still accounts for 40-50% of spontaneous "primary" intraparenchymal hemorrhages in middle-aged and older adults. hICH is 5-10x less common than cerebral ischemia-infarction, accounting for ~ 10-15% of all strokes.

**Demographics.** HTN is associated with a 4x increase in the risk of ICH. Older adult males are the demographic group most at risk for hICH with a peak prevalence between 45-70 years. African Americans are the most commonly affected ethnic group in North America.

**Presentation.** Large hICHs present with sensorimotor deficits and impaired consciousness. Patients may—or may not—have a history of longstanding untreated systemic HTN.

**Natural History.** Neurologic deterioration after hICH is common. HE is frequent in the first few hours and is highly predictive of neurologic deterioration, poor functional outcome, and mortality. For each 10% increase in ICH size, there is a 5% increase in mortality and an additional 15% chance of poorer functional outcome.

Mortality rate approaches 80% in patients with large hemorrhages. Of hICH survivors, between 1/3 and 1/2 are moderately or severely disabled.

## Imaging

**CT Findings.** NECT scans typically show a round or ovoid hyperdense mass centered in the lateral putamen/external capsule or thalamus **(5-34)**. In the presence of active bleeding or coagulopathy, the hemorrhage may appear inhomogeneously hyperdense with lower density areas and even fluid-fluid levels. Intraventricular extension is common. Acute hICH does not enhance on CECT.

**MR Findings.** Signal intensity on MR changes with clot age and varies from a large acute hematoma to a slit-like hemosiderin "scar." White matter hyperintensities on T2/FLAIR are common findings in patients with hICH. T2* sequences (GRE, SWI) frequently demonstrate multifocal "blooming" black dots, especially in the basal ganglia and cerebellum **(5-37)**.

**Angiography.** Most hICHs are avascular on CTA **(5-34)**. However, an enhancing spot sign with contrast extravasation can sometimes be identified in actively bleeding lesions **(5-35)**.

### hICH

**Location**
- Putamen/basal ganglia (60-65%)
- Thalamus (15-25%)
- Pons/cerebellum (10%)
- Lobar hemispheric (5-10%)

**Clinical Issues**
- 10-15% of all "strokes"
- 40-50% of spontaneous hemorrhages in older adults
- Age, hematoma volume early predictors of death/disability

**Imaging**
- Classic = hyperdense clot in putamen/external capsule
- Look for old hemosiderin "scar," microbleeds on T2*

**Differential Diagnosis**
- Cerebral amyloid angiopathy
- Hemorrhagic neoplasm
- Internal cerebral vein thrombosis
- Drug abuse (e.g., cocaine use)

## Differential Diagnosis

The major differential diagnosis for hICH is **cerebral amyloid angiopathy** (CAA). Patients with CAA are usually normotensive and have moderately impaired cognition. Although there is some overlap with hICH, the distribution of hemorrhages in CAA is typically lobar and peripheral more often than striatocapsular and central. Cerebellar hemorrhages are common in hICH but rare in CAA.

**Hemorrhagic neoplasms** (e.g., glioblastoma multiforme or metastasis) are more common in the white matter or gray matter-white matter junction and less common in the basal ganglia and cerebellum.

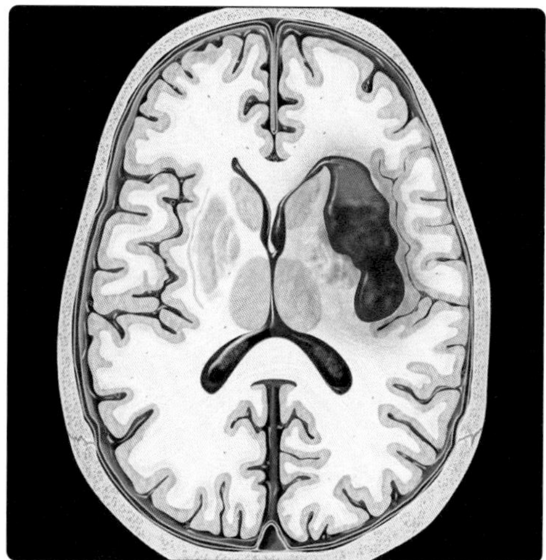

***(5-33)*** *Graphic depicts acute hypertensive striatocapsular hemorrhage with edema, dissection into the lateral and 3rd ventricles.*

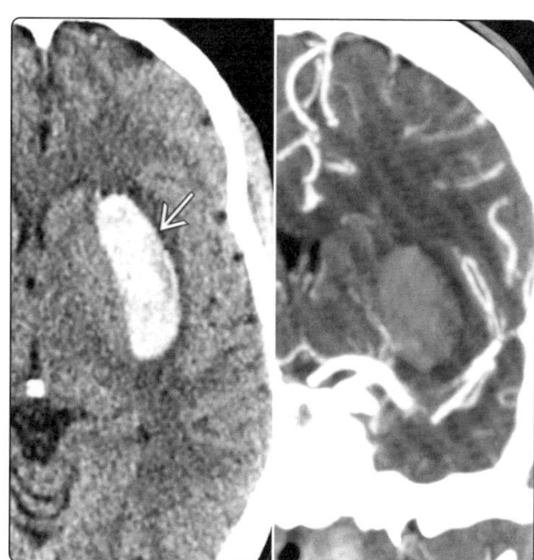

***(5-34)*** *(L) NECT in a hypertensive 57-yo woman shows classic left striatocapsular hemorrhage ➡. (R) Coronal MIP CTA shows no spot sign.*

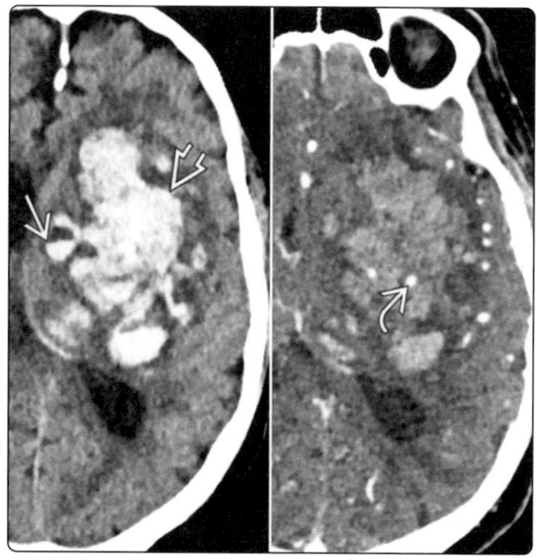

***(5-35)*** *(L) NECT in 73-yo hypertensive man shows acute basal ganglionic hemorrhage ➡, fluid-fluid levels ➡. (R) CTA shows spot sign ➡.*

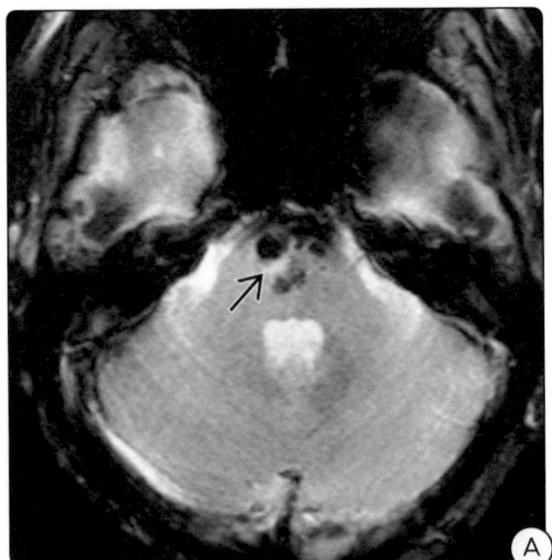

*(5-37A) T2* GRE MR in a patient with chronic hypertension shows multiple "blooming" microbleeds in the pons.*

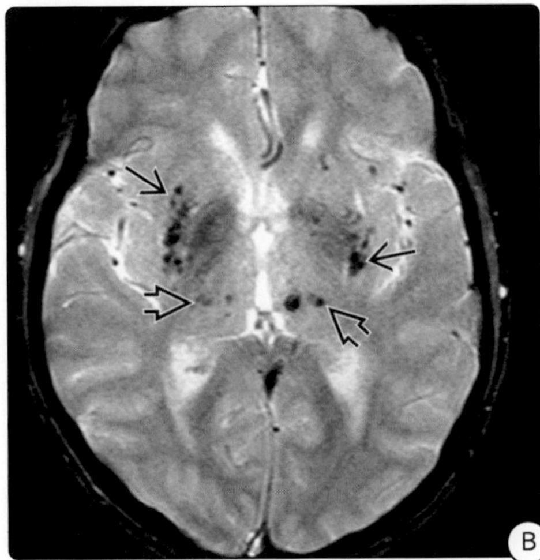

*(5-37B) More cephalad T2* GRE MR shows multiple microbleeds in the putamina and both thalami.*

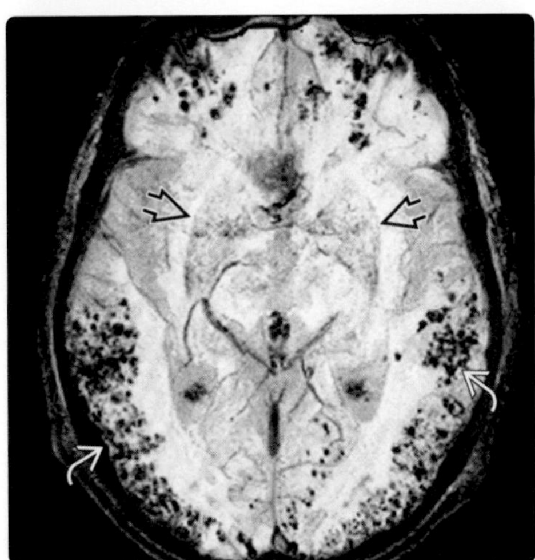

*(5-38) T2* SWI MR in CAA shows innumerable cortical/subcortical "blooming" black dots. Note sparing of basal ganglia.*

With the exception of dAVF, first-time hemorrhage from an underlying **vascular malformation** is unusual in middle-aged and older adult patients. **Coagulopathy** can cause or exacerbate sICH. Coagulation-related hemorrhages are typically lobar, not striatocapsular.

In younger patients, **drug abuse** (e.g., cocaine use) with extreme HTN can cause putamen/external capsule hemorrhage.

**Internal cerebral venous thrombosis** can occur at all ages. These hemorrhages tend to be bilateral, thalamic, and more medially located than the striatocapsular bleeds of hICH.

## Cerebral Amyloid Angiopathy

CAA is one of three morphologic varieties of cerebral amyloid deposition disease. Because CAA—a.k.a. congophilic angiopathy—is a common cause of spontaneous lobar hemorrhage in older adult patients, we discuss it briefly here. The full spectrum of cerebral amyloid disease is discussed in greater detail in the chapter on vasculopathy (Chapter 10).

MR is the most sensitive study to detect CAA. Multifocal and confluent areas of white matter hyperintensity on T2/FLAIR scans are common. At least 1/3 have petechial microhemorrhages, seen as multifocal "blooming" black dots on T2* (GRE, SWI) sequences **(5-38)**. Cortical superficial siderosis is also common and predictive of future lobar hemorrhages.

## Remote Cerebellar Hemorrhage

### Terminology and Etiology

Remote cerebellar hemorrhage (RCH) is a less well recognized and often misdiagnosed cause of spontaneous posterior fossa parenchymal hemorrhage in postoperative patients. Most reported cases occur a few hours following supratentorial craniotomy. RCH also occurs as a rare complication of foramen magnum decompression or spinal surgery.

The etiology of RCH is most likely CSF hypovolemia with inferior displacement or "sagging" of the cerebellar hemispheres. Tearing or occlusion of bridging tentorial veins is thought to result in superficial cerebellar hemorrhage with or without hemorrhagic necrosis.

### Clinical Issues

RCH is relatively rare, occurring in 0.1-0.6% of patients with supratentorial craniotomies, most often for aneurysm clipping, temporal lobe epilepsy, or tumor resection. There is a slight male predominance, and the median age is 51 years.

Many—if not most—cases of RCH are asymptomatic and discovered incidentally at postoperative imaging. The most common symptoms are delayed awakening from anesthesia, decreasing consciousness, and seizures.

Prognosis is generally excellent. Treatment is generally conservative, as hematoma removal is rarely indicated.

### Imaging

NECT demonstrates stripes of hyperdense blood layered over the cerebellar folia, the zebra sign. Hemorrhage can be uni- or bilateral, ipsi- or contralateral to the surgical site **(5-40A)**.

MR findings are variable, depending on the age/stage of hematoma evolution. "Blooming" black stripes are seen on T2* (GRE, SWI) **(5-39B)**.

# Microhemorrhages

Cerebral microbleeds (CMBs) are perivascular collections of hemosiderin-containing macrophages. CMBs are usually small and have many etiologies ranging from trauma to vasculopathy and metastases. Each is discussed in detail in the chapters that deal with the specific pathologic groupings.

In this section, we briefly summarize two distinct but related differential diagnoses: (1) Entities that cause multiple brain microbleeds and (2) the differential diagnosis of nonhemorrhagic "blooming" black dots on T2* MR.

## Multifocal Brain Microbleeds

A number of entities can cause diffuse brain microhemorrhages **(5-41)**. CMBs are best identified as multiple hypointensities on T2* SWI. These can be faint or even invisible on standard GRE sequences.

Trauma with hemorrhagic vascular or axonal injury is the most common cause of CMBs in children and young adults. Chronic HTN and amyloid angiopathy are the two most common pathologies responsible for multiple CMBs in older adults.

**"Critical illness-associated microbleeds"** has been associated with COVID-19, acute respiratory failure, and mechanical ventilation or extracorporeal membrane oxygenation (ECMO) **(5-45)**. **DIC, sepsis, acute hemorrhagic leukoencephalopathy**, and **high-altitude cerebral edema** are other reported causes of CMBs **(5-43)**.

Nonhemorrhagic entities that can cause multifocal "blooming" black dots on T2* imaging include calcifications and pneumocephalus.

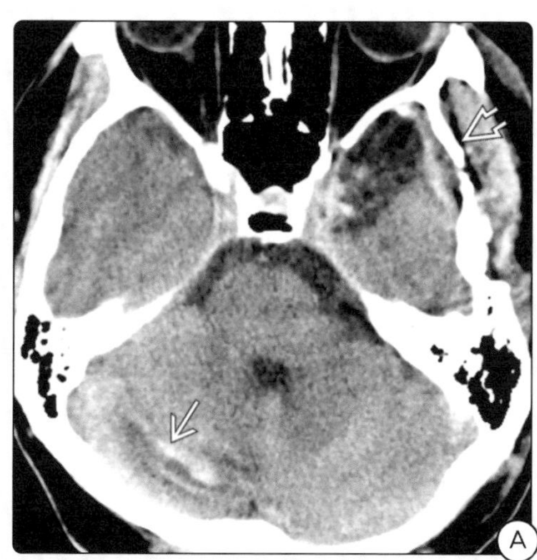
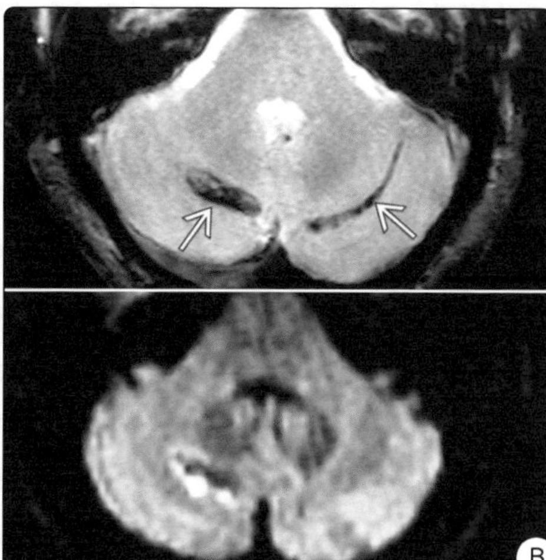

***(5-40A)** NECT after supratentorial craniotomy ➡ shows linear "zebra stripes" ➡ of alternating hyperdensity (blood) and low density (edema) in the right cerebellum, consistent with remote cerebellar hemorrhage. **(5-39B)** Bilateral remote cerebellar hemorrhage followed resection of a supratentorial neoplasm. (Top) T2* GRE shows bilateral "blooming" lesions ➡. (Bottom) DWI shows some restriction in right acute hemorrhage.*

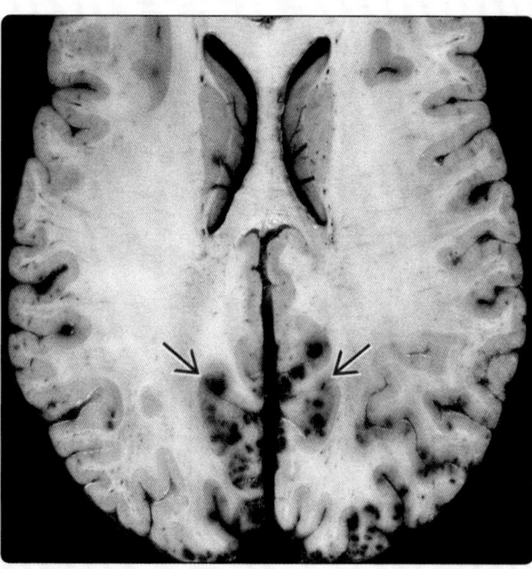
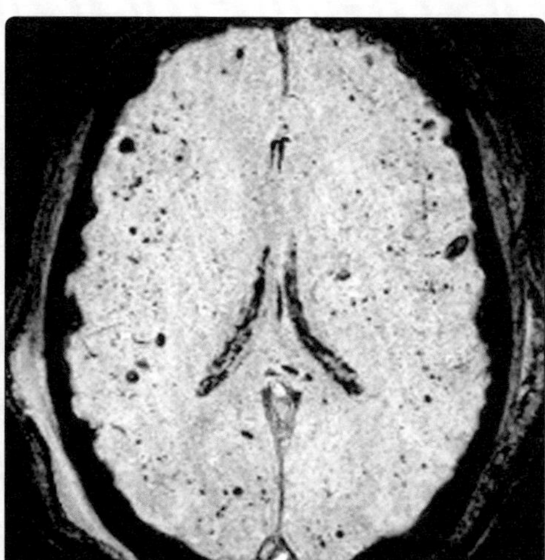

***(5-41)** Autopsy in a septic, immunocompromised patient shows multiple cortical microhemorrhages ➡. **(5-42)** T2* SWI MR in a 33-yo woman with meningococcemia, septic shock, and purpura fulminans shows innumerable microbleeds ("blooming" black dots) scattered throughout both hemispheres.*

## BRAIN MICROBLEEDS: ETIOLOGY, COMMON

**Common**
- Diffuse axonal/vascular injury
- CAA
- Chronic hypertensive encephalopathy
- Hemorrhagic metastases

**Less Common**
- Multiple cavernous malformations
- Septicemia
- Critical illness associated
  - Hypoxemia, acute respiratory distress syndrome
- Fat emboli
- Vasculitis
  - Fungal
  - Sickle cell
- Coagulopathy

## BRAIN MICROBLEEDS: ETIOLOGY, RARE

**Rare but Important**
- Acute hemorrhagic leukoencephalopathy
- Intravascular lymphoma
- Leukemia
- Radiation/chemotherapy
  - Radiation-induced telangiectasias
  - Mineralizing microangiopathy
- Thrombotic microangiopathy
  - Malignant HTN
  - DIC
  - Hemolytic uremic syndrome (HUS), atypical HUS
  - Thrombotic thrombocytopenic purpura
- High-altitude cerebral edema
- Cerebral malaria

*Selected References: The complete reference list is available on the eBooks+ version included with purchase.*

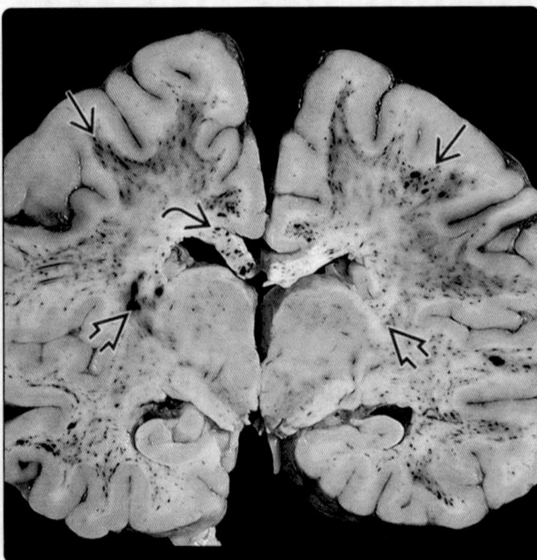

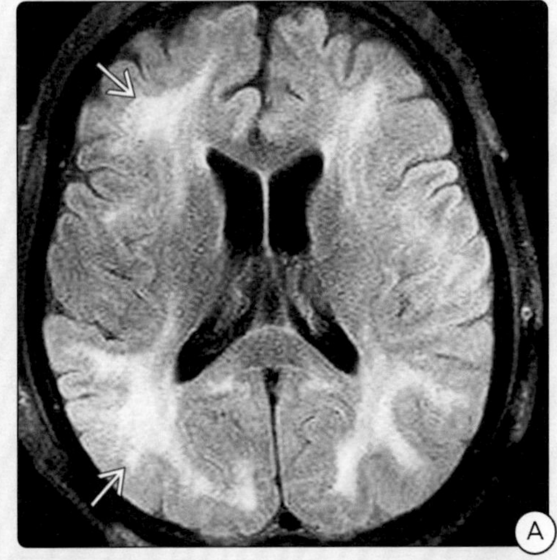


***(5-43)** Coronal autopsy shows innumerable tiny microhemorrhages in the subcortical ➙, deep ➙ WM in a patient with respiratory failure and sepsis. Corpus callosum ➙ is severely affected. (Courtesy R. Hewlett, MD.) **(5-45A)** FLAIR MR in a 55-yo intubated man with acute respiratory distress syndrome shows diffuse confluent symmetric hyperintensity ➙ in the subcortical, deep WM that spares the cortex.*

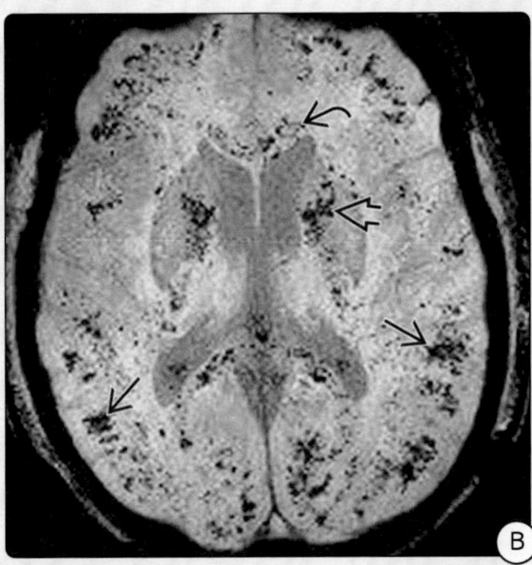


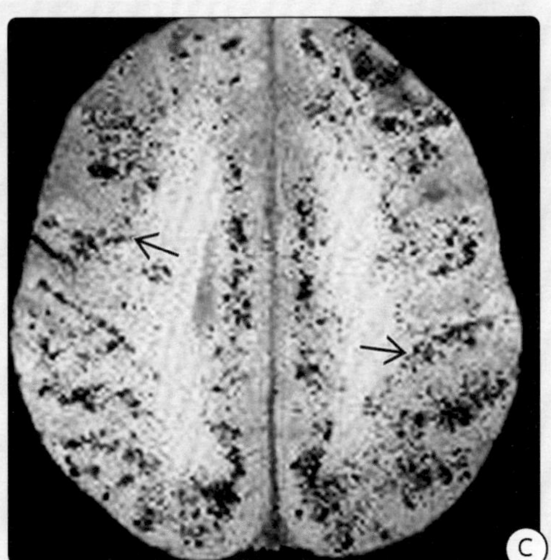


***(5-45B)** T2* SWI MR shows innumerable microbleeds in the subcortical, deep WM ➙, including the corpus callosum ➙ and internal capsules ➙. **(5-45C)** More cephalad SWI MR shows the diffuse subcortical microbleeds ➙ with striking sparing of the overlying cortex. This is a striking case of critical illness-associated cerebral microbleeds. (Courtesy M. Jhaveri, MD.)*

# Subarachnoid Hemorrhage and Aneurysms

*Trauma is, by far, the most common cause of intracranial subarachnoid hemorrhage. Traumatic subarachnoid hemorrhage occurs when blood from contused brain or lacerated vessels extends into adjacent sulci; it was discussed in connection with craniocerebral trauma (Chapter 2). This chapter focuses on nontraumatic subarachnoid hemorrhage and aneurysms.*



## Subarachnoid Hemorrhage

Spontaneous (i.e., nontraumatic) subarachnoid hemorrhage (SAH) accounts for 3-5% of all acute "strokes." Approximately 80% of these are caused by a ruptured intracranial saccular aneurysm (SA). Other identifiable causes of nontraumatic SAH (ntSAH) include a variety of entities, such as dissections, venous hemorrhage or thrombosis, vasculitis, amyloid angiopathy, and reversible cerebral vasoconstriction syndrome (RCVS). No identifiable origin is found in 10-12% of patients presenting with ntSAH.

Neuroimaging plays a central role in the diagnosis and management of SAH. We begin this discussion with imaging **aneurysmal SAH** (aSAH) and its most devastating complications, vasospasm and secondary cerebral ischemia.

We then review two special types of nontraumatic, nonaneurysmal SAHs: **Perimesencephalic SAH** and an unusual pattern of SAH called convexity or **convexal SAH (cSAH)**. Lastly, we discuss chronic repeated SAH and its rare but important manifestation, **superficial siderosis (SS)**.

### Aneurysmal Subarachnoid Hemorrhage

#### Terminology

aSAH is an extravasation of blood into the space between the arachnoid and pia. The typical location of aSAH (basal cisterns and sylvian and inferior interhemispheric fissures) usually helps distinguish it from other causes of ntSAH (see shaded box, p. 99).

#### Etiology

aSAH is most often caused by rupture of a saccular ("berry") or (rarely) a blood blister-like aneurysm (BBA) **(6-1)**. Other less common causes of aSAH include intracranial dissections and dissecting aneurysms.

## Pathology

**Location.** Because most SAs arise from the circle of Willis or middle cerebral artery (MCA) bifurcation, the most common locations for aSAH are the suprasellar cistern and sylvian fissures **(6-2)** **(6-3)**.

Occasionally, an aneurysm ruptures directly into the brain parenchyma rather than the subarachnoid space. This occurs most frequently when the apex of an anterior communicating artery (ACoA) aneurysm points upward and bursts into the frontal lobe.

**Gross Pathology.** The gross appearance of aSAH is typically characterized by blood-filled basal cisterns **(6-17)**. SAH may extend into the superficial sulci and ventricles.

## Clinical Issues

**Demographics.** The overall incidence of aSAH increases with age and peaks between 40-60 years old; M:F = 1:2.

aSAH is rare in children. Regardless of their relative rarity, however, cerebral aneurysms cause the majority of spontaneous (nontraumatic) SAHs in children and account for ~ 10% of all childhood hemorrhagic "strokes."

**Presentation.** At least 75% of patients with aSAH present with sudden onset of the "worst headache of my life." The most severe form is a "thunderclap" headache, an extremely intense headache that comes on "like a boom of thunder" and typically peaks within minutes or even seconds. There are many causes of "thunderclap" headache. The most serious and life threatening is aSAH, although it accounts for just 4-12% of these severe headaches.

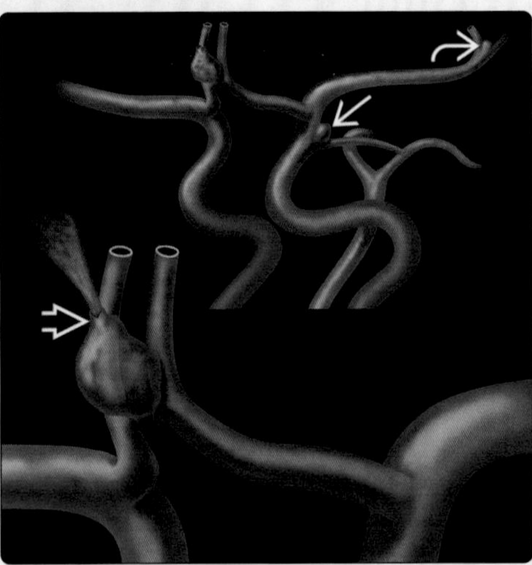

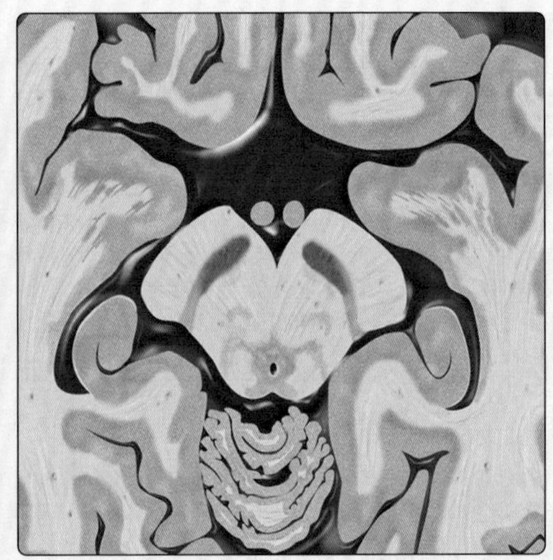

***(6-1)** Graphic shows a saccular aneurysm (SA) of the anterior communicating artery (ACoA) with active extravasation from a superiorly directed bleb ("tit") ➡. Note additional small aneurysms at the ICA-PCoA junction ➡ and MCA bifurcation ➡. **(6-2)** Graphic through the midbrain shows aneurysmal subarachnoid hemorrhage (aSAH) in red, evenly distributed throughout the basal cisterns.*

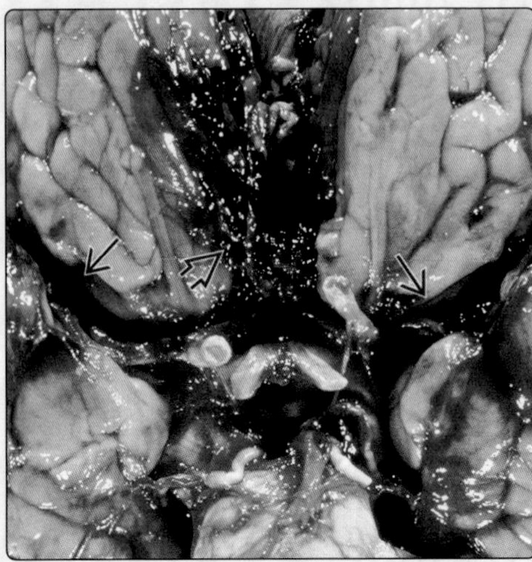

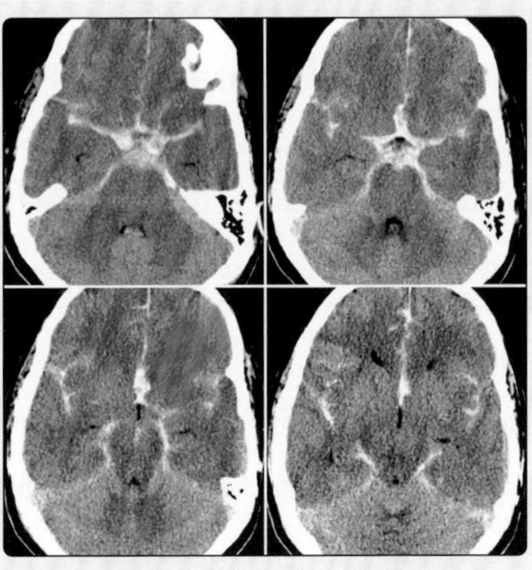

***(6-3)** Autopsy shows blood filling the suprasellar cistern ➡ and sylvian fissures ➡ from a ruptured ACoA aneurysm. **(6-4)** NECT scans show the typical appearance of aSAH. Hyperdensity filling the basilar cisterns, sylvian fissures is typical.*

1/3 of patients with aSAH complain of neck pain and 1/3 report vomiting. 10-25% experience a "sentinel headache" days or up to two weeks before the onset of overt SAH. These "sentinel headaches" are sudden, intense, persistent, and may represent minor bleeding prior to aneurysm rupture.

## SCREENING FOR SUSPECTED ANEURYSMAL SUBARACHNOID HEMORRHAGE

**Clinical Issues**

- Causes 3-5% of "strokes"
- "Thunderclap" headache [aneurysmal subarachnoid hemorrhage (aSAH): 4-12%]
- Peak age = 40-60 years; M:F = 1:2

**NECT**

- Sensitivity: ~ 100% if performed in first 6 hours
- Lumbar puncture unnecessary *if*
    - CT negative
    - Neurologic examination normal

**CTA**

- If NECT shows aSAH

**Natural History.** Although aSAH causes just 3-5% of all "strokes," nearly 1/3 of all stroke-related years of potential life lost before age 65 are attributable to aSAH. The mean age at death in patients with aSAH is significantly lower than in patients with other types of strokes.

Despite significant advances in diagnosis and management, aSAH is fatal or disabling in > 2/3 of patients. Massive SAH can cause coma and death within minutes. Approximately 1/3 of patients with aSAH die within 72 hours; another 1/3 survive but with disabling neurologic deficits.

**Treatment Options.** The goals of aSAH treatment in patients who survive their initial bleed are (1) to obliterate the aneurysm (preventing potentially catastrophic rebleeding) and (2) to prevent or treat vasospasm.

## Imaging

**General Features.** NECT is an excellent screening examination for patients with "thunderclap" headache and suspected aSAH. In the first six hours after ictus, the sensitivity of modern CT scanners approaches 100%. Lumbar puncture is now considered unnecessary if the NECT is negative and the neurologic examination is normal.

The best imaging clue to aSAH is hyperdense cisterns and sulci on NECT.

**CT Findings.** The basal cisterns—especially the suprasellar cistern—are generally filled with hyperdense blood **(6-4)**. Although SAH distribution generally depends on location of the "culprit" aneurysm, it is also somewhat variable and not absolutely predictive of aneurysm location.

ACoA aneurysms often rupture superiorly into the interhemispheric fissure. MCA bifurcation aneurysms usually rupture into the sylvian fissure. Internal carotid-posterior communicating artery (ICA-PCoA) aneurysms generally rupture into the suprasellar cistern **(6-6A)**. Vertebrobasilar aneurysms often fill the fourth ventricle, prepontine cistern, and foramen magnum with blood.

Intraventricular hemorrhage (IVH) is present in nearly 1/2 of all patients with aSAH. Focal parenchymal hemorrhage is uncommon but, if present, is generally predictive of aneurysm rupture site.

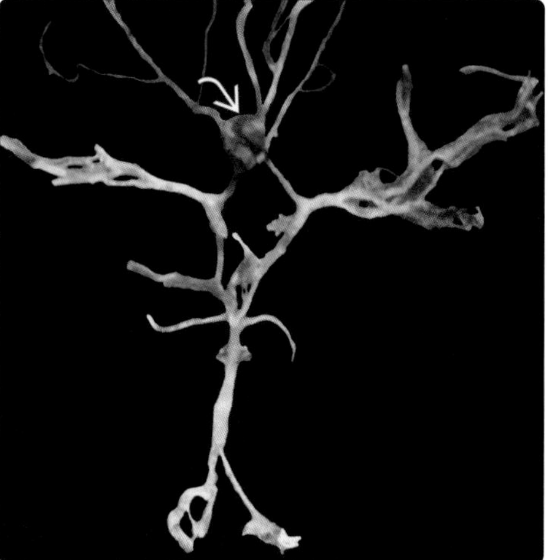

***(6-5)** Autopsy after ACoA aneurysm ➡ ruptured, causing aSAH, shows diffuse vasospasm.*

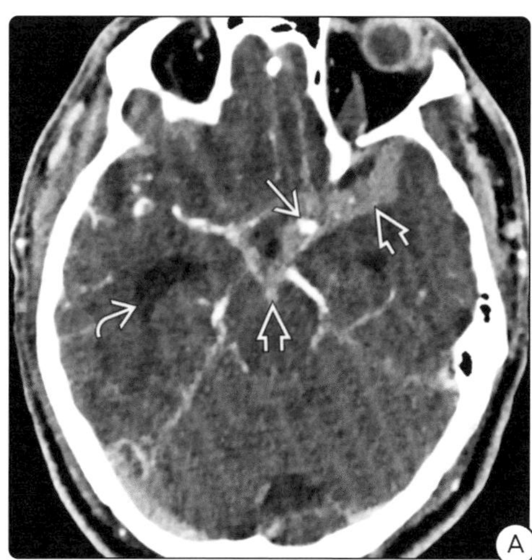

***(6-6A)** CTA in "thunderclap" headache shows aSAH ➡ and 8-mm bilobed ICA-PCoA aneurysm ➡. Note obstructive hydrocephalus ➡.*

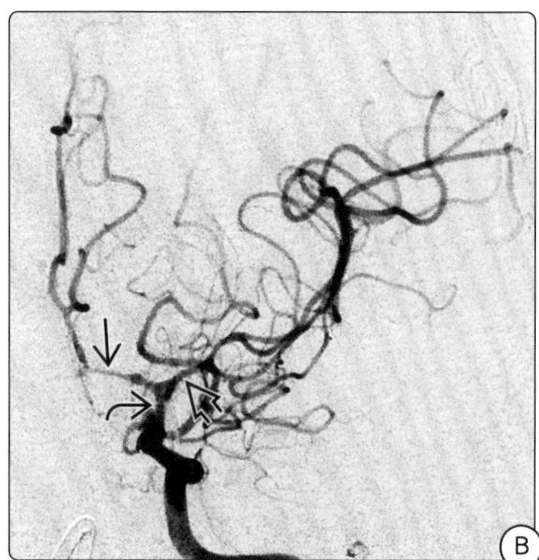

***(6-6B)** DSA 4 days after clipping shows moderate vasospasm involving the distal ICA ➡, proximal A1 ➡, and M1 ➡ segments.*

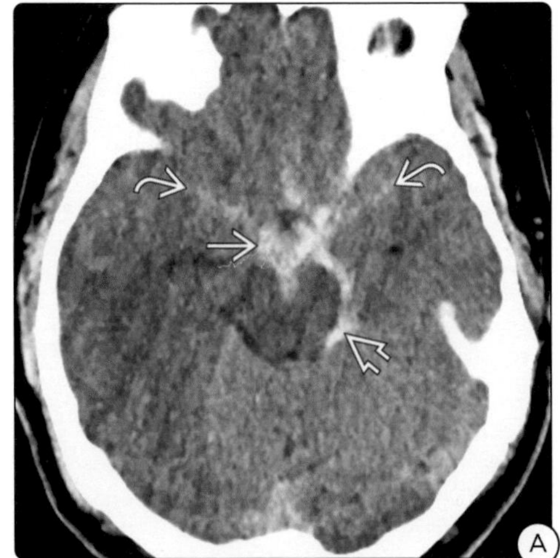

*(6-7A) Hyperdense SAH fills the suprasellar cistern ➡, extends into both sylvian fissures ➡ and around the midbrain ➡.*

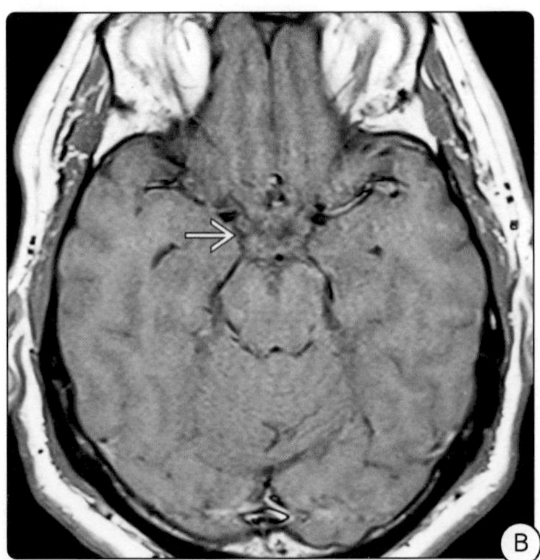

*(6-7B) T1WI shows the suprasellar cistern is filled with acute blood ➡, which, instead of CSF-like, is virtually isointense with brain.*

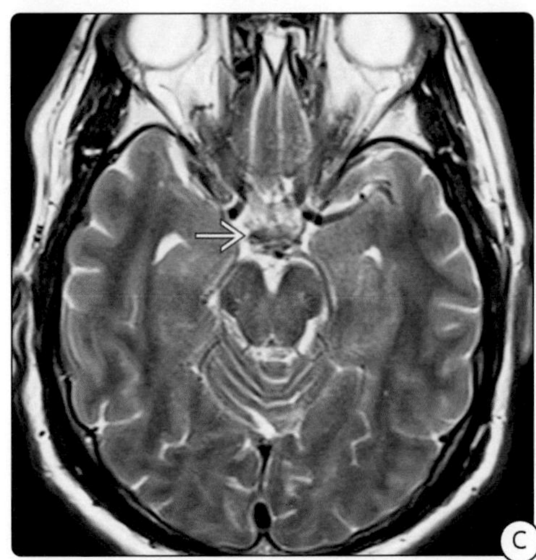

*(6-7C) The acute suprasellar hemorrhage is hypointense compared to normal CSF on T2WI ➡. No aneurysm was found on CTA and DSA.*

**MR Findings.** Acute aSAH is isointense with brain on T1WI **(6-7B)** **(6-8C)**. The CSF cisterns may appear smudged or "dirty" **(6-8D)**. Hyperacute aSAH is isointense with CSF and may be difficult to identify. Acute aSAH is generally hypointense relative to CSF on T2WIs **(6-7C)** **(6-8E)**.

FLAIR is the best sequence to depict acute aSAH. Hyperintensity in the sulci and cisterns is present **(6-8F)** but nonspecific. Other causes of "bright" CSF on FLAIR include hyperoxygenation, meningitis, neoplasm, and artifact.

**Angiography.** CTA is positive in 93% of aSAH cases if the "culprit" aneurysm is 3 mm or larger **(6-6A)**. The addition of 3D postprocessing tools can improve detection of small saccular or BBAs on CTA.

Many patients with aSAH and positive CTA undergo surgical clipping without DSA. DSA identifies vascular pathology in 7-13% of patients with CTA-negative SAH, so such patients should be considered candidates for DSA.

So-called angiogram-negative SAH is found in ~ 15% of cases **(6-8)**. With the addition of 3D rotational angiography and 3D shaded surface displays, the rate of "angiogram-negative" SAH decreases to 4-5% of cases. If the initial DSA is negative, many experts recommend repeat angiography in 2-4 weeks to exclude aneurysm as the cause of the SAH.

### IMAGING OF ANEURYSMAL SUBARACHNOID HEMORRHAGE

**NECT**
- Hyperdense basal cisterns, sulci
- Hydrocephalus common, onset often early

**MR**
- "Dirty" CSF on T1WI
- Hyperintense cisterns, sulci on FLAIR

**Angiography**
- CTA positive in 95% if aneurysm ≥ 2 mm
- DSA reserved for complex aneurysm, CTA negative
- "Angiogram-negative" SAH (15%; 5% if 3D used)
- Repeat "2nd look" DSA positive (5%)

## Differential Diagnosis

The major differential diagnosis of aSAH is **traumatic SAH (tSAH)**. aSAH is generally much more widespread, often filling the basal cisterns. tSAH typically occurs adjacent to cortical contusions or lacerations and is therefore most common in the superficial sulci.

**Perimesencephalic nonaneurysmal SAH** (pnSAH) is much more limited than aSAH and is localized to the interpeduncular, ambient, and prepontine cisterns. Occasionally, pnSAH spreads into the posterior aspect of the suprasellar cistern. It rarely extends into the sylvian fissures.

**Convexal SAH (cSAH)** is, as the name implies, localized to superficial sulci over the cerebral convexities. Often, only a single sulcus is affected. Causes of cSAH are numerous and include cortical vein occlusion, amyloid angiopathy, vasculitis, and RCVS.

**Pseudo-SAH** is caused by severe cerebral edema. The hypodensity of the brain makes blood in the cerebral arteries and veins appear dense, mimicking the appearance of SAH.

**Sulcal-cisternal FLAIR hyperintensity** on MR is a nonspecific imaging finding. It occurs with hemorrhage, meningitis, carcinomatosis, hyperoxygenation, stroke, and gadolinium contrast (blood-brain barrier

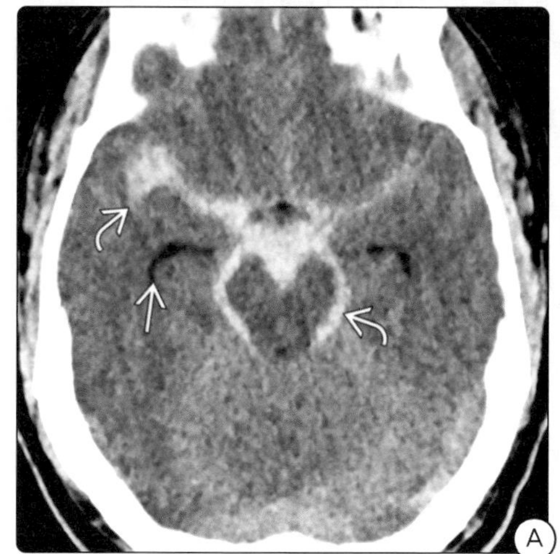

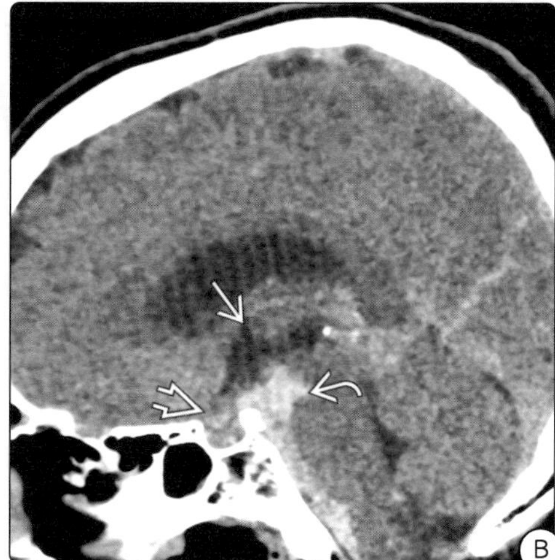

***(6-8A)** NECT in a 58-yo man with "thunderclap" headache shows typical pattern of aSAH filling the basal cisterns, sylvian fissures ➡. Early obstructive hydrocephalus ➡ is present. **(6-8B)** Sagittal reformatted NECT shows iso- ➡ and hyperdense ➡ blood filling the suprasellar, interpeduncular, and prepontine cisterns. Note contrast with normal low-density CSF in the 3rd ventricle ➡.*

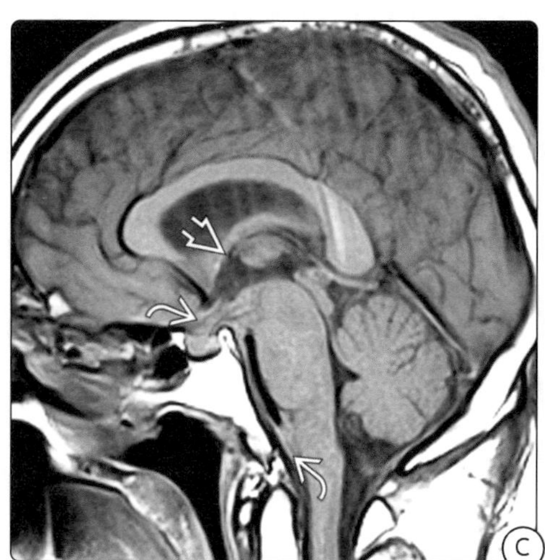

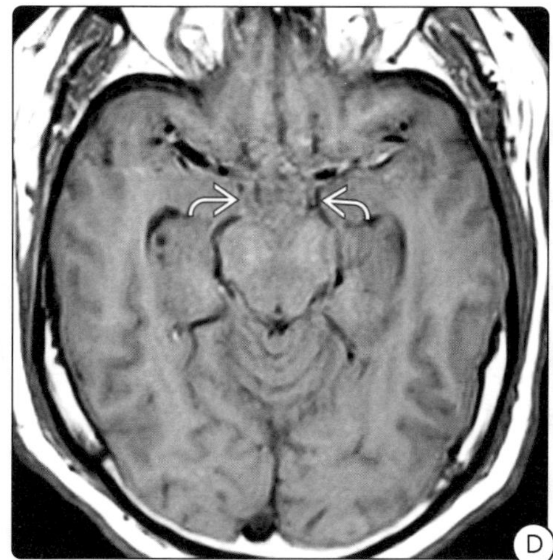

***(6-8C)** Because CTA and DSA were negative, MR was obtained several hours later. Sagittal T1WI shows that "dirty" CSF ➡ surrounds basilar artery "flow void" and is nearly isointense with adjacent brain. Note contrast with normal hypointense CSF in the 3rd ventricle ➡. **(6-8D)** Axial T1WI MR shows that the suprasellar cistern is filled with "dirty" CSF ➡ that is nearly isointense with the surrounding brain.*

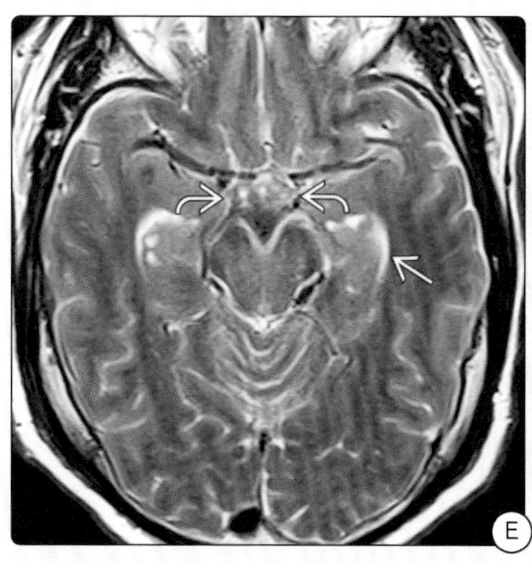

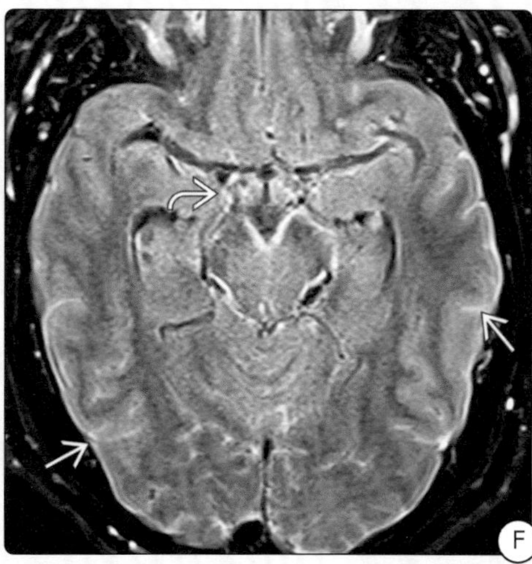

***(6-8E)** T2WI MR shows that CSF in the suprasellar cistern is hypointense ➡, as it is mixed with acute hemorrhage. Note contrast with normal hyperintense CSF in the temporal horns of the lateral ventricles ➡. **(6-8F)** CSF in the suprasellar cistern exhibits incomplete suppression on FLAIR ➡. Note hyperintense, nonsuppressing fluid in the superficial sulci from the SAH ➡.*

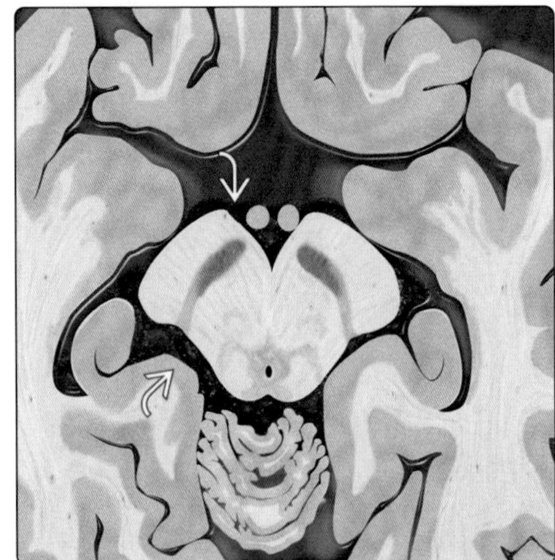
(6-9) In pnSAH, hemorrhage is confined to the interpeduncular fossa and ambient (perimesencephalic) cisterns ➪.

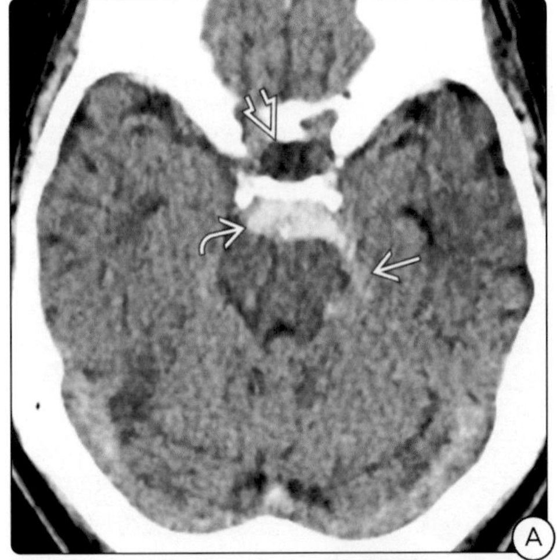
(6-10A) Axial NECT shows pnSAH with blood in the prepontine ➪, left lateral mesencephalic ➪ cisterns. Suprasellar ➪ cistern is normal.

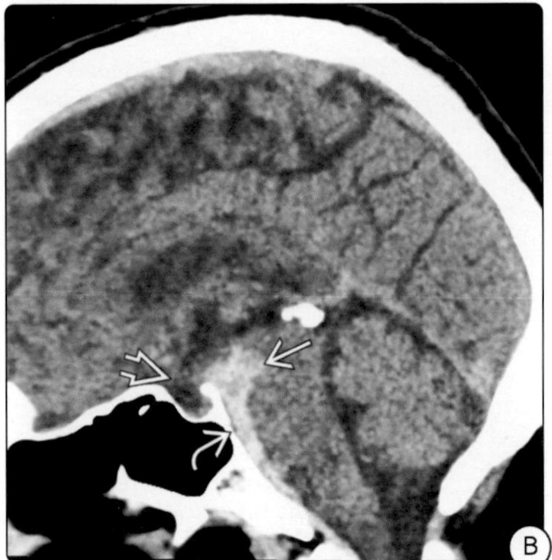
(6-10B) Sagittal NECT shows prepontine ➪, interpeduncular ➪ blood. Anterior suprasellar cistern is clear ➪. DSA was negative. pnSAH.

leakage or chronic renal failure). FLAIR "bright" CSF can also result from flow disturbances and technical artifacts (e.g., incomplete CSF nulling).

Pyogenic meningitis, meningeal carcinomatosis, and high inspired oxygen concentration may also cause CSF hyperintensity on FLAIR. Prior administration of gadolinium chelates (with or without decreased renal clearance) can result in diffuse delayed CSF enhancement.

Other etiologies of sulcal-cisternal FLAIR hyperintensity include hyperintense vessels with slow flow (e.g., acute arterial strokes, pial collaterals developing after cerebral ischemia-infarction, Sturge-Weber syndrome, moyamoya, and RCVS).

## Post Aneurysmal Subarachnoid Hemorrhage Cerebral Ischemia and Vasospasm

Published data suggests delayed cerebral ischemia affects 20-40% of patients who survive their initial SAH and is the major cause of morbidity and death in this group. Cerebral vasospasm (CVS) is the most common cause of cerebral ischemia and typically occurs 4-10 days after aSAH **(6-5)**. Recent studies have also shown that inflammation and microthromboembolism also contribute significantly to ischemic complications following aSAH.

### Imaging Post Aneurysmal Subarachnoid Hemorrhage Complications

Noninvasive methods to detect early-stage post-aSAH complications include transcranial Doppler ultrasound, CTA, and MR/MRA. Multiple segments of vascular constriction and irregularly narrowed vessels are typical findings on CTA and DSA **(6-6)**. MR with DWI and pMR is most sensitive for detecting early ischemic changes following aSAH.

DSA is typically performed if endovascular treatment or intraarterial administration of antispasmolytic agents, such as nicardipine, is anticipated.

### Differential Diagnosis

The differential diagnosis of vasospasm within the context of existing SAH is limited. If the patient has a known aneurysm with recent SAH, the findings of multisegmental vascular narrowing indicate CVS. However, if the SAH is convexal, the differential diagnosis includes **RCVS** and **vasculitis**.

## Other Complications of Aneurysmal Subarachnoid Hemorrhage

**Obstructive hydrocephalus** commonly develops in patients with aSAH, sometimes within hours of the ictus **(6-6A)**, and may be exacerbated by the presence of IVH. Imaging studies show increased periventricular extracellular fluid with "blurred" lateral ventricle margins.

## Perimesencephalic Nonaneurysmal Subarachnoid Hemorrhage

### Terminology

pnSAH is also known as benign perimesencephalic SAH. pnSAH is a clinically benign SAH subtype that is anatomically confined to the perimesencephalic and prepontine cisterns **(6-9)**.

### Etiology

The precise etiology of pnSAH is unknown, although recent studies suggest it can be triggered by physical exertion in nearly 80% of cases. The bleeding source in pnSAH is usually undetermined; most investigators implicate venous—not aneurysmal—rupture as the most likely cause.

### Clinical Issues

pnSAH is the most common cause of nontraumatic, nonaneurysmal SAH. The typical presentation is mild to moderate headache. Occasionally, patients experience severe "thunderclap" headache with meningismus.

The peak age of presentation in patients with pnSAH is between 40-60 years—identical to that of aSAH. There is no sex predilection.

Most cases of pnSAH follow a clinically benign and uneventful course, although MR demonstrates acute—and usually asymptomatic—ischemic lesions in nearly 1/2 of all cases. Rebleeding is uncommon (< 1%). In contrast to aSAH, vasospasm and delayed cerebral ischemia are rare.

### Imaging

pnSAH has well-defined imaging features. NECT scans show focal accumulation of subarachnoid blood around the midbrain (in the interpeduncular and perimesencephalic cisterns) **(6-10)** and in front of the pons. High-resolution CTA is used to rule out underlying aneurysm or dissection **(6-11)**. If the initial CTA is negative, there is no significant additional diagnostic yield from DSA.

### Differential Diagnosis

The major differential diagnosis of pnSAH is **aSAH**. aSAH is significantly more extensive, spreading throughout the basal cisterns and often extending into the interhemispheric and proximal sylvian fissures.

**tSAH** would be suggested both by history and imaging appearance. tSAH occurs adjacent to contused brain. It is usually more peripheral, lying primarily within the sylvian fissure and over the cerebral convexities. During closed head injury, the midbrain may be suddenly and forcibly impacted against the tentorial incisura. In such cases, the presence of perimesencephalic blood can mimic pnSAH. In contrast to pnSAH, interpeduncular and prepontine hemorrhage is usually absent.

**cSAH** is found over the cerebral convexities, not in the perimesencephalic cisterns. Blood within a single sulcus or immediately adjacent sulci is common.

## Convexal Subarachnoid Hemorrhage

### Terminology

Isolated spontaneous ntSAH that involves the sulci over the brain vertex is called *convexal* or *convexity SAH* (cSAH). cSAH is a unique type of SAH with a very different imaging appearance from either aSAH or pnSAH. True cSAH is confined to the cortical surfaces, sparing the basal and perimesencephalic cisterns without extending into the sylvian or hemispheric fissures **(6-12)**.

### Etiology

A broad spectrum of vascular and even nonvascular pathologies can cause cSAH. These include dural sinus and cortical vein thrombosis (CoVT), arteriovenous malformations, dural arteriovenous fistulas, arterial dissection/stenosis/occlusion, mycotic aneurysm, vasculitides, amyloid

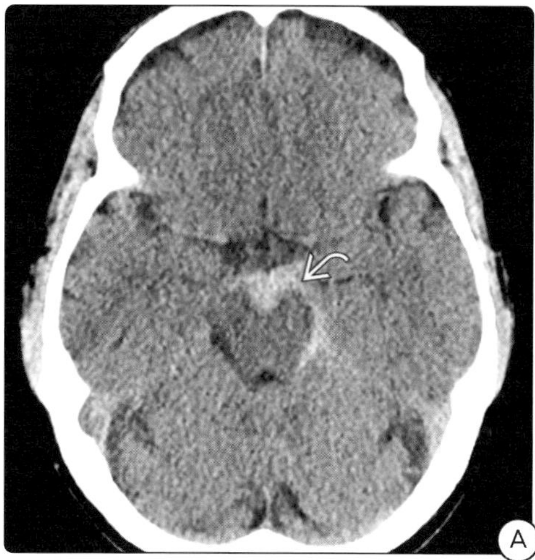


***(6-11A)** NECT in a 64-yo man with "thunderclap" headache after heavy exercise shows classic pnSAH ➡.*

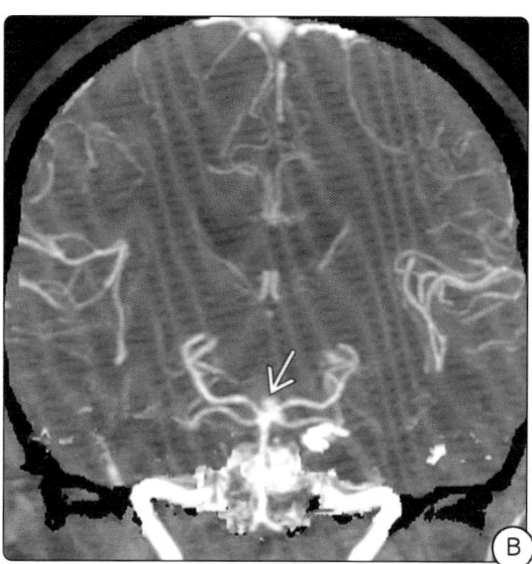


***(6-11B)** Coronal MIP CTA in the same case shows a tiny basilar tip SA ➡.*

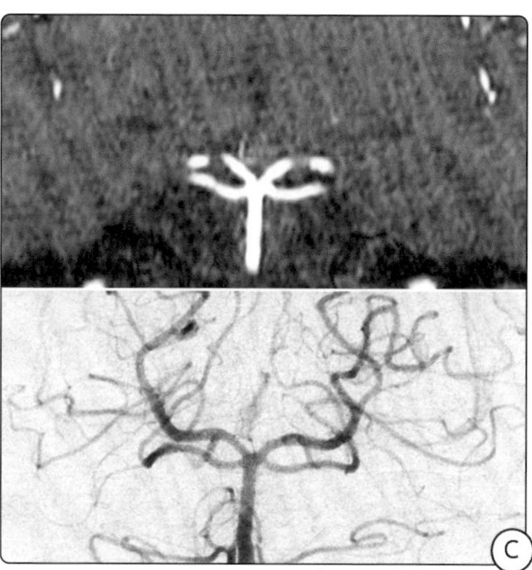


***(6-11C)** Coronal MRA (top), DSA (bottom) 12 hours later show the aneurysm has thrombosed completely. CT/CTA 1 year later was normal.*

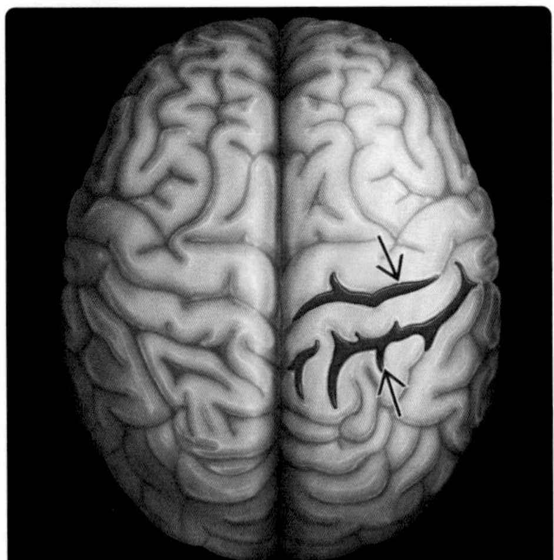

(6-12) Graphic depicts convexal SAH (cSAH) with focal subarachnoid blood ➔ in adjacent sulci along the vertex of the left hemisphere.

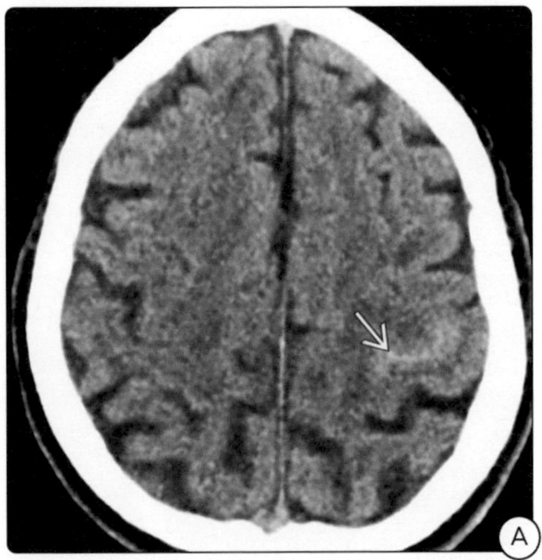


(6-13A) NECT in a 78-yo man with headaches shows subarachnoid blood in a convexity sulcus ➔.

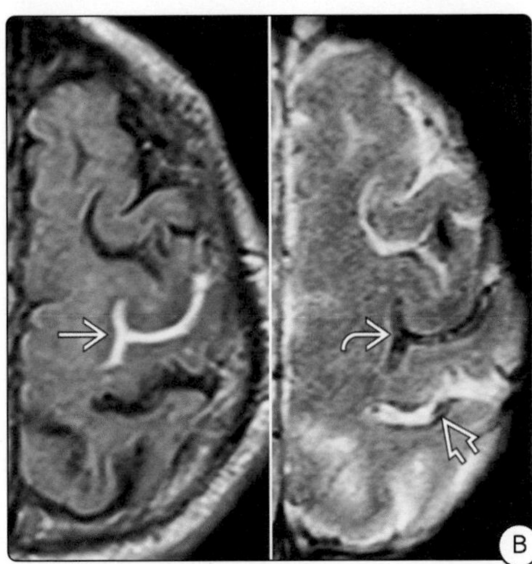


(6-13B) FLAIR (L) shows hyperintensity in the convexity sulcus ➔. T2* (R) shows "blooming" of the hemorrhage ➔ and pial siderosis (CAA) ➔.

angiopathy, coagulopathies, reversible cerebral vasoconstriction syndrome (RCVS), and posterior reversible encephalopathy syndrome (PRES).

Age is a significant predictor of cSAH etiology. In people over 60 years old, cerebral amyloid angiopathy (CAA) is a common cause and the presence of CT-visible cSAH indicates an increased risk for early recurrent ICH. In younger patients, RCVS and PRES are common. Venous occlusions can occur in all age groups. Recent studies show 25% of patients with cerebral venous sinus thrombosis have SAH, mostly in the cerebral convexities.

## Clinical Issues

Although cSAH can occur at virtually any age, most patients are between 4th-8th decades. Peak age is 70 years.

The clinical presentation of cSAH varies with etiology but is quite different from that of aSAH. Most patients with cSAH have nonspecific headache without nuchal rigidity. Some present with focal or generalized seizures or neurologic deficits.

Patients with cSAH secondary to RCVS may present with a "thunderclap" headache. The vast majority are middle-aged women. cSAH caused by venous thrombosis or vasculitis may have milder symptoms with more insidious onset. Mean age of CoVT accompanied by cSAH is 33 years.

### ETIOLOGY OF NONTRAUMATIC CONVEXAL SUBARACHNOID HEMORRHAGE

**Common**
- Reversible cerebral vasoconstriction syndrome (RCVS)
  - Mean age ≈ 50 years
  - Typical presentation = "thunderclap" headache
- Cerebral amyloid angiopathy (CAA)
  - Mean age ≈ 70 years
  - Symptoms = confusion, dementia, sensorimotor dysfunction

**Less Common**
- Endocarditis
- Cortical vein thrombosis ± dural sinus occlusion

**Rare**
- Vasculitis

CAA is the major cause of cSAH in older adult patients. Worsening dementia and headache are the common presentations. cSAH in this age cohort is associated with cognitive impairment and CAA as well as APOE-ε4 overrepresentation compared with age-matched health controls. Between 40-45% experience recurrent cSAH and subsequent lobar hemorrhage (see Chapter 10).

The outcome of cSAH *itself* is generally benign and depends primarily on underlying etiology. Vasospasm and DCI are rare.

## Imaging

**CT Findings.** Most cases of cSAH are unilateral, involving one **(6-13A)** or several dorsolateral convexity sulci. The basal cisterns are typically spared.

**MR Findings.** Focal sulcal hyperintensity on FLAIR is typical in cSAH **(6-13B)**. T2* (GRE, SWI) shows "blooming" in the affected sulci **(6-16C)**. If the etiology of the cSAH is dural sinus or cortical vein occlusion, a hypointense "cord" sign may be present. Patients with CAA have multifocal cortical and pial microbleeds ("blooming black dots") on T2*. They may also show evidence of siderosis and prior lobar hemorrhages of differing ages.

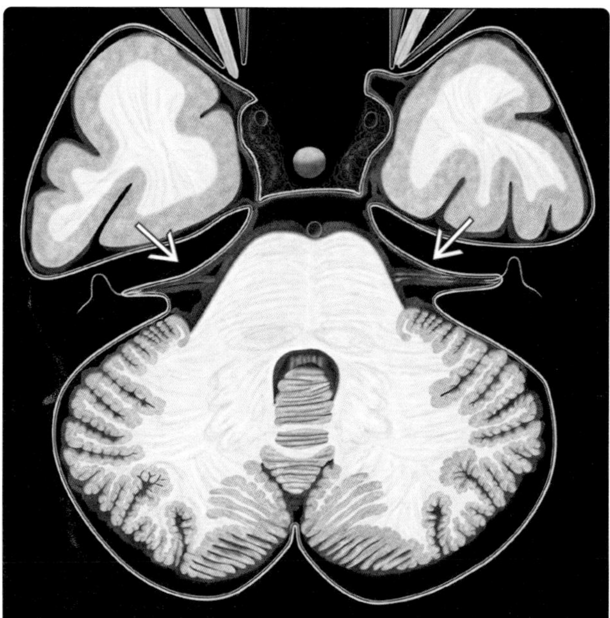

(6-14) Graphic of superficial siderosis shows darker brown hemosiderin staining on surfaces of the brain, meninges, cranial nerves. Notice that CNVII and CNVIII in the CPA-IAC ➡ are particularly affected.

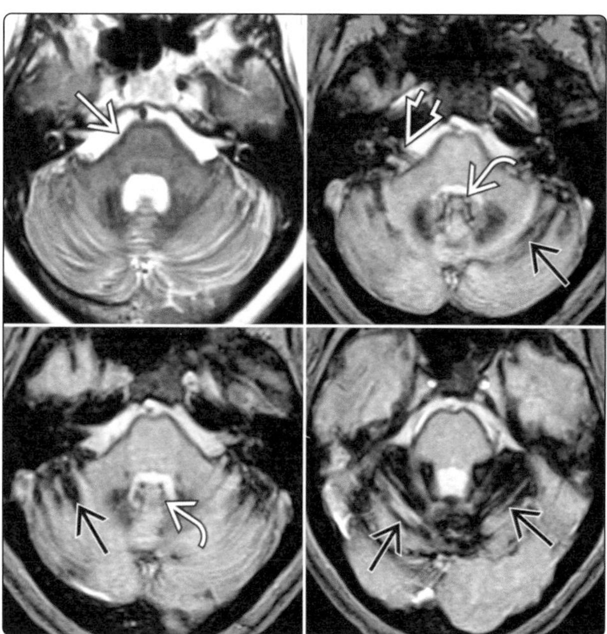

(6-15) FSE T2 shows hypointensity around pons, cerebellum ➡. T2* shows "blooming" along pons, cerebellar hemispheres ➡. Note siderosis along CNVII, CNVIII ➡, hemosiderin deposition in the choroid plexus of the 4th ventricle ➡. cSS.

**NONTRAUMATIC SUBARACHNOID HEMORRHAGE: ANEURYSMAL VS. NONANEURYSMAL**

**Aneurysmal Subarachnoid Hemorrhage**
- Widespread; basal cisterns
- Arterial origin
- Complications (vasospasm, ischemia) common

**Perimesencephalic Nonaneurysmal Subarachnoid Hemorrhage**
- Focal; perimesencephalic, prepontine cisterns
- Probably venous origin
- Clinically benign; complications, recurrence rare

**Convexal Subarachnoid Hemorrhage**
- Superficial (convexity) sulci
- ≥ 60 years? Think CAA!
- ≤ 60 years? Think RCVS!
- All ages: Venous occlusions, vasculitis

## Superficial Siderosis

### Terminology

Linear hemosiderin deposition along brain surfaces, cranial nerves, &/or the spinal cord defines the condition known as **superficial siderosis (SS)** **(6-14)**. There are two subtypes of siderosis that are distinguished by their anatomic distribution, causes and clinical features: Classic or infratentorial SS and cortical SS.

**"Classic" SS** of the CNS primarily affects the infratentorial regions and spinal cord. Classic *infratentorial* SS sometimes also affects the supratentorial regions.

The term **"cortical" SS** (cSS) describes a distinct pattern of iron-bearing blood-breakdown product deposition limited to cortical sulci over the convexities of the cerebral hemispheres. In *cortical* SS, the brainstem, cerebellum, and spinal cord are spared.

### Etiology

SS is a consequence of chronic intermittent or continuous minor hemorrhage into the subarachnoid space. Trauma and surgery are the most common causes of classic SS. Other reported etiologies include hemorrhagic neoplasm, vascular malformations, venous obstruction(s) and intracranial hypotension with spinal CSF leaks, including CSF-venous fistulae. SS due to repeated aSAH is relatively uncommon.

Cortical SS has many potential causes, but, in older individuals, cortical SS is most often associated with CAA.

### Pathology

**Location.** Although it can occur anywhere in the CNS, *classic* SS has a predilection for the posterior fossa (cerebellar folia and vermis, CNVIII) and brainstem.

*Cortical* SS is seen in 60% of patients with CAA but is rare in non-CAA forms of intracerebral hemorrhages.

**Gross Pathology.** Brownish yellow and blackish gray encrustations cover the affected structures, layering along the sulci and encasing cranial nerves.

### Clinical Issues

Patients with classic SS often present with slowly progressive gait ataxia, dysarthria, and bilateral sensorineural hearing loss.

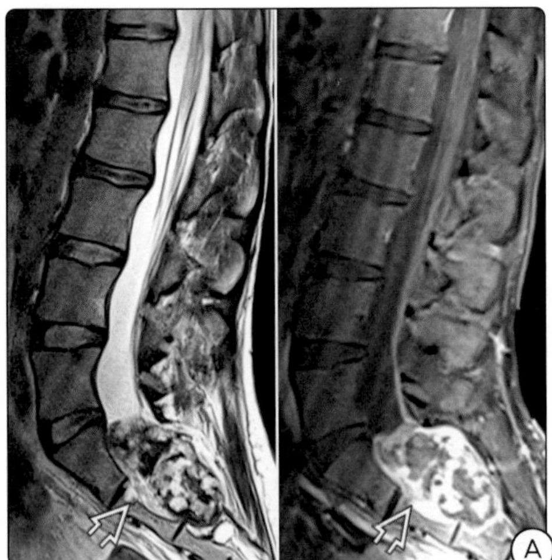

***(6-16A)** (L) T2WI and (R) T1 C+ in a 30-yo man with severe back pain shows enhancing hemorrhagic intradural mass ➲ in distal spine.*

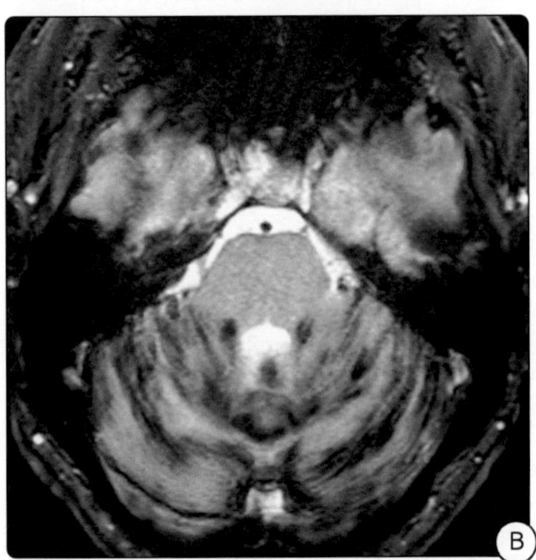

***(6-16B)** T2* GRE in the same case shows extensive classic siderosis over the cerebellar hemispheres and vermis.*

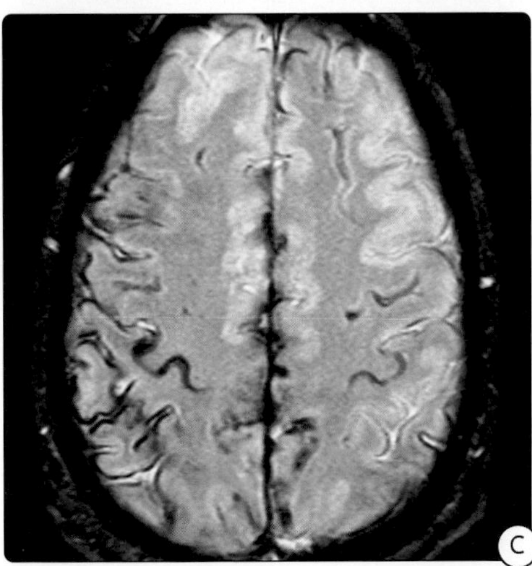

***(6-16C)** T2* GRE through the vertex shows extensive bilateral cSS.*

Some patients present with progressive myelopathy. Often, decades pass between the putative event that causes SS and the development of overt symptoms.

As cortical SS most commonly occurs in the setting of CAA, progressive dementia and cognitive decline are common.

In contrast, a rare, relatively "acute" rapidly progressive SS syndrome can present as a consequence of ongoing and extensive intracranial hemorrhages.

## Imaging

CT is usually normal in patients with SS.

SS on MR is best identified on T2* (GRE, SWI) imaging and is seen as a hypointense rim that follows along brain surfaces and coats the cranial nerves &/or spinal cord **(6-15)** **(6-16)**. A characteristic bilinear track-like appearance is common with cortical SS **(6-13B)**.

Despite extensive neuroimaging, the source of the SS often remains occult. In 50% of classic SS, a hemorrhage source is never identified despite extensive investigation of the entire neuraxis.

## Differential Diagnosis

The major imaging mimic of classic SS is **"bounce point" artifact**, which makes the posterior fossa surfaces appear artifactually dark.

Most cortical SS mimics contain deoxygenated blood or blood products. **Cerebral veins** appear markedly hypointense on SWI but do not run parallel to the convexity sulci. Slow flow in sulcal arteries (pial collaterals in stroke or moyamoya) can appear hypointense on SWI as well.

In Sturge-Weber syndrome, hypointensity due to gyriform calcifications may be linear and cortical but can be easily identified on NECT and T1 C+ MR. Rare causes of cortical SS include **hemorrhagic subarachnoid metastases, neurocutaneous melanosis** (hyperintense on T1WI), and **meningioangiomatosis** (thickened enhancing, sometimes calcified and infiltrating proliferations of meningeal cells and blood vessels).

### SUPERFICIAL SIDEROSIS

**Classic Superficial Siderosis**

- Posterior fossa
  - Occasionally affects supratentorial areas
- Brain (typically cerebellum), cranial nerves coated with hemosiderin
- Chronic repeated SAH
- May occur with spinal dural leaks, including CSF-venous fistulae
- Cause undetermined in ≈ 50%
- Sensorineural hearing loss

**Cortical Superficial Siderosis**

- Cortex over hemisphere convexities
  - Posterior fossa typically spared
- Most common etiology = CAA
- Transient focal neurologic episodes
- Parallel track-like hypointensities on T2*
- High risk of future intracerebral hemorrhage
- Lobar hemorrhages, microbleeds

# Aneurysms

## Overview

Intracranial aneurysms are classified by their gross phenotypic appearance. The most common intracranial aneurysms are called **saccular** or **"berry" aneurysms** because of their striking sac- or berry-like configuration **(6-17)**. Saccular aneurysms (SAs) are acquired lesions that arise from branch points of major cerebral arteries in which hemodynamic stresses are maximal. SAs lack some of the arterial layers (usually the internal elastic lamina and media) found in normal vessels. More than 90% of SAs occur on the "anterior" (carotid) circulation **(6-18)**.

**Pseudoaneurysms (PSAs)** (also sometimes called "false" aneurysms) are focal arterial dilatations that are not contained by any layers of the normal arterial wall. They are often irregularly shaped and typically consist of a paravascular, noncontained blood clot that cavitates and communicates with the parent vessel lumen. Extracranial PSAs are more common than intracranial lesions. Intracranial PSAs usually arise from mid-sized arteries distal to the circle of Willis. Trauma, drug abuse, infection, and tumor are the usual etiologies.

**Blood blister-like aneurysms** (BBAs) are a special type of aneurysm recently recognized in the neurosurgical literature. BBAs are eccentric hemispherical arterial outpouchings that are covered by only a thin layer of adventitia. These dangerous lesions are both difficult to detect and difficult to treat. They have a tendency to rupture at a much smaller size and relatively younger age compared with SAs. Although BBAs can be found anywhere, they have a distinct propensity to occur along the supraclinoid ICA.

**Fusiform aneurysms** (FAs) are *focal* dilatations that involve the entire circumference of a vessel and extend for relatively short distances. FAs are more common on the vertebrobasilar ("posterior") circulation. FAs can be atherosclerotic (more common) or nonatherosclerotic in origin. Nonatherosclerotic FAs (nASVD FAs) are often associated with collagen-vascular disorders, such as Marfan or Ehlers-Danlos type IV.

## Saccular Aneurysm

### Terminology

Saccular ("berry") aneurysms (SAs) are sometimes called "true" aneurysms (to contrast them with PSAs).

An SA is a pathologic outward bulge that affects only part of the parent artery circumference. Most SAs lack two important structural components of normal intracranial arteries—the internal elastic lamina and the muscular layer ("media")—and often have a focally thinned wall that is prone to rupture.

### Etiology

**General Concepts.** Very few SAs are congenital (i.e., present at birth). SAs are *acquired* lesions that develop from abnormal extracellular matrix (ECM) maintenance and excessive hemodynamic stress. SA formation begins with endothelial dysfunction followed by inflammatory cascades, pathologic remodeling, and degenerative changes in vessel walls.

**Genetics.** Modeling studies have shown a distinct familial predisposition to forming SAs. Persons with first-degree relatives with known aSAH are at risk for developing unruptured intracranial aneurysms. Aneurysm risk at five years is 2-12%, 4-28% at 10 years and 7-40% at 15 years.

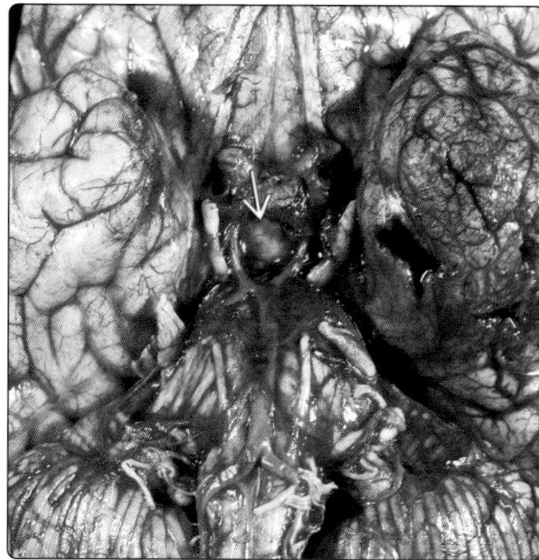

***(6-17)** Ruptured basilar bifurcation aneurysm ➡ has massive SAH extending throughout all the basilar cisterns. (Courtesy R. Hewlett, MD.)*

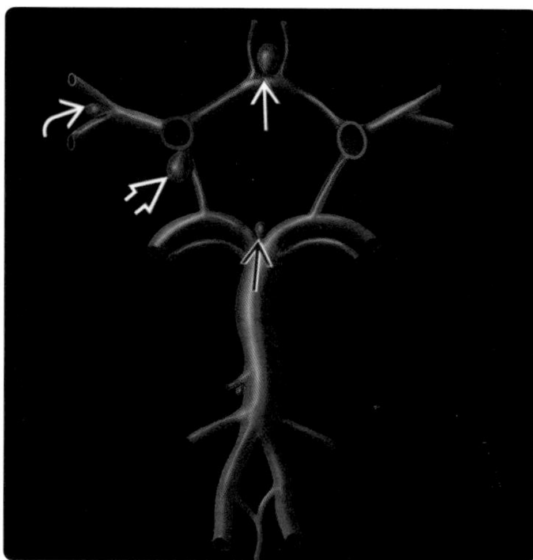

***(6-18)** Common SA sites are ACoA ➡ and the ICA-PCoA junction ➡. Other locations include the MCA bifurcation ➡ and the basilar tip ➡.*

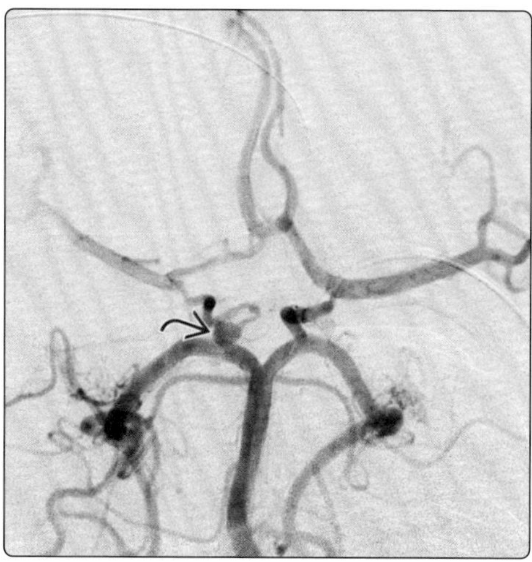

***(6-19)** Submentovertex DSA shows entire circle of Willis. A small SA ➡ arises from the junction of the right PCoA and the P1 PCA segment.*

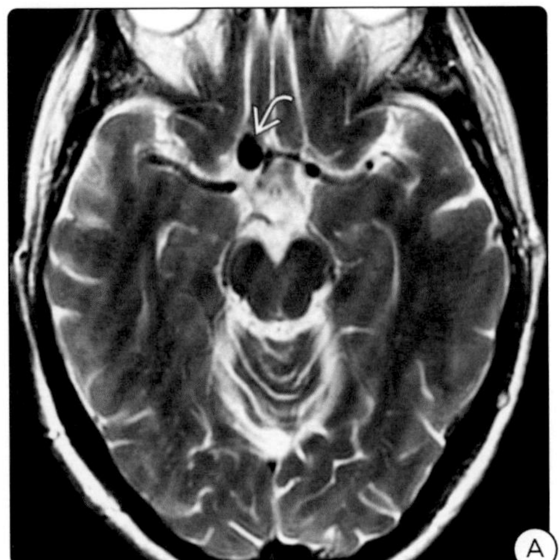

***(6-20A)*** *T2WI in a 70-yo woman shows an unruptured supraclinoid ICA aneurysm* ➢.

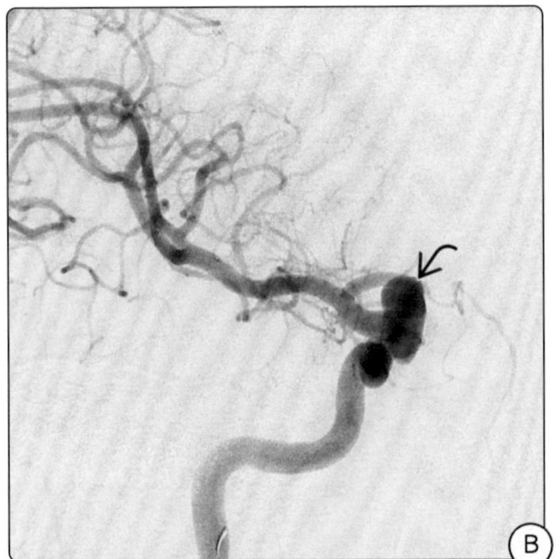

***(6-20B)*** *AP DSA shows the large, lobulated supraclinoid ICA aneurysm* ➢.

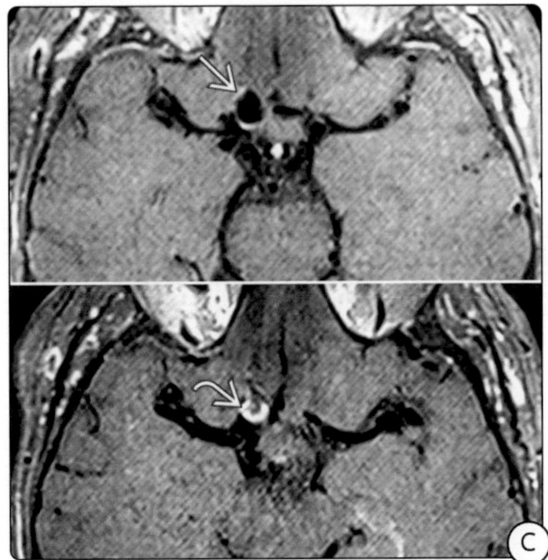

***(6-20C)*** *(Top) Vessel wall imaging shows aneurysm wall enhances* ➢. *(Bottom) 3 months after pipeline stenting, aneurysm* ➢ *is smaller.*

Autosomal dominant polycystic kidney disease (ADPCKD), inherited connective tissue disorders, anomalous blood vessels, familial predisposition, and "high-flow" states (i.e., vessels supplying an arteriovenous malformation) all increase the risk of SA development.

Systemic hypertension, smoking, and heavy alcohol consumption also contribute significantly to the risk of developing SAs and may augment any underlying genetic propensities.

**Anomalous Blood Vessels.** Bicuspid aortic valves, aortic coarctation, persistent trigeminal artery, and congenital anomalies of the anterior cerebral artery (ACA) (i.e., A1 asymmetries or infraoptic course of the A1 segment) all carry an increased risk of SA.

**Inherited Vasculopathies and Syndromic Aneurysms.** Some heritable connective tissue disorders (such as **Marfan** and **Ehlers-Danlos II and IV** syndromes or **fibromuscular dysplasia**) are associated with increased risk of intracranial aneurysms. Arteriopathy—not necessarily with aneurysm formation—is common in patients with **neurofibromatosis type 1** (NF1). **ADPCKD** carries an increased lifetime risk (9-11.5%) of developing an SA, but aneurysm rupture is a rare event (0.04 per 100 patient years).

### SACCULAR ANEURYSM: ETIOLOGY

**General Concepts**
- Acquired, not congenital!
- Abnormal hemodynamics, shear stresses → weakened artery wall
- Underlying genetic alterations common

**Increased Risk of Saccular Aneurysm**
- Anomalous vessels
  - Persistent trigeminal artery
  - Fenestrated anterior communicating artery (ACoA)
- Vasculopathies, syndromes
  - Abnormal collagen (Marfan, Ehlers-Danlos)
  - Fibromuscular dysplasia
  - Autosomal dominant polycystic kidney disease
- Familial intracranial aneurysm
  - 4-10x ↑ risk if 1st-order family member with aSAH

**Familial Intracranial Aneurysms.** A positive family history represents the strongest known risk factor for aSAH (4-10x general population). Up to 20% of patients with SAs have a family history of intracranial aneurysms. SAs in "clusters" of related individuals without any known heritable connective tissue disorder are termed **familial intracranial aneurysms** (FIAs).

## Pathology

**Location.** Most intracranial SAs occur at points of maximal hemodynamic stress. The vast majority arise from major blood vessel bifurcations or branches **(6-17)**. The circle of Willis and the MCA bifurcations are the most common sites **(6-18)** **(6-1)**. Aneurysms beyond the circle of Willis are uncommon. Many peripheral aneurysms are actually PSAs secondary to trauma, infection, or tumor.

***Anterior Circulation Aneurysms.*** 90% of SAs occur on the "anterior" circulation **(6-18)**. The anterior circulation consists of the ICA and its terminal branches, the ACA, and MCA. Approximately 1/3 of SAs occur on the ACoA with another 1/3 arising at the junction of the ICA and the PCoA. Approximately 20% of SAs occur at the MCA bi- or trifurcation.

***Posterior Circulation Aneurysms.*** 10% of SAs are located on the vertebrobasilar ("posterior") circulation. The basilar artery bifurcation is the most common site, accounting for ~ 5% of all SAs **(6-17)**. The posterior inferior cerebellar artery is the second most common location.

**Size and Number.** In autopsy studies, the reported prevalence of unruptured SAs across all age groups is 0.3-4%. Minute SAs (< 2 mm), diagnosed microscopically at autopsy, are present in 10-20% of the general population. Recent reviews suggest these minute unruptured SAs occur at a high rate. However, only a few (10%) of these small SAs enlarge to ≥ 2 mm, and 10% of these will eventually rupture within 10 years.

SAs vary in size from tiny (2-3 mm) **(6-19)** to large lesions > 1 cm **(6-21)**. SAs that are ≥ 2.5 cm are called "giant" aneurysms. Between 15-20% of aneurysms are multiple and significantly more common in women.

**Gross Pathology.** The gross configuration of an SA changes with time as the arterial wall is remodeled in response to hemodynamic stresses. As it becomes progressively weakened, the wall begins to bulge outward, forming an SA. The opening (ostium) of an SA can be narrow or broad based. One or more lobules or an apical "tit" may develop. These outpouchings are the most vulnerable rupture site.

**Microscopic Features.** SAs demonstrate a disrupted or absent internal elastic lamina. The smooth muscle cell layer (media) is generally absent. The wall of an SA is usually quite fragile, consisting of intima and adventitia in a degraded ECM. Variable amounts of thrombus and atherosclerotic changes may also be present, especially in larger "giant" SAs. Inflammatory cell infiltration is a histologic hallmark of SAs.

**SACCULAR ANEURYSM: PATHOLOGY**

**Location**
- 90% anterior circulation
  - Circle of Willis, middle cerebral artery (MCA) bifurcation
  - ACoA, internal carotid artery (ICA)/posterior communicating artery (PCoA) junction most common
- 10% posterior circulation (basilar bifurcation)

**Size, Number**
- Tiny (1-2 mm) to giant (≥ 2 cm)
- 15-20% multiple (> 2, F:M = 10:1)

**Gross, Microscopic Features of Saccular Aneurysm Walls**
- Saccular aneurysms lack internal elastic lamina, media
- Variable thrombus
- Inflammatory changes common

## Clinical Issues

**Epidemiology.** Unruptured intracranial aneurysms (UIAs) are found in 3% of the adult population and are increasingly detected due to more frequent cranial imaging. Asymptomatic unruptured SAs are at least 10x more prevalent than ruptured SAs.

**Demographics.** Peak presentation is between 40-60 years of age. There is a definite female predominance, especially with multiple SAs. SAs are rare in children, accounting for < 2% of all cases. Childhood aneurysms lack female predominance and are more often associated with trauma or infection.

**Presentation.** Between 80-90% of all ntSAHs are caused by ruptured SAs. The most common presentation is sudden onset of severe, excruciating headache ("thunderclap" or "worst headache of my life").

Cranial neuropathy is a relatively uncommon presentation of SA. Of these, a pupil-involving CNIII palsy from a PCoA aneurysm is the most common.

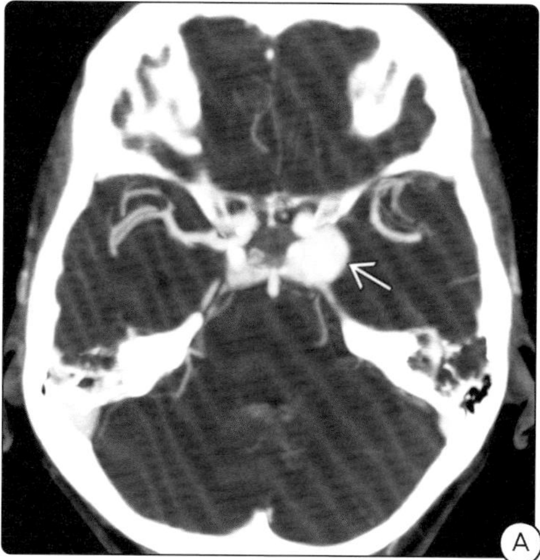


***(6-21A)** MIP of CTA in an 82-yo woman with diplopia shows a well-delineated, intensely enhancing mass ➡ in the left cavernous sinus.*

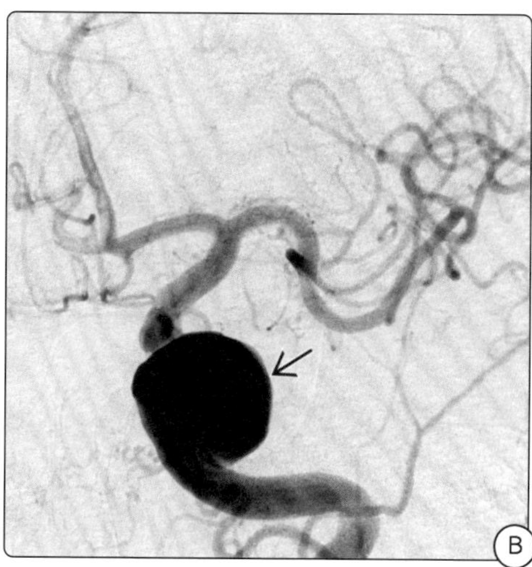


***(6-21B)** Oblique DSA of the left carotid angiogram shows a cavernous ICA aneurysm ➡, but details are difficult to appreciate.*

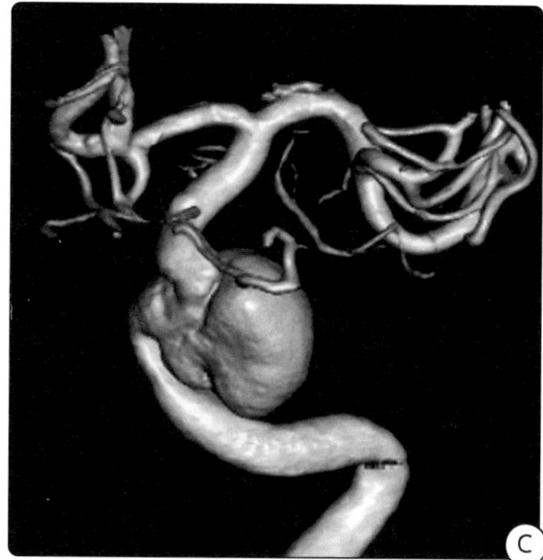


***(6-21C)** 3D rotational DSA with shaded surface display allowed full delineation of the aneurysm and its relationship to the parent vessel.*

***(6-22A)*** *NECT shows a round, well-delineated suprasellar mass causing obstructive hydrocephalus.* ***(6-22B)*** *CT angiogram in the same case shows a large basilar tip aneurysm.*

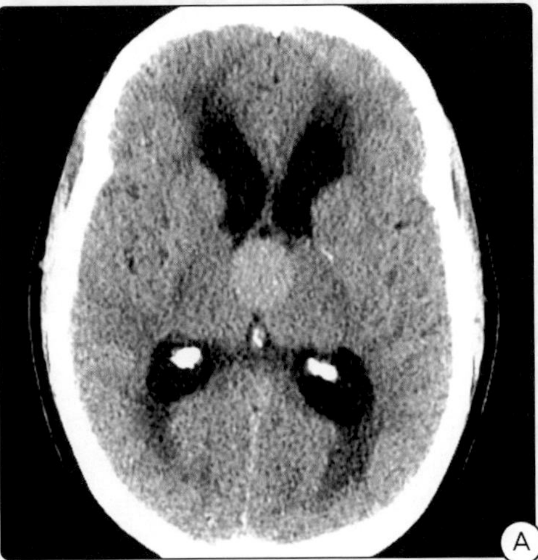
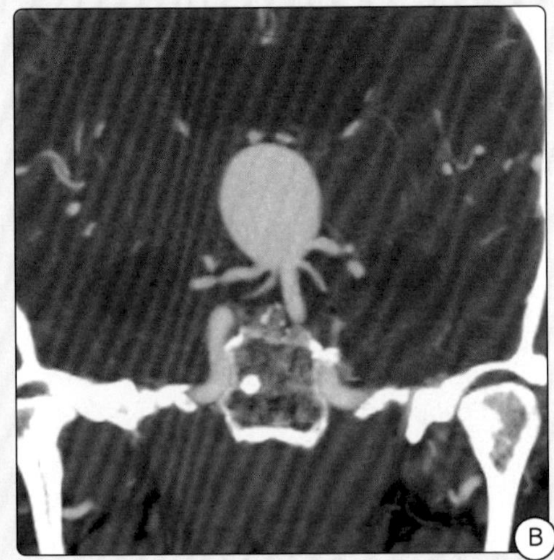

***(6-23)*** *Gross pathology shows mostly thrombosed giant SA. The small patent lumen ➯ is surrounded by concentric rings of various-aged hemorrhages.* ***(6-24A)*** *T1WI shows an enormous mostly thrombosed ACoA aneurysm ➡ containing multiple concentric rings of different-aged hemorrhages with a tiny residual lumen ➯.*

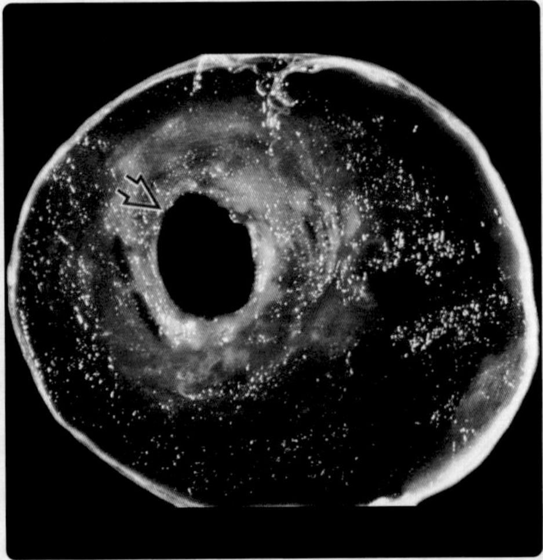
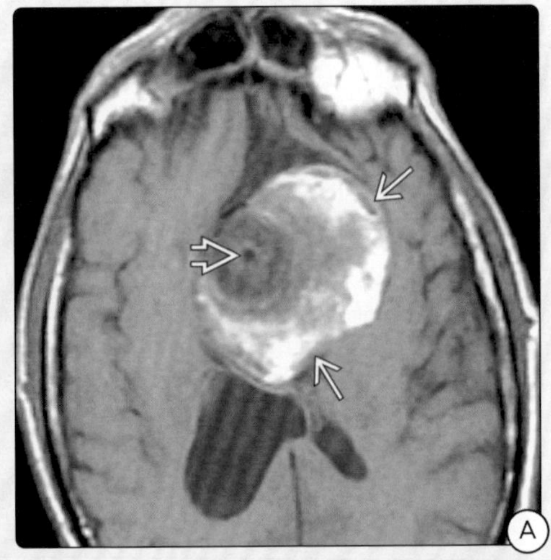

***(6-24B)*** *T2WI in the same case nicely shows the laminated rings of subacute and chronic thrombus.* ***(6-24C)*** *T1 C+ FS shows enhancement ➯ in the small patent lumen of the mostly thrombosed giant SA.*

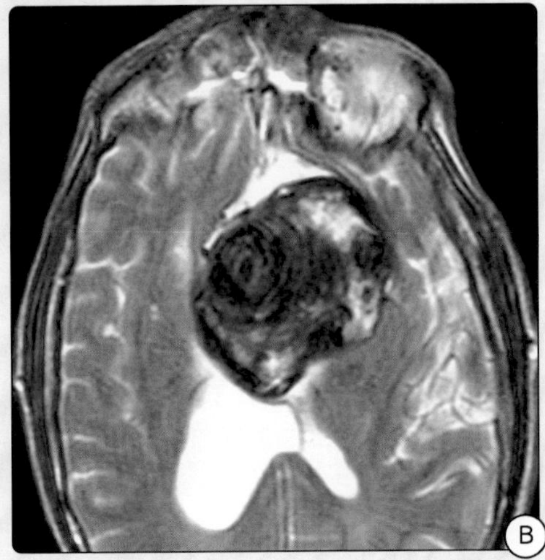
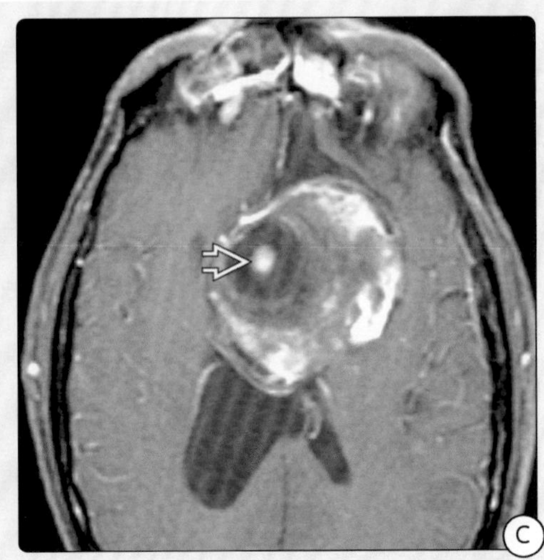

Occasionally, patients with partially or completely thrombosed aneurysms present with a transient ischemic attack (TIA) or stroke.

**Natural History.** The overall annual rupture rate of all SAs is 1-2%. However, the rupture risk varies according to size, location, and shape of the aneurysm.

***Size and Rupture Risk.*** Aneurysms that are ≥ 5 mm are associated with a significantly increased risk of rupture compared with 2- to 4-mm aneurysms. Demonstrable growth on surveillance imaging is also associated with an increased rupture risk.

***Shape/Configuration and Rupture Risk.*** In addition to size, shape and configuration also matter. Nonsaccular (nonspherical) shape increases rupture risk. The presence of a "bleb" (irregular wall protrusion) or elongated aspect ratio (length compared with width) are independent predictors of rupture risk.

Formation of a "bleb" is, in turn, related to the presence of strong and concentrated inflow jets, high speed, complex and unstable flow patterns and heterogeneous wall stress shear patterns. More distorted shapes are also associated with bleb formation.

***Location and Rupture Risk.*** Vertebrobasilar artery aneurysms have a significantly higher rupture risk, as do ICA-PCoA aneurysms. MCA and ACA aneurysms are associated with modest risk. Bifurcation aneurysms are more prone to growth than sidewall aneurysms.

**Treatment Options.** aSAH is a catastrophic event with high mortality and significant morbidity. Approximately 1/3 of patients die and 1/3 survive with significant residual neurologic deficits. Only 1/4-1/3 of patients with aSAH recover with good functional outcome.

***Ruptured SAs.*** Virtually all *ruptured* SAs are treated. Neuroendovascular options, such as coiling (with or without balloon/stent assistance) and flow diversion, are increasingly more common. The percentage of patients with cerebral aneurysms treated with craniotomy and clip ligation is decreasing.

***Unruptured SAs.*** The management of *unruptured* SAs (UIAs) is controversial because of their unpredictable natural history. Initial size and multiplicity are significant factors related to aneurysm growth. Recent studies have shown that the growth rate for 7-mm UIAs is significantly faster than that for < 3-mm UIAs.

**CLINICAL FEATURES OF SACCULAR ANEURYSMS**

**Epidemiology**
- 3% of population; F > M
- Peak age of presentation: 40-60 years (rare in children)

**Presentation**
- Most common = SAH
  - Sudden, severe "thunderclap" headache
  - Mass effect (cranial nerve palsy) less common

**Natural History**
- Most saccular aneurysms do not rupture!
- Incidental finding of saccular aneurysm on imaging increasingly common

**What Increases Risk of Rupture?**
- Size matters!
  - Rupture risk increases with size
  - ≥ 5 mm greater risk than 2-4 mm
- Shape, configuration matter!
  - Nonround (nonsaccular shape) = ↑ rupture risk!
  - "Daughter" sac or "tit" = ↑ rupture risk!
- Location affects rupture risk!
  - Vertebrobasilar, ICA-PCoA location highest rupture risk
  - MCA, anterior cerebral artery (ACA) moderate risk; non-PCoA-ICA aneurysms lowest
- **Type**
  - Blood blister-like aneurysms rupture at smaller size

## Imaging

**General Features.** SAs are round or lobulated arterial outpouchings that are most commonly found along the circle of Willis and at the MCA bifurcation. Imaging features depend on whether the aneurysm is unruptured or ruptured (with aSAH) and whether the aneurysm sac is patent or partially or completely thrombosed.

**CT Findings.** Very small unruptured SAs may be invisible on standard NECT scans. Larger lesions appear as well-delineated masses that are slightly hyperdense to brain **(6-22A)**. Rim or mural calcification may be present.

Acutely ruptured SAs present with aSAH, which is often the dominant imaging feature and frequently obscures the "culprit" aneurysm. Occasionally, an SA appears as a well-delineated, relatively hypodense filling defect within a pool of hyperdense subarachnoid blood.

A partially or completely thrombosed SA is typically hyperdense compared with the adjacent brain on NECT scans.

Patent SAs show strong, uniform enhancement of the aneurysm lumen **(6-22B)**. A partially thrombosed SA shows enhancement of the residual lumen. Completely thrombosed SAs do not enhance, although longstanding lesions may demonstrate rim enhancement secondary to reactive inflammatory changes.

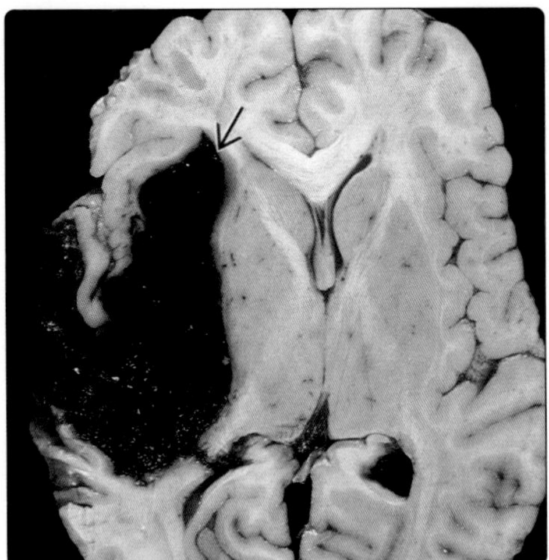

***(6-25)** Large focal right temporal lobe hematoma ⇒ was caused by a ruptured mycotic pseudoaneurysm of the MCA (not shown).*

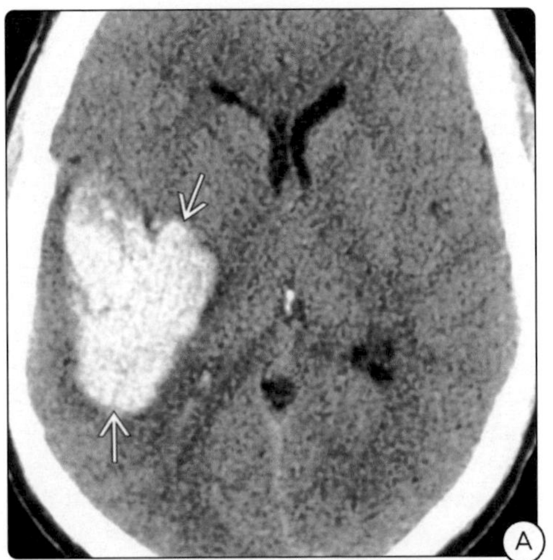

***(6-26A)** NECT shows nontraumatic ICH ➡ in patient with bacterial endocarditis, suggesting mycotic pseudoaneurysm as underlying etiology.*

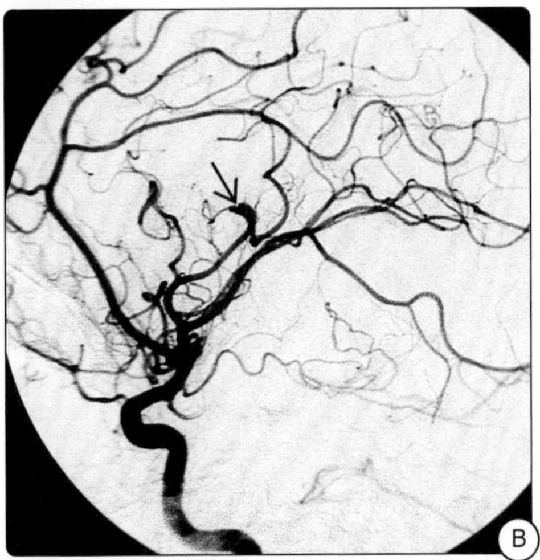

***(6-26B)** DSA demonstrates an irregular fusiform dilatation of an M2 MCA branch ⇒. Mycotic pseudoaneurysm was confirmed at surgery.*

**MR Findings.** MR findings vary with pulse sequence, flow dynamics, and the presence as well as the age of associated hemorrhage (either in the subarachnoid cisterns or within the aneurysm itself).

About 1/2 of all patent SAs demonstrate "flow voids" on T1WI and T2WI **(6-20A)**. The other 1/2 exhibit heterogeneous signal intensity secondary to slow or turbulent flow, saturation effects, and phase dispersion. Propagation of pulsation artifacts in the phase-encoding direction is common. FLAIR scans may show hyperintensity in the subarachnoid cisterns secondary to aSAH.

If the aneurysm is partially or completely thrombosed, laminated clot with differing signal intensities is often present **(6-23)** **(6-24)**. "Blooming" on susceptibility-weighted images (GRE, SWI) is common. Contrast-enhanced scans may show T1 shortening in intraaneurysmal slow-flow areas. High-resolution contrast-enhanced MR may demonstrate inflammatory changes in the aneurysm wall and adjacent brain.

DWI sequences may show ischemic areas secondary to vasospasm or embolized thrombus.

Postcontrast 3DT1 FSE vessel wall imaging emphasizes pathology in the vessel wall itself rather than the vessel lumen. Aneurysm wall enhancement on high spatial resolution "black-blood" sequences, such as DANTE (**d**elay **al**ternating with **n**utation for **t**ailored **e**xcitation), has been associated with instability (i.e., growing or symptomatic aneurysms) **(6-20C)**. Lack of wall enhancement is more predictive of aneurysm stability.

**Angiography.** High-resolution CTA is a common screening procedure in patients with suspected aSAH. The sensitivity of CTA is > 95% for aneurysms > 2 mm in diameter **(6-11B)**.

Deep learning based on a convolutional neural network reports overall sensitivity and positive predictive value for detecting intracranial aneurysms from CTA images are 92.3% and 100%, respectively. Detection sensitivity is closely related to size, diminishing to 66.7% for small aneurysms (≤ 3 mm) while rising to 100% for medium (3-10 mm) and large (> 10 mm) aneurysms.

Although many patients with aSAH and an SA that has been convincingly demonstrated on either CTA or MRA go directly to surgery, conventional DSA is still considered the gold standard for detecting intracranial SAs—especially if endovascular treatment is considered.

Multiple intracranial aneurysms are shown in 15-20% of cases. When more than one aneurysm is identified in aSAH patients, determining which aneurysm ruptured is essential for presurgical planning. Angiographic features suggesting rupture include lobulation or presence of an apical "tit," size (the largest aneurysm is generally, though not always, the one that ruptured), and presence of focal perianeurysmal clot on CT or MR.

## Differential Diagnosis

The major differential diagnosis of intracranial SA is a **vessel loop**. Intracranial arteries curve and branch extensively. CTA/DSA with multiple projections, MIP views, and 3D shaded surface displays are helpful in sorting out overlapping or looping vessels from SA.

The second most common differential diagnosis is an **arterial infundibulum**. An infundibulum is a focal, symmetric, conical dilatation at the origin of a blood vessel that can easily be mistaken for a small SA. An infundibulum is small, typically < 3 mm in diameter. The distal vessel typically arises from the apex—not the side—of the infundibulum. The PCoA is the most common location for an infundibulum.

A **PSA** may be difficult to distinguish from an SA. PSAs are more common on vessels distal to the circle of Willis and are often fusiform or irregular in shape. Focal parenchymal hematomas often surround intracranial PSAs.

A **BBA** may also be difficult to distinguish from a small, wide-necked SA. Although they can be found in virtually any part of the intracranial circulation, BBAs typically arise along the greater curvature of the supraclinoid ICA, not at its terminal bifurcation or PCoA origin.

## Pseudoaneurysm

PSA are complex vascular lesions that are a rare but important underdiagnosed cause of intracranial hemorrhage. PSAs account for just 1-6% of all intracranial aneurysms. Delayed onset and continued deterioration of neurologic symptoms are common.

### Terminology

PSA—also sometimes called a "false" aneurysm to distinguish it from a "true" SA—is an arterial dilatation with complete disruption of the arterial wall. PSAs are classically characterized by disruption of all three vessel wall layers, resulting in a thin-walled paravascular hematoma that communicates directly with the vessel lumen.

### Etiology

PSAs are usually caused by a specific inciting event—e.g., trauma, infection, drug abuse, neoplasm, or surgery—that initially weakens and then disrupts the normal arterial wall. PSAs are contained only by relatively fragile, friable cavitated clot and variable amounts of fibrous tissue.

The defective side wall architecture of PSAs renders them prone to rapid expansion and rupture, often leading to intracerebral hemorrhage and SAH within a few weeks of the inciting event.

### Pathology

**Location.** Approximately 80% of PSAs affecting the carotid and vertebral arteries are extracranial, whereas 20% involve their intracranial segments. Patients with traumatic cavernous/paraclinoid ICA PSAs often have skull base fractures. PSAs distal to the circle of Willis are usually infectious (mycotic), drug related, neoplastic (oncotic), or traumatic in origin.

**Gross Pathology.** PSAs are purplish masses typically contained only by thinned, discontinuous adventitia and organized hematoma. Hematomas associated with PSAs are often large **(6-25)** and may contain clots of varying ages.

### Clinical Issues

As they lack normal vessel wall components, PSAs are especially prone to hemorrhage. The interval between the initial injury and neurologic deterioration varies from a few days up to several months.

Although PSAs account for < 1% of all intracranial aneurysms, they account for nearly 20% of pediatric intracranial aneurysms. Head trauma—direct, closed, or penetrating—accounts for > 60% of cases.

### Imaging

**CT Findings.** A paravascular parenchymal hematoma is common **(6-26)**. CTA sometimes shows a spot sign (focus of contrast enhancement) within a rapidly expanding hematoma **(6-28)**.

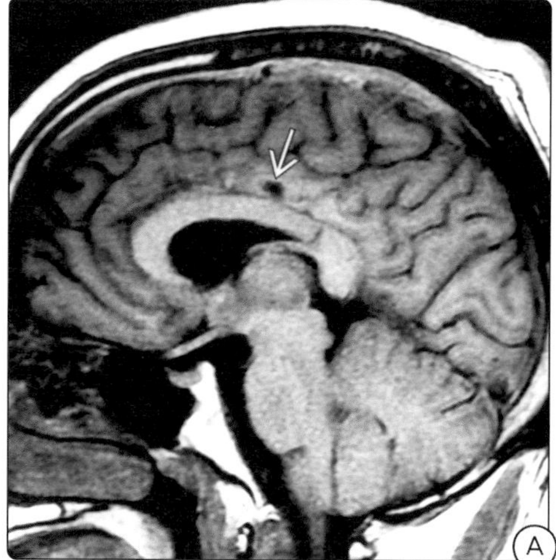


***(6-27A)** Sagittal T1WI in a 23-yo man with headaches, remote history of head trauma shows a "flow void" ➡ above the corpus callosum.*

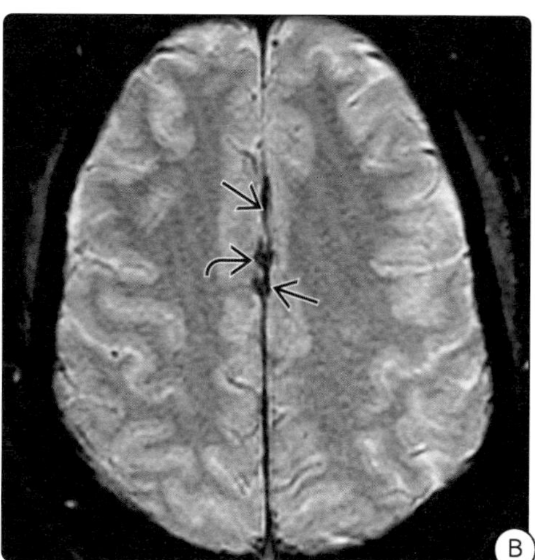


***(6-27B)** T2* GRE shows some hemosiderin staining along the falx cerebri ⇨ adjacent to the flow void ⮕.*

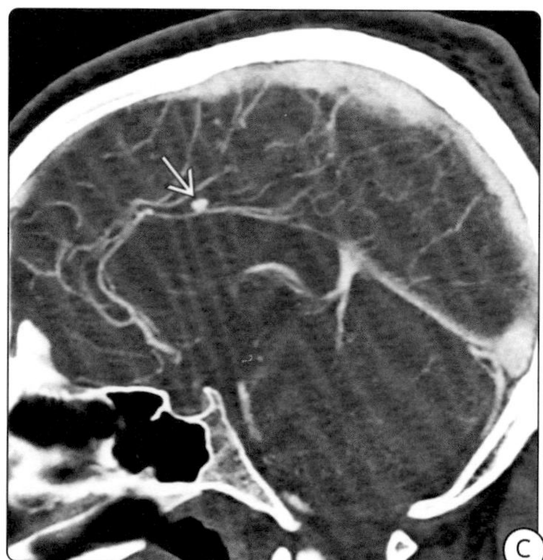


***(6-27C)** Sagittal CTA shows a pericallosal artery pseudoaneurysm ➡. The ACA was impacted against the falx during closed head injury.*

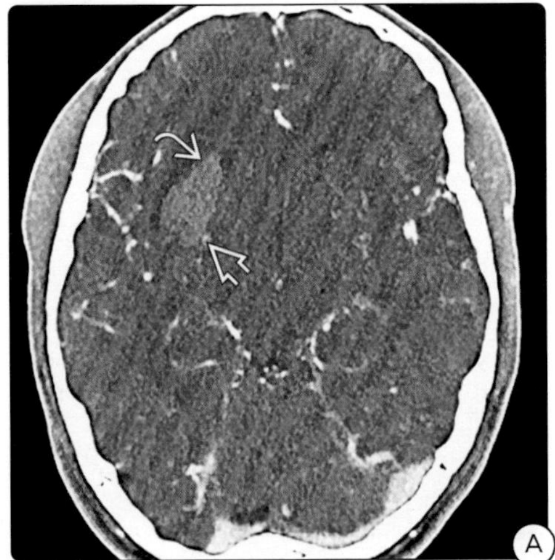

*(6-28A) CTA in an 18-yo male cocaine user with hypertensive stroke shows hematoma ➲, subtle spot sign ➲ adjacent to the hematoma.*

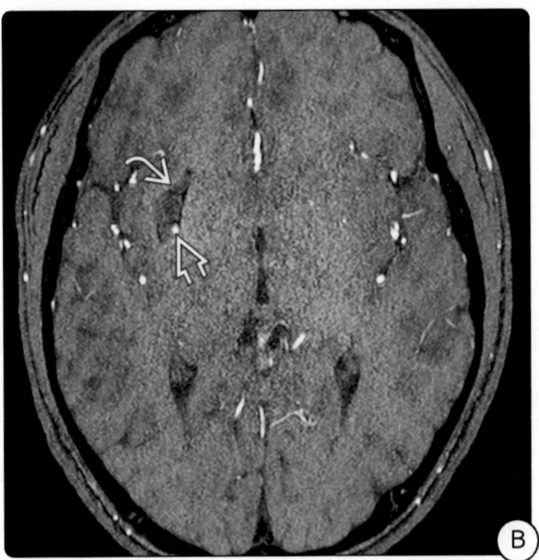

*(6-28B) MRA 2 weeks later shows a rounded vascular-appearing focus ➲ immediately adjacent to the resolving hematoma ➲.*

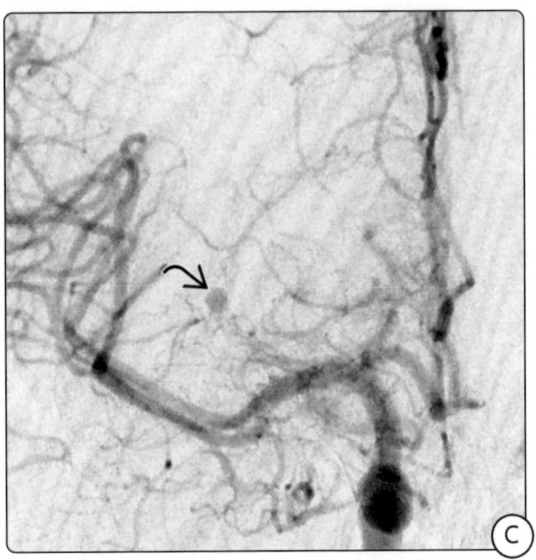

*(6-28C) AP DSA shows a "Charcot-Bouchard" microaneurysm ➲ of the lenticulostriate arteries. This is drug-related pseudoaneurysm.*

**MR Findings.** Hematoma signal varies with clot age and sequence. A "flow void" representing the residual lumen may be present within the hematoma. Intravascular enhancement represents the slow, delayed filling and emptying often seen with PSAs.

**Angiography.** DSA shows a globular, fusiform, or irregularly shaped "neckless" aneurysm with delayed filling and emptying of contrast agent **(6-29)**. Endovascular occlusion with a flow-diverting stent, such as the Pipeline embolization device, is now the method of choice to treat most intracranial PSAs.

## Differential Diagnosis

The major differential diagnosis of PSA is a "true" aneurysm or **SA**. Location is a helpful feature, as SAs typically occur along the circle of Willis and at the MCA bifurcation.

### PSEUDOANEURYSM: IMAGING AND DIFFERENTIAL DIAGNOSIS

**Imaging Features**

- Irregularly shaped outpouching
  - "Neck" usually absent
  - ± surrounding avascular mass effect (cavitated hematoma)
- CTA
  - May show spot sign
  - Pseudoaneurysms often small, easily overlooked
  - DSA may be required if CTA is negative
- MR: Look for distal emboli

**Differential Diagnosis**

- Blood blister-like aneurysm
  - May be form of pseudoaneurysm
- Saccular aneurysm
- Dissecting aneurysm
- Fusiform aneurysm

# Blood Blister-Like Aneurysm

BBA, a.k.a. blister or "dorsal variant blister" aneurysm, is an uncommon but potentially lethal subtype of intracranial PSA. BBAs can be difficult to diagnose and treacherous to treat. They represent ~ 1% of all intracranial aneurysms and 0.5-2.0% of all ruptured aneurysms.

BBAs are small, broad-based hemispheric bulges that typically arise at nonbranching sites of intracranial arteries (most commonly the supraclinoid ICA) **(6-30)**. BBAs have different clinical features and pose special diagnostic and treatment challenges compared with those of typical SAs. Preoperative recognition of a BBA is essential for proper management.

## Pathology

Hemodynamic stress and atherosclerosis seem to be the most important factors in formation of a BBA. BBAs are often covered with only a thin, fragile fibrin layer or a friable cap of fibrous tissue. Although BBAs can arise anywhere in the intracranial circulation, the anterosuperior (dorsal) wall of the supraclinoid ICA is the most common site.

## Clinical Issues

BBAs exhibit more aggressive behavior compared with SAs. They tend to rupture at an earlier patient age and at a significantly smaller size compared with typical SAs. They are also extremely fragile lesions that lack a definable neck and easily tear during surgical clipping. Intraprocedural rupture is common, occurring in nearly 50% of cases.

Most BBAs are now treated with stent-assisted coiling or stent-only therapy.

**BLOOD BLISTER-LIKE ANEURYSM**

**Pathology**
- Broad-based "blister" covered by thin friable tissue cap
- Usually solitary
- Can occur almost anywhere
- Dorsal wall of supraclinoid ICA most common site

**Clinical Issues**
- Easily rupture, may cause catastrophic aSAH
- Compared with saccular aneurysms
  - Rupture at earlier age
  - Rupture at smaller size

**Imaging**
- Small, easy to miss on CTA
- DSA with 3D shaded surface display best

**Treatment**
- Endovascular > surgical clipping
  - Flow-diverting stent
  - Stent-assisted coil embolization

## Imaging

BBAs are small, often subtle lesions that are easily overlooked. A slight irregularity or small focal hemispheric bulge of the arterial wall may be the only finding **(6-31)**. 3D DSA with shaded surface display has been helpful in identifying these difficult, dangerous lesions.

# Fusiform Aneurysm

FAs can be atherosclerotic (common) or nonatherosclerotic (rare). In contrast to SAs, FAs usually involve long, nonbranching vessel segments and are seen as focal circumferential outpouchings from a generally ectatic, elongated vessel.

Atherosclerotic FAs (ASVD FAs) are typically seen in older adults. vASVD FAs can be seen at any age but are most common in children and younger adults.

# Atherosclerotic Fusiform Aneurysm

## Terminology

ASVD FAs are also called aneurysmal dolichoectasias, distinguishing them from the more generalized nonfocal vessel elongations seen as a common manifestation of intracranial atherosclerosis.

## Pathology

Arteriectasis is common with advanced atherosclerosis of the cerebral arteries. Fusiform dilatation is a frequent complication. Generalized ASVD with a focally dilated fusiform enlargement is the typical gross manifestation of an ASVD FA.

ASVD FAs are more common in the vertebrobasilar (posterior) circulation and usually affect the basilar artery **(6-32)**. Atherosclerotic plaques of foam cells with thickened but irregular intima and extensive loss of elastica and

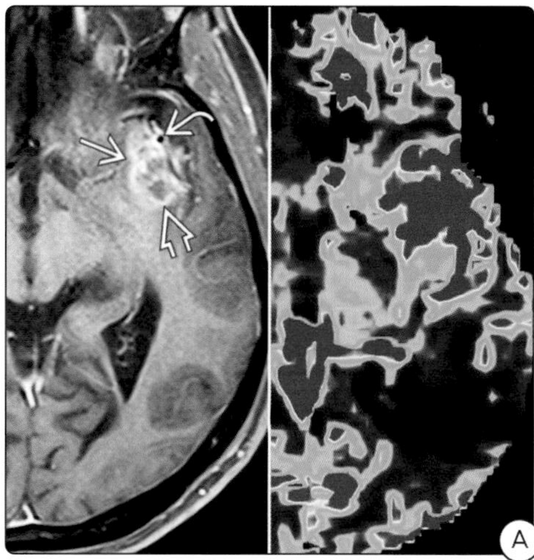

***(6-29A)** (L) T1 C+ FS in a 59-yo woman with TIAs shows enhancing mass ➡ encasing MCA ➡. Note focal dilatation ➡; (R) pMR. Glioblastoma.*

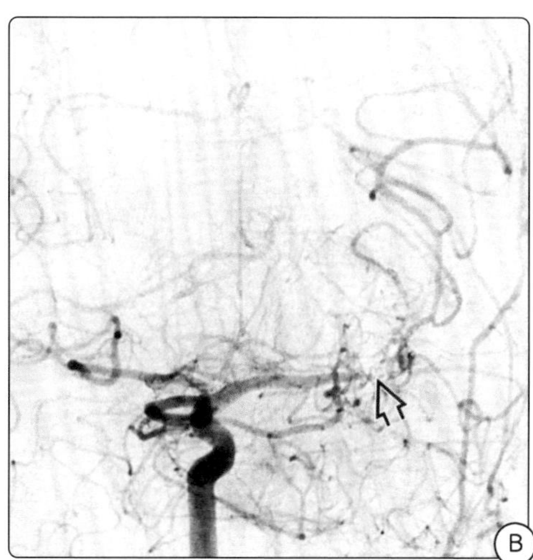

***(6-29B)** AP DSA shows extremely narrowed M2/M3 MCA junction ➡.*

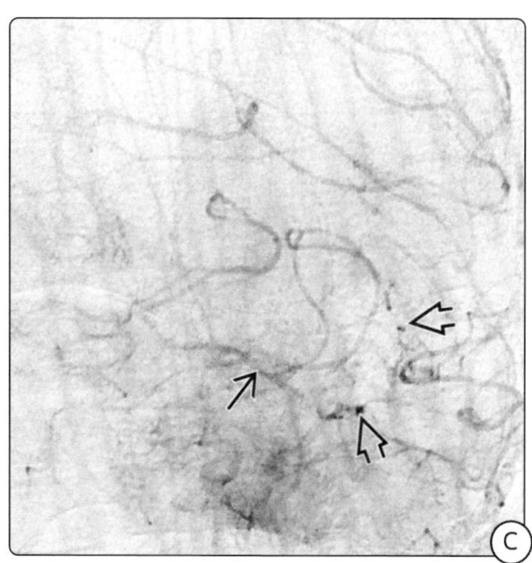

***(6-29C)** Late arterial phase shows multiple irregularities ➡, tiny MCA branch mycotic pseudoaneurysms ➡ caused by glioblastoma.*

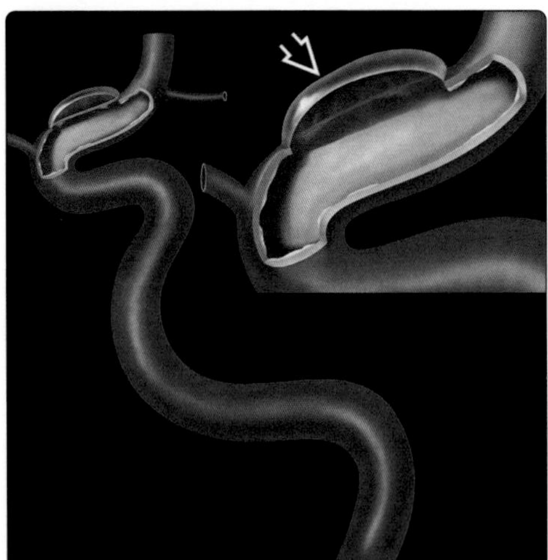

***(6-30)** BBA is seen here as a broad-based hemispheric bulge covered with a tissue paper-thin layer of adventitia ➡.*

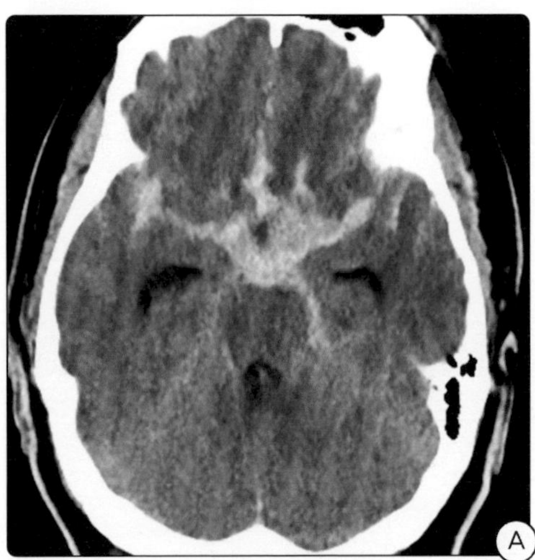

***(6-31A)** NECT in a 38-yo man with "worst headache of his life" shows diffuse SAH, early hydrocephalus.*

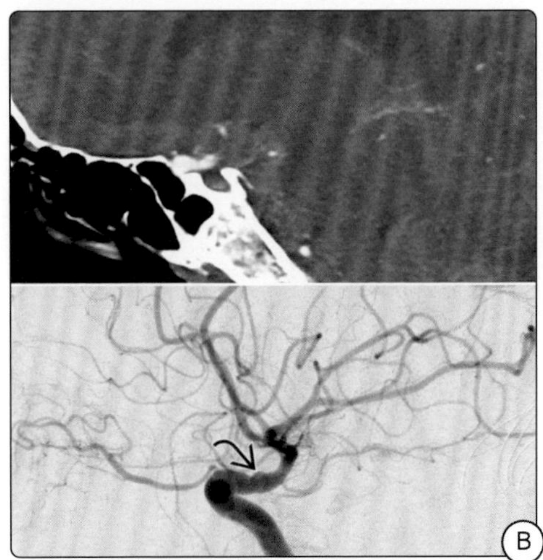

***(6-31B)** (Top) Sagittal CTA shows no definite abnormality. (Bottom) Lateral DSA shows tiny BBA ➡. Treated with pipeline.*

media are present. Layers of organized thrombus surrounding a patent residual lumen are common.

## Clinical Issues

Peak age of presentation is the 7th-8th decades. Posterior circulation TIAs and stroke are the most common presentation. Cranial neuropathy is relatively uncommon.

## Imaging

**General Features.** ASVD FAs are often large (> 2.5 cm in diameter) fusiform or ovoid dilatations that are superimposed on generalized vascular dolichoectasias **(6-33)**.

**CT Findings.** ASVD FAs are often partially thrombosed and frequently demonstrate mural calcification. Heterogeneously hyperdense clot is often present. The residual lumen enhances intensely following contrast enhancement.

**MR Findings.** Signal intensity of FAs varies with pulse sequence, degree and direction of flow, and the presence and age of clot within the FA. Slow, turbulent flow in the residual lumen causes complex, sometimes bizarre signal.

FAs are often very heterogeneous on T1WI and strikingly hypointense on T2WI. The residual lumen can be seen as a rounded "flow void" surrounded by complex thrombus that varies from hypointense to hyperintense. Intense enhancement of the residual lumen with prominent phase artifact is common following contrast administration.

Inflammatory changes are common in the walls of ASVD FAs. Vessel wall imaging may show variable enhancement. The enhancement is typically patchy, short segment, and discontinuous.

**Angiography.** CTA and DSA show generalized enlargement and ectasia of the parent vessel with a focal, round or fusiform, somewhat irregular contour **(6-33A)**. In some cases, the residual lumen resides within a larger mass caused by mural thrombus.

## Differential Diagnosis

The major differential diagnosis of an ASVD FA is **dolichoectasia**. Dolichoectasias are fusiform elongations of vessels—usually in the posterior circulation—without focal fusiform or saccular dilatations. Vertebrobasilar dolichoectasia is defined as a diameter > 4.5 mm, tortuous basilar artery lying lateral to the clivus or dorsum sellae, or basilar artery protruding above the suprasellar cistern.

**nASVD FAs** are seen in younger patients who often have an inherited vasculopathy or immune deficiency (see following section). Like ASVD FAs, intracranial **dissecting aneurysms** are most common on the vertebrobasilar (posterior) circulation. Findings of generalized ASVD are usually absent.

### ATHEROSCLEROTIC FUSIFORM ANEURYSM

**Terminology**
- AVSD with focally dilated fusiform enlargement
- a.k.a. aneurysmal dolichoectasias

**Pathology**
- More common in vertebrobasilar artery
- Affects long nonbranching segment
- ASVD with irregular intima
- Extensive loss of elastica, media
- Layers of organized mural, intraluminal thrombus
  - Clot often much larger than residual lumen

**Clinical Issues**
- Middle-aged, older patients
  - Peak = 60-80 years
  - Most common = posterior circulation TIAs, stroke

**Imaging**
- CT, CTA
  - Generalized changes of ASVD present
  - Elongated vessel + fusiform or ovoid dilatation
  - Mural calcification
  - Partial thrombosis common
- MR
  - Layered thrombus in wall, lumen
  - Signal intensity often complex
  - Clot surrounds variably sized residual "flow void"

**Differential Diagnosis**
- Dolichoectasia
  - Elongated artery
  - No focal fusiform or saccular dilatation
- Dissection, dissecting aneurysm
  - Often younger patients
  - Also posterior circulation
  - ASVD changes minimal/absent
- Nonatherosclerotic fusiform aneurysm
  - Younger patients (including children)
  - Inherited vasculopathy (e.g., Marfan, Ehlers-Danlos type IV)
  - Vascular neurocutaneous syndrome (e.g., neurofibromatosis type)
  - Acquired immune deficiency

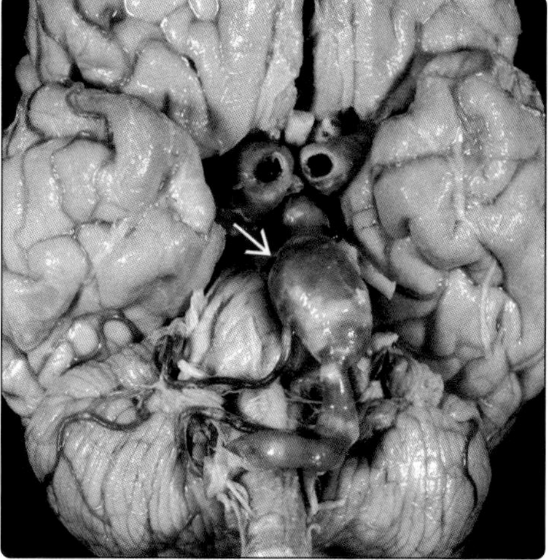

***(6-32)** Autopsy case shows giant atherosclerotic fusiform aneurysm ➡ of the vertebrobasilar artery.*

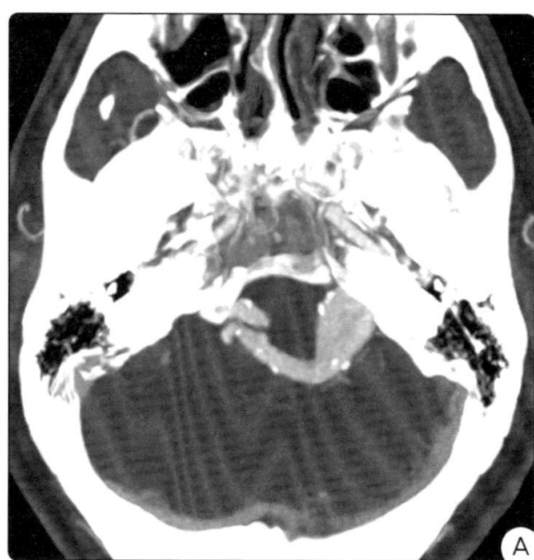

***(6-33A)** Axial MIP of CTA shows a fusiform vertebrobasilar aneurysm with wall calcifications.*

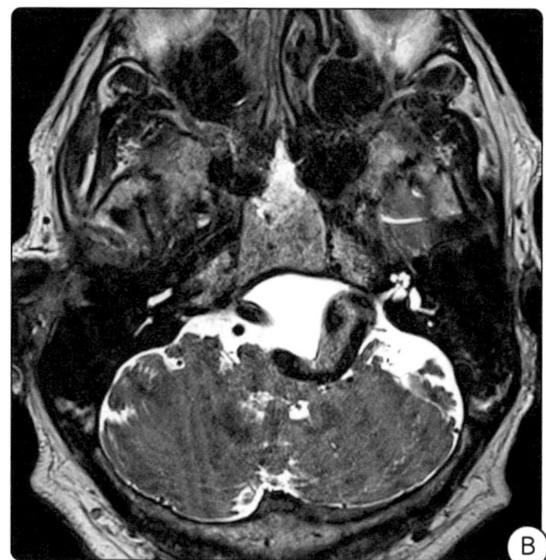

***(6-33B)** T2 FS shows the aneurysm nicely.*

## Nonatherosclerotic Fusiform Aneurysm

### Terminology

nASVD FAs are fusiform elongations that occur in the absence of generalized intracranial ASVD.

### Etiology

nASVD FAs occur with collagen vascular disorders (e.g., lupus), inherited vasculopathies (e.g., Marfan, Ehlers-Danlos), and vascular neurocutaneous syndrome (NF1, tuberous sclerosis). Viral infections (varicella, HIV) can also cause nonatherosclerotic vasculopathy.

### Pathology

nASVD FAs are focally dilated fusiform arterial ectasias that often involve nonbranching segments of intracranial arteries. Multiple lesions are common. The carotid (anterior) and vertebrobasilar circulations are equally affected.

## Clinical Issues

Patients tend to be younger than those with ASVD FAs. nASVD FAs are most common in children and young adults. HIV-associated aneurysmal arteriopathy carries an especially high morbidity.

## Imaging

Long segments of tubular, fusiform, or ovoid arterial dilatations are seen in the absence of generalized ASVD **(6-34)**. Circumferential involvement of the affected vessels is typical, as is extension into proximal branches.

## Differential Diagnosis

Fusiform intracranial dilatations in relatively young patients should suggest the possibility of nASVD vasculopathy and FA with or without accompanying dissection. **Vertebrobasilar dolichoectasia** is seen in older patients with generalized changes of ASVD.

*Selected References: The complete reference list is available on the eBooks+ version included with purchase.*

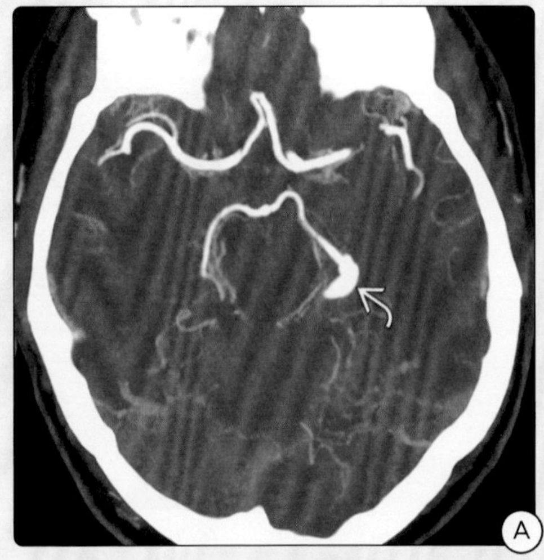

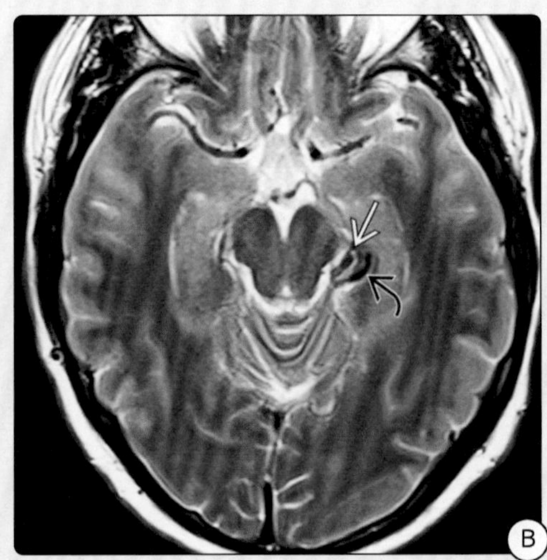

***(6-34A)** MIP of CTA in a 39-yo man with headaches shows fusiform enlargement of the P2 and P3 segments of the left PCA. **(6-34B)** T2WI shows a large fusiform hypointensity along the P3 PCA segment with a central hyperintensity.*

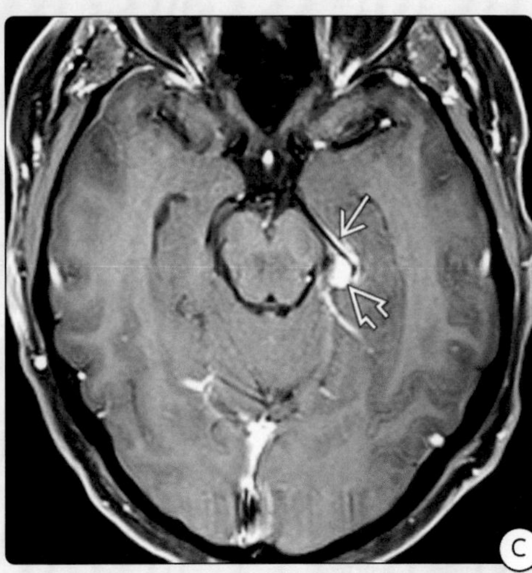

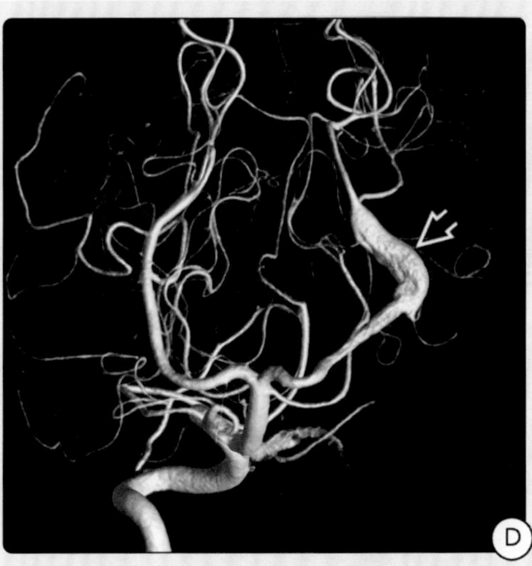

***(6-34C)** T1 C+ FS shows enhancement along the thickened P2 segment wall. Some enhancement is seen in enlarged P2-P3 junction. **(6-34D)** 3D shaded surface display of a right vertebral angiogram shows fusiform enlargement of the distal P2/proximal P3 PCA segment. Note lack of ASVD in the vertebrobasilar system, indicating this is a nonatherosclerotic fusiform aneurysm.*

# Vascular Malformations

*Brain vascular malformations, a.k.a. cerebrovascular malformations, are a heterogeneous group of disorders that exhibit a broad spectrum of biologic behaviors. Some cerebrovascular malformations (e.g., capillary malformations) are almost always clinically silent and found incidentally on imaging studies. Others, such as arteriovenous malformations and cavernous angiomas, may hemorrhage unexpectedly and without warning.*



In this chapter, we begin with an overview of cerebrovascular malformations (CVMs), starting with a discussion of terminology, etiology, and classification. CVMs are grouped according to whether or not they exhibit arteriovenous shunting, and then each type is discussed individually.

## Terminology

Two major groups of vascular anomalies in the central nervous system are recognized: Vascular *malformations* and *hemangiomas*. All CVMs—the entities considered in this chapter—are nonneoplastic lesions. CVMs are sometimes referred to as angiomas.

In contrast, "hemangiomas" are benign neoplastic vascular lesions that can be isolated, solitary or multiple, or occur as part of a *PIK3CA*-related overgrowth syndrome. In the most recent WHO classification of CNS tumors, hemangiomas are grouped with other soft tissue tumors and designated as mesenchymal, nonmeningothelial CNS tumors. Hemangiomas are discussed in Chapter 28.

## Classification

CVMs have been traditionally classified by histopathology into four major types: (1) Arteriovenous malformations (AVMs), (2) venous angiomas (developmental venous anomalies), (3) capillary telangiectasias (sometimes simply termed "telangiectasia" or "telangiectasis"), and (4) cavernous malformations.

Many interventional neuroradiologists and neurosurgeons group CVMs by function, not histopathology. In this functional classification, CVMs are divided into two basic categories: (1) CVMs that display arteriovenous shunting and (2) CVMs without arteriovenous shunting **(Table 7-1)**. The former are potentially amenable to endovascular intervention; the latter are either treated surgically or left alone.

## Cerebrovascular Malformations

| Type | Etiology | Pathology | Number | Location | Prevalence | Age | Hemorrhage Risk | Best Imaging Clues |
|---|---|---|---|---|---|---|---|---|
| **CVMs With AV Shunts** | | | | | | | | |
| AV malformations | Congenital (dysregulated angiogenesis) | Nidus + arterial feeders, draining veins; no capillary bed | Solitary (< 2% multiple) | Parenchyma (85%); supratentorial (15%); posterior fossa | 0.04-0.50% of population; 85-90% of CVMs with AV shunting | Peak: 20-40 years (25% by age 15 years) | Very high (2-4% per year, cumulative) | "Bag of worms," "flow voids" on MR |
| Dural AV fistula | Acquired (trauma; dural sinus thrombosis) | Network of multiple AV microfistulas | Solitary | Skull base; dural sinus wall | 10-15% of CVMs with AV shunting | Peak: 40-60 years | Varies with venous draining (increased if cortical veins involved) | Enlarged meningeal arteries with network of tiny vessels in wall of thrombosed dural venous sinus |
| Vein of Galen malformation | Congenital (fetal arterial fistula to primitive precursor of vein of Galen) | Large venous pouch | Solitary | Behind 3rd ventricle | < 1% of CVMs with AV shunting | Newborn > > infant, older child | Low (but hydrocephalus brain damage common) | Large midline venous varix in neonate with high-output congestive heart failure |
| **CVMs Without AV Shunts** | | | | | | | | |
| Developmental venous anomaly | Congenital (arrested fetal medullary vein development) | Dilated WM veins; normal brain in between | Solitary (unless BRBNS) | Deep WM, usually near ventricle | Most common CVM (60% of all), between 2-9% of population | Any age | Extremely low unless mixed with cavernous malformation | "Medusa head" of dilated WM veins converging on enlarged collector vein |
| Sinus pericranii | Congenital | Bluish blood-filled subcutaneous scalp mass | Solitary | Scalp | Rare | Any age (usually childhood) | Extremely low unless direct trauma | Vascular scalp mass connecting through skull defect to intracranial venous circulation |
| Cavernous malformation | Congenital (CCM, *KRIT1* gene mutations in familial autosomal dominant syndrome; "de novo" lesions continue to form) | Collection of blood-filled "caverns" with no normal brain; complete hemosiderin rim | 2/3 solitary (sporadic); 1/3 multiple (familial) | Throughout brain | | Any age (peak: 40-60 years; younger in familial CCM syndrome) | High (0.25-0.75% per year; 1% per lesion per year in familial) | Varies; most common is solitary "popcorn ball" (locules with blood-fluid levels, hemosiderin rim); multifocal "black dots" in familial |
| Capillary telangiectasia | Congenital | Dilated capillaries; normal brain in between | Solitary > > > multiple | Anywhere but pons; medulla most common | 15-20% of all CVMs | Any age (peak: 30-40 years) | Extremely low unless mixed with cavernous malformation | Faint brush-like enhancement; becomes hypointense on T2* |

***(Table 7-1)*** *AV = arteriovenous; BRBNS = blue rubber bleb nevus syndrome; CCM = cerebral cavernous malformation; CVM = cerebrovascular malformation; WM = white matter.*

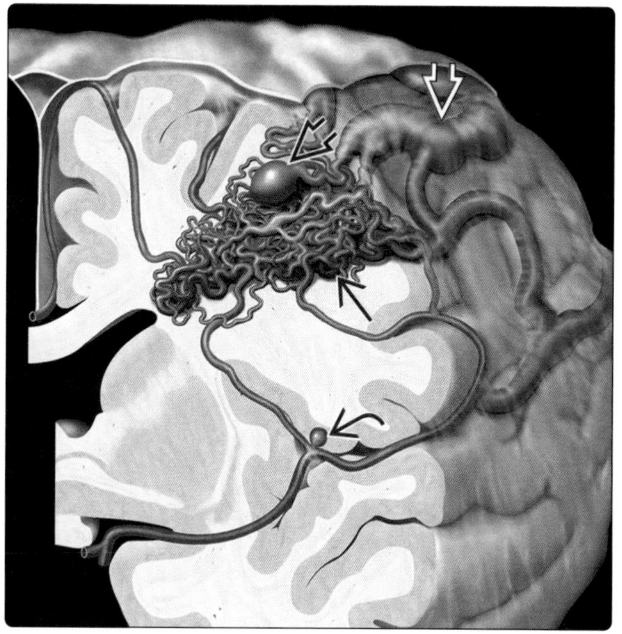

(7-1) Graphic depicts pyramid-shaped arteriovenous malformation (AVM) nidus ➙ with broad base toward cortical surface. Intranidal aneurysm ➙, feeding artery ("pedicle") aneurysm ➙, and enlarged draining veins ➙ are shown.

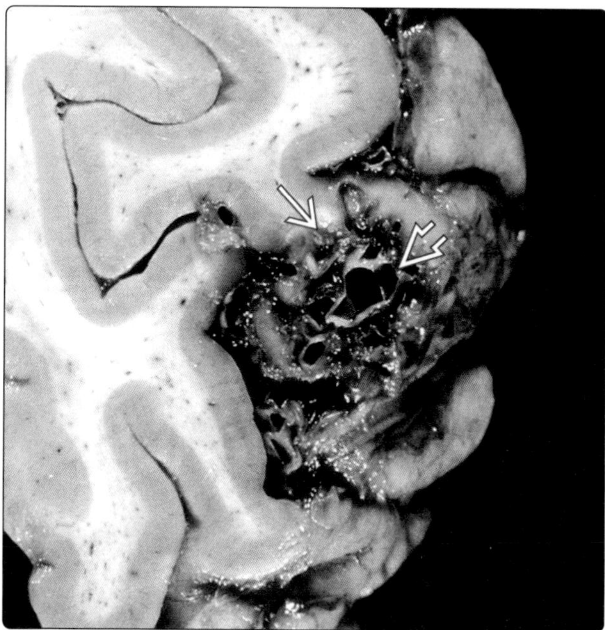

(7-2) Autopsy case demonstrates a classic AVM. The nidus ➙ contains no normal brain. An intranidal aneurysm ➙ is present. (Courtesy R. Hewlett, MD.)

# Cerebrovascular Malformations With Arteriovenous Shunting

## Arteriovenous Malformation

### Terminology

A brain AVM (BAVM) is a tightly packed tangle of serpiginous, thin-walled vessels without an intervening capillary bed.

### Etiology

**Genetics.** Most BAVMs are solitary and nonsyndromic. Recent evidence suggests that germline and somatic mutations are crucial for AVM development and that aberrant angiogenesis might be the key mechanism. Somatic *KRAS* mutations activating the MAPK-ERK signaling pathway in brain endothelial cells have recently been identified as playing a key role in BAVM development.

Multiple BAVMs are almost always syndromic. Less than 5% of all BAVMs occur in autosomal dominant inherited genetic syndromes, such as **hereditary hemorrhagic telangiectasia** (HHT) or capillary malformation-AVM syndrome. Inherited vascular neurocutaneous syndromes are discussed in detail in Chapter 44.

### Pathology

**Location.** Over 85% of AVMs are supratentorial, located in the cerebral hemispheres **(7-1)**. Only 15% are found in the posterior fossa.

**Size.** AVMs vary from tiny lesions to giant malformations that can occupy an entire cerebral lobe or hemisphere. Most are intermediate in size with a nidus ranging from 2-6 cm in diameter. Both the feeding arteries and draining veins are usually enlarged.

"Micro"-AVMs have a nidus ≤ 1 cm; feeding arteries and draining veins are usually normal in size. Micro-AVMs are typically associated with HHT.

**Gross Pathology.** AVMs appear as a *focal*, compact, ovoid or wedge-shaped mass of malformed arteries and veins of varying caliber and thickness that connect through a nidus instead of a normal capillary bed **(7-2)**. Their broadest surface is at or near the cortex with the apex pointing toward the ventricles **(7-1)**. Dilated draining veins are often found on the cortical surface overlying an AVM.

The brain surrounding an AVM often appears abnormal due to ischemic "steal" and tissue rarefaction. Hemorrhagic residua, such as gliosis and secondary ischemic changes, are common, as are siderotic changes in the overlying pia. Occasionally, an AVM presents with large, obliterating hemorrhage, often secondary to rupture of an intranidal aneurysm or sudden, catastrophic thrombosis of outlet draining veins.

**Microscopic Features.** There are no capillaries within an AVM nidus. Parenchyma within the nidus itself is minimal and gliotic. The nidus contains dysplastic, hyalinized, thin-walled vessels with "arterialized" veins, varying amounts of laminated thrombus, dystrophic calcifications, and hemorrhagic residua.

### AVM: ETIOLOGY AND PATHOLOGY

**Etiology**

- Congenital defect
  - Abnormal vascular development
  - Dysregulated angiogenesis
- **Genetics**
  - Sporadic BAVMs have somatic activating *KRAS* mutations
  - Syndromic BAVMs (e.g., HHT) have known specific mutations

**Pathology**

- Gross pathology
  - Ovoid or wedge-shaped with broad base toward cortex
  - 3 components: Feeding arteries, nidus (center), draining veins
- Microscopic features
  - Dysplastic thin-walled vessels
  - Ectatic "arterialized" veins
  - Only nonfunctional gliotic brain in nidus

## Clinical Issues

**Epidemiology.** Almost all AVMs are sporadic and solitary. With very rare exceptions ("de novo" AVMs), most are considered congenital lesions. Sporadic (nonsyndromic) AVMs are found in 0.15% of the general population.

**Presentation.** Peak presentation occurs between 20-40 years of age, although 25% of patients harboring an AVM become symptomatic by 15 years of age. There is no sex predilection.

Headache with parenchymal hemorrhage is the most common presentation, occurring in ~ 1/2 of all patients. Seizure and focal neurologic deficits are the initial symptoms in 25% each. Small micro-AVMs in patients with vascular neurocutaneous syndromes, such as HHT, are often asymptomatic and only discovered when screening imaging studies are performed.

**Natural History.** A growing body of gene expression and polymorphism-based research studies support the involvement of localized inflammation in BAVM disease and rupture.

The annual hemorrhage risk is ~ 3%, but, depending on the clinical and anatomic features of the AVM, the risk may be as low as 1% per year (in patients whose initial presentation was nonhemorrhagic) or as high as 33% in hemorrhagic lesions with deep brain or brainstem location and exclusively deep venous drainage. Other features associated with bleeding include feeding artery aneurysm and venous outflow restriction.

Several grading systems have been devised to characterize AVMs and estimate the risks of surgery. The most widely used is the **Spetzler-Martin scale**. Here, AVMs are graded on a scale from 1-5 based on the sum of "scores" calculated from lesion size, location (eloquent vs. noneloquent brain), and venous drainage pattern (superficial vs. deep).

### AVM: CLINICAL ISSUES

**Demographics**

- Peak age: 20-40 years (mean: 33 years)
- 25% symptomatic by 15 years

**Presentation**

- Headache with intracranial hemorrhage (ICH) in 50-60%
- Seizure in 25%, neurologic deficit in 25%

**Natural History**

- Overall annual ICH risk is 3% but wide variation

**Treatment Options.** Embolization, surgery, stereotactic radiosurgery, or a combination of treatments are all current options in treating ruptured (i.e., hemorrhagic) BAVMs. Stereotactic radiosurgery is an option in patients with small unruptured AVMs (< 3 cm) &/or low Spetzler-Martin grades.

### SPETZLER-MARTIN AVM GRADING SCALE

**Size**

- Small (< 3 cm) = 1
- Medium (3-6 cm) = 2
- Large (≥ 6 cm) = 3

**Location**

- In noneloquent brain = 0
- In eloquent brain = 1

**Venous Drainage**

- Superficial veins only = 0
- Deep veins (e.g., internal cerebral veins) = 1

## Imaging

The imaging diagnosis of an uncomplicated AVM is relatively straightforward. However, the presence of hemorrhage or thrombosis can complicate its appearance. Acute hemorrhage may obliterate any typical findings of an AVM. Residua of previous hemorrhagic episodes, such as dystrophic calcification, gliosis, and blood in different stages of degradation, may also complicate its appearance.

**General Features.** AVMs are complex networks of abnormal vascular channels consisting of three distinct components: (1) Feeding arteries, (2) a central nidus, and (3) draining veins **(7-1)**.

**CT Findings.** AVMs generally resemble a bag of worms formed by a tightly packed tangle of vessels with little or no mass effect on adjacent brain. NECT scans typically show numerous well-delineated, slightly hyperdense serpentine vessels **(7-3)**. Calcification is common. Enhancement of all three AVM components (feeding arteries, nidus, draining veins) is typically intense and uniform on CECT scans.

CTA is commonly included as part of the initial evaluation in patients who present with nontraumatic "spontaneous" intracranial hemorrhage (sICH) and may be helpful in

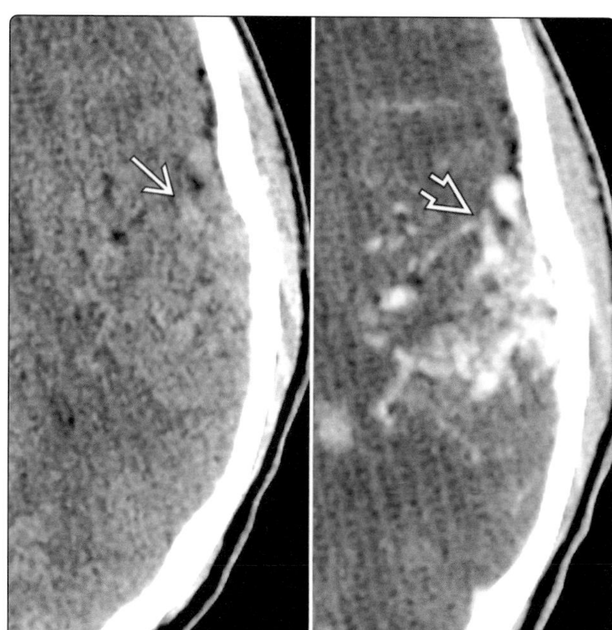

*(7-3) (L) NECT shows serpentine hyperdensities ➡. (R) CECT shows strong uniform enhancement ➡. Wedge-shaped configuration is typical for AVM. Roughly 85% of AVMs are supratentorial.*

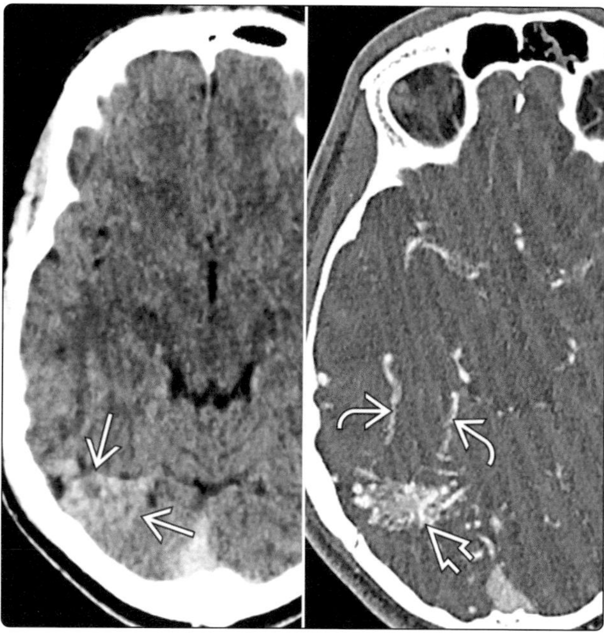

*(7-4) (L) Axial NECT in a 19-yo man with acute visual migraine symptoms shows a slightly hyperdense, wedge-shaped lesion ➡ in R occipital lobe. (R) CTA shows a tightly packed nidus of enhancing vessels ➡ with some enlarged draining veins ➡.*

delineating the feeding arteries and draining veins of an underlying AVM **(7-4)**.

**MR Findings.** The typical appearance of a BAVM is a tightly packed mass or a "honeycomb" of "flow voids" on both T1 **(7-5A)** and T2 **(7-5B)** scans. Any brain parenchyma within an AVM is typically minimal, gliotic, and hyperintense on T2WI and FLAIR **(7-5C)**.

Contrast enhancement of AVMs is variable, depending on flow rate and direction. Draining veins typically enhance strongly and uniformly **(7-5D)**.

Hemorrhagic residua are common. T2* sequences often show foci of "blooming" both within and around AVMs as well as siderosis in the adjacent pia.

**Angiography.** The pial **feeding arteries** that supply an AVM are often enlarged and tortuous **(7-5E)**. A flow-induced **"pedicle" aneurysm** is seen in 10-15% of cases.

The **nidus**, the core of the AVM, is a tightly packed tangle of abnormal arteries and veins without an intervening capillary bed **(7-6)**. Up to 50% contain at least one aneurysmally dilated vessel **("intranidal aneurysm")**.

As there is no intervening capillary bed, direct arteriovenous shunting within the nidus occurs. **Draining veins** typically opacify in the mid to late arterial phase ("early draining" veins) **(7-5F)**. Veins draining an AVM may become so prominent that they form varices and even exert local mass effect on the adjacent cortex. Stenosis of one or more "outlet" draining veins may elevate intranidal pressure and contribute to AVM hemorrhage.

Approximately 25% of superficially located, large, or diffuse AVMs have some transdural arterial contributions, so thorough evaluation of the dural vasculature should also be part of the complete angiographic delineation of AVM arterial supply.

**AVM: IMAGING**

**NECT**
- Slightly hyperdense "bag of worms"
- Tightly packed
- Little/no mass effect

**CECT**
- Strong serpentine enhancement

**MR**
- "Honeycomb" of "flow voids"
- No normal brain inside

**Differential Diagnosis**
- Highly vascular neoplasm (e.g., glioblastoma multiforme)
- Cerebral proliferative angiopathy

## Differential Diagnosis

Occasionally, a highly vascular neoplasm, such as **glioblastoma** (GBM), displays such striking neoangiogenesis that it can mimic an AVM. Most GBMs contain significant amounts of neoplasm interposed between the enlarged vessels. Sometimes, densely calcified neoplasms, such as oligodendroglioma, can mimic the "flow voids" of an AVM on MR.

*(7-5A) Sagittal T1 MR in a 32-yo man with headaches shows a wedge-shaped mass of "flow voids" ➡ in the parietal lobe. Note prominent angular branch of the middle cerebral artery (MCA) in the sylvian fissure ➡. (7-5B) T2 MR in the same case shows a wedge-shaped collection of "flow voids" ➡ in the left parietal lobe.*

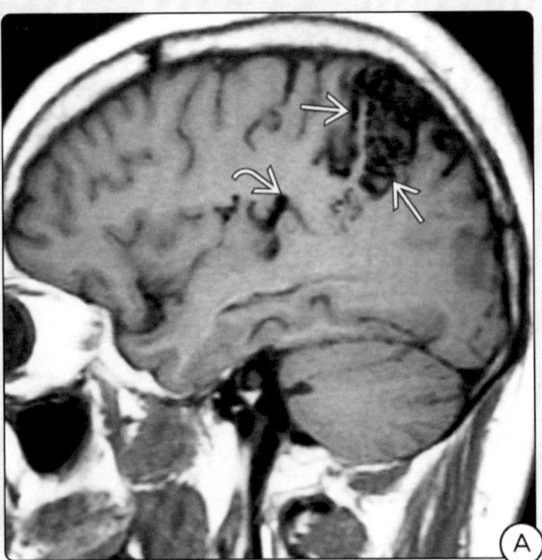

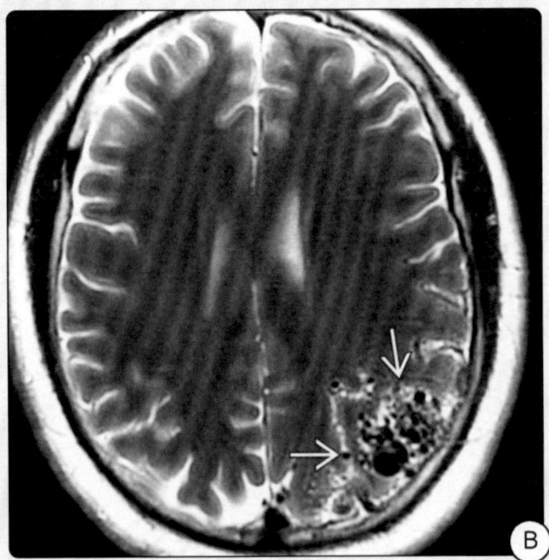

*(7-5C) FLAIR MR in the same case shows the tightly packed "snarl" of vessels ➡ and some prominent sulcal "flow voids" ➡ adjacent to the vascular lesion. Note absence of mass effect. (7-5D) T1 C+ MR in the same case shows some enhancement within the nidus ➡ as well as in the adjacent enlarged draining veins ➡.*

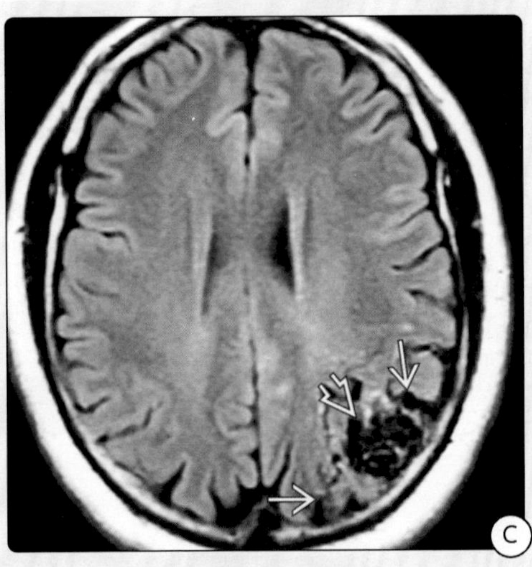

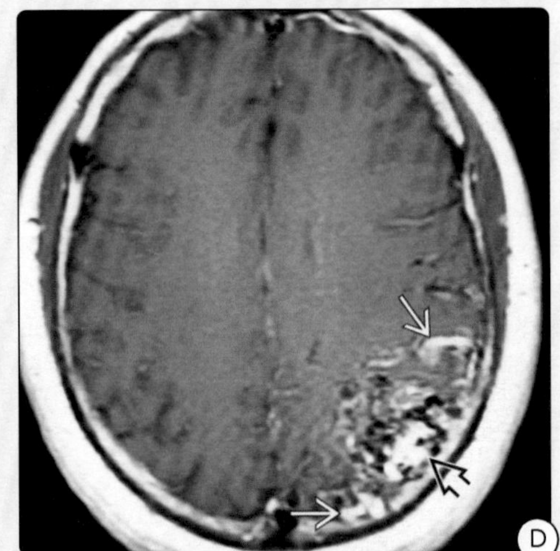

*(7-5E) Left internal carotid DSA shows enlarged cortical branches of the anterior cerebral artery (ACA) and MCA ➡ feeding the nidus of the lesion ➡. Note some pseudophlebitic vessels in the adjacent parenchyma ➡ outside of the nidus. (7-5F) Late arterial phase of DSA shows early appearance of contrast in dilated veins ➡ draining nidus that then opacify the adjacent superior sagittal sinus (SSS) ➡. This is classic unruptured cerebral AVM.*

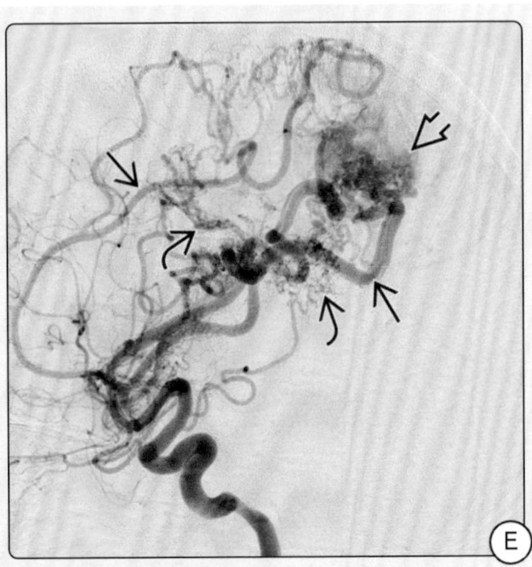

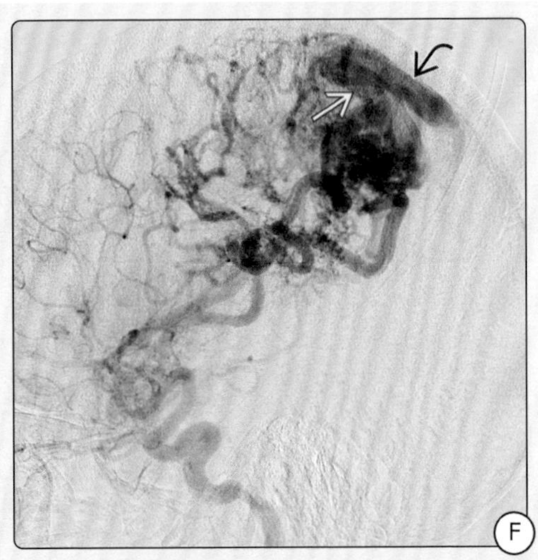

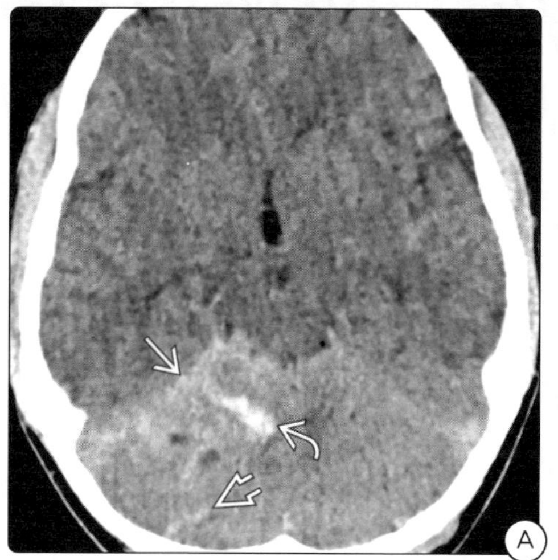

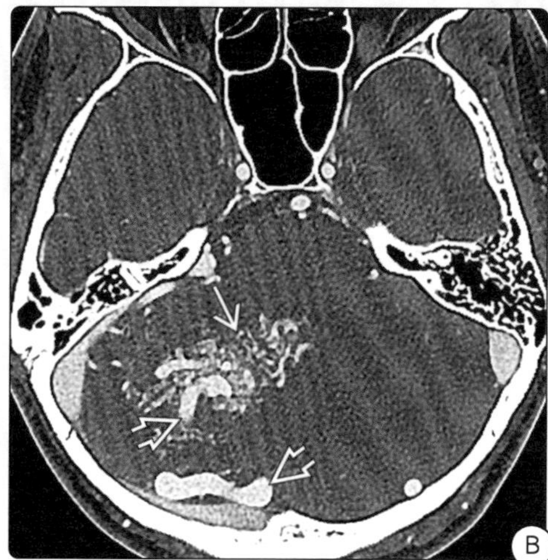

***(7-6A)** NECT in a 21-yo man with the "worst headache of his life" shows a moderately hyperdense mass in the right cerebellar hemisphere ➡. Note acute hemorrhage ↪ as well as a tubular hyperdense vessel ➡. **(7-6B)** CTA shows a wedge-shaped tangle of vessels in the right cerebellum and vermis ➡ with several prominent draining veins ➡.*

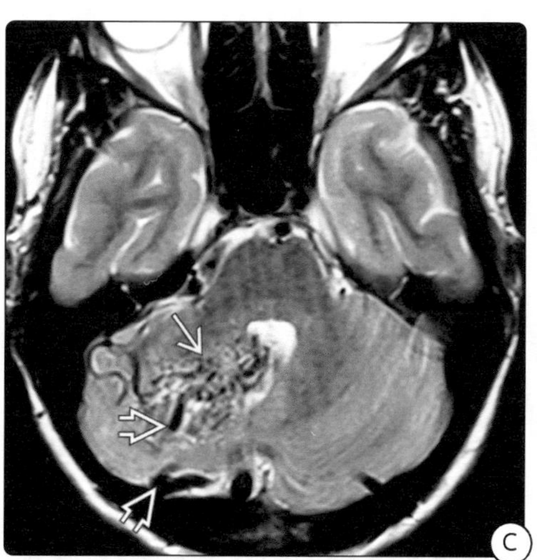

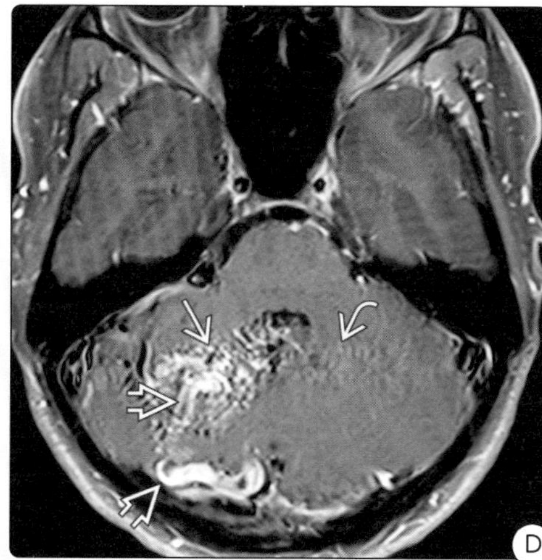

***(7-6C)** T2 MR in the same case shows a wedge-shaped "tangle" or "snarl" of "flow voids" ➡ with some prominent draining veins ➡. No normal cerebellar parenchyma is seen within the tightly packed mass. **(7-6D)** T1 C+ FS MR shows vessels ➡ within the AVM intensely enhance. Note prominent draining veins ➡ and flow artifact ↪.*

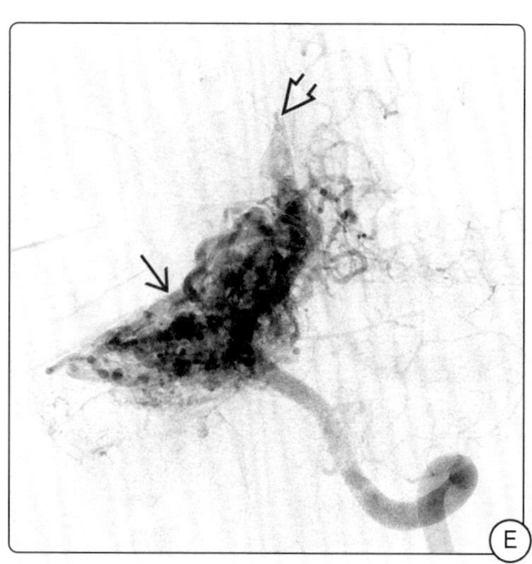

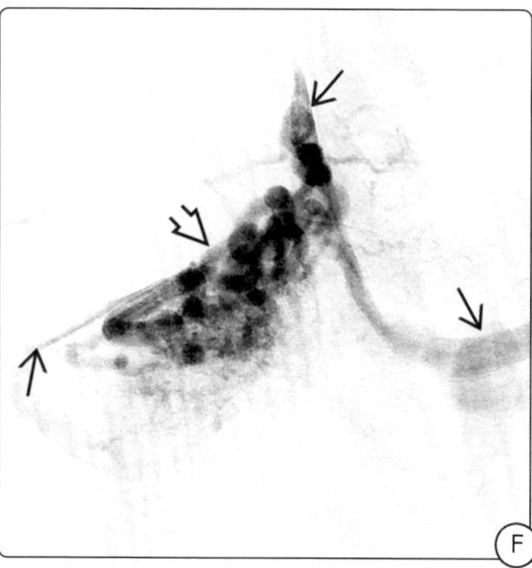

***(7-6E)** AP DSA of the left vertebral angiogram shows the wedge-shaped, tightly packed tangle of vessels ➡ with early contrast in the straight sinus ➡. **(7-6F)** Late capillary phase of the DSA shows multiple enlarged draining veins ➡ and early opacification of the adjacent dural venous sinuses ➡. This is classic AVM with sentinel hemorrhage.*

**Cerebral proliferative angiopathy** (see below) is a large, diffuse vascular malformation that has innumerable small feeding vessels, no definable nidus, and *normal brain interposed between the proliferating vascular channels.*

## Cerebral Proliferative Angiopathy

### Terminology

Cerebral proliferative angiopathy (CPA), formerly considered a variant of AVM known as "holohemispheric giant cerebral AVM" or "diffuse AVM," is now recognized as a separate entity with distinct imaging features and natural history unlike classic AVMs.

### Pathology

CPA is characterized by diffuse abnormal vessels with intermingled brain parenchyma. Feeding arteries are numerous, and draining veins are prominent. In contrast to classic AVMs, there is no nidus and there are no high-flow arteriovenous shunts present. Intralesional hemorrhage is uncommon.

### Clinical Issues

While CPA is a progressive disorder, its natural history is quite different from a classic AVM. CPA typically presents with seizure (45%) or headache (40%). Only 15-15% present with neurologic deficits or TIAs.

Mean age at diagnosis is 22 years with a 2:1 female predominance.

Long-term prognosis in CPA is poor. Unlike classic AVMs, CPA is characterized by ongoing angiogenesis and progressive hypervascular shunting. Over time, CPA may demonstrate progressive lesion enlargement with extension into previously uninvolved normal brain parenchyma.

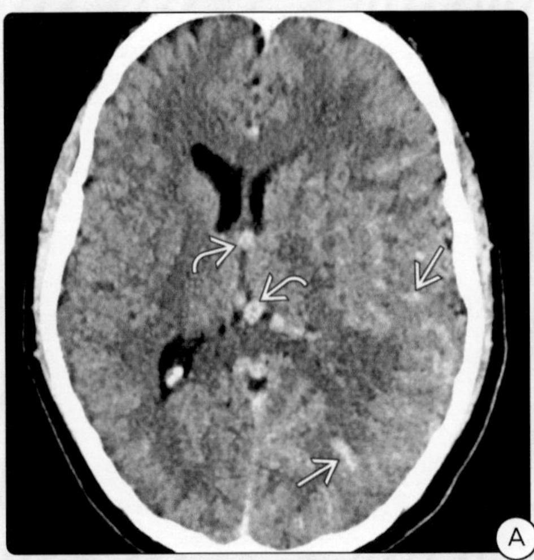


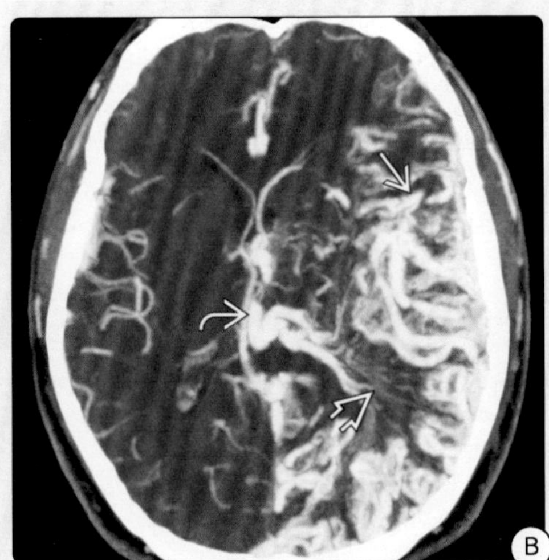


***(7-7A)** NECT in a 40-yo man with severe intractable headache shows multiple hyperdense, enlarged veins ➡ and tubular structures ➡ that are likely prominent arteries. Note mild mass effect on the left lateral ventricle. **(7-7B)** MIP of CTA in the same case shows enlarged medullary ➡ and deep periventricular veins ➡. The MCA and PCA cortical branches ➡ are diffusely enlarged. Note normal parenchyma between the veins and enlarged cortical arteries.*

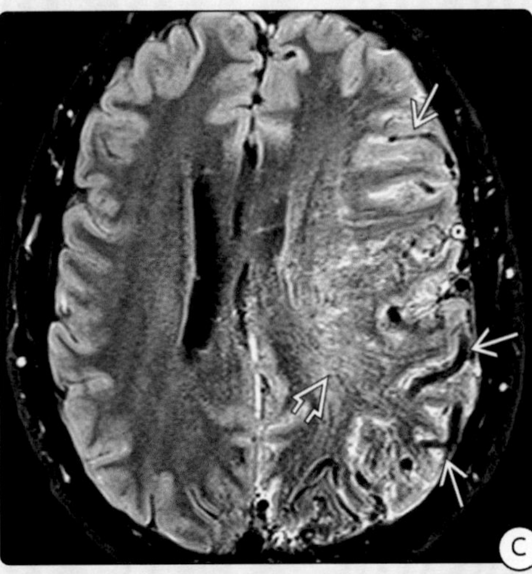


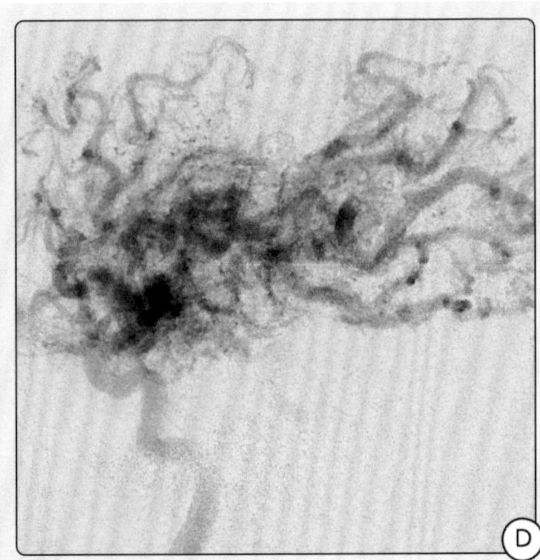


***(7-7C)** FLAIR MR in the same case shows prominent medullary veins ➡ and multiple dilated vessels in the superficial sulci ➡. Note normal cortex and white matter (WM) between the enlarged vessels. **(7-7D)** Lateral view of the left internal carotid DSA in the same case shows diffusely enlarged cortical arteries. Initial diagnosis was diffuse AVM, but this is cerebral proliferative angiopathy.*

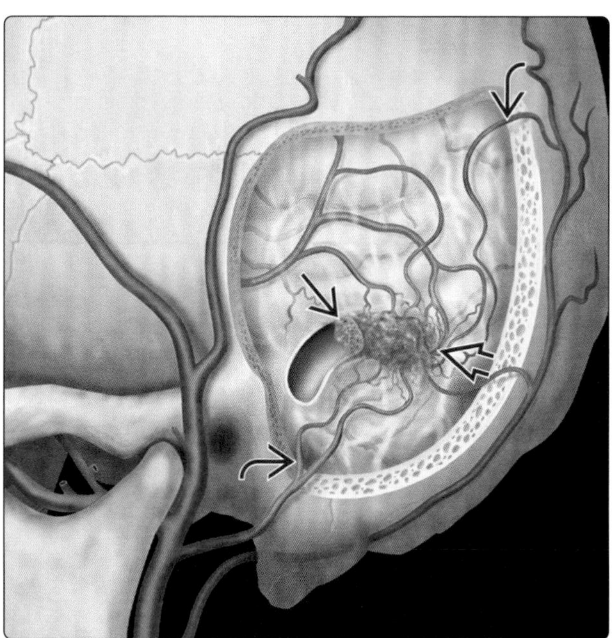

***(7-8)** Graphic shows dural arteriovenous fistula (dAVF) with thrombosed transverse sinus (TS) ⇨ and multiple tiny arteriovenous vessels in dural wall ⇨. Lesion is mostly supplied by transosseous feeders ⇨ from external carotid artery (ECA).*

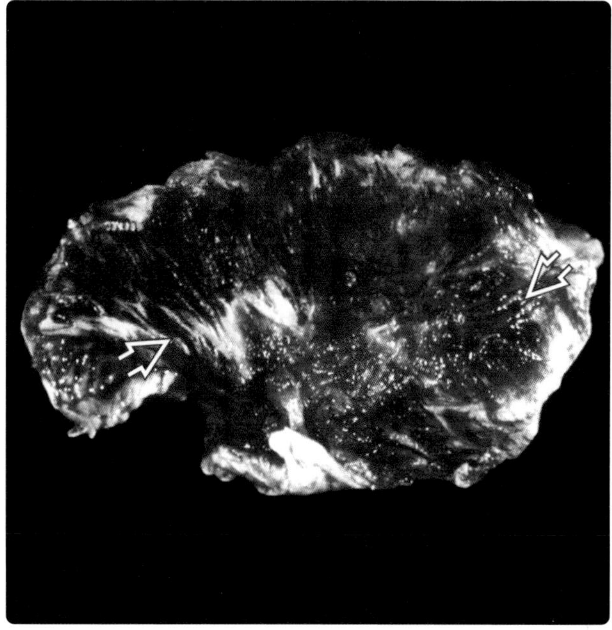

***(7-9)** Mass-like surgical specimen from a resected dAVF in a chronically thrombosed TS wall shows a mass-like thrombotic lesion with innumerable crack-like vessels ⇨. (Courtesy R. Hewlett, MD.)*

## Imaging

CPA is seen on MR as a large (usually > 6 cm) diffusely dispersed network of innumerable dilated vascular spaces intermingled with normal brain parenchyma **(7-7)**. Dense enhancement following contrast administration is typical. Reflecting the hypervascularity, pCT and pMR may demonstrate increased cerebral blood flow (CBF) and cerebral blood volume (CBV), although the brain parenchyma itself is typically hypoperfused. SPECT and PET may demonstrate hypometabolism within the lesion.

DSA and CTA show numerous small feeding arteries, usually with no dominant arterial supply. Recruitment of dural and even transosseous feeders is common. There is no discernible nidus **(7-7D)**, and flow-related aneurysms on feeding vessels are absent. A dense, prolonged vascular "staining" of the affected parenchyma is common. In contrast to AVMs, veins draining CPA are only moderately enlarged relative to the large extent of the abnormality. In further contrast to AVMs, hemorrhage is rare.

## Differential Diagnosis

The major differential diagnosis is a large, so-called **"diffuse" cerebral AVM**. It is crucial to differentiate the two entities because there is lack of dominant feeding arteries and normal functioning brain within a CPA. Unlike AVM, hemorrhage is a rare occurrence in CPA.

**Moyamoya disease** is an idiopathic progressive occlusive (not proliferative) angiopathy characterized by stenosis of the distal (supraclinoid) internal carotid artery (ICA) with development of an abnormal "telangiectatic" vascular network at the base of the brain.

# Dural Arteriovenous Fistula

Dural arteriovenous fistula (dAVF) is the second major type of CVM that exhibits arteriovenous shunting. Much less common than AVMs, dAVFs exhibit a spectrum of biologic behavior that ranges from relatively benign to catastrophic ICH.

A special type of dAVF, carotid-cavernous fistula (CCF), has its own classification schema, distinctive clinical findings, and unique imaging features that differ from dAVFs elsewhere. CCF is discussed separately in this chapter.

## Terminology

Intracranial dAVFs are abnormal direct vascular communications between arteries that supply the dura and one or more draining cortical veins or dural venous sinuses. An intervening capillary network is absent.

## Etiology

Unlike parenchymal AVMs, adult dAVFs are usually acquired (not congenital). Although the precise etiology is controversial, upregulated angiogenesis in the wall of a thrombosed dural venous sinus with concomitant venous hypertension is the most commonly cited mechanism.

## Pathology

**Location.** Most dAVFs are found in the posterior fossa and skull base. Between 1/3 and 1/2 occur at the transverse/sigmoid sinus junction. Less common sites are the cavernous sinus (CS) and superior petrosal sinus. dAVFs involving the superior sagittal sinus are rare.

**Size and Number.** dAVFs account for 10-15% of all intracranial vascular malformations with arteriovenous shunting. Most are solitary. Size varies from tiny single vessel shunts to massive complex lesions with multiple feeders and arteriovenous shunts in the sinus wall.

**Gross Pathology.** Multiple enlarged dural feeders converge in the wall of a thrombosed dural venous sinus **(7-8)**. A network of innumerable microfistulas connects these vessels directly to arterialized draining veins. These crack-like vessels may form a focal mass within the occluded sinus **(7-9)**.

## Clinical Issues

**Presentation.** Most dAVFs occur in adults. The peak age is 40-60 years, roughly 20 years older than the peak age for AVMs.

Clinical presentation varies with location and venous drainage pattern. Uncomplicated dAVFs in the transverse/sigmoid sinus region typically present with either bruit &/or tinnitus. dAVFs in the CS cause pulsatile proptosis, chemosis, retroorbital pain, bruit, and ophthalmoplegia.

"Malignant" dAVFs [lesions with cortical venous drainage (CVD)] may cause focal neurologic deficits, seizures, and progressive dementia.

**Natural History.** Prognosis depends on location and venous drainage pattern. Most lesions without CVD follow a benign clinical course. Hemorrhage is rare in such cases (~ 1.5% per year). "Malignant" dAVFs often have an aggressive clinical course with high risk for ICH (risk: ~ 7.5% per year).

**Treatment Options.** Endovascular treatment with embolization of arterial feeders with or without coil embolization of the recipient venous pouch/sinus is most common. Surgical resection of the involved dural sinus wall, used either alone or in combination with endovascular treatment, is another option.

***(7-10A)** CTA source image in a patient with right-sided tinnitus shows no obvious abnormality, although the right sigmoid sinus ➡ looks peculiar. **(7-10B)** Bone CT in the same patient shows multiple enlarged transosseous vascular channels ➡ in the squama of the right occipital bone.*

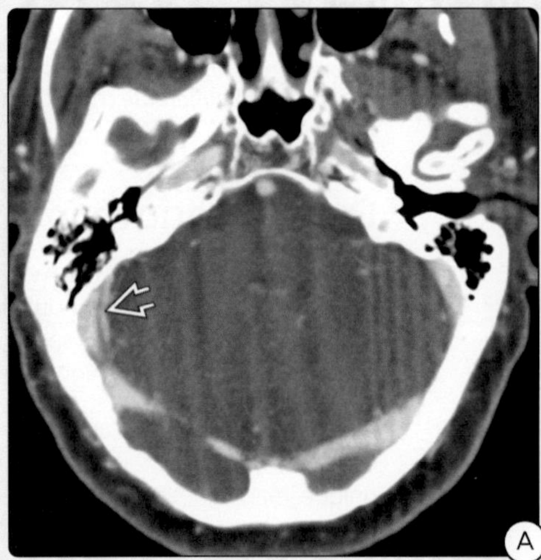



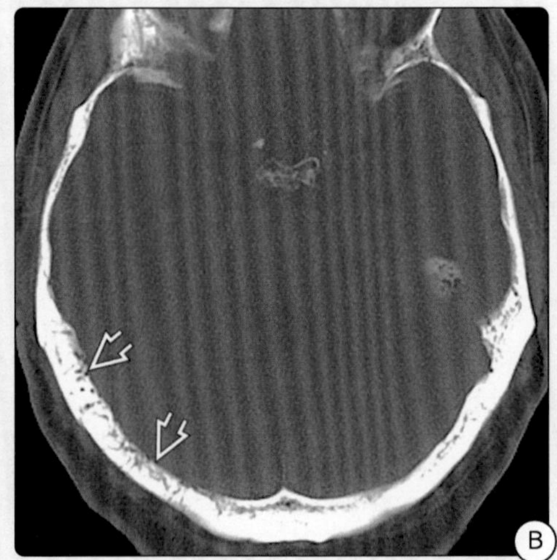



***(7-10C)** Contrast-enhanced MRA source image shows dural sinus thrombosis ➡, multiple enhancing vascular channels ➡ characteristic of posterior fossa dAVF. **(7-10D)** MRA in the same patient shows innumerable tiny feeding arteries ➡ supplying a dAVF at the transverse-sigmoid sinus junction. The sinus has partially recanalized ➡, and the distal sigmoid sinus ➡ and jugular bulb are partially opacified.*

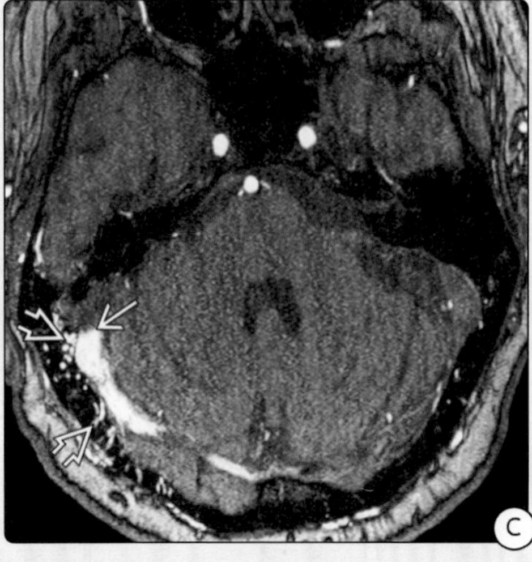



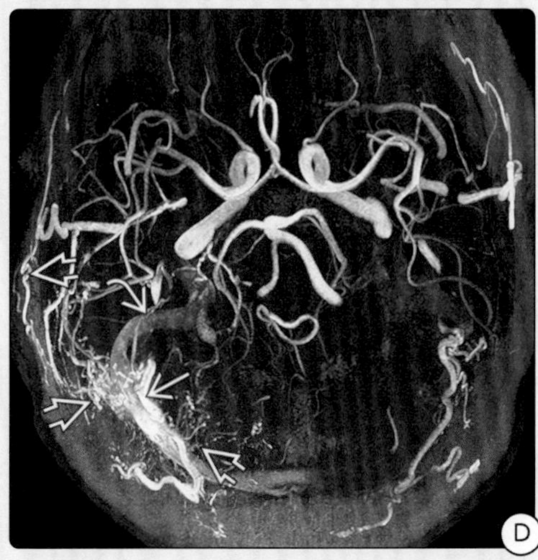

## Imaging

**CT Findings.** CT findings vary from none to striking. Parenchymal hemorrhage is uncommon in the absence of CVD. An enlarged dural sinus or draining vein can sometimes be identified on NECT scans. Dilated transcalvarial channels from enlarged transosseous feeding arteries can occasionally be seen on bone CT images in patients with pulsatile tinnitus **(7-10A)** **(7-10B)**.

Contrast-enhanced scans may demonstrate enlarged feeding arteries and draining veins. The involved dural venous sinus is often thrombosed or stenotic.

**MR Findings.** A thrombosed dural venous sinus containing vascular-appearing "flow voids" is the most common finding **(7-10C)** **(7-10D)**. Thrombus is typically isointense with brain on T1 and T2 scans and "blooms" on T2* sequences. Chronically thrombosed, fibrotic sinuses may enhance.

Parenchymal hyperintensity on T2WI and FLAIR indicates venous congestion or ischemia, usually secondary to retrograde CVD.

**Angiography.** As most dAVFs arise adjacent to the skull base, multiple enlarged dural and transosseous branches arising from the external carotid artery (ECA) are usually present **(7-11A)** **(7-11B)**. Dural branches may also arise from the ICA **(7-11C)** and vertebral arteries **(7-11D)**.

Identifying venous drainage is important. dAVFs with normal antegrade venous drainage or minimal reflux into a dural sinus without drainage into cortical veins are considered low-risk lesions. The presence of dural sinus thrombosis, flow reversal with drainage into cortical (leptomeningeal) veins and tortuous engorged pial veins (pseudophlebitic pattern) **(7-13)** are common in patients with progressive brain disease **(7-12)**.

Angiographic classification of dAVFs helps stratify risk of dAVF rupture and predict clinical course. The Cognard and Borden

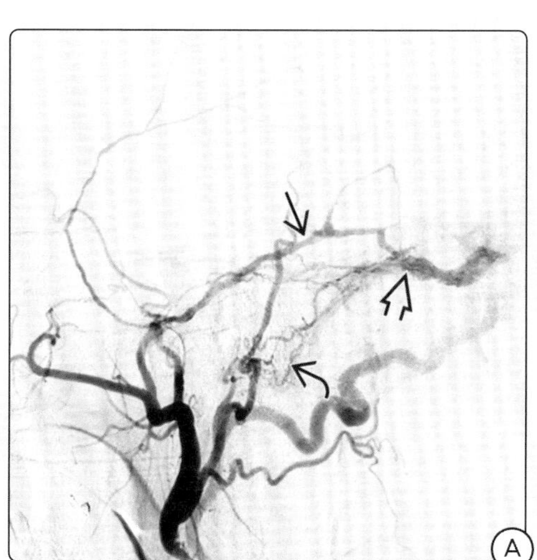


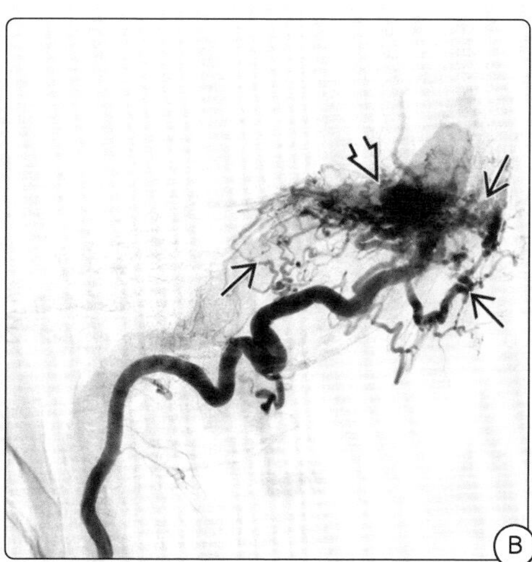


***(7-11A)** Lateral DSA of the ECA in a patient with pulsatile tinnitus shows a dAVF to a partial recanalized TS ⇒. Numerous ECA branches, including the posterior, auricular, ➪ and middle meningeal arteries →, supply the fistula. **(7-11B)** Superselective DSA of the occipital artery shows that it is the major contributor to the dAVF in the wall of the TS ⇒ through innumerable transosseous perforating branches →.*

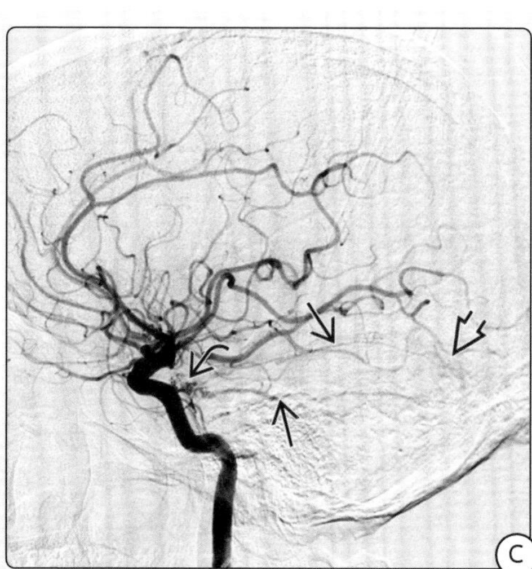


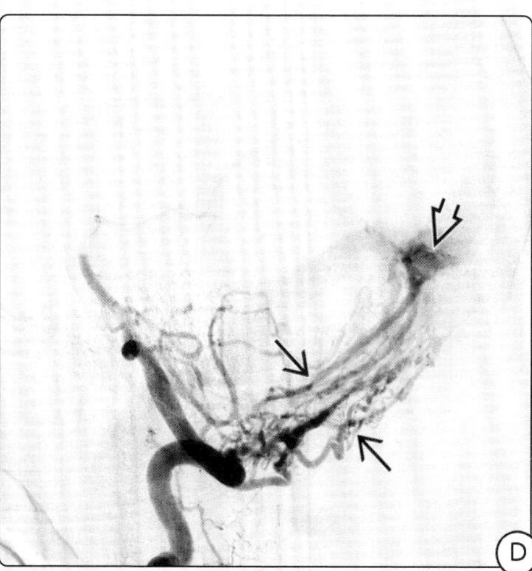


***(7-11C)** Lateral DSA of the left internal carotid artery (ICA) shows a markedly enlarged meningohypophyseal trunk ➪ with several marginal tentorial branches → supplying the dAVF ⇒. **(7-11D)** Lateral DSA of the left vertebral injection shows numerous enlarged posterior meningeal branches → that arise from the V3 segment and supply the dAVF ⇒.*

*(7-12A) NECT in an older woman with headaches, confusion, gait disturbance, and altered mental status shows hypodense right cerebellar mass ➡ and a smaller mass ➡ in left cerebellar hemisphere. (7-12B) NECT shows enlarged lateral ventricles with periventricular hypodensity ➡ suggesting acute obstructive hydrocephalus. Clinical diagnosis was normal pressure hydrocephalus (NPH).*

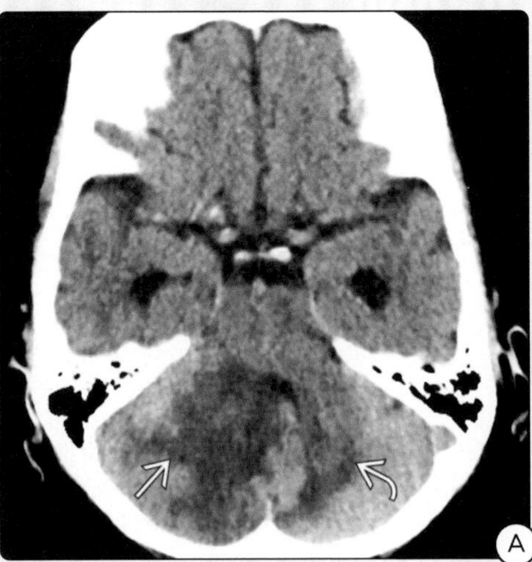

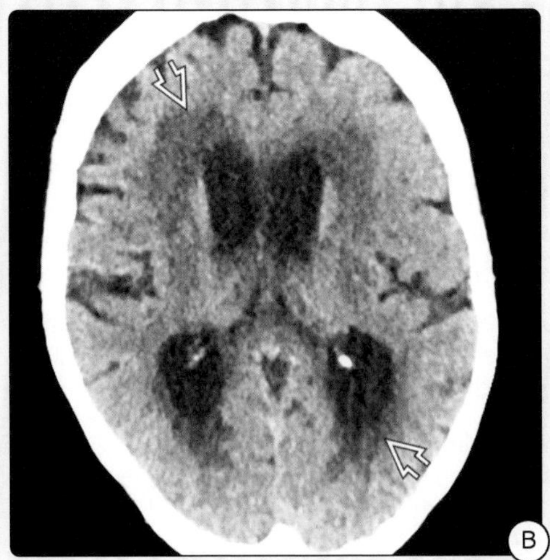

*(7-12C) MIP of CTA in the same case shows a tangle of vessels ➡ draining into the distal right TS ➡. The proximal segment of the TS ➡ appears occluded. (7-12D) T2 SPACE sequence from vessel wall imaging study shows hyperintense bicerebellar lesion ➡ with a mass-like hypodense lesion ➡ adjacent to the right TS. Note prominent "flow voids" ➡ within the mass.*

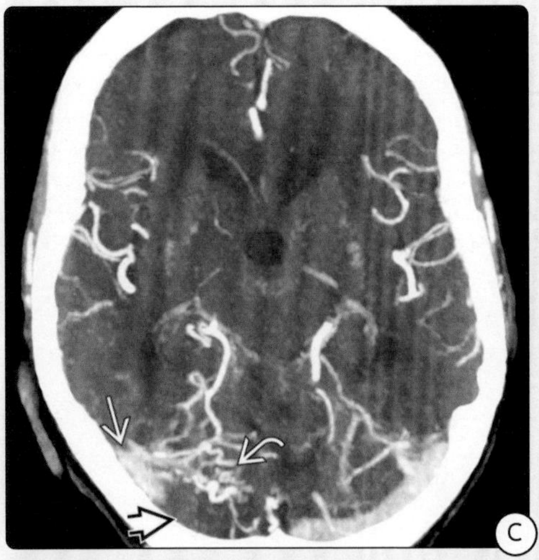

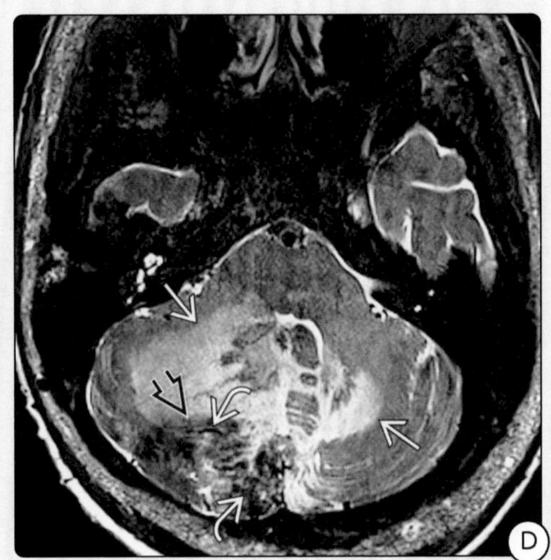

*(7-12E) T1 C+ FS MR shows partial patchy, linear enhancement ➡ of the mass adjacent to the torcular Herophili. No "flow void" is seen in the adjacent right TS. (7-12F) Vertebral angiogram, venous phase shows a tangle of vessels ➡ draining into a partially recanalized distal right TS ➡. Note the presence of spinal perimedullary venous drainage ➡. Mass-like, mostly thrombosed Cognard grade 5 dAVF mimics NPH.*

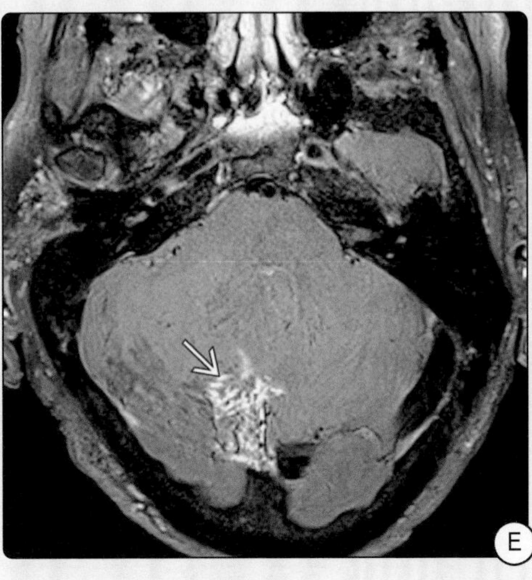

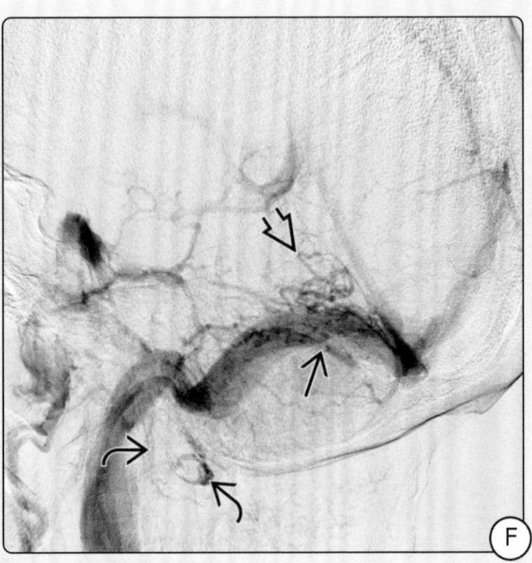

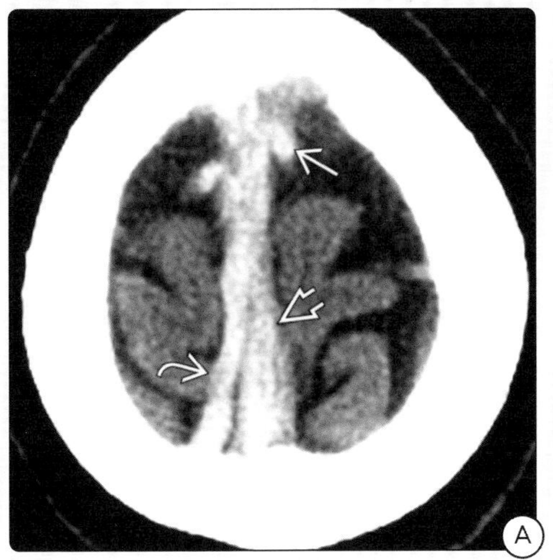

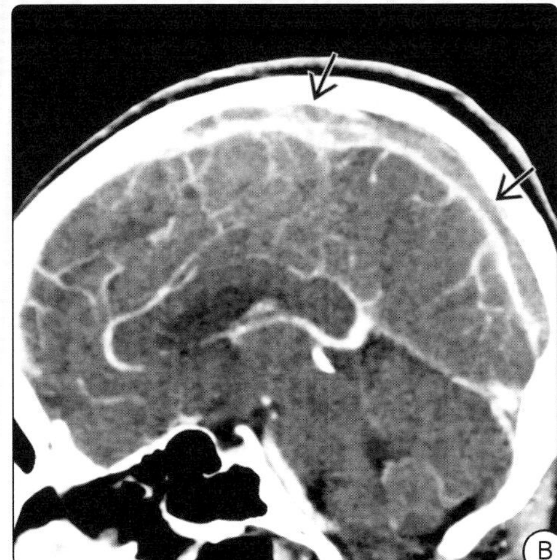

***(7-13A)** NECT in a 62-yo woman with headaches shows thrombosis of the SSS ➡ and multiple cortical veins ➡, including a prominent vein of Trolard ➡. **(7-13B)** Sagittal CT venogram shows long-segment ➡ thrombosis of nearly the entire SSS.*

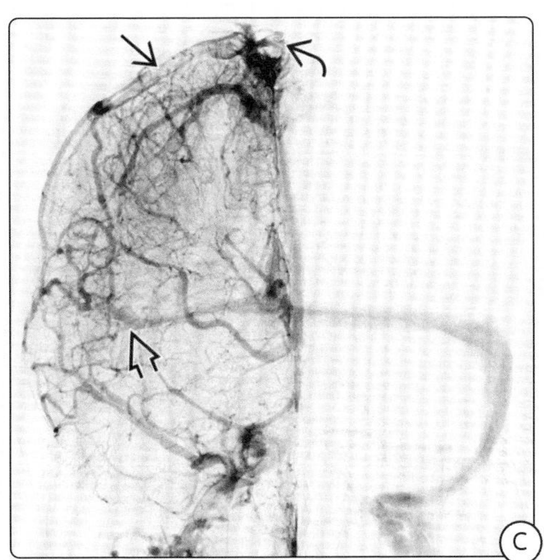

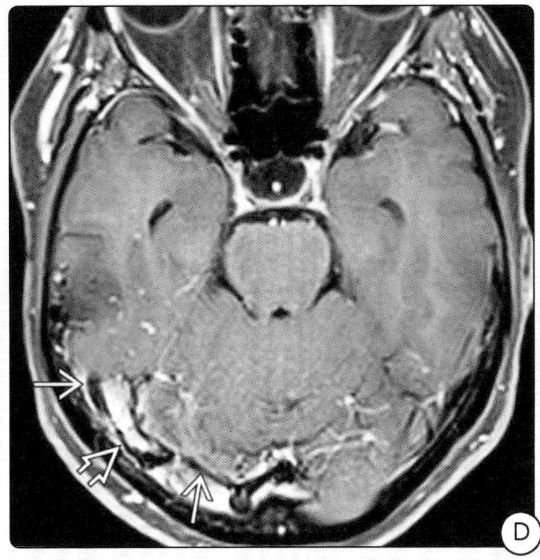

***(7-13C)** AP DSA in the same case shows thrombosis of the right TS ➡ and SSS ➡. Note the clot in the vein of Trolard outlined by contrast ➡. **(7-13D)** Two years later, the patient developed pulsatile tinnitus. T1 C+ FS MR shows enhancing, chronically thrombosed right TS ➡ with partially recanalized venous channels ➡.*

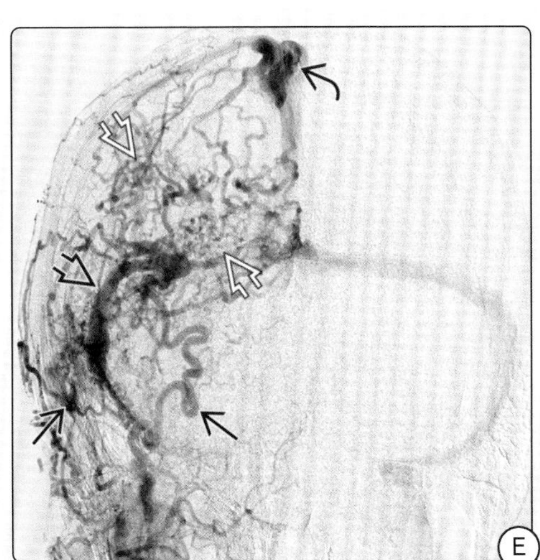

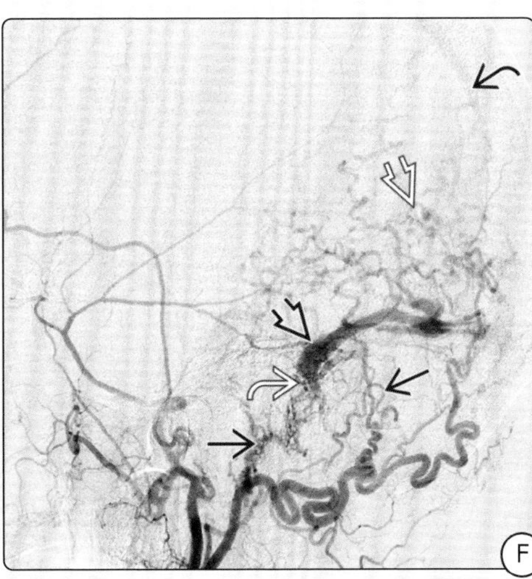

***(7-13E)** Venous phase of AP DSA shows the partially recanalized right TS ➡ with enlarged fistulous arterial feeders arising from the ECA ➡. Innumerable pseudophlebitic tortuous veins ➡ drain into the TS and SSS ➡, which is now patent. **(7-13F)** DSA shows partially recanalized TS ➡ with transosseous branches from the ECA ➡ supplying a dAVF in its wall ➡. Pseudophlebitic veins ➡ drain into SSS ➡.*

*(7-14A) NECT in a 59-yo with headache, increasing weakness, lethargy, confusion, and rapidly declining mental status shows multiple curvilinear calcifications ➡ in the left cerebellum. (7-14B) T2 MR shows numerous vascular "flow voids" around the cervicomedullary junction ➡ and cerebellum ➡. The left cerebellar hemisphere is relatively hypointense ➡ compared to the normal right hemisphere, likely reflecting venous stasis.*

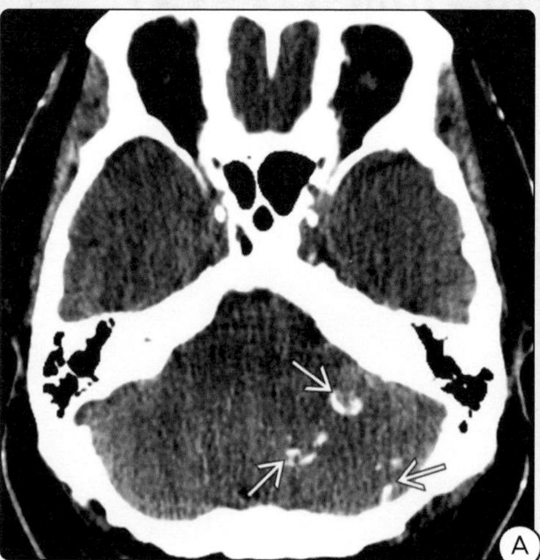

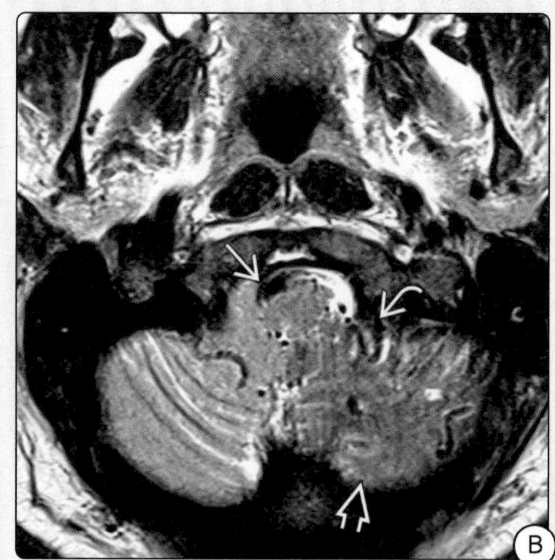

*(7-14C) More cephalad T2 MR shows numerous additional abnormal "flow voids" ➡ and edema ➡ in the left cerebellum. (7-14D) T1 C+ MR in the same case shows enhancement of numerous enlarged vessels in the cerebellar folia ➡ and around the cervicomedullary junction ➡.*

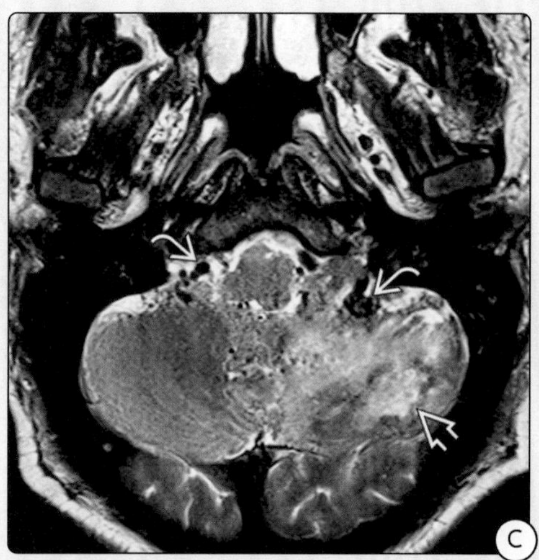

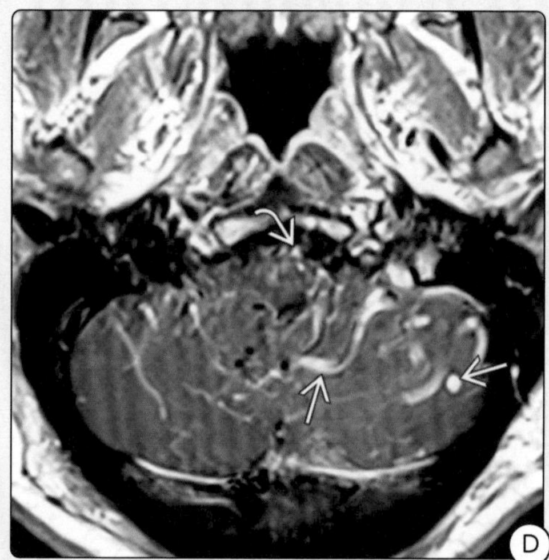

*(7-14E) Coronal T1 C+ MR shows numerous enhancing tortuous vessels ➡ intermixed with several "flow voids" ➡ in both cerebellar hemispheres. (7-14F) DSA of the left common carotid artery shows enlarged dural branches from the petrous ICA and middle meningeal artery ➡ draining directly into dilated variceal medullary veins ➡. This is a Cognard type V dAVF.*

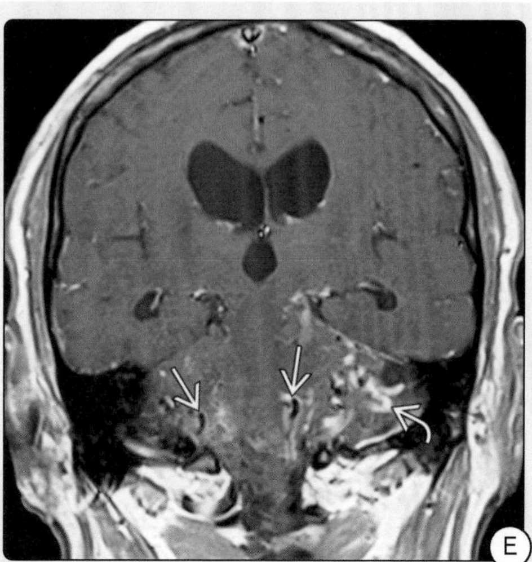

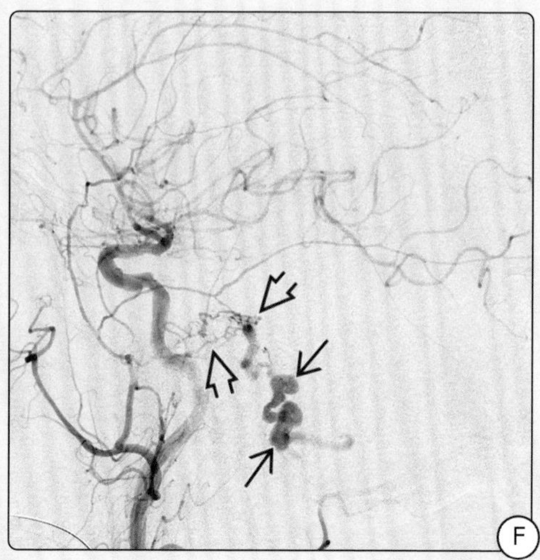

classifications are the most commonly used systems **(7-14)**. In either classification, *the presence of CVD puts a dAVF into a higher grade category with increased risk of parenchymal hemorrhage.* Note that dAVFs are dynamic lesions and may spontaneously regress or progress.

**COGNARD/BORDEN CLASSIFICATION OF dAVFs**

**Benign Venous Drainage Patterns**

- Borden
  - I: Drains to dural sinus; no cortical venous reflux (CVR)
- Cognard
  - I: Drains to dural sinus without reflux; no CVR
  - IIa: Drains to dural sinus with reflux; no CVR

**Aggressive Venous Drainage Patterns**

- Borden
  - II: Drains to dural sinus; CVR present
  - III: Direct drainage to cortical veins or to isolated dural sinus segment
- Cognard
  - IIb: Drains to dural sinus, no sinus reflux; CVR present
  - III: Direct drainage to cortical veins; no venous ectasia
  - IV: Direct drainage to cortical veins + venous ectasia
  - V: Spinal perimedullary venous drainage

## Carotid-Cavernous Fistula

### Terminology

Carotid-cavernous fistulas (CCFs) are a special type of arteriovenous shunt that develops within the CS **(7-15)**. CCFs are divided into two subgroups, direct and indirect fistulas.

**"Direct" CCFs** are typically *high-flow* lesions that result from rupture of the cavernous ICA directly into the CS with or without a preexisting ICA aneurysm. **"Indirect" CCFs** are usually *slow-flow, low-pressure* lesions that represent an AVF between dural branches of the cavernous ICA and the CS.

### Etiology

CCFs are almost always acquired lesions and can be traumatic or nontraumatic. Most *direct* CCFs are traumatic, usually secondary to central skull base fractures. A single-hole laceration/transection of the cavernous ICA with direct fistulization into the CS is the typical finding. Spontaneous (i.e., nontraumatic) rupture of a preexisting cavernous ICA aneurysm is a less common etiology.

*Indirect* CCFs are nontraumatic lesions and are thought to be degenerative in origin. In contrast to dAVFs elsewhere, indirect CCFs rarely occur as sequelae of dural sinus thrombosis. Most indirect CCFs are found in the dural wall of the CS and supplied by intracavernous branches of the ICA and deep (maxillary) branches of the ECA.

### Clinical Issues

**Epidemiology.** An indirect CCF is the second most common intracranial dAVF. Direct high-flow CCFs are much less common.

**Demographics.** Direct CCFs typically occur with trauma and can occur at any age. Indirect CCFs are most frequent in women 40-60 years of age.

**Presentation.** Direct CCFs may present within hours to days or even weeks following trauma. Bruit, pulsatile exophthalmos, decreasing vision, and

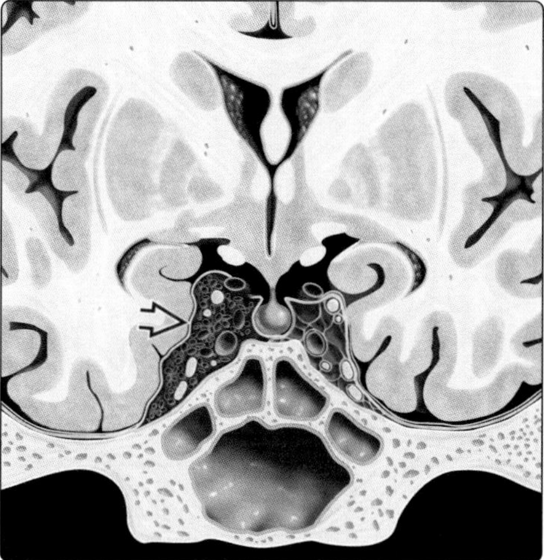

***(7-15)** Graphic shows carotid-cavernous fistula (CCF). Right cavernous sinus (CS) ➩ is enlarged by numerous dilated arterial & venous channels.*

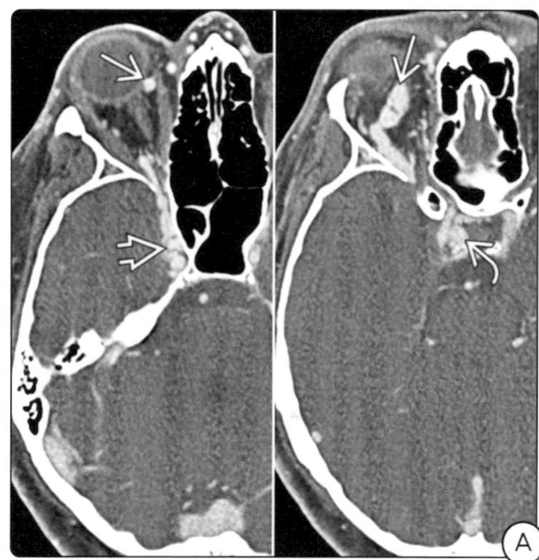

***(7-16A)** CTA of proptosis following skull base fracture and carotid pseudoaneurysm ➡ shows multiple dilated CS ➡ and orbital veins ➡.*

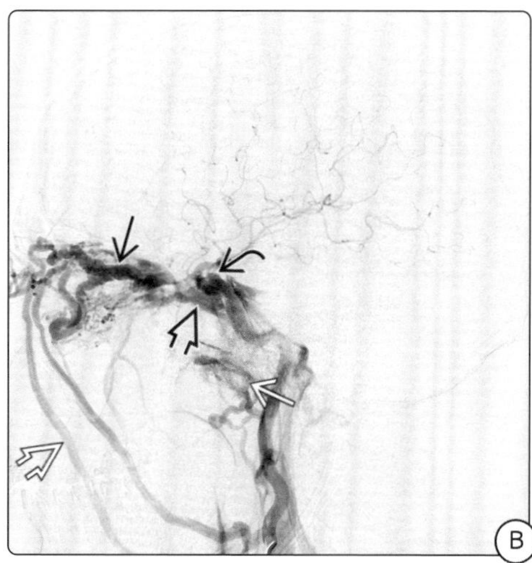

***(7-16B)** Lateral DSA shows a pseudoaneurysm ➩, contrast shunting into CS ➩, orbital ➩ and facial veins ➡, and pterygoid plexus ➡.*

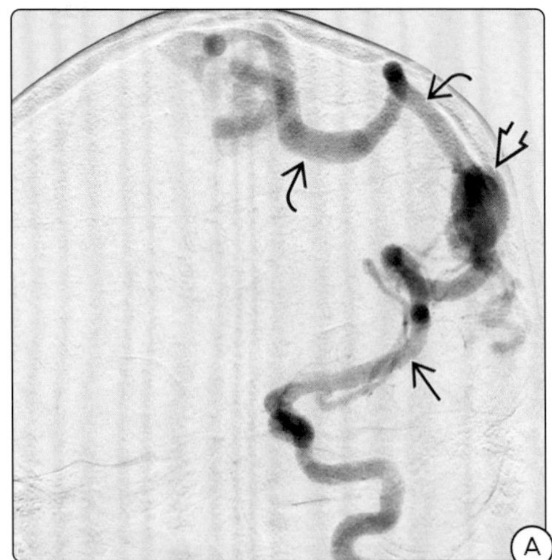


*(7-17A) AP DSA shows an enlarged MCA branch filling the large venous varix that drains into an enlarged cortical vein.*

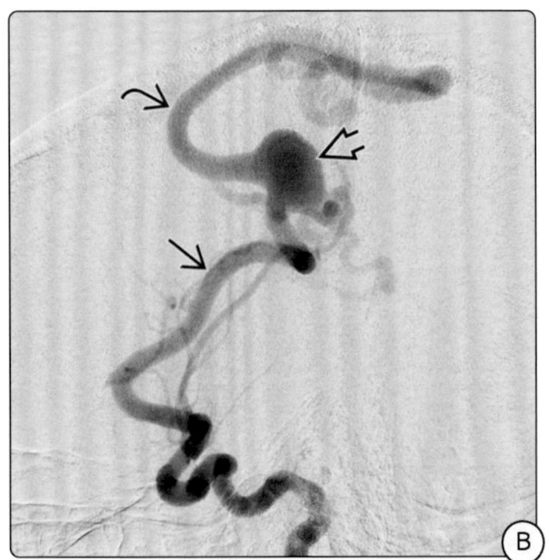


*(7-17B) Early-phase lateral DSA shows enlarged MCA branch fistulizing into a venous varix then a massively enlarged cortical vein.*

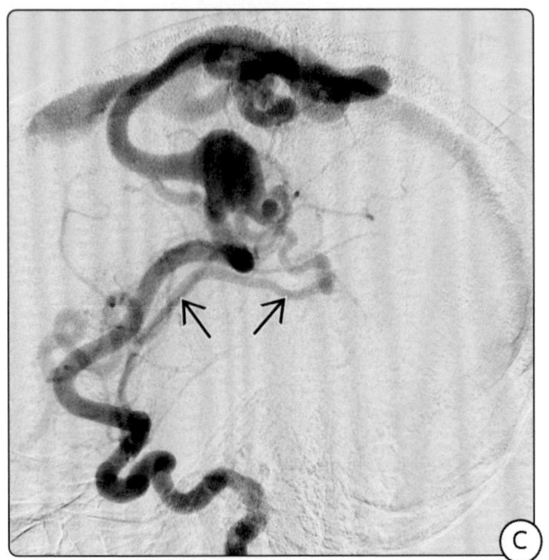


*(7-17C) Later phase shows venous varix also draining into prominent superficial middle cerebral vein. This is direct pial AVF.*

headache are typical. Indirect CCFs cause painless proptosis with variable vision changes.

**Treatment Options.** Direct CCF fistulae are closed with transarterial-transfistula detachable balloon embolization. Indirect CCFs may be treated conservatively or with superselective embolization.

## Imaging

**CT Findings.** NECT scans may demonstrate mild or striking proptosis, a prominent CS with enlarged superior ophthalmic vein (SOV), and enlarged extraocular muscles. "Dirty" fat secondary to edema and venous engorgement may be present.

CECT scans often nicely demonstrate an enlarged SOV and CS. Inferior draining into a prominent pterygoid venous plexus and posterior drainage into an enlarged clival venous plexus are sometimes present.

CTA shows engorgement of the ophthalmic vein and CS **(7-16A)**. Dehiscence of the intracavernous ICA is characteristic for direct CCF.

**MR Findings.** T1WIs may show a prominent "bulging" CS and SOV as well as "dirty" orbital fat. High-flow CCFs may show too many CS "flow voids" on T2WIs. Strong, uniform enhancement of the CS and SOV is typical. Enlarged, tortuous intracranial veins may occur with high-flow, high-pressure shunts.

**Angiography.** DSA is required for definitive diagnosis and treatment. Complete delineation of the arterial supply and venous drainage pattern is the goal.

*Direct* CCFs typically demonstrate rapid flow with very early CS opacification **(7-16B)**. Selective ICA injection with very rapid image acquisition is often necessary to localize the fistula site exactly. A single-hole fistula is usually present, typically between the C4 and C5 ICA segments.

*Indirect* CCFs often have multiple dural feeders from cavernous branches of the ICA (meningohypophyseal and inferolateral trunks) as well as deep branches of the ECA (middle meningeal and distal maxillary branches).

## Differential Diagnosis

The major differential diagnosis with CCFs is **CS thrombosis** (CST). Both CCF and CST may cause proptosis, intraorbital edema, enlarged extraocular muscles, and the appearance of "dirty" fat. In CST, the CS may appear enlarged, but prominent filling defects are present on T1 C+ MR.

# Pial Arteriovenous Fistula

Intracranial pial arteriovenous fistulas (pAVFs), a.k.a. nongalenic pial arteriovenous fistulas, are rare neurovascular malformations. pAVFs account for < 2% of all intracranial AVMs. They can occur in all ages but are most common in children. pAVFs can be congenital or arise from iatrogenic or traumatic injury.

pAVFs usually consist of a single dilated *pial* artery that connects directly to an enlarged cortical draining vein within a *subpial* space. No intervening capillary bed or nidus is present, although a dilated venous pouch ("varix") is common **(7-17)**.

80% of pAVFs are supratentorial. They typically lie on or just within the brain surface under the pia. Supratentorial pAVFs are supplied by the anterior, middle, or posterior cerebral arteries and are usually associated with a venous varix. "Multihole" pAVFs have multiple feeders.

## Vein of Galen Aneurysmal Malformation

Different types of vascular malformations share a dilated vein of Galen as a common feature, but only one of these is a true vein of Galen aneurysmal malformation (VGAM). A VGAM is the most common extracardiac cause of high-output cardiac failure in newborns and comprises 30% of pediatric vascular anomalies.

### Terminology

VGAM is essentially a direct AVF between deep choroidal arteries and a persistent embryonic precursor of the vein of Galen, the median prosencephalic vein (MPV) of Markowski **(7-18)**.

### Etiology

Normally, the developing internal cerebral veins annex drainage of the fetal choroid plexus as the embryonic MPV—the precursor of the vein of Galen—regresses. In a VGAM, a high-flow fistula prevents formation of the definitive vein of Galen. Mutations in Ephrin signaling genes have been identified in nearly 1/3 of VGAMs.

### Clinical Issues

**Demographics.** VGAMs are rare, representing < 1% of all CVMs. Neonatal VGAMs are more common than those presenting in infancy or childhood. There is a definite male predominance (M:F = 2:1).

**Presentation.** In neonates, high-output congestive heart failure and a loud cranial bruit are typical. Older infants may present with macrocrania and hydrocephalus.

**Natural History.** Large VGAMs cause cerebral ischemia and dystrophic changes in the fetal brain. Neonates with untreated VGAMs typically die from progressive brain damage and intractable heart failure. Staged arterial embolization, ideally at 4 or 5 months of age, is the preferred treatment.

### Imaging

**CT Findings.** NECT scans show a well-delineated hyperdense mass at the tentorial apex, usually compressing the third ventricle and causing severe obstructive hydrocephalus. Variable encephalomalacia, hemorrhage, &/or dystrophic calcification in the brain parenchyma are often present. CECT scans show strong uniform enhancement **(7-19)**.

**MR Findings.** Rapid but turbulent flow in the VGAM causes inhomogeneous signal loss and phase artifact. Enlarged arterial feeders are seen as serpentine "flow voids" adjacent to the lesion.

**Angiography.** Multiple branches from the pericallosal, choroidal, and thalamoperforating arteries drain directly into an enlarged, aneurysmally dilated midline venous sac **(7-20)**. In > 50% of all VGAMs, the straight sinus is hypoplastic or absent, and venous drainage is into a persistent embryonic **"falcine sinus" (7-19)**.

### Differential Diagnosis

Typical imaging findings in a neonate with high-output congestive heart failure are virtually pathognomonic of VGAM. A **thalamic AVM with deep venous drainage** may cause secondary enlargement of the vein of Galen but rarely presents in the neonatal period. A high-flow **giant childhood dural AVM (dAVM)** may present in infancy and clinically resemble a VGAM. Involvement of the dural venous sinuses rather than the vein of Galen is typical.

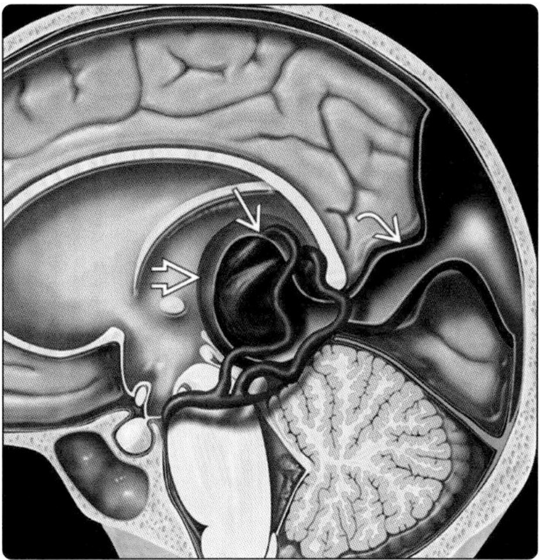

***(7-18)** VGAM shows enlarged choroid arteries ➡ draining into venous pouch (dilated median prosencephalic vein) ➡ and falcine sinus ➡.*

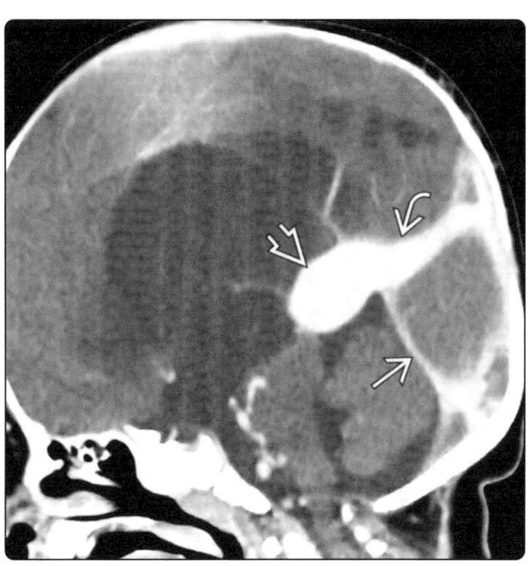

***(7-19)** CTV in a newborn infant shows acute hydrocephalus from a VGAM ➡. Note persistent falcine sinus ➡, hypoplastic straight sinus ➡.*

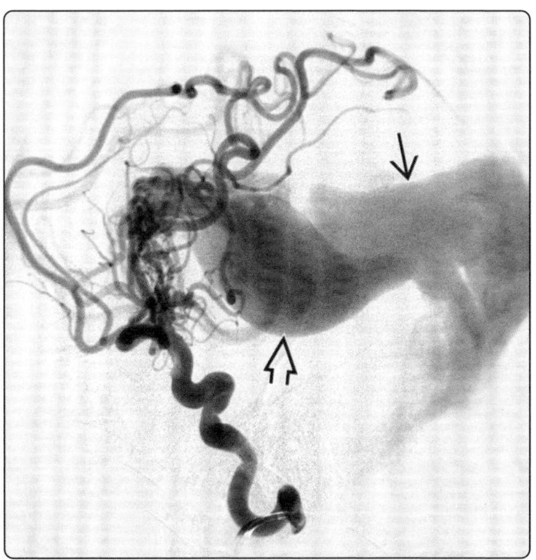

***(7-20)** Lateral DSA shows a VGAM ➡ draining into a massively enlarged falcine sinus ➡. (Courtesy S. Blaser, MD.)*

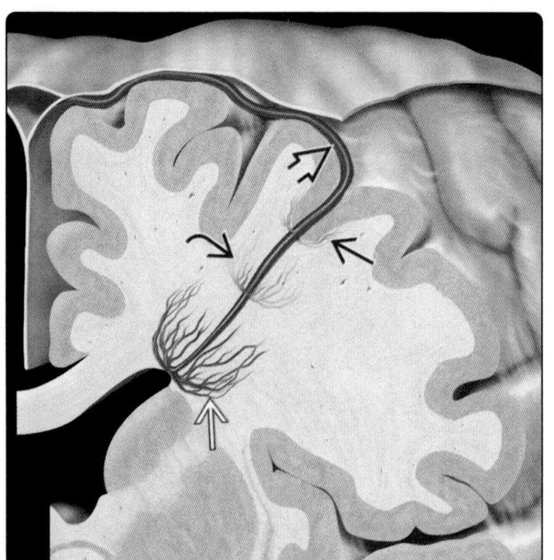

***(7-21)** DVA with enlarged juxtacortical, subcortical, periventricular medullary veins drains into a single transmantle collector vein.*

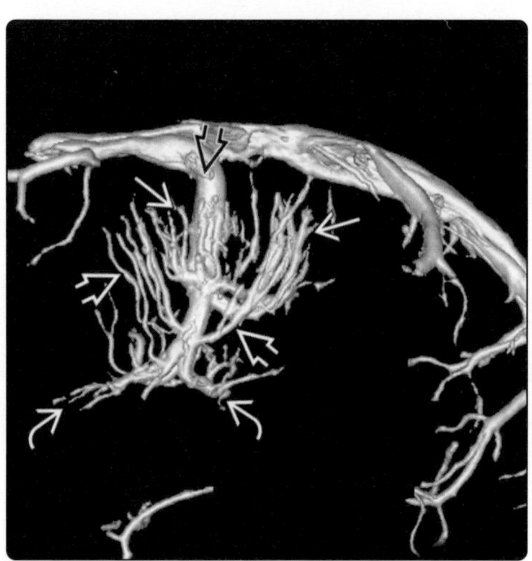

***(7-22)** 3D DSA: DVA with juxta-, subcortical, periventricular medullary veins, collector vein. (Courtesy P. Lasjaunias, MD.)*

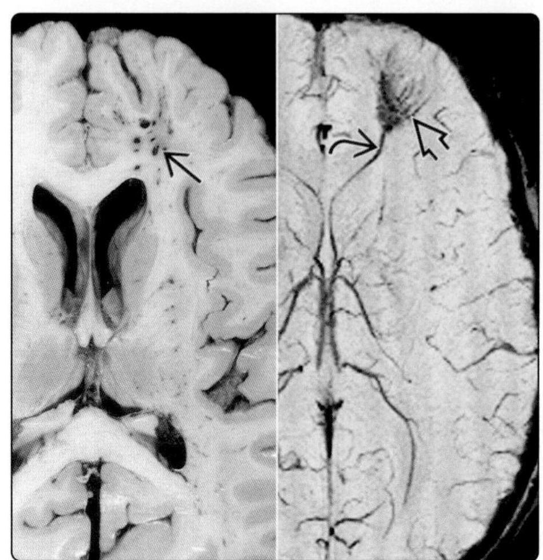

***(7-23)** (L) Frontal DVA autopsy shows normal parenchyma between enlarged venous radicles. (R) T2* SWI shows DVA, collector vein.*

# Cerebrovascular Malformations Without Arteriovenous Shunting

## Developmental Venous Anomaly

### Terminology

**Developmental venous anomaly (DVA)**, a.k.a. **venous "angioma"** or "venous malformation," is an umbrella-shaped congenital cerebral vascular malformation composed of angiogenically mature venous elements. Dilated, thin-walled venous channels lie within (and are separated by) normal brain parenchyma.

### Etiology

The precise etiology of DVAs is unknown. Most investigators believe it is arrested medullary vein development between 8 and 11 gestational weeks that results in DVAs. The underlying genetics involved in DVA development, whether germ-line or somatic, remain to be elucidated.

### Pathology

**Location.** Approximately 70% of DVAs are found in the deep white matter, adjacent to the frontal horn of the lateral ventricle **(7-21)**. The second most common location is next to the fourth ventricle (15-30%).

DVA depth is defined as where the medullary venous radicles converge into the collector vein. Three depths are recognized: Juxtacortical, subcortical, and periventricular **(7-22)**. Some larger DVAs can have dual or even triple convergence sites.

**Size and Number.** DVA size varies from tiny, almost imperceptible lesions to giant venous malformations that involve most of the hemispheric white matter.

Between 6-7% of patients with a DVA have two lesions; multiple DVAs occur in 1%. Multiple DVAs have been reported in **blue rubber bleb nevus syndrome** (BRBNS, a.k.a. Bean syndrome) and other superficial craniofacial venous and venolymphatic malformations.

**Gross Pathology.** DVAs consist of two elements: A cluster of variably sized prominent medullary (white matter) veins (the so-called caput medusa) that converges on an enlarged stem or single "collector vein." A DVA is embedded within and drains grossly normal-appearing brain parenchyma, forming its primary or sole venous drainage pathway **(7-23)**.

Hemorrhage and calcification are uncommon unless the DVA is associated with another vascular malformation or the collecting vein becomes thrombosed. The most common "histologically mixed" CVM is a cavernous-venous malformation found in 10-15% of patients with a DVA.

**Microscopic Features.** Thin-walled, somewhat dilated venous channels are interspersed in normal-appearing white matter. Varying degrees of focal parenchymal atrophy, white matter gliosis, neuronal degeneration, and demyelination may be present within the venous drainage territory of some DVAs.

### Clinical Issues

**Demographics.** DVA is the most common of all intracranial vascular malformations, accounting for 60% of all CVMs. Estimated prevalence on contrast-enhanced MR scans ranges from 2.5-9.0%.

**Presentation.** DVAs occur in patients of all ages. At least 98% of isolated DVAs are asymptomatic and discovered incidentally. About 2% initially present with hemorrhage or infarct, often related to presence of a **coexisting cavernous malformation** or stenosis of the collecting ("outlet") vein, usually at the entrance to the superior sagittal sinus.

DVAs may also coexist with a **sinus pericranii (SP)**. SP is typically the cutaneous sign of an underlying venous anomaly **(7-31)**. DVAs are also associated with HHT (4% of cases). Other reported associations include malformations of cortical development.

Because **multiple sclerosis** (MS) lesions evolve predominantly around venous structures, some studies indicate MS may be associated with an increased prevalence of DVAs. Occasionally, demyelinating disease will occur in conjunction with a DVA. MS-associated DVAs are not associated with significantly altered clinical outcomes or disease progression.

### DEVELOPMENTAL VENOUS ANOMALY

**Terminology**
- DVA is a.k.a. venous "angioma"

**Pathology**
- Solitary > > multiple; small > large
- Enlarged white matter veins interspersed with normal brain
- Usually found adjacent to lateral or fourth ventricle

**Clinical Issues**
- Epidemiology and demographics
  - Most common CVM (60%)
  - Prevalence on T1 C+ MR: 2-9%
  - All ages, no sex predilection

**Natural History**
- Usually benign, nonprogressive
- May hemorrhage if mixed with cavernous malformation or collector vein thrombosis

**Treatment Options.** No treatment is required or recommended for solitary DVAs (they are "leave me alone" lesions). If a DVA is histologically mixed, treatment is determined by the coexisting lesion. Preoperative identification of such mixed malformations is important, as ligating the collector vein or removing its tributaries may result in venous infarction.

## Imaging

**General Features.** DVAs are composed of radially arranged medullary veins that converge on a transcortical or subependymal large collector vein. The classic appearance is that of a Medusa head or upside-down umbrella **(7-21)**.

**CT Findings.** NECT scans are usually normal unless the collector vein is large **(7-27)**. Unilateral basal ganglia calcification has been reported in the drainage territory of some deep DVAs **(7-24A)**.

CECT scans and CTVs show numerous linear &/or punctate enhancing foci that converge on a well-delineated tubular collector vein **(7-24B)** **(7-24C)**. In larger DVAs, perfusion CT may show a venous congestion pattern with increased CBV, CBF, and mean transit time (MTT) in the adjacent brain parenchyma.

**MR Findings.** If the DVA is small, it may be undetectable unless contrast-enhanced scans or susceptibility-weighted sequences are obtained.

***T2/FLAIR.*** Large DVAs can exhibit a "flow void" on T2WI **(7-25A)**. Venous radicles of the caput medusa are often hyperintense on T2/FLAIR. DVA-

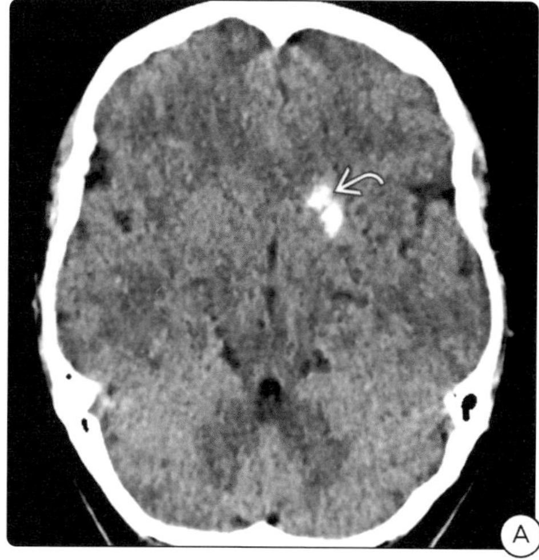


***(7-24A)** NECT in a 34-yo woman with headaches shows calcification in the left basal ganglia.*

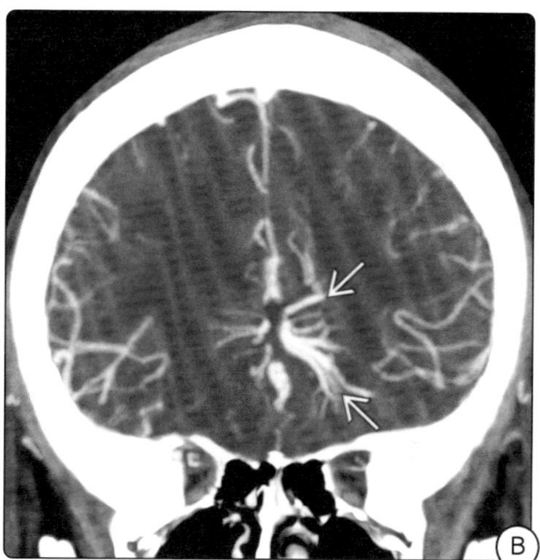


***(7-24B)** Coronal MIP of CT venogram in the same patient shows a large left DVA.*

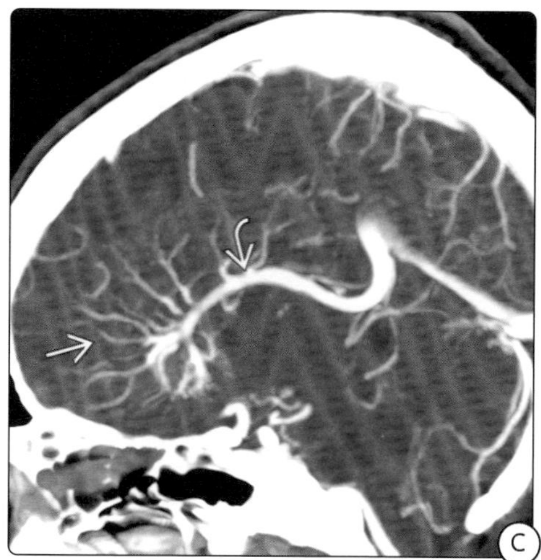


***(7-24C)** Sagittal MIP CTV nicely shows the "Medusa head" of the DVA draining into an enlarged internal cerebral vein.*

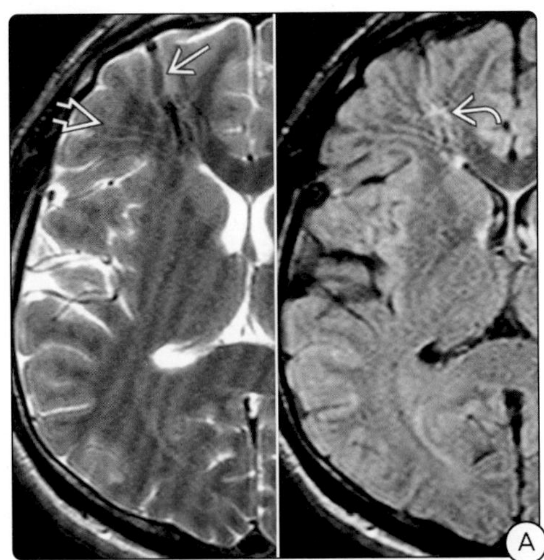

(7-25A) (L) T2 of DVA shows hypointense draining ➡ and enlarged medullary veins ➡. (R) FLAIR shows mild parenchymal hyperintensity ➡.

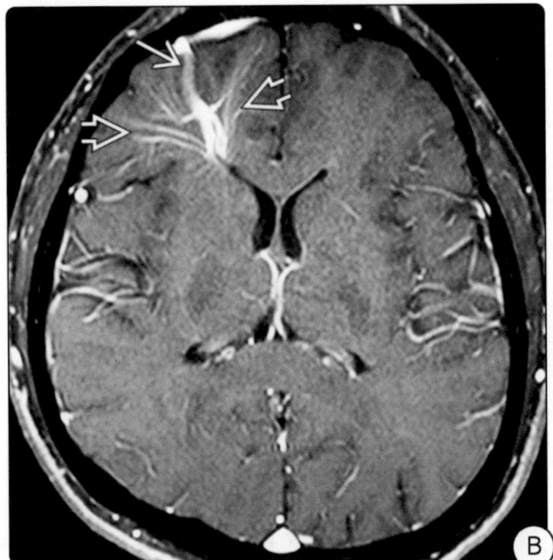

(7-25B) T1 C+ FS MR shows prominent transmantle draining vein ➡, dilated medullary veins forming the classic "Medusa head" ➡.

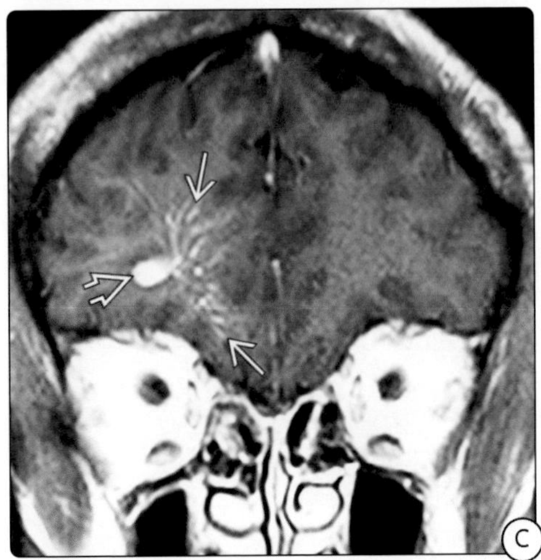

(7-25C) Coronal T1 C+ MR nicely shows an "umbrella" of enlarged medullary veins ➡ converging on the transmantle draining vein ➡.

associated parenchymal abnormalities are common. T2/FLAIR parenchymal abnormalities are present in 10-25% of DVAs **(7-28A)**. The etiology of such associated hyperintensities is unknown but could represent gliosis or hemodynamic stress, such as venous congestion or ischemia, demyelination, or hypomyelination.

***T2* (GRE, SWI).*** Because flow in the venous radicles of a DVA is typically slow, blood deoxygenates and T2* scans (GRE, SWI) show striking linear hypointensities **(7-23)**.

If a DVA is mixed with a cavernous malformation, blood products in various stages of degradation may be present and "bloom" on T2* sequences **(7-30)**. Discrete hypointense foci on 3T SWI are seen in the majority of cases, especially in DVAs that are associated with parenchymal hyperintensities on FLAIR. Venous congestion in a DVA may result in microhemorrhages or possibly promote the formation of small cavernous malformations.

***T1 C+.*** T1 C+ sequences show a stellate collection of linear enhancing structures **(7-26B)** converging on the transparenchymal or subependymal collector vein **(7-25B)** **(7-25C)** **(7-28B)**. The collector vein may show variable high-velocity signal loss **(7-26A)**.

***pMR and fMRI.*** DSC pMR is usually normal in small DVAs. Elevated CBV and CBF with mildly increased MTT are common within larger DVAs. DVAs can strongly resemble neural signal on resting-state fMRI.

**Angiography.** Except in the rare "arterialized" DVA, the arterial phase is normal. The venous phase shows the typical hair-like collection ("Medusa head") of dilated medullary veins within the white matter. A faint, prolonged "blush" or capillary "stain" may be present in some cases.

**Nuclear Medicine Studies.** More than 3/4 of DVAs are associated with hypometabolism in the adjacent brain parenchyma on FDG PET studies, often in the absence of any other structural abnormalities.

## Differential Diagnosis

**A histologically mixed vascular malformation** in which the DVA provides prominent venous drainage is common. The most common combination is a mixed cavernous-venous malformation **(7-30)**. Unusually large ("giant") **capillary telangiectasias** often have a dominant central collector vein and may therefore resemble a DVA **(7-46)**. DVAs have also been reported adjacent to foci of cortical dysplasia and in/adjacent to demyelinating lesions (see Digital-Only images 27-30).

### DEVELOPMENTAL VENOUS ANOMALY: IMAGING

**MR**

- T2/FLAIR
  - Collector vein = flow void on T2WI
  - Radicles of "Medusa head" hyperintense on FLAIR
  - 10-25% have T2/FLAIR parenchymal hyperintensities
- T2* (GRE/SWI)
  - Linear hypointensities in radicles, collector vein
  - "Blooming" foci if mixed with cerebral cavernous malformations
  - 3T SWI may show microbleeds
- T1 C+
  - "Umbrella" of tubular radicles → collector vein
- pMR
  - Increased CBV/CBF, increased MTT

**DSA**

- Classic "Medusa head" in venous phase

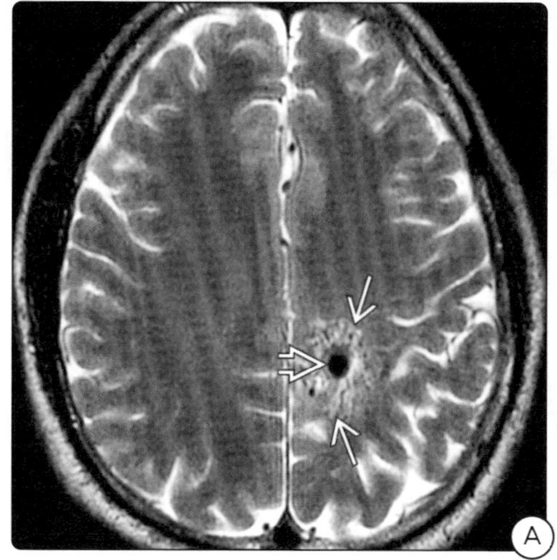

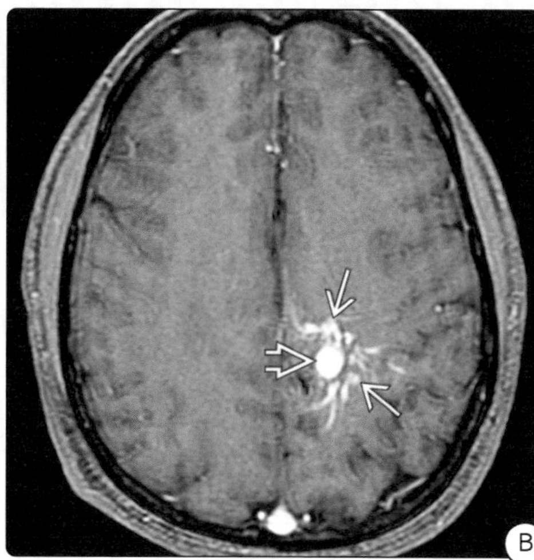

***(7-26A)** Series of images illustrates complex DVA in a 34-yo man. Axial T2 MR shows a large "flow void" ➡ surrounded by many smaller, more tortuous-appearing vessels ➡. **(7-26B)** T1 C+ MR in the same case shows a large well-delineated enhancing vessel ➡ that appears to drain a cluster of smaller, more tortuous vessels ➡.*

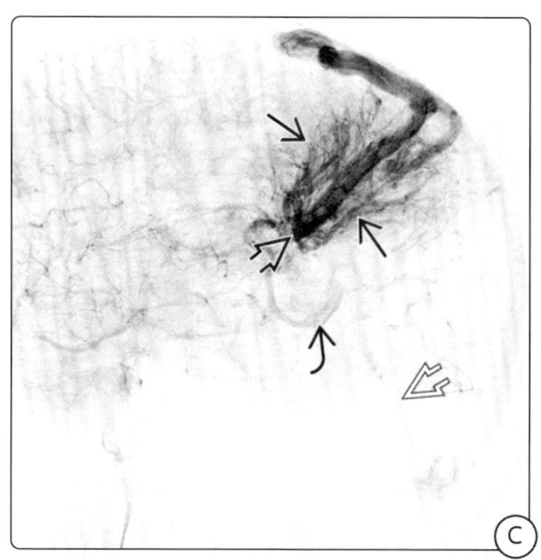

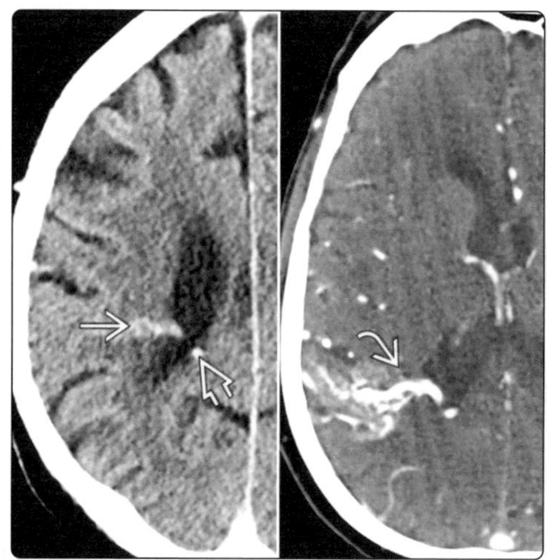

***(7-26C)** Lateral capillary phase of the left ICA DSA in the same case shows a giant "Medusa head" blush of enlarged medullary veins ➡ that drains into a dilated transmantle collector vein ➡. Note AV shunting with early draining vein of Galen ➡ and straight sinus ➡. This is giant "complex" DVA. **(7-27)** (L) NECT shows linear ➡, dot-like hyperdensities ➡. (R) CTA shows large vascular malformation ➡, most likely a "giant" DVA.*

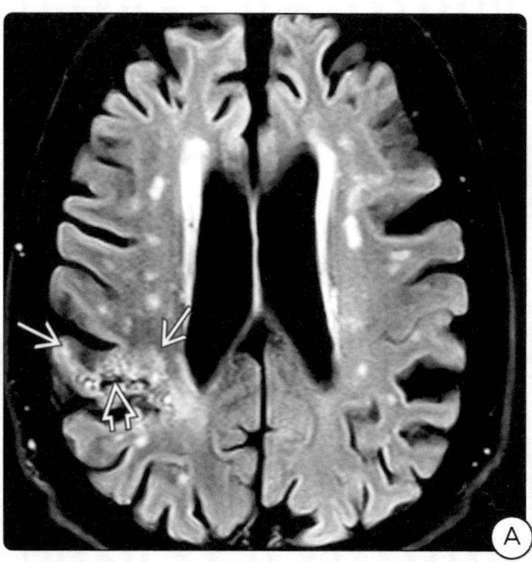

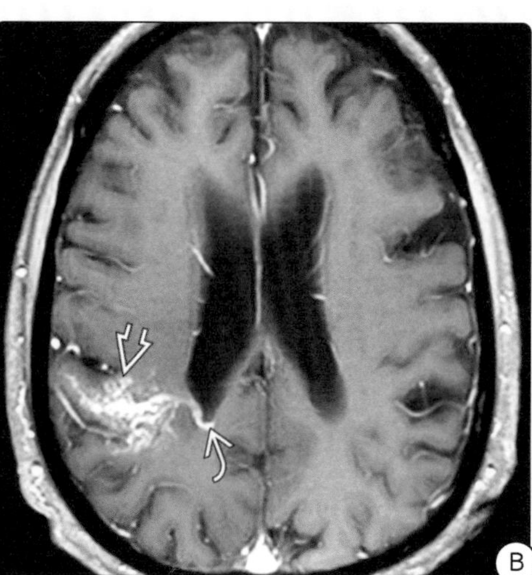

***(7-28A)** Axial FLAIR MR in the same case shows extensive WM hyperintensity ➡ in the same area surrounding a linear "flow void" ➡. **(7-28B)** T1 C+ MR in the same case shows the lesion is a very large DVA ➡ with dominant draining vein ➡ emptying into the subependymal venous system.*

*(7-29A) Sagittal T1 C+ MR shows a bizarre-appearing midline frontal vascular mass that connects to a massively enlarged inferior sagittal sinus (ISS). (7-29B) Venous phase of a left internal carotid DSA in the same case shows dilated medullary veins draining into a large venous varix that connects to an enlarged ISS. The anterior SSS is hypoplastic, and a large frontal superficial cortical vein joins the SSS at the coronal suture.*

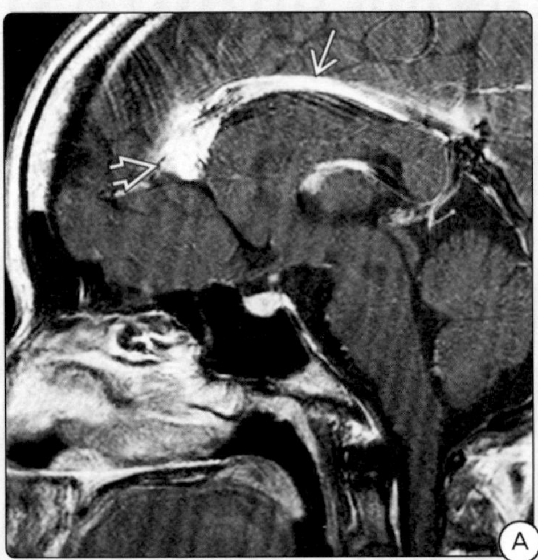

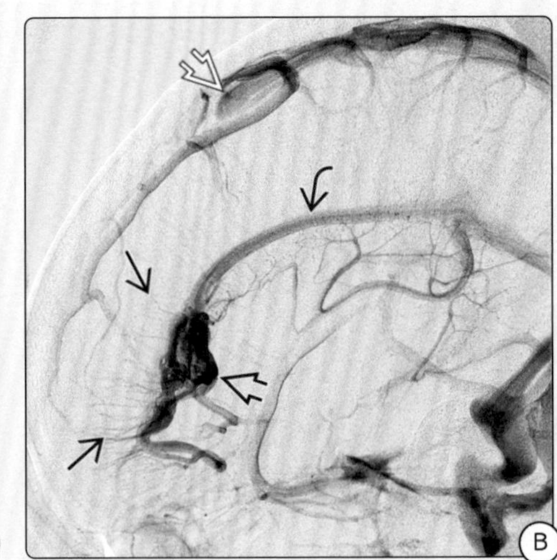

*(7-30A) T1 MR in a 30-yo man with sudden-onset, left-sided weakness shows a mixed-signal, mostly hyperintense mass in the right thalamus. Note subtle fluid-fluid levels in some of the locules. (7-30B) FLAIR MR shows multiple locules with fluid-fluid levels and surrounding vasogenic edema. A smaller, separate mass is seen in the anterior basal ganglia.*

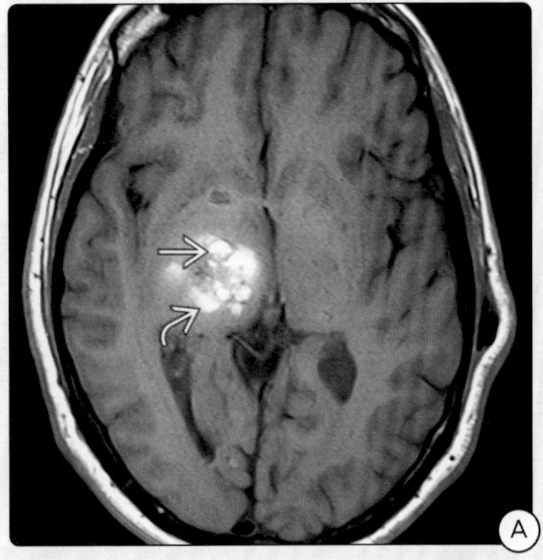

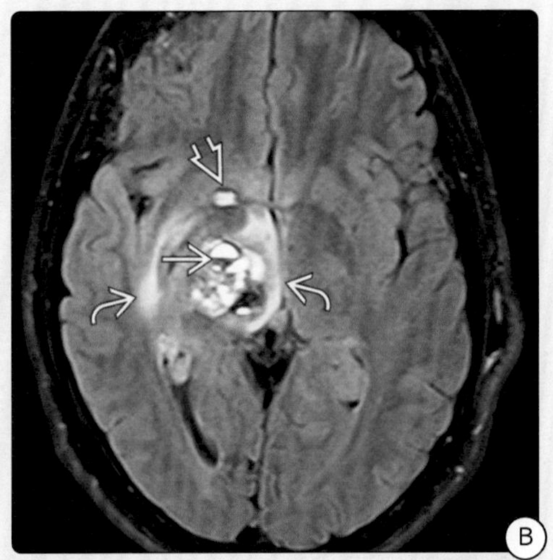

*(7-30C) T2* GRE shows striking "blooming" in 3 separate hemorrhage lesions. (7-30D) T1 C+ FS MR shows some enhancement around the loculated mass. Multiple enlarged bilateral venous channels are present. Multiple giant DVAs are associated with multiple cavernous malformations. Mixed cavernous-venous histology is the most common mixed cerebral vascular malformation.*

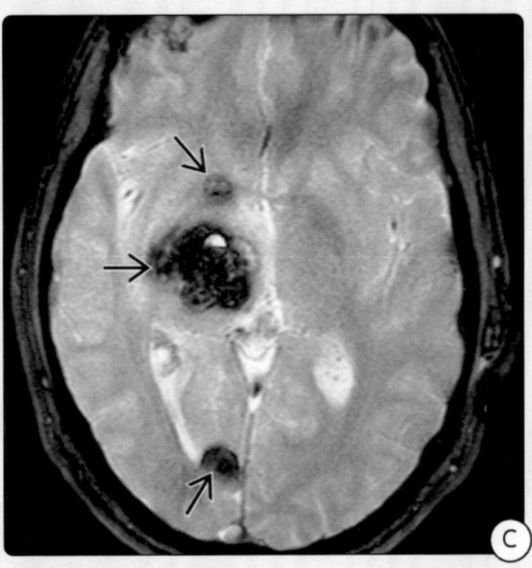

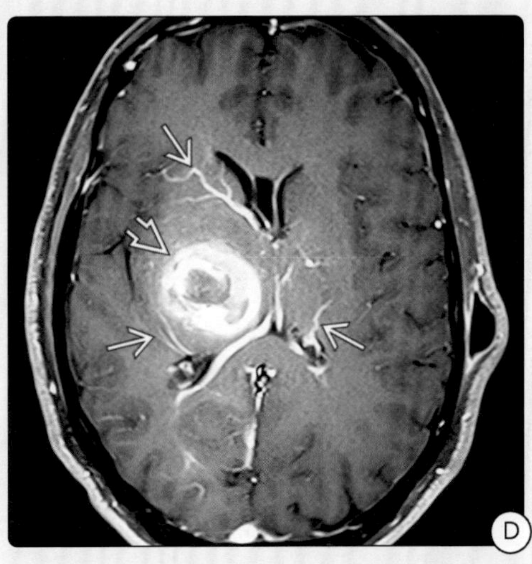

## Sinus Pericranii

### Terminology

Sinus pericranii (SP) is a rare benign venous anomaly that consists of an emissary intradiploic vein that connects an intracranial dural venous sinus with an extracranial venous varix **(7-31)**. The dilated venous pouch hugs the external table of the skull.

### Pathology

A bluish sac beneath or just above the periosteum of the calvarium is typical. The dilated, blood-filled sac connects with the intracranial circulation through a well-defined bone defect **(7-31)**. The frontal lobe is the most common site, followed by the parietal and occipital lobes. SPs in the middle and posterior cranial fossae are rare.

SP may be associated with single or multiple intracranial DVAs. Other reported associations include craniosynostosis and dural sinus hypoplasia. SP with multiple DVAs is associated with BRBNS.

### Imaging

**CT Findings.** An SP shows strong uniform enhancement after contrast administration **(7-32)**. The underlying calvarial defect varies in size but is typically well demarcated.

**MR Findings.** Most SPs are isointense on T1WI and hyperintense to brain on T2WI. "Puddling" of contrast within the SP on T1 C+ is typical unless the lesion is unusually large and flow is rapid. MRV is helpful in delineating both the intra- and extracranial components.

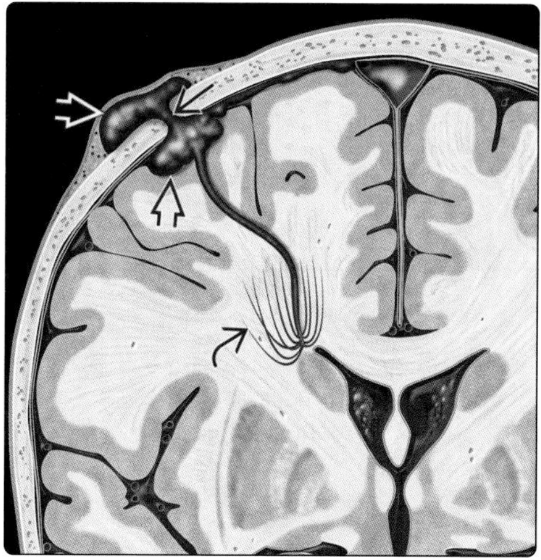

*(7-31) Graphic shows SP with extracranial venous pouch ➡, transcalvarial channel ⇨, intracranial pouch ⇨, and associated DVA ↗.*

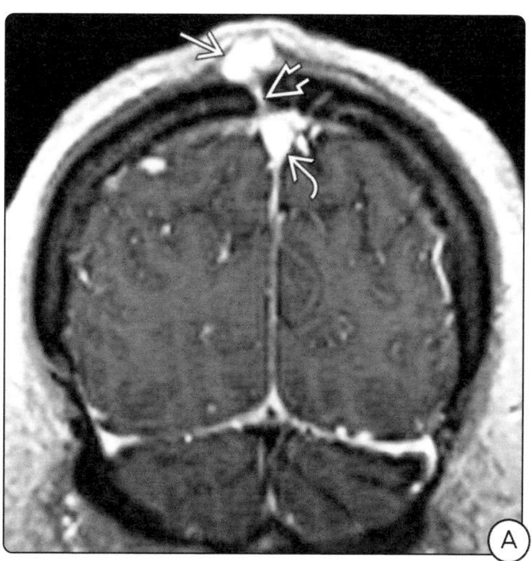


*(7-32A) Coronal T1 C+ SPGR study shows classic SP. An extracranial venous pouch ➡ connects with the SSS ➡ via a transosseous vein ➡.*

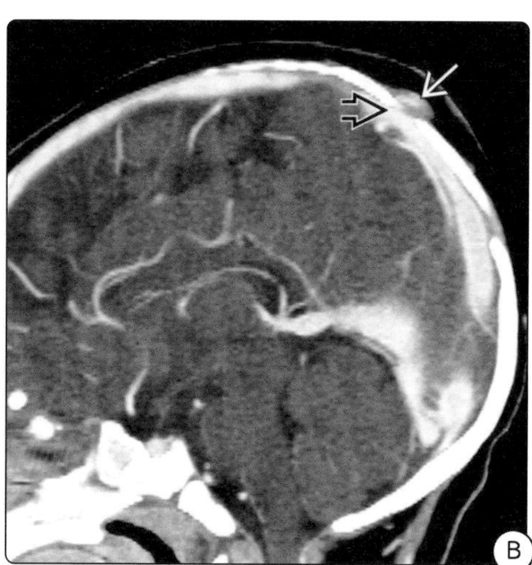


*(7-32B) Sagittal CTV shows a small SP ➡ connecting to the SSS through an adjacent skull defect ⇨.*

## Cerebral Cavernous Malformation

Cerebral cavernous malformations (CCMs) are a distinct type of intracranial vascular malformation characterized by repeated "intralesional" hemorrhages into thin-walled, angiogenically immature, blood-filled locules called caverns. CCMs are discrete, well-marginated lesions that do not contain normal brain parenchyma. Most are surrounded by a complete hemosiderin rim **(7-33)**.

Cavernous malformations exhibit a wide range of dynamic behaviors. They are a relatively common cause of spontaneous nontraumatic ICH in young and middle-aged adults, although they can occur at any age.

### Terminology

CCMs are a.k.a. cavernous "angiomas" or "cavernomas." They are benign malformative vascular hamartomas. CCMs are sometimes erroneously referred to as cavernous hemangiomas. Hemangiomas are benign vascular neoplasms, *not* malformations.

### Etiology

**General Concepts.** CCMs are angiogenically immature lesions with endothelial proliferation and increased neoangiogenesis. They consist of closely clustered, abnormally dilated and leaky capillaries that occur predominately in the central nervous system.

CCMs can be inherited or acquired. Acquired CCMs are rare and usually associated with prior radiation therapy (XRT). Approximately 3.5% of children who have whole-brain XRT develop multiple CCMs with a mean latency interval of ~ 3 years (3-102 months).

**Genetics.** CCMs can be solitary and sporadic (80% of cases) or multiple and familial (20%). Familial CCMs are inherited as an autosomal dominant disease with variable penetrance and are more common in Hispanic Americans of Mexican descent.

Three independent genes have been identified in familial CCMs: *KRIT1*/CCM1, *CCM2*, and *PDCD10*/CCM3. All the mutations in these genes cause a loss of function and compromise the protein functions needed for maintaining vascular barrier integrity.

**Associated Abnormalities.** CCMs are the most common component in mixed vascular malformations. Cavernous-venous and cavernous-capillary are the two most frequent combinations.

## Pathology

**Location and Size.** CCMs can occur anywhere in the CNS and range in size from tiny, near-microscopic lesions to giant malformations that can occupy an entire lobe or most of the cerebral hemisphere.

**Gross Pathology.** A compact, spongy collection of reddish-purple blood-filled "caverns" devoid of intervening neural elements is typical. Most CCMs are surrounded by a rust-colored rim of gliotic, indurated brain.

**Staging, Grading, and Classification.** The most commonly used classification of CCMs, the Zabramski classification, is based on imaging appearance, not histologic findings (see next shaded box).

## Clinical Issues

**Epidemiology.** CCMs are the third most common CVM (after DVA and capillary telangiectasia) and are found in ~ 0.5% of the population. 2/3 occur as a solitary, sporadic lesion; ~ 1/3 are multiple.

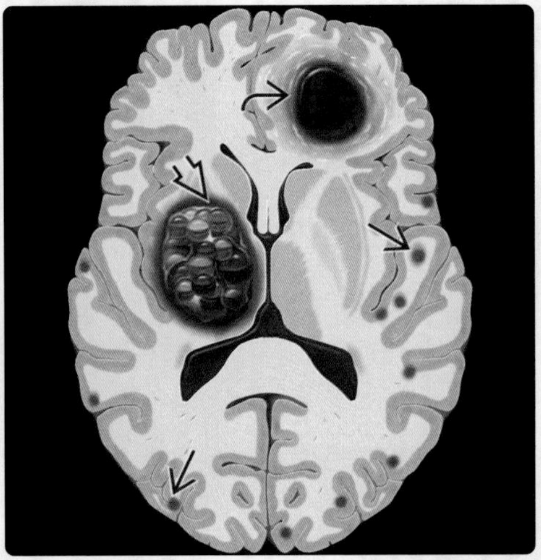

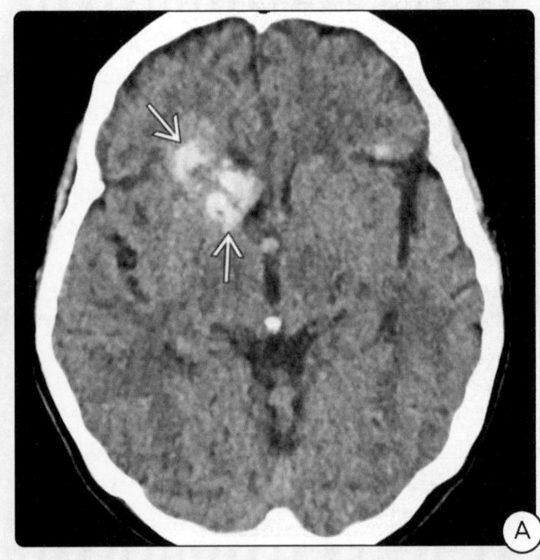

*(7-33) Note subacute ⇨ (Zabramski type I), classic "popcorn ball" ⇨ (Zabramski type II) appearances of cerebral cavernous malformations (CCMs). Microhemorrhages are seen as multifocal "blooming" black dots ⇨ (Zabramski type IV). (7-34A) NECT in a 41-yo woman with headaches shows a heterogeneously hyperdense mass ➡ in the right frontal lobe and caudate nucleus.*

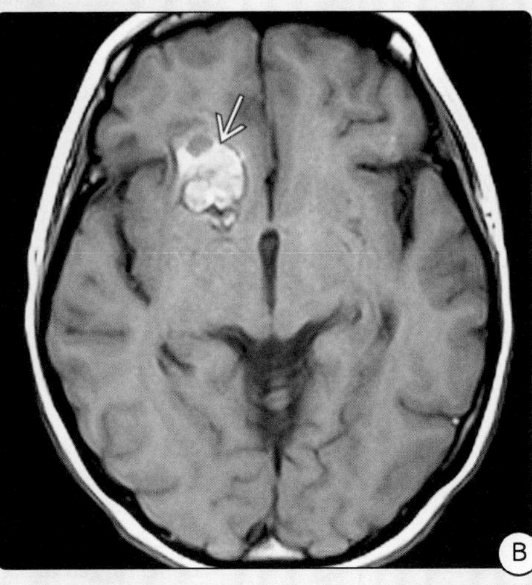

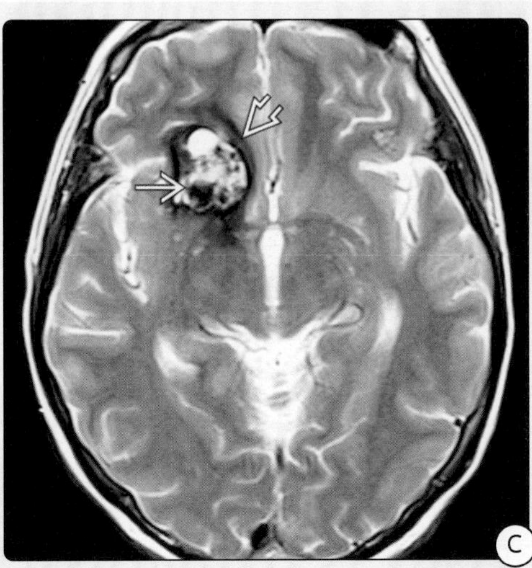

*(7-34B) T1 MR in the same case shows the mass ➡ is well delineated and heterogeneously hyperintense. (7-34C) T2 MR shows the "popcorn ball" mass is surrounded by a complete hemosiderin rim ⇨. The mass itself is composed of mixed hypo- and hyperintense locules. Note fluid-fluid level ➡. This is classic Zabramski type II cavernous malformation.*

## CEREBRAL CAVERNOUS MALFORMATIONS

**Etiology**

- *KRIT1*, *CCM2*, or *PDCD10* mutations in familial CCM

**Pathology**

- Occur throughout CNS
- Solitary (2/3), multiple (1/3, familial)
- Consist of closely clustered, abnormally dilated leaky capillaries
- Multiple thin-walled blood-filled locules ("caverns")
- No normal brain inside; hemosiderin rim outside

**Clinical Issues**

- Can present at any age; peak: 40-60 years
- Course variable, unpredictable
    - Repeated intralesional hemorrhages typical
    - Hemorrhage risk: 0.25-0.75% per lesion per year
    - Higher risk, de novo lesions in familial CCM

**Demographics.** CCMs may occur at any age; they cause 10% of spontaneous brain hemorrhages in children. Peak presentation is 40-60 years (younger in the familial multiple cavernous malformation syndrome). There is no sex predilection.

**Presentation.** 1/2 of all patients with CCMs present with seizures. Headache and focal neurologic deficits are also common. Small lesions, especially microhemorrhages, may be asymptomatic.

**Natural History.** CCMs have a broad range of dynamic behavior, and the clinical course of individual lesions is both highly variable and unpredictable. Repeated spontaneous intralesional hemorrhages are typical. There is a distinct propensity for lesion growth in all patients. Patients with multiple CCM syndrome typically continue to develop de novo lesions throughout their lives.

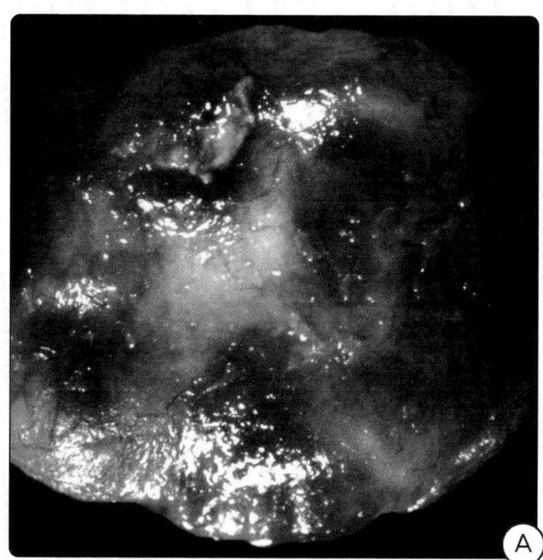


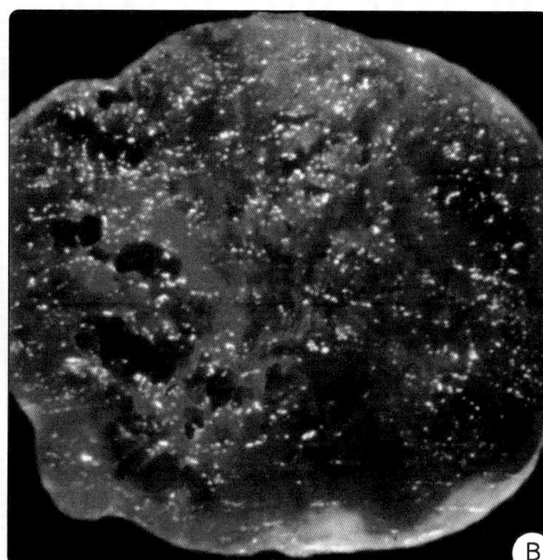


***(7-35A) Resected surgical specimen of cavernous malformation shows the typical well-circumscribed, lobulated, berry-like appearance. (7-35B) Cut section shows multiple locules of various sizes that contain blood in different stages of evolution.***

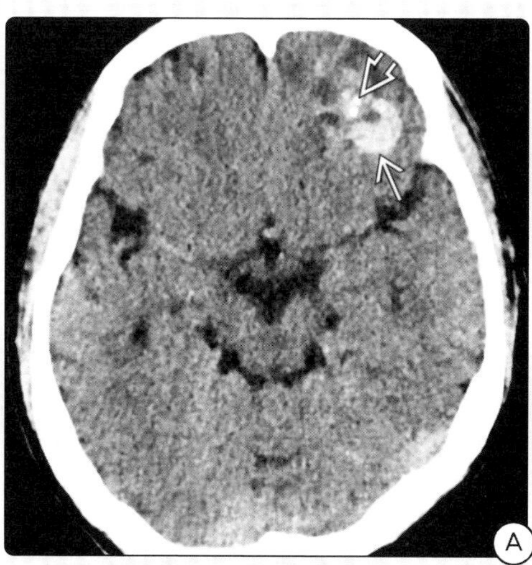


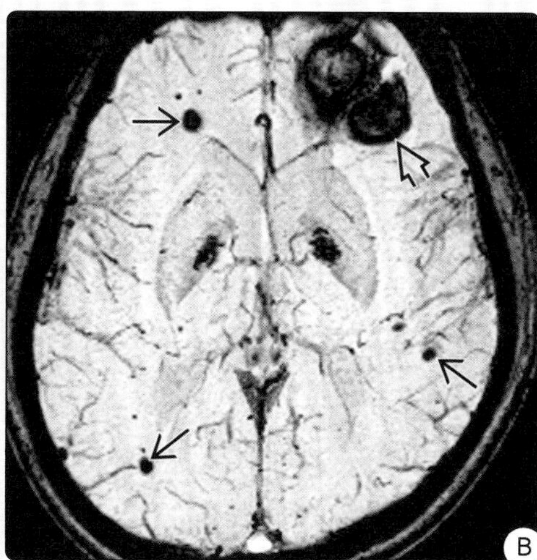


***(7-36A) NECT in a 44-yo man with headaches shows a mixed hypo-, hyper-, and isodense lobulated left frontal mass ➡ with central calcifications ➡. (7-36B) T2* SWI MR in the same case shows the left frontal mass ➡ exhibiting strong susceptibility artifact. Note multiple other "blooming" black dots scattered throughout both hemispheres ➡. Findings are characteristic of multiple CCM syndrome.***

Hemorrhage risk with solitary lesions is estimated at 0.25-0.75% per year, cumulative, and greater for women. In the familial multiple CCM form, hemorrhage risk is much higher, approaching 1-5% cumulative risk per lesion per year.

Hemorrhage rates also vary with imaging appearance based on the Zabramski classification. Zabramski type I and II CCMs have a significantly higher hemorrhage rate than types III and IV.

The presence of acute or subacute blood-degradation products on MR (Zabramski I, II) is the strongest indicator for an increased risk of hemorrhage (mean annual hemorrhage rate of 20-25% vs. 3-4% without signs of acute or subacute blood). Dot-sized CCMs on T2* (GRE or SWI) that are invisible or barely visible on T1WIs and T2WIs (Zabramski type IV) have the lowest mean annual hemorrhage rate (1%).

## Imaging

**General Features.** CCMs occur throughout the CNS. The brain parenchyma is the most common site. A well-circumscribed mixed-density/signal intensity mass surrounded by a complete hemosiderin rim ("popcorn ball") is the classic finding. CCMs can vary from microscopic to giant (> 6 cm) lesions. In rare circumstances, a CCM (often mixed with venous malformations) may occupy an entire lobe of the brain.

**CT Findings.** Large CCMs appear hyperdense **(7-34A)** with or without scattered intralesional calcifications. Most CCMs are well delineated and do not exhibit mass effect unless there is recent hemorrhage.

**MR Findings.** Findings depend on the stage of evolution and pulse sequence utilized. CCMs have been divided into four types based on imaging appearance (Zabramski classification).

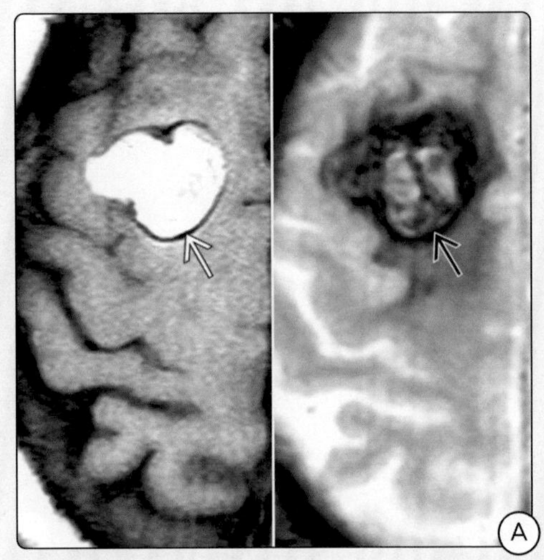

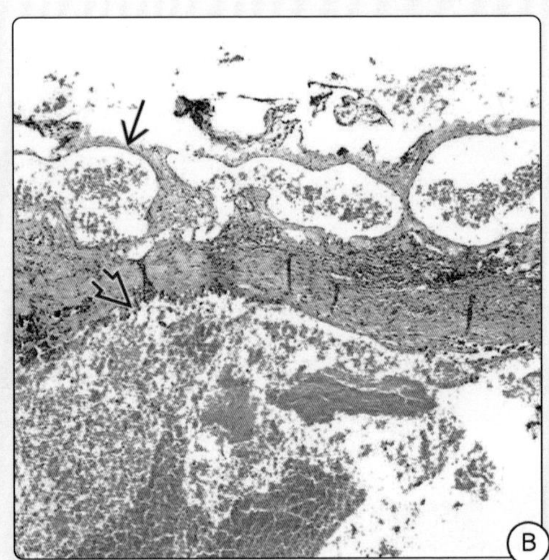

***(7-37A)** Zabramski type I CCM is illustrated. (L) T1 MR shows that the lesion is hyperintense and surrounded by a hypointense hemosiderin rim ➡. (R) T2* GRE shows "blooming" hypointensity both around ➡ and within the lesion. **(7-37B)** Microscopic section from the resected specimen in the same case shows a blood-filled cavity ➡ surrounded by thin endothelium-lined vascular channels ➡. (Courtesy R. Hewlett, MD.)*

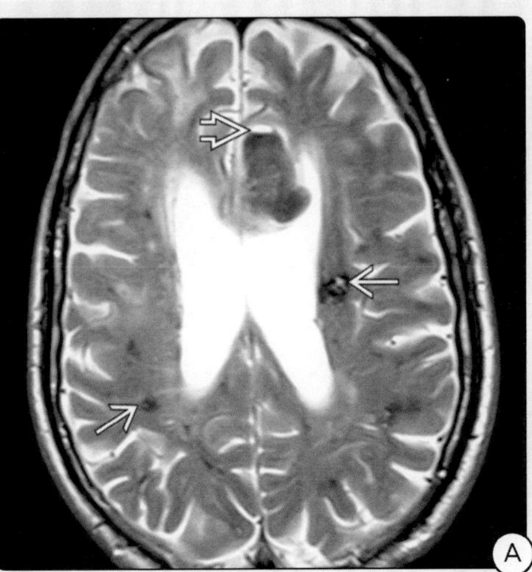

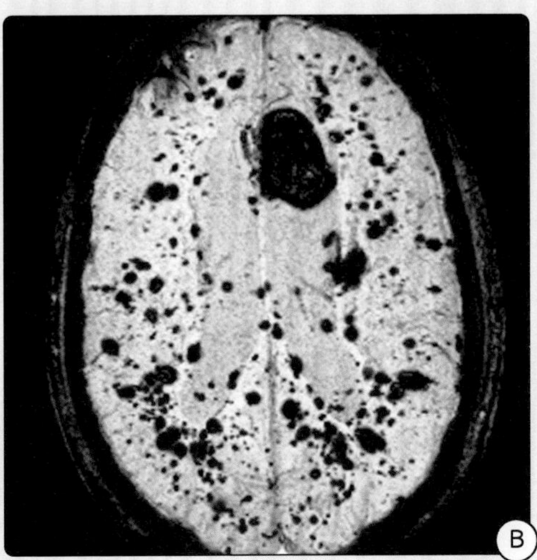

***(7-38A)** T2 MR in a patient with familial multiple CCM syndrome shows multifocal predominately hypointense lesions ➡. A fluid-fluid level ➡ can be seen in the large left frontal lobe mass. **(7-38B)** MIP T2* SWI in the same case shows innumerable "blooming" black dots, each of which represents a separate CCM.*

The classic CCM (Zabramski type II) is a discrete reticulated or "popcorn ball" lesion caused by blood products contained within variably sized "caverns" or "locules." Fluid-fluid levels of differing signal intensities are common **(7-34B)**. The mixed-signal core is surrounded by a complete hemosiderin rim on T2WI that "blooms" on T2* sequences **(7-34C)**. CCMs with subacute hemorrhage (Zabramski type I) are hyperintense on T1WI and mixed hyper-/hypointense on T2WI **(7-37)**.

T2* scans (GRE, SWI) should always be performed to look for additional lesions **(7-36)**. Punctate microhemorrhages are seen as multifocal "blooming" black dots (Zabramski type IV) in many cases with familial CCM **(7-38)**.

Enhancement following contrast administration varies from none (the usual finding) to mild or moderate. If a CCM coexists with a DVA, the venous "angioma" may show strong enhancement.

**Angiography.** CCMs have no identifiable feeding arteries or draining veins. DSA, CTA, and MRA are usually negative unless the CCM is mixed with another vascular malformation (most commonly a DVA).

## Differential Diagnosis

The most common differential diagnosis is a **mixed vascular malformation** in which a CCM is the dominant component **(7-39)**. Occasionally, a **hemorrhagic** or **densely calcified neoplasm** (such as a GBM or oligodendroglioma, respectively) can mimic a CCM.

Multifocal "black dots" on T2* scans can be seen in a number of lesions besides type IV CCMs. Chronic hypertensive encephalopathy, amyloid angiopathy, axonal stretch injury, and cortical contusions may have similar appearances.

**Hemangiomas** are true benign vasoformative neoplasms and should not be mistaken for CCMs. Most are found in the skin and soft tissues of the head and neck. Hemangiomas within the CNS are rare and most commonly found in dural venous sinuses and cranial meninges, not the brain parenchyma.

### CEREBRAL CAVERNOUS MALFORMATIONS: IMAGING

**CT**

- NECT
  - Hyperdense ± scattered $Ca^{++}$
  - Variable hemorrhage
- DSA

**MR (Zabramski Classification)**

- Type I: Subacute hemorrhage
  - Hyperintense on T1
  - Hyper-/hypointense on T2
- Type II: Differently aged hemorrhages
  - Mixed signal with hyper-/hypointensity on both T1 and T2
  - Classic: "Popcorn ball"
  - Look for blood-filled locules with fluid-fluid levels
- Type III: Chronic hemorrhage
- Type IV: Punctate microhemorrhages
  - "Blooming" black dots on T2* (GRE, SWI)

**DSA**

- Usually negative (unless mixed with DVA)

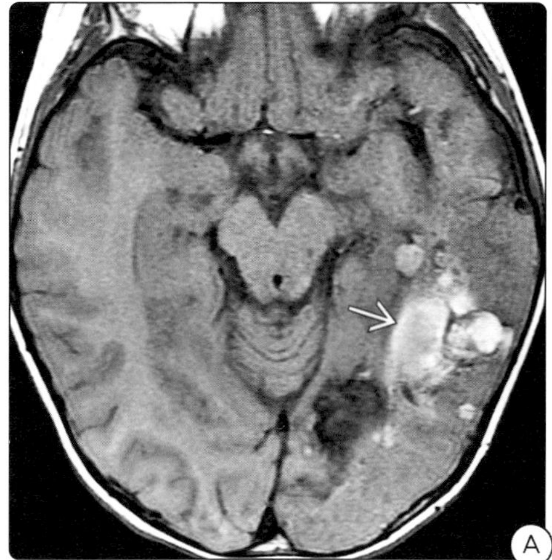


***(7-39A)** Axial T1 MR shows a mixed signal intensity lesion ➡ occupying most of the posterior temporal/occipital lobes.*

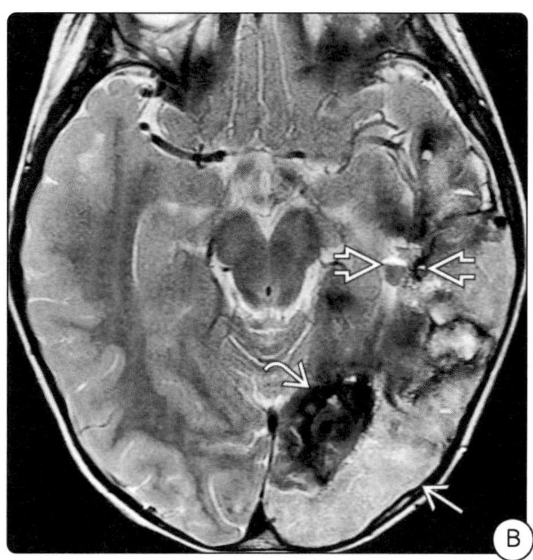


***(7-39B)** T2 MR shows several locules with fluid-fluid levels ➡ and areas of parenchymal hyper- ➡ and hypointensity ➡.*

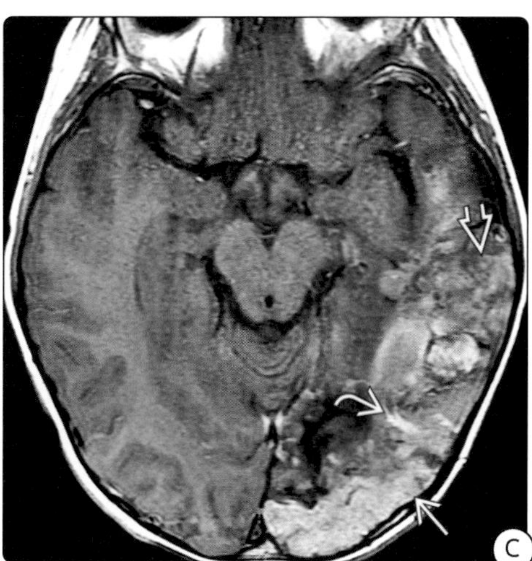


***(7-39C)** T1 C+ MR of giant capillary-cavernous venous malformation shows diffuse ➡, patchy ➡ enhancement, large vein ➡. (W. Fang, MD.)*

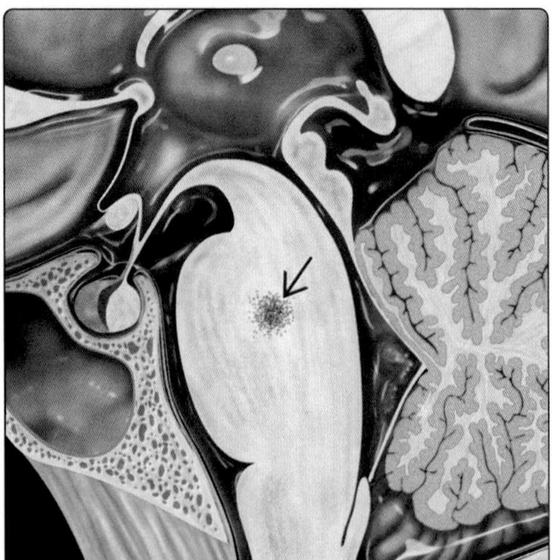

***(7-40)** Graphic depicts pontine capillary telangiectasia ➡ with tiny dilated capillaries interspersed with normal brain.*

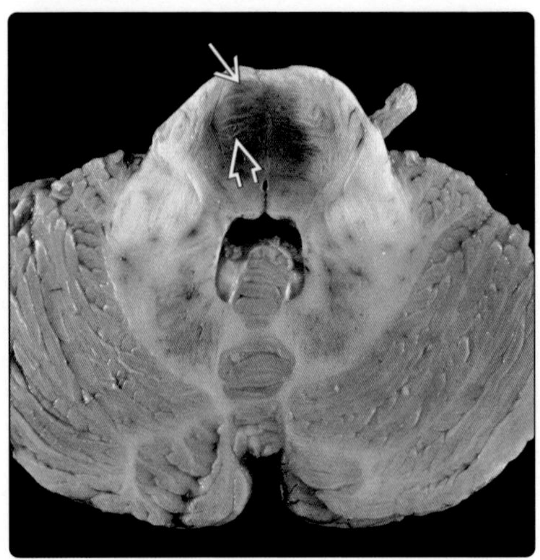

***(7-41)** Autopsy shows large pontine capillary telangiectasia ➡ with pontine fibers ➡ passing through the lesion. (Courtesy B. Horten, MD.)*

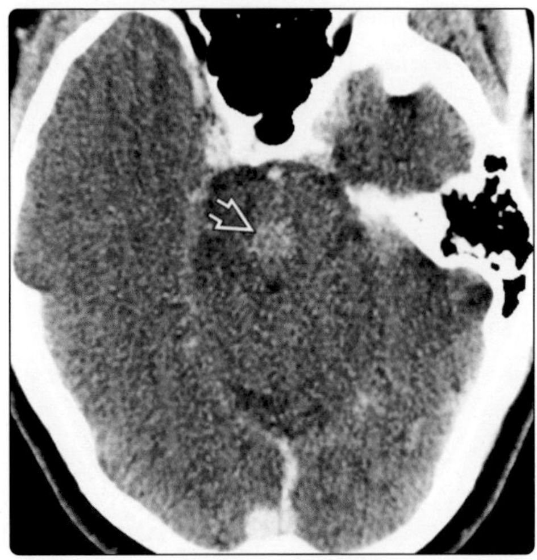

***(7-42)** Axial CECT of the cervical soft tissues shows incidental, asymptomatic large capillary telangiectasia ➡ in the upper pons.*

# Capillary Telangiectasia

## Terminology

A brain capillary telangiectasia (BCT) is a collection of enlarged, thin-walled vessels resembling capillaries. The vessels are surrounded and separated by normal brain parenchyma.

## Etiology

**General Concepts.** Although their exact pathogenesis is unknown, capillary telangiectasias are probably congenital lesions. BCTs have been reported with HHT.

Cranial irradiation may cause vascular endothelial damage and induce development of multiple cavernous or telangiectatic-like lesions in the brain parenchyma. Patients with radiation-induced capillary telangiectasias typically present with seizures several years after whole-brain XRT. Mean age of onset is 11-12 years, and mean latency period is nearly nine years.

**Genetics.** No known genetic mutations have been identified for solitary BCTs. BCTs are the most common vascular malformation in HHT, occurring in 60% of patients.

## Pathology

**Location and Size.** BCTs can occur anywhere in the CNS. The pons, cerebellum, and spinal cord are the most common sites **(7-40)**. Solitary lesions are much more common than multiple BCTs. Although "giant" capillary telangiectasias do occur, the vast majority of BCTs are small, typically < 1 cm in diameter.

**Gross Pathology.** Most BCTs are often invisible to gross inspection. Only 5-10% of BCTs are > 1 cm in diameter. Occasionally, lesions up to 2 cm occur. These can be seen as areas of poorly delineated pink or brownish discoloration in the parenchyma **(7-41)**.

**Microscopic Features.** A cluster of dilated, somewhat ectatic but otherwise normal-appearing capillaries interspersed within the brain parenchyma is characteristic **(7-43)**. Unless mixed with other malformations (such as cavernous angioma), BCTs do not hemorrhage and do not calcify. Gliosis and hemosiderin deposition are absent.

## Clinical Issues

**Epidemiology.** Capillary telangiectasias are the second most common cerebral vascular malformation, representing between 10-20% of all brain vascular malformations. Skin and mucosal capillary telangiectasias are even more common than brain telangiectasias.

**Demographics.** BCTs may occur at any age, but peak presentation is between 30-40 years. There is no sex predilection.

**Presentation.** Most BCTs are asymptomatic and discovered incidentally. A few cases with headache, vertigo, and tinnitus have been reported.

**Natural History.** Sporadic BCTs are quiescent lesions that do not hemorrhage. BCTs in patients with HHT also have a benign natural history. Isolated BCTs do not require treatment.

## Imaging

**General Features.** Because normal brain is interspersed between the dilated capillaries of a BCT, no mass effect is present. Unless they are histologically mixed with other CVMs (such as a cavernous malformation), BCTs lack edema, do not incite surrounding gliosis, and neither hemorrhage nor calcify.

**CT Findings.** Both NECT and CECT scans are usually normal unless the telangiectasia is unusually large **(7-42)**.

**MR Findings.** BCTs are inconspicuous on conventional precontrast MRs **(7-45A)**. T1 scans are typically normal. Large BCTs may show faint stippled hyperintensity on T2WI **(7-44)** or FLAIR.

T2* (GRE, SWI) is the best sequence for demonstrating a BCT **(7-44D)**. Because blood flow in the dilated capillaries is slow, oxyhemoglobin is converted to deoxyhemoglobin and is visible as an area of poorly delineated grayish hypointensity.

BCTs typically show faint stippled or poorly delineated brush-like enhancement on T1 C+ **(7-45)** **(7-44)**. Larger lesions may demonstrate a linear focus of strong enhancement within the lesion, representing a draining collector vein **(7-46)** **(7-47)**.

## Differential Diagnosis

Because they show mild enhancement on T1 C+, BCTs are often mistaken for **neoplasms**, yet they do not exhibit mass effect or surrounding edema. Signal intensity loss on T2* and focal brush-like enhancement in a lesion that is otherwise unremarkable on standard sequences easily distinguish BCT from neoplasm.

**Radiation-induced vascular malformations** are seen as multifocal "blooming" black dots on T2* (GRE, SWI) sequences. Most are cavernous malformations with microhemorrhages, not capillary telangiectasias.

### CAPILLARY TELANGIECTASIAS

**Pathology**
- Cluster of thin-walled, dilated capillaries
  - Normal brain between vascular channels
- Location
  - Pons, cerebellum, spinal cord most common sites
  - **However,** can be found anywhere

**Clinical Issues**
- 10-20% of all CVMs
- All ages
  - Peak: 30-40 years
- Rarely symptomatic
  - Most discovered incidentally at imaging

**Imaging**
- MR
  - T1/T2 usually normal unless unusually large
  - T2* key sequence (dark gray hypointensity on GRE)
  - May become very hypointense on SWI
  - Brush-like enhancement on T1 C+
  - ± prominent central draining vein

*Selected References: The complete reference list is available on the eBooks+ version included with purchase.*

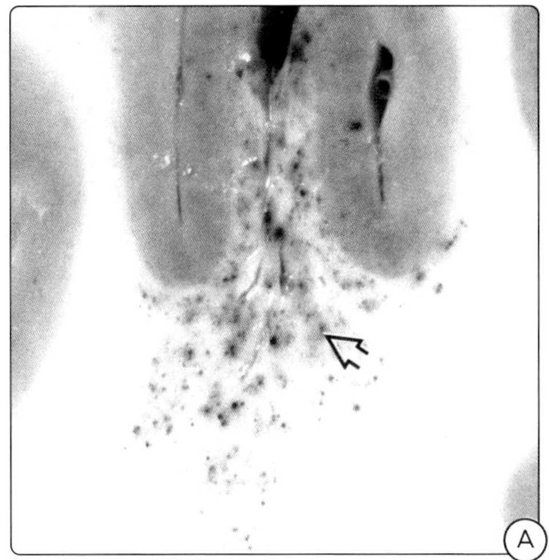


***(7-43A)** Subcortical capillary telangiectasia shows innumerable enlarged pink foci ⇒ in the subcortical WM produced by enlarged capillaries.*

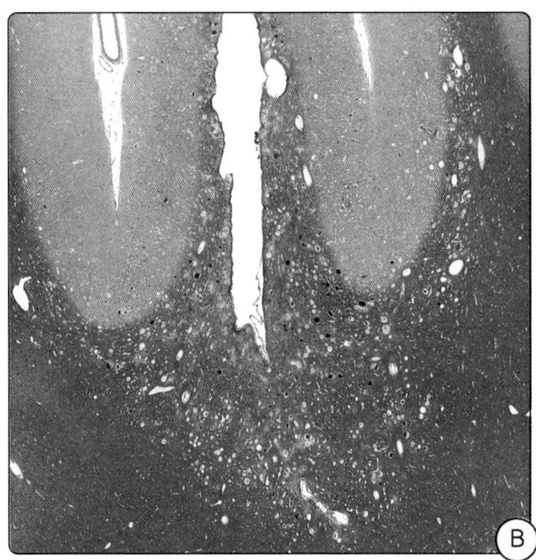


***(7-43B)** Blue myelin stain shows enlarged capillaries in subcortical WM with normal blue-staining WM between the vessels.*

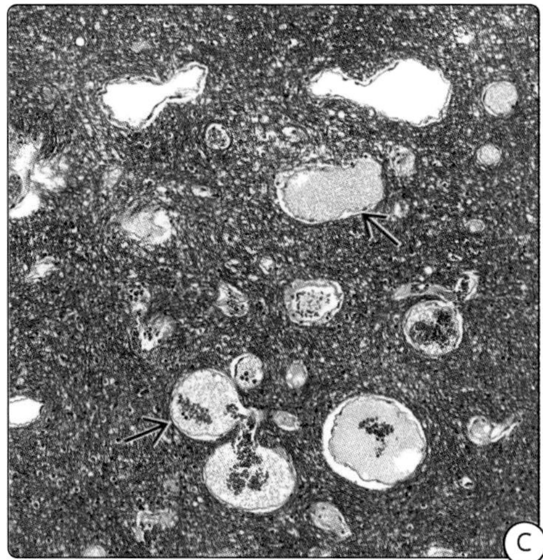


***(7-43C)** Micrograph shows blood-filled, thin-walled enlarged capillaries ⇒, the hallmark of capillary telangiectasia. (Courtesy P. Burger, MD.)*

*(7-44A) T2 MR in a 59-yo man screened for intracranial metastases shows a patchy hyperintense lesion ➡ without mass effect in the pons. (7-44B) The pontine lesion is hyperintense on FLAIR. Note strands of isointense parenchyma ➡ coursing through the hyperintense lesion.*

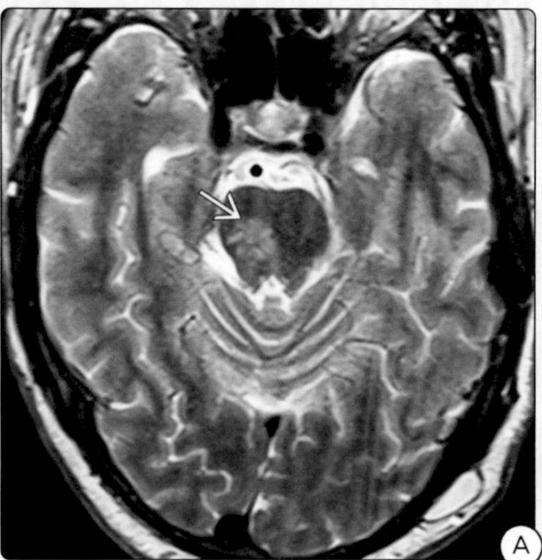

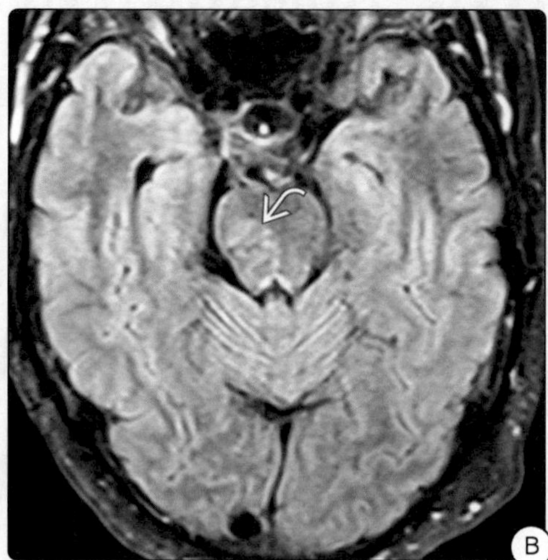

*(7-44C) The lesion ➡ enhances moderately on T1 C+ FS MR. (7-44D) The lesion shows strong "blooming" artifact ➡ on T2* GRE. This is an incidental capillary telangiectasia, not a metastasis from the patient's known systemic primary cancer.*

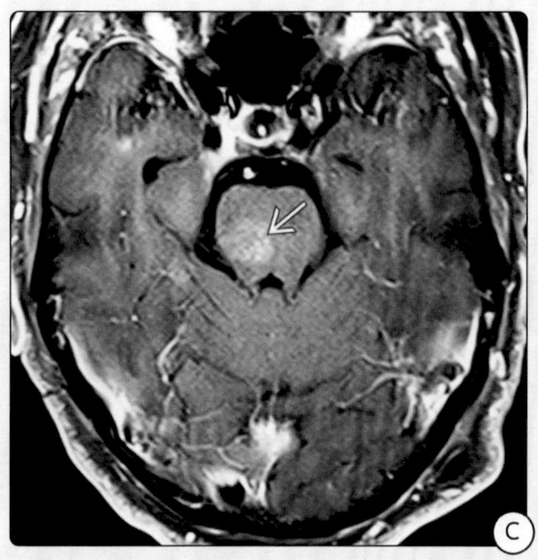

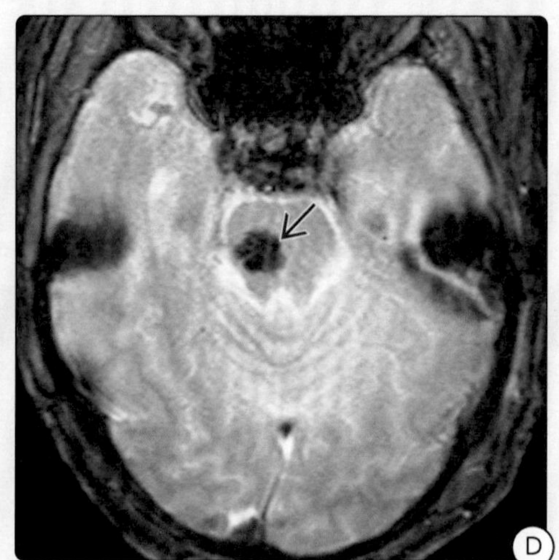

*(7-45A) T2 MR in a 47-yo man with headaches is normal. (7-45B) Thin-section T1 C+ MR in the same case shows a faint but definite stippled vascular "blush" ➡ in the right inferior basal ganglia. Note focus of tubular enhancement ➡ in the center of the lesion, indicating a central draining vein. This is incidental giant capillary telangiectasia.*

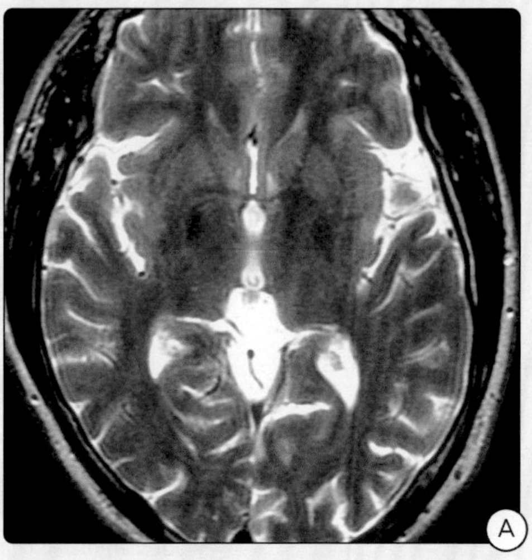

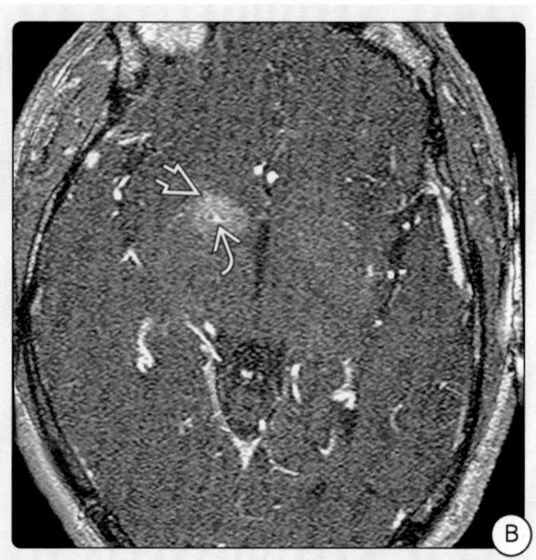

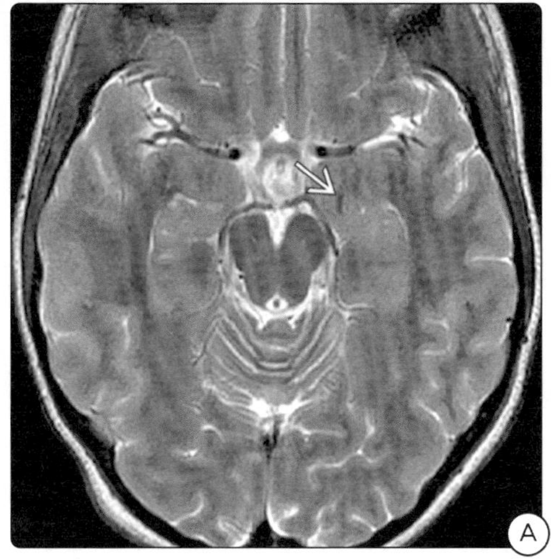

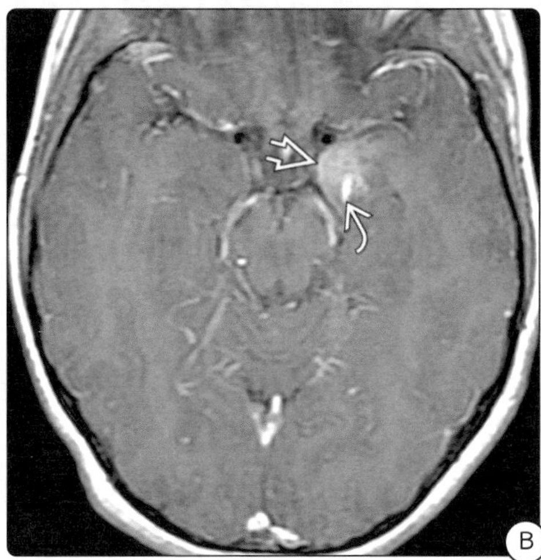

***(7-46A)*** *Axial T2 MR in a 17-yo girl with headaches and dizziness shows an odd tubular "flow void" ➡ in the left medial temporal lobe.* ***(7-46B)*** *T1 C+ MR in the same case shows a diffuse vascular "blush" ➡ of enhancement in the uncus with a prominent tubular draining vein ➡.*

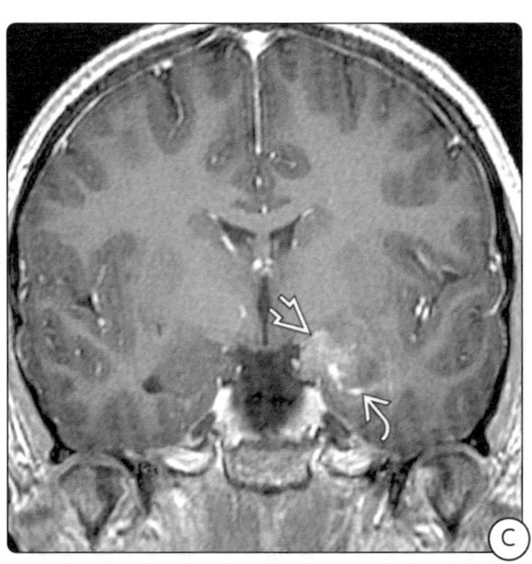

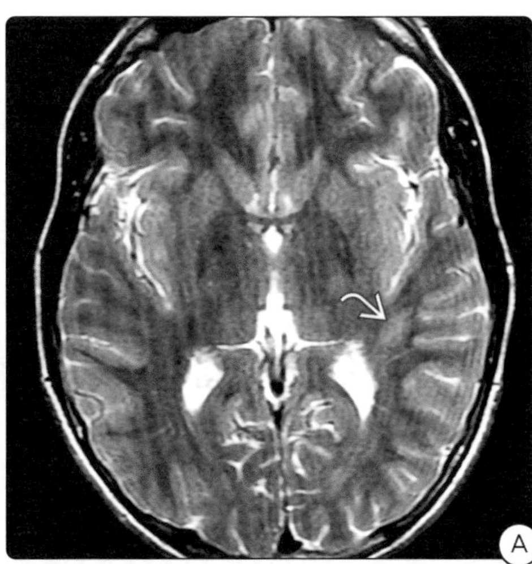

***(7-46C)*** *Coronal T1 C+ MR shows the prominent vascular blush ➡ and draining vein ➡. There is no mass effect. This is giant capillary telangiectasia, which is considered an incidental finding.* ***(7-47A)*** *Axial T2 MR in a 16-yo boy with headaches shows a faint, ill-defined hyperintensity ➡ in the left parietal WM.*

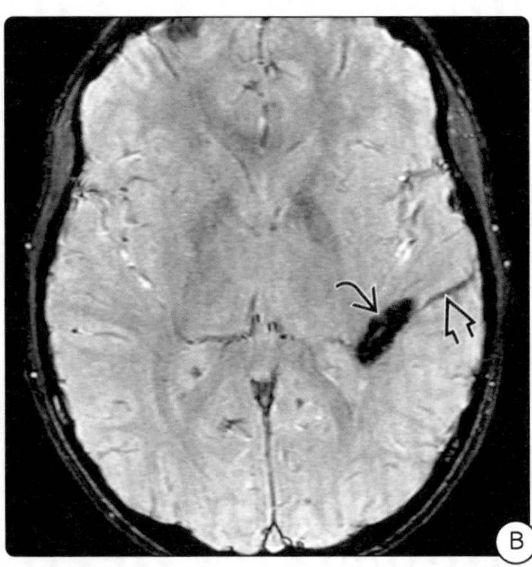

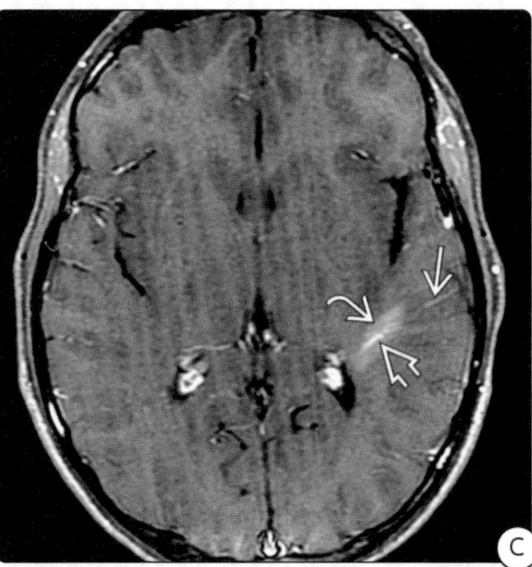

***(7-47B)*** *T2* SWI MR in the same case shows "blooming" hypointensity in the lesion ➡ and a prominent draining vein ➡.* ***(7-47C)*** *T1 C+ FS MR shows a brush-like area of enhancement ➡ surrounding a prominent central draining vein ➡. A superficial cortical vein ➡ also drains the lesion. This is incidental capillary telangiectasia.*

# Arterial Anatomy and Strokes

*"Stroke" is a generic term that describes a clinical event characterized by sudden onset of a neurologic deficit. However, not all strokes are the same! Stroke syndromes have significant clinical and pathophysiologic heterogeneity that is reflected in their underlying gross pathologic and imaging appearances. Arterial ischemia/infarction—the major focus of this chapter—is by far the most common cause of stroke, accounting for 80% of all cases.*



The remaining 20% of strokes are mostly hemorrhagic, divided between primary "spontaneous" intracranial hemorrhage (sICH), nontraumatic subarachnoid hemorrhage (SAH), and venous occlusions. Both sICH and SAH were discussed extensively in preceding chapters, and venous occlusions will be discussed in the following chapter.

We begin by briefly reviewing the normal intracranial arteries and their vascular distributions. With this solid anatomic foundation, we then turn our attention to the etiology, pathology, and imaging manifestations of arterial strokes.

## Normal Arterial Anatomy and Vascular Distributions

### Intracranial Internal Carotid Artery

#### Normal Anatomy

The **intracranial internal carotid artery (ICA)** follows a complex course with several vertical or horizontal segments connected by three curved genus. There are six intracranial segments: The petrous (C2), lacerum (C3), cavernous (C4), clinoid (C5), ophthalmic (C6), and communicating (C7) segments **(8-1)** **(8-2)**. C1 is the ICA within the neck known as the cervical ICA.

The **petrous (C2) segment** is contained within the carotid canal of the temporal bone. As the ICA enters the skull at the carotid canal, it lies just anterior to the internal jugular vein. At this point, the ICA goes from being mobile in the neck, to relatively fixed in the bone, where it is more vulnerable to traumatic shearing forces and dissection.

The C2 segment is surrounded by the extensive sympathetic plexus. The C2 subsegments are joined at the genu. There is a short vertical segment, a genu, where the petrous ICA turns anteromedially in front of the cochlea, and a longer horizontal segment. The ICA exits the carotid canal at the petrous apex.

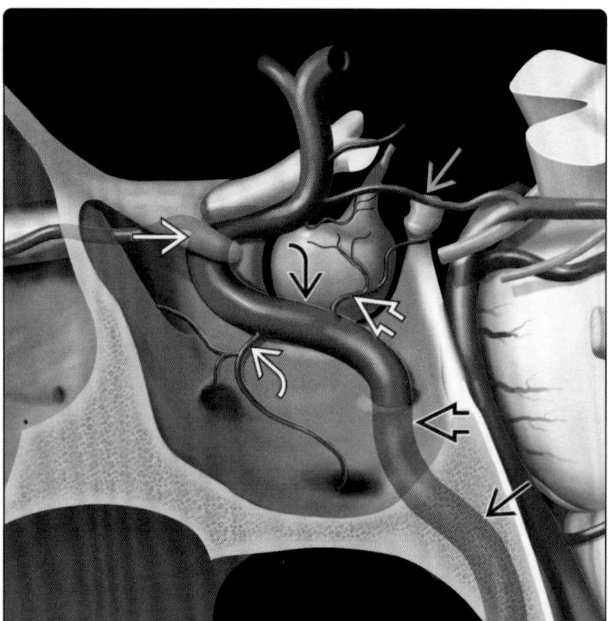

***(8-1)** Intracranial ICA & major branches. C2 segment is within carotid canal ➡. C3 ➡ lies between C2 & cavernous ICA (C4). C4 ➡ branches are the meningohypophyseal ➡ & inferolateral trunk ➡. C5 ➡ is last extradural segment. PCoA ➡.*

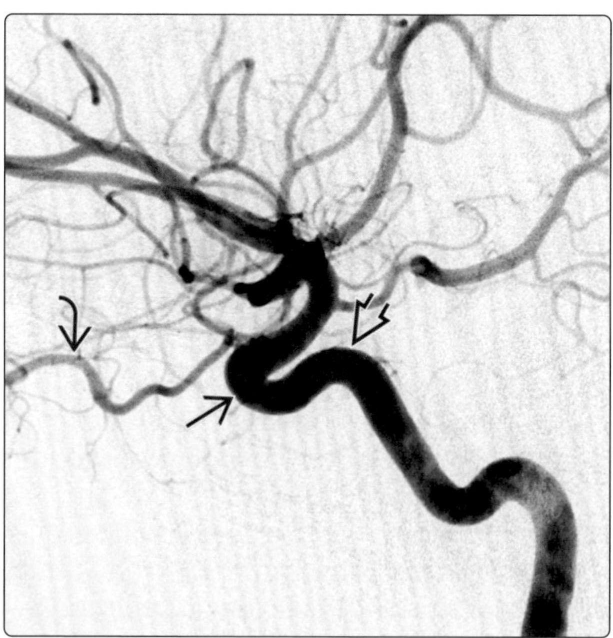

***(8-2)** Lateral ICA DSA injection shows all ICA segments. The cavernous (C4) segment has anterior ➡ & posterior ➡ genus & forms the carotid "siphon." The ophthalmic artery ➡ arises from the ophthalmic (C6) segment, just above clinoid (C5) segment.*

The C2 segment has two small but important branches. The **vidian artery**, a.k.a. the artery of the pterygoid canal, anastomoses with external carotid artery (ECA) branches, most commonly the internal maxillary artery. The second branch is the small **caroticotympanic** artery, which supplies the middle ear.

The **lacerum (C3) segment** is a short segment that extends from the petrous apex just above foramen lacerum, curving upward toward the cavernous sinus. It is covered by the trigeminal ganglion and has no branches.

The **cavernous (C4) segment** has three subsegments joined by two genus. There is a posterior vertical (ascending) portion, a posterior (more medial) genu, a horizontal segment, an anterior (more lateral) genu, and an anterior vertical (subclinoid) segment. The C4 segment is covered by trigeminal ganglion posteriorly.

The **abducens nerve** (CNVI) is inferolateral to the C4 segment. The major branches include the **meningohypophyseal trunk**, which arises from the posterior genu and supplies the pituitary, tentorium, and clival dura. The **inferolateral trunk** arises from the horizontal segment and supplies the cavernous sinus dura and cranial nerves. The inferolateral trunk anastomoses with the ECA branches through foramen rotundum, spinosum, and ovale.

The **clinoid (C5) segment** is a short segment between the proximal and distal dural rings of the cavernous sinus. The C5 segment terminates as the ICA exits the cavernous sinus and enters the subarachnoid space near the anterior clinoid process. There are no important branches unless the ophthalmic artery arises within the cavernous sinus.

The **ophthalmic (C6) segment** is the first ICA segment that lies completely within the subarachnoid space. It extends from the distal dural ring at the superior clinoid to just below the posterior communicating artery (PCoA) origin.

There are two important branches that arise from the ophthalmic ICA segment. The **ophthalmic branch** originates from the anterosuperior C6 ICA, passes through the optic canal to the orbit. The ophthalmic artery gives off ocular, lacrimal, and muscular branches. There are extensive anastomoses with the ECA. The **superior hypophyseal artery** courses posteromedially and supplies the anterior pituitary, infundibulum, and optic nerve and chiasm.

The **communicating (C7) segment** is the last ICA segment and extends from just below the PCoA origin to the terminal ICA bifurcation into the anterior cerebral artery (ACA) and middle cerebral artery (MCA). The C7 segment passes between the optic (CNII) and oculomotor (CNIII) nerves.

The major branches of the C7 segment are the **PCoA** and the **anterior choroidal artery**. The PCoA joins the anterior to the posterior circulation. The anterior choroidal artery courses posteromedial and then turns superolateral in the suprasellar cistern. It enters the temporal horn at the choroidal fissure. It supplies the choroid plexus, medial temporal lobe, basal ganglia, and posteroinferior internal capsule. The anterior choroidal artery is reciprocal with the posterior choroidal arteries, which are branches of the posterior cerebral artery (PCA).

### Variants and Anomalies

There are three important ICA vascular anomalies: An aberrant ICA, a persistent stapedial artery, and an embryonic carotid-basilar anastomosis.

An **aberrant ICA** is a congenital vascular anomaly that enters the posterior middle ear cavity from below and hugs the cochlear promontory as it crosses the middle ear **(8-3)**. An aberrant ICA is important to recognize, as it may mimic a middle ear tumor, the glomus tympanicum paraganglioma. Approximately 30% of aberrant ICAs have an associated persistent stapedial artery.

Appearance of an **aberrant ICA** on thin-section (< 1-mm) temporal bone CT or CTA is diagnostic **(8-4)**. The artery appears as a tubular structure crossing the middle ear from posterior to anterior. There may be an enlarged inferior tympanic canaliculus. The location of the aberrant ICA is posterior and lateral to the expected site of the petrous carotid canal. It is typically unilateral and may be discovered at the time of routine physical examination, during middle ear surgery, or as an incidental imaging finding. It has been associated with pulsatile tinnitus and conductive hearing loss.

A **persistent stapedial artery** is a rare congenital vascular anomaly where the embryonic stapedial artery persists. This anomaly is typically found incidentally and is associated with an aberrant ICA. On temporal bone CT or CTA, there is absence of the foramen spinosum. The persistent stapedial artery may be seen as a tiny linear vessel in the medial aspect of the middle ear. There is typically enlargement of the anterior tympanic segment of the facial nerve canal. It is often a bilateral lesion.

**Embryonic carotid-basilar anastomoses** are abnormal connections between the carotid and basilar system related to persistence of normally transient embryonic-type arterial supply. There are four types, named according to their anatomic relationship to specific cranial or spinal nerves. From superior to inferior, these are a persistent trigeminal artery (CNV), persistent otic artery (CNVIII), persistent hypoglossal artery (CNXII), and proatlantal intersegmental artery (C1-C3) **(8-5)**.

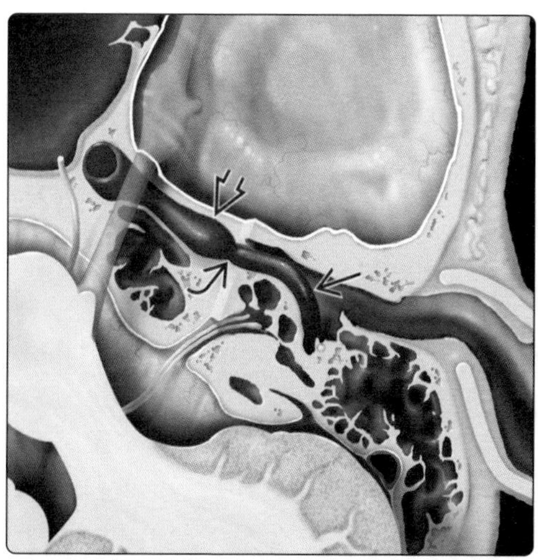

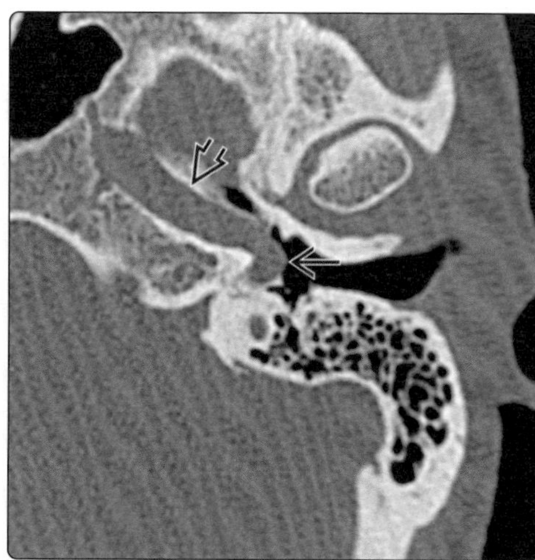

***(8-3)*** *Axial graphic shows an aberrant ICA ➡ along the posterior cochlear promontory, at medial middle ear to rejoin the horizontal petrous ICA ➡. At point of connection to the petrous ICA, stenosis ➡ is often present.* ***(8-4)*** *Axial temporal bone CT shows aberrant ICA ➡ on the low cochlear promontory, a typical location for glomus tympanicum. Its tubular shape can help prevent misdiagnosis. Note normal horizontal ICA ➡.*

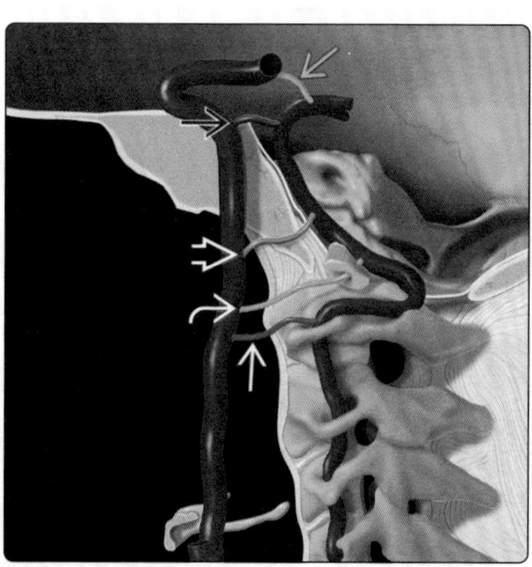

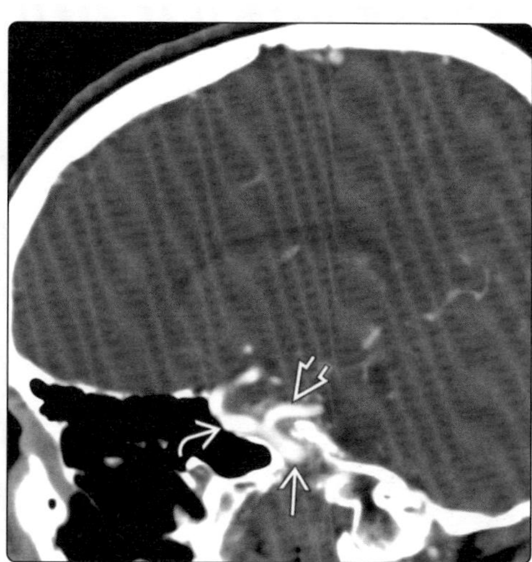

***(8-5)*** *Graphic shows anastomoses between ICA & VA. Normal PCoA ➡ connects PCA with supraclinoid ICA. PTA ➡ connects cavernous ICA & BA. POA ➡ connects petrous ICA to BA at IAC. PHA ➡ connects cervical ICA & VA at hypoglossal canal. Proatlantal artery ➡ connects cervical ICA & VA at C1-C3.* ***(8-6)*** *Sagittal CTA shows a PTA ➡ as a classic trident formed by the ascending ➡ & horizontal ➡ segments of the cavernous ICA & PTA.*

The **persistent trigeminal artery** (PTA) arises from the intracavernous ICA and connects with the basilar artery (BA) and parallels the course of the trigeminal nerve. On lateral DSA and sagittal CTA and MRA, it often forms a trident shape **(8-6)**. It is the most common of the persistent anastomoses and is identified in 0.1-0.2% of cases. Nearly 25% of patients with PTA have associated vascular anomalies, such as aneurysm, moyamoya, aortic coarctation, and arterial fenestrations.

The **persistent otic artery** (POA) arises from the petrous ICA to connect with the BA through the internal auditory canal. It is very rare with only a few cases reported. The **persistent hypoglossal artery** arises from the cervical ICA at the C1-C2 level and connects to the BA. It is a rare lesion with a prevalence of ~ 0.03-0.09%. The **proatlantal intersegmental artery** arises from the cervical ICA at the C2-C3 level, or, rarely, from the ECA to connect with the vertebral artery (VA) between C1 and the occiput.

# Circle of Willis

## Normal Anatomy

The circle of Willis (COW) has 10 components: Two ICAs, two proximal or horizontal (A1) ACA segments, the anterior communicating artery (ACoA), two PCoAs, the BA, and two proximal or horizontal (P1) segments of the PCAs **(8-7)** **(8-8)**. The MCA is *not* part of the COW.

## Vascular Territory

Important perforating branches arise from all parts of the COW and supply most of the basilar brain structures. COW *variants* are the rule, not the exception. One or more components of the COW is hypoplastic or absent in the majority of cases. A hypoplastic or absent PCoA is the most common COW variant.

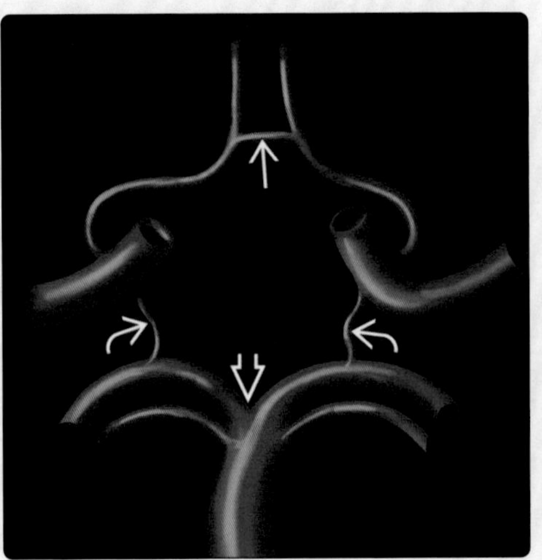
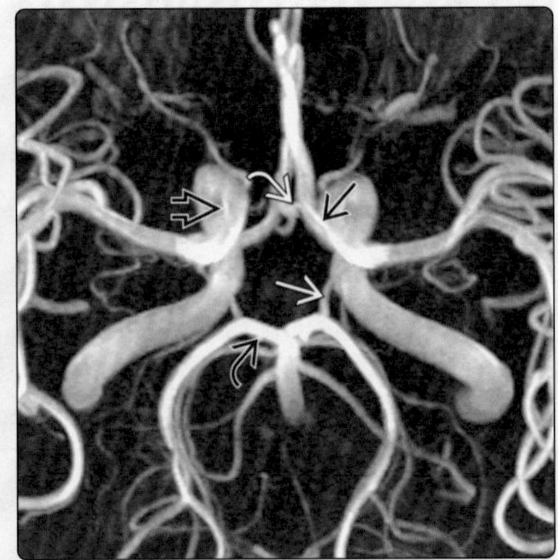

***(8-7)** Graphic depicts the COW with the ACoA & PCoAs connecting the anterior (carotid) circulation to the posterior (vertebrobasilar) circulation. **(8-8)** Submentovertex 3T MRA shows COW with ACoA & PCoAs. A1s, P1s, & ICAs are shown.*

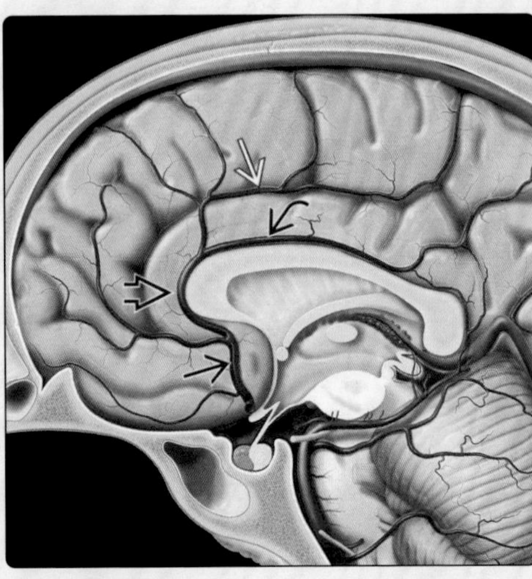
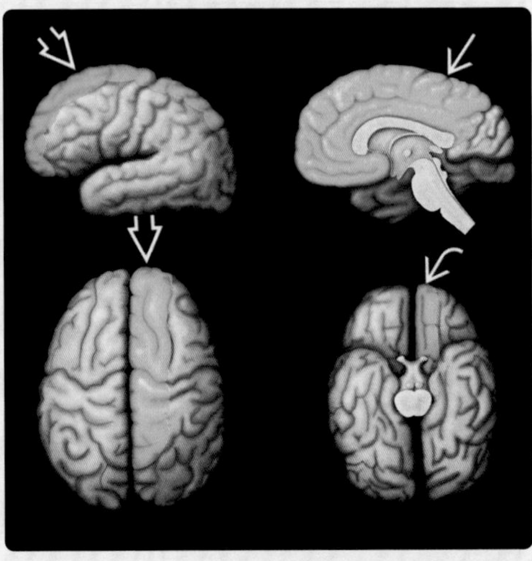

***(8-9)** Midline graphic shows A2 ascends in front of 3rd ventricle. A3 curves around corpus callosum genu. Pericallosal, callosomarginal arteries are major terminal ACA branches. **(8-10)** Cortical ACA territory (green) includes the anterior 2/3 of the medial surface of the hemisphere, a thin strip of cortex over the top of the hemisphere vertex, & a small wedge along the inferomedial frontal lobe.*

## Anterior Cerebral Artery

### Normal Anatomy

The ACA is the smaller, more medial terminal branch of the supraclinoid ICA. Its first (horizontal) ACA segment is also termed **A1**. Small perforating vessels arise from A1 and supply the medial basal ganglia.

The **A2** or vertical ACA segment extends from the A1-ACoA junction to the corpus callosum rostrum **(8-9)**. The **A3** (callosal) segment curves anteriorly around the corpus callosum genu then divides into two terminal ACA branches, the pericallosal and callosomarginal arteries.

### Vascular Territory

Cortical ACA branches supply the anterior 2/3 of the *medial* hemispheres and corpus callosum, the inferomedial surface of the frontal lobe, and the anterior 2/3 of the cerebral convexity adjacent to the interhemispheric fissure **(8-10)**. Penetrating ACA branches (mainly the medial lenticulostriate arteries) supply the medial basal ganglia, corpus callosum genu, and anterior limb of the internal capsule.

## Middle Cerebral Artery

### Normal Anatomy

The MCA has four defined segments. The **M1** MCA (horizontal) segment extends laterally from the ICA bifurcation toward the sylvian (lateral cerebral) fissure. Lateral lenticulostriate and anterior temporal arteries arise from the M1 **(8-11)**. The lateral lenticulostriates supply the lateral putamen, caudate nucleus, and external capsule. The M1 segment usually bifurcates or trifurcates just before it enters the sylvian fissure. The postbifurcation trunks enter the sylvian fissure then turn upwards. In current stroke trials, the M1/M2 junction is considered the MCA as it turns upwards in the

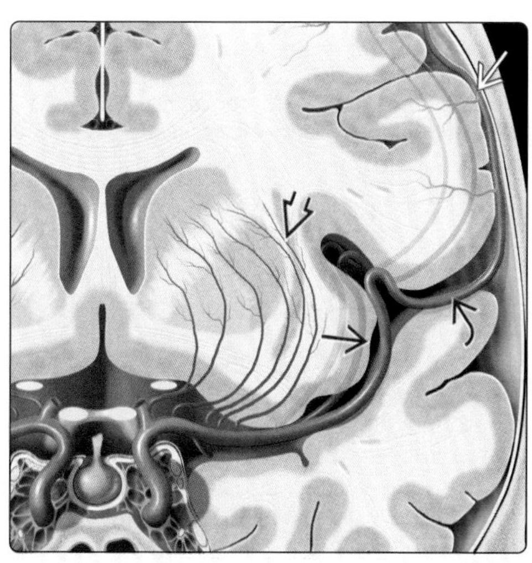

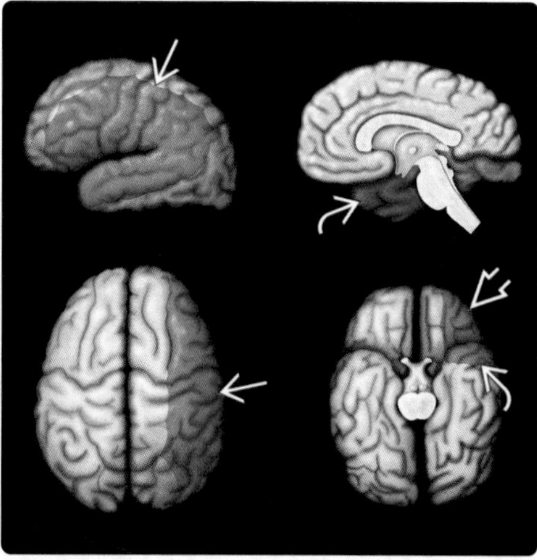

***(8-11)** Coronal graphic shows the lateral lenticulostriate arteries ➾, M2 segments over the insula ➾, M3 segments ➾ running laterally in the sylvian fissure, & M4 (cortical) branches ➡ coursing over the lateral surface of the hemisphere. **(8-12)** Cortical MCA territory (red) supplies most of the lateral surface of the hemisphere ➡, the anterior tip of the temporal lobe ➡, & the inferolateral frontal lobe ➡.*

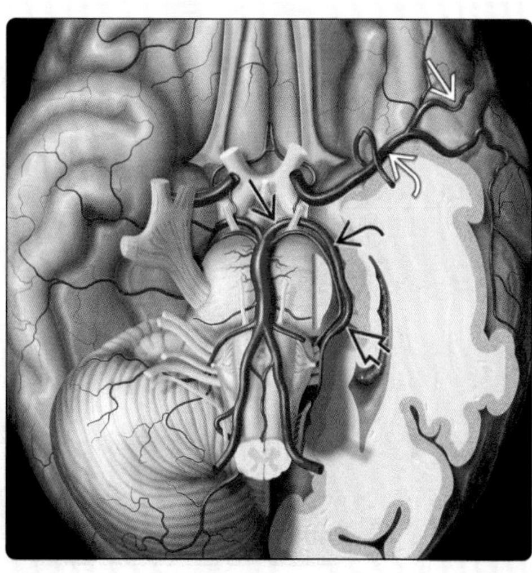

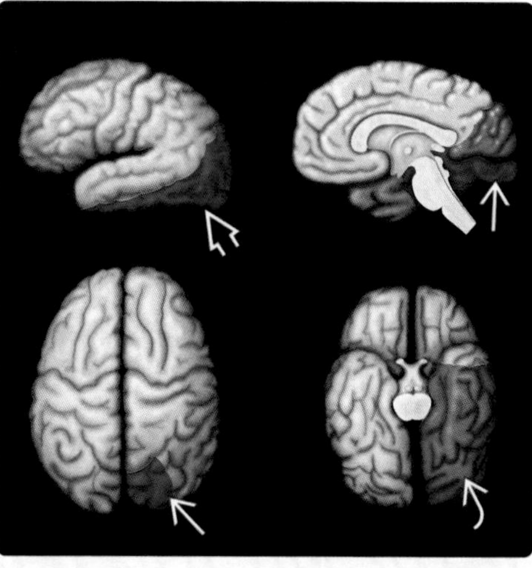

***(8-13)** Submentovertex graphic shows COW, basal brain vessels in relationship to cranial nerves. P1 ➾, P2 ➾, P3 ➾ PCA segments are shown, as are the M1 ➡ (horizontal) & M2 (insular) MCA segments ➡. **(8-14)** Cortical PCA territory (purple) includes the occipital lobe & posterior 1/3 of the medial ➡ & the posterolateral surfaces of the hemisphere ➡, as well as almost the entire inferior surface of the temporal lobe ➡.*

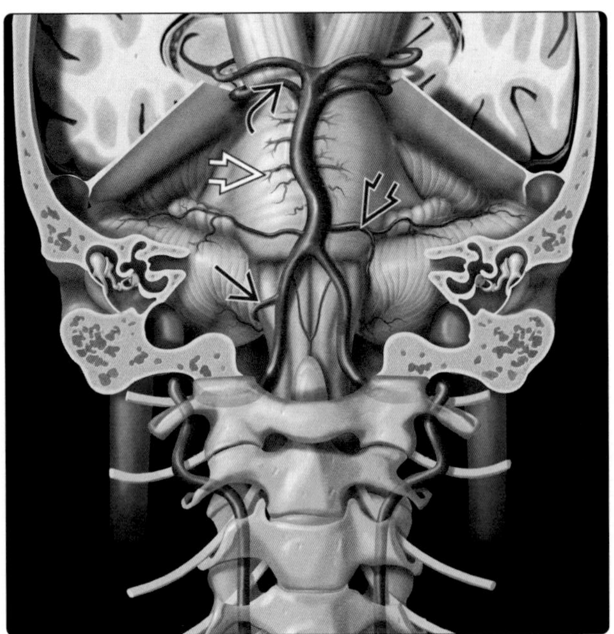

***(8-15)** Vertebrobasilar system: PICAs ➙ arise from VAs before the basilar junction, curve posteriorly around the medulla. AICAs ➙ course laterally to the CPAs. SCAs ➙ arise from the distal BA. Perforating BA branches ➙ supply most of the pons.*

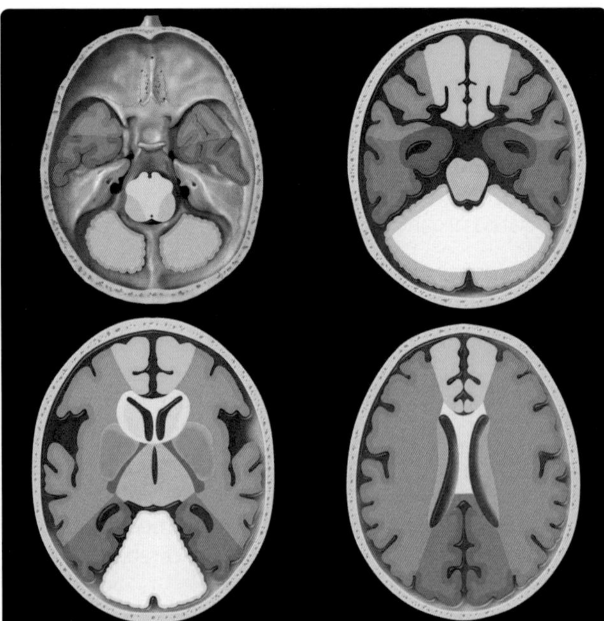

***(8-16)** Graphic shows penetrating artery territories. Medulla (light green) is supplied by VAs, pons & thalami (light purple) by BA, caudate & medial basal ganglia, corpus callosum by ACAs (light green), putamen/globi pallidi by MCAs (blue).*

sylvian fissure. Classic teaching of the location of the M1/M2 junction has been at the bifurcation/trifurcation. It is important to be descriptive when discussing the location of an intraluminal thrombus, as it may directly impact patient care.

The **M2** (insular) branches turn posterosuperiorly in the sylvian fissure, following a gentle curve (the genu or "knee" of the MCA). Several branches sweep upward over the surface of the insula. The insular M2 segments end at the top of the sylvian fissure.

MCA branches loop at or near the top of the sylvian fissure, then course laterally under the parts ("opercula") of the frontal, parietal, and temporal lobes that hang over and enclose the sylvian fissure. These are the **M3** or opercular segments. MCA branches become the **M4** segments when they ramify over the lateral surface of the cerebral hemisphere.

### Vascular Territory

The MCA has the largest vascular territory of any of the major cerebral arteries. The MCA supplies most of the *lateral* surface of the cerebral hemisphere with the exception of a thin strip at the vertex (supplied by the ACA) and the occipital and posteroinferior parietal lobes (supplied by the PCA) **(8-12)**. Its penetrating branches supply most of the lateral basal brain structures.

## Posterior Cerebral Artery

### Normal Anatomy

The two PCAs are the major terminal branches of the distal BA.

The **P1** segment extends laterally from the BA bifurcation to the junction with the PCoA. The P1 segment has perforating branches that course posterosuperiorly in the interpeduncular fossa to enter the undersurface of the midbrain.

The **P2** segment extends from the P1-PCoA junction, running in the ambient (perimesencephalic) cistern as it sweeps posterolaterally around the midbrain **(8-13)**. **P3** (quadrigeminal) is a short segment that lies entirely within the quadrigeminal cistern. It begins behind the midbrain and ends where the PCA enters the calcarine fissure of the occipital lobe. The **P4** segment terminates within the calcarine fissure, where it divides into the terminal PCA trunks, including the calcarine artery.

### Vascular Territory

The PCA supplies most of the *inferior* surface of the cerebral hemisphere with the exception of the temporal tip and frontal lobe. It also supplies the occipital lobe, posterior 1/3 of the medial hemisphere and corpus callosum, and most of the choroid plexus **(8-14)**. Penetrating PCA branches are the major vascular supply to the midbrain and posterior thalami.

### Variants and Anomalies

A common normal variant is the **"fetal" origin of the PCA.** Here, the proximal PCA arises from the ICA instead of from the basilar bifurcation. "Fetal" PCA origin is seen in 10-30% of cases. This variant is easily recognized on CTA, MRA, and DSA.

A rare but important PCA variant is an **artery of Percheron** (AOP). Here, a single dominant thalamoperforating artery arises from the P1 segment and supplies the rostral midbrain and bilateral medial thalami.

## Vertebrobasilar System

### Normal Anatomy

The vertebrobasilar system consists of the two VAs, the BA, and their branches. Four VA segments are identified. Only one—the V4 segment—is intracranial **(8-15)**.

The **V1** (extraosseous segment) arises from the ipsilateral subclavian artery and courses posterosuperiorly to enter the C6 transverse foramen. The **V2** segment courses superiorly through the C6-C3 transverse foramina until it reaches C2, where it first turns superolaterally through the "inverted L" of the transverse foramen and then turns upward to pass through the C1 transverse foramen.

**V3** begins after the VA exits the C1 transverse foramen. The **V4** (intracranial) segment extends from the foramen magnum to its junction with the BA. The VAs unite at or near the pontomedullary junction to form the **BA**. After giving off pontine and cerebellar branches, the BA terminates by dividing into the two **PCAs**.

### Vascular Territory

The vertebrobasilar system normally supplies all of the posterior fossa structures as well as the midbrain, posterior thalami, occipital lobes, most of the inferior and posterolateral surfaces of the temporal lobe, and upper cervical spinal cord **(8-16)**.

# Arterial Infarcts

## Acute Cerebral Ischemia-Infarction

Imaging is *the* basis of rapid stroke triage. Because of speed and accessibility, NECT and CTA (with or without CT perfusion) are the most commonly used modalities.

There are four "must know" questions in acute stroke triage that need to be answered rapidly and accurately. (1) Is intracranial hemorrhage or a stroke "mimic" present? (2) Is a large vessel occluded? (3) Is part of the brain irreversibly injured (i.e., is there a core of critically ischemic, irreversibly infarcted tissue)? (4) Is there a *clinically relevant* "penumbra" of ischemic but potentially salvageable tissue?

**4 "MUST KNOW" ACUTE STROKE QUESTIONS**

- (1) Is there intracranial hemorrhage (or stroke "mimic")?
- (2) Is large vessel occluded?
- (3) Is part of brain irreversibly injured?
- (4) Is ischemic "penumbra" present?

### Terminology

Stroke—a generic term meaning sudden onset of a neurologic event—is also referred to as a cerebrovascular accident (CVA) or "brain attack."

The distinction between cerebral ischemia and cerebral infarction is subtle but important. In cerebral *ischemia*, the affected tissue remains viable, although blood flow is inadequate to sustain normal cellular function. In cerebral *infarction*, frank cell death occurs with loss of neurons, glia, or both.

Timing is important in patient triage. *Hyperacute* stroke designates events within the first six hours following symptom onset. In hyperacute stroke, cell death has not yet occurred, so the combined term *acute cerebral ischemia-infarction* is often used. *Acute* strokes are those 6-48 hours from onset.

### Etiology

**Stroke Subtypes. Atherosclerotic (ASVD) strokes** are the most common type of acute arterial ischemia/infarction, representing ~ 40-45% of cases.

Most large artery territorial infarcts are embolic, arising from thrombi that develop at the site of an "at-risk" ASVD plaque. The most common site is the carotid bifurcation. The most frequently occluded intracranial vessel is the MCA.

**Small vessel disease** represents 15-30% of all strokes. Small artery occlusions, a.k.a. **lacunar infarcts**, are defined as lesions measuring < 15 mm in diameter. Many are clinically silent, although a strategically located lesion (e.g., in the internal capsule) can cause significant neurologic impairment.

Lacunar infarcts can be embolic, atheromatous, or thrombotic. Most involve penetrating arteries in the basal ganglia/thalami, internal capsule, pons, and deep cerebral white matter (WM).

**Cardioembolic disease** accounts for another 15-25% of major strokes.

**Pathophysiology.** An estimated two million neurons are lost each minute when a major vessel, such as the MCA, is suddenly occluded. CBF falls precipitously. The center of the affected brain parenchyma—the densely **ischemic core**—typically has a CBF < 6-8 $cm^3$/100 g/min.

Neuronal death with irreversible loss of function occurs in the core of an acute stroke. A relatively less **ischemic penumbra** surrounding the central core is present in ~ 1/2 of all patients. CBF in the penumbra is significantly reduced, falling from a normal of 60 $cm^3$/100 g/min to 10-20 $cm^3$/100 g/min. This ischemic but not-yet-doomed-to-infarct tissue represents physiologically "at-risk," but potentially salvageable, tissue.

### Pathology

**Location.** The MCA is the most common site of large artery thromboembolic occlusion **(8-17)** followed by the PCA and vertebrobasilar circulation. The ACA is the least commonly occluded major intracranial vessel.

**Size and Number.** Acute infarcts can be solitary or multiple and vary in size from tiny lacunar to large territorial lesions that can involve much of the cerebral hemisphere.

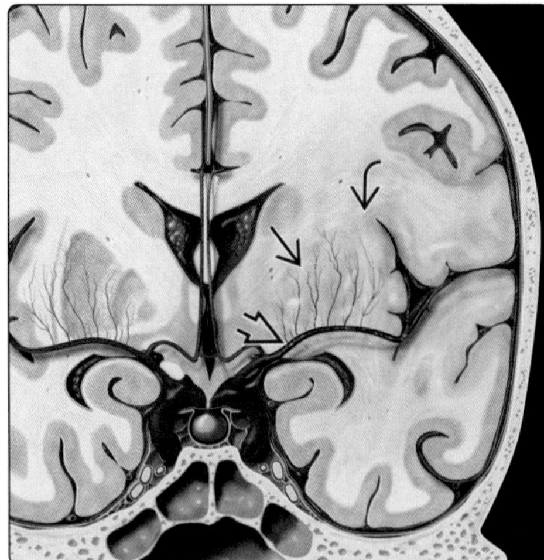

***(8-17)** Graphic shows M1 occlusion ➡. Acute ischemia is seen as subtle loss of GM-WM interfaces ➡ & "blurred" basal ganglia ➡.*

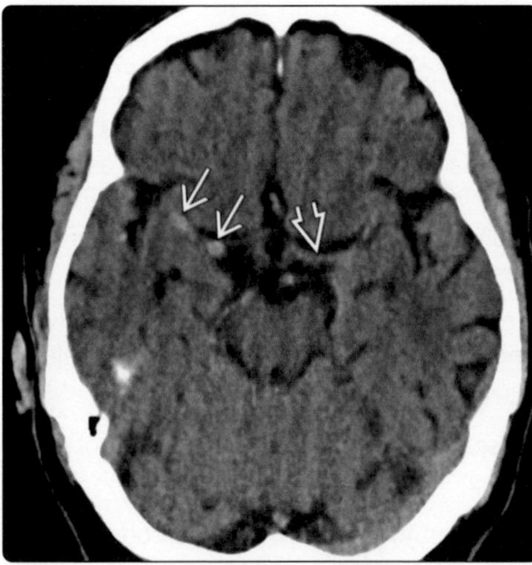

***(8-18)** NECT shows hyperdense MCA sign ➡ (thrombus in the right MCA) compared to the normal, mild hyperdensity of the left MCA ➡.*

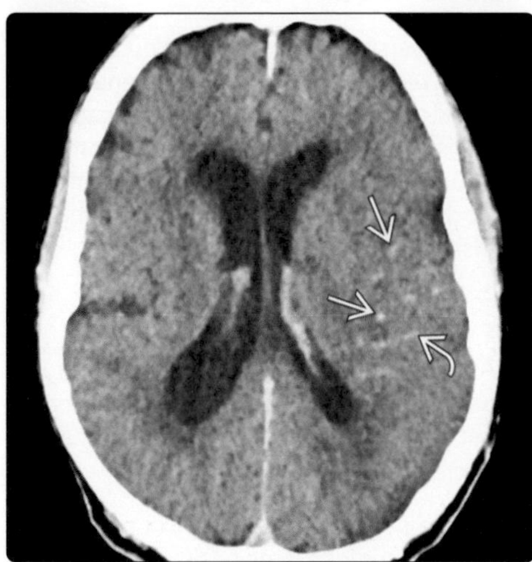

***(8-19)** NECT in acute onset of right hemiparesis shows hyperdense thrombus in the left M2 (dot sign) ➡ & M3 ➡ MCA branches.*

**Gross Pathology.** An acutely thrombosed artery is filled with soft purplish clot that may involve the entire vessel or just a short segment.

Gross parenchymal changes are minimal or absent in the first 6-8 hours, after which edema in the affected vascular territory causes the brain to appear pale and swollen. The gray matter (GM)-WM boundaries become less distinct and more "blurred." As the gyri expand, the adjacent sulci are compressed, and the sulcal-cisternal CSF space is effaced.

## Clinical Issues

**Epidemiology and Demographics.** Stroke is the third leading cause of death in industrialized countries and is the major worldwide cause of adult neurologic disability.

Strokes affect patients of all ages—including newborns and neonates—although most occur in middle-aged or older adults. Children with strokes often have an underlying disorder, such as right-to-left cardiac shunt, sickle cell disease, or inherited hypercoagulable syndrome. Strokes in young adults are often caused by dissection (spontaneous or traumatic) or drug abuse.

**Presentation.** Sudden onset of a focal neurologic deficit, such as facial droop, slurred speech, paresis, or decreased consciousness, is the most common presentation. The NIH Stroke Scale (NIHSS) is a 15-item neurologic examination scale to assess stroke severity and changes in clinical status. The score ranges 0-42 with higher scores indicating greater stroke severity.

**Natural History.** Stroke outcome varies widely. Between 20-25% of strokes are considered "major" occlusions and cause 80% of adverse outcomes. Six months after stroke, 20-30% of all patients are dead, and a similar number are severely disabled.

Prognosis in individual patients depends on a number of contributing factors, i.e., which vessel is occluded, the presence or absence of robust collateral blood flow, and whether there is a significant ischemic penumbra.

Uncontrolled brain swelling with herniation and death can result from so-called malignant MCA infarction. In such cases, emergent craniectomy may be the only treatment option.

**Treatment Options.** Ultrafast stroke triage is essential with the goal of a "door to needle" time (i.e., from arrival in the emergency department to intervention) < 60 minutes.

The single most important factor in successful intervention is patient selection with the two most important considerations being (1) elapsed time from symptom onset and (2) imaging findings.

Once hemorrhage has been excluded by NECT, *intravenous* recombinant tissue plasminogen activator (rTPA) may be administered, as patients are often transferred to a major stroke center ("drip and ship"), especially if elapsed time is less than three hours from ictus (the so-called golden hours). Most centers have expanded the treatment window for IV tPA to four and 1/2 hours from onset of symptoms.

Several large studies have shown that the most effective treatment for acute large vessel occlusion (LVO) by thrombus is endovascular mechanical thrombectomy. Endovascular therapy (EVT) significantly improves outcomes and reduces long-term disability after ischemic stroke. Stent retriever and clot aspiration are the two most currently used EVT techniques with continued improvements leading to very high reperfusion rates.

Evaluating endovascular success is done with a modified thrombolysis in cerebral infarction (TICI) grading system. The TICI score ranges 0-3 with grade 0 = no reperfusion, grade 1 = limited distal filling past the initial occlusion, grade 2 = further reperfusion with subdivisions based on the amount of reperfused MCA territory (2a: < 50%; 2b: > 50%; 2c: 90-99%), and grade 3 indicates complete reperfusion **(8-26)**. Grade ≥ 2b is considered "successful" reperfusion.

## Imaging

**"Brain Attack" Protocols.** The primary goals of emergent stroke imaging are (1) to distinguish "bland" or ischemic stroke from intracranial hemorrhage and (2) to select/triage patients for possible reperfusion therapies.

Most protocols begin with emergent NECT to answer the *first* "must know" question in stroke imaging: Is intracranial hemorrhage or a stroke "mimic" (such as subdural hematoma or neoplasm) present? If a typical hypertensive hemorrhage is identified on the screening NECT and the patient has a history of systemic hypertension, no further imaging is generally required. CTA is sometimes requested to evaluate for active bleeding (spot sign).

Once intracranial hemorrhage is excluded, the *second* critical issue is determining whether a major cerebral vessel is occluded. CTA can be obtained immediately following the NECT scan and is the noninvasive procedure of choice for depicting potentially treatable major vessel occlusions. MRA is more susceptible to motion artifact, which is accentuated in uncooperative patients. DSA is typically reserved for patients undergoing EVT.

The *third* and *fourth* questions can be answered with either CT or MR perfusion (pCT, pMR) studies. Both can depict what part of the brain is irreversibly damaged (i.e., the unsalvageable core infarct) and determine whether there is a clinically relevant ischemic penumbra (potentially salvageable brain).

**CT Findings.** A complete multimodal acute stroke CT protocol includes nonenhanced head CT, an arch-to-vertex CTA, and

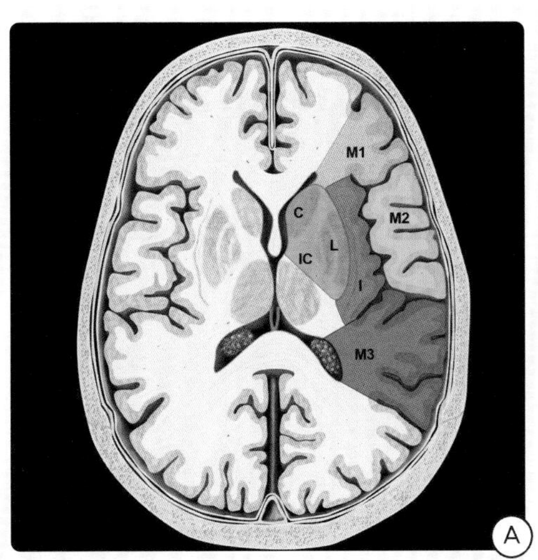


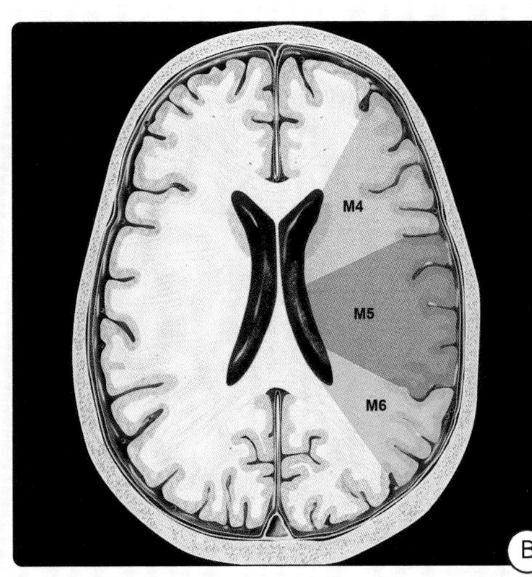


***(8-20A)** Anatomic regions for calculating ASPECTS are illustrated. M1-M3 represent the MCA cortex with each area allotted 1 point. The insular cortex (I), lentiform nuclei (L), caudate head (C), & internal capsule are scored with 1 point each. **(8-20B)** More cephalad graphic shows the superior 3 MCA territories. ASPECTS is calculated by subtracting 1 point for each affected area from 10 (normal total score).*

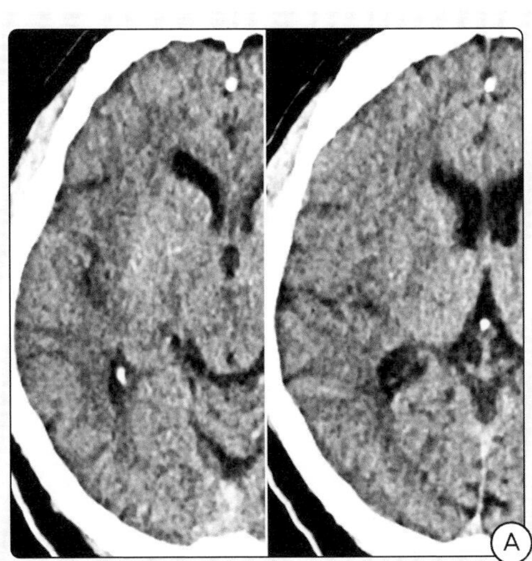


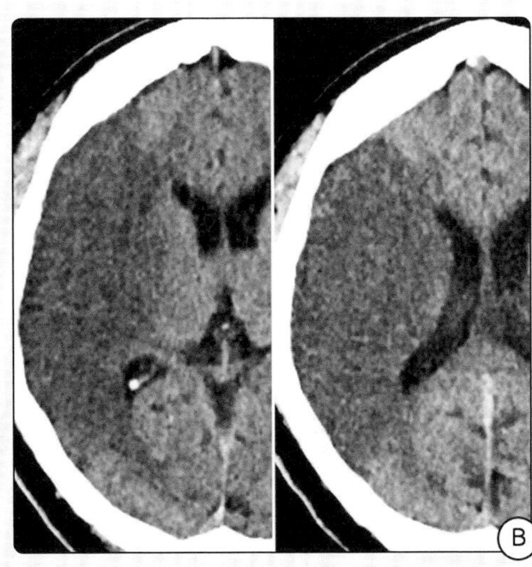


***(8-21A)** Axial NECTs in a 60-year-old man with acute stroke symptoms show (L) hypodensity in the right insular cortex, M1, M2, & M3 cortical areas. The caudate, lentiform nucleus, & internal capsule are spared. (R) More cephalad NECT shows hypodensity in the M4-M6 cortical regions. ASPECTS is 3. **(8-21B)** At 24 hours, the wedge-shaped infarction is sharply delineated. ASPECTS of 3 has a poor prognosis.*

dynamic first-pass pCT. With helical acquisition, the entire protocol can be completed within 15 minutes as a single examination with separate contrast boluses. CTA with pCT improves diagnostic accuracy compared with NECT alone and does not delay intravenous tPA or EVT.

***NECT.*** Initial NECT scans—even those obtained in the first six hours—are abnormal in 50-60% of acute ischemic strokes if viewed with narrow window width.

The most specific, but least sensitive, sign is a hyperattenuating vessel filled with acute thrombus. A **dense MCA sign** is seen in 30% of cases with documented M1 occlusion **(8-18)**. Less common sites for a hyperdense vessel sign are the intracranial ICA, BA, and MCA branches in the sylvian fissure (dot sign) **(8-19)**.

Uncommon but important NECT findings that indicate vascular occlusion include one or more calcified emboli **(8-34)**, most likely from an "at-risk" ulcerated atherosclerotic plaque in the cervical or cavernous ICA. It is critically important to identify calcified cerebral emboli, as they carry a near 50% risk of repeat ischemic stroke.

Blurring and indistinctness of GM-WM interfaces can be seen in 50-70% of cases within the first three hours following occlusion. Loss of the insular cortex **(insular ribbon sign)** **(8-21A)** and decreased density of the basal ganglia **(disappearing basal ganglia sign)** are the most common findings.

**Wedge-shaped parenchymal hypodensity** with indistinct GM-WM borders and **cortical sulcal effacement** develops in large territorial occlusions **(8-21B)**. If > 1/3 of the MCA territory is initially involved, the likelihood of a "malignant" MCA infarct with severe brain swelling rises, as does the risk of hemorrhagic transformation with attempted revascularization.

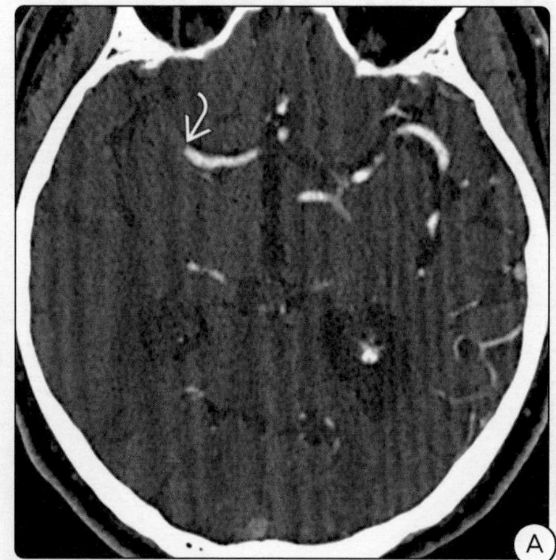


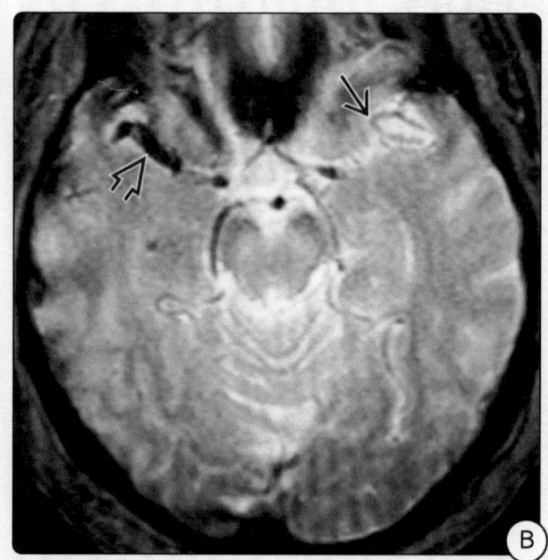


***(8-22A)** CTA in a 65-year-old in the ER with rapid stroke evaluation shows an abrupt cut-off of the right MCA ➡ related to an acute thrombus. CTA is a vital part of "brain attack" protocols to evaluate for a large vessel thrombosis that may be amenable to EVT. **(8-22B)** T2* GRE shows striking "blooming" of a right M1 & proximal M2 MCA thrombus ⇨. Compare to the normal signal intensity in the left MCA genu ⇨.*

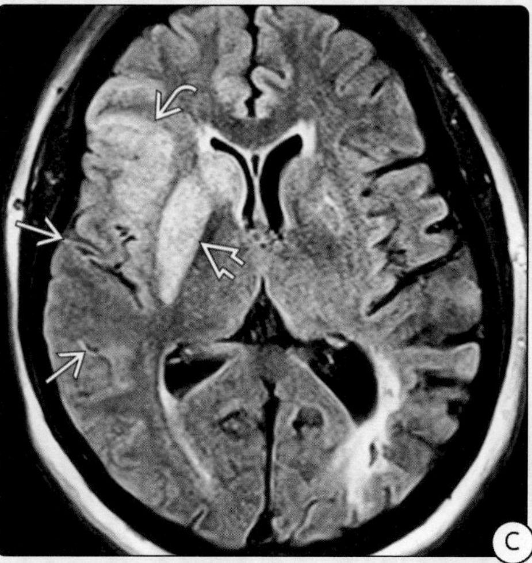


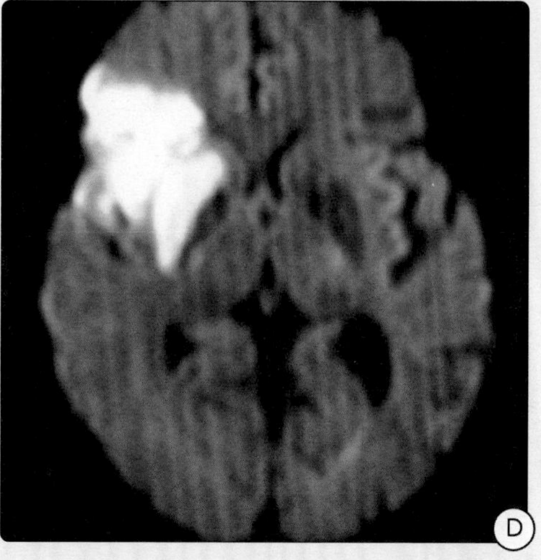


***(8-22C)** FLAIR shows hyperintensity in the right basal ganglia ➡ & insular/frontal cortex ➡. Note intravascular signal in the distal cortical branches ➡, indicating slow flow. **(8-22D)** DWI trace MR shows restricted diffusion in the basal ganglia, right frontal lobe. The territory supplied by the posterior division of the right MCA is not affected, indicating that the slow collateral flow seen on FLAIR was sufficient to avoid ischemia.*

The **A**lberta **S**troke **P**rogram **E**arly **C**omputed **T**omographic **S**core (ASPECTS) is a straightforward, quick, and reproducible measure of early ischemic change **(8-20)**. ASPECTS is calculated by subtracting one point for each of 10 regions affected. ASPECTS ≤ 6 equates to > 1/3 of the MCA territory and has been associated with increased risk of hemorrhage and poor outcome **(8-21)**.

In the past, most trials excluded patients with ASPECTS of < 5 or a core infarct volume of > 70 mL. These patients, however, have poor outcomes. Therefore, newer trials have expanded the treatment windows to include patients with lower ASPECTS. These stroke trials have continued to show improved patient outcomes with EVT in patients with lower ASPECTS, 3-5.

***CTA.*** CTA (with or without CT perfusion) quickly answers the *second* "must know" stroke question **(8-22A)**, i.e., is a major vessel occlusion with a "retrievable" intravascular thrombus present? CTA defines the intravascular thrombus and assesses collateral blood flow.

***pCT.*** The *third* and *fourth* "must know" questions can be answered with whole-brain pCT. pCT depicts the effect of vessel occlusion on the brain parenchyma itself, offering a rapid assessment of cerebral hemodynamics and parenchymal viability that is key to acute stroke management **(8-23)**.

Classic pCT has three major parameters: Cerebral blood volume (**CBV**), **CBF**, and mean transit time **(MTT)**. CBV is the volume of flowing blood in a given volume of brain. CBF is the volume of flowing blood moving through a given volume of brain in a specified amount of time. MTT is the average time it takes blood to transit through a given volume of brain. Parameters similar to MTT often used in pCT include time to peak (TTP) and time to drain (TTD).

All three pCT parameters can also be depicted either visually or on a color scale. The standard color scale is graduated from

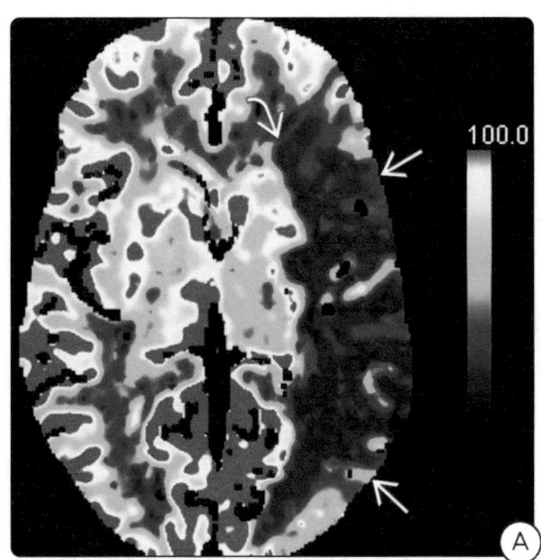


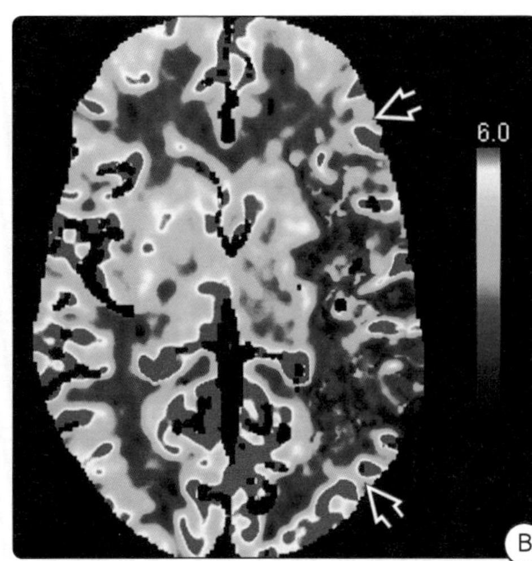


***(8-23A) Patient with large left MCA infarct from distal M1 thrombus is shown. pCT shows markedly reduced CBF in the lateral basal ganglia/insula ➡ & the entire cortical territory ➡. (8-23B) CBV in the same case shows small areas of preserved blood volume ➡ around the margins of the core infarct.***

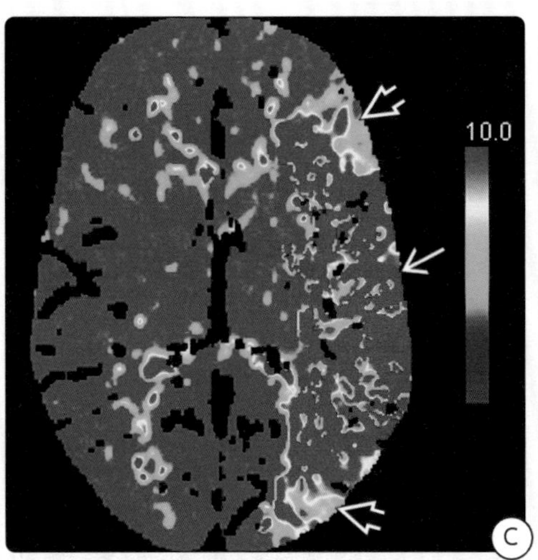


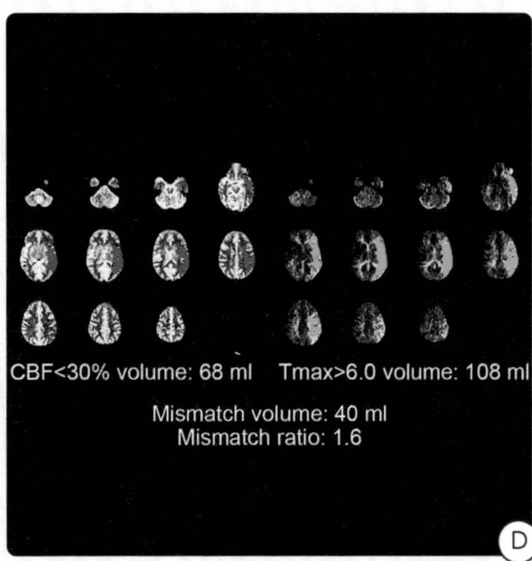


***(8-23C) MTT shows severely prolonged transit time in the core infarct ➡. Less severely ↑ MTT is present at the lesion margins ➡. (8-23D) Automated pCT calculation shows volume with CBF < 30% (pink, representing severely ischemic core infarct) is 68 mL. Volume with Tmax > 6.0 seconds (green) is 108 mL. The mismatch volume is 40 mL & the mismatch ratio is 1.6. Thrombectomy was unsuccessful.***

shades of red and yellow to blue and violet. With CBV and CBF, perfusion is portrayed in red/yellow/green (highest) to blue/purple/black (lowest). Well-perfused GM appears red/yellow, WM appears blue, and ischemic brain is blue/purple.

The densely ischemic **infarct core**—the irreversibly injured brain—shows **matched** reduction in *both* **CBV** and **CBF** and is seen as a dark blue/purple or black area **(8-23A)**. Prolonged MTT is seen as a red area in contrast to the blue brain, in which transit time is normal **(8-23C)**.

An **ischemic penumbra** with potentially salvageable tissue is seen as a "mismatch" between markedly reduced CBV in the infarcted core and a surrounding area (penumbra) characterized by decreased CBF with normal or even transiently increased CBV. Thus, the potentially salvageable brain tissue is equivalent to CBV - CBF. Between 15-20% of large MCA infarcts cause hypoperfusion with reduced CBF in the *contralateral* cerebellum, a phenomenon called **crossed cerebellar diaschisis**.

Parameters present on automated processing maps include CBF, time to maximum of the tissue residue function (Tmax), CBV, and MTT. Only **CBF** and **Tmax** have been widely studied in randomized clinical trials. Automated pCT software estimates **core infarct volume** on the basis of a < 30% threshold for CBF reduction and penumbral volume on the basis of a threshold > 6 seconds for prolongation of Tmax. Automated processing can quickly measure volumes with **CBF < 30%** (ischemic core infarct) and **Tmax > 6 seconds** (penumbra) as well as calculate mismatch volumes and ratios **(8-23D)**.

Management of acute ischemic stroke is continually evolving. The initial target mismatch profile for those patients who may benefit from EVT included an ischemic core volume < 70 mL, a mismatch ratio > 1.8, and a mismatch volume > 15 mL **(8-25)**.

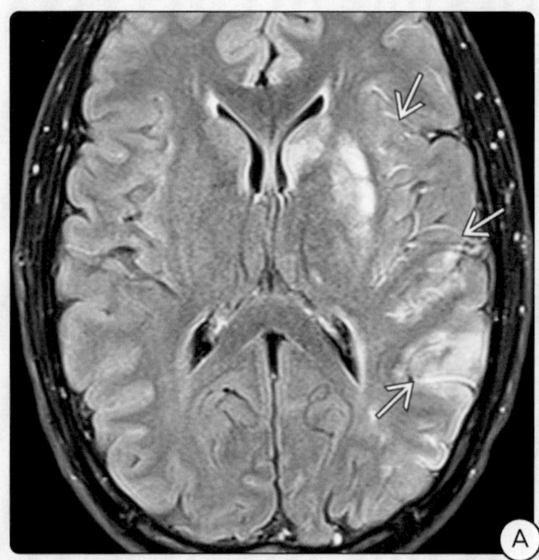


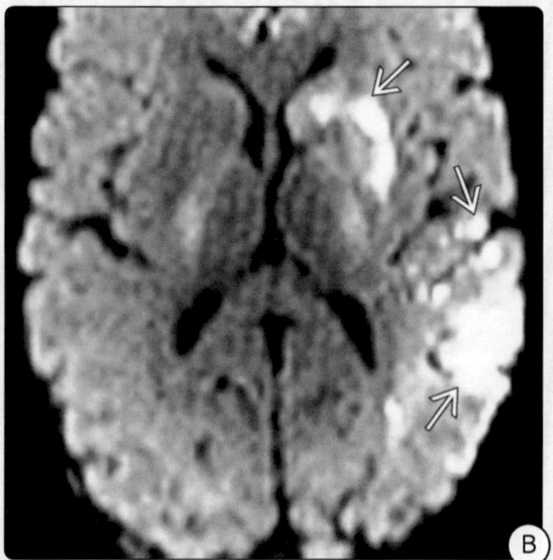


***(8-24A)** Acute stroke in a 47-year-old man shows patchy hyperintensity in the left caudate nucleus, lateral putamen, & parietal cortex. Note multiple linear foci of intravascular hyperintensity ➡, consistent with slow flow in the MCA distribution.* ***(8-24B)** DWI trace MR in the same patient shows multiple patchy foci of diffusion restriction ➡, consistent with acute cerebral infarct.*

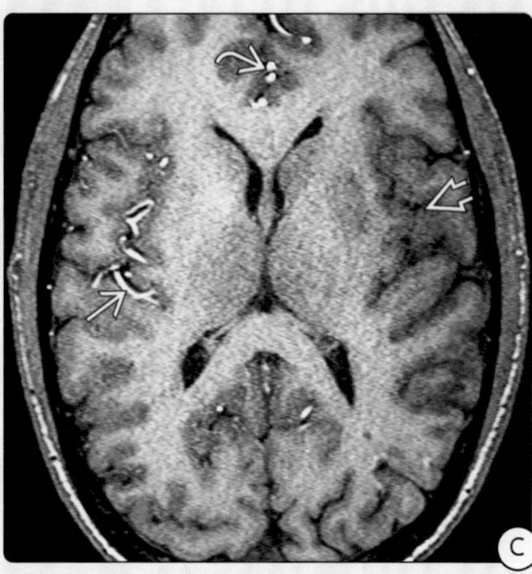


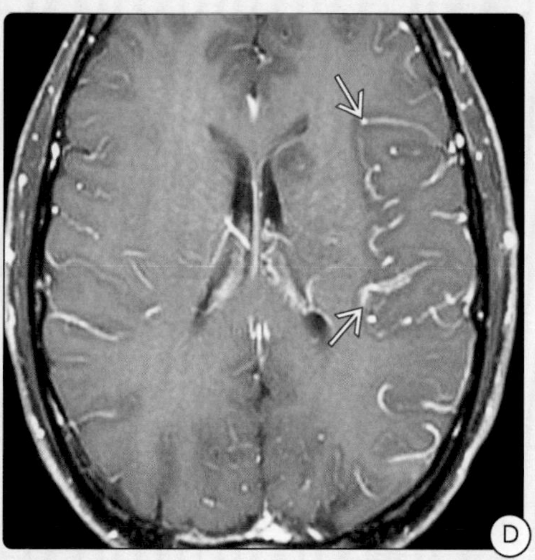


***(8-24C)** Axial source image from 2D TOF MRA shows normal signal intensity in the right MCA ➡ & both ACA branches ➡ but no flow in the left MCA vessels ➡.* ***(8-24D)** Axial T1 C+ FS MR shows striking intravascular enhancement in the left MCA branches ➡, consistent with slow flow in patent (nonthrombosed) vessels.*

New studies are changing these values to be more inclusive of patients eligible for EVT with favorable results.

**MR Findings.** Although CT/CTA/pCT is often preferred because of accessibility and speed, "expedited" rapid stroke protocols with only fast FLAIR, T2*, DWI, and pMR can be used. MR is superior to CT in detecting small ischemic and lacunar strokes.

***T1WI.*** T1WI is usually normal within the first 3-6 hours. Subtle gyral swelling and hypointensity begin to develop within 12-24 hours and are seen as blurring of the GM-WM interfaces. With large vessel occlusions, loss of the expected "flow void" in the affected artery can sometimes be identified.

***T2/FLAIR.*** Only 30-50% of acute strokes show cortical swelling and hyperintensity on FLAIR scans within the first four hours. Nearly all strokes are FLAIR positive by seven hours following symptom onset **(8-22C)**. Intraarterial hyperintensity on FLAIR is an early sign of stroke and indicates slow flow, either from delayed antegrade flow or, more commonly, retrograde collateral filling across the cortical watershed (WS) **(8-24A)**. FLAIR-DWI "mismatch" (negative FLAIR, positive DWI) has been suggested as a quick indicator of viable ischemic penumbra and eligibility for thrombolysis.

***T2* GRE.*** Intraarterial thrombus can sometimes be detected as "blooming" hypointensity on T2* (GRE, SWI) **(8-22B)**. Large MCA infarcts sometimes exhibit increased hypointensity in deep medullary veins due to prolonged transit time and increased deoxyhemoglobin. Although hemorrhagic transformation may sometimes occur as early as 24-48 hours following ictus, it is more typical of late acute and early subacute infarcts.

***T1 C+.*** Postcontrast T1 scans show intravascular enhancement **(8-24D)**. Parenchymal enhancement is uncommon in acute/hyperacute ischemia.

***DWI and DTI.*** Around 95% of hyperacute infarcts show diffusion restriction on DWI with hyperintensity on DWI **(8-22D)** **(8-24B)** and corresponding hypointensity on ADC. DTI is even more sensitive than DWI, especially for small pontine and medullary lesions.

***pMR.*** Restriction on DWI generally reflects the densely ischemic core of the infarct, whereas pMR depicts the surrounding "at-risk" penumbra. A **DWI-PWI mismatch** is one of the criteria used in determining suitability for EVT.

**Angiography.** Findings include abrupt vessel cut-off, a meniscus sign, tapered or "rat-tail" narrowing, or tram-track appearance (contrast around intraluminal thrombus) **(8-26)**. Others are "bare" or "naked" area(s) of nonperfused brain, slow antegrade filling with intraarterial contrast persisting into the capillary or venous phase, and pial collaterals with retrograde filling across the cortical WS.

Less common signs are hyperemia with a vascular "blush" around the infarcted zone (so-called luxury perfusion) and "early draining" veins.

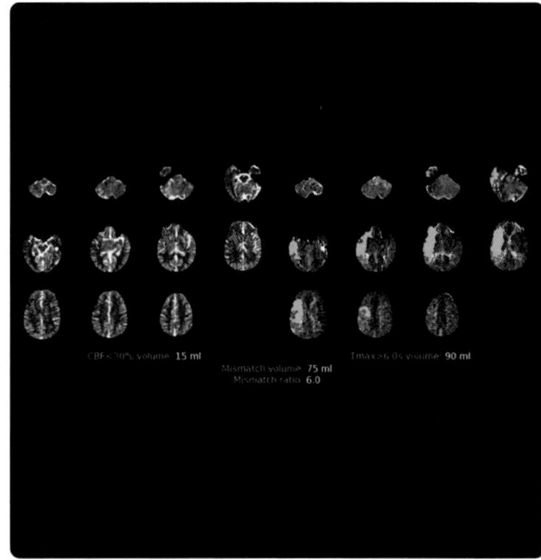

***(8-25)** Automated pCT maps show CBF < 30% (core infarct) 15 mL. Tmax > 6.0 seconds (green) is 90 mL. pCT suggests benefit from EVT.*

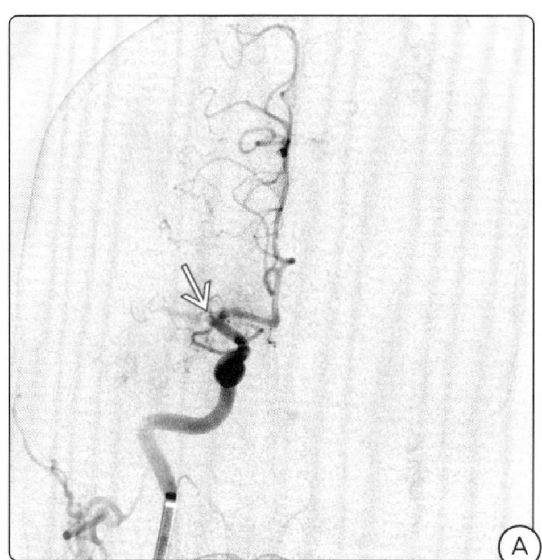


***(8-26A)** MCA cut-off ➡ related to acute thrombus. Proximal location results in loss of lenticulostriate arteries supplying basal ganglia.*

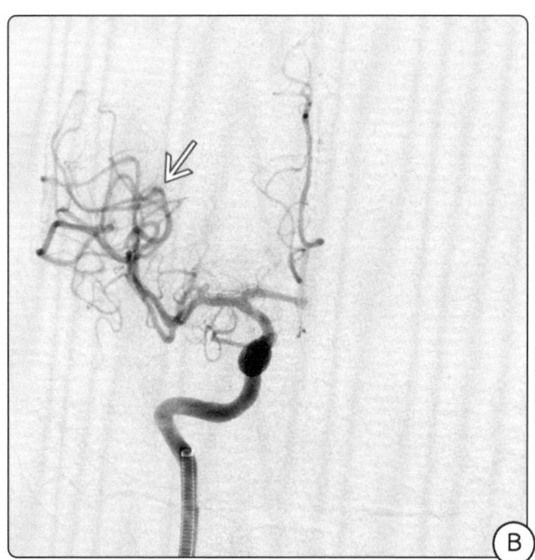


***(8-26B)** DSA after a single-pass thrombectomy with a stent retriever shows complete reperfusion of the MCA branches ➡, TICI 3.*

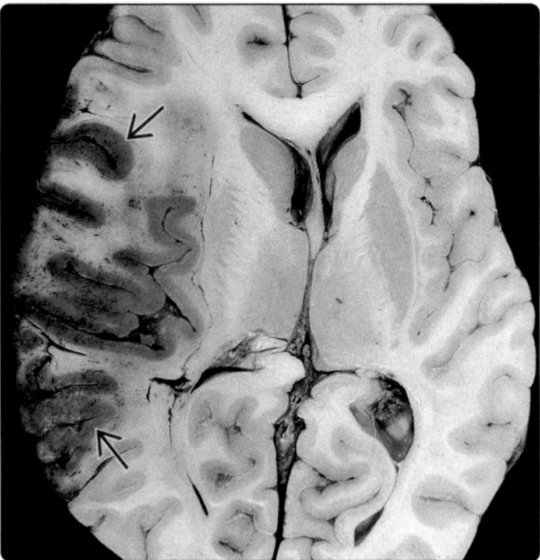

*(8-27) Late acute/early subacute stroke with gyriform HT ⇒ & mass effect. (Courtesy R. Hewlett, MD.)*

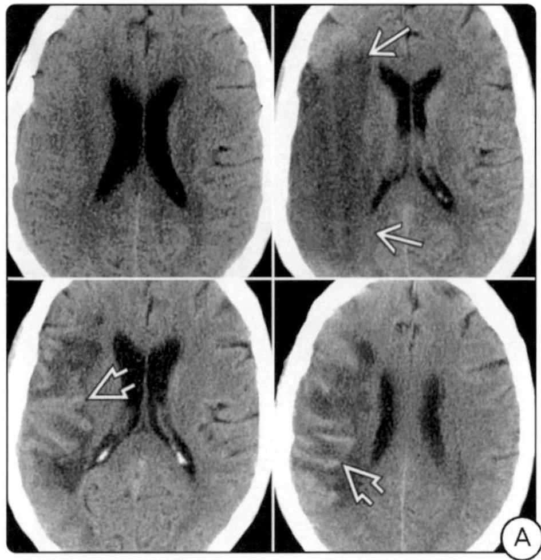

*(8-28A) (Top) NECT at 2 h shows mild sulcal effacement. At 48 h, wedge-shaped hypodensity ⇒ involves GM, WM. (Bottom) HT ⇒ at 1 week.*

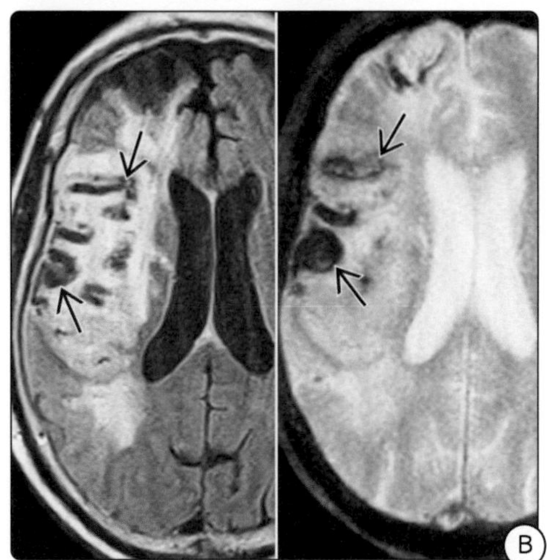

*(8-28B) FLAIR (L) & GRE (R) in the same case show HT ⇒ in this example of subacute stroke.*

## ACUTE STROKE IMAGING

**NECT**
- Hyperdense vessel ± dot sign
- "Blurred," effaced GM-WM borders
  - Insular ribbon sign
  - "Disappearing" basal ganglia
- Wedge-shaped hypodensity
  - Involves both cortex, WM
- Look for $Ca^{++}$ emboli (≈ 50% risk of future stroke)

**CECT**
- ± enhancing vessels (slow flow, collaterals)

**CTA**
- Shows site, length of major vessel thrombus
- ASVD
  - Extracranial: Aorta, carotid bifurcation
  - Intracranial: Cavernous ICA, COW + branches

**pCT**
- Infarct core (irreversibly damaged brain)
  - Matched perfusion (CBV, CBF both decreased)
  - CBF < 30% (automated)
- Ischemic penumbra
  - Perfusion "mismatch" (decreased CBF but normal CBV)
  - Tmax > 6 (automated)

**T1WI/T2WI**
- Usually normal in first 4-6 hours
- ± loss of expected "flow void"

**FLAIR** (use narrow windows)
- 50% positive in first 4-6 hours
  - Cortical swelling, gyral hyperintensity
  - Intraarterial hyperintensity (usually slow flow, not thrombus)

**T2* (GRE, SWI)**
- Thrombus may "bloom"
- Large infarcts may show prominent hypointense medullary veins
- Microbleeds (chronic hypertension, amyloid)

**DWI and DTI**
- > 95% restriction within minutes
  - Hyperintense on DWI trace
  - Hypointense on ADC map
- "Diffusion-negative" acute strokes
  - Small (lacunar) infarcts
  - Brainstem lesions
  - Rapid clot lysis/recanalization
  - Transient/fluctuating hypoperfusion

**pMR**
- DWI-PWI "mismatch" estimates penumbra
- CBV-CBF, DWI-FLAIR mismatches estimate penumbra

**DSA**
- Vessel "cut-off," meniscus sign, tapered/"rat-tail" narrowing
- "Bare" area of unperfused brain
- Slow antegrade or retrograde filling
- Delayed intraarterial contrast washout
- Luxury perfusion
  - "Blush" around "bare area"
  - "Early draining" veins

## Differential Diagnosis

Stroke "mimics" with restricted DWI include **infection, status epilepticus**, and acute **hypoglycemia**. These typically affect cortex in a nonvascular distribution while sparing the underlying subcortical WM.

Normal circulating blood is always slightly hyperdense compared with brain on NECT. A hyperdense vessel sign can be simulated by **elevated hematocrit** (all the vessels appear dense, not just the arteries), arterial wall **microcalcifications**, and **hypodense brain** parenchyma (e.g., diffuse cerebral edema).

# Subacute Cerebral Infarcts

## Terminology

Strokes evolve pathophysiologically with corresponding changes reflected on imaging studies. Although there are no firm divisions that demarcate the various stages of stroke evolution, most neurologists designate infarcts as acute, subacute, and chronic.

"Subacute" cerebral ischemia/infarction generally refers to strokes that are between 48 hours and two weeks following the initial ischemic event.

## Pathology

**Edema** and **increasing mass effect** caused by cytotoxic edema become maximal within 3-4 days following stroke onset. Frank tissue necrosis with progressive influx of microglia and macrophages around vessels ensues with reactive astrocytosis around the perimeter of the stroke. Brain softening and then cavitation proceeds over the next two weeks.

Most thromboembolic strokes are initially "bland," i.e., nonhemorrhagic. **Hemorrhagic transformation** of a previously ischemic infarct occurs in 20-25% of cases between two days and a week after ictus **(8-27)**. Ischemia-damaged vascular endothelium becomes "leaky," and blood-brain barrier permeability increases. When reperfusion is established—either spontaneously or following treatment with tissue plasminogen activator—exudation of red blood cells through the damaged blood vessel walls causes parenchymal hemorrhages. Petechial hemorrhages are more common than lobar bleeds and are most common in the basal ganglia and cortex.

## Clinical Issues

Hemorrhagic transformation itself, when small, generally does not cause clinical deterioration. Hemorrhagic transformation is actually related to favorable outcome, probably reflecting early vessel recanalization and better tissue reperfusion.

## Imaging

**General Features.** There are significant variations within the subacute time period. Early subacute strokes have significant mass effect and often exhibit hemorrhagic transformation, whereas edema and mass effect have mostly subsided by the late subacute period.

**CT Findings.** On NECT, the wedge-shaped area of decreased attenuation seen on initial scans becomes more sharply defined. Mass effect initially increases, then begins to decrease by 7-10 days following stroke onset. Hemorrhagic transformation develops in 15-20% of cases and is seen as gyriform cortical or basal ganglia hyperdensity **(8-28A)**.

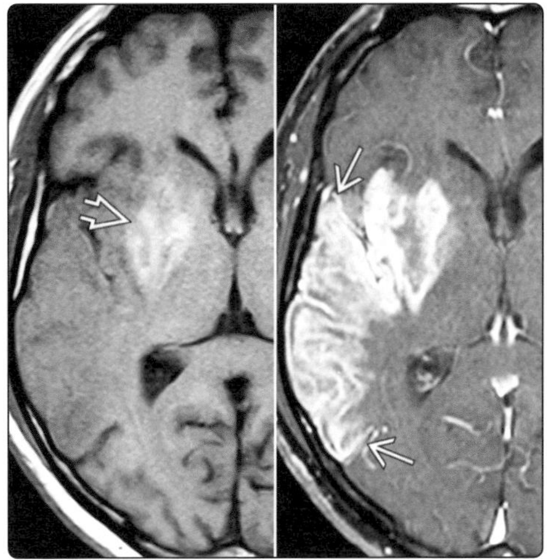

***(8-29)*** *MR 2 weeks after right MCA stroke shows HT ➾ (L) & the intense enhancement ➾ characteristic of subacute infarction (R).*

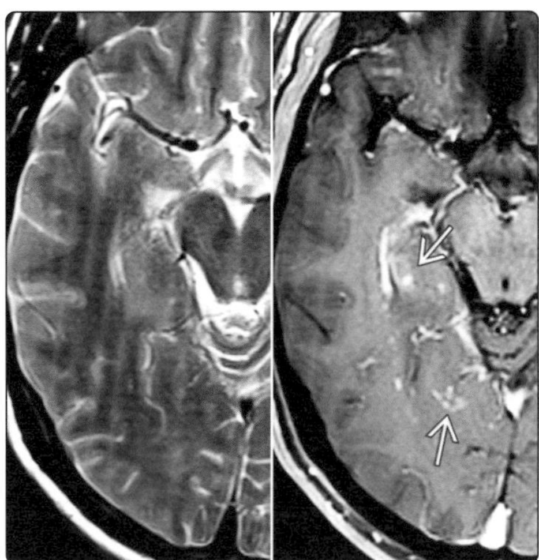

***(8-30)*** *T2 "fogging effect" 2 weeks after stroke is shown. (L) T2 appears normal. (R) T1 C+ FS shows patchy enhancement ➾ in PCA infarct.*

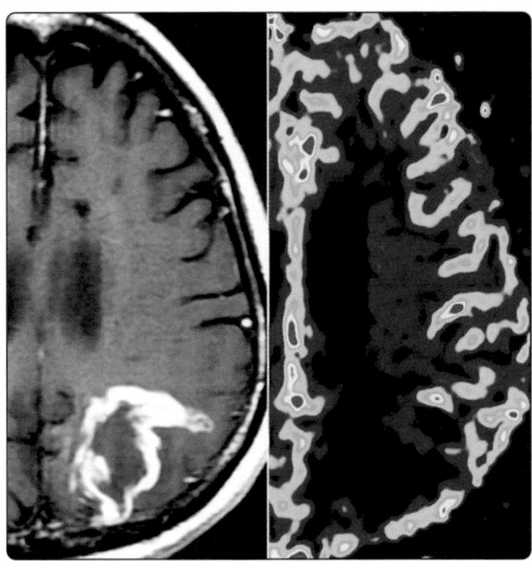

***(8-31)*** *(L) Subacute infarct with ring enhancement mimics neoplasm. (R) pMR shows "cold" lesion with profoundly ↓ rCBV.*

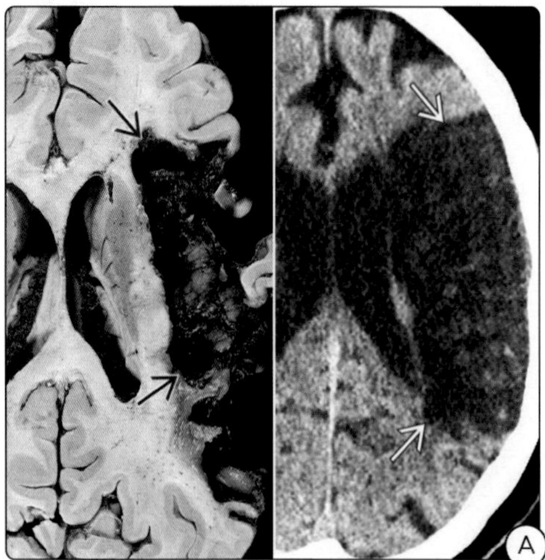
(8-32A) (L) Old MCA infarct with HT ➡. (R) NECT shows encephalomalacia, old MCA infarct ➡. (Courtesy R. Hewlett, MD.)

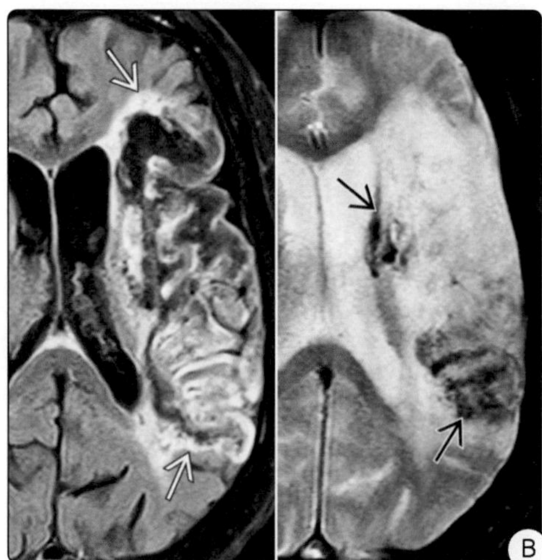
(8-32B) FLAIR (L) shows hyperintensity ➡ around the cavitated, encephalomalacic area, whereas T2* GRE (R) shows some HT ➡.

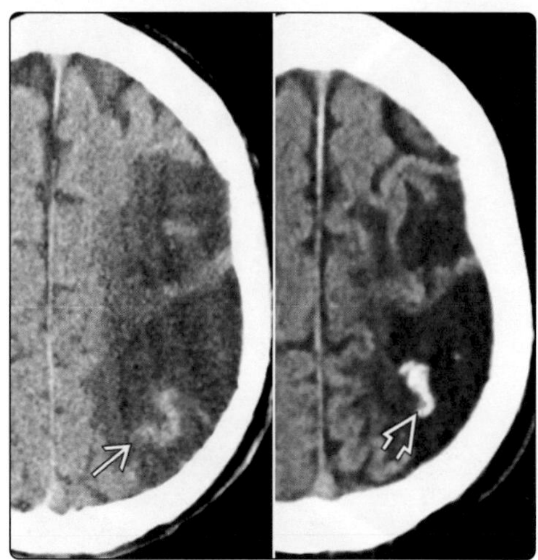
(8-33) (L) Small focus of HT ➡ in late subacute MCA infarct. (R) Gyriform calcification ➡ is present in same area 3 years later.

CECT follows a "2-2-2" rule. Patchy or gyriform enhancement appears as early as two days after stroke onset, peaks at two weeks, and generally disappears by two months.

## SUBACUTE STROKE

**Pathology**

- Edema, mass effect initially increase
- Vessel damage → hemorrhagic transformation in 25%

**CT**

- Hypodensity sharply defined
- Gyriform enhancement 2 days to several weeks

**MR**

- T1WI
  - Iso- to hypointense
  - May see T1 shortening (cortex, basal ganglia)
- T2WI
  - "Fogging effect" (isointensity)
  - ± early wallerian degeneration
- FLAIR
  - Hyperintensity corresponds to final infarct
- T2*
  - "Blooming" hemorrhagic transformation
  - Prominent medullary veins
- DWI
  - Pseudonormalization
  - T2 "shine-through"
- T1 C+
  - Enhances (gyriform, even ring-like)

**Differential Diagnosis**

- Neoplasm
- Infection
  - Cerebritis
  - Encephalitis

**MR Findings.** Signal intensity in subacute stroke varies depending on (1) time since ictus and (2) the presence or absence of hemorrhagic transformation.

***T1WI.*** Nonhemorrhagic subacute infarcts are hypointense on T1WI and demonstrate moderate mass effect with sulcal effacement. Strokes with hemorrhagic transformation are initially isointense with cortex and then become hyperintense **(8-29)**.

***T2WI.*** Subacute infarcts are initially hyperintense compared with nonischemic brain. Signal intensity decreases with time, reaching isointensity at 1-2 weeks (the T2 "fogging effect") **(8-30)**. Early wallerian degeneration can sometimes be identified as a well-delineated hyperintense band that extends inferiorly from the infarcted cortex along the corticospinal tract.

***FLAIR.*** Subacute infarcts are hyperintense on FLAIR **(8-28B)**. By one week after ictus, "final" infarct volume corresponds to the FLAIR-defined abnormality.

***T2* (GRE, SWI).*** Petechial or gyriform "blooming" foci are present if hemorrhagic transformation has occurred in the infarcted cortex **(8-28B)**. Basal ganglia hemorrhages can be confluent or petechial.

Prominent ipsilateral medullary veins on SWI in MCA territory strokes within 3-7 days of ictus are a significant predictive biomarker of poor clinical outcome. Prominent medullary veins in the contralateral (normal) hemisphere may indirectly reflect increased CBF and are associated with good clinical outcome.

***T1 C+.*** The intravascular enhancement often seen in the first 48 hours following thromboembolic occlusion disappears within three or four days and is replaced by leptomeningeal enhancement caused by persisting pial collateral blood flow. Patchy or gyriform parenchymal enhancement can occur as early as two or three days after infarction **(8-29)** and may persist for 2-3 months, in some cases, mimicking neoplasm **(8-31)**.

***DWI and pMR.*** Restricted diffusion with hyperintensity on DWI and hypointensity on ADC persists for the first several days following stroke onset, then gradually reverses to become hypointense on DWI and hyperintense with T2 "shine-through" on ADC. pMR with arterial spin labeling shows crossed cerebellar diaschisis in 50% of patients with subacute ischemic strokes.

## Chronic Cerebral Infarcts

### Terminology

Chronic cerebral infarcts are the end result of ischemic territorial strokes and are also called postinfarction encephalomalacia.

### Pathology

The pathologic hallmark of chronic cerebral infarcts is volume loss with gliosis in an anatomic vascular distribution. A cavitated, encephalomalacic brain with strands of residual glial tissue and traversing blood vessels is the usual gross appearance of an old infarct **(8-32A)**.

### Imaging

NECT scans show a sharply delineated wedge-shaped hypodense area that involves both GM and WM and conforms to the vascular territory of a cerebral artery. The adjacent sulci and ipsilateral ventricle enlarge secondary to volume loss in the affected hemisphere **(8-32A)**. Dystrophic calcification occurs but is uncommon **(8-33)**.

Wallerian degeneration with an ipsilateral small, shrunken cerebral peduncle is often present with large MCA infarcts. Look for atrophy of the contralateral cerebellum secondary to crossed cerebellar diaschisis.

Chronic infarcts older than 2-3 months typically do not enhance on CECT.

MR scans show cystic encephalomalacia with CSF-equivalent signal intensity on all sequences. Marginal gliosis or spongiosis around the old cavitated stroke is hyperintense on FLAIR **(8-32B)**. DWI shows increased diffusivity (hyperintense on ADC).

## Multiple Embolic Infarcts

Brain emboli are less common but important causes of stroke. Most consist of clots containing fibrin, platelets, and red blood cells. Less common emboli include air, fat, calcium, tumor, and foreign bodies (e.g., debris from metallic heart valves).

### Cardiac and Atheromatous Emboli

**Pathoetiology.** Simultaneous small acute infarcts in multiple different vascular distributions are the hallmark of embolic cerebral infarcts **(8-35)**. The heart is the most common source; cardiac emboli can be septic or aseptic **(8-37)**. Peripheral signs of emboli, such as splinter hemorrhages, are sometimes present. Echocardiography may demonstrate valvular

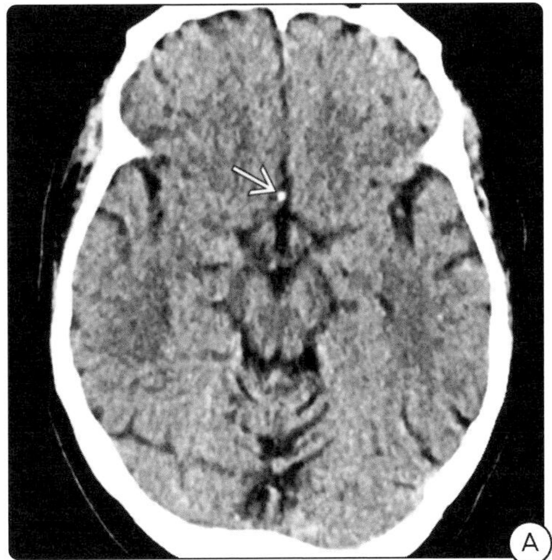


***(8-34A) NECT in a 65-year-old with altered mental status shows a 2-mm, rounded calcification ➡ in the interhemispheric fissure.***

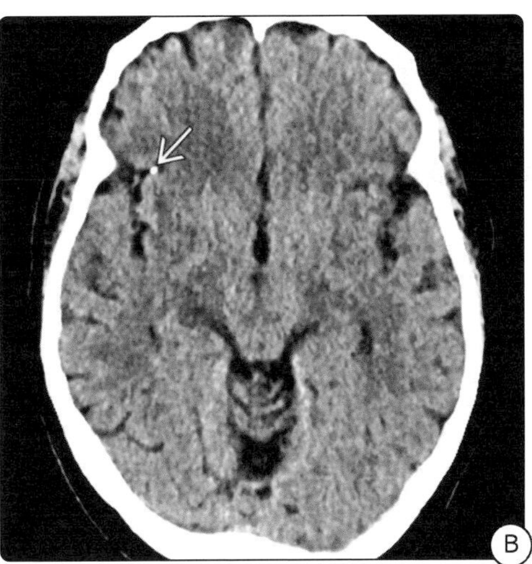


***(8-34B) More cephalad image shows a rounded hyperdensity in the sylvian fissure ➡. Calcified cerebral emboli in distal arterial branches.***

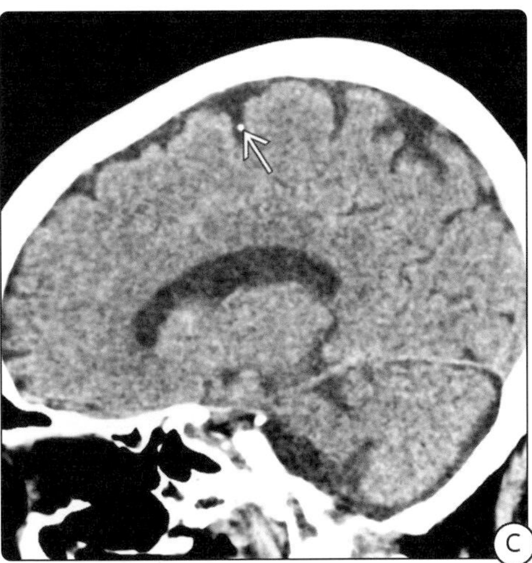


***(8-34C) Sagittal NECT shows calcification within a vertex sulcus ➡. This patient had a calcified mitral valve. High risk for recurrent strokes.***

vegetations, intracardiac filling defect, or atrial or ventricular septal defect.

Ipsilateral hemispheric emboli are most commonly due to atheromatous ICA plaques. Many are clinically silent but convey a high risk for subsequent overt stroke.

**Imaging.** In contrast to large artery territorial strokes, embolic infarcts tend to involve terminal cortical branches. The GM-WM interface is most commonly affected.

NECT scans show low-attenuation foci, often in a wedge-shaped distribution. Calcified emboli (usually from heart valves or atherosclerotic plaques) are seen as small round or ovoid calcifications within sulci **(8-34)**. These are important to identify, as they carry a high risk of recurrent stroke. Septic emboli are often hemorrhagic. CECT scans may demonstrate multiple punctate or ring-enhancing lesions.

MR scans show multifocal peripheral T2/FLAIR hyperintensities. Hemorrhagic emboli cause "blooming" on T2* sequences **(8-36)**. The most sensitive sequence is DWI. Small peripheral foci of diffusion restriction in several different vascular distributions are typical of multiple embolic infarcts **(8-37B)**. T1 C+ imaging may show multiple punctate enhancing foci. Septic emboli often demonstrate ring enhancement, resembling microabscesses.

**Differential Diagnosis.** The major differential diagnosis of multiple embolic infarcts is **hypotensive cerebral infarction**. Hypotensive infarcts are usually caused by hemodynamic compromise and tend to involve the deep internal WS zones. **Parenchymal metastases** have a predilection for the GM-WM interface, as do embolic infarcts, but generally do not restrict on DWI.

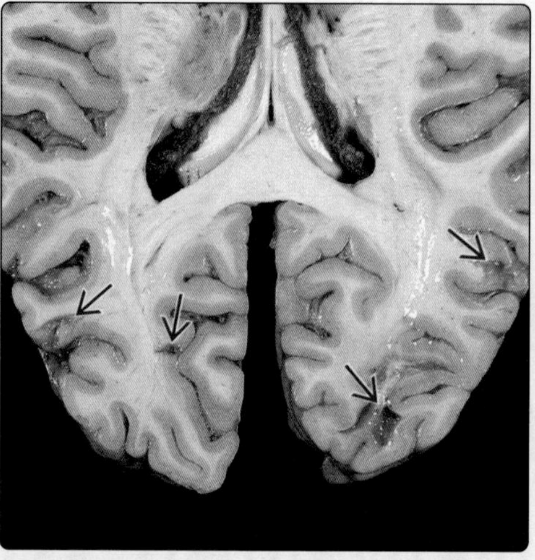

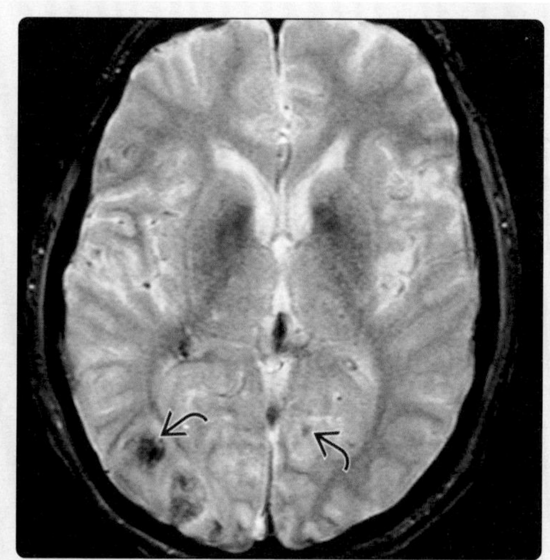

***(8-35)** Autopsy specimen shows multiple old healed infarcts at the GM-WM junctions ⇒. Embolic infarcts tend to involve terminal cortical branches. (Courtesy R. Hewlett, MD.) **(8-36)** T2* GRE in a 70-year-old with decreasing mental status with multiple septic & hemorrhagic embolic infarcts shows multiple areas of "blooming" related to petechial hemorrhages ⇒. GM-WM interface is most commonly affected.*

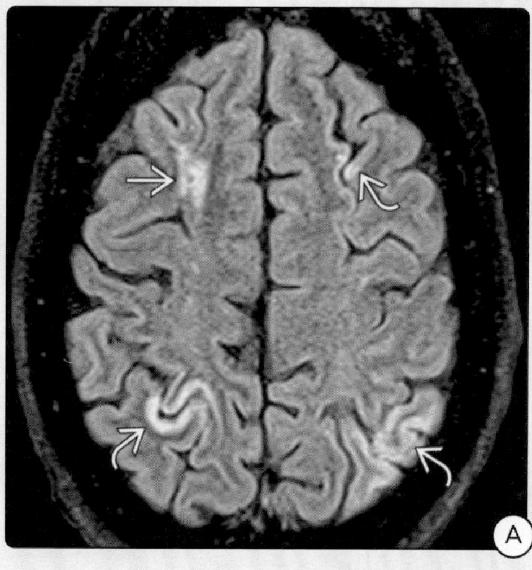



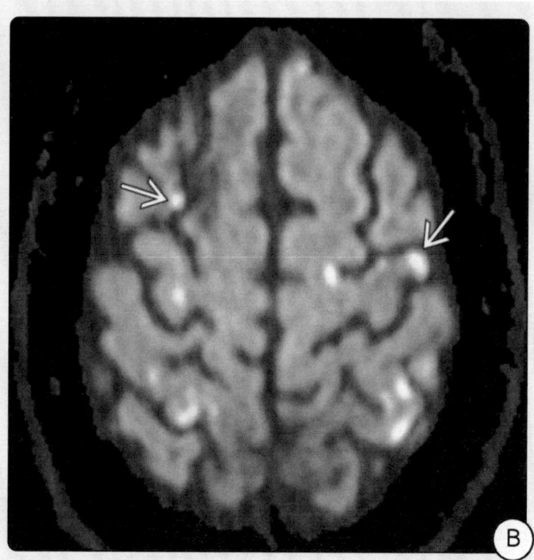



***(8-37A)** Axial FLAIR MR in a 39-year-old man with altered mental status shows multifocal cortical ⇒ & subcortical WM ⇒ hyperintensities. **(8-37B)** Axial DWI trace MR in the same patient shows multiple bilateral hyperintense foci ⇒ of acute ischemia in multiple vascular territories typical of embolic disease. This patient was found to have mitral valve vegetations at echocardiogram.*

## Fat Emboli

Fat embolism syndrome (FES) is an uncommon disorder that presents as hypoxia, neurologic symptoms, &/or a petechial rash in the setting of severely displaced lower extremity long bone fractures. The term cerebral fat emboli (CFE) refers to the neurologic manifestations of FES.

**Pathoetiology.** Two mechanisms have been proposed to explain the effects of FES: (1) Small vessel occlusions from fat particles and (2) inflammatory changes in surrounding tissue initiated by breakdown of fat into free fatty acids and other metabolic byproducts.

The pathologic hallmark of CFE is arteriolar fat emboli with perivascular microhemorrhages **(8-38)**.

**Epidemiology and Clinical Issues.** The overall incidence of FES in patients with long bone fractures—most commonly the femoral neck—is 1-2%. FES also occurs with pelvic fractures, elective orthopedic procedures (e.g., total hip arthroplasty), cardiac surgery, anesthesia, and systemic illness (e.g., pancreatitis). FES in patients with bone marrow necrosis secondary to sickle cell crisis has also been reported.

CFE occurs in up to 80% of patients with FES. Signs and symptoms vary in severity and include petechial rash, headache, seizure, drowsiness, altered mental status, and coma. Focal neurologic deficits are less common. Onset is from two hours up to two days after trauma or surgery with a mean of 29 hours. However, many cases are subclinical and remain undiagnosed.

**Imaging.** Imaging findings reflect the *effect* of the fat emboli (i.e., multifocal tiny strokes and microhemorrhages) on brain tissue, not the fat itself. NECT scans are, therefore, usually normal.

MR shows numerous (average = 50) punctate or confluent hyperintensities in the cerebellum, basal ganglia,

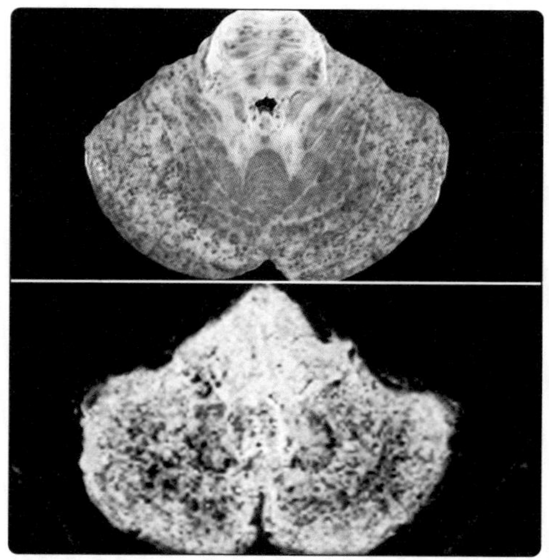

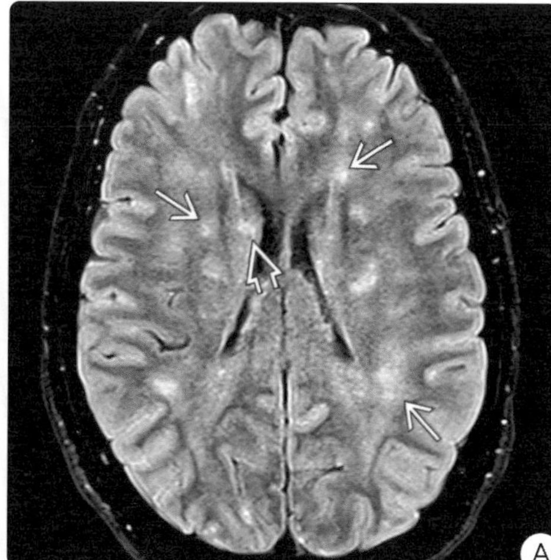


***(8-38)** (Top) Autopsy case of fat embolism shows innumerable small microbleeds throughout the pons & cerebellum. (Courtesy Klatt, Robbins, & Cotran, Atlas of Neuropathology, 2015.) (Bottom) MIP SWI in fat embolism shows multiple "blooming black dots." **(8-39A)** FLAIR in a 45-year-old with altered mental status after fractured hip repair surgery shows multiple hyperintense foci ➔ in periventricular, subcortical WM & basal ganglia ➲.*

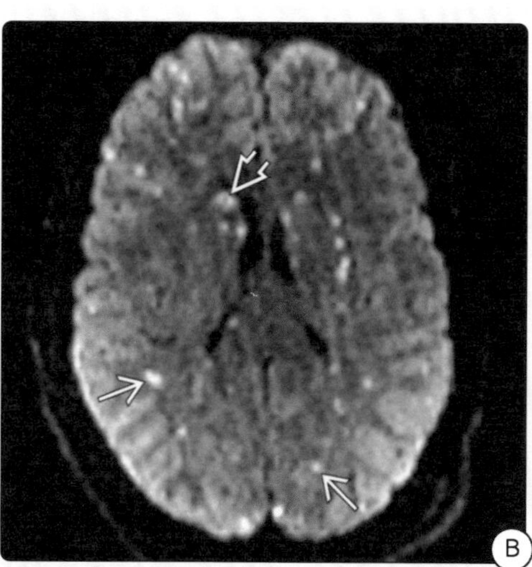


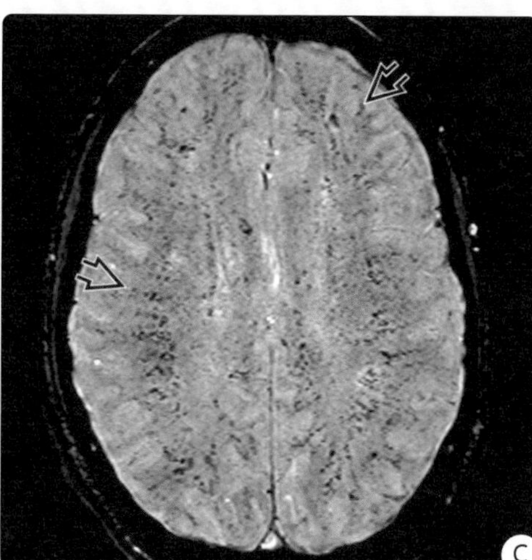


***(8-39B)** DWI trace image in the same patient shows innumerable tiny foci of diffusion restriction in the WM ➔ & GM ➲, the so-called star field pattern characteristic of cerebral FES. **(8-39C)** T2* SWI in the same patient shows thousands of tiny "blooming" hypointense foci throughout the hemispheres ➲, characteristic of microbleeds related to cerebral FES.*

periventricular WM, and GM-WM junctions on T2/FLAIR **(8-39A)**. DWI shows innumerable tiny punctate foci of diffusion restriction in multiple vascular distributions, the star field pattern **(8-39B)**. The deep WS border zones are commonly involved.

Solitary or multiple small hypointense "blooming" foci can be identified in up to 1/3 of all FES cases on T2* GRE. SWI discloses innumerable (> 200) tiny "black dots" in the majority of patients **(8-39C)**.

**Differential Diagnosis.** The major differential diagnosis of cerebral FES is **multiple embolic infarcts**. Multiple cardiac or atheromatous embolic infarcts rarely produce the dozens or even hundreds of lesions seen with CFE. Embolic infarct lesions tend to involve the basal ganglia and corticomedullary junctions more than the WM.

Multifocal "blooming" hypointensities on T2* can be seen with severe **diffuse axonal injury (DAI)** or **diffuse vascular injury (DVI)**. As patients with CFE often have polytrauma, the distinction may be difficult on the basis of imaging studies alone. DAI and DVI tend to cause linear as well as punctate microbleeds.

## Cerebral Gas Embolism

**Pathoetiology.** Minor amounts of air in the intracranial venous systems is usually iatrogenic, introduced during intravenous catheter placement.

Massive cerebral gas embolism (CGE) is a potentially catastrophic complication of central venous catheter (CVC) manipulation/disconnection and has been reported with cardiac procedures.

Other etiologies of arterial or venous air embolism include lung biopsy, craniotomy in the sitting position, and

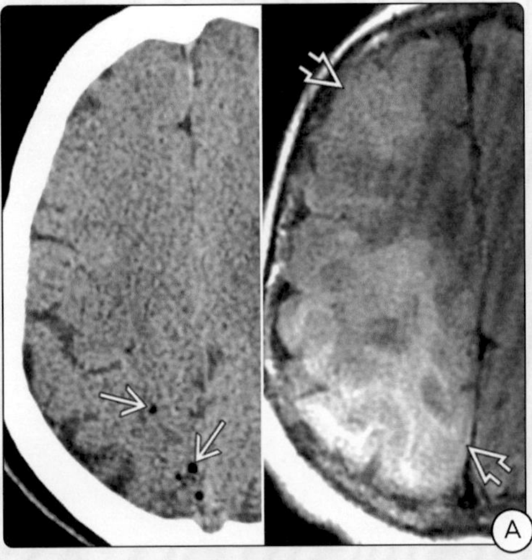


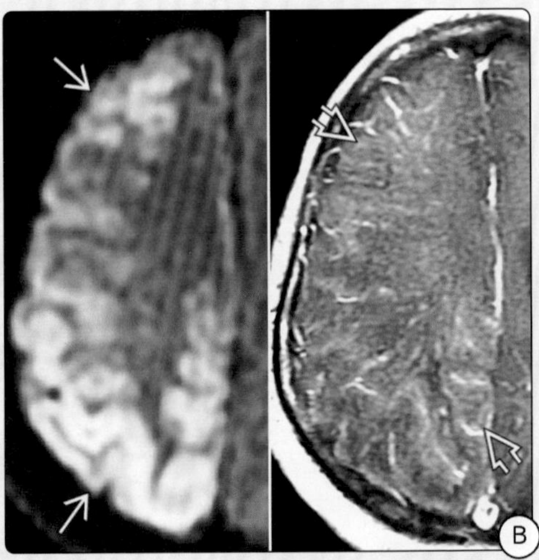


***(8-40A)** 55-year-old experienced left hemiparesis after esophageal dilatation. (L) Axial NECT of cerebral gas embolism shows multiple "dots" of air in the brain ➡. (R) FLAIR shows a much more extensive area of diffuse cortical/subcortical WMH ➡. **(8-40B)** (L) DWI shows restricted diffusion ➡ in the cortex. (R) T1 C+ shows extensive patchy, linear enhancement ➡ in the cortex & subcortical WM. (Courtesy P. Hildenbrand, MD.)*

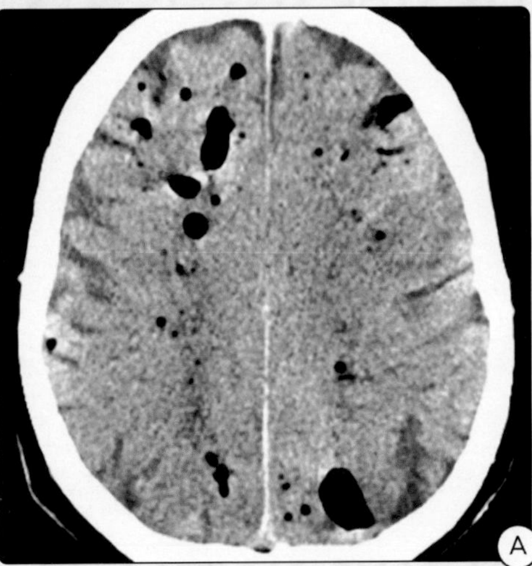


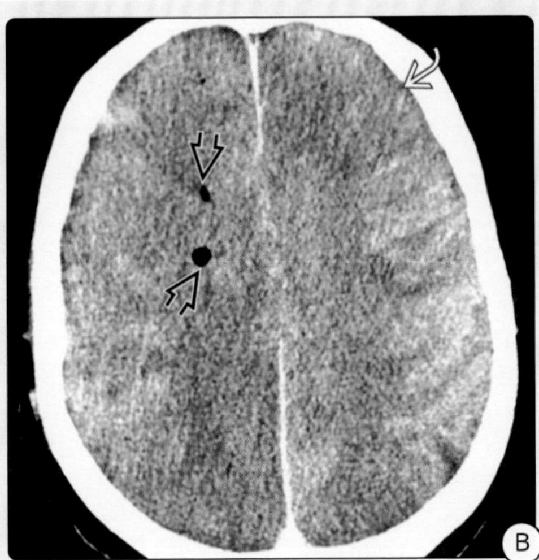


***(8-41A)** Axial NECT scan in a 69-year-old with altered mental status immediately after cardiac ablation shows massive cerebral gas embolism. **(8-41B)** NECT in the same case 1 h later shows that most of the air has been resorbed with only 2 small parenchymal dots of air ➡ remaining. Severe diffuse cerebral edema ➡ is now present with effacement of the sulci & blurring of the corticomedullary junctions.*

angiography. Penetrating trauma, decompression sickness, and hydrogen peroxide ingestion are other causes of gas embolism.

**Clinical.** Small amounts of CGE may be asymptomatic or mild and transient. In more severe cases, focal neurologic deficit, coma, seizures, and encephalopathy may ensue. Reported mortality of CGE associated with CVCs approaches 20%.

**Imaging.** Asymptomatic air following intravenous catheter placement is most commonly observed as an incidental finding, typically as dots of air in the cavernous sinus.

Intracranial air bubbles can be identified in 70% of symptomatic CGE cases, appearing on NECT as transient small intravascular rounded or curvilinear hypodensities, typically located at the depths of sulci **(8-40A)**. Intraparenchymal air is less common.

Air is quickly absorbed and can rapidly disappear **(8-41)**. If massive air embolism occurs, cerebral ischemia or diffuse brain swelling typically ensues **(8-41)**.

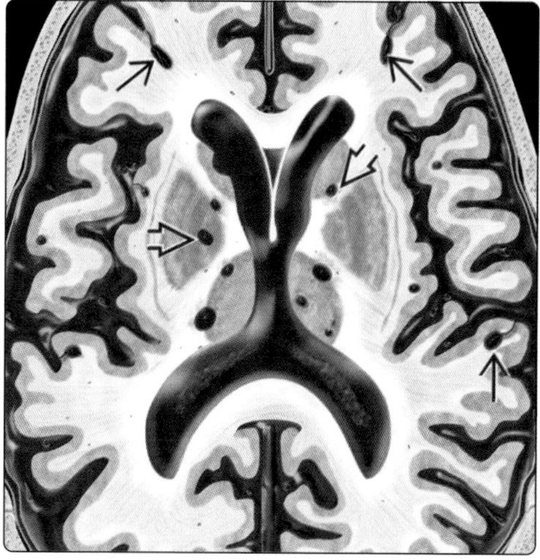

***(8-42)** Graphic shows lacunar infarctions in thalami, basal ganglia ⇨. Note also prominent perivascular (Virchow-Robin) spaces →.*

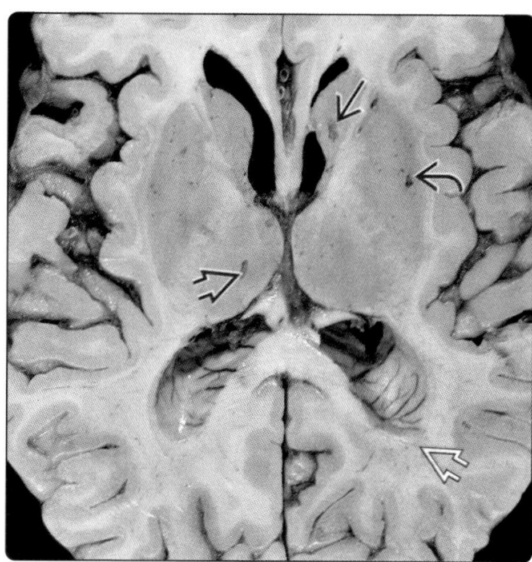

***(8-43)** Old lacunar infarcts are in the caudate →, putamen ⇨, thalamus ⇨, periatrial WM rarefaction ➡. (Courtesy R. Hewlett, MD.)*

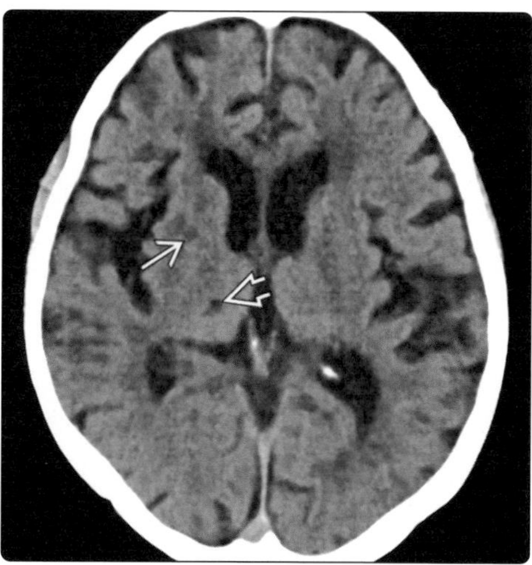

***(8-44)** NECT in an 83-year-old shows typical old thalamic ➡ & basal ganglia ➡ lacunar infarcts as hypodense, slightly irregular lesions.*

EMBOLIC INFARCTS

**Cardiac and Atheromatous Emboli**
- Small, simultaneous; multiple lesions
- Bilateral, multiple vascular distributions
- Typically involve cortex, GM-WM interfaces
- May be $Ca^{++}$
- ± punctate/ring enhancement
- Usually not hemorrhagic unless septic

**Fat Emboli**
- 12-72 hours after long bone trauma, surgery
- Less commonly from bone marrow necrosis (e.g., sickle cell crisis)
- Arteriolar/capillary fat emboli
- Cause multiple tiny microbleeds
- Multiple foci of restricted diffusion in star field pattern (bright spots on dark background)
- Microbleeds best seen on T2* SWI > > GRE
- Deep WM > cortex

**Cerebral Gas Embolism**
- Usually iatrogenic (procedural) or traumatic
- Can occur with hydrogen peroxide ingestion
- NECT may show transient round or curvilinear air densities in sulcal vessels
- Quickly absorbed, disappear
- If massive, lethal brain swelling ensues rapidly

# Lacunar Infarcts

## Terminology

The terms "lacuna," "lacunar infarct," and "lacunar stroke" are often used interchangeably. **Lacunae** are 3- to 15-mm, CSF-filled cavities or "holes" that most often occur in the basal ganglia or cerebral WM **(8-42)**. They are often observed coincidentally on imaging studies in older patients but are not clearly associated with discrete neurologic symptoms, i.e., they are subclinical strokes. Lacunae are sometimes called "silent" strokes, a misnomer, as subtle neuropsychologic impairment is common in these patients.

**Lacunar stroke** means a clinically evident stroke syndrome attributed to a small subcortical or brainstem lesion that may or may not be evident on brain

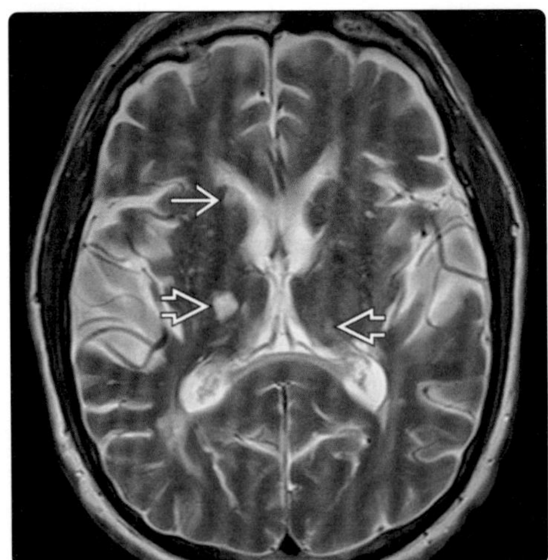

***(8-45)** Axial T2 MR shows multiple rounded & irregular hyperintensities in the basal ganglia ➡ & thalami ➡ related to lacunar infarcts.*

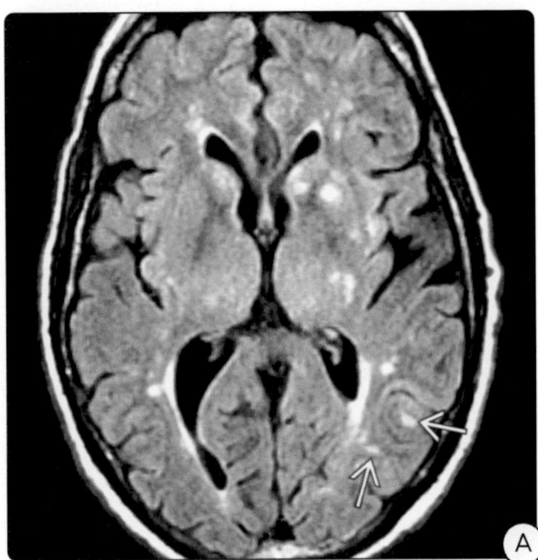


***(8-46A)** FLAIR MR shows multiple hyperintensities in both hemispheres. Some small subcortical lesions ➡ are also present.*

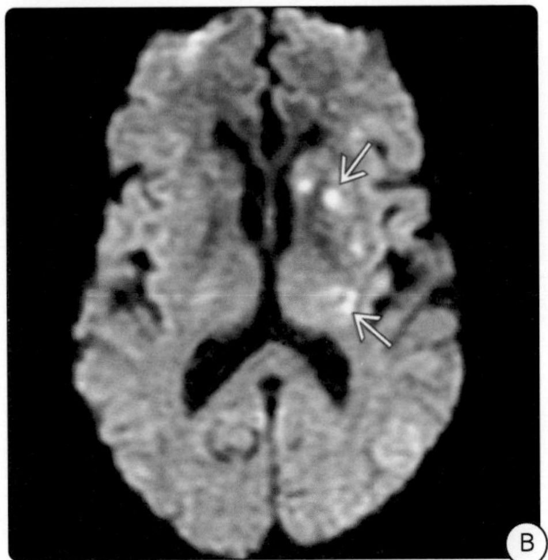


***(8-46B)** Some lesions demonstrate acute restriction ➡. DWI is helpful in distinguishing acute from chronic lacunar infarcts.*

imaging. The term "état lacunaire" or **lacunar state** designates multiple lacunar infarcts.

## Epidemiology and Etiology

Approximately 25% of all ischemic strokes are lacunar-type infarcts. Lacunae are considered macroscopic markers of cerebral small vessel ("microvascular") disease. There are two major vascular pathologies involving small penetrating arteries and arterioles: (1) Thickening of the arterial media by lipohyalinosis, fibrinoid necrosis, and atherosclerosis, causing luminal narrowing and (2) obstruction of penetrating arteries at their origin by large intimal plaques in the parent arteries.

The *MTHFR* C677T genotype is correlated with lacunar stroke.

## Pathology

**Location.** Penetrating branches that arise from the COW and peripheral cortical arteries are small end arteries with few collaterals, so lacunar infarcts are most common in the basal ganglia (putamen, globus pallidus, caudate nucleus), thalami, internal capsule, deep cerebral WM, and pons.

**Size and Number.** Lacunae are, by definition, ≤ 15 mm in diameter. Multiple lesions are common. Between 13-15% of patients have multiple simultaneous acute lacunar infarcts.

**Gross and Microscopic Appearance.** Grossly, lacunae appear as small, pale, irregular but relatively well-delineated cystic cavities **(8-43)**. Brown-staining siderotic discoloration can be seen in old hemorrhagic lacunae. Microscopically, ischemic lacunar infarcts demonstrate tissue rarefaction with neuronal loss, peripheral macrophage infiltration, and gliosis.

## Clinical Issues

Independent risk factors for lacunar infarcts include age, hypertension, and diabetes. Other contributing factors include smoking and atrial fibrillation.

Outcome of lacunar stroke is highly variable. Although most lacunae are asymptomatic, "little strokes" can mean "big trouble." A single subclinical stroke—often a lacuna—is associated with increased likelihood of having additional "little strokes" as well as developing overt clinical stroke &/or dementia. Nearly 20% of patients > 65 years old with WM hyperintensities (WMHs) on T2/FLAIR MR will develop new lacunae within three years.

Between 20-30% of patients with lacunar stroke experience neurologic deterioration hours or even days after the initial event. The pathophysiology of "progressive lacunar stroke" is incompletely understood, and no treatment has been proven to prevent or halt progression.

## Imaging

Imaging findings vary with whether the lacuna is acute or chronic.

**Acute Lacunar Infarcts.** Most acute lacunar infarcts are invisible on NECT scans. Acute lacunar infarcts are hyperintense on T2/FLAIR and may be difficult to distinguish from foci of coexisting chronic microvascular disease **(8-45)** **(8-46A)**. Acute and early subacute lacunae restrict on DWI **(8-46B)** and also usually enhance on T1 C+.

DWI overestimates the eventual size of lacunar infarcts. Cavitation and lesion shrinkage are seen in > 95% of deep symptomatic lacunar infarcts on follow-up imaging.

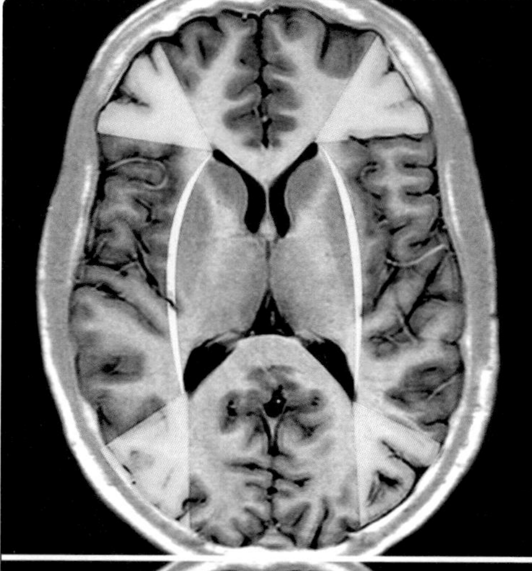
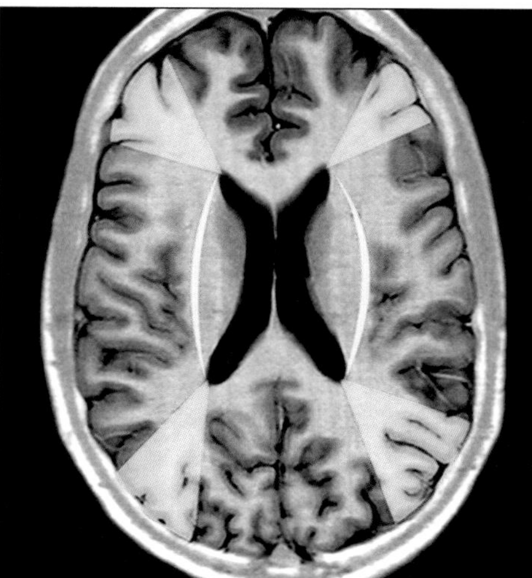
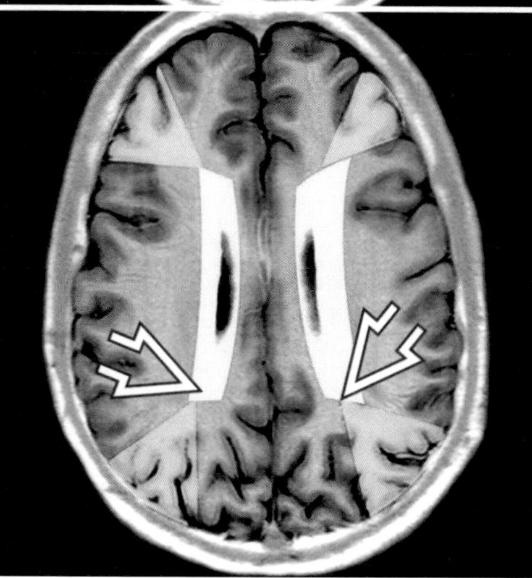
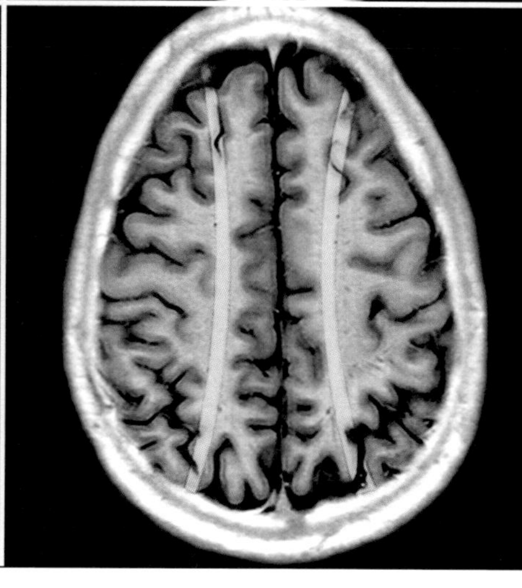

***(8-47)** T1-weighted images show 2 vascular WS zones with external (cortical) WS zones in turquoise. Wedge-shaped areas between the ACAs, MCAs, & PCAs represent "border zones" between the 3 major terminal vascular distributions. Curved blue lines (lower right) represent subcortical WS zone near the vertex. The external WS infarcts are more common & are often embolic. The triple "border zones" ➡ represent confluence of all 3 major vessels. Involvement of the triple "border zones" is often related to global hypoperfusion. Bilateral involvement is often related to acute hypotension. Yellow lines indicate the internal (deep WM) WS zone between perforating arteries & the major territorial vessels. Internal WS infarcts are most often related to regional hypoperfusion secondary to hemodynamic compromise, i.e., ipsilateral carotid stenosis. There are located parallel to & slightly above the lateral ventricles.*

### LACUNAR INFARCTS

**Etiology and Pathology**

- Macroscopic markers of small vessel disease
- Atherosclerosis, lipohyalinosis
- Along small penetrating arteries (few collaterals)
- Most common in basal ganglia, deep WM

**Imaging**

- Acute lacunae often invisible on NECT
- T2/FLAIR hyperintense
- Use DWI to distinguish from WMHs of chronic microvascular disease
- Chronic lacunae irregular, CSF-like
- May be surrounded by gliotic rim

**Chronic Lacunar Infarcts.** Old lacunae appear as well-defined but often somewhat irregular CSF-like "holes" in the brain parenchyma on NECT scans **(8-44)**.

Chronic lacunar infarcts are hypointense on T1WI and hyperintense on T2WI. The fluid in the cavity suppresses on FLAIR, whereas the gliotic periphery remains hyperintense. Multifocal WM disease, seen as WMHs, is also common in patients with frank lacunar infarcts.

Most lacunae are nonhemorrhagic and do not "bloom" on T2* sequences. However, parenchymal microbleeds—multifocal "blooming black dots" on T2* (GRE, SWI)—are common comorbidities in patients with lacunar infarcts and chronic hypertension.

## Differential Diagnosis

The major differential diagnosis of lacunar infarct is **prominent perivascular spaces** (PVSs). Also known as Virchow-Robin spaces, prominent PVSs are pia-lined, interstitial fluid-filled spaces. Prominent PVSs can be found in virtually all locations and in patients of all ages, although they tend to increase in size and frequency with age. The most common locations for PVSs are the inferior 1/3 of the basal ganglia (clustered around the anterior commissure), subcortical WM (including the external capsule), and the midbrain (see Chapter 32).

PVSs are sharply marginated and ovoid, linear, or round; lacunae tend to be more irregularly shaped. PVSs faithfully follow CSF signal intensity on all MR sequences and suppress completely on FLAIR. The adjacent brain is typically normal, although a thin rim of FLAIR hyperintensity around the PVSs is present in 25% of cases.

**Embolic infarcts** are typically peripheral (cortical/subcortical) rather than the usual central and deep location of typical lacunae.

WS or **"border zone" infarcts** grossly resemble lacunar infarcts on imaging studies. However, "border zone" infarcts occur in specific locations—along the cortical and subcortical WM WS zones—whereas lacunae are more randomly scattered lesions that primarily affect the basal ganglia, thalami, and deep periventricular WM.

The WMHs associated with **microvascular disease** (primarily lipohyalinosis and arteriolosclerosis) are less well defined and usually more patchy or confluent than the small (< 15-mm) lesions that represent true lacunar infarcts. WMHs tend to cluster around the occipital horns and periventricular WM, not the basal ganglia and thalami.

A few scattered T2/FLAIR hyperintensities are common in the **normal aging brain**. A general guideline is "one white spot per decade" until the age of 50, after which the number and size of WMHs increase at accelerated rates.

## Watershed ("Border Zone") Infarcts

### Terminology and Epidemiology

Watershed (WS) infarcts, a.k.a. "border zone" infarcts, are ischemic lesions that occur in the junction between two nonanastomosing distal arterial distributions. WS infarcts are more common than generally recognized, constituting 10-12% of all brain infarcts.

### Anatomy of Cerebral "Border Zones"

WS zones are defined as the "border" or junction where two or more major arterial territories meet. Two distinct types of vascular "border zones" are recognized: An external (cortical) WS zone and an internal (deep) WS zone **(8-47)**.

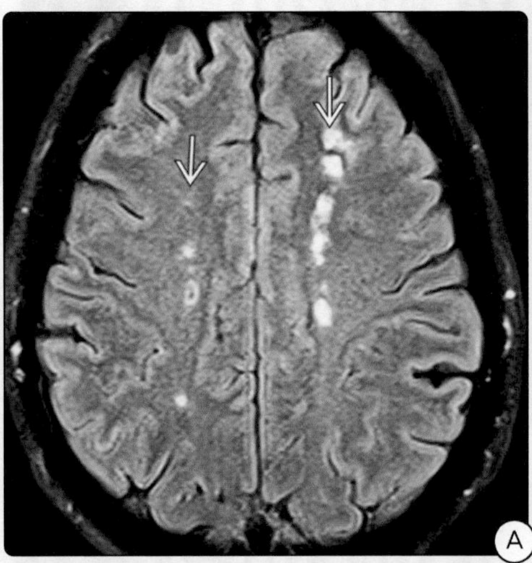
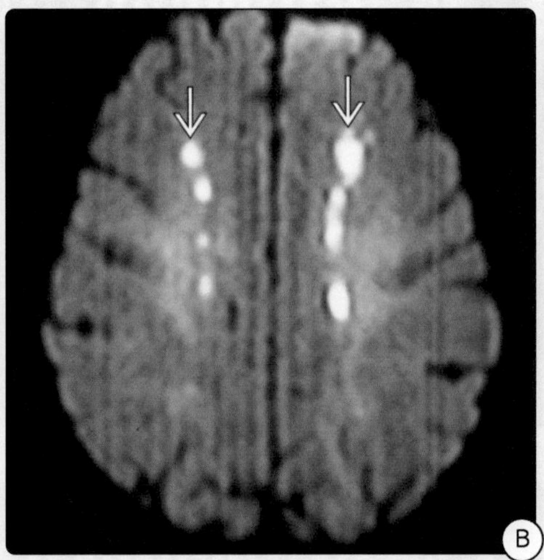

***(8-48A)** FLAIR MR demonstrates classic findings of internal WS zone ischemia. WMHs ➡ are not randomly distributed; they lie just above the lateral ventricles & line up from front to back. They often resemble a line of beads extending from front to back in the deep WM. **(8-48B)** The lesions ➡ restrict on DWI MR. High-grade stenoses were found in both proximal ICAs.*

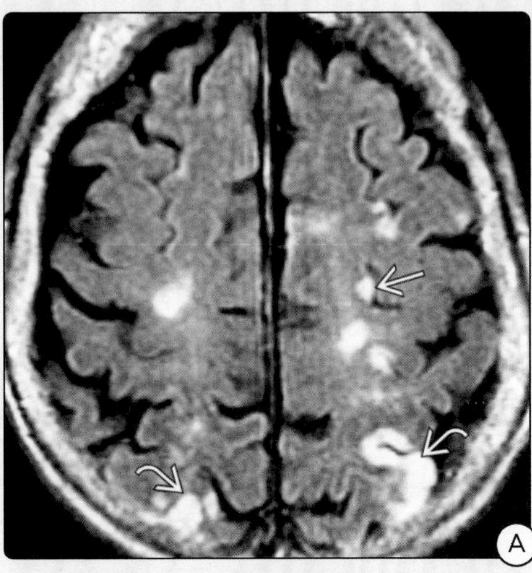
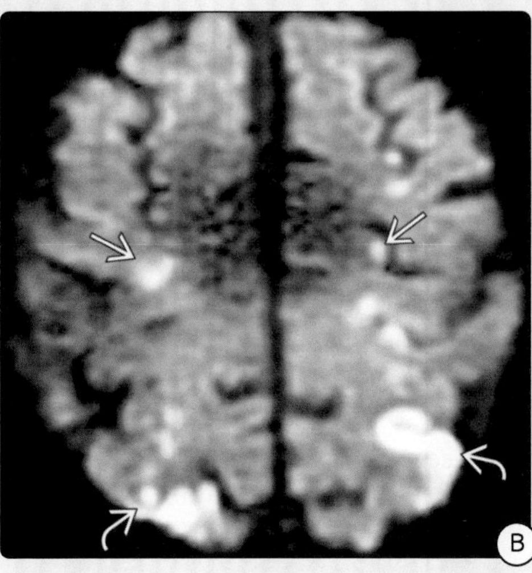

***(8-49A)** FLAIR MR demonstrates external WS zone ischemia. The WMHs are more peripheral & largely cortical ➡. Some are distinctly gyriform ➡ & lie at the "triple WS" zone between the ACA, MCA, & PCA cortical distributions. **(8-49B)** DWI MR shows multiple punctate ➡ & gyriform ➡ foci of restricted diffusion in the cortex related to hypotension with global hypoperfusion in this patient with external WS infarcts.*

The two major **external WS zones** lie in the frontal cortex (between the ACA and MCA) and parietooccipital cortex (between the MCA and PCA). A strip of paramedian subcortical WM near the vertex of the cerebral hemispheres is also considered part of the external WS.

The **internal WS zones** represent the junctions between penetrating branches (e.g., lenticulostriate arteries, medullary WM perforating arteries, and anterior choroidal branches) and the major cerebral vessels (MCA , ACA, and PCA).

## Etiology

Maximal vulnerability to hypoperfusion is greatest where two distal arterial fields meet together. *Hypotension with or without severe arterial stenosis or occlusion can result in hemodynamic compromise.* Flow in the affected WS zone can be critically lowered, resulting in ischemia or frank infarction. The most susceptible "border zone" is the "triple WS" where the ACA, MCA, and PCA all converge.

**External WS infarcts** are the more common type. Most external WS infarcts are *embolic*. Anterior cortical WS embolic infarcts often occur in concert with internal carotid atherosclerosis. External WS infarcts in all three "border zones" are less common and usually reflect *global hypoperfusion*.

**Internal WS infarcts** are rarely embolic. They represent 35-40% of all WS infarcts and are most often caused by *regional hypoperfusion* secondary to hemodynamic compromise (e.g., ipsilateral carotid stenosis).

## Pathology

**Location.** Internal WS infarcts tend to "line up" in the WM, parallel to and slightly above the lateral ventricles. Cerebellar WS infarcts occur at the borders between the posterior inferior, anterior inferior, and superior cerebellar arteries.

External (cortical) WS infarcts show a bimodal spatial distribution. Anteriorly, they center in the posterior frontal lobe near the junction of the frontal sulcus with the precentral sulcus. Posterior WS infarcts center in the superior parietal lobule posterolateral to the postcentral sulcus. The prevalence of WS infarcts decreases between these two areas. WS infarcts spare the medial cortex.

**Size and Number.** WS infarcts vary in size from tiny lesions to large wedge-shaped ischemic areas. Multiple lesions are common and can be uni- or bilateral. Bilateral lesions are often related to global reduction in perfusion pressure, usually an acute hypotensive event **(8-50)**.

## Imaging

**Internal WS Infarcts.** Internal "border zone" infarcts can be confluent or partial. Confluent infarcts are large, cigar-shaped lesions that lie alongside or just above the lateral ventricles. Partial infarcts are more discrete, rosary-like lesions. They resemble a line of beads extending from front to back in the deep WM **(8-48)**.

Stenosis or occlusion of the ipsilateral ICA or MCA is common with unilateral lesions. The presence and degree of hemodynamic impairment can be determined using a number of methods, including pCT, pMR, SPECT, and PET.

**External (Cortical) WS Infarcts.** Cortical (external) WS infarcts are wedge- or gyriform-shaped **(8-49)** **(8-51)**.

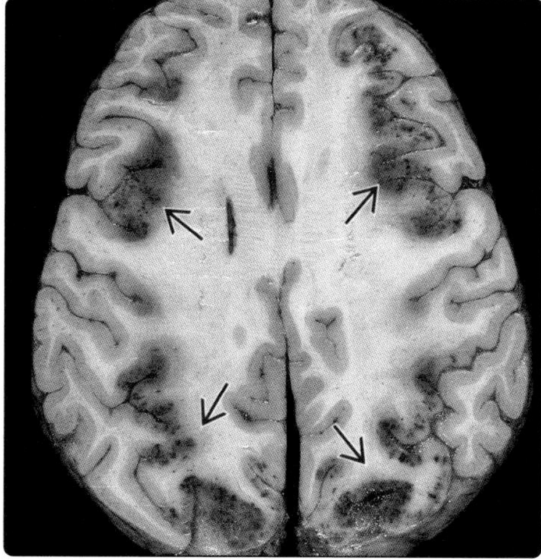

***(8-50)** Autopsy case shows classic external (cortical) WS infarcts ⇨ with areas of petechial hemorrhage.*

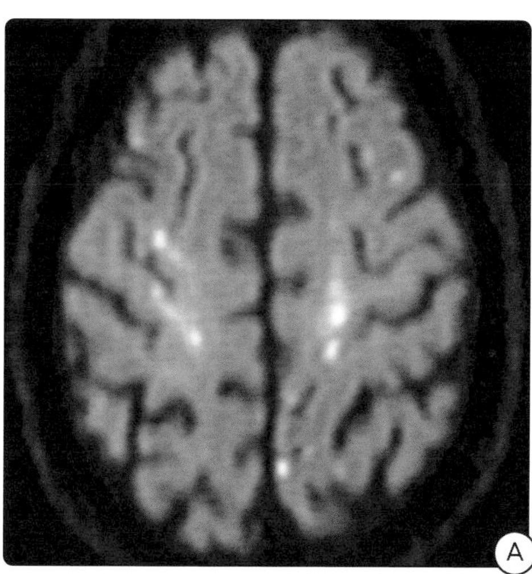


***(8-51A)** Axial DTI MR in a 59-year-old man with acute ICA occlusion shows bilateral foci of restriction in a WS distribution.*

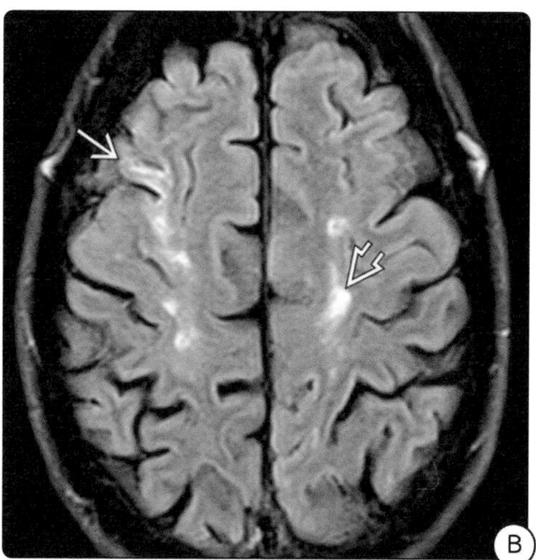


***(8-51B)** Axial FLAIR MR in the same patient shows cortical ➡ & subcortical ⇨ regions of hyperintensity related to hypoperfusion.*

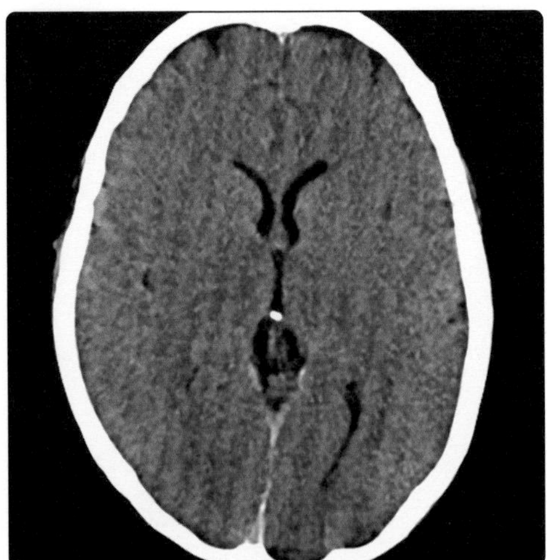

*(8-52) NECT in 36-year-old after cardiac arrest shows diffuse loss of GM-WM differentiation related to HII. Note "disappearing" basal ganglia.*

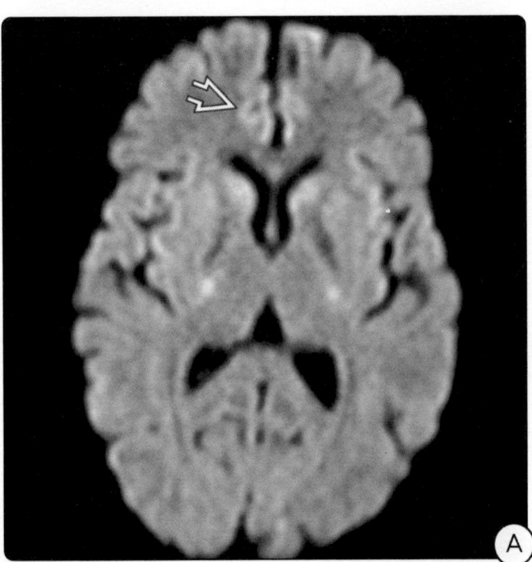

*(8-53A) Axial DTI MR in a 40-year-old immediately after a cardiac arrest shows subtle hyperintensity in the frontal lobe cortex ➲.*

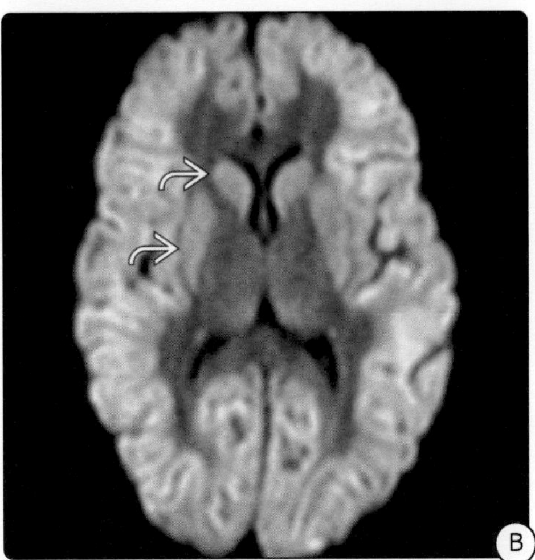

*(8-53B) Axial DTI MR in the same patient 3 days later shows diffuse cortical & basal ganglia ➲ diffusion restriction related to severe HII.*

## Differential Diagnosis

The major differential diagnosis of WS infarction is **lacunar infarcts**. Lacunar infarcts typically involve the basal ganglia, thalami, and pons and appear randomly scattered. Multiple **embolic infarcts** can also closely resemble WS infarcts. Emboli are often bilateral and are present in multiple territories but can also occur at vascular "border zones."

**Posterior reversible encephalopathy syndrome (PRES)** typically occurs in the setting of acute hypertension. The cortex/subcortical WM in the PCA distribution is most commonly affected, although PRES can also involve "border zones" and the basal ganglia. PRES rarely restricts on DWI (vasogenic edema), whereas "border zone" infarcts with cytotoxic edema show acute restriction.

### WATERSHED ("BORDER ZONE") INFARCTS

**Anatomy and Etiology**

- 2 types of vascular "border zones"
  - External (cortical): Between ACA, MCA, PCA
  - Internal (deep WM): Between perforating branches, major arteries
- Etiology
  - Emboli (cortical more common)
  - Regional hypoperfusion (deep WM common)
  - Global hypoperfusion (all 3 cortical WS zones)

**Imaging**

- External: Wedge or gyriform
- Internal: Rosary-like line of WMHs

# Hypoxic-Ischemic Injury

## Terminology and Etiology

Hypoxic-ischemic injury (HII) includes global HII, global anoxic injury, and cerebral hypoperfusion injury. The typical etiologies include cardiac arrest, cerebrovascular disease, drowning, and asphyxiation.

Brain-damaging effects of HII are age dependent but do not increase linearly with advancing age and development. The immature brain is less resistant to HII than its adult counterpart. Intermediate age groups are more tolerant to HII than either very young or more mature ages.

## Pathology

There is a common underlying process regardless of the cause of HII. There is decreased CBF and decreased blood oxygenation. There is a switch from oxidative phosphorylation to anaerobic metabolism. Glutamate-related cytotoxic processes also play a role. Brain ischemia is typically due to cardiac arrest or cerebrovascular disease and secondary to hypoxia due to decreased blood flow.

Sites of brain injury is determined by the maturity of brain as well as the severity and duration of hypoxic-ischemic insult. There is selective vulnerability with patterns of injury reflecting dysfunction of selected excitatory neuronal circuits depleted most rapidly. The areas with the highest concentrations of glutamate or excitatory amino acid receptors (GM) are more susceptible to injury.

## Clinical Issues

HII may result in death or profound long-term neurologic disability. Neurologic sequela, such as cerebral palsy and epilepsy, are often common. Basal ganglia involvement often leads to movement disorders.

There is a type of delayed WM injury known as postanoxic leukoencephalopathy that typically presents 2-3 weeks after the HII event in 2-3% of patients **(8-56)**. Patients with this leukoencephalopathy often have initial clinical stability followed by an acute neurologic decline. The majority of these patients, ~ 75%, recover.

## Imaging

Injury patterns of HII are highly variable depending on brain maturity as well as the severity and length of the insult **(8-53)**. Mild to moderate HII typically results in WS zone infarcts.

With severe HII, there is typically involvement the deep GM structures, including the basal ganglia, thalami, cortex, cerebellum, and hippocampi **(8-54)**.

CT may be normal initially. Depending on severity and timing of imaging, there may be bilateral symmetric hypodensity in the basal ganglia, thalami, &/or cerebral cortex. Other patterns may include diffuse cerebral edema with loss of normal GM-WM differentiation and effacement of the sulci with "disappearing" basal ganglia **(8-52)**. If severe, there may be a "white" cerebellum, sometimes called cerebellar reversal sign, where the cerebellum appears relatively hyperdense compared to diffuse supratentorial hypodensity.

MR is the best to assess overall extent of injury within hours after the HII event. DWI/DTI is often the first modality to show abnormalities, typically within hours of the event. Classically, DWI/DTI shows restriction in the deep nuclei with or without cortical involvement. T2/FLAIR MR shows hyperintense signal

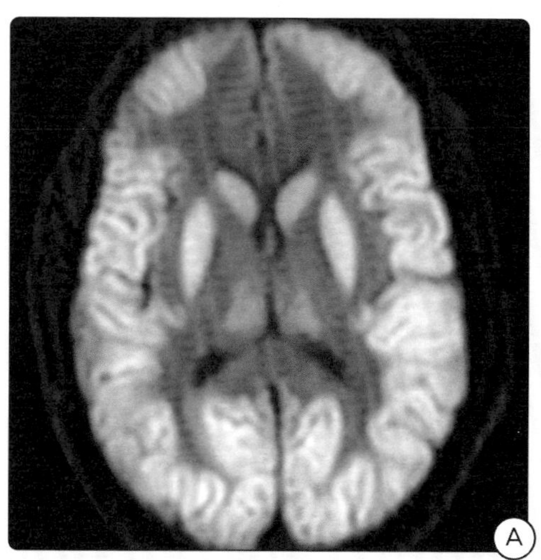


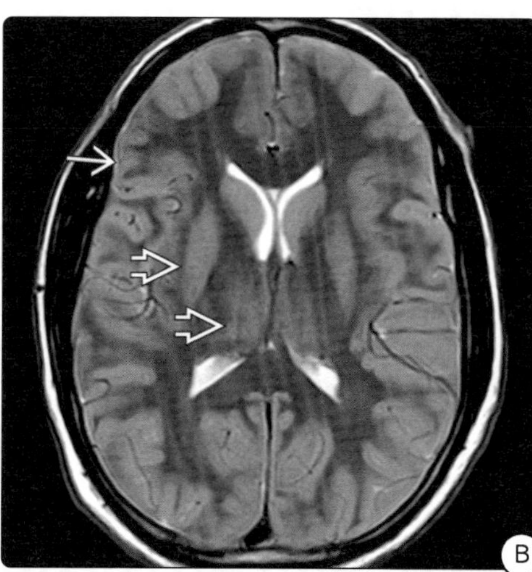


***(8-54A)** Axial DTI trace MR in a patient with severe HII related to severe hypoxia shows symmetric hyperintensity in the cortex & deep gray nuclei. The diffusion abnormalities often "pseudonormalize" within 1 week. **(8-54B)** Axial T2 MR in the same patient shows diffuse hyperintensity in the cortex ➡ & deep gray nuclei, including the basal ganglia & thalami ➡. There is also cortical swelling & mild diffuse sulcal effacement.*

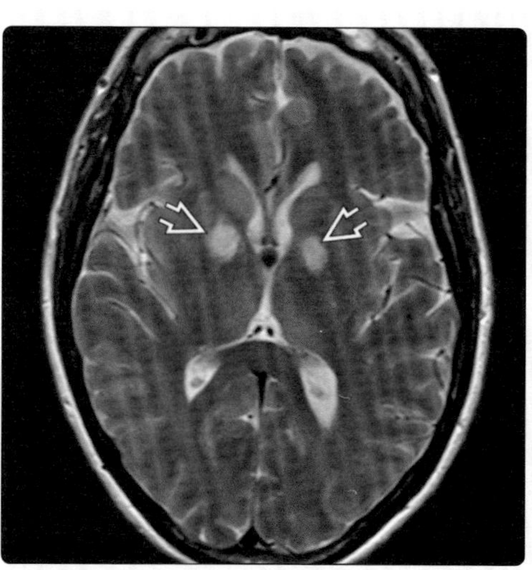

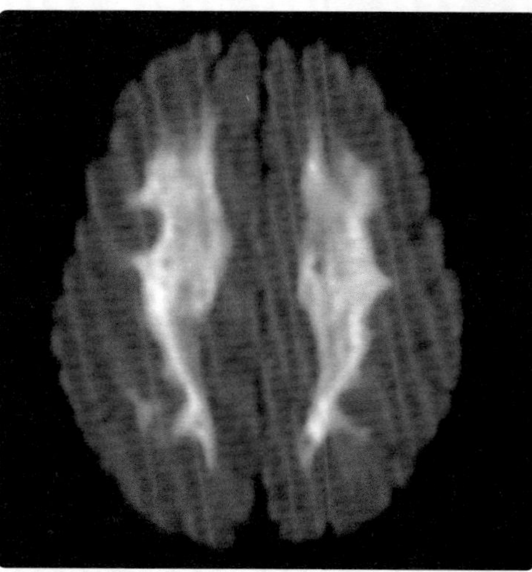

***(8-55)** Axial T2 MR in a 45-year-old patient with HII shows symmetric hyperintensity within the globus pallidus ➡. Imaging mimics toxic metabolic lesions, including carbon monoxide poisoning. **(8-56)** Axial DTI MR in a patient "found down" shows diffuse WMH related to postanoxic leukoencephalopathy. This delayed WM injury may develop 2-3 weeks following the initial insult.*

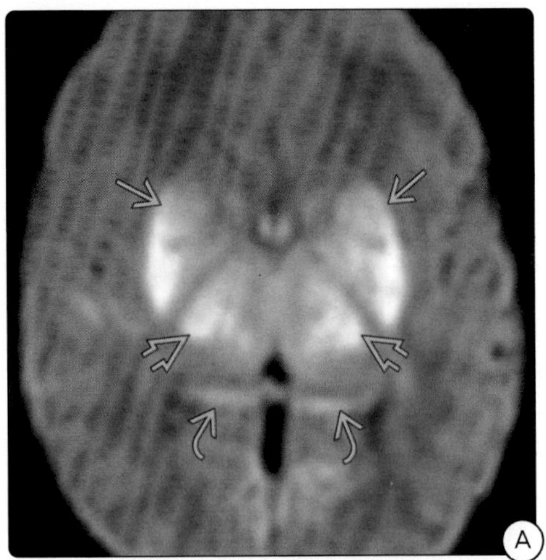


***(8-57A)*** *Axial DWI in a 3-day-old with acute profound HIE shows injury to the putamina →, thalami →, & hippocampi →.*

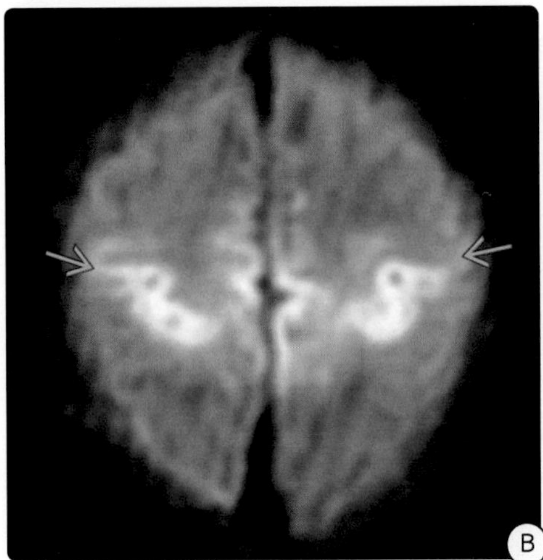


***(8-57B)*** *Axial DWI in the same patient at the vertex shows selective injury to the perirolandic cortex → in this acute profound injury pattern.*

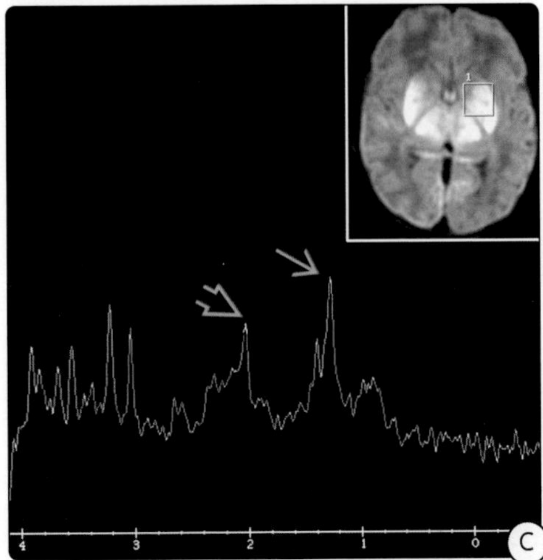


***(8-57C)*** *Single-voxel short-echo MRS centered in the left basal ganglia shows an ↑ lactate peak → at 1.3 ppm & a ↓ NAA → peak at 2.0 ppm.*

in the cerebellum, basal ganglia, and cortex **(8-54)** **(8-55)**. Acute changes are not reliably identified with T2 MR.

In chronic HII, T1 MR may show gyriform hyperintense signal related to cortical laminar necrosis of the involved cortex.

**HYPOXIC-ISCHEMIC INJURY**

**Etiology and Pathology**
- Global HII, anoxic injury, cerebral hypoperfusion injury
- Cardiac arrest, cerebrovascular disease, drowning, asphyxiation

**Imaging**
- Mild to moderate: WS zone infarcts
- Severe: Basal ganglia, thalami, cortex, cerebellum, and hippocampi
- DWI/DTI positive acutely

## Differential Diagnosis

The major differential diagnosis of HII is **acute infarcts** related to **thromboembolic disease** or **WS** ischemia. The clinical history can often help differentiate these etiologies as well as the imaging pattern. Emboli are often bilateral and are present in multiple territories but can also occur at vascular "border zones."

Other differential considerations include **toxic and metabolic** etiologies. These entities often involve the deep gray nuclei symmetrically and show DWI/DTI restriction acutely. For example, **carbon monoxide poisoning** shows T2/FLAIR symmetric, hyperintense globus pallidus often with subcortical WM involvement. DWI/DTI is positive acutely.

Lastly, **Creutzfeldt-Jakob Disease (CJD)** may mimic HII. However, the clinical history in CJD is that of a patient with progressive dementia. MR shows T2/FLAIR hyperintensity in the basal ganglia, thalamus, and cortex. DWI/DTI shows restriction in the deep gray nuclei and cortex, similar to HII.

# Neonatal Hypoxic-Ischemic Encephalopathy

## Terminology

Hypoxic-ischemic encephalopathy (HIE) is a clinical syndrome of disturbed neurologic function due to an HII. For the purposes of this discussion, we will focus on HII in the term neonate. While HII in the preterm neonate shares many of the same principles, many of the injury types and patterns are quite different in the preterm vs. the term neonate.

## Etiology

HII is a brain injury due to a combination of decreased blood flow and oxygen over a sustained period of time. The underlying causes of HII may occur in the antepartum, intrapartum, and postpartum periods, but the overwhelming majority of cases occur in the intrapartum period. The specific causes of HII are numerous but include maternal (e.g., uterine rupture), fetal (e.g., anemia, cardiac disease), and placental (e.g., placental abruption) disease processes, among many others. Multiple risk factors may combine to increase the risk for any given newborn to suffer HII.

If the degree of hypoperfusion and hypoxia is severe, such injuries will occur within a shorter period of time and will typically result in an "acute profound" or "deep" pattern of brain injury. This acute profound pattern of injury occurs when metabolically active areas of the brain (deep gray nuclei and perirolandic cortex) cannot be protected due to ineffectual cerebral autoregulatory mechanisms in the face of severely decreased blood flow. If the degree of hypoperfusion and hypoxia is mild to moderate, the injury takes longer to develop and will result in a "partial-prolonged" or "peripheral" pattern of injury. This partial-prolonged pattern of injury occurs when the cerebral autoregulatory mechanisms are successful in shunting blood to the most metabolically active areas of the brain, leaving the WS cortex and beyond with relatively less blood flow and susceptible to injury.

## Clinical Issues

HII is a relatively common neurologic disease of newborns with ~ 1-8 of every 1,000 births affected worldwide. It is less common in resource-rich nations but remains a significant source of infant morbidity and mortality.

Clinical manifestations of HIE in early life include abnormal fetal heart tracings, low apgar scores, poor umbilical cord gases, and need for resuscitative measures immediately following birth.

When the clinical history and patient examination fulfill criteria for HII and the newborn is within the therapeutic time window, therapeutic hypothermia has been shown to reduce the risk of mortality and neurologic disability.

## Imaging

Cranial US is often employed within the first few hours and days following suspected HIE, primarily to exclude intracranial hemorrhage or other acute processes. US findings are usually not evident within the first day following HII, and, depending on the severity and location of injury, US is often insensitive for detection of HII. US findings of HII include increased brain parenchymal echogenicity and exaggerated cortical GM-WM differentiation.

CT is not typically employed in the setting of HIE unless birth trauma or intracranial hemorrhage are the primary diagnostic considerations.

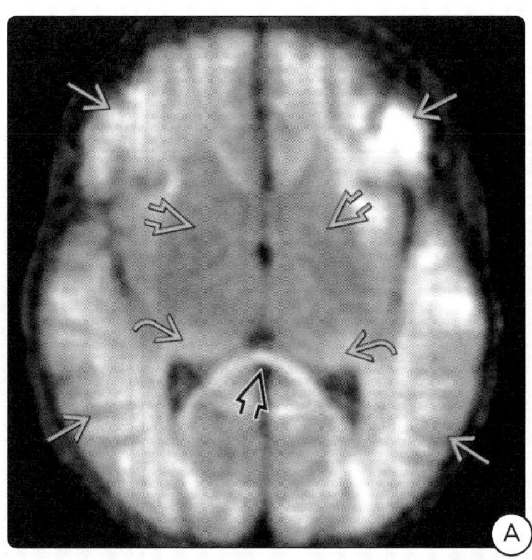


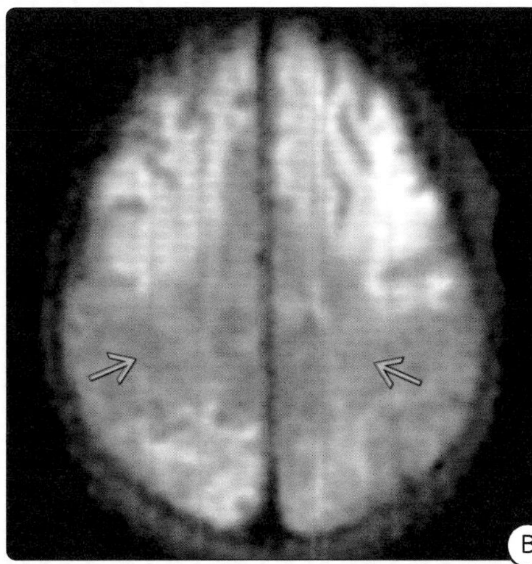


***(8-58A)** Axial DWI MR in a 5-day-old with partial prolonged HIE shows symmetric diffusion restriction throughout the visualized cortex with sparing of the deep gray nuclei. Diffusion restriction in the corpus callosum & dorsal thalami represents secondary or network injury. **(8-58B)** Axial DWI MR in the same patient shows sparing of the perirolandic cortex, which is typical for a partial-prolonged pattern of injury.*

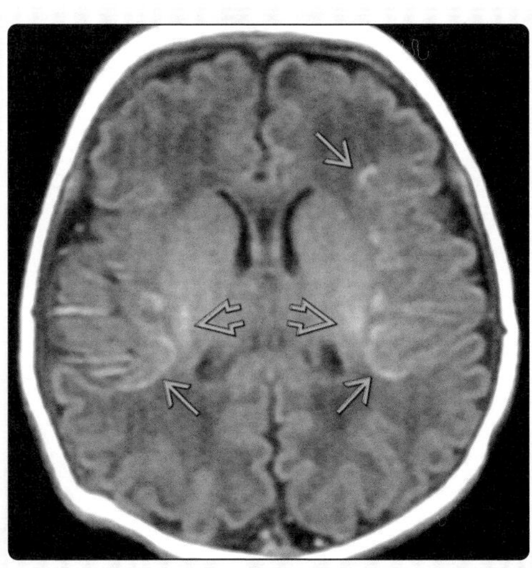

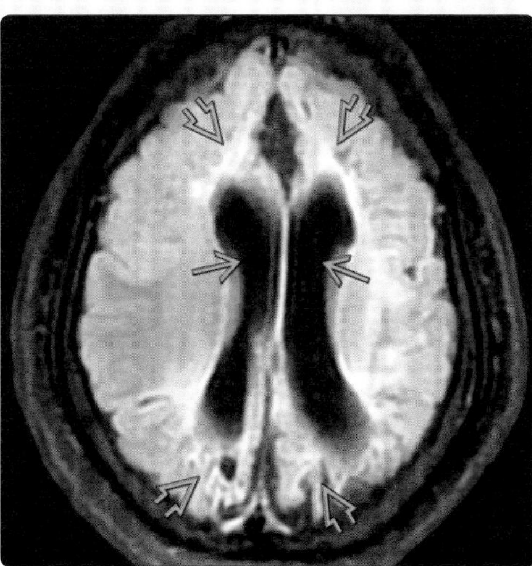

***(8-59)** Axial T1 MR in a 5-day-old with HIE shows T1 signal hyperintensity in the bilateral insular cortex, consistent with early cortical laminar necrosis. Note the normal T1-hyperintense posterior limbs of internal capsule. **(8-60)** Axial FLAIR MR in a 14-year-old with remote history of neonatal HIE shows nearly symmetric encephalomalacia in the WS regions. There is associated ex vacuo ventricular enlargement.*

MR is the gold standard for identifying HII and defining the extent of injury, The most sensitive sequence for detection of HII is DWI. The most characteristic finding of HII is symmetric or nearly symmetric diffusion restriction of injured brain parenchyma **(8-57A)**. Studies have shown that diffusion restriction in neonatal HII peaks at ~ 4-5 days after the brain injury occurrence. Therefore, because most infants with suspected HIE undergo therapeutic hypothermia for ~ 72 hours and diffusion restriction peaks at ~ 4-5 days after the brain injury, this is the ideal time window to image neonates with MR. Diffusion restriction in the primary areas of brain injury begins to "pseudonormalize" approximately one week following the injury. Areas of network or secondary injury (e.g., corpus callosum and corticospinal tracts) may continue to show diffusion restriction up to ~ 10 days after injury. In the setting of therapeutic hypothermia, the time to "pseudonormalization" of diffusion abnormality is extended by a few days.

Conventional T1WI and T2WI often become abnormal in the first few days following the injury. Areas of injured brain typically show hyperintense T2 signal and often subtle T1 hypointensity. Depending on the severity of the injury and degree of cortical involvement, loss of GM-WM differentiation is common **(8-61C)**. Later in the first week, following injury, areas of T2 signal hypointensity and T1 signal hyperintensity **(8-59)** may develop.

MRS is often employed as an adjunct evaluation tool. MRS may show elevated lactate and decreased NAA in areas of injury **(8-57C)**.

HII preferentially affects supratentorial brain structures with sparing of the brainstem and cerebellar hemispheres except in the most severe cases. Injury to the cerebellar vermis is seen with some frequency.

"Acute profound" or "deep" pattern of injury is characterized by involvement of metabolically active areas of the newborn

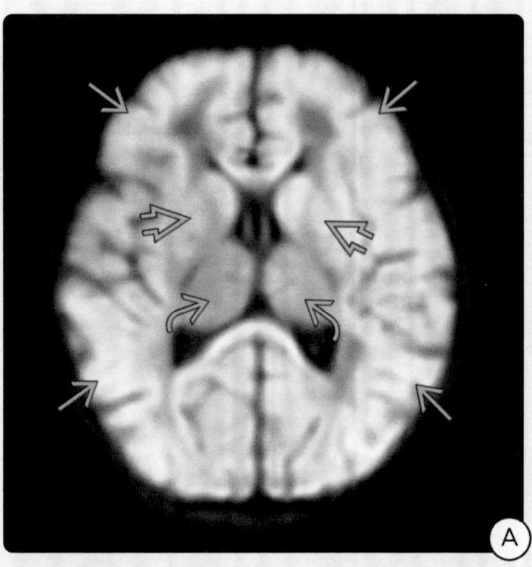

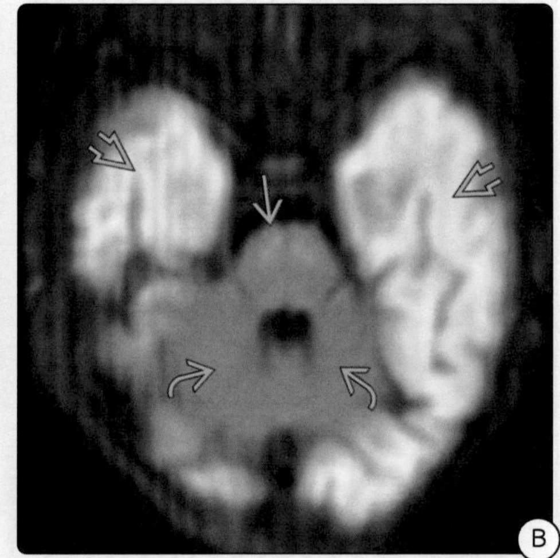

***(8-61A)** Axial DWI in a 5-day-old with severe mixed pattern HIE shows symmetric marked diffusion restriction throughout the cerebral hemispheres, ➡ basal ganglia ➡, & thalami ➡. **(8-61B)** Axial DWI in the same patient shows the normal signal within the cerebellar hemispheres ➡ in comparison to the severely injured supratentorial brain ➡. Also note the mild cytotoxic edema in the brainstem ➡.*

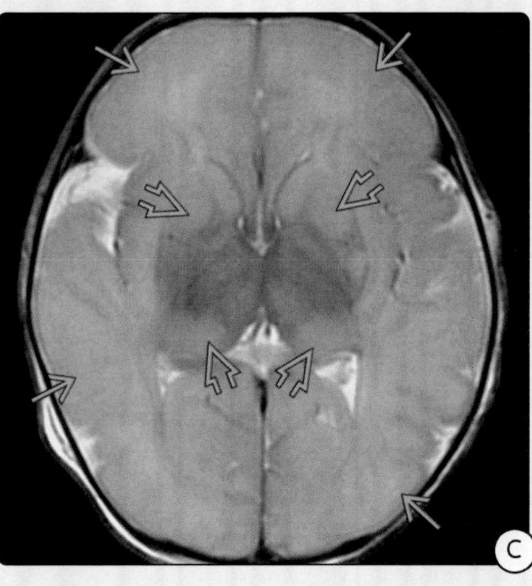

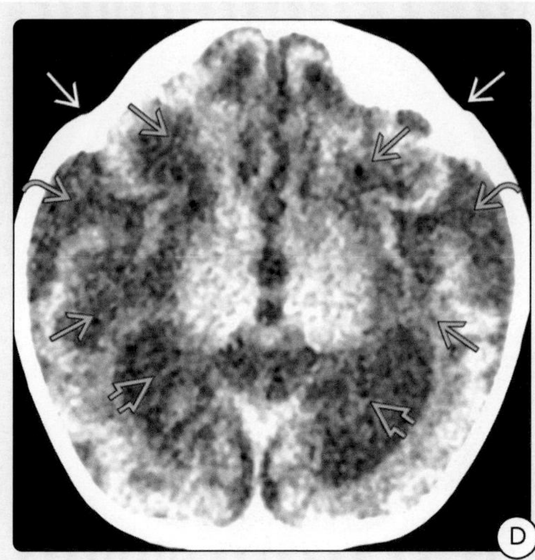

***(8-61C)** Axial T2 MR in the same patient shows diffusely ↑ T2 signal throughout the cerebral hemispheres, resulting in loss of GM-WM differentiation ➡. Also note the ↑ T2 signal within the deep gray nuclei ➡. **(8-61D)** Axial NECT in the same patient at 7 months shows severe encephalomalacia ➡ with resultant expansion of the subarachnoid spaces ➡ & ventricles ➡. Also note the frontal bone depression & sutural overlap ➡.*

brain, including the thalami, basal ganglia, perirolandic cortex, and hippocampi **(8-57)**.

"Partial-prolonged" or "peripheral" pattern of injury is characterized by preferential injury to WS cortex in mild injuries and more extensive cortical involvement as the severity &/or duration of injury increases **(8-58)**.

It is important to note that a significant proportion of HII injuries will show a combination of these patterns or a "mixed" pattern of injury. This should not be surprising, as many intrapartum hypoxic-ischemic events begin with mild to moderate reduction in blood flow/oxygenation followed by gradually worsening conditions that eventually become severe.

Chronic imaging findings of HII include volume loss, cystic and noncystic encephalomalacia, ex vacuo ventricular enlargement, and microcephaly **(8-61D)**. Ulegyria (mushroom-shaped gyri) are a commonly seen imaging sequela of HII. T2/FLAIR is the most sensitive sequence for detection of chronic sequelae of HIE once brain is fully myelinated (approximately two years old) **(8-60)**.

**NEONATAL HYPOXIC-ISCHEMIC ENCEPHALOPATHY**

**Etiology and Pathology**
- Newborn brain injury due to decreased blood flow/oxygenation
- Diverse causes: Maternal, fetal, placental

**Clinical**
- Major cause of neurologic disability worldwide
- Risk factors: Abnormal fetal heart tracings, low apgars, poor cord gases
- Primary treatment: Therapeutic hypothermia

**Imaging**
- US: Insensitive depending on timing and severity
  - Increased echogenicity in areas of injury
- MR: Gold standard for imaging evaluation
  - DWI: Most sensitive when performed within 1st week
  - T2: Increased signal common; decreased signal may develop later
  - T1: Increased signal develops days after injury and may persist
  - FLAIR: Most sensitive for detection of chronic injury once brain is myelinated
  - MRS: Increased lactate, decreased NAA in injured areas
- Acute profound or deep pattern
  - Thalami, basal ganglia, perirolandic cortex
- Partial-prolonged or peripheral pattern
  - WS cortex

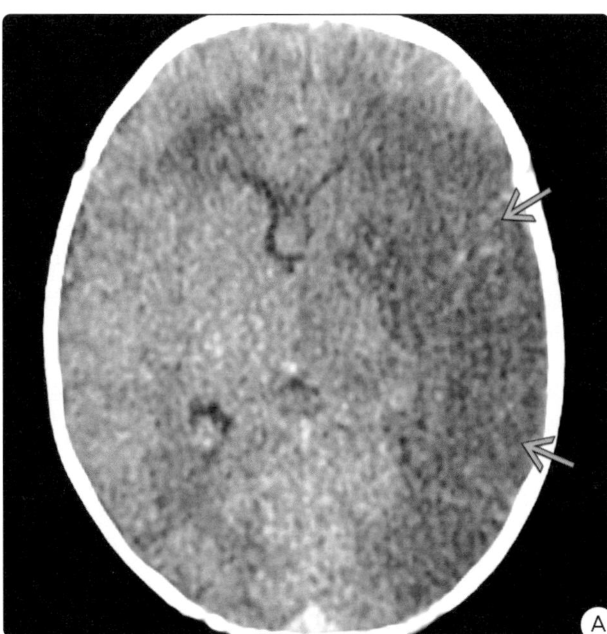


***(8-62A)** Axial NECT in a 5-day-old with unremarkable delivery presenting with seizures shows ↓ attenuation & loss of GM-WM differentiation throughout the left MCA territory ➡. This is NAIS.*

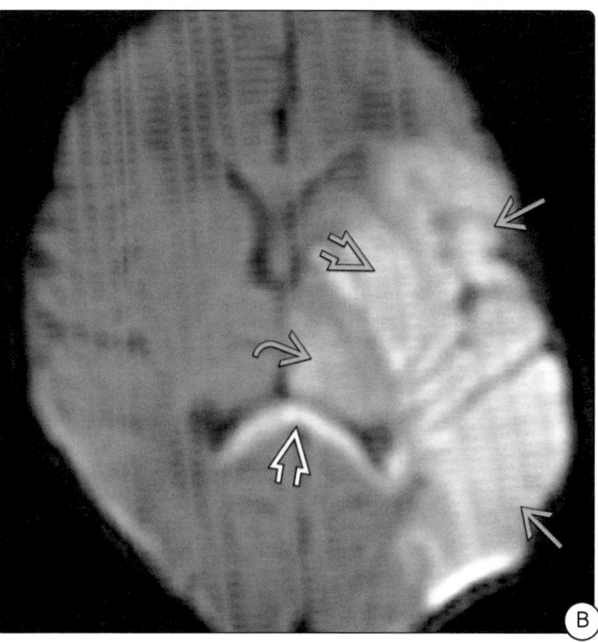


***(8-62B)** Axial DWI in the same patient shows diffusion restriction throughout the left MCA territory ➡, including the putamen ➡. Cytotoxic edema in the left thalamus ➡ & corpus callosum ➡ represents network or secondary injury.*

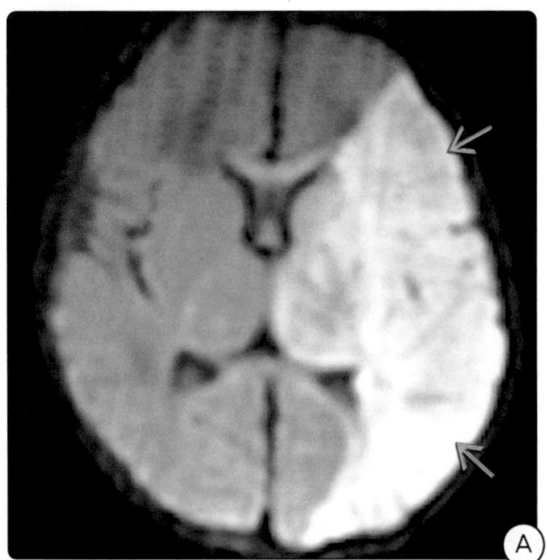

*(8-63A) Axial DWI MR in a 4-day-old term neonate with NAIS shows diffusion restriction ➡ throughout the left MCA territory.*

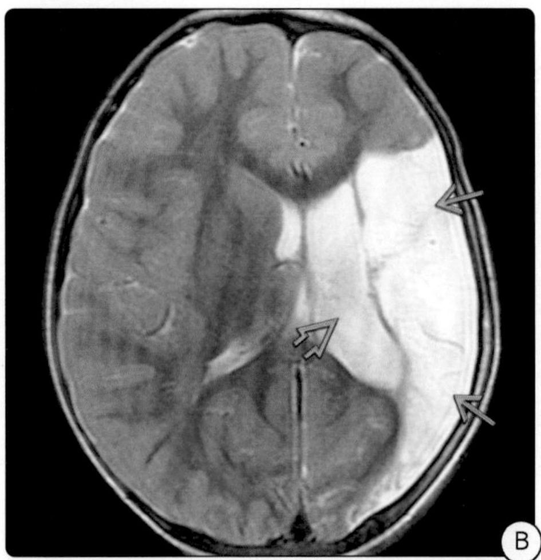

*(8-63B) Axial T2 MR 2 years later shows cystic encephalomalacia throughout left MCA territory ➡ & ex vacuo ventriculomegaly ➡.*

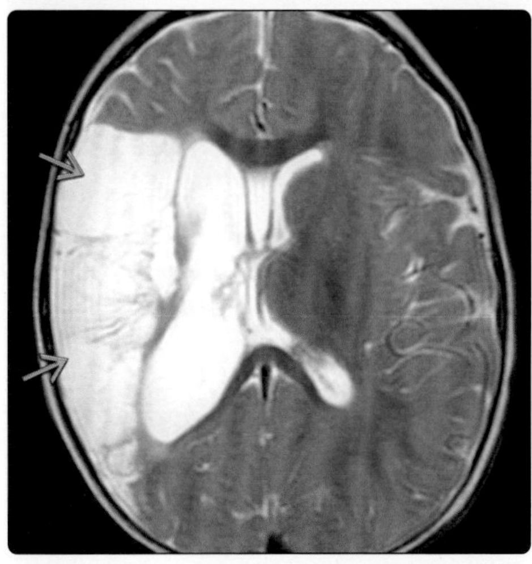

*(8-64) Axial T2 in a 9-month-old with left-sided weakness shows presumed perinatal arterial ischemic stroke in the right MCA territory ➡.*

## Differential Diagnosis

Primary differential considerations include viral encephalitides and metabolic disease.

Viral infectious mimics of HIE include **human parechovirus encephalitis (HPeV)** and **neonatal herpes simplex encephalitis (HSE)**. HPeV infection typically manifests as symmetric deep and periventricular diffusion restriction with or without thalamic involvement. Cortical injury has not been reported in HPeV. Symptoms of HPeV (e.g., seizures, fever) are usually delayed by days or weeks after birth. Neonatal HSE typically shows diffusion restriction of affected cortex, WM, and sometimes deep gray nuclei. Findings are often unilateral, and, when bilateral, is typically asymmetric in its involvement. The vast majority of HSE present weeks after birth with seizure.

Metabolic diseases that may mimic HIE include **isolated sulfite oxidase deficiency, molybdenum cofactor deficiency**, and **nonketotic hyperglycinemia**, among others.

# Neonatal Arterial Ischemic Stroke

## Terminology

Neonatal arterial ischemic stroke (NAIS) is diagnosed in either term or preterm infants after birth on or before day of life 28.

## Etiology

Cause is not definitively understood, but the most commonly accepted etiology is emboli from a placental or fetal source causing cerebral artery occlusion and subsequent infarction. Risk factors are numerous and include maternal (e.g., smoking, preeclampsia, maternal fever), fetal (e.g., congenital heart disease, infection), and placental (e.g., chorioamnionitis). These risk factors are only a few examples of the much longer list of risk factors for NAIS.

## Clinical Issues

Incidence is 20-35/100,000. Perinatal stroke accounts for 25% of strokes in children. These strokes are the most common etiology for hemiparesis in children. NAIS almost always presents with seizure when detected in the neonatal period, and NAIS is the cause of up to 15% of all neonatal seizures. If seizure does not occur in the neonatal period, the diagnosis is not typically made until years later when motor development reveals early hand preference or hemiplegia of varying degrees.

### NEONATAL ARTERIAL ISCHEMIC STROKE

**Etiology and Clinical**
- Most common theory is placental or fetal embolic stroke
- 25% of all childhood stroke; usually presents with seizure in days after birth

**Imaging**
- DWI: Cytotoxic edema confined to arterial territory
    - MCA most common; predominantly unifocal
- T2: Hyperintense signal, loss of GM-WM differentiation
- T1: ± cortical laminar necrosis
- MRA: Usually normal but may show arterial occlusion

## Imaging

Cranial US is often employed as the initial test in neonates but is not sensitive for detection of peripheral or smaller infarcts. Areas of infarction typically are hyperechogenic to adjacent brain parenchyma.

CT will typically show wedge-shaped areas of low attenuation confined to an arterial territory with loss of GM-WM differentiation **(8-62A)**.

MR is the most sensitive and specific examination for detection of NAIS. MR findings of NAIS are well defined. NAIS shows diffusion restriction typically confined to a cerebral arterial territory, or sometimes involving the entire territory **(8-62B)** **(8-63A)**. The MCA is most often involved. The majority of neonatal strokes are unifocal, but occasionally they may be multifocal. T1WI and T2WI shows loss of GM-WM differentiation within days of the stroke. In the subacute phase, T1-hyperintense cortex representing cortical laminar necrosis may be evident. MRA is most often normal but may demonstrate cerebral artery occlusion.

Imaging in the chronic phase will demonstrate typically severe cystic and noncystic encephalomalacia confined to an arterial territory **(8-63B)** **(8-64)**.

# Cerebral Hyperperfusion Syndrome

## Terminology

Cerebral hyperperfusion syndrome (CHS) is a rare but potentially devastating disorder. It is sometimes called luxury perfusion or post carotid endarterectomy (CEA) hyperperfusion and is defined as a major increase in CBF well above normal metabolic demands. It most commonly occurs as a complication of cerebral revascularization **(8-65)**. CHS is reported in ~ 3-4% of post-CEA patients.

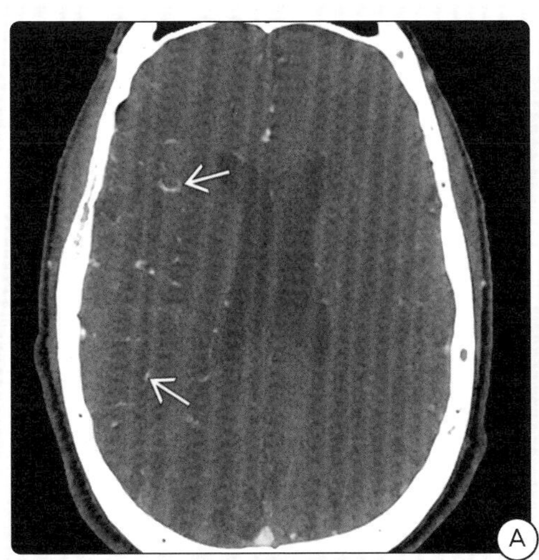

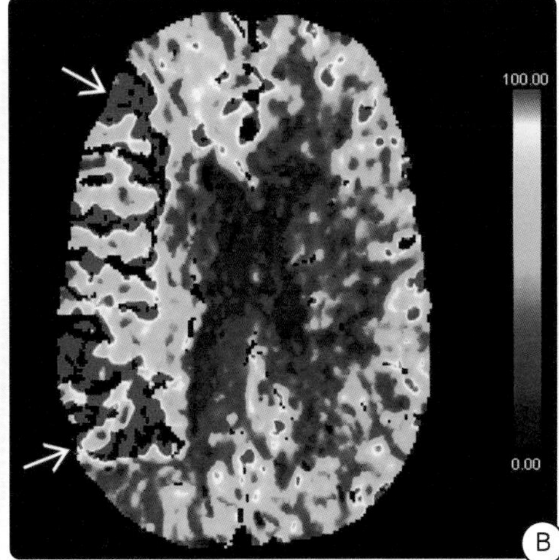


***(8-65A)** Axial CTA in a 74-year-old status post mechanical thrombolysis for a prior right M1 occlusion shows ↑ vascularity ➡ with engorged vessels in the right hemisphere. There was no large vessel occlusion. **(8-65B)** The pCT in the same patient shows elevated CBF ➡ in the right MCA distribution compared with the left. MTT was ↓ on the right. Cerebral hyperperfusion typically occurs within 12 hours of a revascularization procedure.*

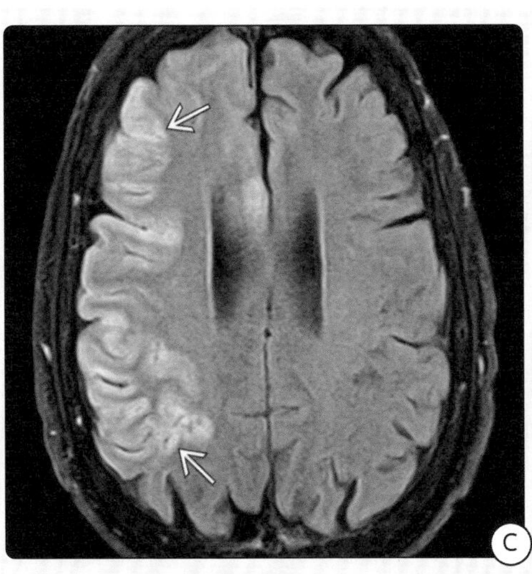

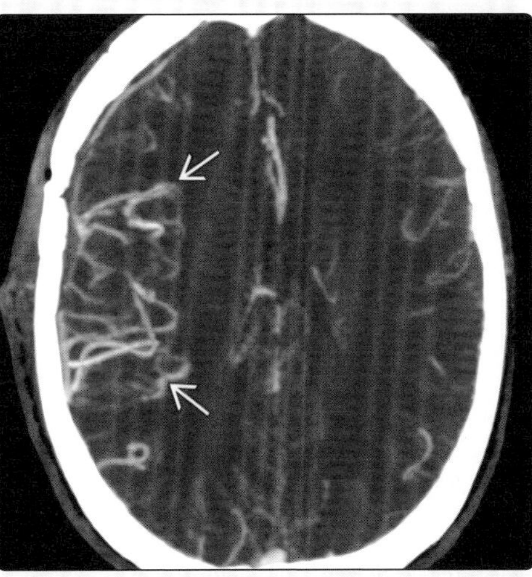

***(8-65C)** Axial FLAIR MR in the same patient shows hyperintense cortex ➡ in the MCA distribution. DWI is classically normal in CHS. **(8-66)** Axial CTA MIP in a patient status post STA-MCA revascularization procedure with severe right-sided headaches shows marked engorgement of the right MCA branches ➡. CBF was also elevated. CHS is a rare complication seen in ~ 3-4% of post-CEA patients.*

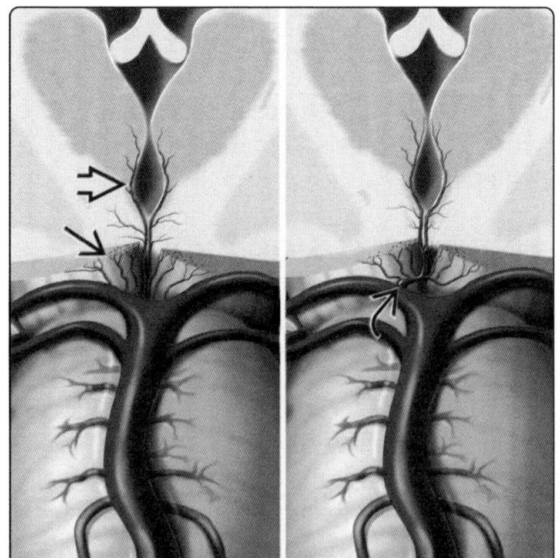

***(8-67) (L) Normal BA with perforating arteries supplying midbrain ⇨, medial thalami ⇨. (R) AOP has single dominant trunk ⇨.***

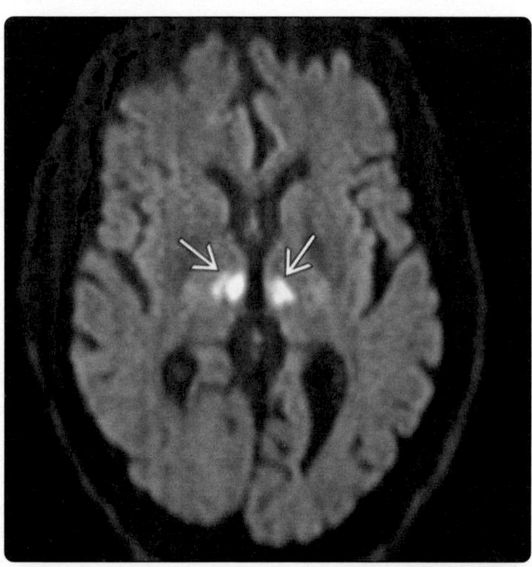

***(8-68) Axial DTI MR in a patient with acute visual changes shows an AOP infarct with involvement of the bilateral medial thalami ➡.***

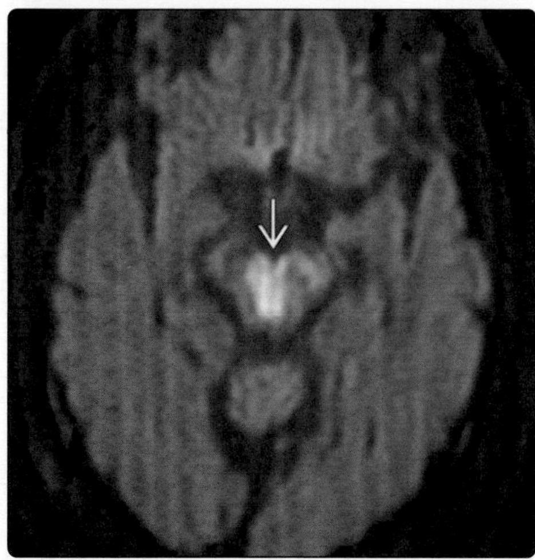

***(8-69) Axial DTI shows a typical V-shaped hyperintensity ➡ involving the medial cerebral peduncles & midbrain in an AOP infarct.***

## Etiology

CHS has been reported in patients status post CEA, angioplasty with stenting, and after thrombolysis. It has also been reported after superficial temporal artery (STA)-MCA anastomosis in moyamoya disease, status epilepticus, hypercapnia, and **m**itochondrial **e**ncephalopathy, **l**actic **a**cidosis, and **s**troke-like episodes (MELAS) as well as after drainage of chronic subdural hematomas.

## Pathology

Cerebral hyperperfusion syndrome is likely caused by maladaptive autoregulatory mechanisms and altered cerebral hemodynamics. There is rapid restoration of normal perfusion following revascularization, which leads to hyperperfusion in previously underperfused brain.

## Clinical Issues

Patients may be asymptomatic in mild cases. In severe cases, they present with ipsilateral headache, neurologic deficits, &/or seizures. Patients may also have cognitive impairment or face or eye pain. Symptoms may happen hours to days after revascularization. Typically, symptoms occur 12 hours after the procedure.

## Imaging

NECT may show mild gyral swelling and cortical effacement. Patchy or diffuse WM edema may be present. Hemorrhage is a rare complication occurring in < 1%. CTA shows an increase in vascularity with congested, dilated vessels **(8-65A)** **(8-66)**. pCT shows elevated CBF **(8-65B)** and decreased mean transit time (MTT) and time to peak (TTP).

T2/FLAIR MR shows hyperintense cortex **(8-65C)**. Postcontrast FLAIR may also show hyperintensity in the subarachnoid secondary to blood-brain barrier disruption. DWI is typically normal.

The major differential diagnosis of CHS is **acute infarct**. With acute infarcts, there is typically a large vessel occlusion with decreased vascularity of the affected hemisphere on CTA. pCT shows the MTT as increased instead of decreased. DWI shows restriction acutely.

# Strokes in Unusual Vascular Distributions

## Artery of Percheron Infarction

The **artery of Percheron** (AOP) is a vascular variant in which a single large midbrain-perforating artery arises from the P1 PCA segment to supply the midbrain and medial thalami **(8-67)**. AOP occlusion can cause obtundation, oculomotor and pupillary deficits, vertical gaze palsy, ptosis, and lid retraction.

MR with DWI is the imaging study of choice **(8-68)**. T2/FLAIR images show round or ovoid hyperintensities in the medial thalami, lateral to the third ventricle. In slightly more than 1/2 of the cases, a V-shaped hyperintensity involves the medial surfaces of the cerebral peduncles and rostral midbrain **(8-69)**. DWI/DTI shows diffusion restriction.

The major differential diagnosis of the AOP occlusion is **"top of the basilar" infarct**. These uncommon infarcts involve more extensive areas of the brain, typically all or part of the rostral midbrain, occipital lobes, superior vermis, and thalami. The other differential consideration is **deep cerebral venous thrombosis** involving the internal cerebral veins or great vein of Galen. These venous infarcts typically involve the basal ganglia, posterior limb of the internal capsule, and the entire thalami. Hemorrhage is common with venous infarcts.

## "Top of the Basilar" Infarction

The **"top of the basilar" infarct** is a clinical syndrome characterized by visual, oculomotor, and behavioral abnormalities caused by thrombosis of the distal BA **(8-70)**. "Locked-in" syndrome is a rare but devastating manifestation of the top of the basilar thrombosis.

There is typically occlusion of the proximal PCAs as well as distal perforators that supply the rostral midbrain and thalami. Both occipital lobes are usually infarcted. Depending on the extent of the thrombus, pontine perforators and one or both superior cerebellar artery territories may be affected.

NECT may show a dense BA sign **(8-71)**. Hypodensity in the occipital lobes &/or thalami may be present.

MR shows T2/FLAIR hyperintensity within the midbrain, thalami, upper pons, and superior cerebellar hemispheres commonly. DWI/DTI shows restricted diffusion in the affected areas **(8-72)**.

*Selected References: The complete reference list is available on the eBooks+ version included with purchase.*

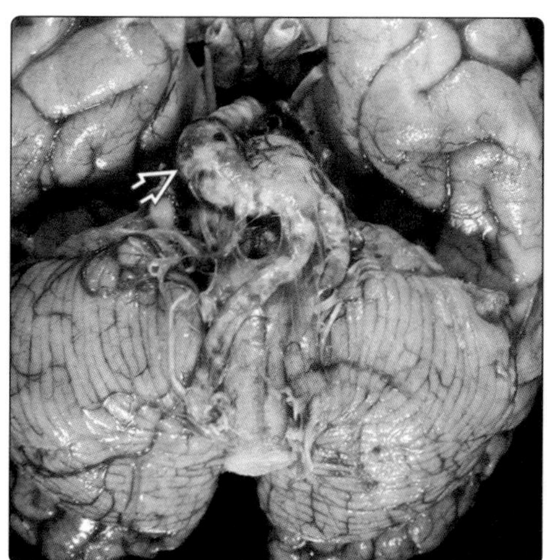

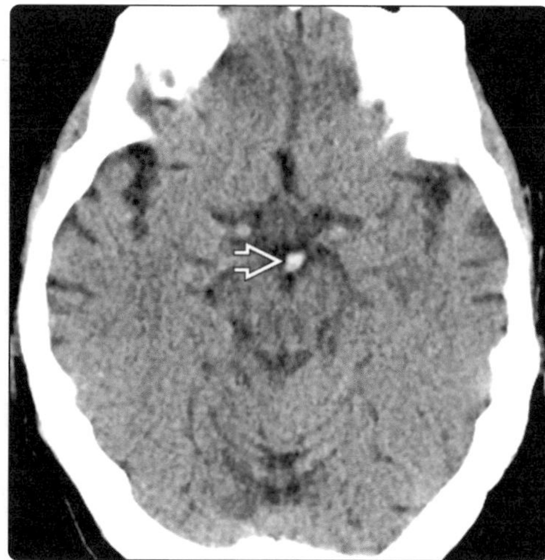

***(8-70)** Autopsy shows a BA thrombosis ➡ in a patient with dolichoectasia of the vertebrobasilar system. (Courtesy R. Hewlett, MD.) **(8-71)** Axial NECT shows a hyperdense BA ➡ related to an acute thrombus. These infarcts typically involve the brainstem, thalami, occipital lobes, and cerebellum. They may result in a "locked-in" syndrome.*

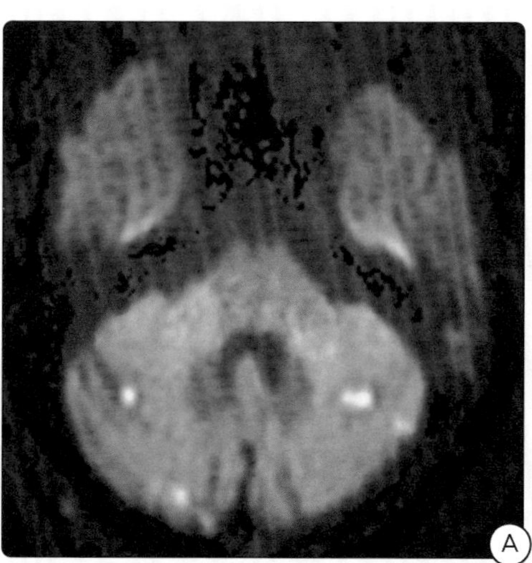


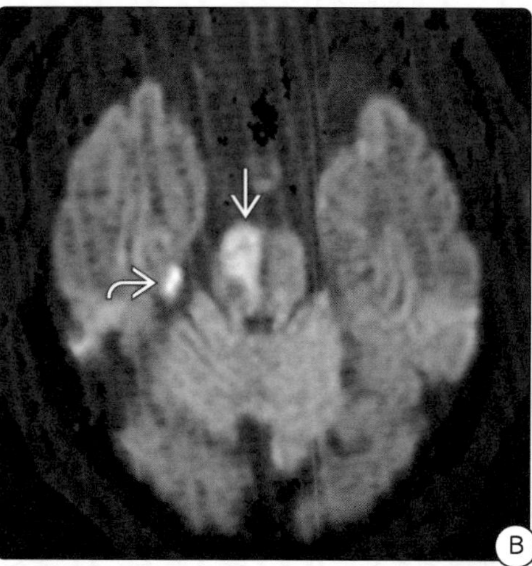


***(8-72A)** Axial DWI in a 70-year-old man shows bilateral superior cerebellar infarcts. Top of the basilar infarcts involve SCAs, PCAs, & perforator arteries. **(8-72B)** Axial DWI in the same patient shows a right pons acute infarct ➡ & part of a right medial temporal lobe infarct ➡, PCA territory. Patients with top of the basilar infarcts often present with visual, oculomotor, and behavioral abnormalities.*

# Venous Anatomy and Occlusions

*Dural venous sinus and cerebral vein occlusions are relatively rare, accounting for only 1% of all strokes. They are notoriously difficult to diagnose clinically and are frequently overlooked on imaging studies, as attention is focused on the arterial side of the cerebral circulation.*



Familiarity with both normal venous anatomy and drainage patterns is essential for understanding the imaging appearance of sinovenous occlusive disease. Therefore, in this chapter, we first briefly review the normal gross and imaging anatomy of the cerebral venous system. Because ~ 1/2 of all venous occlusions result in parenchymal infarcts, we also discuss their drainage territories.

## Normal Venous Anatomy and Drainage Patterns

The intracranial venous system has two major components, the **dural venous sinuses** and the **cerebral veins**.

### Dural Venous Sinuses

Dural sinuses and venous plexuses are endothelium-lined channels that are contained between the outer (periosteal) and inner (meningeal) dural layers.

#### Superior Sagittal Sinus

The superior sagittal sinus (SSS) is a large, curvilinear sinus that parallels the inner calvarial vault. It runs posteriorly in the midline at the junction of the falx cerebri with the calvarium **(9-1)**. The SSS increases in diameter as it courses posteriorly, collecting a number of unnamed, small, superficial cortical veins and the larger anastomotic vein of Trolard (VofT).

#### Inferior Sagittal Sinus

Compared with the SSS, the inferior sagittal sinus (ISS) is a much smaller and more inconstant curvilinear channel that lies in the bottom of the falx cerebri. It terminates at the falcotentorial junction where it joins the vein of Galen (VofG) and basal veins of Rosenthal to form the straight sinus (SS).

#### Straight Sinus

The SS is formed by the junction of the ISS and VofG. It runs posteroinferiorly from its origin at the falcotentorial apex to the venous sinus confluence.

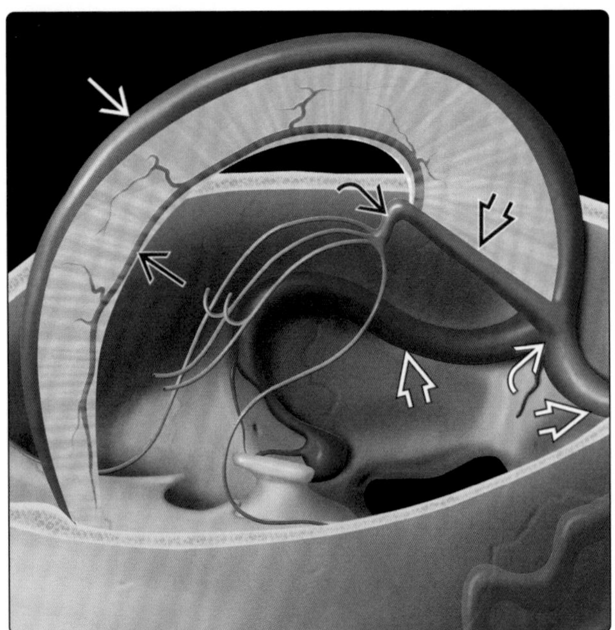

***(9-1) Falx cerebri extends from the crista galli to the falcotentorial junction and holds the SSS ➡ and the ISS ➡. VofG ➡ receives the ICVs and BVR. Straight sinus (SS) ➡, sinus confluence ➡, and transverse sinuses (TSs) ➡ are shown.***

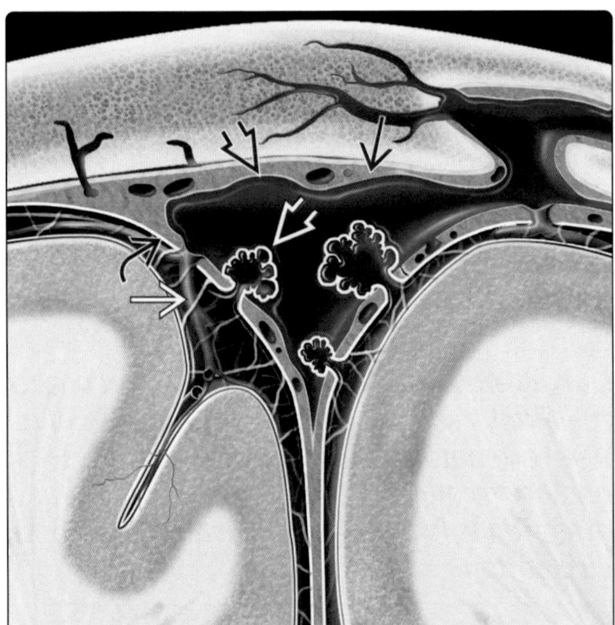

***(9-2) The SSS ➡ is between the outer ➡ and inner ➡ dural layers. CSF-containing projections [arachnoid granulations (AGs)] ➡ extend from the subarachnoid space (SAS) into the SSS. Cortical veins ➡ also enter the SSS.***

SS variants are relatively uncommon. A **persistent falcine sinus** is an unusual variant that is identified on 2% of normal CTAs. Here, a midline venous structure—the persistent falcine sinus—connects the ISS or VofG directly with the SSS.

### Sinus Confluence and Transverse Sinuses

The SS terminates by joining the SSS and transverse sinuses (TSs) to form the **venous sinus confluence** (torcular Herophili). The TSs are contained between attachments of the tentorium cerebelli to the inner table of the skull. The TSs curve laterally and then turn inferiorly to become the sigmoid sinuses.

The two TSs are frequently asymmetric with the right side typically larger than the left. Hypoplastic or stenotic segments are present in 1/3 of the general population. Filling defects caused by arachnoid granulations (AGs) and fibrous septa are also common.

### Sigmoid Sinuses and Jugular Bulbs

The sigmoid sinuses are the inferior continuations of the TSs. They follow a gentle S-shaped curve, descending behind the petrous temporal bone to terminate by becoming the internal jugular veins (IJVs). Side-to-side asymmetry of the sigmoid sinuses is common and normal.

### Cavernous Sinus

The cavernous sinuses (CSs) are irregularly shaped, heavily trabeculated/compartmentalized venous sinuses that lie along the sides of the sella turcica and extend from the superior orbital fissures anteriorly [where they receive the superior ophthalmic veins (SOVs)] to the clivus and petrous apex posteriorly. The two CSs communicate extensively with each other via intercavernous venous plexuses.

The CSs contain the two cavernous internal carotid arteries (ICAs) and abducens (CNVI) nerves. CNIII, CNIV, CNV1, and CNV2 are actually **within** the lateral dural wall, not inside the CS proper **(9-3)**.

The size and configuration of the CSs are relatively constant on imaging studies. The lateral walls normally appear straight or concave (not convex), and the venous blood enhances quite uniformly.

### Arachnoid Granulations

The dural sinuses frequently contain **AGs**, CSF-containing projections that extend from the subarachnoid space (SAS) into dural venous sinuses **(9-2)**. Although AGs can occur in all dural venous sinuses, the most common locations are the TS and SSS.

## Cerebral Veins

The cerebral veins are subdivided into three groups: (1) Superficial ("cortical" or "external") veins, (2) deep cerebral ("internal") veins, and (3) brainstem/posterior fossa veins.

### Superficial Cortical Veins

Between 8-12 unnamed superficial cortical veins course over the cerebral convexities, cross the SAS, pierce the arachnoid membrane and inner (meningeal) layer of the dura, and drain directly into the SSS **(9-4)**. A dominant anastomotic superficial cortical vein, the **vein of Trolard** (VofT), may be present. The

VofT courses upward from the sylvian fissure and over the convexity of the brain to join the SSS.

The **superficial middle cerebral vein** (SMCV) lies over the sylvian fissure and drains the brain surrounding the lateral cerebral fissure. The SMCV also collects tributaries from the temporal, frontal, and parietal operculae that overhang the sylvian fissure.

The **deep middle cerebral vein** (DMCV) collects tributaries from the insula and basal ganglia, then anastomoses with the **basal vein of Rosenthal** (BVR) **(9-5)**. The BVR then curves laterally around the midbrain, courses posterosuperiorly, and then joins with the internal cerebral vein (ICV) to drain into the VofG **(9-9A)**.

A prominent posterior anastomotic vein, the **vein of Labbé**, courses inferolaterally over the temporal lobe to drain into the TS **(9-4)**.

All three named superficial anastomotic veins—the VofT, vein of Labbé, and SMCV—vary in size, maintaining a reciprocal relationship with each other. If one or two are dominant, the third anastomotic vein is usually hypoplastic or absent.

## Deep Cerebral Veins

The deep cerebral ("internal") veins are themselves subdivided into three groups: (1) Medullary veins, (2) subependymal veins, and (3) deep paramedian veins.

**Medullary Veins.** Innumerable small veins originate between 1-2 cm below the cortex and course straight through the white matter toward the ventricles where they terminate at right angles in subependymal veins **(9-10)**. These veins are generally inapparent on CTV, but DSA **(9-9)** and contrast-enhanced MR may show faint linear stripes of contrast coursing toward the ventricles. 3T T2* susceptibility-weighted imaging (SWI) best depicts the medullary veins because the deoxygenated blood is paramagnetic. Here, they are seen as

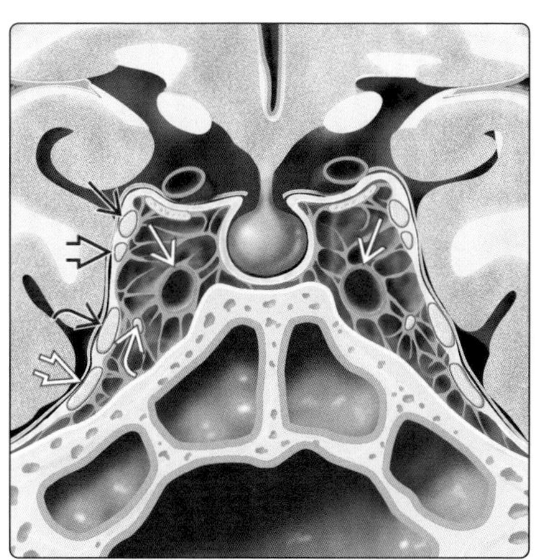

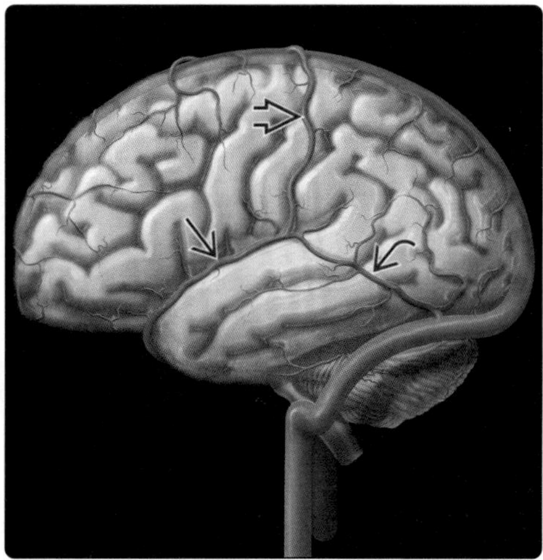

***(9-3)** Coronal graphic shows the trabeculated CSs and their contents. Internal carotid arteries ➡ and CNVI ➡ are inside the CSs. CNIII ➡, CNIV ➡, CNV1 ➡, and CNV2 ➡ lie in the lateral dural wall. **(9-4)** Lateral graphic depicts the superficial cortical veins. The 3 named anastomotic veins—Trolard ➡, Labbé ➡, and the superficial middle cerebral vein ➡ —are depicted. 1 or 2 of the superficial cortical veins are usually dominant.*

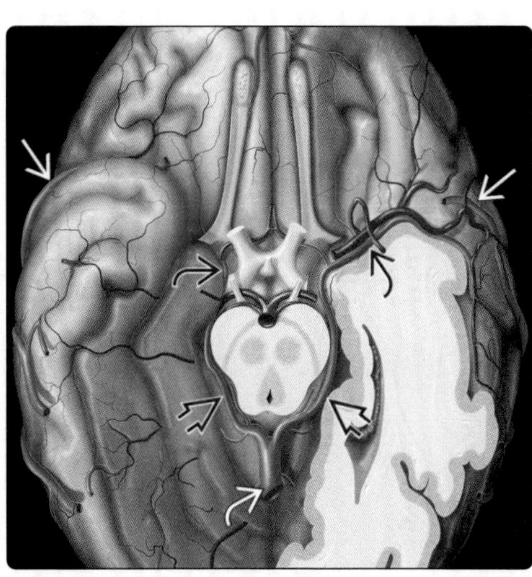

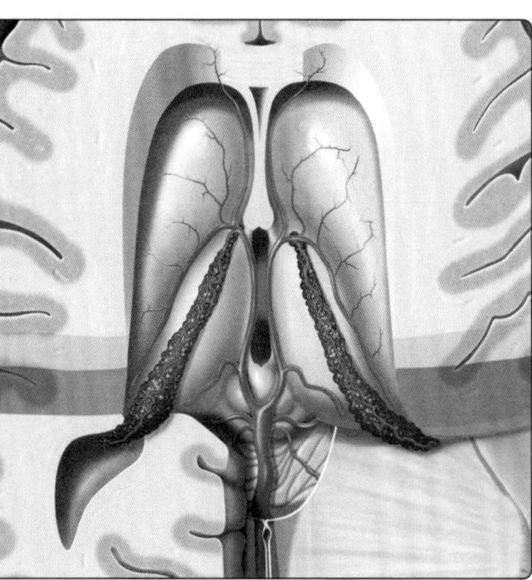

***(9-5)** Graphic shows superficial middle cerebral veins ➡. Deep middle cerebral veins ➡ collect tributaries from medial temporal lobes and drain into BVRs ➡. BVRs join with ICVs to form the VofG ➡. **(9-6)** Deep venous drainage is seen from the top down. Septal, caudate veins converge near the foramen of Monro to form ICVs. ICVs drain into the VofG and SS.*

parallel hypointense black lines converging on subependymal veins that outline the lateral ventricles **(9-11)**.

**Subependymal Veins.** These veins course under the ventricular ependyma, collecting blood from the basal ganglia and deep white matter (via the medullary veins) **(9-6)**. Prominent, named veins include the septal veins, thalamostriate veins, and ICVs. The **thalamostriate veins** receive tributaries from the caudate nuclei and thalami, curving medially to unite with the **septal veins** near the foramen of Monro to form the paired **ICVs** **(9-9)**.

**Deep Paramedian Veins.** The **ICVs** and **VofG** provide drainage for most of the deep brain structures. The ICVs are paired paramedian veins that course posteriorly in the cavum velum interpositum, the thin invagination of SAS that lies between the third ventricle and the fornices. The ICVs terminate by uniting with each other and the BVR to form the VofG. The VofG (great cerebral vein) curves posterosuperiorly under the corpus callosum splenium, uniting with the ISS to form the SS **(9-1)**.

## Venous Drainage Territories

The cerebral venous drainage territories are both less familiar and somewhat more variable than the major arterial distributions. Intracranial venous drainage follows four basic patterns: A peripheral (brain surface) pattern, a deep (central) pattern, an inferolateral (perisylvian) pattern, and a posterolateral (temporoparietal) pattern **(9-12)**. Accurately diagnosing and delineating venous occlusions depends on understanding these specific venous drainage territories.

### Peripheral (Surface) Brain Drainage

Most of the mid and upper surfaces of the cerebral hemispheres, together with their subjacent white matter, drain centrifugally (outward) via cortical veins into the SSS.

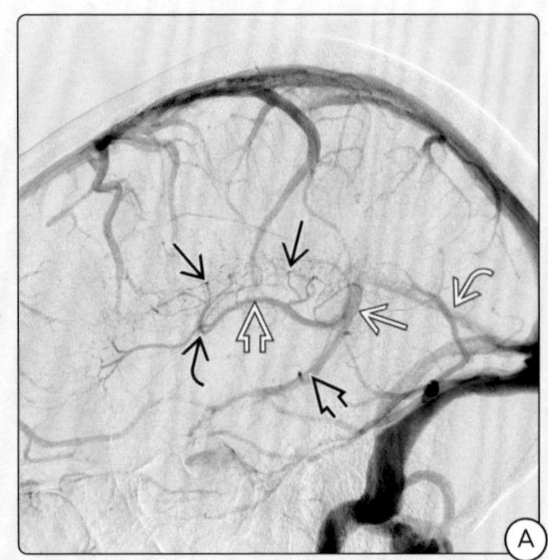


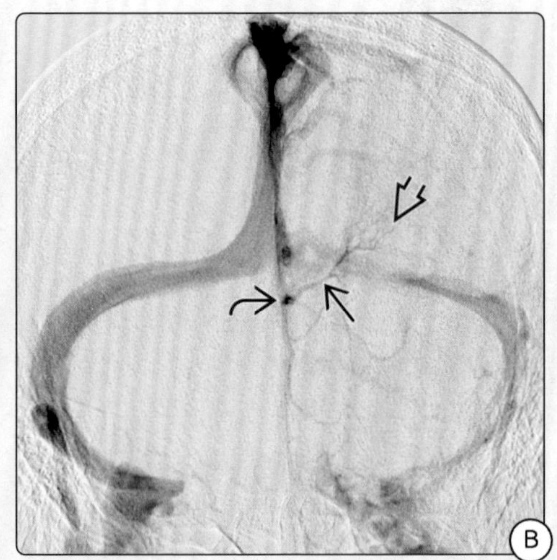


***(9-9A)** Venous-phase DSA, lateral view, shows septal, thalamostriate veins converging near the foramen of Monro ➲ to form the ICV ➡. Subependymal veins ⇨ outline the lateral ventricle. BVR ⇨ joins the VofG ➡ to form the SS ➡. **(9-9B)** AP view of DSA, late venous phase, shows SSS draining into a dominant right TS. Medullary veins ⇨, thalamostriate vein ⇨ drain around, outline the lateral ventricle, and form the midline ICV ➲.*

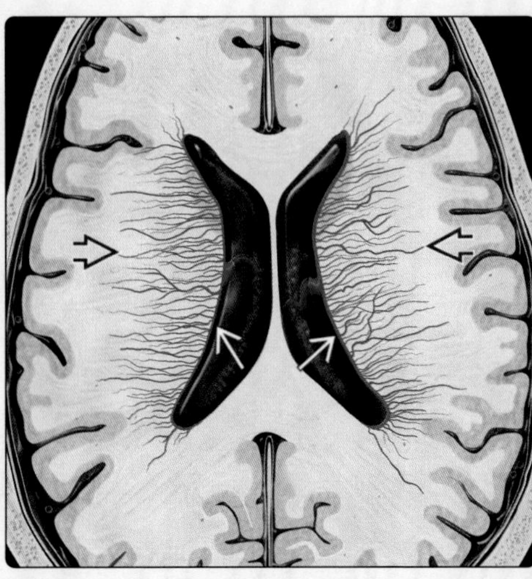

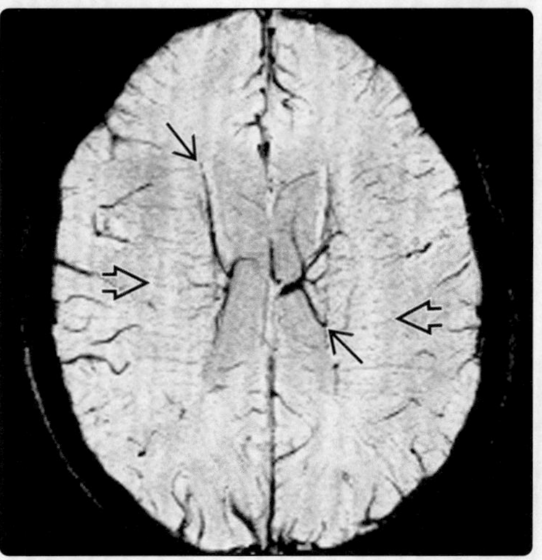

***(9-10)** Graphic through lateral ventricles shows medullary veins ⇨ draining hemispheric white matter (WM). Veins are perpendicular to ventricular margins, empty into subependymal veins ➡, eventually into ICVs. **(9-11)** T2* SWI shows medullary veins ⇨ converging at right angles on outer margins of lateral ventricles, draining into subependymal veins ⇨, and outlining the bodies of the lateral ventricles.*

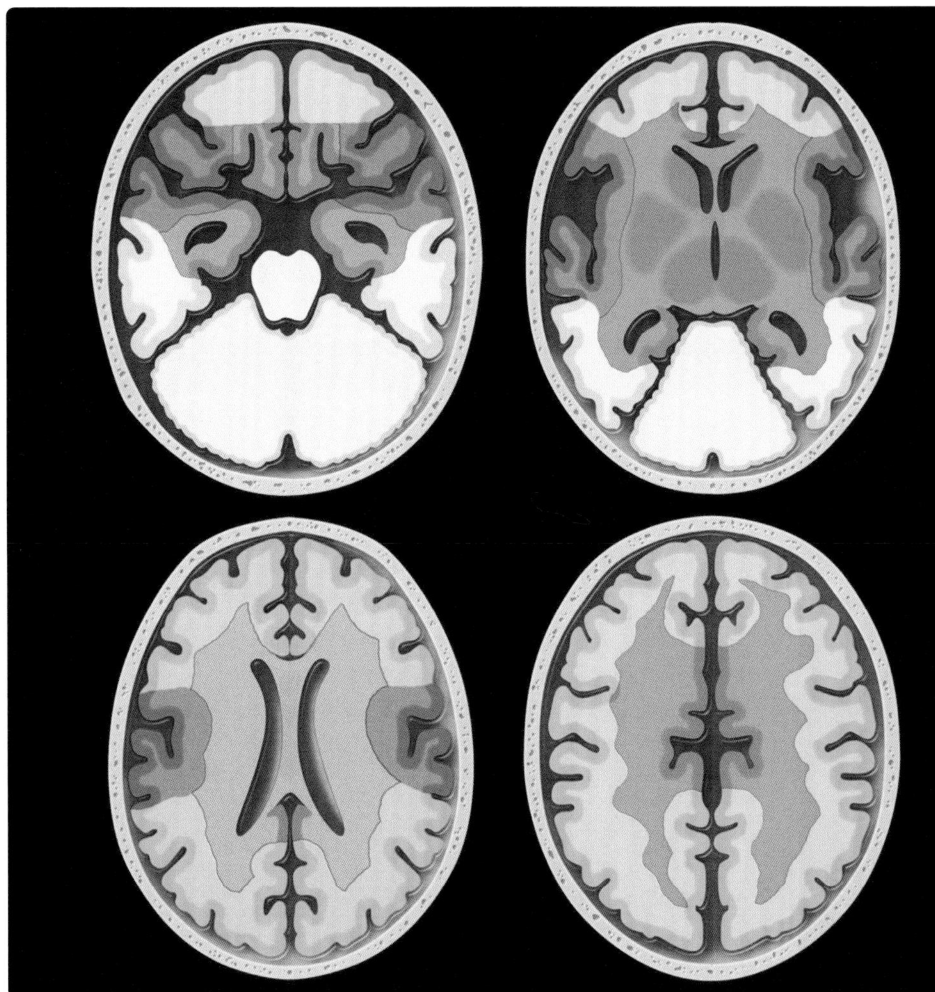

*(9-12) Color-coded anatomic diagram depicting brain venous drainage territories is shown at 4 representative levels: The base of the brain (upper left), basal ganglia and internal capsules (upper right), middle of the lateral ventricles (lower left), and upper corona radiata above the level of the corpus callosum (lower right). Superficial parts of the brain (cortex, subcortical WM) are drained by cortical veins [including the vein of Trolard (VofT)] and SSS (shown in green). Central core brain structures (basal ganglia, thalami, internal capsules, lateral and 3rd ventricles) and most of the corona radiata are drained by the deep venous system (ICVs, VofG, SS) (red). The veins of Labbé and the TSs drain the posterior temporal, inferior parietal lobes (yellow). The sphenoparietal sinus and CS drain the area around the sylvian fissures (purple).*

### Deep (Central) Brain Drainage

The basal ganglia, thalami, and most of the hemispheric white matter all drain centripetally (inward) into the deep cerebral veins. The ICVs, VofG, and SS together drain virtually the entire central core of the brain.

The most medial aspects of the temporal lobes, primarily the uncus and the anteromedial hippocampus, also drain into the galenic system via the DMCVs and BVR.

### Inferolateral (Perisylvian) Drainage

Parenchyma surrounding the sylvian (lateral cerebral) fissure consists of the frontal, parietal, and temporal opercula plus the insula. This perisylvian part of the brain drains via the SMCV into the sphenoparietal sinus and CS.

### Posterolateral (Temporoparietal) Drainage

The posterior temporal lobes and inferolateral aspects of the parietal lobes drain via the sphenoparietal sinuses and anastomotic vein of Labbé into the TSs.

# Cerebral Venous Thrombosis

Dural venous sinus, superficial (cortical) vein, and deep vein occlusions are collectively termed cerebral venous thrombosis (CVT). CVT is an elusive diagnosis with a great diversity of causes and clinical presentations; it is also easily overlooked on imaging studies.

We begin with the most common intracranial venous occlusion: Dural sinus thrombosis (DST). We next discuss superficial vein thrombosis and follow with deep cerebral occlusions. We conclude the discussion with a consideration of CS thrombosis/thrombophlebitis.

## Dural Sinus Thrombosis

### Terminology

Cerebral DST is defined as thrombotic occlusion of one or more intracranial venous sinuses **(9-13)**. DST can occur either in isolation or in combination with cortical &/or deep venous occlusions.

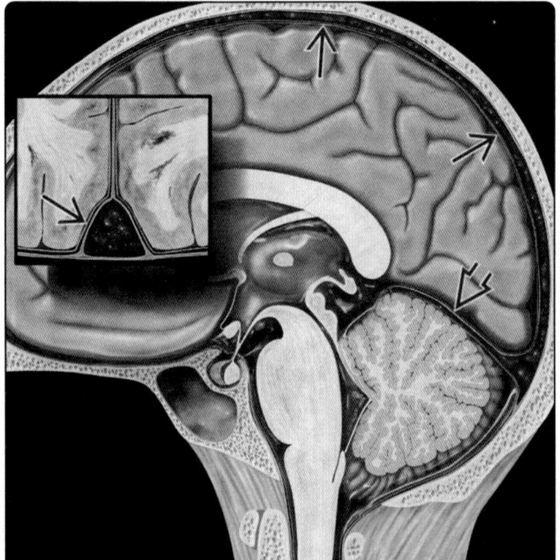

*(9-13) Sagittal graphic shows SSS and SS thrombosis. Insert shows the pathologic basis of the empty delta sign.*

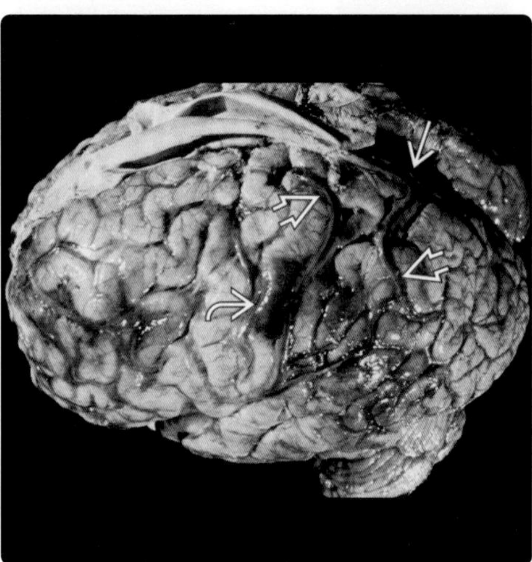

*(9-14) Autopsy case demonstrates acute SSS, cortical vein thrombosis, and venous infarcts.*

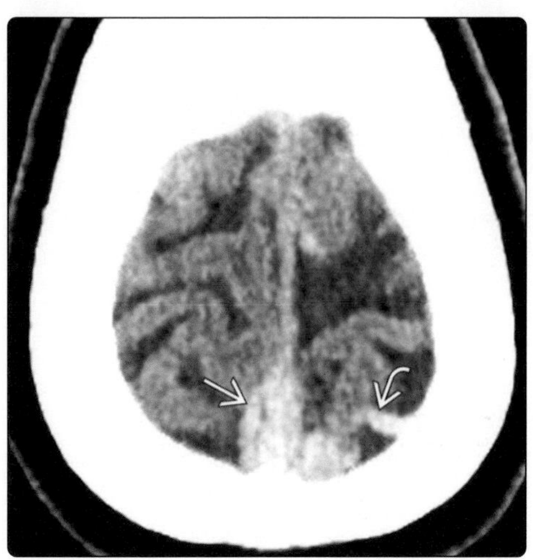

*(9-15) NECT shows hyperdense thrombus fills, expands SSS. Note hyperdensity in the adjacent cortical vein (cord sign).*

## Etiology

The majority of CVTs are acquired disorders. Oral contraceptive use and pregnancy/puerperium are the most common causes. Others include trauma, infection (including COVID-19), inflammation, hypercoagulable states, such as heparin-induced thrombocytopenia and vaccine-induced immune thrombotic thrombocytopenia, elevated hemoglobin levels, severe dehydration, collagen-vascular disorders (such as antiphospholipid syndrome), vasculitis (such as Behçet syndrome), drugs, and Crohn disease. Between 20-35% of all patients with CVT have genetic thrombophilic disorders.

### CEREBRAL VENOUS THROMBOSIS: CAUSES

**Common**

- Oral contraceptives
- Prothrombotic conditions
  - Deficiency of proteins C, S, or antithrombin III
  - Resistance to activated protein C (V Leiden)
  - Prothrombin gene mutations
  - Antiphospholipid, anticardiolipin antibodies
  - Hyperhomocysteinemia
- Puerperium, pregnancy
- Metabolic (dehydration, thyrotoxicosis, etc.)

**Less Common**

- Infection
  - Mastoiditis, sinusitis
  - Meningitis
- Trauma
- Neoplasm-related causes

**Rare but Important**

- Collagen-vascular disorders (e.g., antiphospholipid antibody syndrome)
- Hematologic disorders (e.g., polycythemia)
- Inflammatory bowel disease
- Vasculitis (e.g., Behçet disease)
- Rare hypercoagulable states
  - Heparin-induced thrombocytopenia
  - Autoimmune heparin-induced thrombocytopenia
  - Vaccine-induced immune thrombotic thrombocytopenia

## Pathology

When thrombus forms in a dural sinus, venous outflow is restricted. This results in venous congestion, elevated venous pressure, and hydrostatic displacement of fluid from capillaries into the extracellular spaces of the brain. The result is blood-brain barrier breakdown with vasogenic edema. If a frank venous infarct develops, cytotoxic edema ensues.

**Location.** The TS is the most commonly thrombosed dural venous sinus followed by the SSS.

**Gross Pathology.** In acute DST, the affected dural sinus appears distended by a soft, purplish clot that can be isolated to the sinus or may extend into adjacent cortical veins **(9-14)**. In chronic DST, firm proliferative fibrous tissue fills the sinus and thickens the dura-arachnoid. Associated brain injury in DST varies from venous congestion to ischemia to petechial hemorrhages and frank hemorrhagic infarcts.

## Clinical Issues

**Epidemiology.** CVTs represent between 1-2% of all acute strokes. Although CVT can occur at any age (from neonates to older adults), it is most commonly seen in young individuals. Nearly 80% of patients are younger than 50 years of age.

**Demographics.** CVT predominantly affects women (F:M = 3:1). A sex-specific risk factor (oral contraceptives, pregnancy, puerperium, and hormone replacement therapy) is present in nearly 2/3 of all women with CVT. Mean age at presentation is nearly a decade younger in women compared with men (34 years vs. 42 years).

**Presentation.** CVT causes two distinct pathophysiologic entities: Cortical venous infarction with focal neurologic symptoms and elevated intracranial pressure.

Nonfocal headache is the most common symptom, occurring in 70-90% of cases. Headache often slowly increases in severity over several days to weeks. Nearly 25% of patients present without focal neurologic findings.

**Natural History.** Many DSTs recanalize spontaneously without long-term sequelae. In some cases, a thrombosed or partially recanalized venous sinus forms an arteriovenous fistula in the adjacent dural wall.

Prompt recognition of DST has a significant impact on clinical outcome. Diagnostic delay—averaging seven days in large series—is associated with increased death and disability.

## Imaging

Keys to the early neuroradiologic diagnosis of DST are (1) a high index of suspicion, (2) careful evaluation of dural sinus density/signal intensity and configuration, and (3) knowledge of normal venous drainage patterns.

**CT Findings.** *NECT is normal in up to 25-30% of CVT cases, so a normal NECT scan does* **not** *exclude the diagnosis of CVT!* Early signs are often subtle. Slight hyperdensity **(9-17A)** compared with the carotid arteries is seen in 50-60% of cases. Density measuring ≥ 70 HU is highly suggestive of DST **(9-20A)**.

When present, a hyperattenuating vein (cord sign) **(9-31)** **(9-32)** or dural venous sinus sign **(9-15)** is both a sensitive and specific sign of cerebral venous occlusive disease. Parenchymal edema with or without petechial hemorrhage in the territory drained by the thrombosed sinus is a helpful but indirect sign of DST.

In 70% of cases, CECT scans show an **empty delta sign** caused by enhancing dura surrounding nonenhancing thrombus **(9-34)** **(9-23A)**. "Shaggy," enlarged, or irregular veins suggest collateral venous drainage.

**MR Findings.** Diagnosing CVT on MR can be challenging because thrombus and normal venous flow can have similar signal intensities. The imaging appearance of DST also varies significantly with imaging sequence and clot age.

***Acute DST.*** An acutely thrombosed sinus often appears moderately enlarged (fat sinus sign) and displays abnormally convex—not straight or concave—margins. The "flow void" of rapidly moving blood typically seen in large venous sinuses disappears **(9-20C)**. Acute DST appears **isointense** with the underlying cortex on **T1WI** **(9-20B)**.

As hemoglobin in blood clots rapidly desaturates to deoxyhemoglobin, it becomes very **hypointense** relative to brain on **T2WI** **(9-20D)**. Therefore, the acute T2 "dark" DST mimics normal intrasinus "flow void." Most acute

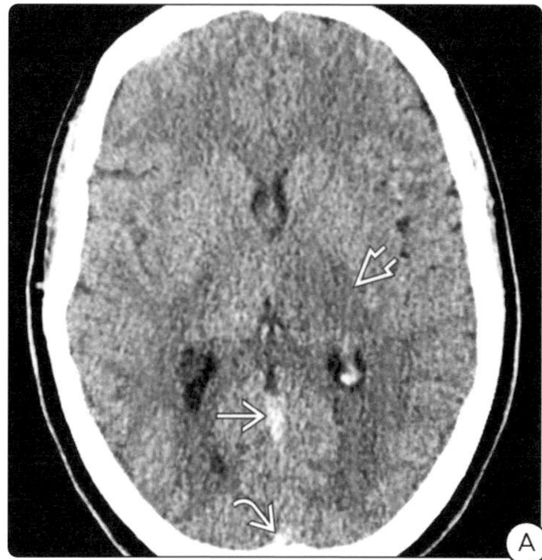


***(9-17A)** NECT in "thunderclap" headache shows hyperdensity of SS ➡, and torcular ➡. The left thalamus also appears hypodense ➡.*

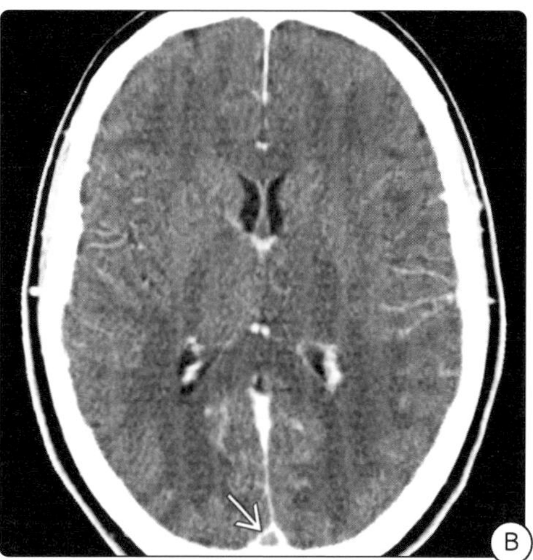


***(9-17B)** CECT in the same patient shows classic empty delta sign ➡ formed by enhancing dura around nonenhancing thrombus.*

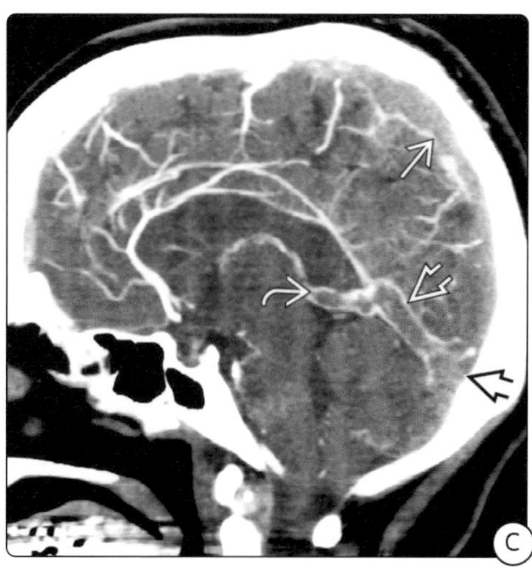


***(9-17C)** Sagittal CTV shows extensive thrombus filling the SSS ➡, SS ➡, VofG ➡, and torcular (sinus confluence) ➡.*

thrombi are hyperintense on FLAIR. Venous congestion may cause brain swelling with hyperintense parenchymal changes on T2/FLAIR.

Acute venous clots **"bloom"** on **T2* (GRE, SWI)**. SWI shows the profoundly hypointense clot and slow flow with deoxygenated blood in dilated cortical veins. The appearance may nonetheless be confusing, as normal-flowing but deoxygenated venous blood also appears hypointense.

Extensive acute (or longstanding chronic) DST may result in collateral venous drainage through the medullary (white matter) veins into the deep subependymal veins. The medullary veins enlarge and contain desaturated hemoglobin; thus, they are seen on T2* sequences as prominent linear hypointensities entering the subependymal veins at right angles.

When seen in cross section, **T1 C+** scans demonstrate an **empty delta** sign, similar to the appearance on CECT and CTA/CTV. Intrasinus thrombi usually appear as elongated **cigar-shaped** nonenhancing filling defects on axial T1 C+.

Coronal 2D unenhanced TOF **MRV** may demonstrate **absent flow**, especially if the thrombus is in the SSS. As the TSs often have hypoplastic segments, a "flow gap" must be interpreted with caution. **Contrast-enhanced MRV** has the highest sensitivity of all MR sequences for visualizing acute DST.

***Late Acute DST.*** As the intrasinus thrombus organizes, the clot begins to exhibit T1 shortening and becomes progressively hyperintense.

With T2 prolongation, a thrombosed sinus progresses from appearing very hypointense to iso- and then hyperintense with brain on both T2WI and FLAIR. T2* can be misleading, as clot signal gradually approaches that of normal sinuses. Late acute DST continues to exhibit an empty delta sign on T1 C+.

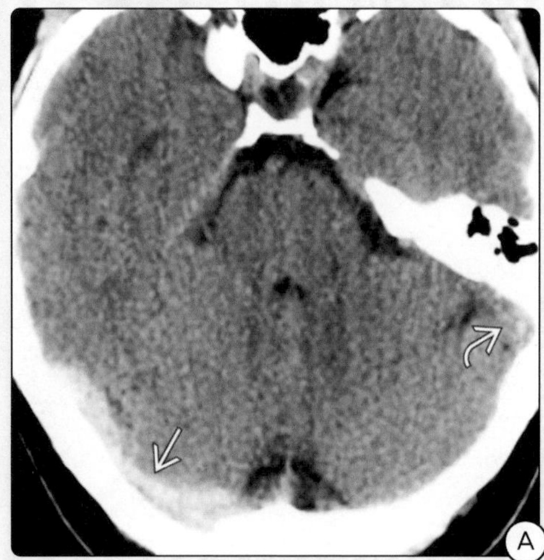


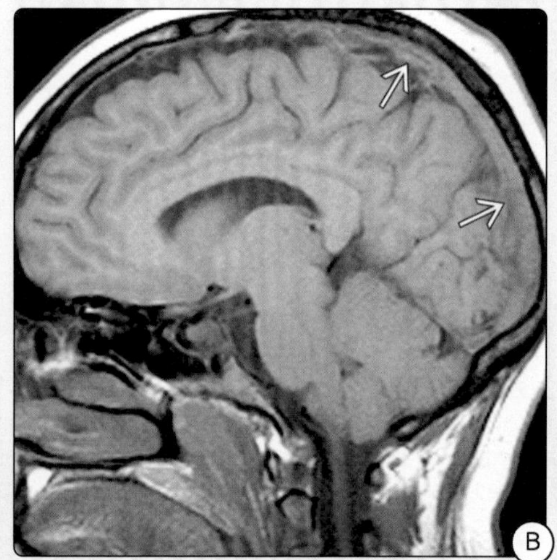


***(9-20A) Axial NECT in a 29-year-old pregnant woman with headaches, papilledema shows hyperdense right TS ➡ compared with the left sigmoid sinus ➡. (9-20B) Sagittal T1 MR in the same patient shows the SSS ➡ is also acutely thrombosed and is exactly the same signal intensity as the underlying brain.***

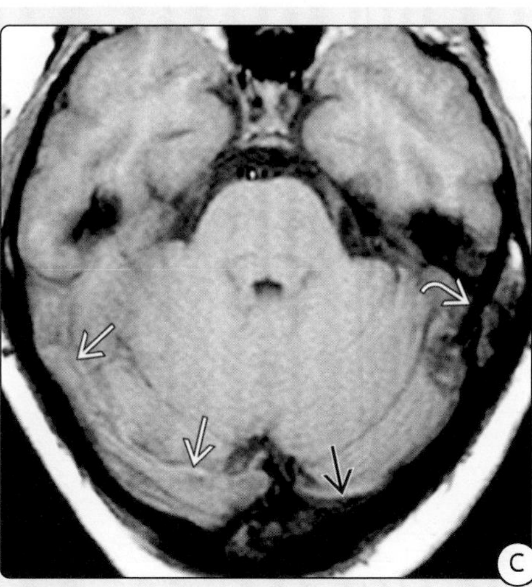


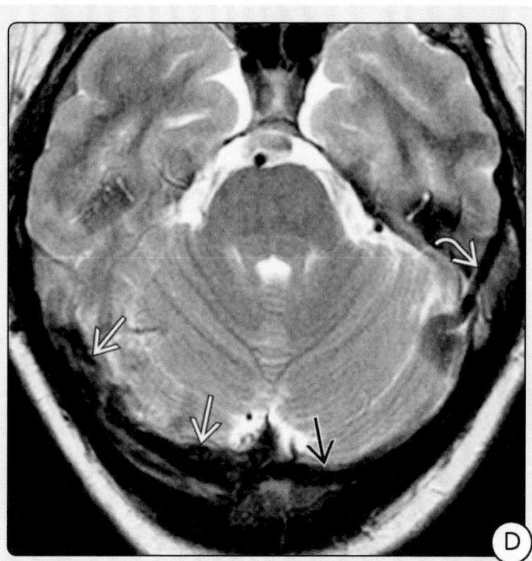


***(9-20C) Axial T1 MR in the same patient shows an enlarged right TS that appears filled with an isointense clot ➡. Compare with the normal "flow void" in the left vein of Labbé ➡ and TS ➡. (9-20D) Axial T2 MR in the same patient shows that the thrombosed right TS ➡ appears very hypointense and mimics the "flow voids" of the patent left TS ➡ and vein of Labbé ➡; this is acute dural sinus thrombosis (DST).***

***Subacute DST.*** Subacute thrombus is hyperintense on all sequences (T1, T2, FLAIR, T2*) **(9-26)** **(9-21)**.

***Chronic DST.*** Clot signal in chronic DST is quite variable and depends on the degree of clot organization. Chronic organized, fibrotic thrombus eventually becomes isointense with brain on T1WI and remains isointense to moderately hyperintense on T2WI. As blood has resorbed and largely disappeared, there is little or no T2* "blooming." CTA/CTV readily demonstrates nonenhancing thrombus within the intensely enhancing dura.

Longstanding cerebral venous sinus thrombosis may develop significant collateral drainage through the medullary veins. This is seen as tortuous, corkscrew, or "squiggly" white matter vessels on CTV and intraparenchymal "flow voids" on T2WI that enhance on T1 C+ scans. The enlarged collateral veins sometimes become so prominent that they mimic an arteriovenous malformation on SWI and DSA **(9-28)**.

Dura-arachnoid thickening is also common in longstanding chronic DST. In some cases, the dural thickening becomes so pronounced that it appears very hypointense on T2WI.

## Differential Diagnosis

**Normal dura** and **circulating blood** are mildly hyperdense on NECT scans. If a dural venous sinus appears unusually hyperdense, compare it to density of the ICAs. A dural sinus measuring > 70 HU is likely thrombosed.

Asymmetry of the TSs is common. A **hypoplastic segment** is seen in 1/4 to 1/3 of imaged cases and may mimic DST. A **high-splitting torcular** can mimic an empty delta sign on CECT.

**Giant AGs** are focal, round or ovoid, CSF-like filling defects in the sinuses, whereas clots tend to be elongated, cigar-shaped lesions (see "Venous Occlusion Mimics" section later in the chapter).

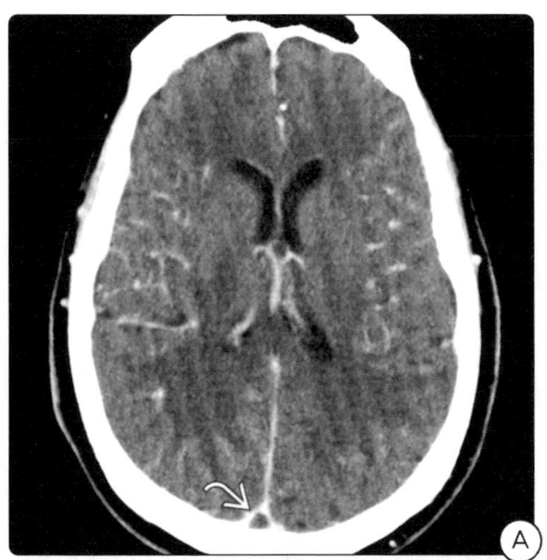

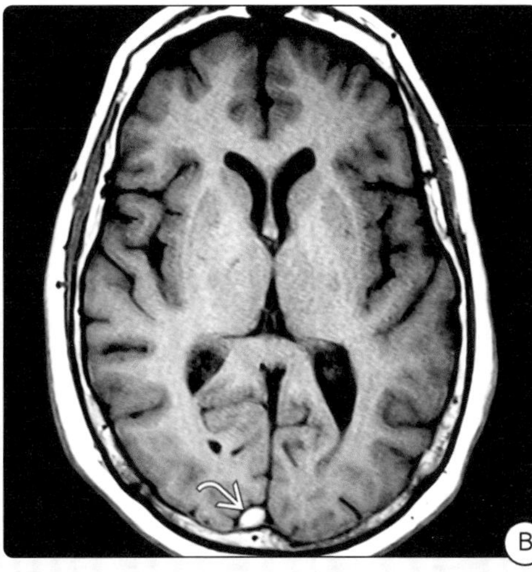

***(9-23A)** Axial CT venogram in a patient with 8 days of increasing headache shows an empty delta sign ➲ in the SSS, indicating enhancing dura around nonenhancing thrombus. **(9-21B)** T1 MR in the same patient shows subacute thrombus in the sinus is hyperintense ➲.*

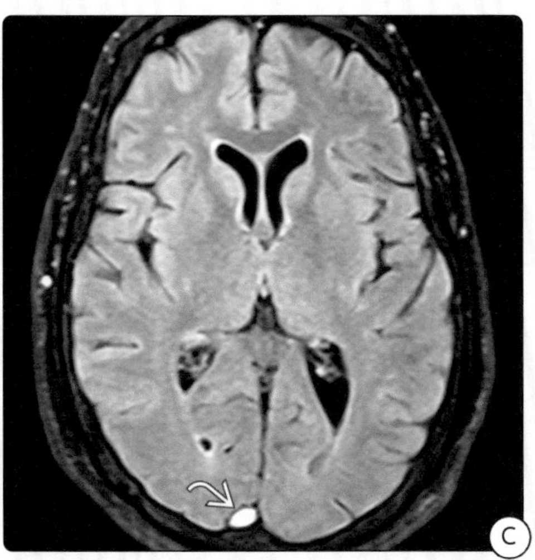

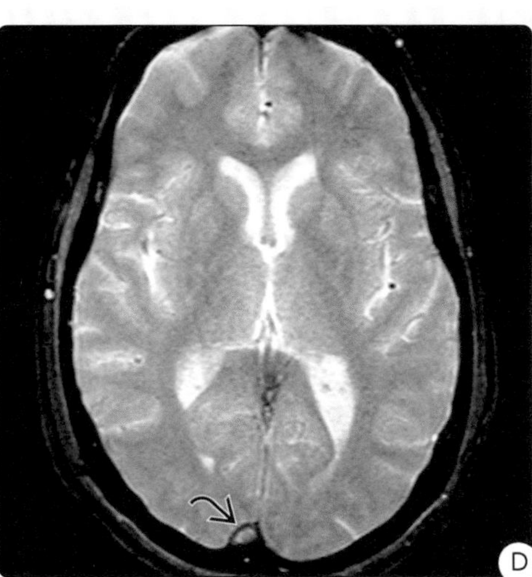

***(9-21C)** The subacute thrombus remains hyperintense on FLAIR ➲. **(9-21D)** T2* GRE shows the clot ➲ is mildly hyperintense and does not show gradient "blooming."*

**DURAL SINUS THROMBOSIS: MR**

**Acute**
- "Fat" sinus with bulging convex walls
- T1 isointense, T2 profoundly hypointense
- T2* "blooms," T1 C+ shows empty delta sign

**Late Acute**
- T1 mixed isointense, mildly hyperintense
- T2/FLAIR mildly hypointense/isointense
- T2* "blooms"

**Subacute**
- T1 hyperintense, T2/FLAIR hyperintense
- T2* hyperintense

**Chronic**
- T1 isointense, T2/FLAIR moderately hyperintense
- T2*, T1 C+ show "squiggly" parenchymal enhancement
- T1 C+ shows thick, enhancing dura

## Superficial Cerebral Vein Thrombosis

Superficial cerebral vein thrombosis (SCVT) can occur with **(9-32)** **(9-41)** or without DST.

### Superficial Vein Thrombosis *With* DST

Imaging findings of SCVT with accompanying DST are similar to those of DST alone. Thrombus extends from the affected dural sinus into one or more draining cortical veins **(9-35)**.

SSS occlusion with SCVT usually causes variable amounts of edema and petechial hemorrhage involving the cortex and subcortical white matter **(9-48)**. If the anastomotic **VofT** is dominant, its occlusion may result in lobar hemorrhage. TS occlusion that extends into a dominant **vein of Labbé** often causes extensive posterior temporal and anterior parietal hemorrhage **(9-42)** **(9-45)**.

***(9-26A)** Axial T1 MR shows classic early subacute hyperintense thrombus ➡ in an occluded right TS. **(9-26B)** Axial T2 MR shows that subacute thrombus is hyperintense ➡. Contrast with normal "flow void" in the hypoplastic left TS ➡.*

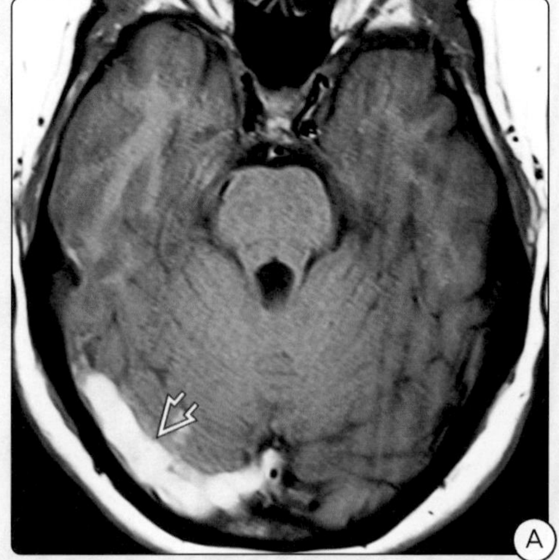


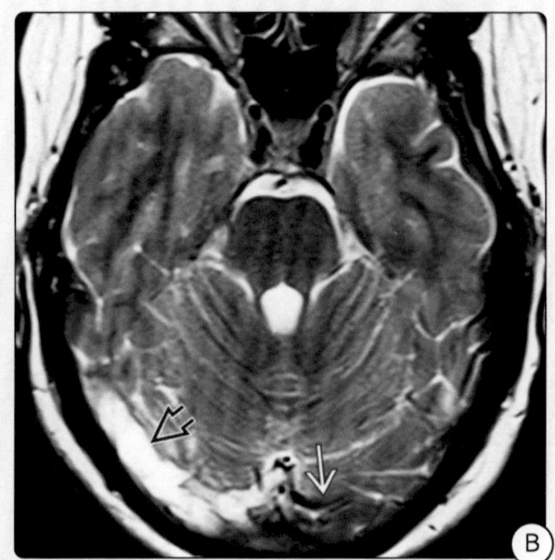


***(9-26C)** T2* GRE shows that the thrombus is mostly hyperintense ➡ with some residual "blooming" in the right TS ➡, tentorial tributary veins ➡. **(9-26D)** T1 C+ FS MR shows the intensely enhancing dura ➡ surrounding the nonenhancing, slightly less hyperintense subacute thrombus ➡. The left TS is hypoplastic but patent with a normal "flow void" ➡. This is subacute DST.*

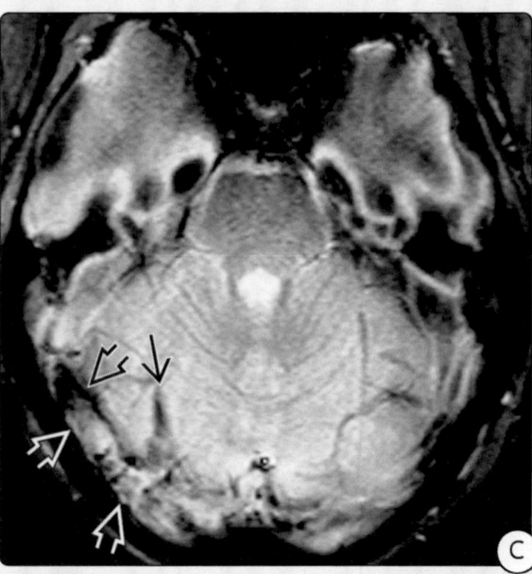


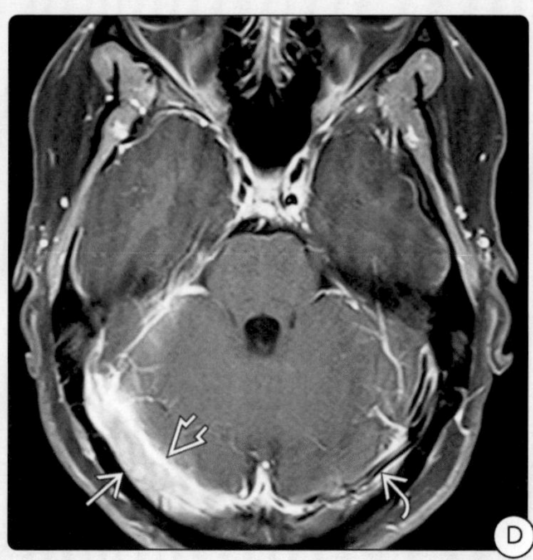

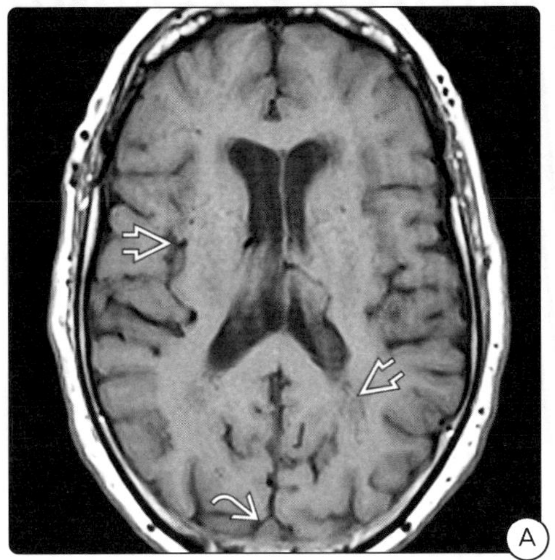

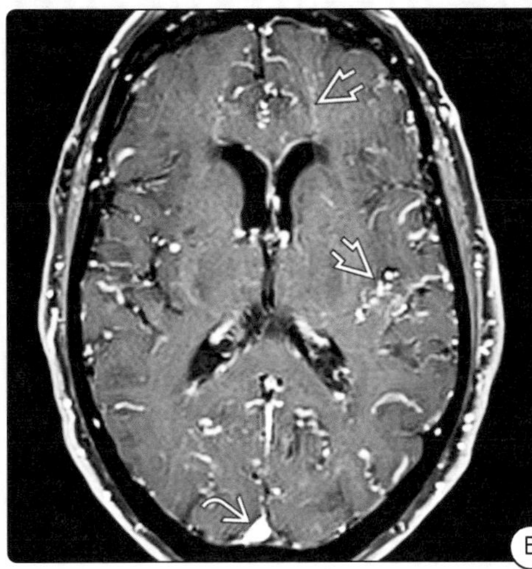

***(9-30A)*** *T1 MR in an 82-yo man with confusion, multiple falls, and altered mental status shows absence of normal "flow void" in the SSS ➔, which is isointense with brain. Note multiple unusually prominent tortuous "flow voids" in the sulci, parenchyma ➔.* ***(9-29B)*** *Axial T1 C+ FS MR shows a chronically thrombosed SSS that enhances intensely ➔. Tortuous, corkscrew vessels in the parenchyma and sulci also enhance intensely ➔.*

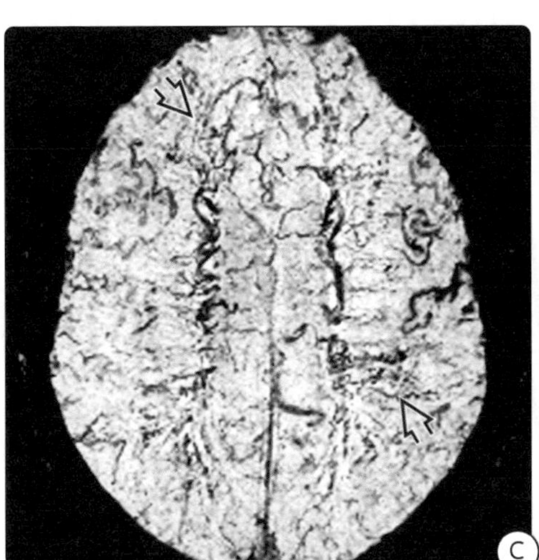

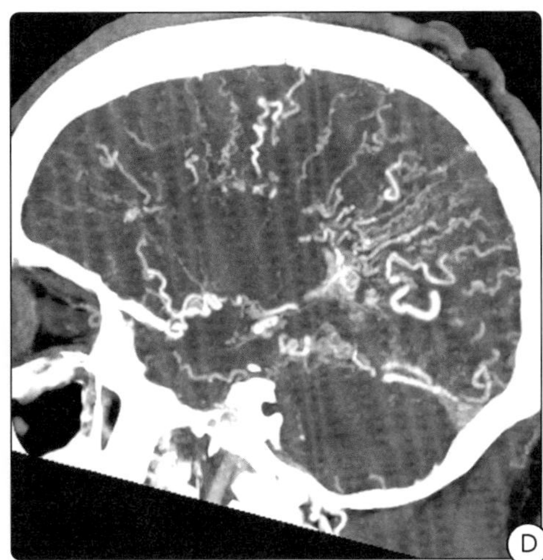

***(9-28C)*** *Axial T2* SWI shows prominent tortuous, corkscrew, "squiggly" medullary veins in both cerebral hemispheres ➔.* ***(9-28D)*** *Sagittal MIP of CT venogram shows innumerable corkscrew, enlarged, tortuous medullary veins that are providing collateral venous drainage.*

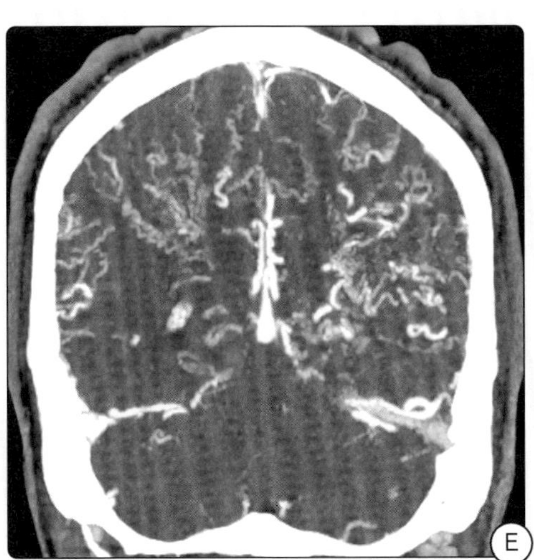

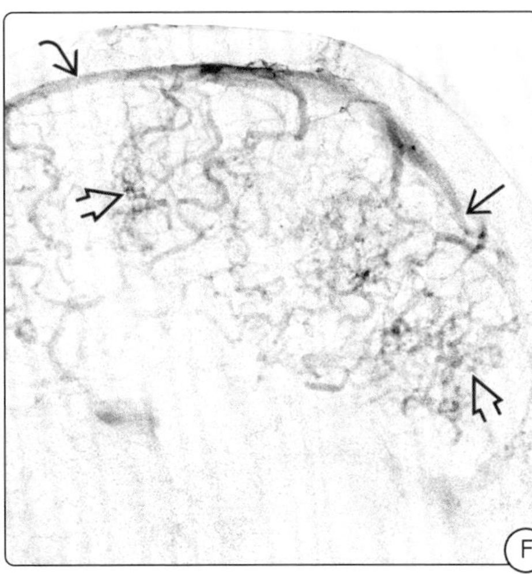

***(9-28E)*** *Coronal CT venogram shows the absence of a normal SSS and cortical draining veins. The tortuous corkscrew vessels are massively enlarged medullary veins.* ***(9-27F)*** *Venous DSA shows distal SSS is occluded ➔, but proximal, middle segments are patent ➔. Note enlarged corkscrew medullary veins ➔. Chronic SSS occlusion with striking medullary collateral venous ("pseudophlebitic") drainage.*

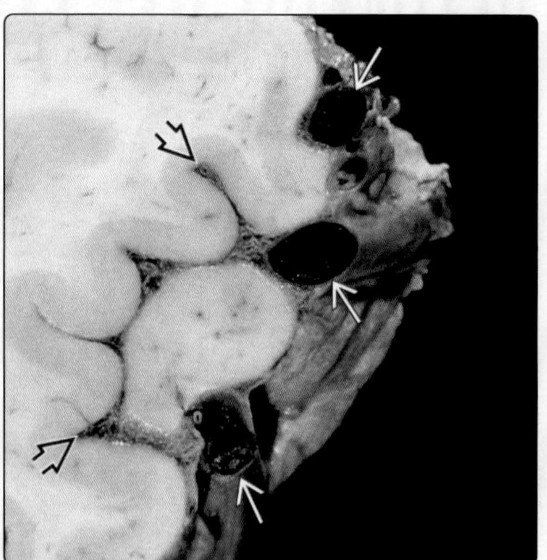

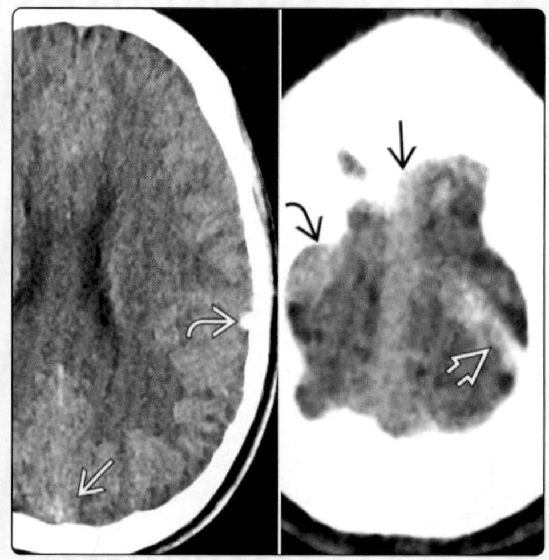

***(9-31)** Autopsy case shows thrombus in several cortical veins ➡ (cord sign) and adjacent convexal subarachnoid hemorrhage ⇨. **(9-32)** (L) NECT shows cord sign ➡ caused by a thrombosed cortical vein (VofT). SSS ➡ is normal. (R) More cephalad scan through the SSS shows it ⇨ and the right VofT ⇨ are normal density. The right VofT ➡ is hyperdense. This is isolated cortical vein thrombosis.*

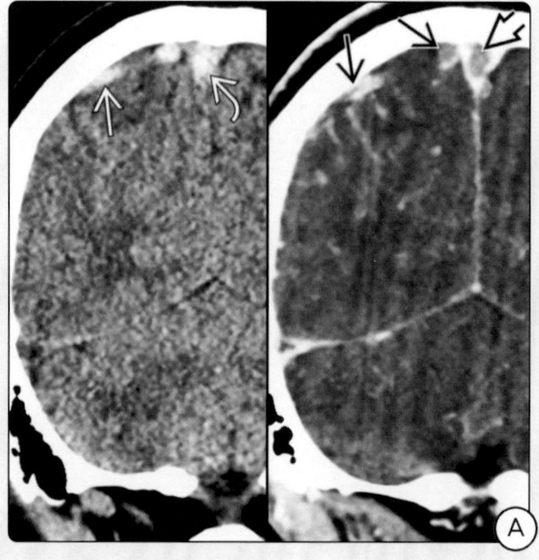

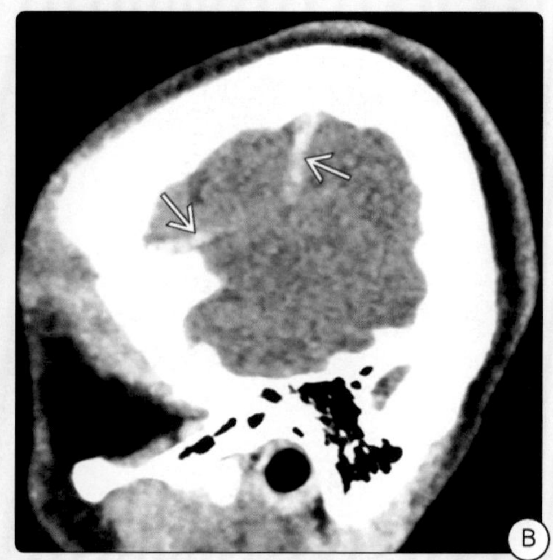

***(9-35A)** In this 62-yo woman in the ER with headache, left-sided weakness, (L) coronal NECT shows hyperdense SSS ➡, thrombosed VofT ➡. (R) CTV shows empty delta sign in SSS ⇨ and filling defects ⇨ in VofT. **(9-35B)** Sagittal CT venogram in the same patient shows hyperdense VofT ➡.*

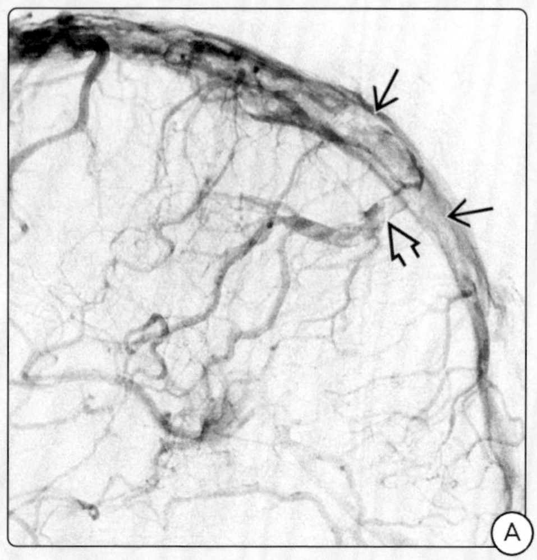

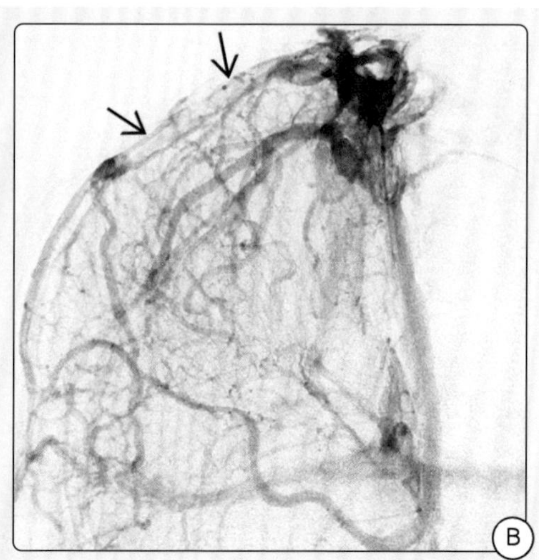

***(9-38A)** Lateral view of DSA in the same patient shows filling defects in a partially opacified VofT ⇨. The SSS is also partially thrombosed ⇨. **(9-38B)** AP DSA in the same patient shows filling defect ⇨ in the VofT caused by intraluminal thrombus.*

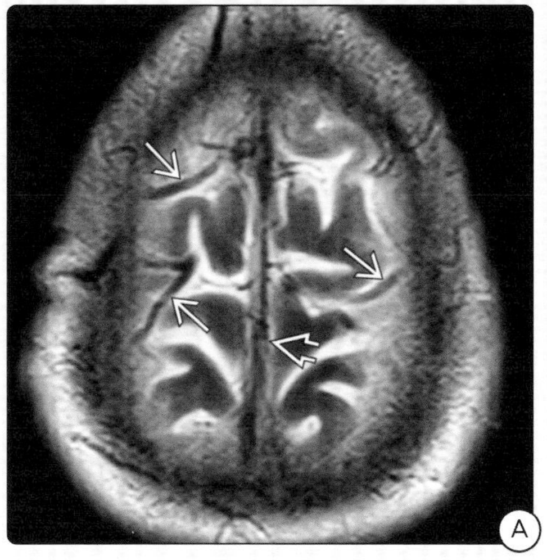

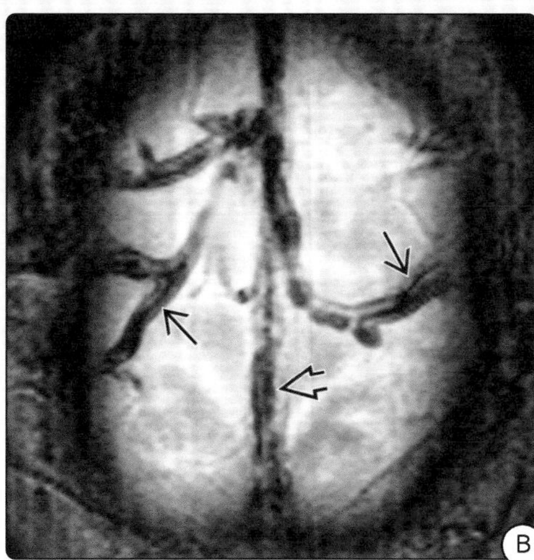

*(9-41A) Axial T2 MR in a patient with headache shows that acute hypointense thrombus in the cortical veins ➡ and SSS ➡ mimic normal "flow voids." (9-41B) T2* GRE shows acutely thrombosed cortical veins, seen here as curvilinear hypointensities ➡. The adjacent SSS is also occluded ➡. In very acute DST and cortical vein thrombosis, it is easy to overlook subtle MR findings, but T2* sequences are extremely helpful.*

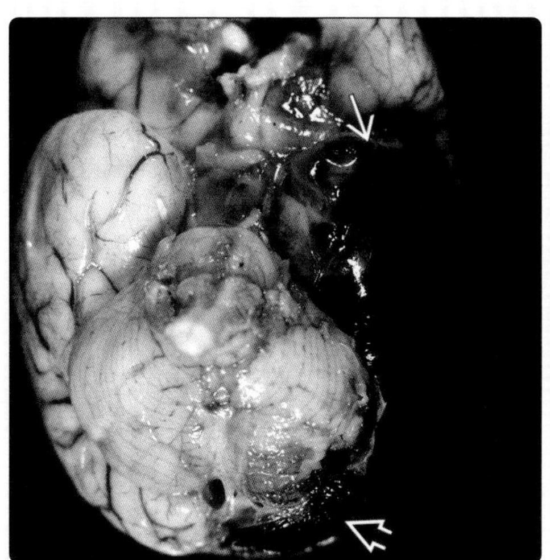

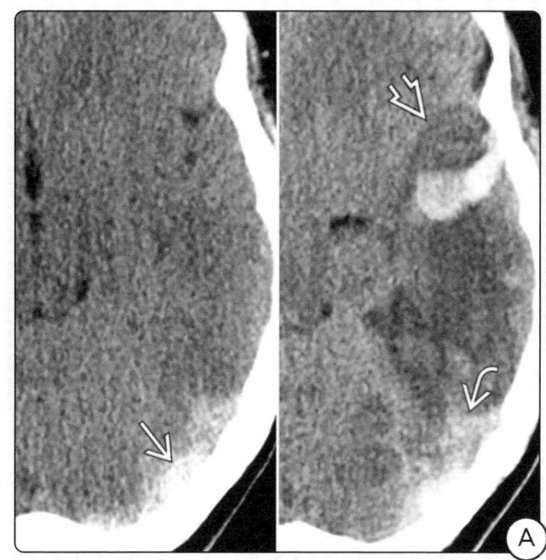

*(9-42) Autopsy shows acutely thrombosed TS ➡ that caused a large temporal lobe hemorrhagic infarct ➡. (9-45A) (L) In this 23-yo woman with migraine, left TS thrombosis ➡ was missed. (R) 24 hours later, VofT ➡ has also thrombosed, causing hemorrhagic infarct ➡.*

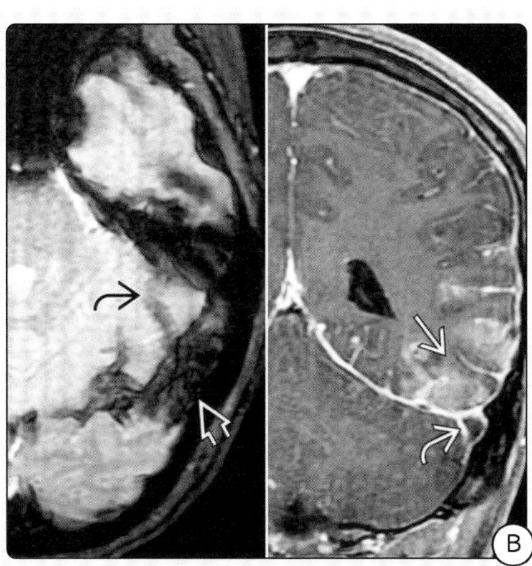

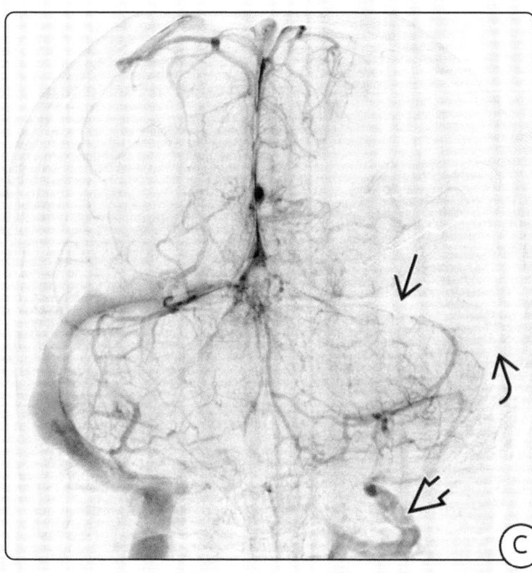

*(9-45B) (L) T2* GRE shows a thrombosed left TS ➡. The vein of Labbé is also thrombosed, seen here as hypointense linear "blooming" ➡. (R) Coronal T1 C+ FS MR shows empty delta sign ➡ and some parenchymal enhancement ➡ from venous ischemia. (9-45C) AP DSA in the same patient shows occlusion of the left TS ➡ and sigmoid sinus ➡. Note nonocclusive clot in a extracranial collateral draining vein ➡.*

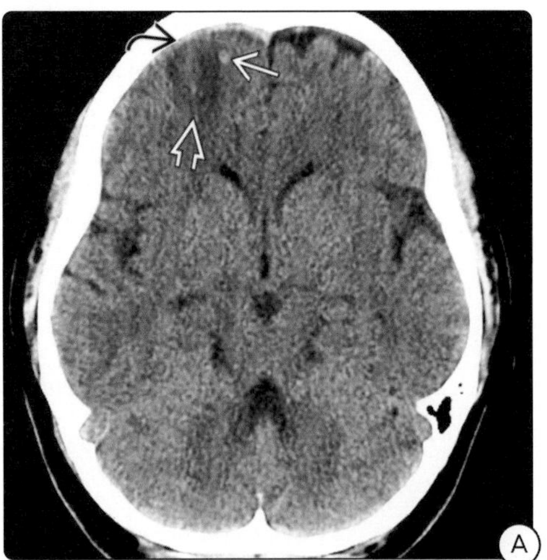


***(9-48A) NECT in 36-yo woman with seizure shows hypodense R frontal mass , hemorrhage . Cortical vein thrombosis was overlooked.***

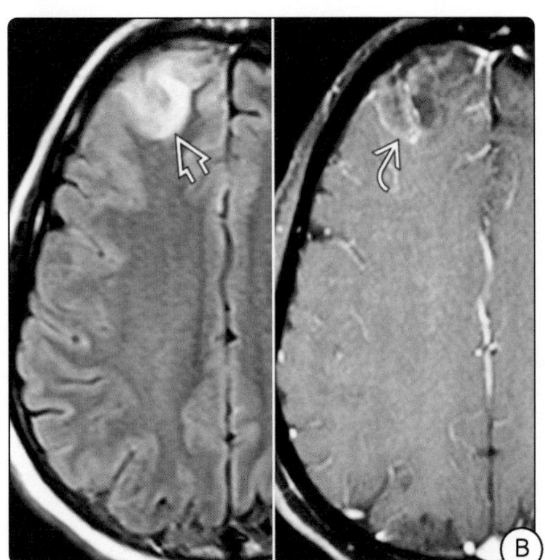


***(9-48B) (L) FLAIR shows cortical/subcortical mass . (R) T1 C+ MR shows patchy enhancement (called neoplasm vs. cerebritis).***

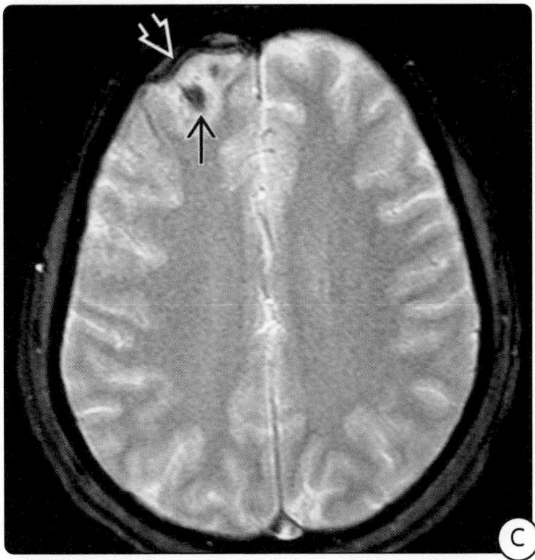


***(9-48C) T2* GRE shows hemorrhage . Note adjacent thrombosed cortical vein . Venous occlusion mimics neoplasm.***

SUPERFICIAL CORTICAL VEIN THROMBOSIS

**Superficial Thrombosis Without DST**

- Rare (5% of all CVTs)
- May cause convexal subarachnoid hemorrhage
- May see cord sign
- Deoxygenated thrombus can mimic normal "flow voids" on T2WI
- T2* (GRE, SWI) key to diagnosis
  - "Blooming" thrombus in vein(s)

**Superficial Thrombosis With DST**

- DST extends into adjacent veins
- Edema, hemorrhage in cortex, adjacent white matter
- Can be extensive if VofT or Labbé occluded

## Superficial Vein Thrombosis *Without* DST

Isolated SCVT (iSVCT) without DST is rare, representing only 2-5% of all sinovenous occlusions. The clinical outcome of iSVCT is generally good.

iSCVT usually presents with a nonspecific headache. Approximately 10% of patients report sudden onset of a "thunderclap" headache that clinically mimics aneurysmal subarachnoid hemorrhage.

Symptoms, such as focal neurologic deficits, seizures, and impaired consciousness, are less common than with dural sinus or deep vein thrombosis.

The imaging diagnosis of iSCVT can be problematic. NECT is usually negative, although some cases may demonstrate focal **convexal subarachnoid hemorrhage** or a **cord sign**, representing a hyperdense thrombosed vein.

CTA/CTV or DSA may show a thin, round or tubular layer of contrast surrounding the thrombus.

The MR diagnosis of SCVT—whether with or without dural sinus involvement—is difficult to establish using only standard T1- and T2-weighted sequences. Acute thrombi are isointense with brain on T1WI and hypointense on T2WI, making them difficult to distinguish from normal "flow voids."

FLAIR may demonstrate focal convexal subarachnoid hemorrhage seen as hyperintense sulcal CSF. Cortical-subcortical hyperintensities consistent with vasogenic edema are common associated findings.

Intraluminal thrombus can sometimes be seen as a linear hyperintensity on FLAIR or DWI. Venous ischemia may result in transient diffusion restriction.

T2* (GRE, SWI) sequences are key to the noninvasive diagnosis of SCVT **(9-48)**. With a sensitivity of > 95%, they are by far the best imaging sequences for detecting thrombosed cortical veins. A well-delineated tubular hypointensity with "blooming" of hemoglobin degradation products within the clot is observed at all stages of evolution, persisting for weeks. Patchy or petechial hemorrhages in the underlying cortex and subcortical white matter are common, as is associated convexal subarachnoid hemorrhage.

Superficial vein thrombosis in the absence of DST can be problematic to diagnose. If the thrombosed vein is overlooked, iSCVT can mimic neoplasm, infection, or other more ominous pathologies.

## Cavernous Sinus Thrombosis/Thrombophlebitis

Cavernous thrombosis/thrombophlebitis is the most common form of septic cerebral venous sinus thrombosis, a rare but potentially lethal condition with significant morbidity and high mortality.

### Terminology

CS thrombosis (CST) is a blood clot in the CS. If it occurs in conjunction with sinus infection, it is termed CS thrombophlebitis **(9-51)**.

### Etiology and Pathology

The CS is composed of numerous heavily trabeculated venous spaces that have numerous valveless communications with veins in the orbit, face, and neck. Infection can thus spread easily through these venous conduits into the CS.

CST usually occurs as a complication of sinusitis or other midface infection. *Staphylococcus aureus* is the most frequent pathogen. Other less common agents include anaerobes and angioinvasive fungal infections.

Otomastoiditis, odontogenic disease, trauma, and neoplasm are less frequent causes of CST.

### Clinical Issues

**Epidemiology.** CST without trauma, infection, or multiple other dural venous sinus occlusions is extremely rare.

**Presentation.** Headache, especially in the CNV1 and CNV2 distributions, and fever are usually the earliest symptoms. Orbital pain with edema, chemosis, proptosis, ophthalmoplegia, and visual loss is present in 80-100% of cases.

**Natural History.** Untreated CST can be fatal. Even with antibiotics, the mortality rate of CS thrombophlebitis is 25-30%.

### Imaging

**CT Findings.** CS thrombophlebitis causes proptosis, "dirty" orbital fat, periorbital edema, sinusitis, and lateral bulging of the CS walls and may demonstrate a thrombosed superior ophthalmic vein (SOV) on NECT. CECT scans demonstrate multiple irregular filling defects in the expanded CS and SOVs **(9-51A)**.

**MR Findings.** MR scans show enlarged CSs with convex lateral margins. Acute thrombus is isointense with brain on T1WI and demonstrates variable hypointensity on T2WI **(9-51B)**. Nonenhancing filling defects within the enhancing dural walls of the CS and thrombosed orbital veins on T1 C+ are the definitive imaging findings in CST **(9-51C)**.

Look for the normal intracavernous carotid artery "flow void," as CS thrombophlebitis can lead to thrombosis or pseudoaneurysm formation.

**Angiography.** Nonvisualization of the CS on DSA can be a normal finding and does not indicate the presence of CST.

### Differential Diagnosis

The differential diagnosis of CST includes neoplasm, carotid-cavernous fistula, and inflammatory disorders. **Neoplasms** (e.g., lymphoma, metastases) enhance uniformly. **Carotid-cavernous fistula** causes "flow

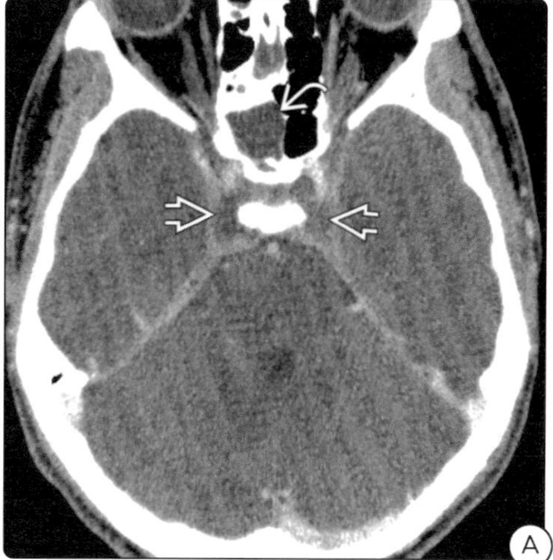


***(9-51A)** Axial CECT in a 16-yo boy with severe sphenoid sinusitis ➡ shows nonopacification of most of the CS ➡.*

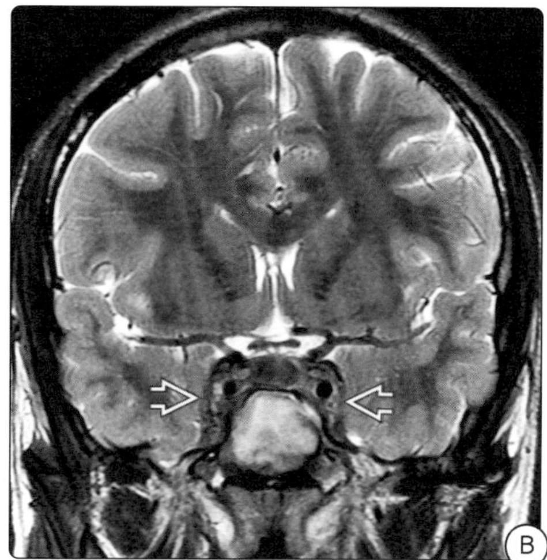


***(9-51B)** Coronal T2 MR shows hypointense thrombus bulging the CS walls laterally ➡.*

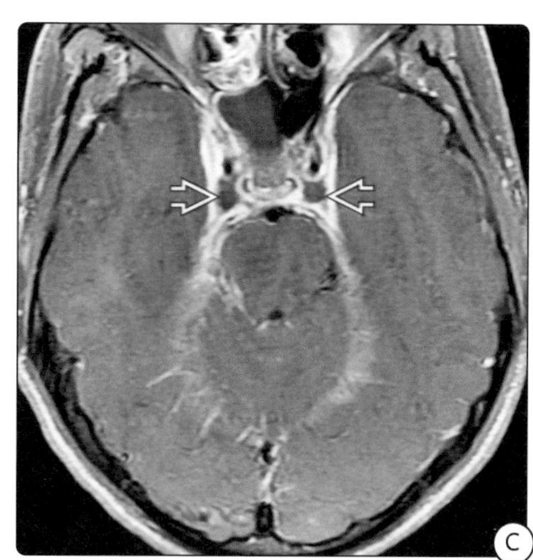


***(9-51C)** T1 C+ FS MR shows intensely enhancing dura surrounding foci of nonenhancing thrombus ➡. This is septic CS thrombophlebitis.*

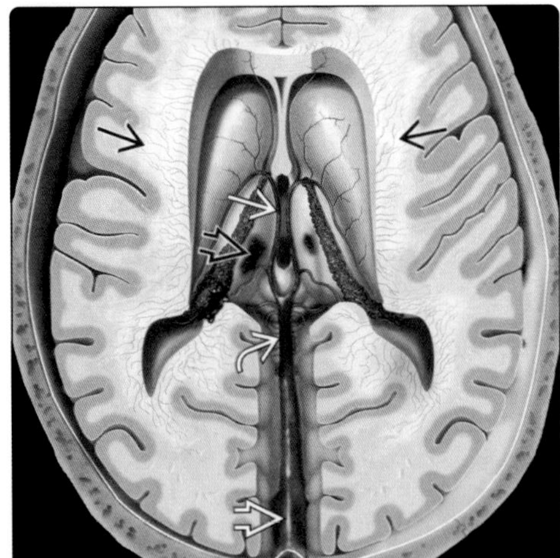

(9-52) Thrombosis of both ICVs ➡, VofG ➡, SS ➡ are shown. Note thalamic hemorrhages ➡ and engorgement of WM medullary veins ➡.

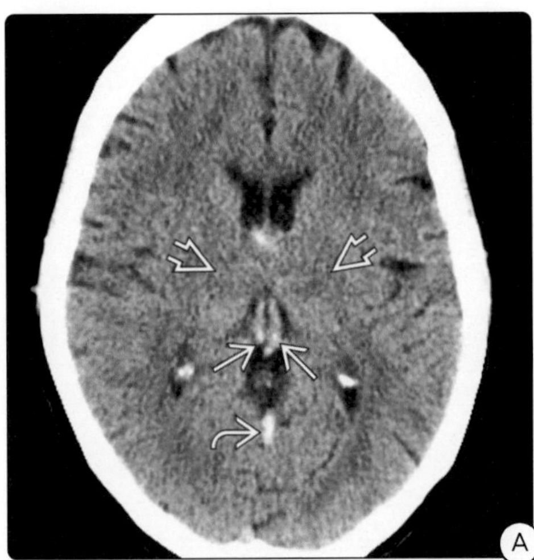

(9-55A) NECT in deep vein thrombosis shows hyperdense ICVs ➡, SS ➡, and hypodense edematous thalami ➡.

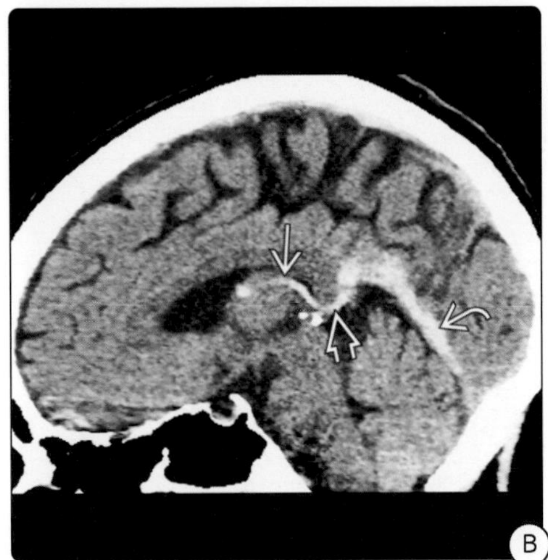

(9-55B) Sagittal reformatted NECT shows a hyperdense thrombus in the ICV ➡, VofG ➡, and SS ➡.

voids," and **inflammatory disorders** (e.g., sarcoid, inflammatory pseudotumors) enhance strongly and uniformly.

**CAVERNOUS SINUS THROMBOSIS/THROMBOPHLEBITIS**

**Pathoetiology**
- Numerous valveless communications between CS, orbit, face
- CST secondary to sinusitis, dental disease > trauma, neoplasm
- Spontaneous, isolated CST rare

**Clinical Issues**
- Headache, cranial neuropathy
- Proptosis, chemosis common

**Imaging**
- NECT may be normal early
  - Look for sinusitis, "dirty" orbit fat
  - Lateral bulging of CS walls
- CECT/CTV
  - Nonenhancing filling defects on CECT
  - Nonopacification on early-phase CTV
- MR
  - T1WI isointense, laterally bulging walls
  - T2 iso-/hypointense
  - Look for cavernous carotid thrombosis (loss of "flow void")
  - T1 C+ shows nonenhancing filling defects

## Deep Cerebral Venous Thrombosis

Deep CVT (DCVT) is a potentially life-threatening disorder with a combined mortality/disability rate of 25%.

### Etiology and Pathology

The deep cerebral venous system (the ICVs and BVR, together with their tributaries, the VofG, and SS) is involved in ~ 10-15% of all patients with cerebral venoocclusive disease **(9-52)**.

DCVT can occur either alone or in combination with other sinovenous occlusions. Because the cerebral venous system lacks valves and tunica muscularis, thrombosis in one sinus can easily extend to adjacent sinuses. Isolated DCVT is present in 20% of cases while 80% have additional thrombi in other sinuses. DCVT is almost always bilateral and results in symmetric venous congestion/infarction of the basal ganglia and thalami.

### Clinical Issues

Initial symptoms of DCVT are variable and nonspecific, making diagnosis difficult. Most patients present with headache (80%) followed by rapid neurologic deterioration and impaired consciousness (70%). Focal neurologic findings are frequently absent, and subacute presentation is the rule, not the exception.

Deep system involvement, either isolated or in association with other venous sinuses, is an independent predictor of death and disability.

### Imaging

Early NECT findings may be subtle. Hyperdense ICVs and SSs resemble a contrast-enhanced scan **(9-58A)**. Hypodense "fading" or "disappearing" thalami with effacement of the border between the deep gray nuclei and internal capsule are key but nonspecific findings of DCVT **(9-55A)**.

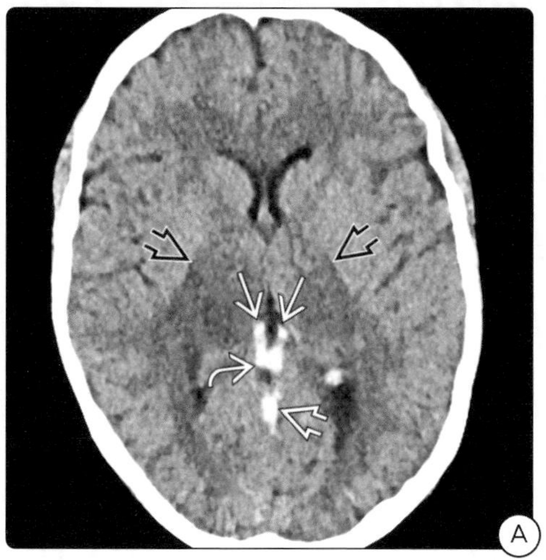

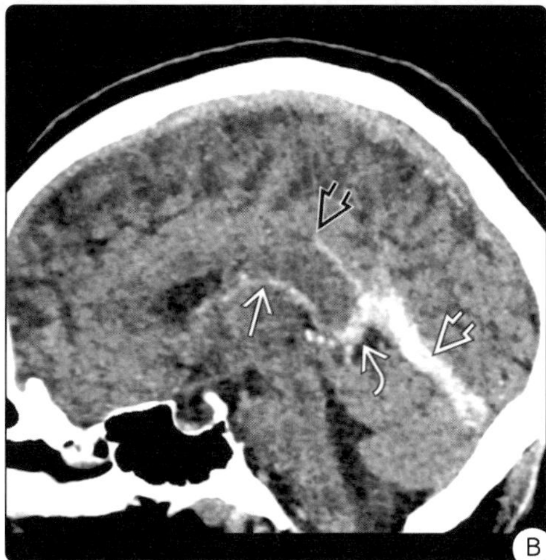

***(9-58A)** NECT in a 19-yo woman on birth control pills who came to the ER after 3 days of increasingly severe headaches shows hyperdense thrombus in both ICVs ➡, VofG ➡, and SS ➡. Note hypodensity in both thalami ➡, which appear swollen and mass-like. **(9-58B)** Sagittal reformatted CT shows hyperdense clot in the ICVs ➡, VofG ➡, SS ➡, and even the ISS ➡.*

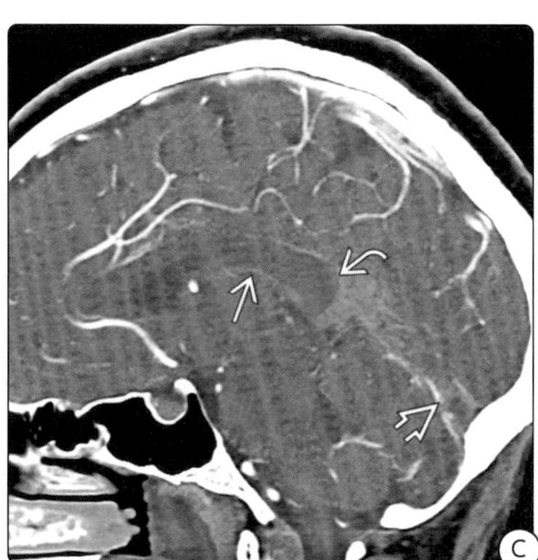

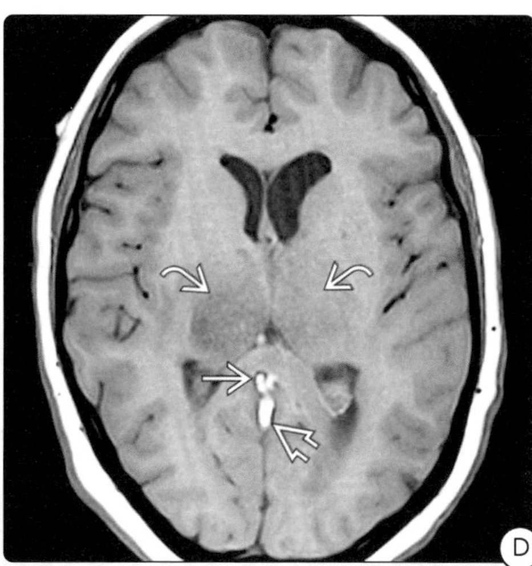

***(9-58C)** Sagittal CTV shows no filling of the slightly hyperdense thrombosed ICVs ➡, VofG ➡, SS ➡, and ISS. **(9-58D)** MR was obtained 4 days later after the patient's condition worsened. Hyperintense thrombus is present in the ICVs ➡ and VofG/proximal SS ➡. Note hypointensity in both thalami ➡.*

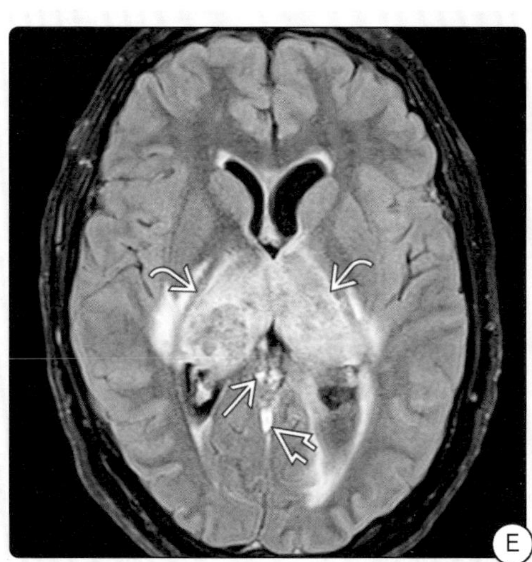

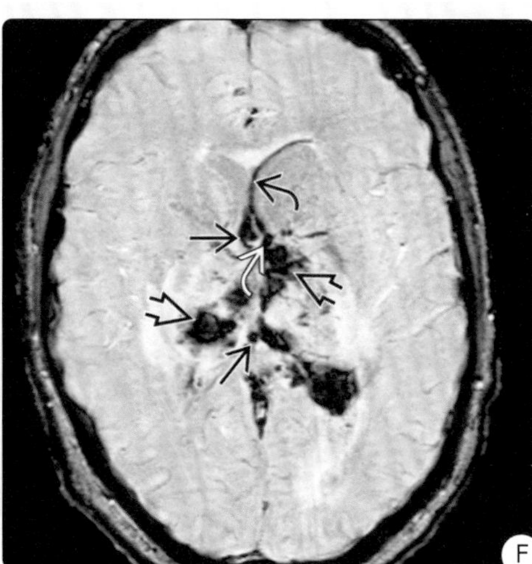

***(9-58E)** FLAIR MR in the same patient shows enlarged, hyperintense thalami ➡. Note that the thrombus in the ICVs ➡ and SS ➡ is hyperintense. **(9-58F)** T2* GRE shows patchy hemorrhage in the thalami ➡. Note "blooming" thrombus in the left septal vein ➡, both ICVs ➡, and the left thalamostriate vein ➡. The patient expired shortly after the scan was obtained.*

MR is the imaging modality of choice. Acute thrombus is isointense on T1WI and hypointense on T2WI (pseudo-"flow void"). Venous congestion causes hyperintensity with swelling of the thalami and basal ganglia on T2/FLAIR in 70% of cases **(9-58A)**.

The most sensitive sequence is T2* GRE on which acute clots show distinct "blooming." Venous congestion in the medullary and subependymal veins is also hypointense due to slow flow and hemoglobin deoxygenation.

CTA/CTV and DSA show absent opacification in deep venous drainage system **(9-58C)**, and MRV shows absence of flow.

## Differential Diagnosis

### DEEP VENOUS THROMBOSIS

**Pathology**
- Uncommon (15% of CVTs)
- Usually both ICVs ± VofG, SS involved

**Imaging**
- Hyperdense ICVs (may look like CECT scan)
- Bithalamic edema common
- Variable hemorrhage
- CTV shows nonopacification of deep (Galenic) veins
- DSA shows absent visualization of ICVs ± VofG, SS
- Differential diagnosis
  - Neoplasm (bithalamic glioma)
  - Top of basilar, artery of Percheron thrombosis
  - Wernicke encephalopathy

# Venous Occlusion Mimics

We conclude this chapter on venous anatomy and occlusions with a brief discussion of conditions that can mimic—or obscure—venous thrombosis.

## Sinus Variants

The major differential diagnosis of CVT is a **congenital anatomic variation**. The right TS is usually the dominant venous sinus and is often significantly larger than the left side. A **hypoplastic TS** segment is present in 1/4 to 1/3 of all imaged cases and is **especially** common in the nondominant sinus (usually the left TS) **(9-61A)**. In such instances, the ipsilateral jugular bulb is typically small. Correlation with bone CT can also be helpful in demonstrating a small bony jugular foramen or sigmoid sinus groove. A hypoplastic TS or sigmoid sinus is also often—but not invariably—associated with alternative venous outflow pathways, such as a persistent occipital sinus or prominent mastoid emissary veins.

The absence of occluded draining veins, enlarged venous collateral channels, or abnormally thick dural enhancement supports the diagnosis of TS sinus hypoplasia or anatomic variant vs. true cerebral venous sinus thrombosis.

## Flow Artifacts

A **"flow gap"** on 2D TOF MRV can result from a number of factors, including slow intravascular or in-plane flow or complex blood flow patterns. Flow parallel to the plane of acquisition (in-plane flow) can cause signal loss on MR venography and is most prominent in vertically oriented structures, such as the distal sigmoid sinus. Use of inferior

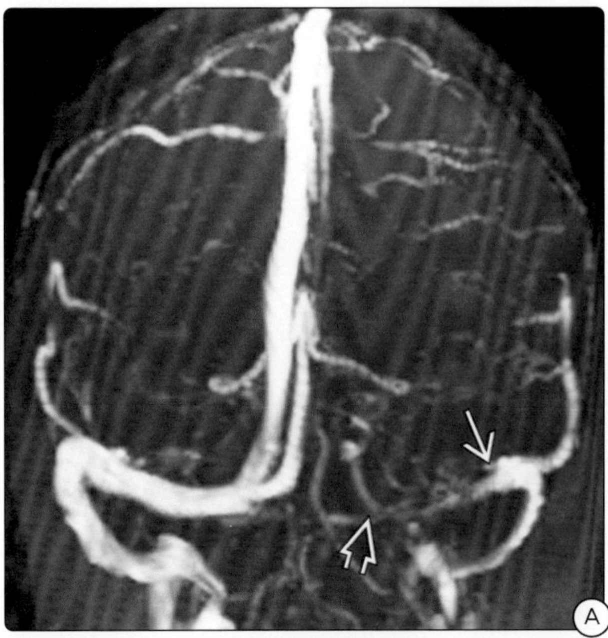

*(9-61A) MR venogram in a 22-yo woman shows a dominant right TS. The left TS shows a "missing" segment ➡ and possible filling defect ➡.*

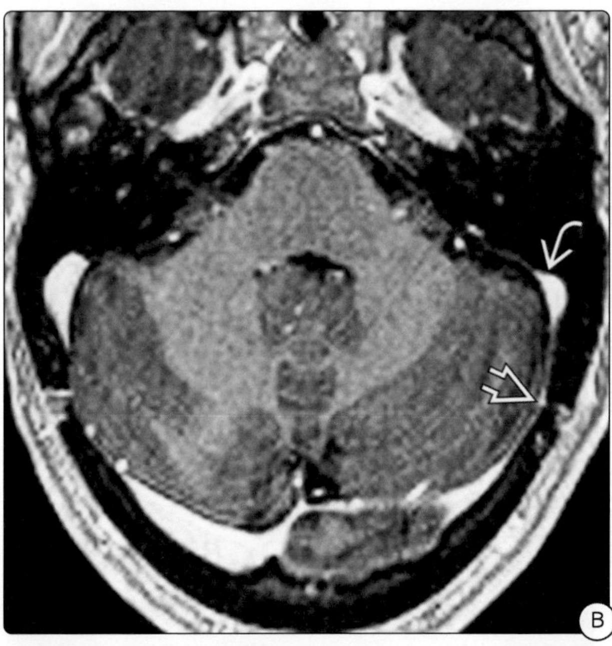

*(9-61B) Axial MP-RAGE shows hypoplastic but patent left TS ➡ and a small sigmoid sinus ➡.*

saturation pulses with axial 2D TOF MRV can saturate flow in parts of the curving SSS but can be avoided by imaging in the coronal plane.

## Arachnoid Granulations and Septations

Another key differential diagnosis of DST is **giant AG**. Giant AGs are round or ovoid short-segment filling defects that exhibit CSF-like attenuation on NECT and do not enhance on CECT scans.

MR appearance of AGs is more problematic than its CT findings. Giant AGs often do not follow CSF signal intensity (SI) on all sequences. CSF-incongruent SI is seen on at least one sequence (usually FLAIR) in 80% of MRs. Even large AGs do not fill the entire sinus, as most thrombi do, and, unlike clots, may show central linear enhancement. Brain tissue may **herniate** into the dural venous sinuses, often part of a complex giant AG **(9-62)**.

**Septations** or **trabeculations** are fibrotic bands looking like linear filling defects in dural venous sinuses. Between 1-5 septa are in 30% of TSs, most often the right TS.

## Physiologic Hyperdensity

On NECT scans, all dural venous sinuses normally appear mildly hyperdense compared to adjacent brain and CSF. This appearance can be accentuated by relatively decreased attenuation in the adjacent brain (e.g., edema or, in the case of neonates and infants, physiologic polycythemia and immature myelination, respectively).

Elevated hematocrit (physiologic, e.g., high altitude, or polycythemic) can also cause this appearance. When in doubt, compare density in the dural venous sinus to the ICA. Dural venous sinus density should be ≤ 70 HU.

Dehydration and hypovolemia, "low flow" states (e.g., shock, cardiac failure), and some hemoglobinopathies (e.g., sickle cell disease, thalassemia) may all cause equally increased density in dural venous sinuses and intracranial arteries.

### DURAL VENOUS THROMBOSIS MIMICS

**Sinus Variants**
- Small/hypoplastic transverse sinus
  - "Flow gaps" common in MRV

**Flow Artifacts**
- "Flow gaps" common on 2D TOF MRV
- Imaging in coronal plane helpful

**Arachnoid Granulations and Septations**
- Common
- Round/ovoid, short segment
- "Giant" AGs often do not follow CSF on MR
- May contain brain tissue

**Physiologic Hyperdensity**
- Intracranial arteries, veins normally hyperdense relative to brain
- Dural sinuses should be ≤ 70 HU
- High altitude, dehydration, polycythemia
- Low-density brain (edema, immature myelination)

*Selected References: The complete reference list is available on the eBooks+ version included with purchase.*

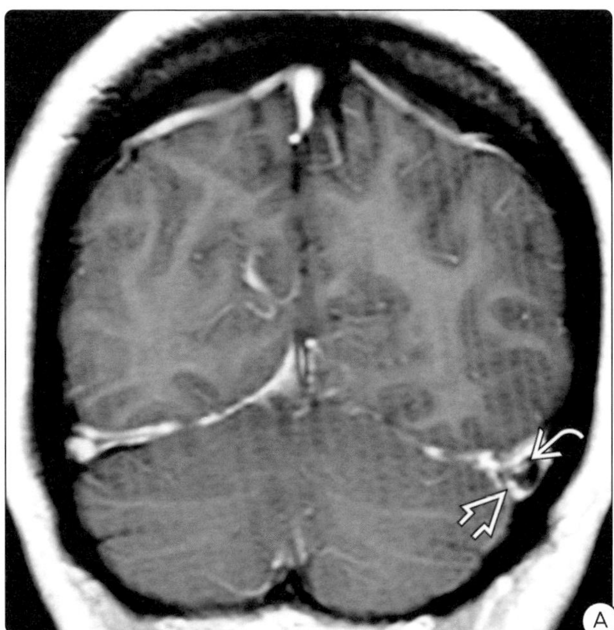


***(9-62A)** Coronal T1 C+ MR in a 23-yo woman shows a large, hypointense filling defect in the left TS. Note linear enhancement within the well-delineated, ovoid, CSF-like lesion. Is this a thrombus or normal variant?*

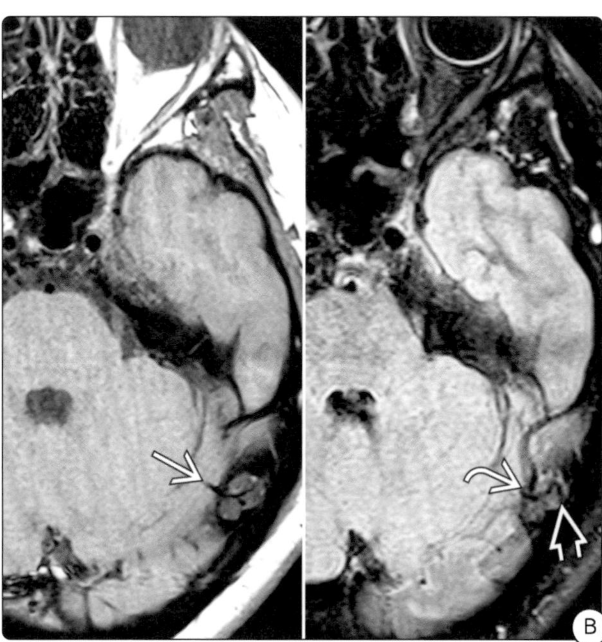


***(9-62B)** (L) T1 MR shows a Y-shaped "flow void" entering the lesion. (R) FLAIR MR shows the signal in giant AG is isointense with brain and does not suppress. Note "flow voids" within AG. This is a normal variant, not thrombus.*

# Vasculopathy

*The generic term "vasculopathy" literally means blood vessel pathology—of any kind, in any vessel (artery, capillary, or vein). Evaluating the craniocervical vessels for vasculopathy is one of the major indications for neuroimaging. Large vessel atherosclerotic vascular disease is the single most prevalent vasculopathy in the head and neck, whereas carotid stenosis or embolization from atherosclerotic vascular disease plaques are the most common causes of ischemic strokes.*



In this chapter, we discuss diseases of the craniocervical arteries, first laying a foundation with normal anatomy. We then review atherosclerosis, starting with a general discussion of atherogenesis. Extracranial atherosclerotic vascular disease (ASVD) and carotid stenosis are followed by a brief overview of intracranial large and medium artery ASVD. We conclude the discussion with arteriolosclerosis, the most common brain "microvascular disease."

The broad spectrum of nonatheromatous vasculopathy is then addressed. Finally, we devote the last section of this chapter to non-ASVD diseases of the cerebral macro- and microvasculature. While arteriolosclerosis is by far the most common cause of small vessel vascular disease, nonatherogenic microvasculopathies, such as amyloid angiopathy, can have devastating clinical consequences.

## Normal Anatomy of Extracranial Vessels

### Aortic Arch and Great Vessels

The aorta has four major segments: The ascending aorta, transverse aorta [primarily consisting of the aortic arch (AA)], aortic isthmus, and descending aorta.

#### Aortic Arch

The **AA** lies in the superior mediastinum. It begins at the level of the second right sternocostal articulation. It then curves backward and to the left over the pulmonary hilum. The AA has two curves, one convex upward anterior to posterior and another that is right to left in the superior mediastinum.

The AA is anatomically related to a number of important structures. The cervical sympathetic plexus branches and left vagus nerve, CNX, lie in front of the AA. The trachea, left recurrent laryngeal nerve, esophagus, thoracic

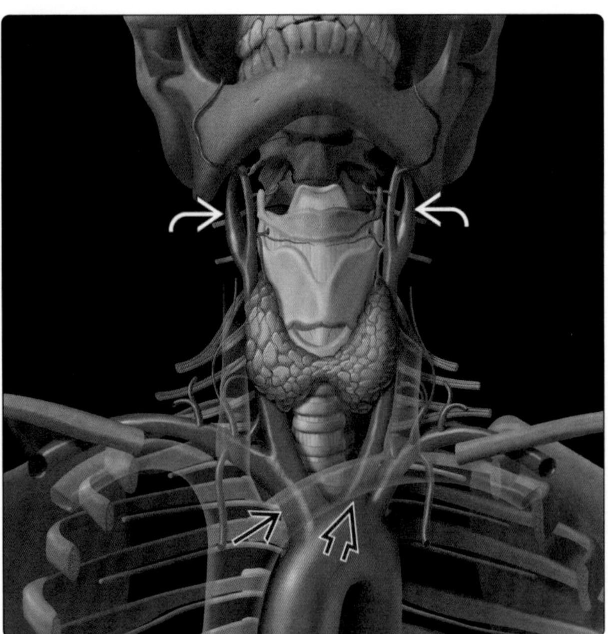

***(10-1)** AP graphic shows the normal aortic arch, its relationship to adjacent structures. The right CCA arises from the BCT ➡, while the left CCA ➡ arises from arch. CCA bifurcations are at ~ C3-C4 with ICAs ➡ lateral to ECAs.*

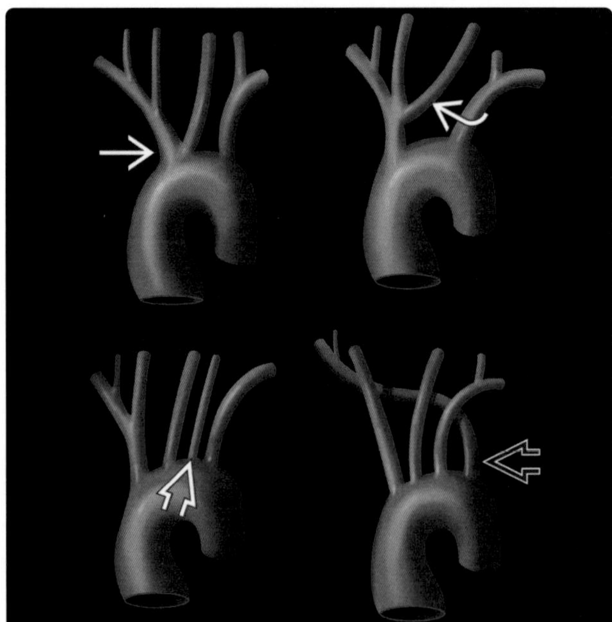

***(10-2)** Four arch variants: BCT & right ICA arise from a V-shaped common origin ➡; left ICA arises from BCT ➡; left VA arises directly from arch ➡; aberrant right subclavian arises from arch as 4th great vessel ➡.*

duct, and vertebral column lie behind the arch. The great vessels lie above the AA, as does the left brachiocephalic vein. The pulmonary bifurcation, ligamentum arteriosum, and left recurrent laryngeal nerve lie below the arch.

### Great Vessels

Three major vessels arise from the AA. From right to left, there are the **brachiocephalic trunk** (BCT), the **left common carotid artery** (CCA), and the **left subclavian artery** (SCA) **(10-1)**. The BCT, a.k.a. the **innominate artery**, is the first and largest branch of the AA. It bifurcates into the **right SCA** and the **right CCA**.

The major branches of the right SCA are the right **internal mammary** (thoracic) artery, right **vertebral artery** (VA), right **thyrocervical trunk**, and right **costocervical trunk**. The right CCA bifurcates into its two terminal branches, the right **internal carotid artery** (ICA) and the right **external carotid artery** (ECA).

The **left CCA** arises from the AA just distal to the BCT origin. The left CCA bifurcates in the left ICA and left ECA near the upper border of the thyroid cartilage. The left CCA lies anterior and medial to the internal jugular vein.

The left SCA arises from the AA distal to the left CCA origin. It ascends into the neck, lateral to the medial border of the anterior scalene muscle. The major branches are the left **internal mammary** (thoracic) artery, the left **VA**, left **thyrocervical trunk** and the left **costocervical trunk**.

### Normal Variants

The "classic" AA has the **three** "great vessel" branching pattern, which is present in 80% of patients **(10-1)**. Normal variants are seen in ~ 20% of patients. In 10-25% of cases, the left CCA shares a common V-shaped origin with the BCT. This is sometimes called a bovine configuration, which is a misnomer. The left CCA arises from the proximal BCT in 5-7% of cases. The left CCA and left SCA share a common origin, a left BCT, in 1-2% of cases. Finally, the left VA arises directly from AA in 0.5-1% of cases **(10-2)**.

## Cervical Carotid Arteries

The CCAs and their branches provide the major blood supply of much of the neck, all of the face, and the entire brain. The right CCA arises at the sternoclavicular level. The left CCA originates from the AA and ascends in front of and then lateral to the trachea. The CCAs course superiorly in the carotid space, anteromedial to the internal jugular vein. The CCA bifurcations are typically at C3-C4 or C4-C5.

### Internal Carotid Artery

The cervical ICA is entirely extracranial and is designated as the C1 segment. In 90% of cases, the cervical ICA arises from the CCA posterolateral to the ECA.

The C1 has two parts, the carotid bulb and the ascending segment. The **carotid bulb** is the most proximal aspect of the cervical ICA and is seen as a focal dilatation with a cross-sectional area nearly twice as large as that of the distal ICA. Flow reversal occurs in carotid bulb normally. The **ascending ICA** segment courses cephalad in the carotid space, a fascially defined tubular sheath that contains all three layers of deep cervical fascia. The cervical ICA has no normal branches in the neck. It enters the carotid canal at the skull base in the petrous temporal bone.

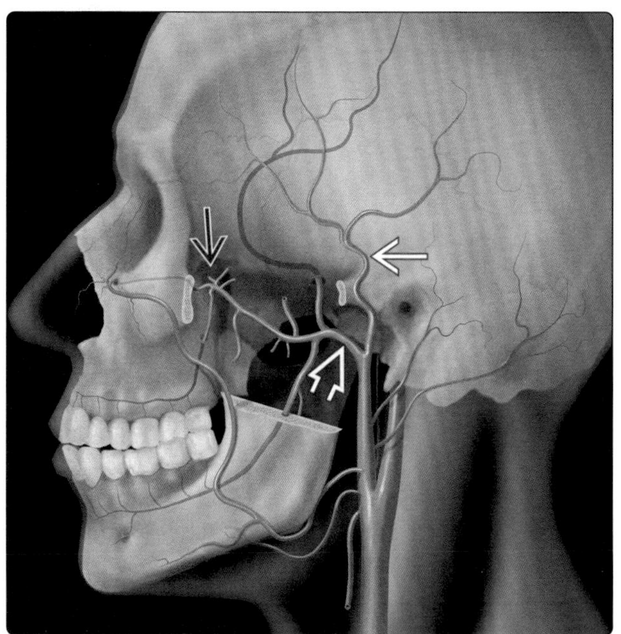

***(10-3)** Graphic shows the ECA branches, including its 2 terminal branches: The superficial temporal ➡ & maxillary arteries ➡. The maxillary artery divides into its distal branches in the pterygopalatine fossa ➡.*

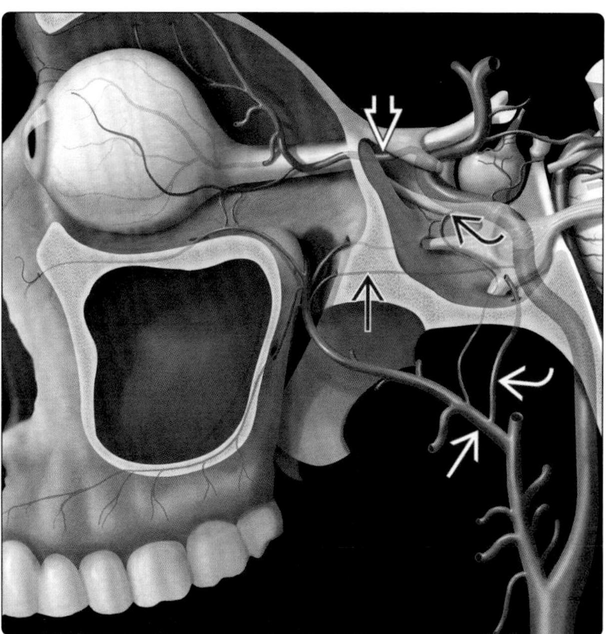

***(10-4)** Anastomoses between ECA & ICA branches. ECA, orbital & cavernous branches of ICA provide potential sources for collateral blood flow. Maxillary a. ➡, middle meningeal a. ➡, inferolateral trunk ➡, vidian a. ➡, ophthalmic a. ➡.*

## External Carotid Artery

Each ECA has eight major branches **(10-3)** and is smaller and lies medial to the ICA. The first ECA branch is usually the **superior thyroid artery**, which may also arise from the CCA bifurcation. The superior thyroid artery arises anteriorly from the ECA and courses inferiorly to supply the superior thyroid and larynx. The **ascending pharyngeal artery** arises posteriorly from the ECA (or CCA bifurcation) and courses superiorly between the ECA and ICA to supply the nasopharynx and oropharynx, middle ear, eustachian tube dura, and CNIX-XI.

The **lingual artery** is the third ECA branch. It loops anterior and inferiorly, then courses superiorly to supply the tongue, oral cavity, and submandibular gland. The **facial artery** arises just above the lingual artery, curving around the mandible before it passes anterior and superiorly to supply the face, palate, lips, and cheek.

The **occipital artery** originates from the posterior aspect of the ECA and courses posterosuperiorly between the occiput and C1. It supplies the scalp, upper cervical musculature, and posterior fossa meninges. The occipital artery has extensive anastomoses with muscular VA branches.

The **posterior auricular artery** arises from the posterior ECA above the occipital artery. It courses superiorly to supply the pinna, scalp, external auditory canal, and chorda tympani. The **superficial temporal artery (STA)** is the smaller of the two terminal ECA branches. It runs superiorly behind the mandibular condyle, across the zygoma. It supplies the scalp and gives off the transverse facial artery.

The **maxillary artery** is the larger of the two terminal ECA branches. The maxillary artery arises within the parotid gland, behind the mandibular neck. It gives off the **middle meningeal artery**, which supplies the cranial meninges and runs anteromedially in the masticator space. Within the pterygopalatine fossa, it sends off terminal branches to the deep face and nose.

Numerous **anastomotic channels** exist between nearly all of the extracranial branches of the ECA (except the superior thyroid and lingual arteries) and the intracranial branches of the ICAs or musculospinal branches of the VAs **(10-4)**. These anastomoses both provide an important pathway for collateral blood flow and pose a potential risk for intracranial embolization during neurointerventional procedures.

The major anastomoses include the ascending pharyngeal artery with the middle/accessory meningeal artery and caroticotympanic artery. The facial artery has anastomoses with the ophthalmic artery (ICA branch) and other ECA branches. The occipital artery has extensive anastomoses with muscular VA branches. The maxillary artery has anastomoses with the inferolateral trunk of the cavernous ICA, the ophthalmic artery, vidian artery, and the recurrent meningeal arteries.

# Atherosclerosis

**Atherosclerotic vascular disease** (ASVD) is by far the most common cause of mortality and severe long-term disability in industrialized countries, so it is difficult to overemphasize its importance. It affects all arteries, of all sizes, in all parts of the body.

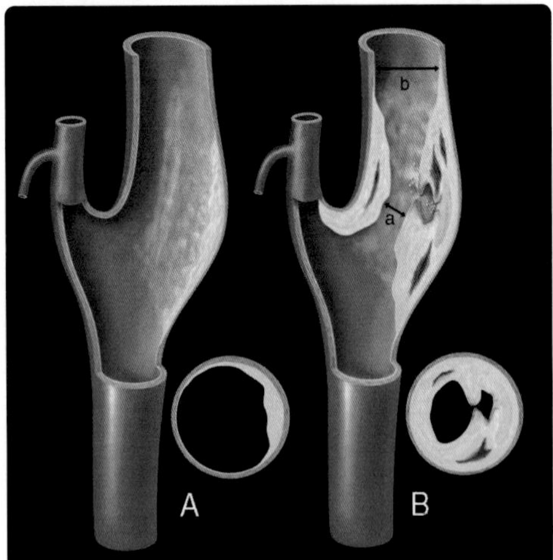


***(10-5)** (A) Mild ASVD with "fatty streaks." (B) Severe ASVD; percent of stenosis = (b - a)/b x 100; b = normal lumen, a = residual lumen diameter.*

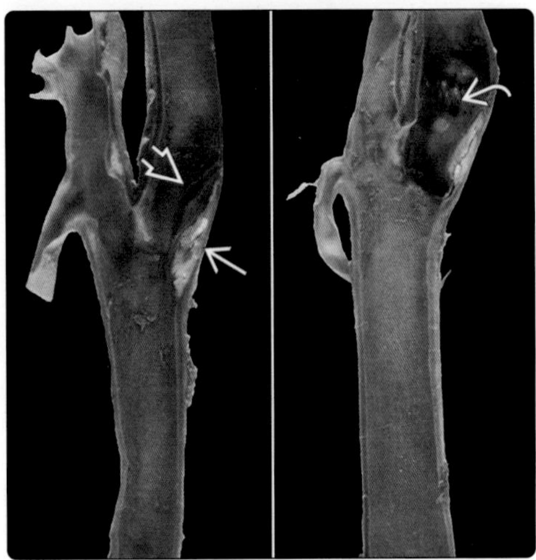

***(10-6)** (L) Stable ASVD shows fatty plaque ➡, intact intima ➡. (R) Initially "at-risk" plaque now shows ulceration ➡, disrupted intima.*

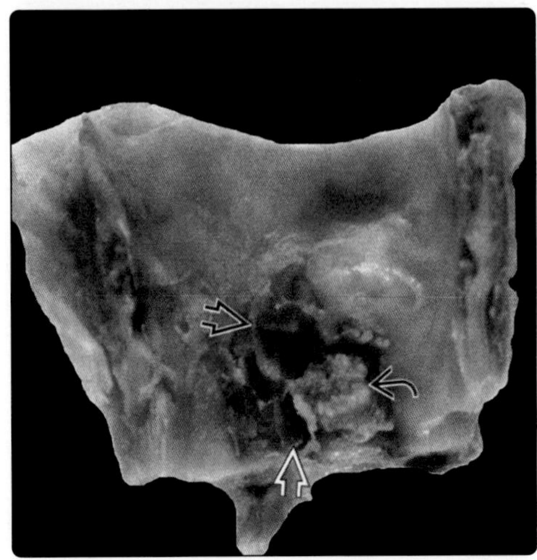

***(10-7)** Carotid endarterectomy shows ulcerated intima ➡, calcification ➡, IPH ➡. (Courtesy J. Townsend, MD.)*

The principal cause of cerebral infarction is atherosclerosis and its sequelae. Over 90% of large cerebral infarcts are caused by thromboemboli secondary to ASVD. We begin with extracranial ASVD before concluding with a brief discussion of the clinical and imaging manifestations of intracranial ASVD, including its microvascular manifestations.

## Atherogenesis and Atherosclerosis

### Terminology

The term "atherosclerosis" was originally coined to describe progressive "hardening" or "sclerosis" of blood vessels. The term "atheroma" (Greek for "porridge") designates the material deposited on or within vessel walls. "Plaque" is used to describe a focal atheroma together with its epiphenomena, such as ulceration, platelet aggregation, and hemorrhage.

**Atherogenesis** is the degenerative process that results in atherosclerosis. **Atherosclerosis** is the most common pathologic process affecting large elastic arteries (e.g., the aorta) and medium-sized muscular arteries (e.g., the carotid arteries and VAs). **Arteriolosclerosis** describes the effects of atherogenesis on smaller arteries (and is treated separately at the end of this section). **ASVD** is the generic term describing atherosclerosis in any artery, of any size, in any area of the body.

### Etiology

**General Concepts.** Plasma lipids, connective tissue fibers, and inflammatory cells accumulate at susceptible sites in arterial walls, forming focal atherosclerotic plaques. Angiogenic factors cause vasa vasorum proliferation, formation of immature vessels, and loss of capillary basement membranes. Neoangiogenesis is closely associated with plaque progression and is likely the primary source of intraplaque hemorrhage.

### Pathology

**Location.** ASVD occurs preferentially at highly predictable locations. In the extracranial vasculature, the most common sites are the proximal ICAs and CCA bifurcations, followed by the AA and great vessel origins.

**Size and Number.** ASVD plaques vary in size from small, almost microscopic lipid deposits to large, raised, fungating, ulcerating lesions that can extend over several centimeters and dramatically narrow the parent vessel lumen. Multiple lesions in multiple locations are common.

**Gross Pathology.** ASVD plaques develop in stages **(10-5)**. The first detectable lesion is lipid deposition in the intima, seen as yellowish "fatty streaks." Other than "fatty streaks" and slightly eccentric but smooth intimal thickening, visible changes at this early stage are minimal.

**Microscopic Features.** ASVD plaques are classified histopathologically as "stable," "vulnerable," or "ulcerated."

***Stable Plaques.*** Uncomplicated **stable plaques**—the basic lesions of atherosclerosis—consist of cellular material, lipid, and an overlying fibrous cap. The intima covering a stable plaque is thickened, but its exterior surface remains intact. No ulceration or intraplaque hemorrhage is present **(10-6)**.

***Vulnerable Plaques.*** As a necrotic core of lipid-laden foam cells, cellular debris, and cholesterol gradually accumulates under the elevated fibrous cap, the cap thins and becomes prone to rupture **("vulnerable" plaque) (10-6)**.

Proliferating small blood vessels also develop around the periphery of the necrotic core. **Neovascularization** can lead to **subintimal**

**hemorrhage**, which enlarges the necrotic core, further weakening the overlying fibrous cap.

***Ulcerated Plaques.*** Plaque **ulceration** occurs when the fibrous cap weakens and ruptures through the intima, releasing necrotic debris **(10-7)** **(10-8)**. Plates and fibrin aggregate within the ulcerated denuded endothelium. These aggregates can be pulled into the rapidly flowing main artery slipstream, causing arterioarterial embolization to distal intracranial vessels.

## Clinical Issues

**Epidemiology and Demographics.** Most patients with symptomatic lesions are middle-aged or older adults. However, atherosclerosis is increasingly common in younger patients, contributing to the rising prevalence of strokes in patients < 45 years old.

**Presentation.** Many ASVD lesions remain asymptomatic until they cause hemodynamically significant stenosis or thromboembolic disease. Transient ischemic attacks (TIAs) and "silent strokes" are common precursors of large territorial infarcts.

**Natural History.** The natural history of ASVD is also highly variable. ICA occlusion poses an especially high risk for eventual stroke with > 70% of these patients eventually experiencing ischemic cerebral infarction.

**Treatment Options.** Treatment options include prevention, medical therapy (lipid-lowering regimens), and surgery or endovascular therapy.

# Extracranial Atherosclerosis

Extracranial ASVD is the single largest risk factor for stroke. That risk starts with the AA, an underrecognized source of intracranial ischemic strokes. Complete imaging evaluation of patients with thromboembolic infarcts in the brain should include investigation of the AA.

## Aortic Arch/Great Vessels

Aortic ASVD is more common in the descending thoracic aorta than in the ascending aorta or arch **(10-8)**. However, late diastolic retrograde flow from complex plaques in the proximal descending aorta distal to the left SCA origin can reach all supraaortic arteries. Retrograde flow extends to the left SCA orifice in nearly 60% of cases, the left CCA in 25%, and the BCT in 10-15%.

Aortic emboli involve the left brain in 80% of cases and show a distinct predilection for the vertebrobasilar circulation. This striking geographic distribution is consistent with thromboemboli arising from ulcerated plaques in the descending aorta that are then swept by retrograde flow into left-sided arch vessels.

## Carotid Bifurcation/Cervical Internal Carotid Arteries

Between 20-30% of all ischemic infarcts are caused by carotid artery stenosis. Therefore, determining the degree of carotid stenosis on imaging studies is now both routine and required.

Using data from the North American Symptomatic Carotid Endarterectomy Trial (NASCET), carotid stenosis is classified as moderate (50-69%), severe (70-93%), and "preocclusive" or critical (94-99%) **(10-9)**. Patients with critical stenosis are at high risk for embolic stroke as long as the ICA lumen is patent.

In addition to stenosis degree, several recent studies have demonstrated the importance of also assessing the morphologic features of ASVD plaques. Rupture of an "at-risk" plaque with a large, necrotic core under a thin, fibrous

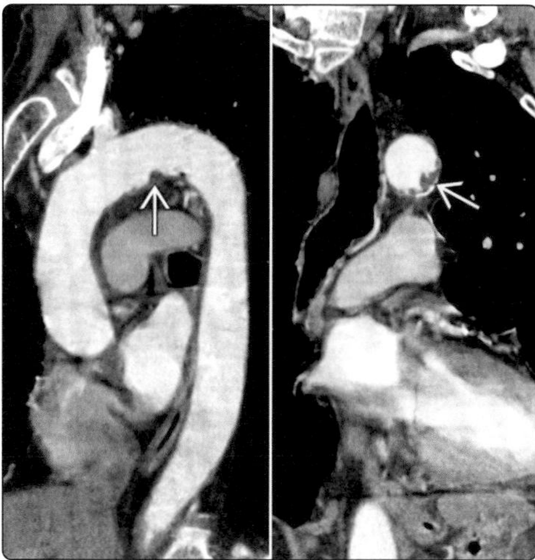

***(10-8)** Oblique, coronal views show ulcerated atherosclerotic plaque ➡ along lesser curvature of the aortic arch. (Courtesy G. Oliveira, MD.)*

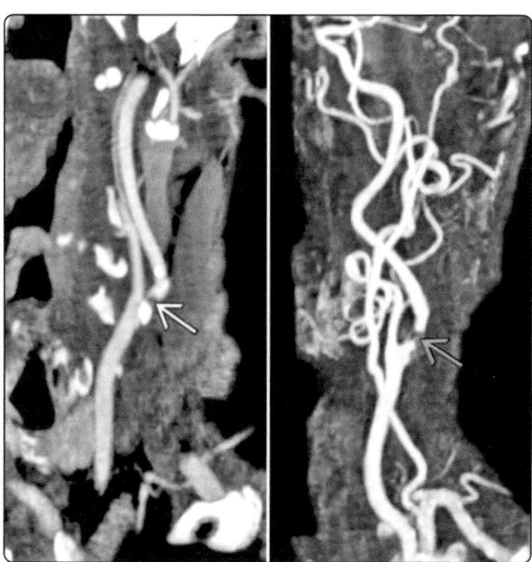

***(10-9)** (L) CTA ➡ & (R) MRA show critical ICA stenosis with a "flow gap" ⇨, characteristic of a high-grade, flow-limiting lesion.*

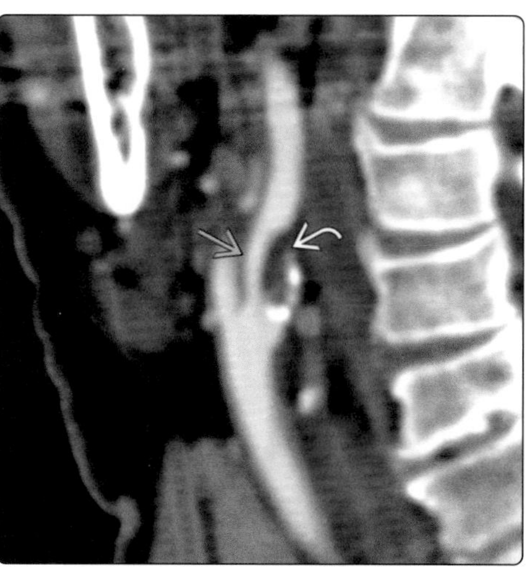

***(10-10)** Sagittal CTA reformatted image in a 62-yo with acute stroke shows ICA stenosis ⇨ related to soft & calcified plaque ⮌.*

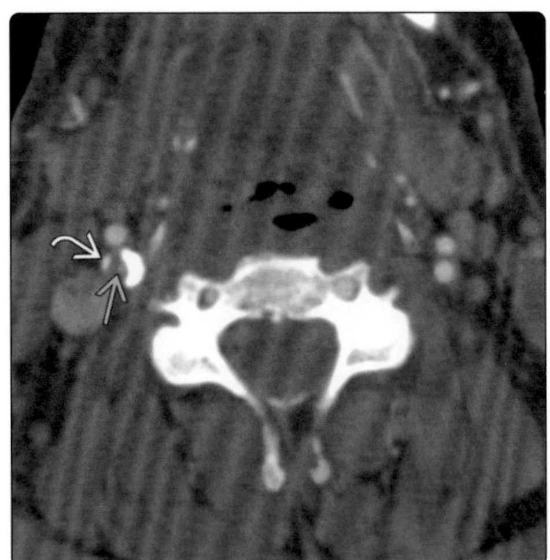

***(10-11) Axial CTA shows severe ICA stenosis ⇨ with calcified & soft ASVD plaque. CT rim sign ➡ suggests IPH.***

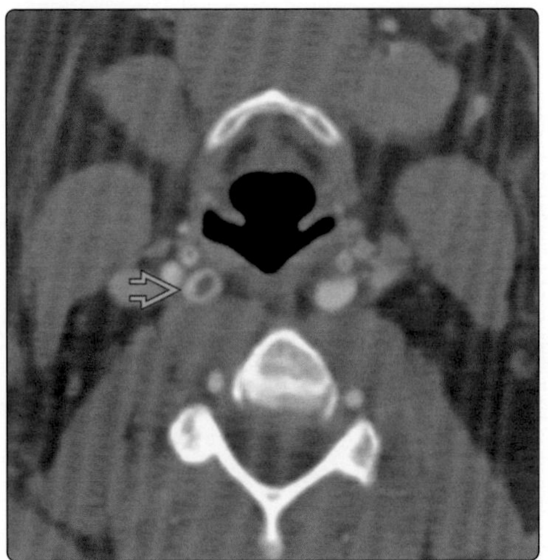

***(10-12) Axial CTA in a young adult with stroke shows a classic intraluminal thrombus ⇨ in the right ICA, a doughnut sign.***

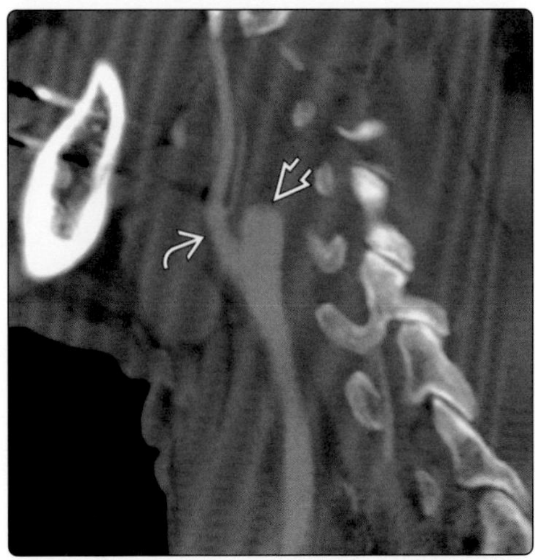

***(10-13) Sagittal CTA in an acute stroke patient shows carotid occlusion ➡ as the carotid bulb ending blindly in a rounded pouch. ECA ➡.***

cap is responsible for the majority of acute thrombi. As distal embolization from proximal ASVD-related clots is a common cause of cerebral ischemia/infarction, *identifying rupture-prone "vulnerable" plaques is at least as important as determining stenosis!*

**CT Findings.** The most common imaging findings in extracranial ASVD are mural calcifications, luminal irregularities, varying degrees of vessel stenosis, occlusion, and thrombosis **(10-10)**. Elongation, ectasia, and vessel tortuosity can occur with or without other changes of ASVD.

NECT scans easily show vessel wall calcifications. Large atherosclerotic plaques may demonstrate one or more subintimal low-density foci. These represent the lipid-rich core of a "soft" plaque. High-density subintimal foci indicate intraplaque hemorrhage. Both findings carry increased risk of plaque rupture and concomitant distal embolization.

CTA source images display the carotid lumen in cross section **(10-11)**. CTA is as accurate as DSA for ICA stenosis measurements. Smooth luminal narrowing is the most common finding in ASVD. The percent of stenosis is typically measured with NASCET criteria. However, there are also single-diameter thresholds for CTA: 2.2 mm (50% stenosis) and 1.3 mm (70% stenosis). Ulcerations—seen as irregularly shaped contrast-filled outpouchings from the lumen—are detected with 95% sensitivity and 99% specificity. Intraluminal thrombi are also readily demonstrated (doughnut sign) **(10-12)**. Carotid occlusion is seen as contrast ending blindly in a blunted, rounded, or pointed pouch in the proximal ICA **(10-13)**.

In addition to calculating percentage of stenosis **(10-5)**, plaque morphologic characteristics should be described in detail, as stenosis alone does not define complete stroke risk in symptomatic patients. Intraplaque hemorrhage has been identified as an independent risk factor for ischemic stroke at *all* degrees of stenosis, including symptomatic patients with low-grade lesions (< 50%). CTA rim sign of adventitial calcification with internal soft plaque is highly predictive of carotid intraplaque hemorrhage. Therefore, accurate characterization of plaque morphology is important for patient management.

**MR Findings.** High-resolution MR imaging can be used to characterize carotid plaques, allowing identification of individual plaque components, including lipids, hemorrhage, fibrous tissue, and calcification.

High signal intensity on T1-weighted fat-suppressed scans, MRA source images, or MP-RAGE sequences represents hemorrhage into complicated "vulnerable" atherosclerotic plaques, not lipid accumulation **(10-14)**. Unlike intraparenchymal brain bleeds, plaque hemorrhages may remain hyperintense for up to 18 months. Vulnerable plaques are usually hyperintense on T2WI, whereas stable plaques are isointense on both T1- and T2WI.

T1 C+ FS scans may show enhancement around plaque margins, consistent with neovascularity in a vulnerable "at-risk" plaque.

Contrast-enhanced or unenhanced 2D TOF MRA is 80-85% sensitive and 95% specific for the detection of ICA > 70% ICA stenosis. Signal loss with a "flow gap" occurs if the stenosis is > 95%. Compared with CTA and DSA, MRA tends to overestimate the degree of stenosis.

## Vertebral Arteries

ASVD in the extracranial VAs accounts for up to 20% of all posterior circulation ischemic strokes. Although mid- and distal cervical segment lesions occur, extracranial ASVD is most common at or near the VA origin **(10-15)**.

A special type of VA pathology is called **subclavian steal**. Here, the SCA or BCT is severely stenotic or occluded *proximal* to the VA origin. Flow reversal in the affected VA occurs as blood is recruited (i.e., "stolen") from the opposite VA, crosses the basilar artery (BA) junction, and flows in retrograde fashion down the VA into the SCA to supply the shoulder and arm distal to the stenosis/occlusion **(10-16)**.

Noninvasive imaging of subclavian steal can be problematic. Because superior saturation bands are applied in 2D TOF MRA, reversed flow direction in a VA can mimic occlusion. Standard TOF MRA alone may not be adequate to differentiate *reversed* flow from *absent* flow, so confirmation and quantification with additional imaging is usually required.

## Differential Diagnosis

The major differential diagnoses of extracranial ASVD include dissection, dissecting aneurysm, vasospasm, and fibromuscular dysplasia (FMD). All usually spare the carotid bulb.

**Dissection** (either traumatic or spontaneous) is more common in young/middle-aged patients and occurs in the *middle* of extracranial vessels. Extracranial dissections typically terminate at the exocranial opening of the carotid canal. Most are smooth or display minimal irregularities, whereas calcifications and ulcerations—common in carotid plaques—are absent.

Midsegment vessel narrowing with a focal mass-like outpouching of the lumen is typical of **dissecting aneurysm**. **Vasospasm** is more common in the intracranial vessels. When it involves the cervical carotid arteries or VAs, it also typically spares the proximal segments.

**FMD** spares the carotid bulb and usually affects the middle or distal aspects of the extracranial carotid arteries and VAs. A

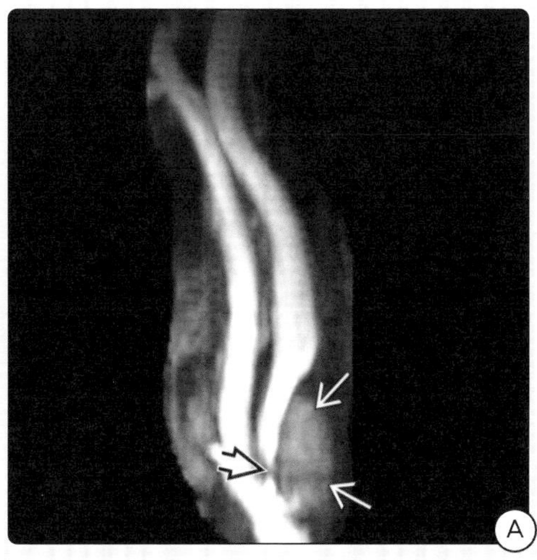


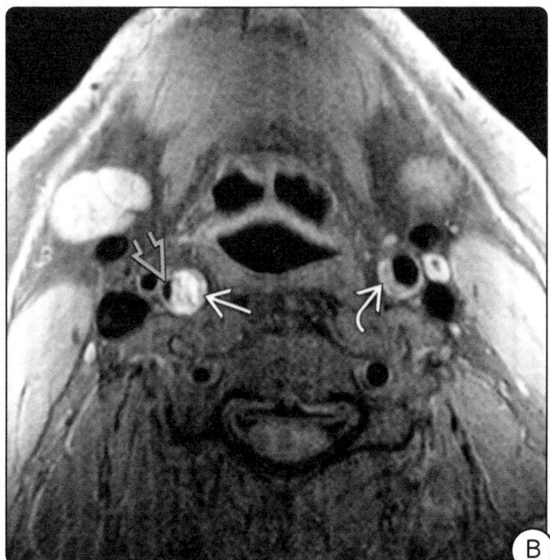


***(10-14A)** Oblique 3T MRA in a patient with an acute stroke shows very high-grade (> 95%) stenosis of the right carotid artery with a "flow gap" ⇨ caused by a large ASVD plaque ➡. **(10-14B)** MP-RAGE shows IPH ➡ as T1 hyperintensity with tiny residual lumen ⇨ in the right ICA, subintimal hemorrhage ➦ in the left ICA. Note hemorrhage is brighter than muscle. IPH is an independent stroke risk factor.*

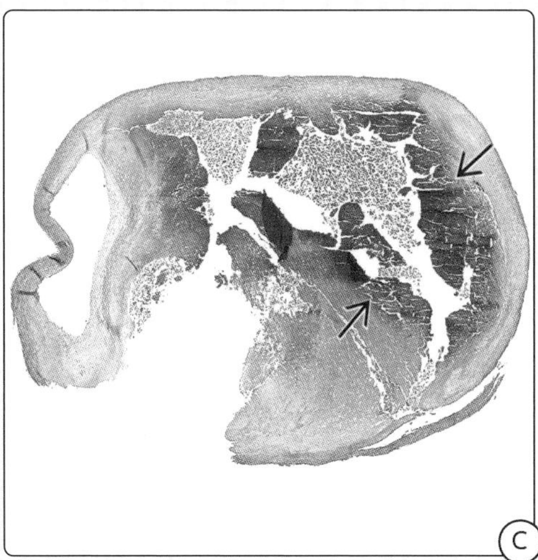


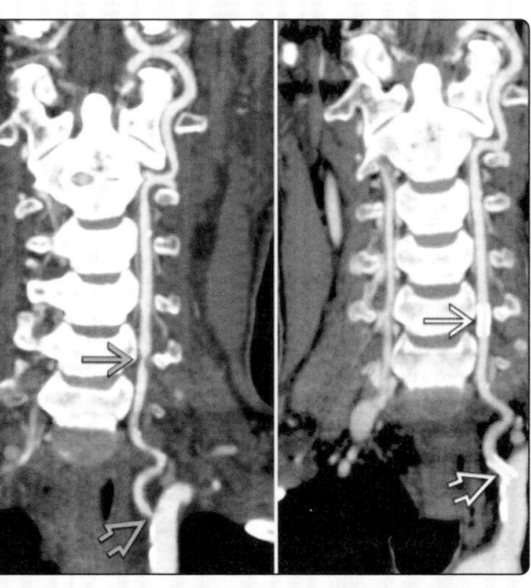

***(10-14C)** Right ICA endarterectomy specimen shows that plaque hyperintensity is due to acute hemorrhage ➡, not lipid. (Courtesy S. McNally, MD, PhD.) **(10-15)** CTA shows severe vertebral artery origin ASVD stenosis ⇨ & moderate midcervical stenosis ⇨. Right CTA shows poststent placement at the origin ➡ & midcervical VA ➡. Extracranial VA ASVD is commonly at or near the VA origin. (Courtesy C. Baccin, MD.)*

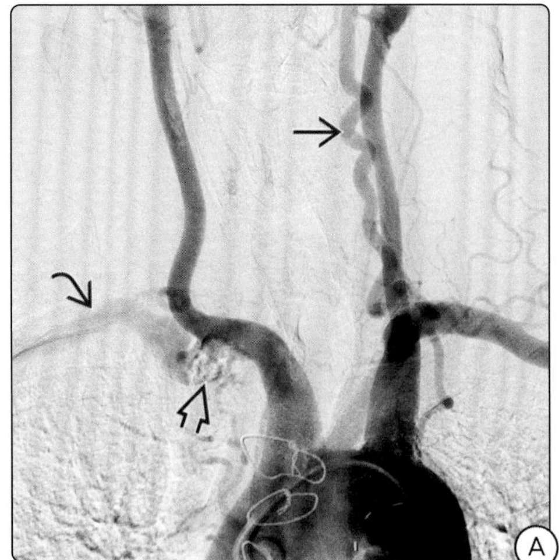


***(10-16A)** DSA shows calcification, faint contrast in distal SCA. The right VA is unopacified. Left VA is enlarged & tortuous.*

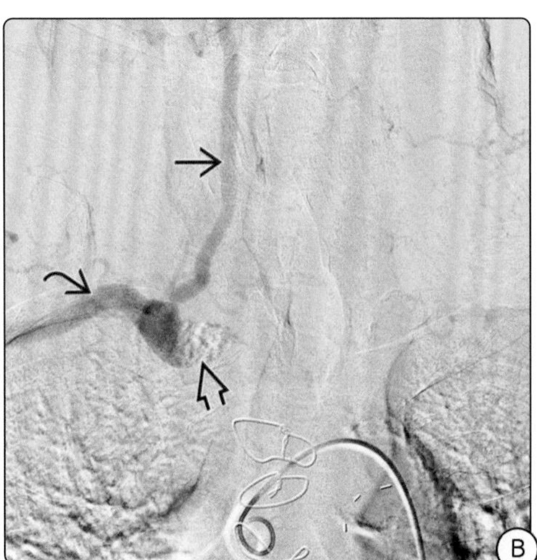


***(10-16B)** Retrograde filling of right VA & SCA distal to calcification & high-grade stenosis shows classic subclavian steal.*

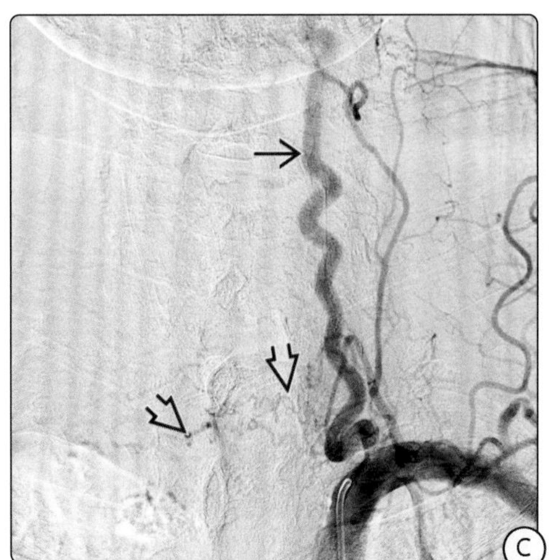


***(10-16C)** Left SCA angiogram shows prominent VA & muscular branches collateralizing to the right SCA vascular distribution.*

string of beads appearance is typical. Long-segment tubular narrowing is less common and may reflect coexisting dissection.

**EXTRACRANIAL ATHEROSCLEROSIS**

**Etiology**
- Multifactorial, progressive disease
- Plasma lipids accumulate in susceptible sites
- Lipids incite inflammatory response

**Pathology**
- Predictable locations
  - Carotid bifurcation, proximal ICA (carotid bulb)
  - Aortic arch, great vessel origins
- 1st sign = "fatty streaks," intimal thickening
- Stable plaque
  - Subintimal smooth muscle cells, macrophages accumulate
  - Fibrous cap formed under intact intima
- "Vulnerable" plaque
  - Necrotic core of cellular debris, cholesterol ± calcifications
  - Plaque thins, becomes prone to rupture
  - Neovascularization, subintimal hemorrhage
- Ulcerated plaque
  - Fibrous cap ruptures through intima
  - Denuded intima → platelet, fibrin aggregates
  - May embolize to intracranial circulation

**Clinical Issues**
- Identifiable risk factors in patients with ischemic stroke
  - Older age (> 60 years)
  - Diabetes mellitus
  - Elevated LDL
  - Hypertension
  - ± history of heart disease

## Intracranial Atherosclerosis

One of the most serious and disabling manifestations of ASVD is stroke. Most acute ischemic strokes are thromboembolic, most often secondary to cardiac sources or plaques in the cervical ICA.

Many clinicians focus on extracranial carotid artery disease, considering intracranial ASVD a relatively infrequent cause of stroke. However, intracranial ASVD accounts for 5-10% of all ischemic strokes. Nearly 1/2 of all patients with fatal cerebral infarction have at least one intracranial plaque-associated luminal stenosis at autopsy **(10-17)**.

### Ectasia

Generalized nonfocal vessel elongation is called "ectasia," "dolichoectasia," "arteriectasis," or "dilative arteriopathy." Ectasias can involve any part of the intracranial circulation but are most common in the vertebrobasilar arteries ("vertebrobasilar dolichoectasia") and supraclinoid ICA.

### Atherosclerotic Fusiform Aneurysm

Atherosclerotic fusiform aneurysms (FAs) are focal arterial enlargements that are usually superimposed on an ectatic artery. ASVD FAs were discussed in detail in Chapter 6. ASVD FAs are most common in the vertebrobasilar circulation. When they occur in the anterior circulation, they can produce a rare but dramatic manifestation called a giant "serpentine" aneurysm.

## Intracranial Stenoocclusive Disease

Atherosclerosis that causes large artery intracranial occlusive disease (LAICOD) is now a well-defined yet relatively neglected and poorly understood stroke subtype. Recent studies have shown that the overall prevalence of intracranial ASVD in patients with concurrent extracranial disease varies between 20-50%, and 12% of patients have diffuse (multifocal) intracranial ASVD **(10-20)**.

Overall, symptomatic patients with moderate to severe stenosis (i.e., 70-99%) in the intracranial circulation have a 25% two-year risk for recurrent stroke.

The availability of endovascular techniques, such as intracranial angioplasty, has opened new treatment avenues for LAICOD. A variety of balloon-expandable, drug-eluting, and self-expanding stents are also now available as options.

**Imaging.** Mural calcifications are common on NECT with patterns varying from scattered stippled foci to thick continuous linear ("railroad track") deposits. CTA or DSA may show solitary or multifocal stenoses alternating with areas of poststenotic dilatation **(10-19)**. When ASVD affects distal branches of the major intracranial vessels, the appearance can mimic that of vasculitis (see below).

High-resolution "black blood" vessel wall imaging on MR directly depicts intracranial ASVD and is a reliable tool for identifying intracranial ASVD and measuring plaque burden **(10-18)**. Intramural hemorrhage and irregular, noncircumferential short-segment enhancing foci are common findings.

### INTRACRANIAL ATHEROSCLEROSIS

**Epidemiology**
- Found in 1/3 of patients in population-based imaging studies
  - Causes 8-10% of strokes in USA, Europe
  - > 50% in Asia

**Clinical Issues**
- Moderate/severe stenosis → 25% 2-year stroke risk

**Imaging**
- Mural calcifications
- Irregular narrowing ± ulcerations
- Deep watershed ischemia, lacunae
- High-resolution vessel wall imaging
  - Wall hemorrhage
  - Enhancement irregular, short segment, noncircumferential

**Differential Diagnosis.** The major differential diagnoses of intracranial ASVD are vasculitis, vasospasm, and dissection.

**Vasculitis** occurs at all ages but is more common in middle-aged patients. Vasculitis and ASVD appear virtually identical on angiography (MRA, CTA, or DSA). Remember: The most common cause of a vasculitis-like pattern in an older patient is not vasculitis; it is ASVD!

**Vasospasm** spares the cavernous ICA and is usually more diffuse than ASVD. A history of trauma, subarachnoid hemorrhage (SAH), or drug abuse (typically with sympathomimetics) is common. **Intracranial dissection**—especially in the anterior circulation—is rare and usually occurs in young patients.

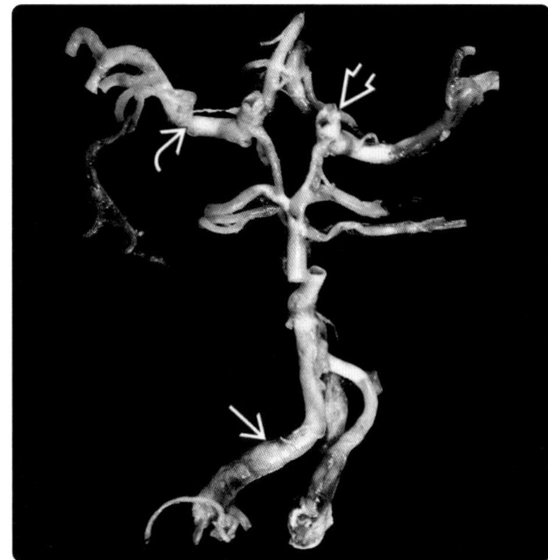

***(10-17)** Intracranial ASVD. Most severe disease is in the vertebrobasilar system ➡, ICAs ➡, & proximal MCAs ➡. (Courtesy R. Hewlett, MD.)*

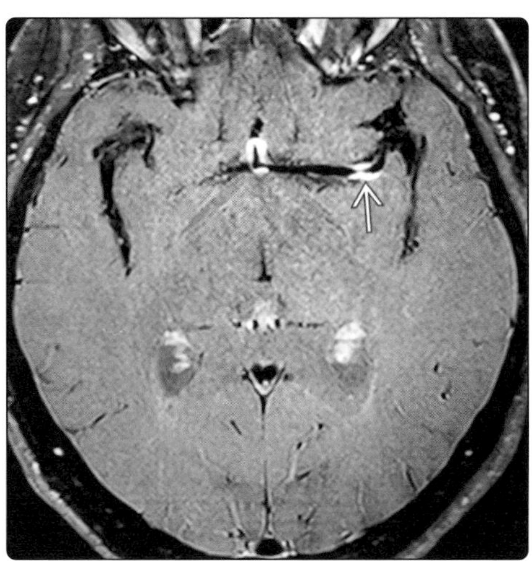

***(10-18)** T1 C+ "black blood" vessel wall imaging in a patient with cryptogenic stroke shows stenosis, enhancement around distal M1 MCA ➡.*

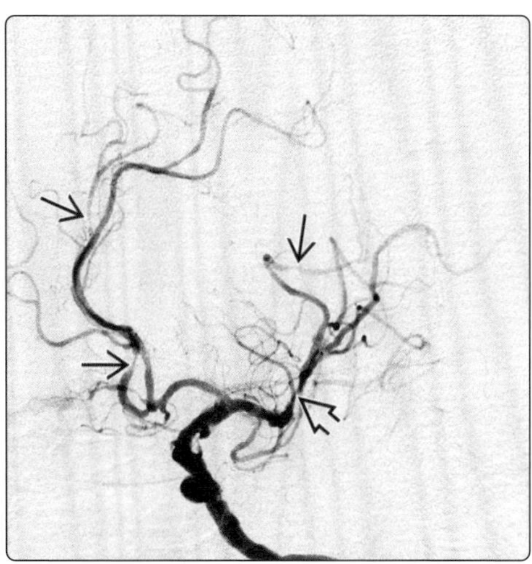

***(10-19)** DSA in a patient with deep watershed infarcts shows severe ASVD ➡. High-grade stenosis ➡ of the M2 MCA is present.*

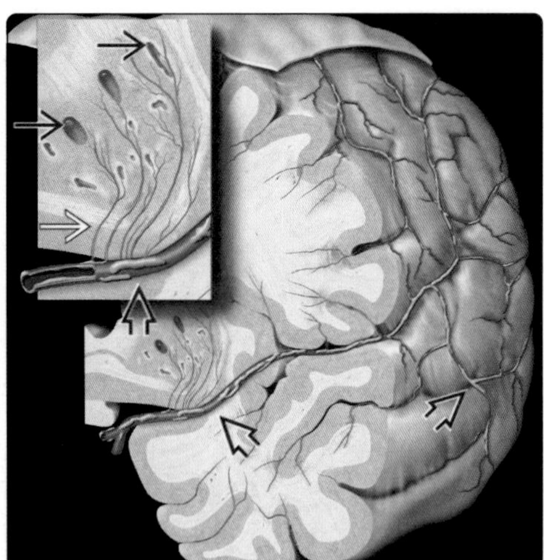

*(10-20) ASVD involves the MCA ➲ & its branches, including penetrating (lenticulostriate) arteries ➡. Note lacunar infarcts ➲.*

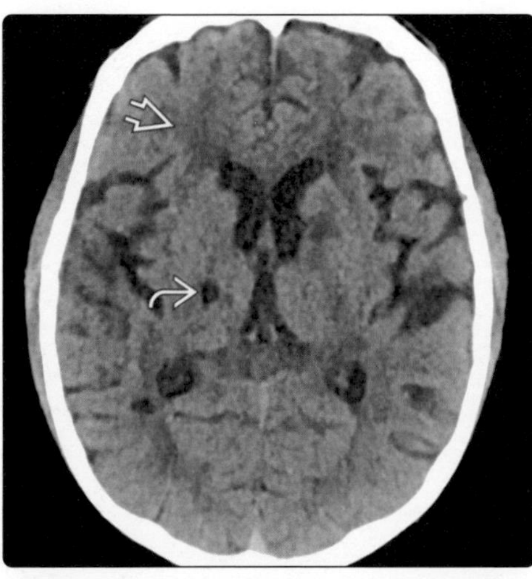

*(10-21) NECT in chronic hypertension shows confluent ➡ hypodensities in the subcortical & deep periventricular WM & lacunar infarcts ➡.*

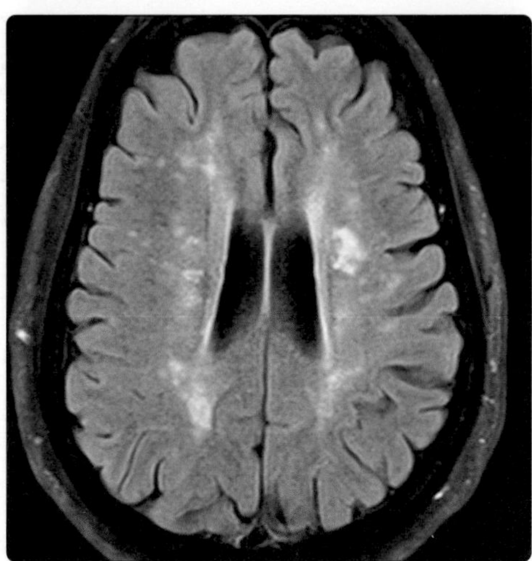

*(10-22) Axial FLAIR MR shows hyperintensities with cortical sparing, typical of "microvascular disease" (arteriolosclerosis & lipohyalinosis).*

## Arteriolosclerosis

Arteriolosclerosis, also known less specifically as cerebral "microvascular disease," is a microangiopathy that typically affects small arteries (i.e., arterioles), especially in the subcortical and deep cerebral white matter (WM). Aging, chronic hypertension, hypercholesterolemia, and diabetes mellitus are the most common factors that predispose to cerebral microvascular disease.

### Pathology

Generalized volume loss, multiple lacunar infarcts, and deep WM spongiosis are typical. Stenosis or occlusion of small vessels by arteriolosclerosis and lipohyalinosis probably results in WM microinfarctions.

### Imaging

CT scans show patchy &/or confluent subcortical and deep WM hypodensities **(10-21)**. Periventricular lesions have a broad or confluent base with the ventricular surface and are especially prominent around the atria of the lateral ventricles.

MR shows patchy or confluent periventricular and subcortical WM hypointensities on T1WI. The lesions are hyperintense on T2WI and are especially prominent on FLAIR **(10-22)**. T2* (GRE, SWI) sequences often demonstrate multifocal "blooming" hypointensities, especially in the presence of chronic hypertension.

### Differential Diagnosis

The major differential diagnosis is **age-related hyperintensities** in the periventricular WM. Scattered T2/FLAIR WM hyperintensities are almost universal after age 65. **Enlarged perivascular (Virchow-Robin) spaces** (PVSs) can be seen in patients of all ages and in virtually all locations, although they do increase with age. Unlike arteriolosclerosis, PVSs suppress on FLAIR.

**Demyelinating disease** typically causes ovoid or triangular periventricular lesions that abut the callososeptal interfaces, which are rarely involved by arteriolosclerosis.

# Nonatheromatous Vascular Diseases

Although atherosclerotic vascular disease (ASVD) is by far the most common disease to affect the craniocervical vasculature, a number of other nonatheromatous disorders can affect the brain, causing stroke or stroke-like symptoms. In this section, we briefly discuss some of the most important entities, including fibromuscular dysplasia (FMD), vasculitis, and non-ASVD noninflammatory vasculopathies, such as cerebral amyloid disease.

## Fibromuscular Dysplasia

### Terminology

FMD is an uncommon segmental nonatherosclerotic, noninflammatory disease of unknown etiology. FMD is a polyvascular disease that affects medium and large arteries in many areas of the body.

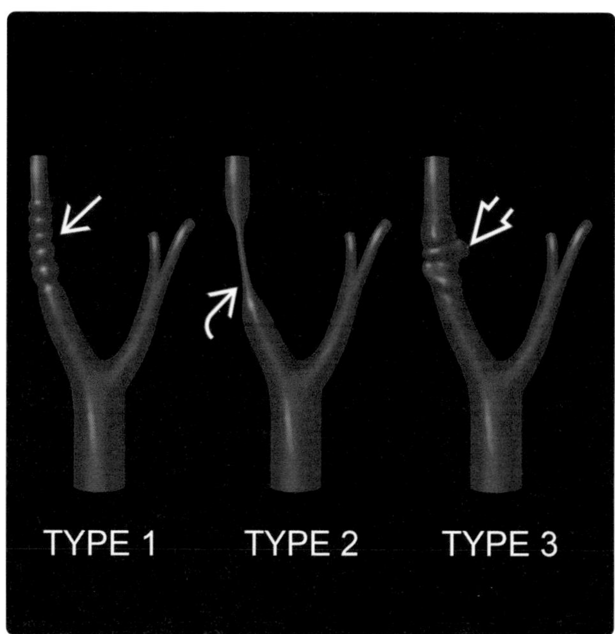


*(10-23) Carotid bifurcation shows the classic subtypes of fibromuscular dysplasia (FMD): Type 1 FMD (80-90% of patients) = "string of beads" or "corrugated" ➡, type 2 as tubular stenosis ➡, type 3 as focal corrugations ± diverticulum ➡.*

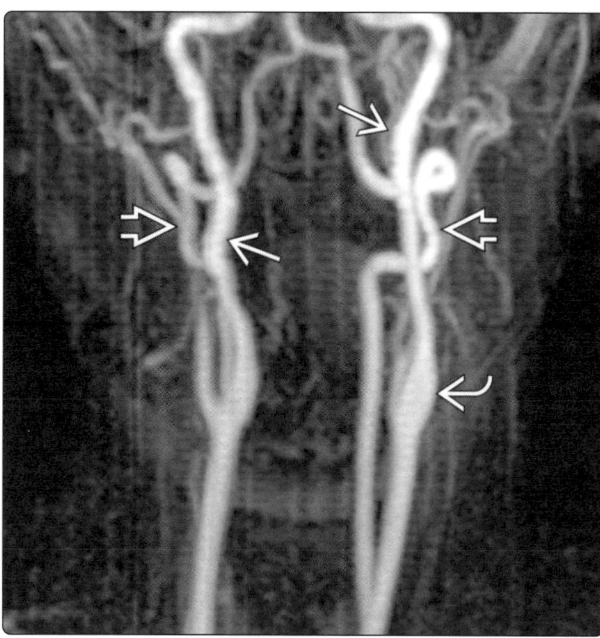

*(10-24) Coronal MR MIP image shows type 1 FMD in bilateral cervical ICAs ➡ with sparing of the carotid bulbs ➡. Subtle FMD is also noted in the VAs ➡. These patients are at high risk for dissection & aneurysms.*

## Pathology

**Location.** Although virtually any artery in any location can be affected, FMD affects some arteries far more than others. The renal arteries are affected in 75% of cases; ~ 35% of these are bilateral. Patients with known renal artery FMD often have cerebrovascular disease (and vice versa).

The cervicocephalic vessels are involved in up to 75% of cases. The ICA is the most common site; FMD typically involves the middle of the ICA and spares the bifurcation. VA FMD is seen in 20% of cases. Approximately 1/2 of all cervicocephalic FMD cases involve more than one artery (usually either both ICAs or one ICA and one VA). Intracranial FMD is very rare.

Multiple arterial systems are involved in 25-30% of cases. When multisystem disease is present, the renal arteries are almost always involved.

FMD carries an increased risk of developing intracranial saccular aneurysms. Intracranial saccular aneurysms are present in ~ 7-10% of patients with cervical FMD.

**Staging, Grading, and Classification.** FMD is classified histologically into three categories according to which arterial wall layer is affected (media, intima, or adventitia) **(10-23)**.

By far, the most common type **(type 1)** is **medial fibroplasia**, accounting for ~ 60-85% of all FMD cases. The media has alternating thin and very thick areas formed by concentric rings of extensive fibrous proliferations and smooth muscle hyperplasia.

**Intimal fibroplasia (type 2)** accounts for < 10% of FMD cases. The intima is markedly thickened, causing smooth, long-segment narrowing.

**Adventitial (periarterial) fibroplasia (type 3)** is the least common type of FMD, accounting for < 5% of cases. Dense collagen replaces the delicate fibrous tissue of the adventitia and may infiltrate the adjacent periarterial tissues.

## Clinical Issues

**Epidemiology.** Once thought to be a relatively rare vasculopathy, overall prevalence of FMD is estimated between 4-6% in the renal arteries and 0.3-3.0% in the cervicocephalic arteries. FMD is identified in 0.5% of all patients screened with CTA for ischemic neurologic symptoms.

FMD primarily affects individuals between 20-60 years of age. Sex disparity in FMD is striking with a 9:1 female predominance.

**Presentation.** Sudden onset of high blood pressure in a young woman is a classic presentation of renal FMD. FMD is found in ~ 1% of hypertensive patients and is the second leading cause of renovascular hypertension (after ASVD).

Cervical FMD can present with headache, pulsatile tinnitus/bruit, dizziness, neck pain, TIA, stroke, or dissection (often with Horner syndrome, i.e., ptosis, pupil constriction, and facial anhidrosis). Between 5-6% of patients are asymptomatic at the time of diagnosis.

**Natural History.** The natural history of FMD is unclear, as many cases are now discovered incidentally on imaging studies. Overall, 1 in 5 patients with FMD will have dissections and 1 in 5 patients will have aneurysms.

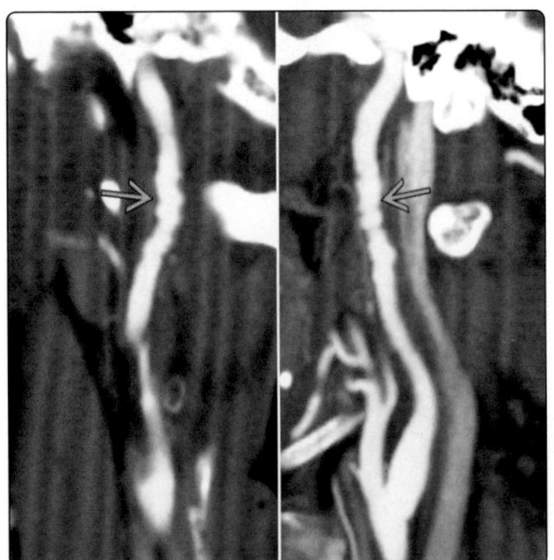

*(10-25) CTA images show the classic "string of beads" ⮕ of type 1 FMD involving the cervical ICAs.*

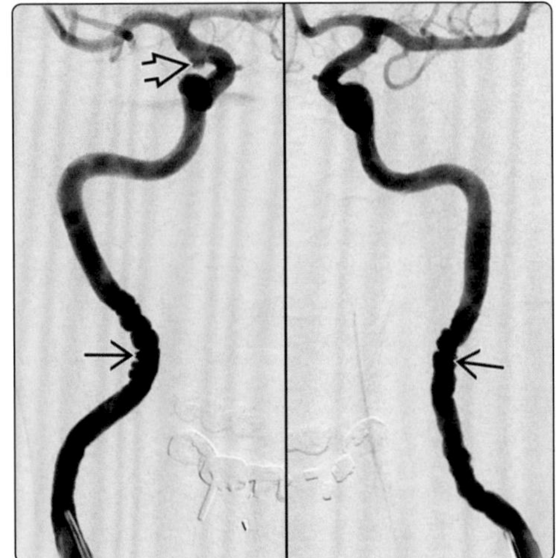

*(10-26) DSA shows type 1 FMD in midcervical segments ⮕ & small unruptured saccular aneurysm ⮕ of the right supraclinoid ICA.*

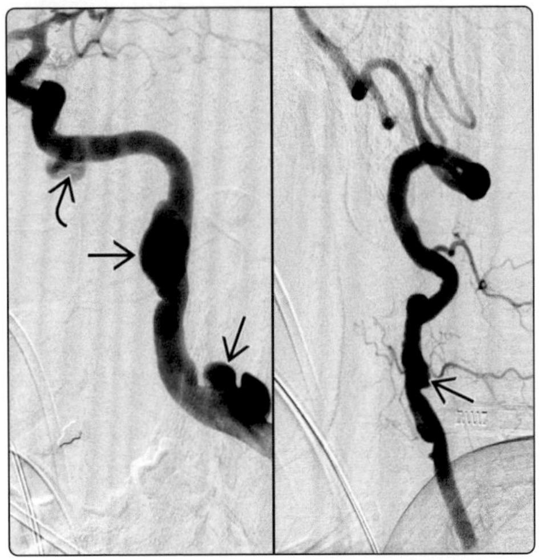

*(10-27) (L) DSA of ICA, (R) VA with type 3 FMD show diverticulum-like outpouchings ⮕ & saccular aneurysm ⮕.*

## Imaging

**Technical Considerations.** CTA is noninvasive and accurately depicts FMD in the cervicocephalic arteries **(10-25)**. Visualization of the intracranial vessels should be included to detect the presence of associated aneurysms. TOF MRA can be problematic, as artifacts caused by patient motion or in-plane flow and susceptibility gradients can mimic the appearance of FMD.

Because multisystem disease is common, patients with newly diagnosed carotid &/or vertebral FMD should also have their renal arteries examined. The prevalence of renal FMD is 40-45% in patients with cephalocervical disease.

**Imaging Findings.** Type 1 FMD (medial fibroplasia) is seen as an irregular corrugated or string of beads appearance with alternating areas of constriction and dilatation **(10-24)** **(10-26)**. In type 2 (intimal fibroplasia), a smooth, long-segment tubular narrowing is present. In type 3 (adventitial) FMD, asymmetric diverticulum-like outpouchings from one side of the artery are present **(10-27)**.

All three cervical FMD subtypes spare the carotid bifurcations and great vessel origins, involve the middle segments, and are most common at the C1-C2 level. Complications of cervicocephalic FMD include dissection, intracranial aneurysm with or without SAH **(10-27)**, and arteriovenous fistulas. Other less common manifestations of FMD include vascular loops and fusiform vascular ectasias.

## Differential Diagnosis

The major differential diagnosis of FMD is **atherosclerosis**. FMD is most common in young women, a group that is generally at low risk for ASVD. FMD involves the middle to distal portions of the affected arteries, sparing the carotid bifurcation. Atherosclerosis is typically short-segment stenosis at or above the carotid bifurcation with mural calcifications.

**Arterial standing waves** are a form of transient vasospasm that can be misinterpreted as type 1 FMD on catheter angiograms. The regular corrugated appearance contrasts with the irregular "string of beads" of FMD **(10-33)**. Standing waves resolve spontaneously on repeat angiography (including CTA or MRA) or after the administration of vasodilators.

The smooth, tapered "tubular" narrowing of type 2 (intimal FMD) can be difficult to distinguish from **spontaneous dissection**, which also occurs as a complication of FMD. The asymmetric, diverticulum-like outpouchings sometimes seen in FMD can mimic **traumatic cervical pseudoaneurysms**.

Other **nonatherosclerotic vasculopathies**, such as Takayasu arteritis and giant cell arteritis, can mimic tubular (i.e., intimal) FMD.

**FIBROMUSCULAR DYSPLASIA**

**Pathology**
- Nonatherosclerotic, noninflammatory arteriopathy
- 10% familial
- Commonly affects medium-sized/large arteries
  - Renal: 75%
  - Cervical arteries: 75%
  - ICA: 50%
  - VA: 20-25%
  - Multiple vessels: 50%
  - Intracranial very rare
- Classified by affected arterial wall layer
  - Type 1: Medial fibroplasia
  - Type 2: Intimal fibroplasia
  - Type 3: Adventitial (periarterial) fibroplasia

**Clinical Issues**
- Any age
  - But 20-60 years most common
- F:M = 9:1
- Presentation
  - Can be asymptomatic, incidental (0.5% of cervical CTAs)
  - Most common = renovascular hypertension
  - Headache, pulsatile tinnitus
  - Neck pain, Horner syndrome
  - Stroke
- Natural history
  - 1 in 5 patients will have dissection
  - 1 in 5 patients will develop saccular aneurysm

**Imaging**
- Midsegments of cervical ICA, VA affected
- Spares carotid bulbs, artery origins
- Usually terminates before entering skull base
- Appearance
  - String of beads (type 1): 60-85%
  - Smooth, long-segment narrowing (type 2): 10%
  - Adventitial (periarterial narrowing): ≤ 5%

**Differential Diagnosis**
- Atherosclerosis
  - Involves bulb > midsegment
- Arterial "standing waves"
  - Type of vasospasm occurs with catheter angiograms
- Dissection (can occur with FMD)

## Dissection

Craniocervical arterial dissection (CAD) is strongly associated with ischemic events, primarily artery-to-artery embolism, so early diagnosis and appropriate treatment are essential.

### Terminology

A **dissection** is a tear in at least one layer of the vessel wall that permits blood to penetrate into and delaminate (split apart or "dissect") wall layers **(10-28)**.

A **dissecting aneurysm** is a dissection characterized by an outpouching that extends beyond the vessel wall. Most occur with subadventitial dissections and are more accurately designated as **pseudoaneurysms** (i.e., they lack all normal vessel wall components).

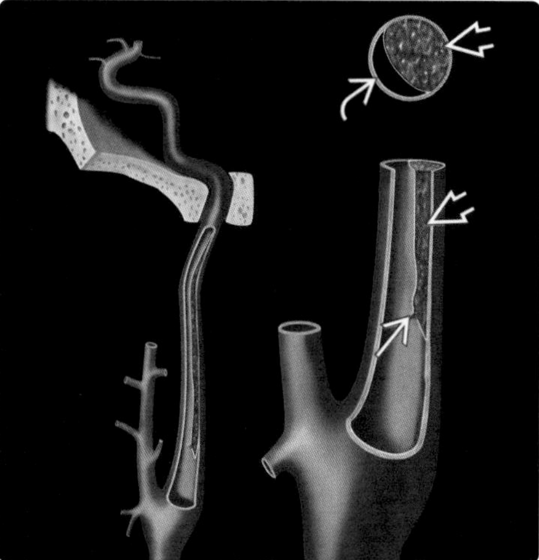

***(10-28)** Extracranial ICA dissection shows intimal tear ➡ & subintimal thrombus ➡ compressing residual lumen ➡. Bulb is spared.*

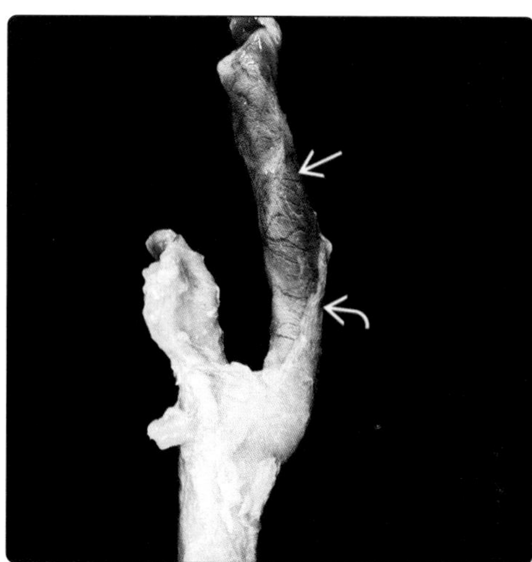

***(10-29)** Extracranial ICA dissection shows extensive mural thrombus ➡. Dissection begins ➡ distal to the bulb. (Courtesy R. Hewlett, MD.)*

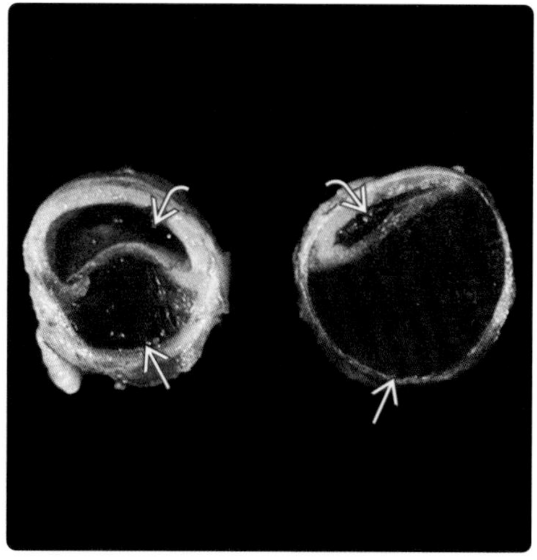

***(10-30)** Axial sections show carotid dissection with subintimal hematoma ➡, compressed residual lumen ➡. (Courtesy R. Hewlett, MD.)*

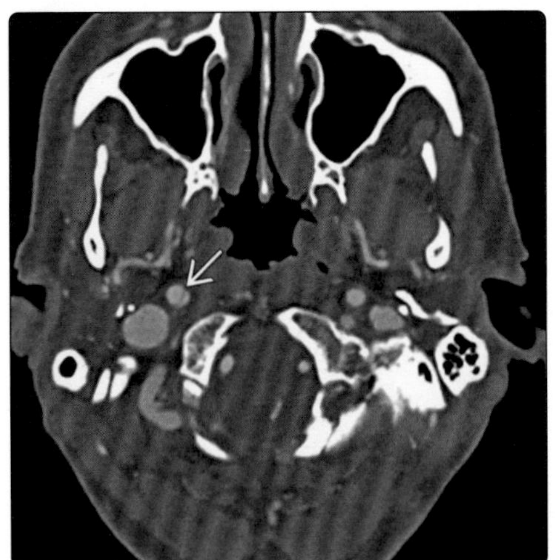

***(10-31)** Axial CTA in a 54-yo trauma patient with FMD shows an acute ICA dissection flap ➡. FMD increases dissection risk.*

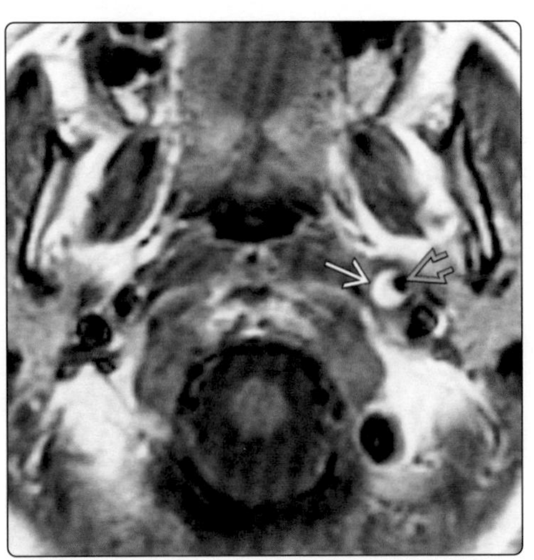

***(10-32)** Axial T1 MR shows subacute subintimal hematoma, crescent-like hyperintensity ➡ around narrow "flow void" ➡ of midcervical ICA.*

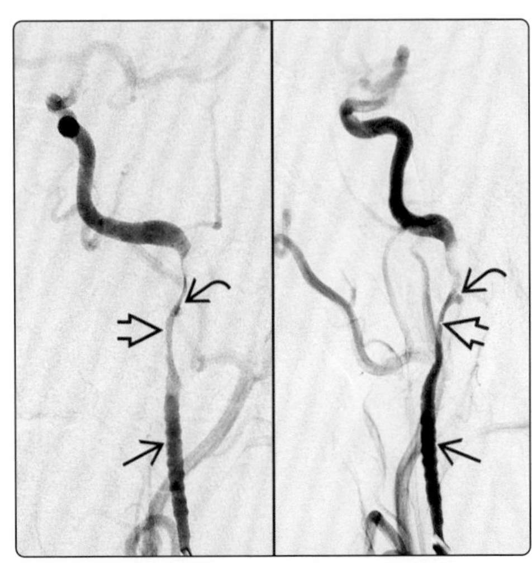

***(10-33)** (L) AP, (R) lateral DSA show cervical ICA dissection ➡ to skull base, pseudoaneurysm ➡, arterial "standing waves" ➡.*

## Etiology

Extracranial CAD is more common than intracranial dissection. Almost 60% of *extracranial* dissections are "spontaneous," i.e., nontraumatic. Most have an underlying vasculopathy, such as FMD, Marfan syndrome, or other connective tissue disorder (e.g., Ehlers-Danlos type 4) **(10-34)**. Less common predisposing conditions include hypertension, migraine headaches, vigorous physical activity, hyperhomocysteinemia, and recent pharyngeal infection.

Traumatic extracranial dissections occur with blunt or penetrating injury, but sports (e.g., wrestling) or chiropractic manipulations have also been implicated **(10-31)** **(10-35)**.

*Intracranial* dissections can be either traumatic or spontaneous. Iatrogenic dissections (typically secondary to endovascular procedures) are becoming increasingly common.

## Pathology

**Location.** Extracranial dissections typically occur in the most mobile segment of a vessel, often starting or ending where the vessel transitions from a relatively free position to a position fixed by an encasing bony canal. The extracranial ICA is the most common overall site in the head and neck. Extracranial ICA dissections spare the carotid bulb and often extend up to—but only occasionally into—the skull base **(10-33)**. Vertebral dissections are most common between the skull base and C1 and between C1 and C2 **(10-36)**.

The most frequently involved intracranial site is the VA. Dissections in the anterior circulation are even less common. They almost always involve the supraclinoid ICA with or without extension into the proximal middle cerebral artery (MCA).

**Size and Number.** Dissections can be limited to a focal intimal tear and small subintimal hematoma. Most are solitary, long-segment lesions that extend for several centimeters. Approximately 20% involve two or more vessels. Multiple dissections are more common if an underlying vasculopathy, such as Marfan, Ehlers-Danlos type 4, or FMD, is present **(10-34)**.

**Gross Pathology.** An intimal tear permits dissection of blood into the vessel wall, resulting in a medial or subendothelial hematoma that may narrow or occlude the vessel lumen **(10-30)**. Occasionally, dissections—especially in the VA—extend through the adventitia and present with SAH.

## Clinical Issues

**Epidemiology and Demographics.** CAD is the most common cause of ischemic stroke in young and middle-aged adults **(10-35)**. Peak age is 40 years.

**Presentation.** Neck pain and headache are the most common symptoms. One or more lower cranial nerve palsies, including postganglionic Horner syndrome, may occur.

**Natural History.** The natural history of most *extracranial* CADs is benign. Approximately 90% of stenoses resolve and 60% of all occlusions recanalize. Recurrent dissection is rare. *Intracranial* CAD is much more problematic. Stroke is more common, and spontaneous recanalization is less frequent.

## Imaging

**General Features.** Dissections can present as stenosis, occlusion, or aneurysmal dilatation.

**CT Findings.** NECT may show crescent-shaped thickening caused by the wall hematoma. Posterior fossa SAH is seen in 20% of intracranial VA dissections.

**MR Findings.** Fat-saturated T1WI is the best sequence for demonstrating CAD. A hyperintense crescent of subacute blood adjacent to a narrowed "flow void" in the patent lumen is typical **(10-32)**. T2WI may show laminated thrombus that "blooms" on T2*.

At least 1/2 of all patients with cervicocephalic dissections have cerebral or cerebellar infarcts, best depicted on DWI. Multiple ipsilateral foci of diffusion restriction are typical findings.

**Angiography.** *Extracranial* ICA dissections typically spare the carotid bulb, beginning 2-3 cm distal to the bifurcation and terminating at the exocranial opening of the carotid canal **(10-33)** **(10-35)**. Vertebral dissections are most common around the skull base and upper cervical spine.

CTA and MRA demonstrate an eccentrically narrowed lumen surrounded by a crescent-shaped mural thickening **(10-32)**. A dissection flap can sometimes be identified **(10-31)**. Pseudoaneurysms are common. An opacified double lumen ("true" + "false" lumen) occurs in < 10% of cases.

The most common finding on DSA is a smooth or slightly irregular, tapered midcervical narrowing **(10-33)** **(10-35)**. Craniocervical dissections with occlusion shows a tapered "rat-tail" termination **(10-36)**. Occasionally, a subtle intimal tear or flap, a double lumen, narrowed or occluded true lumen, or pseudoaneurysm can be identified. If the dissection is subadventitial and does not narrow the vessel lumen, DSA can appear entirely normal; the paravascular hematoma must be detected on cross-sectional imaging.

*Intracranial* dissections are more difficult to diagnose than their extracranial counterparts. They are significantly smaller and findings are often subtle.

## DISSECTION

### Terminology

- Vessel wall tear → blood penetrates into, splits layers apart
  - Intramural hematoma formed
  - ± pseudoaneurysm

### Pathoetiology

- "Spontaneous" (nontraumatic): 60%; traumatic: 40%
  - Underlying vasculopathy (FMD, Marfan, etc.): 40%
- Location
  - Extracranial ICA (spares bulb, usually terminates at skull base)
  - VA (skull base-C1, C1-C2 most common)
  - Intracranial = extracranial (vertebral > > carotid)
  - Multiple arteries: 20% (look for underlying vasculopathy)

### Clinical Issues

- Most common cause of stroke in young, middle-aged adults
  - Occurs at all ages but peak = 40 years
- Neck pain, headache

### Imaging Findings

- Eccentric, crescent-shaped mural hematoma
  - Hyperintense on T1 FS
  - "Blooms" on T2*
  - Look for infarcts on DWI
- Long-segment, smooth narrowing of vessel lumen typical
- ± pseudoaneurysm

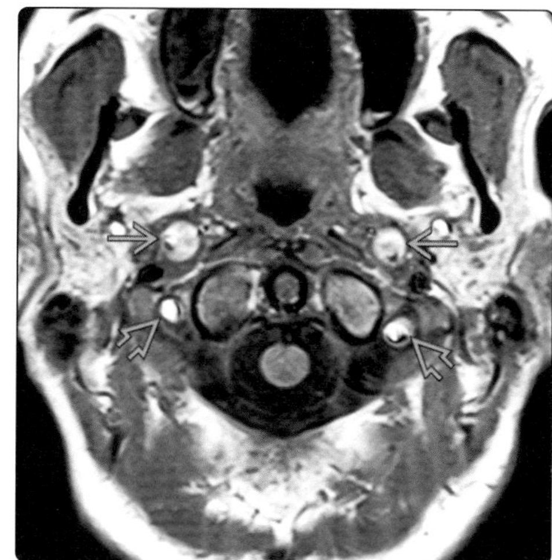

***(10-34)** Axial T1 MR in Marfan shows dissection of both cervical ICAs ➡ & VAs ➡ with mural thrombus around small residual flow voids.*

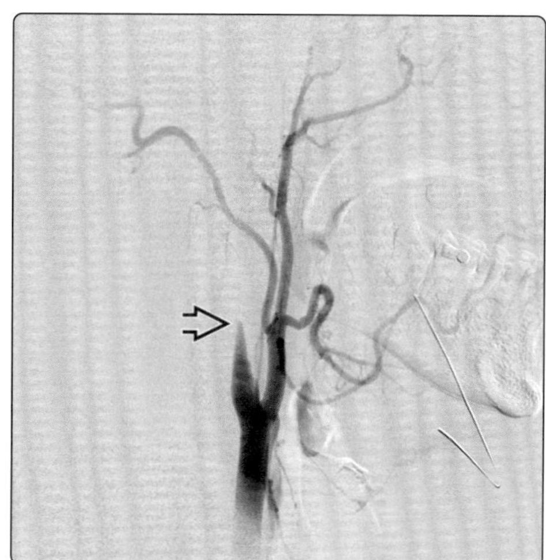

***(10-35)** Lateral angiogram shows a classic flame-shaped, tapered occlusion of the ICA ➡ due to acute dissection.*

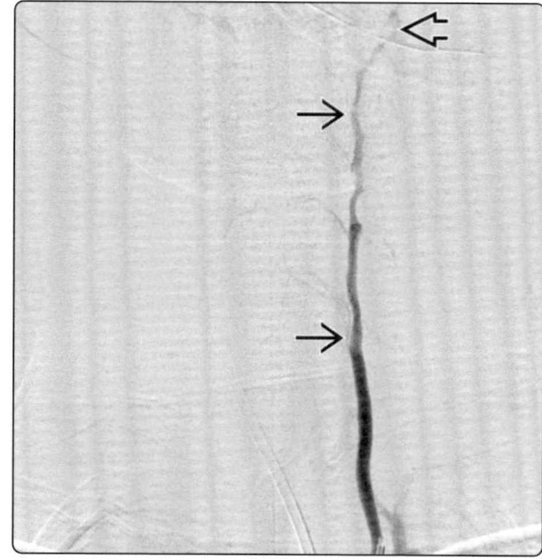

***(10-36)** AP DSA shows acute long-segment VA dissection ➡ & occlusion ➡ in a young adult with an acute stroke following MVA.*

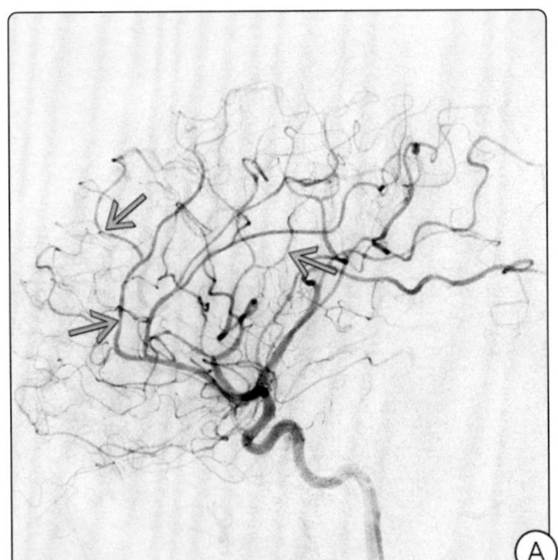

***(10-37A)** DSA in a 35-yo woman with "thunderclap" headache shows multifocal "beaded" arterial segments ➾.*

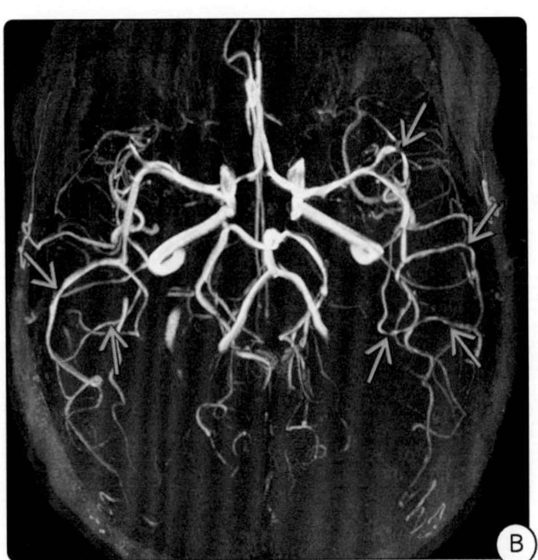

***(10-37B)** DSA 3 days later shows dramatic worsening with multiple bilateral "beaded" 2nd- & 3rd-order MCA branches ➾.*

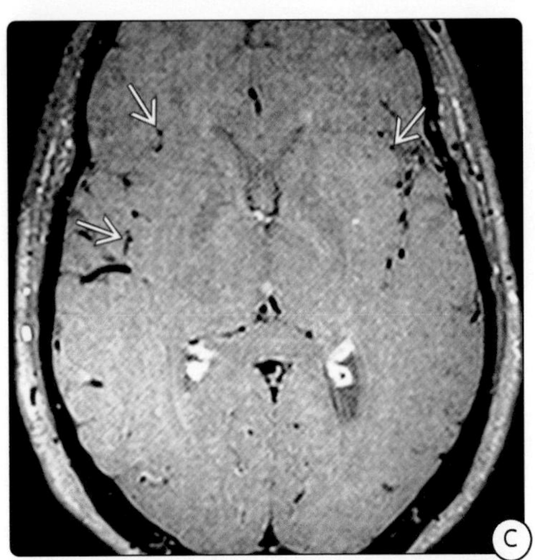

***(10-37C)** High-resolution "black blood" contrast-enhanced vessel wall imaging shows constricted vessels with no wall enhancement ➡; RCVS.*

## Differential Diagnosis

The major differential diagnosis of *extracranial* arterial dissection is type 2 (intimal) **FMD**. A common complication of FMD is dissection, so the two conditions may be indistinguishable and may occur in the same patient.

**Atherosclerosis** is more common in older patients. ASVD typically involves the great vessel origins and carotid bulb, sites that are almost always spared by dissection. Multiple vessels are usually affected. Dissections are usually solitary unless an underlying vasculopathy is present.

# Vasoconstriction Syndromes

Vasospasm with multifocal foci of arterial constriction and dilation is a common, well-recognized complication of aneurysmal SAH (aSAH) and is the most common cause of severe cerebral vasoconstriction (see Chapter 6). Vasospasm and vasospasm-like arterial constrictions can also occur in the absence of aSAH, trauma, or infection.

## Terminology

**Reversible cerebral vasoconstriction syndrome (RCVS)** now encompasses what was once considered a group of distinct clinical entities, including Call-Fleming syndrome, postpartum angiopathy, drug-induced angiopathy, migrainous vasospasm, and "thunderclap" headache with reversible vasospasm.

The International Headache Society diagnostic criteria for RCVS include severe acute headache, a uniphasic disease course, no evidence for *a*SAH [*convexal* (cortical) SAH (cSAH) is common], normal/near-normal CSF, and imaging demonstration of segmental cerebral artery vasoconstrictions that resolve within three months.

## Etiology

The exact etiology of RCVS is unknown. Some authors posit that, rather than representing a single specific disease entity, the broad heterogeneity of clinical and imaging manifestations associated with RCVS suggests that it may represent a common end point of numerous diverse disease processes.

RCVS may result from deregulation in vascular tone induced by sympathetic overactivity (including sympathomimetic medications and recreational drugs), endothelial dysfunction, and oxidative stress.

Brain biopsies have demonstrated no histopathologic evidence for vasculitis or inflammatory infiltrates within the constricted, diffusely thickened vessel walls often associated with RCVS.

## Clinical Issues

RCVS most commonly affects patients between the ages of 20-50 years, although cases have also been reported in children and older adults. There is a slight female predominance (2.5:1.0).

Although "thunderclap" headache is characteristic, it is not specific for RCVS. A waxing and waning course with repeated episodes for 1-3 weeks is common.

A history of migraine headaches is elicited in 20-40% of cases. An exogenous "trigger," such as vasoactive medications and postpartum state, is reported in 25-60% of cases.

## Imaging

The diagnosis of RCVS requires demonstration of multifocal segmental arterial constrictions in multiple vascular territories on CTA, MRA, or DSA **(10-37)**. A beaded appearance with multifocal areas of narrowing interspersed with normal segments is typical. Initial imaging may be unremarkable during the first week after symptom onset, so repeat examination may be necessary.

High-resolution vessel wall imaging typically shows no or minimal enhancement **(10-37)**.

cSAH is identified in ~ 1/3 of cases **(10-38A)** **(10-38B)**, whereas strokes are seen in 6-39% and concomitant posterior reversible encephalopathy syndrome (PRES) in 9-38% of cases.

### REVERSIBLE CEREBRAL VASOCONSTRICTION SYNDROME

**Terminology**
- Vasospasm with multifocal arterial constrictions
- RCVS now encompasses several entities
  - Call-Fleming syndrome
  - Postpartum angiopathy
  - Drug-induced angiopathies
  - Migrainous vasospasm, etc.

**Pathoetiology**
- Unknown
  - May represent end point of several disease processes
- Dysregulated vascular tone
- No histopathologic evidence for vasculitis, inflammation

**Clinical Issues**
- International Headache Society criteria of RCVS
  - Severe acute headache ("thunderclap" characteristic, nonspecific)
  - Uniphasic course
  - No evidence for aSAH
  - Normal/near-normal CSF
  - Imaging shows segmental vasoconstrictions; resolve in 3 months
- Demographics
  - 20-50 years most common
  - F:M = 2.5:1.0
- Other: Vasoactive medications, pregnancy, etc.: 25-60%

**Imaging Findings**
- Multifocal arterial constrictions
  - Multiple vascular territories involved
- Beaded appearance
  - Characteristic but nonspecific
- High-resolution vessel wall imaging
  - No/minimal enhancement
  - ± thickened wall, reduced lumen
- Other
  - cSAH
  - Strokes

**Differential Diagnosis**
- PRES
  - Overlaps, often coexists with RCVS
- aSAH-related vasospasm
- Vasculitis
  - Concentric, long-segment wall enhancement

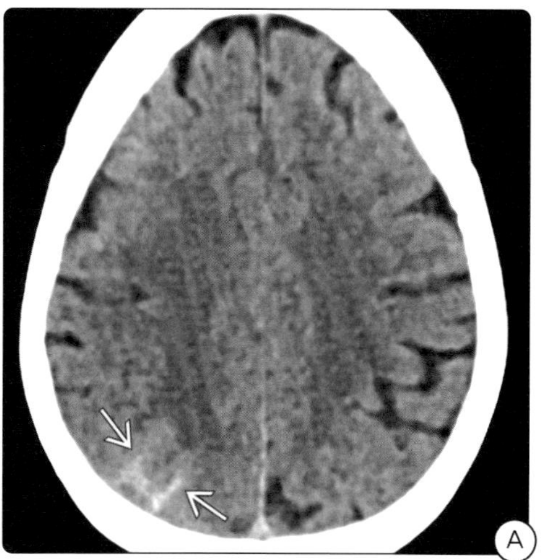


***(10-38A)** Axial NECT in a 50-yo woman with severe headaches shows subtle SAH ➡ in the right parietal convexity.*

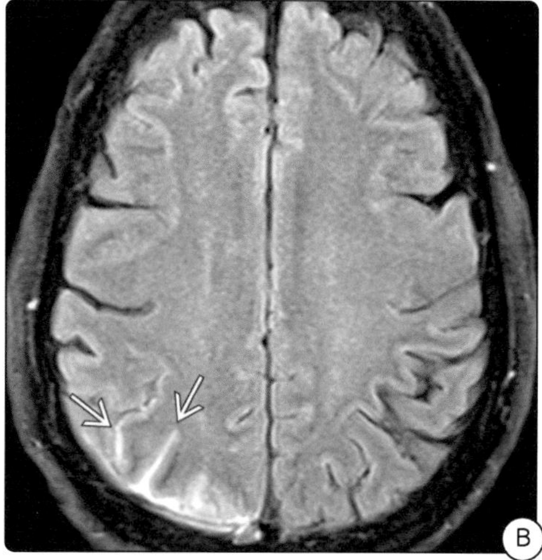


***(10-38B)** Axial FLAIR MR shows the focal SAH ➡. No acute infarct was present on DTI images. VWI can help distinguish RCVS from vasculitis.*

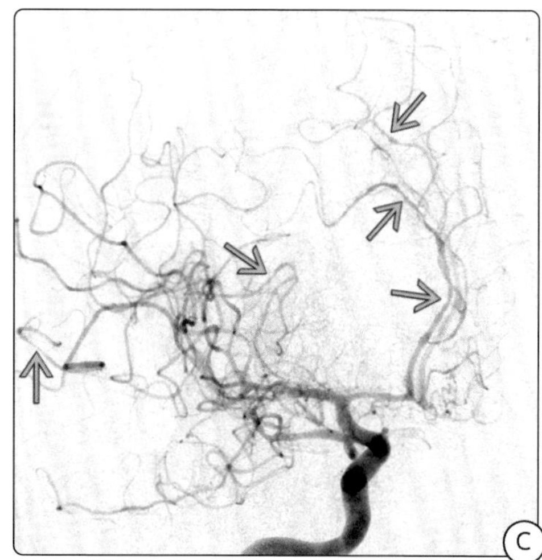


***(10-38C)** DSA shows multifocal irregularity & beading of the ACA & MCA branches ➡. RCVS. Arterial narrowing improved after IA verapamil.*

## Differential Diagnosis

RCVS and **PRES** overlap in both their clinical and imaging features and may occur concurrently. PRES-like reversible cerebral edema is seen in up to 1/3 of RCVS cases, and RCVS-like vasoconstrictions can be identified in the majority of PRES patients.

The other major differential diagnoses of RCVS are **aSAH-related vasospasm** and **CNS vasculitis**. In aSAH, the vasospasm is typically long-segment narrowing of arteries in/around the circle of Willis. In RCVS, the segmental vasoconstrictions preferentially involve the more distal (second- and third-order) branches. Vessel wall imaging can also help distinguish RCVS from vasculitis. Concentric or tram-track wall enhancement is common in vasculitis; it is mild or absent in RCVS.

# Vasculitis and Vasculitides

## Terminology

The generic terms "vasculitis" and "angiitis" denote inflammation of blood vessels affecting arteries, veins, or both. The plural "vasculitides" is a more generic term that is often used interchangeably. "Arteritis" is more specific and refers solely to inflammatory processes that involve arteries.

## Etiology

Vasculitis can be caused by infection, collagen vascular disease, immune complex deposition, drug abuse, and even neoplasms (e.g., lymphomatoid granulomatosis). The general pathologic features of many vasculitides are quite similar **(10-39)**. As a result, the definitive diagnosis depends primarily on hematologic and immunohistochemical characteristics.

*(10-39) Graphic shows vasculitis ➙ with multifocal infarcts, scattered hemorrhages ➙ in the basal ganglia & at the GM-WM junction. (10-40) Coronal T1 C+ MR shows bilateral, prominent linear patterns of enhancement ➙. This is biopsy-proven primary arteritis of the CNS (PACNS). Vasculitis often presents with convexal SAH & small infarcts. VWI may show arterial wall enhancement.*

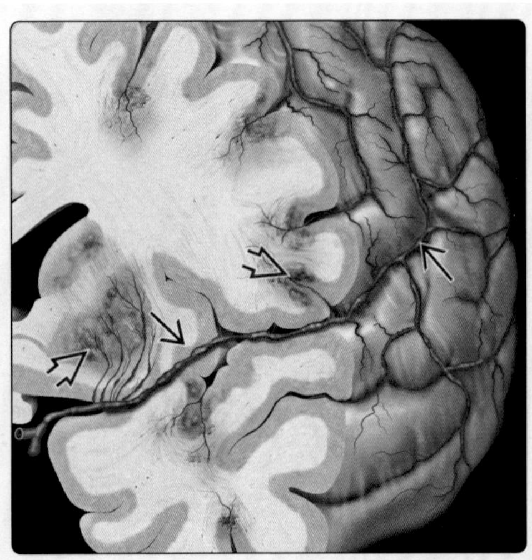

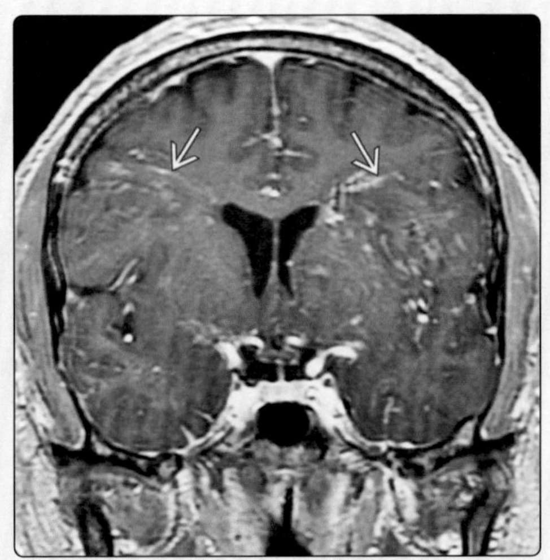

*(10-41) DSA in a patient with streptococcal meningitis & multiple foci of restricted diffusion on MR shows multifocal segmental "beaded" areas of arterial narrowing & dilatation ➙, classic findings of vasculitis (in this case, secondary vasculitis). (10-42) "Black blood" contrast-enhanced VWI in autoimmune vasculitis shows circumferential, linear enhancement in the right MCA ➙. Enhancement in a subacute infarct ➙.*

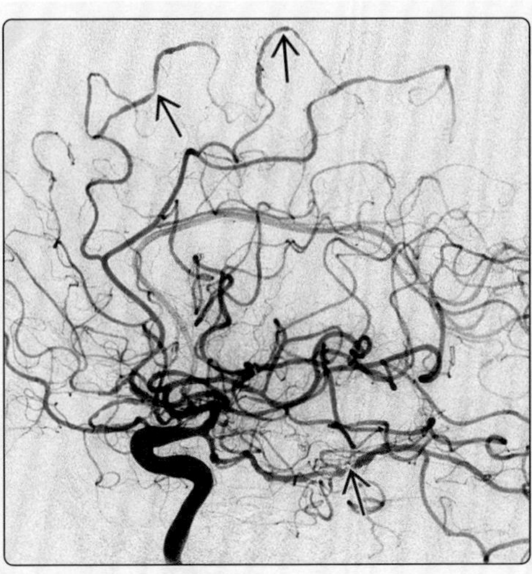

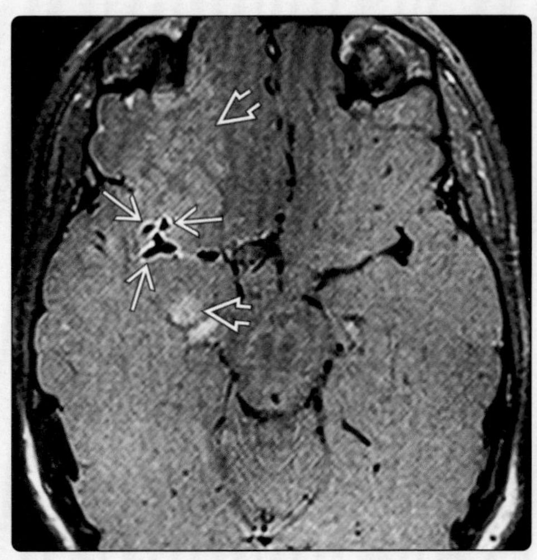

Isolated CNS vasculitis in which thorough clinical and laboratory examination does not identify another disorder causing the vascular inflammation is called **primary arteritis of the CNS (PACNS)**. This contrasts with the many *secondary* causes of CNS vasculitis.

## Pathology

Although the vasculitides are a heterogeneous group of CNS disorders, they are characterized histopathologically by two cardinal features: Inflammation and necrosis in blood vessel walls. Infarcts in multiple vascular distributions are common.

## Imaging

As imaging in most vasculitides is similar regardless of etiology, this discussion will focus on the general features of vasculitis as it affects the brain.

**CT Findings.** NECT scans are relatively insensitive and are often normal. Rarely, vasculitis causes cSAH.

Multifocal hypodensities in the basal ganglia and subcortical WM with or without patchy enhancement on CECT are common.

**MR Findings.** Involvement of the cortex/subcortical WM together with the basal ganglia is strongly suggestive of vasculitis. T1 scans can be normal or show multifocal cortical/subcortical and basal ganglia hypointensities. T2/FLAIR scans demonstrate hyperintensities in the same areas. T2* (GRE, SWI) may show parenchymal microhemorrhages &/or SAH in some cases.

Patchy enhancement with punctate and linear lesions is common on T1 C+ scans. Dural and leptomeningeal thickening/enhancement occur in some cases of granulomatosis with polyangiitis. Acute lesions with cerebral ischemia show multiple foci of diffusion restriction in the cortex, subcortical WM, and basal ganglia.

High-resolution "black blood" vessel wall imaging shows thickening and multifocal homogeneous smooth, intense, concentric enhancement of the vessel wall.

**Angiography.** Findings include multifocal irregularities, stenoses, and vascular occlusions **(10-41)**. Pseudoaneurysm formation and branch occlusions occur but are less common than luminal irregularities. Distal branches are more commonly affected than proximal arterial segments.

## Differential Diagnosis

The major differential diagnosis of vasculitis is ASVD. **ASVD** typically occurs in older patients and involves larger, more proximal intracranial arteries, although it sometimes affects second- and third-order branches. Vessel wall imaging usually shows mild noncircumferential or no wall enhancement.

**Vasospasm** can also mimic vasculitis. Vasospasm most commonly affects the major cerebral vessels. A history of trauma or SAH is common but not invariably present. **RCVS** and **postpartum angiopathy** can be indistinguishable from vasculitis.

# Other Macro- and Microvasculopathies

A broad spectrum of both inherited and acquired noninflammatory, nonatherosclerotic diseases can involve the intracranial vasculature. We briefly review a few of the more important miscellaneous vasculopathies.

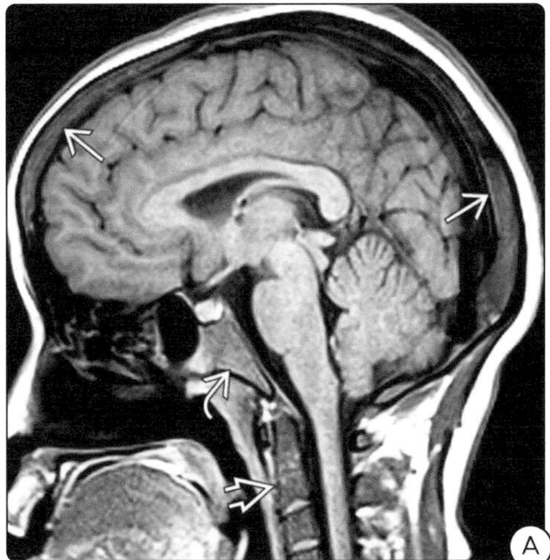


***(10-43A)** T1 MR in 29-yo woman with SCD shows thick calvarium with hypointense marrow ➡. Clivus ➡, vertebral bodies ➡ hypointense.*

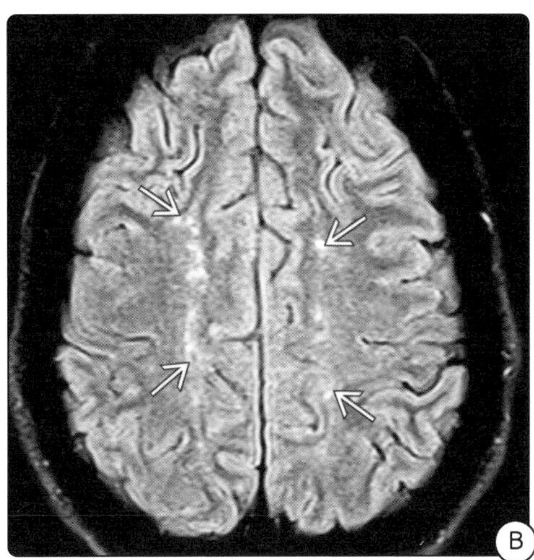


***(10-43B)** FLAIR MR in the same patient shows punctate hyperintensities in both watershed zones ➡, a common finding in SCD.*

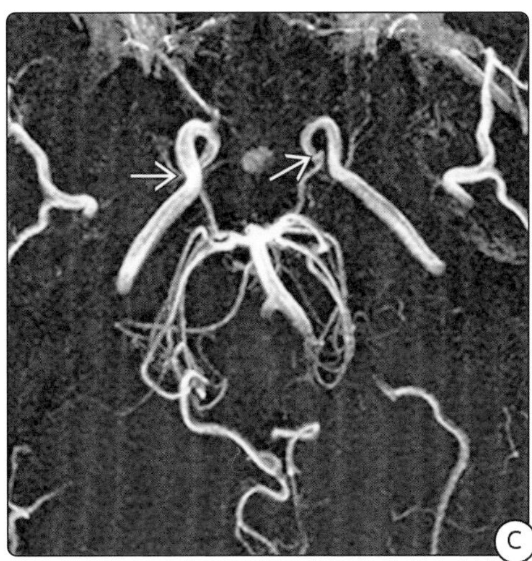


***(10-43C)** Submentovertex MIP of the MRA in the same patient shows occlusion of both supraclinoid ICAs ➡.*

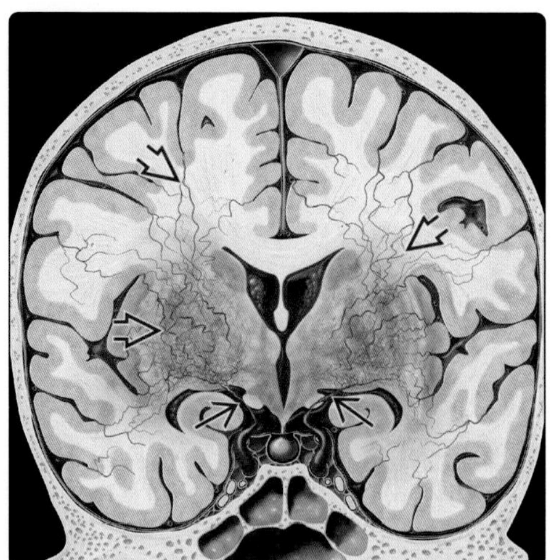

*(10-44) MMD shows severely narrowed supraclinoid ICAs ⇒, striking "puff of smoke" from extensive basal ganglia, WM collaterals ⇒.*

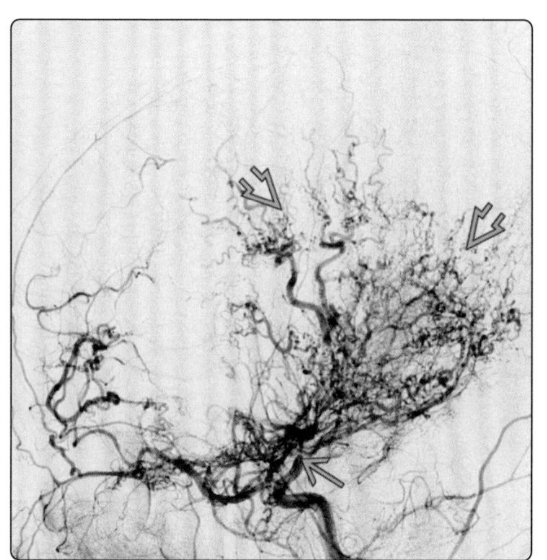

*(10-45) MMD in a 3-yo shows near-total supraclinoid ICA stenosis ⇒ with innumerable tortuous, enlarged moyamoya-like collaterals ⇒.*

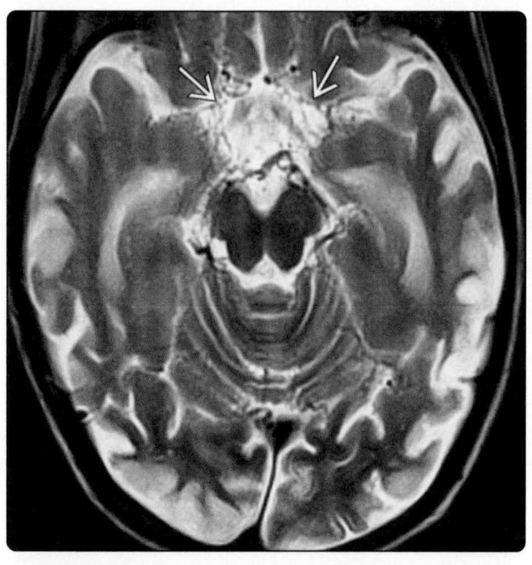

*(10-46) T2WI in MMD shows severely narrowed thread-like supraclinoid ICAs, MCAs ➡ with marked cortical atrophy. (Courtesy H. Els, MD.)*

## Sickle Cell Disease

Sickle cell disease (SCD) is the most common worldwide cause of childhood stroke. African American and African Brazilian children are the most affected children outside of continental Africa.

**Clinical Issues.** The most common CNS complication of SCD is stroke. Stroke risk is highest between 2-5 years of age. Approximately 75% of SCD-related strokes are ischemic and 25% are hemorrhagic. Hemorrhagic strokes are more common in adult-onset SCD.

**Imaging.** MR scans often demonstrate subcortical and WM hyperintensities along the deep watershed zone on T2/FLAIR **(10-43B)**. A moyamoya-like pattern with supraclinoid ICA stenosis may develop with especially severe SCD **(10-43C)**. An ivy sign with serpentine hyperintensities in the cerebral sulci from leptomeningeal collaterals can sometimes be seen on FLAIR.

## Moyamoya Disease

**Terminology.** Moyamoya disease (MMD) is an idiopathic progressive arteriopathy characterized by stenosis of the distal (supraclinoid) ICAs and formation of an abnormal vascular network at the base of the brain **(10-44)**. Multiple enlarged "telangiectatic" lenticulostriate, thalamoperforating, leptomeningeal, dural, and pial arteries develop as compensatory circulation. These "moyamoya collaterals" can become so extensive that they resemble the "puff of smoke" from a cigarette, the Japanese term for which the disease is named **(10-45)**.

**Clinical Issues.** MMD has worldwide distribution but is most prevalent in Japan and Korea. 2/3 of cases occur in children, and at least 1/2 of these occur under the age of 10 years. Between 1/4-1/3 present in adults with peak presentation in the fifth decade.

When MMD presents in childhood, the initial symptoms are usually ischemic. In adults, ~ 1/2 of all patients develop intracranial hemorrhage from rupture of the fragile moyamoya collateral vessels. The other 50% present with TIAs or cerebral infarcts.

MMD is relentlessly progressive. A recently proposed new system, the Berlin grading system, can be used to stratify clinical severity and predict postoperative morbidity in revascularization surgery.

**Imaging.** T1 and T2 scans show markedly narrowed supraclinoid ICAs with multiple tortuous, serpentine "flow voids" **(10-46)**. The appearance of multiple tiny collateral vessels in enlarged CSF spaces has been likened to "swimming worms in a bare cistern." T1 C+ scans often show contrast stagnating in slow-flowing collateral vessels, both in the brain parenchyma and over its surface.

An ivy sign with sulcal hyperintensity from slow flow in leptomeningeal collaterals is sometimes seen on FLAIR and correlates with decreased vascular reserve in the affected hemisphere. Microbleeds on T2* GRE scans are associated with increased risk of overt cerebral hemorrhage.

DSA, CTA, and MRA show predominantly anterior circulation disease with marked narrowing of both supraclinoid ICAs (bottle neck sign). The PCAs are less commonly involved. Prominent lenticulostriate and thalamoperforator collaterals are present, forming the puff of smoke appearance characteristic of moyamoya. Numerous transosseous and transdural collaterals from the extracranial to intracranial circulation may develop.

**MOYAMOYA DISEASE**

**Terminology**
- Moyamoya = "puff of smoke"
- MMD = progressive arteriopathy → stenosis of supraclinoid ICAs

**Clinical Issues**
- Worldwide distribution, most common in Japan
- Children (70%, usually < 10 years)
  - TIAs, stroke
- Adults (30%)
  - Hemorrhage > stroke
- Revascularization (encephalo-duro-arterial-synangiosis, extracranial-intracranial bypass)

**Imaging**
- Stenosis/occlusion of supraclinoid ICAs
- Innumerable basal collaterals
- Strokes (acute, chronic)
- Hemorrhage (SAH, parenchymal)

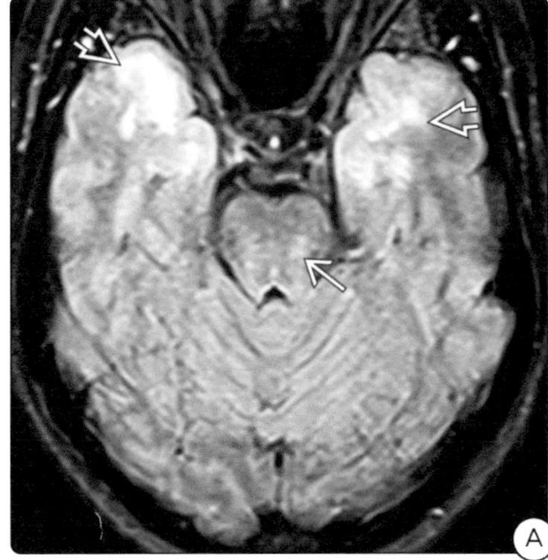

***(10-47A)** FLAIR in 32-yo with repeat strokes shows patchy/confluent WM hyperintensities in her anterior temporal lobes ➡, pons ➡.*

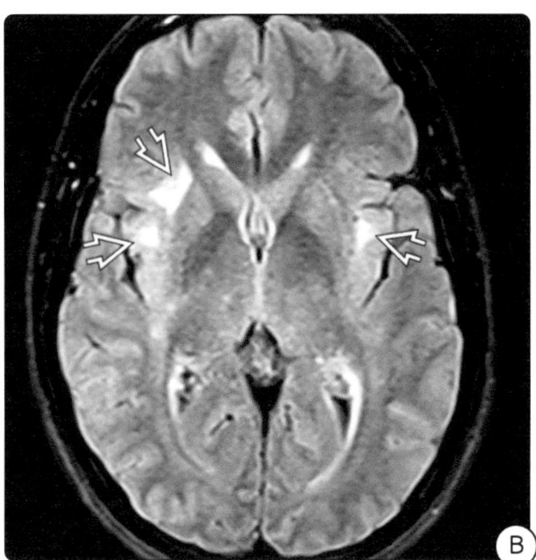

***(10-47B)** More cephalad FLAIR MR in the same patient demonstrates lesions in both external capsules ➡.*

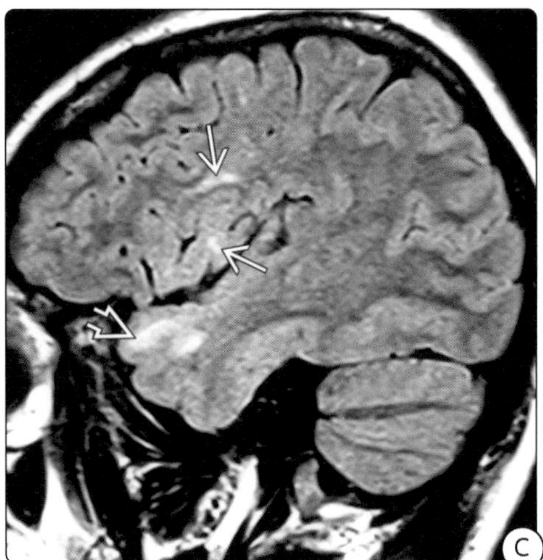

***(10-47C)** Sagittal FLAIR shows anterior temporal subcortical WM ➡, external capsule lesions ➡; proven CADASIL with NOTCH3 mutation.*

**Differential Diagnosis.** Other slowly developing occlusive vasculopathies may develop multiple small moyamoya-like collateral vessels. These include **radiation therapy, neurofibromatosis type 1, trisomy 21, SCD**, and even **atherosclerosis**.

Classic moyamoya typically affects *both* supraclinoid ICAs with relative sparing of the posterior circulation. A unilateral acquired, usually atherosclerotic, **"segmental" high-grade stenosis** or occlusion of the M1 MCA with a network of small vessels bridging the gap between the horizontal and distal segments should be differentiated from MMD.

## CADASIL

CADASIL is the acronym for **c**erebral **a**utosomal **d**ominant **a**rteriopathy with **s**ubcortical **i**nfarcts and **l**eukoencephalopathy. CADASIL is an autosomal dominant disease of the cerebral microvasculature that primarily affects smooth muscle cells in penetrating cerebral and leptomeningeal arteries.

**Etiology and Pathology.** CADASIL is caused by point mutations in the *NOTCH3* gene. 14 distinct familial forms of CADASIL have been identified with mutations in different *NOTCH3* exons.

The pathologic hallmark of CADASIL is accumulation of granular osmiophilic material in the basement membranes of small arteries and arterioles that causes severe fibrotic thickening and stenosis.

**Clinical Issues.** CADASIL is the most common monogenic heritable cause of lacunar stroke and vascular dementia in adults. At initial presentation, only 35% of patients have a first-degree relative with known CADASIL.

The classic clinical presentation involves a young to middle-aged adult without identifiable vascular risk factors ("cryptogenic stroke"). The main manifestations are recurrent ischemic strokes, migraine headache with aura (often the earliest manifestation of the disease), psychiatric disturbances, and progressive cognitive impairment. Symptom onset is generally in the third decade and follows a progressive course, causing disability and dementia in 75% of cases.

**Imaging. Characteristic imaging patterns may precede overt symptoms by more than a decade**. Typical findings are multiple lacunar infarcts in the basal ganglia and high signal intensity lesions in the subcortical and periventricular WM.

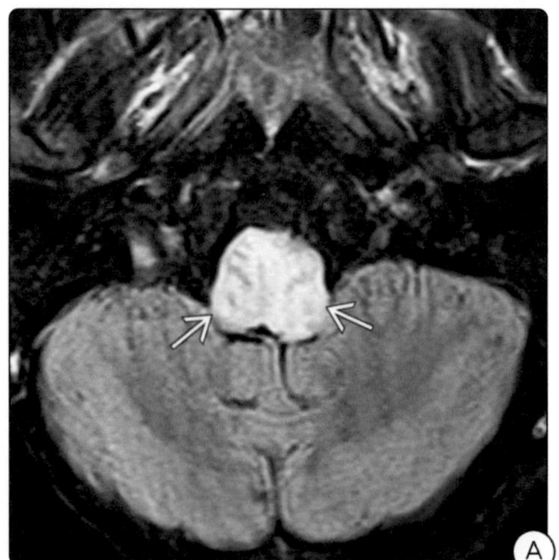


*(10-48A) Axial FLAIR MR in a 33-yo with acute exacerbation of her CNS lupus shows confluent hyperintensity expanding the medulla ➡.*

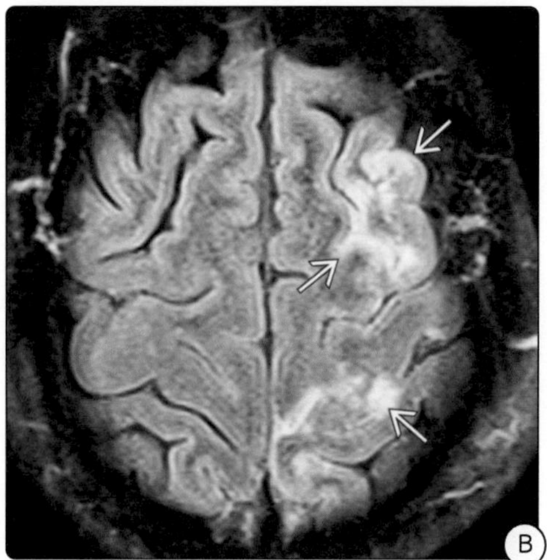


*(10-48B) FLAIR MR in the same patient shows patchy cortical & subcortical hyperintensities in frontal & parietal lobes ➡ with mild mass effect.*

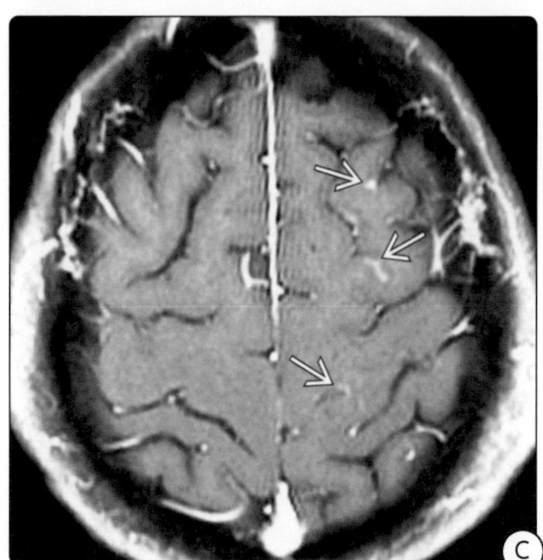


*(10-48C) T1 C+ FS MR in the same patient shows mild patchy enhancement in the cortex & subcortical WM of the left hemisphere ➡.*

Bilateral, multifocal T2 and FLAIR hyperintensities in the periventricular and deep WM begin to appear by age 20. Involvement of the **anterior temporal lobe** and **external capsule** has high sensitivity and specificity in differentiating CADASIL from common cerebral small vessel disease **(10-47A)**.

Lacunar infarcts in the subcortical WM, basal ganglia, thalamus, internal capsule, and brainstem are found in 75% of patients between 30-40 years of age and increase in both number and prominence with age. Mild to moderate generalized cerebral atrophy is a relatively late finding and is independently associated with the extent of cognitive decline.

Cerebral microbleeds (CMBs) are found on T2* scans in 25% of patients between 40-50 years old and are seen in nearly 50% of patients over 50. Cortical superficial siderosis is absent.

**Differential Diagnosis.** The imaging differential diagnosis of CADASIL includes **ASVD** (usually spares the anterior temporal lobe WM), mitochondrial encephalomyopathy with lactic acidosis and stroke-like episodes **(MELAS), vasculitis**, and **antiphospholipid syndromes** (APSs).

**Other hereditary small vessel diseases** that can mimic CADASIL include **CARASIL** (**c**erebral **a**utosomal **r**ecessive **a**rteriopathy with **s**ubcortical **i**nfarcts and **l**eukoencephalopathy).

## Systemic Lupus Erythematosus

**Terminology.** Systemic lupus erythematosus (SLE or "lupus") is a multisystem complex autoimmune disorder. When overt CNS symptoms are present, the disorder is termed CNS lupus (CNS SLE) or neuropsychiatric SLE (NPSLE).

**Etiology.** SLE is an autoimmune disorder characterized by immune complex deposition, vasculitis, and vasculopathy. Circulating autoantibodies may be present years before overt clinical SLE symptoms emerge.

CNS SLE is generally considered an angiopathic disease, although neural autoimmune damage, demyelination, and thromboembolism may be contributing factors. Lupus-related cerebral ischemia/infarction can result from coagulopathy (secondary to APS), accelerated atherosclerosis (often associated with corticosteroid treatment), thromboembolism (secondary to Libman-Sacks endocarditis), or a true primary lupus vasculitis.

**Clinical Issues.** CNS SLE occurs in 30-40% of lupus cases and can be a serious, potentially life-threatening manifestation of SLE. It occurs at all ages with peak onset between 2nd-4th decades. In adults, > 90% of patients are female. In children, the F:M ratio is 2-3:1.

**Imaging.** Initial NECT scans are often normal or show scattered patchy cortical/subcortical hypodensities. Large territorial infarcts and dural sinus occlusions occur but are less common. Spontaneous intracranial hemorrhages can occur in SLE patients with uremia, thrombocytopenia, and hypertension.

MR findings vary from normal to striking. The most common finding, seen in 25-50% of newly diagnosed NPSLE patients, is that of multiple small subcortical and deep WM hyperintensities on T2/FLAIR **(10-48)**. Large, confluent lesions that resemble acute disseminated encephalomyelitis (ADEM) occur but are generally seen only in patients with CNS symptoms **(10-49)**. Diffuse cortical, basal ganglia, and brainstem lesions—suggestive of vasculopathy or vasculitis—are also common.

Acute lesions demonstrate transient enhancement on T1 C+ studies and restricted diffusion. pMR in patients with NPSLE shows elevated cerebral blood volume and cerebral blood flow.

Dural venous sinus and cortical/deep venous thrombosis occur in 20-30% of NPSLE cases. Systemic hypertension is common in SLE patients. PRES is a rare but treatable manifestation of CNS lupus.

**Differential Diagnosis.** The imaging differential diagnosis of NPSLE is broad and includes **arteriolosclerosis** ("small vessel disease"), **multiple sclerosis (MS), Susac syndrome**, non-lupus **APSs, Lyme disease**, and **other vasculitides**, such as primary angiitis of the CNS.

There is a significant overlap of lupus with APS; between 25-40% of SLE patients have APS. While there are no universally accepted diagnostic imaging criteria for NPSLE, the presence of multifocal infarcts and "migratory" edematous areas is suggestive of the disease.

## Behçet Disease

**Etiology and Pathology.** Behçet disease is a chronic, idiopathic, relapsing-remitting, multisystem vascular-inflammatory disease characterized by recurrent orogenital ulcerations and uveitis. The CNS is involved in 20-25% of patients.

CNS involvement is divided into parenchymal and nonparenchymal lesions. Parenchymal disease is mainly a meningoencephalitis primarily affecting the brainstem. Additional areas of involvement are the basal ganglia, thalami, and hemispheres.

The nonparenchymal manifestations include dural sinus thrombosis, arterial occlusion, &/or aneurysm.

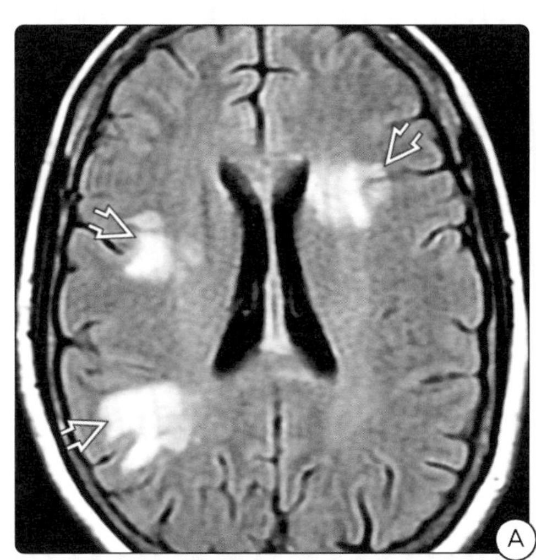


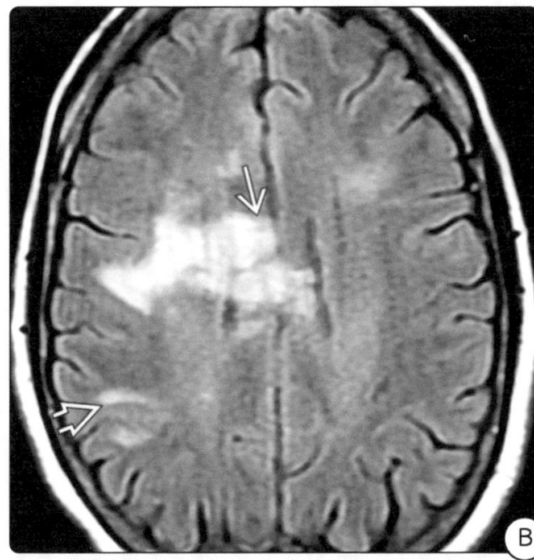


***(10-49A)** Axial FLAIR MR in a 55-yo woman with unusual neuropsychiatric symptoms shows patchy & confluent hyperintensities in the subcortical & deep periventricular WM ➲. **(10-49B)** Axial FLAIR MR in the same patient shows subcortical WM lesions ➲ in addition to "fluffy" confluent lesions that cross the corpus callosum ➲ & resemble acute disseminated encephalomyelitis (ADEM).*

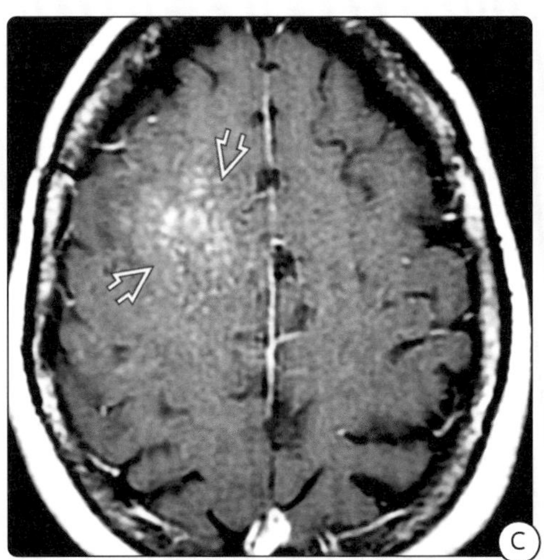


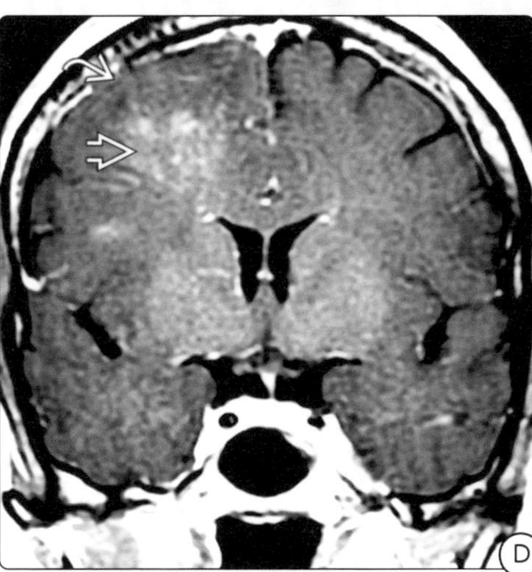


***(10-49C)** Coronal T1 C+ MR in the same patient shows mild punctate & linear foci of enhancement in the subcortical & deep cerebral WM ➲. **(10-49D)** Coronal T1 C+ MR shows patchy & linear enhancing foci in the subcortical WM ➲. Note the burr hole ➲ from biopsy. Histopathologic examination disclosed CNS lupus vasculitis.*

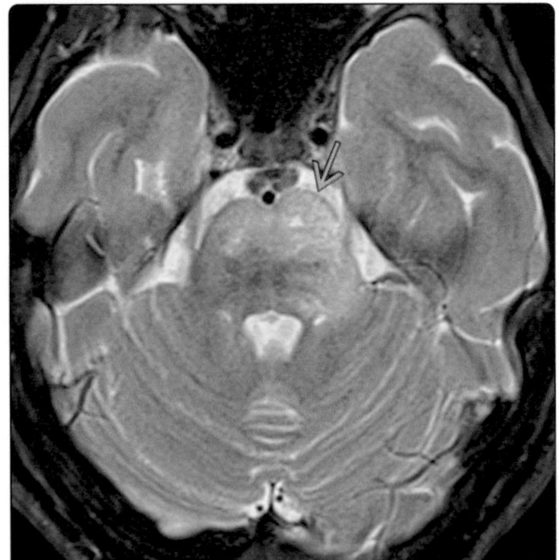

*(10-50) Axial T2 MR shows hyperintensity & mild expansion of the pons ⇒ in this young adult with Behçet disease.*

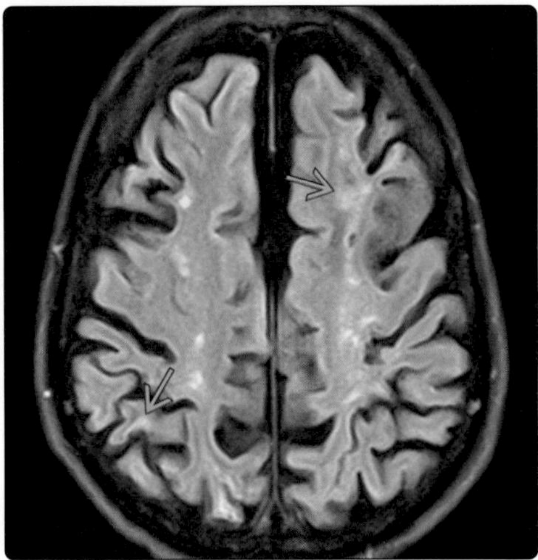

*(10-51) Axial FLAIR MR in a 44-yo woman with APS shows volume loss & multiple areas of prior ischemic infarcts ⇒.*

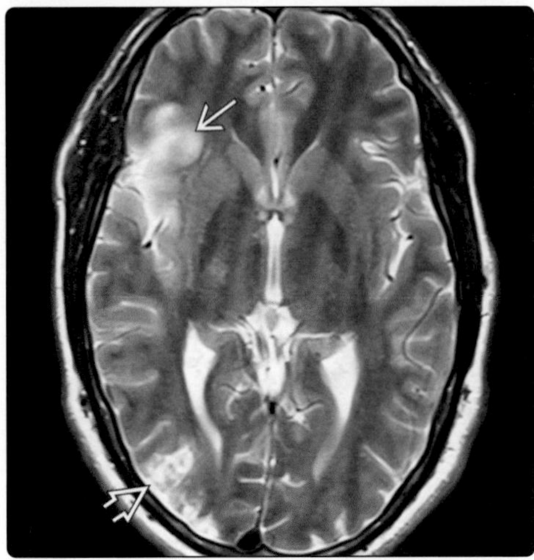

*(10-52) Axial T2 MR in a 36-yo man with APS & multiple strokes shows acute gyral edema ➡, parietal encephalomalacia ➡.*

**Clinical Issues.** Behçet disease is most common in the Mediterranean region, the Middle East, and East Asia, though it has a worldwide distribution. It typically affects young adults between 20-40 years old, and has a moderate male predominance.

The clinical course is often chronic and may span up to a decade, though fulminant disease with rapid clinical deterioration has been reported. Neurologic involvement typically occurs months to years following systemic disease. Treatment involves corticosteroids and immunosuppressive therapy.

**Imaging.** Brainstem involvement, particularly the cerebral peduncles, with T2/FLAIR hyperintensity occurs in 50% of cases **(10-50)**. The deep gray nuclei are the next most commonly involved sites followed by the hemispheric WM. Spinal cord lesions have been reported.

Enhancement of the lesions is typically mild to moderate and patchy. There may be associated mass effect, which may mimic a neoplasm.

**Differential Diagnosis.** Other imaging differential considerations include demyelination, specifically **ADEM**, which often affects the middle cerebellar peduncles and WM more often than the deep gray nuclei. Other systemic inflammatory disease, such as **SLE** and **APS**, may resemble Behçet disease.

## Antiphospholipid Syndrome

**Terminology and Etiology.** APS is a multisystem disorder characterized by arterial or venous thrombosis, early strokes, cognitive dysfunction, and pregnancy loss.

**Clinical Issues.** The diagnosis of APS requires the presence of at least one clinical criterion (e.g., vascular thrombosis or pregnancy morbidity) and one laboratory finding, i.e., persistently positive lupus anticoagulant, antiphospholipid antibodies (e.g., anticardiolipin antibodies), or anti-β2 glycoprotein 1 antibody.

Mean age of onset is 50 years. There is a 2:1 female predominance (women with APS are often initially diagnosed because of pregnancy loss).

CNS involvement in APS is common. Manifestations of CNS APS include cerebrovascular disease with arterial thrombotic events (early-onset TIA, stroke) or venous occlusions, MS-like syndromes, seizure, headache, and cognitive dysfunction.

**Imaging.** Mixed-age multifocal cortical/subcortical infarcts, parietal-dominant atrophy with relative sparing of the frontal and temporal lobes, and "too many for age" deep WM hyperintensities on T2/FLAIR scans are typical findings in APS **(10-51)** **(10-52)**. Both arterial and venous thromboses are common.

**Differential Diagnosis.** APS in the CNS can be difficult to distinguish from **MS**. **Multiinfarct ("vascular") dementia** usually lacks the parietal-dominant atrophy of APS. **SLE** commonly occurs with APS and may present with similar clinical and imaging findings.

## Cerebral Amyloid Disease

**Terminology.** Cerebral amyloid disease occurs in several forms. The most common is an age-related microvasculopathy termed **cerebral amyloid angiopathy** (CAA). Rarely, cerebral amyloid disease presents as an **amyloid β-related angiitis** (ABRA) with diffuse inflammatory changes that primarily affect the WM.

**Etiology.** Imbalance between amyloid β (Aβ) production and clearance is considered the key element causing formation of CNS amyloid deposits in small cerebral vessels. Aβ is normally cleared through the brain's "glymphatics." Failure to clear Aβ from the brain has two major consequences: (1) Intracranial hemorrhages associated with rupture of Aβ-laden vessels in CAA and (2) altered neuronal function caused by pathologic accumulation of Aβ and other soluble metabolites in Alzheimer disease (AD). The most frequent vascular abnormality seen in AD is CAA.

**Genetics.** CAA can be primary or secondary, sporadic or familial. Sporadic CAA is much more common than familial CAA and is strongly associated with presence of the *APOE-ε4* allele.

Hereditary forms of CAA are generally familial and occur as an autosomal dominant disorder with several recognized subtypes. Hereditary CAA is generally more severe and earlier in onset compared with the sporadic disease form.

**Pathology.** Gross pathologic findings include major lobar hemorrhages of different ages, cortical petechial hemorrhages ("microbleeds"), small cerebral infarcts, and WM ischemic lesions **(10-53)**.

On Congo red stains, CAA vessels have a salmon-colored "congophilic" appearance. A characteristic yellow-green color ("birefringence") appears when the affected vessels are viewed using polarized light.

ABRA demonstrates mural and perivascular inflammatory changes with necrosis, variable numbers of multinucleated giant cells, epithelioid histiocytes, eosinophils, and lymphocytes. ABRA is a type of inflammatory CAA but is distinct from CAA-related inflammation, which is limited to the perivascular region without destructive vasculitis.

**Clinical Issues.** Advancing age is the strongest known risk factor for developing CAA. Sporadic CAA usually occurs in patients older than 55 years, whereas the hereditary forms present one or two decades earlier.

CAA causes 5-20% of all nontraumatic cerebral hemorrhages and is now recognized as a major cause of spontaneous intracranial hemorrhage and cognitive impairment in older adults.

The most common clinical manifestations of CAA are focal neurologic deficits (with recurrent lobar hemorrhages) and cognitive impairment (with multiple chronic microbleeds).

Patients with ABRA also tend to be younger than those with sporadic, noninflammatory CAA. The clinical presentation of patients with CAA-related inflammation (e.g., ABRA) differs, usually resembling an autoimmune-mediated vasculitis or a subacute meningoencephalitis. The most common symptoms include focal neurologic deficits, seizures, acute to subacute cognitive dysfunction, and headaches.

### Imaging

***CT.*** NECT scans in patients with acute manifestations of CAA typically show a hyperdense lobar hematoma with varying peripheral edema **(10-55A)**. Multiple irregular confluent WM hypointensities together with generalized volume loss are common.

Occasionally, patients with CAA can present with so-called **convexal SAH** (cSAH). In cSAH, one or more adjacent convexity sulci demonstrate curvilinear hyperdensity consistent with blood.

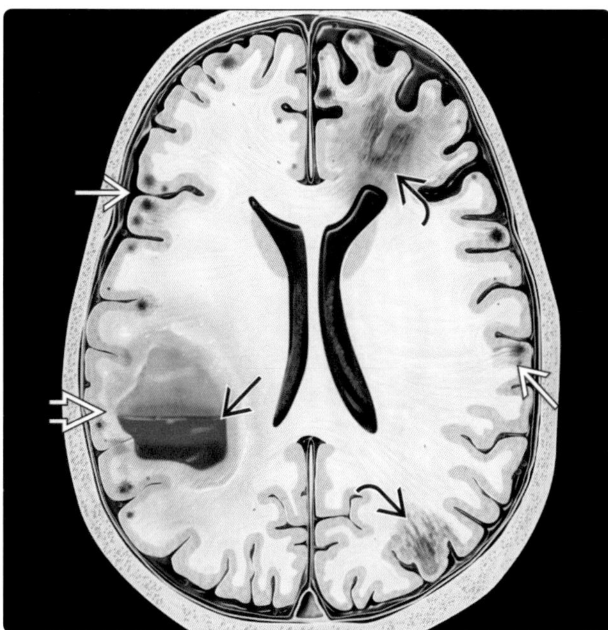

***(10-53)** Acute hematoma ➡ with fluid level ➡ is shown. Microbleeds ➡ & old lobar hemorrhages ➡ are typical findings in cerebral amyloid disease.*

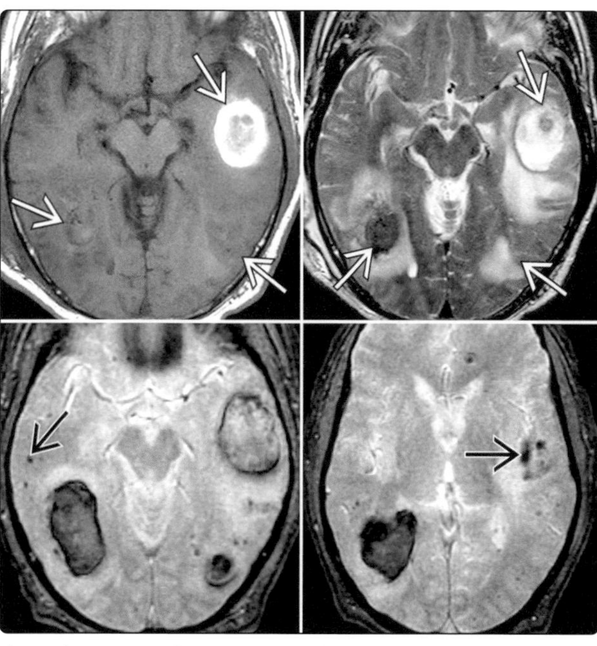

***(10-54)** MR scans demonstrate multiple lobar hemorrhages of different ages ➡, multifocal peripheral "blooming black dots" ➡ that are classic for CAA.*

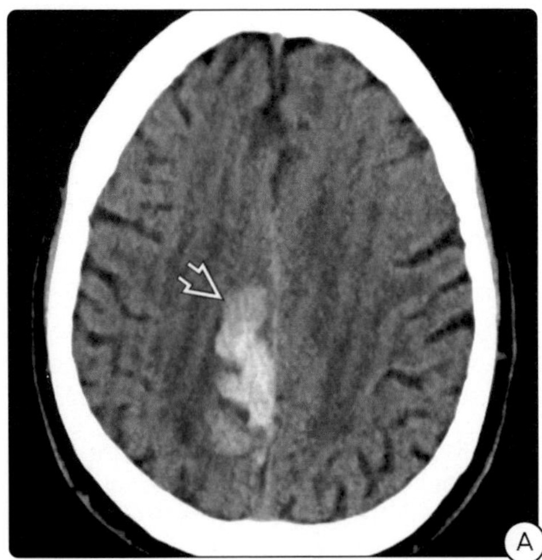


***(10-55A)** Axial CT in a 77-yo man with confusion shows a lobar hemorrhage ➡ with surrounding edema, typical for CAA.*

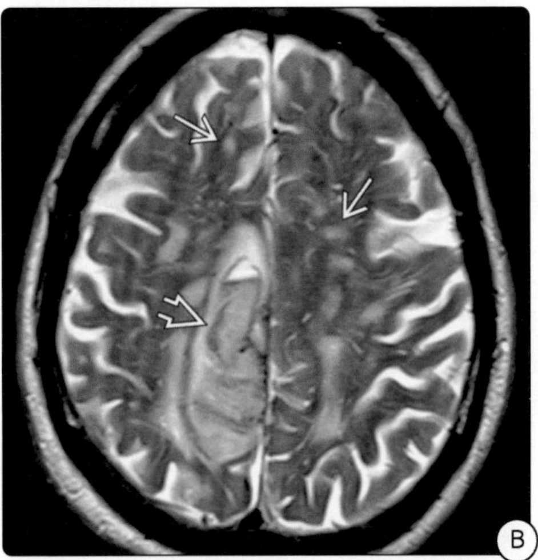


***(10-55B)** T2 MR in the same patient shows the hemorrhage ➡ & multiple additional foci of T2 hyperintensity ➡ in both hemispheres.*

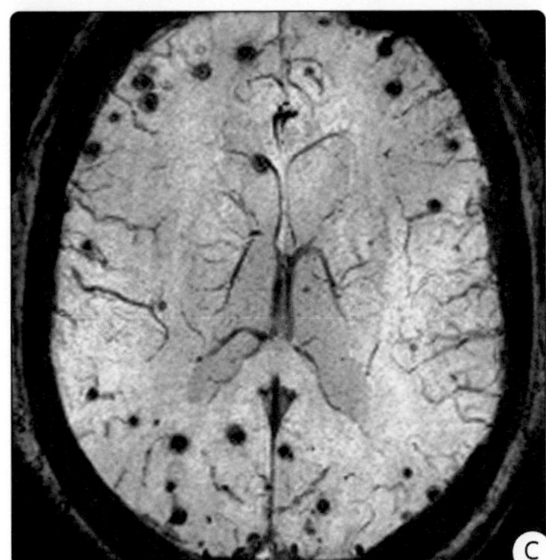


***(10-55C)** Axial SWI shows multiple hypointense foci located peripherally, typical for CAA. Chronic hypertensive encephalopathy may mimic CAA.*

***MR.*** Signal intensity of a CAA-associated lobar hematoma varies with clot age **(10-54)**. Acute hematomas are isointense on T1WI and iso- to hypointense on T2WI.

The vast majority of patients with CAA have focal or patchy confluent WM hyperintensity on T2/FLAIR **(10-55B)**. Lobar lacunae are present in 25% of cases. Larger, asymmetric areas of confluent WM hyperintensity related to vasogenic edema on T2/FLAIR with or without microhemorrhages are characteristic of ABRA **(10-56A)**. Mass effect is typically absent unless ABRA **(10-56)** or a focal amyloid mass ("amyloidoma") is present.

In addition to residua from lobar hemorrhages **(10-54)**, T2* (GRE, SWI) sequences demonstrate multifocal punctate "blooming black dots" in the leptomeninges, cortex, and subcortical WM **(10-55C)** **(10-56B)**. The basal ganglia and cerebellum are relatively spared.

Both ABRA and amyloidoma may show such striking enhancement on T1 C+ that they mimic meningitis, encephalitis, or neoplasm. Vessel wall imaging has shown vessel wall enhancement in patients with inflammatory amyloid.

### CEREBRAL AMYLOID DISEASE

**Pathology**

- Aβ40 deposited in meningeal, cortical arterioles
  - "Congophilic" angiopathy
  - Mural, perivascular inflammation common
- Vessel walls thicker but weaker
- Lobar bleeds
- Perivascular microhemorrhages

**Clinical Issues**

- Causes 5-20% of spontaneous intracranial hemorrhages in older adult patients
  - Increased age = strongest risk factor
  - Most patients > 55 years old
- Normotensive, demented older adult typical

**Imaging**

- Classic NECT findings
  - Lobar hemorrhages of different ages
  - cSAH
- MR shows multifocal microbleeds
  - "Blooming" hypointensities on T2*
  - Typically cortical, meningeal (pial)
  - Cerebellum, brainstem, basal ganglia generally spared
  - Cortical superficial siderosis common
- Less common = Aβ-related inflammatory angiitis
  - T2/FLAIR parenchymal hyperintensity
  - Edema, mass effect
  - ± T2* "blooming" microbleeds
  - ± sulcal-cisternal enhancement
- Rare = intracerebral amyloidoma (focal mass)

***Differential Diagnosis.*** The major differential diagnosis of CAA is **chronic hypertensive encephalopathy** (CHtnE). The microbleeds associated with CHtnE often involve the basal ganglia and cerebellum. Peripheral microbleeds occur but are less common than CAA-related microhemorrhages, which typically affect the cortex and leptomeninges.

**Hemorrhagic lacunar infarcts** can demonstrate "blooming" hemosiderin deposits. The basal ganglia and deep cerebral WM are the most common sites, helping distinguish these infarcts from the peripheral microbleeds of CAA.

**Multiple cavernous angiomas** (Zabramski type 4) typically involve the subcortical WM, basal ganglia, and cerebellum. The cortex is a less common site. "Locules" of blood with fluid-fluid levels and hemorrhages at different stages of evolution are often present in addition to multifocal "blooming black dots" on T2*.

**Hemorrhagic metastases** at the gray matter-WM junction can resemble CAA. The multifocal microbleeds typical of CAA lack mass effect, peripheral edema, and enhancement.

**Neurocysticercosis** may result in multiple foci of "blooming" hemosiderin deposits. These are often located at the convexity subarachnoid spaces but may occur throughout the brain.

The major differential diagnosis for ABRA includes **CAA-related inflammation**, which has imaging features that mimic ABRA and may require biopsy to differentiate.

**Vasculitis** is another consideration, though typically presents as multiple cerebral infarcts of variable ages in different vascular territories, often with blood products. Angiography shows multifocal vascular narrowing involving small- and medium-sized vessels.

With the new therapies for AD, including amyloid-lowering monoclonal antibodies, **amyloid-related imaging abnormalities (ARIA)** may mimic ABRA. ARIA includes ARIA-E and ARIA-H. **ARIA-E** is parenchymal or sulcal FLAIR hyperintensities related to parenchymal edema &/or CSF effusions. **ARIA-H** is characterized by hypointense foci of "blooming" hemosiderin on T2*/GRE/SWI.

*Selected References: The complete reference list is available on the eBooks+ version included with purchase.*

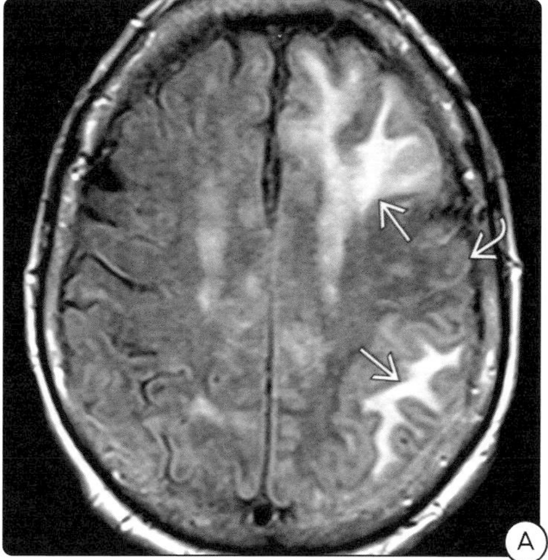


***(10-56A)** FLAIR shows confluent WM hyperintensity ➡ with mild mass effect, sulcal effacement, & lack of FLAIR suppression ➡.*

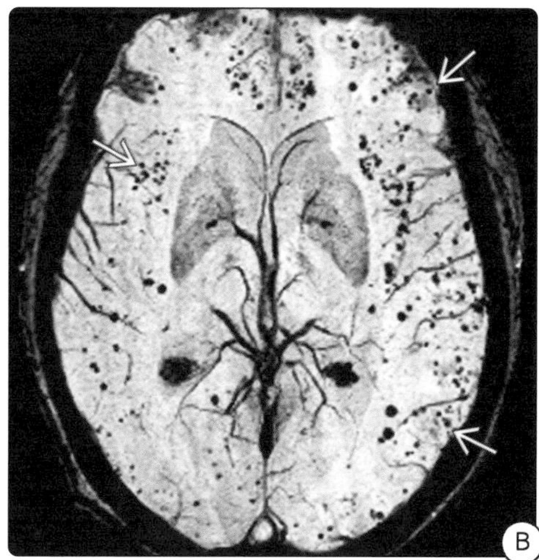


***(10-56B)** T2* SWI shows innumerable peripheral "blooming black dots" in both hemispheres ➡ with sparing of the basal ganglia & thalami.*

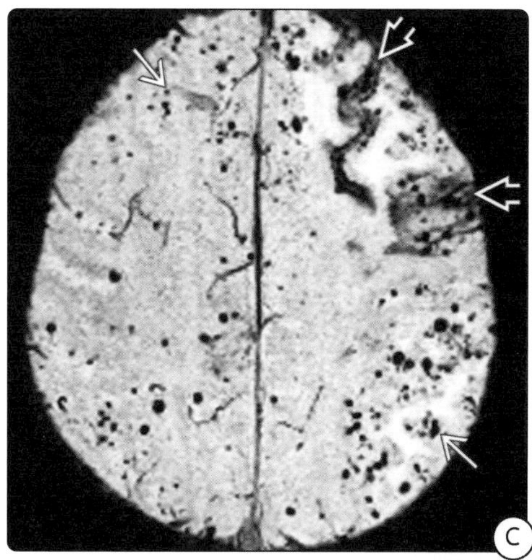


***(10-56C)** Cephalad T2* shows of siderosis ➡ & numerous microhemorrhages ➡. CAA-related inflammation [amyloid β-related angiitis (ABRA)].*

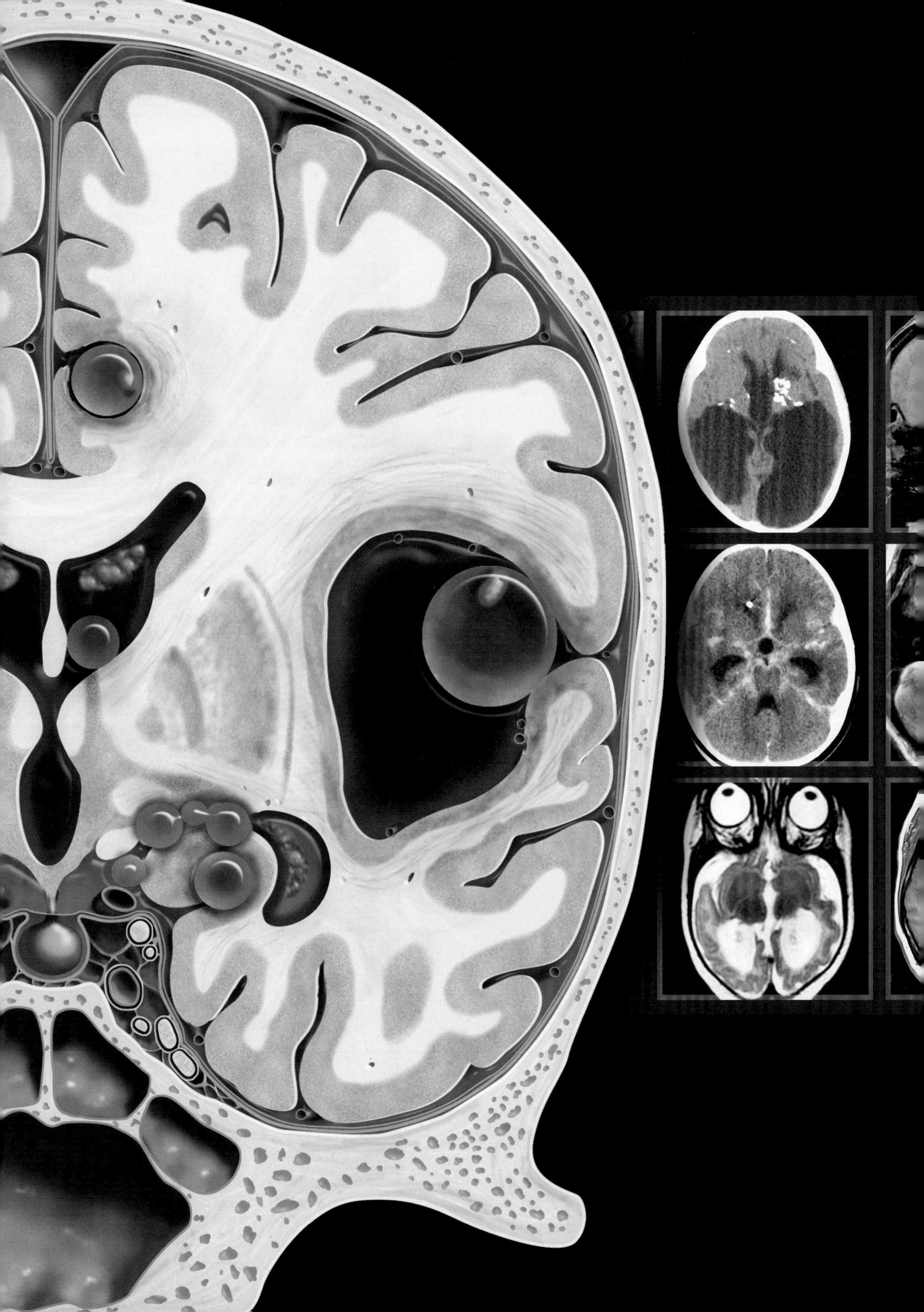

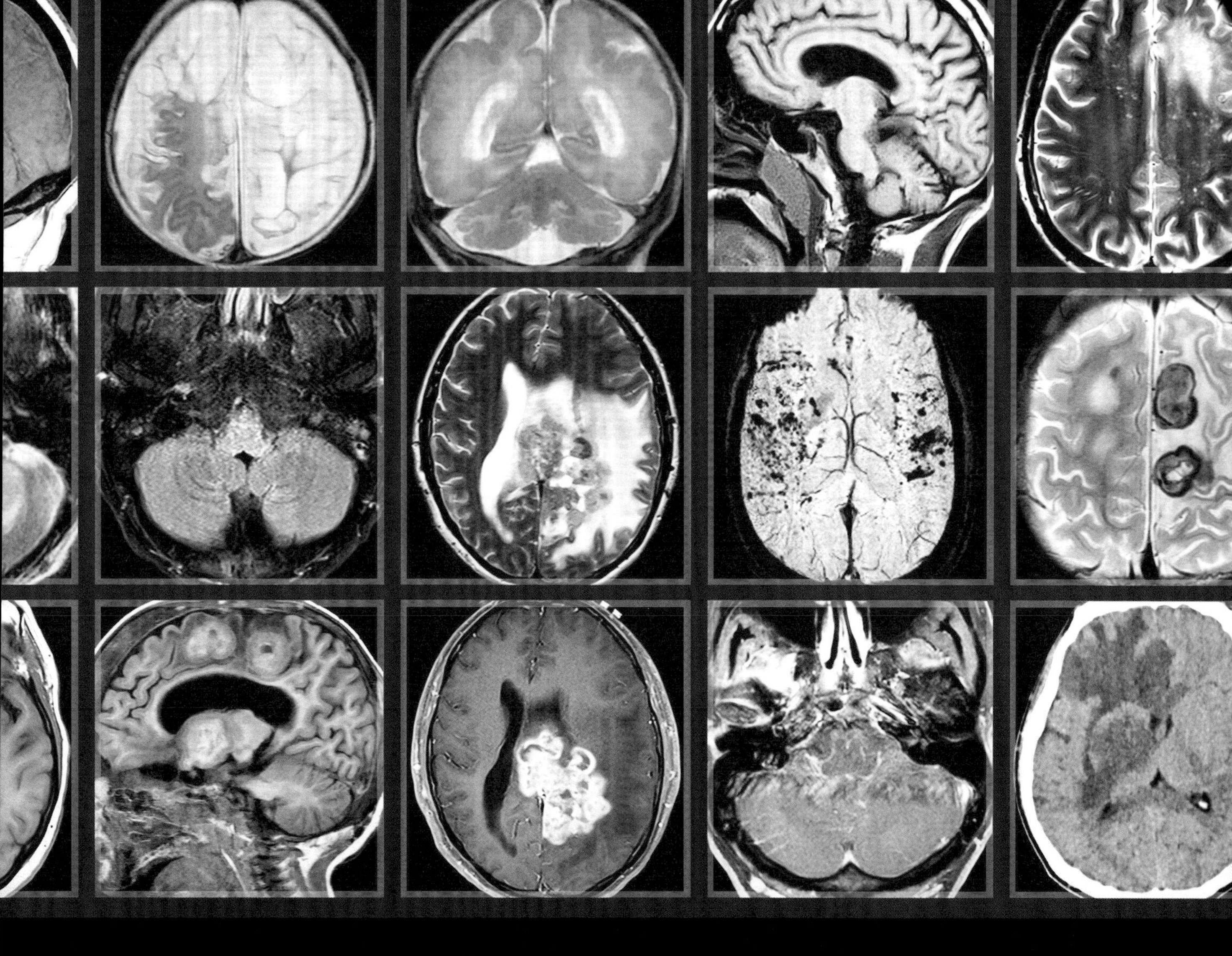

SECTION 3

# Infection, Inflammation, and Demyelinating Diseases

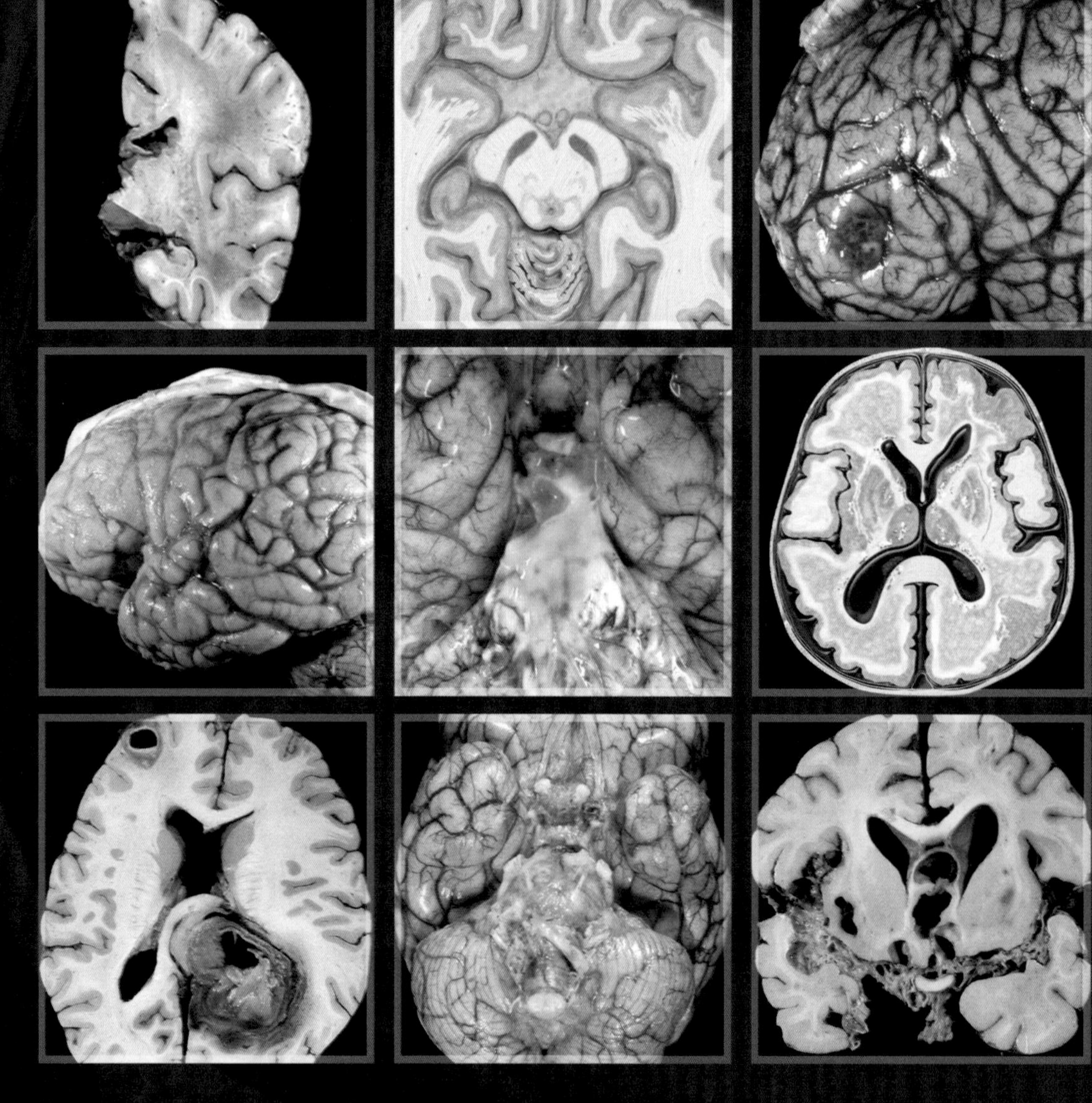

SECTION 3

# Infection, Inflammation, and Demyelinating Diseases

# Approach to Infection, Inflammation, and Demyelination

*Although any part of the human body can become inflamed or infected, the brain has long been considered an "immunologically protected" site because of the blood-brain barrier. While CNS infections are considerably less common than their systemic counterparts, the brain is by no means invulnerable to onslaught from pathogenic organisms.*



The role of medical imaging in the emergent evaluation of intracranial infection ideally should be supportive, not primary. But in many health care facilities worldwide, triage of acute CNS disease frequently uses brain imaging as an initial noninvasive "screening procedure." Therefore, the radiologist may be the first—not the last—to recognize the presence of possible CNS infection.

In this part, we devote Chapters 12 and 13 to CNS infections. HIV/AIDS is covered in Chapter 14. The last chapter, Chapter 15, considers the surprisingly broad spectrum of noninfectious idiopathic inflammatory and demyelinating disorders that affect the CNS.

## CNS Infections

The concept that the brain was an "immune-privileged" organ in which the blood-brain barrier (BBB) was a relative fortress that restricted pathogen entry and limited inflammation has recently undergone significant revision. Lymphocytes circulate through the normal healthy brain, immune responses can occur without lasting consequence, and cross-talk between the brain and extra-CNS organs is both extensive and robust.

Evidence has also recently emerged that there is extensive CSF and interstitial fluid (ISF) exchange throughout the brain, a process now termed "glymphatics."

A pathway of waste removal from the CNS does exist and is facilitated by CSF entering the brain parenchyma and spinal cord via aquaporin-4 water channels on astrocytes that surround the brain vasculature. This wave of CSF entry drives ISF toward the perivenous space where it collects and drains through lymphatic channels in the dural sinuses through foramina at the skull base to the deep cervical lymph nodes. The process flushes extracellular debris (including β-amyloid) from the parenchyma.

The presence of these drainage systems within the CNS is evidence that there is a constant flow and exchange of proteins within the brain and the blood. CD4(+) central and effector memory T cells are found in healthy CSF. The brain is therefore not a "privileged organ" that is immunologically isolated from the rest of the body but rather is actively monitored by—and accessible to—blood-borne lymphocytes and their mediators.

A surprisingly large number of pathogens, including many neurotropic viruses, can infect the CNS. Well over 200 different organisms have been described as causing CNS infections of one type or another. Most recently, the importance of recognizing brain disorders in patients infected with SARS-CoV-2 virus has become paramount. Patients with COVID-19 infections may experience an array of neurologic manifestations ranging in severity from headaches to life-threatening strokes and brain bleeds. Awareness of neurologic involvement in SARS-CoV-2 infection and the broad spectrum of its potential imaging manifestations is essential for clinical neuroimaging.

In this text, we divide infections into congenital and acquired disorders. Congenital infections are briefly covered in Chapter 12. Because this is a relatively short discussion, we combine these with acquired pyogenic and viral infections.

Our discussion of pyogenic infections begins with meningitis followed by a consideration of focal brain infections (cerebritis, abscess), ventriculitis **(11-1)**, and pus collections in the extraaxial spaces (subdural/epidural empyemas) **(11-2)**. We close the chapter with CNS manifestations of acquired viral infections.

The pathogenesis and imaging of tuberculosis (TB), fungal infections, and parasitic and protozoal infestations are considered in Chapter 13.

# HIV/AIDS

In the more than four decades since AIDS was first identified, the disease has become a worldwide epidemic. With the development of effective combination antiretroviral

*__(11-1)__ Note the small, well-encapsulated frontal lobe abscess ➡ has a larger, less well-defined lesion in the contralateral hemisphere. A larger abscess ➡ ruptured into the ventricle ➡, causing pyocephalus and death. __(11-2)__ Autopsy shows the dura ➡ reflected up to reveal purulent-appearing collection in the underlying subdural space ➡, typical findings for pyogenic subdural empyema. (Courtesy R. Hewlett, MD.)*

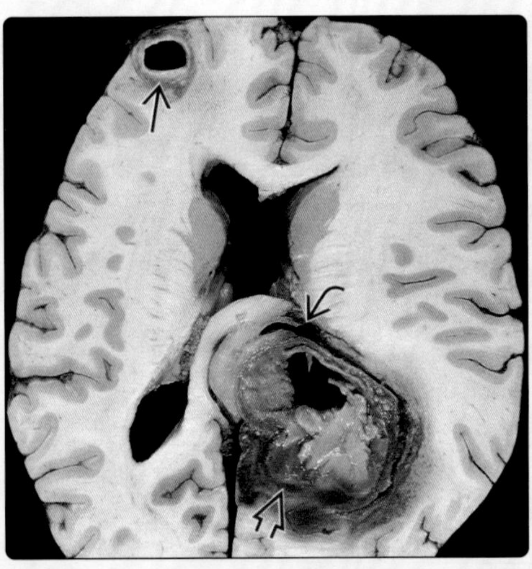

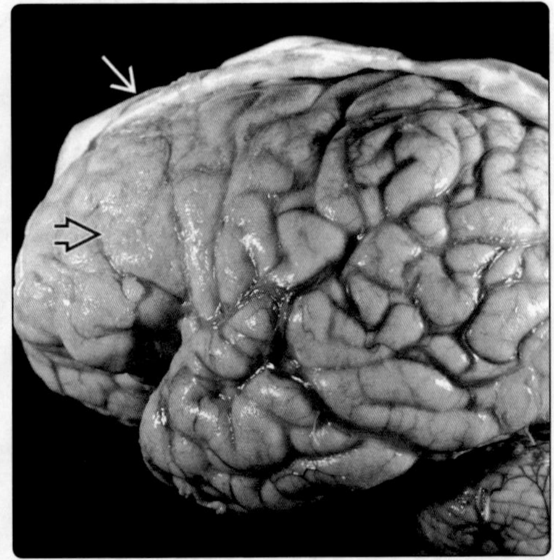

*__(11-3)__ Autopsy case of tuberculous meningitis shows thick exudate filling the basal cisterns ➡ and covering the pial surfaces of the frontal/temporal lobes and cerebellum ➡. (Courtesy R. Hewlett, MD.) __(11-4)__ Axial cut section of an autopsied brain in a patient with septicemia shows multifocal petechial hemorrhages, primarily in the cortex and gray matter-white matter interfaces. (Courtesy R. Hewlett, MD.)*

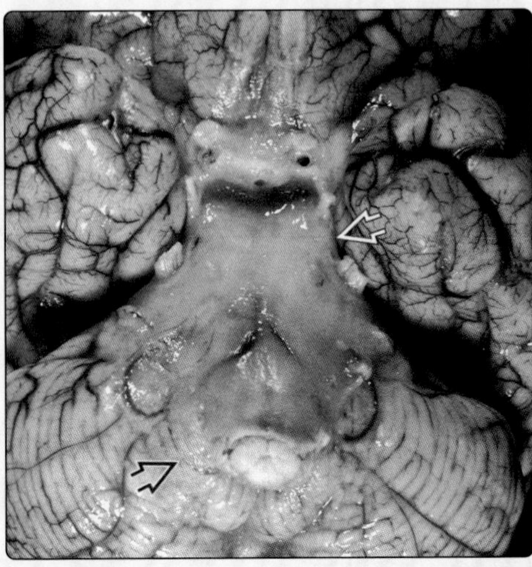

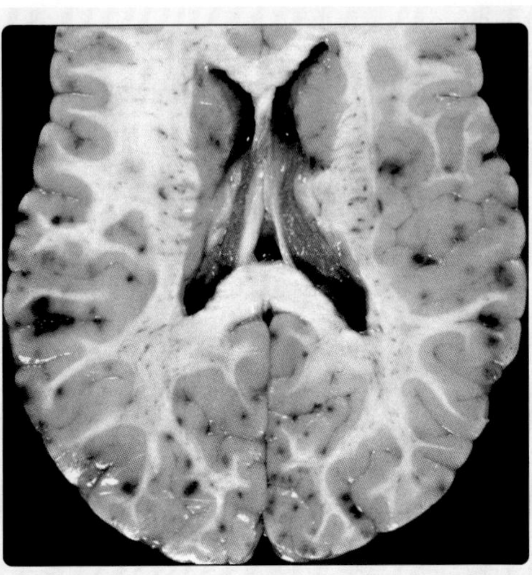

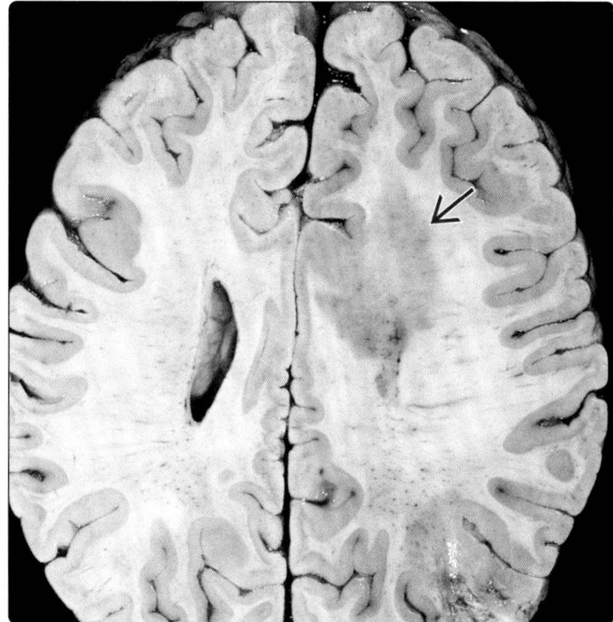

***(11-5) Axial autopsied brain shows a solitary "horseshoe" postinfectious tumefactive demyelinating lesion ⇒.***

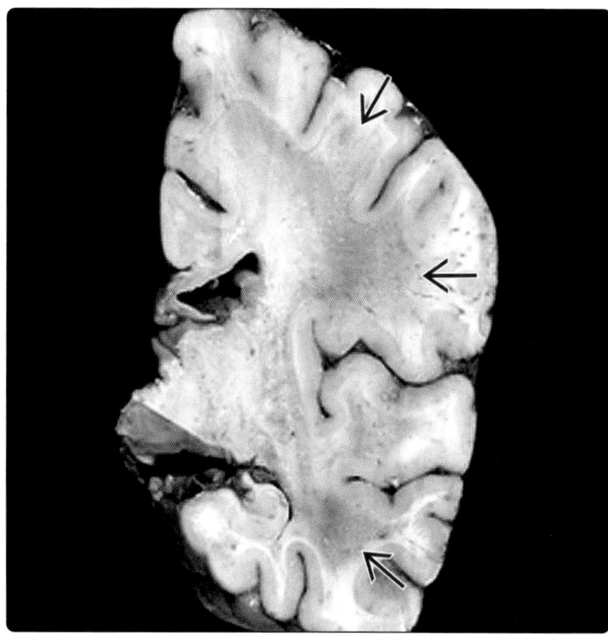

***(11-6) Coronal gross pathology in a case of severe multiple sclerosis shows confluent demyelination in the subcortical white matter ⇒. Note sparing of the subcortical U-fibers.***

therapies, HIV/AIDS has evolved from a virtual death sentence to a chronic but manageable disease if the treatment is (1) available and (2) affordable. As treated patients with HIV/AIDS now often survive for a decade or longer, the imaging spectrum of HIV/AIDS has also evolved.

Treated HIV/AIDS as a chronic disease looks very different from HIV/AIDS in so-called high-burden regions of the world. In such places, HIV in socioeconomically disadvantaged patients often behaves as an acute, fulminant infection. Comorbid diseases, such as TB, malaria, or overwhelming bacterial sepsis, are common complications and may dominate the imaging presentation.

Complications of HAART treatment have created their own set of recognized disorders, such as immune reconstitution inflammatory syndrome (IRIS). In Chapter 14, we consider the effect of HIV itself on the CNS (HIV encephalitis) as well as opportunistic infections, IRIS, miscellaneous manifestations of HIV/AIDS, and HIV-associated neoplasms.

# Demyelinating and Inflammatory Diseases

The final chapter in this section is devoted to demyelinating and noninfectious inflammatory diseases of the CNS **(11-5)**.

*Inflammation* is not synonymous with infection. Inflammation (from Latin, meaning "to ignite" or "set alight") is the response of tissues to a variety of pathogens (which may or may not be infectious microorganisms). The inflammatory "cascade" is complex and multifactorial. It involves the vascular system, immune system, and cellular responses, such as microglial activation, the primary component of the brain's innate immune response.

The CNS functions as a unique microenvironment that responds differently than the body's other systems to infiltrating immune cells. The brain white matter is especially susceptible to inflammatory disease. Inflammation can be acute or chronic, manageable or life threatening. Therefore, imaging plays a central role in the identification and follow-up of neuroinflammatory disorders.

The bulk of Chapter 15 is devoted to multiple sclerosis (MS) **(11-6)**. Also included is a discussion of MS variants and the surprisingly broad spectrum of idiopathic (noninfectious) inflammatory demyelinating diseases (IIDDs), such as neuromyelitis optica. Susac syndrome is a retinocochleocerebral vasculopathy that is often mistaken for MS on imaging studies, so it is also discussed in the context of IIDDs.

Postinfection, postvaccination, autoimmune-mediated demyelinating disorders are considered next. Acute disseminated encephalomyelitis (ADEM) and its most fulminant variant, acute hemorrhagic leukoencephalitis (AHLE), are delineated in detail.

We close the chapter with a discussion of neurosarcoid and inflammatory pseudotumors, including the rapidly expanding category of IgG4-related disorders.

*Selected References: The complete reference list is available on the eBooks+ version included with purchase.*

# Congenital, Acquired Pyogenic, and Acquired Viral Infections

*Infectious diseases can be conveniently divided into congenital/neonatal and acquired infections. There are unique infectious agents that affect the developing brain. The stage of fetal development at the time of infection is often more important than the causative organism. The clinical manifestations of fetal and neonatal infection and long-term neurologic consequences compared with infections that affect the more mature or fully developed brain will be emphasized.*

We then delineate the first major category of acquired infections, i.e., pyogenic infections. We start with meningitis, the most common of the pyogenic infections. Abscess, together with its earliest manifestations (cerebritis), is discussed next, followed by considerations of ventriculitis (a rare but potentially fatal complication of deep-seated brain abscesses) and intracranial empyemas.

We close the chapter with a discussion of the pathologic and imaging manifestations of acquired viral infections.



## Congenital Infections

Parenchymal calcifications are the hallmark of most congenital infections **(12-1)** and have been reported with cytomegalovirus (CMV) **(12-1)**, toxoplasmosis, congenital herpes simplex virus (HSV) infection, rubella, congenital varicella-zoster virus (VZV), Zika virus, and lymphocytic choriomeningitis virus (LCMV).

Infections of the fetal brain result in a spectrum of injury and malformation that depends more on the timing of infection than the infectious agent itself. Infections early in fetal development (e.g., during the first trimester) usually result in miscarriage, severe brain destruction, &/or profound malformations, such as anencephaly, agyria, and lissencephaly.

When infections occur later in pregnancy, encephaloclastic manifestations and myelination disturbance (e.g., demyelination, dysmyelination, and hypomyelination) predominate. Microcephaly with frank brain destruction and widespread encephalomalacia are common.

With few exceptions (toxoplasmosis and syphilis), most congenital/perinatal infections are viral and usually secondary to transplacental passage of the infectious agent. Zika virus is a relative newcomer to the list of viruses recognized as a cause of congenital CNS infection and is capable of causing profound brain destruction and resultant microcephaly. Zika virus infection

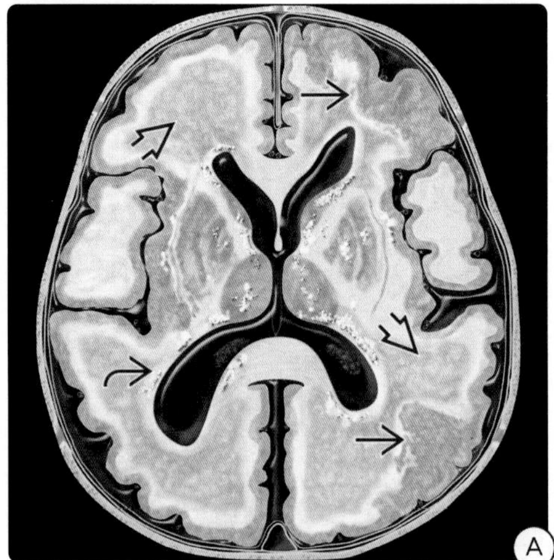

(12-1A) Congenital CMV is shown with periventricular parenchymal $Ca^{++}$ ➩, damaged WM ➩, and dysplastic cortex ➩.

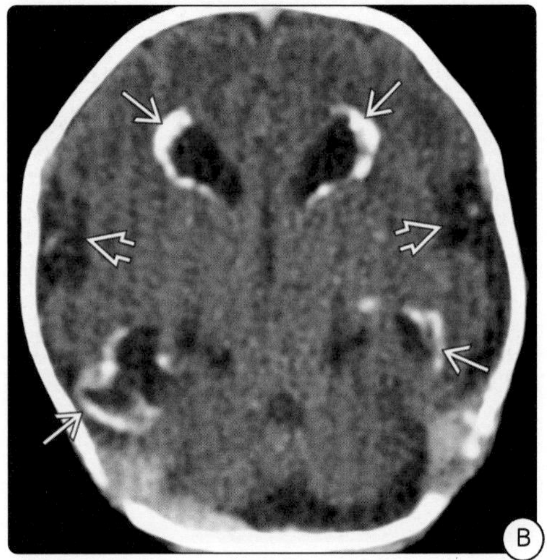

(12-1B) NECT in a newborn with CMV shows broad sylvian fissures ➩ and periventricular $Ca^{++}$ ➩.

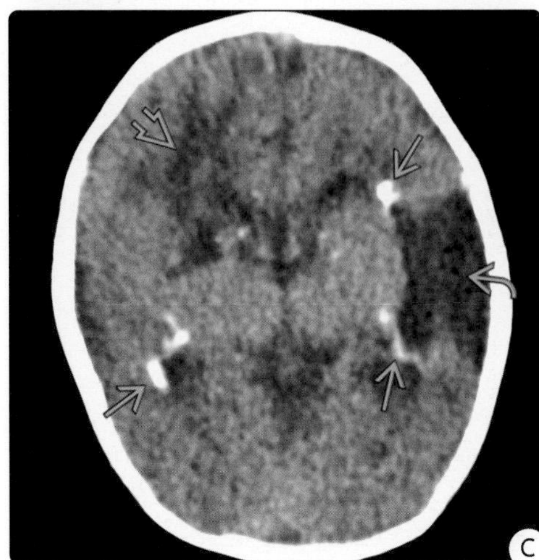

(12-1C) Axial NECT in a 2-month-old shows periventricular $Ca^{++}$ ➩, WM hypoattenuation ➩, and left opercular encephalomalacia ➩.

represents the first reported congenital CNS infection to be mostly transmitted by mosquitoes.

Six members of the herpesvirus family cause neurologic disease in children: HSV-1, HSV-2, VZV, Epstein-Barr virus (EBV), CMV, and human herpesvirus 6 (HHV-6). Aside from CMV, HSV-2, Zika virus, and congenital HIV (vertically transmitted), congenital CNS infections have become less common due to immunization programs, prenatal screening, and global infection surveillance.

We begin the chapter with an overview of TORCH infections and important non-TORCH congenital/perinatal CNS infections. We start with the most globally common of the congenital infections: Congenital CMV infection.

## TORCH Infections: Overview

### Terminology

Congenital infections include diverse bacteria, viruses, and parasites. They are often grouped together and simply called **TORCH** infections—the acronym for **to**xoplasmosis, **r**ubella, **C**MV, and **h**erpes. The TORCH pneumonic provides a limited description of the expanding list of pathogens that can be associated with congenital infection.

### Etiology

The placenta normally restricts vertical transmission but some pathogens access the intraamniotic space and can overcome placental defenses. In addition to the recognized "classic" TORCH(S) infections, a host of new organisms have been identified as causing congenital and perinatal infections. These include Zika virus, LCMV, human parvovirus B19, human parechovirus, hepatitis B, VZV, tuberculosis, HIV, and the parasitic infection toxocariasis.

Sequelae of congenital infections range from asymptomatic infection to severe debilitating disease and still birth.

### Imaging

CMV, toxoplasmosis, rubella, Zika virus, VZV, LCMV, and HIV may all cause parenchymal calcifications **(12-1A)**. The location and distribution of the calcifications may strongly suggest the specific infectious agent. CMV—the most common congenital infection in resource-rich countries—causes periventricular calcifications **(12-1B)**, cysts, cortical clefts **(12-1C)**, polymicrogyria (PMG), schizencephaly, and white matter (WM) injury.

Early CNS infection with Zika virus leads to severe microcephaly and calcifications at the gray matter (GM)-WM junction. Rubella and HSV cause lobar destruction, cystic encephalomalacia, and nonpatterned calcifications. Congenital syphilis is relatively rare, causing basilar meningitis, arterial strokes, and scattered dystrophic calcifications. Congenital HIV is associated with basal ganglia calcification, atrophy, and aneurysmal arteriopathy.

TORCH(S), Zika virus, and LCMV infections should be considered in newborns and infants with microcephaly, parenchymal calcifications, chorioretinitis, and intrauterine growth restriction.

The timing of the gestational infection determines the magnitude and appearance of the brain insult. For example, early gestational CMV infection causes germinal zone necrosis with subependymal cysts and dystrophic calcifications. WM volume loss occurs at all gestational ages and can be diffuse or multifocal. Malformations of cortical development are very common, and PMG has the greatest prevalence.

## Congenital Cytomegalovirus Infection

Congenital CMV is the leading cause of nonhereditary deafness in children and is the most common cause of congenital brain infection in resource-rich countries.

### Terminology

Congenital CMV infection is also called CMV encephalitis. CMV is a ubiquitous DNA virus that belongs to the HHV family. Human CMV is ubiquitous, present in 40-100% of the population worldwide.

### Pathology

Timing of the gestational infection determines the magnitude of brain insult. Early gestational CMV infection causes germinal zone necrosis with subependymal cysts and dystrophic calcifications. WM volume loss occurs at all gestational stages and can be diffuse or multifocal. Malformations of cortical development are common, and PMG has the greatest prevalence.

### Clinical Issues

**Epidemiology.** CMV is the most common of congenital infection in the resource-rich world. Between 0.25-1% of newborn infants shed CMV in their urine or saliva at birth. 10-15% of infected newborns develop CNS or systemic symptoms and signs.

**Presentation and Natural History.** Symptomatic newborns and infants may exhibit microcephaly, jaundice, hepatosplenomegaly, chorioretinitis, and rash. Asymptomatic newborns may show microcephaly but otherwise initially appear developmentally normal. Sensorineural hearing loss, seizures, and developmental delay are the major long-term risks.

### Imaging

Advances in fetal MR now permit antenatal detection of PMG, germinolytic cysts, and cerebellar dysgenesis. Postnatal manifestations are protean and include microcephaly, ventriculomegaly, germinolytic cysts, malformations of cortical development, calcifications, cerebellar and hippocampal dysgenesis, and WM abnormalities.

**CT Findings.** NECT shows intracranial calcifications and ventriculomegaly in the majority of symptomatic infants. Calcifications are predominately periventricular with a predilection for the germinal matrix zones along the caudostriatal interfaces **(12-1)**. Some gross abnormalities, such as cortical clefting and GM anomalies, may be demonstrable on NECT.

**MR Findings.** Ventriculomegaly is almost universal. Cortical migrational anomalies, such as PMG, are common **(12-2)**. Germinal zone and anterior temporal cysts, parenchymal calcifications, WM abnormalities (dysplastic and demyelinating), hippocampal dysgenesis, and cerebellar malformations are common.

Cortical migrational and organizational abnormalities range from minor dysgenesis with focal cortical clefting, simplified gyral pattern and "open" (i.e., shallow) sylvian fissures to more severe manifestations, including agyria, lissencephaly, and schizencephaly.

T1WIs show microcephaly, enlarged ventricles and germinal zone or anterior temporal cysts. Cerebellar and hippocampal dysgenesis are common. WM hypointensities corresponding to regions of demyelination and dysplasia are common. Brain calcifications are typically best demonstrated on SWI (or to a lesser degree, GRE) **(12-3)**, but may also be evident as hyperintense T1 and hypointense T2 foci.

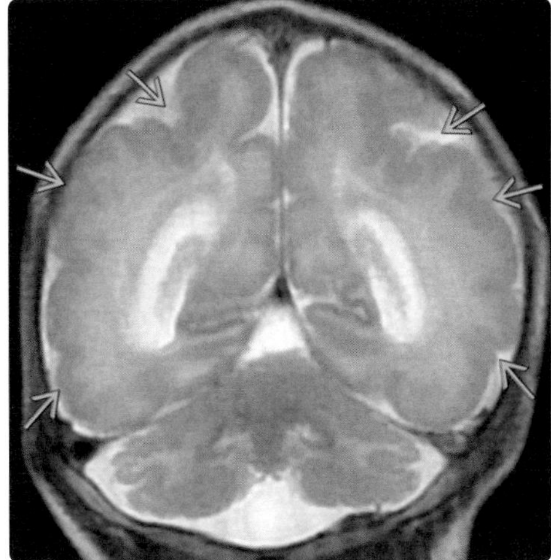

***(12-2)** Coronal T2WI in a neonate with CMV shows symmetric bilateral perisylvian polymicrogyria ➔.*

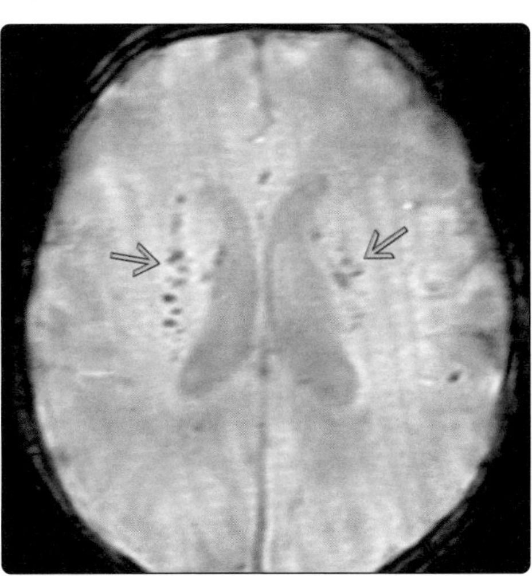

***(12-3)** Axial SWI in a neonate with congenital CMV shows caudostriatal $Ca^{++}$ ➔.*

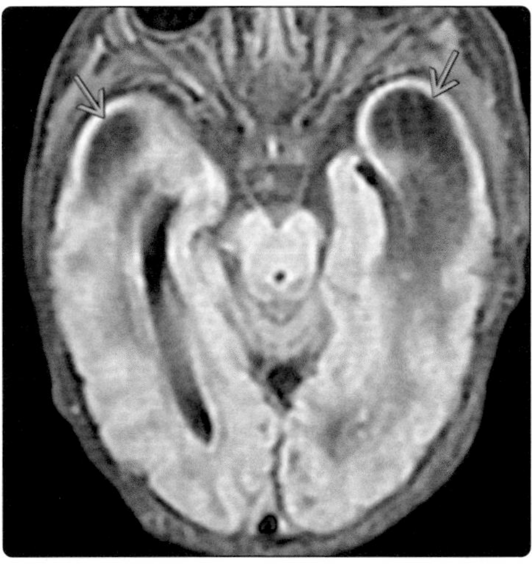

***(12-4)** Axial FLAIR in a newborn with CMV shows bilateral anterior temporal lobe cysts ➔.*

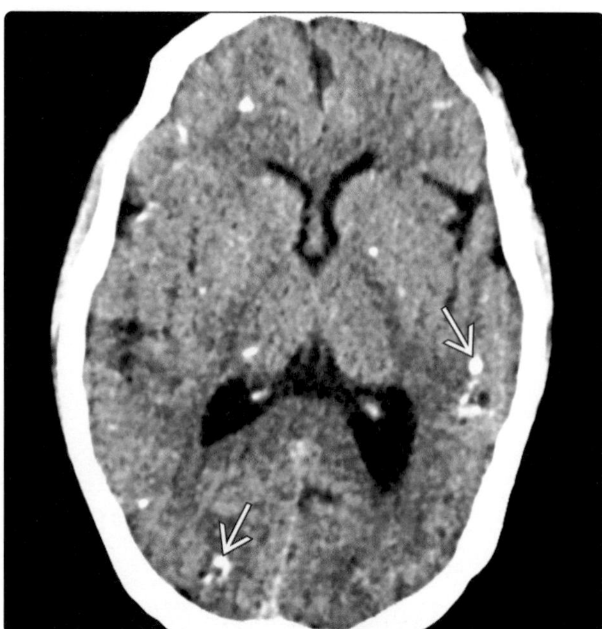

***(12-5) NECT in a 29-yo with known congenital toxoplasmosis, intellectual disability, and seizures shows multiple Ca$^{++}$ that are mainly peripheral, in the cortex or at the GM-WM interfaces ➡.***

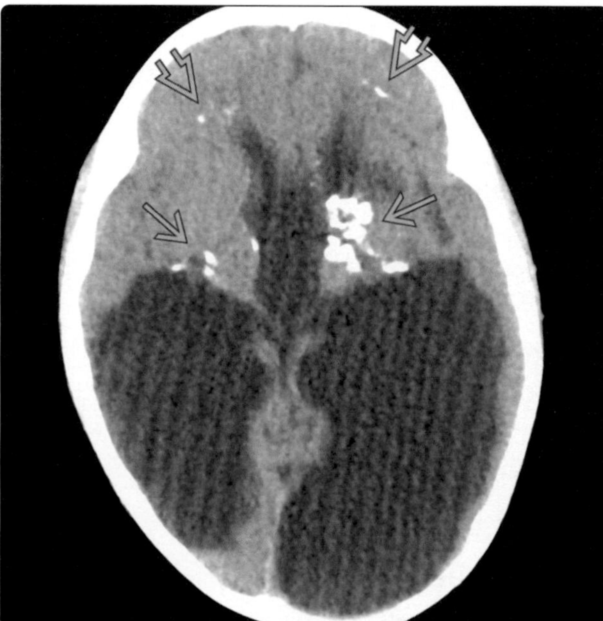

***(12-6) Axial NECT in a 6-yo with congenital toxoplasmosis shows deep nuclear ➡ and WM ➡ Ca$^{++}$ as well as ventricular enlargement, reflecting a combination of volume loss and hydrocephalus.***

T2WI and FLAIR show delayed myelination, WM injury, anterior temporal cysts **(12-4)**, and volume loss with focal, patchy or confluent periventricular abnormalities. Malformations of cortical organization and migrational disturbances are common. Coronal FLAIR/T2WIs may show vertically oriented, dysmorphic hippocampi and cerebellar dysgenesis.

## Differential Diagnosis

The differential diagnosis of congenital CMV includes other TORCH and non-TORCH infections, including toxoplasmosis, Zika virus, and lymphocytic choriomeningitis (LCMV).

**Toxoplasmosis** is much less common than CMV and typically causes scattered parenchymal calcifications, not the dominant subependymal pattern observed in CMV. **Zika virus** infection can also cause multiple peripherally located calcifications. However, Zika generally causes much more severe microcephaly with overlapping sutures and striking craniofacial disproportion. Sulcation-migration disorders with PMG and lissencephaly are also common.

Some genetic disorders called **pseudo-TORCH syndromes** mimic the imaging abnormalities of congenital infections, such as CMV. Diseases, such as Aicardi-Goutières and Coats plus syndrome, are rare, mostly autosomal recessive degenerative disorders. Basal ganglia and brainstem calcifications are more common than the subependymal pattern characteristic of CMV, Zika, or LCMV infections. Pseudo-TORCH syndromes also typically lack the cortical malformations so common in many of the congenital infections.

# Congenital Toxoplasmosis

## Etiology

Congenital toxoplasmosis is the second most common of the congenital infections. Intrauterine infection is caused by ingestion of water or food contaminated by *Toxoplasma gondii*, one of the world's most common obligate intracellular parasites. The infection is usually acquired by direct contact with the feces of an infected cat.

## Pathology

Ependymitis leading to aqueductal obstruction and hydrocephalus with resultant macrocephaly is seen in ~ 50% of congenital toxoplasmosis. Diffuse inflammation of the meninges is typical. Unlike CMV, malformations of cortical development are rare.

## Clinical Issues

Congenital toxoplasmosis causes severe chorioretinitis, jaundice, hepatosplenomegaly, growth restriction, and brain damage. Infants with subclinical infection at birth are at risk for seizures and delayed cognitive and motor development. Visual defects from chorioretinitis are common.

## Imaging

With some exceptions, imaging features resemble those of CMV, Zika, and LCMV. NECT shows extensive parenchymal calcifications that appear scattered throughout the brain parenchyma **(12-5)**, unlike the germinal zone calcifications of CMV or subcortical calcifications of Zika virus infection.

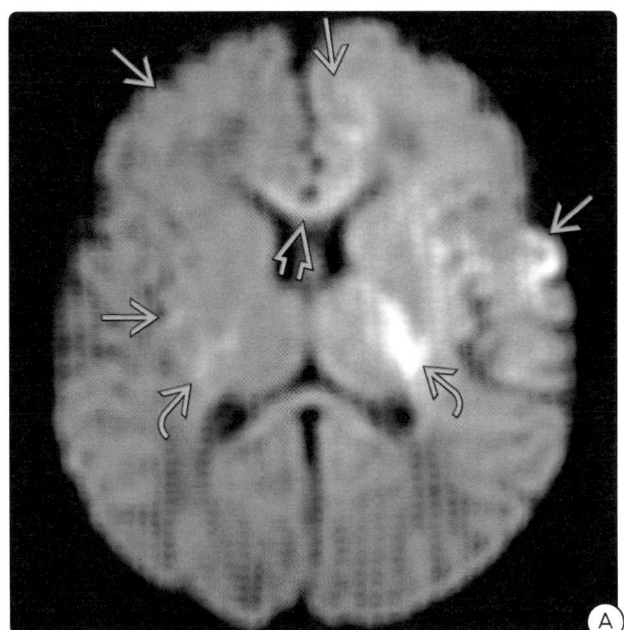

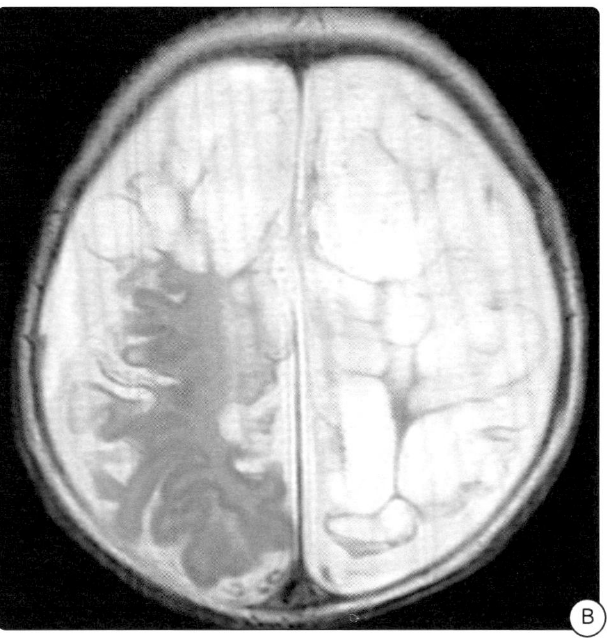

***(12-7A) Axial DWI in a 4-week-old with seizures and neonatal herpes encephalitis shows diffusion restriction involving the L > R frontal lobe cortex ⮕, corpus callosum ⮕, and internal capsules ⮕. T1 and T2 were normal.***

***(12-7B) Axial T2WI in the same patient at 4 months shows near-complete loss of affected cerebral hemispheres with development of severe cystic encephalomalacia.***

MR may show multiple subcortical cysts, ventriculomegaly **(12-6)**, and porencephaly. Malformations of cortical development are uncommon.

### Differential Diagnosis

The major differential diagnosis is **congenital CMV** infection. Here, the calcifications are deep in the periventricular zone and cortical dysplasias are common.

## Herpes Simplex Virus: Congenital and Neonatal Infections

### Terminology

CNS involvement in HSV infection is called **congenital** or **neonatal HSV** when it involves neonates. In contradistinction, herpes simplex encephalitis (HSE) (which is also sometimes called HSV encephalitis) describes encephalitis in individuals beyond the first postnatal month. In this section, we discuss neonatal HSV. HSE is discussed subsequently with other acquired viral infections.

### Etiology

Approximately 2,000 infants in the USA annually are diagnosed with either HSV-1 or HSV-2 neonatal infection. The vast majority (85%) of cases are acquired at parturition while 10% are contracted postnatally. Only 5% of cases are due to **in utero** transmission.

### Pathology

Neonatal HSV encephalitis is a diffuse disease without the predilection for the temporal lobes and limbic system seen in older children and adults. Early changes include meningoencephalitis with necrosis and hemorrhage. Atrophy with gross cystic encephalomalacia and parenchymal calcifications is typical of late-stage HSV. Near-total loss of brain substance with hydranencephaly is seen in severe cases.

### Clinical Issues

**Epidemiology.** Approximately 2,000 infants in the USA are diagnosed with neonatal HSV-1 or HSV-2 infections each year. HSV-2 is one of the most prevalent sexually transmitted infections worldwide. The majority are asymptomatic and most are completely unaware of the disease.

Neonatal HSV infections are vertically transmitted. The vast majority (85%) are acquired at parturition while 10-15% is acquired postnatally. Only 5% of cases are due to in utero transmission.

**Presentation.** Neonatal HSV infection causes three clinicopathologic disease patterns: (1) Skin, eye, and mouth disease; (2) encephalitis; and (3) disseminated disease with or without CNS disease. Approximately 50% of all infants with neonatal HSV will have CNS infection.

As most (~ 85%) HSV is transmitted at time of parturition, the onset of symptoms usually occurs ~ 2-4 weeks after delivery. Symptoms include lethargy, poor feeding, jaundice, and seizures. The definitive diagnosis is based on serum or CSF PCR, although up to 25% of neonates with HSV encephalitis have negative PCR studies.

**Natural History.** Death by one year of age occurs in ~ 50% of untreated neonates with overt CNS disease and 85% with disseminated infection. Surviving infants are at high risk for permanent deafness, vision loss, cerebral palsy, &/or epilepsy.

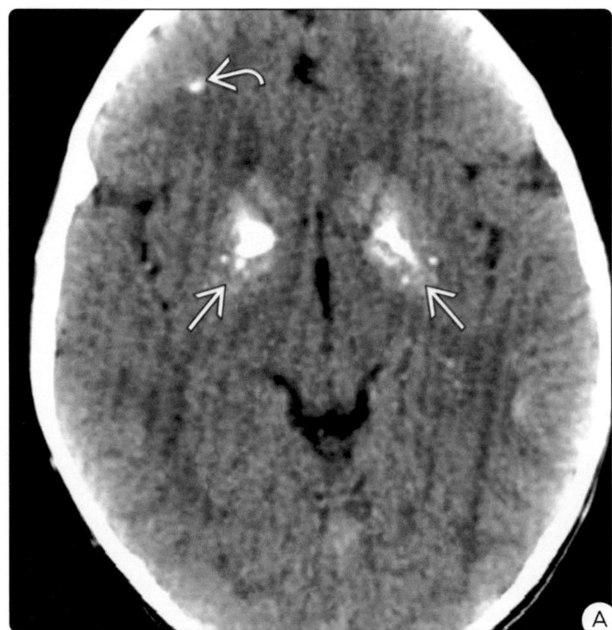

*(12-8A) NECT in a 5-yo child with congenital (perinatal) HIV shows bilateral symmetric $Ca^{++}$ in the basal ganglia ➡, subcortical WM ➡.*

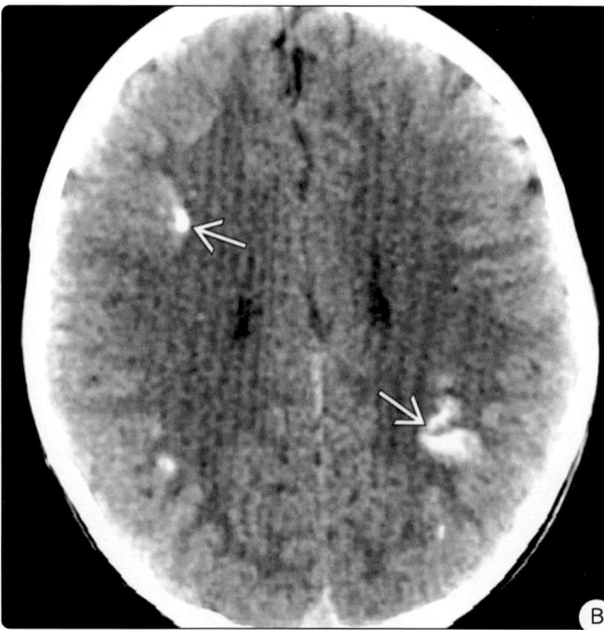

*(12-8B) More cephalad NECT shows punctate and curvilinear calcifications ➡ at the GM-WM junctions caused by mineralizing microangiopathy. With HAART, congenital HIV has become much less common. (Courtesy V. Mathews, MD.)*

Prompt treatment with antiviral agents significantly reduces morbidity.

## Imaging

Unlike childhood or adult HSE, neonatal HSV CNS infection is much more diffuse. Both GM and WM are affected. Radiologists should strongly consider neonatal HSV encephalitis when cranial imaging at 2-4 weeks of neonatal life shows unexplained diffuse cerebral edema with leptomeningeal enhancement, without or with cerebral parenchymal hemorrhage. Early MR with diffusion is advised.

**CT Findings.** NECT may be normal early in the disease or show diffuse hypoattenuation involving both cortex and subcortical WM, reflecting cerebral edema. Hemorrhages may present as multifocal punctate, patchy, and curvilinear regions of hyperattenuation in the basal ganglia, WM, and cortex.

**MR Findings.** In the acute and subacute stages of neonatal HSV, multifocal lesions (67%), deep GM involvement (58%), hemorrhage (66%), "watershed" pattern of injury (40%), and the occasional involvement of the brainstem and cerebellum may occur. It is important to note that T1WI and T2WI may be normal in the early stages of disease. DWI is the most sensitive early imaging marker of disease **(12-7A)**. T1WI may show hypointensity in affected areas. T2WIs may be show hyperintensity in the cortex, WM, and basal ganglia. Hemorrhagic foci on T2* or SWI sequences are common. Late-stage disease shows severe volume loss with enlarged ventricles and multicystic encephalomalacia **(12-7B)**.

DWI is key for the initial diagnosis of neonatal HSV encephalitis. DWI is the first sequence to become abnormal and typically is the most accurate sequence in determining the extent of brain involvement. In most patients, DWI demonstrates bilateral or significantly more extensive disease than seen on conventional MR.

FLAIR sequences at under eight months of age underestimate parenchymal pathology, particularly within the hemispheric WM.

Foci of patchy enhancement, typically a meningeal pattern of enhancement, are common on T1 C+. In later stages, T1 shortening and T2 hypointensity with "blooming" on T2* GRE/SWI secondary to hemorrhagic foci may develop.

MRS in early HSV encephalitis shows elevated lactate, lipids, choline, and excitatory neurotransmitters. NAA is reduced.

## Differential Diagnosis

The major differential diagnoses for neonatal HSV are **other TORCH and non-TORCH infections**. Because the initial imaging features of acute and subacute HSV encephalitis are often so nonspecific and may manifest with generalized cerebral edema, metabolic, toxic, and hypoxic-ischemic insults must also be considered in the differential diagnosis.

In some cases, HSV causes watershed distribution ischemic injury in areas remote from the primary herpetic lesions. Findings may be difficult to distinguish from partial protracted or mild to moderate **hypoxic-ischemic injury**. Hemorrhage with "blooming" on T2* GRE or SWI is uncommon in neonatal hypoxic-ischemic injury.

# Congenital (Perinatal) HIV

The imaging presentation of congenital HIV infection is quite different from the findings in acquired HIV/AIDS. The most striking and consistent finding is atrophy, particularly in the frontal lobes. Bilaterally symmetric basal ganglia calcifications are common **(12-8)**. Ectasia and fusiform enlargement of intracranial arteries are found in 3-5% of cases.

### Differential Diagnosis

The differential diagnosis of congenital HIV is other TORCH infections. **CMV** is characterized by periventricular calcifications, microcephaly, and cortical dysplasia. Other than volume loss, the brain in congenital HIV appears normal. **Toxoplasmosis** is much less common than CMV and causes scattered parenchymal calcifications, not symmetric basal ganglia lesions. **Pseudo-TORCH** calcifications involve cortex and WM, basal ganglia, brainstem, and cerebellum.

## Zika Virus Infection

### Etiology

Zika virus is a single-stranded RNA *Flavivirus*, closely related to dengue fever, yellow fever, West Nile virus, and chikungunya. The virus is mostly transmitted by infected female mosquito bites. It can also be transmitted through blood contamination perinatally and sexually.

### Pathology

Zika virus has been directly linked to severe fetal microcephaly in infants born to infected mothers. Like CMV, Zika virus crosses the fetal-placental barrier. Studies have confirmed the tropism of Zika virus for neural progenitor stem cells. Zika virus elicits a deleterious inflammatory response that compromises neurogenesis and brain formation.

### Clinical Issues

**Presentation.** Up to 80% of infected individuals are asymptomatic. Zika virus causes severe fetal brain damage, resulting in extreme microcephaly with overlapping sutures, closed fontanelles, seizures, poor feeding, and lethargy.

### Imaging

**CT Findings.** Microcephaly with craniofacial disproportion can be severe. By comparison to the small brain, the eyes can appear enlarged.

Cerebral parenchymal calcifications—typically at the hemispheric GM-WM junctions—are universally present **(12-9A)**. Calcifications may also occur in the basal ganglia/thalami, brainstem, and cerebellum. Ventriculomegaly and microcephaly are typical. Migrational disorders, such as polymicrogyria (PMG), lissencephaly, and pachygyria, are present in the majority of cases.

**MR Findings.** MR is the most comprehensive tool to depict parenchymal calcifications (SWI is more sensitive than GRE sequences). Malformations of cortical development, disturbed WM myelination, and ventriculomegaly are almost universal **(12-9)**.

### Differential Diagnosis

**Congenital CMV** can present with microcephaly and PMG. Calcifications along the caudostriatal groove are more common than those at the GM-WM interfaces. **Congenital toxoplasmosis** presents with macrocephaly, hydrocephalus, scattered calcifications, and lack of cortical malformations.

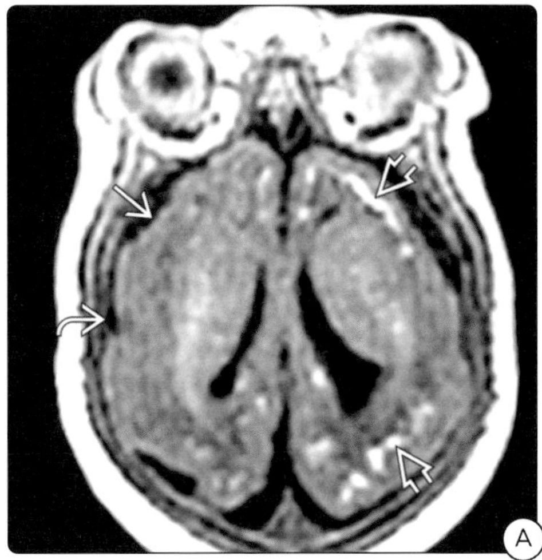

***(12-9A)** Congenital Zika virus infection shows smooth brain ➡, shallow sulci ➡, multiple Ca$^{++}$ at the GM-WM junction ➡.*

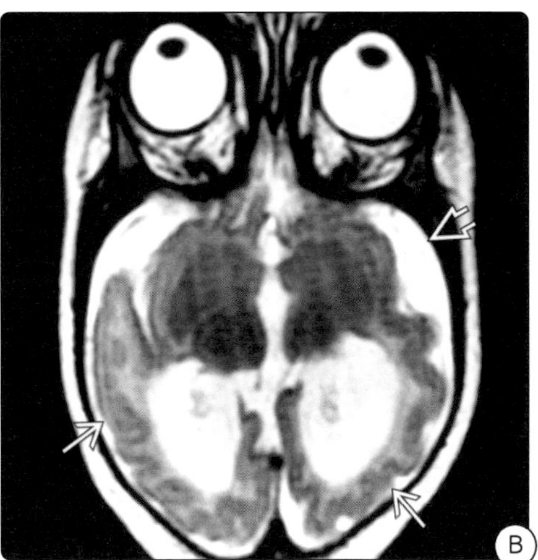

***(12-9B)** T2WI shows extreme craniofacial disproportion, shallow sylvian fissures ➡, simplified gyral pattern with polymicrogyria ➡.*

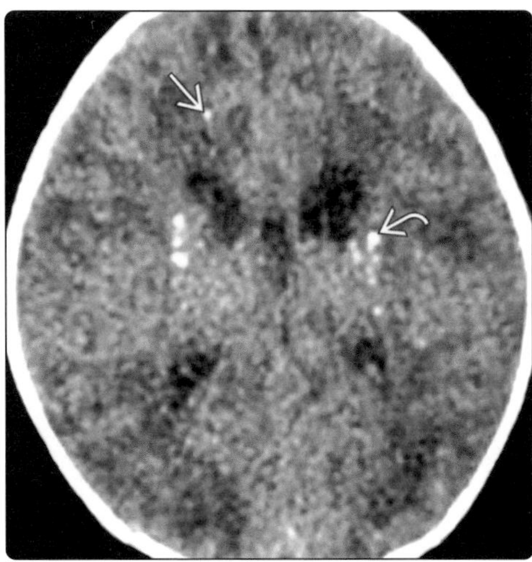

***(12-10)** NECT in an infant with congenital lymphocytic choriomeningitis shows focal parenchymal ➡, periventricular Ca$^{++}$ ➡.*

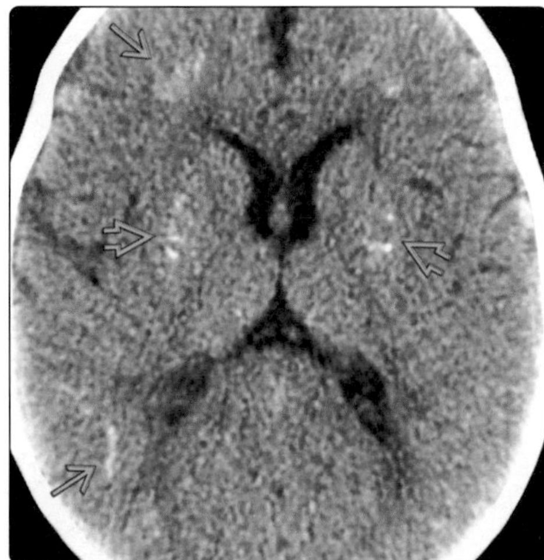

*(12-11) NECT in an 18-month-old boy with congenital rubella shows subcortical → and basal ganglia ⇒, $Ca^{++}$.*

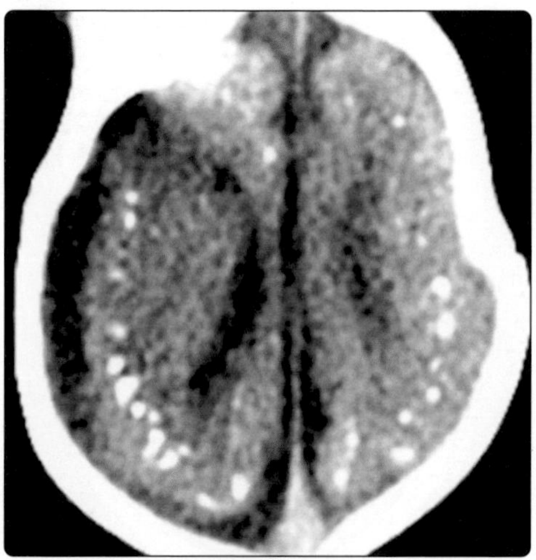

*(12-12) NECT shows microcephaly, subcortical $Ca^{++}$, and extremely undersulcated brain in congenital VZV infection.*

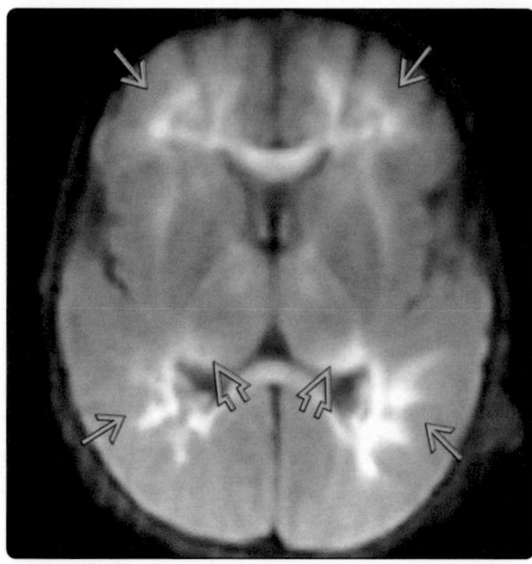

*(12-13) Axial DWI in a 14-day-old with human parechovirus shows cytotoxic edema in the WM → and portions of the thalami ⇒.*

## Lymphocytic Choriomeningitis Virus

### Etiology

Congenital lymphocytic choriomeningitis virus (LCMV) is an arenavirus with rodents as its typical vector. Many, but not all, cases are reported from rural environments.

### Pathology

LCMV causes a necrotizing ependymitis similar to congenital toxoplasmosis. Microcephaly, periventricular calcifications, hydrocephalus, and cortical migrational anomalies are common.

### Clinical Issues

In contrast to other congenital CNS infections, hepatosplenomegaly, jaundice, and skin rashes are absent in congenital LCMV. Definitive diagnosis requires LCMV-specific serologic responses, as they are often not routinely evaluated in TORCH(S) laboratory assessments. Mortality rate is high and survivors often have severe neurologic sequelae.

### Imaging

LCMV causes no pathognomonic imaging findings and can mimic CMV or toxoplasmosis **(12-10)**. Hydrocephalus and malformations of cortical development are typical. The diagnosis of LCMV should be considered when imaging findings mimic CMV, Zika, or toxoplasmosis and the clinical and serologic evaluation is reported as "normal."

### Differential Diagnosis

**Toxoplasmosis** lacks cortical malformations, **congenital CMV** typically shows caudostriatal groove or periventricular calcification and PMG. **Zika virus** calcification is most common at the GM-WM junction and **pseudo-TORCH** calcification involves the brainstem, basal ganglia, WM, and cortex and lacks cortical malformations.

## Other Congenital Infections

Congenital **rubella** infection is rare. With the widespread advent of effective vaccination, the prevalence of congenital rubella syndrome has decreased dramatically. Humans are the only known reservoir for the **rubella** virus.

Reported imaging findings include microcephaly, parenchymal calcifications **(12-11)**, including cortical calcifications, delayed myelination, periventricular and basal ganglia cysts, frontal-dominant WM lesions (NECT hypoattenuating and MR T2 hyperintense), and atrophy, and, in severe cases, total brain destruction has been described. Imaging findings are nonspecific. Late infection causes generalized brain volume loss, dystrophic calcifications, and regions of demyelination &/or gliosis.

Congenital **VZV** infection ("chickenpox") causes microcephaly, parenchymal calcifications **(12-12)**, ventriculomegaly, and PMG with nonpatterned necrosis of WM, lobar cortical and subcortical tissues, and deep gray nuclei.

Congenital/perinatal human **parechovirus** infection causes bilateral confluent WM abnormalities, often with involvement of the internal/external capsules and thalami **(12-13)**. The symmetric pattern of injury to the WM and thalami is often mistaken for hypoxic-ischemic injury in the neonate. These patients typically present later than perinatal asphyxia, usually with symptom onset and subsequent imaging investigation occurring many days or sometimes even weeks after birth. Chronic appearance is that of deep and periventricular leukomalacia.

**SELECTED CONGENITAL AND PERINATAL INFECTIONS: NEUROIMAGING FINDINGS AND COMMON CAUSES**

**Cytomegalovirus**
- Microcephaly, calcification at caudostriatal groove, PMG, cysts, WM abnormalities, cerebellar hypoplasia, vertical hippocampi

**Toxoplasmosis**
- Macrocephaly, hydrocephalus, scattered calcifications, lack of cortical malformations

**Herpes Simplex Virus**
- Early-diffuse cerebral edema, multifocal lesions, DWI abnormalities, hemorrhage, watershed infarctions, leptomeningeal enhancement, late cystic encephalomalacia

**Lymphocytic Choriomeningitis Virus**
- May precisely mimic features of CMV, negative routine TORCH testing

**Zika Virus**
- Microcephaly, ventriculomegaly, calcification at GM-WM junctions, cortical malformations

**Rubella Virus**
- Microcephaly, calcification (basal ganglia, periventricular, and cortex) may cause lobar destruction

**Varicella-Zoster Virus**
- Necrosis of WM, deep GM nuclei, cerebellum ventriculomegaly, cerebellar aplasia, PMG

**Syphilis**
- Basilar meningitis, stroke, scattered calcifications

**HIV**
- Atrophy, basal ganglia calcification, fusiform arteriopathy

**Human Parechovirus**
- Symmetric WM and thalamic involvement, best seen on DWI in acute setting

**Human Parvovirus B19**
- WM, cortical, and basal ganglia injury in setting of severe fetal anemia

# Acquired Pyogenic Infections

## Meningitis

Meningitis is a worldwide disease that leaves up to 1/2 of all survivors with permanent neurologic sequelae. Despite advances in antimicrobial therapy and vaccine development, bacterial meningitis represents a significant cause of morbidity and mortality. Infants, children, and older adults or immunocompromised patients are at special risk. In this section, we focus on the etiology, pathology, and imaging findings of this potentially devastating disease.

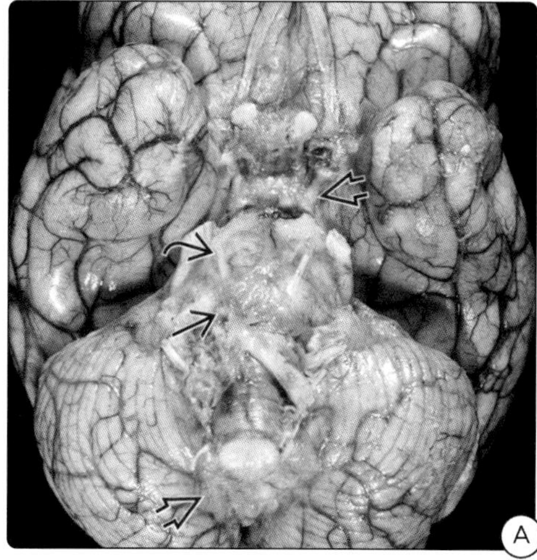


***(12-14A)** Severe meningitis with dense purulent exudate covering the pons ⇨, coating the cranial nerves ⇨, and filling the basal cisterns ⇨.*

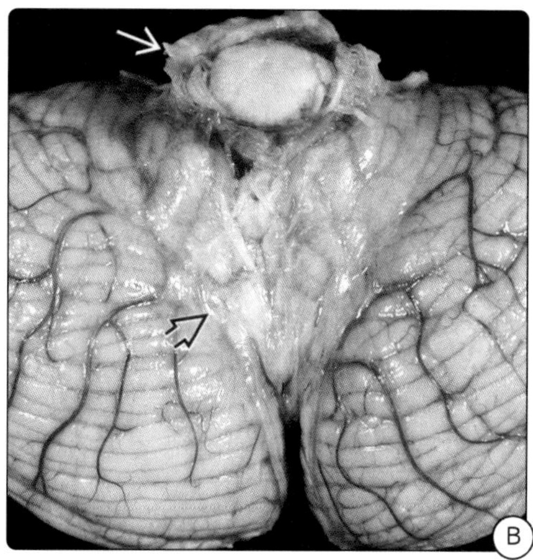


***(12-14B)** Exudate coats the medulla ➡ and completely fills the cisterna magna ⇨. (Courtesy R. Hewlett, MD.)*

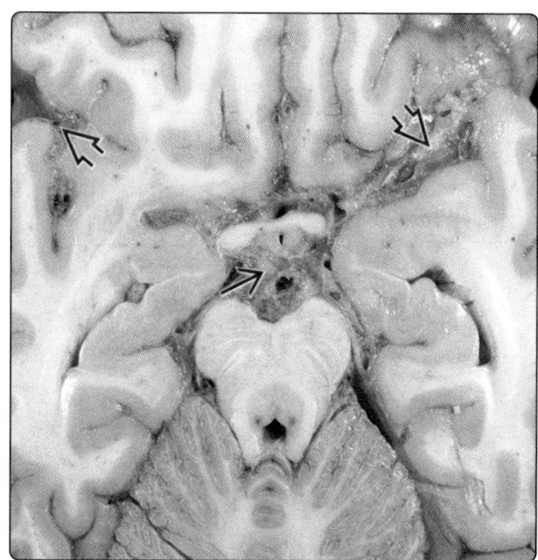

***(12-15)** Meningitis with exudate completely filling the suprasellar cistern ⇨ and sylvian fissures ⇨ is shown. (Courtesy R. Hewlett, MD.)*

(12-16) Meningitis graphic shows purulent exudate involving the leptomeninges and filling the basal cisterns and sulci ➡.

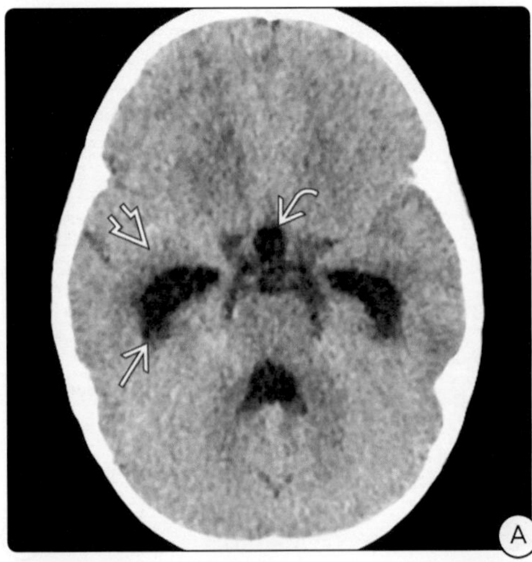

(12-17A) NECT shows prominent temporal horns ➡, dilated 3rd ventricle ➡. Note periventricular "hazy" hypodensity ➡.

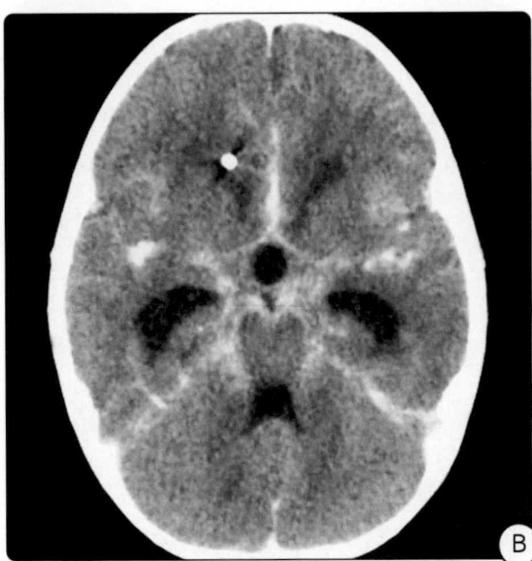

(12-17B) CECT shows diffuse enhancement throughout the basilar subarachnoid cisterns. This is TB meningitis. (Courtesy S. Candy, MD.)

## Terminology

Meningitis is an acute or chronic inflammatory infiltrate of meninges and CSF. **Pachymeningitis** involves the dura-arachnoid; **leptomeningitis** affects the pia and subarachnoid spaces.

## Etiology

Most cases are caused by acute pyogenic (bacterial) infection. Meningitis can also be acute lymphocytic (viral) or chronic (tubercular or granulomatous).

The most common responsible agent varies with age, geography, and immune status. The three most common causes of community-acquired bacterial meningitis worldwide are *Streptococcus pneumoniae, Neisseria meningitidis*, and *Haemophilus influenzae* type B. Group B β-hemolytic streptococcal meningitis is the leading cause of neonatal meningitis in resource-rich countries.

Vaccination has significantly decreased the incidence of *H. influenzae* meningitis, so the most common cause of childhood bacterial meningitis is now *N. meningitidis*. The tetravalent meningococcal vaccine used to vaccinate adolescents in the USA does not contain serotype B, the causative organism of 1/3 of all cases of meningococcal disease in industrialized countries.

*Listeria monocytogenes, S. pneumoniae*, gram-negative bacilli, such as *Escherichia coli*, and *N. meningitidis*, affect pregnant women, older adults, and transplant recipients.

Tuberculous meningitis is common in resource-limited countries and in immunocompromised patients (e.g., HIV/AIDS patients and solid organ transplant recipients).

## Pathology

Cloudy CSF initially fills the subarachnoid spaces followed by development of a variably dense purulent exudate that covers the pial surfaces **(12-14)**. The basal cisterns and subarachnoid spaces are the most commonly involved sites by meningitis **(12-15)** **(12-16)** followed by the cerebral convexity sulci. Vessels within the exudate may show inflammatory changes and necrosis.

## Clinical Issues

**Presentation.** Presentation depends on patient age. In adults, fever (≥ 38.5 °C) and either headache, nuchal rigidity, or altered mental status are the most common symptoms. Fever, lethargy, poor feeding, and irritability are common among infected infants. Seizures occur in 30% of patients.

**Natural History.** Despite rapid recognition and effective therapy, meningitis still has significant morbidity and mortality rates. Death rates from 15-25% have been reported in disadvantaged children with poor living conditions.

Complications are both common and numerous. **Extraventricular obstructive hydrocephalus** is one of the earliest and most common complications. The choroid plexus can become infected, causing choroid plexitis and then **ventriculitis**. Infection can also extend from the pia along the perivascular spaces into the brain parenchyma itself, causing **cerebritis** and then **abscess**.

SDEs and epidural **empyemas** (EDEs) or sterile **effusions** may develop. **Cerebrovascular complications** of meningitis include vasculitis, thrombosis, and occlusion of both arteries and veins.

## Imaging

**General Features.** Remember: **Imaging is neither sensitive nor specific for the detection of meningitis**! Imaging (CT &/or MR) should be used in conjunction with—and not as a substitute for—appropriate clinical and laboratory evaluation. CSF analysis remains the mainstay of diagnosis.

**CT Findings.** Initial NECT may be normal or show only mild ventricular enlargement **(12-17A)**. "Blurred" ventricular margins indicate acute obstructive hydrocephalus with accumulation of extracellular fluid in the deep WM. Bone CT should be carefully evaluated for sinusitis and otomastoiditis.

Cellular inflammatory exudate replaces the normally clear CSF. Subtle effacement of surface landmarks may occur as sulcal-cisternal CSF becomes almost isodense with brain on NECT. CECT may show intense enhancement of the inflammatory exudate as it covers the brain surfaces, extending into and filling the sulci **(12-17B)**.

**MR Findings.** The purulent exudates of acute meningitis are isointense with underlying brain on T1WI, giving the appearance of "dirty" CSF **(12-18A)**. The exudates are isointense with CSF on T2WI and do not suppress on FLAIR **(12-18B)**. Hyperintensity in the subarachnoid cisterns and superficial sulci on FLAIR is a typical but nonspecific finding of meningitis (see box on p. 246).

DWI is especially helpful in meningitis, as the purulent subarachnoid space exudates usually show restriction. pMR may demonstrate multiple regions of increased cerebral blood flow.

Pia-subarachnoid space enhancement occurs in 50% of patients. A curvilinear pattern that follows the gyri and sulci (the pial-cisternal pattern) is typical **(12-18C)** and more common than dura-arachnoid enhancement. Postcontrast T2-weighted FLAIR and delayed postcontrast T1-weighted sequences may be helpful additions in detecting subtle cases.

**Complications of Meningitis.** Other than hydrocephalus **(12-19)**, complications from meningitis are relatively uncommon **(12-20)**. Postmeningitis reactive **effusions**—sterile CSF-like fluid pockets—develop in 5-10% of children treated for acute bacterial meningitis. NECT shows bilateral crescentic extraaxial collections that are iso- to slightly hyperdense compared with normal CSF.

Effusions are iso- to slightly hyperintense to CSF on T1WI and isointense on T2WI. They are often slightly hyperintense relative to CSF on FLAIR. Effusions usually do not enhance on T1 C+ and do not restrict on DWI, differentiating them from subdural empyemas (SDEs).

Less common complications include pyocephalus (ventriculitis), empyema, cerebritis &/or abscess, venous occlusion, and ischemia. All are discussed separately.

## Differential Diagnosis

The major differential diagnosis of infectious meningitis is noninfectious meningitis. Other causes of meningitis include **noninfectious inflammatory disorders** (e.g., rheumatoid or systemic lupus erythematosus-associated meningitis, IgG4-related disease, drug-related aseptic meningitis, and multiple sclerosis) and neoplastic or **carcinomatous meningitis**. All can appear identical on imaging, so correlation with clinical information and laboratory findings is essential. Remember: **Sulcal/cisternal FLAIR hyperintensity is a nonspecific finding and can be seen with a number of different entities**.

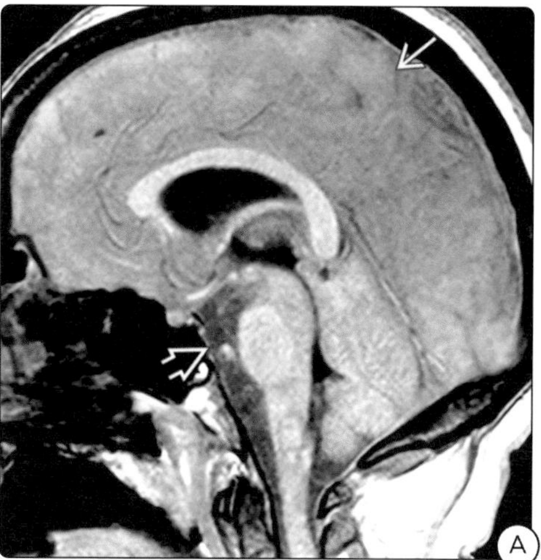


***(12-18A)** Sagittal T1WI in severe meningitis shows grayish CSF in basal cisterns ➯. CSF in sulci ➡ is isointense with brain, nearly invisible.*

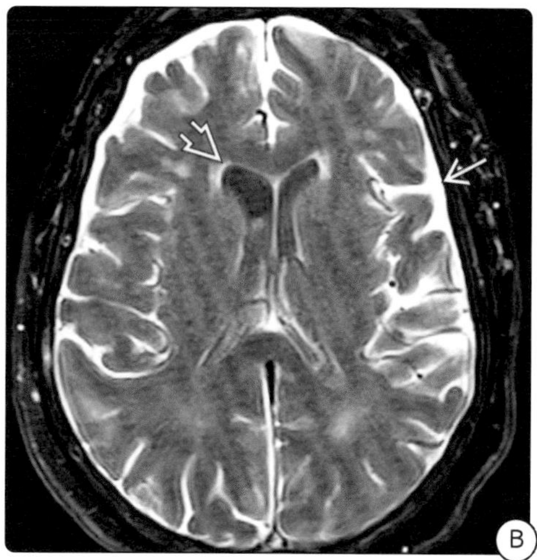


***(12-18B)** FLAIR in the same case shows nearly normal CSF suppression in ventricles ➯. Pus-filled sulci ➡ are extremely hyperintense.*

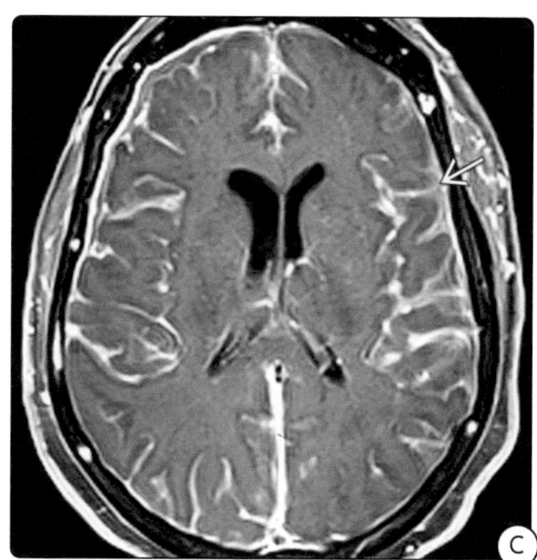


***(12-18C)** T1 C+ FS shows striking sulcal-cisternal enhancement ➡ from inflammatory exudate. This is TB meningitis.*

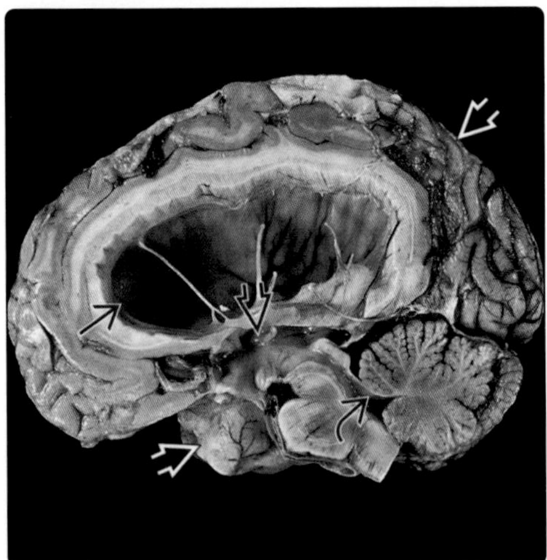

*(12-19) Autopsy of meningitis ➡ with EVOH shows lateral ➡, 3rd ➡, 4th ventricular ➡ aqueductal dilation. (From DP: Neuro.)*

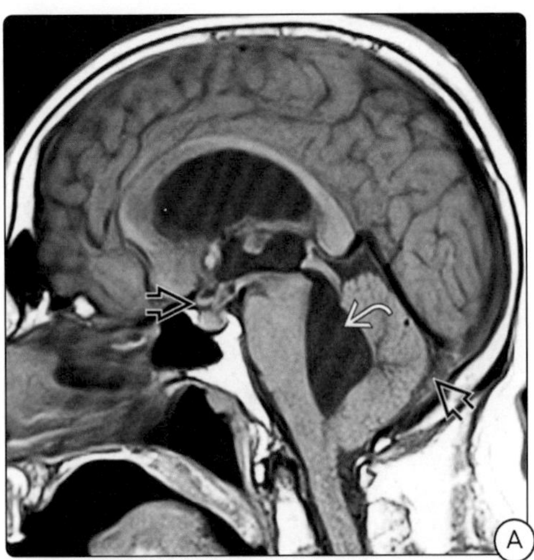

*(12-20A) Sagittal T1 MR shows basilar meningitis ➡. Lateral, 3rd ventricles are enlarged; 4th ventricle ➡ appears "ballooned" or obstructed.*

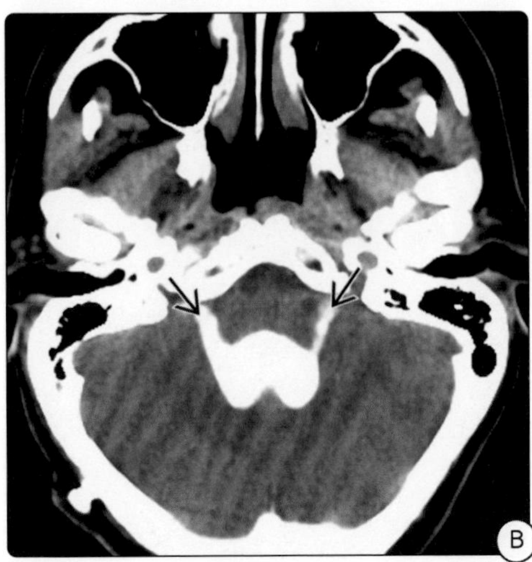

*(12-20B) CT ventriculogram shows dilated 4th ventricle, obstructed outflow at foramina of Luschka ➡. EVOH is secondary to meningitis.*

### CAUSES OF HYPERINTENSE CSF ON FLAIR

**Common**

- Blood
  - Subarachnoid hemorrhage
- Infection
  - Meningitis
- Artifact
  - Susceptibility; flow
- Tumor
  - CSF metastases

**Less Common**

- High inspired oxygen
  - 4-5x signal with 100% $O_2$
- Prominent vessels
  - Stroke (pial collaterals); ivy sign (moyamoya); pial angioma (Sturge-Weber)

**Rare but Important**

- Fat (ruptured dermoid)
- Gadolinium in CSF
  - Renal failure; blood-brain barrier leakage

# Abscess

## Terminology

A cerebral abscess is a localized infection of the brain parenchyma.

## Etiology

Most abscesses are caused by hematogenous spread from an extracranial location (e.g., lung or urinary tract infection and endocarditis). Abscesses may also result from penetrating injury or direct geographic extension from sinonasal and otomastoid infection. These typically begin as extraaxial infections, such as empyema or meningitis, and then spread into the brain itself.

Abscesses are most often bacterial, but they can also be fungal, parasitic, or (rarely) granulomatous. Although myriad organisms can cause abscess formation, the most common agents in immunocompetent adults are *Streptococcus* species, *Staphylococcus aureus*, and pneumococci. *Enterobacter* species like *Citrobacter* are a common cause of cerebral abscess in neonates. *Streptococcus intermedius* is emerging as an important cause of cerebral abscess in immunocompetent children and adolescents. In 20-30% of abscesses, cultures are sterile, and no specific organism is identified.

Proinflammatory molecules, such as tumor necrosis factor-α and interleukin-1β, induce various cell adhesion molecules that facilitate extravasation of peripheral immune cells and promote abscess development.

Bacterial abscesses are relatively uncommon in immunocompromised patients. *Klebsiella* is common in diabetic patients, and fungal infections by *Aspergillus* and *Nocardia* are common in transplant recipients. In patients with HIV/AIDS, toxoplasmosis and tuberculosis are the most common opportunistic infections.

In children, predisposing factors for cerebral abscess formation include meningitis, uncorrected cyanotic heart disease, sepsis, suppurative pulmonary infection, paranasal sinus or otomastoid trauma, or suppurative infections, endocarditis, and immunodeficiency or immunosuppression states.

## Pathology

Four general stages are recognized in the evolution of a cerebral abscess: (1) Focal suppurative encephalitis/early cerebritis, (2) focal suppurative encephalitis/late cerebritis, (3) early encapsulation, and (4) late encapsulation. Each has its own distinctive pathologic appearance, which, in turn, determines the imaging findings.

**Focal Suppurative Encephalitis.** Sometimes also called the **"early cerebritis"** stage of abscess formation, in this earliest stage, suppurative infection is focal but not yet localized **(12-21)**. An unencapsulated, edematous, hyperemic mass of leukocytes and bacteria is present for 1-3 days after the initial infection **(12-22)**.

**Focal Suppurative Encephalitis With Confluent Central Necrosis.** The next stage of abscess formation is also called **"late cerebritis"** and begins 2-3 days after the initial infection **(12-23)**. This stage typically lasts between a week and 10 days.

Patchy necrotic foci within the suppurative mass form, enlarge, and then coalesce into a confluent necrotic mass. By days 5-7, a necrotic core is surrounded by a poorly organized, irregular rim of granulation tissue consisting of inflammatory cells, macrophages, and fibroblasts. The surrounding brain is edematous and contains swollen reactive astrocytes.

**BRAIN ABSCESS: PATHOLOGY AND EVOLUTION**

**Stages**

- Focal suppurative encephalitis (days 1-2)
  - Edematous, suppurative mass
  - No visible necrosis or capsule
- Focal suppurative encephalitis with confluent central necrosis (days 2-7)
  - Necrotic foci form, begin to coalesce
  - Poorly organized irregular rim
- Early encapsulation (days 5-14)
  - Coalescent core
  - Well-defined wall of fibroblasts, collagen
- Late encapsulation (> 2 weeks)
  - Wall thickens, then shrinks
  - Inflammation; edema decreases/disappears

**Early Encapsulation.** The **"early capsule"** stage starts around one week. Proliferating fibroblasts deposit reticulin around the outer rim of the abscess cavity. The abscess wall is now composed of an inner rim of granulation tissue at the edge of the necrotic center **(12-26)** and an outer rim of multiple concentric layers of fibroblasts and collagen **(12-27)**. The necrotic core liquefies completely by 7-10 days, and newly formed capillaries around the mass become prominent.

**Late Capsulation.** The **"late capsule"** stage begins several weeks following infection and may last for several months.

With treatment, the central cavity gradually involutes and shrinks. Collagen deposition further thickens the wall, and the surrounding vasogenic edema disappears. The wall eventually contains densely packed reticulin and is lined by sparse macrophages. Eventually, only a small gliotic nodule of collagen and fibroblasts remains.

## Clinical Issues

**Demographics.** Brain abscesses are rare. Only 2,500 cases are reported annually in the USA. Brain abscesses occur at all ages but are most common

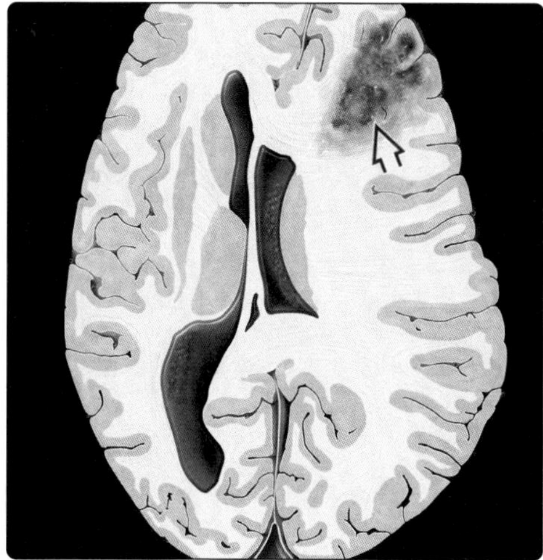

***(12-21)** Graphic of early cerebritis shows focal unencapsulated mass of petechial hemorrhage, inflammatory cells, and edema ➡.*

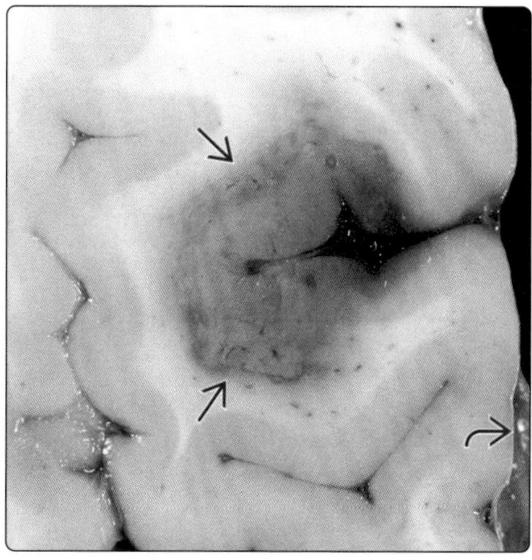

***(12-22)** Pathology shows meningitis ➡ with unencapsulated mass of edema, petechial hemorrhages ➡. This is early cerebritis.*

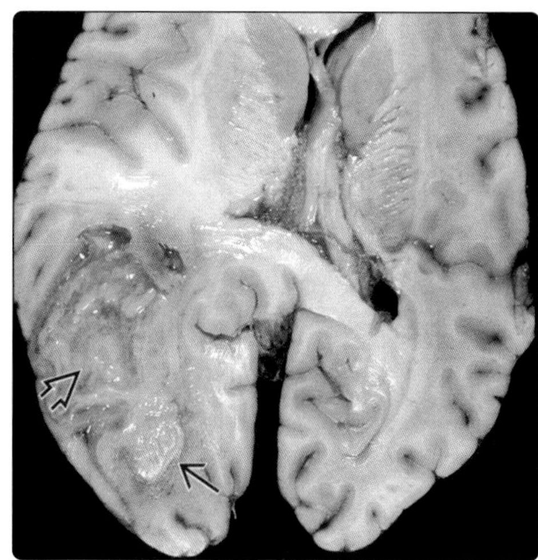

***(12-23)** Autopsied late cerebritis demonstrates coalescing lesion with some central necrosis ➡, the beginnings of an ill-defined abscess rim ➡.*

in patients between 3rd-4th decades. Almost 25% occur in children under the age of 15 years. The M:F ratio is 2:1 in adults and 3:1 in children.

**Presentation and Prognosis.** Headache, seizure, and focal neurologic deficits are the typical presenting symptoms. Fever is common but not universal. CSF cultures may be normal early in the infection.

Brain abscesses are potentially fatal but treatable lesions. Rapid diagnosis, stereotactic surgery, and appropriate medical treatment have reduced mortality to 2-4%.

## Imaging

**General Features.** Imaging findings evolve with time and are related to the stage of abscess development. MR is more sensitive than CT and is the procedure of choice.

**Early Cerebritis.** Very early cerebritis may be invisible on CT. A poorly marginated cortical/subcortical hypodense mass is the most common finding **(12-24A)**. Early cerebritis often shows little or no enhancement on CECT.

Early cerebritis is hypo- to isointense on T1WI and hyperintense on T2/FLAIR. T2* GRE may show punctate "blooming" hemorrhagic foci. Patchy enhancement may or may not be present. DWI shows diffusion restriction **(12-24B)**.

**Late Cerebritis.** A better-delineated central hypodense mass with surrounding edema is seen on NECT. CECT typically shows irregular rim enhancement **(12-25A)**.

Late cerebritis has a hypointense center and an iso- to mildly hyperintense rim on T1WI. The central core of the cerebritis is hyperintense on T2WI, whereas the rim is relatively hypointense. Intense but somewhat irregular rim enhancement is present on T1 C+ images **(12-25B)**.

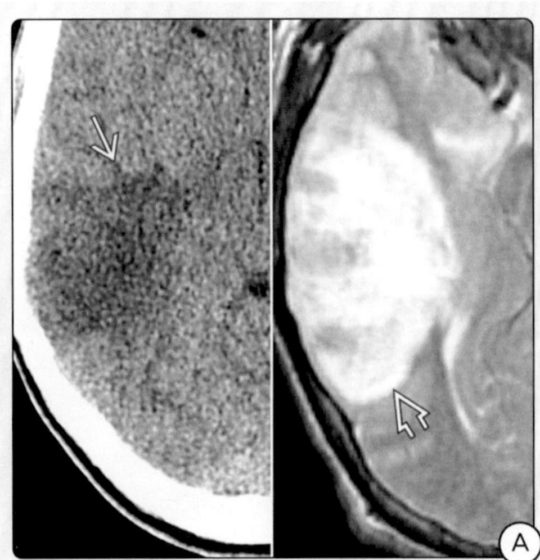


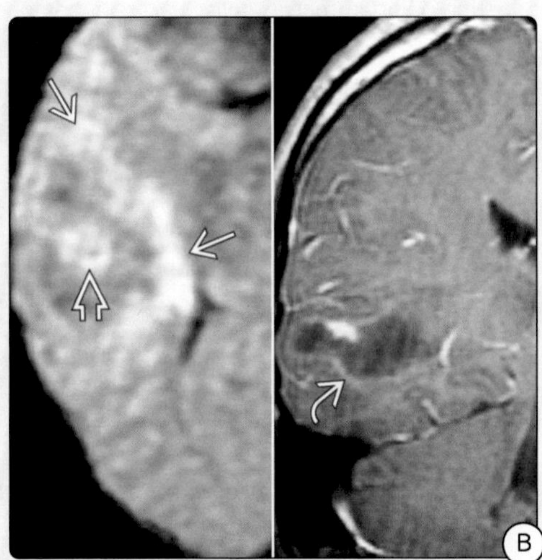


***(12-24A) (L) NECT shows ill-defined hypoattenuation ➡ and mass effect within the right temporal lobe. Arterial infarction was suspected. (R) T2 MR shows a hyperintense right temporal lobe mass ➡. (12-24B) (L) DWI MR shows restricted diffusion at the periphery ➡, center ➡ of the lesion. (R) Coronal T1 C+ MR shows a faint rim of peripheral enhancement ➡. This is the early cerebritis stage of abscess formation.***

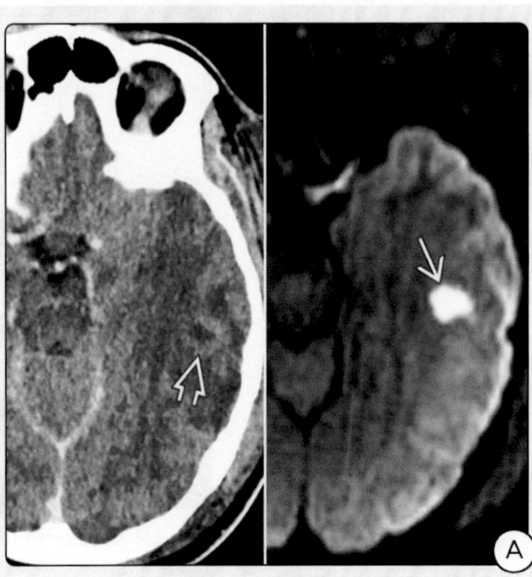


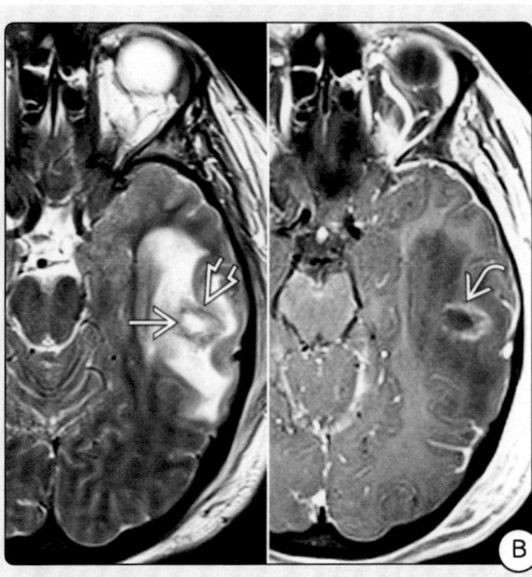


***(12-25A) (L) CECT shows faint, ill-defined left temporal lobe ring-enhancing lesion with peripheral edema ➡. (R) DWI MR shows strong diffusion restriction ➡ in the center of the mass. (12-25B) (L) The mass exhibits a hyperintense center ➡, hypointense periphery ➡ on T2WI. (R) Irregular, poorly defined enhancing rim ➡ is seen on T1 C+ FS. This is the late cerebritis stage of abscess formation.***

Late cerebritis restricts strongly on DWI **(12-25A)**. MRS shows cytosolic amino acids (0.9 ppm), lactate (1.3 ppm), and acetate (1.9 ppm) in the necrotic core **(12-29D)**. The abscess wall demonstrates low rCBV on pMR.

**BRAIN ABSCESS IMAGING: CEREBRITIS STAGES**

**Early Cerebritis**
- CT
  - Ill-defined hypodense mass on NECT
  - Usually no enhancement
- MR
  - T2/FLAIR heterogeneously hyperintense
  - T2* ± petechial hemorrhage; DWI+ (often mild)
  - T1 C+ may show patchy enhancement

**Late Cerebritis**
- CT
  - Round/ovoid hypodense mass on NECT
  - ± thin, irregular ring on CECT
- MR
  - T2-/FLAIR-hyperintense center, hypointense irregular rim
  - T2* GRE-hypointense rim; restricts on DWI
  - Moderate/strong but irregular enhancing rim

**Early Capsule.** Abscesses are now well-delineated, round or ovoid masses **(12-28)** with liquefied, hyperintense *cores* on T2/FLAIR **(12-29A)**. The *rims* of abscesses are usually thin, complete, smooth, and hypointense on T2WI. A double rim sign demonstrating two concentric rims, the outer hypointense and the inner hyperintense relative to cavity contents, is seen in 75% of cases **(12-29A)**.

The necrotic core of encapsulated abscesses restricts strongly on DWI **(12-29C)**. T1 C+ sequences show a strongly enhancing rim **(12-29B)** that is thinnest on its deepest (ventricular) side **(12-30B)** and "blooms" on T2*.

**Late Capsule.** With treatment, the abscess cavity gradually collapses while the capsule thickens even as the overall mass diminishes in size. The shrinking abscess often assumes a crenulated appearance, much like a deflated balloon **(12-30A)**.

Contrast enhancement in the resolving abscess may persist for months, long after clinical symptoms have resolved **(12-30C)**.

**BRAIN ABSCESS IMAGING: CAPSULE STAGES**

**Early Capsule**
- Well-defined mass + strongly enhancing rim
- Core: T2/FLAIR hyperintense, restricts on DWI
- Wall: Double rim sign (hyperintense inner, hypointense outer)

**Late Capsule**
- Wall thickens, cavity and edema reduce
- Enhancing focus may persist for months

## Differential Diagnosis

The differential diagnosis of abscess varies with its stage of development. Early cerebritis is so poorly defined that it can be difficult to characterize and can mimic many lesions, including **cerebral ischemia** or neoplasm.

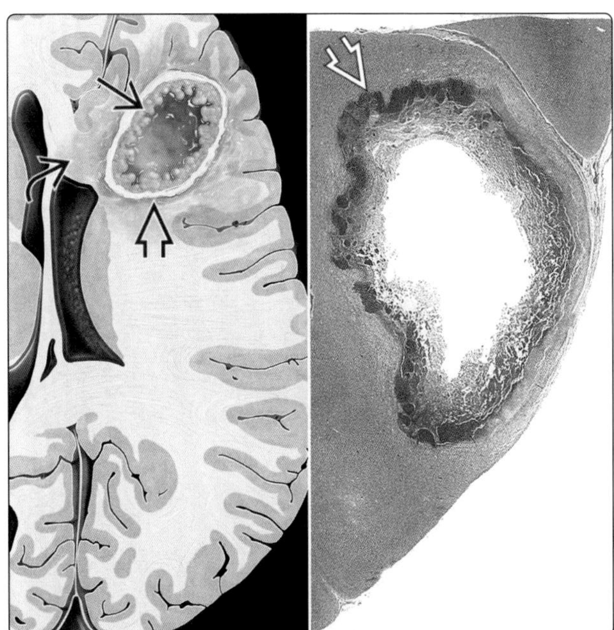

***(12-26) (L) Graphic shows edema ⇨ surrounding early capsule abscess. Well-defined, double-layered wall ⇨ surrounds a central core of necrosis, inflammatory debris ⇨. (R) Micrograph shows double-layered abscess wall ⇨. (From DP: Neuro.)***

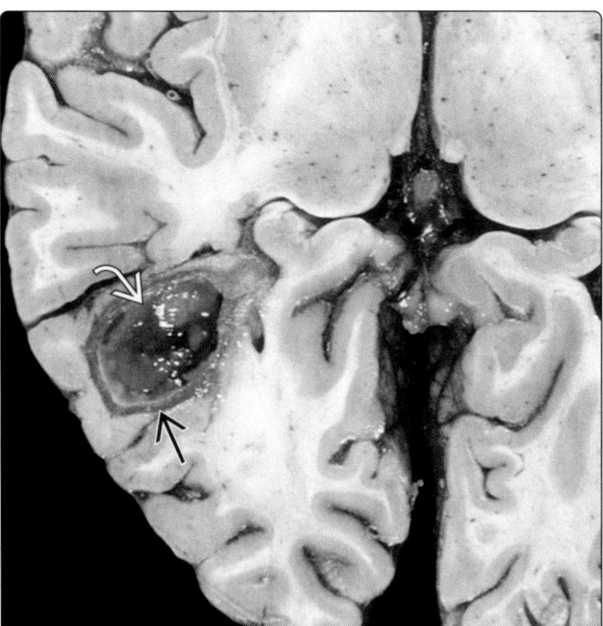

***(12-27) Abscess at early capsule stage is shown. Necrotic core ⇨ is surrounded by a double-layered, well-developed capsule ⇨. (Courtesy R. Hewlett, MD.)***

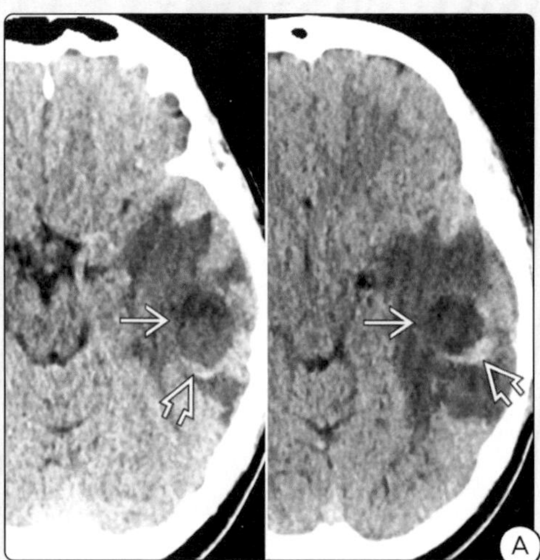

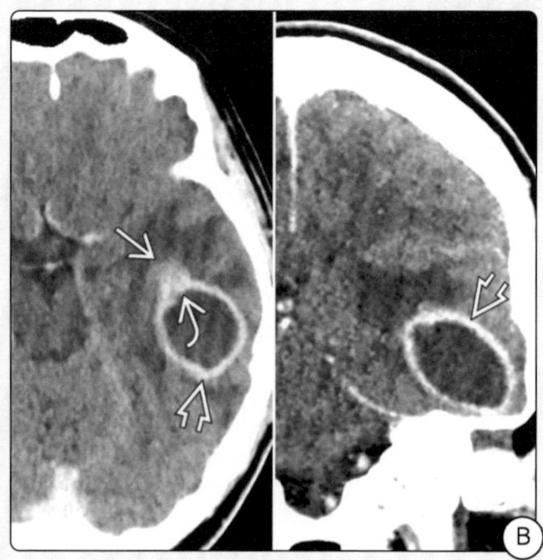

*(12-28A) NECT scans show large, well-defined lesion with hyperdense rim ➡ and a hypodense center ➡. (12-28B) Axial (L), coronal (R) CECT scans show complete, well-delineated rim enhancement ➡. The abscess has progressed from late cerebritis to the early capsule stage. Note the wall defect ➡ with the adjacent area of new cerebritis ➡.*

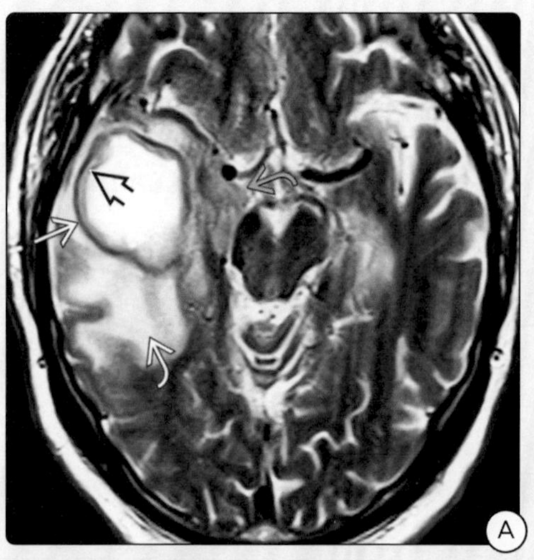

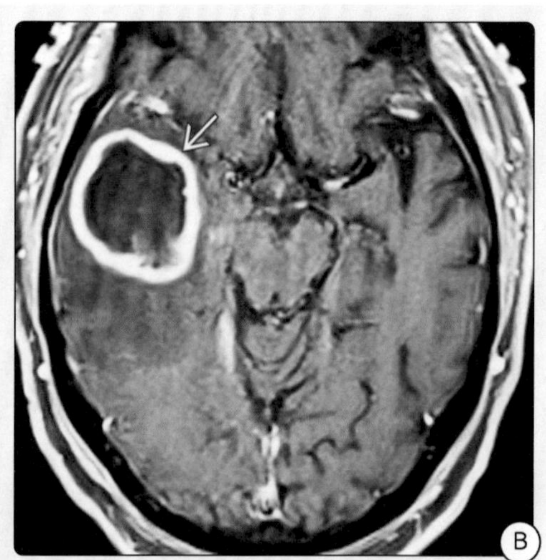

*(12-29A) T2 MR in the early capsule stage of abscess development shows the classic double rim sign with a hypointense outer rim ➡ and a mildly hyperintense inner rim ➡ surrounding a very hyperintense necrotic core. Note the peripheral edema ➡ and mass effect (uncal herniation) ➡. (12-29B) T1 C+ FS MR in the same case shows intense enhancement ➡ of the well-developed abscess capsule.*

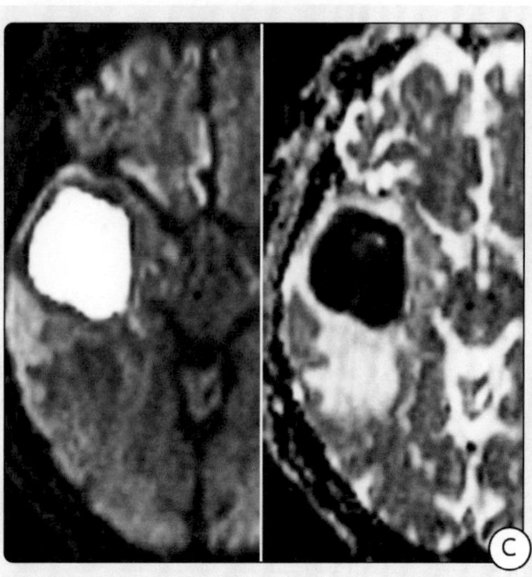

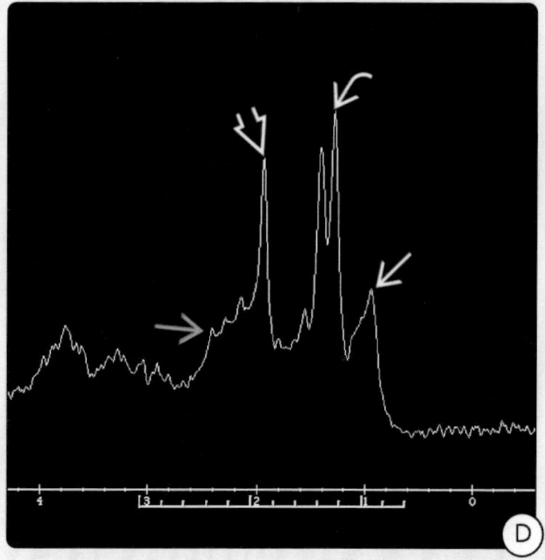

*(12-29C) DWI MR (L) and ADC map (R) in the same case show that necrotic contents of the abscess cavity restrict strongly, whereas the wall of the capsule itself does not. (12-29D) MRS in another late cerebritis/early capsule abscess with TR 2,000 TE 35 shows amino acids (valine, leucine, isoleucine) at 0.9 ppm ➡, acetate at 1.9 ppm ➡, lactate at 1.3 ppm ➡, and succinate at 2.4 ppm ➡.*

Once a ring develops around the necrotic center, the differential diagnosis is basically that of a generic ring-enhancing mass. Although there are many ring-enhancing lesions in the CNS, the most common differential diagnosis is infection vs. **neoplasm (glioblastoma or metastasis)**.

Tumors have increased rCBV in their "rind," usually do not restrict (or if they do, not as strongly as an abscess), and do not demonstrate cytosolic amino acids on MRS.

Less common entities that can appear as a ring-enhancing mass include **demyelinating disease**, in which the ring is usually incomplete and "open" toward the cortex. Resolving hematomas can exhibit a vascular, ring-enhancing pattern.

### BRAIN ABSCESS: DIFFERENTIAL DIAGNOSIS

**Early Cerebritis**

- Encephalitis (may be indistinguishable)
- Stroke
  - Vascular distribution
  - Usually involves both cortex, WM
- Neoplasm (e.g., diffusely infiltrating low-grade astrocytoma)
  - Usually does not enhance or restrict

**Late Cerebritis/Early Capsule**

- Neoplasm
  - Primary (glioblastoma)
  - Metastasis
- Demyelinating disease
  - Incomplete ("horseshoe") enhancement

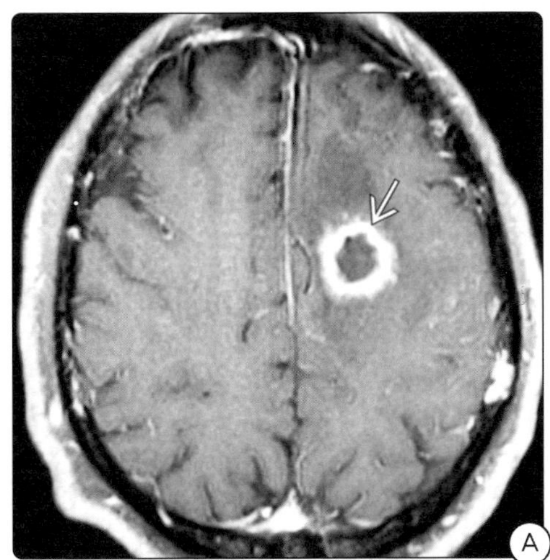


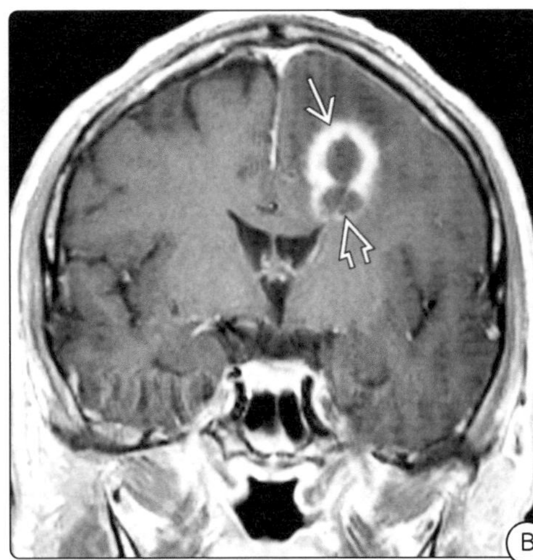


***(12-30A)** Axial T1 C+ FS MR in a 65-yo man with a history of dental abscess and headaches for 2-3 weeks shows a left posterior, frontal, thick-walled, ring-enhancing mass ➡. Findings are consistent with late capsule stage of abscess development. **(12-30B)** Coronal T1 C+ FS MR in the same case shows the abscess wall ➡ is thinnest on its deepest side ➡ next to the lateral ventricle. Note edema and mass effect on the ventricle.*

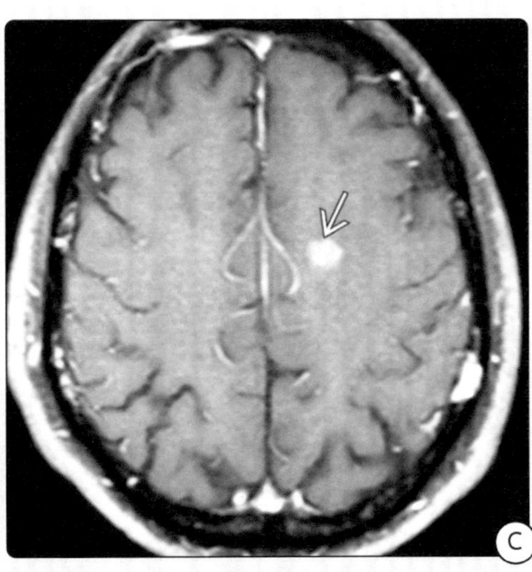


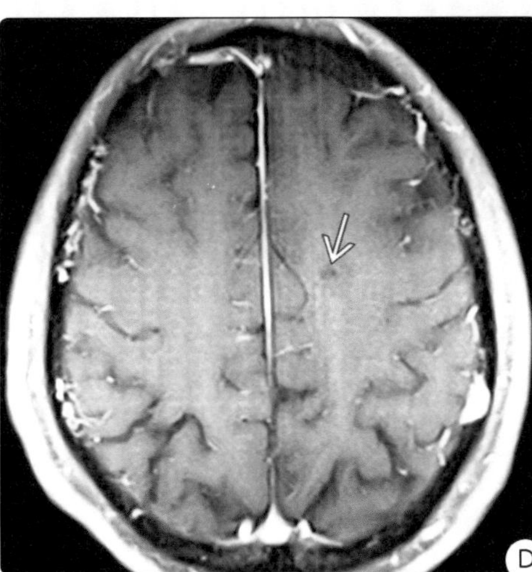


***(12-30C)** The patient was treated with IV antibiotics for 6 weeks. Follow-up scan at the end of treatment shows a small residual enhancing nodule ➡ with almost complete resolution of the surrounding edema. **(12-30D)** Follow-up T1 C+ FS MR 1 year later shows that only a small hypointense nonenhancing focus ➡ remains.*

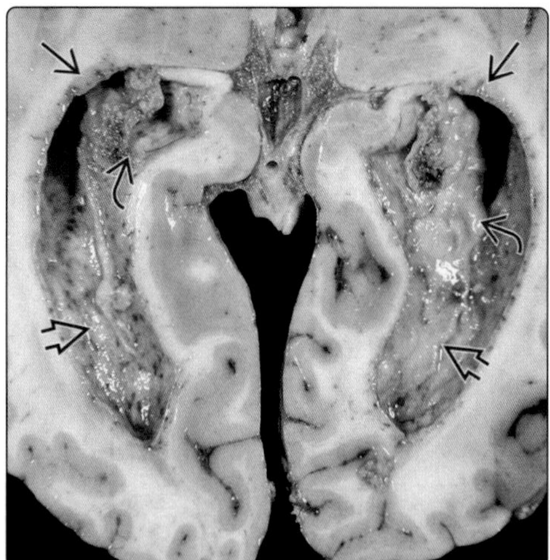

*(12-31) Autopsy of IVRBA shows ependymal infection ➡, choroid plexitis ➡, pus adhering to ventricular walls ➡. (Courtesy R. Hewlett, MD.)*

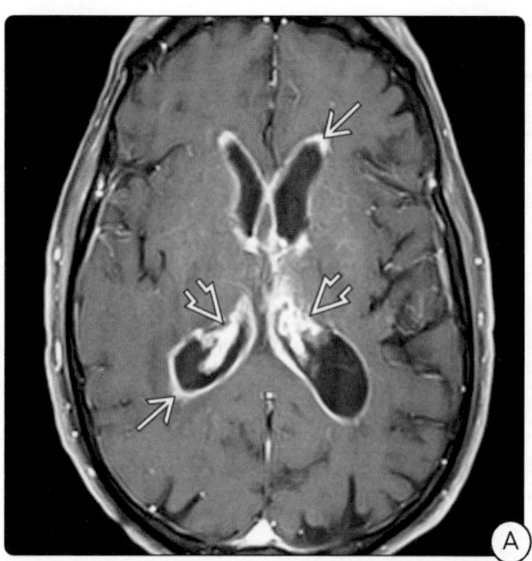

*(12-32A) T1 C+ FS shows diffuse ependymal enhancement along the lateral ventricle walls ➡, enlarged enhancing choroid plexi ➡.*

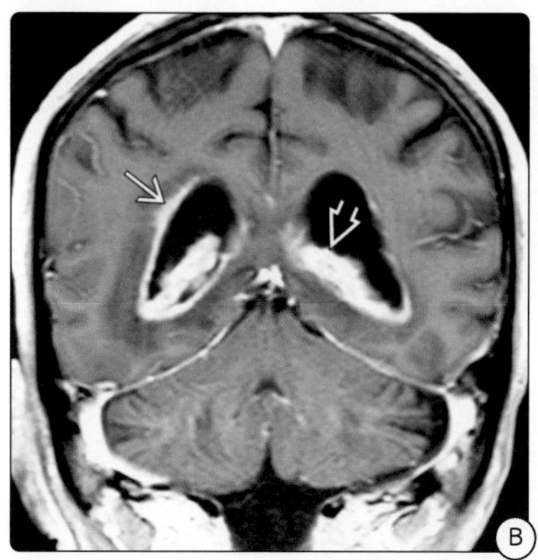

*(12-32B) Coronal T1 C+ shows diffuse ependymal thickening and enhancement ➡, enlarged choroid plexi ➡. Ventriculitis, choroid plexitis.*

# Ventriculitis

Primary intraventricular abscess is rare. A collection of purulent material in the ventricle is more likely due to intraventricular *rupture* of a brain abscess (IVRBA), a catastrophic complication. Ventriculitis also occurs as a complication of meningitis and neurosurgical procedures, such as external ventricular drainage (so-called "health care-associated ventriculitis"). Recognition and prompt intervention are necessary to treat this highly lethal condition.

## Terminology

Ventriculitis is also called **ependymitis, pyocephalus**, and (less commonly) ventricular empyema.

## Etiology

Infection of the ventricular ependyma most often occurs when a pyogenic abscess ruptures through its thin, medial capsule into the adjacent ventricle. Risk of IVRBA increases if an abscess is deep seated, multiloculated, &/or close to the ventricular wall. The most common pathogens causing ventriculitis are *Staphylococcus*, *Streptococcus*, and *Enterobacter*. Infections are often multidrug resistant and difficult to treat.

## Pathology

Autopsy examination shows that the ependyma, subependymal region, and choroid plexus are congested and covered with pus **(12-31)**. Hemorrhagic ependymitis may be present. Hydrocephalus with pus obstructing the aqueduct is common.

## Clinical Issues

Overall mortality is 25-85%. Only 40% of patients survive with good functional outcome.

## Imaging

MR should be the first-line imaging modality in cases of suspected ventriculitis. Irregular ventricular debris that appears hyperintense to CSF on T1WI **(12-34A)** and hypointense on T2WI with layering in the dependent occipital horns is typical **(12-33)**.

The most sensitive sequences are FLAIR and DWI. A "halo" of periventricular hyperintensity is usually present on both T2WI and FLAIR **(12-34C)**. DWI shows striking diffusion restriction of the layered debris **(12-34)**.

Ependymal enhancement is seen in only 60% of cases and varies from minimal to moderate **(12-32)**. When present, ependymal enhancement tends to be relatively smooth, thin, and linear rather than thick and nodular.

## Differential Diagnosis

Thin, linear ependymal enhancement of the periventricular and ependymal veins is normal, especially around the frontal horns and bodies of the lateral ventricles.

Primary neoplasms, such as **glioblastoma, primary CNS lymphoma, and germinoma**, can spread along the ventricular ependyma. Rarely, **metastases** from an extracranial neoplasm can cause irregular ependymal thickening and enhancement.

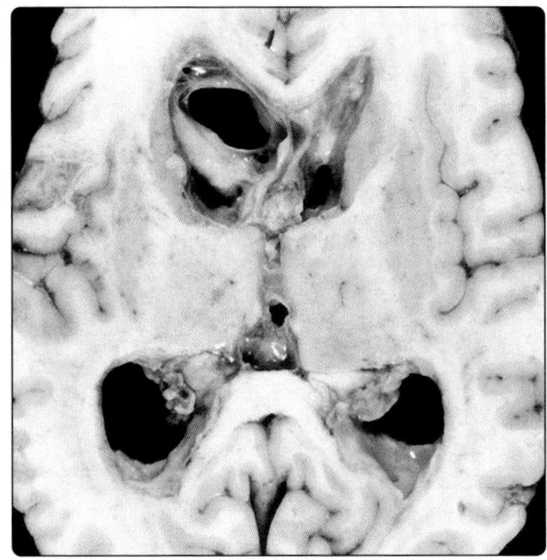

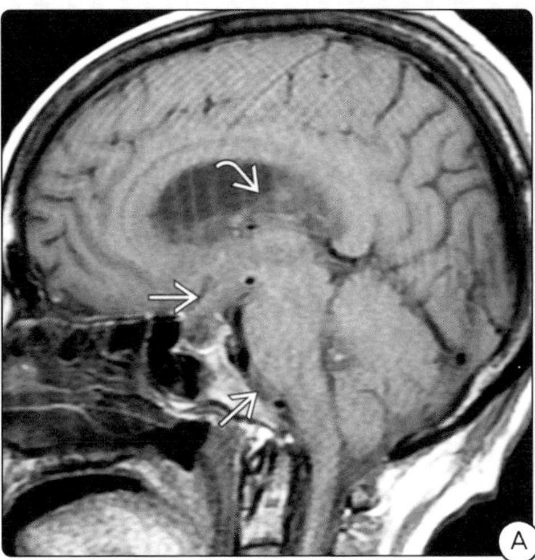

*(**12-33**) Gross pathology illustrates ventriculitis with ependymal inflammation, purulent contents within the frontal and occipital horns. Note swollen, discolored choroid plexi from plexitis. (**12-34A**) Sagittal T1WI in a 51-yo woman with Escherichia coli pyelonephritis, altered mental status, and renal failure shows "dirty" CSF in the basal cisterns ➡ and lateral ventricle ➡.*

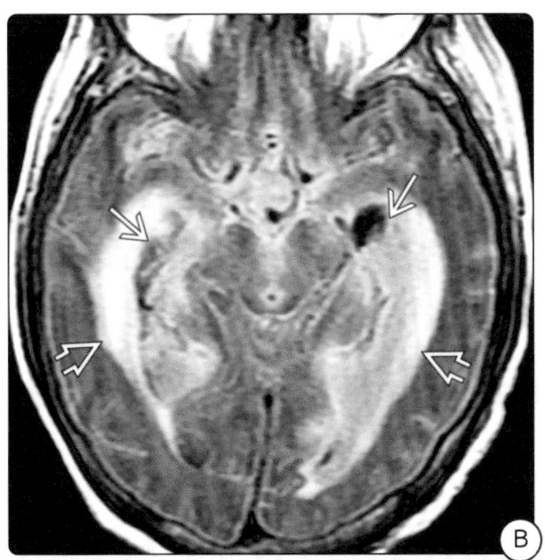

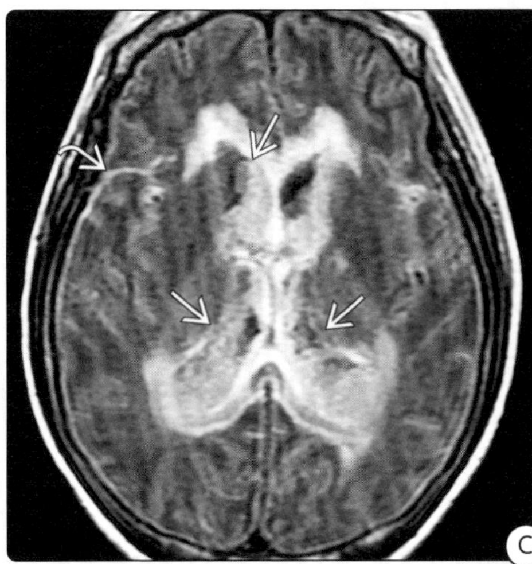

*(**12-34B**) FLAIR in the same case shows very heterogeneous, nonsuppressing material in both temporal horns ➡. Periventricular "halo" ➡ indicates acute obstructive hydrocephalus. (**12-34C**) More cephalad FLAIR shows mixed signal intensity of the debris ➡ almost completely filling both lateral ventricles. Sulcal hyperintensity ➡ indicates meningitis.*

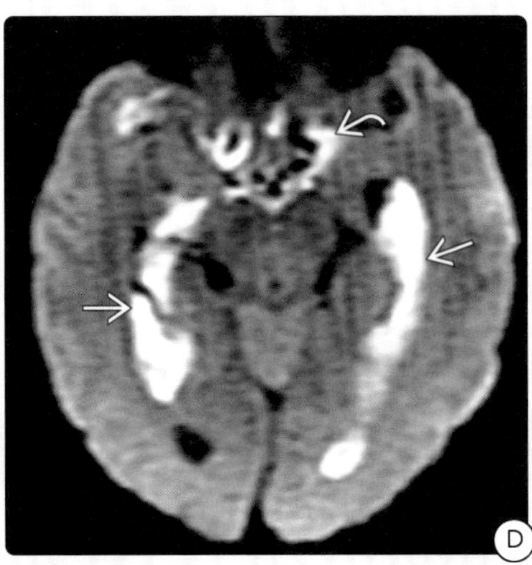

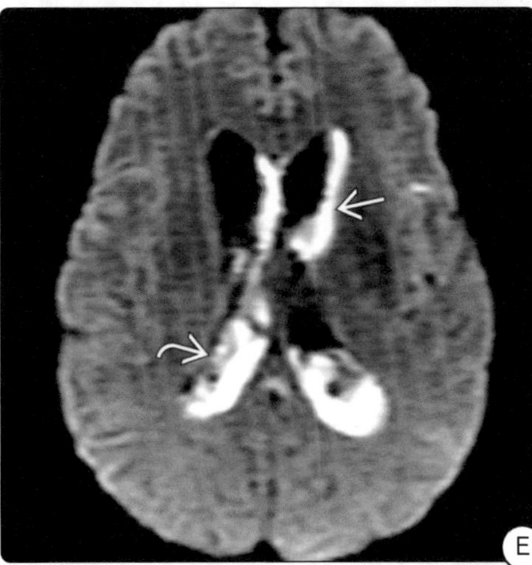

*(**12-34D**) DWI shows the intraventricular debris restricts strongly ➡ as does the meningitis in the basal cisterns ➡. (**12-34E**) More cephalad DWI shows intraventricular debris ➡ restricts strongly. No contrast was administered because of the renal failure. Meningitis, pyocephalus/ventriculitis ➡, and choroid plexitis. The patient expired shortly after the scan was obtained.*

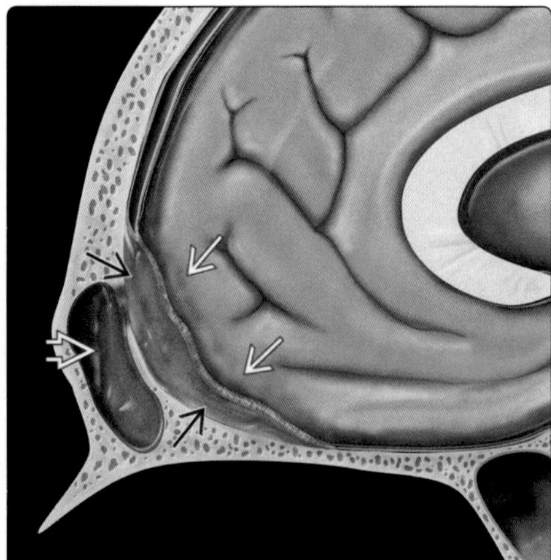

***(12-35) Purulent frontal sinusitis ➡ with extension into epidural space causes epidural empyema ⇨ and frontal lobe cerebritis ➡.***

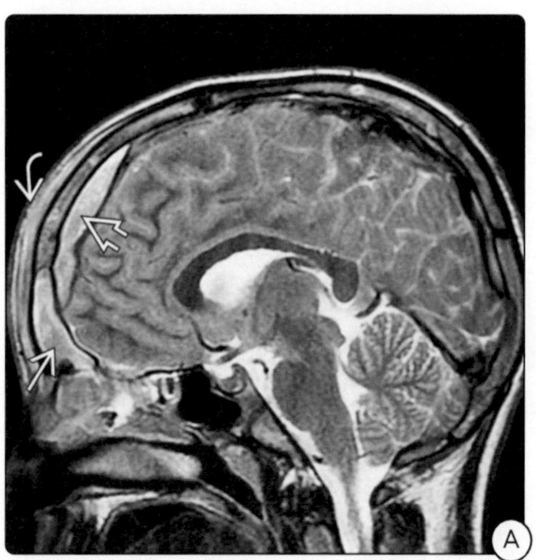

***(12-36A) Sagittal T2 MR is from a child with frontal sinusitis ➡ causing scalp cellulitis ➡ and epidural empyema ➡.***

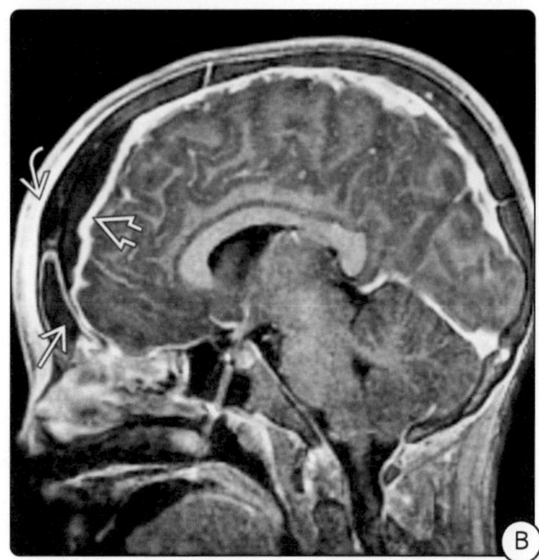

***(12-36B) T1 C+ MR shows the frontal sinusitis ➡, cellulitis ➡, and enhancing endosteal dura ➡ displaced by the epidural empyema.***

## Empyemas

Extraaxial infections of the CNS are rare but potentially life-threatening conditions. Early diagnosis and prompt treatment are essential to maximize neurologic recovery.

### Terminology

Empyemas are pus collections that can occur in either the subdural or epidural space.

### Etiology

Empyemas in infants and young children are most commonly secondary to bacterial meningitis, otitis media, or sinusitis. The *Streptococcus anginosus* group (SAG; *S. anginosus*, *S. intermedius*, and *Streptococcus constellatus*) is the most frequently isolated cause and is associated with substantial morbidity.

In older children and adults, > 2/3 occur as an extension of infection from paranasal sinus disease, while 20% are secondary to otomastoiditis. Rare causes include penetrating head trauma, neurosurgical procedures, or hematogenous spread of pathogens from a distant extracranial site.

### Pathology

Empyemas are extraaxial pus collections **(12-35)**. Subdural empyemas (SDEs) are much more common than epidural empyemas (EDEs). Empyemas range from small, focal epidural collections to extensive subdural infections that spread over most of the cerebral hemisphere and extend into the interhemispheric fissure. The most common locations are the frontal and frontoparietal convexities.

### Clinical Issues

**Presentation.** Empyemas can occur at any age. The most common clinical presentation is headache followed by fever. Preceding symptoms of sinusitis or otomastoiditis are common. Meningismus, seizures, and focal motor signs are also frequent.

"Pott puffy tumor"—a fluctuant ("doughy"), tender, erythematous swelling of the frontal scalp—is considered a specific sign for frontal bone osteomyelitis with a subperiosteal abscess. Most occur in the setting of untreated frontal sinusitis that breaches the posterior table of the sinus.

**Natural History.** Untreated empyemas can spread quite rapidly, extending from the extraaxial spaces into the subjacent brain. Besides cerebritis and abscess formation, the other major complication of empyema is cortical vein thrombosis with venous ischemia.

### Imaging

Imaging is essential to the early diagnosis of empyema. NECT may be normal or show a hypodense extraaxial collection that demonstrates peripheral enhancement on CECT. Bone CT should be evaluated for signs of sinusitis and otomastoiditis.

MR is the procedure of choice for evaluating potential empyemas. T1 shows an extraaxial collection that is mildly hyperintense relative to CSF. SDEs are typically crescentic and lie over the cerebral hemisphere. The extracerebral space is widened, and the underlying sulci are compressed by the collection. SDEs often extend into the interhemispheric fissure but do not cross the midline.

EDEs are biconvex and usually more focal than SDEs. The inwardly displaced dura can sometimes be identified as a thin, hypointense line between the epidural collection and the underlying brain **(12-36A)**. In contrast to SDEs, frontal EDEs may cross the midline, confirming their epidural location.

Empyemas are iso- to hyperintense compared with CSF on T2WI and are hyperintense on FLAIR. Hyperintensity in the underlying brain parenchyma may be caused by cerebritis or ischemia (either venous or arterial) **(12-37A)**.

SDEs typically demonstrate striking diffusion restriction on DWI **(12-37C)**. EDEs are variable but usually have at least some restricting component.

Empyemas show variable enhancement depending on the amount of granulomatous tissue and inflammation present **(12-36B)**. The encapsulating membranes, especially on the outer margin, enhance moderately strongly **(12-37B)**.

## Differential Diagnosis

The major differential diagnosis of extraaxial empyema is a nonpurulent extraaxial collection, such as subdural effusion, subdural hygroma, and chronic subdural hematoma (cSDH).

A **subdural effusion** is usually postmeningitic, typically bilateral, and does not restrict on DWI. Because of its increased proteinaceous contents, effusions are typically hyperintense to CSF on FLAIR.

A **subdural hygroma** is a sterile, nonenhancing, nonrestricting CSF collection that occurs with a tear in the arachnoid, allowing escape of CSF into the subdural space. Hygromas are usually posttraumatic or postsurgical and behave exactly like CSF on imaging studies.

A **cSDH** is hypodense on NECT. Signal intensity varies with chronicity. Early cSDHs are hyperintense compared with CSF on both T1WI and T2/FLAIR. They may show some residual blood that "blooms" on T2* (GRE, SWI). The encapsulating membranes enhance and may show diffusion restriction. In contrast to SDEs, the cSDH contents themselves typically do not restrict on DWI. Very longstanding cSDHs look similar to CSF and may show little or no residual evidence of prior hemorrhage.

### EMPYEMAS

**Pathology**
- SDEs > > EDEs
- EDE focal (usually next to sinus, mastoid)
- SDE spreads diffusely along hemispheres, tentorium/falx

**Imaging**
- Bone CT: Look for sinus, ear infection
- EDE is focal, biconvex; can cross midline
- SDE is crescentic, covers hemisphere, may extend into interhemispheric fissure
- SDEs restrict strongly on DWI; EDEs variable

**Differential Diagnosis**
- cSDH
- Subdural hygroma
- Subdural effusion

# Acquired Viral Infections

A number of both familiar and less well-known but emerging viruses can cause CNS infections. In this section, we focus on neurotropic herpesvirus

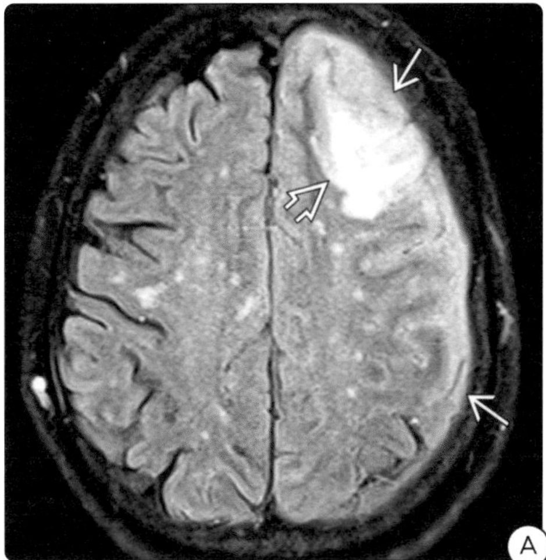


***(12-37A)** FLAIR in a 63-yo man with seizure shows heterogeneously hyperintense parenchymal mass with crescentic subdural fluid collection .*

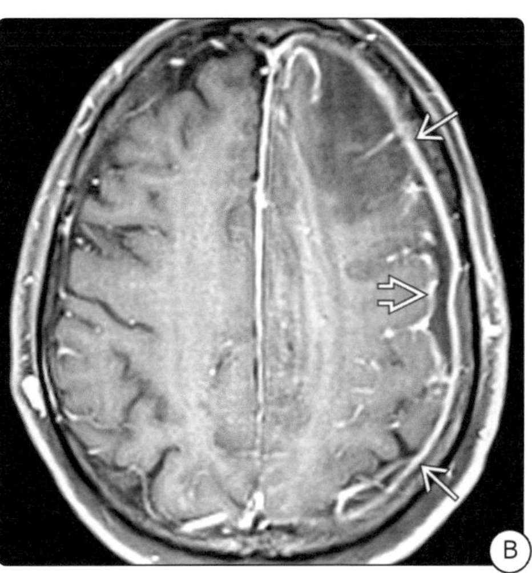


***(12-37B)** T1 C+ FS shows near holohemispheric fluid collection between thickened dura , enhancing arachnoid .*

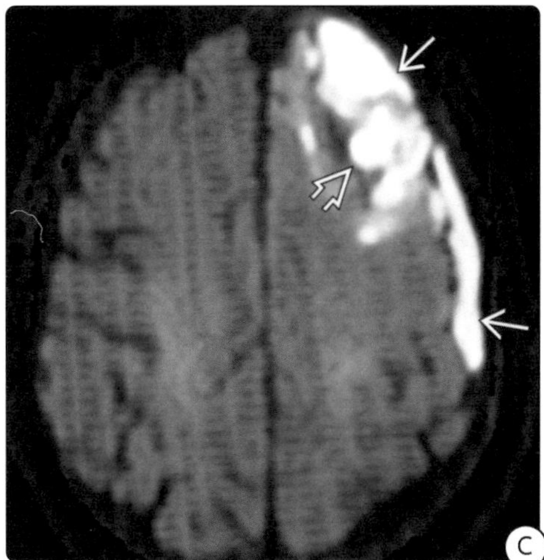


***(12-37C)** DWI shows subdural fluid restricts strongly. Subdural empyema with underlying cerebritis is shown.*

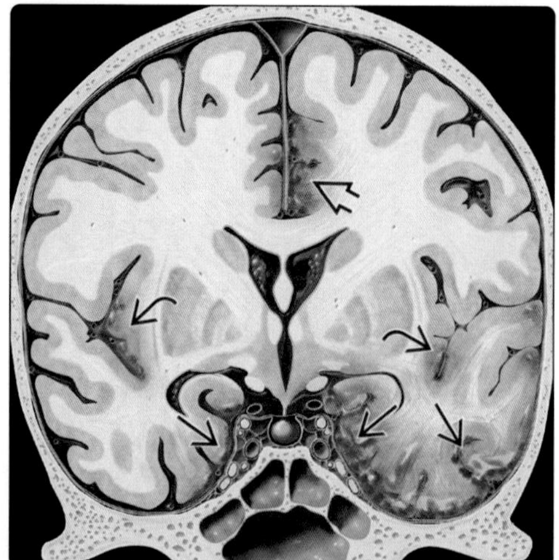

***(12-38)** Graphic shows herpes encephalitis with bilateral, asymmetric involvement of temporal lobes ➡, cingulate gyri ➡, and insula ➡.*

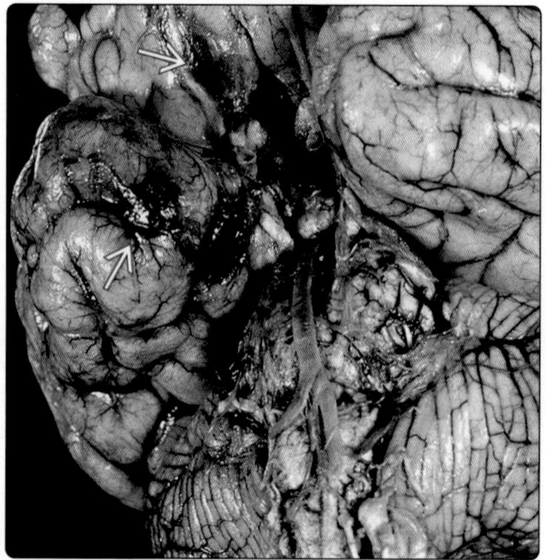

***(12-39)** Autopsy of HSE shows hemorrhagic lesions in the basal medial temporal lobes and subfrontal regions ➡. (Courtesy R. Hewlett, MD.)*

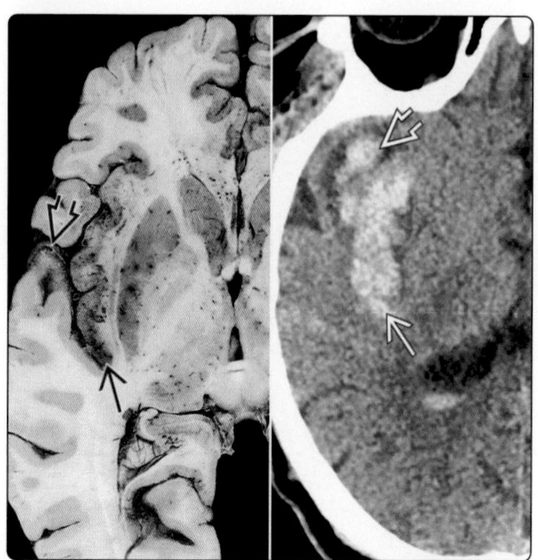

***(12-40)** (L) Autopsy shows insular ➡, temporal lobe ➡ cortical hemorrhage. (R) NECT shows insular ➡, temporal lobe ➡ hemorrhage. HSE.*

infections, which can promote acute fulminant CNS disease and become latent with the potential of reactivation that may last for decades.

Eight members of the herpesvirus family are known to cause disease in humans. These are herpes simplex virus 1 (HSV-1) and HSV-2, varicella-zoster virus (VZV), Epstein-Barr virus (EBV), cytomegalovirus (CMV), and human herpesvirus (HHV)-6, HHV-7, and HHV-8. Each has its own disease spectrum, clinical setting, and imaging findings.

Congenital HSV-2 and CMV were both considered earlier, as their manifestations in newborn infants differ from those of acquired herpesvirus infections. HSV-1 and HHV-6 are discussed in this section. VZV, EBV, and other agents are discussed later in the chapter under "Other Common Acute Viral Encephalitides."

## Herpes Simplex Encephalitis

### Etiology

After the neonatal period, > 95% of HSE is caused by reactivation of HSV-1, an obligate intracellular pathogen. The virus initially gains entry into cells in the nasopharyngeal mucosa, invades sensory lingual branches of the trigeminal nerve, then passes in retrograde fashion into the trigeminal ganglion. It establishes a lifelong latent infection within sensory neurons of the trigeminal ganglion, where it can remain dormant indefinitely.

### Pathology

**Location.** HSE has a striking affinity for the limbic system **(12-38)**. The anterior and medial temporal lobes, insular cortex, subfrontal area, and cingulate gyri are most frequently affected **(12-39)**. Bilateral but asymmetric disease is typical. Extratemporal, extralimbic involvement occurs but is more common in children or in immunocompromised oncology patients. When it occurs, extralimbic HSE most often involves the parietal cortex. Brainstem-predominant infection is uncommon. The basal ganglia are usually spared.

**Gross Pathology.** HSE is a fulminant, hemorrhagic, necrotizing encephalitis **(12-40)**. Massive tissue necrosis accompanied by numerous petechial hemorrhages and severe edema is typical. Inflammation and tissue destruction are predominantly cortical but may extend into the subcortical WM. Advanced cases demonstrate gross temporal lobe rarefaction and cavitation.

### Clinical Issues

**Epidemiology.** HSV-1 is the most common worldwide cause of sporadic (i.e., nonepidemic) viral encephalitis, and HSE may occur at any age. It follows a bimodal age distribution with 1/3 of all cases occurring between the ages of six months and three years and 1/2 seen in patients older than 50. There is no sex predilection.

**Natural History.** Typical initial presentation of an HSE is a viral prodrome followed by fever, headache, seizures, and altered mental status. Mortality rates range from 50-70%. Rapid clinical deterioration with coma and death is typical. Nearly 2/3 of survivors have significant neurologic deficits despite antiviral therapy.

**HERPES SIMPLEX ENCEPHALITIS**

**Etiology**
- > 95% caused by HSV-1

**Pathology**
- Necrotizing, hemorrhagic encephalitis
- Limbic system
  - Anteromedial temporal lobes, insular cortex
  - Subfrontal region, cingulate gyri

**Imaging**
- Bilateral > unilateral; asymmetric > symmetric
- FLAIR most sensitive
- DWI shows restriction

**Differential Diagnosis**
- Acute cerebral ischemia
- Other encephalitides
  - HHV-6 encephalitis
  - Autoimmune/paraneoplastic limbic encephalitis
  - SARS-CoV-2-associated hemorrhagic encephalitis
  - Acute encephalitis of unknown cause
- Neoplasm (diffuse astrocytoma)

## Imaging

**CT Findings.** NECT is often normal early in the disease course. Hypodensity with mild mass effect in one or both temporal lobes and the insula may be present **(12-41A)**. CECT is usually negative, although patchy or gyriform enhancement may develop after 24-48 hours **(12-41C)**.

**MR Findings.** MR is the imaging procedure of choice. T1 shows gyral swelling with indistinct GM-WM interfaces **(12-42A)**. T2 demonstrates cortical/subcortical hyperintensity with relative sparing of the underlying WM. FLAIR is the most sensitive sequence and may be positive before signal changes are apparent on either T1- or T2WI **(12-42B)**. Bilateral but asymmetric involvement of the temporal lobes and insula is characteristic of HSE but not always present.

T2* (GRE, SWI) may demonstrate petechial hemorrhages after 24-48 hours. Gyriform T1 shortening **(12-42E)**, volume loss, and confluent curvilinear "blooming" foci on T2* are seen in the subacute and chronic phases of HSE.

HSE shows restricted diffusion early in the disease course **(12-42D)**, sometimes preceding visible FLAIR abnormalities. Enhancement varies from none (early) to intense gyriform enhancement several days later **(12-42C)**.

## Differential Diagnosis

The major differential diagnoses for HSE are neoplasm, acute cerebral ischemia, status epilepticus, other encephalitides (especially HHV-6), and autoimmune/paraneoplastic limbic encephalitis. **SARS-CoV-2-associated hemorrhagic encephalitis** can mimic herpes encephalitis. **Encephalitis of unknown cause** may represent up to 1/3 of cases with acute encephalitis syndrome.

Primary neoplasms, such as **diffusely infiltrating astrocytoma**, usually involve WM or WM + cortex.

**Acute cerebral ischemia-infarction** occurs in a typical vascular distribution involving both the cortex and WM. **Status epilepticus** is usually unilateral and typically involves just the cortex. The ipsilateral thalamus is often

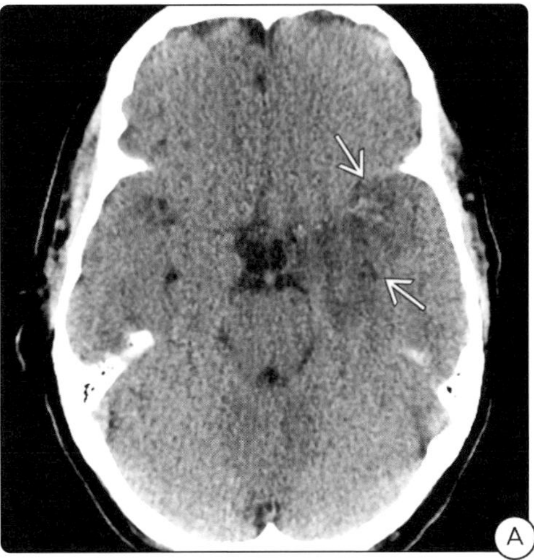


***(12-41A)** NECT in a 60-yo woman with altered mental status shows ill-defined, low-attenuation temporal lobe mass ➡, but it was called normal.*

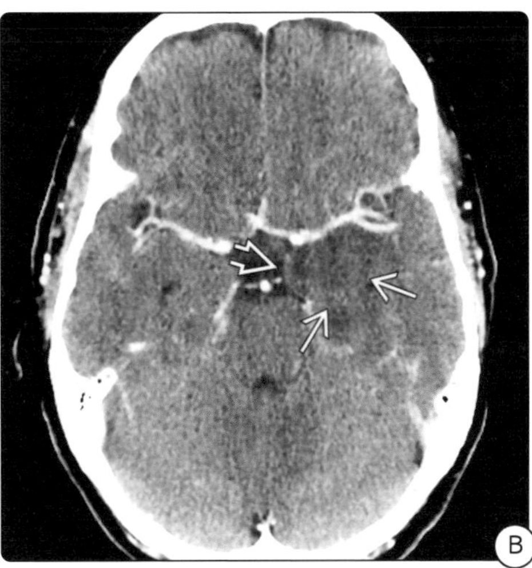


***(12-41B)** CECT in the same case obtained 48 hours later shows a hypoattenuating temporal lobe mass ➡. Note uncal herniation ➡.*

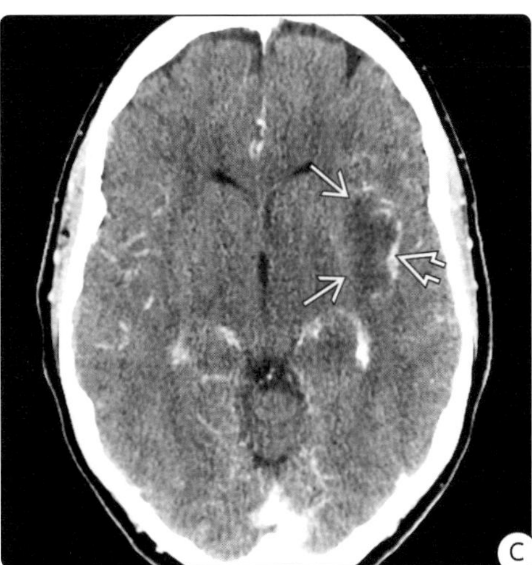


***(12-41C)** More cephalad CECT shows a hypoattenuating insular mass ➡ with superficial gyriform enhancement ➡.*

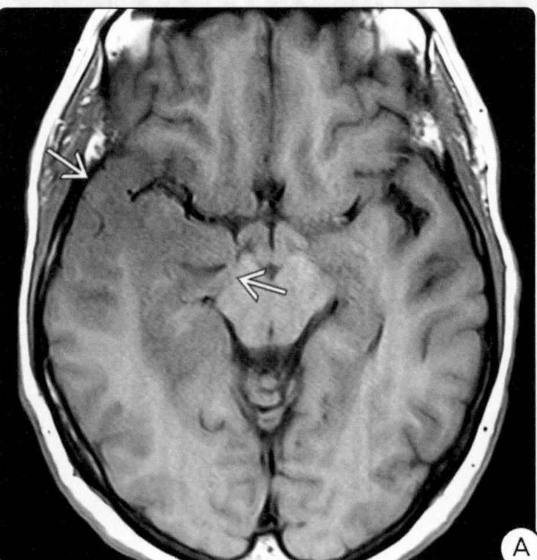

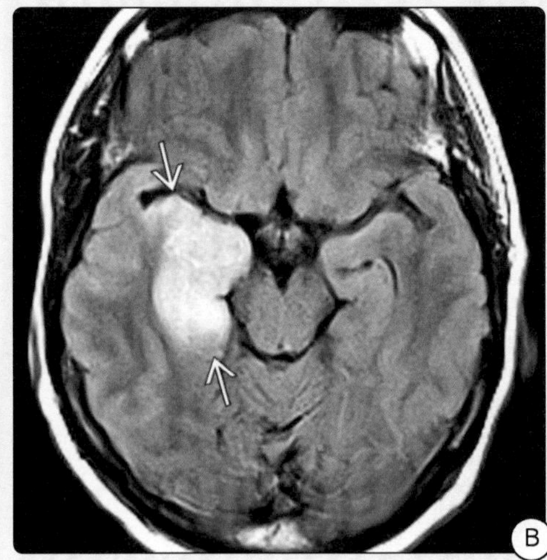

***(12-42A)** T1WI in a 64-yo woman with headache, increasing confusion 1 week after a flu-like episode shows right temporal lobe gyral swelling ➡. **(12-42B)** FLAIR in the same case shows the right temporal lobe cortex is grossly enlarged, hyperintense ➡. The left temporal lobe appears normal.*

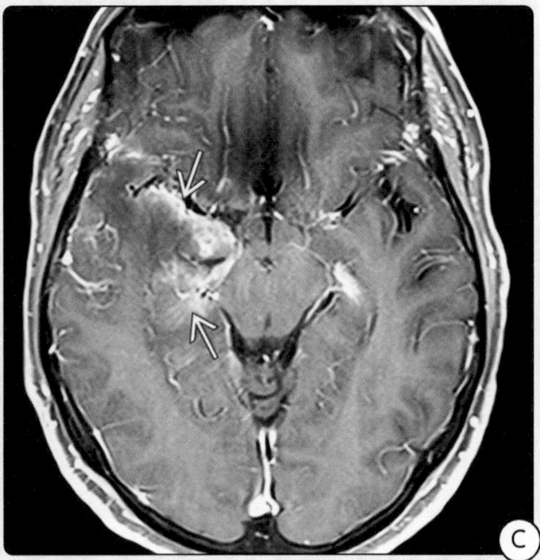

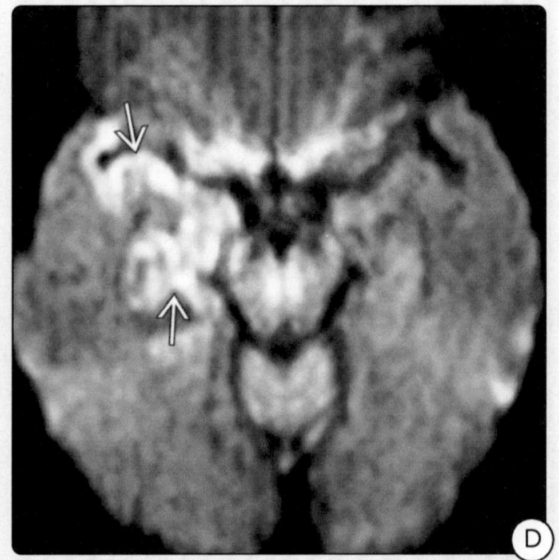

***(12-42C)** T1 C+ FS shows patchy cortical enhancement ➡ in the right anteromedial temporal lobe. **(12-42D)** DTI DWI shows cortical restriction in the right anteromedial temporal lobe ➡.*

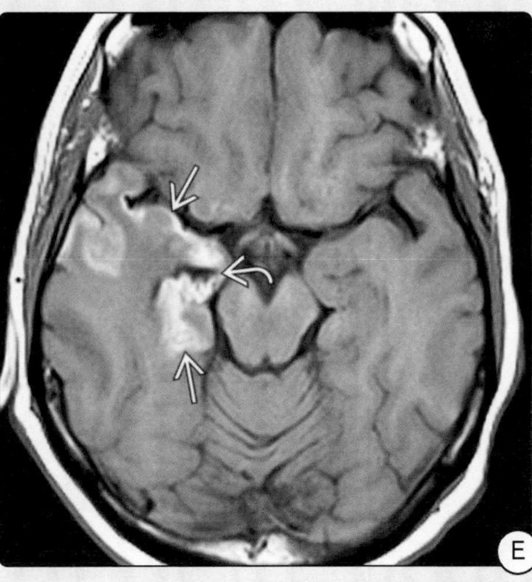

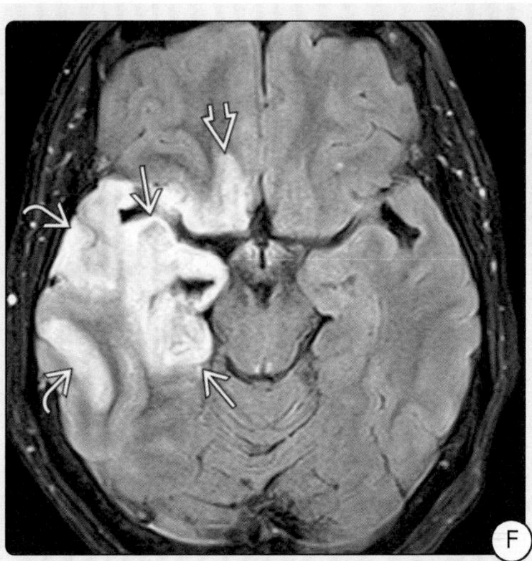

***(12-42E)** T1WI 2 weeks later shows cortical volume loss, hyperintensity ➡ from HSV-induced hemorrhagic necrosis. The temporal horn of the lateral ventricle is enlarged ⤻. **(12-42F)** FLAIR 2 weeks later shows hyperintensity, volume loss in the anteromedial temporal lobe ➡. Note additional cortical edema, hyperintensity in the right subfrontal lobe ⇨, posterolateral temporal lobe ⤻ from ongoing HSE.*

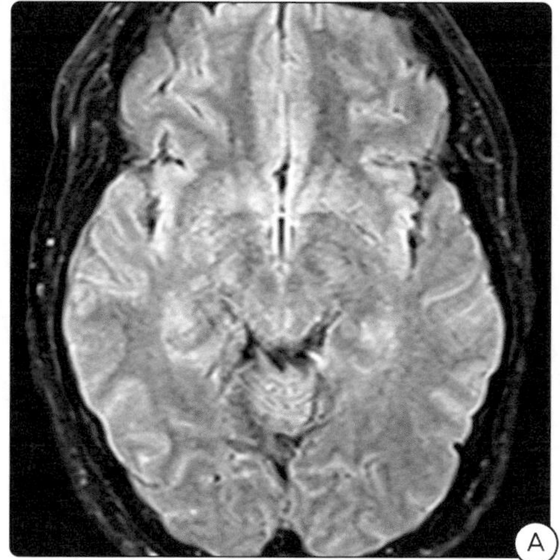

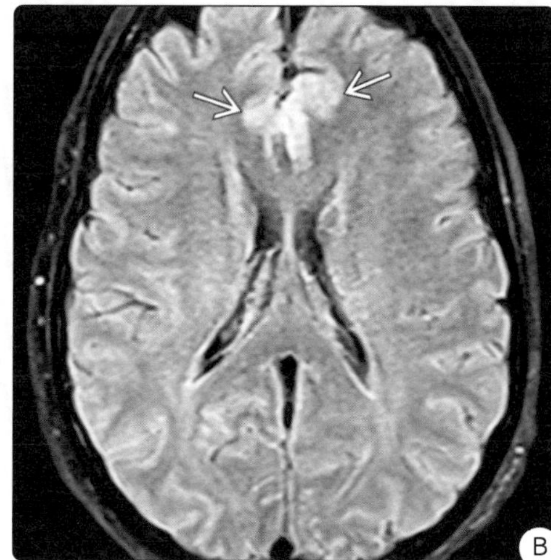

***(12-43A)** FLAIR in a 55-yo woman with 2-day history of headaches, increasing confusion following a flu-like illness shows no definite abnormalities. **(12-43B)** More cephalad FLAIR in the same case shows cortical swelling, hyperintensity in both frontal lobes ➡.*

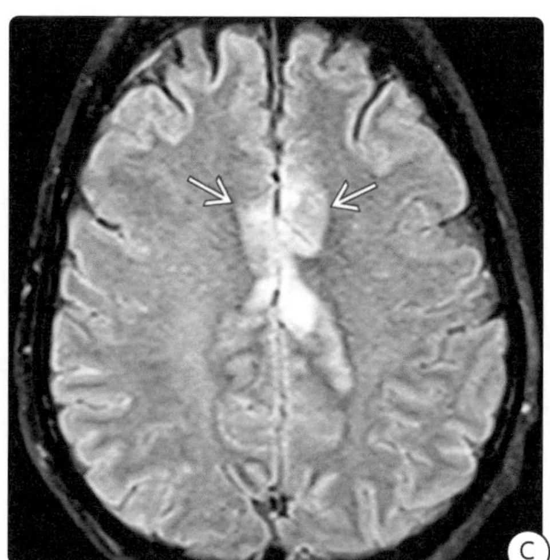

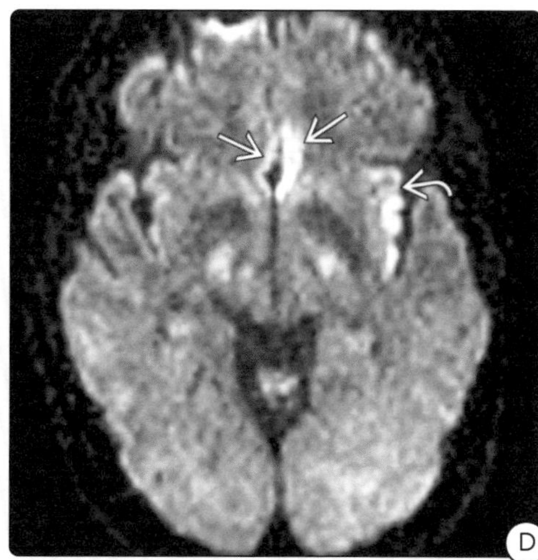

***(12-43C)** More cephalad FLAIR in the same case shows edema, hyperintensity in both cingulate gyri ➡. **(12-43D)** DWI in the same case shows restricted diffusion in the left insula ↪, both subfrontal cortices ➡.*

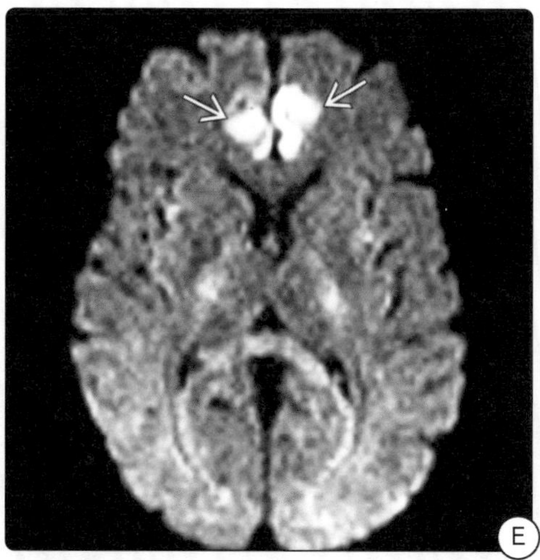

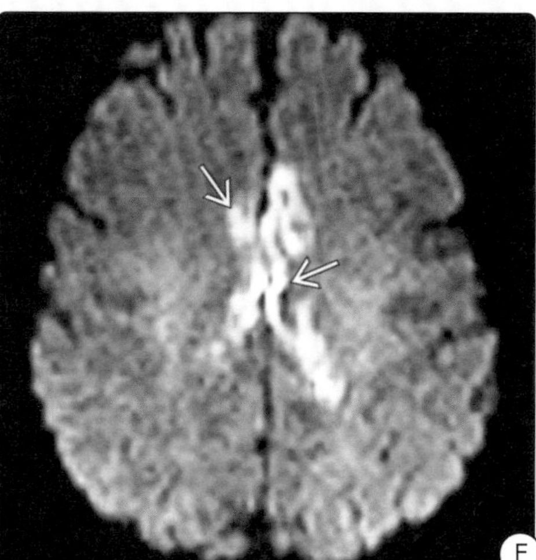

***(12-43E)** More cephalad DWI shows restricted diffusion in the cortex of both frontal lobes ➡. **(12-43F)** More cephalad DWI shows restricted diffusion in both cingulate gyri ➡. Predominately extralimbic HSE was proven by PCR.*

affected. Postictal edema is transient but generally more widespread, often involving most or all of the hemispheric cortex.

**HHV-6 encephalitis** usually involves just the medial temporal lobes, but, if extrahippocampal lesions are present, it may be difficult to distinguish from HSE solely on the basis of imaging findings.

Antibody-mediated CNS disorders, such as **limbic encephalitis** and **autoimmune encephalitis**, often have a more protracted, subacute onset and frequently present with altered mental status of unclear etiology. In some cases, imaging findings may be virtually indistinguishable from those of HSE.

**M**itochondrial myopathy, **e**ncephalopathy, **l**actic **a**cidosis, and **s**troke-like episodes **(MELAS)** occasionally presents with acute onset of fever, headache, and epilepsy similar to HSE. MR demonstrates T2/FLAIR cortical hyperintensity and restricted diffusion in a nonvascular distribution, but MRS shows elevated lactate. Nucleotide 3243 A→G mutation in mitochondrial DNA confirms the diagnosis.

## HHV-6 Encephalitis

### Etiology

More than 90% of the general population is seropositive for HHV-6 by two years of age. Most primary infections are asymptomatic, after which the virus remains latent.

HHV-6 can become pathogenic in immunocompromised patients, especially those with hematopoietic stem cell or solid organ transplantation. The median interval between transplantation and onset of neurologic symptoms is three weeks. Patients typically present with altered mental status, short-term memory loss, and seizures.

*(12-44A) Axial FLAIR MR in a 43-yo man with allogenic stem cell transplant and proven HHV-6 encephalitis shows bilaterally symmetrical hyperintensity in the hippocampi ➡ and anteromedial temporal lobes ↪, including the amygdalae. (12-44B) More cephalad FLAIR MR shows involvement of the hippocampal tails ➡ and left insular cortex ⇨.*

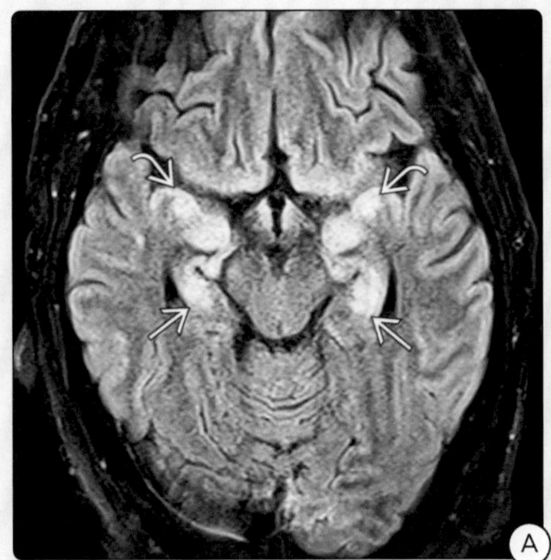


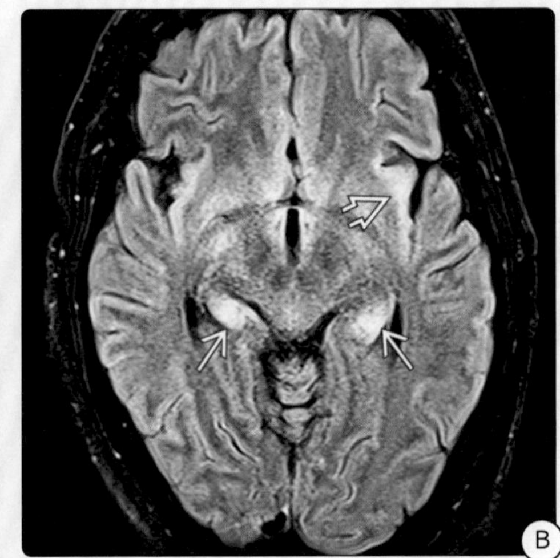


*(12-44C) DWI MR shows strong, symmetric diffusion restriction ➡ in the hippocampi, medial temporal lobes, and amygdalae. (12-44D) DWI MR shows restricted diffusion in the hippocampal tails ➡ and left insular cortex ⇨. There is also mild involvement of the right insular cortex ↪. This is variant HHV-6 encephalitis with extrahippocampal involvement.*

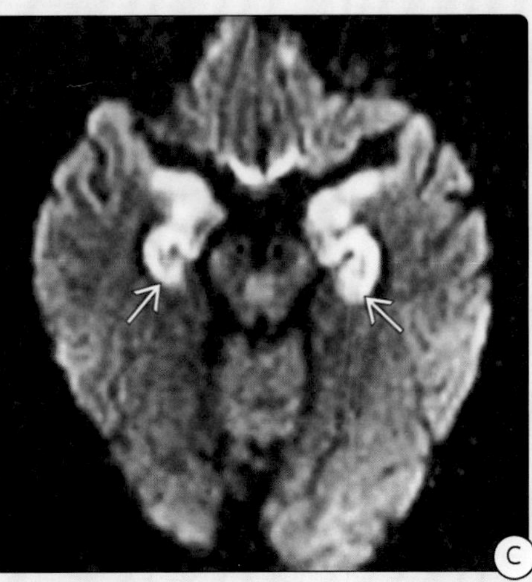


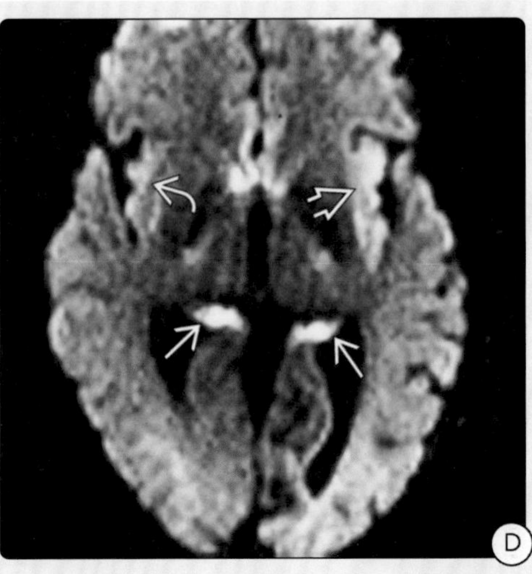

## Imaging

NECT scans are typically normal. MR shows predominant or exclusive involvement of one or both medial temporal lobes (hippocampus and amygdala) **(12-44)**. Extrahippocampal disease is less common than with HSE.

Transient hyperintensity of the mesial temporal lobes on T2WI and FLAIR with restriction on DWI is typical. In contrast to HSE, T2* (GRE, SWI) in HHV-6 encephalopathy shows no evidence of hemorrhage.

## Differential Diagnosis

The major differential diagnosis is **HSE**. The disease course of HSE is more fulminant. Extratemporal involvement and hemorrhagic necrosis are common in HSE but rare in HHV-6 encephalopathy. In contrast to HSE, in HHV-6, MR abnormalities tend to resolve with time. **Postictal hippocampal hyperemia** is transient, and extrahippocampal involvement is generally absent. **Subclinical status epilepticus** may mimic HHV-6 encephalopathy; the posteromedial thalamus is often subtly hyperintense on FLAIR.

**Autoimmune encephalitis** can easily mimic both HSE and HHV-6 encephalopathy. **Encephalitis of unknown cause** can mimic both disorders.

# Other Common Acute Viral Encephalitides

Many viruses can cause encephalitis. Over 100 different viruses in more than a dozen families have been implicated in CNS infection. HSV-1, EBV, mumps, measles, and enteroviruses are responsible for most cases of encephalitis in immunocompetent patients. CSF or serum analysis with pathogen identification by PCR amplification establishes the

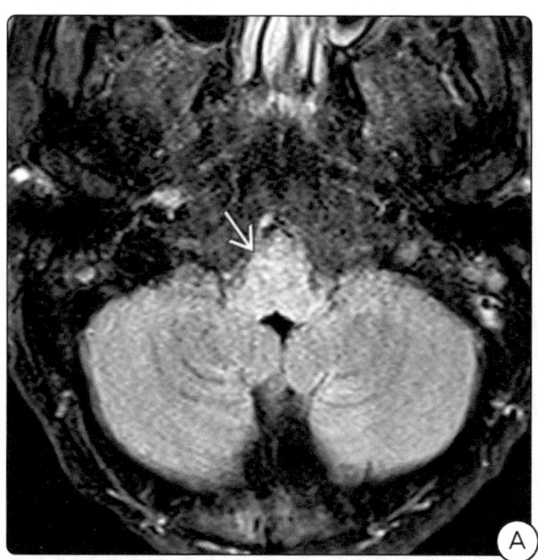

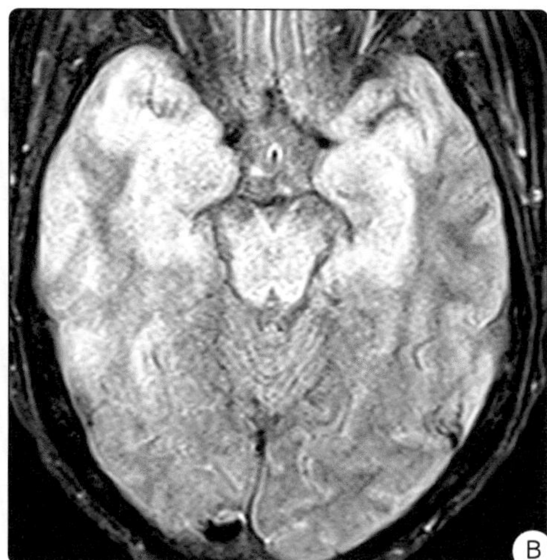

*(12-45A) FLAIR in a 59-yo man with multiple myeloma and autologous marrow transplant shows hyperintensity of the entire medulla ➡. (12-45B) More cephalad FLAIR in the same case shows midbrain hyperintensity, swollen hyperintense cortex in both hippocampi and temporal lobes.*

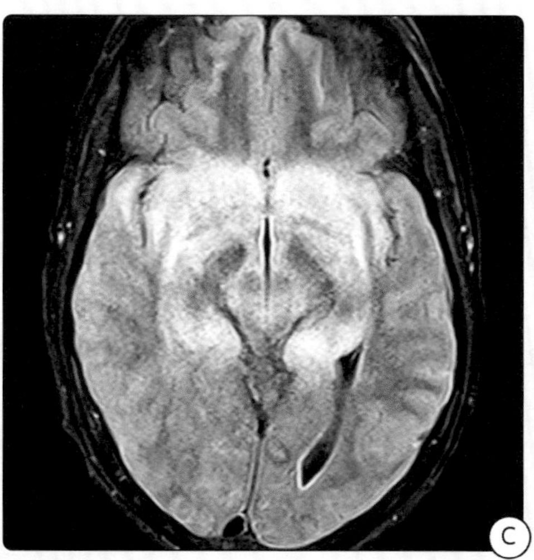

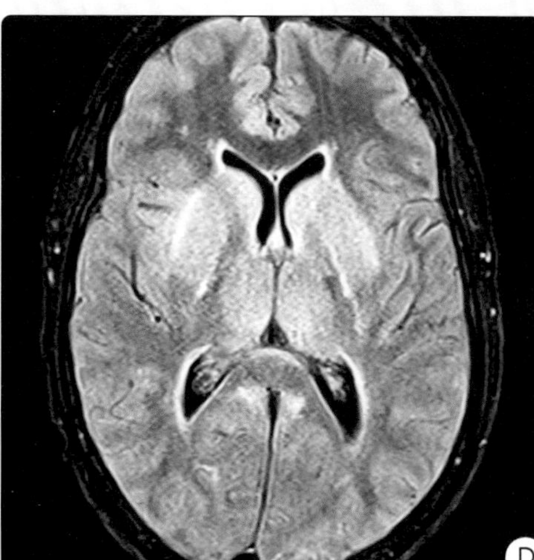

*(12-45C) More cephalad FLAIR shows hyperintensity in the insular cortices, hippocampal tails, and basal ganglia. (12-45D) Both caudate nuclei, basal ganglia, and thalami are hyperintense. No enhancement or restricted diffusion was present. This is atypical HHV6 encephalitis.*

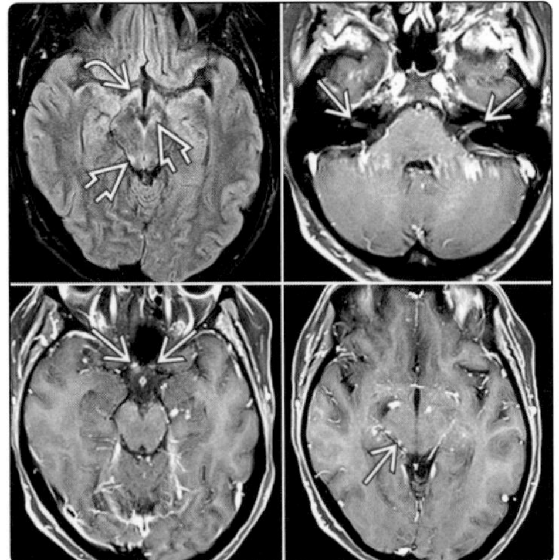

*(12-46) VZV meningitis with optic tract ➡, midbrain FLAIR hyperintensity ➡. Bilateral CNVII/VIII, optic nerves, right CNIV enhance ➡.*

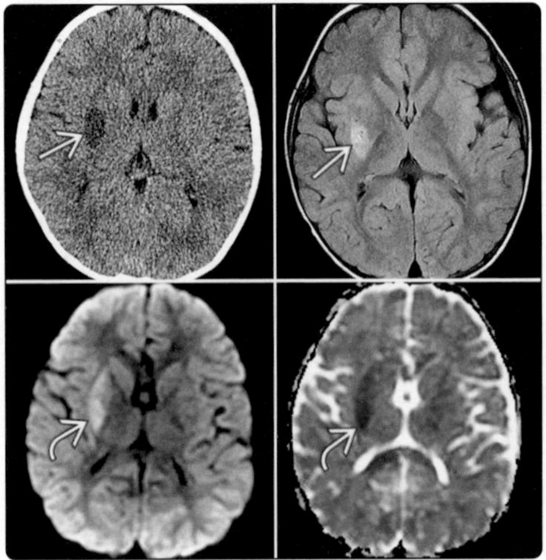

*(12-47) VZV vasculitis with stroke. NECT, FLAIR show right putaminal infarct ➡ that restricts on DWI and ADC ➡.*

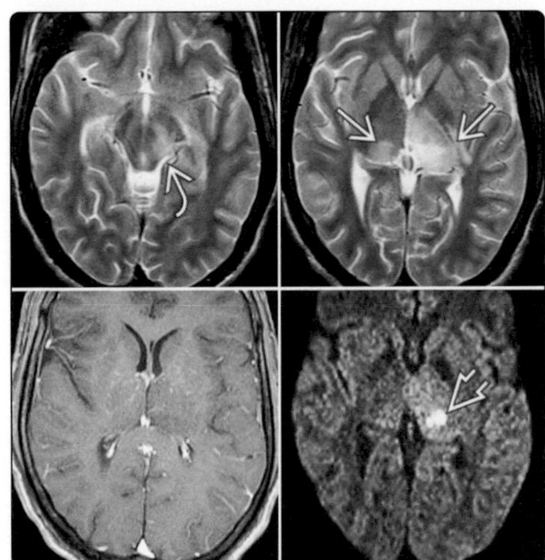

*(12-48) WNV encephalitis with T2-hyperintense lesions in the midbrain ➡ and both thalami ➡. Lesions do not enhance but do restrict ➡.*

definitive diagnosis. Nevertheless, imaging is essential to early diagnosis and treatment.

## Varicella-Zoster Encephalitis

VZV causes chickenpox (varicella) and shingles (zoster). Latent VZV can remain lifelong in ganglionic neurons and the adrenal glands but can be reactivated when VZV-specific cell-mediated immunity declines with age or immunocompromise.

VZV can present with a variety of neurologic and ophthalmic manifestations, which often overlap. Potential neurologic manifestations include herpes zoster ophthalmicus (ophthalmic branch of CNV), Bell palsy (peripheral facial nerve), Ramsay-Hunt syndrome (herpes zoster oticus), meningoencephalitis, myelitis, Reye syndrome, and postherpetic neuralgia. Definitive diagnosis is usually made by VZV PCR in the CSF or serum.

Meningitis is the most frequent overall manifestation (50% of cases) and the most common clinical presentation in immunocompetent patients (90%). Encephalitis is the second overall most common CNS presentation (42%) but is the most common manifestation in immunodeficient patients (67%). The most common presentation in children is acute cerebellitis with diffuse cerebellar swelling and hyperintensity on T2/FLAIR.

Imaging findings include cranial nerve enhancement and sometimes cavernous sinus enhancement (herpes zoster ophthalmicus). Multiple cranial nerves are affected in up to 20% of patients. Detection is limited without postcontrast fat-saturated orbit or skull base sequences.

VZV may also cause both intra- and extracerebral artery vasculopathy. Ischemic or hemorrhagic strokes, aneurysms, subarachnoid and parenchymal hemorrhages, arterial ectasias, and dissections have all been described.

## Epstein-Barr Encephalitis

EBV causes infectious mononucleosis. Neurologic complications occur in < 7% of cases, but, occasionally, CNS disease can be the sole manifestation of EBV infection. Bilateral diffuse T2/FLAIR hyperintensities in the basal ganglia and thalami are common. Patchy WM hyperintensities are seen in some cases. EBV can also cause a transient, reversible lesion of the corpus callosum splenium that demonstrates restricted diffusion.

The differential diagnosis of EBV includes acute disseminated encephalomyelitis (ADEM) and other viral infections, especially West Nile virus and autoimmune encephalitis, as well as posttransplant lymphoproliferative disorder.

## West Nile Virus Encephalitis

West Nile virus CNS infection can result in meningitis, encephalitis, and acute flaccid paralysis/poliomyelitis. The definitive diagnosis is made by PCR. Bilateral hyperintensities on T2/FLAIR in the basal ganglia, thalami, and brainstem are typical **(12-48)**. West Nile virus may cause a transient corpus callosum splenium lesion. Lesions restrict on DWI but rarely enhance.

## Influenza-Associated Encephalopathy

Influenza-associated encephalitis or encephalopathy (IAE) usually affects children younger than five years old. Many viruses have been reported as causing IAE, most recently H3N2 and influenza A (H1N1 a.k.a. swine flu). The morbidity and mortality are particularly impressive among patients with trisomy 21.

Imaging studies are abnormal in the majority of cases. Symmetric bilateral thalamic lesions, hemispheric edema, and reversible lesions in the corpus callosum splenium and WM are common. Findings resembling posterior reversible encephalopathy syndrome (PRES) have also been reported.

## Brainstem Encephalitis/Rhombencephalitis

Brainstem encephalitis/rhombencephalitis (BE) is a rare infectious/inflammatory condition that affects the rhombencephalon (pons, cerebellum, and medulla). The mesencephalon (midbrain) is technically not part of the rhombencephalon, although, because it is continuous with the pons and is often affected, it is included as part of the disease spectrum.

The most common causes of BE are infectious disorders, autoimmune disorders, demyelinating disease, and paraneoplastic syndromes. The most common cause of infectious BE is *L. monocytogenes*. The disease spectrum ranges from meningitis and meningoencephalitis to abscess. On imaging, *Listeria* BE exhibits T2-/FLAIR-hyperintense signal with high affinity for the dorsal brain stem/floor of the fourth ventricle. Ring-enhancing abscess formation is common with central restricted diffusion.

**Enteroviruses** are the second most common infectious cause of BE. EV-A71 is the most common subtype followed by EV-D68. Neurologic manifestations include aseptic meningitis, cerebellar ataxia, and symptoms similar to poliomyelitis (flaccid monoparesis or bulbar polio). Imaging findings include T2/FLAIR hyperintensity in the brainstem. The most common sites are the dorsal pons and medulla, followed by the dentate nuclei, midbrain, and thalami.

**Epstein-Barr virus** (EBV) causes infectious mononucleosis, usually a self-limiting disease. Approximately 1% develop CNS complications, including meningitis, encephalitis, transverse myelitis, and Guillain-Barré syndrome. EBV encephalitis is usually diffuse with nonspecific T2/FLAIR hyperintensity in the GM and WM, deep gray nuclei, and brainstem. Cerebellar involvement is also common.

**Influenza** causes 2-11% of childhood encephalitides. Influenza A and B can cause acute cerebellar syndromes with T2/FLAIR hyperintensities in the cerebellar hemispheres because of cytotoxic edema. H1N1 and H3N2 influenza have also been associated with brainstem/cerebellar encephalitis.

**JC virus** occurs mainly in immunosuppressed patients and occasionally involves the cerebellum, especially the middle cerebellar peduncles.

The imaging differential diagnosis of BE is wide and includes neuro-Behçet disease, autoimmune encephalitis, demyelinating disease (including neuromyelitis optica spectrum disorder), and neurosarcoidosis. Metronidazole can induce a medication-induced encephalopathy that causes symmetric T2/FLAIR hyperintensities in the dentate nuclei, midbrain, and dorsal pons. In ~ 30% of cases, the exact etiology of BE remains unknown despite extensive medical and laboratory work-up.

## Acute Necrotizing Encephalopathy

Acute necrotizing encephalopathy (ANE) is a more severe, life-threatening form of IAE characterized by high fever, seizures, and rapid clinical deterioration within two or three days after onset. The disease is often fatal.

A familial variant of ANE occurs in patients with dominant missense mutations in the *RANBP2* gene. Here, seemingly healthy individuals—often children between 1-3 years of age—develop a cytokine storm in the CNS in response to viral infection. A viral prodrome followed by rapid neurologic deterioration is typical. Untreated, this condition leads to seizures, coma, long-term neurologic damage, and high mortality rate.

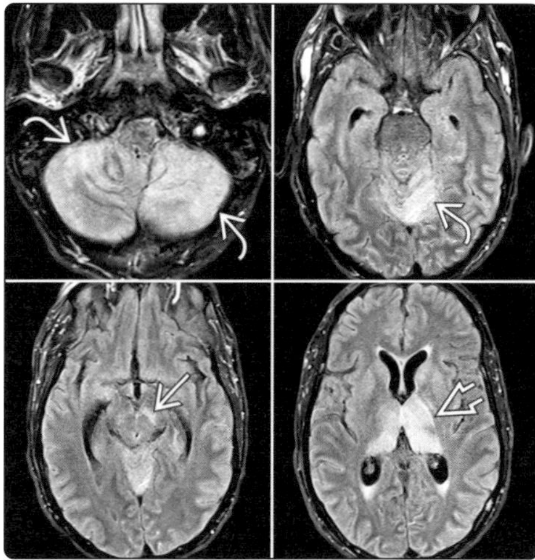

***(12-49)** FLAIR in WNV rhombencephalitis shows bilateral cerebellum, midbrain as well as lesions in both thalami.*

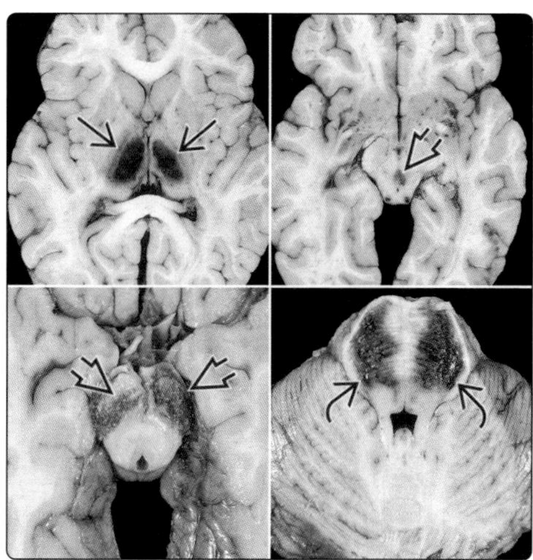

***(12-50)** Autopsied case of ANE shows symmetric, hemorrhagic necrosis in the thalami, midbrain, and pons.*

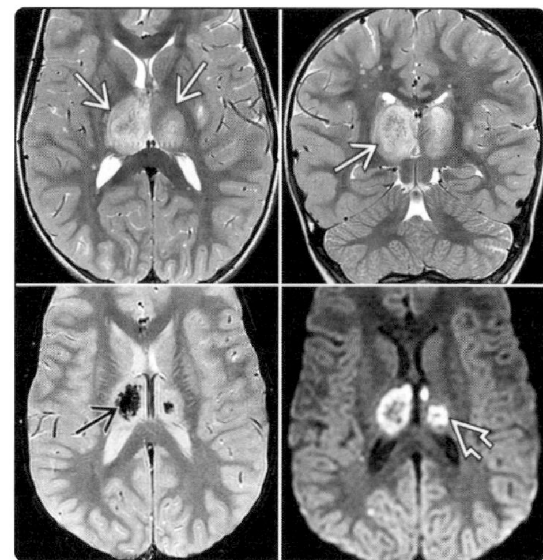

***(12-51)** 4-yo with influenza A shows bithalamic T2-hyperintense lesions, hemorrhage on T2*GRE, restricted diffusion. This is ANE.*

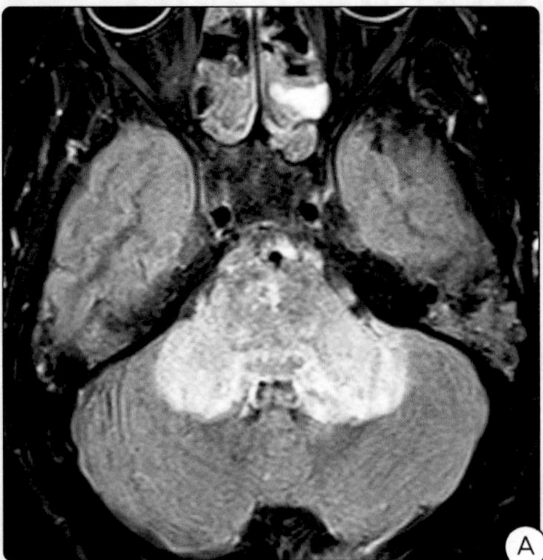


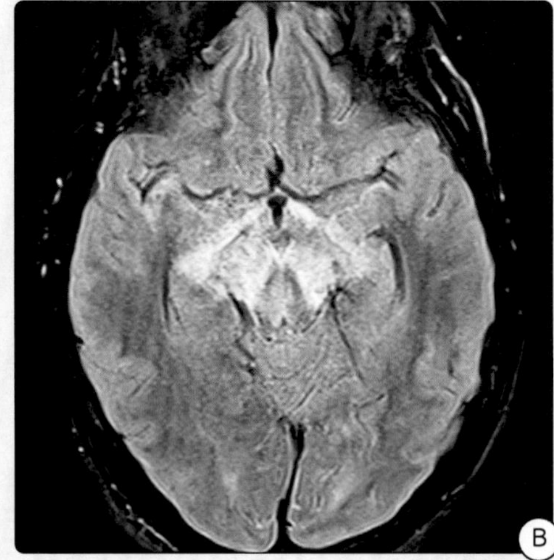


***(12-52A)*** *19-yo man had a 1-week history of skin rash, headache, nausea, and vomiting after which he became somnolent. FLAIR shows diffusely swollen, heterogeneously hyperintense pons with abnormal signal extending into both major cerebellar peduncles.* ***(12-52B)*** *More cephalad FLAIR shows hyperintensity extending into the midbrain as well as both optic tracts.*

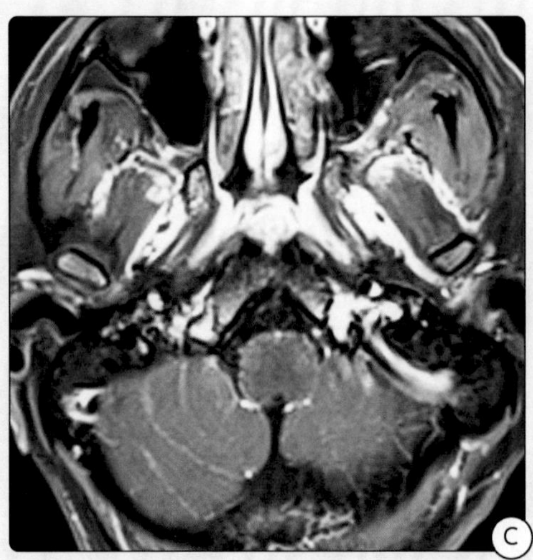


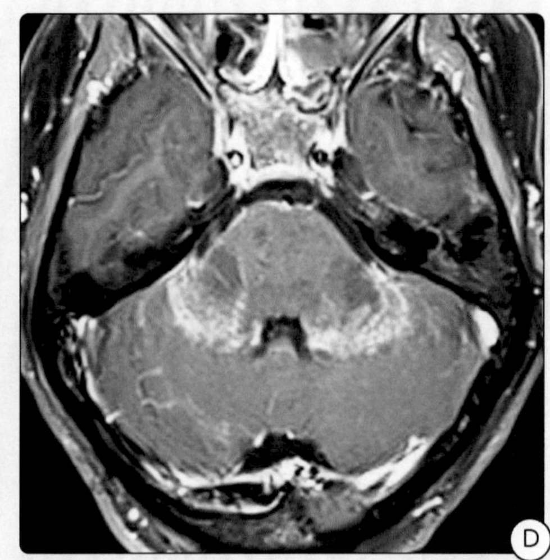


***(12-52C)*** *T1 C+ FS MR shows pial enhancement over the surface of the midbrain that also extends along the cerebellar folia.* ***(12-52D)*** *More cephalad T1 C+ shows meningeal enhancement along the surface of the pons. Note enhancement of the left 6th nerve with faint enhancement of the right CNV. Peripheral enhancement is present around the areas of pontine and peduncular necrosis. Acute necrotizing rhombencephalitis.*

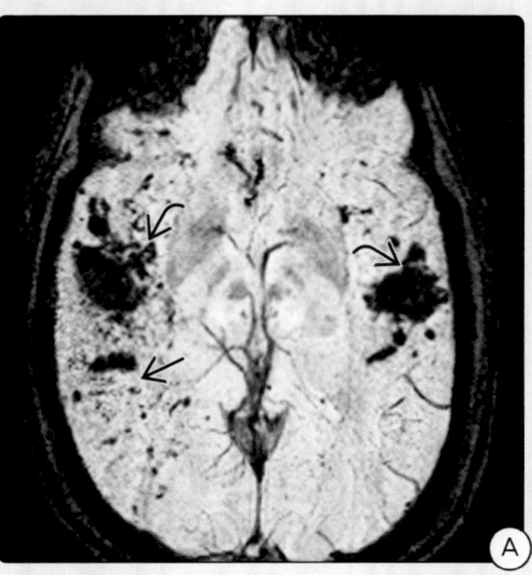


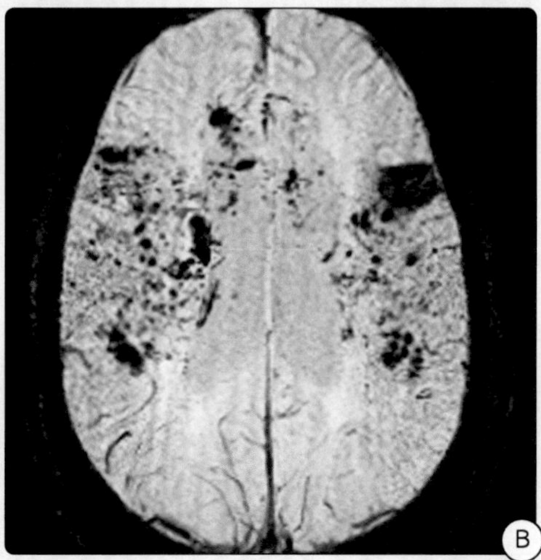


***(12-53A)*** *Axial MIP of T2* SWI in a 38-yo man with fever, altered mental status, and seizures shows multiple confluent ↷ and petechial → hemorrhages in the cortex and subcortical WM.* ***(12-53B)*** *Extensive microbleeds are seen in the cortex and WM with relative frontal/occipital sparing. CSF indicated viral encephalitis but PCR identified no causative organism. This is acute hemorrhagic leukoencephalitis.*

Multifocal symmetric T2-/FLAIR-hyperintense lesions, typically in the thalami, develop during the acute phase.

## Acute Hemorrhagic Leukoencephalitis

Acute hemorrhagic leukoencephalitis (AHLE) may be an unusually severe variant of ADEM. A viral prodrome precedes acute neurologic deterioration and has been reported in a variety of CNS infections, including dengue fever and COVID-19. Multifocal discrete and coalescing WM and deep GM lesions with restricted diffusion and cerebral microbleeds can be seen.

## Less Common Infectious Viral Encephalitides

A host of other viral encephalitides have been identified. While some (such as rotavirus encephalitis) are widespread, others (e.g., Japanese encephalitis, LaCrosse encephalitis, Nipah virus encephalitis) currently have a more restricted geographic distribution.

Arboviruses are zoonotic RNA viruses that involve arthropod vectors. Arthropod-borne (ticks and mosquitoes) viruses represent an underappreciated cause of encephalitis in older pediatric patients and adults. The main emerging arboviruses in the Americas are dengue, Zika, yellow fever (Flaviviridae), and chikungunya (Togaviridae). These infections can cause hemorrhagic encephalitis, myelitis, ADEM, Guillain-Barré syndrome, as well as congenital malformations **(12-9)**.

MR demonstrates a spectrum of imaging features. T2-hyperintense lesions of the thalami, substantia nigra, basal ganglia, brainstem, cerebellum, and cerebral cortical and hemispheric WM.

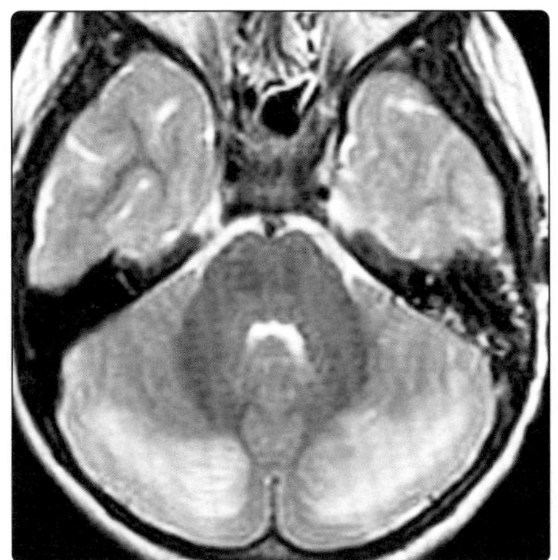

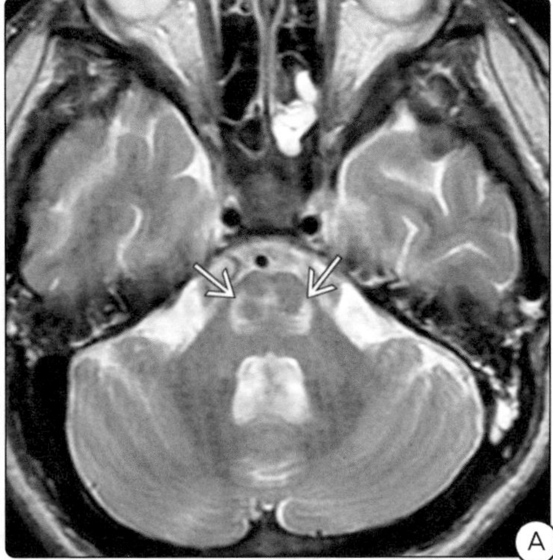

***(12-54)** 6-yo child with influenza cerebellitis shows symmetric hyperintensity in both cerebellar hemispheres. **(12-55A)** T2WI in a 15-yo man with H1N1 influenza (influenza A) shows symmetric hyperintensity in the pons ➡.*

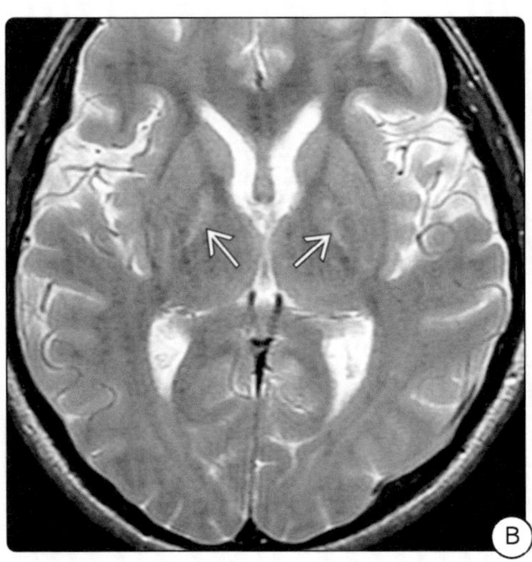

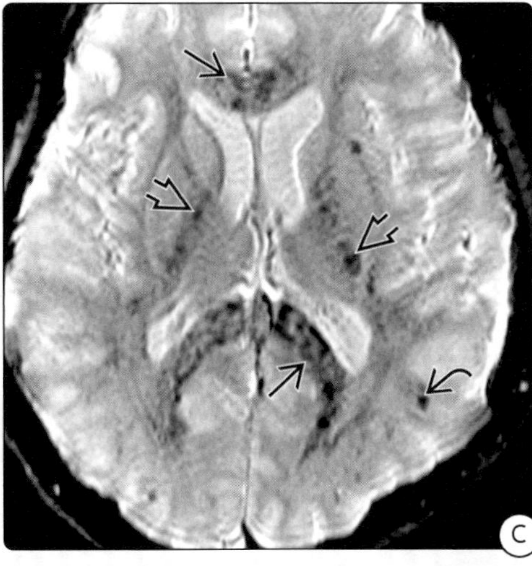

***(12-55B)** More cephalad T2WI shows hyperintensity in both globi pallidi ➡. **(12-55C)** T2* GRE shows numerous WM microhemorrhages in the corpus callosum ➡, internal capsules ➡, and subcortical WM ➡. This is influenza-related acute hemorrhagic encephalitis.*

## Chronic Encephalitides

Some viruses cause acute, fulminating CNS infection. Others have a more insidious onset, producing a "slow" chronic infection with symptoms and imaging manifestations that span months or even years. Some, such as the measles virus, can cause both. In this section, we briefly consider two chronic encephalitides: The measles reactivation syndrome called subacute sclerosis panencephalitis (SSPE) and Rasmussen encephalitis (RE).

### Subacute Sclerosing Panencephalitis

SSPE is a rare progressive encephalopathy that occurs years after measles virus infection. The measles virus infects neurons and remains latent for years. Why and how reactivation occurs is not fully understood but with increasingly insufficient childhood vaccinations, SSPE is reemerging as an archetype of nonvaccination consequences. The disease has no specific cure and is associated with a high degree of disability and mortality.

Symptoms appear an average of six years after measles virus infection. Imaging studies may be initially normal but then show relentless progression. Cortical GM reduction in the frontotemporal cortex occurs relatively early and is followed by diffuse, progressive bilateral volume loss. Bilateral but asymmetric cortical and subcortical WM and periventricular T2/FLAIR hyperintensities are present.

### Rasmussen Encephalitis

RE is a rare, chronic inflammatory disorder that affects only one cerebral hemisphere. The etiology of RE is unknown; no virus is identified on PCR studies and by definition, serologic CSF studies are negative for neurotropic viruses, such as HSV1 and 2, CMV, and EBV. T-cell-mediated cytotoxicity is a key feature of RE.

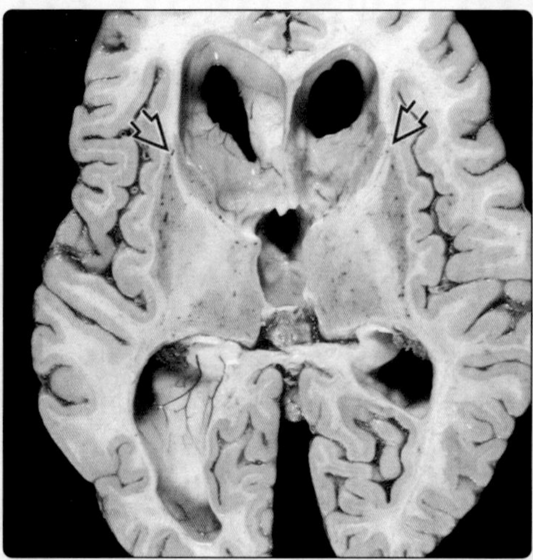

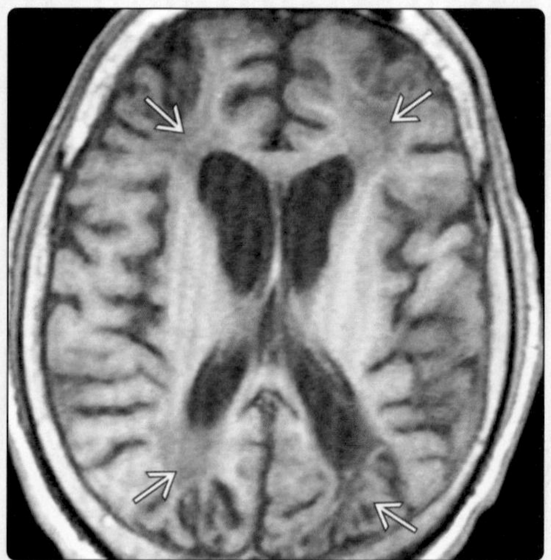

***(12-56)** Autopsy case of SSPE shows grossly enlarged ventricles, superficial sulci with striking volume loss in the basal ganglia ⇨ and cerebral WM. **(12-57)** T1WI in a 16-yo boy with deteriorating school performance shows diffuse atrophy with bifrontal and bioccipital parenchymal hypointensities ➡. CSF was positive for measles antibodies.*

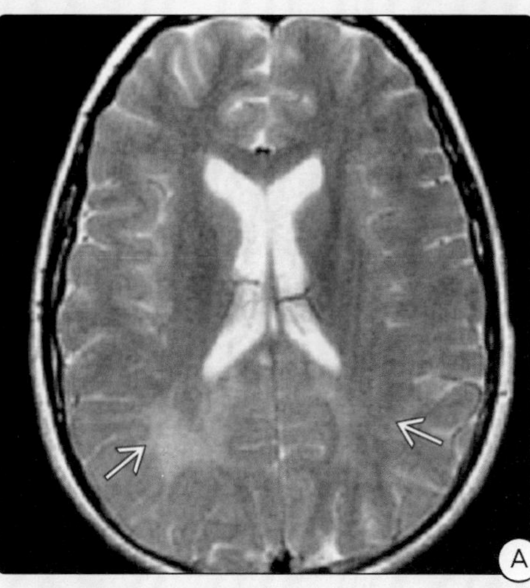


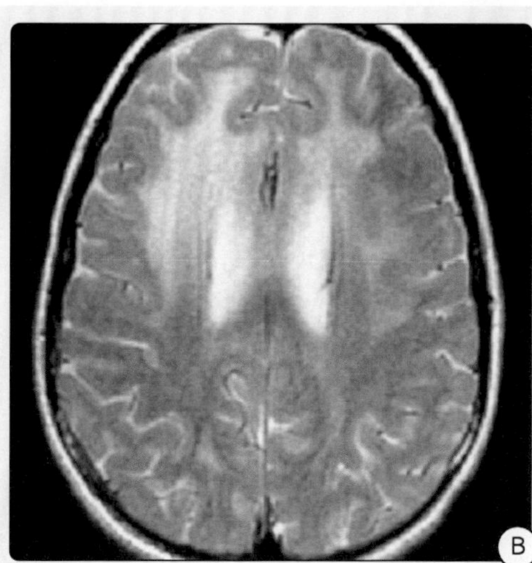


***(12-58A)** T2WI in a 13-yo child with unexplained cognitive decline and progressive motor impairment shows bilateral asymmetric hyperintensities in both occipital lobes ➡. The ventricles are mildly enlarged for the patient's age. **(12-58B)** Six months later, WM hyperintensities have spread to involve both frontal and parietal lobes. CSF was positive for measles antibodies. This is SSPE.*

RE is a disease that primarily affects children. Median age at onset is six years with normal developmental milestones before onset of seizures. Adolescent and adult cases are more protracted, generally occurring with a milder clinical course.

RE is distinguished by progressive unilateral hemispheric atrophy, intractable seizures, and neurologic deterioration. Damage to the hemisphere spreads from frontotemporal to occipital regions over time with the pattern of spread correlating with the progression of epileptic foci across the hemisphere.

RE develops in three clinical stages beginning with a prodromal stage characterized by low frequency seizures and mild hemiparesis. The second or acute stage is marked by frequent seizures. If the dominant hemisphere is affected, progressive hemiparesis, hemianopia, cognitive decline, and aphasia occur. After 8-12 months, children with RE may enter a stage of permanent but stable neurologic deficits, while the disease may progress slowly in adults and adolescents.

Histologic features depend on disease duration. In the earliest stages, perivascular lymphocytic cuffing and microglial clusters with or without neuronophagia are present. Neuronal loss, gliosis, and, eventually, late-stage cavitation and cortical destruction ensue. Surgery is the only cure for RE disease progression, often requiring hemispherectomy.

Initial imaging studies may be normal. Serial MRs show the relentless disease progression. The earliest abnormal MR finding is cortical swelling with increasing T2/FLAIR hyperintensity in the affected hemisphere. In the subacute stage, multifocal T2/FLAIR hyperintensities in the WM may develop. In the chronic phase, atrophy of the affected hemisphere is characterized by sulcal widening, dilatation of the ipsilateral ventricle, and basal ganglia atrophy.

*Selected References: The complete reference list is available on the eBooks+ version included with purchase.*

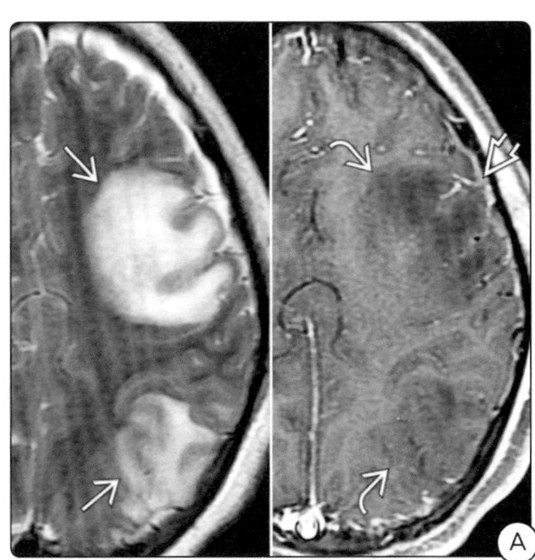


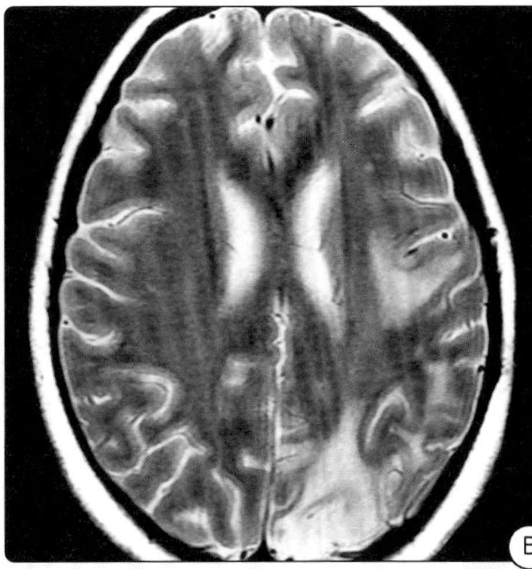


***(12-59A)** (L) T2WI in a 12-yo girl with seizure who then became hemiplegic and aphasic shows cortical/subcortical hyperintense masses in the left hemisphere ➡. (R) T1 C+ FS shows the lesions ➡ are hypointense with mild overlying sulcal-cisternal enhancement ➡. **(12-59B)** T2WI 2 years later shows mild volume loss in the left hemisphere with several cortical/subcortical areas of confluent hyperintensity.*

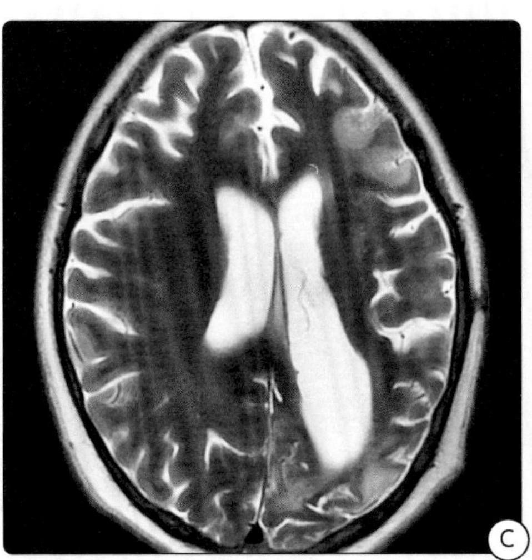


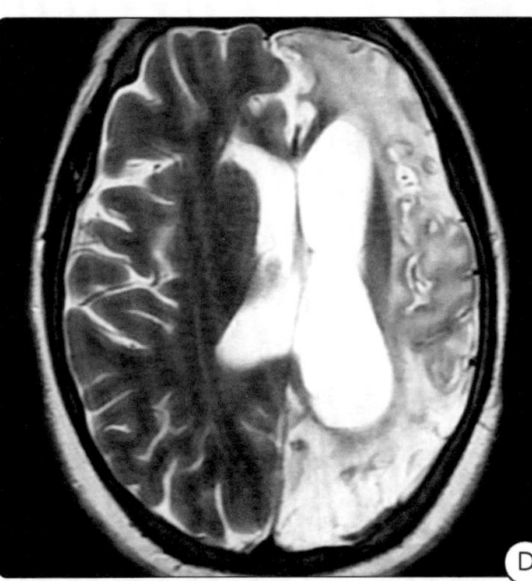


***(12-59C)** Two years after the initial scan, there is more severe volume loss with dilatation of the ipsilateral ventricle and sulci, multiple foci of T2 confluent hyperintensity in the subcortical WM. The overlying cortex, especially in the occipital lobe, is grossly atrophic. **(12-59D)** Four years after the initial scan, the entire left hemisphere is atrophic and gliotic. No positive viral titers or PCR were ever identified. This is Rasmussen encephalitis.*

# Tuberculosis and Fungal, Parasitic, and Other Infections

*In this chapter, we continue the delineation of acquired infections that we began in Chapter 12 with pyogenic and viral CNS infections.*

We first turn our attention to mycobacterial infections, focusing primarily on tuberculosis (TB) followed by a brief discussion of fungal and parasitic infections. We close the chapter with a brief consideration of miscellaneous and emerging CNS infections to remind us that the "hot zone" is right outside our windows, no matter where we live!



## Mycobacterial Infections

Mycobacteria are small, rod-shaped, acid-fast bacilli that are divided into three main groups, each with a different signature disease: (1) *Mycobacterium tuberculosis* (TB), (2) nontuberculous mycobacteria ("atypical" mycobacterial spectrum infections), and (3) *Mycobacterium leprae* (leprosy). *M. tuberculosis* causes > 98% of CNS TB and is therefore the major focus of our discussion.

### Tuberculosis

#### Etiology

Most TB is caused by *M. tuberculosis*. Human-to-human transmission is typical. Animal-to-human transmission via *Mycobacterium bovis*, a common pathogen in the past, is now rarely encountered. Neurotuberculosis is secondary to hematogenous spread from extracranial infection, most frequently in the lungs.

#### Pathology

CNS TB has several distinct pathologic manifestations. Acute/subacute TB **meningitis** (TBM) constitutes 70-80% of cases. An inflammatory reaction ("exudate") with a variable admixture of exudative, proliferative, and necrotizing components in subarachnoid cisterns is typical finding **(13-1)** **(13-2)**.

The second most common manifestation of neurotuberculosis is a focal parenchymal infection with central caseating necrosis (TB granuloma or **tuberculoma**) **(13-3)**. True CNS abscesses are rare. TB **pseudoabscess** is found in 20% of TB patients coinfected with HIV.

**Location.** TBM has a striking predilection for the basal cisterns, although exudates in superficial convexity sulci do occur **(13-2)**. Most tuberculomas occur in cerebral hemispheres, especially frontal and parietal lobes and basal ganglia.

**Size and Number.** Tuberculomas vary in size. The majority are small (< 2.5 cm), and the "miliary" nodules are often just a few millimeters in diameter. "Giant" tuberculomas can reach 4-6 cm.

Tuberculomas also vary in number, ranging from a solitary lesion to innumerable small "miliary" lesions.

**Gross Pathology. TBM** is a dense exudate that coats the brain surfaces and cranial nerves (CNs) **(13-1)**. The suprasellar/chiasmatic region, ambient cisterns, and interpeduncular fossa are most commonly involved **(13-2)**. **Tuberculomas** with "caseating" necrosis have a creamy (cheese-like) necrotic center surrounded by a grayish granulomatous rim **(13-3)**.

## Clinical Issues

**Demographics.** CNS TB occurs in both immunocompetent and immunocompromised patients. Among people with latent TB infection, HIV is the strongest known risk factor for progression to active TB. In TB and HIV/AIDS co-infection, each disease greatly amplifies the lethality of the other.

CNS TB occurs at all ages, but 60-70% of cases occur during the first two decades. There is no sex predilection.

**Presentation.** The most common manifestation of active CNS TB is meningitis (TBM). Presentation varies from fever and headache with mild meningismus to confusion, lethargy, seizures, and coma. Symptoms of increased intracranial pressure and cranial neuropathies are common.

Focal neurologic deficits may occur; **one of the most common "brain tumors" in endemic countries is tuberculoma, which accounts for 10-30% of all CNS mass lesions.**

**Natural History and Treatment.** Prognosis depends on the patient's immune status as well as treatment. Untreated TB can be fatal in 4-8 weeks. Even with treatment, 1/3 of patients

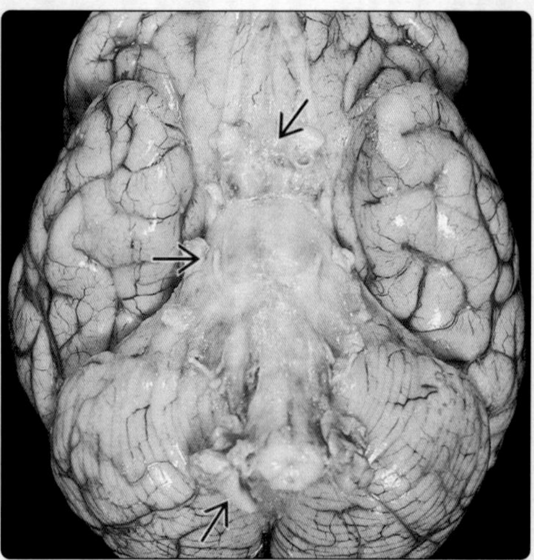

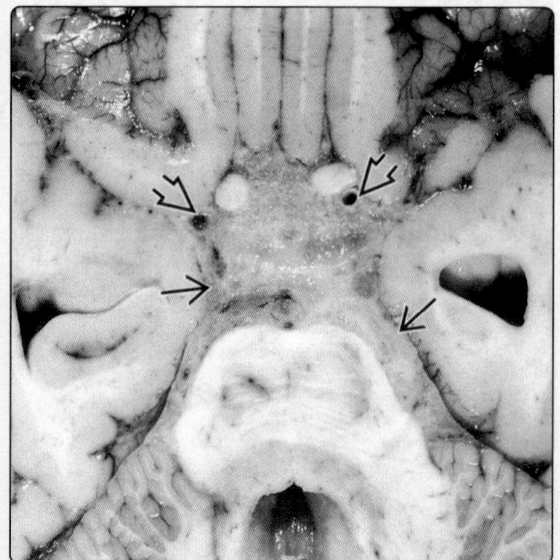

***(13-1)** Autopsy shows typical findings of TBM + dense exudates extending throughout basal cisterns ⇨. Gross appearance is indistinguishable from that of pyogenic meningitis. (Courtesy R. Hewlett, MD.)* ***(13-2)** Axial section through suprasellar cistern in TBM shows thick exudate ⇨ filling suprasellar cistern & coating pons. Note extremely small diameter of supraclinoid ICAs ⇨ due to TB vasculitis. (Courtesy R. Hewlett, MD.)*

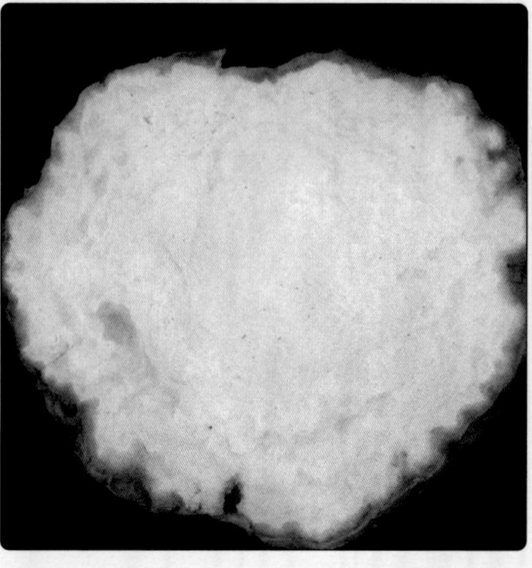

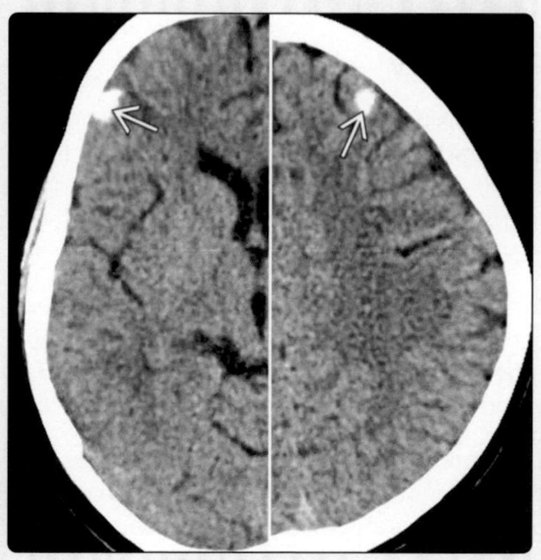

***(13-3)** Surgically resected TB gumma shows the solid cheesy appearance of a caseating granuloma. (Courtesy R. Hewlett, MD.)* ***(13-4)** Two different axial images from a NECT in a patient with CNS TB shows 2 calcified healed granulomas ➡. There was no evidence of active TBM. (Courtesy R. Ramakantan, MD.)*

deteriorate within six weeks. Overall mortality is 25-30% and is even higher in drug-resistant TB. TB is also the leading cause of communicable disease-related deaths in people with HIV.

**Multidrug-resistant TB (MDR TB)** is resistant to at least two of the first-line anti-TB drugs (isoniazid and rifampin). **Extensively drug-resistant TB (XDR TB)** is defined as TB that is resistant to first-line drugs, any fluoroquinolone, and at least one of three injectable second-line drugs (i.e., amikacin, kanamycin, or capreomycin).

Common complications of CNS TB include hydrocephalus (70%) and stroke (up to 40%).

### CNS TUBERCULOSIS: ETIOLOGY, PATHOLOGY, AND CLINICAL ISSUES

**Etiology**

- Most caused by *Mycobacterium tuberculosis*
- Hematogenous spread from extracranial site (e.g., lung)

**Pathology**

- TB meningitis (70-80%)
  - Basal cisterns > convexity sulci
- Tuberculoma (TB granuloma) (20-30%)
  - Caseating necrosis (hemispheres, basal ganglia)

**Clinical Issues**

- All ages, but 60-70% in children < 20 years
- 10-30% of brain parenchymal masses in endemic areas
- Overall mortality: 25-30% (worse with MDR/XDR TB)

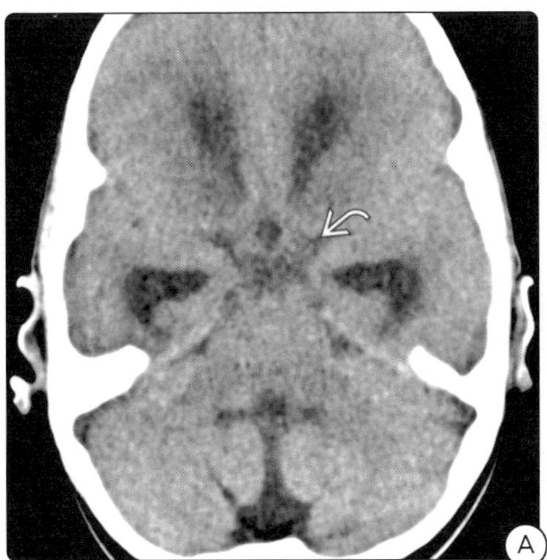


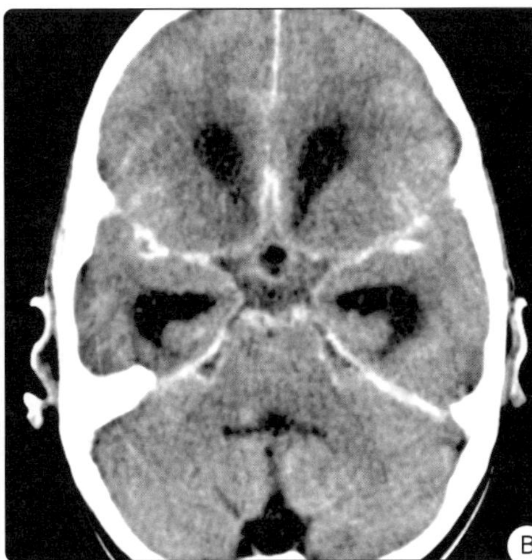


*(13-5A) NECT in a 3-yo boy with TBM shows dilated temporal, frontal horns. Note that the CSF in the suprasellar cistern ➪ is hyperdense compared to more normal CSF in the lateral ventricles.* ***(13-5B)*** *CECT in the same patient shows diffuse enhancement in the basal cisterns and sylvian fissures.*

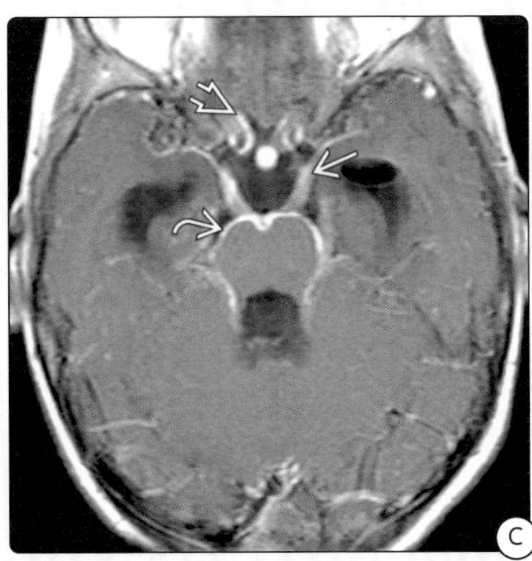


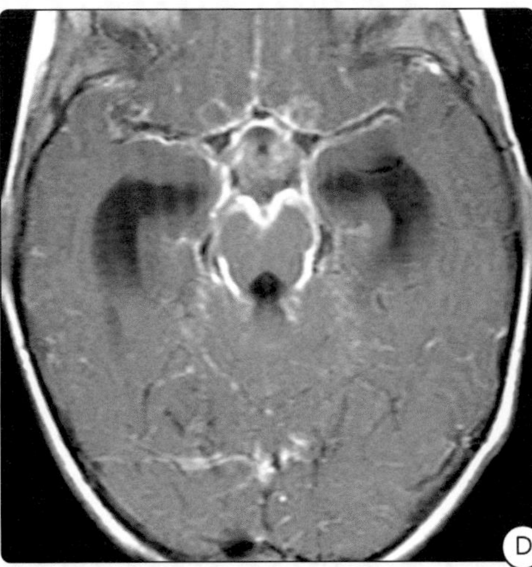


*(13-5C) T1 C+ MR in the same patient shows thick enhancing exudate around the upper pons ➪. Note enhancement covering the surface of the optic ➪ and both 3rd cranial nerves ➪.* ***(13-5D)*** *More cephalad T1 C+ MR shows the diffuse enhancement throughout the basal cisterns. Note thick exudate entirely covering the midbrain. This is TBM.*

## Imaging

### CT Findings

***TB Meningitis.*** Nonspecific hydrocephalus is the most frequent finding on NECT. "Blurred" ventricular margins indicate extracellular fluid accumulation in the subependymal white matter. As the disease progresses, iso- to mildly hyperdense basilar and sulcal exudates replace and efface the normal hypodense CSF **(13-5A)**. CECT usually shows intense enhancement of the basilar meninges and subarachnoid spaces **(13-5B)**.

***Tuberculoma.*** NECT scans show one or more iso- to slightly hyperdense round, lobulated, or crenated masses with variable perilesional edema. Calcification can be seen in healed granulomas **(13-4)**. CECT scans demonstrate punctate, solid, or ring-like enhancement.

### MR Findings

***TB Meningitis.*** Basilar exudates are isointense with brain on T1WI, giving the appearance of "dirty" CSF. FLAIR scans show increased signal intensity in the sulci and cisterns **(13-6A)**. Marked linear or nodular meningeal enhancement is seen on T1 C+ FS sequences **(13-5D)** **(13-6)**. Tuberculous exudates may extend into the brain parenchyma along the perivascular spaces, causing a meningoencephalitis.

Vascular complications occur in 20-50% of cases. The "flow voids" of major arteries may appear irregular or reduced. Penetrating artery infarcts with enhancement and restricted diffusion are common.

CN involvement is seen in 17-40% of cases. The optic nerve and CNs III, IV, and VII are most commonly affected **(13-5C)**. The affected CNs appear thickened and enhance intensely on postcontrast images **(13-5C)**.

***(13-6A)** Axial FLAIR MR in a 41-yo man with proven TBM shows diffuse sulcal-cisternal hyperintensity with thick exudate anterior to the upper pons and in the suprasellar cistern. **(13-6B)** T1 C+ FS MR shows diffuse sulcal enhancement. Note the thick rind of enhancing exudate around the upper pons.*

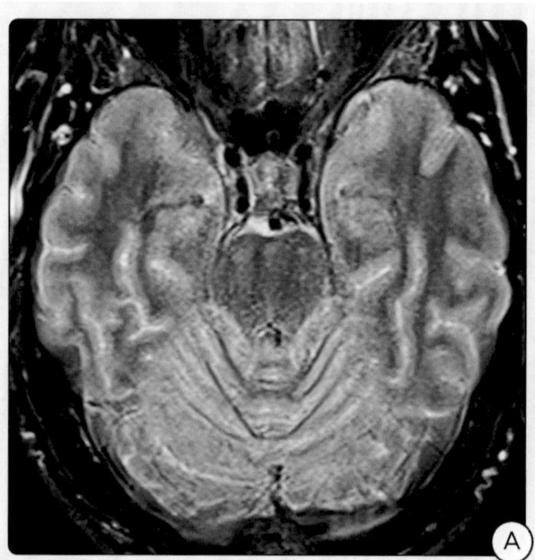


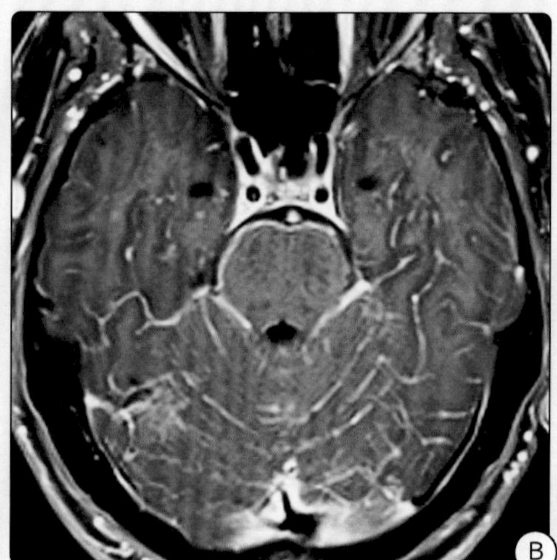


***(13-6C)** More cephalad T1 C+ FS MR in the same patient shows striking, diffuse sulcal enhancement. **(13-6D)** DWI MR shows restriction in the cerebellar hemispheres from TB-induced cerebellitis.*

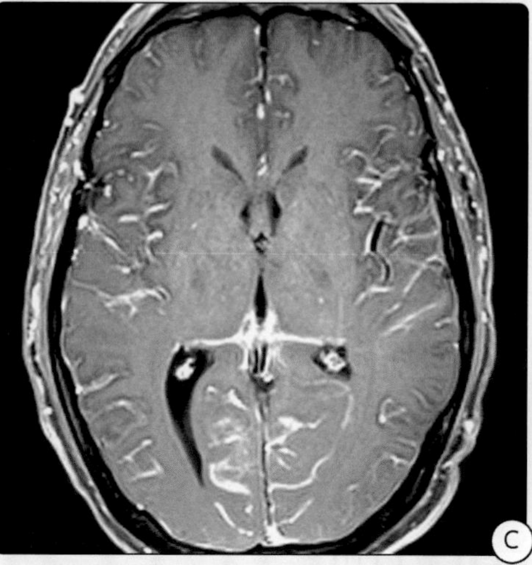


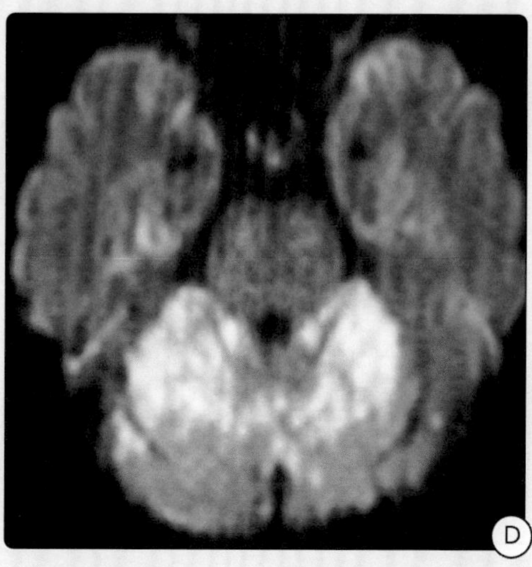

***Tuberculoma.*** Most TB granulomas are solid caseating, necrotizing lesions that appear hypo- or isointense with brain on T1WI **(13-7A)** and hypointense on T2WI **(13-7B)** **(13-8A)**. Liquefied areas may be T2 hyperintense with a hypointense rim and resemble abscess.

Enhancement is variable, ranging from small punctate foci to multiple rim-enhancing lesions. Mild to moderate, round or lobulated ring-like enhancement around a nonenhancing center is the most typical pattern **(13-8C)**.

MRS can be very helpful in characterizing tuberculomas and distinguishing them from neoplasm or pyogenic abscess. A large lipid peak with absence of other metabolites, such as amino acids and succinate, is seen in 85-90% of cases.

**PET/CT.** FDG PET/CT has the unique ability to identify a subset of patients declared cured based on the current standard of care but who still harbor live bacilli capable of causing relapse after therapy is discontinued.

## Differential Diagnosis

The major differential diagnosis of **TBM** is **pyogenic or carcinomatous meningitis**, as their imaging findings can be indistinguishable. **Carcinomatous meningitis** is usually seen in older patients with a known systemic or primary CNS neoplasm.

**Neurosarcoidosis** can also mimic TBM. Infiltration of the pituitary gland, infundibulum, and hypothalamus is common.

The major differential diagnosis of multiple parenchymal **tuberculomas** is **neurocysticercosis** (NCC). NCC usually shows multiple lesions in different stages of evolution. Tuberculomas can also resemble pyogenic **abscesses** or **neoplasms**. Abscesses restrict on DWI. Tuberculomas have a large lipid peak on MRS and lack the elevated Cho typical of neoplasm.

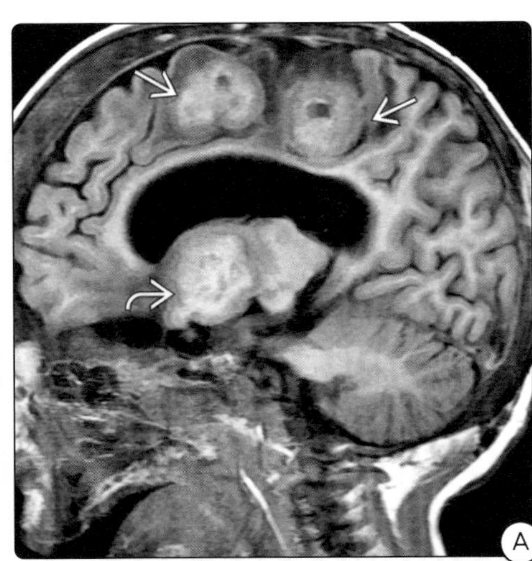


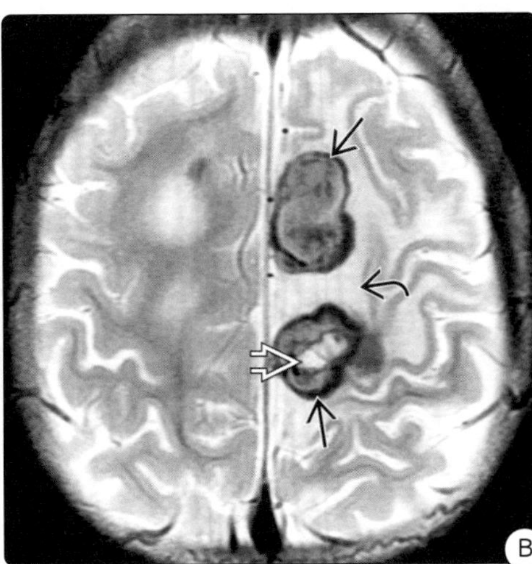


***(13-7A)** Sagittal T1 MR shows several caseating granulomas as mixed iso-, hypo-, and slightly hyperintense nodular masses in the cerebral hemisphere and basal ganglia. **(13-7B)** T2 MR shows that the masses are heterogeneously hypointense. One caseating granuloma has hyperintense central liquefaction. The masses are associated with edema in the hemispheric white matter (WM).*

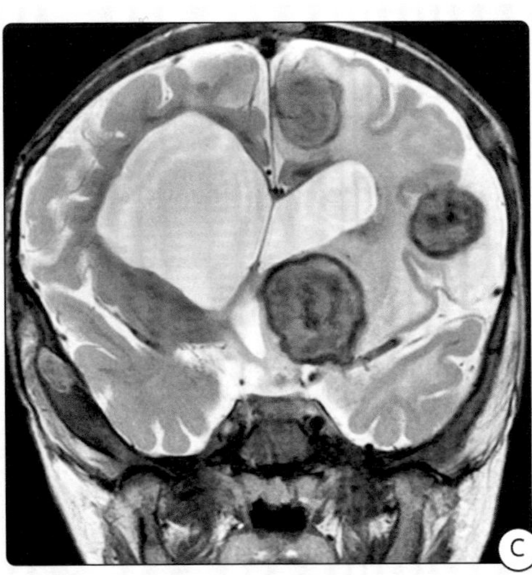


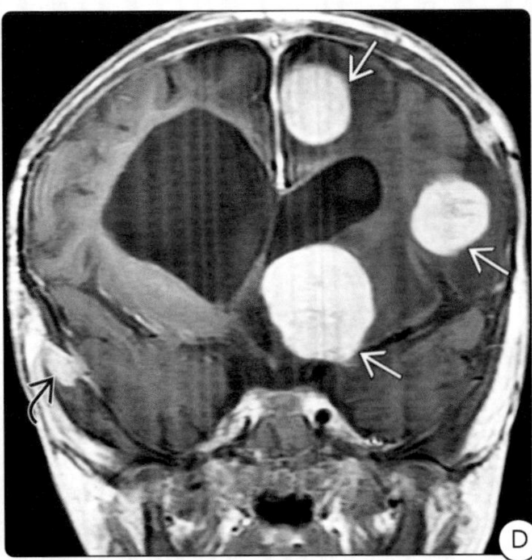


***(13-7C)** Coronal T2 MR shows that the caseating granulomas cause diffuse cerebral edema in the adjacent WM. **(13-7D)** The masses enhance strongly on T1 C+ MR. Note that a small dural-based tuberculoma is present along the right temporal lobe.*

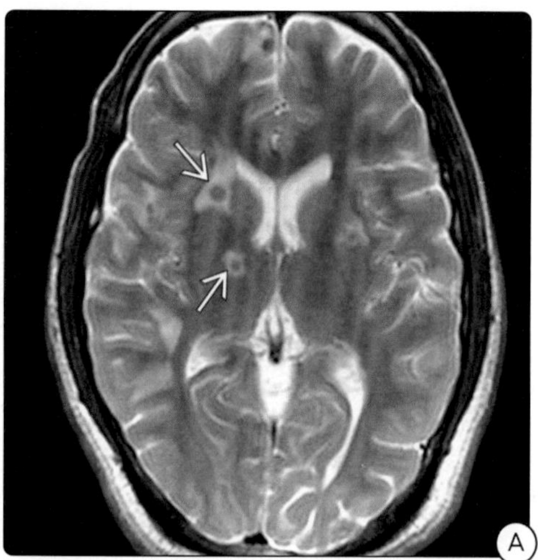


***(13-8A)** T2 MR demonstrates multifocal tuberculomas as hypointense foci surrounded by edema ➡.*

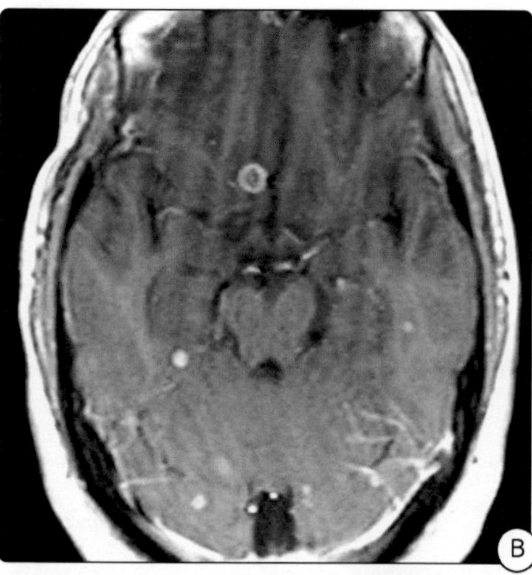


***(13-8B)** T1 C+ FS MR in the same patient shows multiple solid enhancing nodules in addition to a classic ring-enhancing lesion.*

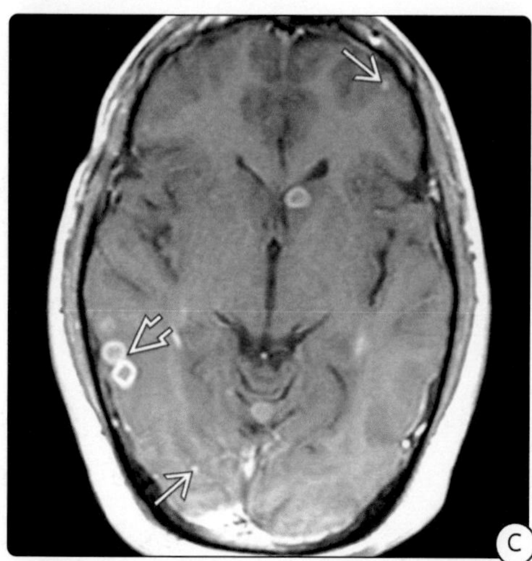


***(13-8C)** T1 C+ MR in the same patient illustrates additional lesions with punctate ➡ and ring enhancement ➡. (Courtesy R. Ramakantan, MD.)*

## CNS TUBERCULOSIS: IMAGING AND DIFFERENTIAL DIAGNOSIS

**General Features**

- Best procedure: Contrast-enhanced MR
- Findings vary with pathology
  - TB meningitis (TBM)
  - Tuberculoma
  - Abscess
- Combination of findings (usually TBM, tuberculoma)

**CT Findings**

- TBM
  - Can be normal in early stages
  - Nonspecific hydrocephalus common
  - "Blurred" ventricular margins
  - Effaced basilar cisterns, sulci
  - Iso-/mildly hyperdense exudates
  - Thick, intense pia-subarachnoid space enhancement
  - Can cause pachymeningopathy with diffuse dura-arachnoid enhancement
  - Look for secondary parenchymal infarcts
- Tuberculoma
  - Iso-/hyperdense parenchymal mass(es)
  - Round, lobulated > irregular margins
  - Variable edema
  - Punctate, solid, or ring enhancement
  - May cause focal enhancing dural mass
  - Chronic; healed may calcify
- Abscess
  - Hypodense mass
  - Perilesional edema usually marked
  - Ring enhancement

**MR Findings**

- TBM
  - Can be normal
  - "Dirty" CSF on T1WI
  - Hyperintense on FLAIR
  - Linear, nodular pia-subarachnoid space enhancement
  - May extend via perivascular spaces into brain
  - Vasculitis, secondary infarcts common
  - Penetrating arteries > large territorial infarcts
- Tuberculoma
  - Hypo-/isointense with brain on T1WI
  - Most are hypointense on T2WI
  - Rim enhancement
  - Rare: Dural-based enhancing mass
  - Large lipid peak on MRS
- Abscess
  - T2/FLAIR hyperintense
  - Striking perilesional edema
  - Rim, multiloculated enhancement

**Differential Diagnosis**

- TBM
  - Pyogenic, carcinomatous meningitis
  - Neurosarcoid
- Tuberculoma
  - Neurocysticercosis
  - Primary or metastatic neoplasm
  - Pyogenic abscess
  - Dural-based mass can mimic meningioma

## Nontuberculous Mycobacterial Infections

Nontuberculous mycobacteria (NTM) are ubiquitous organisms that are widely distributed in water and soil. Human disease is usually caused by environmental exposure, not human-to-human contact.

The most common manifestation of NTM in the head and neck is cervical lymphadenitis, typically occurring in children younger than five years old and immunocompromised patients. CNS involvement is rare. When it occurs, it is usually a manifestation of an immune reconstitution inflammatory syndrome (IRIS).

# Fungal Infections

Fungi are ubiquitous organisms with worldwide distribution. Most CNS fungal infections are opportunistic, acquired by inhaling fungal spores in contaminated dust and soil. Initial pulmonary infection is followed by hematogenous dissemination.

### Terminology

CNS fungal infections are also called cerebral mycosis. A focal "fungus ball" is also called a mycetoma or fungal granuloma.

### Etiology

**Fungal Pathogens.** The specific agents vary with immune status. Candidiasis, mucormycosis, and cryptococcal infections are usually opportunistic infections. They occur in patients with predisposing factors, such as diabetes, hematologic malignancies, and immunosuppression. Coccidioidomycosis and aspergillosis affect both immunocompetent (often older adults) and immunocompromised patients.

Aside from *Candida albicans* (a normal constituent of human gut flora), cryptococcal meningitis is the leading cause of CNS fungal infections in humans.

**Environmental Exposure.** Coccidioidomycosis occurs in areas with low rainfall and high summer temperatures (e.g., Mexico, southwestern United States, some parts of South America), whereas histoplasmosis and blastomycosis occur in watershed areas with moist air and damp, rotting wood (e.g., Africa, around major lakes and river valleys in North America).

**Systemic and CNS Infections.** Hematogenous spread from the lungs to the CNS is the most common route of infection, and cryptococcal meningitis is the most common fungal disease of the CNS.

Fungal sinonasal infections may invade the skull base and cavernous sinus directly. Sinonasal disease with intracranial extension (rhinocerebral disease) is the most common pattern of *Aspergillus* and *Mucor* CNS infection.

Disseminated fungal disease usually occurs only in immunocompromised patients.

### Pathology

CNS mycoses have four basic pathologic manifestations: Diffuse meningeal disease, solitary or multiple focal parenchymal lesions **(13-15)**, disseminated nonfocal parenchymal disease (rare), and focal dura-based masses (rarest).

The most common gross finding is basilar meningitis with congested meninges **(13-13)**. Parenchymal fungal infections can be either focal or disseminated. Fungal abscesses are encapsulated lesions with a soft tan or

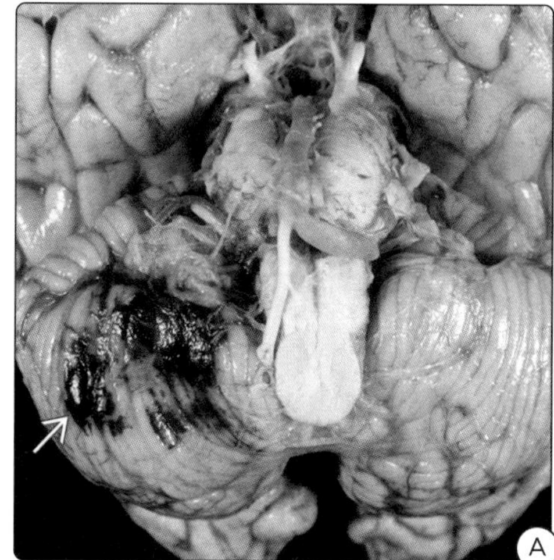


***(13-9A)** Autopsy case demonstrates multiple hemorrhagic infarcts ➡, typical of CNS fungal infections.*

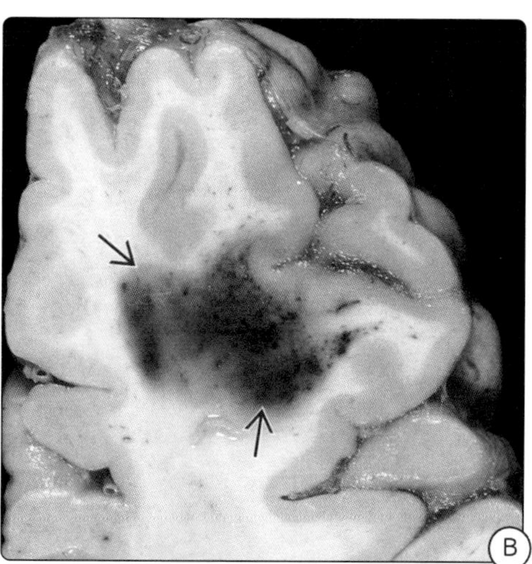


***(13-9B)** Axial section of cerebral hemisphere in the same patient shows a hemorrhagic subcortical infarct ➡. (Courtesy R. Hewlett, MD.)*

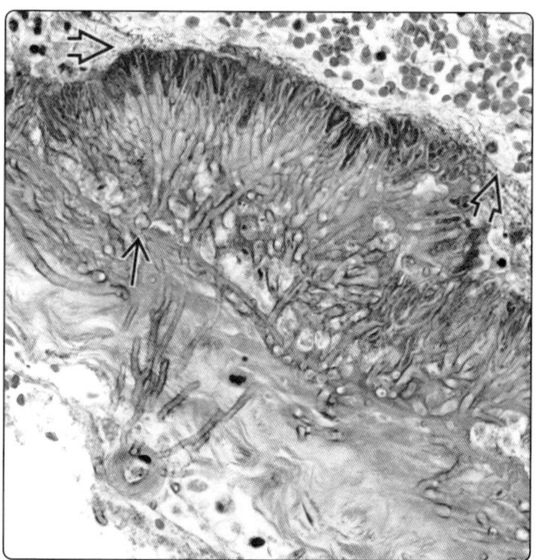

***(13-10)** Corona-like arrays of Aspergillus ➡ penetrate the wall of a leptomeningeal blood vessel ➡. (Courtesy B. K. DeMasters, MD.)*

thick mucoid-appearing center, an irregular reddish margin, and surrounding edema. Disseminated disease is less common and causes a fungal cerebritis with diffusely swollen brain.

Hemorrhagic infarcts **(13-9)**, typically in the basal ganglia or at the gray matter-white matter junction, are common with angioinvasive fungi **(13-10)**. On rare occasions, fungal infections can produce dura-based masses that closely resemble meningioma.

## Clinical Issues

**Epidemiology.** Once uncommon, CNS infections have been rising as the number of immunocompromised patients increases worldwide. Epidemiology varies with the specific fungus. Many infections are both common and asymptomatic (e.g., ~ 25% of the entire population in the USA and Canada are infected with *Histoplasma*).

Candidiasis is the most common nosocomial fungal infection worldwide. Aspergillosis accounts for 20-30% of fungal brain abscesses and is the most common cerebral complication following bone marrow transplantation. *Mucor* is ubiquitous but generally infects only immunocompromised patients.

**Demographics and Presentation.** Immunocompetent patients have a bimodal age distribution with fungal infections disproportionately represented in children and older individuals. There is a slight male predominance. Immunocompromised patients of all ages and both sexes are at risk.

Nonspecific symptoms, such as weight loss, fever, malaise, and fatigue, are common. Many patients initially have symptoms of pulmonary infection. CNS involvement is presaged by headache, meningismus, mental status changes, &/or seizure.

*(13-11) NECT shows multiple bioccipital parenchymal hemorrhages ➲. Angioinvasive aspergillosis was documented at surgery. (13-12A) CECT shows an irregular, crenulated enhancing lesion ➲ with edema and ventriculitis ➲.*

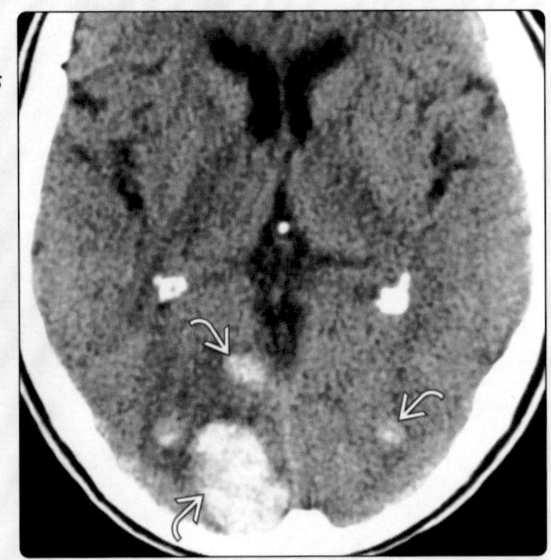

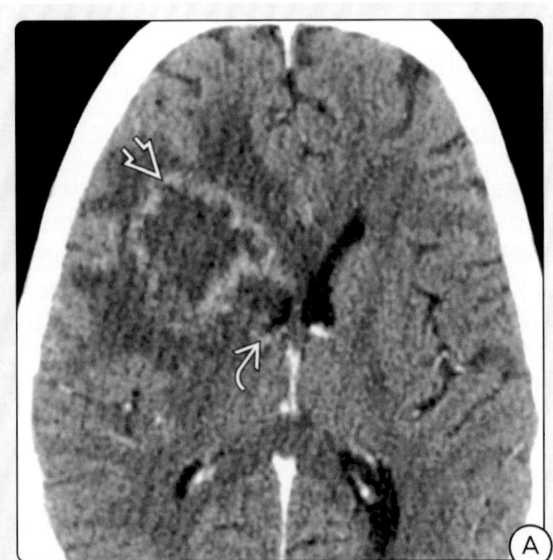


*(13-12B) (L) T2* GRE MR shows multiple punctate "blooming" hemorrhages ➲ within the basal ganglia lesion. (R) T2 MR shows the mass has mixed hyper- and patchy hypointense components ➲. (13-12C) T1 C+ FS MR shows irregular rim enhancement ➲ with ependymal enhancement in the adjacent lateral ventricle ➲. This is aspergilloma.*

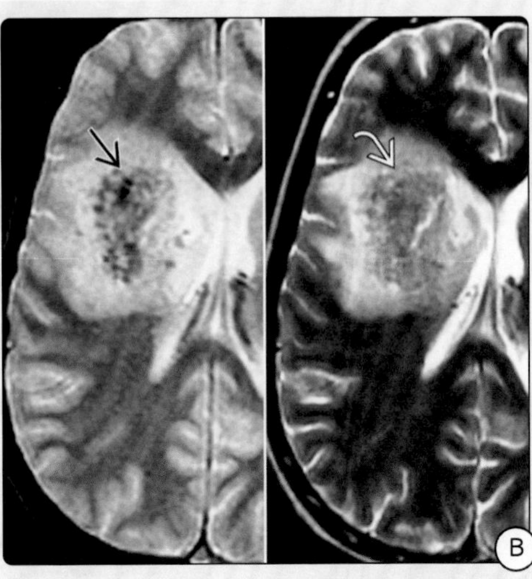


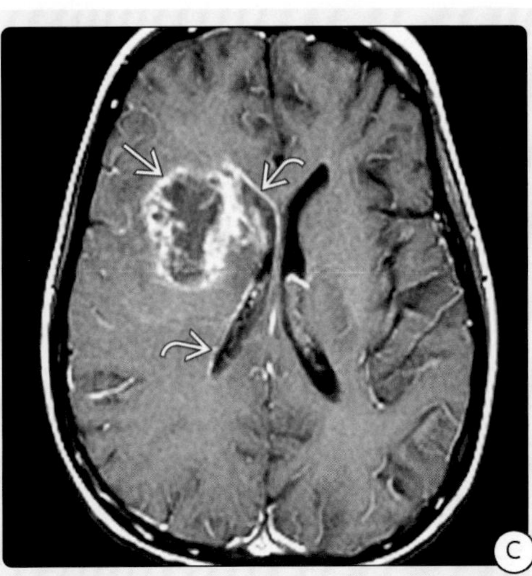

## Imaging

**General Features.** Findings vary with the patient's immune status. Well-formed fungal abscesses are seen in immunocompetent patients. Imaging early in the course of a rapidly progressive infection in an immunocompromised patient may show diffuse cerebral edema more characteristic of encephalitis than fungal abscess.

**CT Findings.** Findings on NECT include hypodense parenchymal lesions **(13-12A)** caused by focal granulomas or ischemia. Hydrocephalus is common in patients with fungal meningitis. Patients with coccidioidal meningitis may demonstrate thickened, mildly hyperdense basal meninges.

Disseminated parenchymal infection causes diffuse cerebral edema. Multifocal parenchymal hemorrhages are common in patients with angioinvasive fungal species **(13-11)**.

Diffuse meningeal disease demonstrates pia-subarachnoid space enhancement on CECT. Multiple punctate or ring-enhancing parenchymal lesions are typical findings of parenchymal mycetomas.

Mycetoma in the paranasal sinuses is usually seen as a single opacified hyperdense sinus that contains fine round to linear calcifications. Fungal sinusitis occasionally becomes invasive, crossing the mucosa to involve blood vessels, bone, orbit, cavernous sinuses, and intracranial cavities **(13-19A)**. Focal or widespread bone erosion with adjacent soft tissue infiltration can mimic neoplasm. Bone CT with reconstructions in all three standard planes is helpful to assess skull base involvement, and T1 C+ FS MR is the best modality to delineate disease spread beyond the nose and sinuses **(13-19)**.

**MR Findings.** Fungal meningitis appears as "dirty" CSF on T1WI. Parenchymal lesions are typically hypointense on T1WI but demonstrate T1 shortening if subacute hemorrhage is

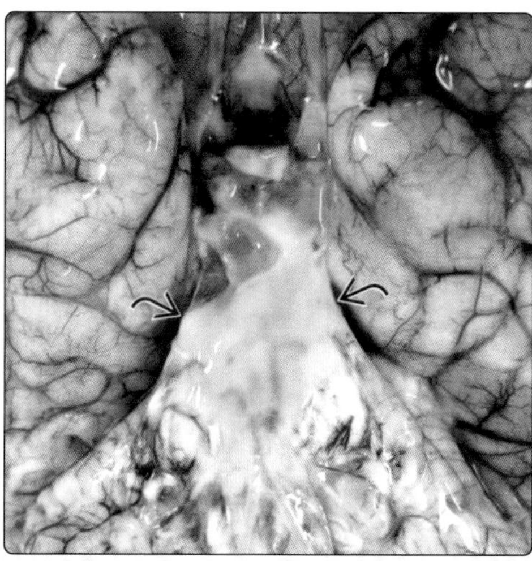

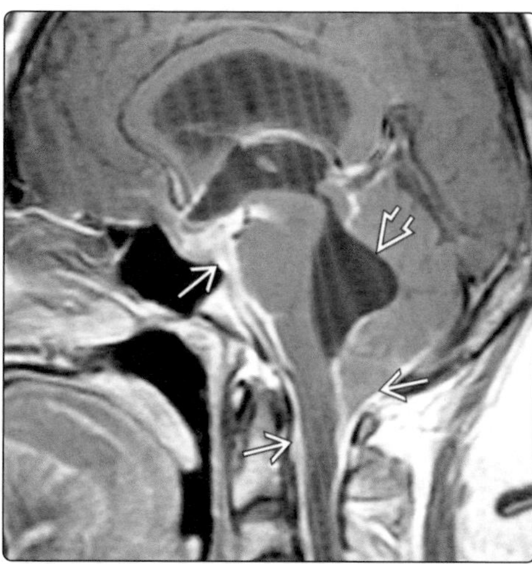

***(13-13)** Coccidioides immitis meningitis is seen in this autopsy case as a dense, exceptionally thick exudate in the basilar cisterns. (From DP: Neuro.) **(13-14)** Sagittal T1 C+ MR of cocci meningitis shows thick enhancing basilar exudate and obstructive hydrocephalus.*

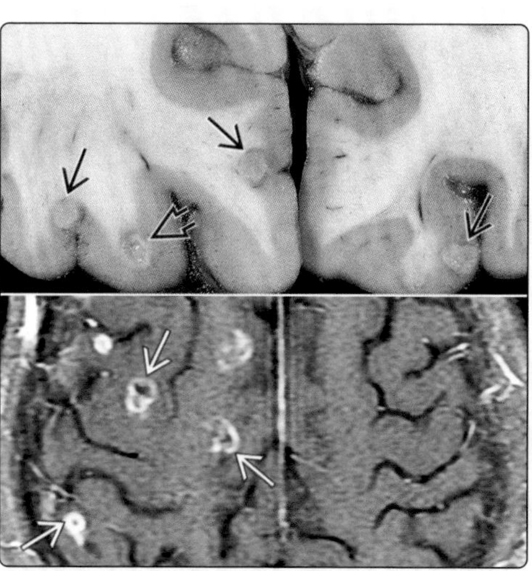

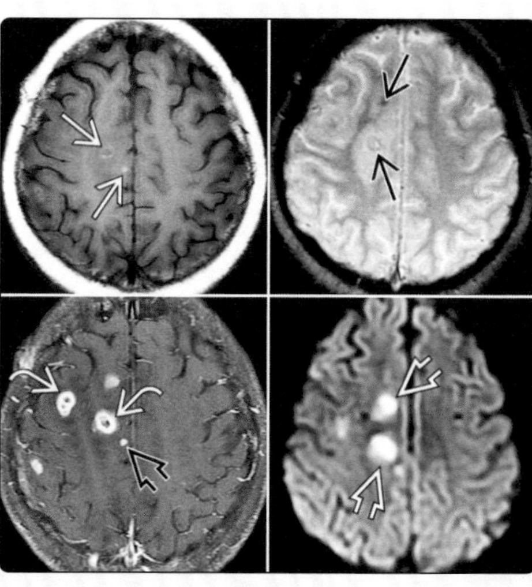

***(13-15)** (Top) Autopsy shows typical solid, necrotic Nocardia abscesses. (Bottom) Note multiple ring-enhancing fungal abscesses. **(13-16)** Aspergillus abscesses are seen in an immunosuppressed patient. T1 MR shows punctate and ring-like hyperintense foci with "blooming" on T2*. Punctate and ring enhancement is seen on T1 C+ FS MR. Lesions restrict on DWI MR.*

present. Irregular walls with nonenhancing projections into the cavity are typical.

T2/FLAIR scans in patients with fungal cerebritis show bilateral but asymmetric cortical/subcortical white matter and basal ganglia hyperintensity **(13-17A)**. Focal lesions (mycetomas) show high-signal foci that typically have a peripheral hypointense rim surrounded by vasogenic edema. T2* scans may show "blooming" foci caused by hemorrhages or calcification **(13-17C)**. Focal paranasal sinus and parenchymal mycetomas usually restrict on DWI.

T1 C+ FS scans usually show diffuse, thick, enhancing basilar leptomeninges **(13-14)** or dura-arachnoid thickening **(13-17D)**. Angioinvasive fungi may erode the skull base, cause plaque-like dural thickening, and occlude one or both carotid arteries **(13-18)** **(13-19)**. Parenchymal lesions show punctate, ring-like, or irregular enhancement **(13-15)** **(13-16)**.

MRS shows mildly elevated Cho and decreased NAA. A lactate peak is seen in 90% of cases, whereas lipid and amino acids are identified in ~ 50%. Multiple peaks resonating between 3.6-3.8 ppm are common and probably represent trehalose.

## Differential Diagnosis

The major differential is **pyogenic abscess(es)** and **tuberculoma**. **TB** can appear similar to fungal abscesses on standard imaging studies. Gross hemorrhage is more common with fungal than either pyogenic or tubercular abscesses. Fungal abscesses have more irregularly shaped walls and internal nonenhancing projections. Resonance between 3.6-3.8 ppm on MRS is typical.

Other mimics of fungal abscesses are primary **neoplasm** (e.g., glioblastoma with central necrosis) or metastases.

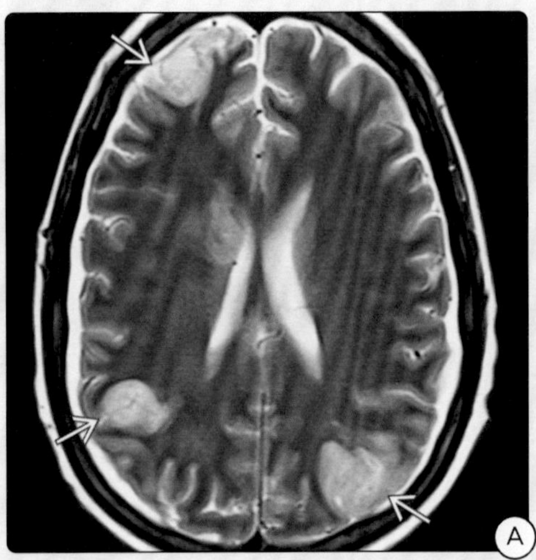


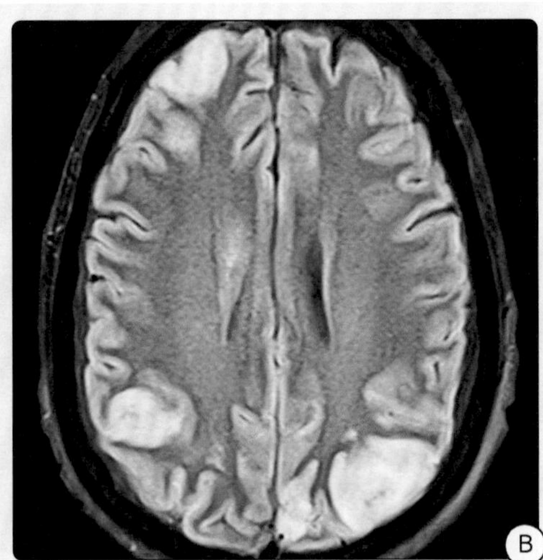


***(13-17A)*** *T2 MR in a 29-yo man with bone marrow transplant shows several cortical-subcortical hyperintense masses* ➡. ***(13-17B)*** *FLAIR MR shows that the lesions are isolated to the cortex and subcortical WM.*

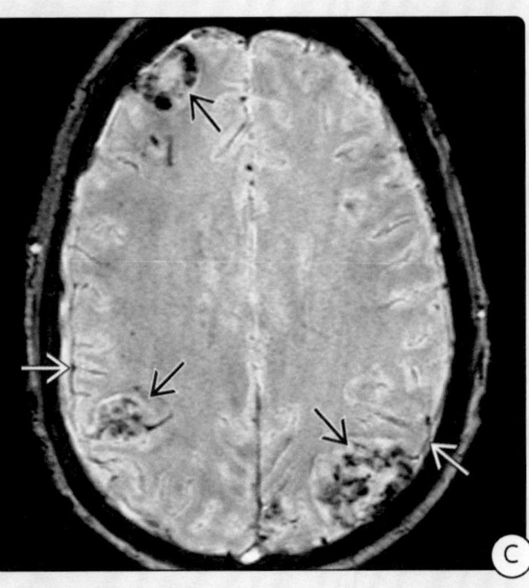


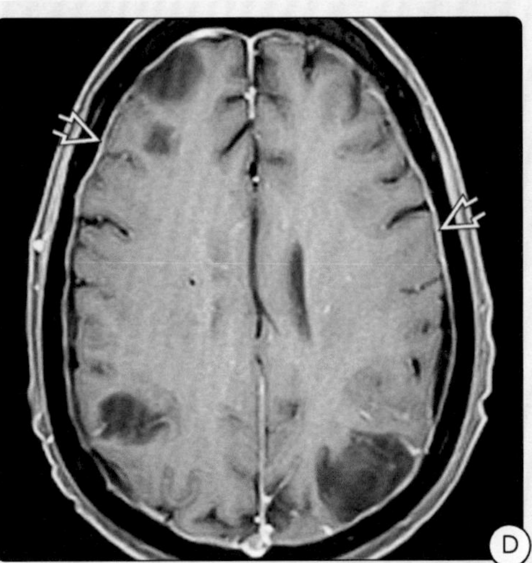


***(13-17C)*** *T2* SWI MR shows "blooming" foci ➡ within the lesions, suggesting hemorrhage. Note subtle hypointensity along the pia* ➡*, extending into the adjacent sulci, suggesting hemorrhagic meningoencephalitis.* ***(13-17D)*** *T1 C+ FS MR shows dura-arachnoid thickening and enhancement* ➡*. This is angioinvasive Aspergillus mycetomas with pachy- and leptomeningitis.*

# Parasitic Infections

Once considered endemic only in countries with poor sanitation and adverse economic conditions, parasitic diseases have become a global health concern, exacerbated by widespread travel and immigration. We begin our discussion of CNS parasitic infections with the most worldwide parasitic infection, cysticercosis. Brain involvement by parasites other than neurocysticercosis (NCC) is relatively uncommon.

## Neurocysticercosis

Cysticercosis is the most common parasitic infection in the world, and CNS lesions eventually develop in 60-90% of patients with cysticercosis.

### Terminology

When cysticercosis infects the CNS, it is termed NCC. A "cysticercus" cyst in the brain is actually the secondary larval form of the parasite. The "scolex" is the head-like part of a tapeworm, bearing hooks and suckers. In the larval form, the scolex is invaginated into one end of the cyst, which is called the "bladder."

### Etiology

Most NCC cases are caused by encysted larvae of the pork tapeworm *Taenia solium* and are acquired through fecal-oral contamination. Humans become infected by ingesting *T. solium* eggs. The eggs hatch and release their larvae that then disseminate via the bloodstream to virtually any organ in the body.

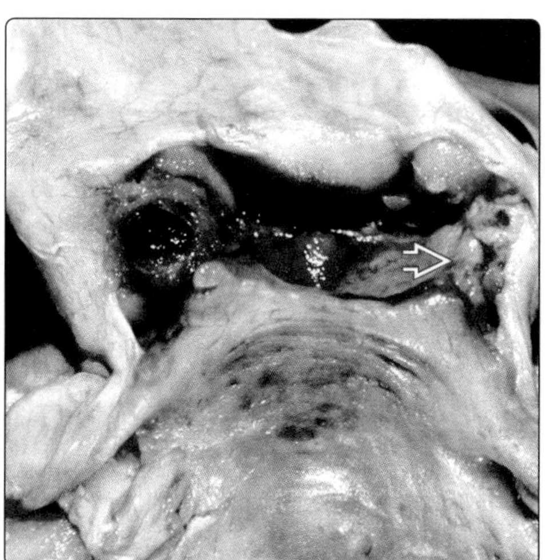

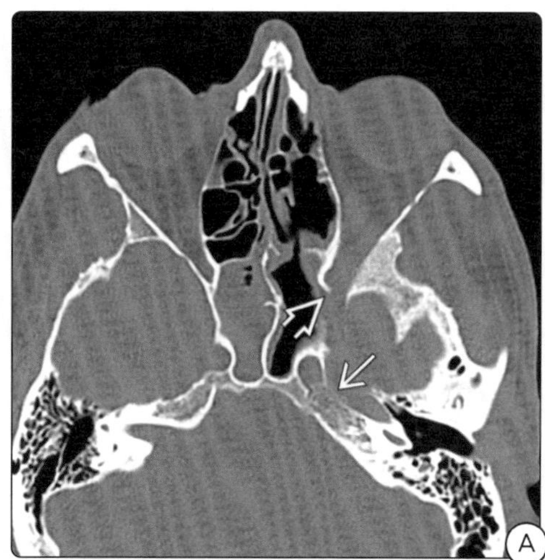

***(13-18)** Close-up view shows autopsied cavernous sinus with invasive fungal sinusitis occluding the left cavernous ICA ➔. (Courtesy R. Hewlett, MD.) **(13-19A)** Bone CT in a patient with poorly controlled diabetes and invasive mucormycosis shows bone invasion, destruction around the orbital fissure and sphenoid sinus ➔, and left petrous apex ➔.*

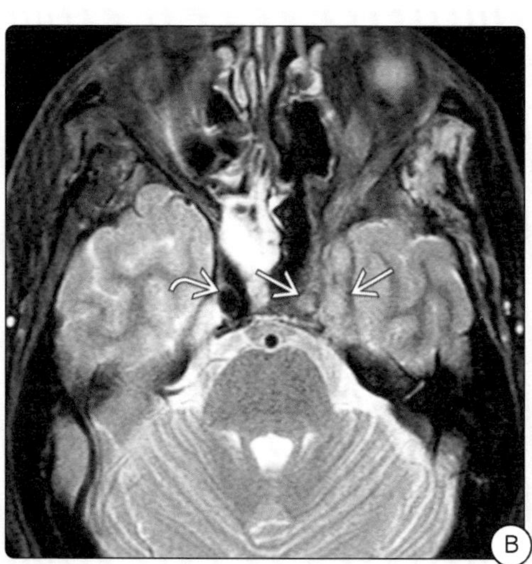

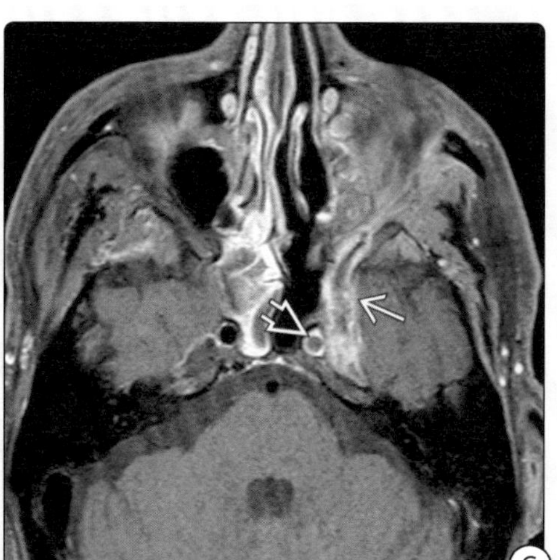

***(13-19B)** Axial T2 FS MR shows normal right cavernous ICA "flow void" ➔ with left cavernous sinus mass and occluded ICA ➔. **(13-19C)** T1 C+ FS MR in the same patient shows the left cavernous sinus invasion ➔ and occluded carotid artery ➔.*

## Pathology

**Location.** *T. solium* larvae are most common in the CNS, eyes, muscles, and subcutaneous tissue. The intracranial subarachnoid spaces are the most common CNS site followed by the brain parenchyma and ventricles (fourth > third > lateral ventricles) **(13-20)**. NCC cysts in the depths of sulci may incite an intense inflammatory response, effectively "sealing" the sulcus over the cysts and making them appear intraaxial.

**Size and Number.** Most parenchymal NCC cysts are small (a few millimeters to 1 cm). Occasionally, multiple large NCC cysts up to several centimeters can form in the subarachnoid space (the "racemose" form of NCC that resembles a bunch of grapes). Either solitary (20-50% of cases) or multiple small cysts may occur.

**Gross Pathology.** Four stages of NCC development and regression are recognized. Patients may have multiple lesions at different stages of evolution.

In the **vesicular stage**, viable larvae (the cysticerci) appear as translucent, thin-walled, fluid-filled cysts with an eccentrically located, whitish, invaginated scolex **(13-21) (13-22)**.

In the **colloidal vesicular stage**, the larvae begin to degenerate. The cyst fluid becomes thick and turbid. A striking inflammatory response is incited and characterized by a collection of multinucleated giant cells, macrophages, and neutrophils. A fibrous capsule develops, and perilesional edema becomes prominent.

The **granular nodular stage** represents progressive involution with collapse and retraction of the cyst into a granulomatous nodule that will eventually calcify. Edema persists, but pericystic gliosis is the most common pathologic finding at this stage.

In the **nodular calcified stage**, the entire lesion becomes a fibrocalcified nodule **(13-23)**. No host immune response is present.

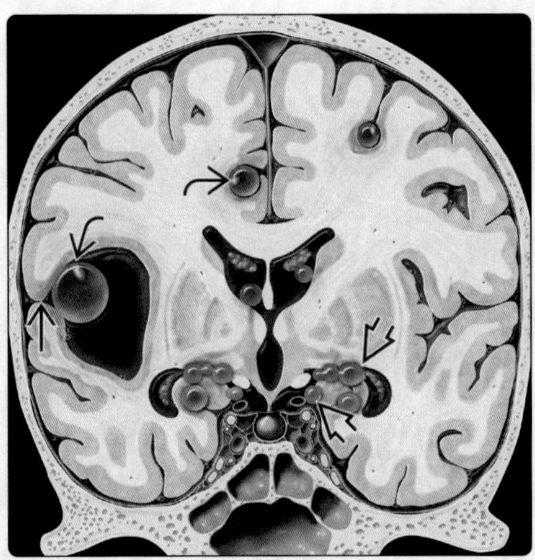

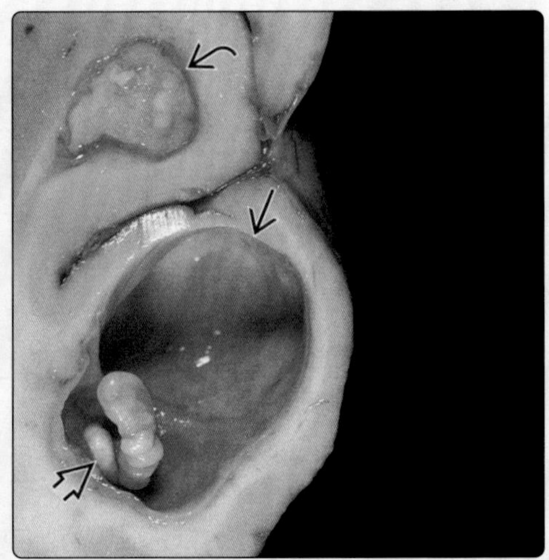

***(13-20)** In this neurocysticercosis (NCC), convexity cysts have scolex and surrounding inflammation, which, around the largest cyst, "seals" sulcus, making it appear parenchymal. "Racemose" cysts without scolices are seen in the basal cisterns. **(13-21)** NCC in the vesicular stage has clear fluid-filled cyst and white, eccentrically positioned scolex. Note 2nd granular nodular lesion. (Courtesy R. Hewlett, MD.)*

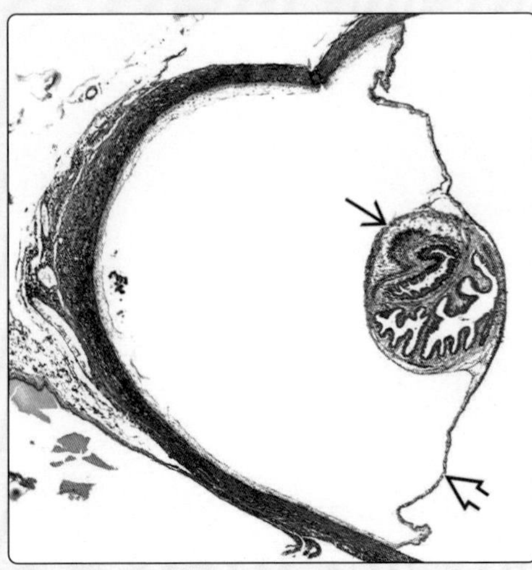

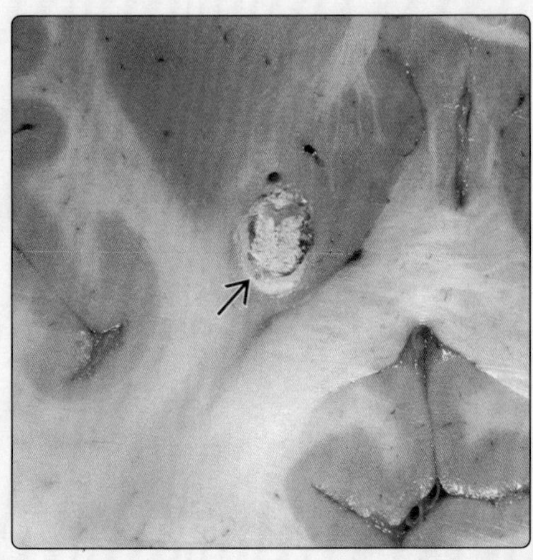

***(13-22)** Low-power photomicrograph of cysticercus shows the invaginated scolex lying within the thin-walled cyst a.k.a. the bladder. (Courtesy B. K. Kleinschmidt-DeMasters, MD.) **(13-23)** Close-up view shows a nodular, calcified NCC cyst. Note the lack of inflammation and lack of mass effect. (Courtesy R. Hewlett, MD.)*

## NEUROCYSTICERCOSIS: GROSS PATHOLOGY

**Location, Size, Number**

- Subarachnoid > parenchyma > ventricles
- Usually < 1 cm
  - Subarachnoid ("racemose") cysts can be giant
- Multiple > solitary
  - Can have multiple innumerable tiny ("miliary") cysts

**Development Stages**

- Vesicular (quiescent, viable larva): Cyst + scolex
- Colloidal vesicular (dying larva)
  - Intense inflammation, edema
- Granular nodular (healing): Cyst involutes, edema ↓
- Nodular calcified (healed)
  - Quiescent, fibrocalcified nodule
  - No edema

## Clinical Issues

**Epidemiology.** In countries where cysticercosis is endemic, calcified NCC granulomas are found in 10-20% of the entire population. Of these, ~ 5% (400,000 out of 75 million) will become symptomatic.

**Demographics.** NCC occurs at all ages, but peak symptomatic presentation is between 15-40 years. There is no sex or race predilection.

**Presentation.** NCC has a range of clinical manifestations. Signs and symptoms depend on the number and location of larvae, developmental stage, infection duration, and presence or absence of host immune response.

Seizures/epilepsy are the most common symptoms (80%) and are a result of inflammation around degeneration cysts. Headache (35-40%) and focal neurologic deficit (15%) are also

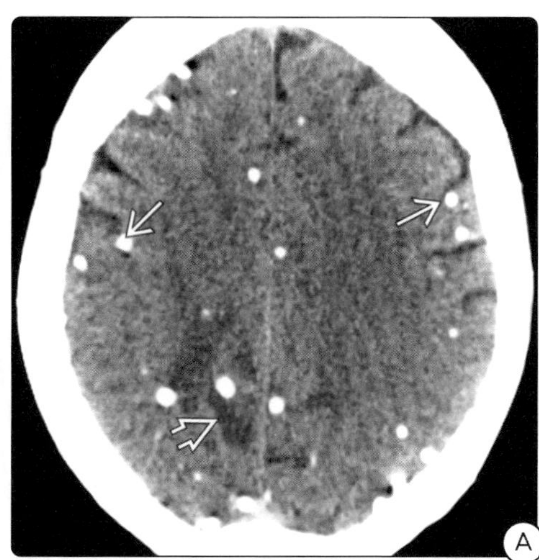


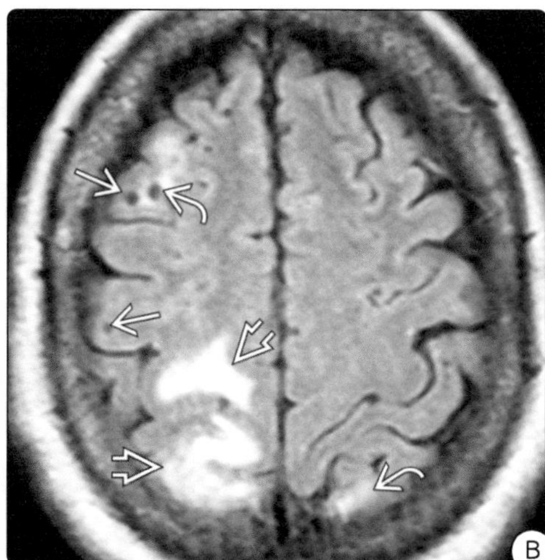


*(13-24A) NECT in a patient with NCC shows multiple nodular calcified lesions ➡. A few demonstrate adjacent edema ➡. (13-24B) FLAIR MR shows a few hypointense foci ➡ caused by quiescent NCC in the nodular calcified stage. Several foci of perilesional edema are apparent around lesions in the colloidal vesicular stage ➡, whereas minimal residual edema surrounds lesions in the granular nodular stage ➡.*

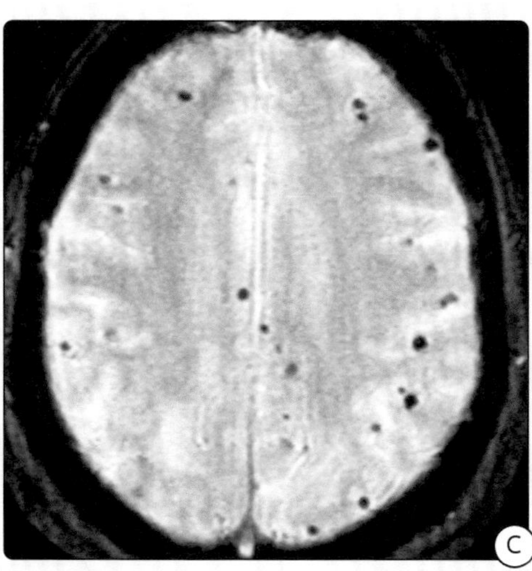


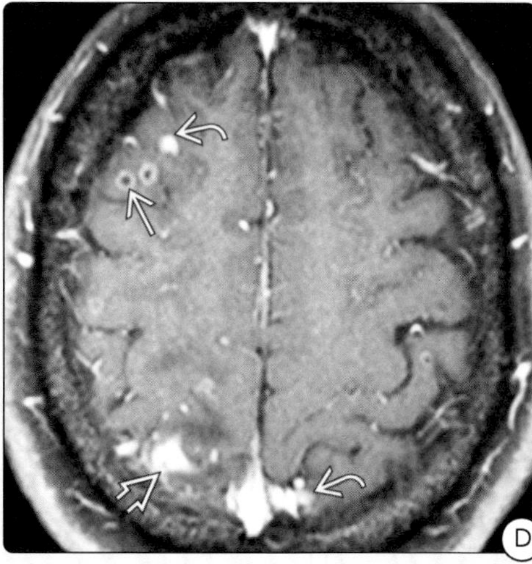


*(13-24C) T2* GRE MR shows multiple "blooming" black dots, characteristic of nodular calcified NCC. (13-24D) T1 C+ FS MR shows faint ring-like ➡ and nodular ➡ enhancement of healing granular nodular NCC cysts. "Shaggy" enhancement with adjacent edema ➡ is characteristic of degenerating larvae in the colloidal vesicular stage. Multiple lesions in different stages of evolution are characteristic of NCC.*

common. Between 10-12% of patients exhibit signs of elevated intracranial pressure.

NCC—particularly the subarachnoid forms—can also cause cerebral vascular diseases. These include cerebral infarction, transient ischemic attacks, and cerebral hemorrhage.

**Natural History.** During the early stages of the disease, patients are frequently asymptomatic. Many patients remain asymptomatic for years. The average time from initial infestation until symptoms develop is 2-5 years. The time to progress through all four stages varies from 1-9 years with a mean of five years.

**Treatment Options.** Oral albendazole with or without steroids, excision/drainage of parenchymal lesions, and endoscopic resection of intraventricular lesions are treatment options.

## Imaging

**General Features.** Imaging findings depend on several factors: (1) Life cycle stage of *T. solium* at presentation, (2) host inflammatory response, (3) number and location of parasites, and (4) associated complications, such as hydrocephalus and vascular disease.

***Vesicular (Quiescent) Stage.*** NECT shows a smooth thin-walled cyst that is isodense to CSF. There is no surrounding edema and no enhancement on CECT.

MR shows that the cyst is isointense with CSF on T1 and T2/FLAIR. The scolex is discrete, nodular, and hyperintense (target or dot in a hole appearance) and may restrict on DWI. Enhancement is typically absent. Disseminated or "miliary" NCC has a striking salt and pepper brain appearance **(13-25)** **(13-26)** with notable lack of perilesional edema.

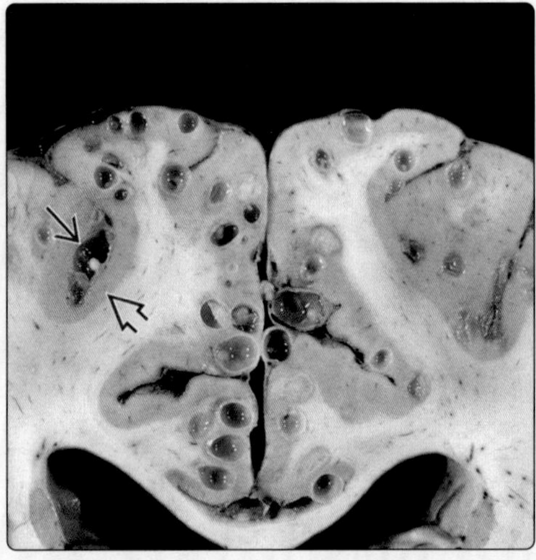

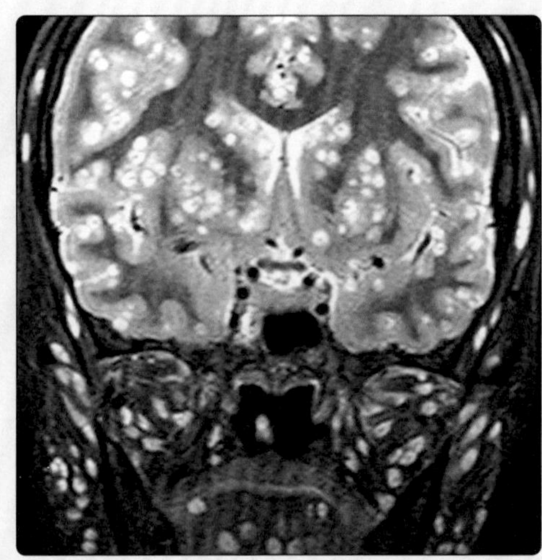

***(13-25)** Disseminated NCC with many cysts, mostly in the subarachnoid space, shows a cyst with scolex in the depth of frontal sulcus ⇒ surrounded by cortex ⇒, making a subarachnoid cyst appear intraparenchymal. **(13-26)** T2 MR shows disseminated vesicular NCC with salt and pepper appearance. Hyperintense cysticerci with scolices (small black dots inside cysts) are present; perilesional edema is absent. Note innumerable cysts in scalp, face muscles.*

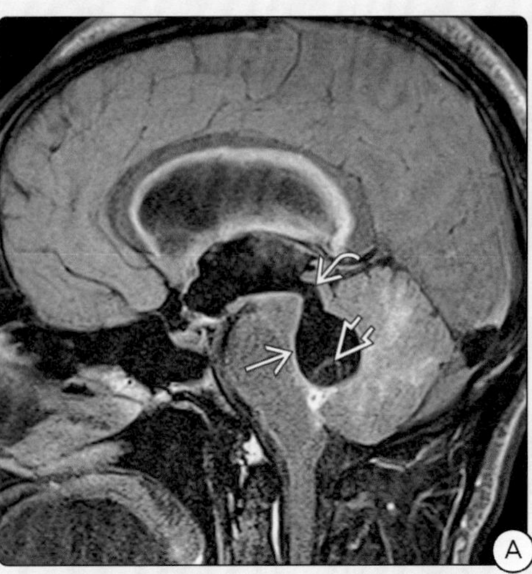


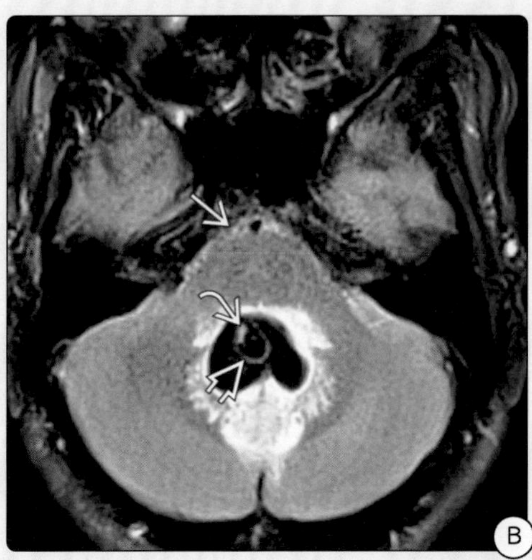


***(13-27A)** Sagittal FLAIR MR in a 26-yo woman with headaches shows obstructive hydrocephalus with enlargement of lateral, 3rd, and 4th ventricles ⇒ as well as aqueduct ⇒. A solitary NCC cyst ⇒ is visible in the bottom of the 4th ventricle. **(13-27B)** Axial FLAIR MR shows cyst wall ⇒, scolex ⇒, and interstitial fluid around the obstructed 4th ventricle. FLAIR hyperintensity ⇒ in the basal cisterns indicates meningitis.*

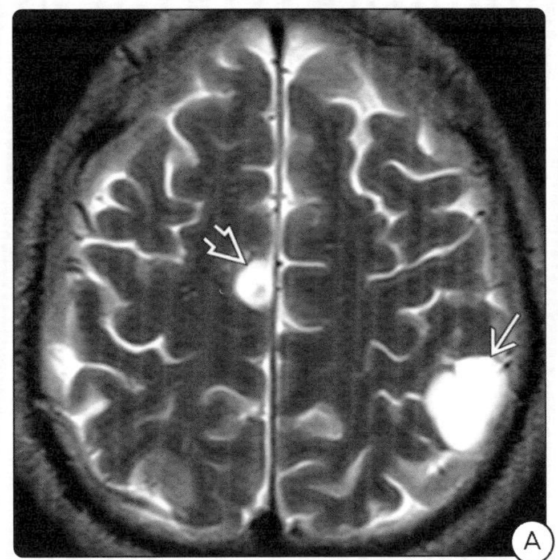

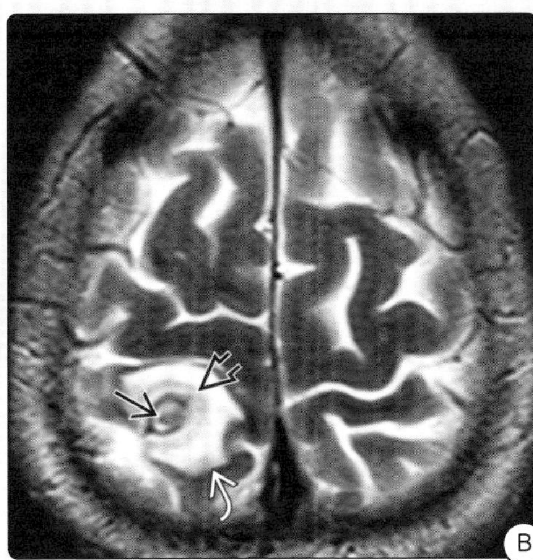

***(13-28A)*** *Series of images in a 41-yo Hispanic man with seizures shows NCC cysts in different stages. Axial T2 MR demonstrates the vesicular stage (cyst + scolex, no edema) ➡ and a cyst in the granular nodular stage ➡.* ***(13-28B)*** *More cephalad scan shows an intrasulcal NCC cyst in the colloidal vesicular stage with a nodule (scolex) ➡ and thick, mixed hypo- and hyperintense intense cyst wall ➡. The surrounding edema ➡ is striking.*

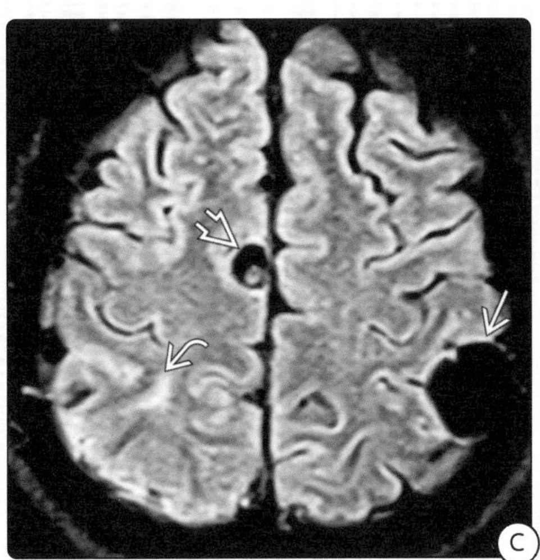

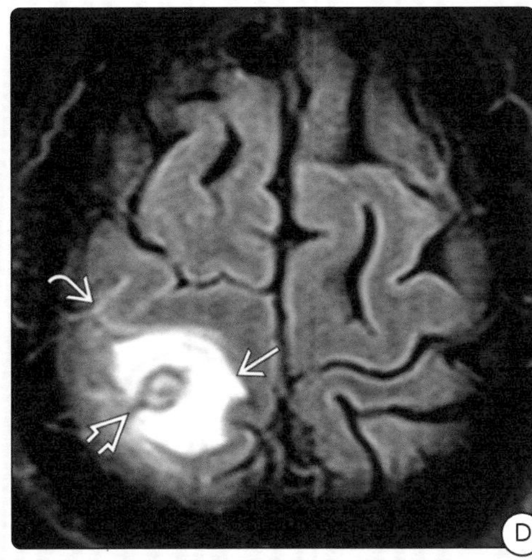

***(13-28C)*** *Axial FLAIR MR shows the vesicular NCC cyst with its scolex ➡. The granular nodular cyst ➡ has minimal residual edema. Group of FLAIR-hyperintense sulci ➡ represents leptomeningeal inflammation from the colloidal vesicular cyst above.* ***(13-28D)*** *More cephalad FLAIR MR shows that the colloidal vesicular cyst + nodule ➡ has striking edema ➡ and adjacent hyperintense sulci ➡.*

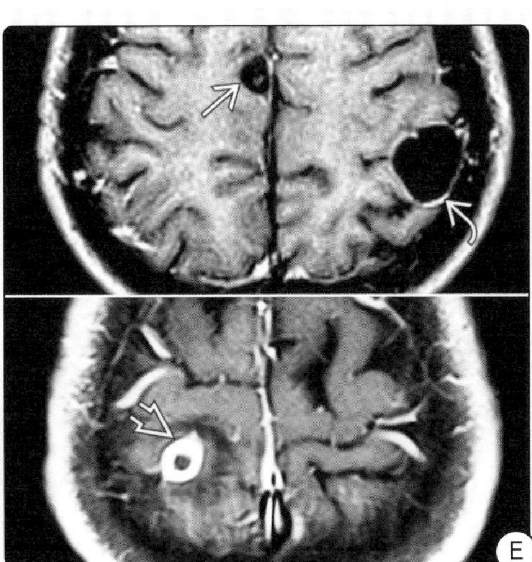

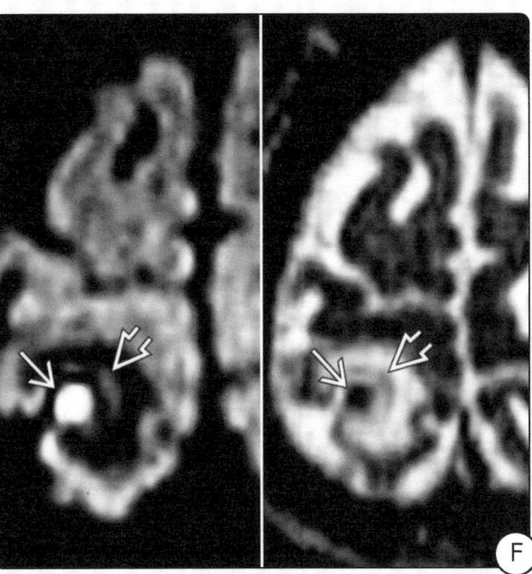

***(13-28E)*** *(Top) Axial T1 C+ FS MR shows no enhancement of vesicular NCC cyst ➡ and faint rim enhancement of granular nodular cyst wall ➡. (Bottom) More cephalad scan shows the granular nodular cyst has thick, intense rim enhancement ➡.* ***(13-28F)*** *Axial DWI MR (L) and ADC map (R) through the colloidal vesicular cyst show that the central viscous cavity of the cyst restricts strongly ➡. Mild restriction in the enhancing capsule ➡ is present.*

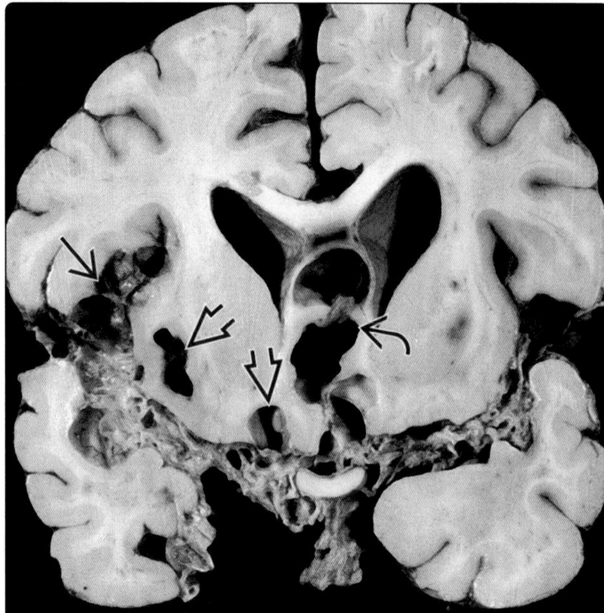

*(13-29) Coronal autopsied case of NCC shows extensive "racemose" cysts throughout the sylvian fissures ➡ and basilar cisterns. Note cysts in perivascular spaces ⇨ and 3rd ventricle ↷.*

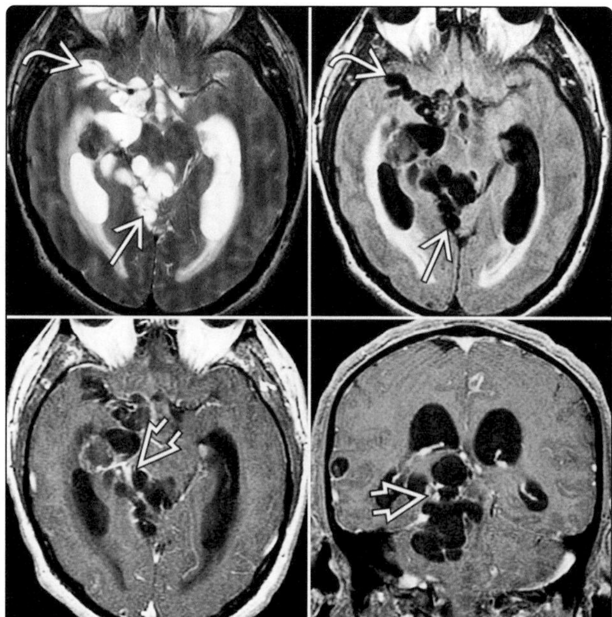

*(13-30) "Racemose" NCC shows numerous variable-sized cysts filling the ambient cistern ➡ and sylvian fissure ↷. Note the hydrocephalus, meningeal reaction with mild/moderate rim enhancement around the "bunch of grapes" cysts ⇨.*

***Colloidal Vesicular Stage (Dying Scolex).*** Cyst fluid is hyperdense relative to CSF on NECT and demonstrates a ring-enhancing capsule on CECT. Moderate to marked edema surrounds the degenerating dying larvae.

MR shows that the cyst fluid is mildly hyperintense to CSF on T1WI and that the scolex appears hyperintense on FLAIR **(13-27)**. Moderate to marked surrounding edema is present **(13-24B)** and may even progress to a diffuse encephalitis.

Enhancement of the cyst wall is typically intense, ring-like, and often slightly "shaggy" **(13-24D)** **(13-28E)**. Restricted diffusion in the scolex and viscous degenerating cyst can be present **(13-28)**.

***Granular Nodular (Healing) Stage.*** NECT shows mild residual edema. CECT demonstrates a progressively involuting, mildly to moderately enhancing nodule.

The cyst wall appears thickened and retracted, and the perilesional edema diminishes substantially, eventually disappearing. Nodular or faint ring-like enhancement is typical at this stage **(13-24D)**.

***Nodular Calcified (Inactive) Stage.*** A small calcified nodule without surrounding edema or enhancement is seen on CT **(13-24A)**. Shrunken, calcified lesions are seen as hypointensities on T1WI and T2WI. Perilesional edema is absent.

"Blooming" on T2* GRE is seen and may show multifocal "Blooming" black dots if multiple calcified nodules are present **(13-24C)**. Quiescent lesions do not enhance on T1 C+.

**Special Features. "Racemose" NCC** shows multilobulated, variably sized, grape-like lesions in the basal cisterns **(13-29)**. Most cysts lack an identifiable scolex. Arachnoiditis with fibrosis and scarring demonstrates rim enhancement around the cysts and along the brain surfaces. Obstructive hydrocephalus is common **(13-30)**.

**NCC-associated vasculitis** with stroke is a rare but important complication of "racemose" NCC that can mimic TB. Most infarcts involve small perforating vessels, although large territorial infarcts have been reported.

**Intraventricular NCC** is associated with poor prognosis. Intraventricular cysts may be difficult to detect on CT. FLAIR and CISS are the most sensitive sequences for detecting the cysts on MR. The fourth ventricle is the most common site (50-55%) **(13-27)** followed by the third ventricle (25-30%), lateral ventricle (10-12%), and aqueduct (8-10%).

## Differential Diagnosis

The differential diagnosis of NCC depends on lesion type and location. Subarachnoid/cisternal NCC can resemble **TB meningitis**. In contrast to NCC, the thick purulent basilar exudates typical of TB are solid and lack the cystic features of "racemose" NCC. **Carcinomatous meningitis** and **neurosarcoid** are also rarely cystic.

**Abscess** and **multifocal septic emboli** can resemble parenchymal NCC cysts but demonstrate a hypointense rim on T2WI and restrict strongly on DWI. A succinate peak on MRS helps distinguish a degenerating NCC cyst from abscess.

A giant parenchymal colloidal-vesicular NCC cyst with ring enhancement can mimic **neoplasm, tuberculoma**, or **toxoplasmosis**. Differential diagnosis of intraventricular cyst includes **colloid cyst** (solid), **ependymal cyst** (cystic but lacks a scolex), and **choroid plexus cyst.**

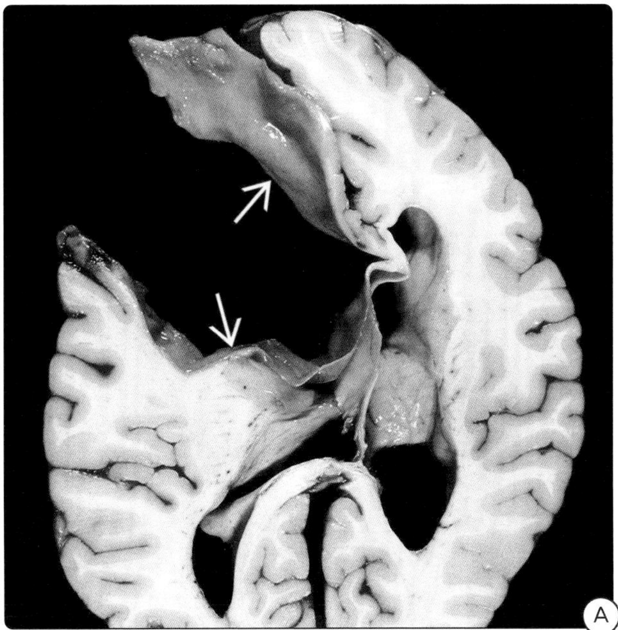

***(13-31A) Autopsy case shows brain after removal of a huge unilocular hydatid cyst. Note well-demarcated border ➡ between the cyst cavity and brain. There is no surrounding edema. Mass effect relative to the size of the cyst is minimal.***

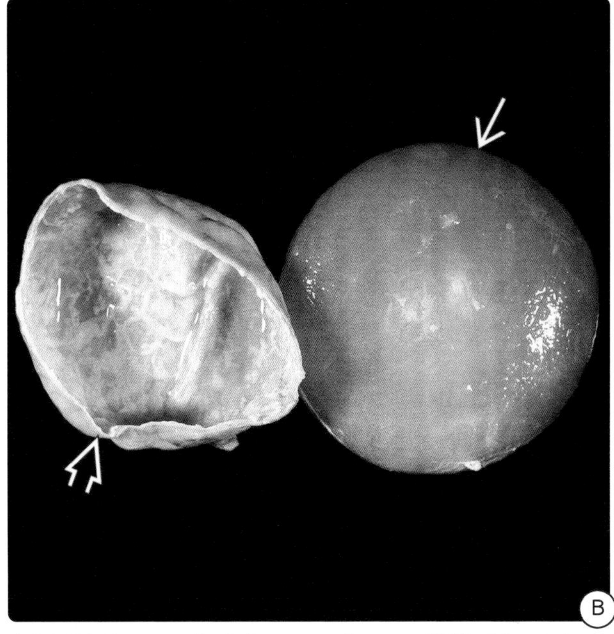

***(13-31B) Photograph of the external cyst wall ➡ with cut view of the cyst ➡ shows the typical thin wall of a classic hydatid cyst. (Courtesy R. Hewlett, MD.)***

NEUROCYSTICERCOSIS: IMAGING AND DIFFERENTIAL DIAGNOSIS

**Imaging**

- Varies with stage (may have lesions in different stages)
  - Vesicular: Cyst with "dot" (scolex), no edema, no enhancement
  - Colloidal vesicular: Ring enhancement, edema striking
  - Granular nodular: Faint rim enhancement, edema decreased
  - Nodular calcified: CT $Ca^{++}$, MR "black dots"

**Differential Diagnosis**

- Parenchymal (colloidal vesicular) cyst: Neoplasm, toxoplasmosis, TB
- "Racemose" (subarachnoid) NCC: Pyogenic/TB meningitis
- Intraventricular cyst: Ependymal, choroid plexus cysts

# Echinococcosis

## Terminology and Etiology

Two species of *Echinococcus* tapeworms, *Echinococcus granulosis* (EG) and *Echinococcus multilocularis/alveolaris* (EM/EA), are responsible for most human CNS infections. EG infection is also called **hydatid disease** or hydatid cyst (HC). Infection with EM/EA is also known as **alveolar echinococcosis**.

## Epidemiology

After NCC, echinococcosis is the second most common parasitic infection that involves the CNS. Humans become accidental intermediate hosts by ingesting eggs in soil contaminated by excrement from a definitive host. Approximately 1-2% of patients with EG and 3-5% of patients with EM/EA develop CNS disease.

EG usually affects children, whereas EM/EA is more common in adults.

## Pathology

EG and EM/EA differ in gross appearance. EG typically produces a well-delineated cyst **(13-31)**. EM/EA has numerous irregular small cysts and appears as an infiltrative, invasive, tumor-like lesion in both the liver and brain.

HCs can be uni- or multilocular with "daughter" cysts. The wall of an HC has three layers: An outer dense fibrous pericyst, a middle laminated membranous ectocyst, and an inner germinal layer (the endocyst). It is the germinal layer that can produce "daughter" cysts.

## Imaging

The most common imaging appearance of HC is that of a large, unilocular thin-walled cyst without calcification, edema, or enhancement on CT and MR **(13-32)**. Occasionally, a single large cyst will contain multiple "daughter" cysts **(13-34)**.

Cyst fluid is generally isointense with CSF on both T1- and T2WIs. Sometimes, a detached germinal membrane and hydatid "sand" can be seen in the dependent portion of the cyst **(13-33)**.

EA consists of numerous irregular cysts that are not sharply demarcated and exhibit irregular peripheral, ring-like, nodular, or even cauliflower-like enhancement **(13-35)**.

## Amebiasis

### Terminology and Etiology

Amebae are species of free-living organisms that are distributed worldwide. *Acanthamoeba* can be found in soil and dust, fresh or brackish water, and a variety of other locations, from hot tubs and hydrotherapy pools to contact lens solutions and dental irrigation units. *Balamuthia mandrillaris* is a soil-dwelling organism. *Naegleria fowleri* is found in both soil and fresh water. *Entamoeba histolytica* occurs in food or water that has become contaminated with feces.

### Pathology

Primary amebic meningoencephalitis (PAM) causes a necrotizing, hemorrhagic meningitis and angiitis **(13-36)**. Granulomatous amebic encephalitis (GAE) demonstrates granulomatous inflammation. Amebic abscesses do occur but are rare.

### Clinical Issues

PAM is an acute, rapidly progressive necrotizing hemorrhagic meningoencephalitis caused by *N. fowleri* and is most often contracted by swimming in fresh but contaminated water, usually in summer. GAE shows no seasonal predilection and is caused by *Acanthamoeba* or *B. mandrillaris*.

### Imaging

A broad spectrum of imaging findings in amebic meningoencephalitis has been described, including meningeal

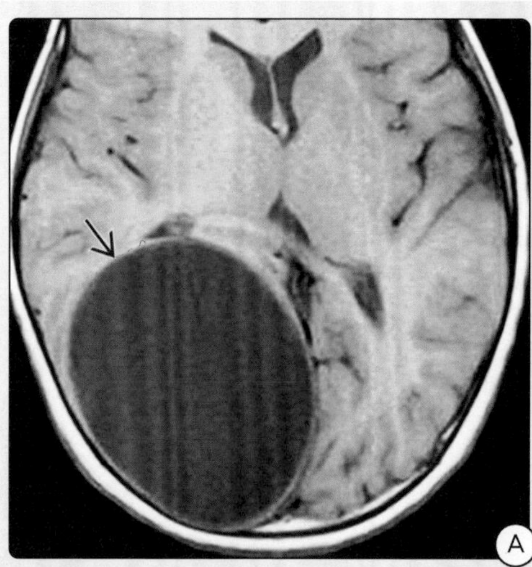


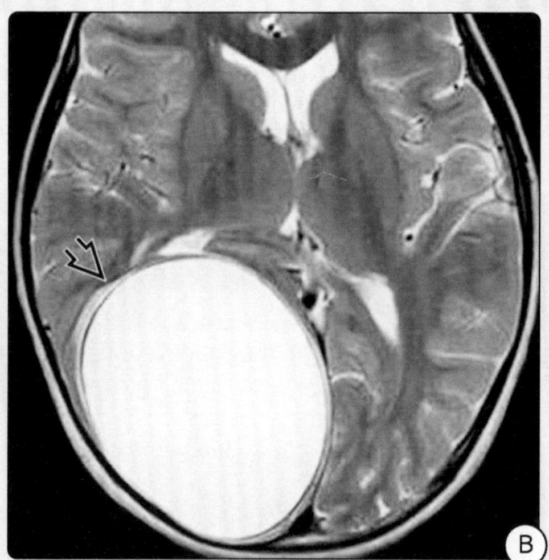


***(13-32A)** Axial T1 MR shows a unilocular hydatid cyst ➡. Note that the mass effect relative to overall cyst size is only moderate. **(13-32B)** T2 MR in the same patient nicely demonstrates the typical 3-layered cyst wall ➡. (Courtesy R. Hewlett, MD.)*

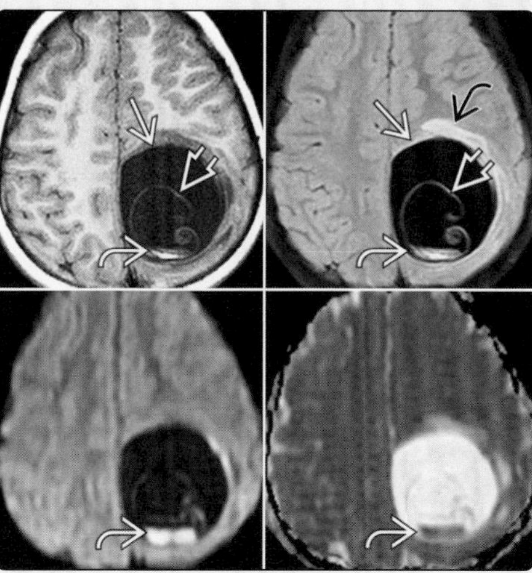

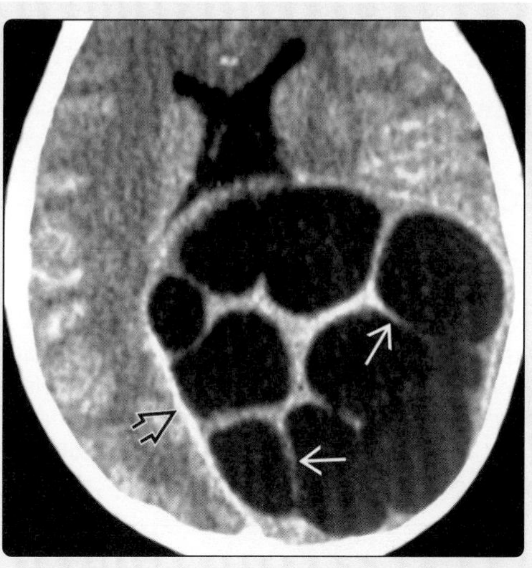

***(13-33)** Series of axial T1, FLAIR, DWI, and ADC images shows a hydatid cyst ➡ with detached germinal membrane ➡ and hydatid "sand" ➡ in the dependent part of the cyst. Surrounding edema ➡ and mass effect are minimal. **(13-34)** CECT shows a multiloculated hydatid cyst ➡ that contains multiple "daughter" cysts ➡ within it. (Courtesy S. Nagi, MD.)*

exudates, multifocal hemorrhagic parenchymal lesions **(13-37)**, and necrotizing angiitis.

## Malaria

### Terminology and Etiology

Cerebral malaria (CM) is caused by infection with the protozoan parasite *Plasmodium* and is transmitted by infected *Anopheles* mosquitoes. Four species cause human disease: *Plasmodium falciparum*, *Plasmodium vivax*, *Plasmodium ovale*, and *Plasmodium malariae*. Of these, *P. falciparum* has the most severe manifestations and causes 95% of all CM cases.

### Pathology

Grossly, the brain appears swollen, and its external surface is often a characteristic grayish or dusky dark red. Petechial hemorrhages are often seen in the subcortical white matter, corpus callosum, cerebellum, and brainstem **(13-40)**.

The major microscopic feature of CM is sequestration of parasitized red blood cells in the cerebral microvasculature **(13-38)**. This causes perivascular ring and punctate microhemorrhages and focal infarcts. Malaria parasites remain intravascular, so encephalitic inflammatory changes are absent.

### Clinical Issues

Between 250-500 million new cases of malaria develop every year, and more than 500,000 people die from the disease.

Malaria is generally restricted to tropical and subtropical areas but may affect travelers or immigrants coming from endemic regions. The incubation period from infection to symptom development is generally 1-3 weeks.

Prognosis is variable. Patients with sickle cell trait generally have milder disease. In other cases, headache, altered sensorium, and seizures develop and can be followed within 1-

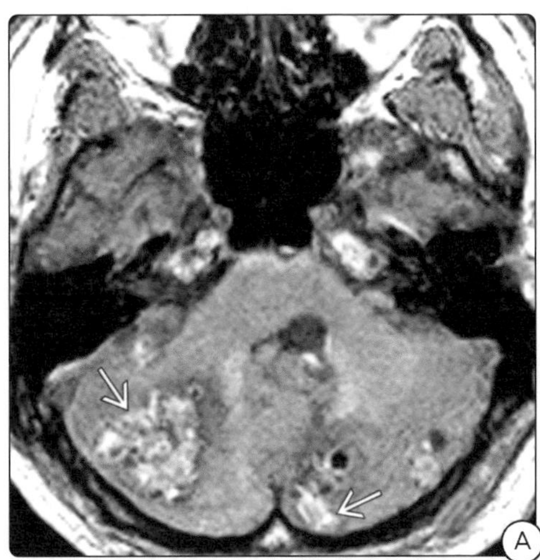


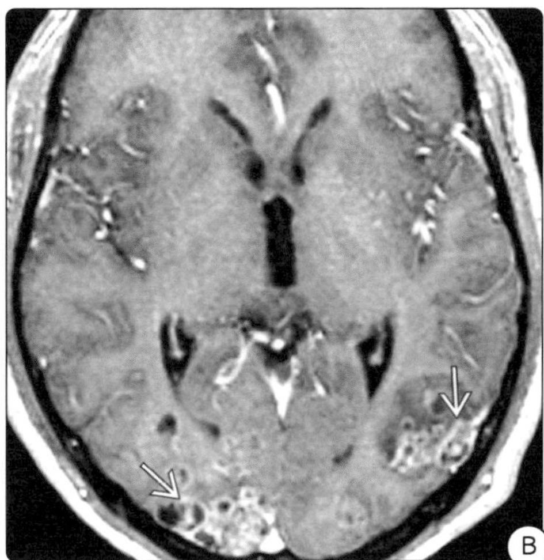


***(13-35A)** T1 C+ MR in a 20-yo man with alveolar echinococcosis demonstrates clusters of multiple small, irregular ring-enhancing cysts ➙. **(13-35B)** More cephalad T1 C+ MR shows additional masses of enhancing cysts ➙. (Courtesy M. Thurnher, MD.)*

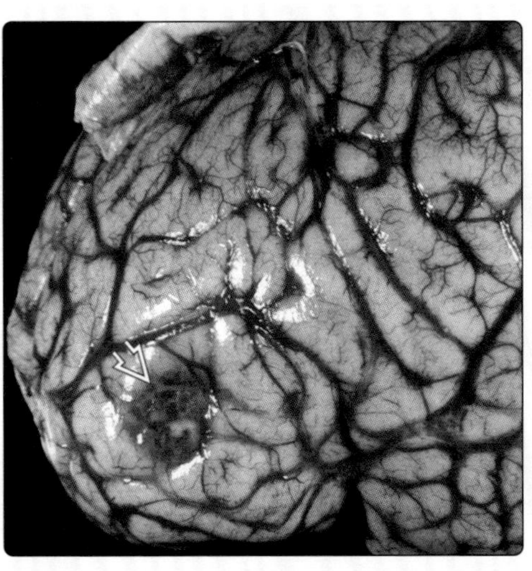

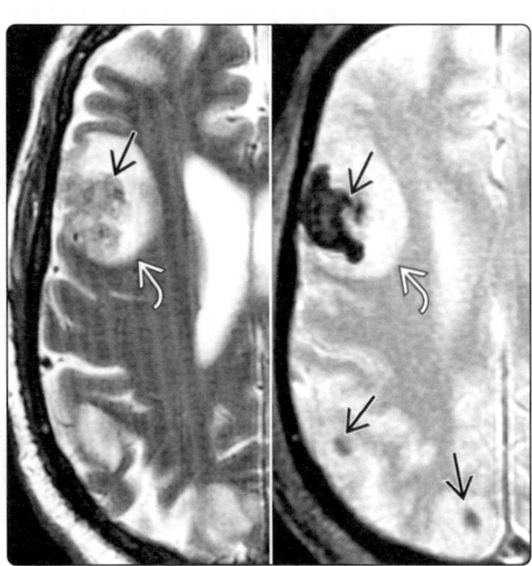

***(13-36)** Autopsied brain in a patient with amebic encephalitis shows a lesion with focal parenchymal hemorrhage ➙. **(13-37)** (L) T2 and (R) T2* GRE MR images in a patient with amebic encephalitis show multiple parenchymal hemorrhages ➙ with edema ➙ and "blooming."*

2 days by impaired consciousness, coma, and death. Mortality in CM is 15-20% even with appropriate therapy.

## Imaging

The most typical finding is focal infarcts in the cortex, basal ganglia, and thalami **(13-39)**. Gross hemorrhage can occur but is rare. Multifocal "blooming" petechial hemorrhages in the basal ganglia and cerebral white matter may be present on susceptibility-weighted imaging **(13-41)**.

## Differential Diagnosis

The major differential diagnosis of CM is multiple cerebral emboli/infarction. Multifocal white matter petechial hemorrhages on T2* and SWI are nonspecific and can be seen in **fat emboli** syndrome, acute **hemorrhagic leukoencephalitis**, trauma with **diffuse vascular injury**, **thrombotic microangiopathies**, **viral infections** (e.g., COVID-19), and **critical-illness associated microbleeds**.

# Other Parasitic Infections

Several less common parasites can invade the CNS, particularly if humans serve as intermediate or nonpermissive hosts. These include schistosomiasis, paragonimiasis, sparganosis, trichinosis, and trypanosomiasis.

Many parasites cause very bizarre-looking masses that can mimic neoplasm **(13-42)**. A history of travel to—or residence in—an endemic area is key to the diagnosis.

"Parasitomas" usually present as mass-like lesions with edema and multiple "conglomerate" ring-enhancing foci **(13-43)**. CNS parasitic infestations can be mistaken for neoplasms like **metastasis** and **glioblastoma**. **Inflammatory granulomas** (e.g., TB granulomas) can also mimic parasitic granulomas and are often endemic in the same geographic areas.

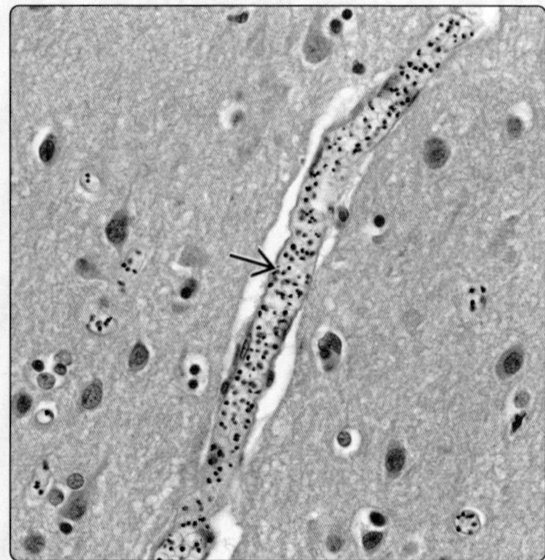

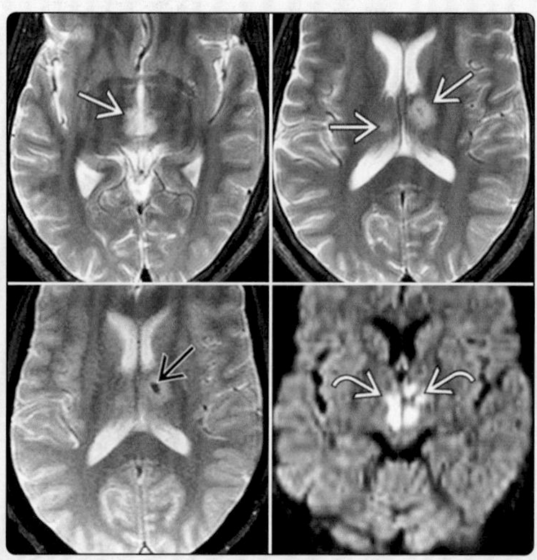

***(13-38)** In cerebral malaria, parasites convert metabolized hemoglobin to hemozoin ("malarial pigment") seen here as tiny black "dots" ➙ in sequestered RBCs in a brain capillary. (Courtesy B. K. Kleinschmidt-DeMasters, MD.) **(13-39)** Scans in a patient with cerebral malaria show T2 basal ganglia hyperintensities ➙ that "bloom" on T2* GRE ➙ and restrict on DWI ➙ MR. (Courtesy R. Ramakantan, MD.)*

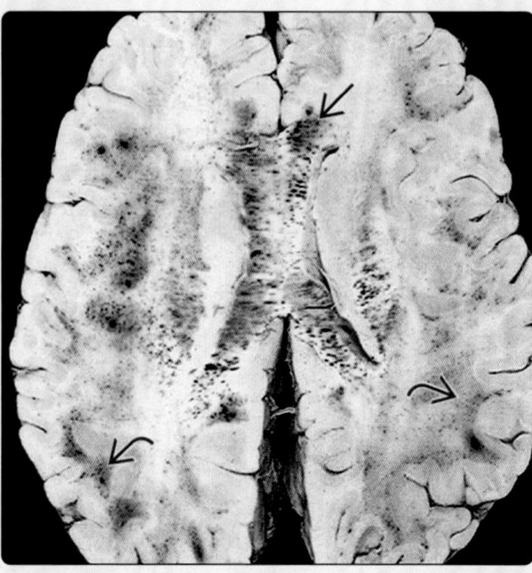

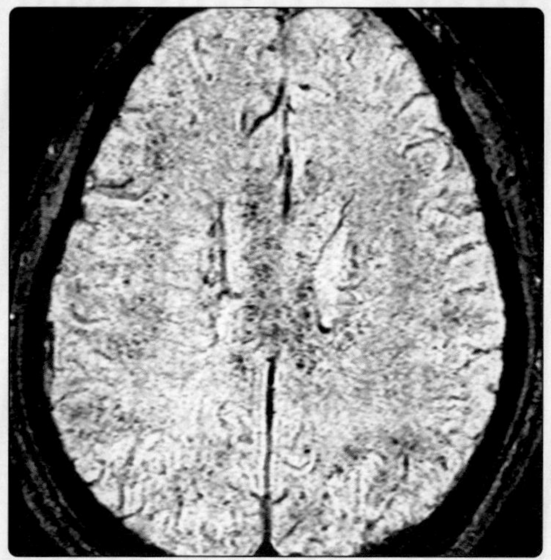

***(13-40)** Cerebral malaria shows innumerable petechial WM hemorrhages in the subcortical ➙, deep WM ➙. (Courtesy L. Chimelli: A morphological approach to the diagnosis of protozoal infections of the CNS. Patholog Res Int., 2011.) **(13-41)** T2* SWI MR in cerebral malaria shows innumerable punctate "blooming" microhemorrhages throughout the WM. (Courtesy K. Tong, MD.)*

# Miscellaneous and Emerging CNS Infections

We begin this section with two important CNS infections caused by spirochetes—Lyme disease (LD) and neurosyphilis (NS)—then turn our attention to emerging CNS infections. We pay special attention to zoonoses (i.e., diseases transmitted from animals to humans) with a focus on the manifestations of COVID-19 and the deadly viral hemorrhagic fevers.

## Spirochete Infections of CNS

Two spirochete species can cause significant CNS disease: *Borrelia* (e.g., LD, relapsing fever borreliosis) and *Treponema* (NS).

### Lyme Disease

**Terminology.** LD is a.k.a. Lyme borreliosis. LD with neurologic disease is called Lyme neuroborreliosis (LNB) or neuro-LD. LD is a multisystem inflammatory disease caused by *Borrelia burgdorferi* in the United States and *Borrelia garinii* or *Borrelia afzelii* in Europe. LD is a zoonosis maintained in animals, such as field mice and white-tailed deer.

**Etiology.** LD is transmitted to humans by *Ixodes* tick bite and requires at least 36 hours of tick attachment as the spirochete moves from the tick midgut to the salivary glands to be transmitted. Most cases result from the bite of an infected nymph (about the size of a poppy seed) and may easily go unnoticed.

**Epidemiology and Demographics.** LD is now the most common tick-borne disease in the United States and Europe with 20,000 new cases reported each year. Prevalence varies significantly with geography. Between 90-95% of cases in the

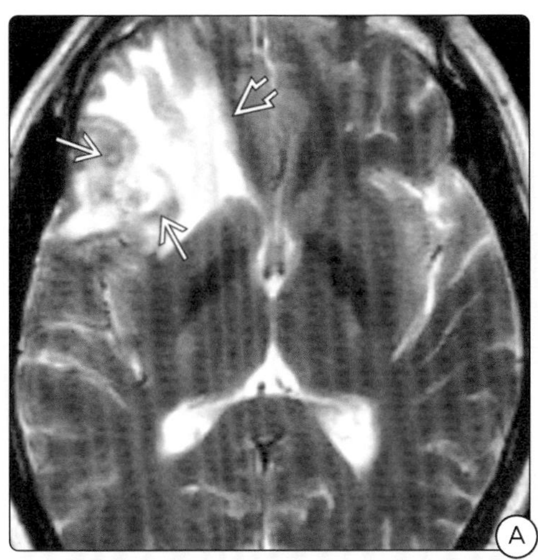

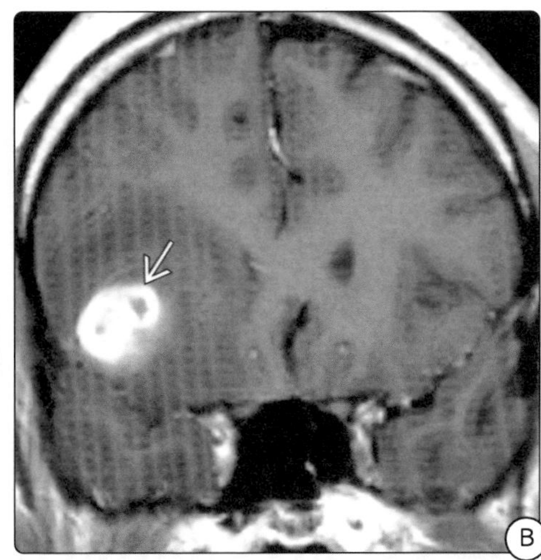

***(13-42A)** Axial T2 MR in a young man from Southeast Asia shows a heterogeneous right frontal lobe mass with intralesional hypointensities ➡, suggesting hemorrhage. Moderate perilesional edema ➡ is present. **(13-42B)** Coronal T1 C+ MR shows conglomerate ring-enhancing lesions ➡. Paragonimiasis granuloma was found at surgery.*

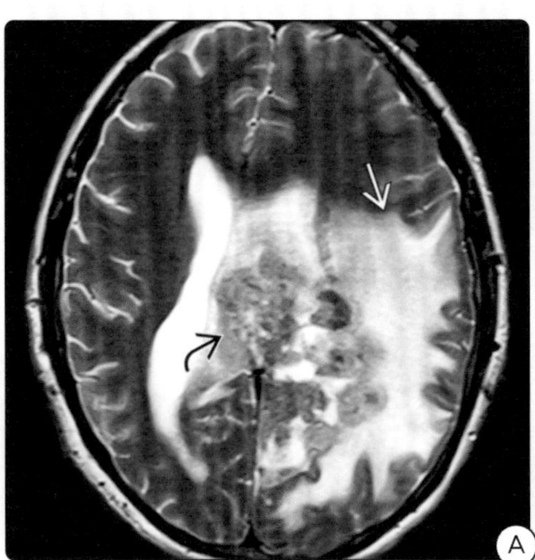

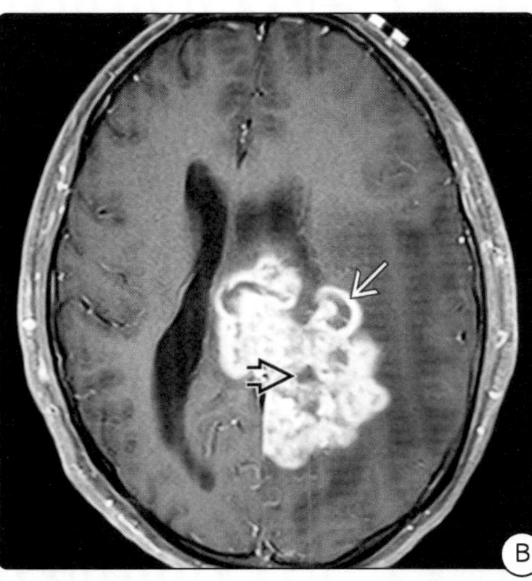

***(13-43A)** Axial T2 MR in a postpartum patient with seizures shows a very bizarre-appearing, mixed signal intensity paraventricular mass ➡ with striking perilesional edema ➡. **(13-43B)** T1 C+ FS MR shows multiple conglomerate enhancing rings ➡ around presumed necrotic foci ➡. No definite causative agent was identified. Initially presumed TB, subsequent considerations include a parasitic mass. Autopsy was declined.*

USA occur in the mid-Atlantic states, the Northeast, and the upper Midwest (primarily Minnesota and Wisconsin). Occurrence peaks during the early summer, especially May and June.

The clinical presentation and imaging features of CNS LD are protean and vary with location. Altered mental status and encephalopathy are the most common manifestations.

**Clinical Features.** LD occurs at all ages, but peak presentation is between 16-60 years. 30% of cases occur in children.

Altered mental status and encephalopathy are the most common general manifestations of LD. The classic triad of LD consists of aseptic (usually lymphocytic) meningitis, cranial neuritis, and radiculoneuritis. In North America, erythema migrans, "Lyme arthritis," and carditis are also common.

**Pathology.** Microscopic features include nonspecific, perivascular, T-lymphocytic cuffing and plasma cell infiltrates. Spirochetes can be identified in the leptomeninges, nerve roots, and dorsal root ganglia but not in the CNS parenchyma.

**Imaging.** Approximately 12-15% of patients with untreated *B. burgdorferi* infection develop CNS involvement. NECT and CECT scans are usually normal.

Multiple small (2- to 8-mm) subcortical and periventricular white matter hyperintensities on T2/FLAIR sequences are typical and identified in ~ 1/2 of all patients **(13-44)**. Enhancement varies from none to moderate. Multiple punctate and ring-enhancing lesions may be present **(13-46)**. Occasionally, "horseshoe" or incomplete ring enhancement occurs and can mimic demyelinating disease.

Cranial nerve (CN) enhancement is seen on T1 C+ but can be clinically occult. CN enhancement is especially common in North American LNB **(13-45)**. CNVII is the most frequently involved followed by CNV and CNIII. Involvement of other CNs is less common.

*(13-44A) Series of axial FLAIR MR images demonstrates the multifocal T2/FLAIR WM hyperintensities persisting 1 year after complete clinical response to treatment. Lesions are present in both middle cerebellar peduncles ➡. (13-44B) More cephalad scan in the same patient shows multifocal punctate ➡, patchy ➡, and confluent ➡ lesions in the subcortical and deep periventricular WM.*

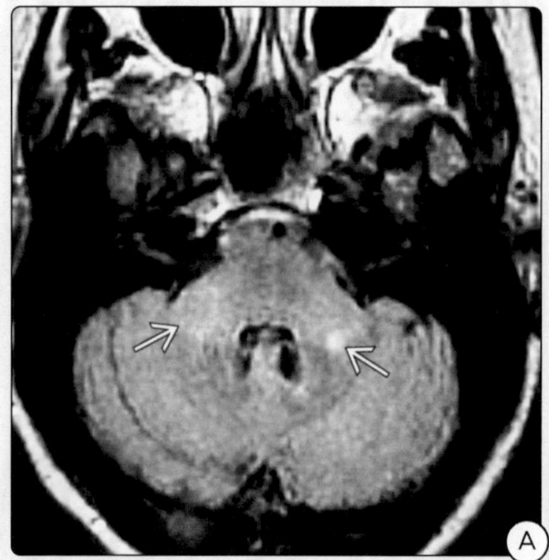


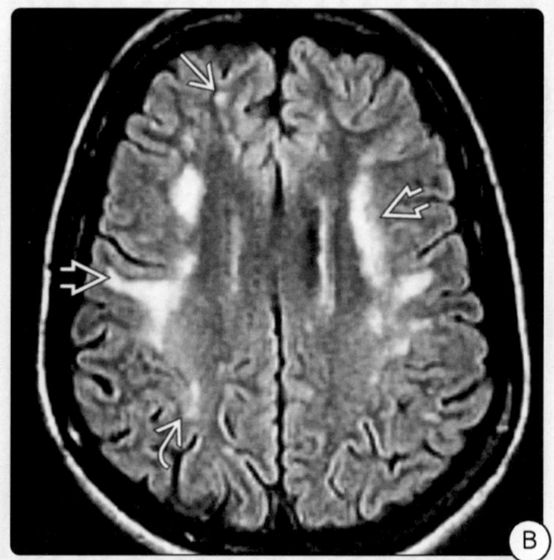


*(13-44C) Midline sagittal FLAIR MR in the same patient shows punctate lesions in the subcortical WM and corpus callosum ➡. A larger confluent lesion in the corpus callosum ➡ is present just anterior to the splenium. (13-44D) More lateral FLAIR MR in the same patient shows multiple punctate ➡ and confluent ➡ lesions in the subcortical WM. Note sparing of the subcortical U-fibers. This is documented Lyme disease.*

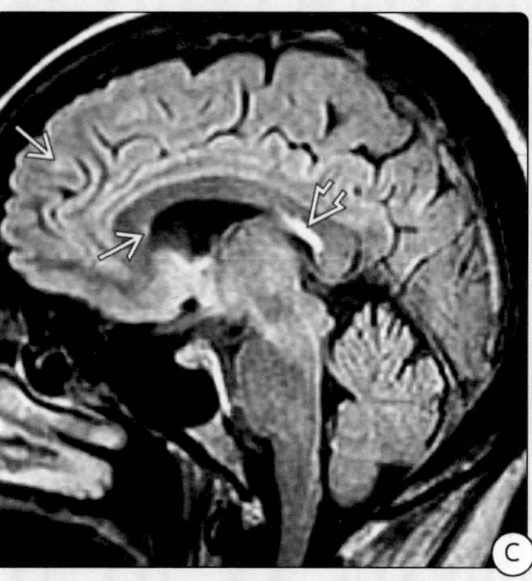


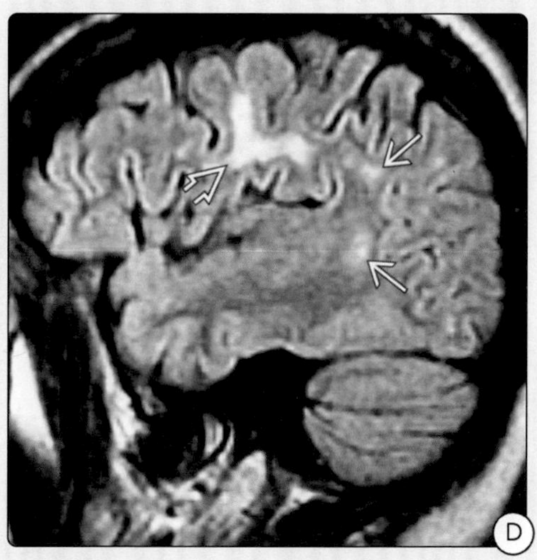

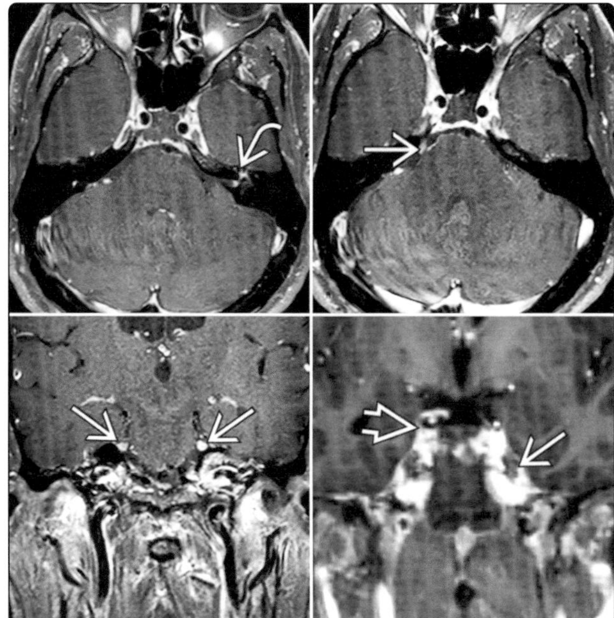

***(13-45)** Axial (top), coronal (bottom) T1 C+ FS MR scans in a patient with Lyme disease demonstrate left CNVII ➡, bilateral CNV ➡, and left CNIII ➡ enhancement. (Courtesy P. Hildenbrand, MD.)*

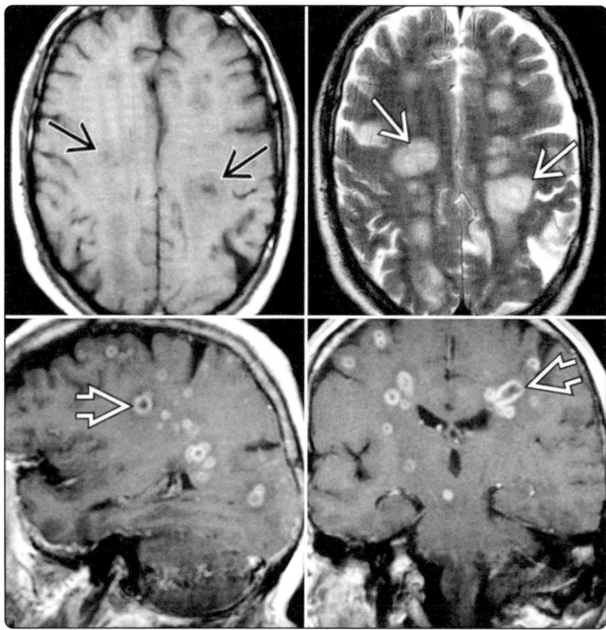

***(13-46)** (Upper L) T1 shows bilateral iso-/hypodense WM lesions ➡. (Upper R) T2 shows bilateral "fluffy" hyperintense lesions ➡ in the corona radiata. Sagittal (lower L) and coronal (lower R) show multifocal ring enhancement ➡; rickettsial encephalitis.*

Myelitis and radiculitis are more common in European LD. Diffuse or multifocal hyperintense lesions on T2WI with patchy cord and linear nerve root enhancement are typical.

**Differential Diagnosis.** The major differential diagnosis of LNB is demyelinating disease. **Multiple sclerosis** (MS) frequently involves the periventricular white matter. Callososeptal involvement is more common in MS compared with LNB. CN enhancement—especially CNVII—is less common than with LNB.

## Neurosyphilis

Syphilis is a chronic systemic infectious disease caused by the spirochete *Treponema pallidum*. Syphilis is usually transmitted via sexual contact. Between 5-10% of patients with untreated syphilis develop neurosyphilis (NS).

Syphilitic gumma is the most common intracranial manifestation. Most are located along the brain subpial surfaces and consist of a dense inflammatory infiltrate surrounding a central caseous necrotic core. Imaging is that of a mixed-density/signal intensity mass with intense ring-like or diffuse enhancement **(13-47)**. Because of their rarity, most syphilitic gummas are initially misdiagnosed as primary or metastatic neoplasms.

### SPIROCHETE CNS INFECTIONS

**Lyme Disease (Neuroborreliosis)**

- 12-15% of infected individuals develop CNS infection
- Cranial neuropathy
  - CNVII > CNV, CNIII; others less common
  - Can affect multiple nerves
- Encephalopathy
  - Punctate T2/FLAIR hyperintensities in 50%
  - Other: Tumefactive lesions ± punctate/ring enhancement

**Neurosyphilis**

- ↑ especially in men having sex with men (MSM)
- "Gumma" = ring or solid enhancement ± meninges
- Meningovascular = infarct

## Emerging CNS Infections

Emerging infections are diseases that are literally emerging to infect humans. Some of these—such as COVID-19—are zoonoses (i.e., diseases transmitted from animals to humans), whereas others are insect borne. Most rarely affect the CNS, but, when they do, the results can be disastrous. Examples of the latter include hemorrhagic viral fevers, such as Korean hemorrhagic fever, Rift Valley fever, hantavirus, dengue **(13-49)**, and Ebola. Most patients are never imaged, but when they are, multifocal brain bleeds are typical findings **(13-48)**.

*Selected References: The complete reference list is available on the eBooks+ version included with purchase.*

*(13-47A) T1 C+ MR in an HIV-positive male patient with right trigeminal neuralgia shows intense enhancement in the pontine lesion ➡ with extension from the root entry zone ➡ along the CNV into the Meckel cave ➡. (13-47B) More inferior T1 C+ FS MR shows leptomeningeal enhancement ➡ along the surface of the medulla. This is biopsy-proven meningovascular syphilis.*

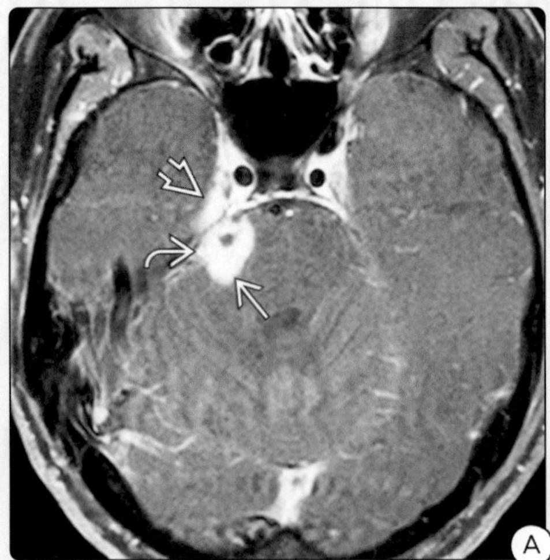

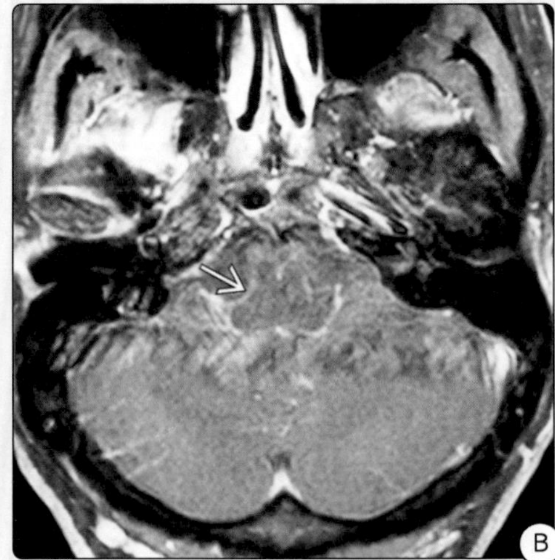

*(13-48A) Axial FLAIR MR in a 38-yo man with high fever, altered mental status, and seizure shows bilateral hyperintense lesions ➡ in the WM of both temporal lobes. (13-48B) SWI MIP shows bilateral lobar hematomas ➡ and numerous petechial microhemorrhages ➡.*

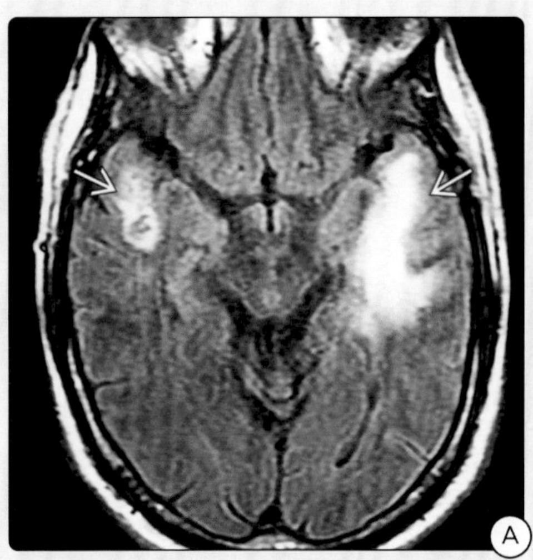

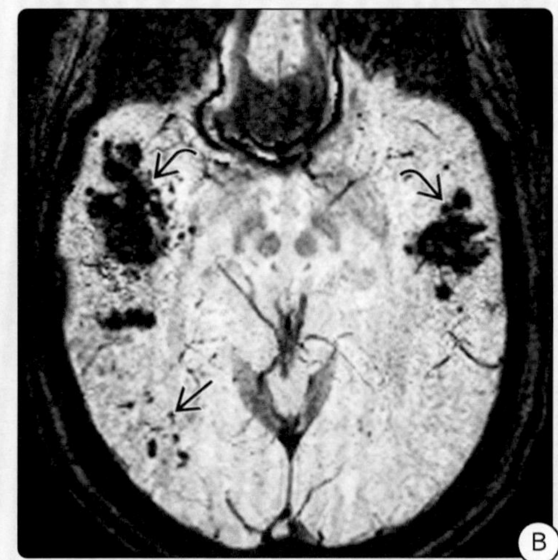

*(13-48C) More cephalad SWI MIP shows additional confluent hemorrhages and scattered microbleeds. Fulminant hemorrhagic encephalitis in this case is most likely viral, although an inciting organism was not identified despite extensive laboratory investigation. (13-49) Dengue fever with lesions in the basal ganglia ➡, medial temporal lobes ➡, midbrain and pons ➡, and hypothalamus ➡ is shown. (Courtesy D. Bertholdo, MD.)*

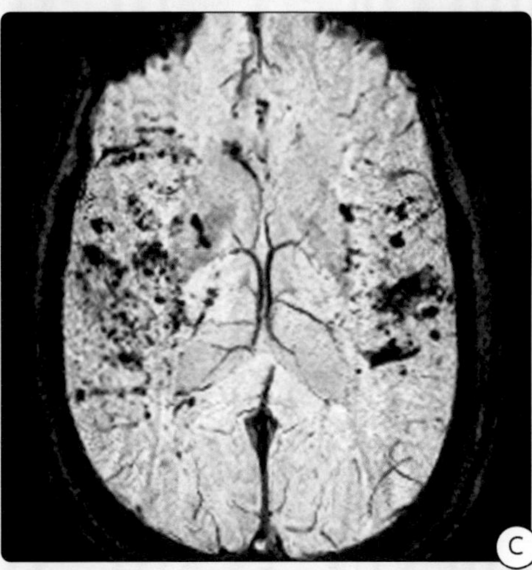

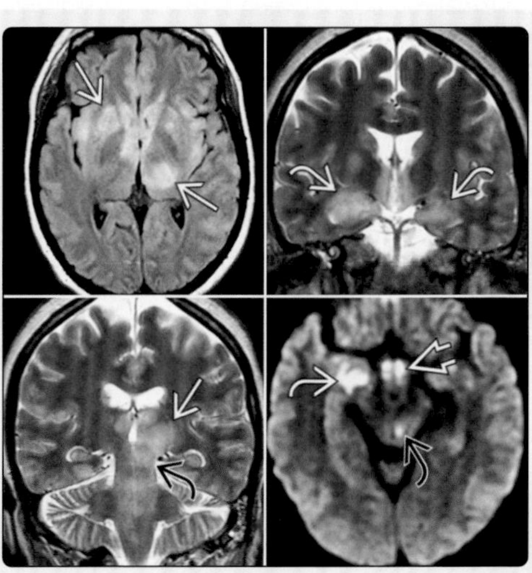

# HIV/AIDS

***In this chapter, we explore the "many faces" of HIV/AIDS as it affects the CNS. We begin by discussing the manifestations of HIV itself in the brain, i.e., HIV encephalitis and the recently described HIV-associated CD8 encephalitis. We follow with a consideration of unusual but important associated findings, such as HIV vasculopathy, HIV-associated bone marrow changes, and benign salivary gland lymphoepithelial lesions.***



We then consider the broad spectrum of opportunistic infections that complicate HIV/AIDS and what happens when an HIV-positive patient is also co-infected with tuberculosis (TB), another sexually transmitted disease, or malaria. Long-term survivors with treated AIDS and the phenomenon of immune reconstitution inflammatory syndrome (IRIS) are then presented. We conclude the chapter by discussing neoplasms that occur in the setting of HIV/AIDS (the so-called AIDS-defining malignancies).

## HIV Infection

HIV is a neurovirulent infection that has both direct and indirect effects on the CNS. Neurologic complications can arise from the HIV infection itself, from opportunistic infections or neoplasms, and from treatment-related metabolic derangements.

In this section, we consider the effects of the HIV virus itself on the brain. Extracranial manifestations of HIV/AIDS may also be identified on brain imaging studies, so we discuss these as well.

### HIV Encephalitis

Between 75-90% of HIV/AIDS patients have demonstrable HIV-induced brain injury at autopsy **(14-1)**. Although many patients remain asymptomatic for variable periods, brain infection is the initial presenting symptomatology in 5-10% of cases. Approximately 25% of treated HIV/AIDS patients develop moderate cognitive impairment despite good virologic response to therapy.

#### Terminology

HIV encephalitis (HIVE) and HIV leukoencephalopathy (HIVL) are the direct result of HIV infection of the brain. Opportunistic infections are absent early, although co-infections or multiple infections are common later in the disease course.

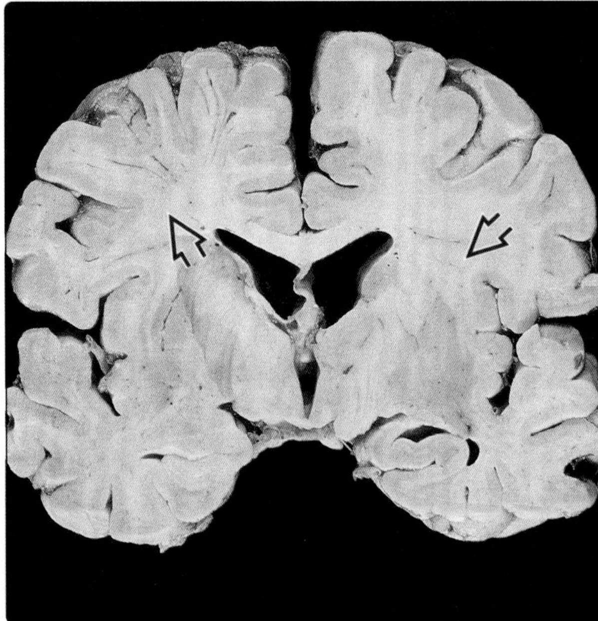

***(14-1)** Coronal autopsy of HIVE shows generalized volume loss with enlargement of the lateral ventricles, sylvian fissures. "Hazy," poorly defined abnormalities are present in WM ➡ but spare the subcortical U-fibers. (Courtesy B. K. DeMasters, MD.)*

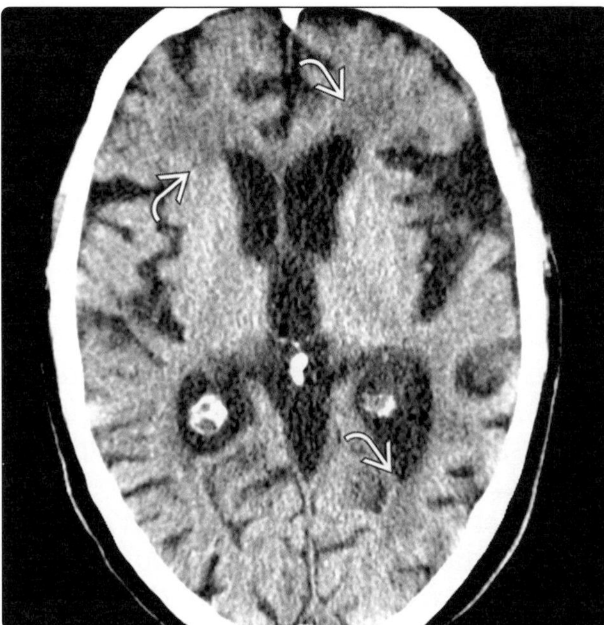

***(14-2)** Axial NECT in a 38-yo man with longstanding HIV/AIDS shows gross cerebral atrophy and multifocal hypodensities ➡ in the subcortical WM.*

## Etiology

HIV is a pathogenic neurotropic human RNA retrovirus. **HIV-1** is responsible for most cases of HIV/AIDS. **HIV-2** infection is found primarily in West Africa. Unless otherwise noted in this discussion, "HIV" or "HIV infection" refers to HIV-1 infection.

The two major targets of viral infection are lymphoid tissue—especially T cells—and the CNS. HIV crosses the blood-brain barrier (BBB) both as cell-free virus and infected monocytes and T cells, which migrate across the intact BBB, penetrating the brain within 24-48 hours after initial exposure.

While HIV does not directly infect neurons, it infects astrocytes and microglia. Recent studies have demonstrated that HIV persists in perivascular macrophages and microglia despite suppression with antiretroviral therapy (ART), thus remaining in a latent "hidden" state that can lead to sustained pathologic inflammatory responses.

Recent studies of cellular silencing mechanisms in microglia show that HIV-1 latency can be reversed by proinflammatory cytokines and signaling from damaged neurons, thus creating intermittent cycles of HIV-1 reactivation and silencing that can lead to sustained pathologic inflammatory responses.

## Pathology

In early stages, the brain appears grossly normal. Advanced HIVE results in generalized brain volume loss ("atrophy") with enlarged ventricles and subarachnoid spaces. Ill-defined, diffuse myelin pallor with poorly demarcated areas of myelin loss ensues. Lesions are most prominent in the deep periventricular white matter (WM) and corona radiata.

Microscopically, HIVE is characterized by gliosis, microglial activation, perivascular inflammation, and multinucleated giant cells containing viral antigens. Lymphocytic infiltrates, predominately T cells [often CD8(+)], are common.

## Clinical Issues

**Epidemiology.** Almost 60% of all AIDS patients eventually develop overt neurologic manifestations. Despite potent suppression of HIV-1 viral replication in the CNS by ART, between 15-60% of patients exhibit ongoing neuroinflammation and symptoms of **HIV-1-associated neurocognitive disorders (HANDs)**.

**Presentation.** Early brain infection with HIV is often asymptomatic, and cognitive and functional performances are both initially normal. HANDs develop as intermediate and long-term complications. A nadir CD4 cell count below 50/mL has the greatest risk of HIV-associated neurocognitive impairment.

## Imaging

**CT Findings.** NECT scans may be normal in the early stages. Mild to moderate atrophy with patchy or confluent WM hypodensity develops as the disease progresses **(14-2)**. HIVE does not cause mass effect and does not enhance on CECT.

**MR Findings.** Generalized volume loss with enlarged ventricles and sulci is best appreciated on T1WI or thin-section inversion recovery sequences. WM signal intensity is generally normal or near normal on T1WI.

T2/FLAIR initially shows bilateral, patchy, relatively symmetric WM hyperintensities. With time, confluent "hazy," ill-defined hyperintensity in the subcortical and deep cerebral WM

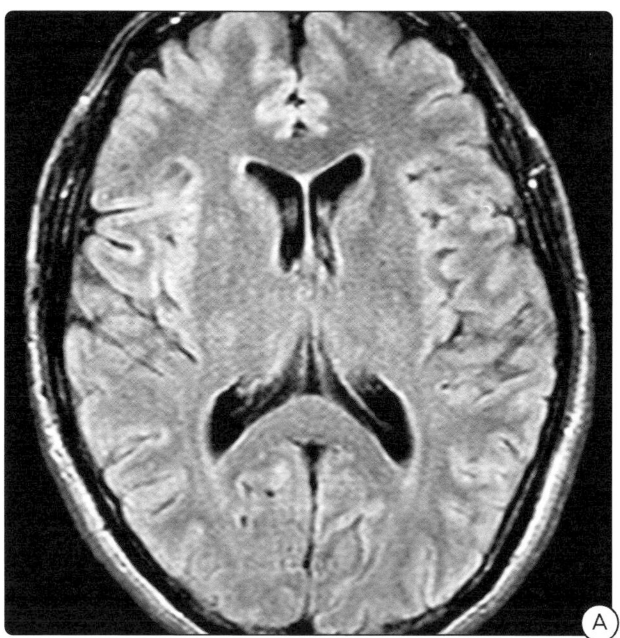

***(14-4A)** Axial FLAIR MR in a 45-yo man recently diagnosed with HIV/AIDS shows mild ventricular prominence but no discernible WM abnormalities.*

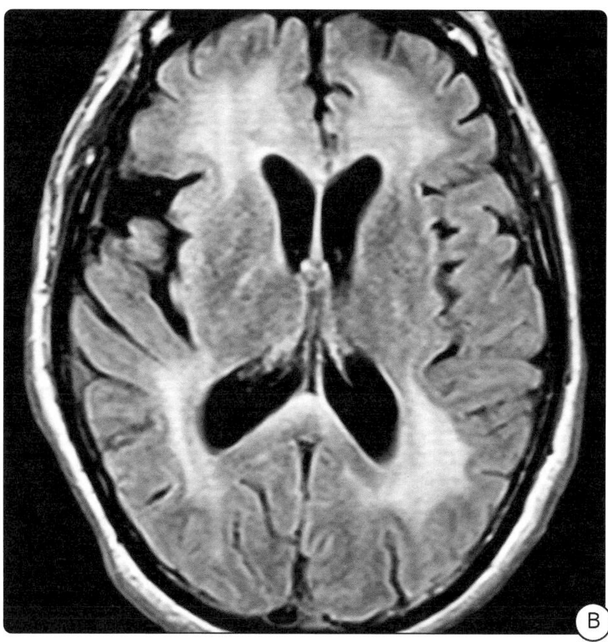

***(14-4B)** Despite being placed on ART, the patient developed HANDs. FLAIR MR 4 years after initial study shows significant brain volume loss and confluent periventricular WM hyperintensity that largely spares the subcortical U-fibers. HIVE.*

develops, and volume loss ensues **(14-4)**. HIVE usually does not enhance on T1 C+ and usually shows no restriction on DWI. In fulminant cases, perivenular enhancement may indicate acute demyelination.

## Differential Diagnosis

**Progressive multifocal leukoencephalopathy** (PML) has strikingly **asymmetric** hyperintensities on T2/FLAIR. Both the hemispheric and posterior fossa WM (often both cerebral peduncles) are commonly affected. PML also often involves the subcortical U-fibers, which are usually spared in HIVE.

Co-infections with other infectious agents are common in HIVE and may complicate its classic imaging appearance. **Cytomegalovirus** (CMV) can also cause a similarly diffuse encephalitis but frequently exhibits ependymal enhancement. **Toxoplasmosis** causes multifocal punctate and "target" or ring-enhancing lesions that are most prominent in the basal ganglia.

**Herpes encephalitis** and **human herpesvirus-6 (HHV-6) encephalitis** both involve the temporal lobes, especially the cortex.

**HIV-associated CD8 encephalitis (HIV-CD8E)** is a distinct disorder characterized by acute brain inflammation and infiltration by CD8(+) T lymphocytes. Imaging shows brain swelling with diffuse T2/FLAIR WM hyperintensity. Enhancement along penetrating arteries, medullary veins, and edges of the WM abnormalities is typical **(14-6)**.

**Immune reconstitution inflammatory syndrome (IRIS)** occurs with and is characterized by other associated infectious agents (e.g., JC virus, TB, fungal infections). HIV viral antigens are inconstant and minimally detected.

### HIV ENCEPHALITIS: MR AND DDx

**MR**
- Volume loss with ↑ sulci, ventricles
- T2/FLAIR "hazy" WM symmetric hyperintensity
  - Spares subcortical U-fibers
- No mass effect
- No enhancement (exception = acute fulminant HIVE)

**Differential Diagnosis**
- PML
  - Usually asymmetric
  - Often involves U-fibers
- Opportunistic infections
  - CMV causes encephalitis, ependymitis
  - Toxoplasmosis: Multiple enhancing rings
- HHV-6 encephalitis
  - Usually involves temporal lobe(s)
- HIV-associated CD8 T-lymphocyte encephalitis
  - Acute, generally diffuse cerebral swelling
  - Multifocal, confluent T2/FLAIR WM hyperintensities
  - Typically more hyperintense, well-defined compared to "hazy" HIVE
  - Variable enhancement (including perivascular, patchy/confluent WM lesions)
- IRIS
  - Minimal/no HIV viral antigens detected
  - Imaging findings related to infectious agent

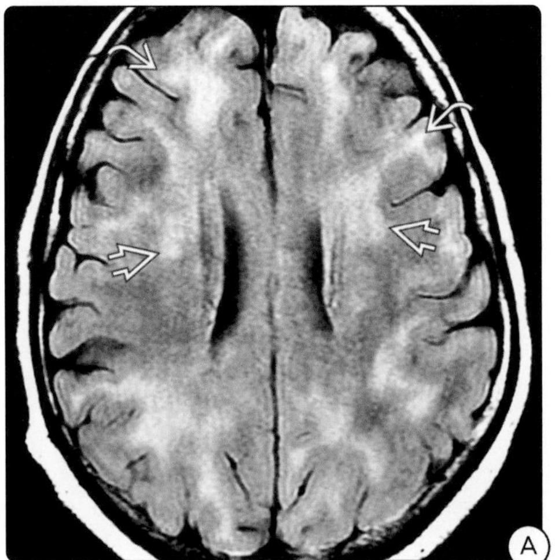


***(14-6A) FLAIR MR in an African female patient with HIV/AIDS shows patchy hyperintensities in subcortical and deep periventricular WM .***

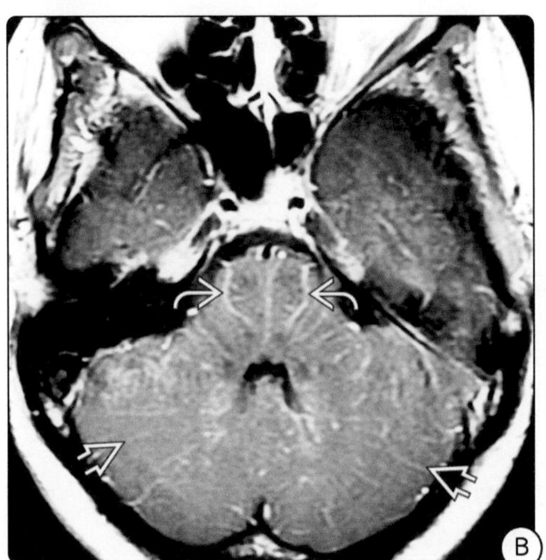


***(14-6B) T1 C+ MR shows striking, symmetric linear enhancement in the pontine and cerebellar WM .***

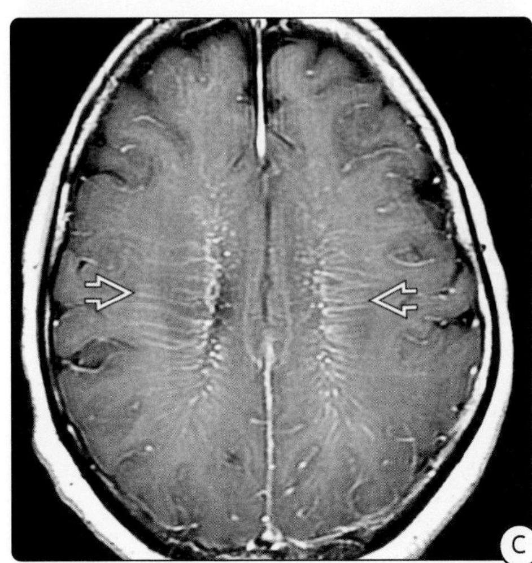


***(14-6C) More cephalad T1 C+ MR shows strikingly enlarged, enhancing medullary veins . CD8(+) T-lymphocyte encephalitis.***

# HIV-Associated CD8 Encephalitis

## Terminology

HIV-associated CD8 encephalitis (HIV-CD8E) is a severe inflammatory disorder with perivascular and diffuse brain infiltration by CD8(+) T lymphocytes. HIV-CD8E is clinically and pathologically distinct from classic HIV encephalitis (HIVE).

## Etiology

HIV viral escape in the CSF has been identified in nearly 70% of HIV-CD8E cases, but the exact pathogenesis of the disorder is unknown. Antiretroviral therapy (ART) and immune reconstitution inflammatory syndrome (IRIS) each occur in 27% of proven cases.

## Pathology

Marked cerebral inflammation and swelling—both supra- and infratentorial—is the hallmark of HIV-CD8E. CD8(+) T cells flood into the brain, causing perivascular and diffuse cerebral infiltrates, almost always in WM. The cerebrum, brainstem, and cerebellum are predominately affected.

Other infectious causes of encephalitis must be excluded. CSF and brain tissue viral studies (HSV, HHV6, HHV8, VZV, EBV, CMV, JC, West Nile, parvovirus) are negative except for HIV-1 ("viral escape").

## Clinical Issues

HIV-CD8E typically occurs when the virus is apparently well controlled by ART and should be considered in an HIV patient whose brain function suddenly deteriorates. Signs and symptoms are related to marked cerebral inflammation and swelling. Coma and death may ensue unless the disease is treated promptly with corticosteroids, which reduces fatality from nearly 70% to 30%.

Black (especially African) ethnicity appears to be a key risk factor in the majority of published cases.

## Imaging

Imaging shows diffuse WM changes and cerebral swelling/edema. The cerebral ventricles and sulci may appear compressed. Multifocal confluent areas of T2/FLAIR hyperintensity in the cerebral and cerebellar WM are typical **(14-6A)**. Multiple enhancing foci are present on T1 C+ sequences **(14-7A)**. Distended, enhancing medullary veins may be striking and are strongly suggestive of the diagnosis **(14-6B)** **(14-6C)**.

## Differential Diagnosis

In **HIVE**, T2/FLAIR confluent hyperintensities are present in the periventricular WM with relative sparing of the subcortical tracts. Mass effect and enhancement are absent.

**Progressive multifocal leukoencephalopathy (PML)** is asymmetric and multifocal, often affecting the subcortical U-fibers, and CSF is positive for JC virus.

Rare cases of CD8E have been reported with progressive hemispheric atrophy, resembling **Rasmussen encephalitis**.

**Primary CNS lymphoma (PCNSL)** is seen as T1-hypointense periventricular/deep WM lesions often occurring with rim enhancement on T1 C+ sequences. Restricted diffusion in the center of the lesion is common.

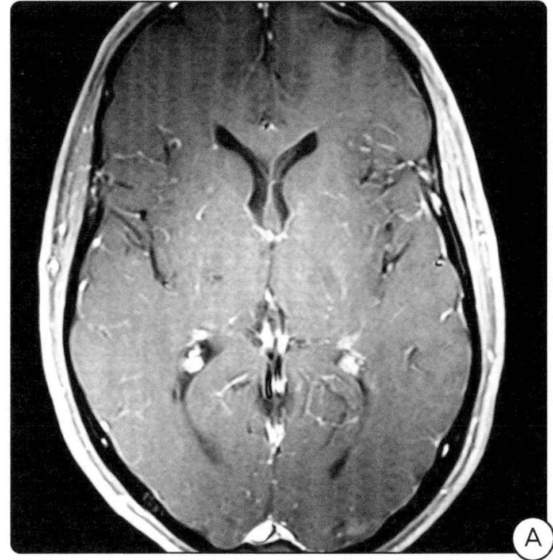

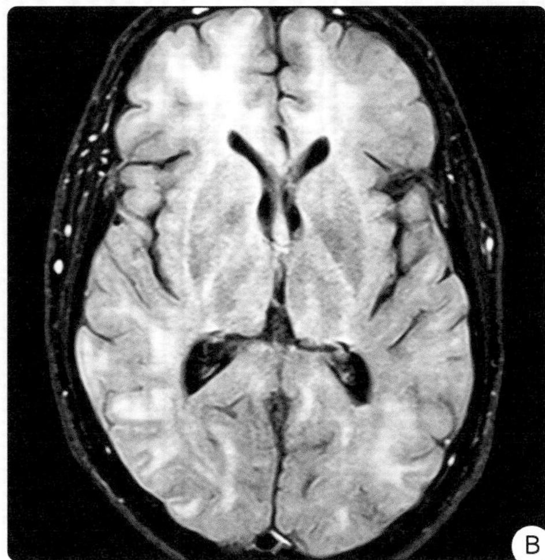

***(14-7A)*** *Initial T1 C+ FS MR in a 45-yo man with newly diagnosed HIV/AIDS appears normal. The patient was placed on ART.* ***(14-7B)*** *Nearly 9 years later, the patient became acutely encephalopathic after recently discontinued ART. Axial FLAIR MR shows confluent WM hyperintensity in the deep, subcortical WM.*

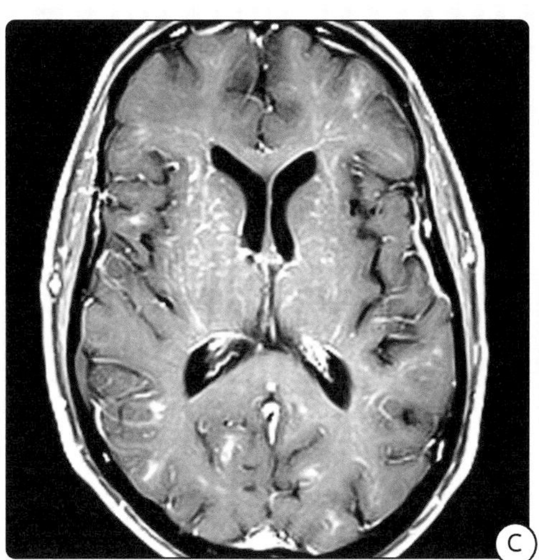

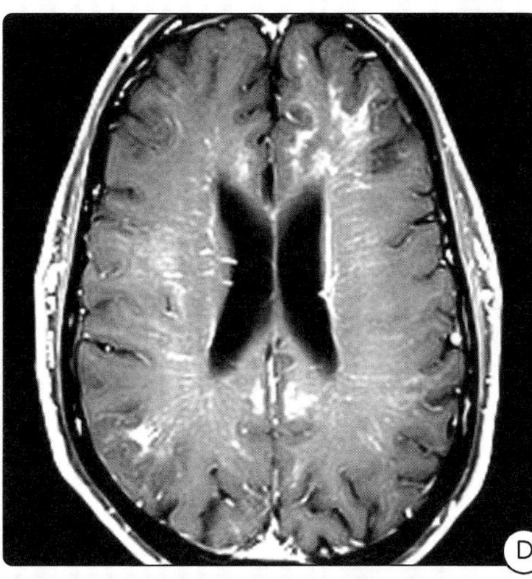

***(14-7C)*** *T1 C+ FS MR shows multiple punctate, linear enhancing foci in a vascular distribution. Patchy enhancement in the subcortical WM is widely scattered.* ***(14-7D)*** *More cephalad T1 C+ FS MR shows enlarged, enhancing medullary veins with more patchy irregular foci of enhancement.*

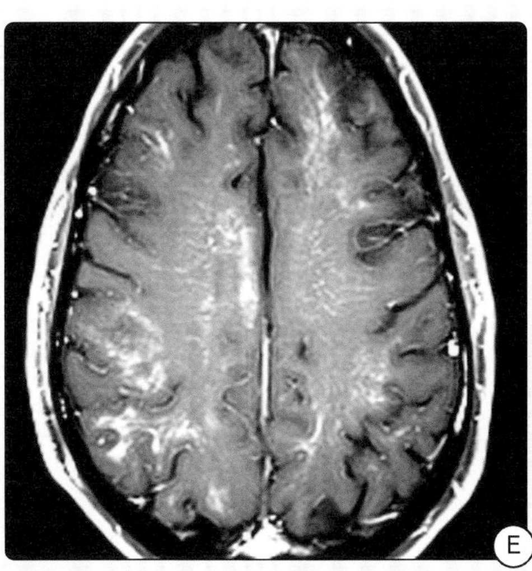

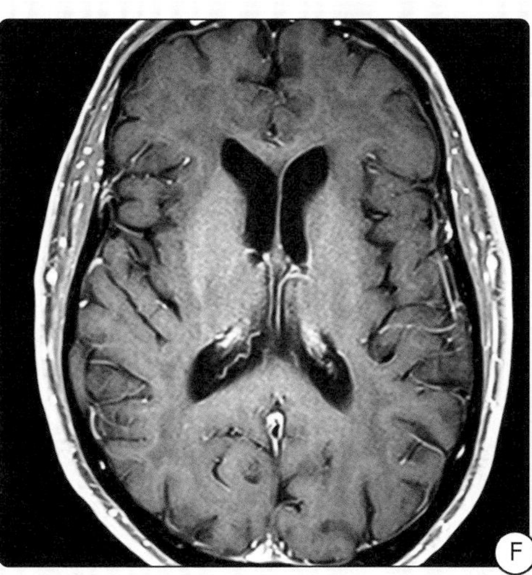

***(14-7E)*** *More cephalad T1 C+ FS MR shows enlarged, enhancing medullary veins. Multiple patchy and confluent enhancing foci are present in the subcortical WM.* ***(14-7F)*** *T1 C+ FS MR after ART was reinstituted shows interval resolution of patchy and perivenular enhancement. Moderate generalized volume loss is present compared to initial imaging (Fig. 14-8A).*

Other differential diagnostic considerations include **HIV vasculitis**, **posterior reversible encephalopathy syndrome**, **acute disseminated encephalitis**, and classic **virus-associated** or **autoimmune encephalitis.**

## Miscellaneous Manifestations of HIV/AIDS

### HIV/AIDS Bone Marrow Changes

Bone marrow alterations are common in HIV/AIDS patients **(14-8)**. Fatty, T1-hyperintense, yellow marrow is replaced with T1-hypointense, active hematopoietic tissue **(14-9)**. The calvarium and clivus appear mottled or gray. The affected vertebral bodies appear hypointense relative to the intervertebral discs (the bright disc sign).

### Lymphoid Hyperplasia

Lymphoid hyperplasia of Waldeyer ring is the most common finding observed on brain MR. Unusually prominent tonsils and adenoids in a patient over 25-30 years of age should raise suspicion of HIV infection **(14-10)**.

### Benign Lymphoepithelial Lesions

Benign lymphoepithelial lesions of HIV (BLL-HIV) are nonneoplastic cystic masses that enlarge salivary glands. Bilateral lesions are common. The parotid glands are most frequently affected **(14-12)**.

NECT scans show multiple bilateral, well-circumscribed cysts within enlarged parotid glands. A thin, enhancing rim is present on CECT scans **(14-13)**. The cysts are homogeneously hyperintense on T2WI and demonstrate rim enhancement on T1 C+ **(14-14)**.

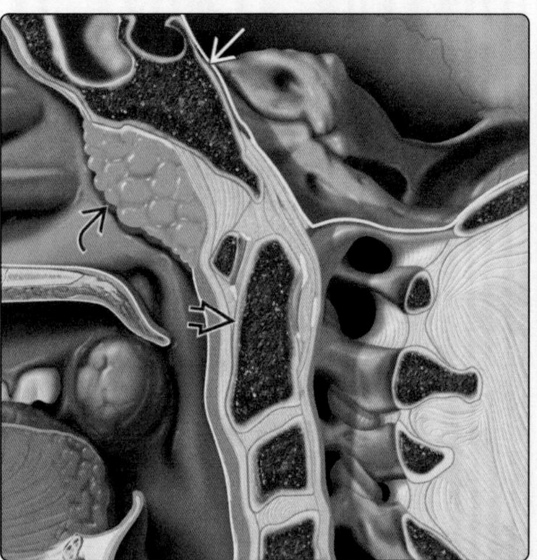

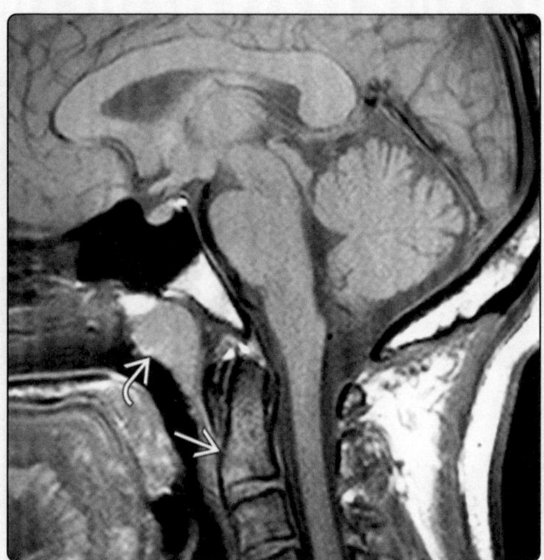

***(14-8) Sagittal graphic in HIV/AIDS depicts ancillary findings of prominent adenoids/tonsils ➩ and active hematopoietic bone marrow with conversion from "yellow" to "red" marrow in the skull ➡ and cervical spine ➩. (14-9) Sagittal T1 MR in a 43-yo man with HIV/AIDS for 20 years shows prominent adenoids ➩ and hypointense marrow ➡ in the upper cervical spine.***

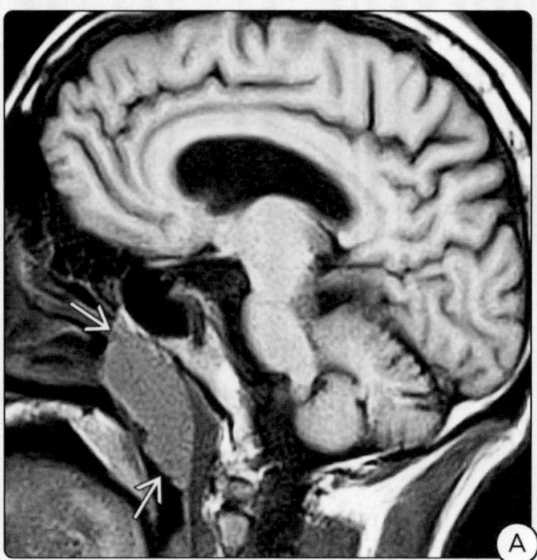

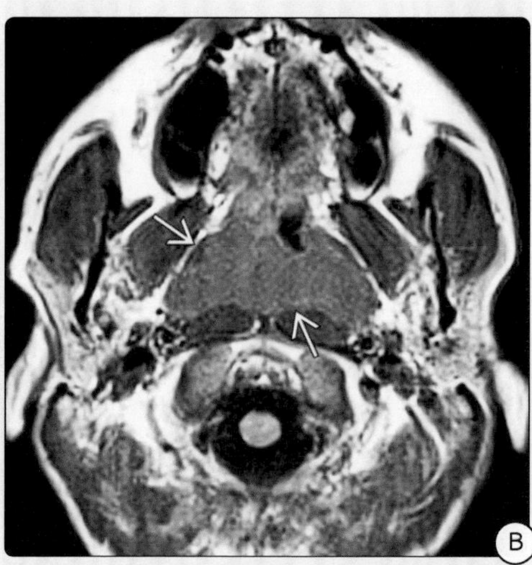

***(14-11A) Sagittal T1 MR in a 43-yo man with longstanding HIV/AIDS shows unusually prominent adenoids ➡. (14-11B) Axial T1 MR in the same patient shows that the upper nasopharynx is almost completely filled with enlarged adenoidal tissue ➡.***

### Vasculopathy

Recurrent strokes are increasingly common in chronic HIV/AIDS. HIV-associated vasculopathy can cause striking fusiform dilatation of the circle of Willis and proximal middle cerebral arteries **(14-15)**.

# Opportunistic Infections

With the advent of effective antiretroviral therapy (ART), the prevalence of CNS opportunistic infections has decreased five- to tenfold. Nevertheless, these infections and HIV co-infections, such as TB, continue to create substantial morbidity.

## Toxoplasmosis

Toxoplasmosis (toxo) is the most common opportunistic infection and most frequent cause of a cerebral mass lesion in patients with HIV/AIDS. As 20-70% of the population is seropositive for *Toxoplasma gondii*, infection in HIV/AIDS patients generally represents activation of latent infection.

With widespread use of ART, the worldwide prevalence of toxo has decreased substantially. In high-income countries, the prevalence is approximately 25%. However, in resource-poor regions, such as Africa, 35-50% of all HIV/AIDS patients develop CNS toxo. Infection most often becomes symptomatic when CD4 counts fall below 200.

CNS toxo most commonly involves the basal ganglia, thalami, corticomedullary junctions, and cerebellum **(14-16)**. Multifocal lesions are more common than solitary ones. In contrast to lymphoma, only 15-20% of toxo lesions present as solitary masses. Although large lesions do occur, most lesions

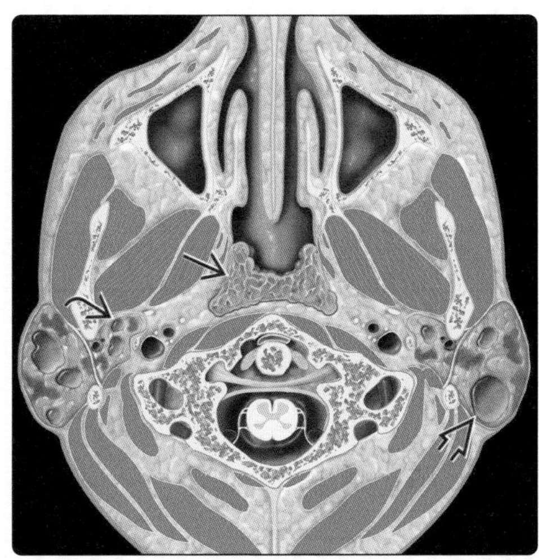

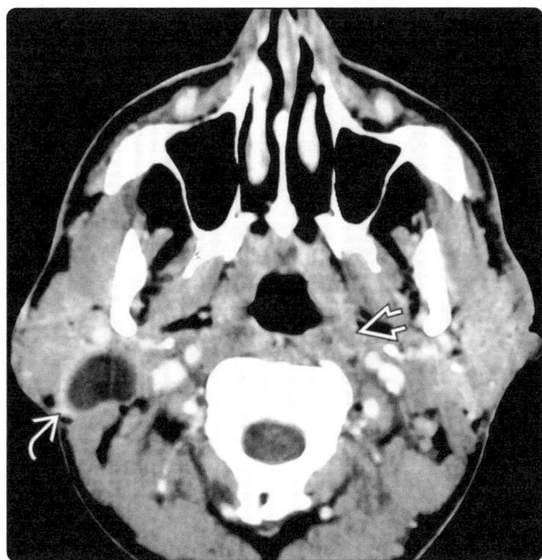

***(14-12)** Axial graphic shows typical lymphoid and lymphoepithelial lesions of HIV/AIDS. Note the hyperplastic tonsils ➔ and multiple cysts in the superficial ➔ and deep ➔ lobes of both parotid glands. **(14-13)** Axial CECT in a 33-yo man with HIV/AIDS shows a large right parotid cyst with enhancing rim ➔ and an enlarged Waldeyer ring ➔.*

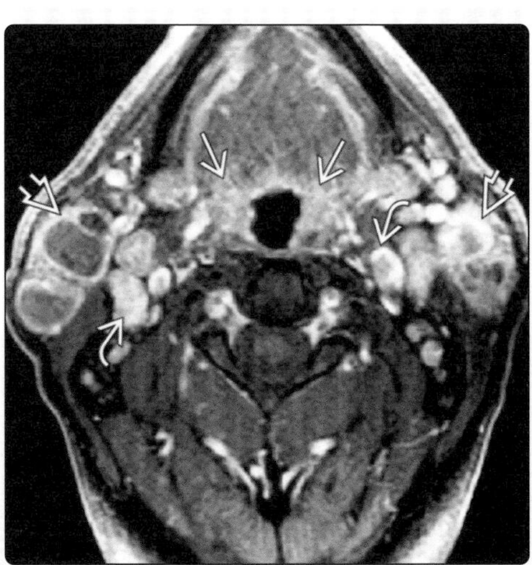

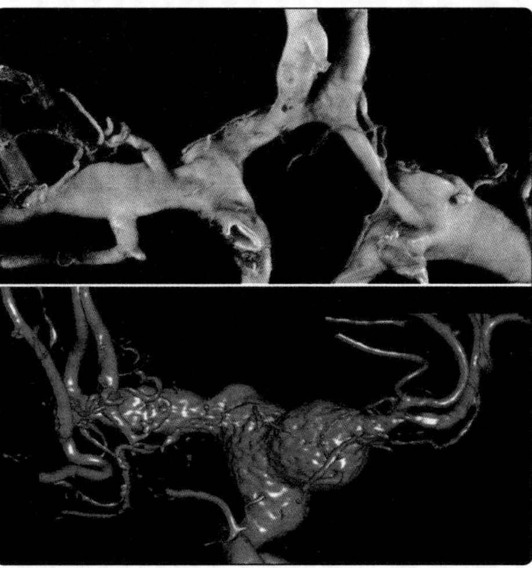

***(14-14)** T1 C+ FS MR in a 31-yo HIV-positive man shows hyperplastic Waldeyer ring ➔, enlarged deep cervical lymph nodes ➔, and rim-enhancing cysts in both parotid glands ➔. **(14-15)** (Top) Autopsied case of HIV-associated vasculopathy shows fusiform dilatation of multiple intracranial arteries. (Courtesy L. Rourke, MD.) (Bottom) 3D DSA shows multiple fusiform dilatations, characteristic of HIV vasculopathy.*

are small and average between 2-3 cm in diameter. The most common finding on NECT scan is multiple ill-defined hypodense lesions in the basal ganglia or thalamus with moderate to marked peripheral edema **(14-17A)**.

MR shows a T1-hypointense mass that occasionally demonstrates mild peripheral hyperintensity caused by coagulative necrosis or hemorrhage. T2WI and FLAIR may exhibit a pattern of concentric zones of hypointensity and hyperintensity **(14-17B)**.

One or more nodular and ring-enhancing masses are typical on T1 C+ **(14-17B)**. A ring-shaped zone of peripheral enhancement with a small, eccentric mural nodule represents the so-called **eccentric target sign** **(14-17C)** and can be identified in approximately 1/3 of cases. The enhancing nodule is a collection of concentrically thickened vessels, whereas the rim enhancement is caused by an inflamed vascular zone that borders the necrotic abscess cavity.

The major differential diagnosis is **primary CNS lymphoma** (PCNSL). Solitary toxo lesions are uncommon; most cases present with multifocal lesions. In contrast, approximately 70% of isolated CNS masses in HIV/AIDS patients are PCNSL **(14-38)**. Mean relative cerebral blood volume (rCBV) in CNS toxo is low (< 1.5) compared to lymphoma. AIDS-related CNS toxo also has positive findings on serology in 80% of cases, and CSF PCR is definitive.

## Cryptococcosis

Fungal infections can be life threatening in immunocompromised patients, especially those with HIV/AIDS. Although many different fungi can cause CNS infection, the most common fungi to affect patients with HIV/AIDS are *Candida albicans*, *Aspergillus* species, and *Cryptococcus neoformans* (crypto). Crypto is the third most common CNS infectious agent in HIV/AIDS patients after HIV and *T. gondii*. Prior to highly active ART (HAART), crypto-CNS

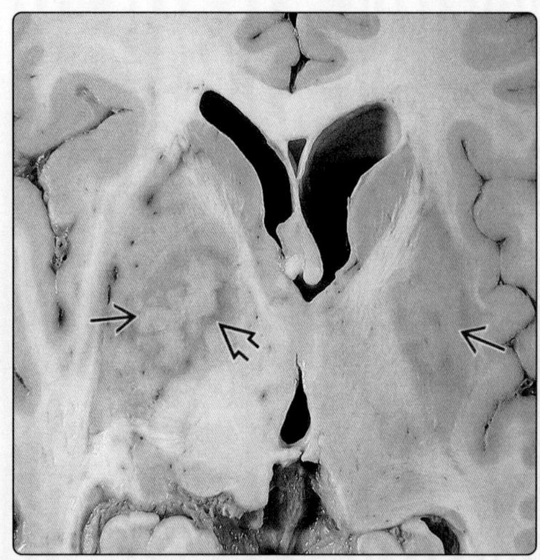

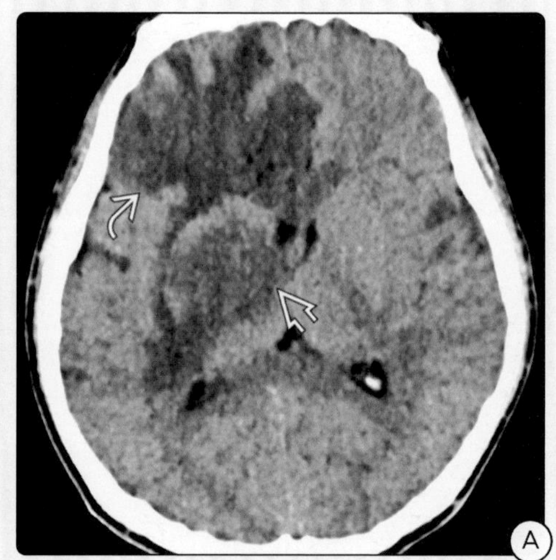


***(14-16) Axial gross pathology from an HIV-positive patient shows ill-defined toxoplasmosis abscesses in both basal ganglia ➡. Note the hemorrhage ➡ surrounding the central necrosis in the right lesion. (Courtesy R. Hewlett, MD.) (14-17A) NECT in a patient with HIV/AIDS and left-sided weakness shows a mostly hypodense mass ➡ in the right basal ganglia. A right frontal mass with significant edema ➡ is also present.***

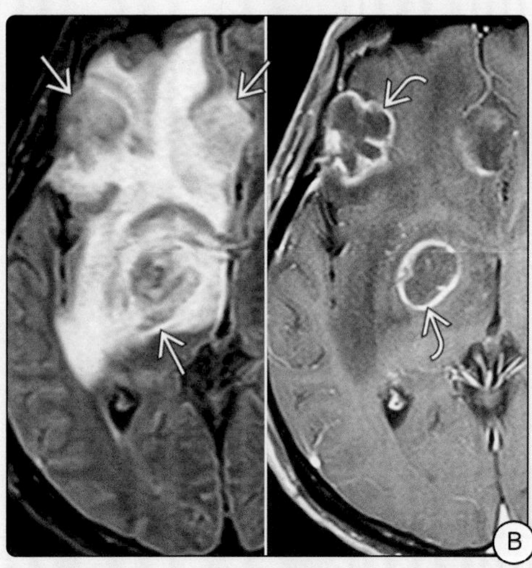


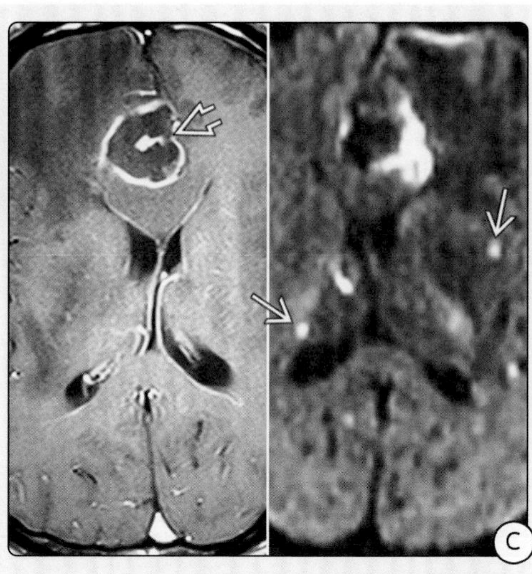


***(14-17B) (L) FLAIR and (R) T1 C+ FS MR images in the same case show 3 separate masses ➡ with confluent surrounding edema, rim enhancement ➡. (14-17C) (L) More cephalad T1 C+ MR shows a classic target sign ➡. (R) DWI MR in the same patient shows multiple small foci of restricted diffusion ➡. Toxoplasmosis is the most common opportunistic infection in patients with HIV/AIDS.***

infections occurred in 10% of HIV patients, but it is now relatively rare in developed countries. Crypto usually occurs when CD4 counts drop below 50-100 cells/µL.

Gelatinous mucoid-like cryptococcal capsular polysaccharides and budding yeast may accumulate within dilated perivascular spaces (PVSs) **(14-18)**, especially in the basal ganglia **(14-19)**, midbrain, dentate nuclei, and subcortical WM **(14-18)**. NECT scans show hypodensity in the basal ganglia. Cryptococcal gelatinous pseudocysts **(14-20)** are hypointense to brain on T1WI and very hyperintense on T2WI **(14-21)**. The lesions generally follow CSF signal intensity and suppress on FLAIR. Perilesional edema is generally absent. Lack of enhancement on T1 C+ is typical, although mild pial enhancement is sometimes observed.

The differential diagnosis includes **prominent PVSs**. Enlarged PVSs do not enhance. In HIV/AIDS patients with CD4 counts under 20, symmetrically enlarged PVSs should be considered cryptococcal infection and treated as such. **Toxoplasmosis** usually has multifocal ring- or target-like enhancing lesions with significant surrounding edema. **TB** usually demonstrates strong enhancement in the basal meninges. Tuberculomas are generally hypointense on T2WI. **PCNSL** in HIV/AIDS patients often shows hemorrhage, necrosis, and ring enhancement. Solitary lesions are more common than multifocal involvement.

## Progressive Multifocal Leukoencephalopathy

Progressive multifocal leukoencephalopathy (PML) is an opportunistic infection caused by the JC virus (JCV), a member of the Papovaviridae family. JCV is a ubiquitous virus that circulates widely. More than 85% of the adult population worldwide has antibodies against JCV. Asymptomatic infection is probably acquired in childhood or adolescence and remains latent until the virus is reactivated.

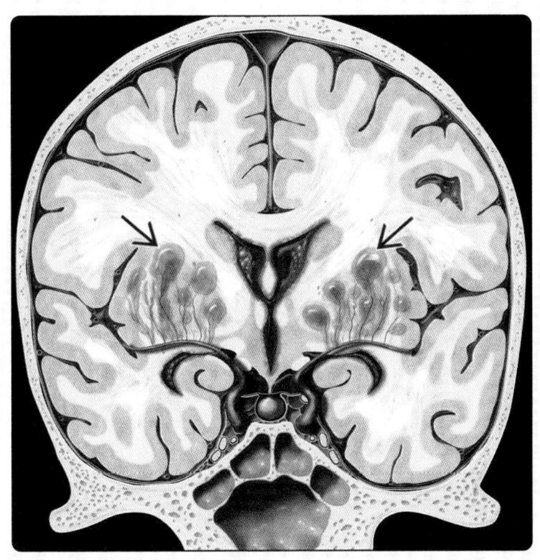

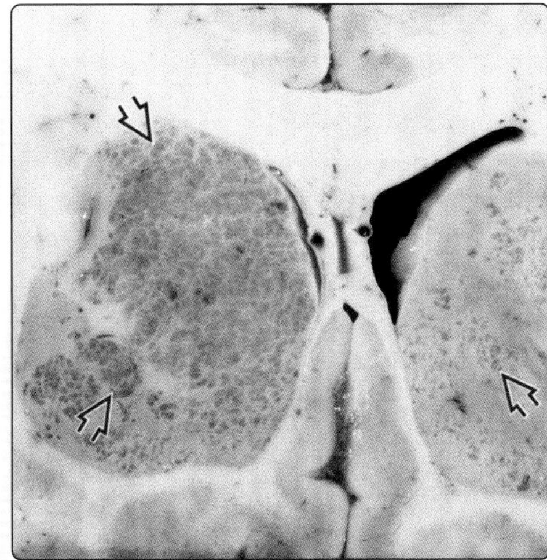

***(14-18)** Coronal graphic shows multiple dilated perivascular spaces ⇒ filled with gelatinous mucoid-appearing material, characteristic of cryptococcal infection in HIV/AIDS patients. **(14-19)** Coronal autopsied brain in HIV/AIDS shows innumerable tiny cryptococcal gelatinous pseudocysts in the basal ganglia ⇒. (Courtesy A. T. Yachnis, Neuropathology, 2014.)*

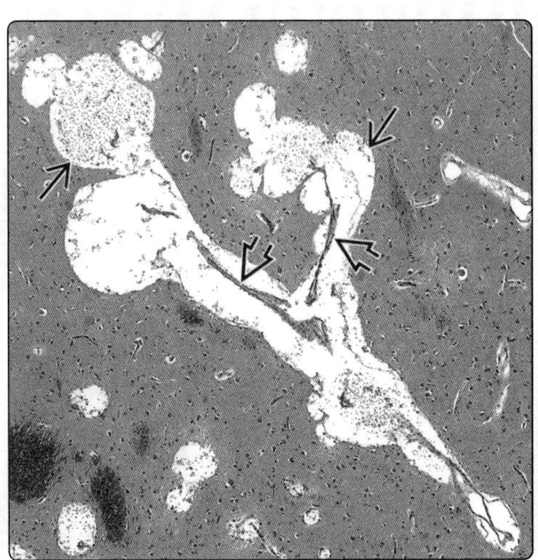

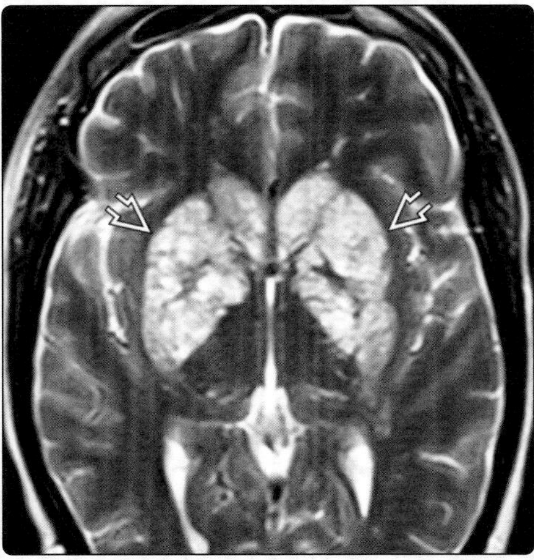

***(14-20)** Photomicrograph shows a branching vessel cut in a longitudinal section ⇒ and surrounded by enlarged perivascular spaces stuffed full of cryptococcal gelatinous pseudocysts ⇒. (Courtesy B. K. DeMasters, MD.) **(14-21)** T2 MR shows lentiform and caudate nuclei are grossly expanded by innumerable hyperintense cysts ⇒, characteristic of cryptococcal gelatinous pseudocysts. (Courtesy N. Omar, MD.)*

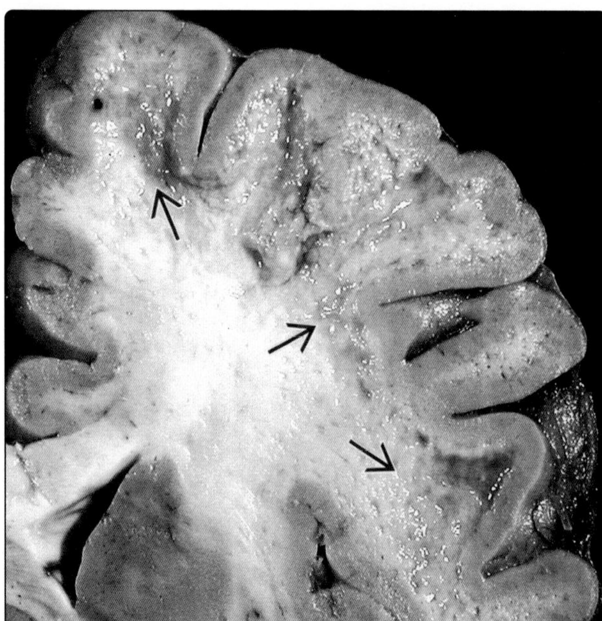

***(14-22) Autopsied case shows PML as distinctly spongy-appearing, punched-out, coalescent WM lesions ⇒ that spare the cortex. (Courtesy B. K. DeMasters, MD.)***

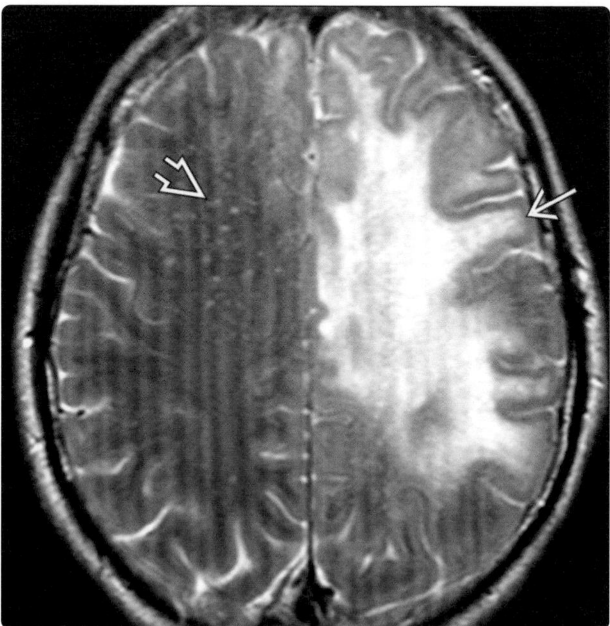

***(14-23) T2 MR in HIV/AIDS shows confluent hyperintensity in the left hemisphere that extends from the corona radiata into the subcortical WM ➡. Note punctate hyperintense foci in the right hemisphere ➡ (Milky Way sign). This is PML.***

Pathologically, early lesions appear as small, yellow-tan, round to ovoid foci at the GM-WM junction. The cortex remains normal. With lesion coalescence, large, spongy-appearing depressions in the cerebral and cerebellar WM appear **(14-22)**.

Imaging plays a key role in the diagnosis and follow-up of JCV infections. Classic PML (cPML) can appear as solitary or multifocal widespread lesions. Any area of the brain can be affected, although the supratentorial lobar WM is the most commonly affected site. The posterior fossa WM—especially the middle cerebellar peduncles—is the second most common location. In occasional cases, a solitary lesion in the subcortical U-fibers is present.

More than 90% of cPML cases show hypodense areas in the subcortical and deep periventricular WM on NECT; 70% are multifocal. Extent varies from small, scattered subcortical foci to large, bilateral but asymmetric confluent WM lesions. In the early acute stage of infection, some mass effect with focal gyral expansion can be present. At later stages, encephaloclastic changes with atrophy and volume loss predominate. PML lesions generally do not enhance on CECT.

MR is the imaging procedure of choice in suspected PML. Multifocal, bilateral but asymmetric, irregularly shaped hypointensities on T1WI are typical. The lesions are heterogeneously hyperintense on T2WI **(14-23)** and typically extend into the subcortical U-fibers all the way to the undersurface of the cortex, which remains intact even in advanced disease. Smaller, almost microcyst-like, very hyperintense foci within and around the slightly less hyperintense confluent lesions represent the characteristic spongy lesions seen in more advanced PML.

Appearance on DWI varies according to disease stage. In newly active lesions, DWI restricts strongly. Slightly older lesions show a central core with low signal intensity and high mean diffusivity (MD) surrounded by a rim of higher signal intensity and lower MD **(14-25)**. Chronic, "burned-out" lesions show increased diffusion due to disorganized cellular architecture.

cPML generally does not enhance on T1 C+ scans, although faint, peripheral rim-like enhancement occurs in 5% of all cases. The exception is hyperacute PML in the setting of IRIS and in multiple sclerosis (MS) patients on natalizumab. In these cases, striking foci with irregular rim enhancement are frequently—but not invariably—present. Peripheral enhancement &/or mass effect decrease with corticosteroids.

The major differential diagnosis of cPML is **HIV encephalitis (HIVE)**. HIVE demonstrates more symmetric WM disease while sparing the subcortical U-fibers. **IRIS** is usually more acute and demonstrates strong but irregular, ring-like enhancement.

## Cytomegalovirus

CNS cytomegalovirus (CMV) is a late-onset disease in immunocompromised patients. With increasing use of HAART, < 2% of HIV/AIDS patients develop overt symptoms of CMV infection.

Acquired CMV in the setting of HIV/AIDS most commonly manifests as meningoencephalitis **(14-26)** and ventriculitis/ependymitis. Typical imaging findings are those of underlying HIVE (atrophy, "hazy" WM disease) with ependymal enhancement around the lateral ventricles **(14-27)**.

## Tuberculosis

TB is one of the most devastating co-infections in immunocompromised patients and is the main cause of morbidity and mortality in HIV-infected patients worldwide.

HIV is the most powerful known risk factor for reactivation of latent TB to active disease. HIV patients who are co-infected with TB have 100x increased risk of developing active TB. In turn, TB co-infection exacerbates the severity and accelerates the progression of HIV.

Patients with prior TB who become HIV positive may also reactivate their disease with old calcified tuberculomas developing new surrounding edema and mass effect **(14-28)**. In severely immunocompromised HIV patients with especially low CD4 counts, fulminant reactivated TB may develop multiple ring-enhancing pseudoabscesses **(14-29)**.

## Immune Reconstitution Inflammatory Syndrome

### Terminology

CNS immune reconstitution inflammatory syndrome (IRIS) is a T-cell-mediated encephalitis that occurs in the setting of treated HIV or autoimmune disease (e.g., MS). CNS IRIS is also called neuro-IRIS. The diagnosis of IRIS is based on evidence of clinical worsening and immune reconstitution in the setting of antiretroviral therapy (ART) initiation.

### Etiology

Most investigators consider neuro-IRIS a dysregulated immune response and pathogen-driven disease whose clinical expression depends on host susceptibility, the intensity and quality of the immune response, and the specific characteristics of the "provoking pathogen" itself.

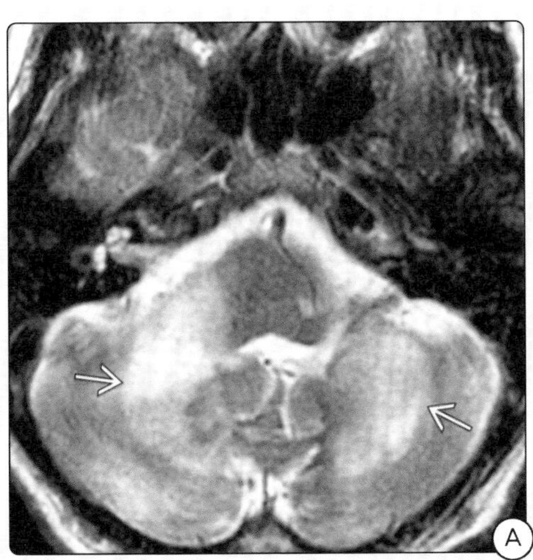


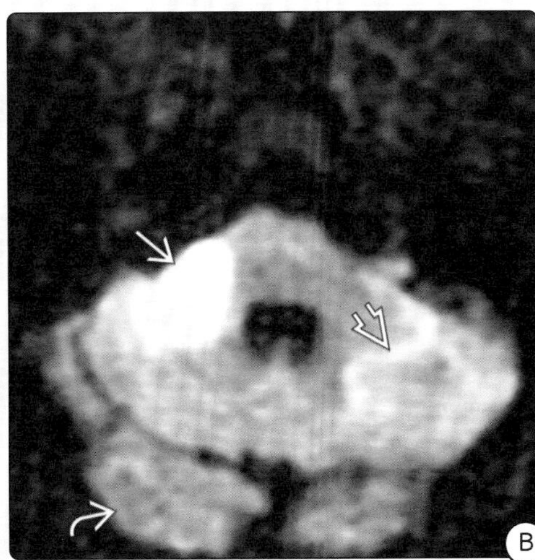


***(14-25A)** T2 MR in HIV/AIDS shows classic cerebellar PML with characteristic involvement of both middle cerebellar peduncles ➡. **(14-25B)** DWI MR in the same patient shows classic PML in different stages. The right posterior cerebellar lesion ➡ shows no restriction, the right middle cerebellar peduncle lesion ➡ restricts strongly and uniformly, and the left cerebellar lesion shows restriction around the lesion's rim ➡.*

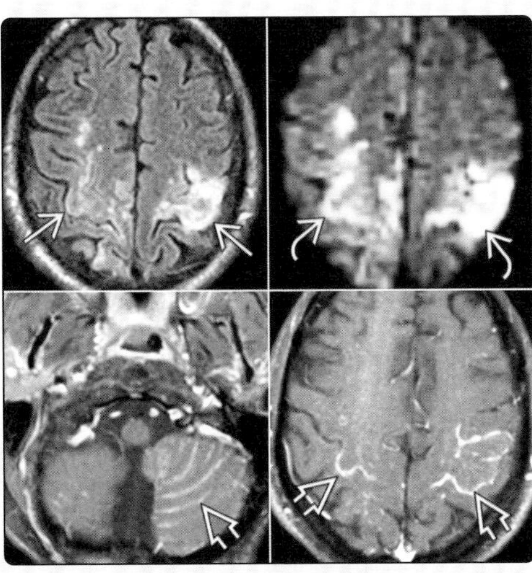

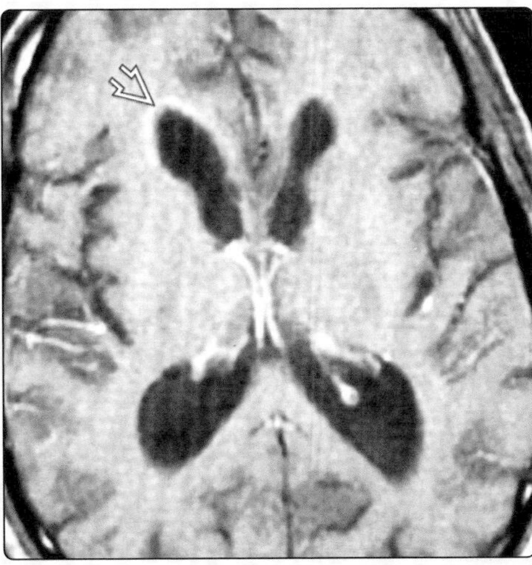

***(14-26)** MR was obtained in a 32-yo HIV-positive man with acute CMV meningoencephalitis. FLAIR shows hyperintensity in both posterior frontal lobes ➡ that restricts on DWI ➡. T1 C+ MR images show pial enhancement ➡. **(14-27)** T1 C+ MR in a patient with HIVE shows generalized volume loss. Note striking ependymal enhancement ➡, atypical for HIVE. This is CMV ventriculitis.*

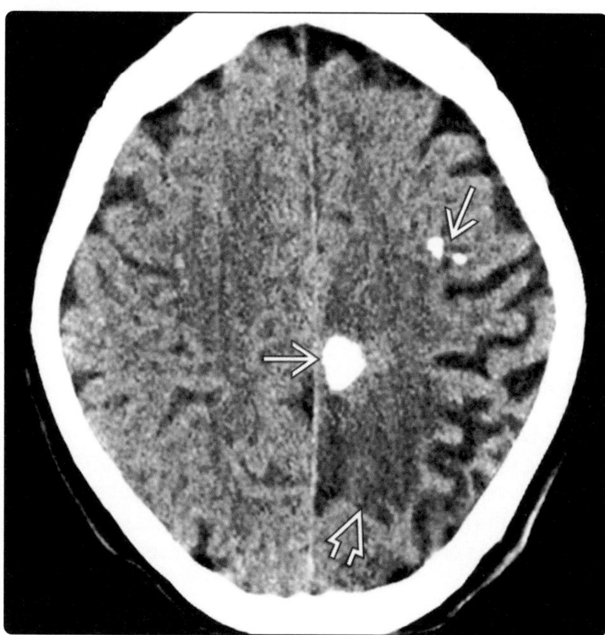

*(14-28) A 30-yo HIV-positive, TB-positive man treated with HAART developed increasing right-sided weakness. NECT shows multiple old calcified granulomas ➡. Note edema surrounding the larger lesion ➡. This is reactivation of latent TB.*

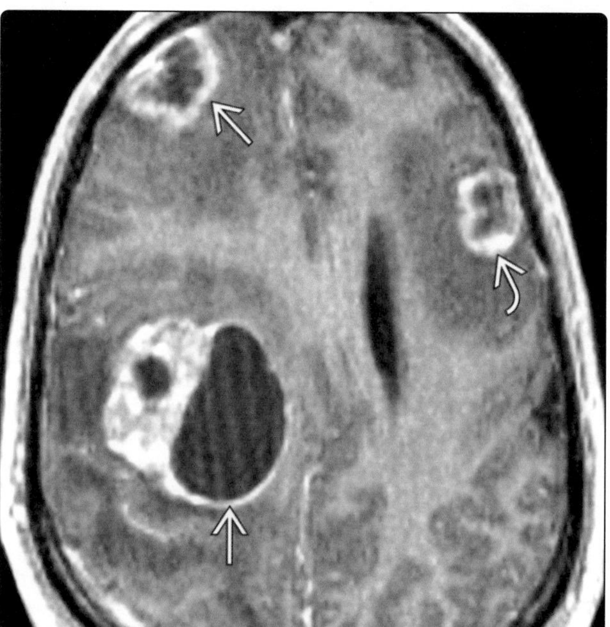

*(14-29) HIV-positive man with a CD4 count < 50 had rapidly decreasing mental status. T1 C+ shows multiple rim-enhancing masses that were both granulomas ➡ and pseudoabscess ➡. This is fulminant reactivated TB. (Courtesy S. Candy, MD.)*

IRIS occurs when forced immune reconstitution causes an exaggerated response to infectious (or sometimes noninfectious) antigens with massive destruction of virus-infected cells. IRIS develops in two distinct scenarios: "Unmasking" IRIS and "paradoxical" IRIS. Both differ in clinical expression, disease management, and prognosis, although their imaging manifestations are similar.

**"Unmasking" IRIS** occurs when ART reveals a subclinical, previously undiagnosed opportunistic infection. Immune restoration leads to an immune response against a living pathogen. Here, brain parenchyma is damaged by both the replicating pathogen and the incited immune response.

**"Paradoxical" IRIS** occurs when a patient who has been successfully treated for a recent opportunistic infection unexpectedly deteriorates after initiation of ART. Here, there is no newly acquired or reactivated infection. The recovering immune response targets persistent pathogen-derived antigens or self-antigens and causes tissue damage.

Several different underlying pathogens have been identified with IRIS. The most common are JCV (PML-IRIS), TB (TB-IRIS), and fungal infections, especially *Cryptococcus* (crypto-IRIS). Some parasitic infections—such as toxoplasmosis—are relatively common in HIV/AIDS patients but rarely associated with IRIS.

Not all neurotropic viruses cause IRIS. HIV itself rarely causes neuro-IRIS. Herpesviruses (e.g., herpes simplex virus, varicella-zoster virus, CMV) are all rarely reported causes of neuro-IRIS.

An unusual type of IRIS occurs in MS patients treated with natalizumab who subsequently develop PML. Natalizumab-related PML is managed by discontinuation of the drug and instituting plasmapheresis/immunoadsorption (PLEX/IA). Neurologic deficits and imaging studies in some patients worsen during subsequent immune reconstitution, causing **natalizumab-associated PML-IRIS**. Two types are recognized: Patients with early PML-IRIS (IRIS develops **before** institution of PLEX/IA) and patients with late PML-IRIS (IRIS develops **after** treatment with PLEX/IA). Neurologic outcome is generally worse in early PML-IRIS with a mortality rate approaching 25%.

## Pathology

There are no specific histologic features or biomarkers for neuro-IRIS; rather, the diagnosis is established on the basis of clinical manifestations, exclusion of other disorders, and imaging or histopathologic evidence of inflammatory reaction.

## Clinical Issues

**Epidemiology.** Between 15-35% of AIDS patients beginning ART develop IRIS. Of these, ~ 1% develop neuro-IRIS. The two most important risk factors are a low CD4 count and a short time interval between treatment of the underlying infection and the commencement of ART. The highest risk is in patients with a count < 50 cells/μL.

While CNS IRIS is thought to be prevalent in resource-limited settings, its identification is constrained by limited data on pretreatment HIV disease and diagnostic testing.

Epidemiology varies according to the specific "provoking pathogen." The most common cause of neuro-IRIS is JCV. Latent virus is reactivated when patients become immunodeficient. The reactivated virus infects oligodendrocytes, causing the lytic demyelination characteristic of PML. Nearly 1/3 of patients with preexisting

PML worsen after beginning HAART and are considered to have "unmasking" **PML-IRIS.**

**TB-IRIS** occurs in 15-18% of patients who are co-infected with TB-HIV if ART is initiated before the TB is adequately treated. Significant increase in CD4 count between ART initiation and IRIS onset supports the diagnosis of IRIS. Almost 20% of TB-IRIS patients develop neurologic involvement characterized by meningitis, tuberculomas, and radiculomyelopathies. TB-IRIS is associated with a mortality rate of up to 30%. Corticosteroids remain the only trial-supported therapy for prevention and management of TB-IRIS.

"Paradoxical" **crypto-IRIS** affects 20% of HIV-infected patients in whom ART was initiated after treatment of neuromeningeal cryptococcosis. The major manifestation of crypto neuro-IRIS is aseptic recurrent meningitis. Parenchymal cryptococcomas are rare.

Despite the high prevalence of parasitic infestations in resource-poor countries, only a few cases of parasite-associated neuro-IRIS have been reported. All have been caused by *T. gondii.*

**Natalizumab-associated IRIS** is rare. To date, ~ 50 cases have been reported. Most are PML-IRIS.

**Presentation.** Neuro-IRIS is a polymorphic condition with heterogeneous clinical manifestations. The most common presentation is clinical deterioration of a newly treated HIV-positive patient despite rising CD4 counts and diminishing viral loads.

**Natural History and Treatment Options.** Given that a low CD4 T-cell count is a major risk factor for developing IRIS, starting HAART at a count of > 350 cells/μL will prevent most cases.

Systemic IRIS is usually mild and self-limited. Prognosis in neuro-IRIS is variable. Corticosteroids and cytokine neutralization therapy have been used for treatment of neuro-IRIS with mixed results and are controversial.

Patients with neuro-IRIS may die within days to weeks. Mortality from PML-IRIS exceeds 40%, whereas that of crypto-IRIS is ~ 20%. TB-IRIS mortality is slightly lower (13%).

## Imaging

A widespread pattern of confluent and linear or "punctate" perivascular hyperintensities on T2/FLAIR is virtually pathognomonic of PML-IRIS. A punctate pattern of enhancement is typical in the acute stage **(14-31)**.

Bizarre-looking parenchymal masses and progressively enlarging lesions can also occur in PML-IRIS. A rind of restricted diffusion and incomplete enhancement likely represent fulminant virus-induced demyelination **(14-32)**.

**IMMUNE RECONSTITUTION INFLAMMATORY SYNDROME**

**Terminology and Etiology**

- Neuro-IRIS
  - "Unmasking" IRIS (HAART "unmasks" existing subclinical opportunistic infection)
  - "Paradoxical" IRIS (treated infection worsens after HAART)
- Pathogens associated with neuro-IRIS
  - JC virus (PML-IRIS) most common
  - TB (TB-IRIS) next most common
  - Fungi (crypto-IRIS)
  - Drugs (natalizumab-associated PML-IRIS)
  - Parasites (rare, except for toxo-IRIS)
  - Neurotropic viruses (e.g., HIV, herpesviruses) rarely cause IRIS

**Epidemiology**

- 15-35% of AIDS patients starting HAART develop IRIS
- Of these, 1% develop neuro-IRIS
- CD4 count < 50 cells/μL = sharply increased risk of IRIS

**Imaging**

- Punctate pattern of T2/FLAIR hyperintensities
  - Punctate pattern of enhancement on T1 C+
- Confluent disease extending into subcortical U-fibers
  - Variable mass-like enhancement, often bizarre and "wild"

**Differential Diagnosis**

- Non-IRIS-associated opportunistic infections
- AIDS-defining malignancies
  - Especially lymphoma

## Differential Diagnosis

The major imaging differential diagnosis of neuro-IRIS is **non-IRIS-associated opportunistic infection**. Contrast enhancement in combination with mass effect is more typical of IRIS but may be absent early in the disease course.

# Neoplasms in HIV/AIDS

In HIV-positive patients, both Epstein-Barr virus (EBV) and human herpesvirus-8 [HHV-8 a.k.a. Kaposi sarcoma-associated herpesvirus (KSHV)] have been implicated in the development of a wide range of tumors.

EBV is associated with several malignancies, including Hodgkin and non-Hodgkin (NHL) lymphomas. EBV plays an especially prominent role in the development of lymphoma in patients with HIV or transplant-related immunosuppression.

KSHV-associated diseases include Kaposi sarcoma (KS), primary effusion lymphoma, and multicentric Castleman disease.

**AIDS-defining malignancies** (ADMs) include NHLs, KS, and cervical cancer. The introduction of antiretroviral therapy (ART) has dramatically modified the natural history of HIV infection, causing a marked decline in the incidence of ADMs.

In the United States and Europe, ADMs peaked in the mid-1990s and have since declined substantially. Recent statistics from South Africa show that if ART is started before advanced immunodeficiency develops, the cancer burden in HIV-positive patients (especially children) can be substantially reduced.

Recent epidemiologic studies have also demonstrated that non-AIDS-defining cancers are an increasingly important cause of morbidity and mortality in patients living with HIV. Deaths from non-AIDS-defining cancers now substantially exceed those attributable to AIDS-defining cancers (9% vs. 5%).

In this text, we briefly discuss the two ADMs that can affect the scalp, skull, and brain: Primary CNS lymphomas (PCNSLs) and KS.

## AIDS-Related Lymphomas

NHLs are the most common ADMs in the CNS and represent the majority of all AIDS-defining cancers, even though they have become less common with the introduction of HAART.

AIDS-related PCNSLs are classified as immunodeficiency-associated CNS lymphomas in the 2021 WHO. Most are EBV related and are the diffuse large B-cell NHL type. Malignancy risk is linked to the patient's immune status and increases with CD4 counts < 50-100 cells/μL.

PCNSLs are the second most common cerebral mass lesion in AIDS (exceeded only by toxoplasmosis) and develop in 2-6% of patients. PCNSLs cause ~ 70% of all **solitary** brain parenchymal lesions in HIV/AIDS patients.

PCNSLs present as single or (less commonly) multiple masses. Multiple lesions and areas of necrosis occur more frequently in immunodeficiency-associated lymphomas than in CNS

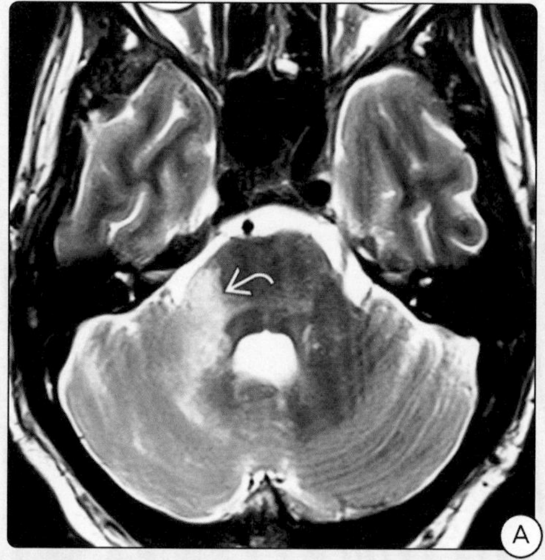


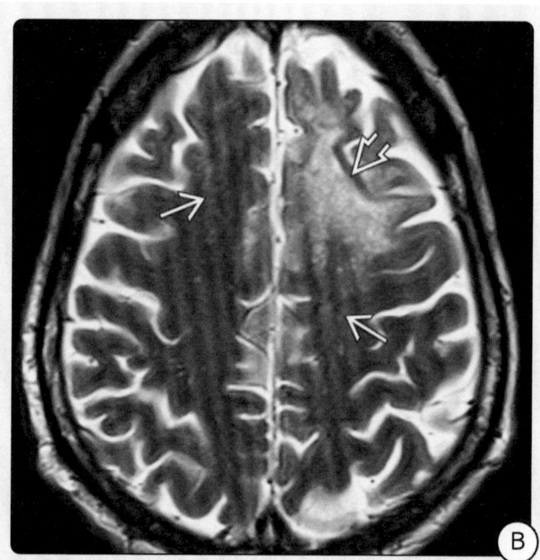


***(14-31A)** Baseline T2 MR in a 40-yo man with untreated HIV/AIDS for 8 years shows a hyperintense, expansile mass in the right cerebellar peduncle ➡. **(14-31B)** More cephalad T2 MR shows diffuse volume loss and bifrontal hyperintense subcortical WM lesions with both patchy confluent ➡ and round ➡ "punctate" lesions. None of the lesions enhanced on T1 C+ MR.*

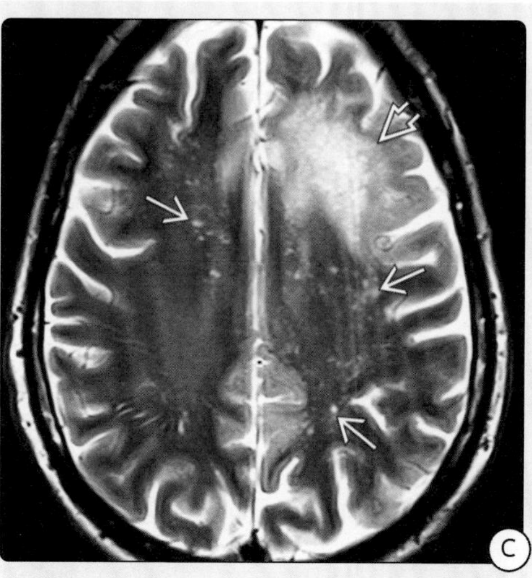


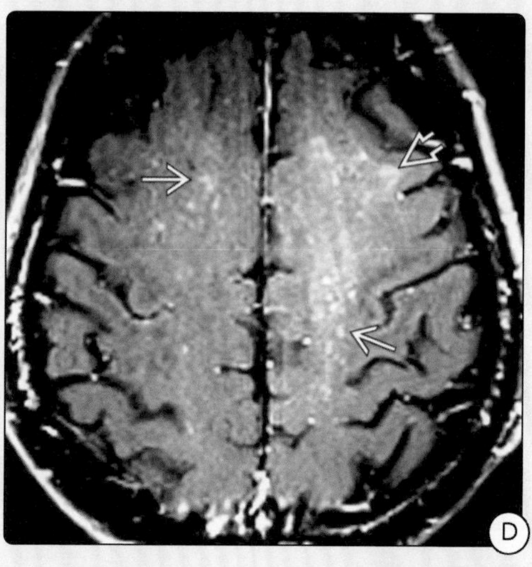


***(14-31C)** The patient deteriorated 5 weeks after beginning ART. Repeat T2 MR shows enlargement of the confluent left frontal lesion ➡ with interval appearance of innumerable punctate hyperintensities ➡ scattered throughout the subcortical and deep WM of both hemispheres. **(14-31D)** T1 C+ FS MR shows that the confluent ➡ and punctate lesions ➡ enhance in a starry-sky pattern. CSF was positive for JC virus. This is PML-IRIS.*

lymphoma of immunocompetent patients. More than 90% are supratentorial with preferential location in the basal ganglia and deep WM abutting the lateral ventricle. PCNSLs often cross the corpus callosum. Central necrosis and hemorrhage are common in AIDS-related lymphomas **(14-34)**, which is reflected in the imaging findings **(14-36)** **(14-37)**.

The major differential diagnosis is **toxoplasmosis**, which can appear similar even in autopsy cases **(14-35)**. Toxoplasmosis is more commonly multiple, and lesions often exhibit the eccentric target sign, i.e., an eccentrically located nodule within a ring-enhancing mass **(14-17C)**. DSC-pMR is helpful in distinguishing PCNSL from toxoplasmosis; lymphoma has typically increased relative cerebral blood volume (rCBV), whereas toxoplasmosis does not. $^{18}$F-FDG PET/CT and SPECT are also helpful imaging adjuncts, as lymphoma is "hot" but toxo is "not."

## Kaposi Sarcoma

KS is the most common sarcoma in immunosuppressed patients. The next most frequent non-KS sarcoma is leiomyosarcoma followed by angiosarcoma and fibrohistiocytic tumors.

KS develops from a combination of factors: HHV-8 infection (a.k.a. KS-associated herpesvirus), altered immunity, and an inflammatory or angiogenic milieu. EBV infection is common in patients with HIV-associated leiomyosarcomas.

There has been a marked decline in the incidence of AIDS-related KS since the advent of ART. Transplant-related KS often resolves after reduction of immunosuppression, highlighting the role of cellular immune response in the control of HHV-8 infection.

KS is the most common neoplasm in untreated AIDS patients. Overall, the most common site is the skin **(14-39)** followed by

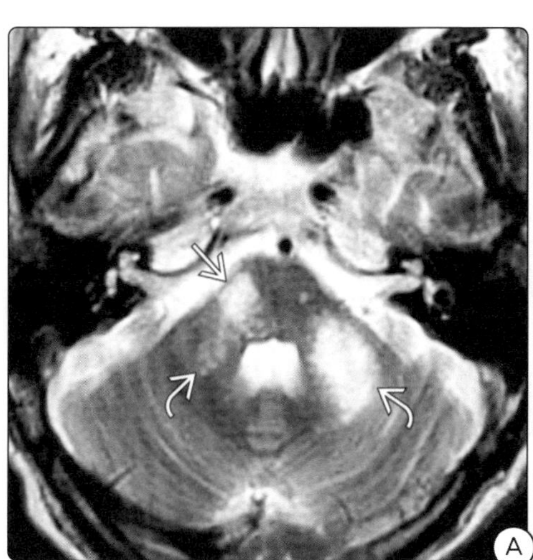


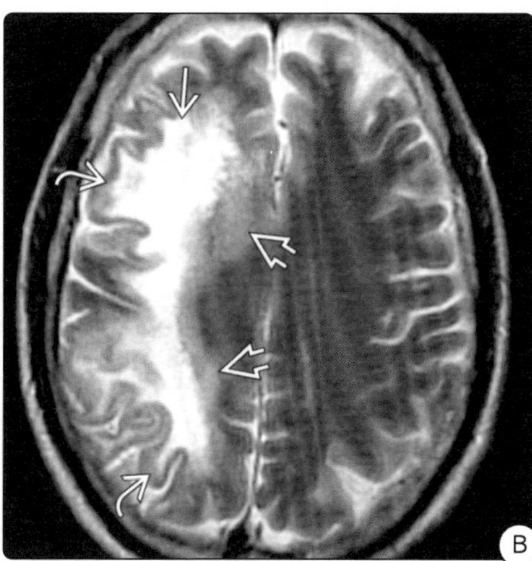


***(14-33A)** Axial T2 MR in a 56-yo man with HIV/AIDS who deteriorated 8 weeks after HAART shows patchy hyperintense lesions in the pons ➡ and major cerebellar peduncles ➡. **(14-33B)** More cephalad T2 MR through the corona radiata shows a confluent hyperintense lesion ➡ surrounded by "hazy," less hyperintensity ➡ in the right cerebral hemisphere. Note involvement of the subcortical U-fibers ➡.*

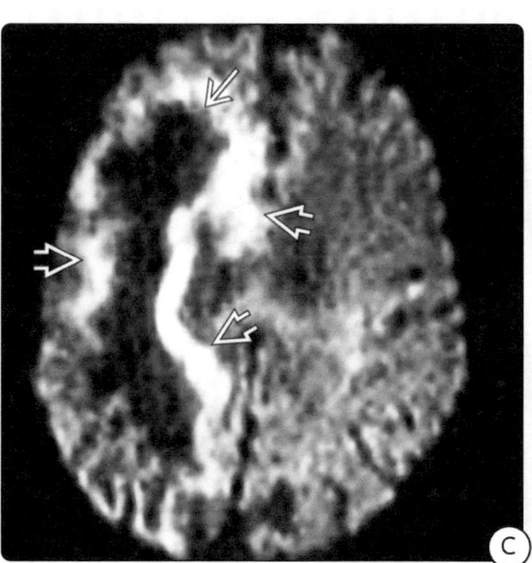


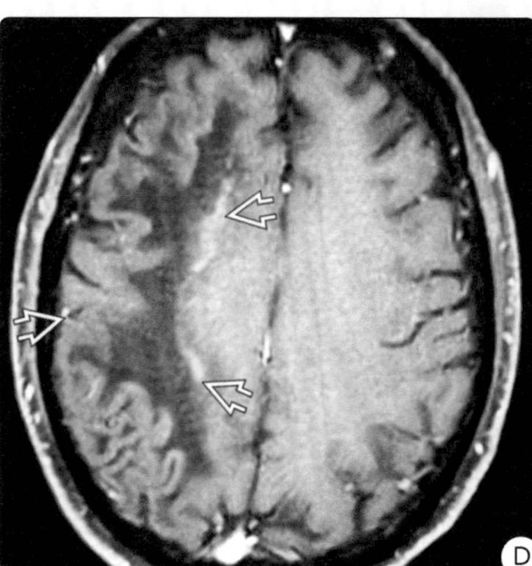


***(14-33C)** DWI MR in the same patient shows a central area of T2 "black out" ➡ surrounded by an irregular area of restricted diffusion ➡ along the periphery of the lesion. **(14-33D)** More cephalad T1 C+ FS MR shows additional areas of strong contrast enhancement ➡. CSF PCR was positive for JC virus, so the imaging diagnosis of PML-IRIS was confirmed.*

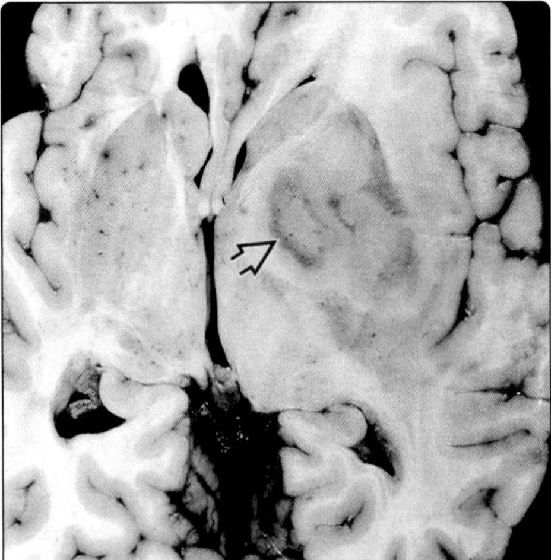

*(14-34) Autopsied AIDS-related PCNSL shows a solitary basal ganglia mass with central necrosis and peripheral hemorrhage ⇒.*

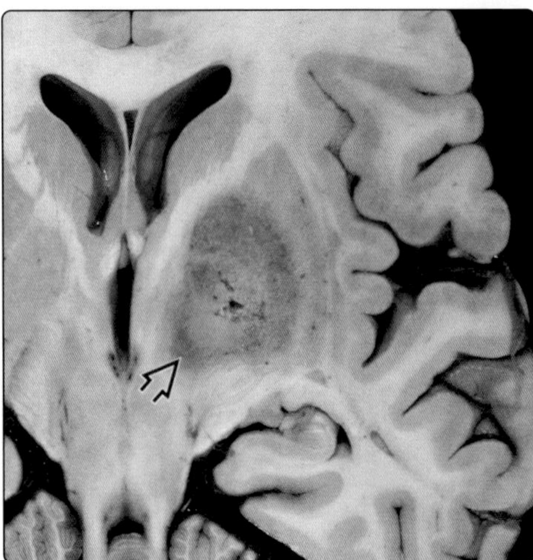

*(14-35) Autopsy shows basal ganglia lesion ⇒ in proven toxoplasmosis. Note resemblance to DLBCL (Fig. 14-34). (Courtesy B. Horten, MD.)*

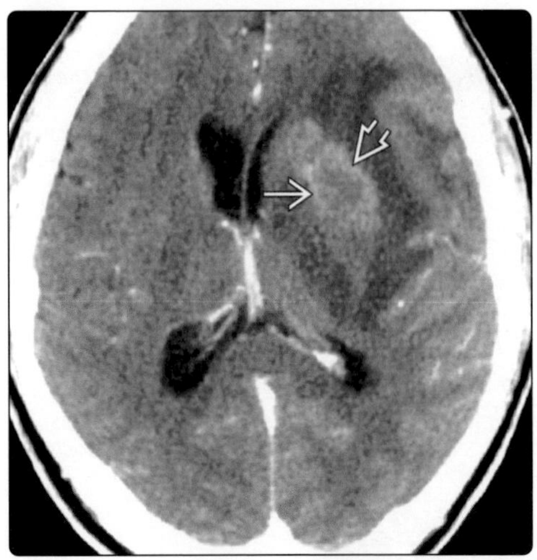

*(14-36) CECT in an HIV-positive patient shows a solitary basal ganglia mass ➡ with mild rim enhancement ➡. Biopsy disclosed PCNSL.*

mucous membranes, lymph nodes, and viscera. Classic KS is an indolent tumor with purplish or dark brown plaques and nodules, usually on the extremities. AIDS-associated KS is much more aggressive. Lesions most commonly occur on the face, genitals, and mucous membranes.

Cranial KS is unusual and much less common than CNS lymphoma. When it occurs, cranial KS is typically seen as a localized scalp thickening **(14-40)** or an infiltrating soft tissue mass in the skin of the face and neck. Calvarial invasion is unusual. KS is isointense with muscle on T1WI, hyperintense on T2WI, and enhances strongly on CECT or T1 C+ MR.

### AIDS-DEFINING MALIGNANCIES

**HIV-Associated Lymphoma**

- Etiology and pathology
  - Often associated with EBV
  - Most are diffuse large B-cell NHL type
- Clinical issues
  - 2nd most common mass lesion in AIDS
  - Occurs in 2-6% of HIV/AIDS patients
  - 70% of solitary CNS masses in HIV(+) patients
  - Multiple lesions more common compared to immunocompetent patients
- Imaging
  - Hemorrhage, necrosis common
  - Supratentorial (90%)
  - Basal ganglia, deep WM (often crosses corpus callosum)
  - Often ring enhancing
  - Increased rCBV

**Kaposi Sarcoma**

- Etiology and pathology
  - Associated with HHV-8
  - Most common sarcoma in immunosuppressed
- Clinical issues
  - Antiretrovirals seriously reduce prevalence
  - Skin, mucous membranes, lymph nodes, scalp
- Imaging
  - Localized scalp thickening
  - Infiltrating soft tissue mass in skin of face or neck

*Selected References: The complete reference list is available on the eBooks+ version included with purchase.*

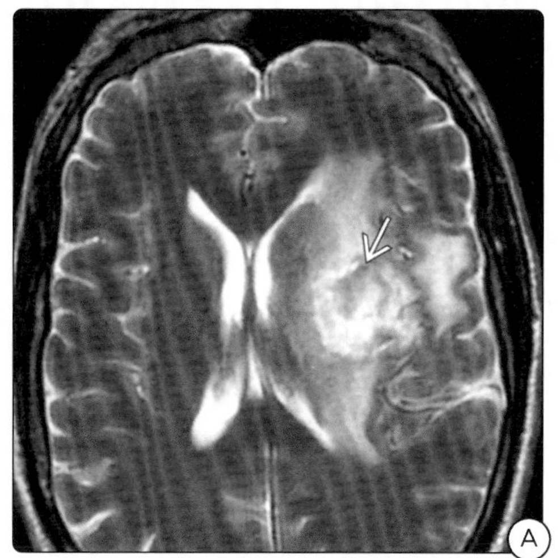

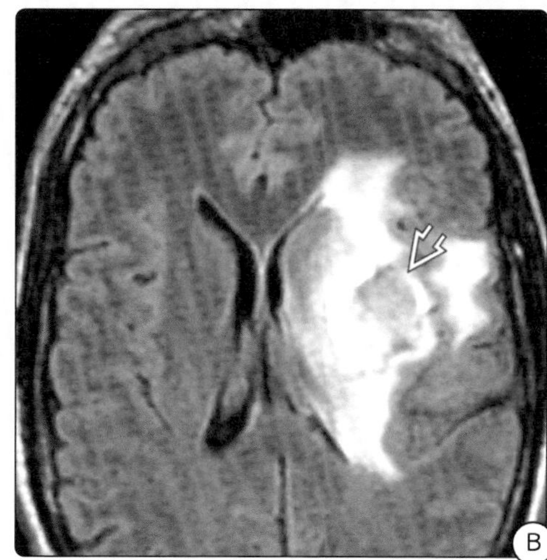

*(14-38A) Axial T2 MR in an HIV/AIDS patient who developed right-sided weakness shows a solitary heterogeneous mass ➡ at the junction of the left basal ganglia and deep WM. (14-38B) The center of the lesion is isointense ➡ with brain on FLAIR MR.*

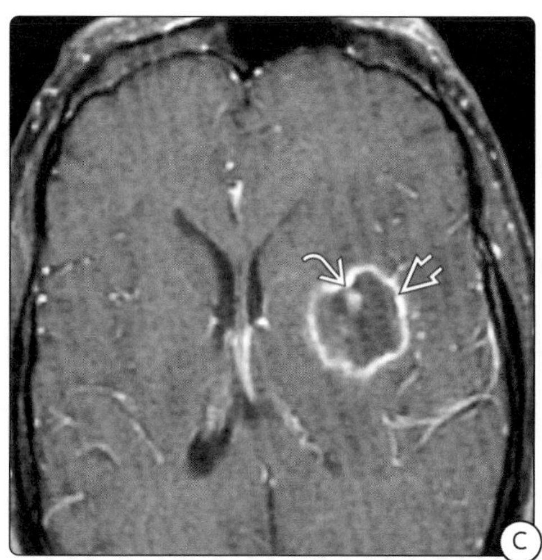

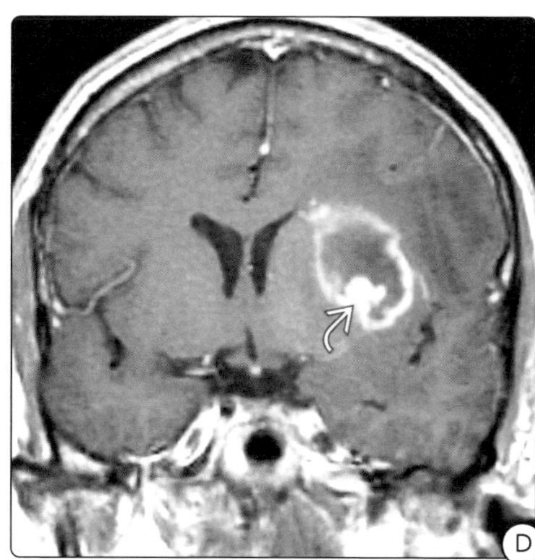

*(14-38C) Axial T1 C+ FS MR shows an irregular rim of enhancement ➡ around the central necrotic area and an eccentric enhancing nodule ➡ within the necrotic mass. (14-38D) Because the coronal T1 C+ MR showed an eccentric target appearance ➡ of the lesion, imaging diagnosis was toxoplasmosis (even though a solitary lesion is statistically more likely to be PCNSL). Anti-toxo therapy was ineffective. Biopsy showed DLBCL.*

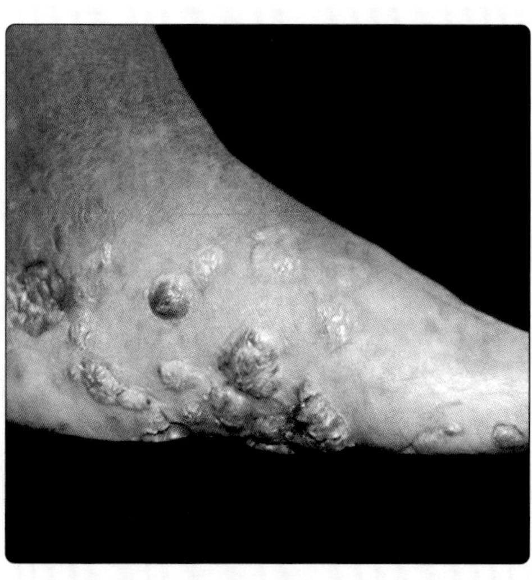

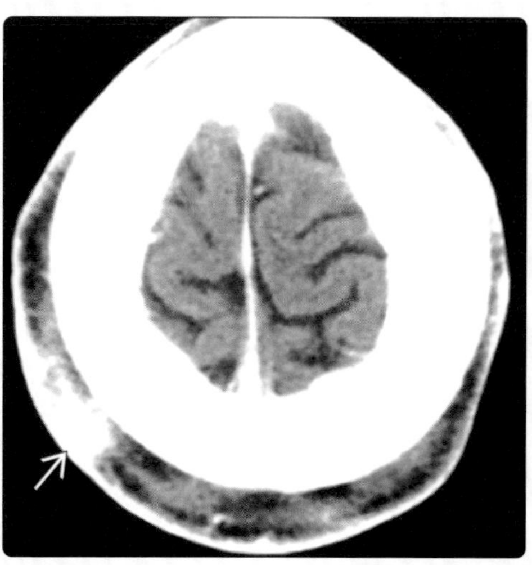

*(14-39) Clinical photograph shows classic Kaposi sarcoma (KS) presenting with multiple nodular skin lesions. (Courtesy T. Mentzel, MD.) (14-40) CECT demonstrates KS of the scalp in this AIDS patient. Note infiltration of the skin and subcutaneous tissues ➡.*

# Demyelinating and Inflammatory Diseases

*Once considered an "immune-privileged" site sequestered beyond the blood-brain barrier, we now know there is active and continuous immunologic surveillance in the CNS. A broad spectrum of noninfectious, inflammatory, autoimmune/autoantibody-mediated disorders can affect the CNS.*



In this chapter, we begin our discussion of autoimmune CNS disorders with **multiple sclerosis** (MS). We follow with a discussion of postinfection and postvaccination inflammatory syndromes, such as **acute disseminated encephalomyelitis** (ADEM). We then discuss the integration of molecular diagnostics into the classification schema with a discussion of antibody-mediated demyelinating diseases, such as **myelin-oligodendrocyte glycoprotein** (MOG) **antibody disease** (MOGAD) and **aquaporin-4** (AQP4) **antibody neuromyelitis optica spectrum disorder** (NMOSD). We then turn our attention to less common inflammatory disorders, such as **autoimmune encephalitis** (AE), an autoantibody-mediated disease, and the rare diagnosis of **acute hemorrhagic leukoencephalitis** (AHLE).

This chapter concludes by discussing uncommon inflammatory-like disorders, such as Susac syndrome (SuS), CLIPPERS, neurosarcoidosis, and idiopathic inflammatory pseudotumors.

## Multiple Sclerosis and Variants

### Multiple Sclerosis

#### Etiology

While the precise pathogenesis of MS remains unknown, the generally accepted hypothesis is that myelin antigens are presented by macrophages, microglia, and astrocytes to T cells. This leads to the release of proinflammatory cytokines and an immune attack on myelin-oligodendrocyte complexes that results in the destruction of myelin, axons, and neurons.

Epstein-Barr virus (EBV) exposure, chemicals, smoking, diet, and geographic variability all contribute to MS risk. MS occurs less often in non-White compared with White patients. MS frequency also increases with increasing latitude and is most common in temperate climates.

#### Pathology

**Location.** Most MS plaques are supratentorial and are primarily (but not exclusively) located in the deep cerebral white matter, oriented perpendicular to the lateral ventricles **(15-5)**. The majority occur at or near the callososeptal interface. Centripetal perivenular extension is common, causing the appearance of so-called Dawson fingers radiating outward from the lateral ventricles **(15-8)**.

Other commonly affected areas include the subcortical U-fibers, brachium pontis, brainstem, and spinal cord **(15-6)**. Gray matter (cortex and basal ganglia) lesions are seen in 10% of cases. Less than 10% occur in the posterior fossa **(15-7)**.

**Gross Pathology.** Acute/subacute MS plaques are linear, round, or ovoid lesions with ill-defined margins. Chronic plaques have more defined borders with excavated, depressed centers.

**Microscopic Features.** Histopathologically, MS plaques typically demonstrate (1) relatively sharp borders **(15-3)**, (2) macrophage infiltrates (both interstitial and perivascular), and (3) perivascular chronic inflammation **(15-4)**. *Acute* lesions are often hypercellular with foamy macrophages and prominent perivascular T-cell lymphocytic cuffing **(15-14)**.

## MULTIPLE SCLEROSIS

**Location**
- Supratentorial (90%), infratentorial (10%) (higher in children)
- Deep cerebral/periventricular white matter
- Predilection for callososeptal interface
- Perivenular extension (Dawson fingers)

**Size and Number**
- Multiple > solitary
- Mostly small (5-10 mm)
- Giant "tumefactive" plaques can be several centimeters
  - 30% of "tumefactive" MS lesions solitary

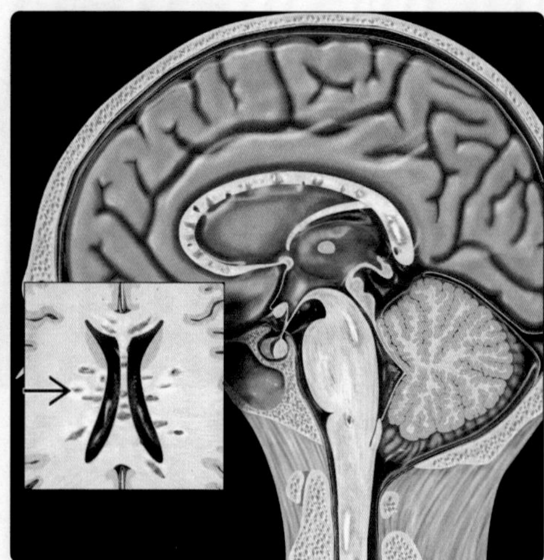

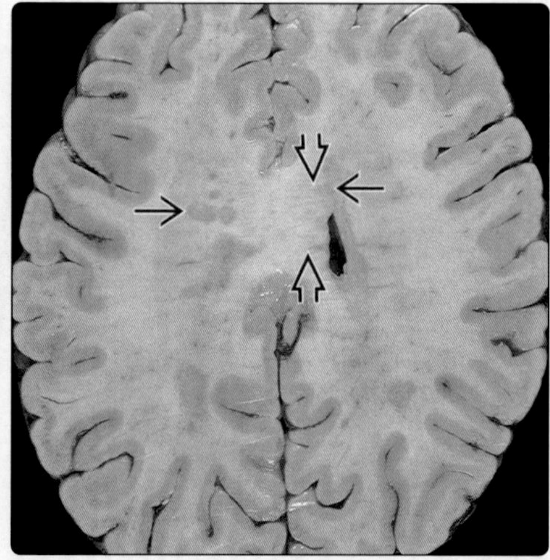

***(15-1)** Sagittal graphic illustrates MS plaques involving the corpus callosum, pons, and spinal cord. Note the characteristic perpendicular orientation of the lesions ➔ at the callososeptal interface along penetrating venules. **(15-2)** Axial autopsy section shows typical ovoid, grayish MS plaques oriented perpendicularly and adjacent to the lateral ventricles ➔, along medullary (deep WM) veins ➩. (Courtesy R. Hewlett, MD.)*

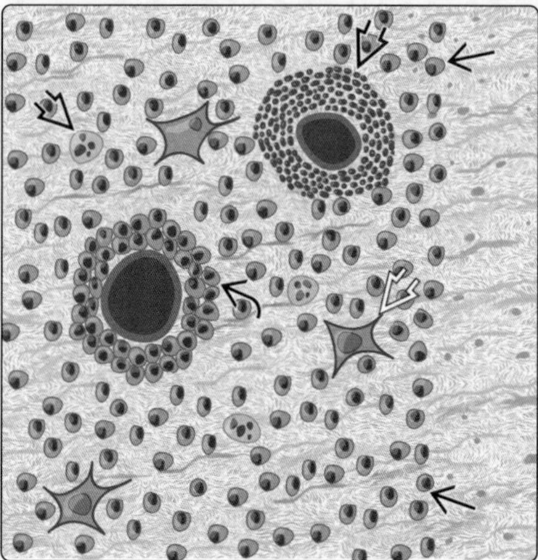

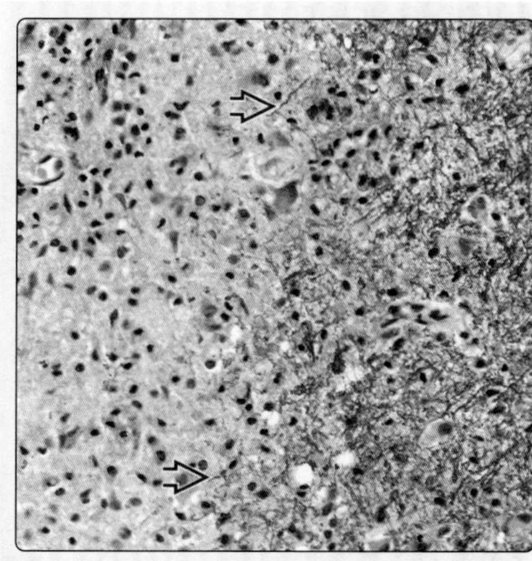

***(15-3)** Graphic of demyelinating plaque shows a sharp border with normal brain ➔ and interstitial and perivascular macrophages ➩. Perivascular chronic inflammation ↗ and scattered stellate reactive astrocytes ➡ are present. **(15-4)** H&E/Luxol fast blue stain of a demyelinating plaque emphasizes sharp interface ➩ between the lesion on the left (pale staining) and normal parenchyma on the right.*

*Chronic* plaques range from chronic active to chronic silent lesions. Chronic active lesions have continuing inflammation around their outer borders. Chronic silent ("burned-out") lesions are characterized by hypocellular regions, myelin loss, absence of active inflammation, and glial scarring.

## Clinical Issues

**Demographics.** MS is the most frequent primary demyelinating pathology in the CNS. Onset typically occurs in young to middle-aged adults from 20-40 years of age. Up to 10% of all patients with MS become symptomatic in childhood.

The overall F:M ratio is 1.77:1.00. White patients of northern European descent living in temperate zones are the most commonly affected ethnic group. MS is significantly less common in Asian and African patients.

**Presentation.** MS presentation varies with heterogeneous neurologic manifestations, evolution, and disability. Intermittent neurologic disturbances followed by progressive accumulation of disabilities are typical.

**Clinical MS Subtypes.** Several major MS subtypes are recognized. From least to most severe, they are radiologically isolated syndrome **(RIS)**, clinically isolated syndrome **(CIS)**, relapsing-remitting MS **(RR-MS)**, relapsing progressive MS **(RP-MS)**, secondary-progressive MS **(SP-MS)**, and primary-progressive MS **(PP-MS)**.

***Radiologically Isolated Syndrome.*** RIS is a new subtype described at the very mildest of the demyelinating disease spectrum. RIS refers to MR findings of T2/FLAIR lesions suggestive of MS in persons with no history of neurologic symptoms and with a normal neurologic examination.

By definition, patients with RIS have dissemination in space (DIS). When a clinical attack occurs in these patients, a

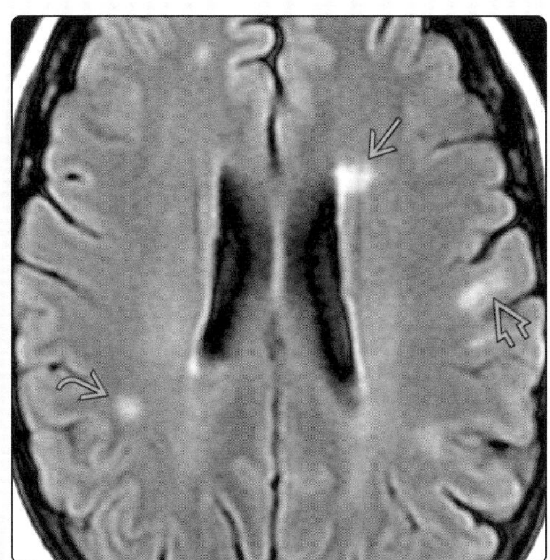

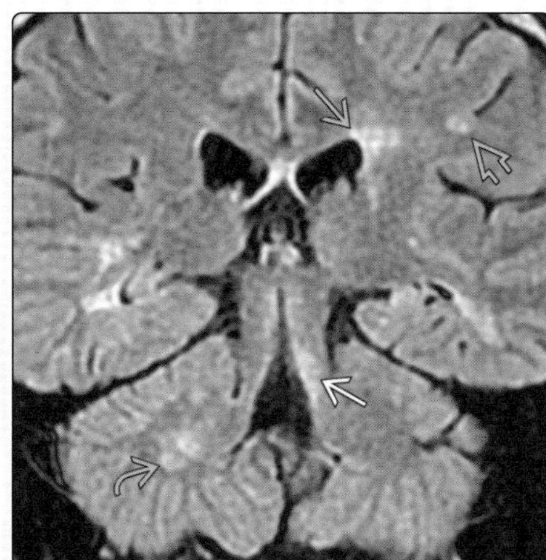

***(15-5)** Axial FLAIR in a woman with MS shows hyperintense demyelinating lesions in characteristic locations of periventricular ➙, deep ➙, and subcortical ➙ WM. **(15-6)** Coronal FLAIR C+ MR in a 22-yo man with MS shows the full extent of locations commonly affected by MS, including periventricular WM ➙, subcortical WM ➙, cerebellum ➙, and brainstem ➙.*

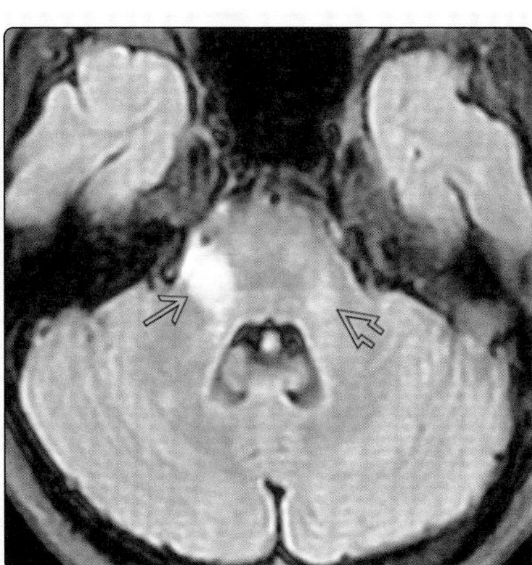

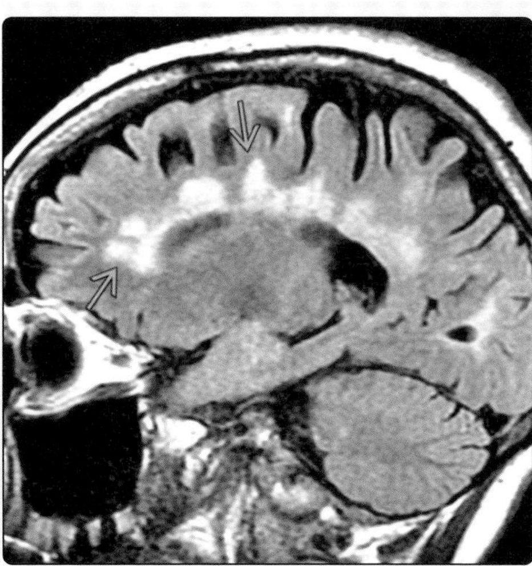

***(15-7)** Axial FLAIR in a 17-yo girl with MS shows a prominent lesion in the right middle cerebellar peduncle ➙. Note the subtle lesion on the left ➙. WM tracts of the brainstem are a common location for MS demyelinating lesions. **(15-8)** Sagittal FLAIR C+ MR in a 47-yo woman with MS shows demyelinating lesions predominantly affecting the pericallosal WM with many lesions ➙ oriented perpendicular to the corpus callosum.*

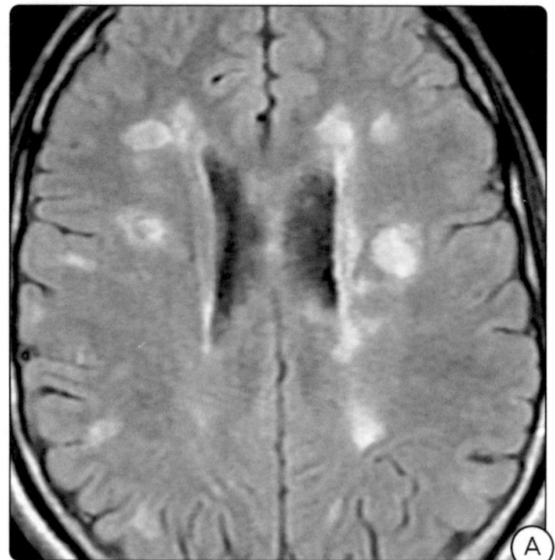
(15-9A) Axial FLAIR in a man with MS shows a moderate burden of demyelinating lesions.

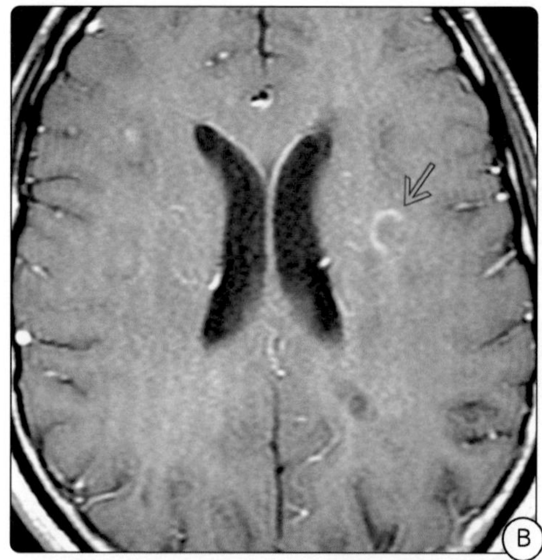
(15-9B) Axial T1 C+ MR in the same patient shows typical incomplete rim enhancement ⇒ often seen in demyelinating lesions.

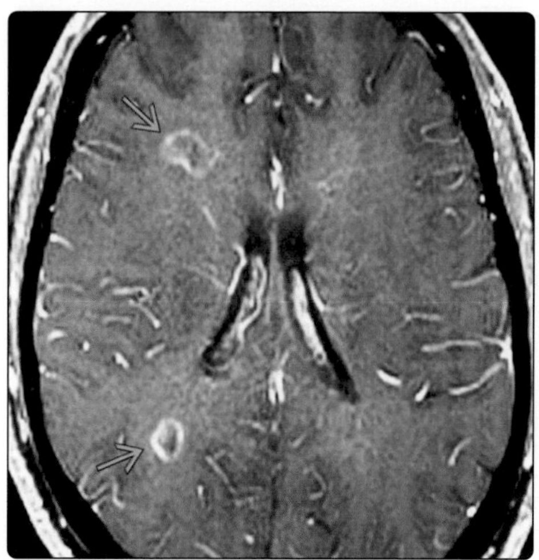
(15-10) T1 C+ FS MR shows irregular rim enhancement, another common enhancement pattern ⇒. This is acute-onset MS.

diagnosis of MS can be made. Until that occurs, most experts agree that MS should **not** be diagnosed solely on the basis of MR findings.

***Clinically Isolated Syndrome.*** The first attack of MS [most commonly optic neuritis (ON), transverse myelitis (TM), or a brainstem syndrome] is known as a clinically isolated syndrome. 1/2 of patients with ON eventually develop MS.

Disease progression to MS varies. Patients with MR-negative CIS have a 20% chance of developing MS. If patients with CIS have MR evidence for typical brain lesions, the chance of developing clinically definite MS is 60-80%. If imaging demonstrates old lesions in a different location, dissemination in time (DIS) is established, and the criteria for establishing MS are fulfilled (see below).

***Relapsing-Remitting MS.*** The vast majority (~ 85%) of all MS patients experience relapses alternating with remission phases and are classified as having RR-MS. Attacks ("relapses" or "exacerbations") are followed by periods of partial or complete recovery. New MR lesions often occur as part of a relapse but may also occur without symptoms.

***Relapsing-Progressive MS.*** RP-MS is also known as SP-MS. In RP-MS, there is progressive worsening of neurologic function (accumulation of disability) over time. Almost 1/2 of RR-MS patients enter an RP-MS stage within 10 years. By 25 years following initial diagnosis, 90% of RR-MS cases become the RP-MS subtype.

***Primary-Progressive MS.*** PP-MS is characterized by worsening neurologic function from the outset and lacks periods of remission. Approximately 5-10% of patients have PP-MS. Patients with PP-MS tend to have fewer brain lesions but more lesions in the spinal cord.

**Diagnosis.** The diagnosis of MS requires (1) elimination of more likely diagnoses and (2) demonstration of dissemination of CNS lesions in space and time. The 2017 revised McDonald diagnostic criteria incorporate clinical presentation (such as clinical presentation in a person with typical attack/CIS at onset) and additional data (e.g., MR evidence for DIS and DIT, characteristic CSF findings) to establish the diagnosis.

### 2017 REVISED MCDONALD CRITERIA FOR MULTIPLE SCLEROSIS DIAGNOSIS

**Clinical Presentation**

- In person with typical attack/CIS at onset
  - Varies with number of attacks, objective clinical evidence
  - May or may not require additional data
  - MR or CSF specific (oligoclonal bands)

**MR: Dissemination in Space**

- ≥ 1 T2-hyperintense lesion(s)
  - Can be symptomatic or asymptomatic
- In ≥ 2 areas
  - Periventricular
  - Juxtacortical/cortical
  - Infratentorial
  - Spinal cord

**MR: Dissemination in Time**

- **Simultaneous** presence of both enhancing, nonenhancing MS-typical lesions
  - Can be symptomatic or asymptomatic
- **New** T2 or enhancing lesion on follow-up MR
  - Compared to baseline scan (without regard to timing of baseline scan)

## Imaging

**General Features.** Most MS plaques are small (5-10 mm), although large lesions can reach several centimeters. Plaques are usually multiple, although 30% of giant "tumefactive" plaques initially occur as solitary lesions and are relatively more common in children and young adults.

**MULTIPLE SCLEROSIS: IMAGING**

CT
- Patchy/confluent hypodensities
- Mild/moderate, patchy, ring enhancement

MR
- Hypointense on T1WI ± faint hyperintense rim
- Very hyperintense center on T2WI, slightly less hyperintense rim
  - Callososeptal interface
  - Triangular on sagittal
  - Ovoid, perivenular on axial
  - Subpial, intracortical lesions common
- Active plaques enhance ("tumefactive" partial rim)
- Steroids suppress enhancement!

**CT Findings.** NECT is often normal early in the disease course, especially with mild cases. Solitary or multiple ill-defined white matter hypodensities may be present. Acute or subacute lesions may show mild to moderate punctate, patchy, or ring enhancement on CECT.

**MR Findings.** Over 95% of patients with clinically definite MS have positive findings on MR scans. Therefore, MR is the procedure of choice for both initial evaluation and treatment follow-up. The 2017 revised McDonald criteria for MS diagnosis allow MR to demonstrate DIS and DIT.

***T1WI.*** Most MS plaques are hypo- or isointense on T1WI. A faint, poorly delineated peripheral rim of mild hyperintensity secondary to lipid peroxidation and macrophage infiltration often surrounds sharply delineated, hypointense "black holes." This gives many subacute and chronic lesions a characteristic beveled or lesion-within-a-lesion appearance **(15-11)**.

Chronic and severe cases typically show moderate volume loss and generalized atrophy. The corpus callosum becomes progressively thinner and is best delineated on sagittal T1WI.

***T2/FLAIR.*** T2WI shows multiple hyperintense, linear, round, or ovoid lesions surrounding the medullary veins that radiate centripetally away from the lateral ventricles **(15-8)**. Larger lesions often demonstrate a very hyperintense center surrounded by a slightly less hyperintense peripheral area and variable amounts of perilesional edema.

MS plaques often assume a distinct triangular shape with the base adjacent to the ventricle on sagittal FLAIR or T2WI images **(15-5)**.

***T1 C+.*** Punctate, nodular, linear, and rim patterns are seen during active demyelination **(15-10)**. A prominent incomplete rim ("horseshoe") of enhancement with the "open" nonenhancing segment facing the cortex can be present **(15-9B)**, especially in large "tumefactive" lesions **(15-12) (15-13)**.

Enhancement disappears within 6 months in > 90% of lesions. **Steroid administration significantly reduces lesion enhancement and conspicuity and may render some lesions virtually invisible!**

***DWI and MRS.*** Although occasionally acute MS plaques can demonstrate restricted diffusion, such an appearance is atypical and should not be

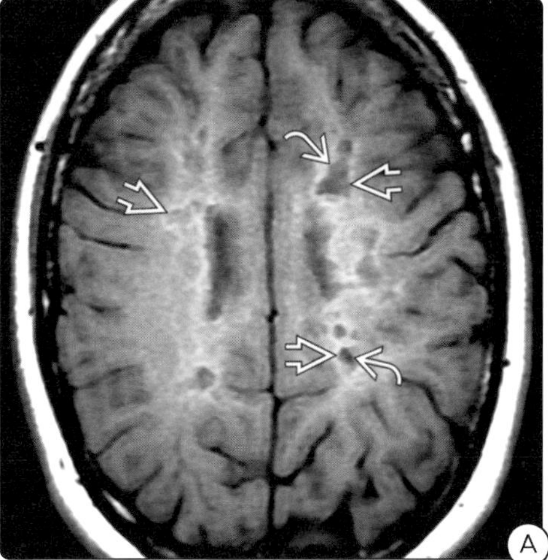


***(15-11A)** T1 MR in chronic MS shows hyperintense rims ➡ surrounding deep WM plaques ➡, giving the distinct lesion-within-a-lesion appearance.*

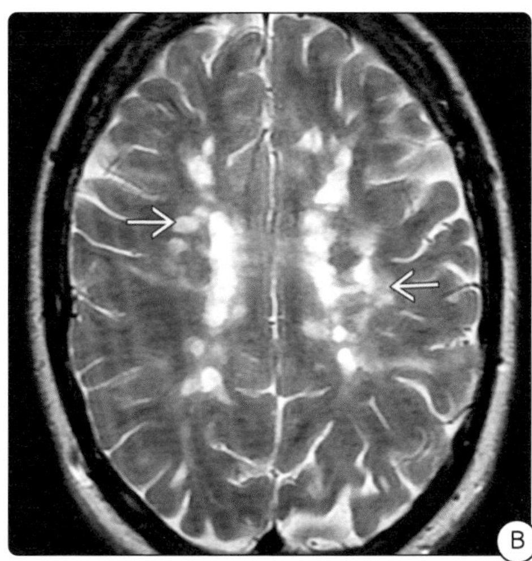


***(15-11B)** T2 MR shows the ovoid perivenular plaques ➡ that are oriented perpendicular to the lateral ventricles, as seen in the axial plane.*

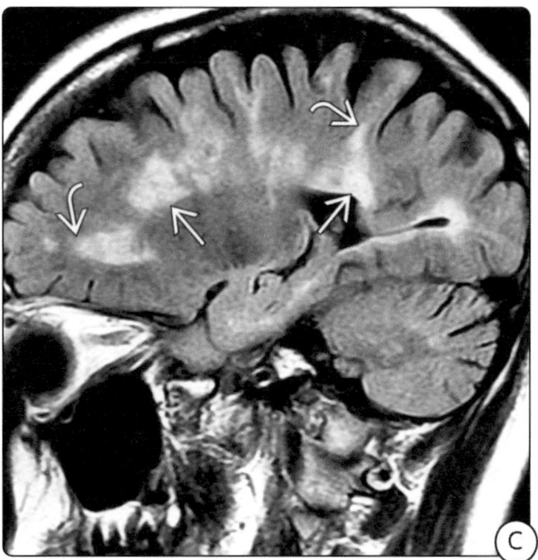


***(15-11C)** FLAIR MR shows broad-based lesions oriented toward ventricular surface ➡ with their apices ➡ pointing toward the cortex.*

considered a reliable biomarker of plaque activity. MRS shows elevated myoinositol in acute lesions. "Tumefactive" MS shows nonspecific findings (elevated choline, decreased NAA, and high lactate).

## Differential Diagnosis

Multifocal nonenhancing T2/FLAIR "white spots" are nonspecific imaging findings and have a broad differential diagnosis. It is helpful to suggest whether such lesions do or do not meet the revised 2017 McDonald criteria for multiple sclerosis.

Multifocal enhancing white matter lesions can be caused by **ADEM, vasculitis, and Lyme disease**. **SuS** (see later discussion) is often mistaken for MS on imaging studies, as both have multifocal T2/FLAIR white matter hyperintensities and both commonly affect young adult women. Lesions in SuS preferentially involve the *middle* of the corpus callosum, not the callososeptal interface **(15-34)**.

"Tumefactive" MS can mimic **abscess** or **neoplasm (glioblastoma** or **metastasis)**. **"Tumefactive" demyelination often has an incomplete or horseshoe pattern of enhancement.**

# Multiple Sclerosis "Variants"

The relationship of atypical demyelinating disorders, such as Marburg disease **(MD)**, Schilder disease **(SD)**, Balo concentric sclerosis **(BCS)**, and progressive solitary sclerosis **(SS)** as well as atypical idiopathic inflammatory demyelinating disorders **(IIDDs)**, to the acute-onset MS spectrum remains uncertain.

## Marburg Disease

MD is generally considered as an acute fulminant MS variant characterized by rapid, relentless progression and an exceptionally severe clinical course that usually leads to death within one year. Patients are typically young adults.

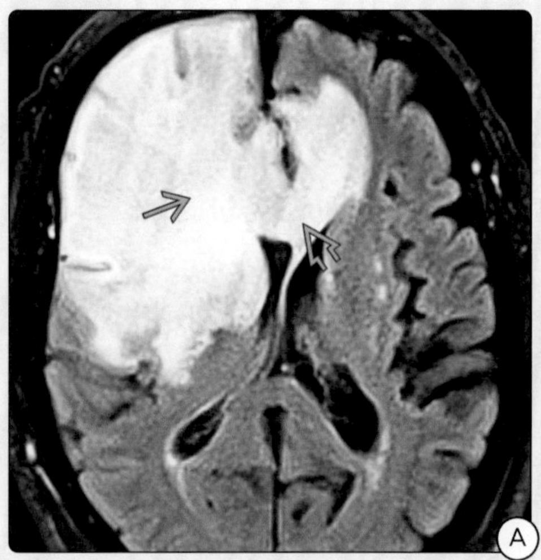


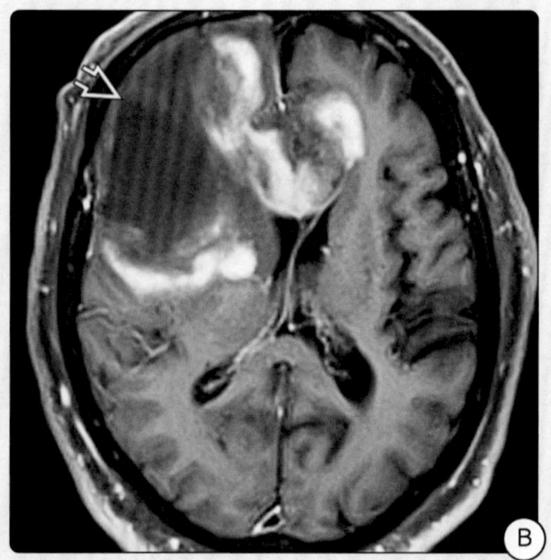


***(15-12A)** Axial FLAIR MR in a 77-yo man with 2 days of progressive confusion shows a large, hypointense right frontal lobe mass ➾ that thickens and crosses the corpus callosum ➾ and extends into the WM of the left frontal lobe. **(15-12B)** T1 C+ FS MR shows that the mass enhances strongly but very heterogeneously with significant nonenhancing areas ➡ near the cortex of the right frontal lobe.*

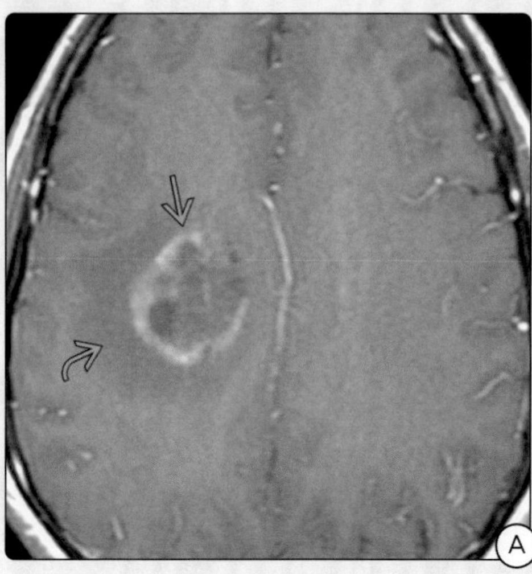


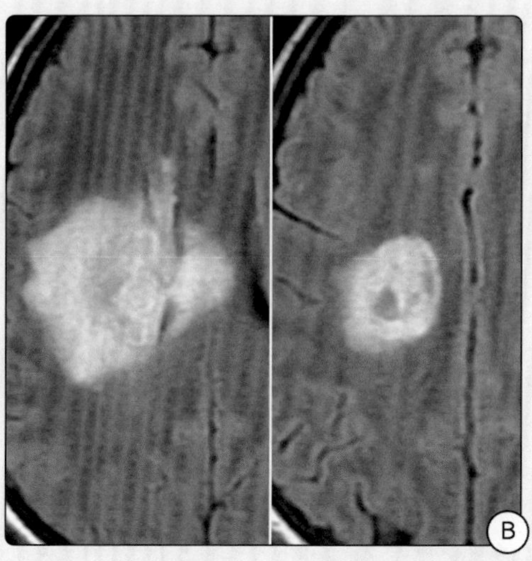


***(15-13A)** Axial FLAIR MR in a 35-yo woman with tumefactive MS shows a large solitary lesion centered in the right centrum semiovale with an incomplete ring of rim enhancement ➾ and adjacent edema ➾. **(15-13B)** Axial FLAIR MR images in the same patient are shown at diagnosis (left) and 6 weeks later (right). Temporal changes in the lesion with treatment help to confirm what was suspected to be a "tumefactive" demyelinating process.*

Marked lymphocytic infiltrates **(15-14)** with inflammatory changes in the perivenular spaces can lead to hyperacute, fulminant demyelination with a "centrifugal" pattern of contrast leakage from medullary veins on T1 C+ imaging **(15-15)**. The presence of developmental venous anomalies (DVAs) seems to predispose to "tumefactive" demyelination centered around the "Medusa head" **(15-16)**.

Imaging shows multifocal diffusely disseminated disease with focal and confluent white matter hyperintensities on T2/FLAIR. Strong patchy enhancement on T1 C+ is typical, and large, cavitating, incomplete, ring-enhancing, "tumefactive" lesions are common **(15-17)**.

## Schilder Disease

SD—a.k.a. myelinoclastic diffuse sclerosis—is a rare subacute or chronic demyelinating disorder characterized by one or more inflammatory demyelinating white matter plaques. SD is typically a disease of childhood and young adults. Median age at presentation is 18 years with a slight female predominance.

Although SD is considered to be a variant of MS, clinical features are atypical for MS, and the disease is usually monophasic with a low rate of recurrence. Signs of increased intracranial pressure, aphasia, and behavioral symptoms are typical. CSF is usually normal, and there is no history to suggest acute disseminated encephalomyelitis (ADEM) (i.e., no fever, infection, or preceding vaccination). Approximately 15% of cases progress to MS.

MR shows a hypointense lesion on T1WI that is hyperintense on T2/FLAIR. Rim enhancement—often the incomplete or open ring pattern—is seen during the acute inflammatory stage. The lesion rim usually restricts on DWI during the acute phase.

The differential diagnosis of SD can be difficult. **"Tumefactive" MS** can appear identical to SD on imaging

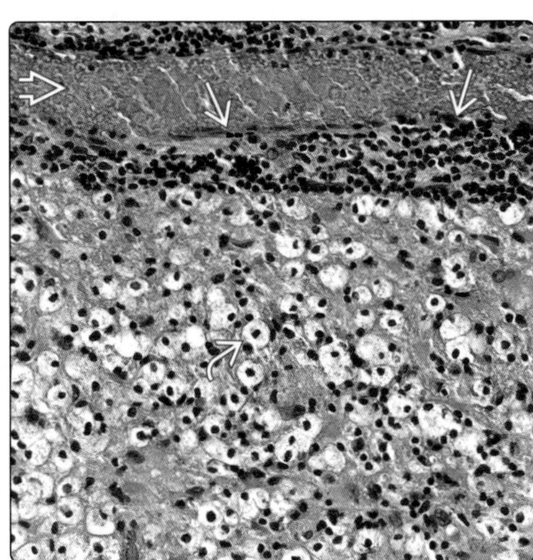

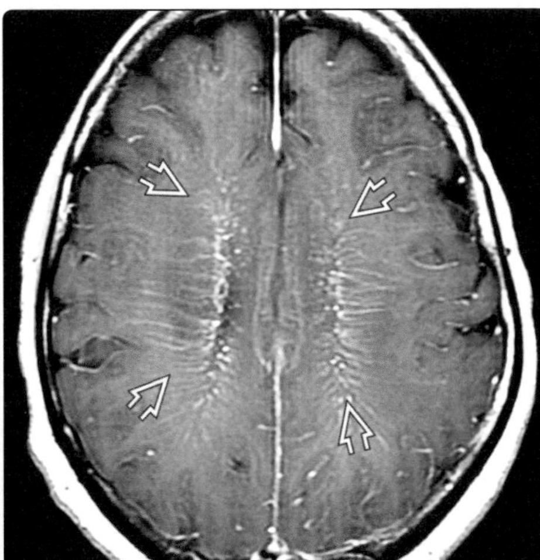

***(15-14)** H&E shows venule with marked perivascular lymphocytic cuffing, striking macrophage infiltrates in acute, fulminant "tumefactive" demyelination. **(15-15)** T1 C+ FS MR in hyperacute demyelination (from fulminant MS or ADEM, PML-IRIS, etc.) can show striking enhancement, enlargement of deep medullary veins. Findings can mimic vasculitis and intravascular lymphoma.*

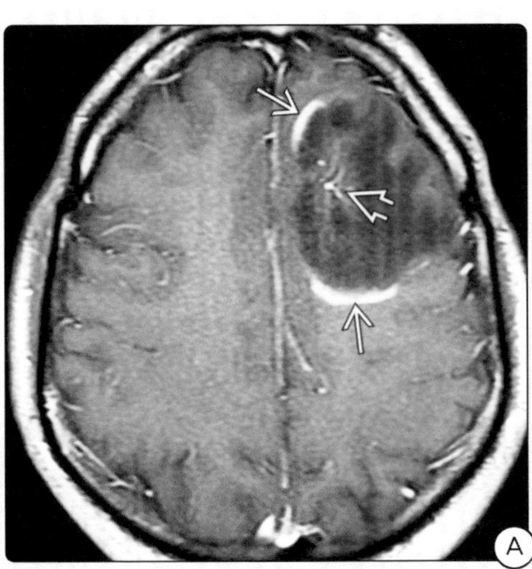


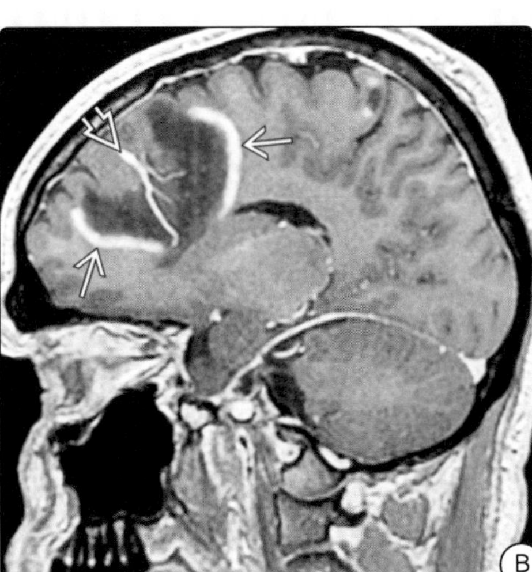


***(15-16A)** T1 C+ MR in a 38-yo man with ON shows "tumefactive" demyelination with partial rim enhancement. Note that the lesion surrounds a classic DVA. **(15-16B)** Sagittal T1 C+ MR shows the DVA surrounded by the incompletely enhancing rim of "tumefactive" MS.*

studies. SD often mimics intracranial neoplasm or abscess both in clinical presentation and on imaging studies. **Pyogenic abscess** generally shows strong diffusion restriction in the lesion core. Perfusion MR may be helpful in distinguishing SD from **metastasis** and **glioblastoma**.

## Balo Concentric Sclerosis

BCS is generally considered an atypical or variant form of MS and occurs as a discrete, concentrically layered white matter lesion. It is often described as having an onion ring or whorled appearance, caused by its peculiar pattern of alternating rims of demyelination and myelin preservation.

BCS is usually characterized by acute onset and rapid clinical deterioration. Peak presentation is between 20-50 years. The F:M ratio is ~ 2:1 and is most common in patients of east Asian origin.

Imaging studies reflect the distinctive gross pathology of BCS and vary with disease stage. Acute lesions have significant surrounding edema **(15-18A)**. The actively demyelinating layers enhance on T1 C+ sequences. Other more typical MS-like plaques can also be present. Lesions in subacute/chronic BCS exhibit alternating bands of differing signal intensities on T2WI and resemble a "whirlpool" of concentric rings **(15-18B)**.

# Other Acquired CNS Demyelinating Syndromes

The system of classification for CNS demyelinating syndromes has been strongly influenced by advances in the molecular diagnosis capabilities developed in the last decade or so. There is a trend towards defining demyelinating syndromes by the antibodies present rather than solely or even predominantly by the clinical and radiologic phenotype.

*(15-17A) T1 C+ FS MR through the ventricles shows the necrotic, cavitating, acutely enhancing right parietal "tumefactive" mass ➡. Other enhancing foci are present ➡. (15-17B) Coronal T1 C+ MR shows extension around the left ventricle ➡ in addition to other enhancing foci ➡. This is the Marburg variant of MS.*

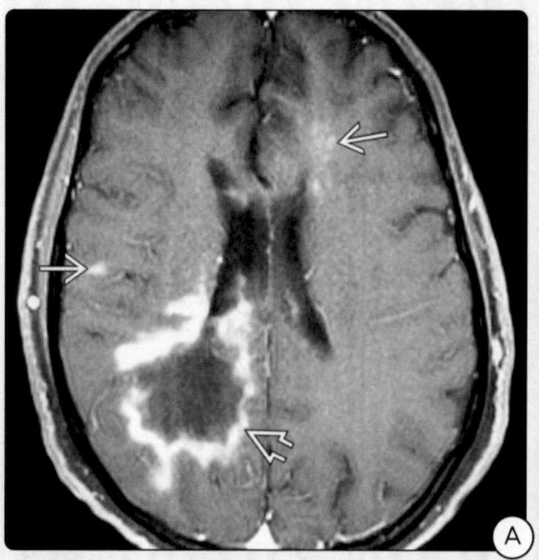


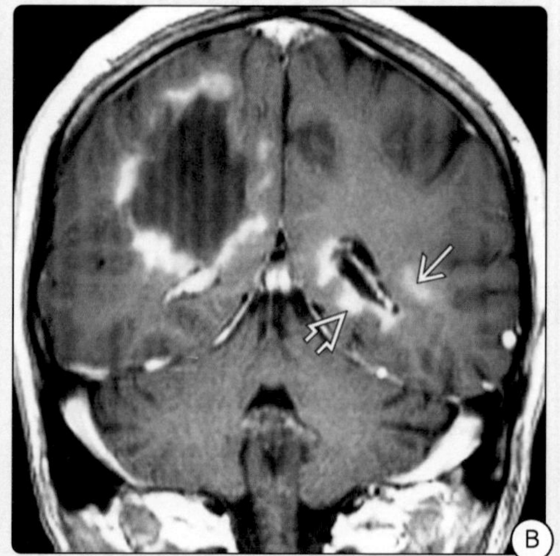


*(15-18A) Acute Balo concentric sclerosis lesions are hyperintense on FLAIR ➡, restrict on DWI ➡, and show concentric "onion bulb" enhancement ➡. (15-18B) Follow-up scans show alternating rings of iso- and hyperintensity on T1 ➡ and T2WI ➡, no enhancement ➡. (Courtesy P. Rodriguez, MD.)*

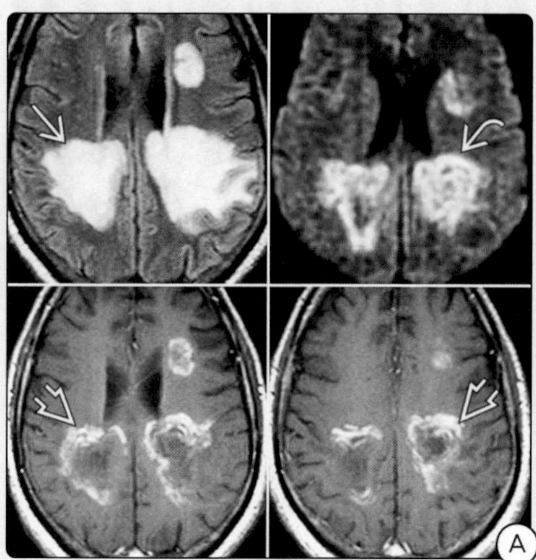


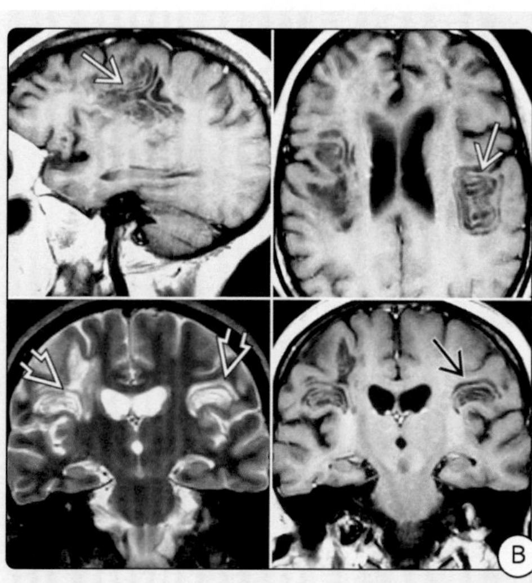

Current clinical recommendations suggest testing for MOG and AQP4 antibodies in patients with acute CNS demyelination of suspected autoimmune origin. The debate continues on whether syndrome-based or biomarker-based criteria should prevail in these classification schemes. It behooves the radiologist to be aware of these important disease biomarkers and their relationship to such imaging-based clinical manifestations, such as **acute disseminated encephalomyelitis (ADEM), optic neuritis (ON), neuromyelitis optica spectrum disorder (NMOSD), and transverse myelitis (TM)**. There is significant overlap in imaging features between MOGAD, AQP4 NMOSD, and MS, but there are important clinical and imaging features that can help us potentially distinguish them. The following discussion will focus on the clinical **(Table 15-1)** and imaging features **(Table 15-2)** that may help distinguish these various clinical entities.

## Acute Disseminated Encephalomyelitis

### Terminology

ADEM is primarily a postinfection, postimmunization disorder that is also called parainfectious encephalomyelitis. Once considered a purely monophasic illness, recurrent and **multiphasic forms (MDEM)** of ADEM are now recognized. Approximately 50% of patients with a clinical and imaging diagnosis of ADEM will have anti-MOG antibodies.

### Etiology

The immunohistopathologic features of ADEM mimic those of experimental allergic encephalitis, an induced autoimmune disease precipitated by myelin antibodies. Therefore, most investigators consider ADEM an immune-mediated CNS demyelinating disorder.

### Pathology

**Location.** As the name implies, ADEM can involve both the brain and spinal cord. White matter lesions usually predominate, but basal ganglia involvement is seen in nearly 1/2 of all cases. Spinal cord lesions are found in 10-30% of cases. When the spinal cord is involved, it often manifests as longitudinally extensive TM (LETM) with lesions extending > 3 vertebral bodies in length. ON is seen in some patients with ADEM, especially those with MOG antibodies.

A rare ADEM variant, acute infantile bilateral striatal necrosis, occurs 1-2 weeks following a respiratory illness. Viral and streptococcal infections have been implicated and cause enlarged hyperintense basal ganglia, caudate nuclei, and internal/external capsules.

**Size and Number.** Lesion size varies from a few millimeters to several centimeters ("tumefactive" ADEM), and lesions have a punctate to flocculent configuration. Multiple lesions are more common than solitary lesions.

**Gross Pathology.** Small lesions are often inapparent on gross examination. Large "tumefactive" lesions cause a gray-pink white matter discoloration and often extend all the way to the cortex-white matter junction **(15-19A)**. Mass effect is minimal compared with lesion size. Gross intralesional hemorrhage is rare and more characteristic of AHLE than ADEM.

**Microscopic Features.** "Sleeves" of pronounced perivenular demyelination with macrophage-predominant inflammatory infiltrates are typical. The outer margins of ADEM lesions are indistinct compared with the relatively well-delineated edges of MS plaques. Viral inclusion bodies are generally absent, unlike viral encephalitis.

**Clinical Features of MOG Antibody Disease, APQ4 Neuromyelitis Optica Spectrum Disorder, and Multiple Sclerosis**

| Clinical Feature | MOG Antibody Disease | APQ4 Antibody Neuromyelitis Optica Spectrum Disorder | Multiple Sclerosis |
|---|---|---|---|
| Age | Children > adults | Mostly adults (< 5% in children) | Mostly adults (< 5% in children) |
| Recent infection/vaccination | Common | Rare | Rare |
| Clinical phenotype | ADEM in younger children; opticospinal (ON/LETM) phenotype in older children/adults | ON, LTEM | Unifocal or polyfocal neurologic event, usually without encephalopathy |
| Serum biomarker | MOG antibody | AQP4 antibody | N/A |
| F:M sex ratio | 3:1 | 3:1 | ~ 2:1 |
| Disease course | Monophasic or relapsing | Typically relapsing (> 90%) | Majority relapsing-remitting |
| Prognosis | Good (best with monophasic course) | Moderate to poor (especially with relapses) | Depends on subtype and relapse |

***(Table 15-1)*** *ADEM = acute disseminated encephalomyelitis; LTEM = longitudinally extensive transverse myelitis; ON = optic neuritis.*

Alonso AS et al: Understanding pediatric neuroimmune conflicts: a neuroradiologic approach in the molecular era. Radiographics. 2020.

## Imaging Features of MOG Antibody Disease, APQ4 Neuromyelitis Optica Spectrum Disorder, and Multiple Sclerosis

| Imaging Feature | MOG Antibody Disease | APQ4 Antibody Neuromyelitis Optica Spectrum Disorder | Multiple Sclerosis |
|---|---|---|---|
| Brain lesions | Poorly defined lesions in white matter and deep gray matter, often enhancing | Large subcortical white matter lesions and propensity to involve area postrema and adjacent to 3rd/4th ventricles | Scattered white matter lesions with propensity for periventricular and corpus callosum; decreased T1 lesions |
| Cortical/leptomeningeal lesions | Frequent leptomeningeal enhancement/lesions | Frequent leptomeningeal lesions | Less common |
| Optic nerve lesions | Frequently bilateral<br>Long lesions, anterior > posterior<br>Perineural orbital fat enhancement common | Frequently bilateral<br>Long lesions, posterior > anterior<br>Long enhancement pattern confined to optic nerve | Bilateral or unilateral<br>Short lesions<br>Short enhancement pattern confined to optic nerve |
| Spinal cord lesions | 2/3 LETM; 1/3 short segment<br>> 1 lesion common<br>Cervical = thoracic<br>Usually centrally located in cord<br>H-shaped central gray common<br>Usually nonenhancing | LETM > > short segment (~ 15%)<br>Usually single lesion<br>Cervicomedullary junction common<br>Usually centrally located in cord<br>H-shaped central gray less common<br>Enhancement common | Short segment > > LETM (~ 15%)<br>Multiple lesions common<br>Cervical > thoracic<br>Peripheral cord location common<br>H-shaped central gray rare<br>Enhancement common |

***(Table 15-2)*** *LTEM = longitudinally extensive transverse myelitis.*

Alonso AS et al: Understanding pediatric neuroimmune conflicts: a neuroradiologic approach in the molecular era. Radiographics. 2020.

### ACUTE DISSEMINATED ENCEPHALOMYELITIS

**Etiology and Pathology**

- Post infection, post immunization
- Immune-mediated perivenular demyelination
- ~ 50% have anti-MOG antibodies

**Clinical Issues**

- 2nd only to MS as acquired demyelinating disease
- No female predominance
- Occurs at all ages, but children 5-8 years old are most affected
- Course, outcome vary (recurrence more likely with MOG antibody)
  - Monophasic ADEM: Most common (> 70%)
  - Recurrent ADEM: 2nd episode, same site (10%)
  - MDEM: Multiple episodes, different sites (10%)
- Recover completely (> 50%)
- Mortality (1-2%)

## Clinical Issues

**Epidemiology and Demographics.** ADEM is second only to MS as the most common acquired idiopathic inflammatory demyelinating disease. Unlike MS, there is no female predominance. ADEM occurs most commonly in spring and autumn.

ADEM can occur at any age but—perhaps because of the frequency of immunizations and antigen exposure—is more common in childhood with peak occurrence between 5-8 years of age. The overall estimated incidence is 0.8 per 100,000 persons annually. The incidence of childhood ADEM is estimated at 2-10 cases per million children per year.

Approximately 50% of patients with a clinical and imaging diagnosis of ADEM will have anti-MOG antibodies. Nearly all ADEM patients with MDEM and those with ON (ADEM-ON) will have anti-MOG antibodies.

**Presentation.** Symptoms typically occur a few days to a few weeks following antigenic challenge (e.g., infection or vaccination). The majority of children with ADEM have a nonspecific febrile illness preceding onset. Viral exanthema is usually absent.

**Natural History.** Disease course and outcome vary. **Monophasic ADEM** is the most common type. However, the disease sometimes follows an atypical course, waxing and waning over a period of several months.

Approximately 25% of patients initially diagnosed with ADEM experience a relapse. **Recurrent ADEM** is characterized by a second episode occurring within two years after the initial illness and involving the *same* anatomic area(s) as the original illness. Patients with persistently elevated anti-MOG antibodies on clinical follow-up are more likely to have recurrent demyelinating episodes.

**MDEM** is characterized by one or more subsequent events that involve a *different* anatomic area as demonstrated by a new lesion on MR or a new focal neurologic deficit. MDEM is usually associated with MOG antibodies.

More than 1/2 of all patients recover completely within one or two months after onset, whereas ~ 20% experience some residual functional impairment. Overall mortality in recent series is low.

**ACUTE DISSEMINATED ENCEPHALOMYELITIS: IMAGING**

**Brain**
- Multifocal T2/FLAIR hyperintensities
  - Bilateral but asymmetric white matter lesions
  - Hazy, flocculent "cotton balls" (> 2 cm, usually in children)
  - ± basal ganglia, posterior fossa, cranial nerves
- Enhancement varies from none to striking
  - Multifocal punctate, linear, partial ring
  - Can be perivenular
  - Large lesions ("tumefactive") less common

**Spinal Cord**
- Patchy/longitudinally extensive T2 hyperintensity
- Strong but patchy enhancement

## Imaging

**CT Findings.** NECT is usually normal. CECT may show multifocal punctate or partial ring-enhancing lesions.

**MR Findings.** Multifocal hyperintensities on T2/FLAIR are the most common findings and vary from small round/ovoid foci to flocculent "cotton ball" lesions with very hyperintense centers surrounded by slightly less hyperintense areas with "fuzzy" margins **(15-22A)**. Bilateral but asymmetric involvement is typical. Basal ganglia **(15-20)** and posterior fossa lesions are common.

Enhancement varies from minimal to striking. Punctate, linear, ring, and incomplete horseshoe patterns all occur **(15-22B)**. Large "tumefactive" lesions with horseshoe-shaped enhancement resemble "tumefactive" MS. Leptomeningeal/pial enhancement is often seen, especially in MOGAD **(15-21)**. Cranial nerve enhancement is relatively common. Acute lesions may show restriction on DWI. ON is

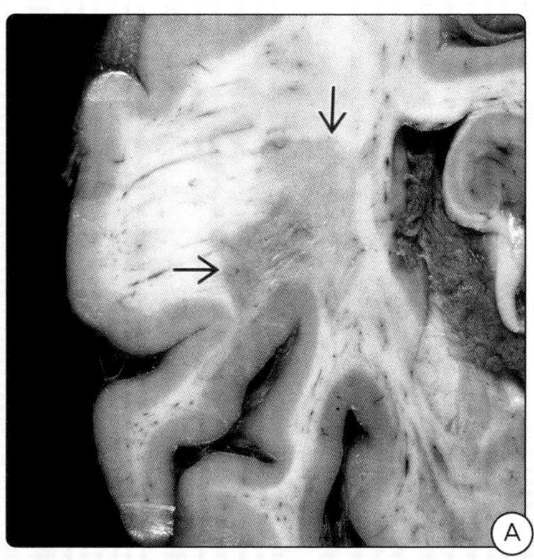

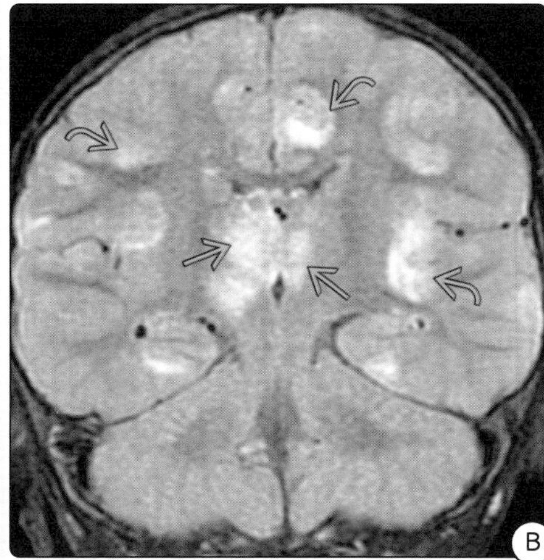

***(15-19A)** Autopsy shows necrotizing demyelination ➔, typical of postinfection, postvaccination disorders. (Courtesy R. Hewlett, MD.) **(15-19B)** Coronal FLAIR in the same patient shows the diffuse extent of the lesions involving subcortical WM ➔ and deep gray nuclear structures ➔.*

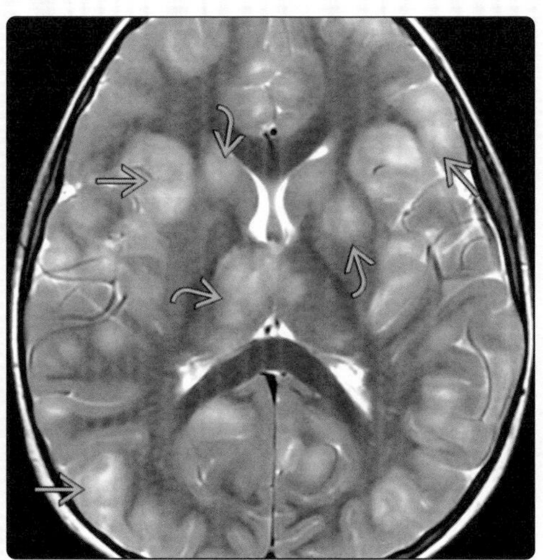

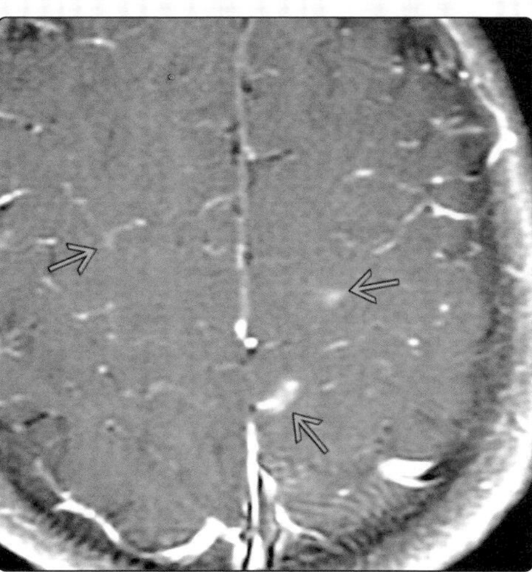

***(15-20)** Axial T2 MR in a 22-month-old with ADEM and positive for MOG antibodies is shown. This is a characteristic appearance for ADEM with numerous cortical/subcortical lesions ➔ and deep gray nuclei ➔. **(15-21)** Axial T1 C+ MR in an 11-yo boy with MOGAD shows areas of leptomeningeal and pial enhancement ➔, which is a common finding in MOGAD.*

uncommon at initial presentation but frequently accompanies MDEM **(15-23)**. Involvement of the spine is seen with regular frequency, especially in those ADEM patients with associated MOGAD. Long-segment myelitis is most common **(15-24)**.

## Differential Diagnosis

The major differential diagnosis of ADEM is **MS**. "Tumefactive" lesions—including those with incomplete ring enhancement—occur in both disorders. ADEM is more common in children and often has a history of viral infection or immunization. MS more commonly involves the callososeptal interface and typically has a relapsing-remitting course, whereas most cases of ADEM are monophasic. Spinal lesions, when present, tend to be short segment in MS, whereas, in ADEM, they are more likely to be long segment (> 3 vertebral segments).

**NMOSD** may be difficult to distinguish from recurrent ADEM. AQP4-positive NMOSD is more likely to involve the area postrema and is more likely to exhibit ependymal and leptomeningeal enhancement. NMOSD is much more common in adults, whereas ADEM is much more common in children.

Although very rare, **treatment-associated demyelinating diseases** with TNF-α inhibitors, such as etanercept, can mimic ADEM and NMOSD on imaging studies **(15-25)**. Demyelination associated with anti-TNF agents typically develops from one week to 12 months after treatment initiation.

# Neuromyelitis Optica Spectrum Disorder

**Neuromyelitis optica (NMO)** is an autoimmune inflammatory demyelinating disease of the CNS. The diagnostic criteria for NMO have recently been broadened and the disease renamed **NMOSD**.

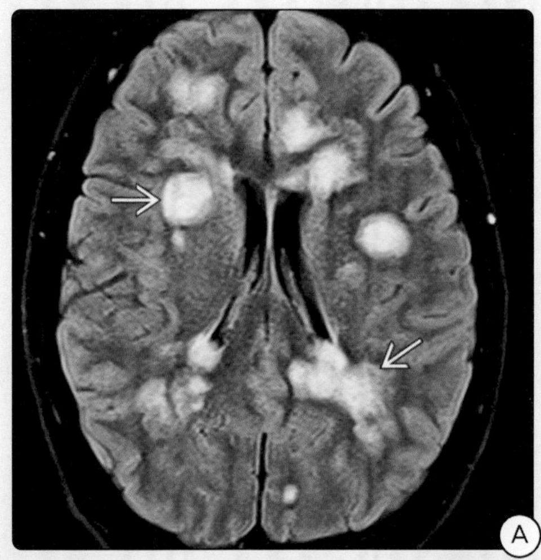


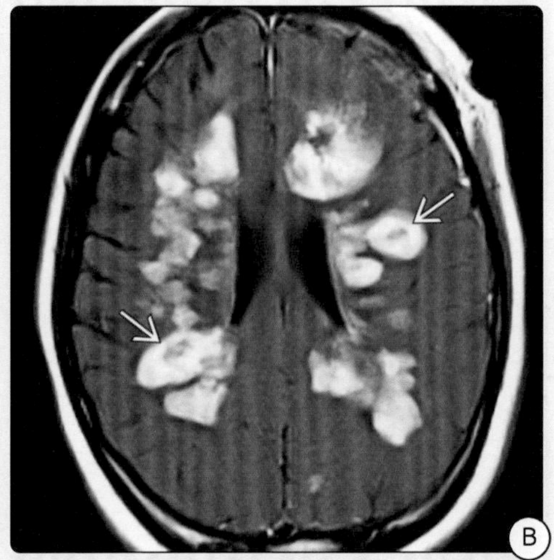


***(15-22A) FLAIR MR following viral infection shows bilateral WM lesions with a fluffy appearance and "fuzzy" margins ➡. (15-22B) T1 C+ MR shows that the lesions enhance intensely but heterogeneously. Some have a ring-like appearance ➡.***

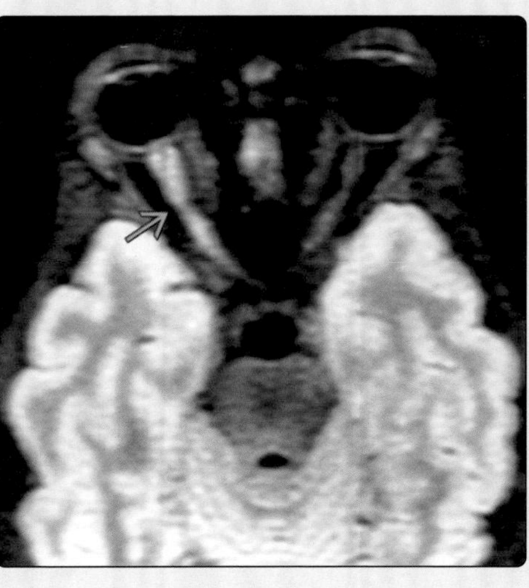

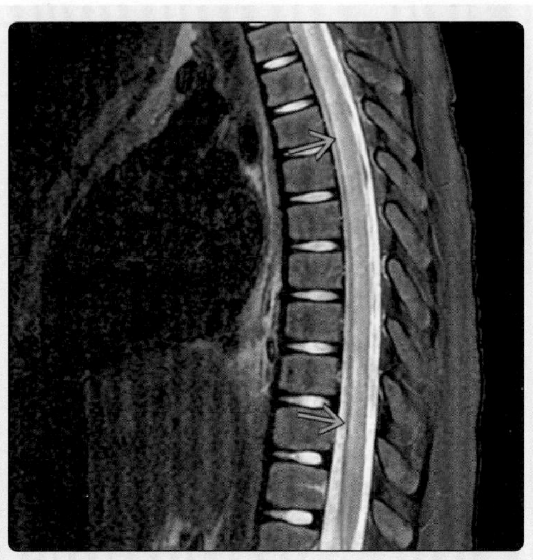

***(15-23) Axial FLAIR in a 10-yo girl with MOGAD shows long-segment ON ➡ involving the entire right intraorbital optic nerve. While ON is uncommon at initial presentation, it is common in those patients with recurrent ADEM. (15-24) Sagittal STIR in a 7-yo girl with MOGAD shows long-segment myelitis ➡. Long-segment myelitis is most often found in MOGAD, although multifocal short-segment myelitis may occur.***

## Etiology

The most common form of NMOSD is an autoimmune-mediated water channelopathy characterized by the presence of autoantibodies to **AQP4**. AQP4 is located in the foot processes of astrocytes and is the most abundant water channel in the CNS. It is especially highly expressed in the circumventricular organs surrounding the third and fourth ventricles.

A specific biomarker of the disease, AQP4-IgG, is 90% specific and 70-75% sensitive for NMOSD. NMOSD can be AQP4-IgG seropositive *or* seronegative (less common). Most seronegative NMOSD is positive for MOG antibodies.

## Pathology

**Location.** In classic NMOSD, one or both optic nerves are involved together with the spinal cord **(15-26)**. The cervical cord is most commonly affected. Lesions usually surround the central canal and classically extend over three or more consecutive segments **(15-26B)**.

Brain lesions may occur anywhere **(15-27)** but frequently cluster around the periependymal surfaces of the ventricles, corpus callosum, cerebral aqueduct, area postrema, and dorsal brainstem **(15-28)**.

Optic nerve lesions are often bilateral, long in extent, and favor the posterior optic nerves and chiasm **(15-26A)**.

**Microscopic Features.** It is the *immunohistochemistry* of AQP4-IgG that is diagnostic. AQP4-IgG binds to the abluminal face of microvessels at sites of immune complex deposition. The active demyelination in NMOSD is characterized by astrocytic injury, vessel hyalinization, and eosinophilic infiltration, findings not typically present in either MS or ADEM.

## Clinical Issues

**Epidemiology and Demographics.** NMOSD is a worldwide disease and does not exhibit the characteristic geographic gradient of MS. Patients with NMOSD are, on average, 10 years older than patients with MS. Mean age at initial diagnosis is ~ 40 years. Pediatric-onset NMOSD does occur and represents 3-5% of cases. The F:M ratio for AQP4-positive NMOSD is ~ 3:1.

Between 10-25% of NMOSD patients are seronegative for AQP4. MOG antibodies are found in 15-40% of seronegative NMO. Seronegative NMO is equally distributed among the sexes.

**Presentation and Natural History.** In adults, NMOSD is classically characterized by severe uni- or bilateral ON and LETM. Involvement of other CNS regions (either by clinical presentation or MR findings) is now recognized as part of the NMOSD spectrum (see box below).

AQP4-seropositive NMOSD patients usually have more severe clinical disease and worse outcome than individuals who are seronegative. The vast majority of cases (85-90%) are relapsing, although monophasic illness may occur.

Almost 30% of NMOSD patients are initially misdiagnosed with MS. Some patients also develop clinical features of anti-N-methyl, D-aspartate receptor (NMDAr) encephalitis.

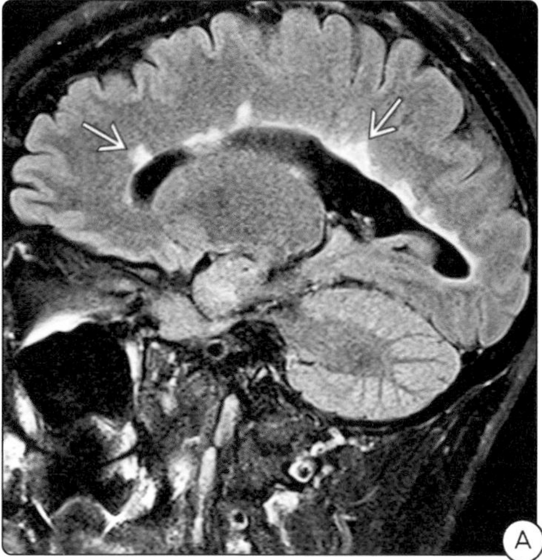


***(15-25A)** FLAIR in 44-yo on etanercept shows classic triangle-shaped demyelinating lesions ➡ along callososeptal interface, ependyma.*

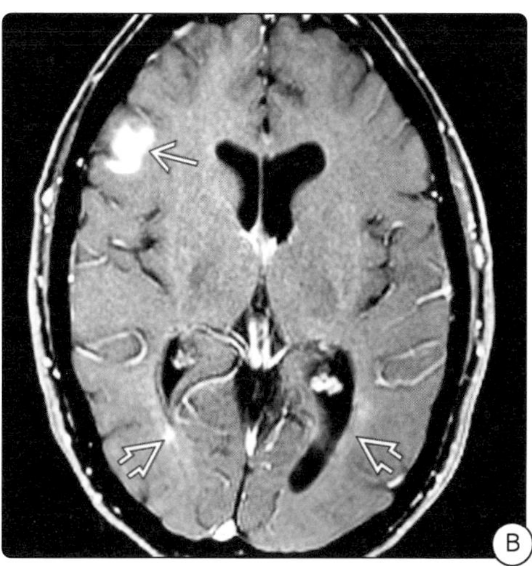


***(15-25B)** T1 C+ FS MR shows a large enhancing lesion in the left frontal subcortical WM ➡, additional ependymal-enhancing foci ⇨.*

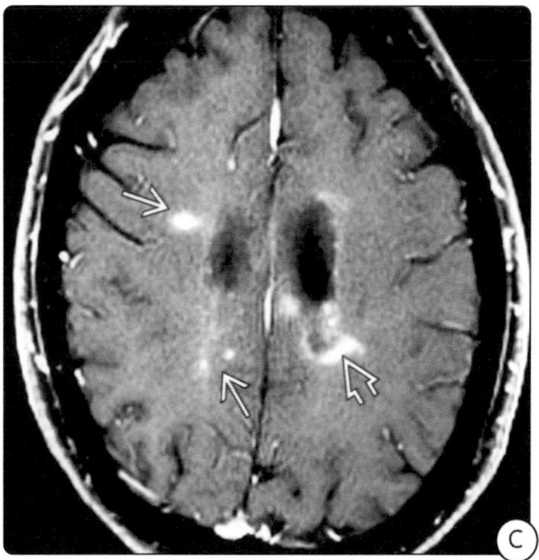


***(15-25C)** T1 C+ FS MR shows additional lesions ➡, partial ring-enhancing mass ⇨. This is anti-TNF treatment-associated demyelination.*

**2015 REVISED NEUROMYELITIS OPTIC SPECTRUM DISORDER DIAGNOSTIC CRITERIA: AQP4-IgG POSITIVITY**

AQP4-IgG positivity + 1 core clinical characteristic

- ON
- Acute myelitis
- Area postrema syndrome
  - Unexplained hiccups or nausea and vomiting
- Acute brainstem syndrome
- Symptomatic narcolepsy or diencephalic syndrome
  - With NMOSD-typical diencephalic MR lesions
- Symptomatic cerebral syndrome
  - With NMOSD-typical brain lesions

**2015 NEUROMYELITIS OPTICA SPECTRUM DISORDER CRITERIA: AQP4-IgG NEGATIVITY**

If AQP4-IgG negative

- At least 2 core clinical characteristics; 1 must be
  - ON, LTEM, or area postrema syndrome
- If **acute ON**, MR with
  - Normal brain or nonspecific white matter lesions
  - Or T2-hyperintense or T1 C+ enhancing ON lesion involving optic chiasm or > 50% of ON
- If **acute myelitis**, MR with
  - Intramedullary lesion over 3 contiguous segments
  - Or focal atrophy of at least 3 contiguous segments
- If **area postrema** syndrome, MR with
  - Dorsal medulla/area postrema lesion(s)
- If **acute brainstem** syndrome, MR with
  - Periependymal brainstem lesions

**Treatment Options.** Accurate diagnosis is essential because some drugs used for MS can worsen NMOSD. Recent studies suggest that the therapeutic options in NMO should be immunosuppressive rather than immunomodulatory drugs. Plasma exchange can be used in severe cases.

## Imaging

MR imaging has become an essential tool for NMOSD diagnosis, particularly for recognition of AQP4-IgG seronegative patients. Radiologists may be the first to recognize the disease.

The most common MR findings are (1) bilateral, longitudinally extensive optic nerve hyperintensity &/or enhancement consistent with acute ON **(15-26)** and (2) hyperintense, enhancing LETM (three or more contiguous vertebral segments). So-called short TM occurs in ~ 15% of patients.

The presence of brain lesions varies. **Between 30-60% of NMOSD patients have nonspecific T2/FLAIR hyperintensities in the cerebral white matter, so this finding does not exclude the diagnosis per se**. However, if lesions are found in areas where AQP4 is highly expressed (e.g., undersurface of the corpus callosum, dorsal brainstem, and periependymal surfaces around the third ventricle) or so-called pencil-thin ependymal enhancement is present, NMOSD should be considered.

## Differential Diagnosis

While there are numerous differential diagnoses, the major differential diagnosis of NMOSD is **MS** in adults and **ADEM** (usually with MOG antibodies) in children. Bilateral, long-segment optic nerve involvement and LETM are more

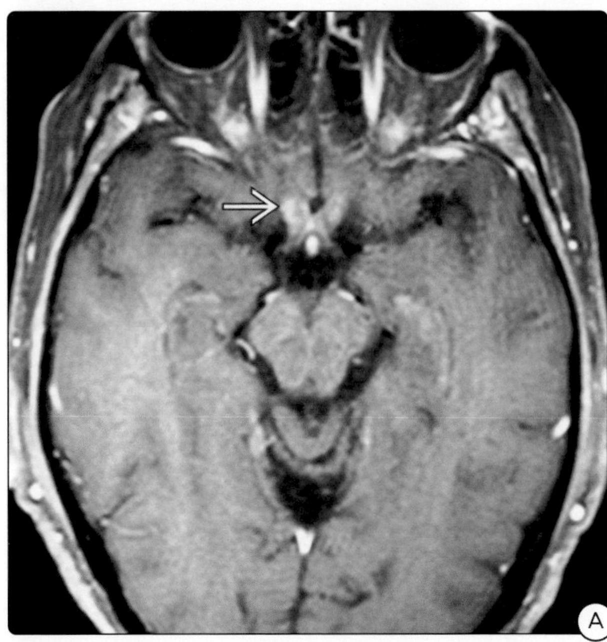

*(15-26A) Axial T1 C+ FS MR in a patient with serologically proven NMO shows posterior optic nerve and chiasm enhancement ➔.*

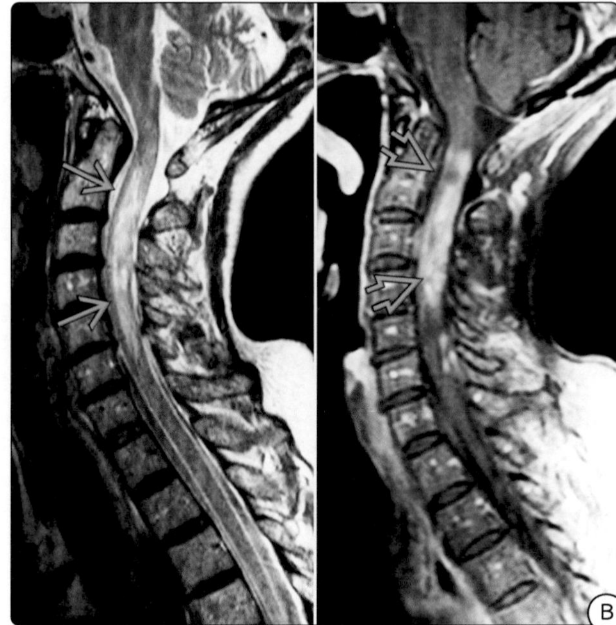

*(15-26B) Sagittal T2 MR (left) in the same case shows longitudinally extensive cord signal and expansion from C1-C5 ➔. T1 C+ MR (right) shows avid associated enhancement ➔.*

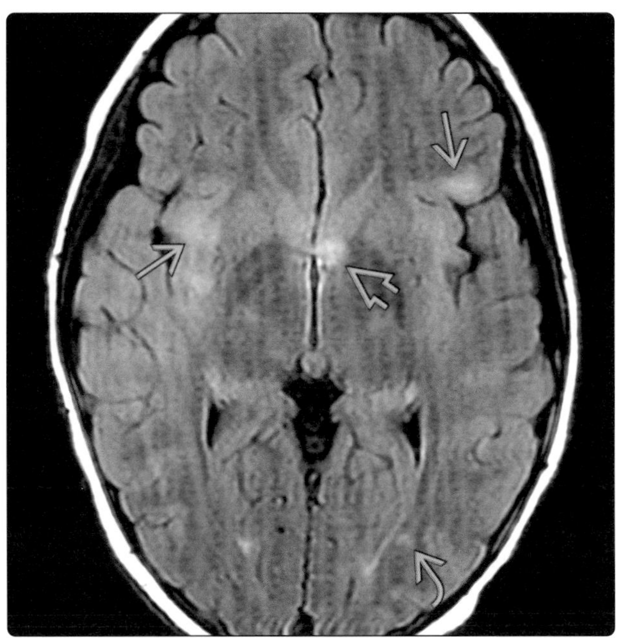

*(15-27) Axial FLAIR MR in an 8-yo girl with antibody-negative NMOSD shows hyperintense lesions in the subcortical WM ➡, periventricular WM ➡, and basal ganglia ➡.*

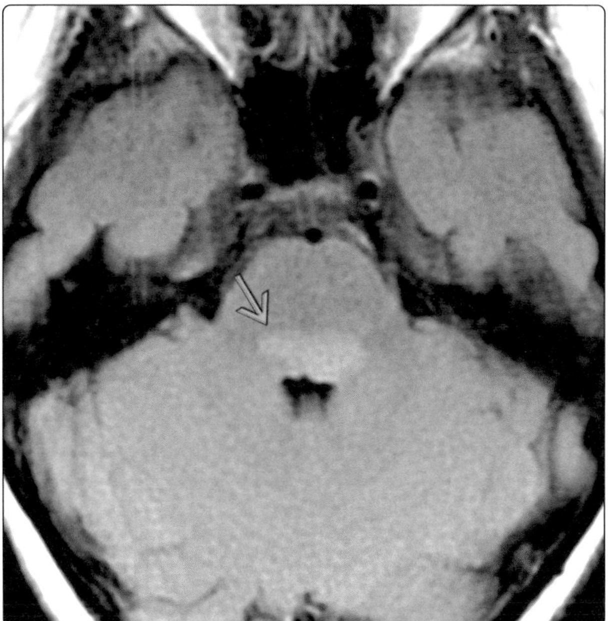

*(15-28) Axial FLAIR MR in the same patient shows hyperintense signal ➡ in the dorsal brainstem, a common location for demyelinating lesions of NMOSD.*

characteristic of NMOSD. The brain is typically more involved in MS. The presence of a cortical or juxtacortical U-fiber lesion is much more characteristic of MS than NMOSD. AQP4-IgG is almost always negative in MS.

Approximately 15-40% of AQP4-IgG seronegative patients have antibodies to MOG. **MOGAD** targets oligodendrocytes, not astrocytes, and most commonly presents with ADEM imaging features in children and NMOSD imaging features in adults.

**ADEM** can have LETM that is identical to NMOSD. "Tumefactive" lesions and gray matter involvement are also more suggestive of ADEM.

Primary CNS **vasculitis** is often multifocal, frequently "blooms" on T2* SWI, and causes cortical/subcortical and basal ganglia infarcts.

**SuS** is characterized classically by bilateral sensorineural hearing loss, branch retinal artery occlusions, and subacute encephalopathy. It involves the middle layers of the corpus callosum, not the periependymal surfaces.

# Other Autoimmune Disorders

In this section, we consider other autoimmune CNS disorders, such as **autoimmune encephalitis** (AE) and **AHLE**. **SuS**—often mistaken for MS—is also considered here.

## Autoimmune Encephalitis

AE is a family of closely related disease processes in which an antibody-mediated attack causes a localized CNS inflammatory response. The prevalence and incidence of AE has been underestimated in the past but may be nearly equal to infectious encephalitis.

AEs share overlapping clinical features and imaging findings and are differentiated by specific antibody subtypes. Most—but not all—are characterized by limbic dysfunction and varying involvement of the temporal lobes and neocortex.

In addition to paraneoplastic and non-tumor-associated disorders, the AEs are further subdivided according to the cellular location of their neuronal antigens.

Group I antibodies target intracellular antigens, whereas group II antibodies target cell surface antigens. Group I antibodies are more closely associated with underlying malignancy, although **anti-glutamic acid decarboxylase (GAD)** disease targets intracellular antigens but is most commonly associated with nonneoplastic conditions, such as type 1 diabetes mellitus.

### Terminology

The AEs are differentiated by—and named according to—specific antibody subtypes that cause immune-mediated attacks on the CNS.

AE can be paraneoplastic or nonparaneoplastic. Paraneoplastic-associated disorders, such as anti-Hu and anti-Ma encephalitis, are discussed in Chapter 31. Nonneoplastic AE is discussed here. Because of its unique imaging findings, AQP4 and NMOSD are discussed separately in this section.

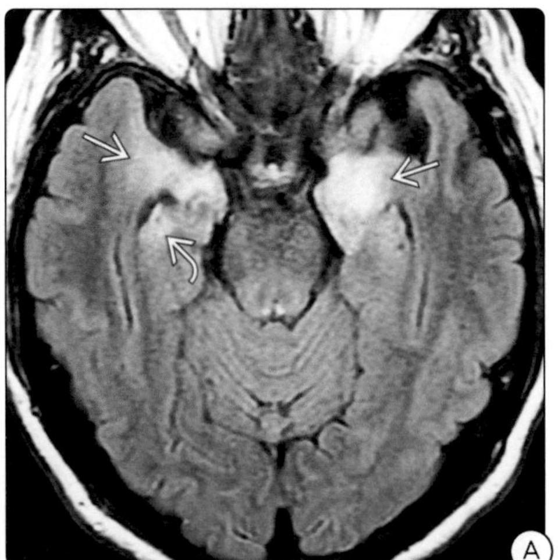

**(15-29A)** *71-yo with subacute encephalopathy shows FLAIR hyperintensity in anteromedial temporal lobes ➡, right hippocampus ↪.*

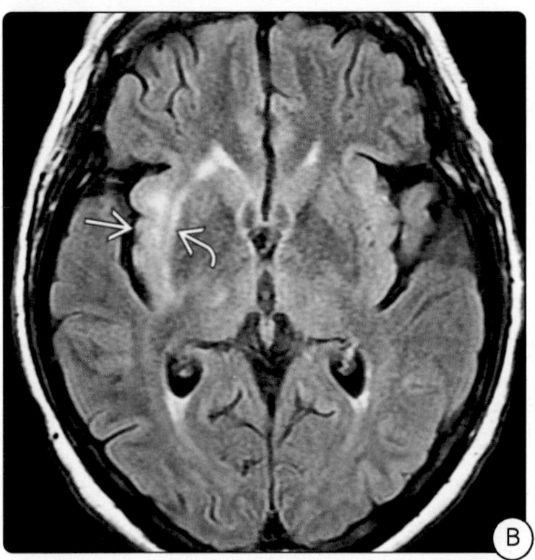

**(15-29B)** *More cephalad FLAIR in the same case shows hyperintensity in the right insular cortex ➡ and external capsule ↪.*

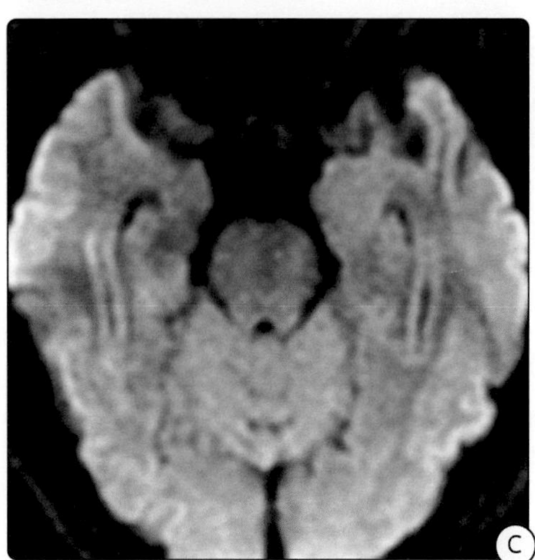

**(15-29C)** *DWI shows no evidence for restricted diffusion. Anti-LGI1 (VKGC) autoantibodies were later detected in her CSF.*

## Etiology

The major antigens responsible for inciting AE are an ever-expanding group of antibodies that is shown in the box below.

Antibodies against cell surface antigens, such as **leucine-rich glioma inactivated 1 (LGI1)**, are among the most common autoantibodies in patients with nonneoplastic autoimmune-mediated CNS disease.

Another common group of autoimmune disorders are those with ion channel antigens. These include the most common AE, **N-methyl, D-aspartate receptor (NMDAR or NMDAr)** and **γ-aminobutyric acid receptor (GABAr)** encephalitis, which has a higher association with malignancies, such as small cell lung cancer, than other group II autoantibodies.

Less common subtypes include **anti-glutamate receptor 3 (GluR3)** autoantibodies (associated with Rasmussen encephalitis) and **voltage-gated calcium channel (VGCC)** encephalitis.

### NONNEOPLASTIC AUTOIMMUNE ENCEPHALITIS

**Group I**

- Intracellular antigens
- Often associated with underlying malignancy
- Examples
  - Anti-Hu (75% due to small cell lung cancer)
  - Anti-Ma (~ 50% due to testicular germ cell tumors)
  - Anti-Ri (breast, small cell lung), anti-Yo (ovarian, breast)
  - Anti-GAD (usually *not* associated with malignancy)

**Group II**

- Cell surface antigens
- Malignancy less common
- Examples
  - NMDAr, GABAr
  - LGI1 (VGKC), VGCC
  - GluR3 (Rasmussen)

## Pathology

Regardless of the etiology and antibody profile, the AEs have a distinct predilection for the limbic system.

## Clinical Issues

Antigenic specificities appear to determine the associated clinical syndromes. Onset is typically *subacute*. The most common presentation is cognitive dysfunction and altered mental status. Seizures and medically intractable epilepsy are also common.

The definitive diagnosis of AE is established by the identification of specific autoantibodies in the CSF &/or sera. **Up to 50% of AE cases are negative, as typical screening panels do not detect all potential autoantibodies!**

## Imaging

Imaging findings are variable; a subset of patients will have no neuroimaging findings despite severe neuropsychiatric dysfunction or subacute cognitive decline.

The most common identifiable pattern is that of limbic encephalitis. T2/FLAIR hyperintensity in one or both medial temporal lobes is typical **(15-29)**. Extralimbic involvement with structures, such as the cortex, striatum, and diencephalon, varies.

Diffusion restriction is variable but usually absent **(15-29C)**. Enhancement on T1 C+ occurs in ~ 25% of cases and is frequently associated with subsequent development of mesial temporal sclerosis.

## Differential Diagnosis

The differential diagnosis of AE includes **herpes simplex encephalitis, HHV-6 encephalitis**, and systemic autoimmune disorders, such as SLE, antiphospholipid antibody syndrome, and thyroid encephalopathy.

# Acute Hemorrhagic Leukoencephalitis

## Terminology

AHLE is also known as acute hemorrhagic leukoencephalopathy, acute hemorrhagic encephalomyelitis (AHEM), and Weston-Hurst disease. Some investigators include AHLE as part of the ADEM spectrum—as a hyperacute, exceptionally severe variant of ADEM.

## Pathology

**Location.** AHLE predominantly affects the white matter. Both the cerebral hemispheres and cerebellum are typically affected. Despite its name, AHLE may affect the gray matter; basal ganglia involvement is common, but the cortical gray matter is generally spared.

**Size and Number.** AHLE has two distinct manifestations: Innumerable petechial microbleeds and macroscopic parenchymal hemorrhages. Some cases have features of both.

**Gross Pathology.** The typical gross appearance is that of marked brain swelling with diffuse confluent **(15-32)** &/or petechial hemorrhages **(15-30)**. Hemorrhages are typically present in the cerebral hemispheres (predominately the white matter) and cerebellum. Fibrinoid necrosis of vessel walls with perivascular hemorrhages and mononuclear inflammatory cell cuffing are the microscopic hallmarks of fulminant AHLE.

## Clinical Issues

**Epidemiology and Demographics.** AHLE is rare. Approximately 2% of all ADEM cases are of the hyperacute hemorrhagic type that could be considered consistent with AHLE. Although AHLE occurs at all ages, most patients are children and young adults.

**Presentation and Natural History.** History of a viral prodrome or flu-like illness followed by rapid neurologic deterioration is typical. Fever and lethargy with increasing somnolence, decreased mental status, impaired consciousness, and long-tract signs are the most common clinical symptoms.

Untreated AHLE has a very poor prognosis. Clinical deterioration and death usually occur within days to a week after symptom onset. Mortality is 60-80%.

AHLE is almost always fatal if untreated. Aggressive treatment with decompressive craniectomy, intravenous high-dose corticosteroids, and plasmapheresis has been associated with survival and even favorable outcome in a few cases.

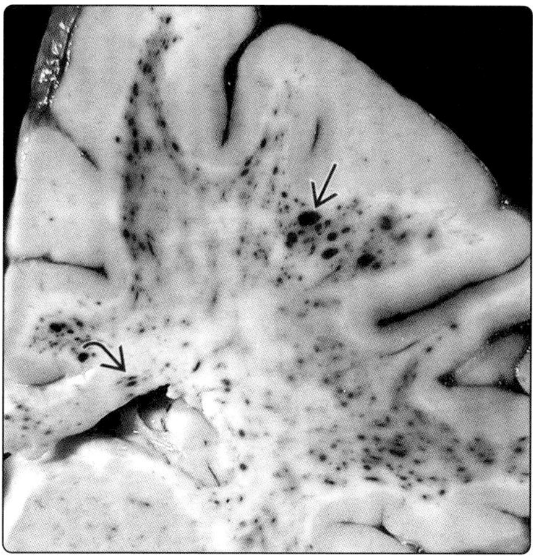

***(15-30)** Autopsied AHLE shows innumerable tiny subcortical WM hemorrhages extending into the corpus callosum. Cortex is spared.*

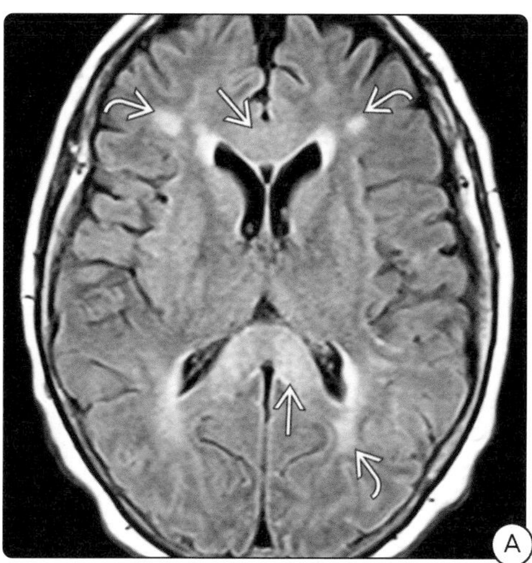

***(15-31A)** FLAIR in a 69-yo with postviral altered mental status shows confluent hyperintensity in corpus callosum, hemispheric WM.*

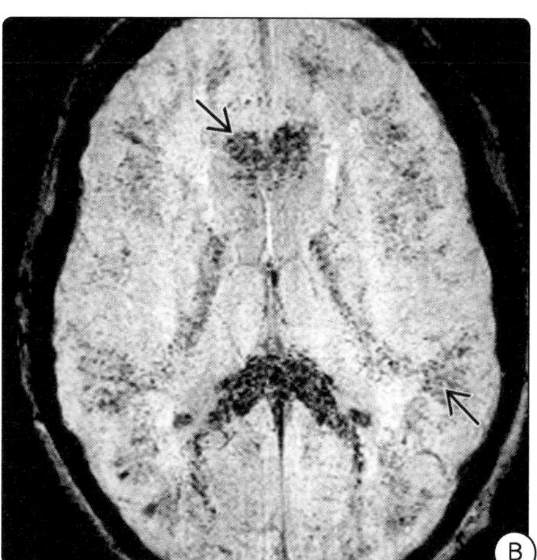

***(15-31B)** SWI 2 weeks later shows "blooming" hypointensities throughout WM. AHLE was diagnosed on imaging and confirmed with biopsy.*

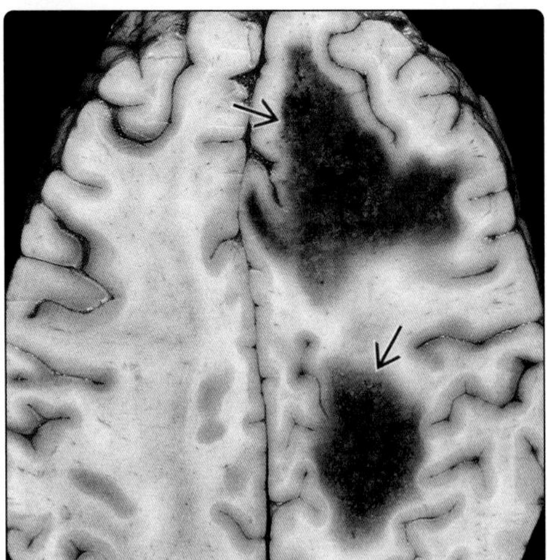

*(15-32) Autopsied fulminant AHLE shows 2 confluent areas of WM hemorrhagic necrosis ➡ with cortical sparing. (Courtesy R. Hewlett, MD.)*

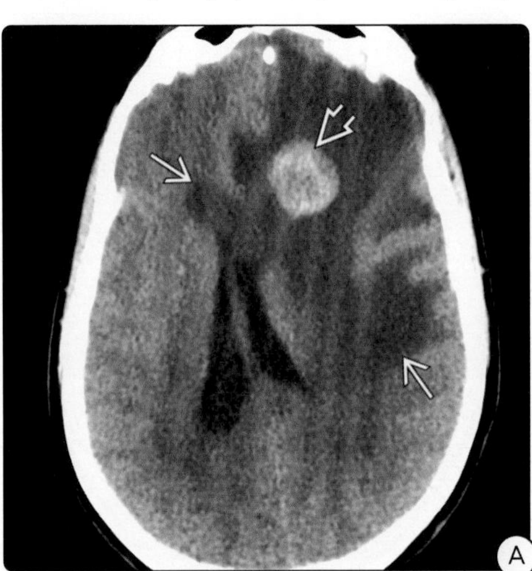


*(15-33A) NECT in a 26-yo woman with biopsy-proven AHLE shows left frontal hematoma ➡ with mass effect, striking perilesional edema ➡.*

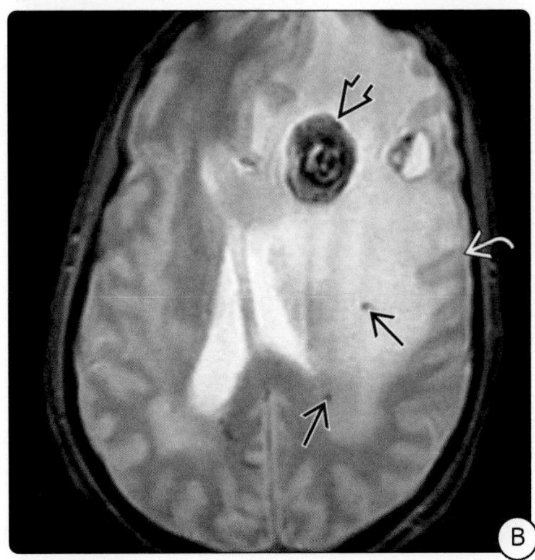


*(15-33B) T2* GRE shows focal hematoma ➡, several "blooming black dots" ➡. Note cortical sparing ➡. (Courtesy M. Preece, MD.)*

**ACUTE HEMORRHAGIC LEUKOENCEPHALITIS**

**Terminology**
- a.k.a. AHEM, Weston-Hurst disease

**Etiology and Pathology**
- Similar to ADEM (viral/postviral autoimmune-mediated condition)

**Clinical Issues**
- Rare; most common in children
- Fever, lethargy, impaired consciousness
- Rapidly progressive, often lethal course

**Imaging**
- General features
  - White matter edema
  - Focal macroscopic hemorrhages or multifocal microbleeds
- MR procedure of choice
  - Multifocal scattered or confluent lesions on T2/FLAIR
  - Corpus callosum, cerebral white matter, pons, cerebellum ± basal ganglia
  - Cortical gray matter generally spared
  - T2* (GRE, SWI) depicts microbleeds

**Differential Diagnosis**
- Severe ADEM
- Critical illness-associated microbleeds

## Imaging

**CT Findings.** NECT may be normal unless confluent lobar hemorrhages are present **(15-33A)**. Petechial microhemorrhages are generally invisible on CT, but white matter edema with diffuse, relatively asymmetric hypodensity in one or both hemispheres may be present.

**MR Findings.** T1 scans are often normal unless lobar hemorrhage is present. T2/FLAIR findings vary from subtle to striking. Multifocal scattered or confluent hyperintensities as well as bilateral confluent hyperintensity of the cerebral white matter are typical but nonspecific findings **(15-31A)**.

T2* scans are the key to diagnosis; SWI sequences are more sensitive than GRE **(15-33B)**. Multifocal punctate and linear "blooming" hypointensities in the corpus callosum that extend through the full thickness of the hemispheric white matter to the subcortical U-fibers are typical findings on T2* **(15-31B)**. Striking sparing of the overlying cortex is common. Additional lesions are frequently present in the basal ganglia, midbrain, pons, and cerebellum.

Enhancement on T1 C+ occurs in 50% of cases and ranges from linear perivascular space enhancement to larger patchy or confluent foci.

## Differential Diagnosis

The major differential diagnosis of AHLE is **ADEM**. Both share a number of similar features; however, ADEM usually follows a much less fulminant course and does not demonstrate the characteristic lobar or perivascular hemorrhages of AHLE.

Petechial microhemorrhages similar to those seen in AHLE can be found in a number of other disorders, including disseminated intravascular coagulopathy, fat emboli, thrombotic thrombocytopenic purpura, sepsis, vasculitis, hemorrhagic viral fevers, malaria, and rickettsial diseases. A recently described entity, **critical illness-associated microbleeds**, may be seen in the setting of acute respiratory failure and appear indistinguishable from AHLE.

## Susac Syndrome

SuS is an autoimmune endotheliopathy that causes microvascular occlusions in the brain. Most patients are young adult females who present with the classic clinical triad of subacute encephalopathy, branch retinal artery occlusions, and sensorineural hearing loss. In 50% of cases, migraine-like headache is a heralding symptom.

### Imaging

SuS is often initially mistaken for MS on imaging studies. Sagittal T1WI in patients with chronic SuS may show typical "punched-out" lesions in the middle layers of the corpus callosum **(15-34)** **(15-36)**. T2/FLAIR shows multiple deep white matter hyperintensities in > 90% of cases. Basal ganglia lesions occur in 70% of cases and brainstem lesions in nearly 1/3 of cases. Acute SuS lesions show punctate enhancement on T1 C+ **(15-35)**.

### Differential Diagnosis

**MS** preferentially involves the undersurface of the corpus callosum, which is usually spared in SuS. **ADEM** and **Lyme disease** also rarely involve the middle layers of the corpus callosum. ADEM is generally monophasic, preceded by a viral prodrome or history of vaccination. **Primary arteritis of the CNS (PACNS)** rarely affects the corpus callosum, whereas cortical lesions and hemorrhages are common.

## CLIPPERS

CLIPPERS is the acronym for **c**hronic **l**ymphocytic **i**nflammation with **p**ontine **p**erivascular **e**nhancement **r**esponsive to **s**teroids.

### Pathology

CLIPPERS is characterized histopathologically by widespread foci of CD4(+) T-cell perivascular inflammation in the brainstem and cerebellum.

### Clinical Issues

Patients typically present with subacute pontocerebellar dysfunction (e.g., gait ataxia) with or without other CNS symptoms (e.g., cognitive dysfunction or myelopathy). Mean age at onset is 40-50 years. Dramatic response to glucocorticosteroids (GCSs) as well as worsening following corticosteroid withdrawal is a hallmark feature of CLIPPERS but does not exclude non-CLIPPERS pathology.

### Imaging

Multifocal T2/FLAIR homogeneously hyperintense lesions with ≤ 3-mm punctate or curvilinear "peppering" enhancement on T1 C+ are typical **(15-37)**. Ring enhancement and mass effect are absent, and the area of T2 signal abnormality typically does not significantly exceed that of the T1 C+ enhancement.

Lesions *outside* the pons and cerebellum are present in 60% of cases and occur in the midbrain, medulla, subcortical white matter, cerebral hemispheres, and spinal cord. There is a clear geographic gradient of lesser inflammation with increasing distance from the brainstem and cerebellum.

Foci of restricted diffusion may occur in the acute phase. Punctate microbleeds in the affected areas are sometimes identified on T2* SWI sequences. Posttreatment atrophy is common.

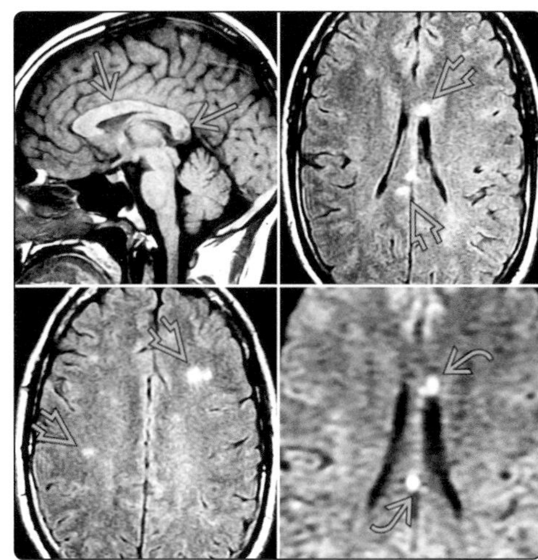

***(15-34)** Susac syndrome (SuS): Middle callosal T1 "holes" ➡, ovoid FLAIR lesions ➡ with increased DWI ➡. (Courtesy P. Rodriguez, MD.)*

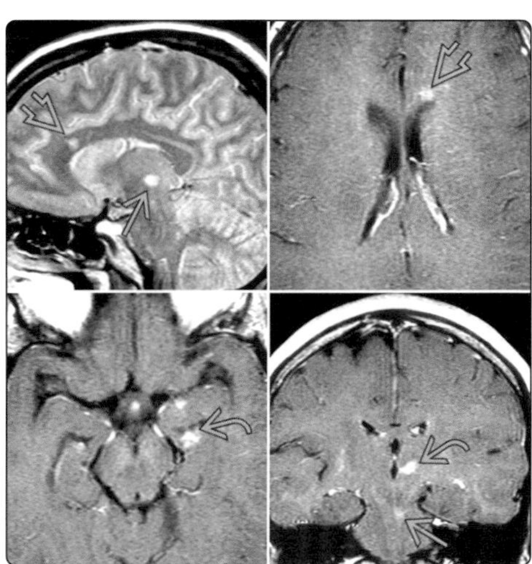

***(15-35)** Findings in SuS: FLAIR-hyperintense and enhancing brainstem lesions ➡, midcallosal lesions ➡, and scattered T1 C+ foci ➡.*

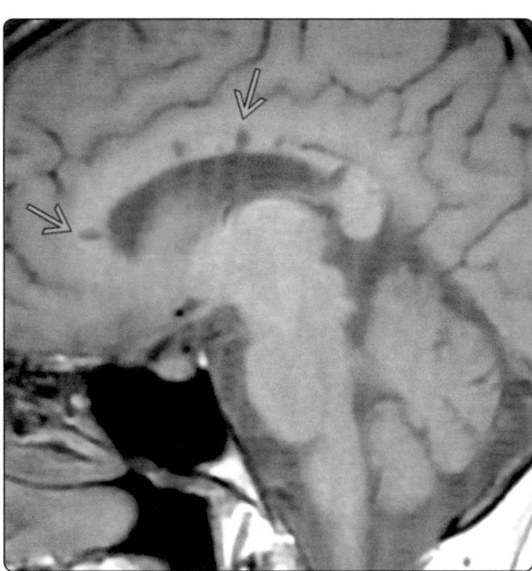

***(15-36)** Sagittal T1 MR in an 18-yo woman with SuS shows typical ovoid areas of "black holes" ➡ within the mid corpus callosum.*

## Differential Diagnosis

Lesion-associated mass effect and lesions with T2/FLAIR signal abnormality much larger than the enhancing foci should suggest non-CLIPPERS etiology, such as **intravascular lymphoma, vasculitis, neurosarcoidosis**, and **MS** or **NMOSD**. GCS therapy failure with lack of complete resolution of enhancing abnormalities should also strongly suggest an alternative diagnosis.

# Inflammatory-Like Disorders

## Neurosarcoidosis

### Terminology

Sarcoidosis ("sarcoid") is a multisystem inflammatory disorder characterized by discrete noncaseating epithelioid granulomas. When sarcoidosis affects the CNS, it is termed neurosarcoidosis (NS).

### Etiology

The etiology of sarcoidosis remains unknown, but the prevailing view is that genetically susceptible individuals develop sarcoidosis following exposure to presently

*(15-37A) Sagittal FLAIR MR in a 52-yo man with diplopia, dysarthria, and facial numbness shows multiple punctate hyperintensities "peppering" the pons ➡, medulla ➡, and extending into the upper cervical spinal cord ➡. (15-37B) T1 C+ FS MR shows punctate ➡ and curvilinear ➡ foci of contrast enhancement. Note extension into the cerebellum ➡ and superior cerebellar peduncle ➡.*

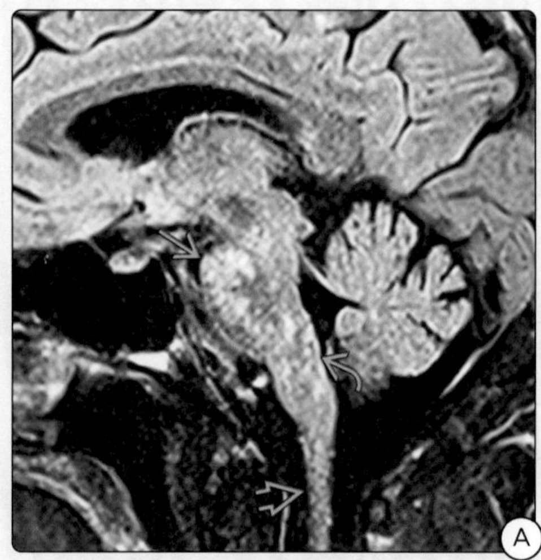


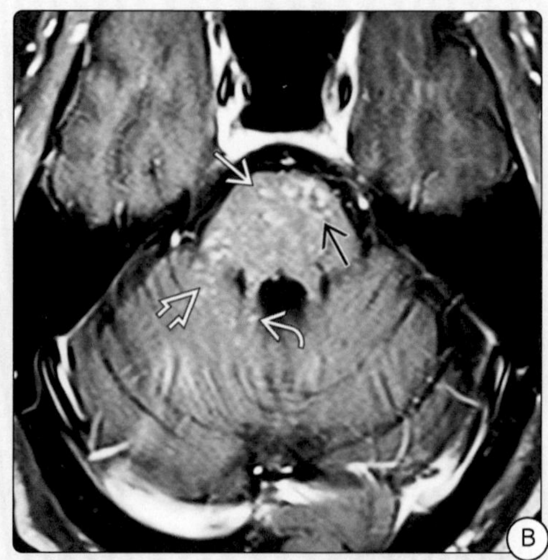


*(15-37C) DWI MR shows scattered foci of restricted diffusion ➡. (15-37D) Axial T2* SWI MIP shows multiple hemorrhagic foci ➡ in the pons. The patient responded dramatically to steroids, but cessation of GCS treatment resulted in disease recurrence. CLIPPERS was diagnosed on the basis of imaging findings and GCS responsiveness.*

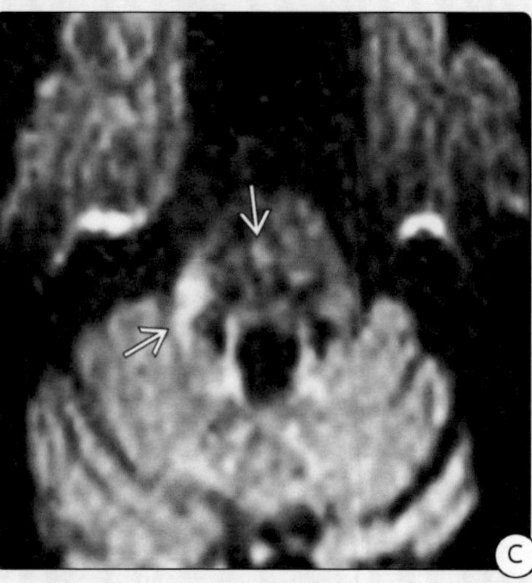


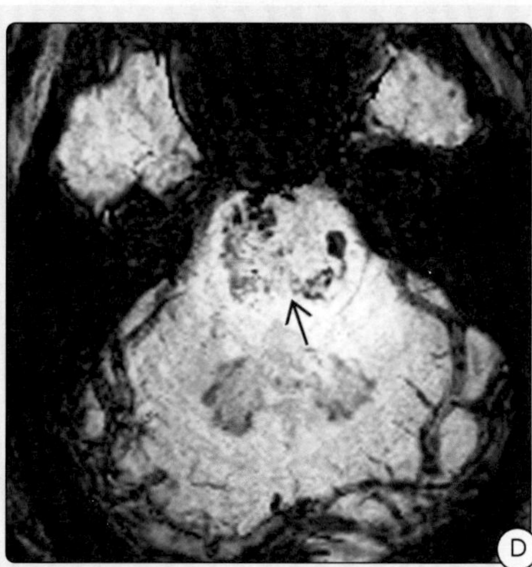

unidentified antigens. A reactive inflammatory cascade ensues that appears to be driven primarily through CD4(+) T cells.

## Pathology

**Location.** The CNS is involved in ~ 5% of cases, usually in combination with disease elsewhere. Only 5-10% of NS cases are confined to the CNS and occur without evidence of systemic sarcoidosis.

Sarcoid can involve any part of the nervous system or its coverings. Lesions vary in size, from tiny granulomas that infiltrate along the pia and perivascular spaces.

The most common location is the meninges, especially around the base of the brain. Diffuse leptomeningeal thickening with or without more focal nodular lesions is seen in ~ 40% of cases **(15-38)**. Large dura-based masses may occur, resembling meningiomas.

The hypothalamus and infundibulum are also favored intracranial sites **(15-39)**. NS can involve cranial nerves, eye and periorbita, bone, the ventricles and choroid plexus, and the brain parenchyma itself. Sarcoid can also involve the spinal leptomeninges, cord, and nerve roots.

## Clinical Issues

**Epidemiology and Demographics.** NS is a worldwide disorder that has a bimodal age distribution. The largest peak occurs during the third and fourth decades with a second smaller peak in patients—especially women—over the age of 50.

**Presentation.** Symptoms vary with location. The most common presentation of NS is isolated or multiple cranial nerve deficits seen in 50-75% of patients. The facial and optic nerves are the most frequently affected. Symptoms of pituitary/hypothalamic dysfunction, such as diabetes insipidus or panhypopituitarism, are seen in 10-15% of cases.

Diagnosing NS may be difficult because the clinical features can be nonspecific, and elevated serum angiotensin-converting enzyme (ACE) levels are seen in < 1/2 of all cases.

**Treatment Options.** Most patients with NS respond to corticosteroids. Second-line treatment with immunosuppressive agents and third-line treatment with monoclonal antibodies against TNF-α have been tried with variable success.

## Imaging

**CT Findings.** Depending on the amount of fibrosis present, NS can appear slightly hyperdense relative to normal brain parenchyma on NECT scan. Well-circumscribed "punched-out" lesions with nonsclerotic margins can be seen on bone CT.

Leptomeningeal disease may enhance on CECT, resembling tuberculosis or pyogenic meningitis. Dura-based masses are typically modestly hyperdense and enhance strongly and uniformly on CECT.

**MR Findings.** NS is isointense with brain on T1WI and hyperintense relative to CSF. Sulci filled with leptomeningeal infiltrates appear effaced, and the border between the sarcoid and brain is indistinct. Dura-based masses resemble meningiomas.

Parenchymal infiltration along the perivascular spaces causes a vasculitis-like reaction with edema, mass effect, and hyperintensity on T2/FLAIR.

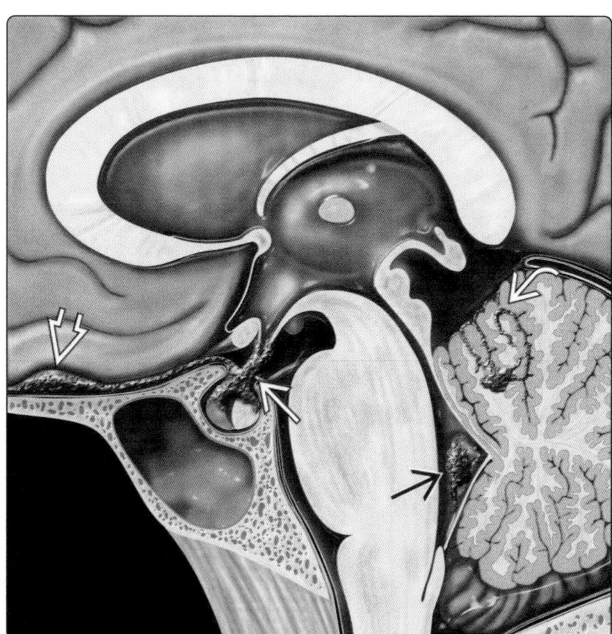

***(15-38)** Graphic illustrates common neurosarcoid locations: (1) Infundibulum, extending into the pituitary ➡, (2) plaque-like dura-arachnoid thickening ➡, and (3) synchronous lesions of the superior vermis ➡ and 4th ventricle choroid plexus ➡.*

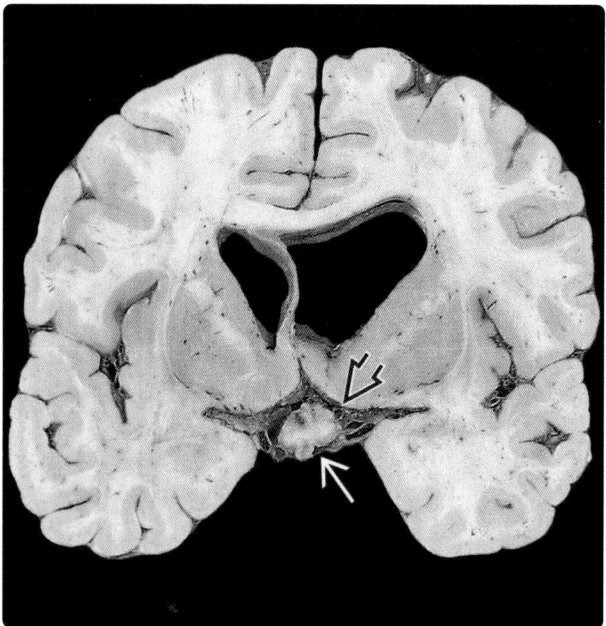

***(15-39)** Autopsy of neurosarcoidosis demonstrates gelatinous infiltration of the leptomeninges ➡ around the thickened hypothalamus and optic chiasm ➡. (From DP: Neuro.)*

The most common finding on T1 C+ scans is nodular or diffuse pial thickening, found in ~ 1/3-1/2 of all cases **(15-40)**.

1/2 of NS patients eventually develop parenchymal disease. Hypothalamic and infundibular thickening with intense enhancement is seen in 5-10% of cases. Multifocal nodular enhancing masses or more diffuse perivascular infiltrates may develop. Solitary parenchymal or dura-based masses are less common. In rare cases, coalescing granulomas form a focal expansile mass ("tumefactive" NS).

NS may cause solitary or multifocal thickened enhancing cranial nerves as well as enhancing masses in the ventricles and choroid plexus.

## Differential Diagnosis

The differential diagnosis of NS depends on lesion location. **Meningitis** can look very similar to NS of the basilar leptomeninges. Dura-based NS may resemble **meningioma** or **lymphoma**; hypothalamic/infundibular/pituitary NS may look like **histiocytosis** or lymphocytic **hypophysitis**.

Multifocal parenchymal enhancing lesions can resemble **MS, metastases, and intravascular lymphoma**. The differential diagnosis of solitary or multiple cranial NS includes infection, demyelinating disease, and neoplasm.

# IgG4-Related Disease

IgG4-related disease (IgG4-RD) is a multisystem, multifocal, fibrosclerotic inflammatory disorder that is primarily tumefactive or mass-like. IgG4-RD most frequently involves the lung and retroperitoneal spaces. The most common head and neck sites are the orbit and salivary glands **(15-41C)**, where IgG4-RD can closely resemble orbital lymphoproliferative disorders.

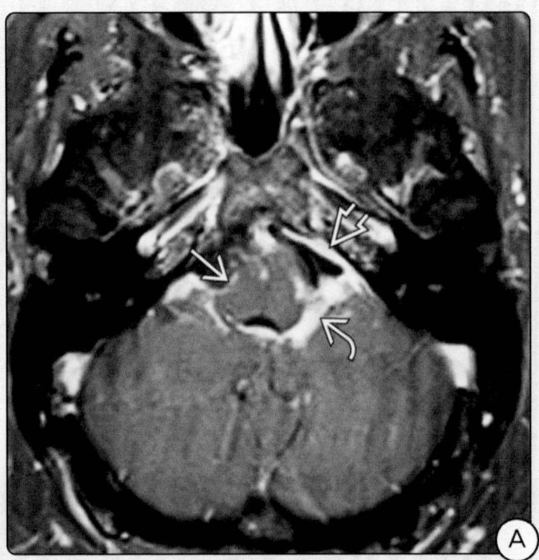


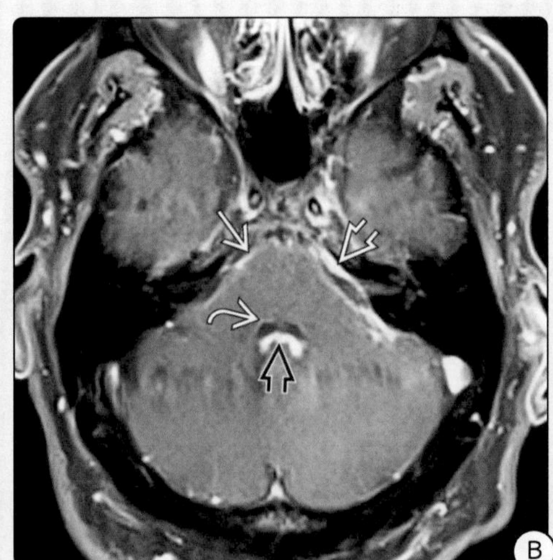


***(15-40A)*** *Axial T1 C+ FS MR in a 56-yo woman with proven neurosarcoid shows thickening and enhancement along the choroid plexus ➡, dura ➡, and pial surface of the medulla ➡.* ***(15-40B)*** *More cephalad T1 C+ FS MR shows a thickened, enhancing dural plaque ➡. Lesions are also present along the pial surface of the pons ➡, the choroid plexus of the 4th ventricle ➡, and the ventricular ependyma ➡.*

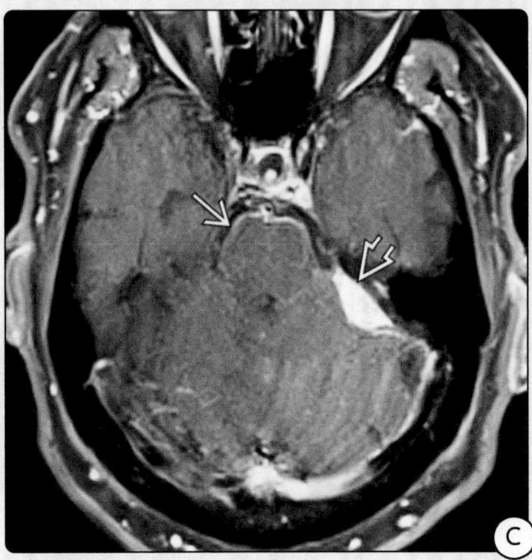


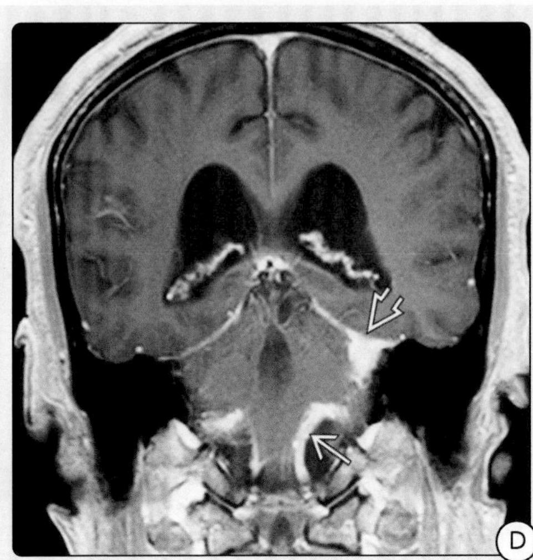


***(15-40C)*** *More cephalad axial T1 C+ FS MR shows the pial involvement ➡. A mass-like enhancing dural plaque at the left cerebellopontine angle (CPA) cistern ➡ resembles a meningioma.* ***(15-40D)*** *Coronal T1 C+ MR in the same case shows the extensive leptomeningeal enhancement ➡ and the CPA dural plaque ➡.*

Intracranial IgG4-RD has been described in the pituitary gland and stalk, cranial nerves, cavernous sinus, and dura **(15-41)**. Isolated intracranial disease occurs but is uncommon.

*Selected References: The complete reference list is available on the eBooks+ version included with purchase.*

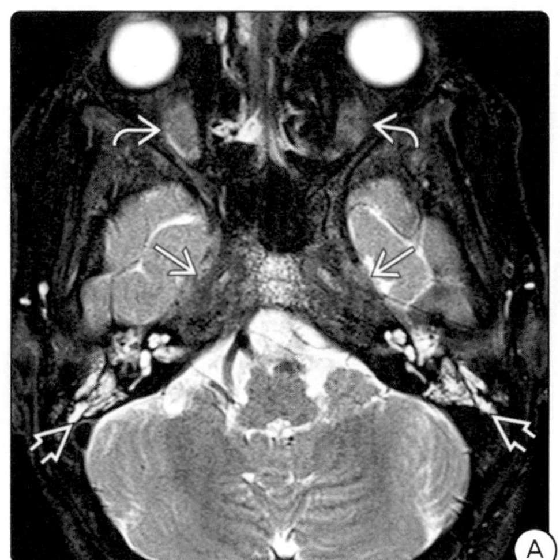


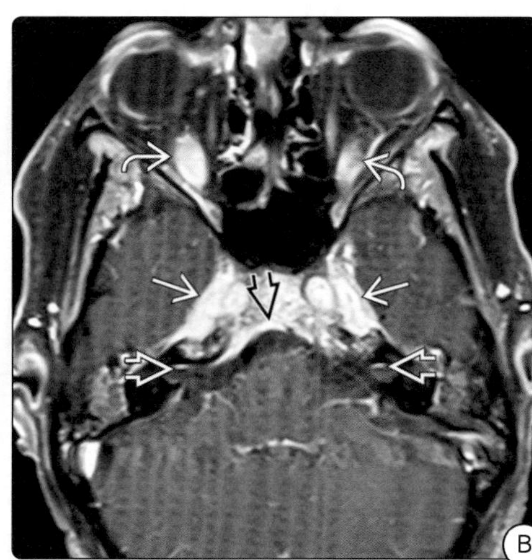


***(15-41A)** Axial T2 FS MR in a 26-yo woman with headache, proptosis, and right CNVI palsy shows hypointense, diffusely infiltrating mass in both cavernous sinuses ➡ and orbital apices ➡. Bilateral serous otitis media is present ➡. **(15-41B)** T1 C+ FS MR in the same case shows that the cavernous sinus ➡ and orbital apex ➡ masses enhance strongly. Also note clival dura-arachnoid ➡ thickening with linear enhancement in both internal auditory canals ➡.*

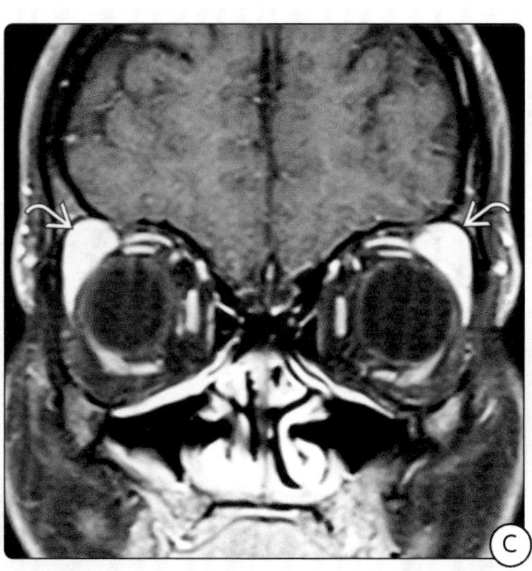


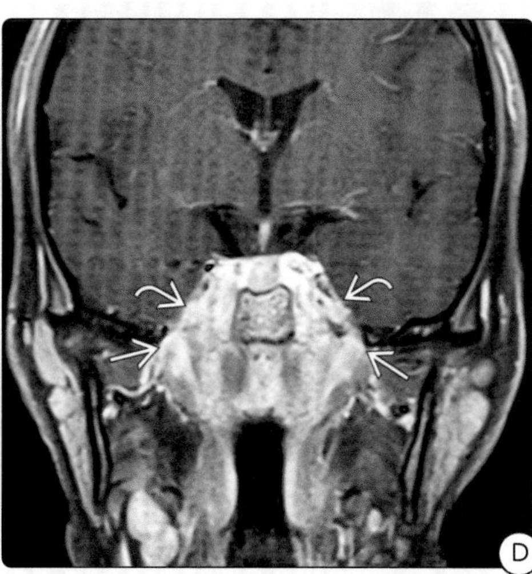


***(15-41C)** Coronal T1 C+ FS MR shows markedly enlarged, intensely enhancing lacrimal glands ➡. **(15-41D)** More posterior T1 C+ FS MR shows that the cavernous sinus-infiltrating mass involves both Meckel caves ➡ and extends through the foramen ovale ➡ into the nasopharynx, obstructing the eustachian tubes. This is biopsy-proven IgG4-related disease.*

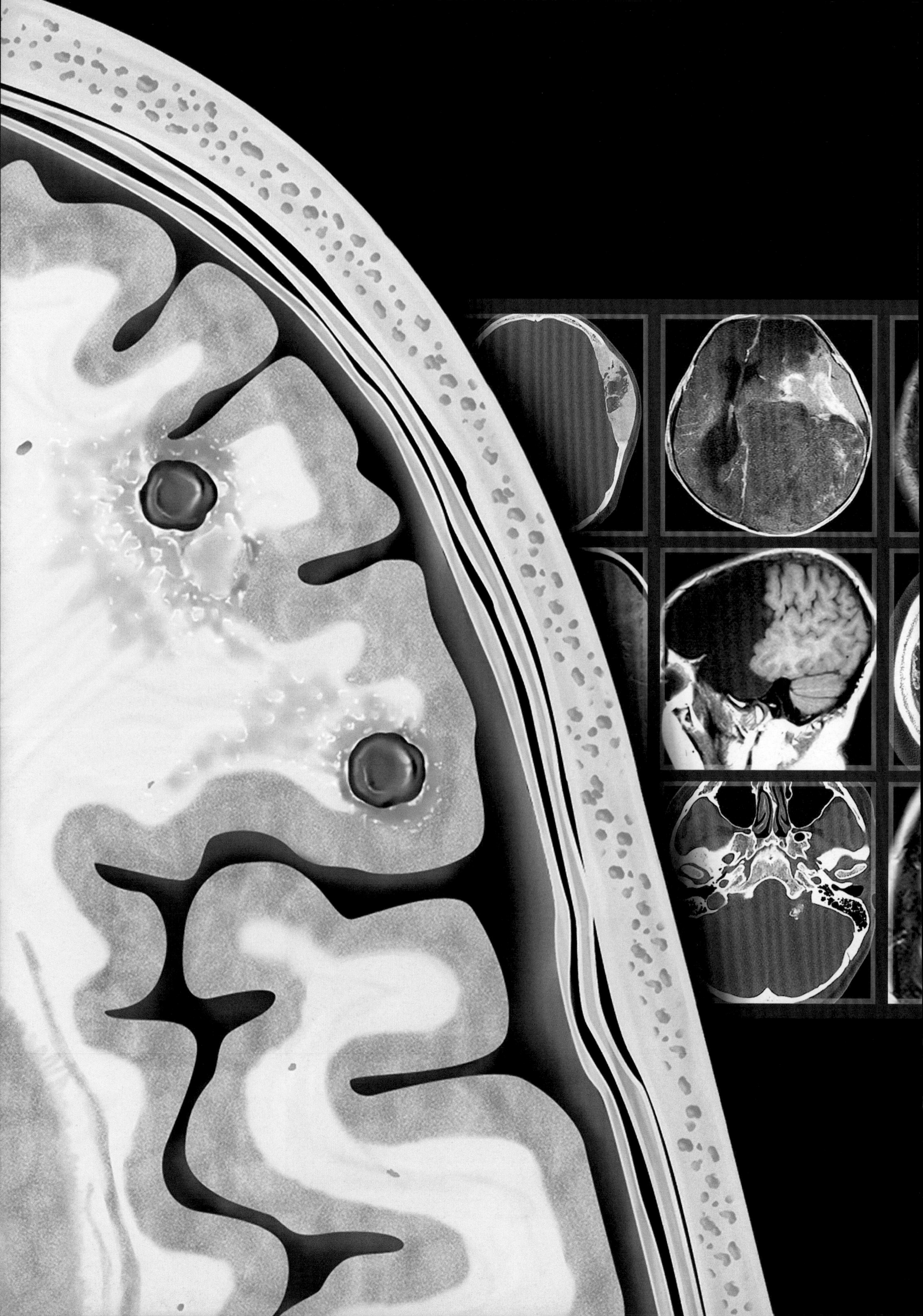

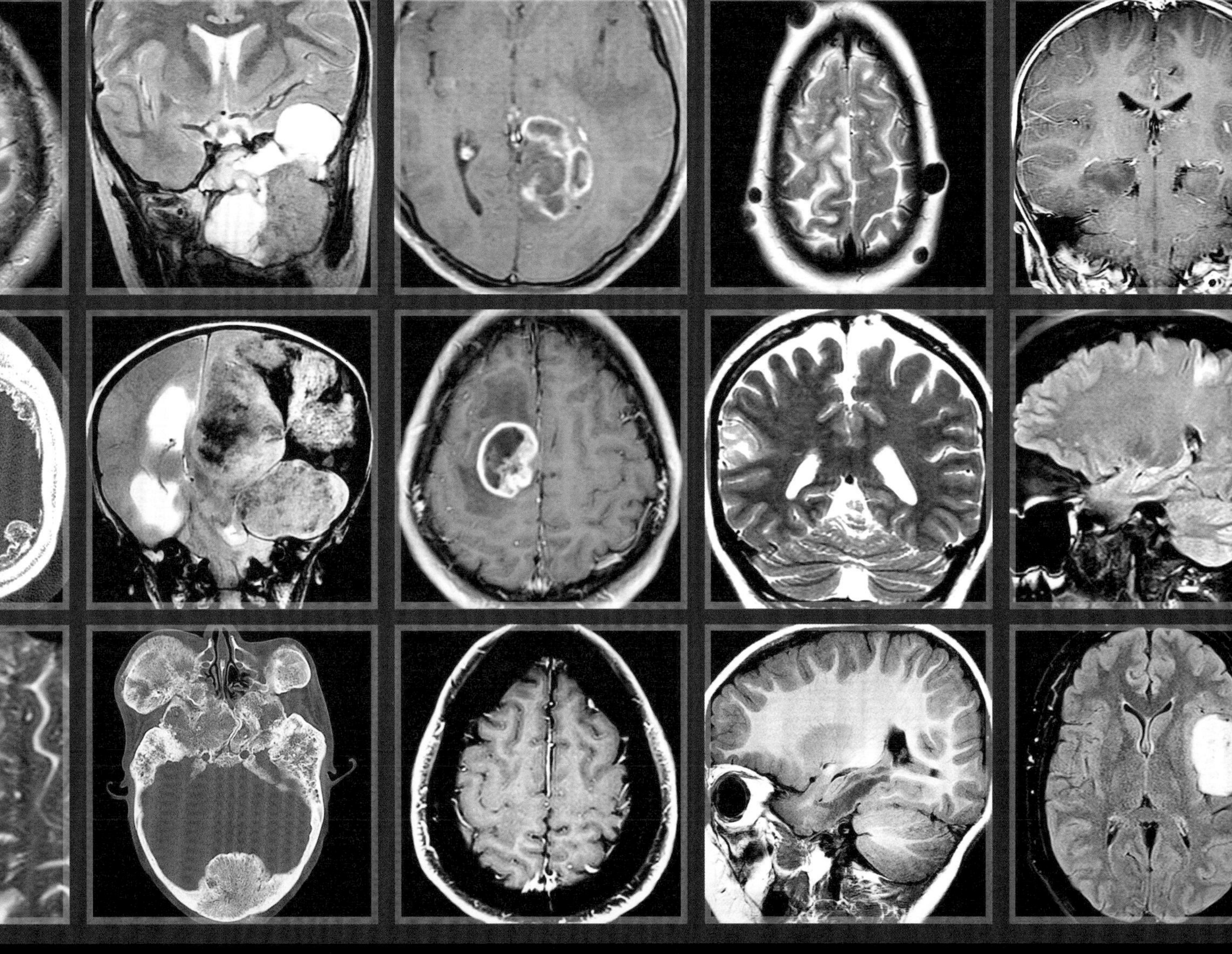

SECTION 4

# Neoplasms, Cysts, and Tumor-Like Lesions

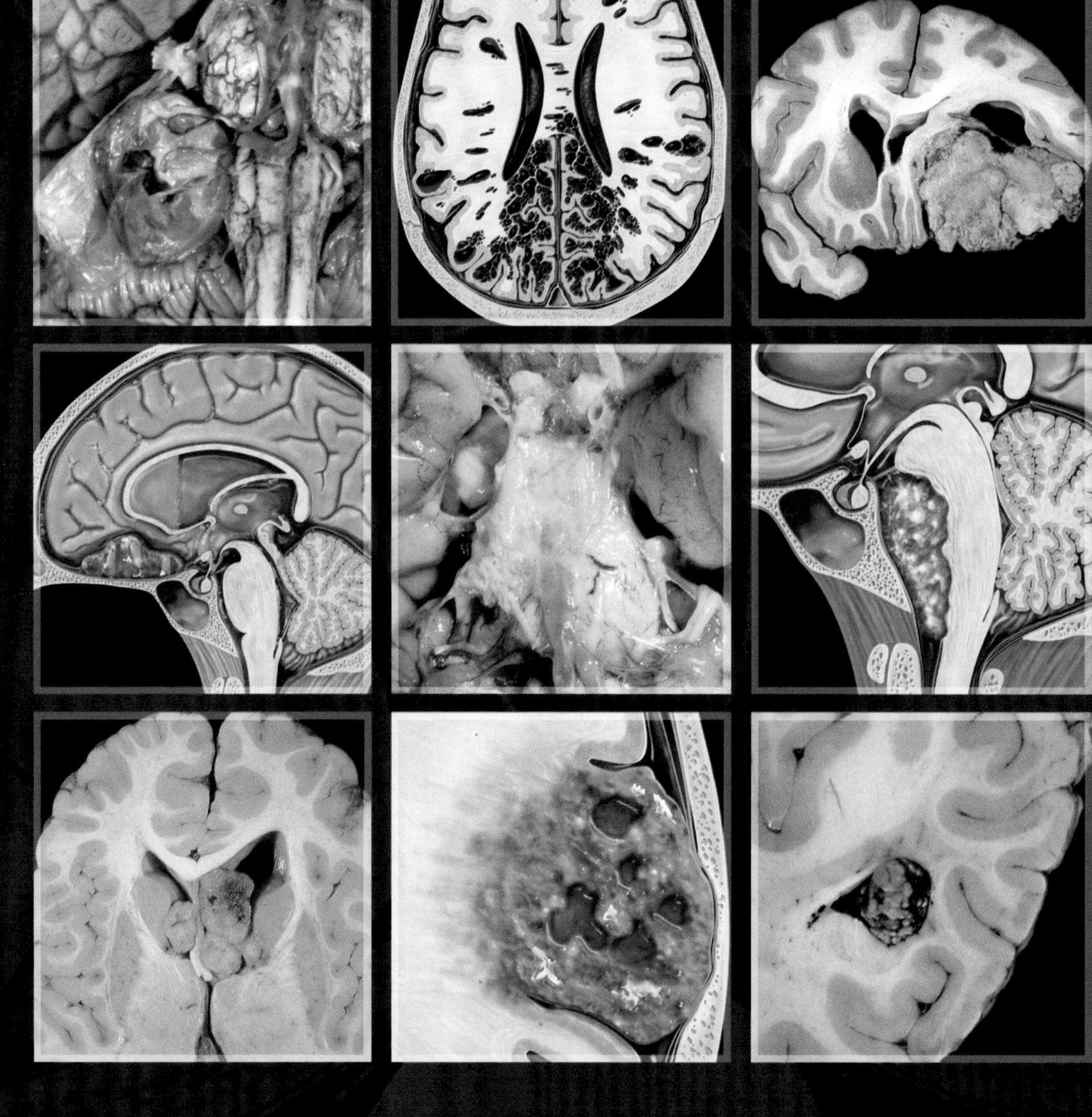

SECTION 4

# Neoplasms, Cysts, and Tumor-Like Lesions

# Introduction to CNS Neoplasms and Nonneoplastic Cysts

*CNS neoplasms are both (1) classified and (2) graded. The universally accepted classification of these tumors is sponsored by the WHO. The 2nd edition of Osborn's Brain was based on the 4th edition of the WHO Classification of Tumours of the Central Nervous System published in 2016. With rapid advancements in the molecular diagnostics of these tumors, a new (5th) edition of the famed "Blue Book" was published in late 2021.*



This introduction presents an overview of major changes incorporated into the 5th edition WHO. We begin with a brief introduction to CNS tumor taxonomy, nomenclature, classification, and grading. We introduce the concept of a pathologic "integrated diagnosis" and emphasize its importance in stratifying patients for treatment.

We close the introduction with a brief summary of the major diagnostic categories/groupings of CNS neoplasms.

## CNS Tumor Taxonomy

CNS neoplasms are both classified and graded. Traditionally, classification assigned CNS neoplasms to discrete categories based on the histologic similarity of tumor cells to normal or embryonic constituents of the nervous system. Hence, terms like "astrocytoma" and "meningioma" were used.

In 2016, the concept of incorporating molecular markers as key aspects of the classification of CNS tumors was introduced. As the molecular foundations of these tumors have been rapidly elucidated, these features have been utilized to group some tumors into families (types) and subtypes. The combination of molecular profiling with histologic features ideally results in an "integrated diagnosis" that can then be used to stratify patients for treatment.

### CNS Tumor Nomenclature and Classification

The 5th edition WHO has made tumor nomenclature generally more consistent and simple. In previous editions, some entities incorporated anatomic site into the entity name, e.g., "chordoid glioma 'of the third ventricle'" is now simply "chordoid glioma."

Some exceptions where location, age, or genetic modifiers have specific diagnostic or clinical utility have been retained in the 5th edition (e.g., "central neurocytoma" and "extraventricular neurocytoma"). In other cases, names retained histopathologic or anatomic features that are characteristically but not invariably present (e.g., myxopapillary ependymomas are not always myxoid or papillary, and diffuse midline gliomas **(16-1)** are usually but not always exactly midline).

Some tumor names with historical associations that are deeply embedded in common usage have also been retained. Thus, the term "medulloblastoma" continues to be used in the 5th edition (even though a medulloblast has never been identified). Genetically defined tumor subtypes with vastly differing prognoses and treatment are grouped together as "medulloblastomas" but are now defined and subtyped by their molecular features (e.g., medulloblastoma, WNT-activated).

Gene and protein nomenclature in the 5th edition mostly utilizes the Human Genome Organization (HUGO) and Human Genome Variation Society (HGVS) systems for gene symbols and gene names. Gene symbols (e.g., *IDH1*) are presented in italics, but proteins and gene groups (e.g., the family of IDH genes) are not italicized.

## CNS Tumor Grading

Tumors are both classified and graded. In the 2016 classification, tumor grading reflected overall expected clinical-biological behavior and represented a combination of histopathology findings and expected natural history. For example, diffuse astrocytic tumors were assigned to three different tumor types: Diffuse astrocytoma (grade II), anaplastic astrocytoma (grade III), and glioblastoma (grade IV).

In the 5th edition, CNS neoplasms are graded **within** tumor types rather than **across** different types. In the current classification, a diffuse adult-type glioma might be identified microscopically and immunohistochemically as an IDH-mutant astrocytoma, then assigned a grade (CNS WHO grades 2-4) according to its molecular profile. Here, all IDH-mutant astrocytomas are considered a single type and graded within that specific tumor type.

Grading is also no longer entirely histologic. As many molecular markers now provide powerful prognostic information, they have been fully incorporated into determining tumor grade in the 5th edition. For example, an IDH-mutant astrocytoma (tumor type) can be designated grade 2, 3, or 4. Modifier terms, such as "anaplastic," have been eliminated. Thus, an "anaplastic astrocytoma" with appropriate histologic and molecular features would now be diagnosed as "astrocytoma, IDH-mutant, CNS WHO grade 3."

Molecular parameters may—and often do—override histologic findings in assigning tumor grade. An adult-type diffusely infiltrating glioma with astrocytic features, *IDH1* or *IDH2* mutation, and absence of 1p/19q codeletion can be a grade 2, 3, or 4 tumor. Presence of homozygous deletion of *CDKN2A* results in the diagnosis of astrocytoma, IDH-mutant, CNS WHO grade 4, even if histologic features like frank anaplasia, microvascular proliferation, and necrosis are absent.

A notable change in the 5th edition is that Arabic numerals (1-4) have now replaced Roman numerals (I-IV). Because CNS tumor grading differs from other (non-CNS) tumor grading, the term "CNS WHO grade _" is now used when assigning tumor grade to a particular entity.

## Integrated ("Layered") Diagnosis

With the increasing importance of molecular information in CNS tumor classification and prognosis, modern neuropathologic reports now combine different data types into a single integrated ("layered") diagnosis. These reports are headed by an integrated diagnosis at the top followed by layers that delineate histologic, molecular, and other key types of information.

Information included in a layered neuropathologic report include tumor site at the top followed by integrated diagnosis (a combination of tissue-based histologic and molecular diagnosis), histopathologic classification, CNS WHO grade, and specific molecular information (listed). An example of such a layered report is shown in the next box.

If complete molecular classification is incomplete or not available, the modifier "NOS" (not otherwise specified) is included in the diagnosis. The modifier "NEC" (not elsewhere classified) is added to denote tumors that have been fully characterized but do not fit within the established classification system.

**CEREBRUM**

**Integrated Diagnosis**
- Diffuse astrocytoma, IDH-mutant, CNS WHO grade 2

**Histopathologic Diagnosis**
- Diffuse astrocytoma

**WHO Grade**
- CNS WHO grade 2

**Molecular Genetics**
- *IDH1* R132H-mutant, *ATRX*-mutant, *TP53*-mutant

# CNS Neoplasm Families

The 5th edition WHO discusses CNS neoplasms in three groups: Primary CNS neoplasms, metastases, and genetic tumor syndromes involving the CNS.

## Primary CNS Neoplasms

Approximately 50% of brain neoplasms are primary tumors. In the 5th edition WHO, primary CNS neoplasms are divided into 11 groups (see next box). For the first time, age is also considered as an integral part in the classification of some primary neoplasms; the new edition differentiates "adult-type" from "pediatric-type" gliomas. Even though some gliomas may appear identical histopathologically, their molecular profiles are distinctly different in different age groups.

Gliomas, glioneuronal tumors, and neuronal tumors are the largest and most varied neoplasms that affect the brain. The 5th edition divides these tumors into six different groups: (1)

Adult-type diffuse gliomas (e.g., astrocytoma, IDH-mutant, oligodendroglioma, and glioblastoma, IDH-wildtype **(16-2)**). These are the most common of all CNS neoplasms. (2) Pediatric-type diffuse low-grade gliomas (much less common and include tumors like angiocentric glioma). (3) Pediatric-type diffuse high-grade gliomas (e.g., H3 K27-altered diffuse midline glioma **(16-1)**). (4) Circumscribed astrocytic gliomas (e.g., pilocytic astrocytoma and subependymal giant cell astrocytoma **(16-3)**). (5) Glioneuronal and neuronal tumors (e.g., ganglioglioma, dysembryoplastic neuroepithelial tumor). (6) Ependymal tumors.

**PRIMARY CNS NEOPLASMS**

- Gliomas, glioneuronal tumors, and neuronal tumors
- Choroid plexus tumors
- Embryonal tumors
- Pineal tumors
- Cranial and paraspinal nerve tumors
- Meningioma
- Mesenchymal, nonmeningothelial tumors involving CNS
- Melanocytic tumors
- Hematolymphoid tumors involving CNS
- Germ cell tumors
- Tumors of sellar region

## Metastases

Approximately 1/2 of all CNS neoplasms are metastatic tumors. CNS metastases are divided into two groups: (1) Metastases to the brain and spinal cord parenchyma and (2) metastases to the meninges. Both are discussed in this section. Metastases to the brain and spinal cord from tumors originating outside the CNS most often spread via a hematogenous route. Direct involvement from adjacent anatomic structures (e.g., the skull, paranasal sinuses) does occur but is significantly less common.

## Genetic Tumor Syndromes Involving CNS

The CNS is frequently involved in genetic tumor predisposition syndromes (formerly designated as "Familial Tumour Syndromes" in the 2016 Classification). Some neoplasms are strongly associated with—or are almost pathognomonic of—certain syndromes (e.g., subependymal giant cell astrocytoma occurs almost exclusively in tuberous sclerosis) **(16-3)**.

The 5th edition WHO added eight additional disorders to the ten syndromes included in the 2016 WHO Classification. These are discussed in the last section of this book ("Congenital Malformations and Genetic Tumor Syndromes"). Vascular neurocutaneous syndromes, such as Sturge-Weber syndrome and PHACES, are included separately in the section.

# Nonneoplastic Intracranial Cysts

Cysts are common findings on neuroimaging studies and, for purposes of discussion, are included in this section of the text. Although our focus here is on neoplasms, CNS cysts can sometimes be confused with neoplasms and are often considered in the differential diagnosis of mass lesions in specific anatomic locations.

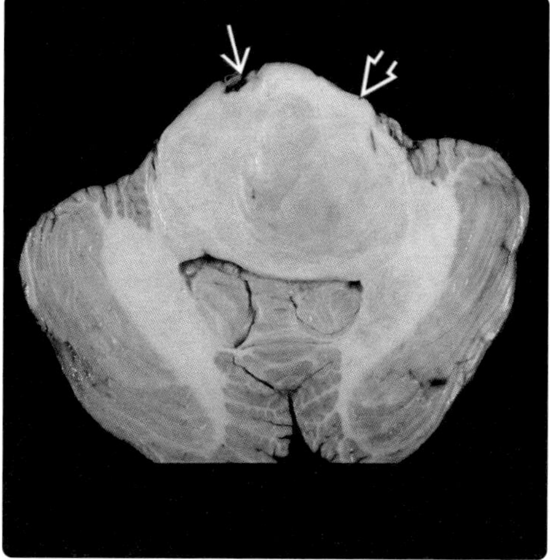

***(16-1)** Pediatric-type diffuse midline glioma enlarges, infiltrates pons ➡, and almost completely envelopes the basilar artery ➡.*

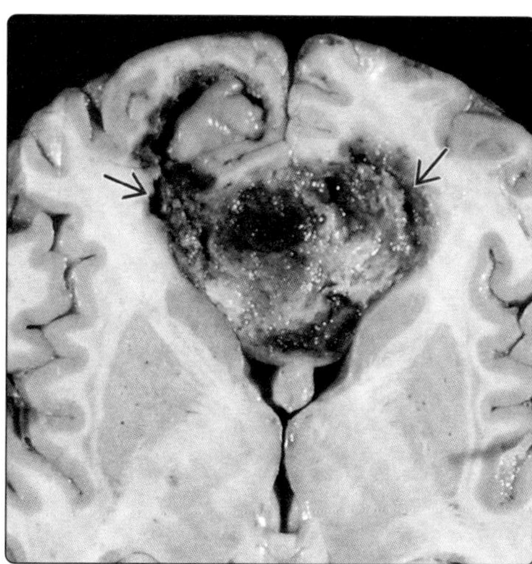

***(16-2)** Autopsy shows infiltrating hemorrhagic, necrotic mass in the corpus callosum genu ➡. Glioblastoma, IDH-wildtype, CNS WHO grade 4.*

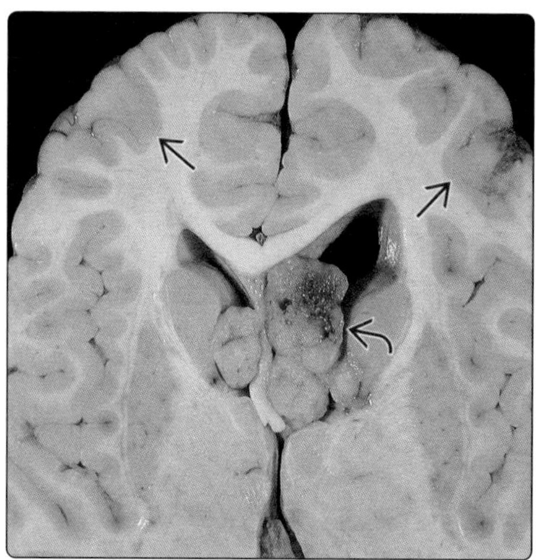

***(16-3)** Tuberous sclerosis with cortical tubers ➡, subependymal giant cell astrocytoma ➡. SEGA obstructs ventricles, does not invade brain.*

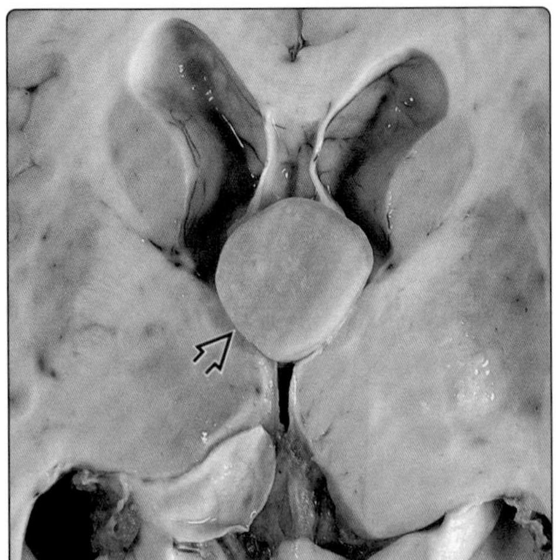

***(16-4)** Colloid cyst ⇨ is tightly wedged into the foramen of Monro, causing sudden obstructive hydrocephalus and death.*

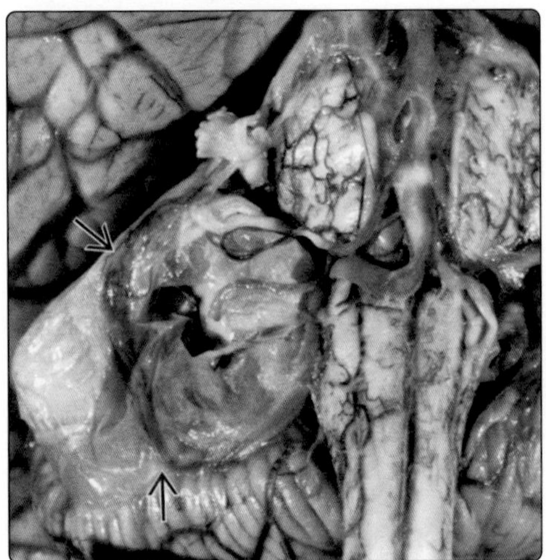

***(16-5)** Coronal autopsied brain shows an arachnoid cyst ⇨ in the cerebellopontine angle cistern. The finding was incidental.*

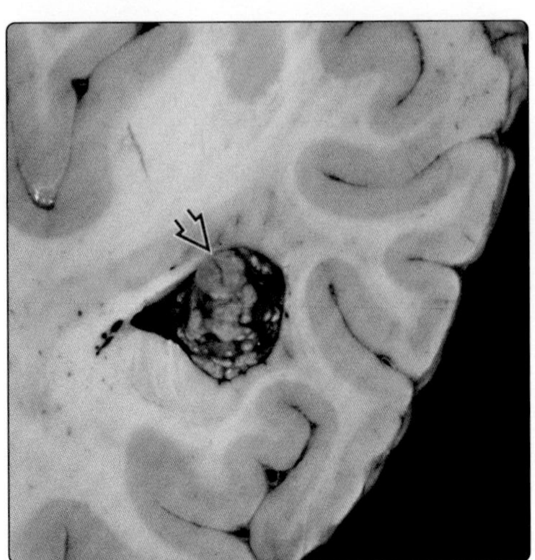

***(16-6)** Close-up view of an autopsied brain with a xanthogranuloma ⇨ in the choroid plexus glomus is shown.*

We therefore take an anatomic- and imaging-based approach to intracranial cysts. Here, the key consideration is not the specific histopathology (as in brain neoplasms) but anatomic location **(16-4)**.

There are four key anatomy-based questions to pose when considering the imaging diagnosis of an intracranial cyst. (1) Is the cyst intra- or extraaxial? (2) Is it supra- or infratentorial **(16-5)**? (3) Is it midline or off-midline? (4) If the cyst is intraaxial, is it in the brain parenchyma or inside the ventricles **(16-6)**?

Although many cysts can be found in multiple locations, each type has its own "preferred" (i.e., most common) site. The three major anatomic sublocations are the extraaxial spaces (including the scalp and skull), the brain parenchyma, and the cerebral ventricles. Some specific locations (e.g., colloid cyst in the foramen of Monro, xanthogranuloma in the choroid plexus) are virtually pathognomonic of their histopathologic diagnoses.

## Extraaxial Cysts

Extraaxial cysts lie outside the brain parenchyma. Scalp cysts are relatively uncommon, typically benign, and are occasionally identified incidentally on imaging studies obtained to visualize intracranial structures. Imaging is important when a scalp lesion is potentially malignant, has a vascular component, or might be in anatomic continuity with intracranial contents.

Age is helpful in the differential diagnosis of nontraumatic scalp masses. Trichilemmal ("sebaceous") cysts are common, cystic-appearing scalp masses in middle-aged and older adults.

If a child has a scalp mass, the most common etiologies are Langerhans cell histiocytosis, epidermoid and dermoid cysts, hemangiomas, and neurofibromas. While less common, it is important to exclude cephalocele and sinus pericranii in this age group.

Most extraaxial cysts are intracranial, lying between the dura and pia. Determining anatomic sublocation (supra- vs. infratentorial, midline vs. eccentric) is helpful in establishing a meaningful differential diagnosis. Arachnoid cysts are the most common of all congenital intracranial cysts.

## Intraaxial Cysts

Intraaxial cysts are the most common of all brain cysts. By definition, they are found in the brain parenchyma or the ventricular system. The most common parenchymal cysts, by far, are enlarged perivascular spaces. Neuroglial (glioependymal) cysts are uncommon, benign, fluid-containing cysts embedded within the cerebral white matter.

Intraventricular cysts are less common. Choroid plexus cysts are the most common intraventricular cysts and are found incidentally when imaging older patients. Colloid cysts—because of their potential to obstruct the lateral ventricles suddenly—are the most important intraventricular cyst to identify on imaging studies.

*Selected References: The complete reference list is available on the eBooks+ version included with purchase.*

# Adult-Type Diffuse Gliomas

*Gliomas, glioneuronal tumors, and neuronal tumors are the most common and most varied neoplasms that affect the brain parenchyma. Of the six different groups that comprise these tumors, the largest is adult-type diffuse gliomas. As noted in the WHO, 5th edition, these neoplasms constitute the bulk of adult neurooncology practice. The most common of all CNS parenchymal neoplasms—glioblastoma, IDH-wildtype—is the prototypical example.*



## Adult-Type Diffuse Gliomas

Historically, diffuse adult gliomas were divided into 15 entities with different grades assigned to different entities. In the 5th edition, classification of adult-type diffuse gliomas was greatly simplified and now includes only three neoplasms: (1) Astrocytoma, IDH-mutant, (2) oligodendroglioma, IDH-mutant and 1p/19q codeleted, and (3) glioblastoma, IDH-wildtype. All three are delineated in detail in this chapter. In addition, we include a discussion of IDH-wildtype diffuse gliomas that do not meet the histologic or molecular definitions of glioblastoma, IDH-wildtype.

### Astrocytoma, IDH-Mutant

#### Terminology

Astrocytoma, IDH-mutant, is a diffusely infiltrating glioma that exhibits *IDH1* or *IDH2* mutations. 1p/19q codeletion (typical of oligodendroglioma) is mutually exclusive and, by definition, absent. *ATRX* &/or *TP53* mutations are common.

#### Etiology

The origin of IDH-mutant astrocytomas is unknown. Astrocytomas have been posited to originate from different cell types, including a distinct population of neural precursor-like cells, oligodendrocyte precursor cells, and astrocytes.

IDH mutations are an early event in gliomagenesis of both astrocytomas and oligodendrogliomas and generally persist during tumor progression. Mutant *IDH1* can induce extensive DNA hypermethylation in gene-promoter regions that may silence expression of cellular differentiation, inducing a stem cell-like state prone to self-renewal and tumorigenesis. *MGMT* encodes a DNA repair protein, and MGMT promoter methylation is commonly observed in IDH-mutant gliomas.

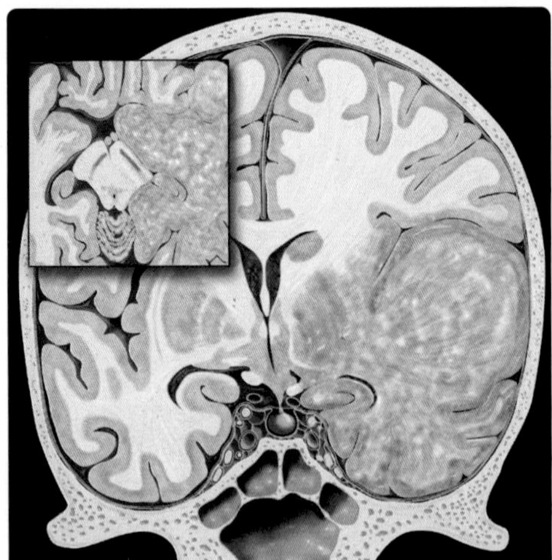

*(17-1) Diffuse astrocytoma, IDH-mutant, is shown expanding the temporal lobe, infiltrating the cortex and subcortical white matter (WM).*

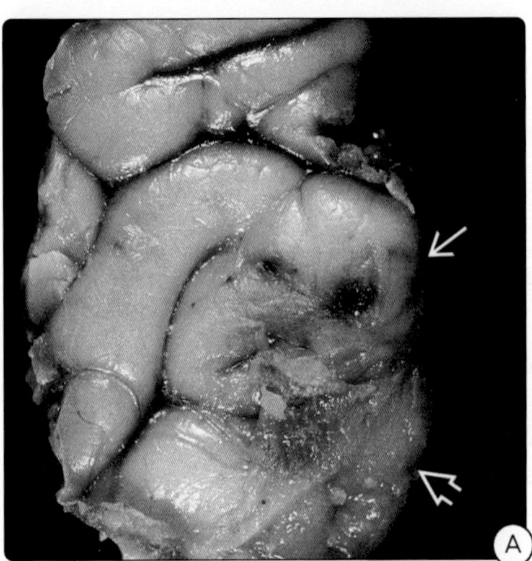


*(17-2A) Surgical specimen from diffuse astrocytoma shows expansion of the cortex ➡ and mass effect on the underlying gyri ⇨.*

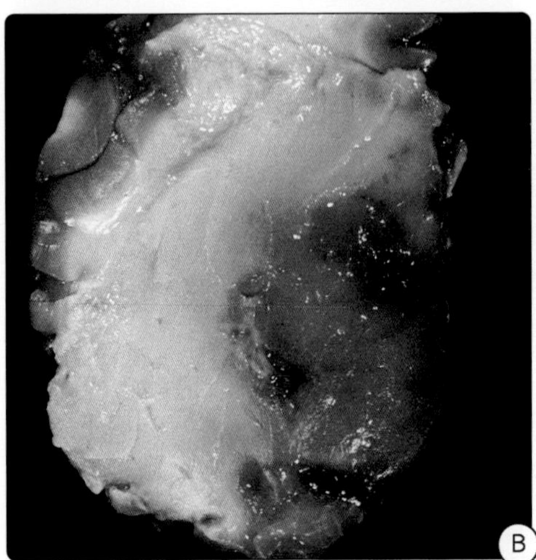


***(17-2B)** Cut section shows tumor infiltrating cortex, subcortical WM without a border between the normal brain and tumor. CNS WHO grade 3.*

Recent studies have shown that over 2/3 of CNS WHO grade 4 IDH-mutant astrocytomas arise de novo rather than occurring as malignant degeneration of a lower grade glioma.

## Pathology

**Location.** Although IDH-mutant diffuse gliomas can arise anywhere, the cerebral hemispheres are the most common overall site with a preferential location in the frontal and temporal lobes **(17-1)**.

**Size and Number.** Frontal lobe IDH-mutant astrocytomas may reach a relatively large size before producing symptoms. Temporal lobe lesions are often smaller at initial presentation because of their propensity to cause partial complex seizures. Most IDH-mutant astrocytomas are solitary lesions.

**Gross Pathology.** Low-grade IDH-mutant astrocytomas are expansile, infiltrating lesions that enlarge, distort, and invade anatomic structures. The gray-white matter interface is often effaced **(17-2)**. Occasional cysts may be present and are sometimes extensive. Calcification is not uncommon in lower grade tumors. Necrosis and gross hemorrhage may be present in higher grade lesions.

**Microscopic Features.** IDH-mutant astrocytomas range from well-differentiated, slow-growing tumors with low mitotic activity (CNS WHO grade 2) to highly anaplastic, hypercellular masses with rapid growth, microvascular proliferation, necrosis, and significant mitotic activity (CNS WHO grade 4).

### Staging, Grading, and Classification

***CNS WHO grade 2.*** Grade 2 IDH-mutant astrocytomas are diffusely infiltrative, well differentiated, and lack histologic anaplasia. Mitotic activity is low. Microvascular proliferation and necrosis are absent.

***CNS WHO grade 3.*** Grade 3 IDH-mutant astrocytomas exhibit focal or dispersed anaplasia and exhibit significant mitotic activity. Microvascular proliferation and necrosis are absent.

***CNS WHO grade 4.*** CNS WHO grade 4 IDH-mutant astrocytomas are diffusely infiltrative tumors that exhibit microvascular proliferation &/or necrosis. If present, homozygous deletions of the cyclin-dependent kinase inhibitor *CDKN2A* &/or *CDKN2B* overrules histologic grade, making a diffuse IDH-mutant astrocytoma a grade 4 lesion regardless of histopathologic features. **Note that in the 5th edition, diffuse astrocytoma, IDH-mutant, CNS WHO grade 4 tumors are NOT called "glioblastoma" (that term is reserved for IDH-wildtype diffuse astrocytomas).**

**Diagnostic Molecular Pathology.** Immunohistochemistry is essential in establishing the diagnosis of IDH-mutant astrocytomas. A routine panel for initial diagnostic work-up of all adult diffuse gliomas includes *IDH1* (codon p.R132H), p53, and ATRX.

Immunostaining for the *IDH1* p.R132H mutation is both sensitive and specific. This mutation accounts for ~ 90% of all IDH mutations in supratentorial astrocytomas. **Identifying IDH2 codon 172 missense mutation and so-called "noncanonical"** *IDH1* **mutations (other than R132H) requires DNA sequencing and should be performed in all WHO grade 4 gliomas in patients < 55 years of age.**

Because IDH-mutant astrocytomas and oligodendrogliomas are both diffusely infiltrating gliomas and share *IDH1* or *IDH2* mutations, loss of nuclear ATRX expression **or** excluding combined whole-arm deletions of 1p and 19q are also required diagnostic criteria for the diagnosis of diffuse astrocytoma, IDH-mutant.

## Clinical Issues

**Epidemiology.** IDH-mutant diffuse astrocytomas account for between 10-15% of astrocytic neoplasms in adults.

**Demographics.** Mean age at presentation is mid-30s (range: 20-50 years). Older age at presentation is more common in CNS WHO grade 4 lesions. IDH-mutant astrocytomas are rare over the age of 55 years.

**Presentation.** Symptoms are location dependent. Seizures are a common presenting sign.

**Natural History.** Younger age and lower grade are associated with increased survival in patients with adult-type IDH-mutant astrocytomas. Resection extent and presence of postoperative residual tumor are strongly associated with overall survival.

Presence of *CDKN2A* &/or *CDNK2B* homozygous deletion is a negative prognostic factor. Therefore, even in the absence of microvascular proliferation or necrosis, tumors with this molecular profile are designated as CNS WHO grade 4 lesions.

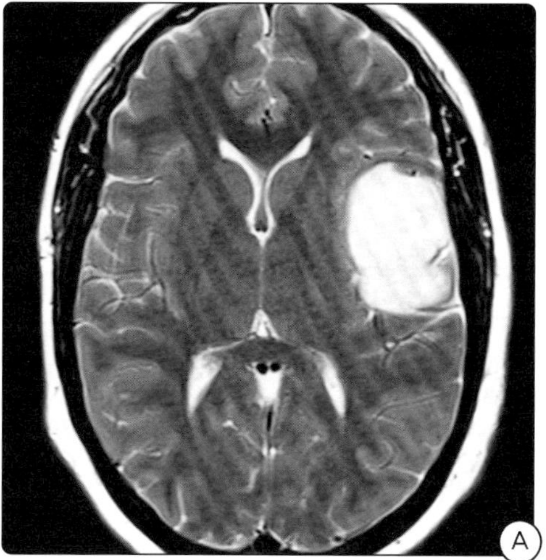

***(17-4A)** T2 MR in a 28-yo man with word-finding difficulty shows uniformly hyperintense left temporal lobe mass.*

**ASTROCYTOMA, IDH-MUTANT**

**Pathology**
- Supratentorial (frontal, temporal lobes most common)
- Diffusely infiltrating, ill-defined borders
- *IDH1* 132 or *IDH2* 172 missense mutation
- No 1p/19q deletions
- CNS WHO grades 2-4
- *CDKN2A* &/or *CDKN2B* homozygous deletion = grade 4
  - Even in absence of microvascular proliferation, necrosis

**Clinical Features**
- 10-15% of astrocytomas
- Age: 20-45 years
  - Older age correlated with ↑ grade
  - Survival ↓ with ↑ grade
- Symptoms are location dependent

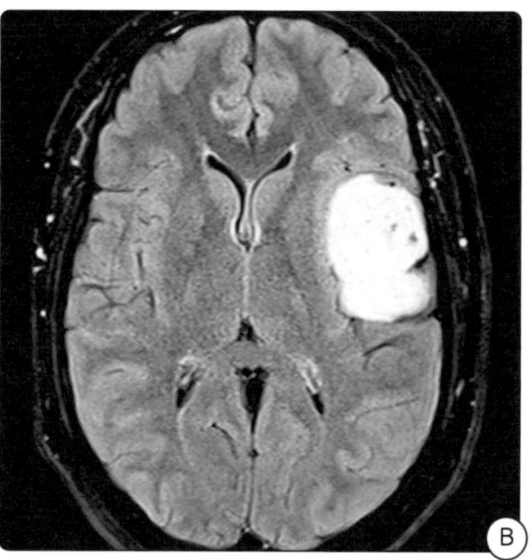

***(17-4B)** The mass is almost uniformly hyperintense on FLAIR MR.*

## Imaging

**CT Findings.** Findings vary with tumor grade. For lower grade IDH-mutant astrocytomas, NECT shows an ill-defined homogeneously hypodense mass. Calcification is seen in 20% of cases. Gross cystic change and hemorrhage are rare but can be seen in grade 4 lesions.

Lower grade lesions typically do not enhance on CECT, but higher grade lesions may exhibit patchy enhancement.

**MR Findings.** IDH-mutant astrocytomas are typically hypointense on T1WI, hyperintense on T2WI **(17-4)**, and hyperintense on FLAIR **(17-4B)**. A hyperintense FLAIR rim with hypointense core is sometimes present **(17-7)** and has been called the T2/FLAIR "mismatch" sign, helpful in identifying IDH-mutant, non-1p/19q codeleted tumors and differentiating them from oligodendroglioma **(17-5C)**. Tumor borders may appear relatively sharp on imaging studies, but these are unencapsulated neoplasms that infiltrate adjacent normal-appearing brain.

Lower grade lesions typically do not enhance or enhance minimally **(17-5)**, but there is a stepwise positive association with WHO grade. Grades 3 and 4 tumors may exhibit some enhancement **(17-7D)** **(17-9)**. Diffusion restriction is absent. ADC is negatively associated with WHO grade.

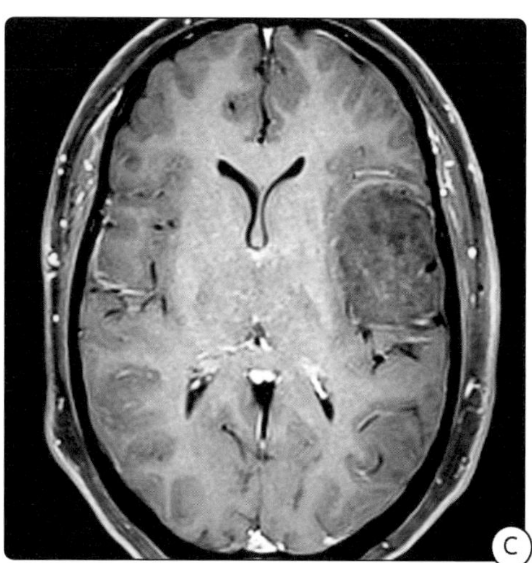

***(17-4C)** T1 C+ FS MR shows no enhancement. This is astrocytoma, IDH-mutant, CNS WHO grade 2.*

MRS shows elevated choline, decreased NAA, and a high mI:Cr ratio. Myoinositol is reduced. 3T MRS may exhibit an elevated 2-hydroxyglutarate (2-HG) peak, resonating at 2.25 ppm.

DCE MR perfusion shows relatively low rCBV in grade 2 lesions. ADC (lower) and rCBV (higher) are with increasing WHO grade.

## Differential Diagnosis

The major imaging differential diagnosis of IDH-mutant astrocytoma is **oligodendroglioma**. Oligodendrogliomas are more often cortically based, more frequently calcify, and may be associated with remodeling of the overlying calvarium. The definitive diagnosis and grading of IDH-mutant astrocytomas require histologic confirmation and diagnostic molecular pathology.

### ASTROCYTOMA, IDH-MUTANT

**Imaging Features**

- CT
  - Ill defined, homogeneously hypodense
  - $Ca^{++}$ in 20% (generally lower grade)
  - No enhancement
- MR
  - T1 hypointense; T2 hyperintense
  - May have hyperintense FLAIR rim, hypointense center
  - Enhancement varies with grade
  - MRS shows 2-HG peak at 2.25 ppm
  - rCBV low but ↑ with higher grade

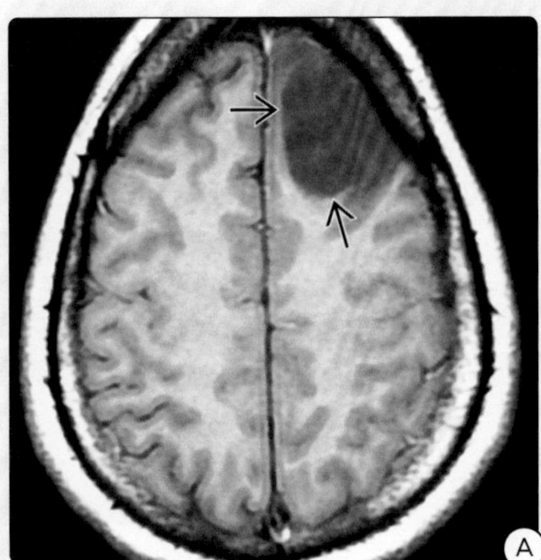


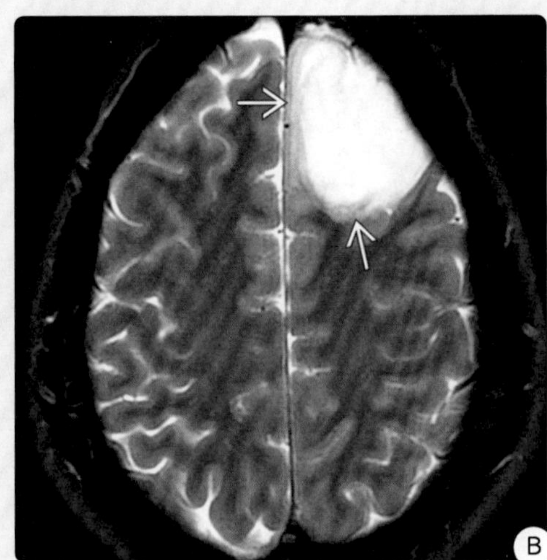


***(17-5A)** Axial T1 MR in a 25-yo man with a 1st-time seizure shows a hypodense mass ➙ in the left frontal lobe. **(17-5B)** The mass ➙ is variably hyperintense on T2 MR.*

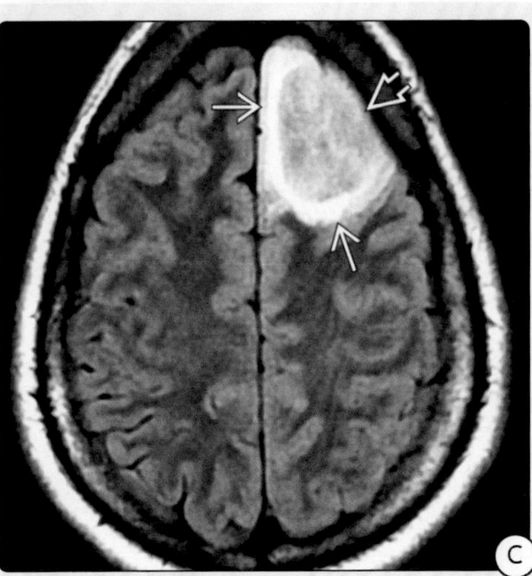


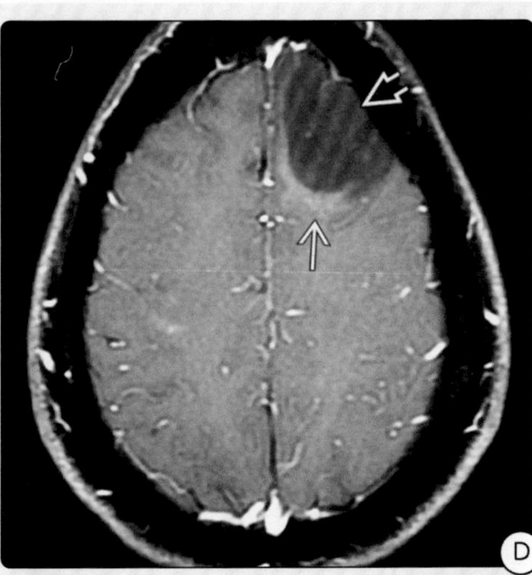


***(17-5C)** FLAIR MR shows a classic T2/FLAIR "mismatch" sign with hyperintense rim ➙ surrounding an iso- to hypointense center ➙. **(17-5D)** T1 C+ FS MR shows the mass ➙ is mostly nonenhancing with a faint, ill-defined, minimally enhancing rim ➙. This is astrocytoma, IDH-mutant, CNS WHO grade 2.*

## Oligodendroglioma, IDH-Mutant and 1p/19q Codeleted

### Terminology

Oligodendroglioma, IDH-mutant and 1p/19q codeleted, is a diffuse glioma with *IDH1* or *IDH2* mutation + codeletion of chromosome arms 1p and 19q. Oligodendrogliomas constitute a spectrum ranging from well-differentiated, relatively indolent tumors to frankly malignant neoplasms with rapid growth.

### Etiology

As with IDH-mutant astrocytomas, the cell of origin remains unknown. Oligodendrogliomas contain malignant oligodendroglial, astrocytic, and neural precursor-like cells.

### Pathology

**Location.** Most oligodendrogliomas arise at the gray-white matter junction **(17-10)**. The vast majority (85-90%) are supratentorial. The most common site is the frontal lobe (50-65%) followed by the parietal, temporal, and occipital lobes. Posterior fossa and spinal cord oligodendrogliomas are uncommon.

**Gross Pathology.** Oligodendrogliomas are solid, fleshy, cortically based tan-to-pink masses **(17-11)**. They are poorly circumscribed and blend gradually into adjacent structures, blurring the gray-white matter boundaries, expanding one or more gyri, and extending into the adjacent brain in a diffuse manner **(17-12)**. Some oligodendrogliomas occasionally spread in a more diffuse, multifocal, gliomatosis cerebri-like pattern.

Calcification is frequent, and zones of cystic degeneration are common, although frank necrosis is rare. Intratumoral

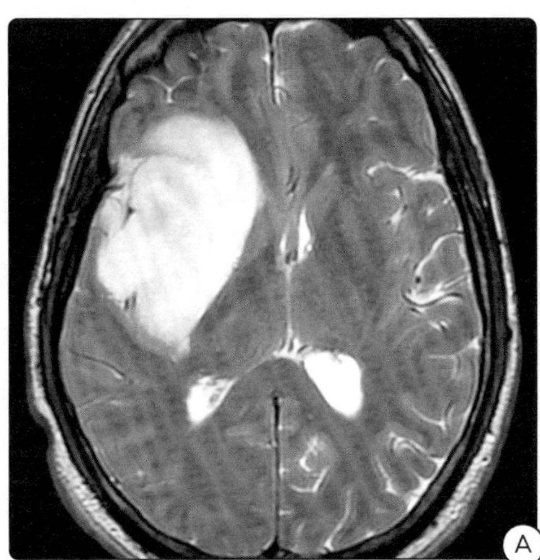
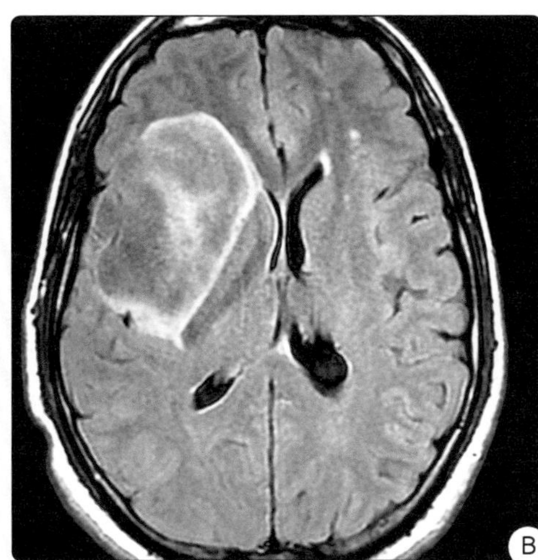

***(17-7A)** T2 MR in a 35-yo man shows a hyperintense right frontotemporal mass. **(17-7B)** FLAIR MR shows a hyperintense rim and hypointense center (T2/FLAIR "mismatch" sign).*

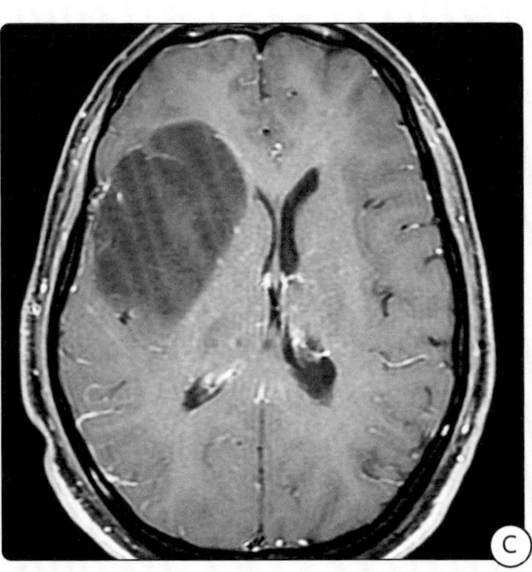
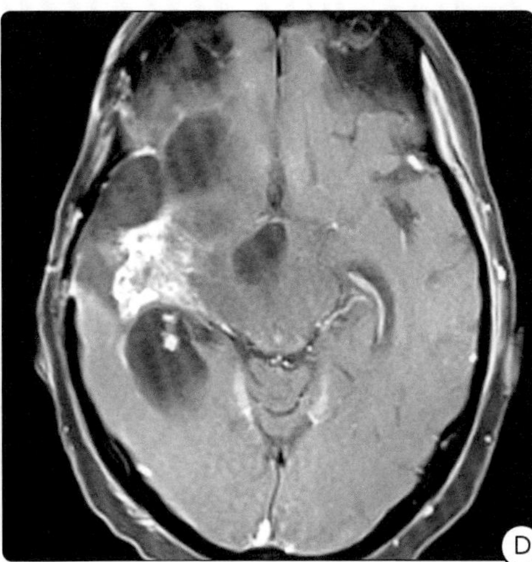

***(17-7C)** T1 C+ FS MR shows no enhancement. Subtotal resection showed diffuse astrocytoma, IDH-mutant, grade 2, but next-generation sequencing (NGS) showed CDKN2A deletion. The tumor was reclassified as astrocytoma, IDH-mutant, grade 4. **(17-7D)** Repeat MR shows enhancing, recurrent tumor. The patient expired 5 years after the initial diagnosis. This is astrocytoma, IDH-mutant, CNS WHO grade 4.*

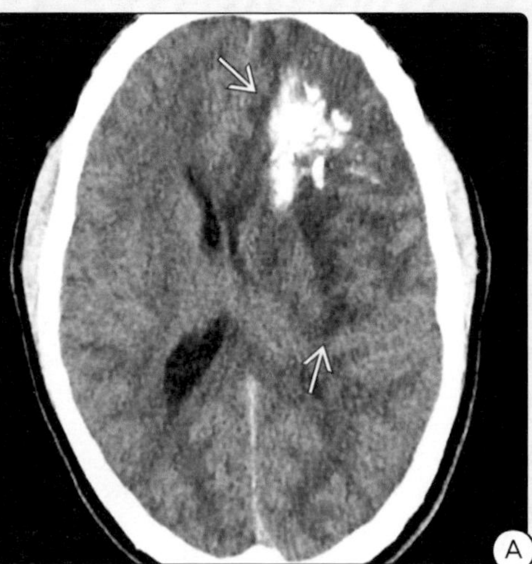

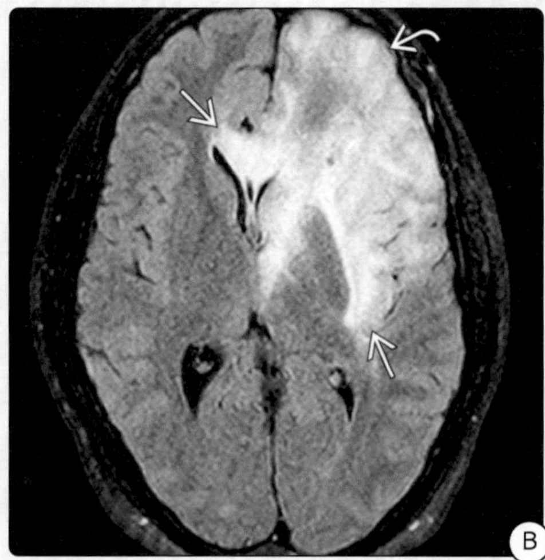

***(17-9A)** Axial NECT in a 25-yo man with 1st seizure shows a partially calcified mass ➡ in the left frontotemporal region. **(17-9B)** FLAIR MR shows the hyperintense mass ➡ diffusely infiltrating the frontotemporal gyri, extending into the internal and external capsules, and crossing the corpus callosum. Note slight bone remodeling of the left frontal bone ↪, indicating a slowly growing expansile mass.*

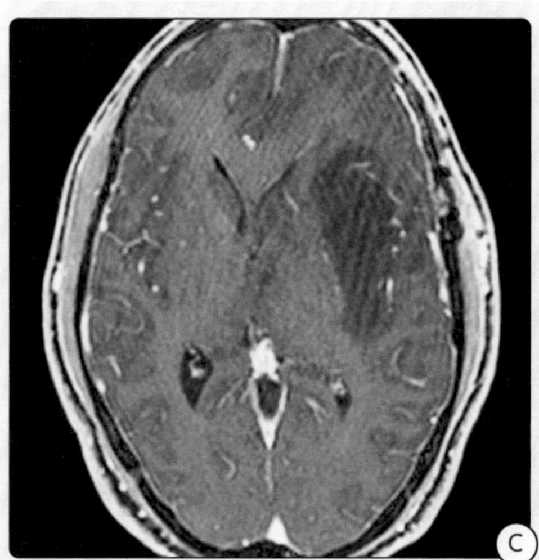

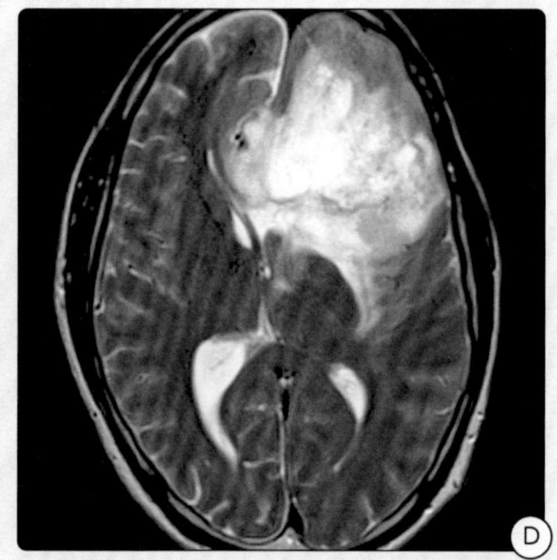

***(17-9C)** T1 C+ SPGR obtained for stereotaxic biopsy showed no enhancement in the mass. Biopsy disclosed a grade 2 IDH-mutant astrocytoma. NGS was not performed at the time. **(17-9D)** T2 MR 3 years later shows that the mass is much more heterogeneous.*

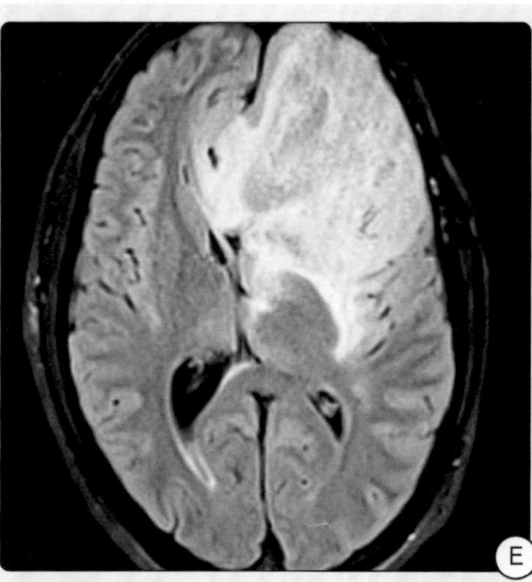

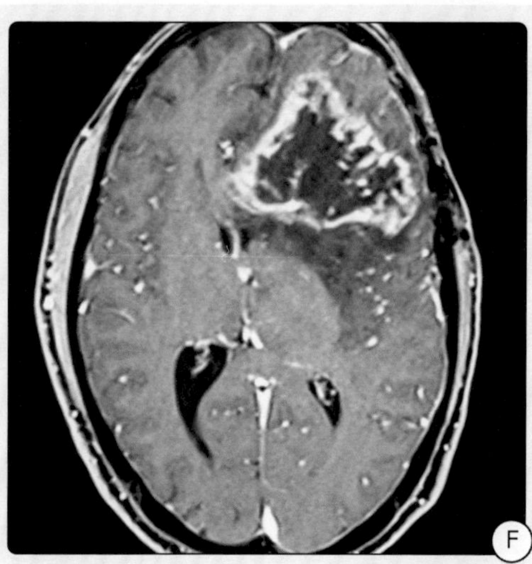

***(17-9E)** FLAIR shows increased mass effect and tumor extension compared to the previous MR. **(17-9F)** T1 C+ SPGR for repeat stereotaxic biopsy shows a necrotic, rim-enhancing mass. Biopsy disclosed necrosis, microvascular proliferation, and brisk mitotic activity. NGS showed CDNK2AB homozygous deletions. Had it been performed initially, the diagnosis would have confirmed CNS WHO grade 4 diffuse astrocytoma, IDH-mutant.*

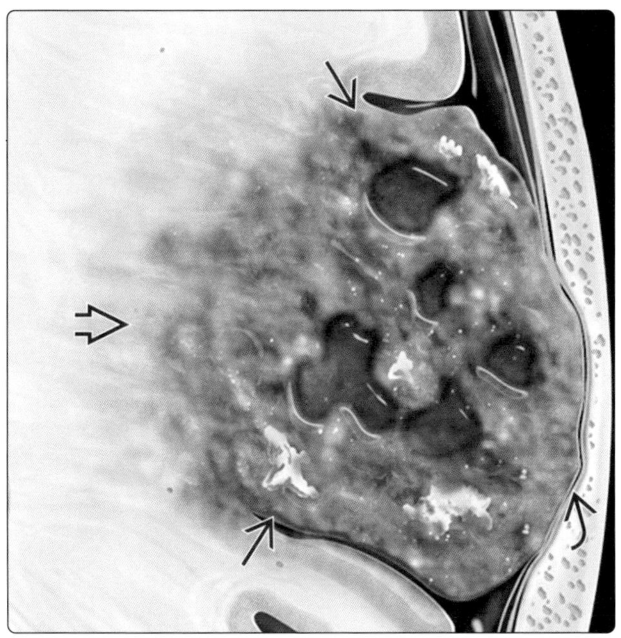

***(17-10) Oligodendrogliomas are poorly demarcated ⇨, cortically based fleshy masses ➡ that infiltrate cortex and subcortical WM. Remodeling of the adjacent bone ↗ is common.***

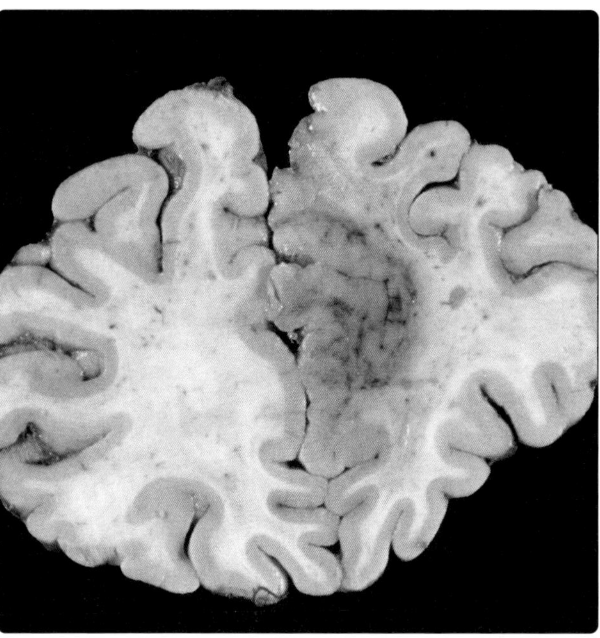

***(17-11) Gross pathology shows a fleshy appearance of oligodendrogliomas. The epicenter is at the GM-WM interface, and the tumor expands the cortex and extends into the subcortical and deep WM.***

hemorrhage is common, especially with larger or higher grade oligodendrogliomas.

**Microscopic Features.** Oligodendrogliomas vary in cellularity. Most are highly cellular lesions with uniform round or slightly oval hyperchromatic nuclei surrounded by a prominent perinuclear "halo." This gives the tumors a classic microscopic fried-egg appearance. Microcalcifications are common.

Oligodendrogliomas typically have a dense network of branching chicken-wire capillaries. Intratumoral hemorrhages are relatively common.

**Staging, Grading, and Classification.** Oligodendrogliomas comprise a continuous spectrum of tumors that ranges from well-differentiated, slow-growing neoplasms to frankly malignant tumors with rapid growth.

Two grades are recognized: CNS WHO grade 2 and grade 3. Mitotic activity is low or absent in CNS WHO grade 2 oligodendrogliomas but is prominent in grade 3 lesions. However, criteria for distinction between these grades remains controversial and poorly defined.

Microvascular proliferation and necrosis are linked to shorter survival; a clear cut-off point for mitotic count is less clear. *CDKN2A* homozygous deletion is generally accepted as designating grade 3 tumor.

**Diagnostic Molecular Pathology.** Oligodendrogliomas are molecularly defined by *IDH1* or *IDH2* mutations and combined whole-arm 1p/19q codeletions. 1p/19q status is decisive for separation of oligodendroglioma from IDH-mutant astrocytoma.

Nearly all oligodendrogliomas have a *TERT* promoter mutation and preserved nuclear *ATRX* expression. Homozygous deletion of *CDKN2A* has been detected in a small proportion of CNS WHO grade 3 oligodendrogliomas.

## Clinical Issues

**Epidemiology.** Oligodendrogliomas account for 1-2% of all primary CNS neoplasms and 5-20% of gliomas. Approximately 2/3 of oligodendrogliomas are CNS WHO grade 2 and 1/3 are grade 3 lesions. The term "anaplastic" oligodendroglioma has been eliminated.

**Demographics.** Oligodendrogliomas are tumors of middle-aged adults. The median age at diagnosis is 43 years. Patients with CNS WHO grade 2 lesions are slightly younger (41 years), while those with grade 3 tumors are slightly older (47 years).

Oligodendrogliomas in children are very rare. Some diffuse gliomas in children have microscopic features that resemble oligodendroglioma but are biologically and molecularly distinct from their adult counterparts. They lack 1p/19q codeletions while *MYB*, *MYBL1*, *FGFR1*, or BRAF alterations are typical.

**Presentation.** Because oligodendrogliomas commonly involve the cortical gray matter, seizures are the most common presenting symptom. Headache is the second most common presentation.

**Natural History.** CNS WHO grade 2 oligodendrogliomas are slow-growing but locally aggressive neoplasms. The five-year survival rate is nearly 80%, and the median survival time is 10-12 years. Local recurrence following resection is very common. Leptomeningeal spread may occur in late-stage disease in some patients.

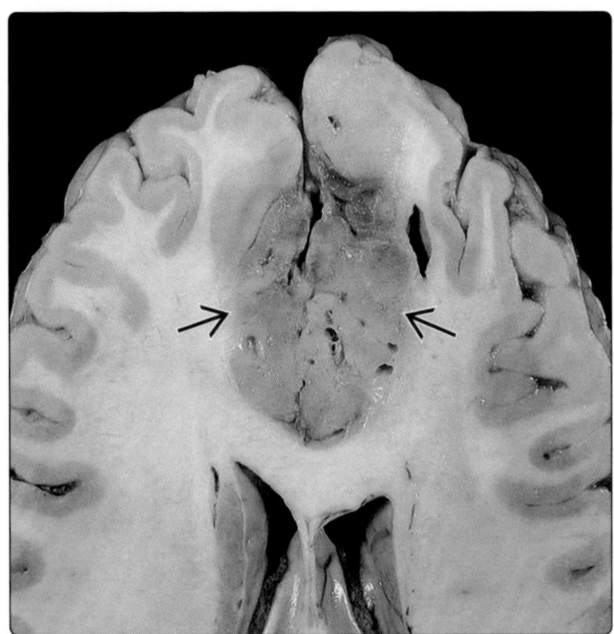

*(17-12) Autopsy of oligodendroglioma shows a fleshy mass ⇨ with preferential involvement of the cortex and subcortical WM.*

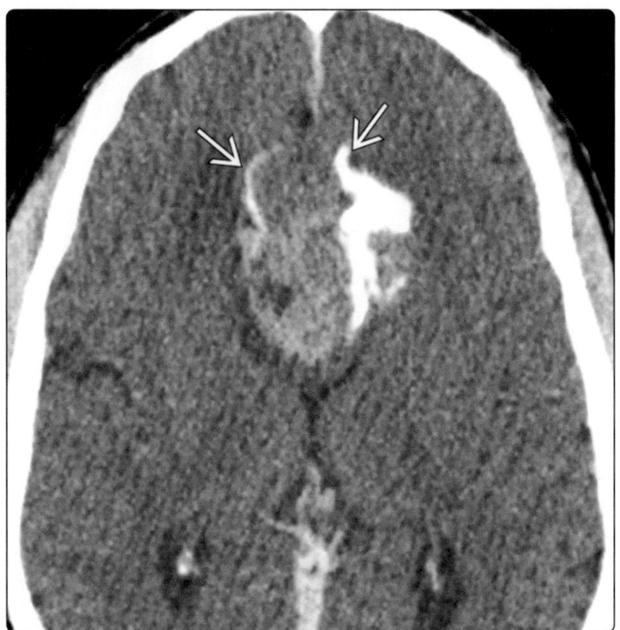

*(17-13) Axial CECT shows an enhancing mass in the corpus callosum genu and cortex of both frontal lobes. Note gyriform calcifications ➡. This is oligodendroglioma, IDH-mutant and 1p/19q codeleted, CNS WHO grade 2.*

**Treatment Options.** Gross total resection is the primary treatment and improves outcome. IDH-mutant 1p/1pq codeleted oligodendrogliomas are generally chemosensitive, so combined radiation and chemotherapy is standard.

## Imaging

**General Features.** Oligodendrogliomas are round or ovoid, relatively sharply delineated masses that involve the cortex and subcortical white matter. Differentiation of CNS WHO grade 2 and grade 3 oligodendrogliomas (formerly called anaplastic oligodendroglioma) on imaging studies is difficult.

**CT Findings.** Typical oligodendrogliomas are peripheral and cortically based lesions, often in the frontal lobe. Focal gyral expansion with thinning and remodeling of the overlying calvarium is common **(17-15)**. Almost 2/3 are hypodense on NECT while 1/3 exhibit mixed-density patterns.

Coarse, nodular, or clumped calcification is seen in 70-90% of cases. Gyriform calcification is very suggestive of oligodendroglioma **(17-13)**. Foci of cystic degeneration are present in 20%. Petechial hemorrhages may be present, but gross hemorrhage and peritumoral edema are less common.

Enhancement varies from none to moderate; ~ 50% of oligodendrogliomas exhibit some degree of enhancement. Contrast enhancement generally correlates with a worse outcome in both CNS WHO grades 2 and 3 oligodendrogliomas.

**MR Findings.** Oligodendrogliomas often appear relatively well delineated and are usually hypointense relative to gray matter on T1WI and heterogeneously hyperintense on T2/FLAIR, and they may exhibit calcified foci or microhemorrhages on T2* sequences **(17-17)**. Oligodendrogliomas do not exhibit a T2/FLAIR "mismatch" sign.

Contrast enhancement varies. Many oligodendrogliomas—especial CNS WHO grade 2 lesions—exhibit little or no enhancement. Approximately 50% exhibit patchy, multifocal contrast enhancement **(17-19)**, which has been associated with higher grade and shorter progression-free survival.

MRS shows moderately elevated Cho and decreased NAA. A 2-HG peak resonating at 2.25 ppm can be detected in some cases. Because of their relatively increased vascularity, oligodendrogliomas may exhibit high rCBV foci that does not necessarily indicate high-grade histopathology.

## Differential Diagnosis

The major differential diagnosis of oligodendroglioma is **astrocytoma, IDH-mutant**. The T2/FLAIR "mismatch" sign, if present, is helpful in distinguishing astrocytoma from oligodendroglioma.

Other cortically based, slow-growing tumors that typically present with seizures include **ganglioglioma** and **dysembryoplastic neuroepithelial tumor** (DNET). Both lack IDH mutation and are more common in children, while oligodendrogliomas are vanishingly rare in this age group.

**IDH-wildtype glioblastoma** and **H3 G34-mutant diffuse hemispheric glioma** can resemble highly cellular CNS WHO grade 3 oligodendrogliomas on imaging studies but can be distinguished by their IDH-wildtype status and other specific molecular markers.

**Extraventricular neurocytoma** is a rare, cortically based tumor that may be indistinguishable from oligodendroglioma on imaging studies.

**OLIGODENDROGLIOMA, IDH-MUTANT AND 1p/19q CODELETED**

**Pathology**
- General features
  - Supratentorial (85-90% in cerebral hemispheres)
  - Most common in frontal lobe
  - Arise at gray-white matter junction
  - Diffusely infiltrate cortex
  - Poorly circumscribed
- Microscopic features
  - "Fried-egg" cells
  - Chicken-wire vascularity
  - CNS WHO grade 2 or 3 (no grade 4)

**Clinical Features**
- Tumor of middle-aged adults
  - Mean age: 41 years (grade 2), 47 years (grade 3)
  - Almost never occur in children (may resemble oligodendroglioma microscopically but completely different molecular features)
- Common presentation: Seizures
- Overall survival: 10-15 years (shorter with grade 3)

**Imaging Features**
- Relatively well circumscribed
- $Ca^{++}$ in 70%
- Gross hemorrhage, edema uncommon
- 50% enhance (may indicate higher grade)

## Glioblastoma, IDH-Wildtype

Glioblastoma (GBM), IDH-wildtype is the most common, most aggressive, and most invasive of primary brain tumors.

### Terminology

GBM is a diffusely infiltrating astrocytic tumor that is IDH-wildtype and H3-wildtype with one or more histologic &/or genetic features specified in the WHO, 5th edition. **In the WHO, 5th edition, the term "glioblastoma" is exclusively for an adult-type, IDH-wildtype grade 4 diffuse glioma**.

### Etiology

As with the other adult-type diffuse gliomas, the precise origin of GBMs is unknown. Genetic sequencing studies suggest that neural precursor cells in the subventricular zone are likely cells of origin. Whether self-renewing glioma stem cell-like elements in GBMs result from transformation of a neural precursor or dedifferentiation of a lineage-restricted cell type is unknown. Recent evidence suggests noncoding RNAs in glioma stem cells may play a key role in tumor development and disease progression.

### Pathology

**Location.** GBMs can occur anywhere in the CNS but are most commonly found in the subcortical white matter of the cerebral hemispheres. Extension into the cortex and through the corpus callosum into the contralateral hemisphere is common. Symmetric involvement of the corpus callosum is common, the so-called butterfly glioma pattern. Tumor spread tends to occur along compact white matter tracts.

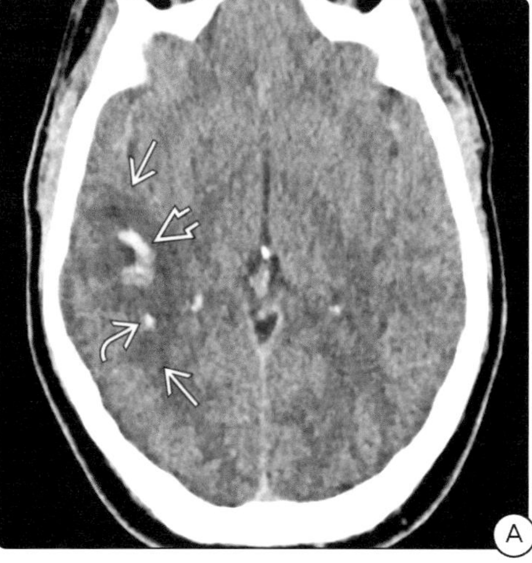

*(17-15A) NECT shows a hypodense mass ➡ in the right temporal lobe. Note punctate ➡ and curvilinear gyriform ➡ calcifications.*

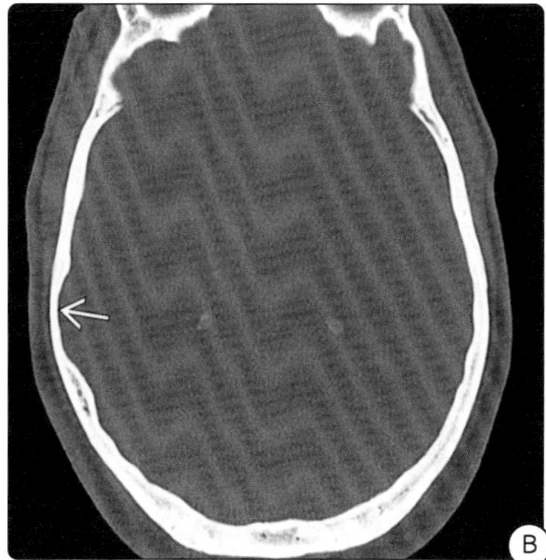

*(17-15B) Bone CT shows smooth thinning, remodeling of the calvarium ➡ overlying the mass, indicating the lesion is slow growing.*

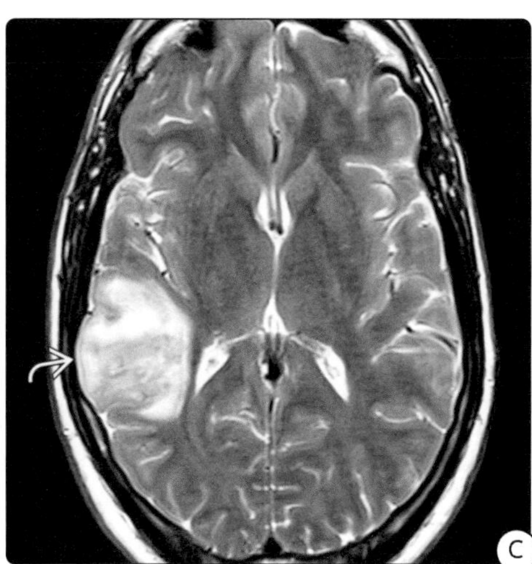

*(17-15C) T2 MR shows a heterogeneously hyperintense mass remodeling bone ➡. This is oligodendroglioma, CNS WHO grade 2.*

*(17-17A) T1 MR in a 64-yo man with seizures shows a mixed signal intensity mass ➡ that diffusely infiltrates the left medial frontal lobe cortex and extends into the subcortical WM. (17-17B) The mass ➡ is heterogeneously hyperintense on T2 MR.*

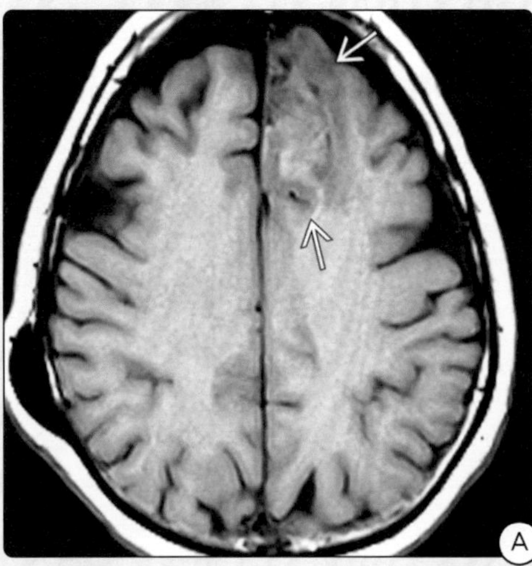

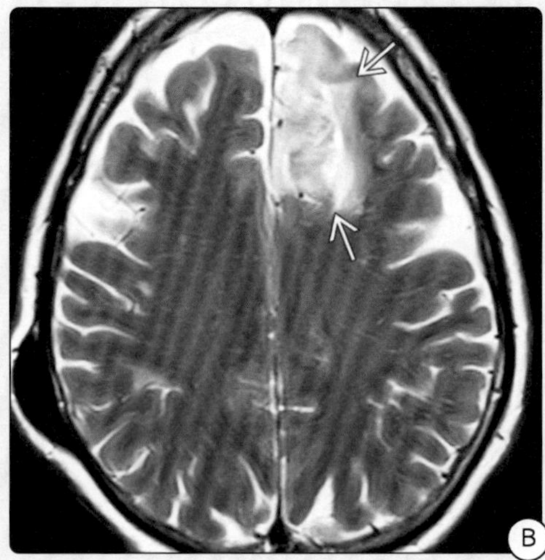

*(17-17C) FLAIR in the same case shows the mass almost uniformly hyperintense. Note somewhat indistinct border between tumor and underlying WM ➡. (17-17D) T1 C+ FS MR shows some gyriform enhancement ➡ in the mass associated with a prominent draining cortical vein ➡. The mass was completely resected, and the patient was still alive 7 years later. This is oligodendroglioma, IDH-mutant and 1p/19q codeleted, CNS WHO grade 3.*

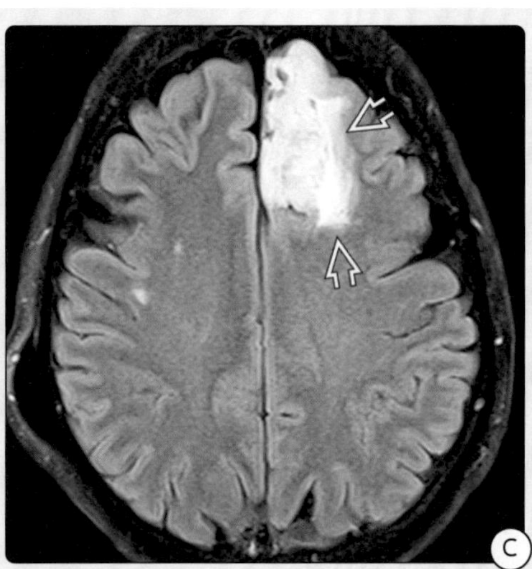

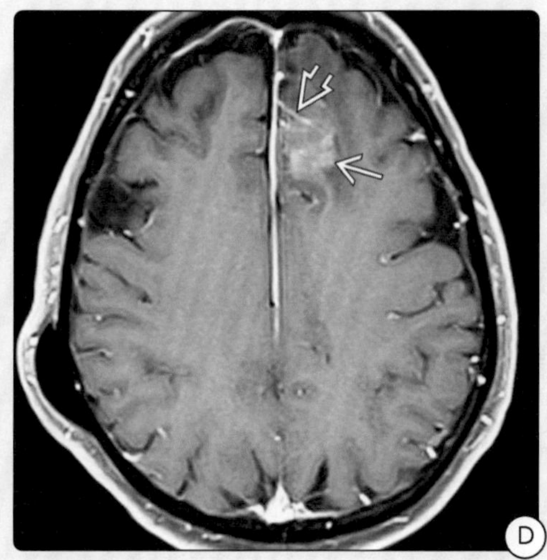

*(17-17E) T2* GRE shows some curvilinear susceptibility in the lesion ➡. (17-17F) MIP T2* SWI MR shows more punctate and curvilinear susceptibility ➡ in the lesion. The tumor was resected and was called anaplastic oligodendroglioma (in the WHO, 5th edition, this tumor would be designated oligodendroglioma, CNS WHO grade 3). The patient was alive 10 years later.*

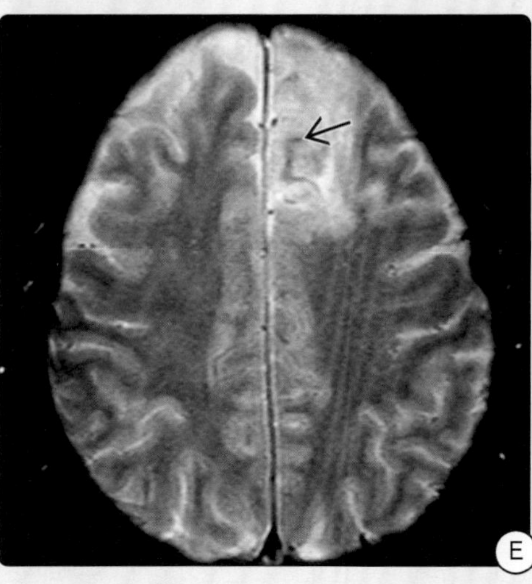

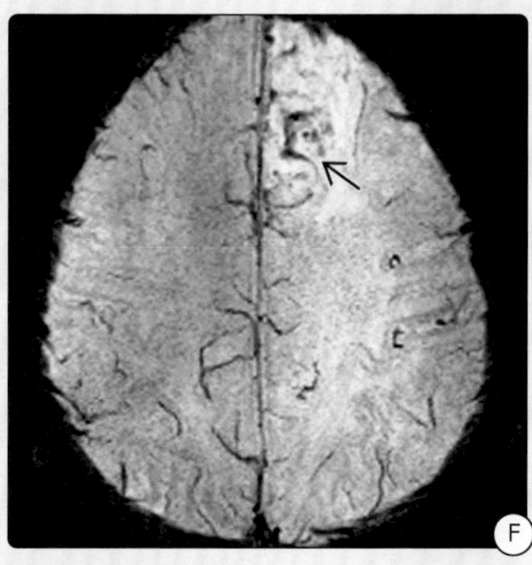

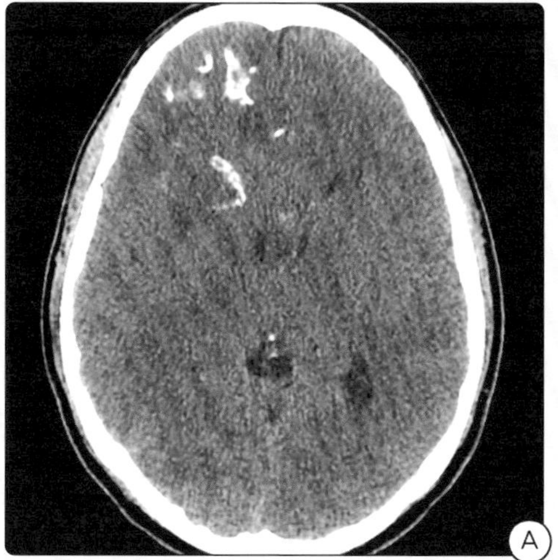

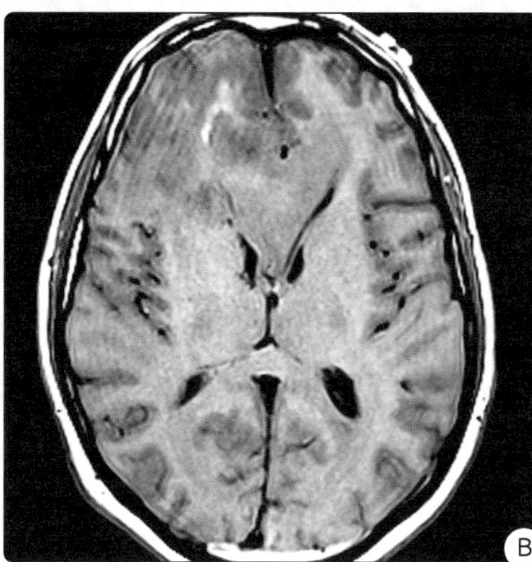

***(17-19A)** NECT in a 27-yo man with new-onset seizures shows an extensive mass in the right frontal lobe that infiltrates and expands the corpus callosum and extends into the left frontal lobe. Note curvilinear calcifications scattered throughout the mass. **(17-19B)** T1 MR in the same case shows the mass is heterogeneously hypointense compared to WM. Curvilinear T1 shortening within the mass probably represents calcification.*

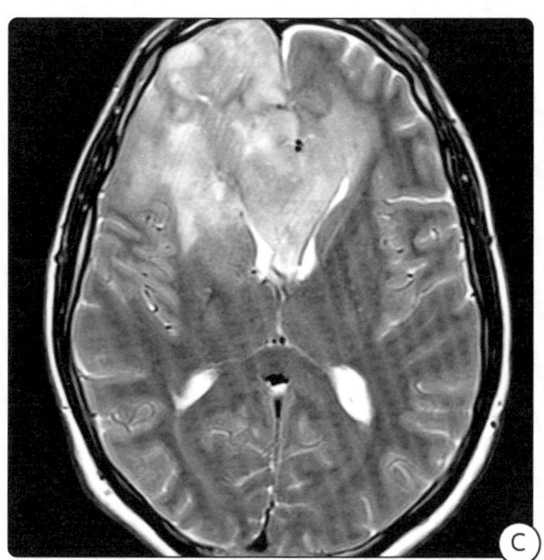

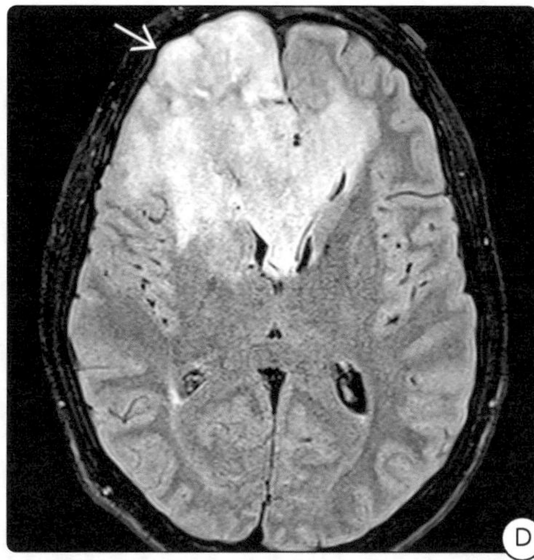

***(17-18C)** T2 MR shows the mass is heterogeneously hyperintense and infiltrates the cortex and WM and crosses the expanded corpus callosum genu into the left frontal lobe. **(17-18D)** The mass is heterogeneously hyperintense on FLAIR MR. Note some subtle remodeling of the adjacent calvarium ➙, suggesting the mass has been growing slowly over a relatively long time.*

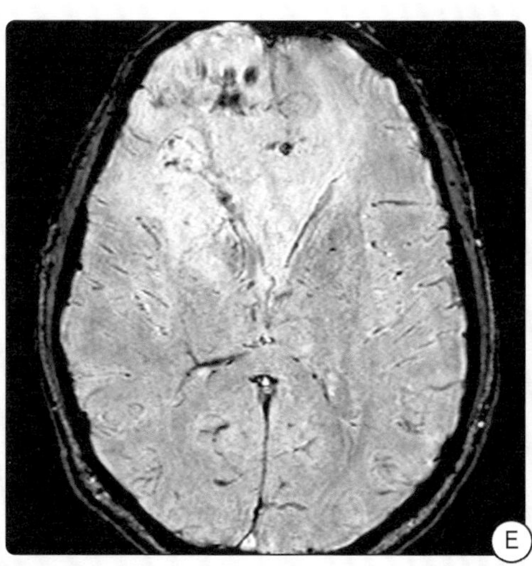

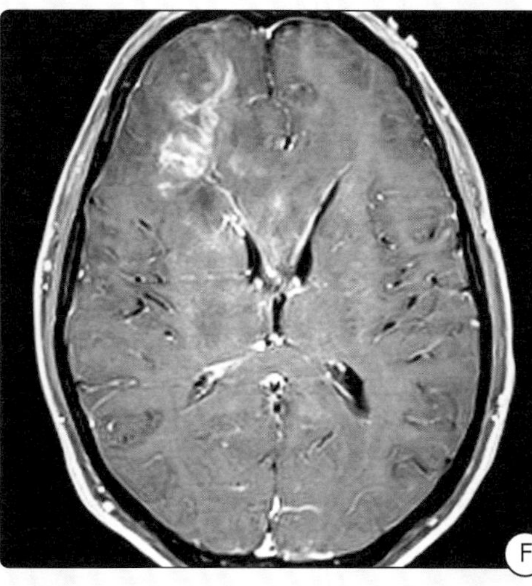

***(17-18E)** T2* SWI MR shows multiple foci of gradient susceptibility. Some are clumped and likely represent calcifications, while others are more linear and may represent enlarged blood vessels. **(17-19F)** T1 C+ FS MR shows patchy and linear enhancing foci within the mass. Note prominent enlarged vessels (probably medullary veins) in the WM. Oligodendroglioma, CNS WHO grade 3 was found at surgery. The patient was alive 4.5 years later.*

GBMs may also occur in the thalami, brainstem, cerebellum, and even the spinal cord. When midline or juxtamidline tumors are identified, diffuse midline glioma, H3 K27-altered should be considered in the differential diagnosis.

**Size and Number.** GBMs vary widely in size from relatively small focal lesions to massive tumors infiltrating multiple lobes in the so-called gliomatosis cerebri pattern. Up to 20% of GBMs appear as multifocal lesions at the time of initial diagnosis, but only 2-5% of multifocal GBMs are true synchronous, independently developing tumors.

**Gross Pathology.** GBMs are poorly delineated masses. The most frequent appearance is a reddish-gray tumor "rind" surrounding a central necrotic core **(17-20)**. Central necrosis can occupy over 80% of tumor volume. Intratumor hemorrhage is common, and macroscopic cysts with liquefied necrotic tumor tissue are often present.

**Microscopic Features.** GBM, IDH-wildtype, is a diffusely infiltrating, highly cellular tumor composed mostly of astrocytic, poorly differentiated tumor cells with nuclear atypia and marked pleomorphism. Necrosis and microvascular proliferation are common throughout the lesion.

Microscopic extension into the so-called peritumoral brain zone bordering the tumor along white matter tracts and seeding of the CSF spaces (e.g., along the ventricular ependyma, pial surfaces, and subarachnoid spaces) is common **(17-23)** **(17-24)**. Extension into the dura and skull are rare, as are systemic metastases.

**Staging, Grading, and Classification.** GBM, IDH-wildtype is a CNS WHO grade 4 neoplasm.

**Diagnostic Molecular Pathology.** IDH-wildtype GBMs lack *IDH1* and *IDH2* mutations and do not carry H3 K27 or H3 G34 mutations. The probability of a noncanonical IDH mutation is <

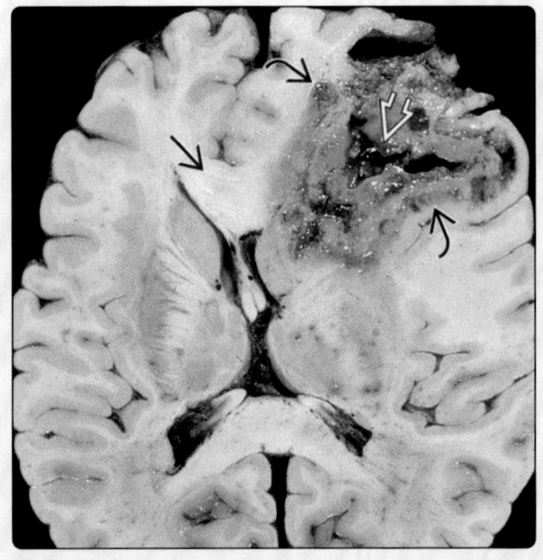

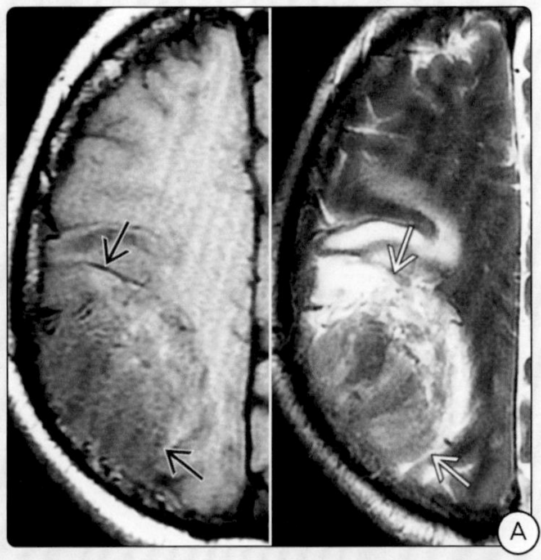

*(17-20) Glioblastoma (GBM), IDH-wildtype exhibits prominent intratumoral hemorrhages and central necrosis ➡. Irregular rim of viable neoplastic tissue ➡ surrounds the necrotic core. The corpus callosum genu is expanded ➡ and infiltrated with tumor. (17-22A) (L) Axial T1 MR shows a hypodense, right parietal infiltrating mass ➡. (R) T2 MR shows that the mass is mixed hyper- and isointense ➡.*

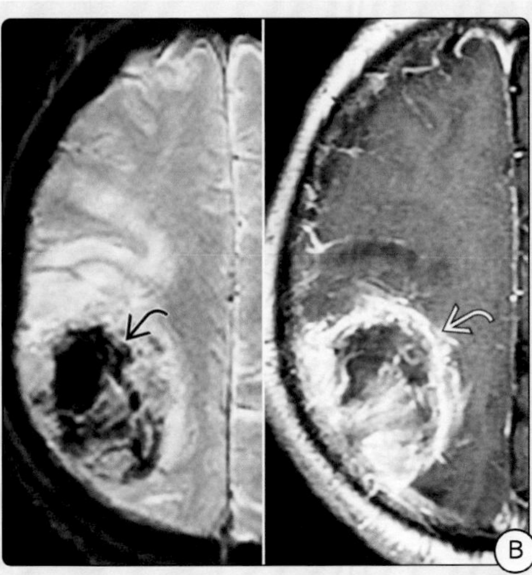

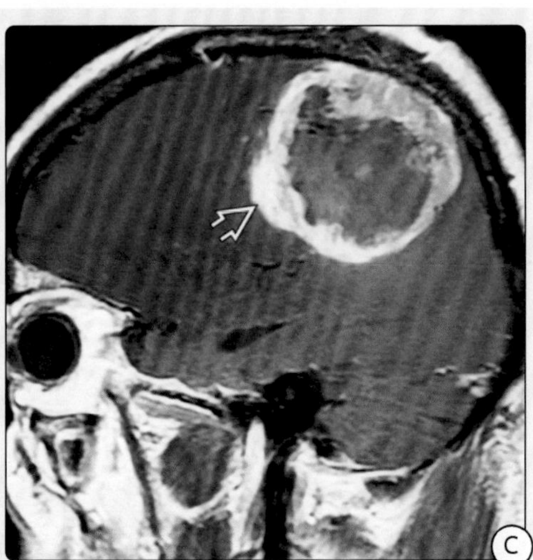

*(17-22B) (L) T2* GRE shows the mass has significant "blooming" ➡. (R) Axial T1 C+ MR shows irregular rim enhancement ➡ around a central nonenhancing core. (17-22C) Sagittal T1 C+ MR shows a thick, irregular "rind" of enhancement ➡ around the central necrotic core. This is GBM, IDH-wildtype, CNS WHO grade 4.*

1% in GBMs in patients ≥ 55 years of age, so further sequencing is generally considered unnecessary.

However, in patients < 55 years or in patients with a history of a lower grade glioma, the WHO, 5th edition recommends negative standard IDH1 immunostaining to be followed by DNA sequencing for less common *IDH1* or *IDH2* mutations. Further, if the tumor is in or adjacent to midline structures, H3 K27-altered mutations should also be excluded.

*TERT* promoter mutations, *EGFR* gene amplification, and a +7/-10 genotype allow for the diagnosis of IDH-wildtype GBM even if microvascular proliferation &/or necrosis is absent. Demonstration of a DNA methylation profile of IDH-wildtype GBM is also sufficient for the diagnosis.

*BRAF* p.V600E mutation is rare but can be identified in up to 50% of GBMs with epithelioid histology. *TP53* mutations are present in ~ 25% of all GBMs but are frequent in giant cell GBMs.

*MGMT* promoter methylation is typically determined in IDH-wildtype GBMs because it is clinically relevant, indicating response to chemotherapy in patients treated with temozolomide.

## DIAGNOSTIC PATHOLOGIC CRITERIA FOR GLIOBLASTOMA, IDH-WILDTYPE

**Essential**

- IDH-wildtype, H3-wildtype diffuse astrocytic glioma

**+1 or More of the Following**

- Microvascular proliferation
- Necrosis
- *TERT* promoter mutation
- *EGFR* gene amplification
- +7/-10 chromosome copy-number alterations

**Supplemental Diagnostic Information**

- DNA methylation profile of GBM, IDH-wildtype

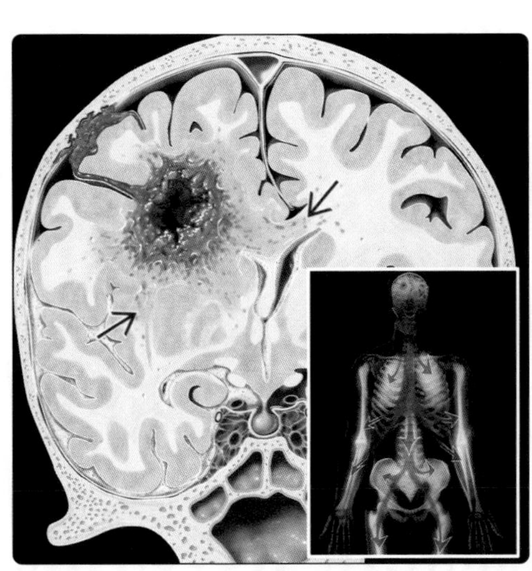

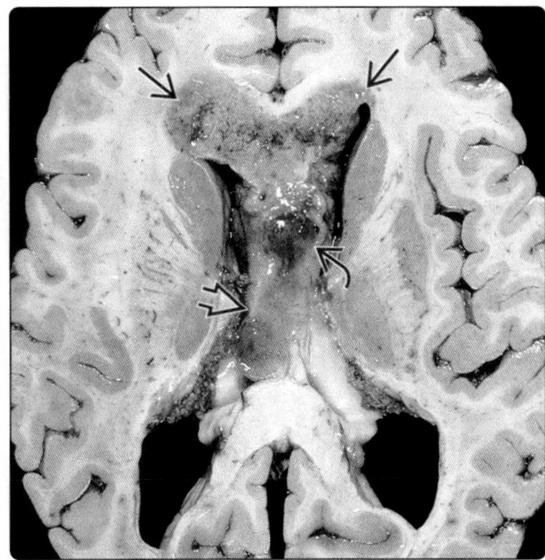

***(17-23)*** *Graphic depicts potential routes of GBM spread. Preferential spread is along WM tracts ➾ but can be ependymal, subpial, diffuse CSF ("carcinomatous meningitis"). Insert shows rare extracranial GBM metastases to lungs and bones.* ***(17-24)*** *Autopsy shows "butterfly" GBM ➾ crossing corpus callosum genu, extending into and enlarging the septum pellucidum ➾ and fornix ➾.*

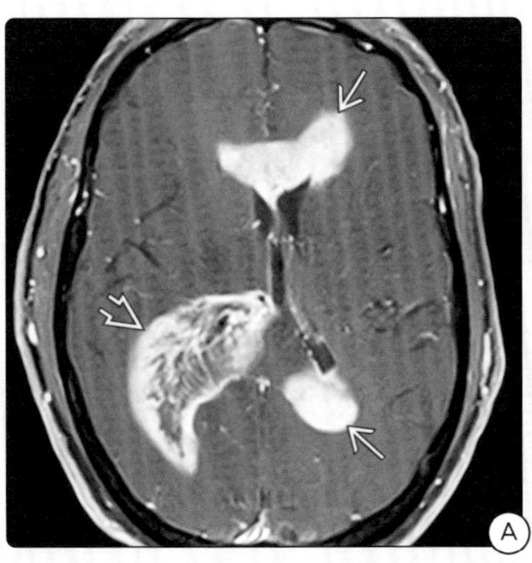


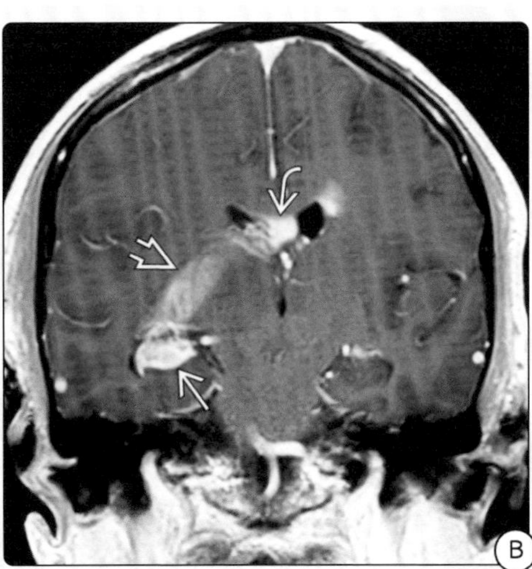


***(17-26A)*** *T1 C+ FS MR shows GBM, IDH-wildtype, CNS WHO grade 4 ➡ with tumor spread throughout the corpus callosum ➡.* ***(17-26B)*** *Coronal T1 C+ MR shows contiguous tumor spread ➡ into the temporal lobe ➡ and fornix ➡.*

## Clinical Issues

**Demographics.** GBM, IDH-wildtype is the most common malignant brain tumor in adults, representing 12-15% of all intracranial neoplasms and 60-75% of astrocytomas.

Most patients with IDH-wildtype GBMs are over the age of 55 years, peaking at 60-75 years. M:F ratio is essentially equal.

**Presentation.** Symptoms vary with tumor location and vary from focal neurologic deficits to seizures. Approximately 2% of GBMs present with sudden stroke-like onset, typically caused by acute intratumoral hemorrhage.

**Natural History.** GBM is a relentless, progressive disease. The disease can progress quickly, leading to rapid clinical decline and death. Median survival is 12 months. Five-year survival is < 10%.

Younger age at diagnosis (≤ 50 years) and complete tumor resection are associated with somewhat prolonged survival.

**Treatment Options.** Standard treatment is radiation and chemotherapy. The efficacy of new techniques, including laser interstitial thermal therapy and targeted immunotherapy, is unproven.

Methylation of the *MGMT* gene promoter is present in approximately 1/2 of GBMs. If methylation status is positive (i.e., the tumor is "methylated"), alkylating chemotherapy (i.e., with temozolomide) may improve survival.

## Imaging

**General Features.** The vast majority of GBMs exhibit a thick, irregular, enhancing "rind" of tumor surrounding a central necrotic core **(17-22)**.

**CT Findings.** Most GBMs demonstrate a hypodense central mass surrounded by an iso- to moderately hyperdense rim on NECT. Hemorrhage is common, and calcification is rare. Peritumoral edema is usually significant and is seen as

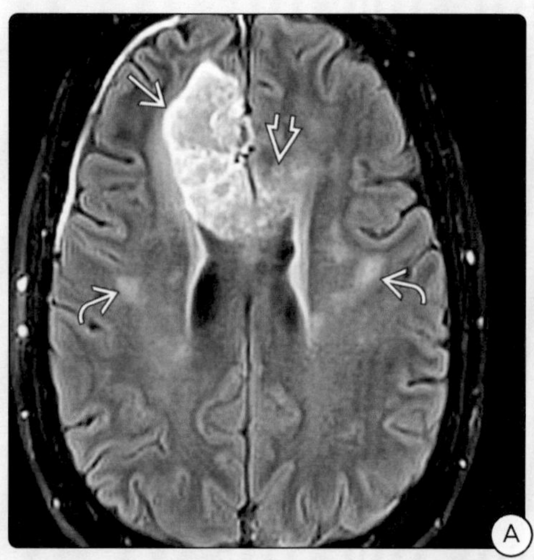


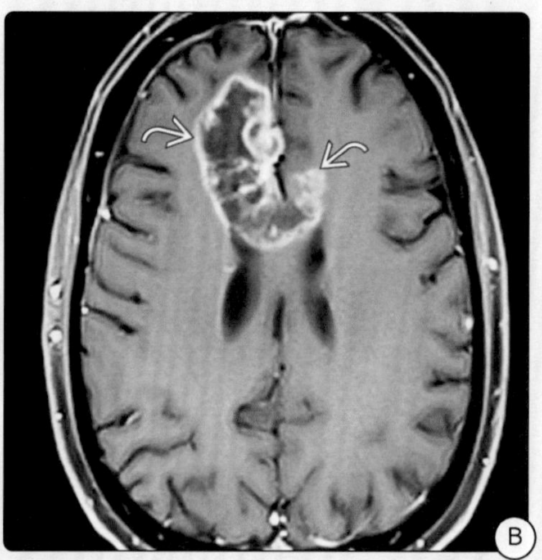


***(17-28A)** FLAIR MR in a 35-yo man with postbiopsy "butterfly" GBM, IDH-wildtype shows the tumor is heterogeneously hyperintense and crosses enlarged corpus callosum genu. Note multiple foci of tumor infiltration into the WM of both cerebral hemispheres. **(17-28B)** T1 C+ FS MR shows enhancing tumor "rind" in this "butterfly" GBM. The WM tumor nodules infiltrating both hemispheres did not enhance.*

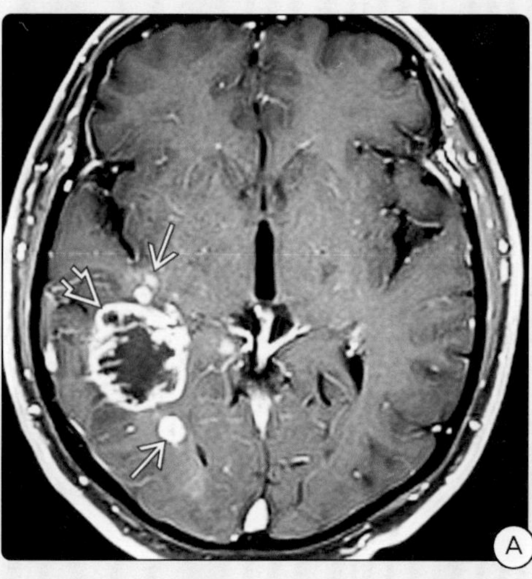


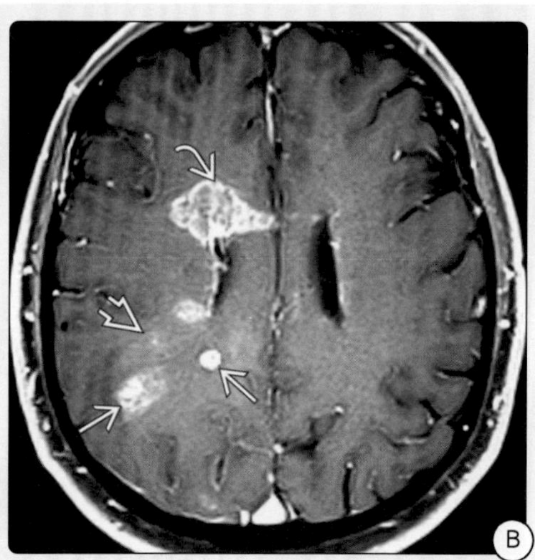


***(17-30A)** T1 C+ FS MR in a 66-yo man with visual problems shows an irregular rim-enhancing mass in the right hemisphere. Note multiple discrete enhancing foci in the adjacent brain. **(17-30B)** More cephalad T1 C+ FS MR shows more tumor crossing the body of the corpus callosum. More discrete tumor nodules are present. Note faint enhancement of WM and medullary veins. "Brain to brain" metastases is from GBM, IDH-wildtype.*

hypodensity surrounding the mass and extending along compact white matter tracts. CECT shows strong but heterogeneous rim enhancement.

**MR Findings.** T1WI shows a poorly marginated mass with mixed signal intensity. Necrosis, intratumoral cysts, and subacute hemorrhage with "blooming" on T2* GRE or SWI is common **(17-22B)**. T2/FLAIR shows heterogeneous hyperintensity with indistinct tumor margins and extensive surrounding vasogenic edema **(17-22A)**. Occasionally, GBMs infiltrate the brain diffusely in a gliomatosis cerebri-like pattern **(17-31) (17-33)**.

T1 C+ shows strong but heterogeneous ring enhancement surrounding a central nonenhancing core of necrotic tumor **(17-22) (17-28) (17-26)**. Nodular, punctate, or patchy enhancement outside the main mass represents macroscopic tumor extension into adjacent structures **(17-30)**. Nonenhancing tumor foci are invariably present, extending at least 2 cm beyond the margins of visible tumor, and CSF dissemination is common **(17-34) (17-36)**.

Most GBMs do not restrict on DWI. DTI may show reduced fractional anisotropy and disrupted white matter tracts surrounding the tumor. DSC pMR shows elevated rCBV in the tumor "rind," and DCE pMR shows evidence of increased vascular permeability. MRS shows reversal of Hunter angle (i.e., increased Cho and decreased Cr and NAA).

**Radiomics.** Recent deep learning models using convolutional neural networks have reported high accuracy, sensitivity, and specificity in predicting IDH status and detecting the presence of *MGMT* promoter methylation preoperatively. Multiparametric machine learning modeling has also been touted as detecting *EGFR* alterations and stratifying patients for targeted chemo- and immunotherapy.

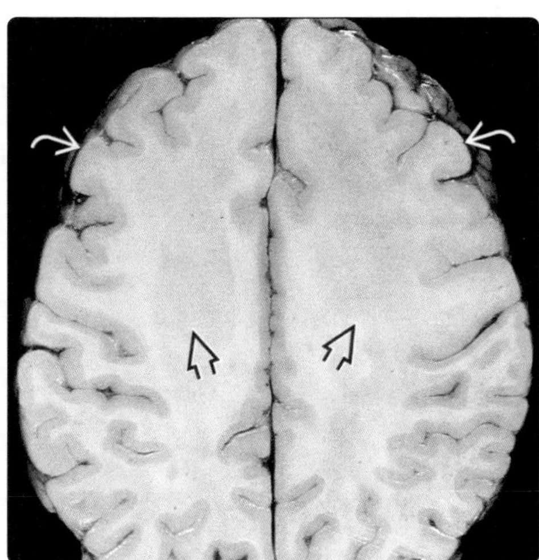

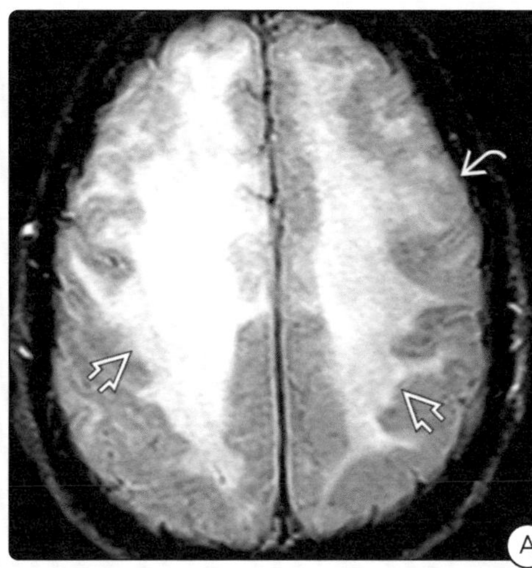


***(17-31)** Autopsy shows that GBM, IDH-wildtype, CNS WHO grade 4 diffusely infiltrates and expands the hemispheric WM ➪. Note extension into adjacent cortex with effacement of GM-WM interfaces ➪. **(17-33A)** FLAIR MR in a 79-yo man with seizures shows diffusely infiltrated WM ➪ and expanded gyri with blurred GM-WM junctions ➪.*

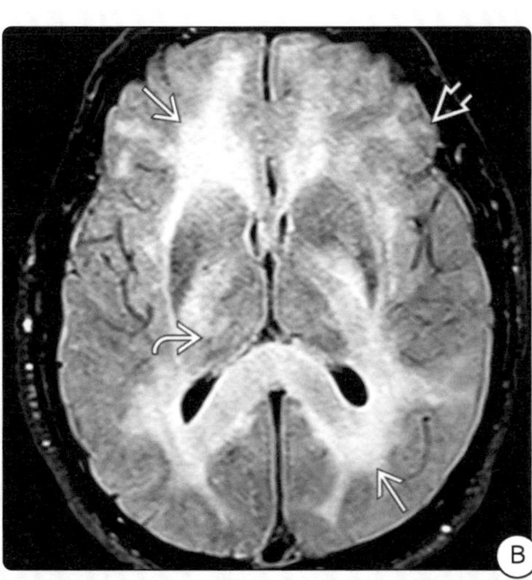


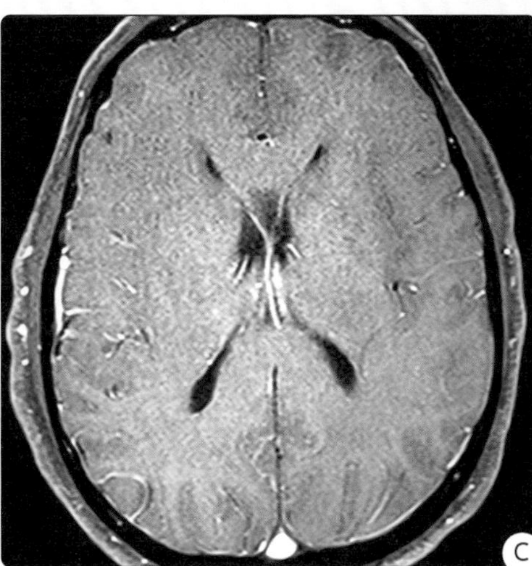


***(17-33B)** FLAIR MR through the lateral ventricles in the same case shows diffuse hyperintensity throughout the hemispheric WM ➪, minimal involvement of the cortex ➪, and deep gray nuclei ➪. **(17-33C)** T1 C+ FS MR shows no enhancement. Biopsy disclosed GBM, IDH-wildtype, CNS WHO grade 4. Occasionally, GBM diffusely infiltrates the brain in a gliomatosis cerebri-like pattern as it did in this case.*

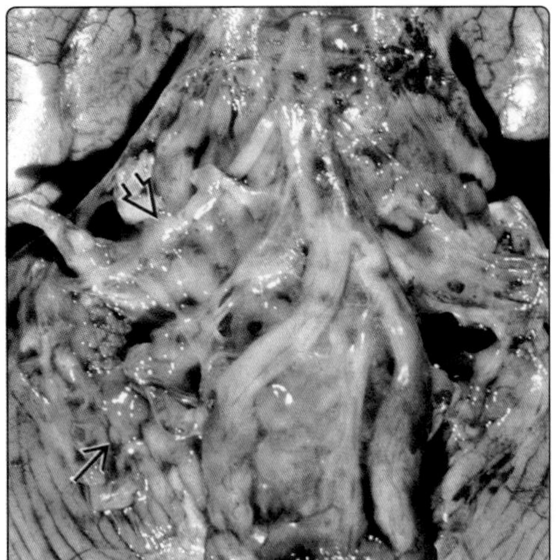

***(17-34)*** *Autopsy illustrates diffuse CSF spread from GBM. Tumor diffusely coats pons ⇨ and cerebellum ⇨ in "carcinomatous meningitis."*

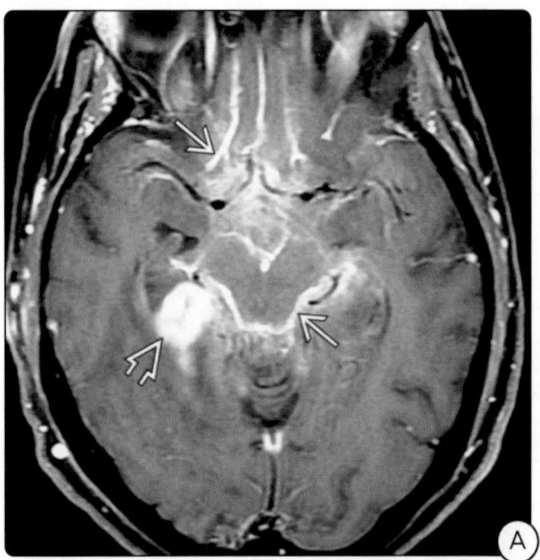

***(17-36A)*** *T1 C+ FS MR of GBM ➡ shows diffuse subarachnoid, pial spread of tumor in a carcinomatous meningitis pattern ➡.*

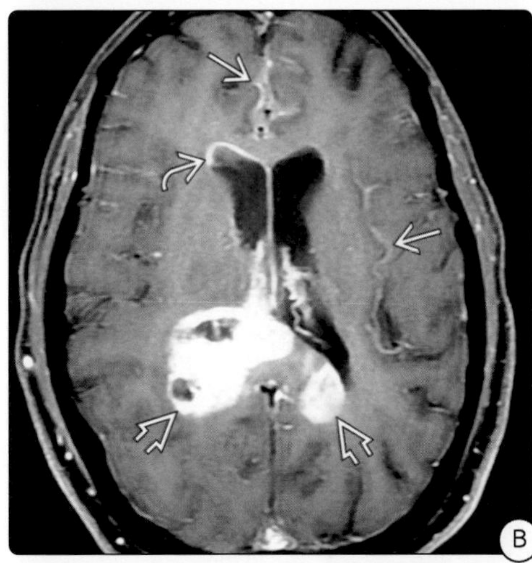

***(17-36B)*** *Tumor also spreads along corpus callosum splenium ➡. Note ependymal metastases in frontal horn ➡, leptomeninges ➡.*

## Differential Diagnosis

The major neoplasm that should be distinguished from GBM is **metastasis** from an extracranial tumor. Metastases are often multiple, more often rounded than diffusely infiltrating, and typically located at the gray-white matter interfaces.

Other potential GBM mimics include **astrocytoma, IDH-mutant, CNS WHO grades 3 and 4**. These tumors are generally less infiltrative, less often necrotic, and generally occur in younger patients. **Oligodendroglioma, CNS WHO grade 3** may be infiltrating and difficult to distinguish from GBM on imaging alone. **Primary CNS lymphoma** often involves the corpus callosum but is rarely necrotic (except in immunocompromised patients) and frequently restricts on DWI.

The major nonneoplastic differential diagnosis of GBM is **abscess**. Abscesses typically have thinner, more regular rims and restrict strongly on DWI. Other GBM "mimics" are rare. Uncommon nonneoplastic brain tumefactions, such as **"tumefactive" vasculitis**, may become necrotic, exhibit intralesional punctate/microhemorrhages on T2* sequences, and resemble GBM. **"Tumefactive" demyelination** in the subcortical white matter may demonstrate partial peripheral ("horseshoe") enhancement and tends to occur in a younger age group.

### GLIOBLASTOMA, IDH-WILDTYPE

**Clinical Issues**

- Most common adult malignant brain tumor
- Age ≥ 55 years
  - Peak: 60-75 years
- Survival: ~ 1 year
- Alkylating chemotherapy if tumor is "methylated"

**Imaging Findings**

- General: Thick, enhancing "rind" around necrotic core
- CT: Hypodense, poorly marginated
  - Striking peripheral edema
  - ± hemorrhage
  - $Ca^{++}$ rare
- MR
  - Mixed signal on T1WI
  - Heterogeneously hyperintense on T2WI, FLAIR
  - Hemorrhage on T2* GRE common
  - Strong, often irregular enhancing tumor "rind" on T1 C+
  - Multifocal, noncontiguous tumors common
  - Tumor extends far beyond imaging margins
  - Usually no restriction on DWI
  - ↑ vascular permeability on pMR
  - ↑ Cho, ↓ Cr, NAA on MRS

## Diffuse Astrocytoma, IDH-Wildtype, Not Elsewhere Classified

In the WHO, 5th edition, all IDH-wildtype diffuse astrocytomas are designated CNS WHO grade 4 neoplasms. To date, there is no officially sanctioned provision for "lower grade" (i.e., grade 2 or 3) adult-type IDH-wildtype diffuse glioma.

Some have reported rare adult low-grade IDH-wildtype astrocytomas that lack the histopathologic features, molecular signatures, and genetic alterations typical of either GBM or pediatric-type high-grade gliomas. In some reports, these tumors exhibited a relatively indolent clinical course with a median overall survival of three years.

The provisional diagnosis of an IDH-wildtype lower grade diffuse astrocytoma assumes (1) there are no molecular changes of a high-grade glioma (e.g., no *TERT* or *EGFR* amplification, +7/-10, or H3 K27 alterations), (2) lower grade tumors have been excluded (e.g., *FGFR1*, *BRAF* mutations are absent), (3) "noncanonical" *IDH1* and other mutations, such as *IDH2*, have been excluded, and (4) genetic sequencing with methylation profiling has been performed and excludes other rare mutations.

In such instances, the tumor is designated as **diffuse astrocytoma, IDH-wildtype, not elsewhere classified** (**NEC**, indicating all molecular testing was performed and it is unclear what the tumor really is). If the histopathology is consistent with a low-grade diffuse astrocytoma but necessary diagnostic tests were either not performed or were negative or inconclusive, the tumor would be designated as **diffuse astrocytoma, IDH-wildtype, not otherwise specified (NOS) (17-38)**.

What to do with these rare IDH-wildtype diffuse astrocytomas that are not grade 4 remains controversial. It is important to distinguish these rare tumors from diffuse astrocytic gliomas in adults who have lower grade histologic features but genomic &/or epigenomic profiling revealing molecular features of GBM, a CNS WHO grade 4 neoplasm. More aggressive patient management in such cases may improve clinical outcome.

*Selected References: The complete reference list is available on the eBooks+ version included with purchase.*

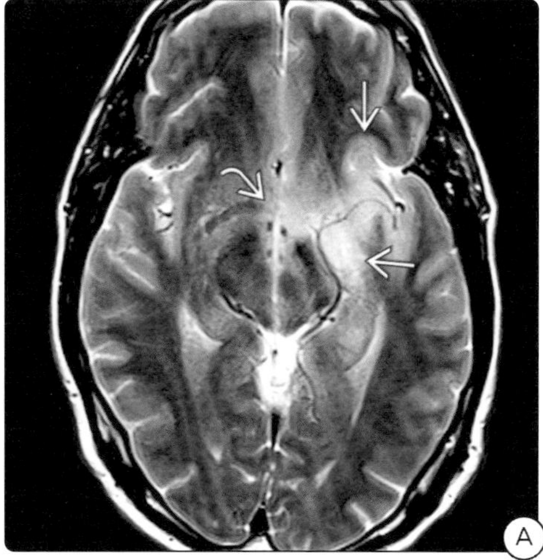


***(17-38A)** Axial T2 MR in a 53-yo man with seizures shows diffusely infiltrating hyperintense mass ➡ crossing into anterior commissure ➡.*

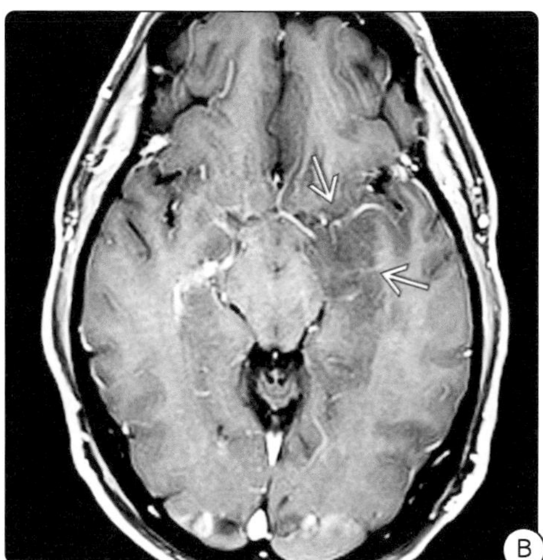


***(17-38B)** T1 C+ FS MR shows that the mass ➡ is hypointense, does not enhance. Biopsy showed grade 2 diffuse astrocytoma, IDH-wildtype.*

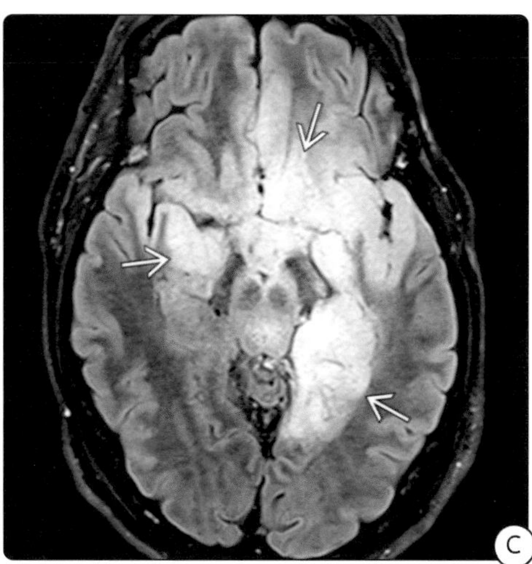


***(17-38C)** FLAIR MR 7 years later shows interval tumor spread ➡. Repeat biopsy showed diffuse astrocytoma, IDH-wildtype, grade 2.*

# Pediatric-Type Diffuse Low-Grade Gliomas

*The 5th edition WHO classification of CNS tumors groups many neoplasms into tumor "families." By far, the largest, most varied tumor family is gliomas, glioneuronal tumors, and neuronal tumors. This tumor "family" is subdivided by age and tumor grade into adult-type diffuse gliomas (the largest single group), pediatric-type diffuse low-grade gliomas, pediatric-type high-grade gliomas, and circumscribed astrocytic gliomas.*



This chapter focuses on the relatively small but important group of pediatric-type diffuse low-grade gliomas (LGGs).

## Pediatric-Type Diffuse Low-Grade Gliomas

There are just four recognized neoplasms in this group of pediatric-type diffuse LGGs: Diffuse astrocytoma, *MYB*- or *MYBL1*-altered; angiocentric glioma (AG); polymorphous low-grade neuroepithelial tumor of the young (PLNTY); and diffuse LGG, MAPK pathway-altered. While these neoplasms are designated as "pediatric-type" tumors, they also occur in adults.

Together with glioneuronal tumors, pediatric-type diffuse LGGs represent nearly 1/3 of pediatric CNS neoplasms. Pediatric-type LGGs are a clinically and biologically distinct group of tumors with a generally favorable outcome. Most are epileptogenic and are often characterized clinically by pharmacologically resistant seizures.

### Diffuse Astrocytoma, *MYB*- or *MYBL1*-Altered

#### Terminology

Diffuse astrocytoma, *MYB*- or *MYBL1*-altered, is a diffusely infiltrative glial neoplasm composed of monomorphic cells with genetic alterations in *MYB* or *MYBL1*.

#### Pathology

Tumors are unencapsulated, soft, gray-white, cortical and subcortical supratentorial masses with monomorphic glial cells in a fibrillar matrix. Histologic features of anaplasia, such as necrosis and microvascular proliferation, are absent, as are IDH, *BRAF* V600E, and H3 mutations. Mitotic activity is absent or low.

*MYB*-altered diffuse astrocytomas are CNS WHO grade 1 neoplasms and account for ~ 2% of pediatric LGGs.

## Clinical Issues

Median age at diagnosis is 29 years, but patients typically have had seizures—often pharmacoresistant—since childhood. Reported cases range from 4-50 years with a 3:1 M:F ratio.

Prognosis is favorable. Most patients become seizure free after complete resection, and malignant progression has not been reported.

## Imaging

CT may show an ill-defined, hypodense, nonenhancing, cortical/subcortical cerebral hemispheric mass.

*MYB*- or *MYBL1*-altered gliomas are typically hypointense on T1WI and heterogeneously hyperintense on T2/FLAIR sequences (some cases report a T2/FLAIR mismatch sign). These tumors do not demonstrate hemorrhage on T2* GRE or SWI and do not enhance following contrast administration **(18-1)**. Restricted diffusion is absent, and pMR shows low rCBV.

## Differential Diagnosis

The major imaging and histopathologic differential diagnosis is **AG**. *MYB*- or *MYB1*-altered diffuse astrocytomas have overlapping histopathologic and imaging features. Almost all AGs have *MYB* rearrangements, most commonly *MYB::QKI* fusions. Both are pediatric-type LGGs, both are CNS WHO grade 1 lesions, and both often present with pharmacoresistant epilepsy. Diffuse astrocytomas, *MYB*- or *MYBL1*-altered, form a distinct methylation cluster on whole-genome methylation profiling.

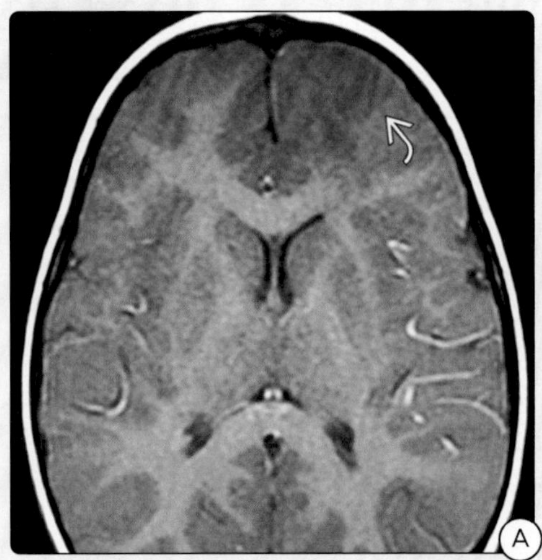

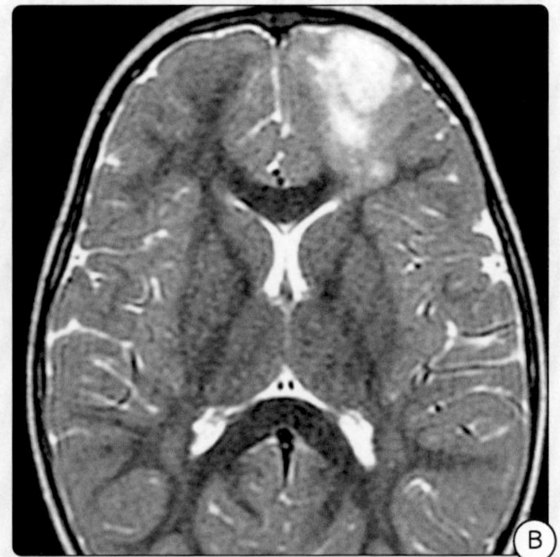

***(18-1A)** T1WI in a boy with complex partial seizures shows an ill-defined, iso-/hypointense left frontal lobe mass ➡ involving the cortex and subcortical white matter. **(18-1B)** The mass is mostly hyperintense on T2WI.*

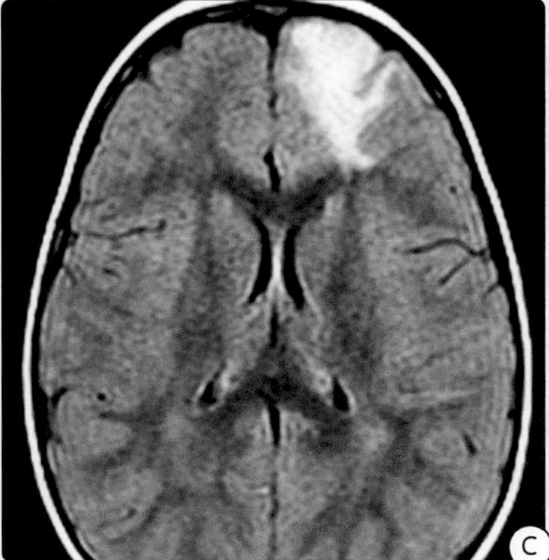

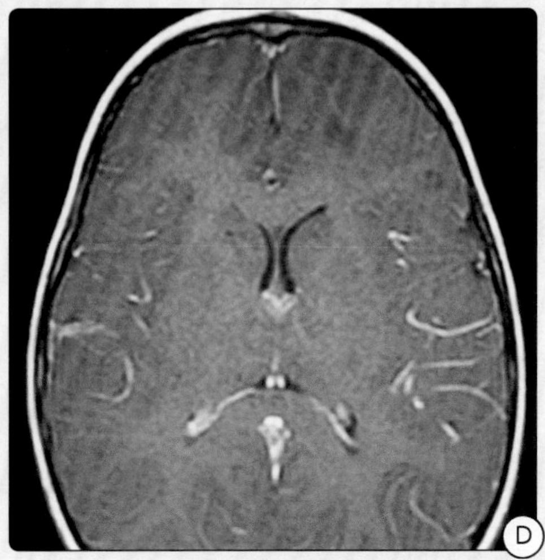

***(18-1C)** The mass is homogeneously hyperintense on FLAIR. **(18-1D)** The mass does not enhance on T1 C+. This is diffuse astrocytoma, MYBL1-altered.*

*MYB*- or *MYBL1*-altered diffuse astrocytomas are relatively indolent tumors and must be distinguished from **adult-type IDH-mutant** and **IDH-wildtype diffuse astrocytic gliomas**.

## Angiocentric Glioma

### Terminology

AG is a diffuse glioma with diffuse growth architecture in a focal angiocentric pattern.

### Pathology

More than 85% of AGs are supratentorial, superficially located, diffuse, expansile neoplasms with angiocentric growth, infiltrative borders, and ependymal differentiation. Involvement of both cortical and subcortical regions is typical. Most AGs are located in the temporal or frontal lobes. Approximately 15% are located in the brainstem.

Almost all AGs have a *MYB::QKI* gene fusion/rearrangement as the driver event in their development. AGs are characterized histopathologically by elongated bipolar spindle cells with a striking angiocentric orientation. Adjacent focal cortical dysplasia (FCD) is common.

Mitoses are sparse or absent; MIB-1 is generally < 1%. Necrosis and microvascular proliferation are absent.

AGs are CNS WHO grade 1 neoplasms.

### Clinical Issues

AGs are typically tumors of children and young adults. Median age at diagnosis is 13 years, although 20-25% of cases are > 20 years of age. There is a 2:1 M:F predominance. More than 90% present with seizures and often have a long history of pharmacoresistant epilepsy.

The majority of AGs are curable with complete surgical resection. If the AG is associated with FCD, fMRI-guided extensive resection may be required for a seizure-free result.

### Imaging

NECT shows a solid, cortically based tumor with variable attenuation. Dystrophic calcification is present in some cases.

Cystoid components are present in ~ 1/2 of all cases **(18-2)**. A rim-like or intratumoral high intensity on T1WI is common. "Blurring" of the gray matter-white matter junction is typical **(18-3)**.

In 20% of cases, T2 and FLAIR demonstrate a stalk-like high-intensity lesion extending through the white matter towards the ventricle **(18-4)**. Focal atrophy of the brain parenchyma near the tumor is common. Heterogeneous, nodular, or rim enhancement occurs in 5-25% of cases. FCD is present in some cases.

### Differential Diagnosis

The major differential diagnoses for AG are other low-grade epileptogenic gliomas, such as **PLNTY** and **FCD type IIA (FCD IIA)**. All three can exhibit stalk-like T2/FLAIR hyperintensity extending through the white matter towards the lateral ventricle, and FCD can coexist with AGs.

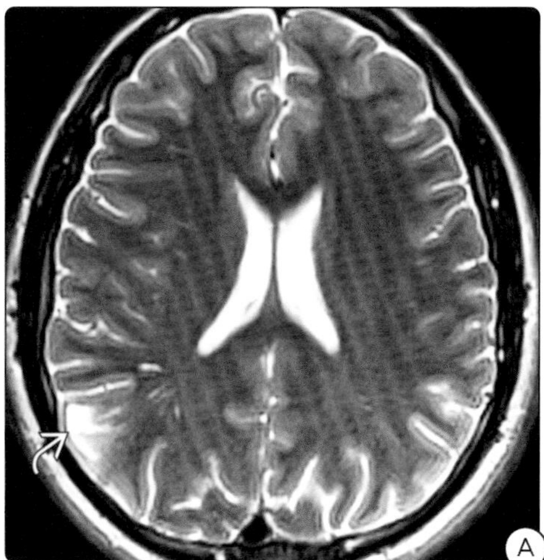


***(18-2A)** Axial T2WI in a patient with intractable seizures shows a wedge-shaped, hyperintense cortical/subcortical mass ➡.*

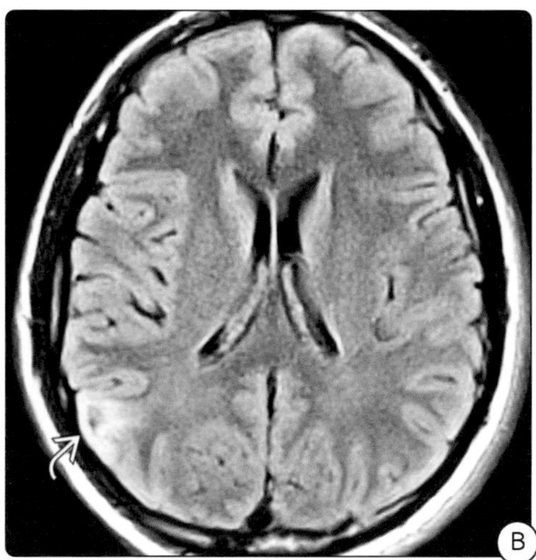


***(18-2B)** The mass ➡ does not suppress on FLAIR.*

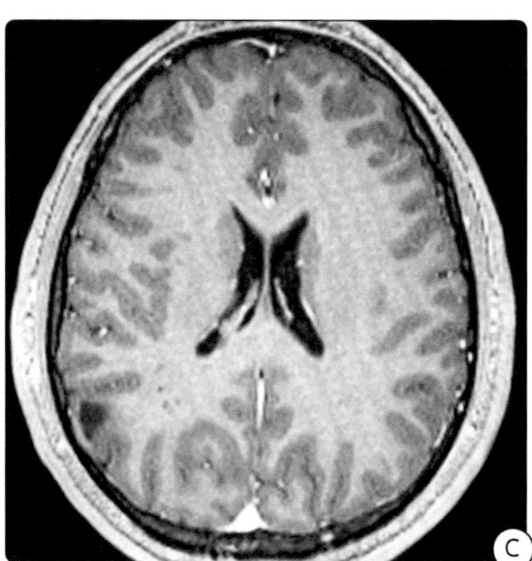


***(18-2C)** No enhancement is seen on T1 C+. This is angiocentric glioma. (Courtesy M. Castillo, MD.)*

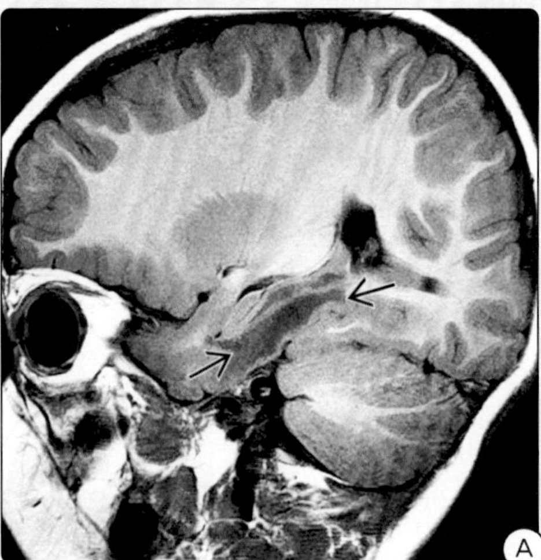

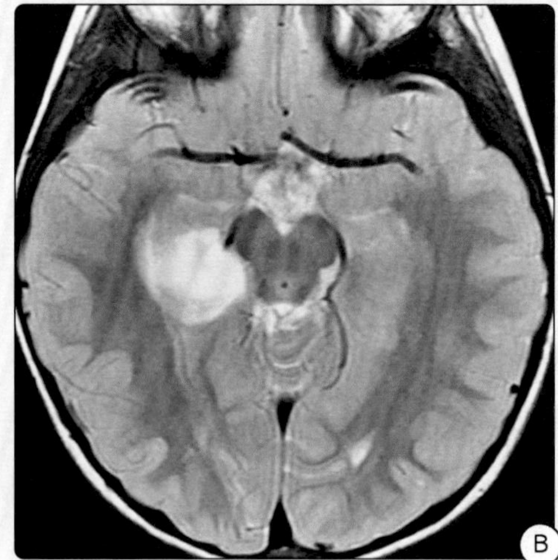

***(18-3A)*** *Sagittal T1WI in a 5-yo boy with temporal lobe epilepsy shows a well-delineated hypointense mass ⇒ in the inferior gyrus of the right temporal lobe.* ***(18-3B)*** *The mass is hyperintense and appears somewhat less well defined on T2WI.*

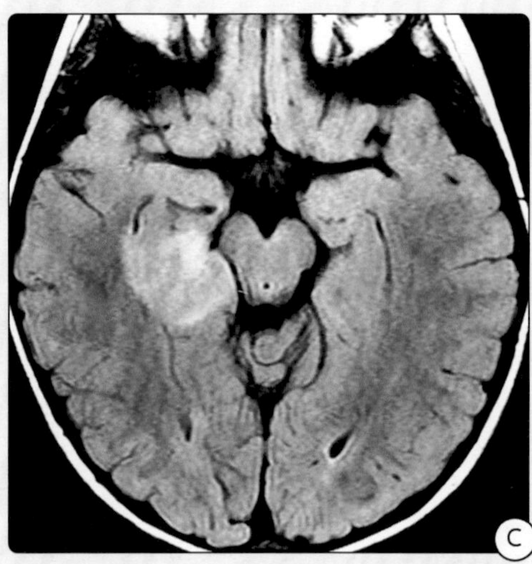

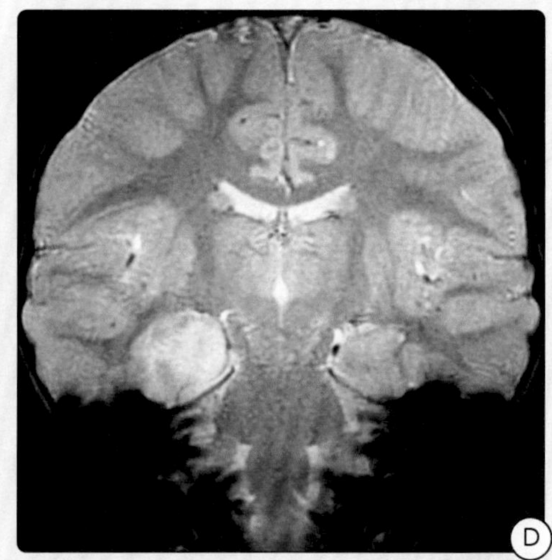

***(18-3C)*** *Axial FLAIR shows the mass is hyperintense and appears somewhat expansile with mass effect on the medial hippocampus and midbrain.* ***(18-3D)*** *Coronal T2* shows no evidence of gradient "blooming" to suggest intralesional hemorrhage or calcification.*

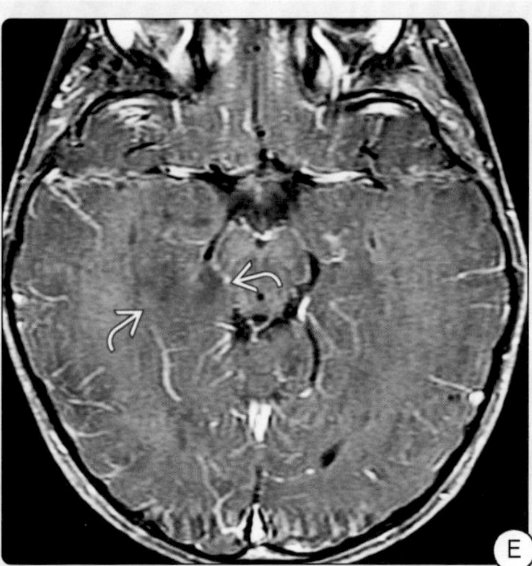

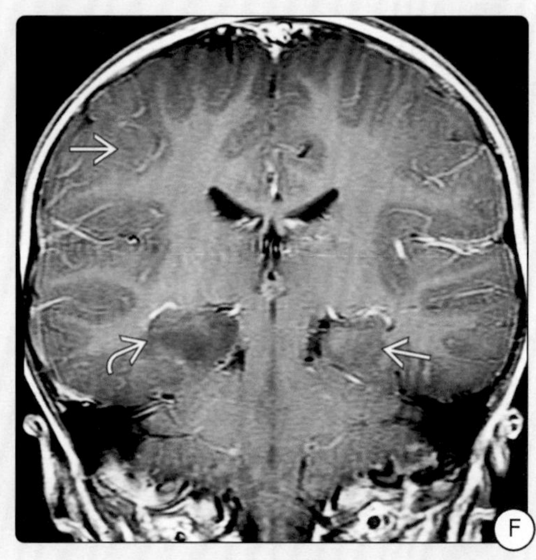

***(18-3E)*** *Axial T1 C+ FS demonstrates that the ill-defined, hypointense mass ➪ shows no evidence for enhancement.* ***(18-3F)*** *Coronal T1 C+ shows the slightly expansile mass ➪ in the right temporal lobe with superomedial displacement of the temporal horn. Compare to the normal left hippocampus ➡. Angiocentric glioma, CNS WHO grade 1, was found at pathologic examination.*

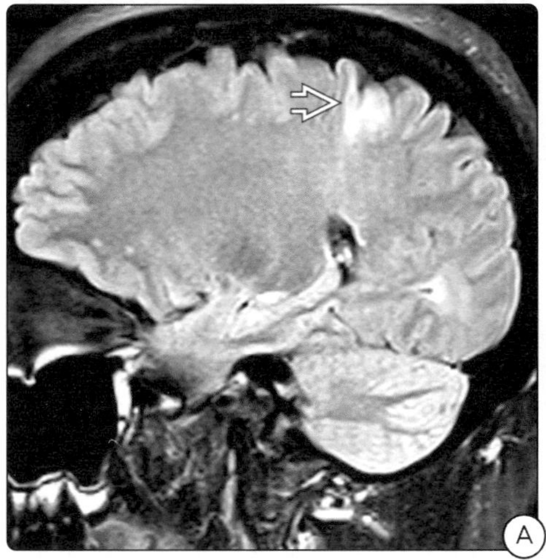

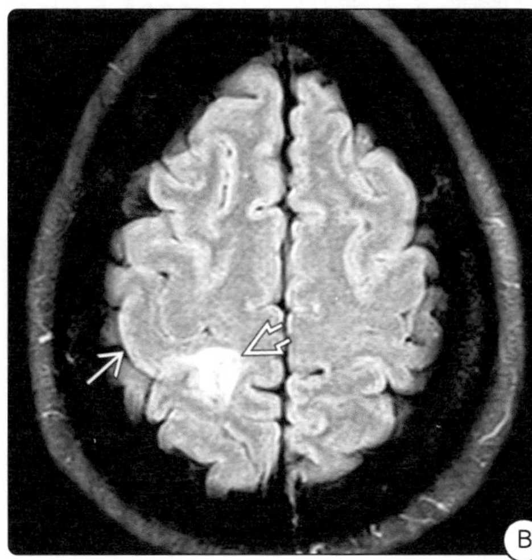

***(18-4A)** Sagittal FLAIR in a patient with longstanding, medically refractory epilepsy shows a hyperintense cortical/subcortical mass in the right parietal lobe. **(18-4B)** Axial FLAIR in the same case shows the hyperintense cortical/subcortical mass with superficial extension into an adjacent thickened postcentral gyrus .*

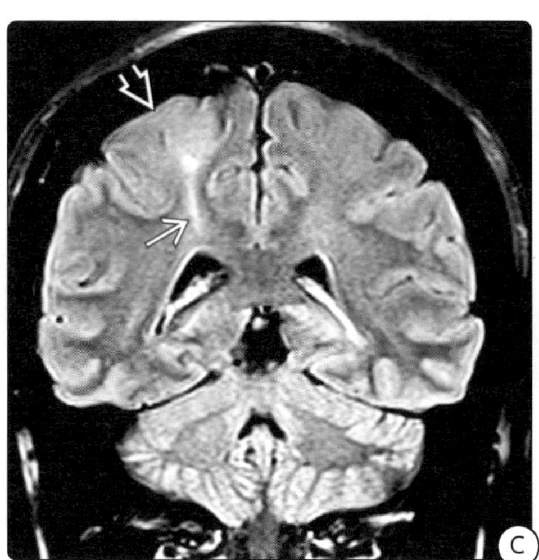

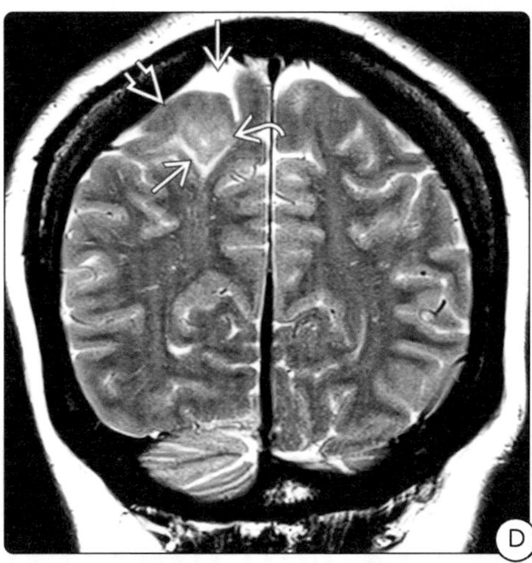

***(18-4C)** Coronal FLAIR shows thickened gyrus , hyperintense cortical/subcortical mass with striking hyperintense, linear stalk-like extension through the white matter of the corona radiata towards the lateral ventricle. **(18-4D)** Coronal T2WI shows focal pachygyria with subcortical hyperintensity . Enlarged CSF-filled sulci around the lesion suggest some focal atrophy.*

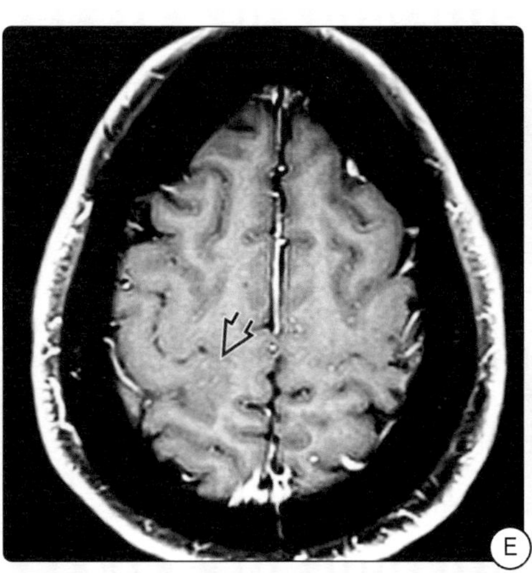

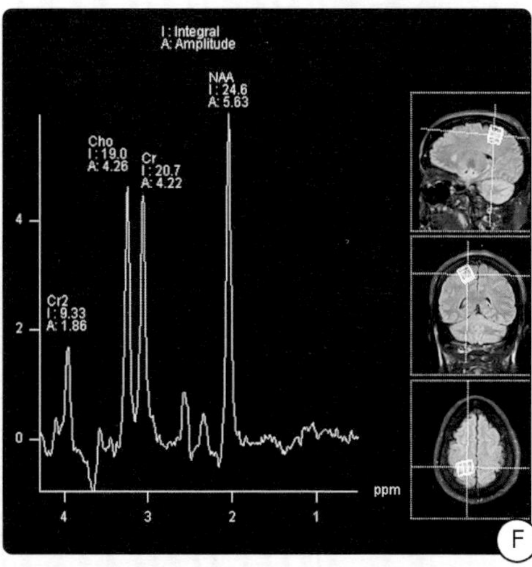


***(18-4E)** T1 C+ FS shows the mass is mildly hypointense relative to white matter and does not enhance. **(18-4F)** Single-voxel MRS in the same case shows mildly decreased NAA and slightly elevated Cho. Pathology disclosed angiocentric glioma with FCD IIA.*

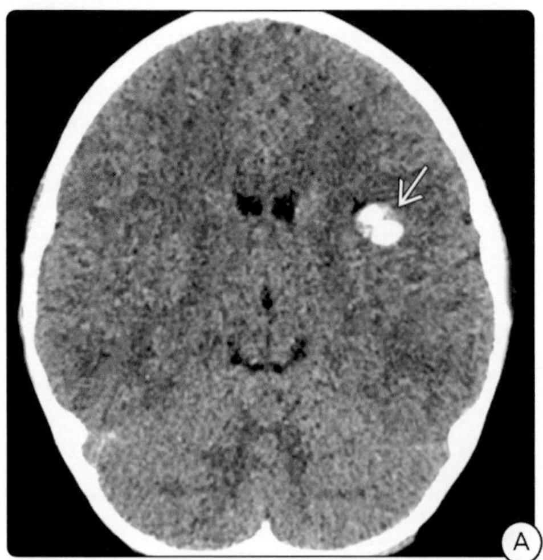


***(18-5A) NECT in a 9-yo boy with seizures shows a well-circumscribed, hyperdense mass with globular calcification ➡.***

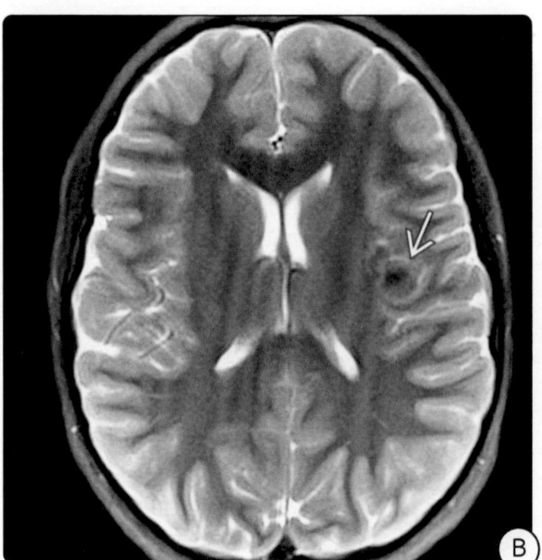


***(18-5B) The mass ➡ is heterogeneously hypointense compared to cortex on T2WI.***

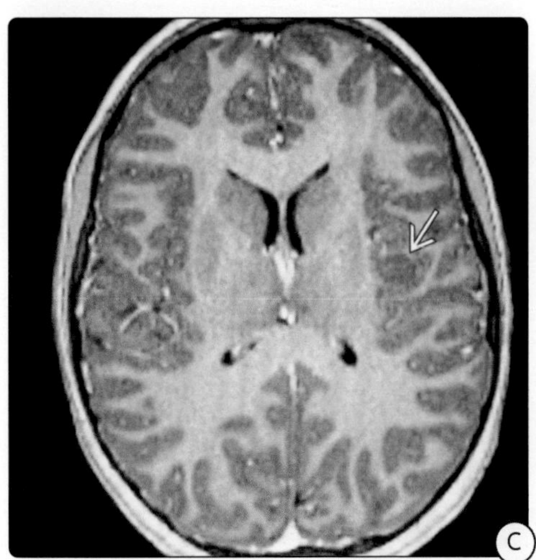


***(18-5C) The mass ➡ does not enhance on T1 C+. PLNTY was found at histopathologic examination. (Courtesy M. Castillo, MD.)***

# Polymorphous Low-Grade Neuroepithelial Tumor of the Young

## Terminology

Polymorphous low-grade neuroepithelial tumor of the young (PLNTY) is classified by the WHO as one of the pediatric-type diffuse LGGs.

## Etiology

PLNTYs are characterized by aberrant CD34 expression and activating alterations in the MAPK pathway. *BRAF* p. V600E mutations, *FGFR2* or *FGFR3* fusions, and other MAPK pathway-driving genetic abnormalities may be present.

## Pathology

PLNTYs are supratentorial, cortical/subcortical masses. 2/3 are found in the temporal lobe.

PLNTYs are characterized by CD34 immunopositive oligodendroglioma-like tumor cells showing a mixed compact and infiltrating growth pattern. Oligodendroglioma-like features, including small round nuclei, "fried egg" perinuclear halos, and branching capillaries, are common, but IDH mutations and 1p/19q codeletion are absent.

Consistent with their name, PLNTYs also often harbor patently astrocytic or histologically ambiguous features in addition to their oligodendroglioma-like appearance. Overtly neoplastic neuronal components are usually absent, although some dysmorphic neurons may be present. Coexistence of FCD is common.

Calcifications are common and range from discrete calcospherules to confluent calcific masses exhibiting osseous metaplasia. Mitoses are few or absent. Necrosis and microvascular proliferation are absent.

PLNTYs are IDH-wildtype, CNS WHO grade 1 lesions. Malignant transformation is exceptionally rare. A single case with *FGFR3::TACC3* fusion with GBM-like disseminated disease has been reported.

## Clinical Issues

PLNTYs are rare. While age at diagnosis ranges from 4-57 years, mean age at presentation is 22 years. The most common presentation is refractory epilepsy. There is a slight female predominance.

Despite its name, PLNTY also occurs in older adults who may present with new-onset headaches and psychiatric symptoms.

Most patients are seizure free after gross total tumor resection.

## Imaging

PLNTYs have wide radiologic variability. They can be well-circumscribed, cystic, or (less commonly) infiltrative lesions. The majority of PLNTYs are well-defined cortical/subcortical masses that are hyperdense on NECT. Between 80-85% are calcified **(18-5A)**. 2/3 of cases are mixed solid and cystic lesions.

Most PLNTYs are iso- to hypointense on T1WI and iso- to hyperintense on T2/FLAIR sequences. A tapered, hyperintense transmantle or stalk-like sign may extend through the white matter towards the lateral ventricles in PLNTYs associated with FCD **(18-6)**. About 1/3 of all reported cases enhance on T1 C+ **(18-5)**. Restricted diffusion is absent, and most PLNTYs show decreased rCBF on dynamic susceptibility pMR.

## Differential Diagnosis

The major imaging and histopathologic differential diagnostic consideration is **oligodendroglioma**. Other low-grade, pediatric-type gliomas and glioneuronal tumors, such as **ganglioglioma, AG**, and **dysembryoplastic neuroepithelial tumor (DNET)**, are common temporal lobe lesions in young patients with refractory epilepsy.

# Diffuse Low-Grade Glioma, MAPK Pathway-Altered

## Terminology

Diffuse LGG, MAPK pathway-altered, is a diffuse astrocytic or oligodendroglial-like tumor of childhood.

## Pathology

MAPK pathway-altered pediatric diffuse LGGs are LGGs with diffuse astrocytic, oligodendroglial, or mixed morphology.

MAPK pathway-altered pediatric diffuse LGGs have mutations in the tyrosine kinase domain (TDK) of *FGFR1* or a *BRAF* p. V600E mutation. These tumors are IDH-wildtype and H3-wildtype. *CDKN2A* homozygous deletions are absent. Cellular atypia is minimal, and mitotic activity is either absent or minimal. Microvascular proliferation and necrosis are absent.

DNA methylation profiling has not demonstrated a single cluster for MAPK pathway-altered pediatric diffuse LGGs. No WHO grade has been formally established.

These tumors occur throughout the neuraxis but are more commonly found in the cerebral hemispheres.

## Clinical Issues

These are rare tumors. Most patients are under 19 years of age and many present with epilepsy. The availability of novel targeted therapies, such as BRAF inhibitors, for MAPK pathway-altered gliomas may significantly alter their disease course.

## Imaging

Imaging findings are nonspecific; diffusely-infiltrating, T2/FLAIR hyperintensity is typical. Enhancement on T1 C+ is variable; nonenhancing infiltrating areas of tumor extension are common **(18-7)**.

## Differential Diagnosis

The main differential diagnoses include pediatric-type diffuse LGGs, such as *MYB*- or *MYBL1*-**altered diffuse astrocytoma**, and circumscribed astrocytic gliomas, such as **pilocytic astrocytoma** and **high-grade astrocytoma with piloid features**.

The imaging differential diagnosis also includes pediatric-type diffuse high-grade gliomas, such as **diffuse hemispheric glioma, H3 G34-mutant, diffuse pediatric-type high-grade glioma, H3- and IDH-wildtype**, and **diffuse midline glioma, H3 K27-altered**.

*Selected References: The complete reference list is available on the eBooks+ version included with purchase.*

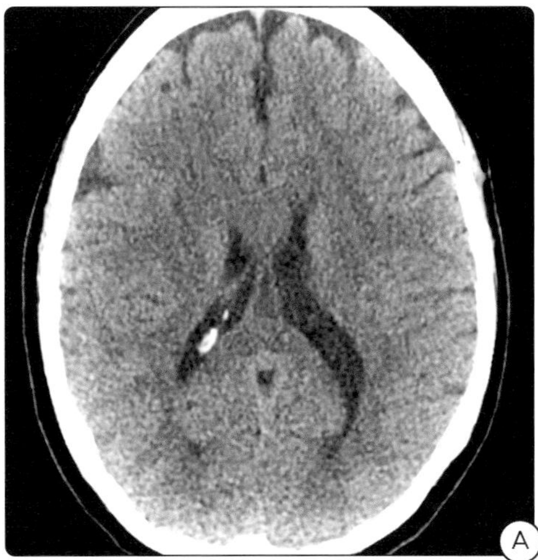

***(18-6A)** NECT in a 30-yo woman with longstanding seizures is normal.*

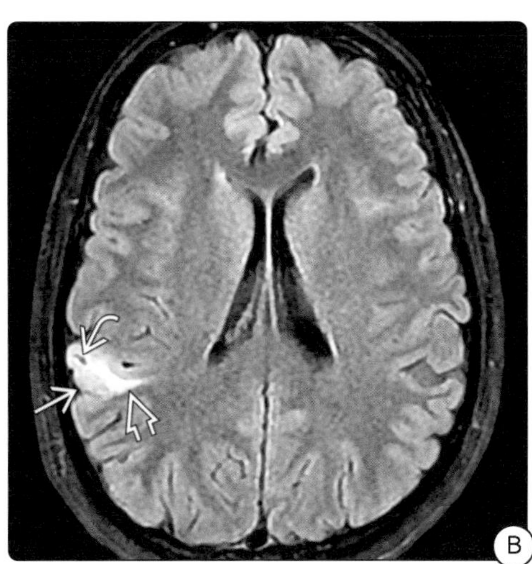

***(18-6B)** FLAIR shows cortical/subcortical mass ➡ with intratumoral cyst ➡ and a transmantle, hyperintense, stalk-like deep extension ➡.*

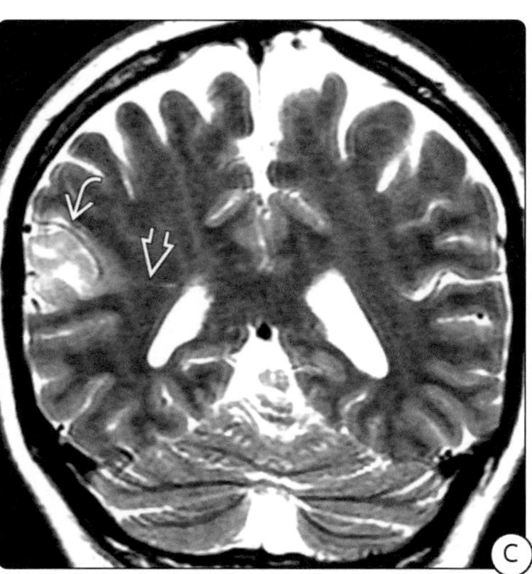

***(18-6C)** Coronal T2WI shows heterogeneously hyperintense mass ➡, transmantle, stalk-like hyperintensity ➡. This is PLNTY.*

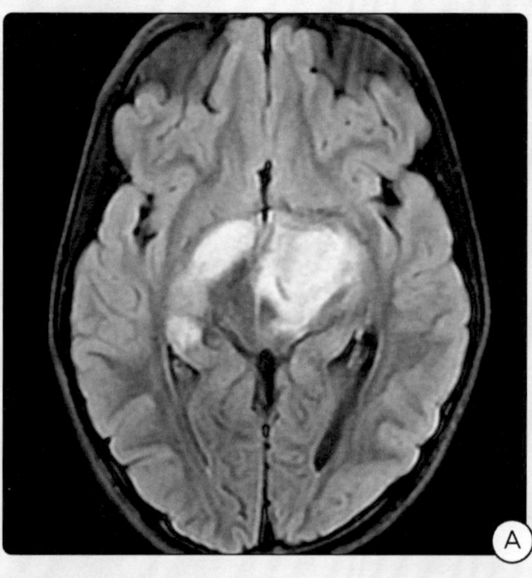


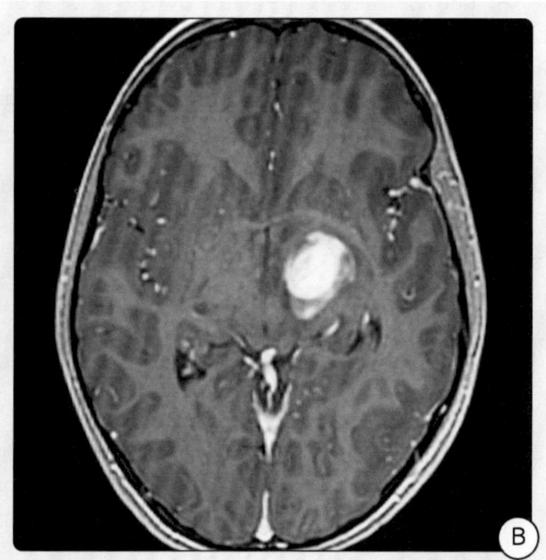


***(18-7A)** Axial FLAIR in a 6-yo shows a hyperintense hypothalamic mass extending into the midbrain. **(18-7B)** T1 C+ SPGR MR in the same case shows intense enhancement in the thalamic portion of the mass. Diffuse low-grade glioma, IDH- and H3-wildtype, MAPK pathway-altered, with a BRAF p.V600E mutation was found at diagnostic molecular examination.*

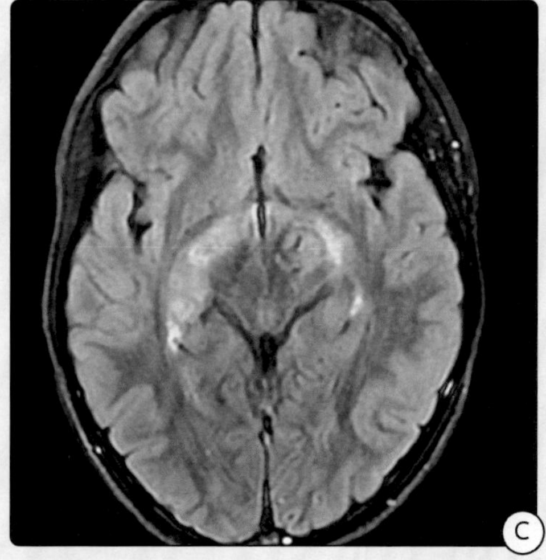


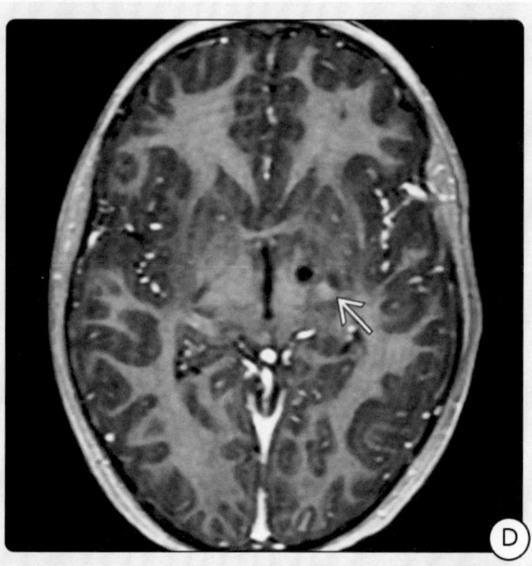


***(18-7C)** Axial FLAIR 6 months after MAPK pathway-targeted BRAF inhibitors shows marked diminution in the size of the tumor. **(18-7D)** T1 C+ SPGR shows dramatic interval diminution in the tumor with only a small residual focus of tumor present ➡.*

# Pediatric-Type Diffuse High-Grade Gliomas

*In recent years, with the advent of molecular diagnosis, our classification of pediatric high-grade gliomas has moved from a histology-based (e.g., "glioblastoma") and location-based (e.g., diffuse intrinsic pontine glioma) scheme to one focused almost exclusively on the genetic and molecular profile of tumors.*



Two tumors that were recently considered distinct based upon their location—diffuse intrinsic pontine gliomas (DIPGs) and thalamic gliomas—are now understood to be biologically similar tumors and are now classified as **diffuse midline gliomas (DMGs)**, most of which harbor an H3K27M mutation.

What would have previously been designated "pediatric glioblastomas" are now classified based upon their molecular profile, including **diffuse hemispheric glioma, H3 G34-mutant; diffuse pediatric-type high-grade glioma, H3-wildtype or IDH-wildtype; and infant-type hemispheric glioma**.

## Pediatric-Type Diffuse High-Grade Gliomas

### Diffuse Midline Glioma, H3 K27-Altered

#### Terminology

DMG is an infiltrative glioma located in a midline location with loss of H3 p.K28me3 (K27me3).

The term DIPG remains an acceptable term to describe these tumors when they arise in the pons.

#### Etiology

Most tumors are due to spontaneous mutations, but some tumor predisposition syndromes (e.g., Li Fraumeni and mismatch repair deficiency) are associated with a small proportion of these tumors.

#### Pathology

DMGs infiltrate adjacent parenchyma in a diffuse fashion. Tumor cells are small and monomorphic and may show astrocytic, piloid, oligodendroglial, giant cell, undifferentiated, or epithelioid cytology. All DMGs are considered CNS WHO grade 4.

Molecular subtypes include DMG, H3.3 K27-mutant; DMG, H3.1 or H3.2 K27-mutant; DMG, H3-wildtype with *EZHIP* overexpression; and DMG, *EGFR*-mutant.

## Clinical Issues

DIPG represents 10-15% of pediatric brain tumors and 75% of all pediatric brainstem tumors. Thalamic DMGs represent 1-5% of pediatric brain tumors and 25% of thalamic tumors. Spinal DMGs represent ~ 40% of spinal astrocytomas.

Most patients with DIPG present with a short clinical history of cranial nerve palsy, pyramidal tract impairment, and ataxia. Thalamic DMGs usually present with intracranial hypertension and motor/sensory deficits.

The prognosis of DMG is poor with a two-year survival of < 10%. Due to their midline location, surgical options are limited.

Historically, DIPG was often treated based upon imaging alone without biopsy, but biopsy is now universal in the age of molecular diagnostics. Radiation therapy remains the mainstay for treatment of DMG.

## Imaging

**General Features.** DIPG typically shows a poorly defined, T2-hyperintense, and expansile lesion centered in the pons. Large tumors often partially or completely surround the basilar artery without narrowing **(19-1) (19-2)**. DMGs in the thalamus and spinal cord have similar imaging features and may be unilateral **(19-3)** or bithalamic **(19-4)**. Metastatic disease may be present at diagnosis but is less common. Despite the fact that DMG has an imaging appearance of a hypocellular tumor (CT hypodensity and bright ADC), these tumors are WHO grade 4 tumors with a very poor prognosis.

**CT Findings.** DMGs typically show expansile and mass-like low attenuation with poorly defined borders. When located in the

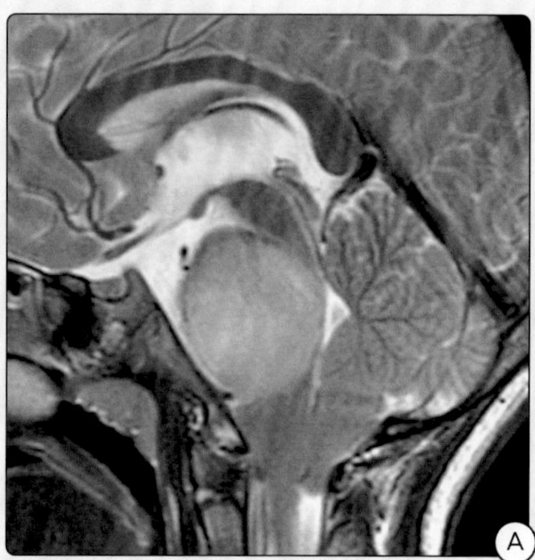

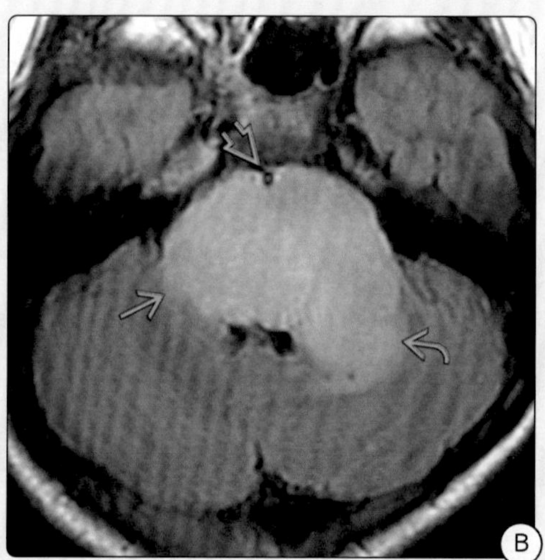

***(19-1A)** Sagittal T2 MR in an 8-year-old with a diffuse midline glioma (DMG), H3K27M-altered, shows expansile, hyperintense signal centered in the pons. When located in the pons, DMGs are often referred to by the former designation, diffuse intrinsic pontine glioma (DIPG). **(19-1B)** Axial FLAIR MR in the same patient shows ill-defined margins ➙, partial encasement of the basilar artery ➙, and infiltrative tumor in the left middle cerebellar peduncle ➙.*

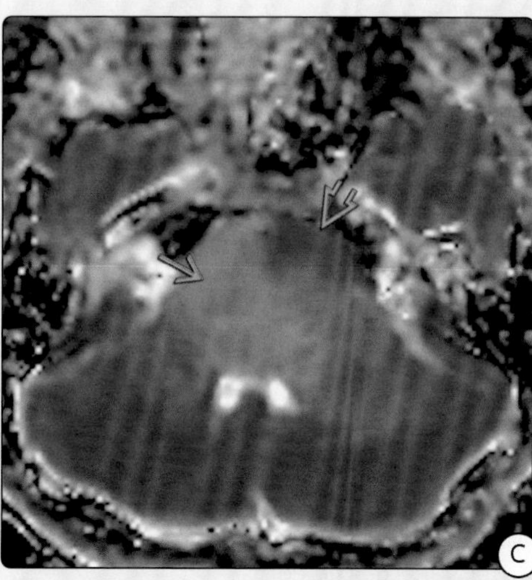

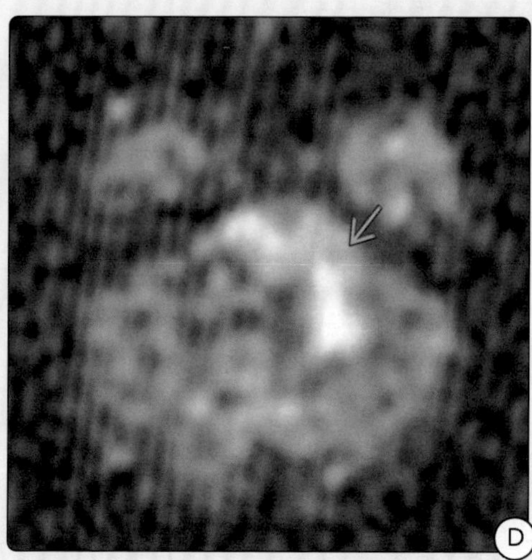

***(19-1C)** Axial ADC in the same patient shows predominantly hyperintense signal ➙, which is common for DIPG. The darker ADC signal in the left anterior pons ➙ is worrisome for a more cellular tumor component. Despite the typical low cellularity appearance of DIPG on imaging, it is WHO grade 4 with poor prognosis. **(19-1D)** Axial ASL MR shows hyperintense signal ➙ corresponding to increased CBF within the tumor.*

pons (DIPG), it can be difficult to distinguish pathologic low attenuation from skull base attenuation artifact—look for effacement of the fourth ventricle and prepontine cisterns.

**MR Findings.** DMGs appear as poorly marginated and expansile masses on MR, often infiltrating adjacent white matter tracts.

T1: Usually fairly homogeneous hypointensity with poorly defined margins.

T2/FLAIR: Typically ill-defined homogeneous hyperintensity with mass effect. Cysts are rare.

DWI: The majority of tumors show facilitated diffusion with ADC greater than adjacent brain. Patchy areas of diffusion restriction at the time of diagnosis may suggest a more aggressive course.

T1 C+: Typically absent or minimal enhancement at diagnosis. Contrast enhancement is more common following therapy or in later stages of the disease.

GRE/SWI: Calcifications and hemorrhage are rare.

PWI: Increased rCBV and CBF are common.

## Differential Diagnosis

Primary differential considerations include **other pediatric-type diffuse high-grade gliomas**, discussed below, circumscribed astrocytic gliomas, such as **pilocytic astrocytoma**, and **embryonal tumors [embryonal tumor with multilayered rosettes (ETMR) and atypical teratoid/rhabdoid tumor (ATRT)]**. **Other pediatric-type diffuse high-grade gliomas** typically are located within the cerebral hemispheres and are more likely to enhance and show diffusion restriction. **Pilocytic astrocytomas** are more likely to enhance, are typically sharply marginated, and are

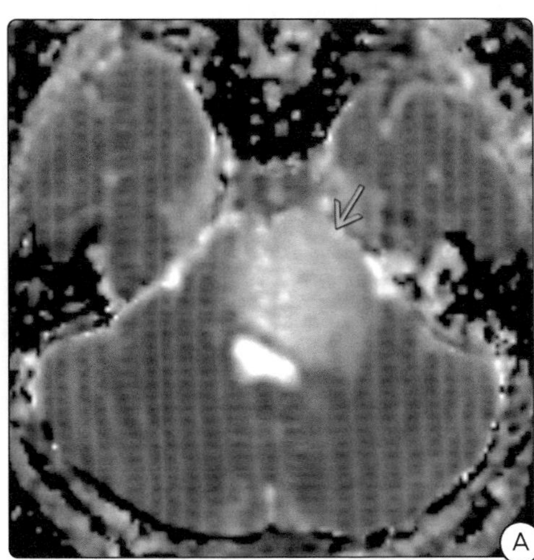


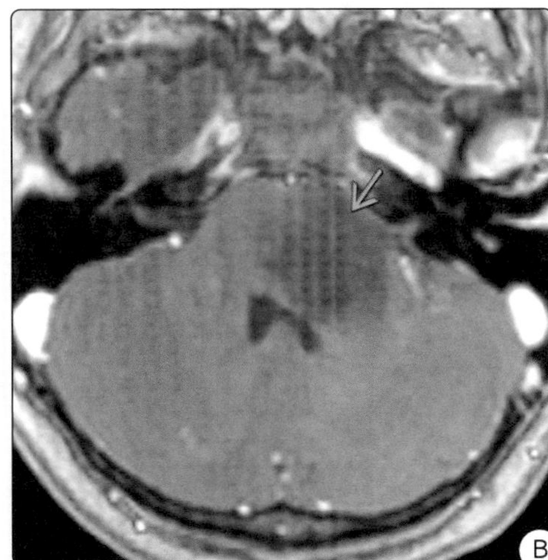


*(19-2A) Axial ADC in a 7-year-old with DIPG (DMG with H3K27M alteration) shows hyperintense signal throughout the tumor ➾, a characteristic appearance for this tumor. (19-2B) Axial T1 C+ in the same patient shows lack of contrast enhancement ➾, also a characteristic appearance for DIPG at time of diagnosis. Heterogeneous enhancement is common following treatment.*

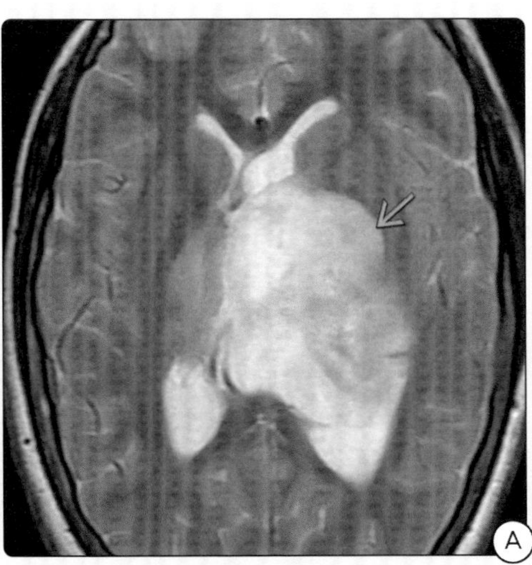


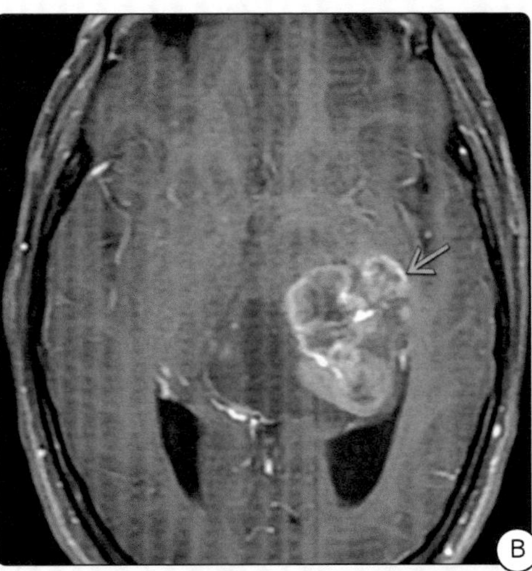


*(19-3A) Axial T2 MR in a 12-year-old with left thalamic DMG with H3K27M alteration shows a large, expansile tumor ➾ centered in the left thalamus. Such tumors may unilaterally involve the thalamus or may be bithalamic. (19-3B) Axial T1 C+ MR in the same patient shows heterogeneous enhancement ➾ of the lateral component of the tumor. Enhancement in thalamic DMG is variable.*

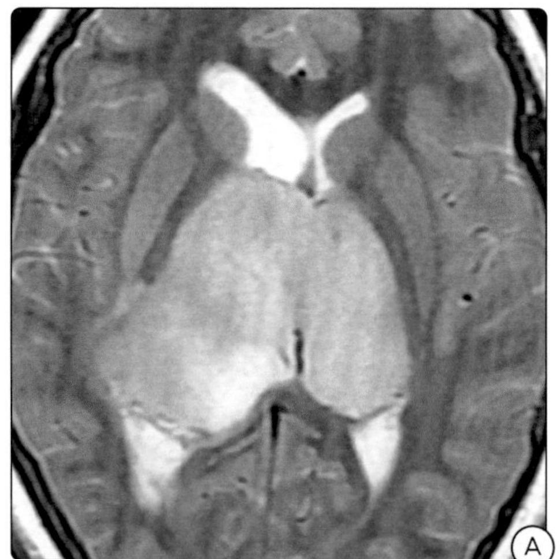

*(19-4A) Axial T2 MR in a child with bithalamic DMG with H3K27M alteration shows expansile T2 signal hyperintensity affecting both thalami.*

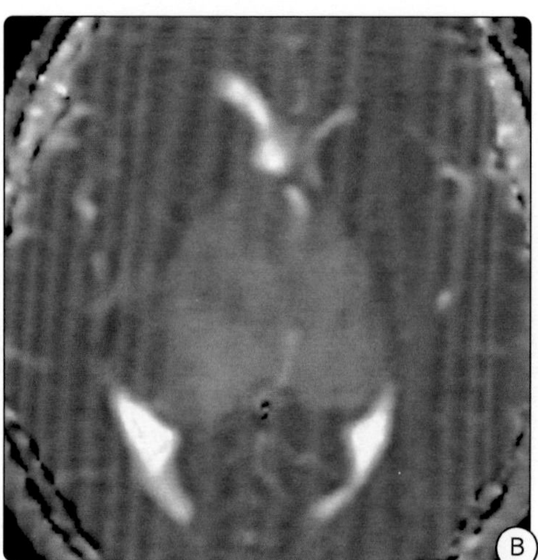

*(19-4B) Axial ADC in the same patient shows predominantly hyperintense signal, a typical appearance for DMG.*

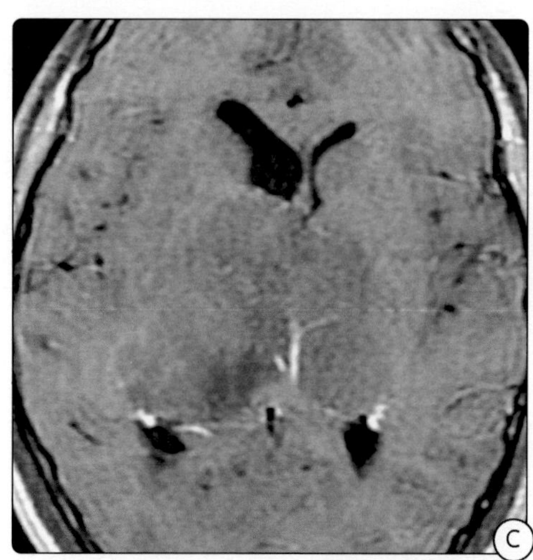

*(19-4C) Axial T1 C+ in the same patient shows no associated enhancement, a typical appearance for DMG.*

more likely to demonstrate cystic change. **Embryonal tumors (ETMR and ATRT)** are usually sharply marginated and show diffusion restriction of solid components, often with minimal or no enhancement. Nonneoplastic differential considerations include **tumefactive demyelinating disease** of the brainstem and **osmotic demyelination syndrome**.

**DIFFUSE MIDLINE GLIOMA, H3 K27-ALTERED: OVERVIEW**

Locations: Pons > thalamus > spinal cord

Pathology: Infiltrative high-grade (WHO grade 4) midline tumor
- DMG, H3.3 K27-mutant
- DMG, H3.1 or H3.2 K27-mutant
- DMG, H3-wildtype with *EZHIP* overexpression
- DMG, *EGFR*-mutant

Imaging:
- CT: Hypointense, expansile lesions; hemorrhage/calcifications rare
- MR
  - T2/FLAIR: Poorly defined margins; cysts are uncommon
  - DWI: Usually bright on ADC (in contrast to other pediatric high-grade gliomas)
  - T1 C+: Usually show no/minimal contrast enhancement
  - PWI: Most tumors show increased perfusion

Clinical:
- Cranial nerve palsies, ataxia, increased intracranial pressure
- Poor prognosis: 2-year overall survival < 10%

Differential Diagnosis
- Embryonal tumors: Occur in very young patients; well-defined margins; diffusion restriction
- Pilocytic astrocytoma: Typically well defined, cystic, with avid enhancement
- Other pediatric high-grade gliomas: Hemispheric location, necrosis, diffusion restriction

## Diffuse Hemispheric Glioma, H3 G34-Mutant

### Terminology

Diffuse hemispheric glioma, H3 G34-mutant, is an infiltrative glioma arising in the cerebral hemispheres with a missense mutation of the *H3-3A* gene.

### Pathology

Infiltration of the brain parenchyma results in expansion and distortion of involved brain ± hemorrhage and necrosis.

The most common histology is a highly cellular and infiltrative astrocytic tumor with increased mitotic activity and a glioblastoma-like pattern. A less common histologic appearance is similar to CNS embryonal tumors with small, monomorphic cells and hyperchromatic nuclei with scant cytoplasm.

The diagnosis is defined by a missense mutation at p.G35 (G34) of the histone variant H3.3. Diffuse hemispheric glioma, H3 G34-mutant, is a WHO grade 4 tumor, regardless of histology.

### Clinical Issues

This tumor has no known genetic susceptibility. It occurs most commonly in adolescents. Prognosis is poor with a median overall survival of 18-22 months.

## Imaging

Due to the typical location within the cerebral hemispheres, many tumors do not present until they are quite large. There is almost universal leptomeningeal contact of tumors.

CT typically demonstrates a cellular lesion sometimes demonstrating hemorrhage &/or calcifications.

MR typically shows a cellular lesion (moderate diffusion restriction in solid portions) with variable contrast enhancement. Tumor margins are variable with some demonstrating ill-defined margins **(19-6A)** and others well demarcated **(19-5)**. Cyst formation and heterogeneity is more likely in larger tumors. Hemorrhage and areas of necrosis are frequently encountered. Few case series suggest that most tumors show increased perfusion.

## Differential Diagnosis

Primary differential considerations include **other diffuse pediatric high-grade gliomas** (pHGGs), for which the imaging feature overlap is broad. **Circumscribed astrocytic tumors** and **gangliogliomas** are an important consideration but typically do not show diffusion restriction or necrosis. The imaging appearance is very similar to many **embryonal tumors (ETMR and ATRT)**, but embryonal tumors typically occur in a much younger population.

**LESS COMMON PEDIATRIC-TYPE DIFFUSE HIGH-GRADE GLIOMAS**

Diffuse Hemispheric Glioma, H3 G34-Mutant
- Pathology: Infiltrative glioma with *H3-3A* gene mutation, WHO grade 4
- Location: Cerebral hemispheres
- Clinical: Adolescents; no known genetic susceptibility
- Imaging: Variable "glioblastoma-like" vs. "diffuse astrocytoma"

Diffuse Pediatric-Type High-Grade Glioma, H3-Wildtype and IDH-Wildtype
- Pathology: Infiltrative glioma; wildtype H3 and IDH genes; WHO grade 4
- Location: > 85% supratentorial; minority in brainstem/cerebellum
- Clinical: Children and young adults; prior XRT or genetic susceptibility
- Imaging: Glioblastoma-like appearance

Infant-Type Hemispheric Glioma
- Pathology: High-grade astrocytoma in infancy
- Location: Cerebral hemispheres
- Clinical: Arise in 1st year of life
- Imaging: Often large and heterogeneous

# Diffuse Pediatric-Type High-Grade Glioma, H3-Wildtype and IDH-Wildtype

## Terminology

Diffuse glioma with histologic features of malignancy found in children and young adults with H3- and IDH-wildtype.

## Etiology

These tumors often arise in the setting of prior radiation therapy and in the context of tumor predisposition syndromes, such as constitutional mismatch repair deficiency syndrome (CMMRD), Lynch syndrome **(19-7)**, and Li-Fraumeni syndrome.

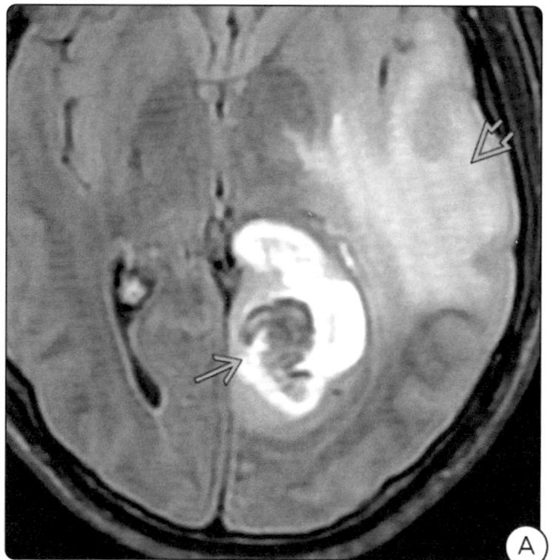


***(19-5A)** Axial FLAIR in a 17-year-old with diffuse hemispheric glioma, H3 G34-mutant, shows occipital tumor ➙, adjacent mass-like signal ➙.*

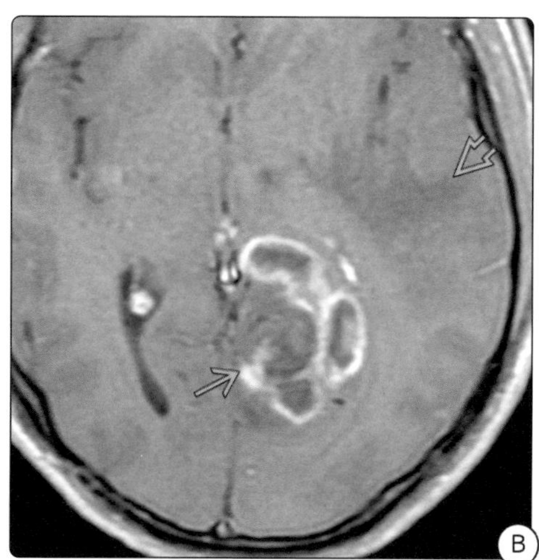


***(19-5B)** Axial T1 C+ shows enhancement of the primary lesion ➙ but no enhancement of the infiltrative signal ➙ in the left temporal lobe.*

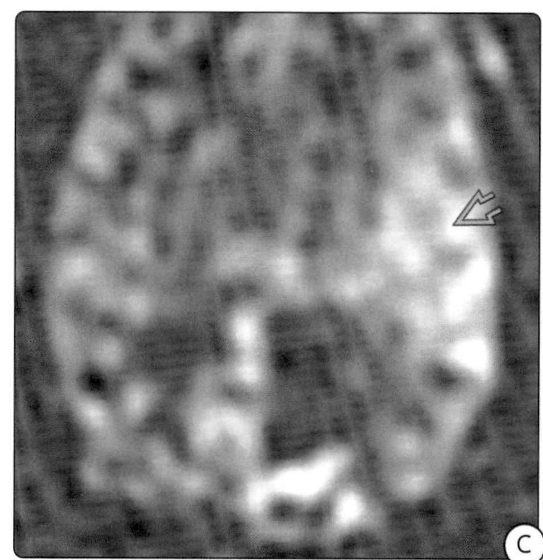


***(19-5C)** ASL perfusion imaging shows increased CBF in the infiltrative left temporal lobe signal ➙, confirming infiltrative tumor.*

*(19-6A) Axial FLAIR in an 18-year-old with diffuse hemispheric glioma, H3 G34-mutant, was obtained 6 months prior to diagnosis. The MR was normal at this time. (19-6B) Axial FLAIR in the same patient at time of diagnosis shows rapid development of the tumor ⇒ over a 6-month period. This rapid change is worrisome for a high-grade glial tumor, such as diffuse hemispheric glioma, H3 G34-mutant.*

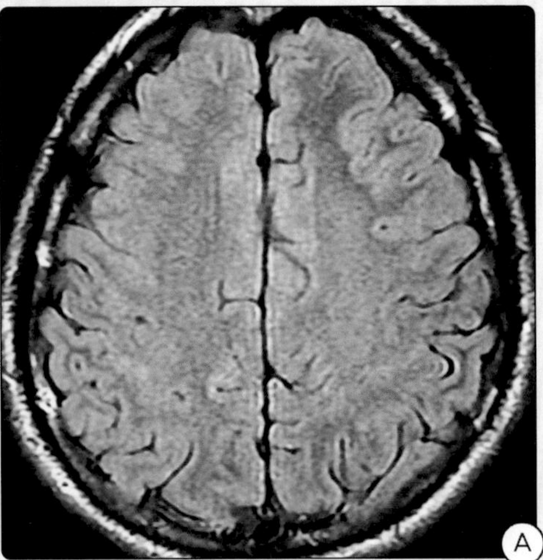

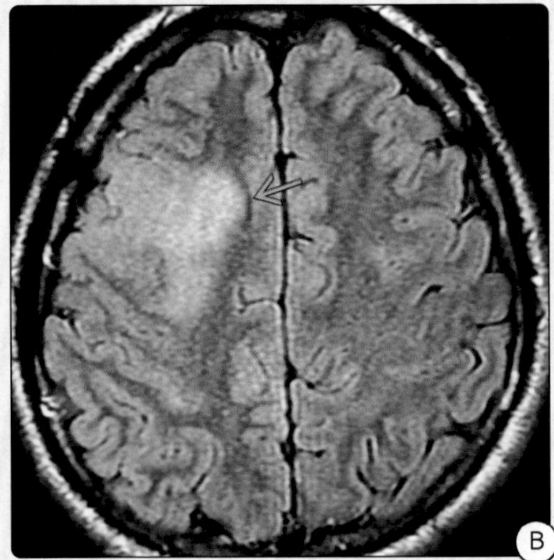

*(19-7A) FLAIR MR in a 26-year-old with Lynch syndrome, pediatric high-grade glioma (pHGG), IDH- and H3-wildtype, shows well-defined paramidline tumor ⇒ centered in posterior frontal cortex with extensive peritumoral edema ⇒. (19-7B) Axial T1 C+ shows an irregular rim of enhancement and central necrosis. Similar to their histologic appearance, pHGG, IDH- and H3-wildtype, typically have a glioblastoma-like imaging appearance.*

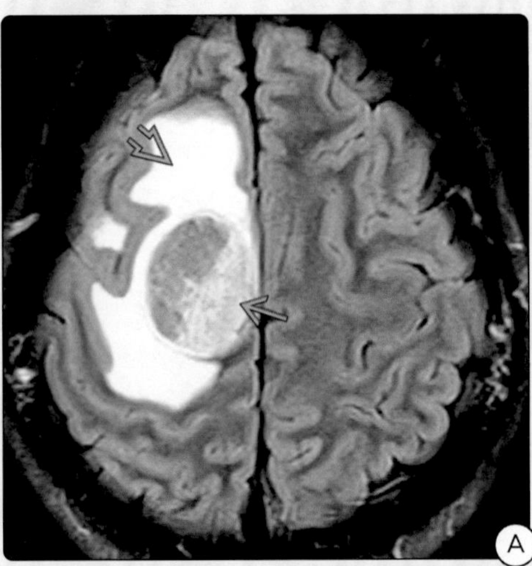

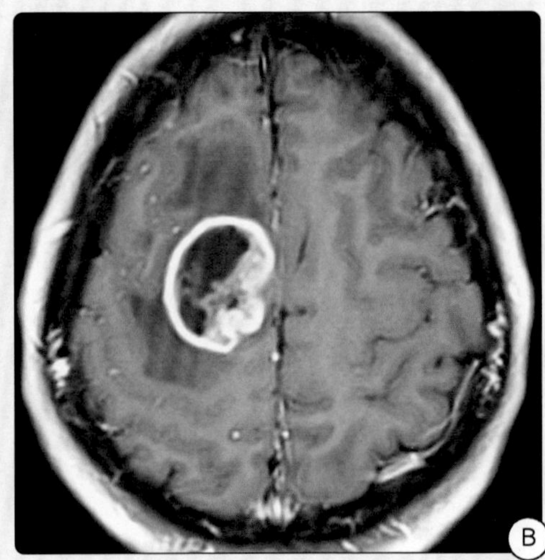

*(19-8A) Axial T1 C+ in a 15-year-old with pHGG, IDH- and H3-wildtype, and EGFR mutation shows a tumor centered in the right thalamus with irregular peripheral enhancement and central necrosis. These tumors can occur anywhere along the neuraxis, but > 85% are located in the supratentorial compartment. (19-8B) Axial ASL perfusion in the same patient shows increased perfusion within the enhancing solid rim ⇒ of the tumor.*

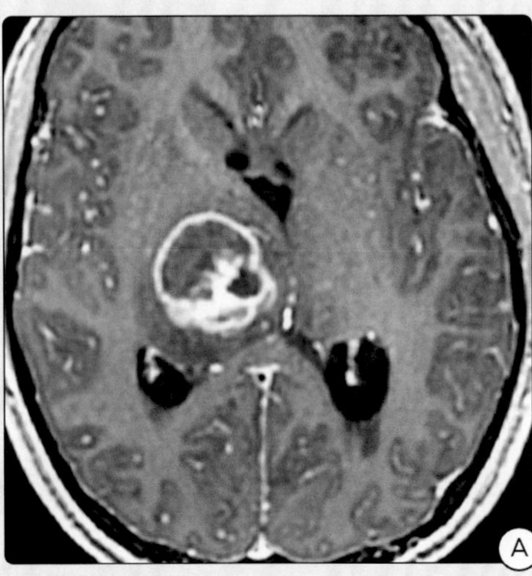

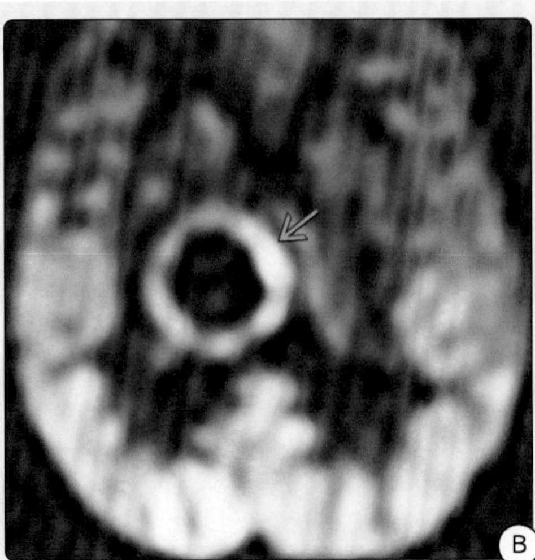

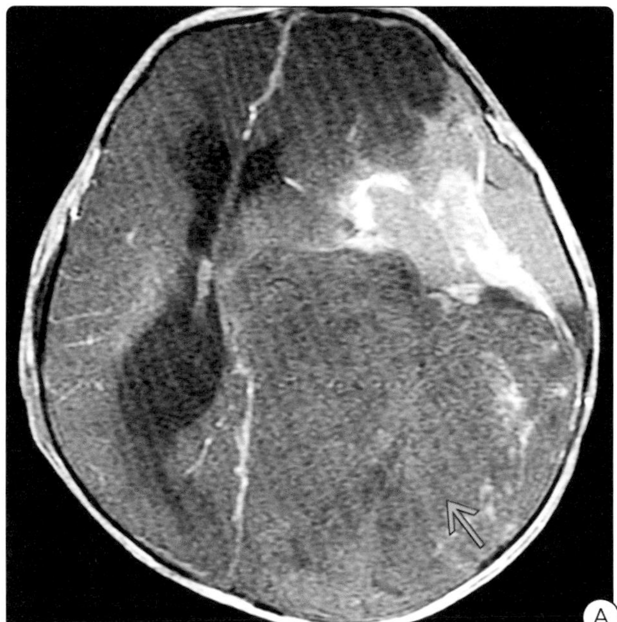

***(19-9A)** Axial T1 C+ in a newborn with an infant-type hemispheric glioma shows a very large left hemispheric mass → that is predominantly nonenhancing.*

***(19-9B)** Coronal T2 MR in the same patient shows a heterogeneous mass with areas of decreased signal →, likely representing hemorrhage.*

## Pathology

Typical histology is that of a glioblastoma-like malignant tumor with vascular proliferation, necrosis, and increased mitotic activity. Some demonstrate a primitive, undifferentiated morphology. This is a WHO grade 4 tumor.

Molecular testing demonstrates no alterations in H3 or IDH. Three molecular subtypes include pHGG RTK1, pHGG RTK2, and pHGG *MYCN*.

## Clinical Issues

Most occur in the setting of prior radiation therapy or tumor predisposition syndromes. pHGGs are aggressive malignant tumors with a median overall survival of 17 months.

## Imaging

The majority (> 85% of cases) are in the supratentorial brain with a minority located in the cerebellum/brainstem.

CT typically shows a iso- or hyperdense mass lesion with occasional intratumoral hemorrhage.

MR shows "glioblastoma-like" imaging features **(19-8)**. Most tumors have some degree of diffusion restriction. Most tumors avidly enhance and many have areas of central necrosis. Leptomeningeal metastatic disease should be carefully evaluated for.

## Differential Diagnosis

Primary differential considerations include other high-grade tumors of the hemispheres, including **other high-grade gliomas, embryonal tumors (ETMR and ATRT), as well as low-grade astrocytic and glioneuronal tumors**. Embryonal tumors mostly occur in very young patients. Low-grade astrocytic and glioneuronal tumors have a relatively low cellularity and mostly show ADC equal to or brighter than adjacent brain parenchyma.

# Infant-Type Hemispheric Glioma

## Terminology

Infant-type hemispheric glioma is a high-grade astrocytoma located in the cerebral hemispheres arising in early childhood.

## Pathology

These tumors are often quite large at diagnosis. On histology, the tumors are typically cellular, often involve the leptomeninges, and tumor margins are usually sharp. There are four molecular subtypes: 1) *NTRK*-altered, 2) *ROS1*-altered, 3) *ALK*-altered, and 4) *MET*-altered. This tumor does not currently have a WHO grade.

## Clinical Issues

Occurs in early childhood, mostly within the first year of life. Infants with this tumor usually present with nonspecific symptoms, such as lethargy, agitation, and macrocephaly. There are no known predisposing factors. Small clinical studies suggest this tumor has a more favorable prognosis compared to typical high-grade gliomas. Prognosis varies between the molecular subgroups with the suggestion that *ALK*-altered is better than *NTRK*-altered is better than *ROS1*-altered.

## Imaging

Case reports of this newly categorized tumor show large hemispheric tumors to be the most typical appearance **(19-9)**. Solid components often have a cellular appearance on conventional and diffusion-weighted imaging.

## Differential Diagnosis

Primary differential considerations include **embryonal tumors (especially ETMR and ATRT)** and **desmoplastic infantile astrocytoma/ganglioglioma**.

*Selected References: The complete reference list is available on the eBooks+ version included with purchase.*

# Circumscribed Astrocytic Gliomas

*In the 2021 5th edition WHO, circumscribed astrocytic gliomas are a separate group within gliomas, glioneuronal and neuronal tumors.*



## Circumscribed Astrocytomas

Six neoplasms comprise the group of circumscribed astrocytic gliomas: Pilocytic astrocytoma (PA), high-grade astrocytoma with piloid features (a newly recognized neoplasm in the 5th edition WHO), pleomorphic xanthoastrocytoma (PXA), subependymal giant cell astrocytoma (SEGA), chordoid glioma (CG), and astroblastoma (AB), *MN1*-altered. For purposes of discussion, we also include an uncommon variant of PA—pilomyxoid astrocytoma (PMA)—and discuss it separately in this group of circumscribed astrocytic gliomas.

Only two of these circumscribed astrocytomas, **PA** and **SEGA**, are designated as CNS WHO grade 1 neoplasms. WHO grade 1 tumors have low proliferative potential, can often be cured with surgical resection alone, and do not display an inherent tendency to malignant progression. Remote metastases are very rare, and, in the uncommon instances when they occur, the metastases generally maintain their bland (i.e., grade 1) histologic features.

### Pilocytic Astrocytoma

The most common of the circumscribed astrocytomas is pilocytic astrocytoma (PA). A rare PA subvariant—pilomyxoid astrocytoma (PMA)—is considered separately.

#### Terminology

PA is a well-circumscribed, typically slow-growing astrocytic neoplasm associated with MAPK pathway gene alterations.

#### Etiology

MAPK pathway mutations are basically universal. Approximately 60% of PAs have *BRAF* duplications or rearrangements, especially p. V600E mutations and *KIAA1549::BRAF* fusions.

Specific alterations in PAs vary with anatomic location. *KIAA1549::BRAF* fusion is more common in cerebellar PAs, whereas *BRAF* p.V600E mutations are common in supratentorial tumors. Less common mutations include *FGFR1* alterations and *NF1* mutations, both found mainly in midline tumors. Approximately 15% of neurofibromatosis type 1 (NF1) patients develop PAs, most commonly in the optic nerves/tracts ("optic pathway gliomas").

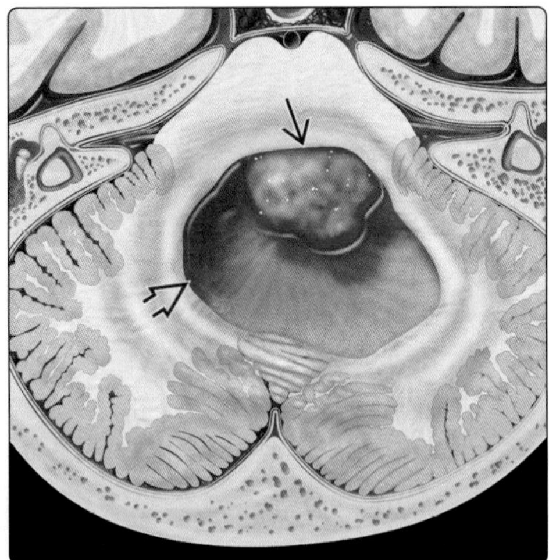

(20-1) Graphic shows typical cerebellar pilocytic astrocytoma with a vascular-appearing tumor nodule ⇨, large nonneoplastic cyst ⇨.

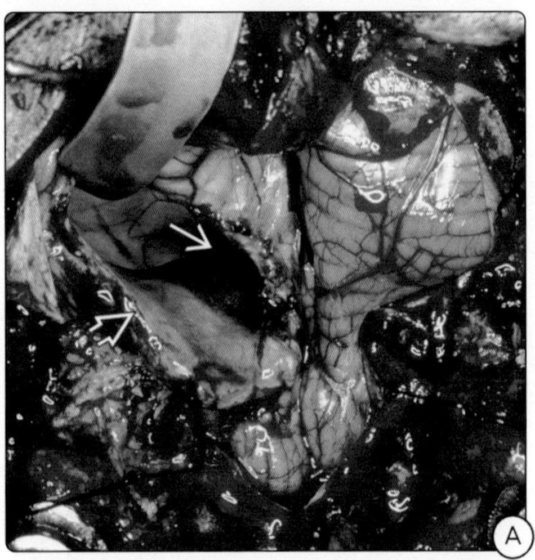

(20-2A) Intraoperative photograph of cerebellar pilocytic astrocytoma shows cyst ➡ with solid, reddish tumor nodule ➡ visible.

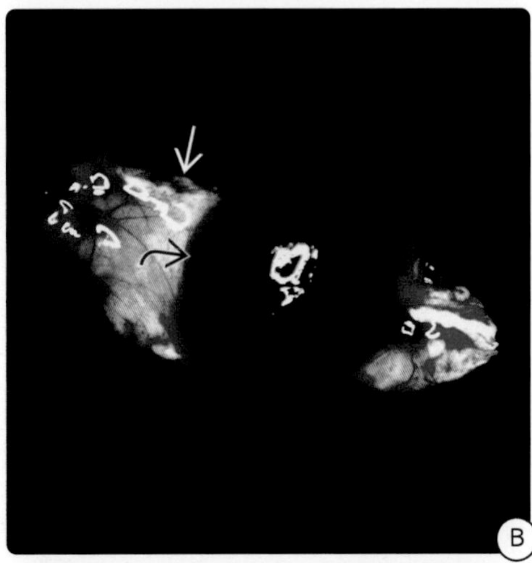

(20-2B) Resection shows a well-delineated vascular nodule ⇨ attached to the cyst wall ➡. Pilocytic astrocytoma, CNS WHO grade 1.

## Pathology

**Location.** PAs may arise anywhere in the neuraxis but have a distinct predilection for certain sites. The cerebellum is the most common location, accounting for nearly 60% of all PAs **(20-1)**.

The second most common site is in and around the optic nerve/chiasm and hypothalamus/third ventricle, which together account for between 1/4 and 1/3 of all PAs. The third most common location is the pons and medulla. PAs also occasionally occur in the tectum, where they may cause aqueductal stenosis.

The cerebral hemispheres are a reported but uncommon location of PA. When they occur outside the posterior fossa, optic pathway, or suprasellar region, PAs tend to be cortically based cysts with a tumor nodule.

**Gross Pathology.** PAs are typically well-circumscribed, grayish tumors with both firm and softer mucoid areas. Focal calcification may be present.

Sometimes PAs form a mural nodule in association with a cyst **(20-1)**. The walls of most PA-associated cysts usually consist of compressed but otherwise normal brain parenchyma with the neoplastic element confined to the mural tumor nodule **(20-2)**. Cyst contents are typically a protein-rich xanthochromic fluid.

Cystic PAs are preferentially located in the cerebellum and (less commonly) the cerebral hemispheres. A solid, more infiltrative appearance is common in the optic pathways and hypothalamus. Frank invasion of surrounding brain is typically absent or limited to a narrow border immediately adjacent to the neoplasm.

**Microscopic Features.** The **classic PA** is composed of a biphasic pattern of two distinct astrocyte populations. The dominant type is composed of compact, hair-like ("pilocytic") bipolar cells with Rosenthal fibers [electron-dense glial fibrillary acidic protein (GFAP)-positive cytoplasmic inclusions]. Intermixed are loosely textured, hypocellular, GFAP-negative areas that contain multipolar cells with microcysts. Telangiectatic or glomeruloid vascular proliferation is common. Myxoid background with microcystic change is common. Ki-67/MIB-1 is typically < 5%, indicating low proliferative potential.

**Staging, Grading, and Classification.** PA is a CNS WHO grade 1 tumor. PAs generally maintain their CNS WHO grade 1 status over many years. Tumor dissemination occasionally occurs but is rare.

PAs with anaplastic features are rare and most commonly occur in adults. These tumors are now considered a distinct type, "high-grade astrocytoma with piloid features" (discussed later in this chapter).

## Clinical Issues

**Epidemiology.** PA accounts for 5-10% of all gliomas and is the most common primary brain tumor in children. PAs represent nearly 25% of all CNS neoplasms and 85% of posterior fossa astrocytomas in this age group. PAs in the cerebral hemisphere are rare and tend to affect an older group of patients than the cerebellar or optic pathway PAs.

**Demographics.** More than 80% of PAs occur in patients under 20 years old. The peak incidence is in "middle-aged" children between the ages of 5-15 years. There is no sex predilection.

**Presentation.** Symptoms vary with location. Cerebellar PAs often present with headache, morning nausea, and vomiting, as intraventricular obstructive hydrocephalus is common. Ataxia, visual loss, and cranial nerve palsies also occur.

Optic pathway PAs typically present with visual loss. An uncommon presentation of a PA involving the hypothalamus is diencephalic syndrome, a rare but potentially lethal cause of failure to thrive despite adequate caloric intake.

Pontine and medullary PAs are uncommon but typically present with multiple cranial nerve palsies.

**Natural History.** PAs generally grow slowly. Ten-year survival exceeds 90%, even with partially resected tumors. Almost 1/2 of residual tumors show spontaneous regression or arrested long-term growth.

PAs generally maintain their CNS WHO grade 1 status over decades **(20-9)**. Anaplastic features rarely develop and predominately occur in adults. These tumors must be distinguished from high-grade astrocytoma with piloid features, a distinct type of neoplasm with a unique DNA methylation profile (discussed later in this chapter).

### PILOCYTIC ASTROCYTOMAS

**Location**
- 60% in cerebellum
- 25-30% optic nerve/chiasm/hypothalamus
- Less common: Pons, medulla, cerebral hemispheres

**Gross Pathology**
- Cyst + mural nodule (cerebellum, hemispheres)
- Solid, infiltrative (optic nerve/chiasm/hypothalamus)

**Histopathology**
- Biphasic
  - Compact with Rosenthal fibers; loose, microcystic areas
  - CNS WHO grade 1 (stable over years)

**Clinical Features**
- 80% < 20 years of age
- Symptoms vary with location
- Grow slowly
  - 10-year survival > 90%
  - Usually maintain grade 1 status over decades
  - Anaplasia rare

## Imaging

Similar to clinical presentation, imaging findings vary with PA location. The most common appearance of a posterior fossa PA is a well-delineated cerebellar cyst with a mural nodule.

PAs in and around the optic nerve, chiasm, third ventricle, and tectum tend to be solid, infiltrating, and less well marginated **(20-4)**. When they occur in these locations, PAs tend to expand the affected structures, which maintain their underlying anatomic configuration.

PAs in the tectum expand the collicular plate and may cause aqueductal obstruction. The rare hemispheric PA typically presents as a cortically based lesion, usually a cyst with a mural nodule **(20-7)**.

**CT Findings.** NECT scans show a mixed cystic/solid or solid lesion with focal mass effect and little, if any, adjacent edema. Calcification occurs in 10-20% of cases. Hemorrhage is uncommon; if present, the tumor may be a PMA rather than PA.

Most PAs enhance on both CT and MR scans. The most common pattern, seen in approximately 1/2 of all cases, is a nonenhancing cyst with a strongly enhancing mural nodule. A solid enhancing mass with central necrosis is seen

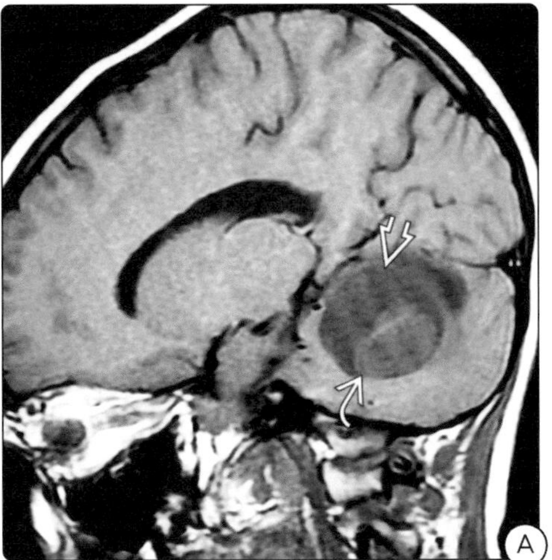


***(20-3A)** Sagittal T1 MR shows hypointense cystic cerebellar mass ➡ with a well-defined nodule ➡ within the cyst.*

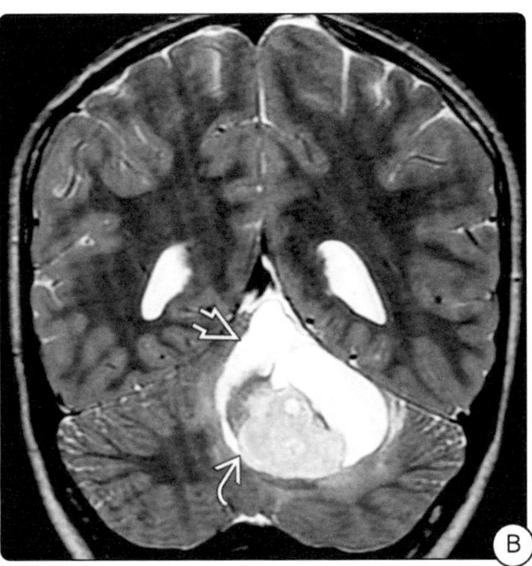


***(20-3B)** Coronal T2 MR shows the hyperintense cyst ➡ with a solid mixed signal intensity nodule ➡.*

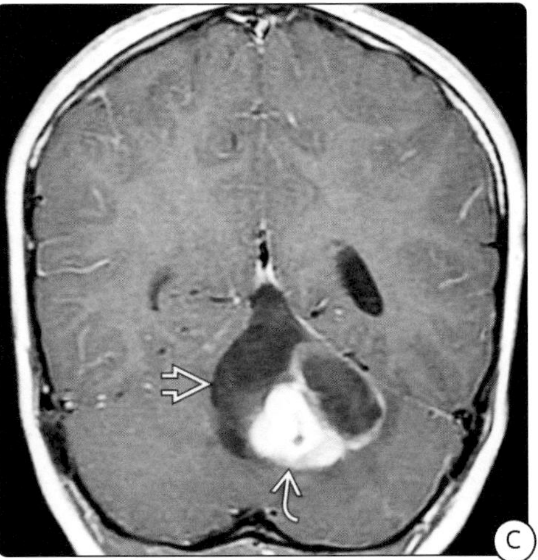


***(20-3C)** T1 C+ shows nonenhancing cyst wall ➡, enhancing cyst nodule ➡. Pilocytic astrocytoma, CNS WHO grade 1, BRAF V600E mutation.*

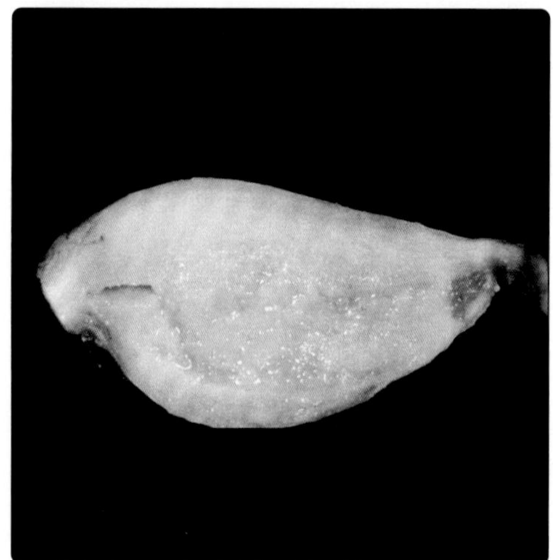

*(20-4) Gross pathology of optic nerve "glioma" shows fusiform enlargement of the optic nerve.*

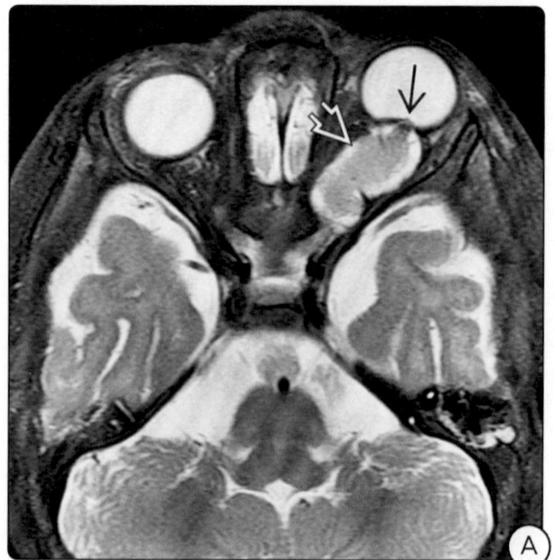


*(20-5A) T2 MR in an infant with NF1 shows a thickened, tortuous left optic nerve ➡ with intraocular protrusion of the optic nerve head ➡.*

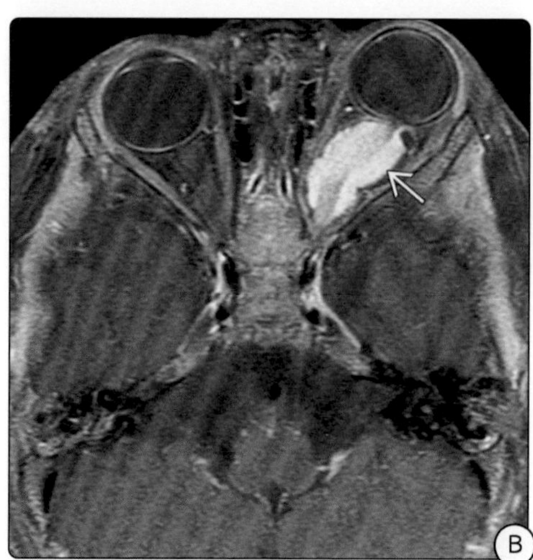


*(20-5B) T1 C+ FS MR shows the left optic nerve is enlarged, infiltrated with enhancing tumor ➡. This is NF1-associated pilocytic astrocytoma.*

in 40%, and 10% show solid homogeneous enhancement. If delayed scans are obtained, a contrast-fluid level may accumulate within the cyst.

**MR Findings.** Cystic PAs are usually well delineated and appear slightly hyperintense to CSF on both T1- and T2WI **(20-6A)**. They do not suppress completely on FLAIR. The mural nodule is iso-/hypointense on T1WI and iso-/hyperintense on T2WI. Solid PAs appear iso- or hypointense to parenchyma on T1WI and hyperintense on T2/FLAIR. Posterior extension along the optic radiations is not uncommon with a suprasellar PA and does not denote malignancy.

PAs contain numerous capillaries with fenestrations and open endothelial tight junctions that permit the escape of large macromolecules across the blood-brain barrier. They may therefore show striking enhancement following contrast administration. Intense but heterogeneous enhancement of the nodule in a cystic PA is typical **(20-3)** **(20-6B)**. Enhancement of the cyst wall itself varies from none to moderate **(20-9)**. A variant pattern is a solid mass with central necrosis and a thick peripherally enhancing "rind" of tumor.

PAs in the optic nerve **(20-4)**, optic chiasm, and hypothalamus/third ventricle show quite variable enhancement (from none to striking) **(20-5)**, whereas hemispheric PAs generally present with a cyst + an enhancing mural nodule **(20-7)**.

MRS in PAs often shows elevated Cho, low NAA, and a lactate peak **(20-8)**. pMR shows low to moderate rCBV.

### IMAGING OF PILOCYTIC ASTROCYTOMA

**Location Dependent**
- Cyst + enhancing nodule
  - Cerebellum (common)
  - Cerebral hemisphere (uncommon)
- Solid, infiltrating
  - Optic nerve/chiasm
  - Hypothalamus/third ventricle
  - Tectum

**CT**
- Cystic/solid or solid mass
- $Ca^{++}$ in 10-20% (hemorrhage rare)

**MR**
- T1/T2 hyperintense
- No suppression on FLAIR
- Variable enhancement
  - None to striking
  - Cyst enhances intensely; wall is variable

## Differential Diagnosis

The differential diagnosis of PA depends on location and imaging appearance. A posterior fossa PA in a child with the classic cyst + tumor nodule appearance is relatively pathognomonic. A cerebellar **hemangioblastoma** (HGBL) can resemble PA, but HGBLs are tumors of middle-aged adults rather than children.

Solid PAs can resemble **medulloblastoma**, especially when they are mostly solid midline tumors. Medulloblastomas typically restrict on DWI, whereas PAs do not. **Ependymoma** is a plastic-appearing tumor that extrudes out the foramen of Magendie and lateral recesses.

The major differential diagnosis of hypothalamic PAs is an **IDH-mutant astrocytoma**. The hypothalamus is a relatively uncommon site for these tumors, which are generally adult-type neoplasms.

The differential diagnosis of a hemispheric PA with a nodule + cyst appearance is **ganglioglioma**. Gangliogliomas are generally cortically based and often calcify. **Pleomorphic xanthoastrocytomas** (PXA) can present with a solid "nodule + cyst" but are tumors of young adults, not children. PXAs often incite meningeal reaction (dural tail sign).

**Pilomyxoid astrocytoma** (PMA) is a subtype/variant of PA. PMAs tend to occur in younger children or infants and are generally larger and more bulky than PAs. Hemorrhage is rare in PA but relatively common in PMA.

Visual pathway PAs must be distinguished from **demyelinating disease** and postviral inflammation.

## Pilomyxoid Astrocytoma

In the 5th edition WHO, pilomyxoid astrocytoma (PMA) is considered a rare subtype of pilocytic astrocytoma (PA). PMAs share many features with classic PA but differ in some important clinicopathologic respects. PMAs are generally noninfiltrative and have a myxoid background with monomorphic piloid cells and angiocentric arrangement. MAPK pathway alterations are common, most often *BRAF* mutations and fusions.

PMAs often present in infancy but have been reported in adults. They are generally more clinically aggressive than PAs with a higher rate of recurrence and propensity for CSF dissemination.

Although PMAs may occur anywhere along the neuraxis, they have a strong geographic predilection for the suprasellar region **(20-10)**. Almost 60-75% center in the hypothalamus/optic chiasm, often extending into both

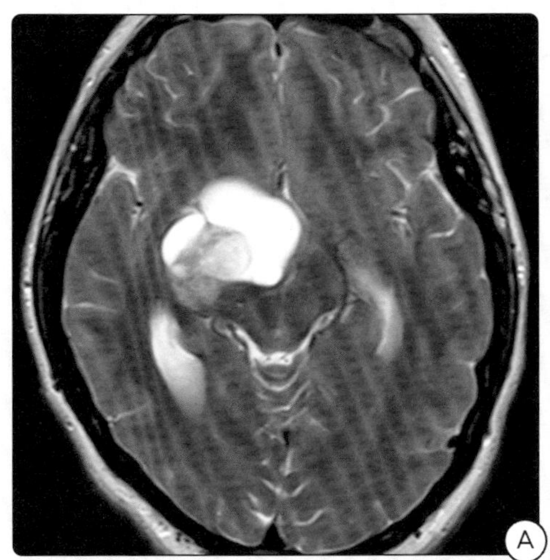

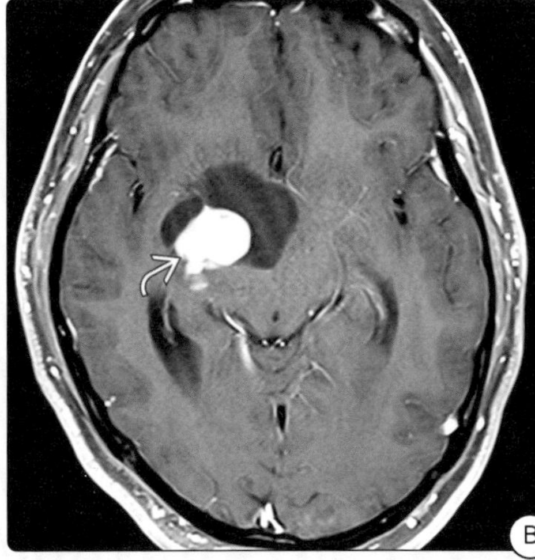

***(20-6A)** T2 MR in a 19-yo woman shows a mixed cystic-solid mass in the right basal ganglia and hypothalamus. **(20-6B)** T1 C+ FS MR shows the solid nodule enhances intensely and quite uniformly ➡. The cyst wall does not enhance. Pathology with next-generation sequencing (NGS) revealed pilocytic astrocytoma, CNS WHO grade 1, with BRAF R506 mutation, methylation subclass midline pilocytic astrocytoma.*

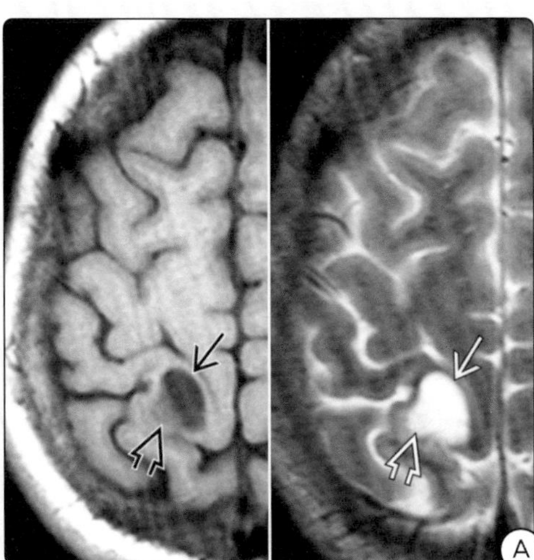

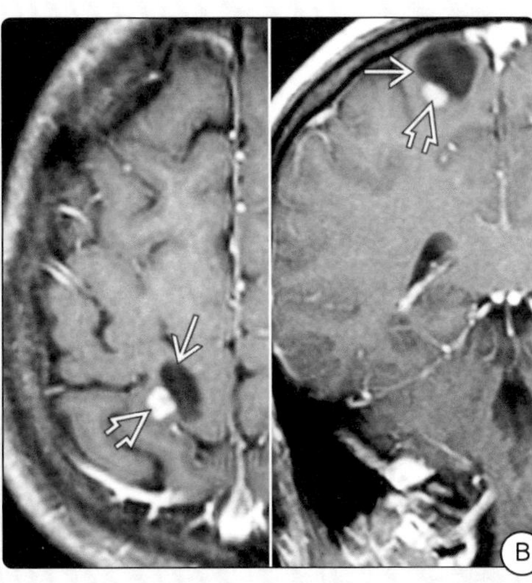

***(20-7A)** (L) T1 MR in a 19-yo man with NF1 shows a cystic lesion in the right parietal lobe ➡ with a small, less hypointense solid component ➡. (R) T2 MR shows that the cyst ➡ and nodule ➡ are both hyperintense. **(20-7B)** (L) Sagittal, (R) coronal T1 C+ MR scans show the solid nodule enhances intensely ➡ while cyst wall does not ➡. Surgery disclosed pilocytic astrocytoma, WHO grade 1. Most common site is the optic chiasm/nerves, especially in NF1.*

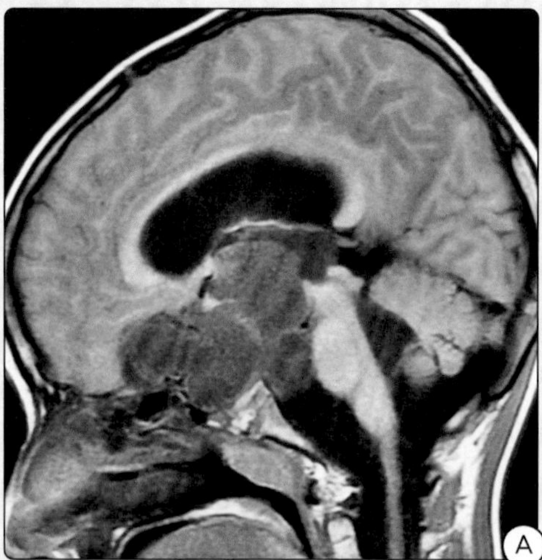


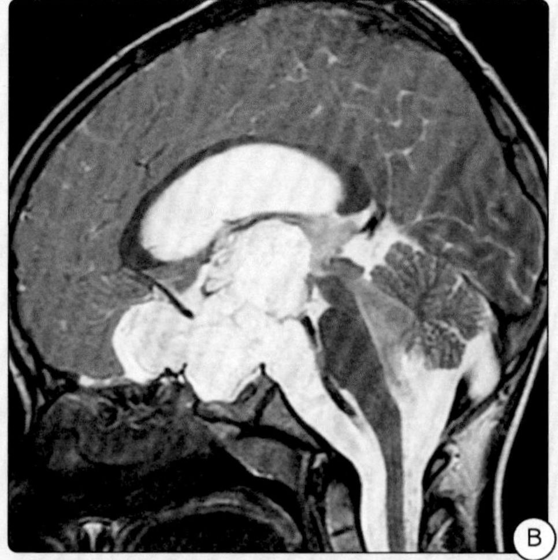


***(20-8A)*** *A 7-yo boy had 2 months of morning vomiting, headache, visual difficulties. NECT showed a large, lobulated suprasellar mass. Sagittal T1 MR shows a hypointense hypothalamic mass that widens and largely fills the sella and extends dorsally in front of the pons. Moderate obstructive hydrocephalus is present.* ***(20-8B)*** *Sagittal T2 MR in the same patient shows that the mass is extremely hyperintense.*

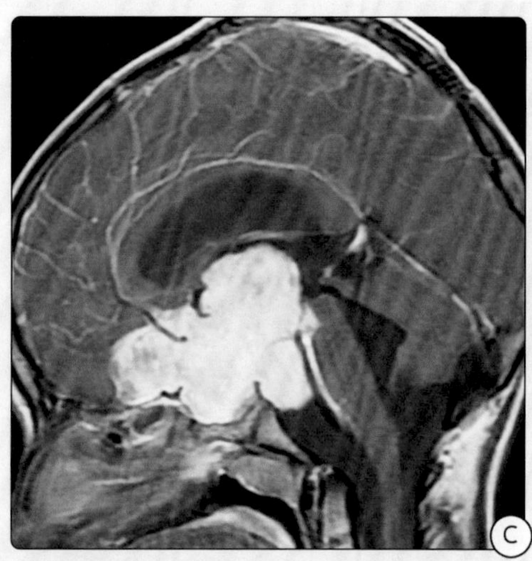


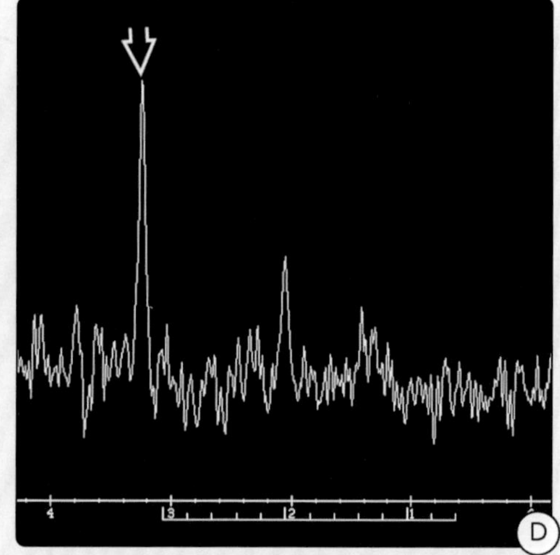


***(20-8C)*** *Sagittal T1 C+ MR shows that the mass enhances intensely and slightly heterogeneously.* ***(20-8D)*** *MRS in the same patient with TR 1500 TE 288 shows a "pseudomalignant" spectrum with a markedly elevated choline peak, a common finding in pilocytic astrocytoma. Imaging diagnosis was chiasmatic-hypothalamic pilocytic astrocytoma. Biopsy confirmed a pilocytic astrocytoma, WHO grade 1.*

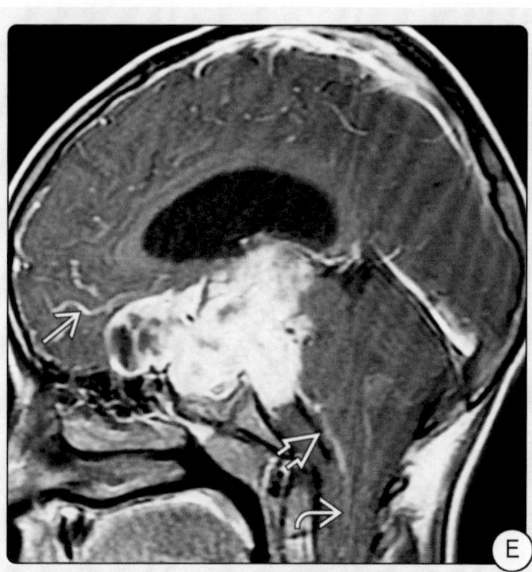


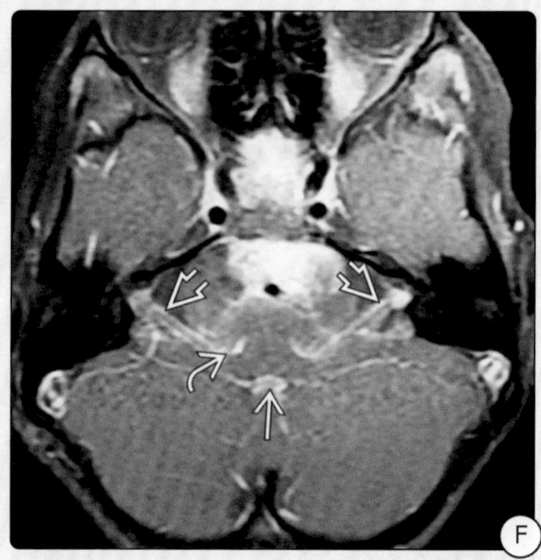


***(20-8E)*** *Sagittal T1 C+ MR obtained 2 months later shows diffuse pial enhancement with tumor along the interhemispheric fissure, coating the brainstem and cervical cord.* ***(20-8F)*** *Axial T1 C+ FS MR shows metastatic tumor in the 4th ventricle, coating the medulla as well as the 7th and 8th cranial nerves. Despite CSF dissemination, the patient is alive 4 years later.*

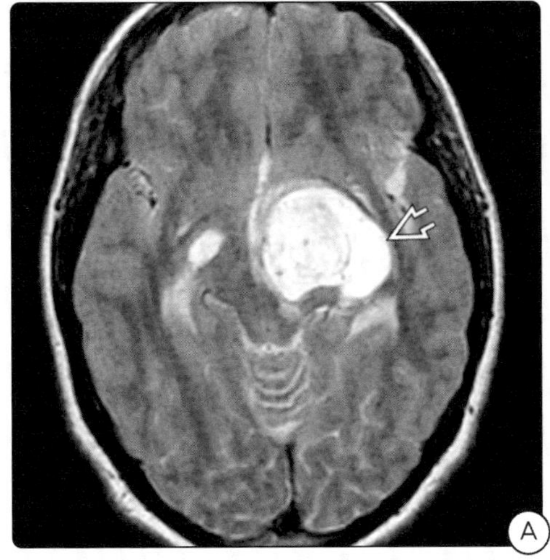

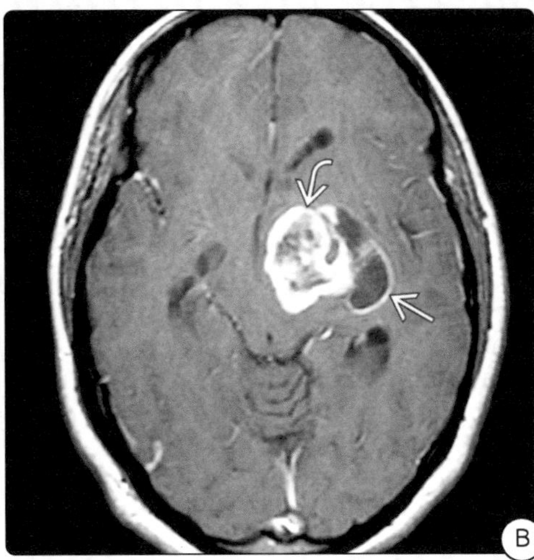

***(20-9A)** T2 MR in a 14-yo girl shows a relatively well-demarcated, heterogeneously hyperintense mass ➡ in the left basal ganglia and hypothalamus. **(20-9B)** T1 C+ FS MR in the same patient shows the mass enhances heterogeneously with mixed solid ➡ and cystic components ➡. The mass was subtotally resected. Pathology disclosed pilocytic astrocytoma.*

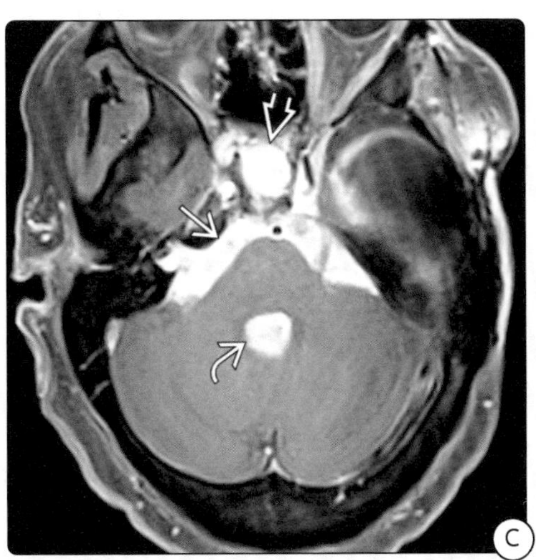

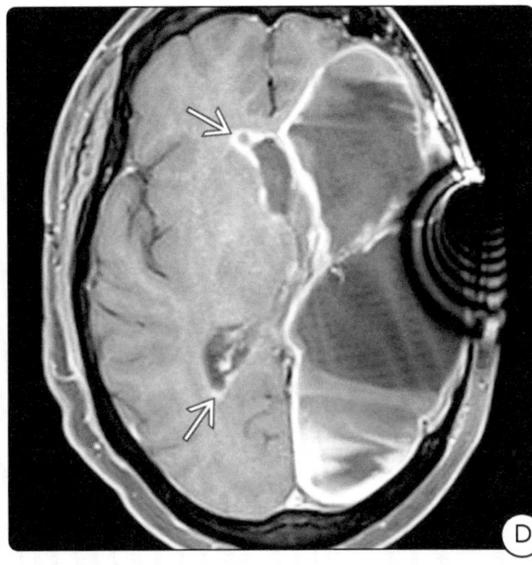

***(20-9C)** The patient experienced multiple recurrences over 20 years before developing diffuse CSF metastases. T1 C+ FS MR through the posterior fossa shows the 4th ventricle ➡ as well as prepontine, suprasellar ➡, and cerebellopontine angle cisterns ➡ are completely filled with enhancing tumor. **(20-9D)** More cephalad T1 C+ FS MR shows ependymal tumor spread around the lateral ventricles ➡.*

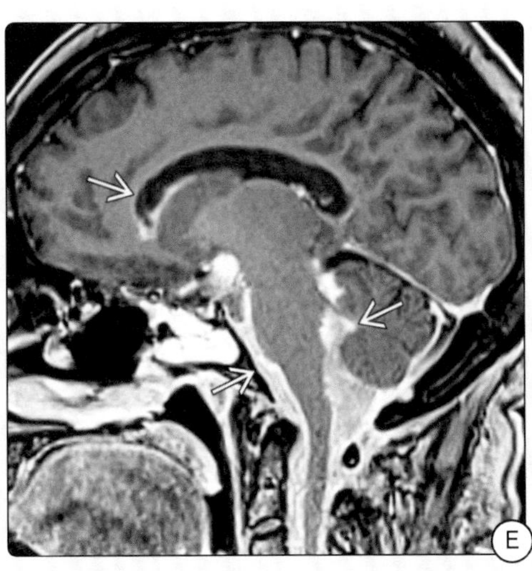

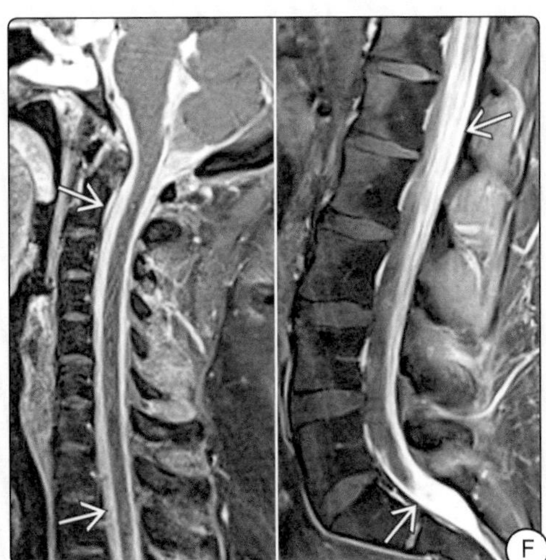

***(20-9E)** Sagittal T1 C+ SPGR shows tumor filling all the CSF spaces ➡. **(20-9F)** Sagittal T1 C+ MR through the cervical (L) and lumbar (R) spine shows intensely enhancing tumor almost completely filling CSF spaces ➡. Rebiopsy showed pilocytic astrocytoma, CNS WHO grade 1 without evidence for histologic anaplasia.*

temporal lobes. PMAs are generally large, bulky, but relatively well-circumscribed masses **(20-11)**. A glistening appearance caused by the myxoid component is common. Hemorrhage and necrosis are more common than with PA.

PMAs look quite different from classic PAs on imaging studies. PMAs are more often solid and are primarily hypodense on NECT. Intratumoral hemorrhage is seen in nearly 1/2 of all cases; calcification is rare.

PMAs are iso- to hypointense on T1WI, and nearly all are hyperintense on T2, reflecting the high proportion of myxoid matrix in these tumors. Peritumoral edema is minimal or absent. Approximately 20% of PMAs demonstrate evidence of intratumoral hemorrhage on T2* (GRE, SWI), which is very rare in PAs.

PMAs demonstrate strong, generally homogeneous enhancement after contrast administration. Occasionally, large lesions may exhibit heterogeneous enhancement **(20-12)**. High ADC values are common, most likely because of the mucinous component. pMR shows higher rCBV compared to PAs.

CSF dissemination is common with PMA, so the entire neuraxis should be imaged prior to surgical intervention.

## High-Grade Astrocytoma With Piloid Features

High-grade astrocytoma with piloid features (HGAP) is a rare astrocytoma with a distinct DNA methylation profile. High-grade piloid &/or glioblastoma-like histologic features are common. In the past, these uncommon neoplasms were called "anaplastic astrocytoma with piloid features" or "anaplastic pilocytic astrocytoma." They are now recognized as a distinct tumor entity in the 5th edition WHO and (perhaps inexplicably) included in the group of circumscribed astrocytomas.

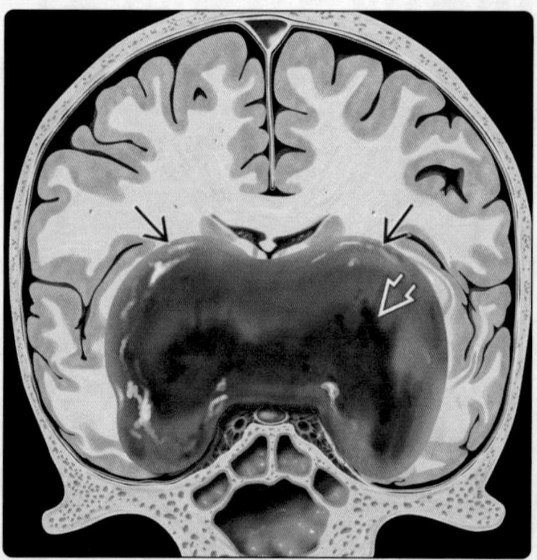

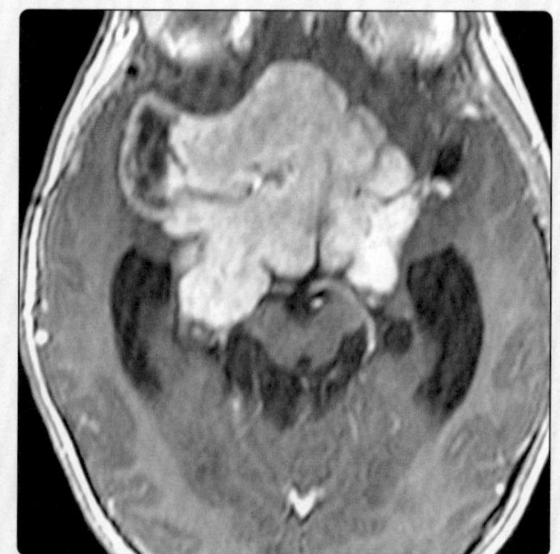

***(20-10)** Pilomyxoid astrocytoma (PMA) has a bulky, H-shaped, hypothalamic/chiasmatic region mass extending to the temporal lobes. Shiny myxoid matrix ➲ and hemorrhage ➲ are seen. **(20-11)** Axial contrast-enhanced MR shows the intensely enhancing H-shaped configuration of a hypothalamic PMA. (Courtesy M. Thurnher, MD.)*

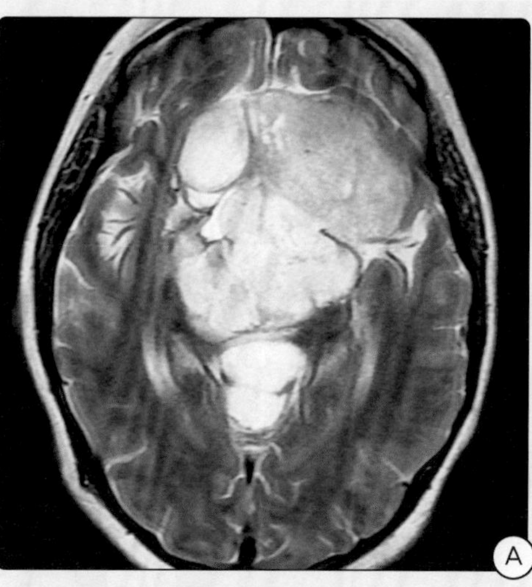


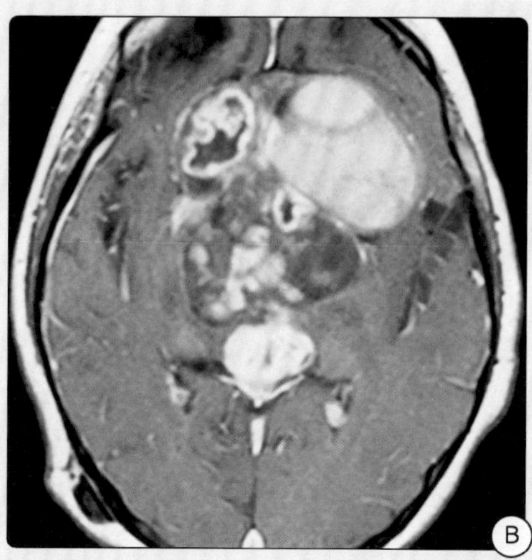


***(20-12A)** T2 MR in a 10-yo girl with recurrent suprasellar mass, weight loss, nausea, and vomiting shows an enormous, heterogeneously hyperintense, suprasellar mass. Original diagnosis at age 2 was pilocytic astrocytoma. **(20-12B)** T1 C+ MR shows heterogeneous enhancement with areas of solid ring enhancement intermixed with nonenhancing foci. Repeat biopsy disclosed PMA in a diffusely myxoid background.*

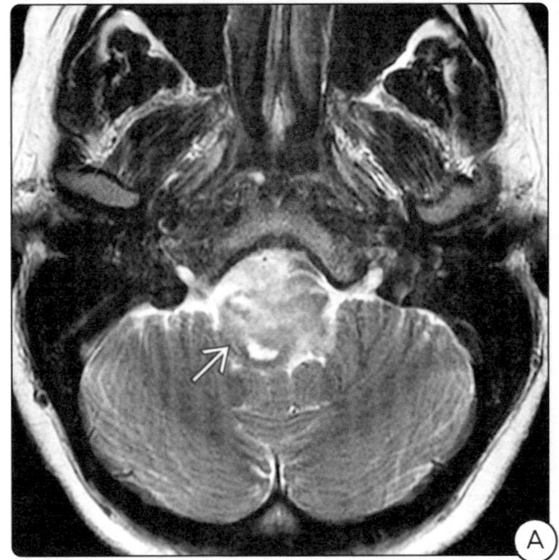

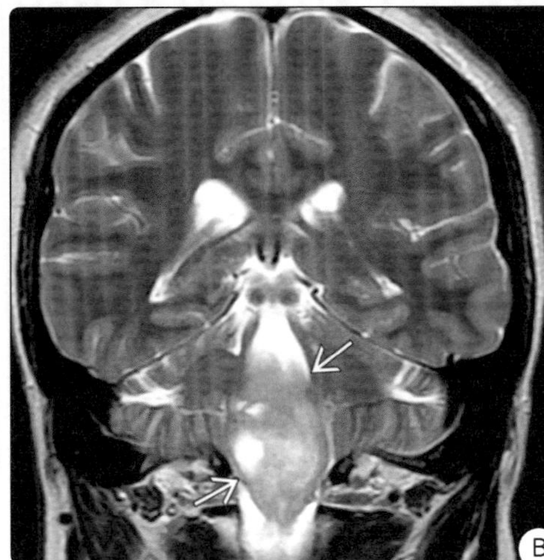

***(20-13A)** Axial T2 MR in a 30-yo woman with sensory changes in her right arm and leg and Lhermitte sign shows a hyperintense mass ➡ infiltrating and expanding the medulla. **(20-13B)** Coronal T2 MR shows that the extensive, heterogeneously hyperintense mass ➡ expands the pons and medulla.*

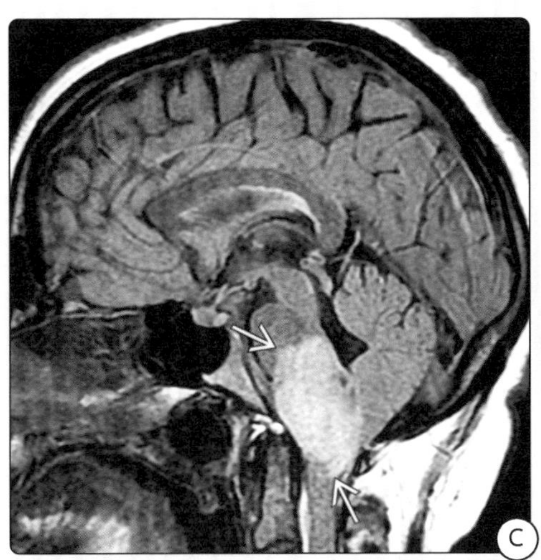

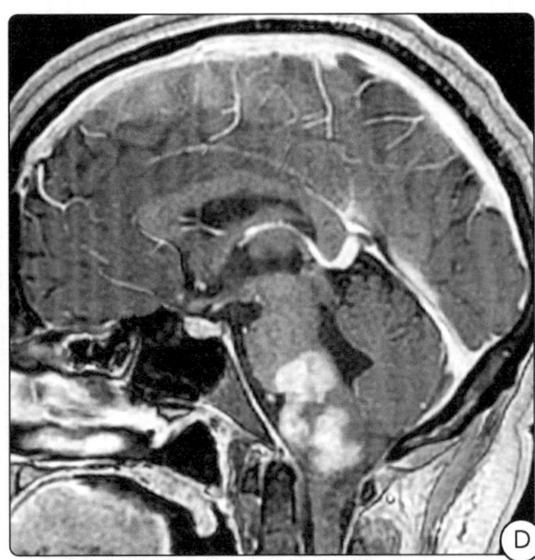

***(20-13C)** Sagittal FLAIR MR shows that the mass ➡ is hyperintense and extends from the midpons into the upper cervical spinal cord. **(20-13D)** T1 C+ FS MR shows strong but patchy enhancement in the mass.*

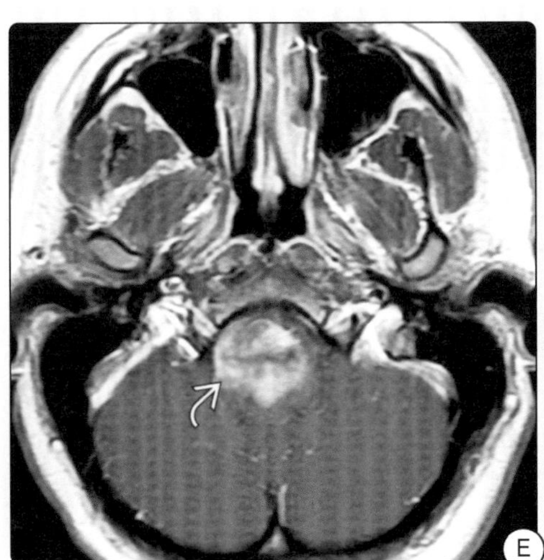

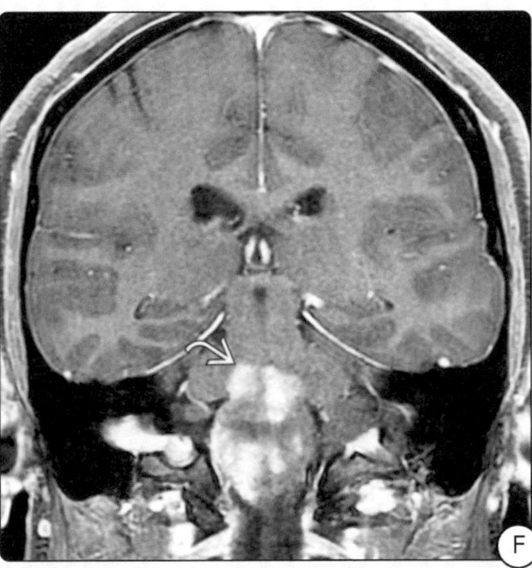

***(20-13E)** Axial T1 C+ MR shows that the mass ➡ expands and infiltrates the medulla and enhances strongly but quite heterogeneously. **(20-13F)** Coronal T1 C+ FS MR shows the patchy enhancement of the mass ➡. Microscopic examination disclosed an anaplastic-appearing pilocytic astrocytoma. Subsequent DNA methylation profile was diagnostic of high-grade astrocytoma with piloid features, CNS WHO grade 3.*

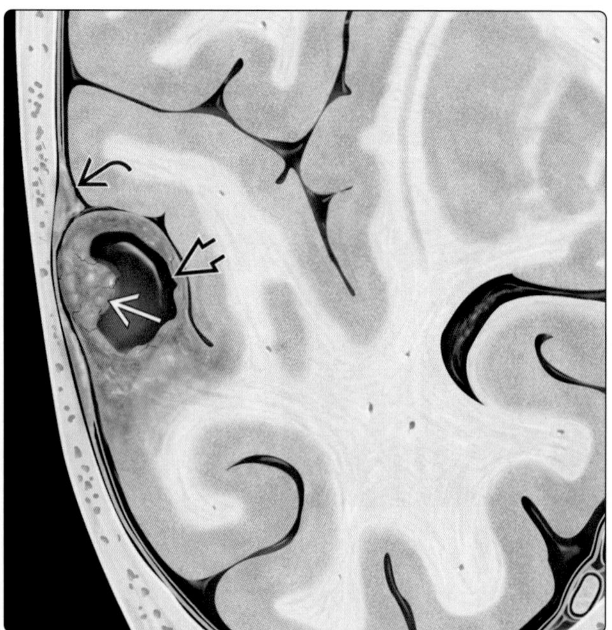

***(20-14)** Coronal graphic depicts pleomorphic xanthoastrocytoma (PXA) with a cyst ➡, a nodule abutting pial surface ➡, and reactive thickening of the adjacent dura-arachnoid ➡.*

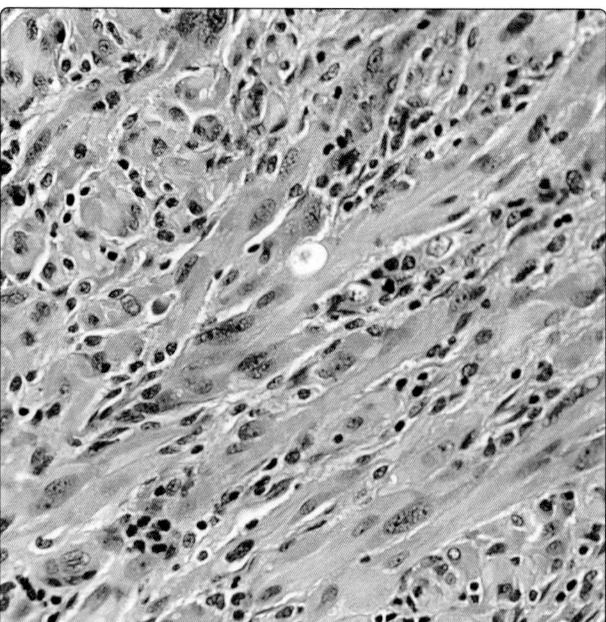

***(20-15)** Classic histologic features of PXA include somewhat fascicular architecture and cells that appear pleomorphic but not "monstrous." The bulk of the lesion is compact and noninfiltrating. (Courtesy P. Burger, MD.)*

In most cases, HGAP occurs as a de novo neoplasm rather than developing from a preexisting lower grade astrocytoma. HGAPs have numerous chromosomal alterations. MAPK pathway activating mutations are common as are *CDKN2A* &/or *CDKN2B* inactivations.

HGAPs are tumors of adults and are vanishingly rare in children. The median age of reported patients is 40 years. The five-year overall survival rate is ~ 50%.

Histopathology shows pleomorphic astrocytic characteristics, often resembling glioblastoma or pleomorphic xanthoastrocytoma. Thin, hair-like "piloid" features may be present. Currently, DNA methylation profiling is the only method for establishing the definitive diagnosis of HGAP.

While a definitive WHO grade for HGAPs has not been assigned, the 5th edition WHO suggests that the clinical behavior roughly corresponds to that of a CNS WHO grade 3 neoplasm.

Imaging shows an infiltrating, poorly marginated neoplasm that is T2/FLAIR hyperintense and generally exhibits strong but heterogeneous enhancement **(20-13)**.

The main differential diagnosis of HGAP is **glioblastoma, IDH-wildtype**. Many adult posterior fossa parenchymal tumors originally diagnosed as "cerebellar glioblastoma" are likely HGAPs. Midline or juxta-midline HGAPs must also be distinguished from **H3 K27-altered diffuse midline glioma.**

## Pleomorphic Xanthoastrocytoma

### Terminology

Pleomorphic xanthoastrocytoma (PXA) is a rare astrocytic glioma that accounts for < 1% of primary CNS tumors. PXAs are characterized by large pleomorphic, frequently multinucleated cells and xanthomatous change.

### Pathology

**Location.** Over 95% of PXAs are supratentorial hemispheric masses. Most are superficial cortically based, seizure-associated neoplasms. The temporal lobe is the most common site (40-50%), and involvement of the adjacent leptomeninges is common. Other frequent locations include the frontal (33%) and parietal (20%) lobes. Cerebellar and spinal cord PXAs have been reported but are very rare.

**Size and Number.** PXAs are usually solitary lesions. Most are small; lesions > 3 cm are uncommon.

**Gross Pathology.** The most common gross appearance is that of a relatively discrete, partially cystic, superficial cortical, yellowish mass with a mural nodule that abuts or is attached to the leptomeninges **(20-14)**. Dural invasion is rare. The deep tumor margins may be indistinct with focal parenchymal infiltration into the adjacent subcortical white matter.

**Microscopic Features.** The most striking features of PXA are its highly pleomorphic histology, dense reticulin network, compact architecture, and lipidization of tumor cells. Fibrillary and giant, multinucleated, neoplastic astrocytes are intermixed with large, lipid-containing, GFAP-positive cells **(20-15)**.

**Staging, Grading, and Classification.** The majority of PXAs are CNS WHO grade 2 tumors. PXAs that display anaplastic features (aPXAs), including higher cellularity and ≥ 5 mitoses/10 HPF, are designated WHO grade 3 tumors (the term "anaplastic pleomorphic xanthoastrocytoma" is not recommended) **(20-17)**.

**Diagnostic Molecular Pathology.** Almost all PXAs have MAPK pathway alterations with 60-80% *BRAF* p.V600E mutations. Up to 95% have homozygous deletion of *CDKN2A* &/or *CDKN2B*.

## Clinical Issues

**Demographics.** PXA is a rare tumor, accounting for slightly < 1% of all astrocytomas. PXAs are generally tumors of children and young adults; mean age at diagnosis is 22 years.

**Natural History.** CNS WHO grade 2 PXAs tend to recur and disseminate in the CSF. Approximately 20% progress to higher grade tumors (CNS WHO grade 3). Resection extent is the most significant prognostic factor. Five-year survival is ~ 70% for grade 2 tumors and 50% for grade 3 lesions.

### PLEOMORPHIC XANTHOASTROCYTOMA

**Pathology**
- Rare; < 1% of astrocytomas
- IDH- and H3-wildtype
  - *BRAF* p. V600E mutations common
- CNS WHO grades 2, 3 (anaplastic PXA)
- Solid or cyst + nodule abutting leptomeninges

**Clinical Features**
- Older children, young adults (mean: 26 years)
- Common presentation: Longstanding epilepsy
- PXAs tend to recur, progress to grade 3
  - CSF dissemination common
  - 5-year survival is 70% (grade 2), 50% (grade 3)

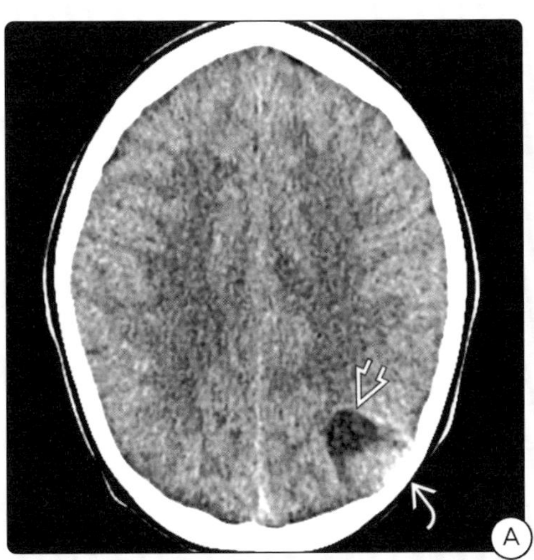


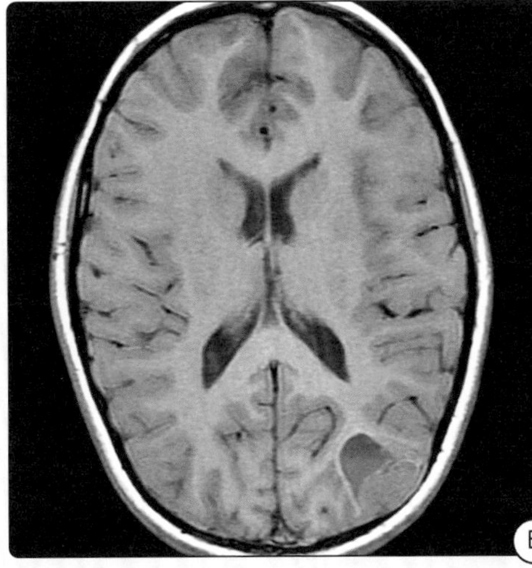


***(20-16A)** NECT in an 11-yo child with seizures shows a mixed cystic/solid mass ➔ in the left parietal lobe. Note slight thinning and remodeling of the overlying calvarium ➔, indicating that the mass is relatively slow growing. **(20-16B)** T1 MR in the same patient shows a solid nodule that is isointense with cortex abutting the calvarium. An associated cystic portion is hypointense.*

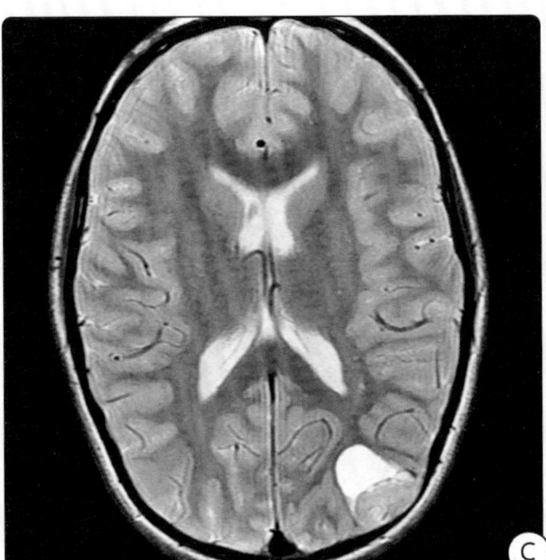


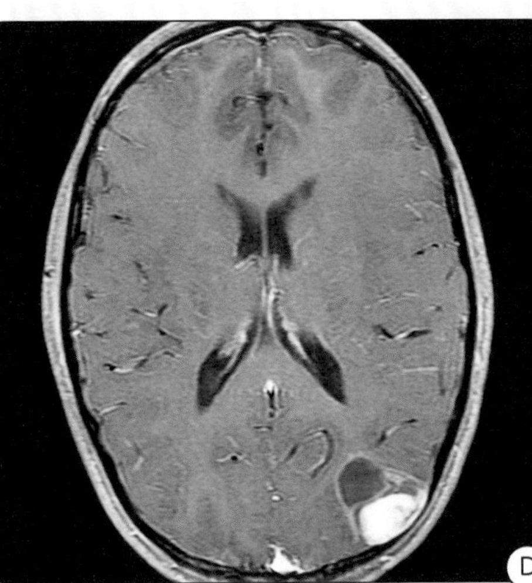


***(20-16C)** T2 MR shows that the cystic portion of the mass is hyperintense compared to CSF while the solid nodule is isointense with cortex. **(20-16D)** T1 C+ FS MR shows that the solid portion of the mass enhances intensely and quite uniformly. An enhancing rim surrounds the nonenhancing tumor-associated cyst. This is PXA, CNS WHO grade 2.*

## Imaging

**CT Findings.** NECT scans show a well-delineated, peripheral, cortically based mass that contacts the leptomeninges. Two imaging patterns are common. A "cyst + nodule" configuration is present in 70% of cases **(20-16A)**, and a predominantly solid mass with intratumoral cysts is seen in 30%. The overlying skull may be thinned and remodeled on bone CT. Calcifications are present in 40% of cases, but gross intratumoral hemorrhage is rare.

The mural nodule of a PXA shows moderate to intense enhancement on CECT.

**MR Findings.** The solid component of a PXA is heterogeneously hypo- or isointense relative to cortex on T1WI **(20-16B)**. Over 90% of the tumor nodules demonstrate heterogeneous hyperintensity on T2WI and FLAIR. If calcifications or hemorrhage is present, "blooming" on T2* can be seen. The cystic portions of PXA are usually hyperintense relative to CSF on T2WI and FLAIR sequences **(20-16C)**.

Moderate enhancement of the tumor nodule is typical following contrast administration **(20-16D)**. Over 90% of PXAs abut the pia and may incite reactive thickening of the adjacent dura. A dural tail sign was seen in 15-50% of cases in a reported series.

## Differential Diagnosis

The major differential diagnosis of PXA is **ganglioglioma**, which has a glial component that may resemble PXAs. A few **gangliogliomas with anaplasia** in the glial component have been reported, but molecular analysis reveals most of these are other neoplasms, most commonly PXA.

**Giant cell glioblastoma** shares many histopathologic features and imaging similarities with PXA but differs in molecular profile.

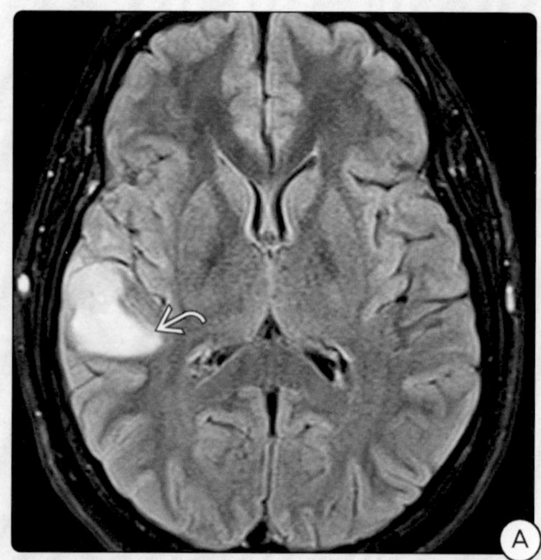


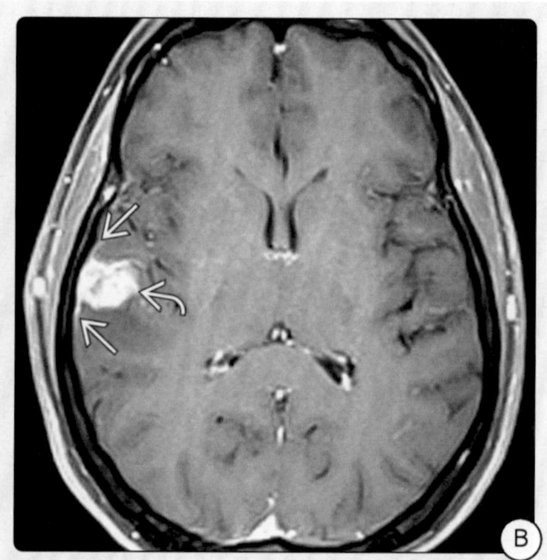


***(20-17A)** FLAIR MR in a 36-yo woman with new onset of seizures shows a hyperintense infiltrating mass ➲ in the right temporal lobe. **(20-17B)** T1 C+ FS MR shows that a solid portion of the mass enhances intensely ➲. Note the presence of subtle "dural tails" ➡ adjacent to the lesion. Pathology disclosed anaplastic PXA by methylation profiling and homozygous loss of CDKN2A/B. This is CNS WHO grade 3.*

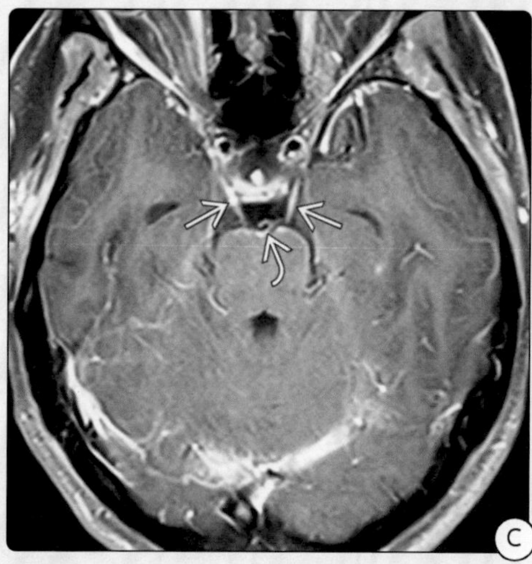


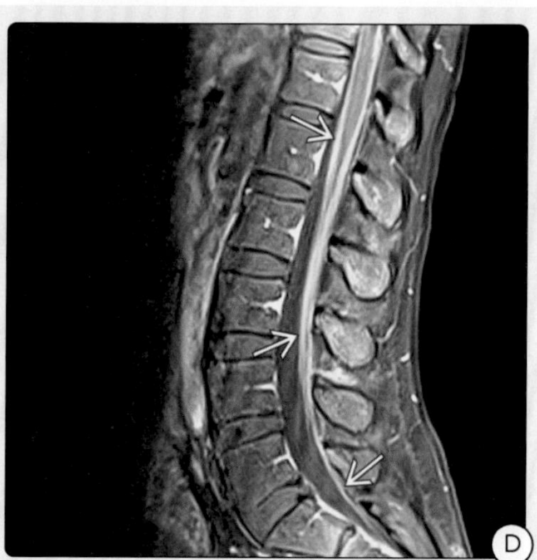


***(20-17C)** Four months later, the patient developed disseminated CSF metastases. Axial T1 C+ FS MR shows enhancement of both oculomotor nerves ➡ and the pontine surface ➲. **(20-17D)** Sagittal T1 C+ FS MR disclosed diffuse leptomeningeal metastases ➡. The patient expired 4 months after the initial diagnosis.*

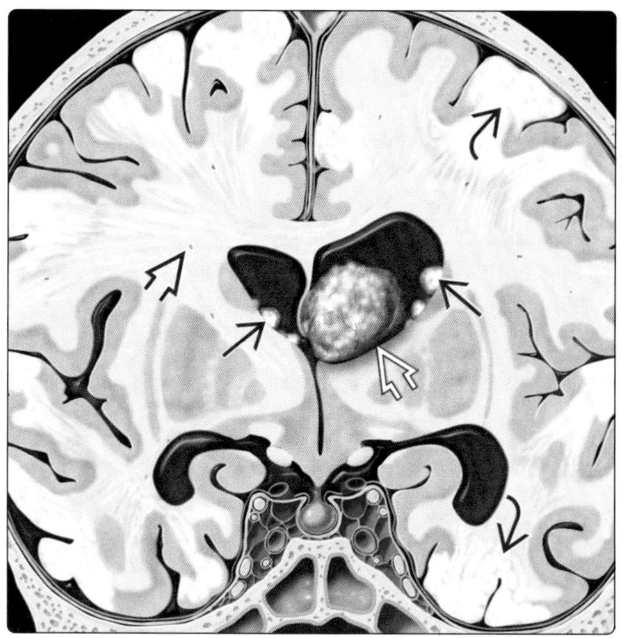

***(20-18)** Coronal graphic shows a SEGA ➡ in a patient with tuberous sclerosis. Note subependymal nodules ➡ and cortical tubers ➡ with "blurring" of the GM-WM interface. Prominent radial glial bands ➡ are also present in the medullary WM.*

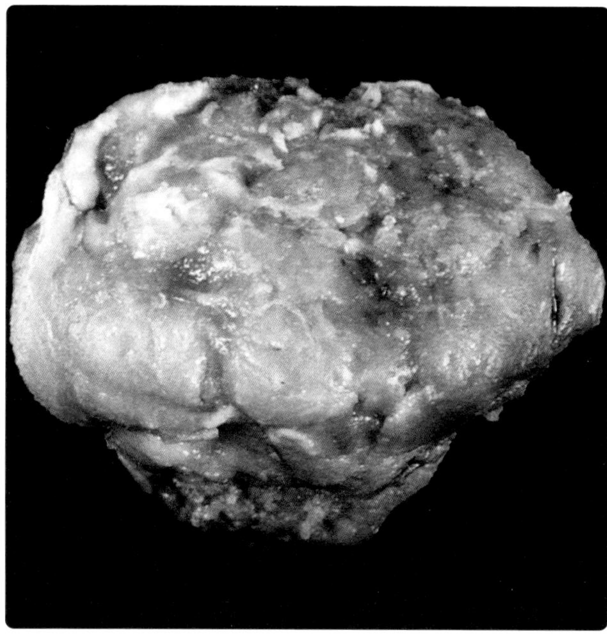

***(20-19)** Gross specimen of SEGA shows that they are resectable, discrete masses that lend themselves to complete or near-complete resection. (From DP: Neuro.)*

**IDH-mutant diffuse astrocytoma** usually involves the white matter and does not involve the meninges.
**Oligodendroglioma** can present as a slow-growing cortical-white matter junction lesion that remodels the adjacent calvaria, but the cyst + nodule pattern is usually absent.

Besides ganglioglioma, other less common tumors with a cyst + nodule appearance that can mimic PXA include hemispheric **pilocytic astrocytoma. Dysembryoplastic neuroepithelial tumor (DNET)** has a similar presentation and age range but typically has a multicystic bubbly appearance.

## Subependymal Giant Cell Astrocytoma

Subependymal giant cell astrocytoma (SEGA) is a localized, circumscribed, periventricular CNS WHO grade 1 astrocytic tumor that is strongly associated with tuberous sclerosis (TS) **(20-18)**.

### Terminology

SEGA is a circumscribed astrocytic glioma that arises from the subependymal tissue of the lateral ventricles adjacent to the foramen of Monro. Rare locations include the third ventricle and the retina.

### Etiology

SEGA has a strong association with TS. Growth of a subependymal nodule (SEN) in TS into a SEGA is a gradual process that generally occurs in the first two decades of life. SEGAs only rarely arise after the age of 20-25 years.

Radiologic evidence supports the evolution of some SENs into SEGAs.

**Genetics.** It is uncertain whether SEGAs can occur outside the setting of TS or if the tumor harbors currently undetectable TS complex (TSC) gene alterations.

***TSC-Associated SEGAs.*** The majority of SEGAs in patients with TSC have biallelic inactivation of the *TSC1* (15%) or *TSC2* (56%) genes. The *TSC1* and *TSC2* genes encode the tumor suppressor proteins hamartin and tuberin, respectively, leading to mammalian target of rapamycin genes (mTOR) upregulation. mTOR upregulation leads to uncontrolled cell growth and protein synthesis.

***Nonsyndromic SEGAs.*** Examples of SEGAs in the absence of other clinical features of TSC have been reported, but these tumors may harbor currently undetectable TSC gene alterations. SEGAs with low levels of *TSC1* or *TSC2* somatic mosaicisms or large deletions may also occur without other clinical manifestations of the disease. In patients with solitary SEGA, mosaic mutations may be present in other organs, and TSC may clinically manifest later in life, so these patients should be followed up for prolonged periods.

Rare isolated nonsyndromic SEGAs have also been reported in patients **without** currently demonstrable germline or tumor mutations in *TSC1* or *TSC2* on sequencing.

### Pathology

**Location.** Nearly all SEGAs are located in the lateral ventricles adjacent to the foramen of Monro **(20-21)**.

**Size and Number.** SEGAs vary in size from tiny to lesions measuring several centimeters in diameter. The average tumor size is 10-15 mm. Most SEGAs are solitary lesions. So-called double SEGAs occur in up to 20% of cases.

**Gross Pathology.** SEGAs are sharply demarcated, well-circumscribed, multilobulated solid intraventricular masses that rarely hemorrhage or undergo necrosis **(20-19)**. Calcification is common. Even large SEGAs generally do not invade the adjacent brain.

**Microscopic Features.** SEGA tumor cells display a wide spectrum of glial phenotypes that may be indistinguishable from SENs. Large pyramidal cells that resemble astrocytes or ganglion cells are typical. Nuclei are large, round, and usually eccentric with open chromatin and prominent nucleoli.

**Staging, Grading, and Classification.** SEGAs are CNS WHO grade 1 neoplasms. The presence of mitoses, vascular proliferation, or necrosis does not indicate anaplastic progression.

**Diagnostic Molecular Pathology.** DNA methylation-based classification studies support SEGA as a distinct tumor entity. Methylome profiling with analyses for *TSC1* or *TSC2* alterations may be helpful in histologically ambiguous cases. However, molecular analyses are usually not needed to establish the diagnosis of SEGA.

## Clinical Issues

**Epidemiology.** SEGAs arise in a relatively small proportion (10-20%) of patients with TSC but cause up to 25% of the morbidity associated with this condition.

**Demographics.** SEGAs generally occur in the setting of TSC and typically develop during the first two decades of life. Mean age at diagnosis is 11 years. Sporadic SEGAs without obvious TS stigmata occur but are extremely rare.

**Presentation.** Epilepsy in TS patients is related to cortical tubers, not SEGAs. SEGAs are generally asymptomatic until

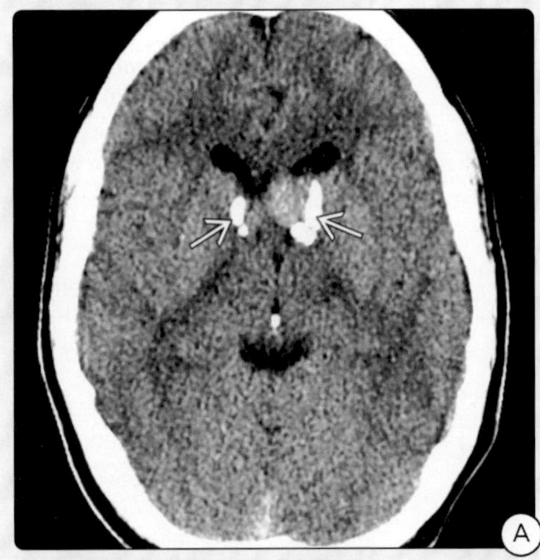


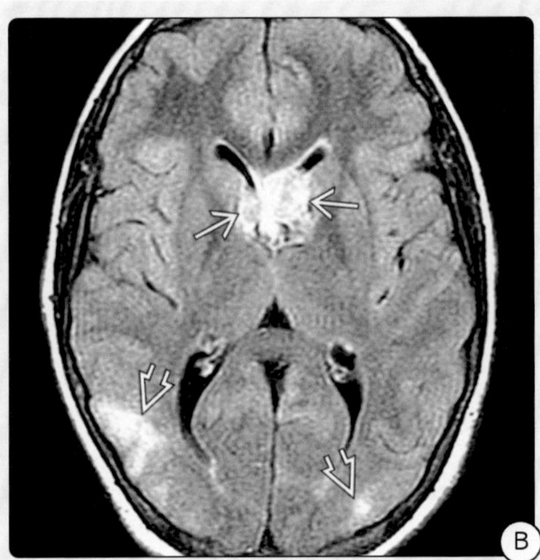


***(20-20A)** NECT in a child with tuberous sclerosis complex shows slightly hyperdense, calcified masses in the frontal horns of both lateral ventricles ➡. **(20-20B)** FLAIR MR in the same patient shows that the masses ➡ are heterogeneously hyperintense. Again note the cortical tubers ➡.*

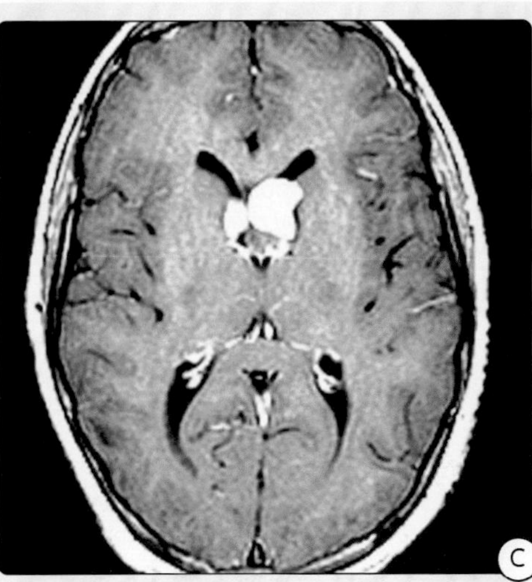


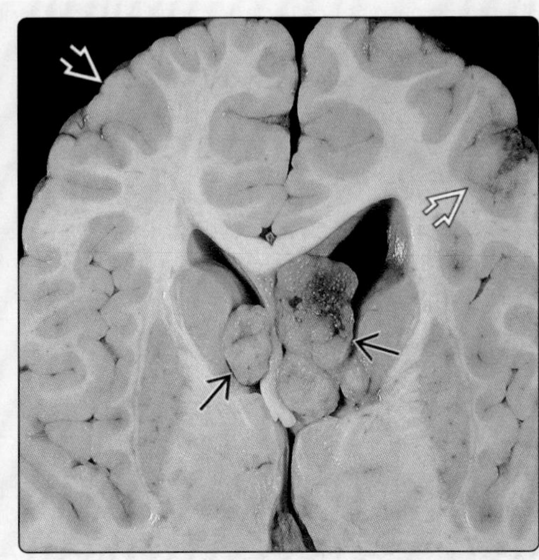

***(20-20C)** T1 C+ MR shows the intense enhancement of the masses. SEGAs are shown in this tuberous sclerosis complex patient. **(20-21)** Axial autopsy in a patient with tuberous sclerosis shows cortical tubers ➡ and bilateral SEGAs ➡. Note that the left frontal horn is enlarged, but the tumor remains circumscribed and noninvasive. (Courtesy R. Hewlett, MD.)*

they cause obstructive hydrocephalus. Headache, vomiting, and loss of consciousness are typical symptoms.

**Natural History.** Prognosis is generally good, as SEGAs are benign lesions that grow slowly and rarely infiltrate adjacent brain. Many patients with SEGAs have small lesions that may remain relatively stable. Median growth rate generally ranges from 2.5-5.6 mm per year.

The clinical course of SEGA, however, is not invariably so benign. The main concern is obstructive hydrocephalus, which may develop suddenly and result in rapidly rising intracranial pressure.

**Treatment Options.** When imaging findings are indeterminate and a lesion near the foramen of Monro cannot be clearly identified as an SEN or SEGA, close interval follow-up imaging (initially every 6 months, then annually if there is no evidence of growth) is recommended. A lesion in this location should be treated as soon as it shows evidence of enlargement.

Surgical resection has been the treatment of choice, as regrowth rates after complete tumor removal are very low. However, not all SEGAs can be resected completely. Biologically targeted pharmacotherapy with mTOR inhibitors, such as sirolimus and everolimus, has provided a safe and efficacious treatment option. SEGAs can recur a few months after drug discontinuation, so continued therapy may be necessary to avoid recurrence.

## Imaging

The most important ancillary imaging findings to identify are those of TSC (see Chapter 44). In the absence of a known family history, intellectual disability, epilepsy, or cutaneous stigmata, imaging may provide the first clues to the diagnosis of TSC.

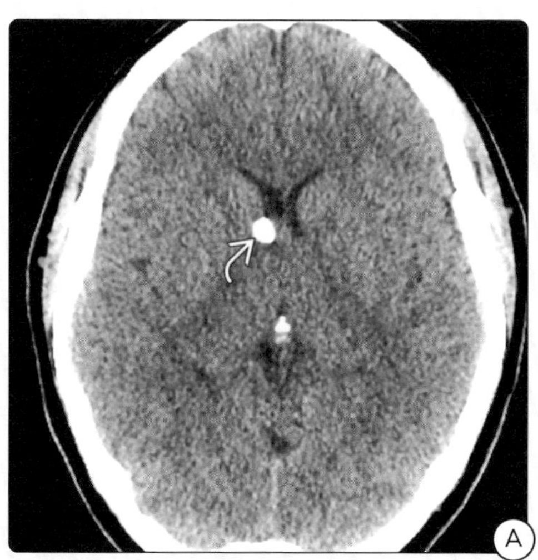


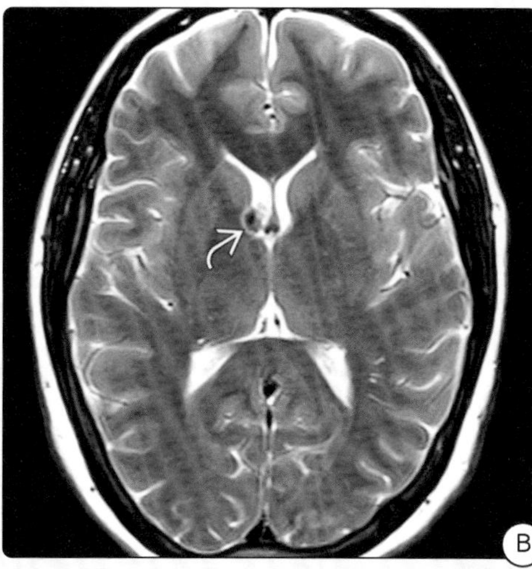


***(20-22A)** NECT in a 28-yo woman with headaches shows a solitary calcification in the right lateral ventricle adjacent to the foramen of Monro. **(20-22B)** T2 MR shows that the mass is very localized and predominately hypointense with a thin, hyperintense rim. No other subependymal nodules were present, and the patient exhibited no stigmata of tuberous sclerosis complex.*

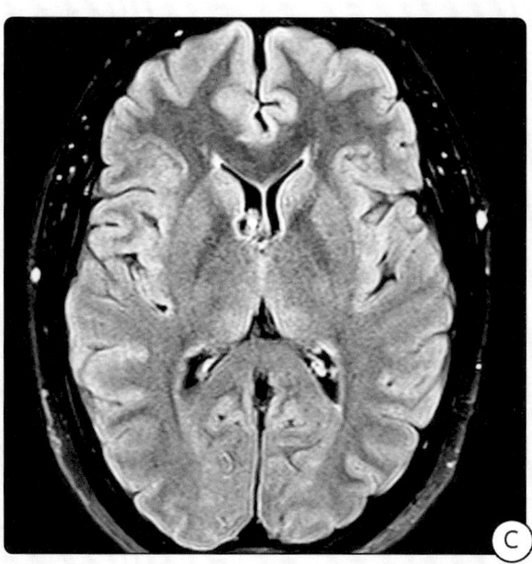


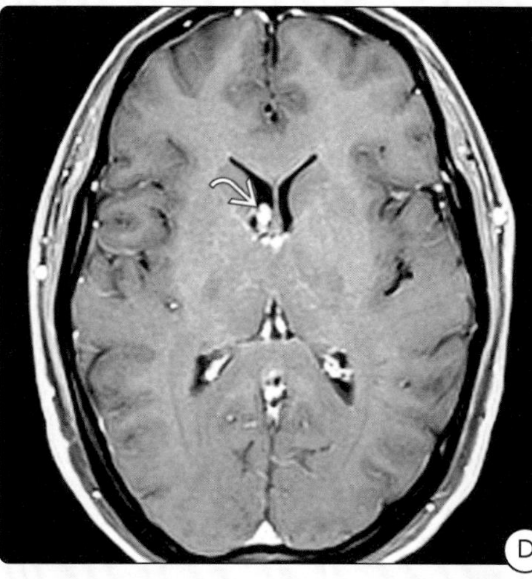


***(20-22C)** FLAIR MR shows no evidence of cortical tubers or other imaging findings of tuberous sclerosis. **(20-22D)** T1 C+ FS MR shows the solid portion and rim of mass enhance. The mass was resected and disclosed SEGA. No evidence for TS1 germline mutation or BRAF p.V600E mutation was present. DNA methylation was indicative of SEGA, and a TSC2 somatic mosaic mutation with loss of heterozygosity was found.*

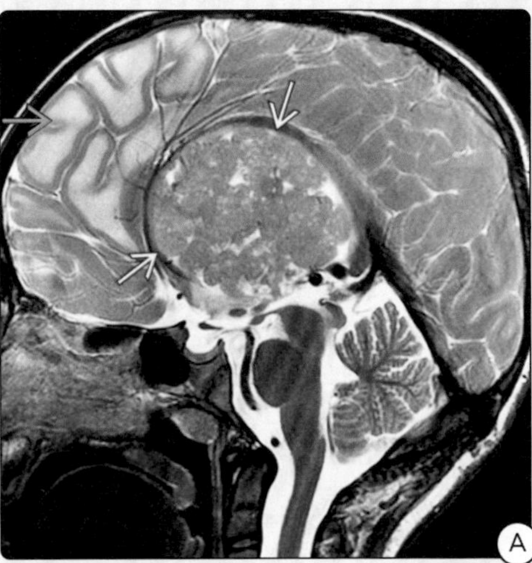
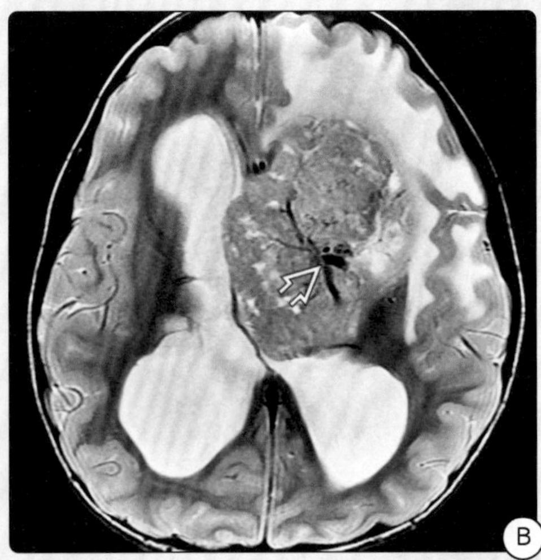

***(20-23A)** Sagittal T2 MR in 7-yo girl with headaches, morning nausea, and vomiting shows heterogeneous, lobulated mass ➡ in lateral ventricle. Note severe obstructive hydrocephalus with upward bowing of corpus callosum ➡. **(20-23B)** Axial T2 MR shows heterogeneous mass with prominent internal "flow voids ➡" obstructs foramen of Monro and causes periventricular fluid accumulation in left frontal lobe.*

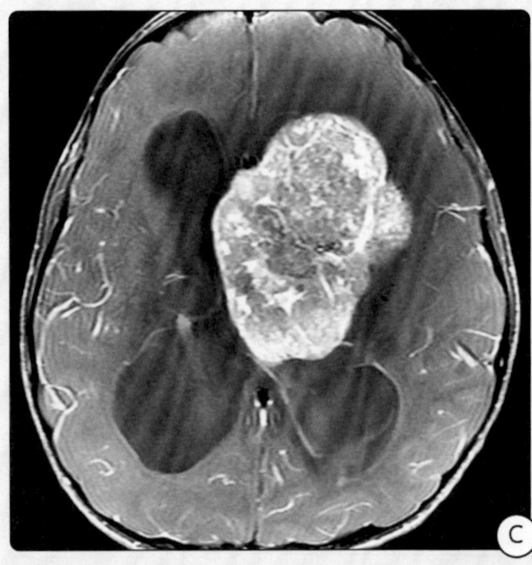
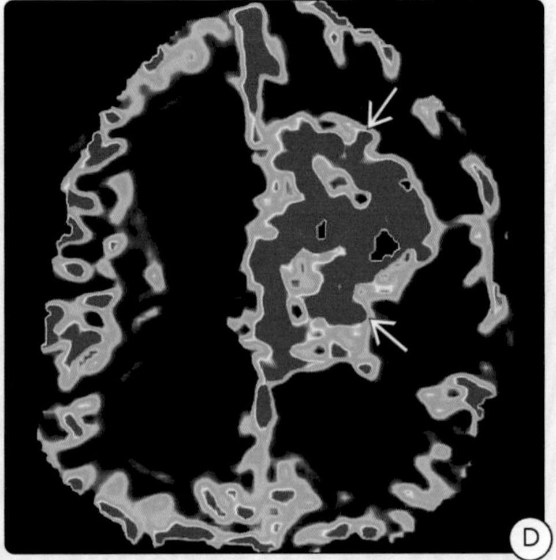

***(20-23C)** T1 C+ FS MR shows that the mass enhances intensely but very heterogeneously. **(20-23D)** Axial pMR shows that the mass exhibits markedly elevated rCBV ➡.*

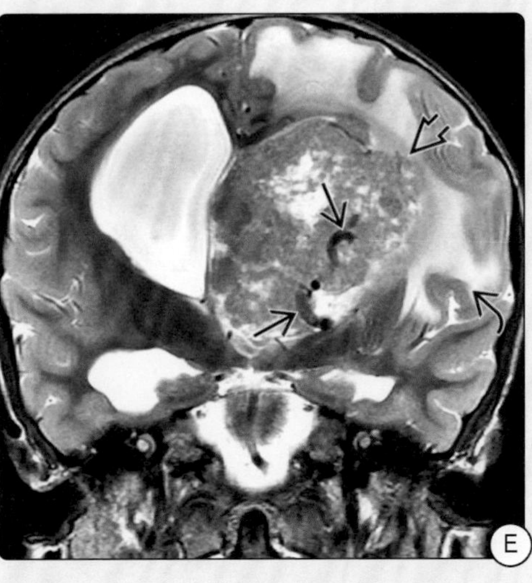
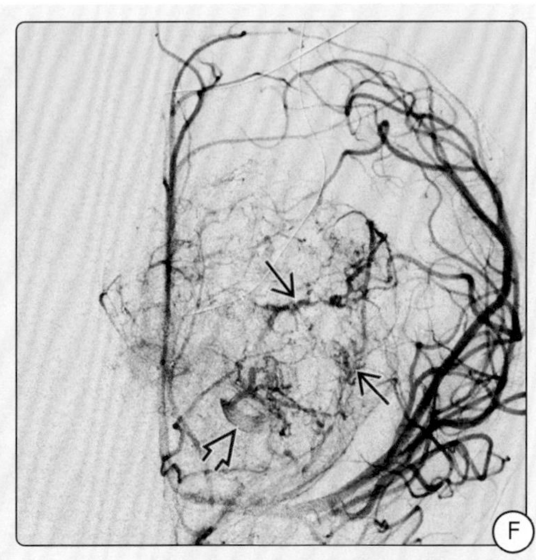

***(20-23E)** Coronal T2 MR shows the prominent vascular "flow voids" ➡ intrinsic to the mass. The margin between the lateral ventricle and brain ➡ is indistinct, and there is significant associated edema ➡. **(20-23F)** AP view of left internal carotid angiogram shows a very hypervascular mass with irregular, enlarged arteries ➡ and early draining veins ➡. A large SEGA without brain invasion was removed at surgery.*

**CT Findings.** SEGAs are hypo- to isodense, variably calcified lesions near the foramen of Monro **(20-20A)**. Calcified SENs may be seen along the lateral ventricle margins, especially the caudothalamic grooves. Hydrocephalus is present in 15% of cases. "Blurred" lateral ventricle margins indicate severe obstructive hydrocephalus with transependymal CSF migration.

SEGAs demonstrate strong but heterogeneous enhancement. An enhancing lesion at the foramen of Monro on CECT scan should be considered SEGA until proven otherwise.

**MR Findings.** SEGAs are hypo- to isointense compared with cortex on T1WI and heterogeneously iso- to hyperintense on T2WI. Larger SEGAs may have prominent "flow voids." Strong but heterogeneous enhancement is typical.

FLAIR is especially useful for detecting subtle CNS features of TSC, such as SENs, cortical tubers, and white matter radial migration lines. Streaky linear hyperintensities extending through the white matter to the subjacent ventricle or wedge-shaped hyperintensities underlying expanded ("clubbed") gyri are typical **(20-20B)**.

SEN enhancement is much more visible on MR than on CT. Between 30-80% of SENs enhance following contrast administration **(20-20C)**, so enhancement alone is insufficient to distinguish a SEN from a SEGA. Although a mass at the foramen of Monro > 10-12 mm in diameter is usually a SEGA **(20-23)**, only progressive enlargement is sufficient to differentiate a SEGA from a SEN.

## Differential Diagnosis

The major differential diagnosis of SEGA in a patient with TSC is a benign nonneoplastic **SEN**. SENs remain stable and do not need to be treated, whereas SEGAs gradually enlarge and eventually require surgical treatment. SEGAs arise only near the foramen of Monro, whereas SENs can be located anywhere around the ventricular wall, especially along the caudothalamic groove. Although SENs are much more common than SEGAs, a partially calcified, enhancing lesion at the foramen of Monro > 5 mm is more likely to be a SEGA than an SEN.

Other lateral ventricle masses that should be included in the differential diagnosis are **subependymoma** (a tumor of middle-aged and older adult patients) and **central neurocytoma** (a "bubbly" tumor that arises in the lateral ventricle body). Low-grade **diffusely infiltrating astrocytoma** can arise in the septi pellucidi or fornices, but these tumors typically neither calcify nor enhance.

### SUBEPENDYMAL GIANT CELL ASTROCYTOMA

**Etiology, Genetics**
- 5-15% of patients with TSC develop SEGA
- Almost all SEGAs are associated with TSC
    - Biallelic inactivation of *TSC1* or *TSC2* genes
    - Loss of hamartin or tuberin immunoexpression
    - Activation of mTOR pathway
- SEGAs without TSC reported but are very rare
    - May have currently undetectable TSC alterations

**Pathology**
- Circumscribed, multinodular mass at foramen of Monro
- Does not infiltrate brain
- CNS WHO grade 1

**Clinical Issues**
- Mean age: 11 years
- Seizures, ↑ intracranial pressure

**Imaging Findings**
- $Ca^{++}$ on NECT, enhance on CECT
- T1 iso-/hypointense, T2/FLAIR hyperintense
- May have prominent vascular "flow voids"
- Strong, heterogeneous enhancement
- Look for ancillary signs of TSC!
    - Cortical tubers (broad expanded gyri)
    - White matter lesions (T2/FLAIR hyperintense radial lines/wedges)

**Differential Diagnosis**
- Benign nonneoplastic SEN
    - Remains stable over years
- Subependymoma (rare in patients < 20 years)
- Central neurocytoma (body of lateral ventricle)

# Chordoid Glioma

Chordoid glioma (CG) is a well-circumscribed glial neoplasm with a stereotypical location in the anterior third ventricle **(20-24)**. CGs are characterized by a novel missense mutation in the *PRKCA* gene.

CGs are rare, accounting for < 0.1% of primary brain tumors and arise from specialized tancytic ependymal cells in the organum vasculosum of the lamina terminalis.

CGs are solid, well-demarcated, slightly lobulated neoplasms with clusters and chords of epithelioid cells in a soft, gray mucinous stroma. CGs are immunopositive for thyroid transcription factor 1 (TTF-1) and classified as CNS WHO grade 2 neoplasms.

CGs are tumors of middle-aged adults (35-60 years). Presentation varies from asymptomatic to aggressive with obstructive hydrocephalus, headache, nausea, and visual field defects. Endocrine disturbances are seen in 10-15% of cases.

CGs are slow-growing tumors, but resection is often subtotal as they are frequently attached to the hypothalamus and floor of the third ventricle. The most common postoperative complication is hypothalamic dysfunction with diabetes insipidus and obesity.

Imaging shows well-demarcated, ovoid, slightly lobulated mass that is confined to the third ventricle and presents as solid (2/3) or mixed cystic-solid (1/3) tumors. CGs are moderately hyperdense compared with brain on NECT. Calcification may be present.

Sagittal T1WIs show the tumor is iso- or hypointense with brain and appears clearly separated from the pituitary gland and infundibular stalk **(20-25)**. CGs are slightly hyperintense on T2WI. Strong but heterogeneous enhancement is typical.

The differential diagnosis is limited. Primary third ventricular tumors in adults are all uncommon. Metastases are rare in this location; a few purely intraventricular pituitary macroadenomas and craniopharyngiomas have been reported. Chordoid meningioma can look just like a CG, but the third ventricle is a very rare site for this uncommon meningioma variant.

As CGs are tumors of adults, childhood hypothalamic masses, such as tuber cinereum hamartomas, craniopharyngiomas, and pilocytic astrocytomas, are not diagnostic considerations.

## Astroblastoma, *MN1*-Altered

Astroblastoma (AB), *MN1*-altered is a rare, circumscribed, glial neoplasm defined by the presence of *MN1* rearrangement (typically *MAMLD1::BEND2*) and occurs almost exclusively in the cerebral hemispheres, although intraventricular, brainstem, and spinal cord ABs have been reported.

ABs account for < 1% of all primary brain tumors. Although they can occur at any age, most ABs are found in children and young adults. Median age at presentation is 15 years (range: three months to 40 years), and there is a striking female predominance.

The histologic hallmark of *MN1*-altered AB is the presence of astroblastic pseudorosettes. Tumors are generally well

***(20-24)** Midline sagittal autopsy specimen shows chordoid glioma as a lobulated mass ⇨ that fills the 3rd ventricle. The whitish, glistening part of the tumor ⇨ represents the chordoid elements of the tumor. (Courtesy P. Burger, MD.) **(20-25A)** Sagittal T1 MR in a 26-yo woman shows a well-demarcated, isointense mass ➡ in the anterior 3rd ventricle attached to the lamina terminalis.*

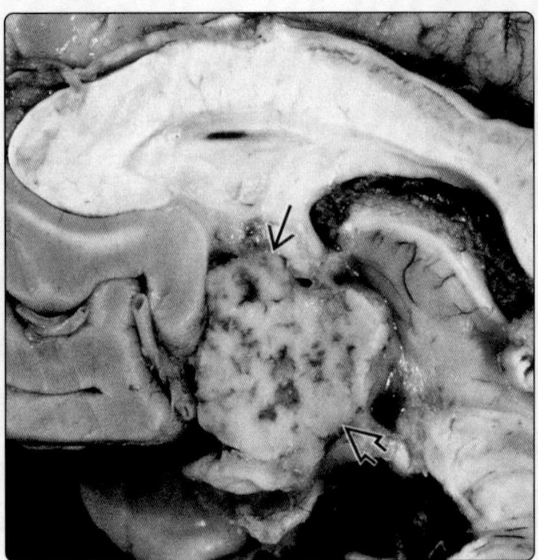

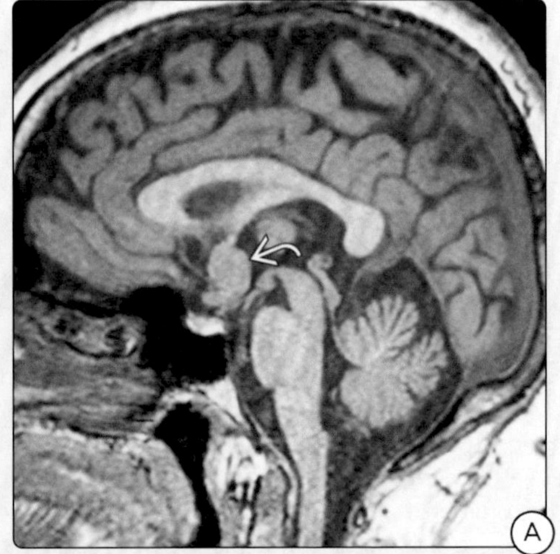


***(20-25B)** The lobulated mass is mixed iso- ➡ to hyperintense on T2 MR ➡. **(20-25C)** T1 C+ MR shows the mass ➡ enhances intensely and uniformly.*

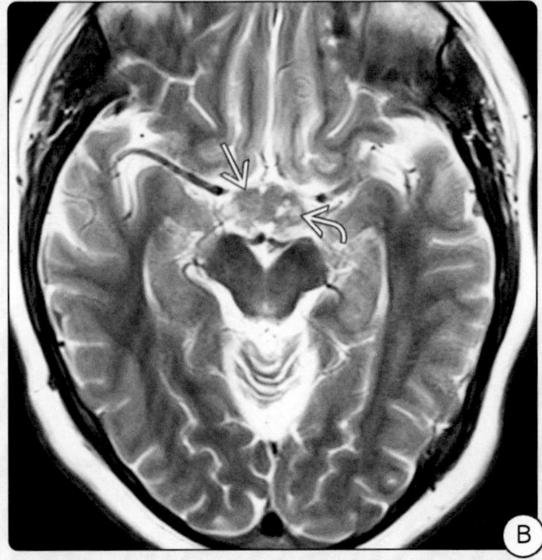


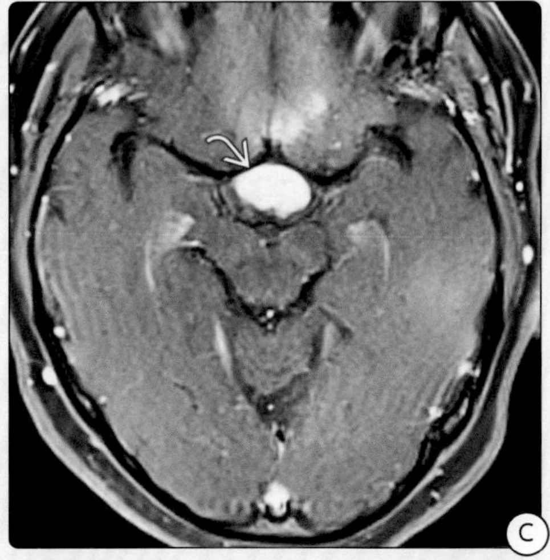

circumscribed with minimal or no invasion of adjacent brain. A definitive CNS WHO grade has not been established.

ABs are superficially located masses that are typically well demarcated **(20-26)**. Most exhibit both solid and cystic components, often giving them a characteristic bubbly appearance on imaging studies **(20-27)**. ABs are hypo- to isointense on T1WI and heterogeneously hyperintense on T2/FLAIR. The combination of peripheral rim and solid nodular enhancement on T1 C+ gives some lesions a signet-ring appearance.

*Selected References: The complete reference list is available on the eBooks+ version included with purchase.*

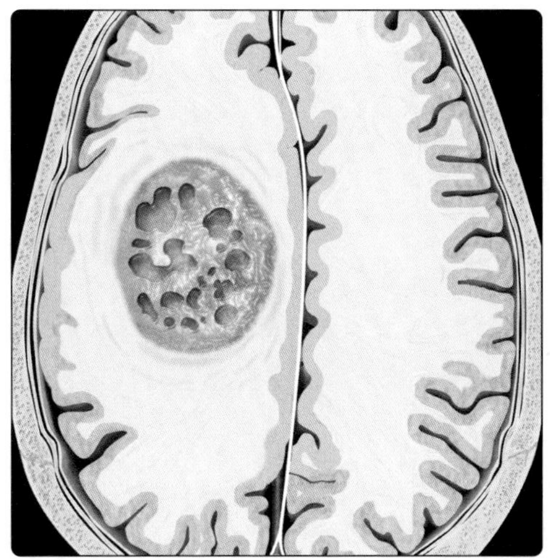

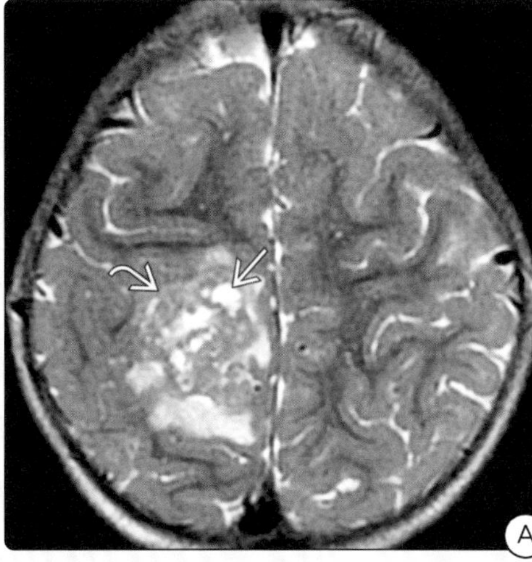


***(20-26)** Graphic depicts astroblastoma, MN1-altered as a relatively well-circumscribed, hemispheric mass with multiple intratumoral cysts and moderate surrounding edema. **(20-27A)** T2 MR shows the mass has a bubbly appearance with isointense solid portions ➙ containing various-sized intratumoral cysts ➙.*

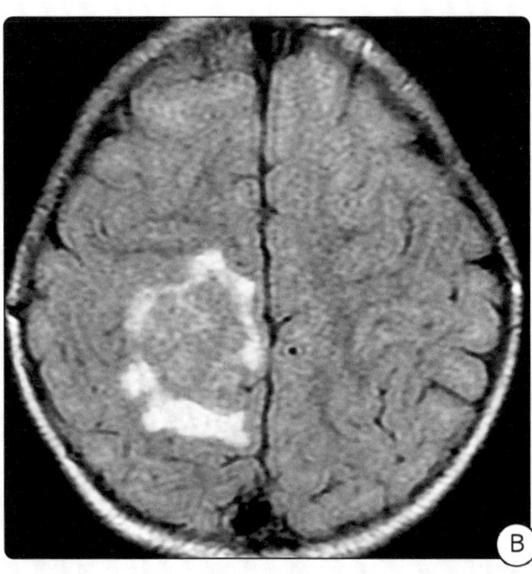


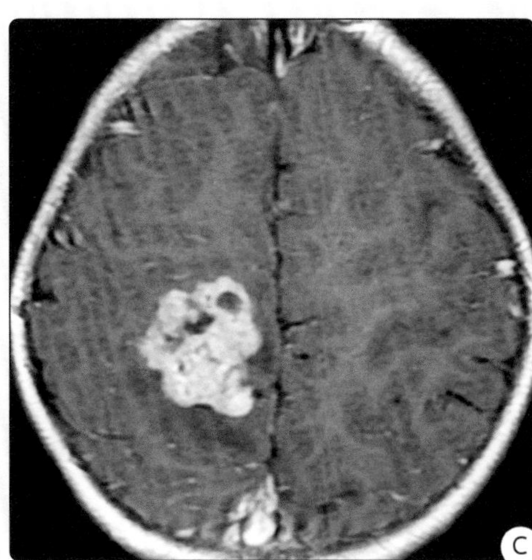


***(20-27B)** The mass is mostly isointense with brain on FLAIR and is surrounded by hyperintense vasogenic edema. **(20-27C)** The solid portions of the mass enhance intensely on T1 C+ MR. This is astroblastoma, MN1-altered.*

# Glioneuronal and Neuronal Tumors

*The 5th edition WHO classification of CNS neoplasms groups gliomas, glioneuronal tumors, and neuronal tumors together. Gliomas are—by far—the largest group of neoplasms in this group. In the previous chapters, we discussed adult-type diffuse gliomas, pediatric-type diffuse low-grade gliomas, pediatric-type diffuse high-grade gliomas, and circumscribed astrocytic gliomas.*

Glioneuronal and neuronal tumors—much less common than the large, very broad group of gliomas discussed in previous chapters—accounts for only 1-2% of all primary brain tumors. This diverse collection of tumors includes both familiar entities, e.g., ganglioglioma as well as a number of newly recognized entities, such as multinodular and vacuolating neuronal tumor (MVNT) and myxoid glioneuronal tumor (MGNT).

Glioneuronal neoplasms are clinically important as they are usually relatively benign, slow-growing tumors that are frequently associated with epilepsy.



## Glioneuronal Tumors

We begin this section with a brief overview of ganglion cell tumors followed by a discussion of the most common histologically mixed glioneuronal neoplasm, **ganglioglioma**. We then turn our attention to **desmoplastic infantile ganglioglioma** followed by a discussion of **dysembryoplastic neuroepithelial tumor (DNET)**, now recognized as one of the more common causes of temporal lobe epilepsy. We close the discussion of glioneuronal tumors with the pathology and imaging of several uncommon neoplasms, such as MVNTs, MGNTs, and rosette-forming glioneuronal tumors.

### Overview of Ganglion Cell Tumors

Ganglion cell tumors are benign, well-differentiated neoplasms characterized by the presence of dysplastic ganglion cells. Two types of ganglion cell tumors are recognized: Gangliogliomas and gangliocytomas.

The vast majority of ganglion cell tumors are histologically mixed lesions that contain **both** neoplastic ganglion cell and glial elements. These neoplasms are called **gangliogliomas** and designated as CNS WHO grade 1.

**Gangliocytomas**—tumors that demonstrate **exclusive** neoplastic ganglion cell composition—are relatively rare and are discussed briefly following the detailed discussion of glioneuronal neoplasms.

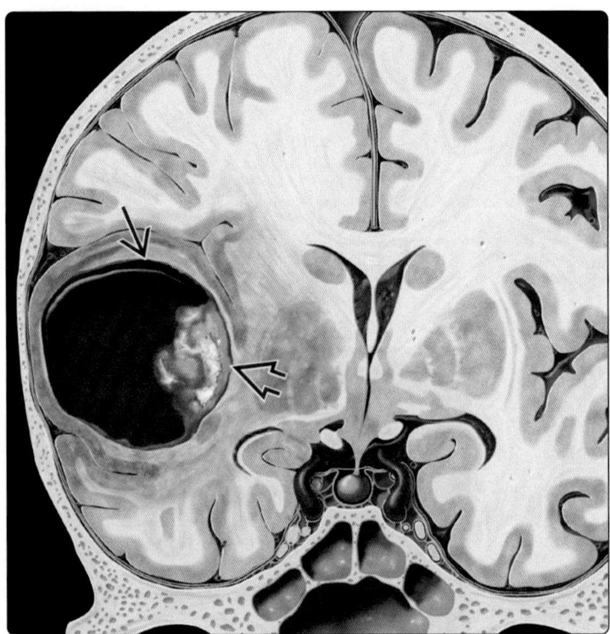

*(21-1) Coronal graphic depicts a typical ganglioglioma (GG) of the temporal lobe with a cyst ⇒ and a partially calcified mural nodule ⇨.*

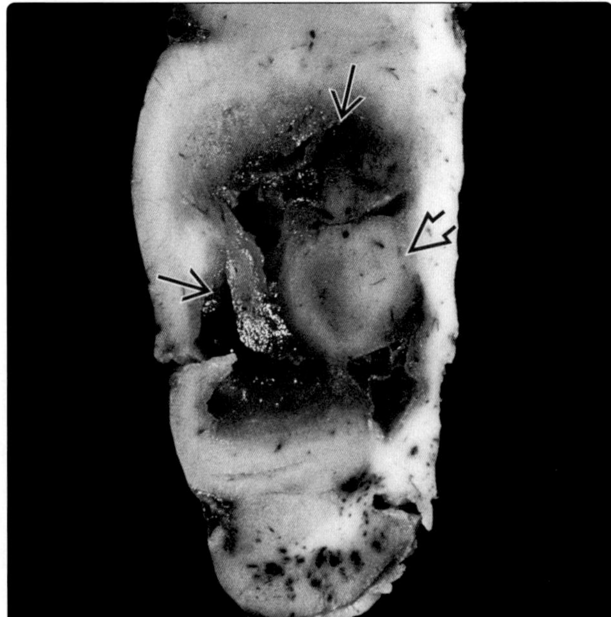

*(21-2) Partial temporal lobectomy specimen with GG shows a tumor nodule ⇨ and a partially collapsed cyst ⇒. Hemorrhage is primarily surgical. (Courtesy R. Hewlett, MD.)*

# Ganglioglioma

## Terminology

Gangliogliomas (GGs) are well-differentiated, slow-growing tumors. They are so-called biphasic tumors that are composed of neuronal and glial elements, most commonly an admixture of dysmorphic ganglion cells and neoplastic glial cells.

## Etiology

The neuronal and glial components in GGs both likely derive from a common precursor cell. The most frequent genetic alterations are MAPK pathway activations, most often *BRAF* V600E mutations (40-60%) or other MAPK pathway alterations, such as *RAF1* fusion, *KRAS* mutation, or *NF1* mutation or deletion.

## Pathology

**Location.** GGs occur throughout the CNS. Most are solitary lesions arising in the cerebral hemispheres. Between 50-75% originate in the temporal lobe. The next most common site is the frontal lobe (10% of GGs). Approximately 15% of GGs are found in the basal ganglia or posterior fossa, usually either in the brainstem or cerebellum. GGs vary in size from 1-6 cm and virtually never metastasize.

**Gross Pathology.** GGs are superficially located, well-delineated neoplasms that often expand the cortex **(21-1)**. The most common appearance is that of a cyst with mural nodule or a solid tumor **(21-2)**. Calcification is common, but gross hemorrhage and frank necrosis are rare.

**Microscopic Features.** The histologic hallmark of GG is its combination of neuronal and glial elements, which can be intermixed or geographically separated. Varying numbers of dysplastic neurons are interspersed with the glial component, which constitutes the proliferative and neoplastic element of the tumor. Astrocytic cells with pilocytic or fibrillary-like features are the most common glial element. GGs are designated as CNS WHO grade 1 neoplasms.

**Grading.** GGs with anaplastic features in the glial component (e.g., conspicuous mitotic activity, necrosis, &/or microvascular proliferation) have been termed **anaplastic gangliogliomas** (AGs) by some authors and provisionally designated as grade 3 lesions. Many reported AGs lack diagnostic molecular pathology to exclude other high-grade glioma subtypes, such as H3 G34-mutant hemispheric glioma. The 2021 WHO concludes further studies are needed to confirm the existence of AG.

GGs are CNS WHO grade 1 neoplasms. Malignant degeneration of a preexisting grade 1 GG is rare, occurring in 1-5% of cases.

Aggressive ganglion cell tumors with anaplasia in the glial component (i.e., those with conspicuous mitotic activity, high Ki-67 index, microvascular proliferation, and occasional necrosis) have been reported both at initial presentation and at the time of recurrence. These tumors have been called **anaplastic gangliomas** by some authors and provisionally designated as grade 3 lesions. However, DNA methylation testing of some tumors reported as AG on initial histopathology and immunohistochemistry shows these tumors often represent other well-defined CNS WHO diagnoses, most often pleomorphic xanthoastrocytoma (PXA), glioblastoma, and other diffuse pediatric-type high-grade gliomas.

## Clinical Issues

GG is predominantly a tumor of children and young adults; 80% of patients are younger than 30 years old. Peak presentation is 15-20 years old. Chronic, pharmacologically resistant temporal lobe epilepsy is present in the majority of cases. Seizures are generally the complex partial type.

GGs are typically very slow-growing neoplasms. Complete surgical resection is generally curative with 80% of patients becoming seizure free after tumor removal.

## Imaging

**General Features.** GGs are cortically based superficial parenchymal lesions that have two general imaging patterns: (1) A well-defined solid or partially cystic mass with mural nodule **(21-2)** and (2) a diffusely infiltrating, less well-delineated mass with ill-defined borders and patchy enhancement (less common).

**CT Findings.** A cystic component is seen in nearly 60% of cases. Approximately 30% have a well-circumscribed hypodense cyst with isodense mural nodule **(21-3A)**, whereas 40% are primarily hypodense. Between 30-50% of GGs calcify. Hemorrhage is rare. Only 50% of GGs enhance following contrast administration. Patterns vary from solid, rim, or nodular to cystic with an enhancing nodule.

**MR Findings.** GGs are hypo- to isointense relative to cortex on T1 and hyperintense on T2/FLAIR **(21-3B)**. Surrounding edema is generally absent. Enhancement varies from none or minimal to moderate. The classic pattern is a cystic mass with an enhancing mural nodule **(21-3)**. Homogeneous solid enhancement also occurs. Ill-defined, patchy enhancement is atypical and associated with a worse clinical outcome **(21-4)**.

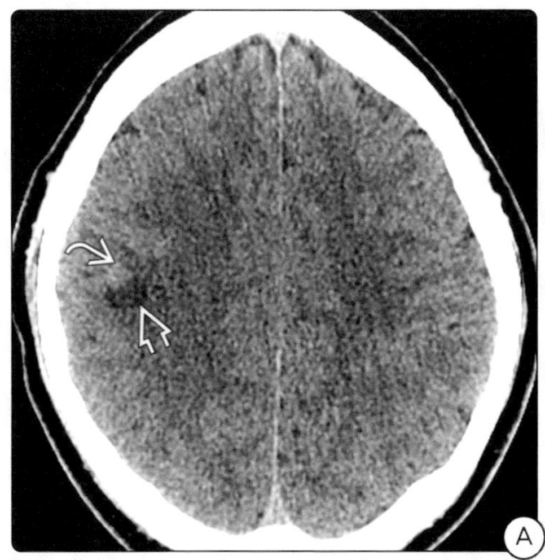


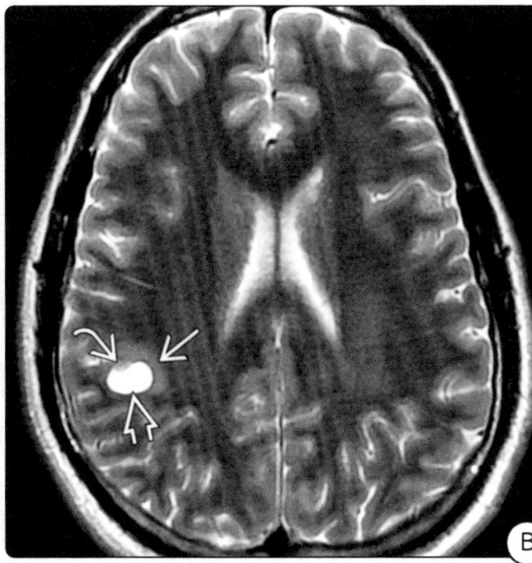


***(21-3A)** NECT in a 24-year-old man with intractable seizures shows a right posterior frontal cyst with a slightly hyperdense nodule. The lesion is located at the cortex in the bottom of a sulcus. **(21-3B)** T2 MR shows that the cyst is extremely hyperintense. The small mural nodule is isointense with cortex, which surrounds the mass completely.*

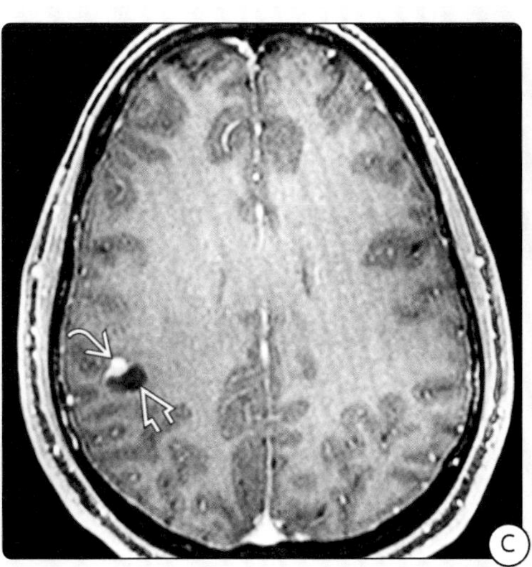


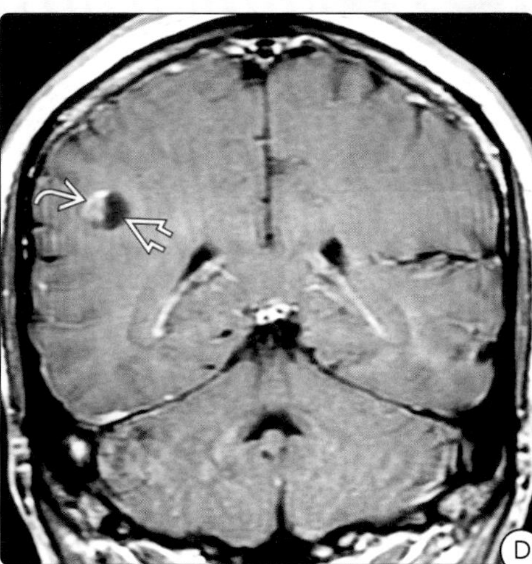


***(21-3C)** T1 C+ SPGR shows that the nodule enhances intensely while the cyst wall does not. **(21-3D)** Coronal T1 C+ MR nicely depicts the classic configuration of a GG with a cyst and an enhancing mural nodule. GG was completely resected, and the patient's longstanding epilepsy resolved.*

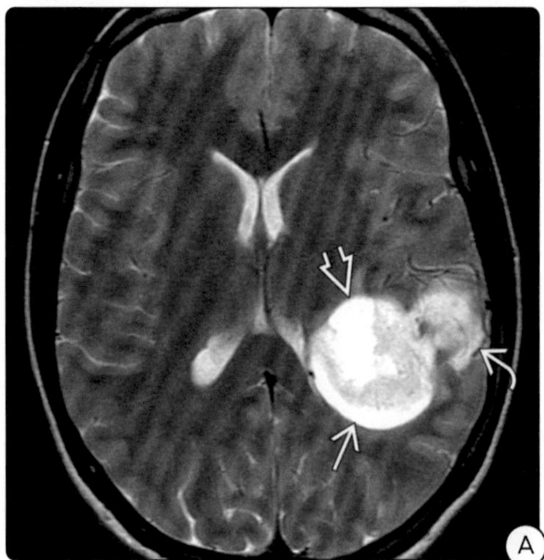


*(21-4A) T2 MR shows a heterogeneously hyperintense left parietal mass and cyst extending superficially toward the cortex.*

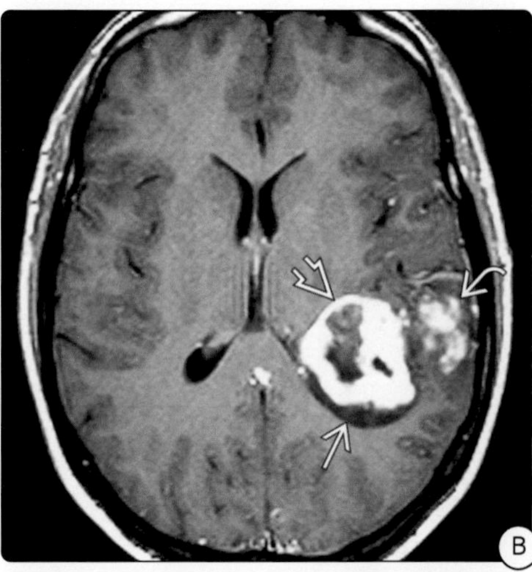


*(21-4B) T1 C+ shows cystic, solid enhancing mass, patchy cortical enhancement; GG grade 1 with "atypical" histopathologic features.*

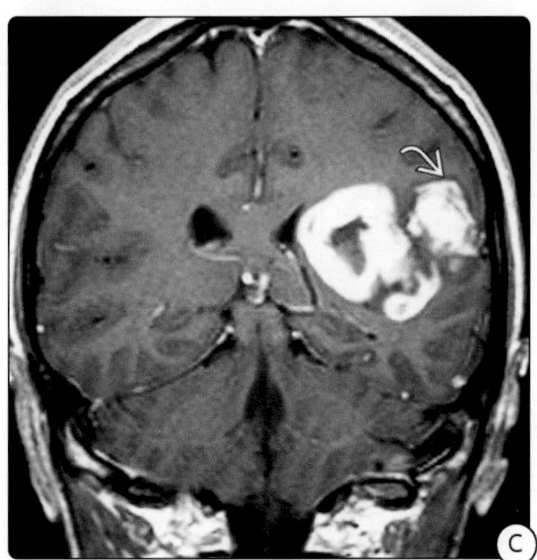


*(21-4C) T1 C+ MR shows deep tumor, ill-defined enhancement. Subtotal resection; recurred later with anaplastic features, WHO grade 3.*

GANGLIOGLIOMAS

**Ganglioglioma**

- Terminology
  - Well-differentiated, slow-growing tumor
  - Variable combination of neuronal, glial elements
- Etiology and genetics
  - *BRAF* V600E mutation
- Pathology
  - Dysplastic ganglion cells + neoplastic glial cells
  - Superficial, corticocentric
  - Solid or mixed cystic/solid, usually noninfiltrative
  - Temporal, frontal lobes > parietal > brainstem, ventricles
  - CNS WHO grade 1
- Clinical issues
  - Most common mixed glial-neuronal neoplasm
  - Children, young adults
  - Common presentation = seizures
- Imaging findings
  - Well-delineated (often temporal lobe) mass
  - Cyst + enhancing nodule most common pattern
- Differential diagnosis
  - Most common: Astrocytoma, IDH-mutant; pilocytic astrocytoma
  - Less common: DNET, polymorphous low-grade neuroepithelial tumor of young
  - Rare but important: Papillary glioneuronal tumor, PXA

**Anaplastic Ganglioglioma**

- Pathology
  - Anaplasia in glial component
  - ↑ mitoses, Ki-67; necrosis; microvascular proliferation
  - Exclude other high-grade gliomas with DNA methylation
  - No CNS WHO grade established
- Imaging findings
  - Atypical location common (i.e., deep rather than cortical)
  - Often larger, more infiltrative/poorly demarcated

## Differential Diagnosis

A supratentorial hemispheric **pilocytic astrocytoma** can present as a cyst with an enhancing nodule. **Polymorphous low-grade neuroepithelial tumor of the young (PLNTY)** often calcifies and can be indistinguishable from GG. **PXA** often has a "cyst + mural nodule" and can resemble GG but frequently has a dural "tail."

**DNET** is a superficial cortical neoplasm that typically has a multicystic bubbly appearance. A hyperintense rim surrounding the mass on FLAIR scan is common. In contrast to GG, enhancement is rare.

Solid, nonenhancing GGs can resemble an **astrocytoma, IDH-mutant**. **Oligodendroglioma** is rare in children; it commonly involves the cortex but is typically more diffuse and less well delineated.

# Desmoplastic Infantile Ganglioglioma/Astrocytoma

Desmoplastic infantile ganglioglioma (DIG) and desmoplastic infantile astrocytoma (DIA) are rare, benign cerebral hemispheric glioneuronal or glial tumors **(21-5)**. The vast majority of DIGs/DIAs occur before the age of two years and typically present with macrocrania, bulging fontanelles, and hemiparesis.

Pathologically, DIGs/DIAs exhibit a biphasic morphology with mixed astrocytic and neuronal (ganglionic) components (DIG) or an astrocytic component only (DIA). Tumor cells are embedded in an extensive peripheral desmoplastic stroma that often adheres to the dura. Mitotic activity is rare. DIG/DIA is a CNS WHO grade 1 tumor.

On imaging studies, DIGs/DIAs are typically large, bulky, superficially located hemispheric tumors with mixed cystic/solid components. The cystic components can be uni- or multilocular, are frequently quite large, and are hypointense on T1WI and hyperintense on T2WI. Peripheral edema is minimal or absent. Intense but heterogeneous enhancement of the solid component is present. The cyst walls and septations also often enhance **(21-6)**.

Despite their ominous-appearing imaging, gross total resection generally results in long-term survival. A few cases of CSF dissemination have been reported.

The imaging differential diagnosis of DIG/DIA is limited. **Infant-type hemispheric gliomas** have an infiltrative growth pattern, are more heterogeneous, often hemorrhage, and have a low ADC. **Embryonal tumor with multilayered rosettes** (ETMR) and **atypical teratoid/rhabdoid tumor** (AT/RT) can occur in the same age group as DIG/DIA but are less often grossly cystic and often appear hyperdense on CT. **Supratentorial ependymoma,** *ZFTA* **fusion positive** occurs in children and young adults (generally not infants). Its cysts are often less complex than DIG/DIA, and the solid portion of the tumor is less peripherally located than DIG/DIA.

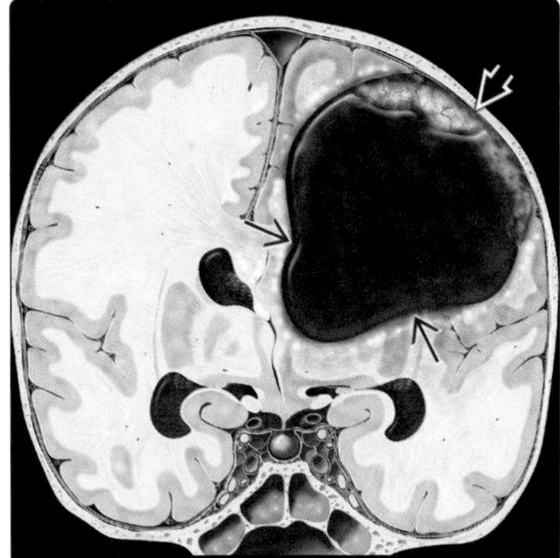

***(21-5)** Desmoplastic infantile astrocytoma/ganglioglioma (DIA/DIG) shows a large, mixed, cystic ➡, solid ➡ component abutting dura.*

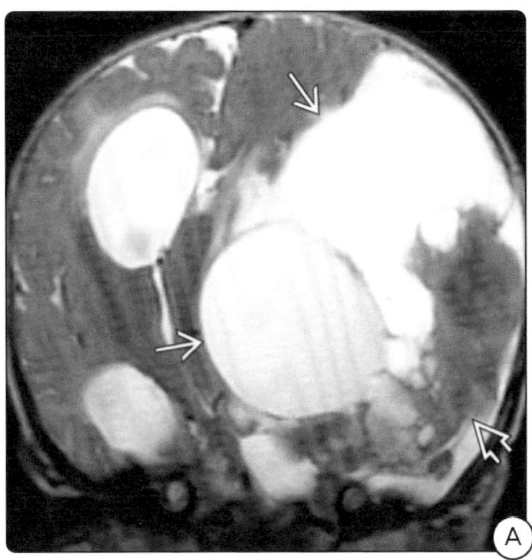


***(21-6A)** Coronal T2 MR in 10-mo infant with a large head, hydrocephalus shows a huge mixed cystic ➡, solid ➡ mass in the left hemisphere.*

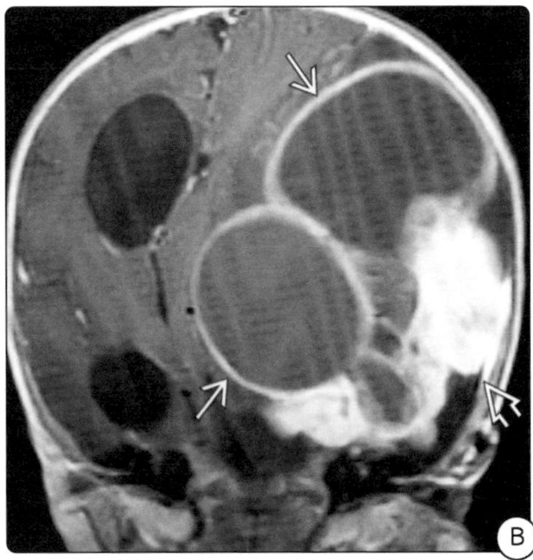


***(21-6B)** T1 C+ MR shows cyst rims enhancing strongly ➡. Solid portion of mass abuts dura ➡, enhances strongly but heterogeneously. DIA/DIG.*

## Dysembryoplastic Neuroepithelial Tumor

Ganglioglioma and dysembryoplastic neuroepithelial tumor (DNET or DNT) are the two most common long-term epilepsy-associated tumors (so-called LEATs).

### Terminology

DNET is a benign, typically cortically based lesion characterized by a lobulated, multinodular architecture with a pathognomonic glioneuronal element **(21-7)**.

### Etiology

*FGFR1* alterations are key events in the pathogenesis of DNET and are present in 40-80% of cases. *BRAF* p.V600E mutations occur in up to 50% cases. DNETs may also occur in RASopathies, such as neurofibromatosis type 1 and Noonan syndrome.

### Pathology

**Location.** DNETs are superficial, cortically based neoplasms. 2/3 are located in the temporal lobes, whereas 1/3 occur in the frontal lobes. Other locations, such as the lateral ventricle, are rare.

**Gross Pathology.** Grossly, DNETs thicken and expand the cortex. Most are solitary, varying in size from millimeters to several centimeters. Mucoid substances, solid areas, and small cysts are present in varying proportions **(21-10)**.

**Microscopic Features.** Microscopic hallmarks of DNETs are its multinodular intracortical growth pattern, "floating neurons" in a mucoid matrix, and a pathognomonic "specific glioneuronal element" (bundles and columns of axons lined by small oligodendroglia-like cells). The adjacent cortex is dysplastic in nearly 80% of DNETs.

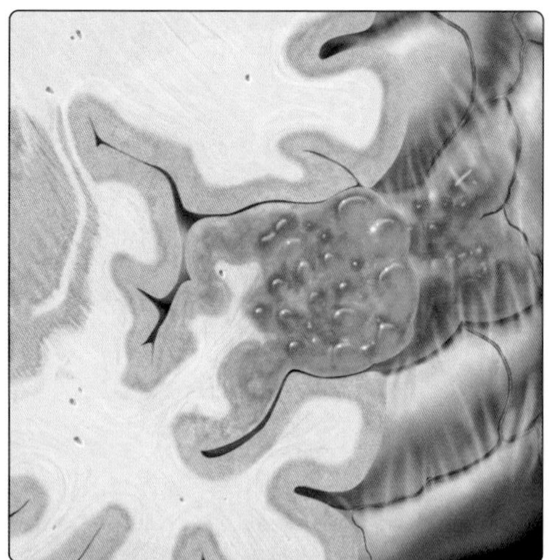

*(21-7) Graphic depicts DNET with multicystic and multinodular components.*

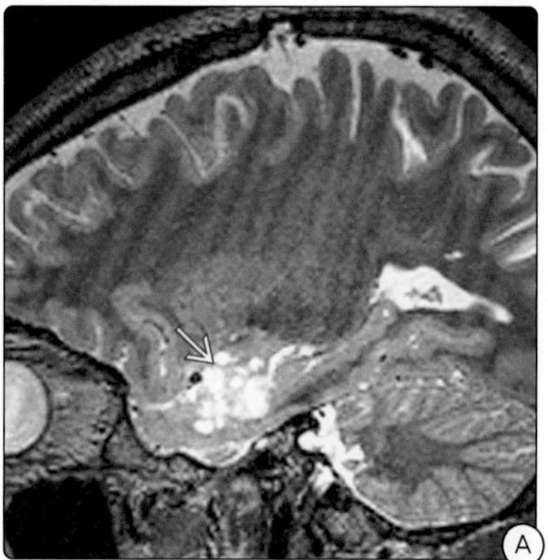

*(21-8A) Sagittal T2 MR shows a "bubbly" temporal lobe mass ➡.*

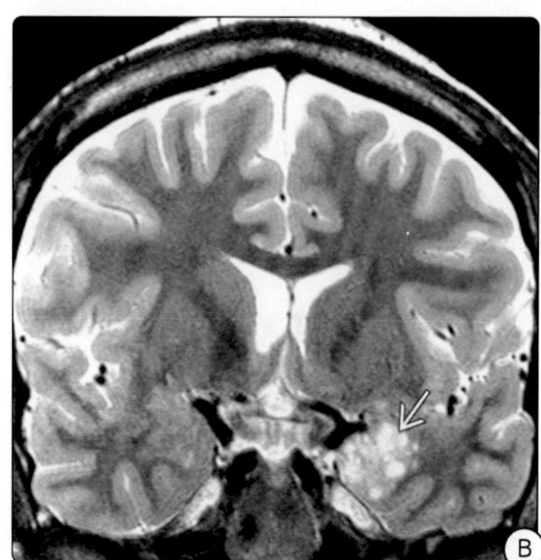

*(21-8B) Coronal T2 MR in the same patient shows a cortically based, "bubbly" mass with the typical appearance of a DNET ➡.*

**Diagnostic Molecular Pathology.** DNETs have a distinct methylation and transcriptional profile. *FGFR1* gene alterations are characteristic of DNETs and found in 40-80% of cases, although not specific to this diagnosis. *BRAF* mutations occur in 50% but should prompt diagnostic consideration of other entities, such as ganglioglioma and MAPK pathway-altered diffuse low-grade glioma.

**Grading.** DNETs are CNS WHO grade 1 neoplasms.

## Clinical Issues

DNET is a tumor of children and young adults. The vast majority present before the age of 20 years, typically with pharmacologically resistant partial complex seizures. Although DNETs account for only 1% of all primary CNS neoplasms, they are second only to ganglioglioma as a cause of temporal lobe epilepsy.

DNETs exhibit little or no growth, but because cortical dysplasia is frequently associated with DNET, a more aggressive resection is often performed. Long-term clinical follow-up usually demonstrates no tumor recurrence, even in patients with subtotal resection. Malignant transformation and CSF dissemination are exceptionally rare.

### DYSEMBRYOPLASTIC NEUROEPITHELIAL TUMOR: ETIOLOGY AND PATHOLOGY

**Etiology**
- *FGFR1* gene alteration

**Pathology**
- Benign (CNS WHO grade 1)
- Rare (< 1% of all 1° CNS tumors)
- Location
  - Supratentorial, superficial
  - Intracortical
  - Temporal lobe most common site
- Frequently associated with cortical dysplasia
  - Classified as International League Against Epilepsy (ILAE) focal cortical dysplasia (FCD) type IIIb

## Imaging

DNET has a distinct appearance on neuroimaging studies. A well-demarcated, triangular or wedge-shaped, "pseudocystic" or "bubbly" cortical/subcortical mass in a young patient with longstanding complex partial epilepsy is highly suggestive of the diagnosis **(21-8)**.

NECT scans disclose a hypodense cortical/subcortical mass **(21-9A)**. Calcification is seen in 20% of cases. Gross intratumoral hemorrhage is rare. Focal bony scalloping or calvarial remodeling is common with tumors adjacent to the inner table of the skull.

A multicystic or septated appearance is typical on MR **(21-11A)**. DNETs are strikingly hyperintense on T2WI **(21-11B)** **(21-9B)**. A FLAIR-hyperintense rim (T2/FLAIR "mismatch" sign) along the tumor periphery is present in 75% of cases **(21-11C)** **(21-9C)** **(21-12)**. Peritumoral edema is absent. "Blooming" on T2* (GRE, SWI) occurs in a few cases, more likely related to calcification than to hemorrhage.

DNETs generally show little or no enhancement on T1WI C+ **(21-9D)**. When present, enhancement is generally limited to a mild nodular or punctate pattern.

## Differential Diagnosis

The main differential diagnoses are **focal cortical dysplasia (FCD)** (often associated), **ganglioglioma**, and **multinodular and vacuolating neuronal tumor of the cerebrum** (MVNT). The bubbly appearance of DNET and FLAIR-hyperintense rim are helpful distinguishing features. MVNTs are typically multifocal and occur in the deep layers of the cortex and white matter, not superficially located like DNET.

A newly recognized tumor, **myxoid glioneuronal tumor** (MGNT) is also T2 hyperintense but occurs primarily in the septum pellucidum, subcallosal area, or juxtaventricular white matter. Similar to DNETs, MGNTs often have a FLAIR-hyperintense rim.

**Polymorphous low-grade neuroepithelial tumor of the young** (PLNTY) more often calcifies and exhibits a somewhat more infiltrative growth pattern. **Angiocentric glioma** closely resembles DNET on imaging, but a hyperintense rim is seen on T1WI, not FLAIR. A stalk-like extension toward the lateral ventricle is common.

### DYSEMBRYOPLASTIC NEUROEPITHELIAL TUMOR: CLINICAL ISSUES AND IMAGING

**Clinical Issues**
- Most patients < 20 years old
- Intractable epilepsy common
- Grows slowly; surgery usually curative

**Imaging**
- Wedge-shaped cortical/subcortical mass
- Tip "points" toward ventricle
- Multicystic/septated bubbly appearance
  - o Hyperintense on T2WI
  - o FLAIR-hyperintense rim
  - o Edema absent
  - o Usually no enhancement

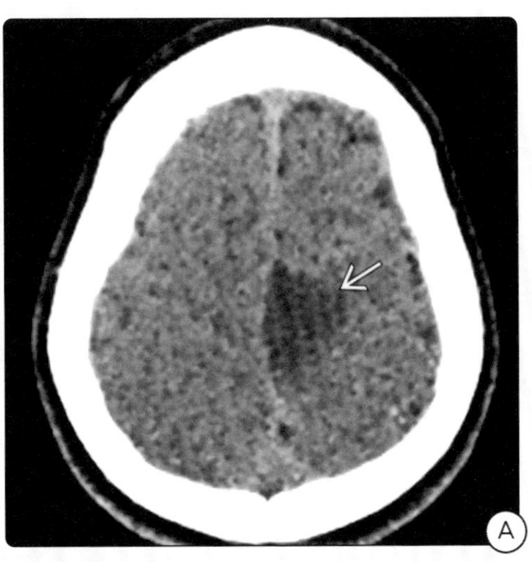


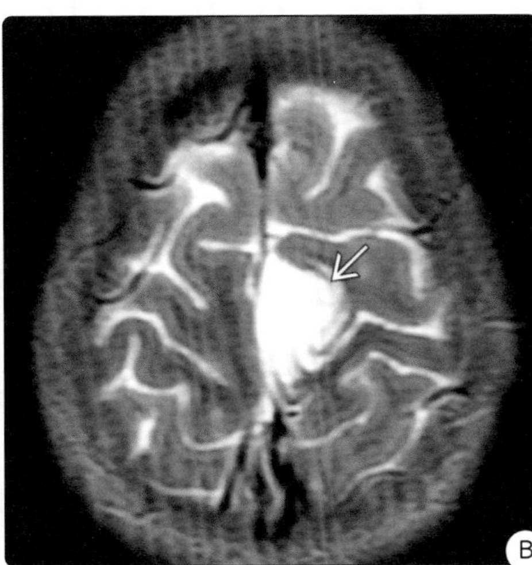


***(21-9A)** NECT in a 6-yo girl with focal seizures in the right arm and leg shows a hypodense cortical/subcortical mass ➡ in the left medial cerebral hemisphere. **(21-9B)** T2 MR in the same patient shows the mass ➡ involves mostly the cortex and is quite uniformly hyperintense.*

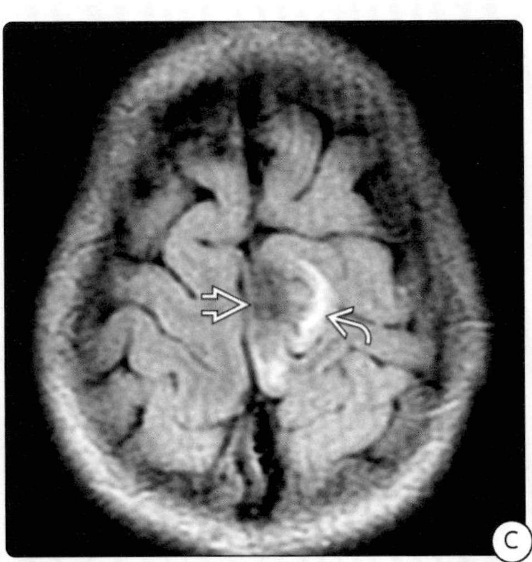


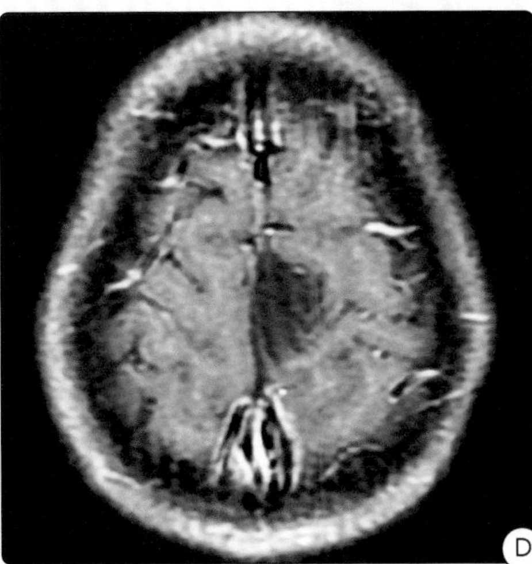


***(21-9C)** The mass has a hypointense center ➡ with a partially hyperintense rim ➡. This T2/FLAIR "mismatch" sign is common in adult IDH-mutant astrocytomas, but these tumors are rare in children. **(21-9D)** T1 C+ FS MR shows no enhancement. DNET was found at surgery.*

***(21-10)** Resected surgical specimen shows the typical nodular, somewhat mucinous-appearing cysts ➡ of a DNET. (Courtesy R. Hewlett, MD.) **(21-11A)** Sagittal T1 C+ MR in a 14-year-old boy with longstanding right body complex partial seizures shows a wedge-shaped, superficially located "bubbly" mass ➡. The mass is hypointense and shows no enhancement. Note the adjacent calvarial remodeling ➡.*

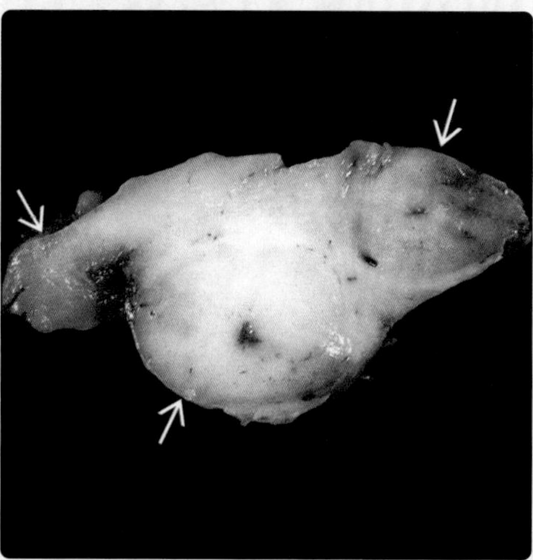

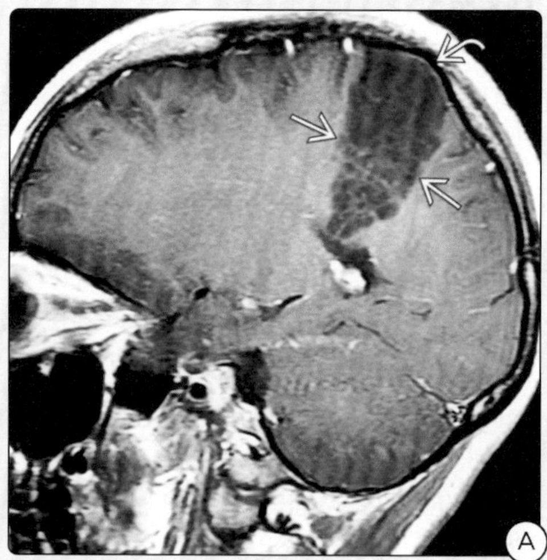

***(21-11B)** T2 MR in the same patient shows that the bubbly-appearing mass ➡ is very hyperintense and sharply demarcated. There is no surrounding edema. **(21-11C)** FLAIR MR in the same patient shows that the mass is heterogeneously hypointense with a hyperintense rim ➡. Classic DNET was found at surgery.*

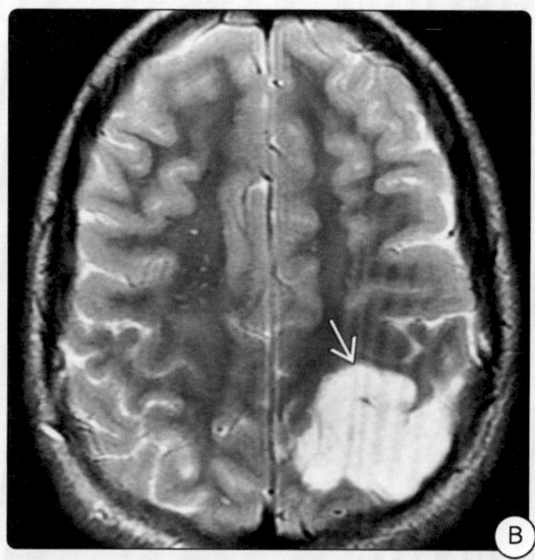

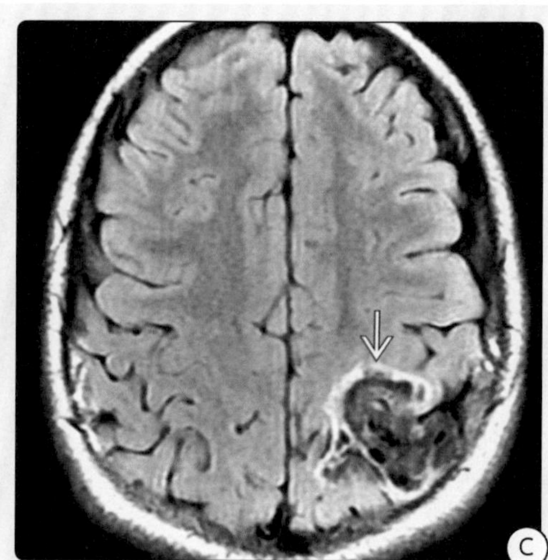

***(21-12A)** T2 MR in an 18-yo woman with seizures shows a well-defined, hyperintense cortical/subcortical mass ➡ in the right frontal lobe. **(21-12B)** FLAIR MR in the same case shows the lesion ➡ exhibits a "mismatch" sign with hyperintense rim, hypointense center. DNET was found after surgical resection.*

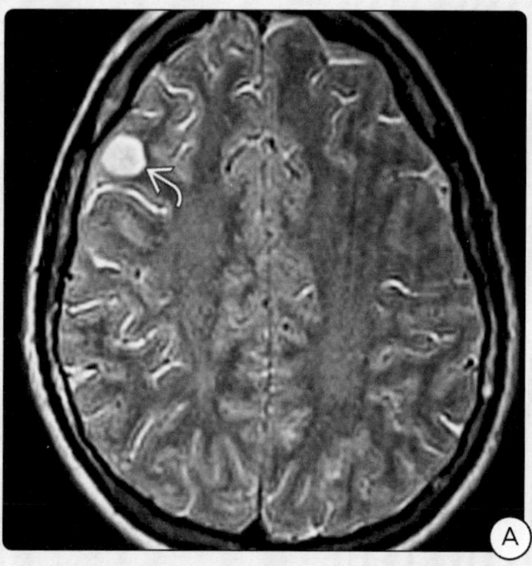

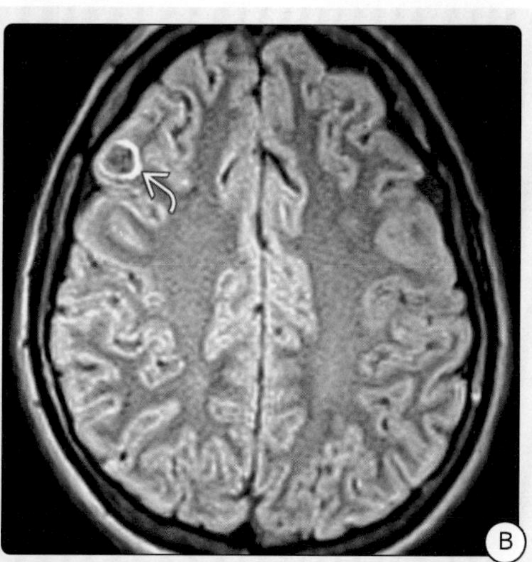

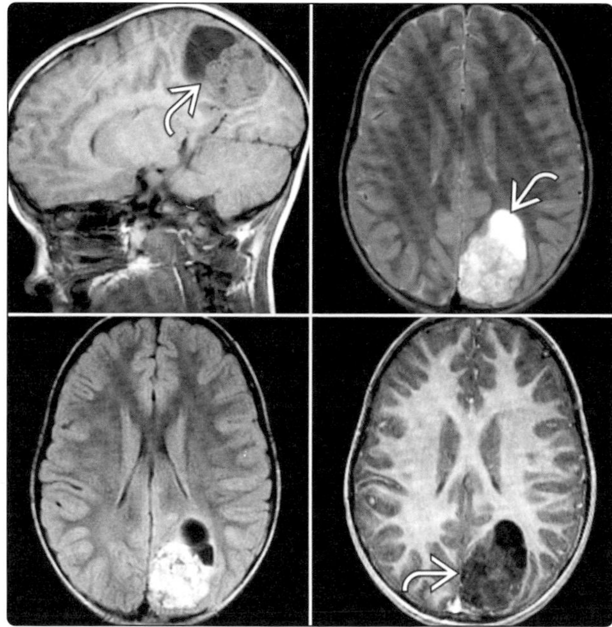

***(21-13)** Sagittal T1 (upper left), axial T2 (upper R), FLAIR (lower L), and T1 C+ (lower R) MR images show a mixed cystic/solid nonenhancing mass ➪ in a child with seizures. This is papillary glioneuronal tumor (PGNT). (Courtesy M. Castillo, MD.)*

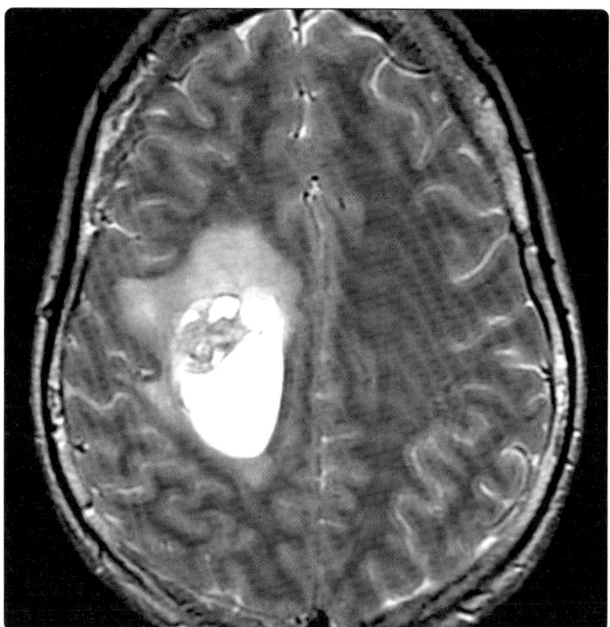

***(21-14)** T2 MR of PGNT shows a well-circumscribed cystic mass with a mural nodule in the deep white matter. (Courtesy F. J. Rodriguez, MD.)*

## Diffuse Glioneuronal Tumor With Oligodendroglioma-Like Features and Nuclear Clusters

Diffuse glioneuronal tumor with oligodendroglioma-like features and nuclear clusters (DGONC) is included in the 2021 5th edition WHO as a provisional, molecularly defined type of neuroepithelial tumor that most often occurs in children with a median age of 9-10 years. The most common presenting symptoms are seizures.

DGONCs are characterized by nuclear clusters of oligodendroglioma-like cells, strong *OLIG2* and synaptophysin expression, and absence of widespread *GFAP* expression. Histology varies from well-differentiated tumors with low mitotic index to undifferentiated cases with brisk mitotic activity. No WHO definitive grade has been established.

A distinct methylation profile of DGONC is currently the only method to clearly identify this neoplasm and is considered essential to establish the provisional diagnosis.

To date, reported cases have been located in the cortex and subcortical white matter of the frontal or temporal lobe. DGONCs adjacent to bone often demonstrate remodeling consistent with a low-grade glioneuronal tumor. DGONCs appear sharply demarcated and are most often hyperintense on T2WI and FLAIR with a ground-glass-like appearance. The presence of internal cysts within the mass is common. Perifocal edema is typically minimal or absent. Enhancement is absent in the majority of cases and, when present, is mild to moderate. Restricted diffusion is uncommon.

## Papillary Glioneuronal Tumor

Papillary glioneuronal tumor (PGNT) is a rare CNS WHO grade 1 neoplasm that primarily affects young adults. PGNTs are characterized by *PRKCA* gene fusion and exhibit a characteristic methylation profile. Histopathologically, PGNTs are biphasic tumors with both pseudopapillary glial structures and interpapillary neuronal components.

PGNTs occur in the cerebral hemispheres, often peripherally located or in the deep periventricular white matter adjacent to the lateral ventricles. The most common imaging presentation is a well-circumscribed T2-/FLAIR-hyperintense cyst with a mural nodule **(21-13)** **(21-14)**. Typically, the nodule enhances intensely; cyst wall enhancement varies.

## Rosette-Forming Glioneuronal Tumor

### Terminology

Rosette-forming glioneuronal tumor (RGNT) is a rare midline/juxtamidline glioneuronal tumor with two distinct components: Neurocytes ("rosette forming") and glial cells (piloid, oligodendroglia-like cells that resemble pilocytic astrocytoma). RGNT was originally described as occurring only in the fourth ventricle but is now recognized as occurring in other anatomic locations as well.

### Etiology

RGNTs are characterized by *FGFR1* mutations with frequent co-occurrence of a *PIK3CA* or *PIK3R1* &/or loss-of-function *NF1* mutation.

## Pathology

**Location.** RGNTs arise in or near midline structures. Initially reported in the fourth ventricle (and therefore designated RGNT "of the fourth ventricle"), the pineal region &/or aqueduct are also common sites. RGNTs can also involve the midbrain, thalami, quadrigeminal plate, brainstem, and cerebellum.

**Size and Number.** Size varies from tiny, nodular lesions to large mixed cystic/solid masses. RGNTs can spread both within the parenchyma and CSF. **In nearly 1/2 of all cases, multiple small satellite lesions in the thalami, vermis, and cerebellum are present at initial diagnosis**. Leptomeningeal (25%) and subependymal (15%) spread are common.

**Gross Pathology.** RGNTs are soft, gelatinous-appearing, well-demarcated tumors.

**Microscopic Features.** RGNTs exhibit biphasic histomorphology with distinct neurocytic and glial elements. The neurocytic elements form a rosette (ring-like array) around neuropil cores. The glial tumor component typically exhibits piloid or oligodendroglia-like histomorphology.

**Diagnostic Molecular Pathology.** Methylation class (MC) RGNT (MC-RGNT) delineates RGNT from other neurocytic CNS tumors with similar histologic features (e.g., pilocytic astrocytoma) or leptomeningeal dissemination [e.g., diffuse leptomeningeal glioneuronal tumor (DLGNT)].

**Staging, Grading, and Classification.** RGNTs are CNS WHO grade 1 neoplasms even if dispersed tumor nodules or leptomeningeal dissemination is present. Malignant transformation has been reported but is exceptionally rare.

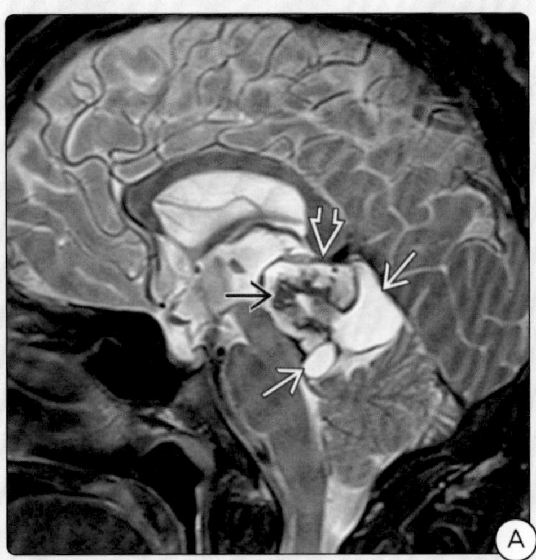

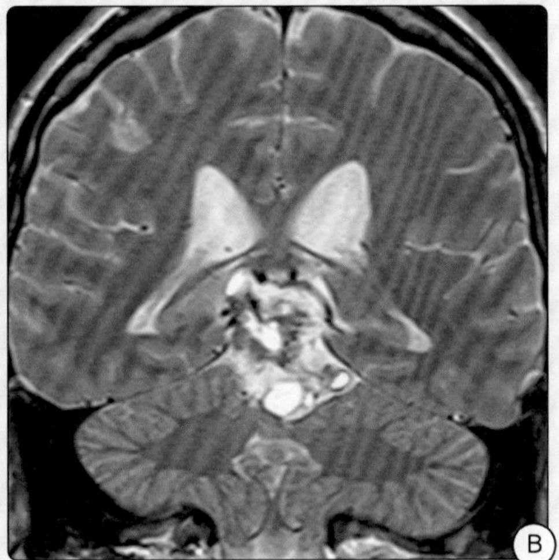

***(21-15A)** Sagittal T2 MR shows a mixed solid/cystic midline mass in the pineal region ➡. Hyperintense cysts ➡ are intermixed with hypointense foci ➡, suggesting hemorrhage. **(21-15B)** Coronal T2 MR shows the large mass exhibits extremely heterogeneous signal intensity varying from very hyperintense (relative to CSF) to strikingly hypointense.*

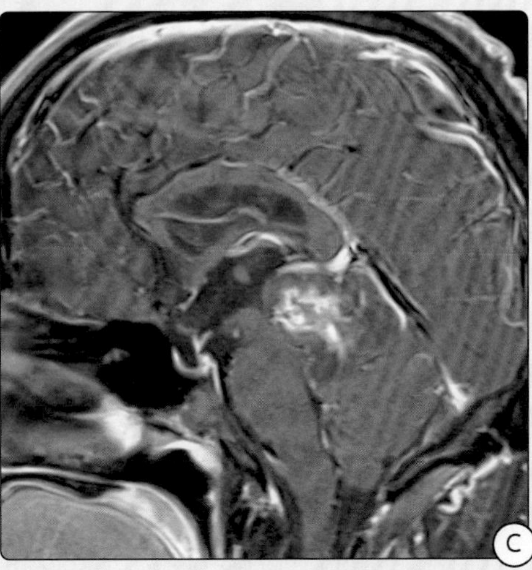

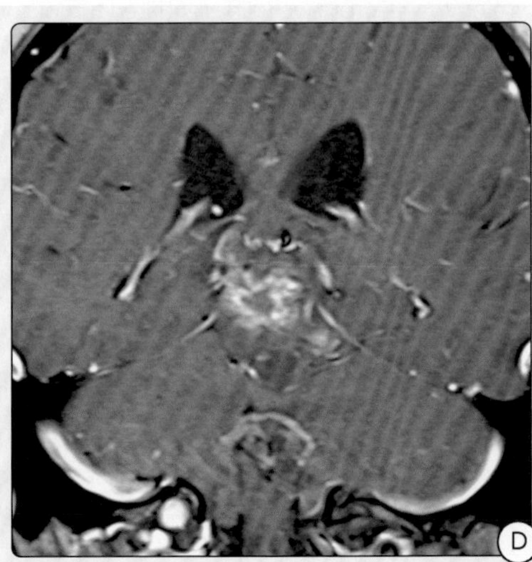

***(21-15C)** Sagittal T1 C+ FS MR shows irregular, crenellated internal enhancement within the mass. **(21-15D)** Coronal T1 C+ MR shows irregular enhancement within the mass that resembles the cut surface of a green pepper (bell pepper sign). This is rosette-forming glioneuronal tumor (RGNT), CNS WHO grade 1.*

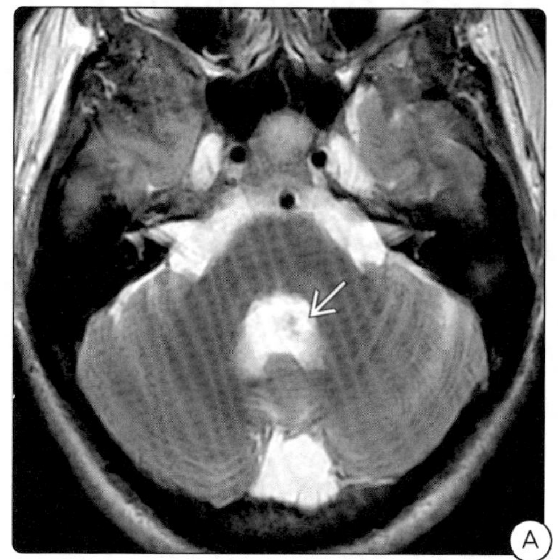


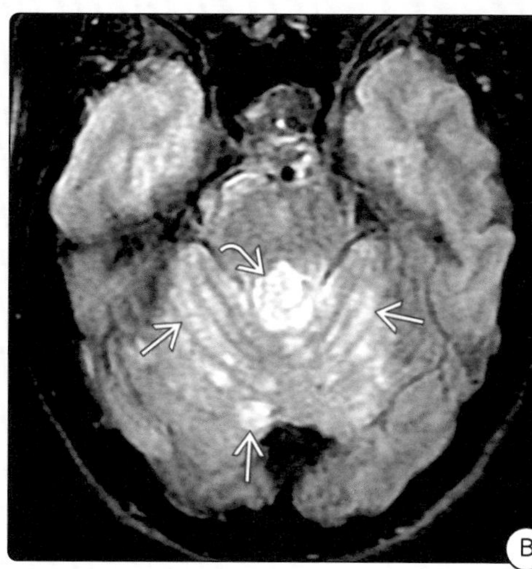


***(21-16A)*** *Axial T2 MR in a 48-yo woman with headaches shows an enlarged 4th ventricle with an ill-defined intraventricular mass ➔.* ***(21-16B)*** *Slightly more cephalad FLAIR shows the hyperintense mass extends into the upper 4th ventricle ➔. Note surfaces of the vermis and both cerebellar hemispheres are studded with innumerable hyperintense nodules ➔.*

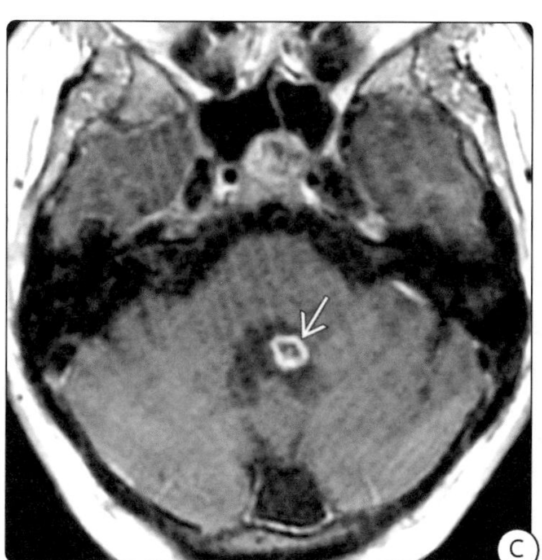


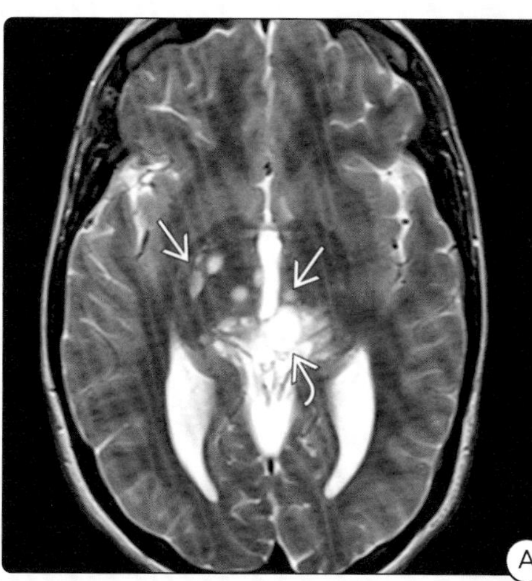


***(21-16C)*** *T1 C+ MR shows ring-like enhancement of the 4th ventricular mass ➔. The satellite lesions did not enhance. Surgery disclosed RGNT of the 4th ventricle.* ***(21-17A)*** *Initial T2 MR in a 34-yo woman with headaches shows a collection of well-demarcated hyperintense nodules scattered throughout both thalami ➔. A large focal mass is present in the left pulvinar ➔. None of the lesions enhanced on T1 C+ MR (not shown).*

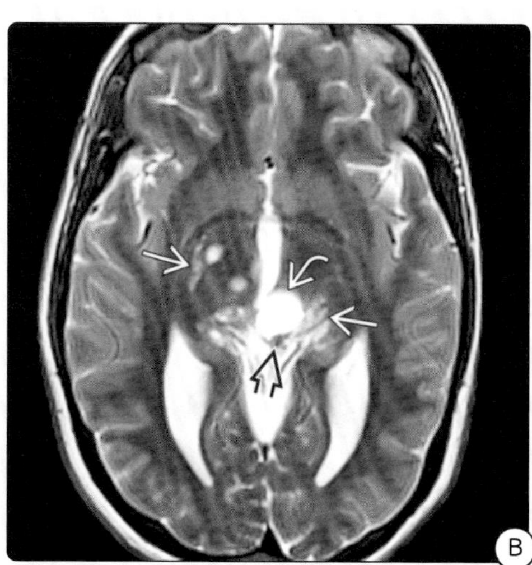


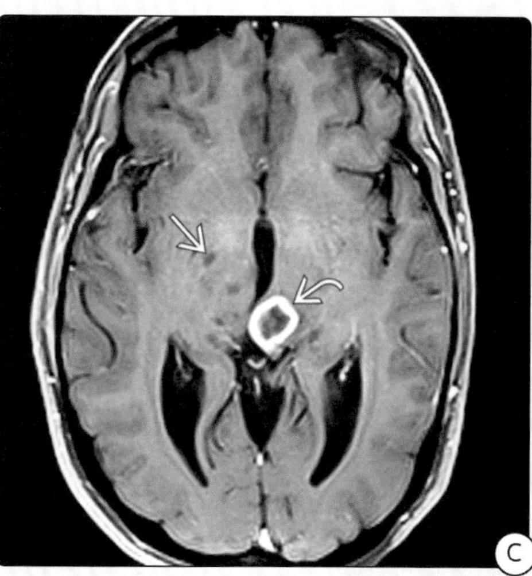


***(21-17B)*** *T2 MR obtained 4 years later shows the pulvinar lesion ➔ has enlarged slightly and now shows focal intracystic hemorrhage ➔. The satellite lesions ➔ appear stable.* ***(21-17C)*** *T1 C+ FS MR shows interval appearance of ring enhancement around the large pulvinar lesion ➔. The other nodules in the thalami ➔ show no enhancement. Biopsy disclosed RGNT, CNS WHO grade 1.*

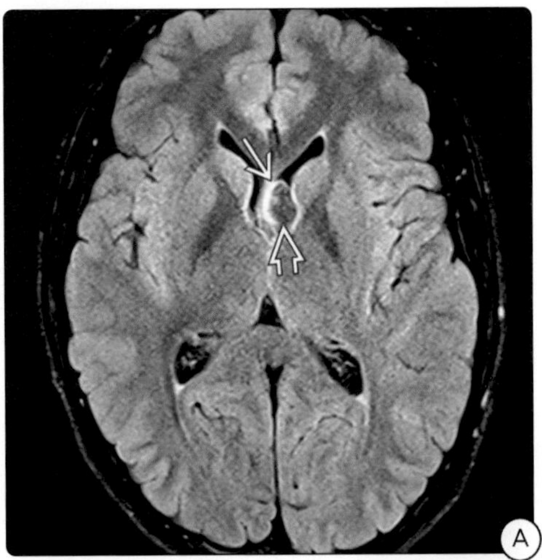


(21-18A) FLAIR MR in an 18-yo woman shows a frontal horn mass with a hyperintense rim ➡ and an isointense center ⇨.

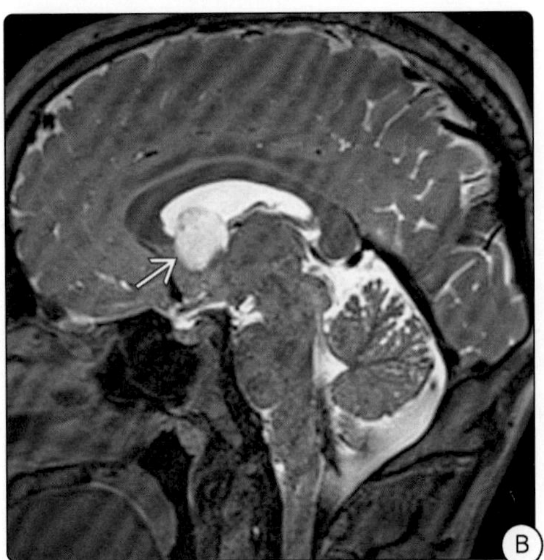


(21-18B) Sagittal T2 SPACE shows the mass ➡ is hyperintense and appears to arise from the septum pellucidum or corpus callosum rostrum.

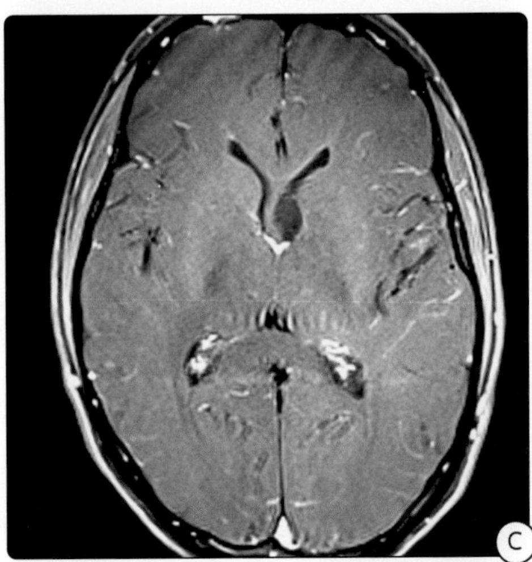


(21-18C) T1 C+ FS MR shows no enhancement. The mass has remained stable over several years. Presumed myxoid glioneuronal tumor (MGNT).

## Clinical Issues

RGNTs are tumors of adolescents and young/middle-aged adults. Headache and ataxia are common presenting symptoms.

## Imaging

**General Features.** A mixed solid/cystic mass in the fourth ventricle, aqueduct, tectum, or thalamus is typical **(21-15)**. Dispersed satellite lesions are present in nearly 50% of cases **(21-16)**.

**CT Findings.** A mixed solid/cystic mass with blood-fluid levels is common. Calcification occurs in 25% of cases.

**MR Findings.** RGNTs are T2/FLAIR heterogeneously hyperintense with variable intratumoral cysts and hemorrhage. Multiple discrete satellite lesions in the thalami and cerebellum are common **(21-16A)**. Enhancement varies from none to ring-like **(21-16C)** **(21-17C)** with a bell pepper configuration reported in some cases **(21-15D)**. If satellite lesions are present, many or most do not enhance, even if the primary tumor mass does **(21-17)**.

## Differential Diagnosis

Solitary neoplasms that can resemble RGNT include **pilocytic astrocytoma**. **Ependymoma** or **subependymoma** in the fourth ventricle can mimic RGNT, although the bell pepper appearance on T1 C+ is highly suggestive of RGNT. RGNT with multifocal satellite lesions can resemble **DLGNT**.

### ROSETTE-FORMING GLIONEURONAL TUMOR

**Etiology**
- *FGFR1* mutation characteristic

**Pathology**
- Location
  - In/near midline structures
  - 4th ventricle ± vermis, cerebellum
  - Pineal region/tectum/quadrigeminal plate
  - Thalami
- Size, number
  - Varies from small to several cm
  - ~ 50% have multiple satellite lesions in adjacent brain
- Gross pathology
  - Well demarcated
  - Soft, gelatinous
- Microscopic features
  - Biphasic neurocytic, glial elements
  - CNS WHO grade 1

**Imaging**
- CT
  - Mixed solid/cystic ± hemorrhage
- MR
  - T2/FLAIR heterogeneously hyperintense
  - Multiple discrete, FLAIR-hyperintense satellite lesions in adjacent brain
  - T1 C+ varies (none to ring-like, bell pepper configuration
- Differential diagnosis
  - In 4th ventricle? Subependymoma, ependymoma
  - In pineal/tectum? Pineal parenchymal tumor of intermediate differentiation
  - Satellite lesions can resemble DLGNT

## Myxoid Glioneuronal Tumor

### Terminology

Myxoid glioneuronal tumor (MGNT) is a CNS WHO grade 1 glioneuronal tumor characterized by *PDGFRA* p.K385 mutation and oligodendrocyte-like tumor cells embedded in a prominent mucoid matrix.

### Pathology

**Location.** MGNTs are classically located in the septum pellucidum (nucleus accumbens or cavum septum pellucidum) or subcallosal area. Less common reported sites include the corpus callosum genu and deep white matter adjacent to the lateral ventricles. CSF spread in/around the ventricles at the time of initial diagnosis is not uncommon. Multifocal dissemination to the spinal cord and nerve roots has also been reported.

**Gross Pathology.** Because of their myxoid stroma, MGNTs are typically well-delineated, soft grayish-white gelatinous masses.

**Microscopic Features.** MGNTs consist of oligodendrocyte-like tumor cells embedded in a prominent myxoid stroma. Floating neurons, neurocytic rosettes, &/or perivascular neuropil resembling DNETs and RGNTs are not uncommon. Mitotic activity is low or absent.

**Staging, Grading, and Classification.** MGNTs are CNS WHO grade 1 tumors.

**Diagnostic Molecular Pathology.** DNA methylation profiling should be performed because of the histologic overlap with other low-grade tumors, such as MGNT, DNET, and pilocytic astrocytoma. Unlike RGNT or DNET, *PIK3CA/PIK3R1* alterations or *BRAF/FGFR1* mutations are absent. Most MGNTs have a *PDGFRA* p.K385L/I dinucleotide mutation. Less common mutations in the extracellular *PDGFRA* domain have been reported.

### Clinical Issues

MGNTs occur across a wide age range (6-65 years), but most typically occur in children and young adults. Some cases are discovered incidentally on imaging. Others present with headache, ataxia, &/or vertigo.

MGNTs are indolent, slow-growing tumors. Prognosis is excellent, and patients do well even with CSF dissemination.

### Imaging

The most common appearance of MGNT is a well-delineated septum pellucidum/corpus callosum mass. MGNTs are hypointense on T1WI and, because of their myxoid stroma, are very hyperintense on T2WIs **(21-18B)**. A T2/FLAIR "mismatch" sign is common with a bright peripheral rim of hyperintensity surrounding an iso-/hypointense center **(21-18A)**. Some cases exhibit intraventricular dissemination at initial presentation **(21-19)**. MGNTs typically do not enhance on T1 C+ **(21-18C)**.

### Differential Diagnosis

MGNTs in the corpus callosum genu/septum pellucidum may resemble **subependymoma**. **Rosette-forming glioneuronal tumor** is rare in the septum pellucidum. **Central neurocytoma** is typically located in the body of the lateral ventricle, not in the septal area. **DNET** shares some imaging features with MGNT but is most common in the superficial cortex, not the white matter. **Colloid cyst** is typically located in the foramen of Monro and splays the fornices. **Ependymal cyst** (of the lateral ventricle) is thin-walled, hyperintense on CISS, and suppresses on FLAIR.

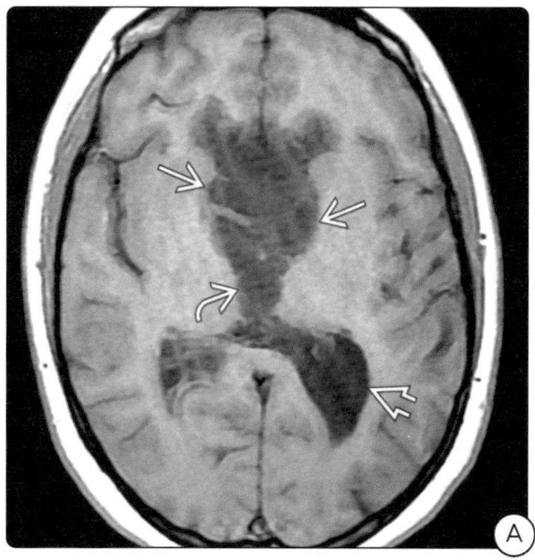


***(21-19A)** T1 MR shows a hypointense mass that fills, expands the lateral ➡ and 3rd ventricles ➡. Compare to normal CSF in the atrium ➡.*

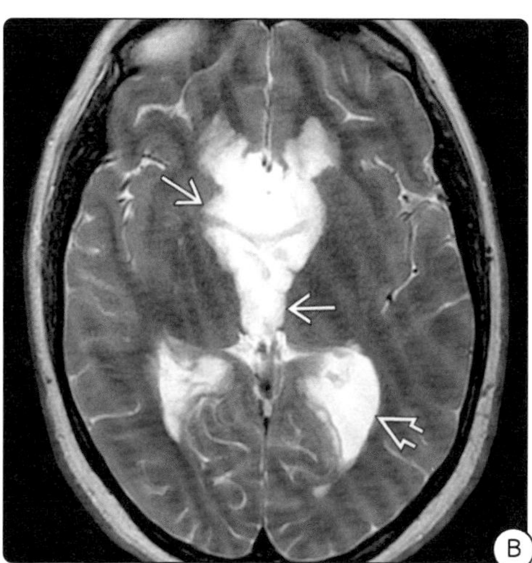


***(21-19B)** Axial T2 MR (same patient) shows the mass ➡ is lobulated, extremely hyperintense, and nearly isointense with normal CSF ➡.*

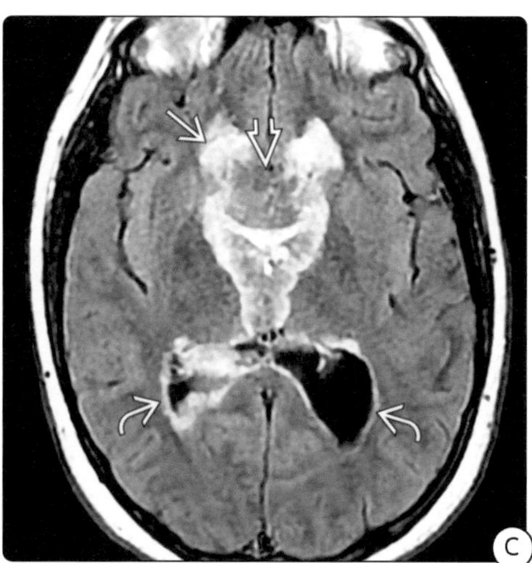


***(21-19C)** FLAIR shows hyperintense rims ➡ around an isointense tumor core ➡. Note tumor spread around ventricular ependyma ➡. MGNT.*

## Diffuse Leptomeningeal Glioneuronal Tumor

### Terminology

Diffuse leptomeningeal glioneuronal tumor (DLGNT) is a mixed glioneuronal neoplasm composed of oligodendrocyte-like cells and is characterized by chromosome 1p loss. More than 80% of cases exhibit *KIAA1549::BRAF* fusion while 1q gain is found in 56%.

### Pathology

**Location.** DLGNTs are most commonly located in the leptomeninges and basal cisterns. Between 70-75% of cases exhibit diffuse nodular leptomeningeal thickening in the suprasellar cistern, sylvian fissures, and posterior fossa. Tumor deposits are frequent in the cerebral ventricles, along cranial nerves and the spinal cord surface **(21-20)**.

Discrete parenchymal lesions are common, typically spreading along the Virchow-Robin (perivascular) spaces (VRSs). Up to 1/3 of cases have an isolated spinal cord mass.

**Size and Number.** Innumerable small, cyst-like tumor nodules are present throughout the basal cisterns. Nodular thickening of the cranial and spinal leptomeninges is typical.

**Gross Pathology.** Diffuse, nodular, glistening, mucoid-appearing leptomeningeal infiltrates along brain/cord surfaces are typical.

**Microscopic Features.** DLGNTs exhibit oligodendroglioma-like morphology. Features of both glial and neuronal differentiation with synaptophysin-positive neurocytes and GFAP-positive glial cells are present. Parenchymal extension along the VRSs is common, and focal mass-like lesions may be present.

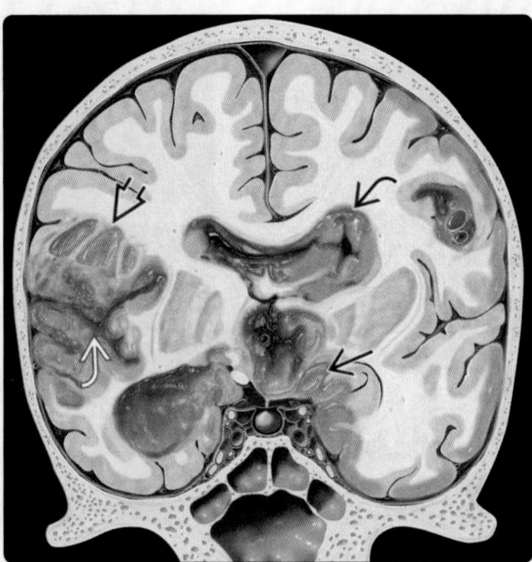

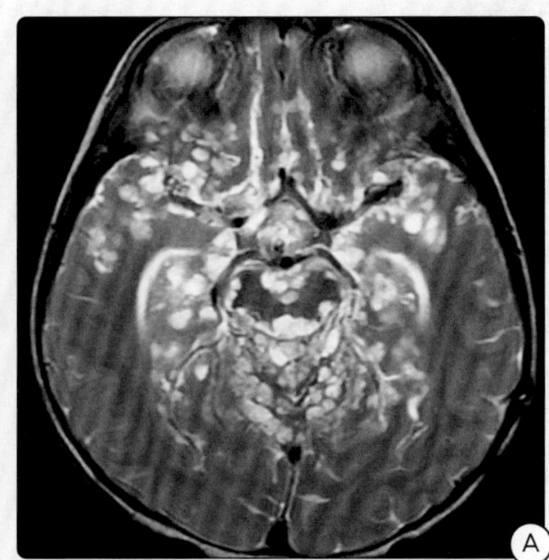

*(21-20) Coronal graphic of diffuse leptomeningeal glioneuronal tumor (DLGNT) shows multiple mucinous-appearing cysts throughout subarachnoid spaces ➡, in ventricles ➡, brain parenchyma ➡. Leptomeninges ➡ are thickened. (21-21A) T2 MR in a child with DLGNT shows innumerable well-demarcated tiny hyperintense cysts throughout basal cisterns, subarachnoid spaces, and along surfaces of midbrain and vermis.*

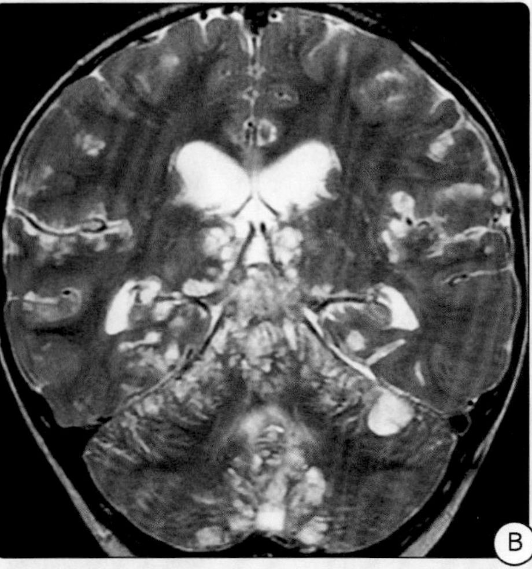

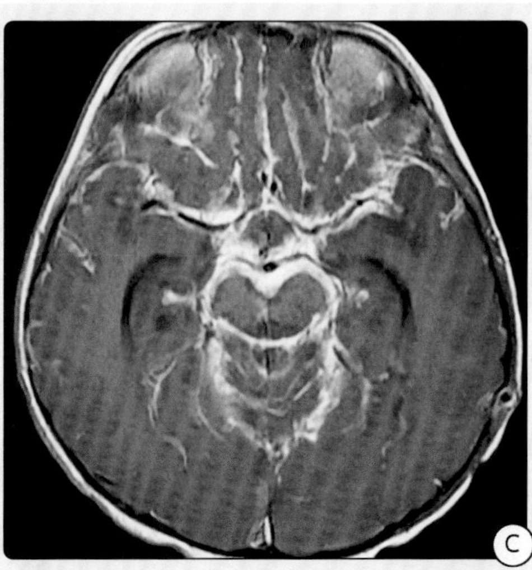

*(21-21B) Coronal T2 MR in the same patient shows the cysts along the surfaces of the cerebellum and sylvian fissures. Some cysts are present in the medial thalami. (21-21C) T1 C+ MR in the same patient shows diffuse leptomeningeal thickening and enhancement. This is DLGNT. (Courtesy T. Poussaint, MD.)*

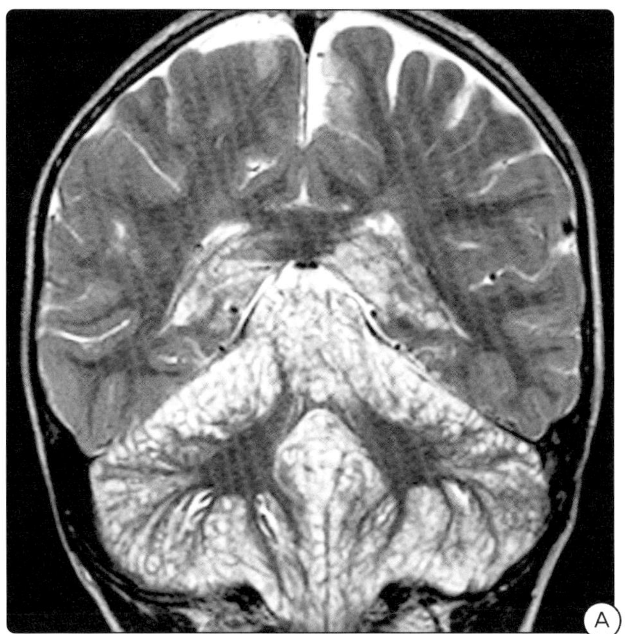


*(21-22A) Coronal T2 MR in a child with DLGNT [originally called disseminated oligodendroglioma-like leptomeningeal neoplasm (DOLN)] shows innumerable hyperintense tumor nodules along surfaces of the cerebellum and lateral ventricles.*

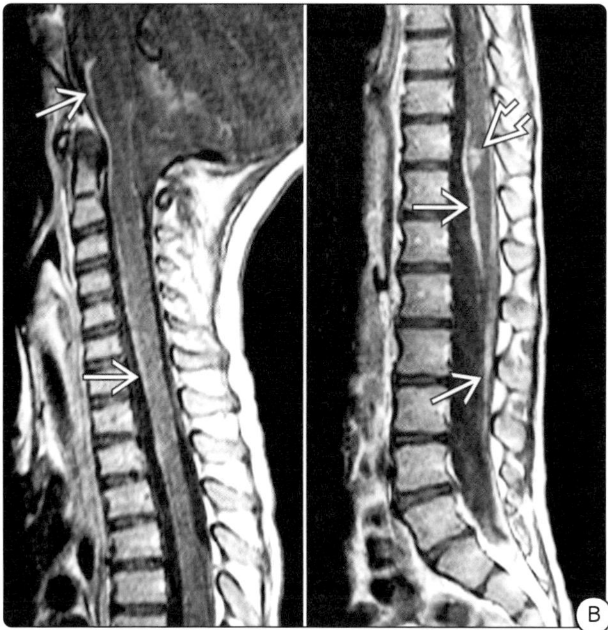


*(21-22B) T1 C+ MR of the cervical (L) and lumbar (R) spine in the same patient shows diffuse pial thickening, enhancement along the brainstem, cord, and spinal nerve roots ➡. Note the lesion within the cord itself ⇨. (Courtesy S. Blaser, MD.)*

**Staging, Grading, and Classification.** DLGNT comprises two distinct methylation classes (MCs): MC-1 and MC-2. Recent studies show that chromosome 1q gain is the only significant prognosticator affecting progression-free survival in DLGNTs, regardless of MC. While no formal CNS WHO grades have been established, DLGNTs without 1q gain have outcomes compatible with CNS WHO grade 1. Most all MC-2 tumors have 1q gain with median time to death of 51 months, an outcome compatible with WHO grade 3 lesions.

## Clinical Issues

**Epidemiology.** DLGNTs are rare and generally occur in childhood (3-14 years with median age of five years). There is a slight male predominance.

**Presentation.** Headaches, seizures, and gait imbalance are common.

**Natural History.** Clinical behavior is variable. Prognosis is strongly associated with 1q status. Tumors with 1q gain are ~ 20x more likely to progress. MC-2 tumors with 1q gain have inferior survival compared to MC-1 tumors (± 1q gain).

## Imaging

**General Features.** Multiple T2-hyperintense cyst-like nodules along the surfaces of the brain &/or spine accompanied by thick/nodular leptomeningeal enhancement are the classic imaging findings

**MR Findings.** Multiple small, T1 hypo- and T2-hyperintense leptomeningeal cysts cover the brain surfaces, especially along the basilar cisterns, sylvian fissures, and cerebellum **(21-21A)** **(21-21B)** **(21-22A)**. The cysts remain hyperintense on FLAIR. Thick, nodular leptomeningeal enhancement along the pial surfaces is typical **(21-21C)**. The entire spine should be imaged, as intraparenchymal lesions are common as is diffuse enhancement along the cauda equina **(21-22)**.

## Differential Diagnosis

**Leptomeningeal carcinomatosis** from diffuse pediatric-type high-grade gliomas, high-grade astrocytoma with piloid features, and occasionally even pilocytic astrocytomas can exhibit leptomeningeal dissemination. The associated T2-hyperintense nodules along the brain and spinal cord that are so characteristic of DLGNTs are absent.

Sulcal-cisternal enhancement from **pyogenic meningitis** is typically smooth rather than nodular. Occasionally, **TB meningitis** can exhibit a nodular configuration. **"Racemose" neurocysticercosis** with T2-hyperintense scolices in the CSF spaces can mimic DLGNT. **Neurosarcoidosis** typically affects older patients, and dural-based focal masses are more common than diffuse nodular meningeal lesions.

# Multinodular and Vacuolating Neuronal Tumor

## Terminology

Multinodular and vacuolating neuronal tumor (MVNT) was codified in the 2021 5th edition WHO as a true clonal neoplasm with MAPK pathway-activating abnormalities.

## Pathology

**Location.** MVNTs are discrete or coalescent clusters of variably sized (usually small) nodules along the inner (deep) surface of the cortical ribbon in a U-shaped configuration **(21-**

23). Scattered discrete nodules extending into the deep white matter toward the lateral ventricles are common. A few cases have been reported in the cerebellar hemispheres and vermis. These have been termed multinodular and vacuolating posterior fossa lesions of unknown significance (MV-PLUS).

**Gross Pathology.** MVNTs are characterized by multiple discrete or coalescent nodules, often with vacuolar changes.

**Microscopic Features.** Discrete tumor nodules with mature-appearing neurons and prominent intracellular, stromal vacuolation are typical **(21-24)**. MVNTs are OLIG2 and synaptophysin positive, GFAO and NeuN negative. Mitotic activity, necrosis, and microvascular proliferation are absent.

**Staging, Grading, and Classification.** MVNTs are CNS WHO grade 1 lesions.

## Clinical Issues

**Presentation.** Most MVNTs are discovered incidentally on imaging studies. Occasionally, patients present with nonfocal headache &/or, rarely, seizures.

**Natural History.** MVNTs are benign, clinically indolent, nonprogressive lesions. The size and imaging appearance are stable over multiple years. Unless proven as epileptogenic (very rare), MVNTs are "leave me alone" lesions that do not need to be biopsied or followed up.

**Demographics.** MVNTs occur at all ages. The mean age of reported cases is 39 years.

## Imaging

**General Features.** The most characteristic MR finding is a cluster of variably sized, usually small (1- to 5-mm), sharply marginated clusters of T2-/FLAIR-hyperintense nodules ("bubbles") hugging the inner surface of the cortical ribbon in a distinct U-shaped configuration **(21-25)**. Discrete nodules may extend into the deep white matter **(21-28)**.

**CT Findings.** CT is usually normal. Larger lesions may appear as a faint, ill-defined wedge or U-shaped subcortical hypodensity **(21-26A)**. Calcification, mass effect, and hemorrhage are absent.

**MR Findings.** MVNTs are isointense with cortex on T1WI, hyperintense on T2WI, and do not suppress on FLAIR **(21-27)**. MVNTs are occasionally bright on DWI/ADC **(21-26B)**, which can be helpful in detecting small/subtle lesions. MVNTs do not enhance on T1 C+ **(21-29)**.

pMR shows slightly decreased cerebral blood volume. MRS can be normal but may show slightly increased Cho and decreased NAA **(21-28C)**.

Most MVNTs are small. Occasionally, larger groups of discrete and coalescent nodules can be seen **(21-28)**. Mass effect is absent, even with larger lesions.

## Differential Diagnosis

The appearance of MVNTs is virtually pathognomonic. Subtle, scattered discrete nodules may extend into the deep white matter toward the lateral ventricle, aiding the diagnosis. Most MVNTs are discovered incidentally on imaging and are almost always asymptomatic.

MVNTs are **not "atypical"** or **"enlarged perivascular spaces"** as perivascular spaces spare the cortical ribbon and suppress on FLAIR.

**Focal cortical dysplasia** affects the superficial, not the deep, cerebral cortex and is generally isointense with gray matter on all sequences. The affected cortex is typically distorted and dysplastic appearing.

MVNTs are sometimes mistaken for low-grade epilepsy-associated tumors, such as **ganglioglioma**, **pleomorphic xanthoastrocytoma**, **pilocytic astrocytoma**, **and DNET**.

### MULTINODULAR AND VACUOLATING NEURONAL TUMOR

**Etiology**

- True clonal neoplasm
    - MAPK pathway-activating abnormalities

**Pathology**

- Discrete tumor nodules
    - Neoplastic neuronal elements
    - Vacuolar changes in fibrillar matrix
- No mitoses, vascular proliferation, or necrosis
- CNS WHO grade 1

**Clinical Features**

- Occur in all ages (mean: 39 years)
- Usually incidental finding on imaging
- Rare cases associated with seizures
- Nonprogressive
    - Stable over multiple years
    - Regarded as "leave me alone" lesions
    - Classic imaging? No need for biopsy or follow-up

**Imaging**

- Cluster of small, discrete, T2-/FLAIR-hyperintense nodules
- Hugs inner surface of cortex
- Scattered nodules may extend into deep WM
- No mass effect
- No enhancement on T1 C+
- ~ 50% hyperintense on DWI and ADC

**Differential Diagnosis**

- DNET
    - Superficial cortex
    - Mass effect
- Focal cortical dysplasia
    - Thickened, distorted cortex
    - Isointense with GM on all sequences
- "Atypical" perivascular spaces? No!
    - CSF-like signal on all sequences
    - Suppress on FLAIR
    - 25% have peripheral hyperintensity
    - Mass effect common

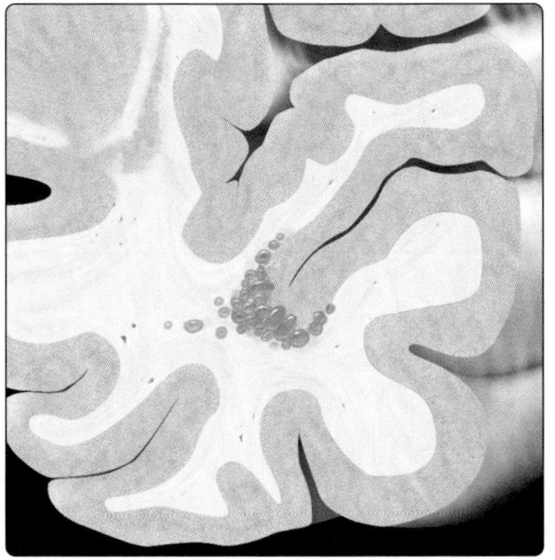

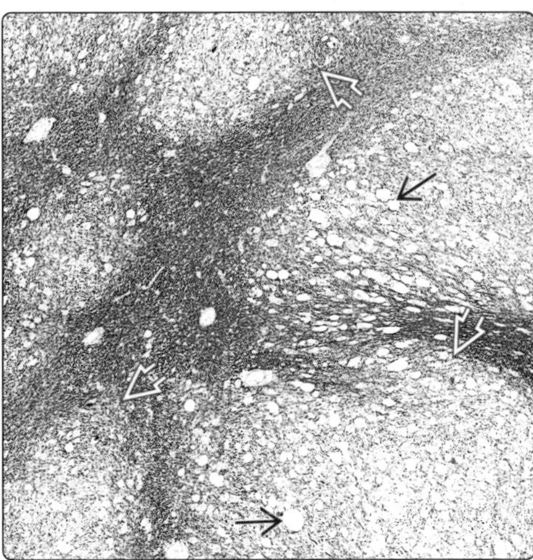

***(21-23)** Graphic of multinodular and vacuolating neuronal tumor (MVNT) shows well-delineated nodules along the inner margin of the cortex with smaller discrete nodules in adjacent white matter.* ***(21-24)** Micrograph of MVNT shows discrete tumor nodules ➡ with vacuolar changes ➡. (Courtesy B. K. Kleinschmidt-DeMasters, MD.)*

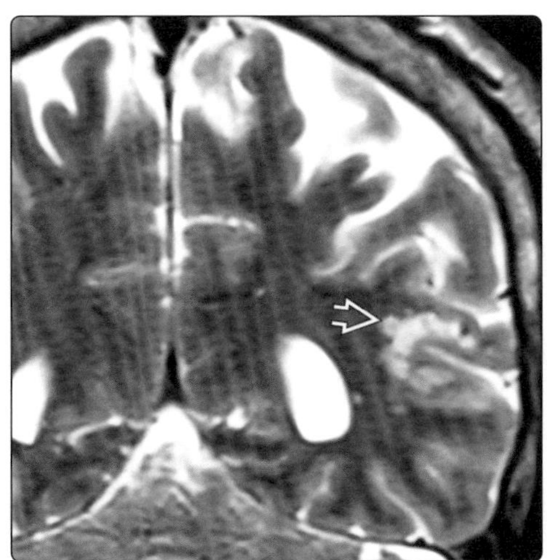

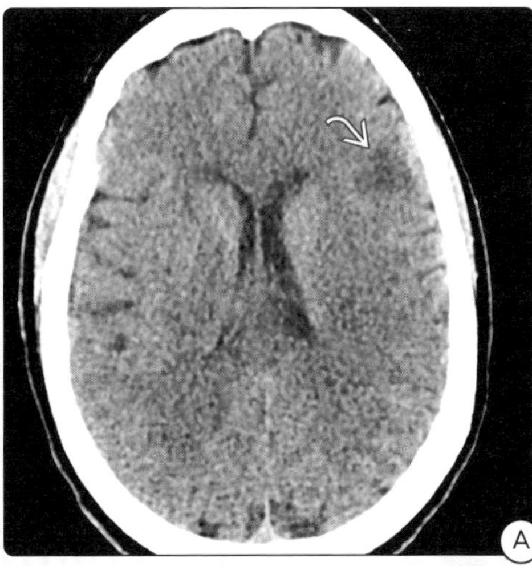

***(21-25)** Coronal T2 MR of MVNT shows hyperintense nodules ➡ cupping the undersurface of the cortex. Lesions did not suppress on FLAIR.* ***(21-26A)** Axial NECT in a patient with minor head trauma shows an ill-defined hypodense area ➡ in the subcortical white matter. No mass effect is present.*

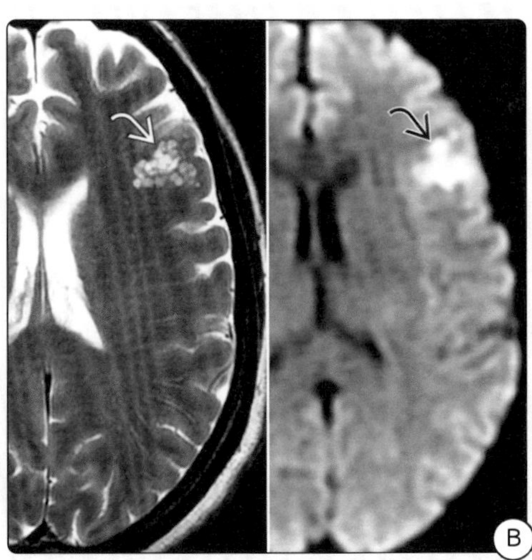

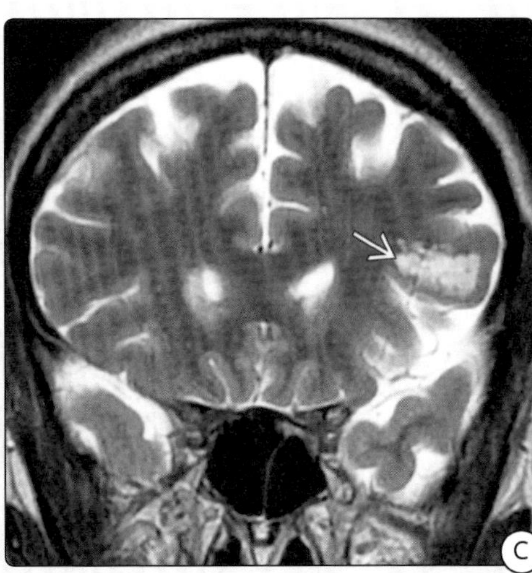

***(21-26B)** (L) T2 MR in the same patient shows a classic "cluster" of hyperintense nodules ➡ in the left frontal subcortical and deep white matter. The lesions did not suppress on FLAIR and did not enhance (not shown). (R) The lesions are hyperintense on DWI ➡ and were hyperintense on ADC (not shown).* ***(21-26C)** Coronal T2 MR shows a cluster of hyperintense "bubbles" in the inner cortex/subcortical white matter ➡. This is biopsy-proven MVNT.*

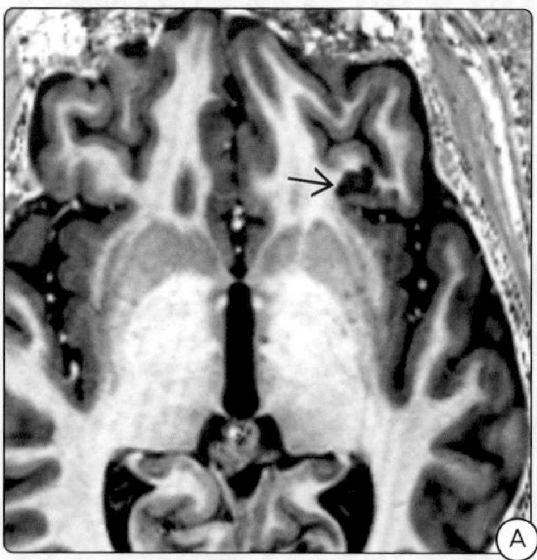

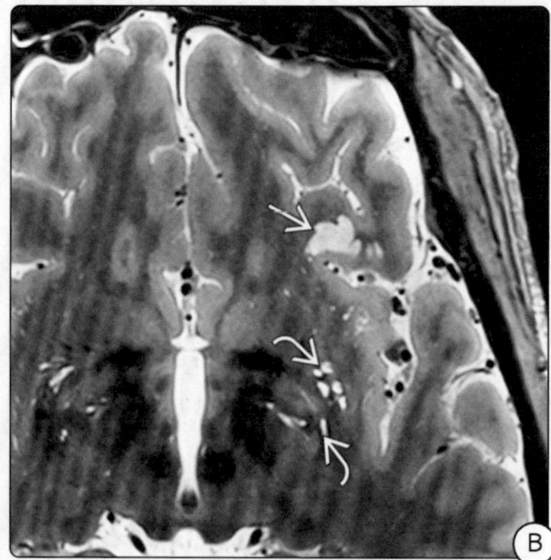

***(21-27A)*** *Axial T1 MR in a normal patient at 7T shows an incidental finding of confluent, rounded, hypointense nodules along the inner surface of the cortex adjacent to the sylvian fissure.* ***(21-27B)*** *T2 MR at 7T in the same patient shows the cluster of well-delineated nodules along the inner cortex is hyperintense and does not exert mass effect. Note typical perivascular spaces in the basal ganglia adjacent to the anterior commissure.*

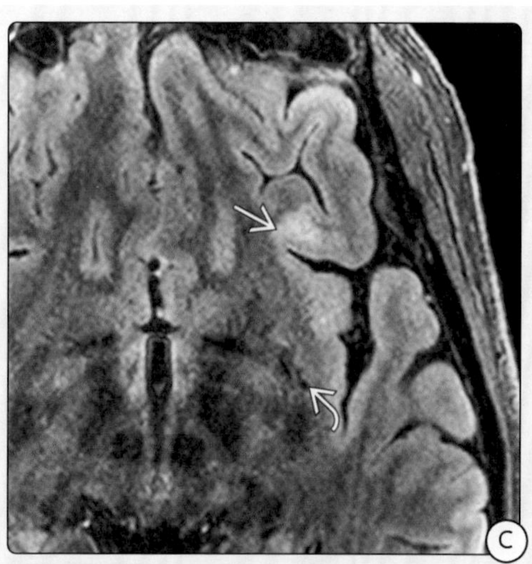

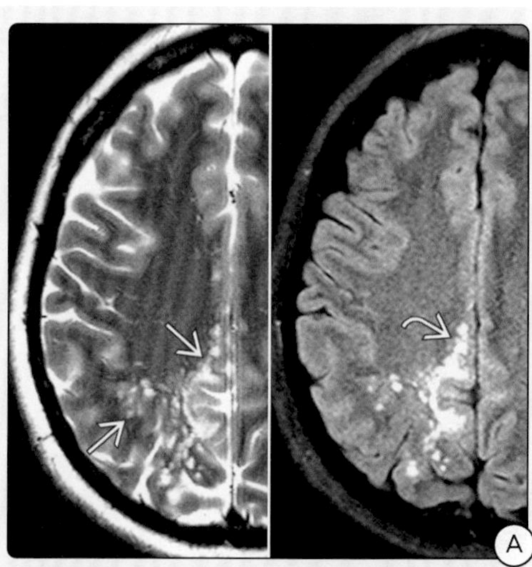

***(21-27C)*** *7T FLAIR shows the collection of coalescent nodules does not suppress while the perivascular spaces around the anterior commissure suppress completely.* ***(21-28A)*** *MR in a 40-yo woman with headaches is shown. (L) Axial T2 shows an odd collection of discrete and confluent hyperintense nodules in the subcortical and deep white matter. (R) The nodules cup the inner cortical surface and do not suppress on FLAIR.*

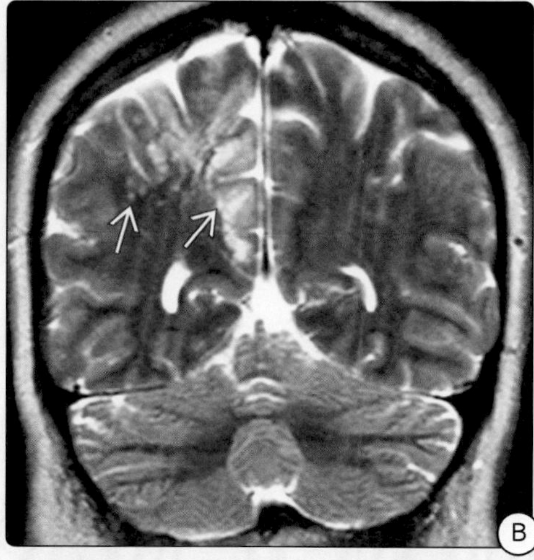

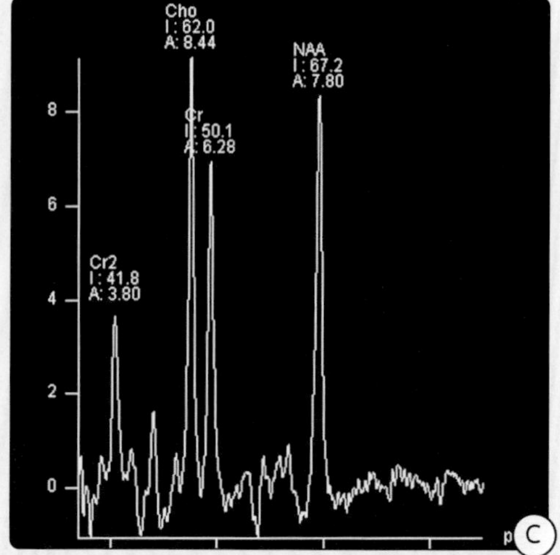


***(21-28B)*** *Coronal T2 MR in the same patient shows numerous discrete, hyperintense nodules extending into the white matter toward the lateral ventricle.* ***(21-28C)*** *MRS shows very slightly elevated choline and mildly decreased NAA. This is presumed MVNT.*

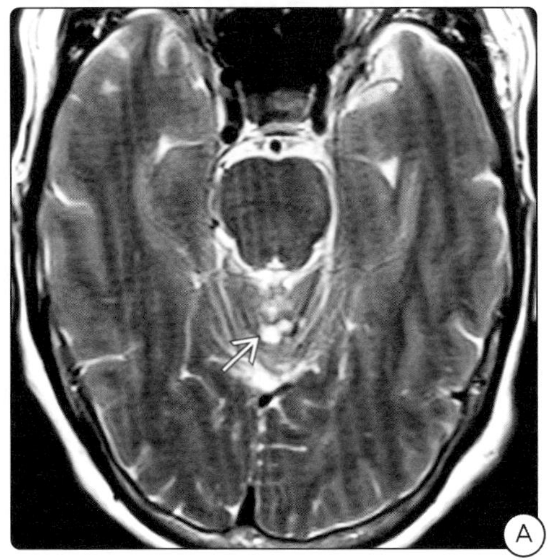

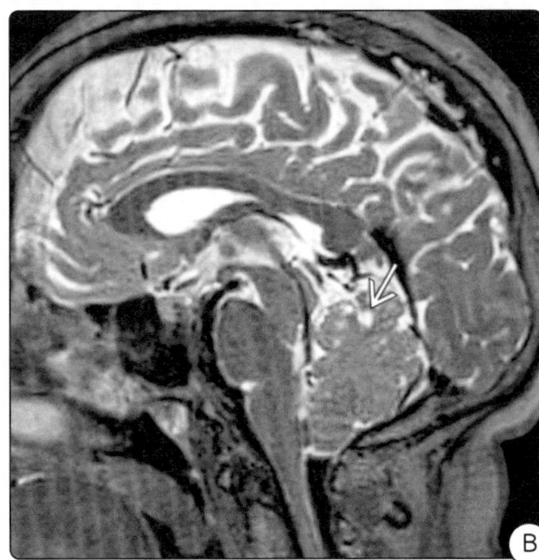

***(21-29A)** T2 MR in a 52-yo woman with headaches and a history of prior head trauma shows a collection of well-delineated, discrete, hyperintense nodules ➡ in the cerebellar vermis. **(21-29B)** Sagittal T2 SPACE shows multiple discrete, hyperintense nodules ➡ in the vermis.*

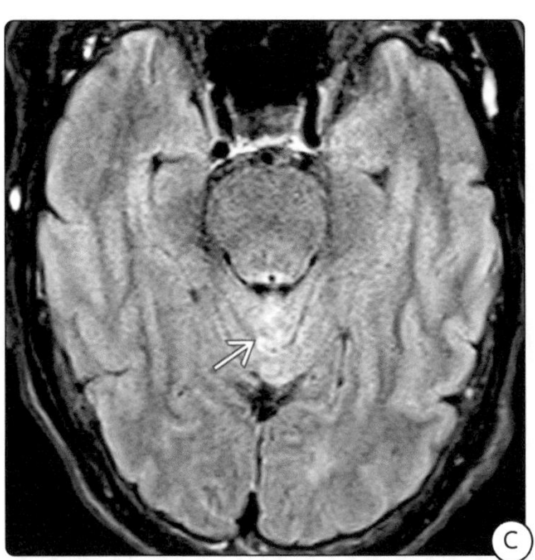

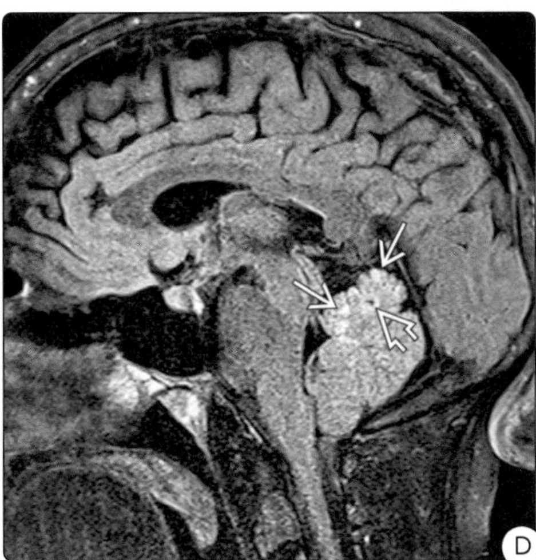

***(21-29C)** The nodules ➡ do not suppress on FLAIR. No mass effect or edema in the adjacent cerebellum is present. **(21-29D)** Sagittal FLAIR shows most of the nodules remain hyperintense ➡. One nodule has a hypointense center with a hyperintense rim ➡.*

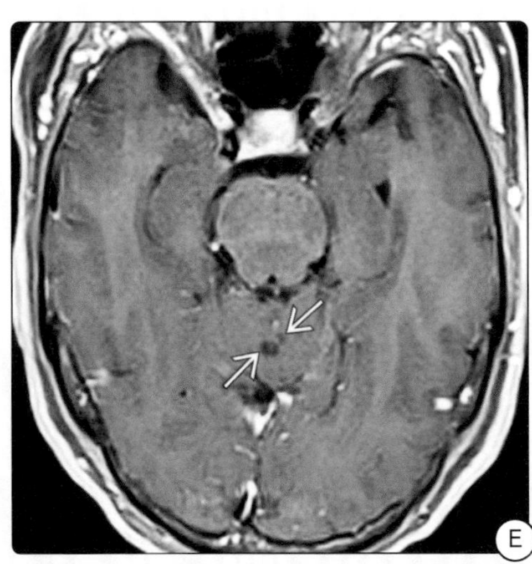

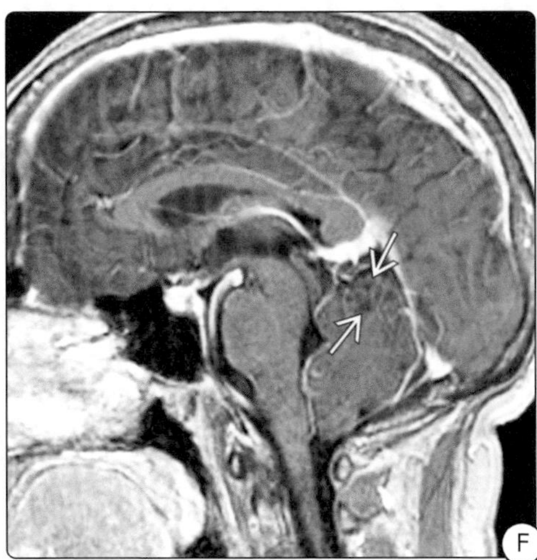

***(21-29E)** Axial T1 C+ FS MR shows no enhancement in the nodules ➡. **(21-29F)** Sagittal T1 C+ MR shows the nodules ➡ are hypointense and do not enhance. Repeat scan 5 years later showed no change. This is presumed MVNT in the posterior fossa (sometimes called MV-PLUS).*

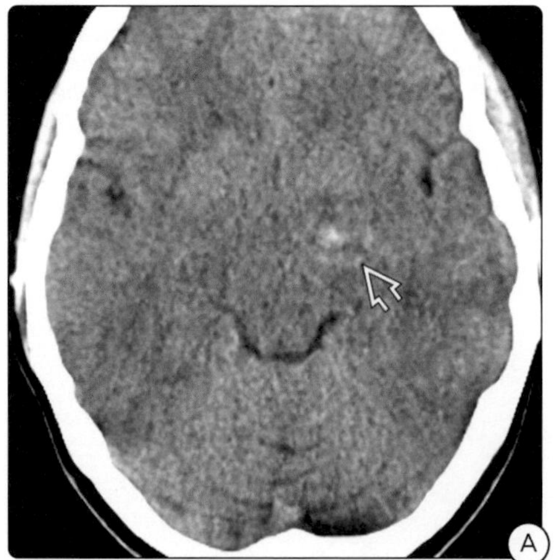

*(21-30A) NECT in a 22-yo woman with seizures shows a partially calcified, mixed-density mass in the left thalamus.*

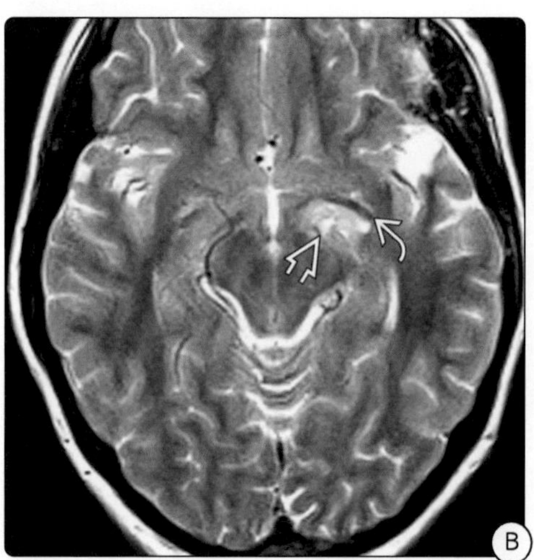

*(21-30B) The mass is heterogeneously hyperintense on T2 MR. Note minimal mass effect on the anterior commissure.*

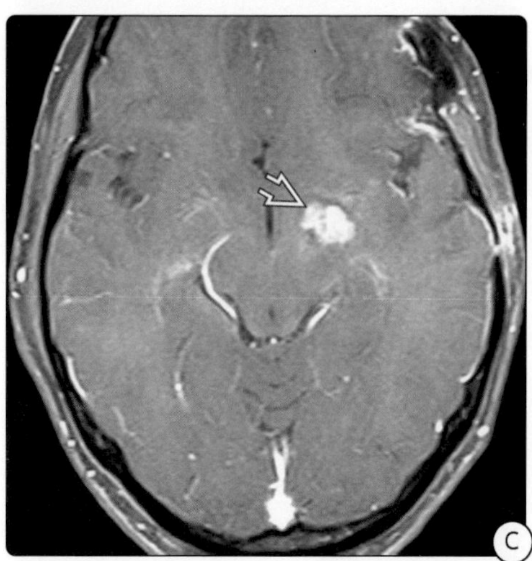

*(21-30C) The mass enhances strongly on T1 C+ FS MR. Biopsy disclosed gangliocytoma, CNS WHO grade 1.*

# Neuronal Tumors

Tumors that exhibit exclusive ganglion cell or neurocytic differentiation are rare. Two general categories of neuronal tumors are recognized: Gangliocytoma and neurocytoma.

We begin our discussion of ganglion cell tumors with a brief consideration of the pure ganglion cell neoplasm, **gangliocytoma**, before discussing dysplastic cerebellar gangliocytoma (better known as **Lhermitte-Duclos disease**). We close this section with a consideration of **neurocytomas** (central neurocytoma, extraventricular neurocytoma, and cerebellar liponeurocytoma).

## Gangliocytoma

### Terminology

Gangliocytoma (GCyt) is a benign, well-circumscribed neuroepithelial neoplasm that contains irregular clusters of mostly mature neoplastic ganglion cells, often with dysplastic features.

### Pathology

GCyts are rare, accounting for < 1% of CNS neoplasms. They have been reported throughout the CNS but are most common in the cerebral hemispheres, especially the temporal lobe. A few cases have been reported in the cerebral ventricles and spinal cord.

GCyts are solid or mixed solid and cystic tumefactive lesions that consist of bizarre-appearing but mature ganglion cells in a matrix that is often indistinguishable from normal brain. Cytoplasmic ballooning or vacuolization is common. Glial elements are rare or absent and free of atypia. Mitotic activity is absent.

GCyts are CNS WHO grade 1 neoplasms.

### Clinical Issues

GCyt occurs most frequently in children and young adults under the age of 30 years. Most patients present with pharmacoresistant epilepsy. GCyts grow slowly, if at all. Surgical resection is generally curative.

Dysplastic **cerebellar** gangliocytoma is associated with Cowden syndrome and is discussed separately.

### Imaging

GCyts are of mixed density on NECT, often containing both cystic and solid components. Calcification is common, occurring in ~ 1/3 of cases **(21-30A)**. Hemorrhage and necrosis are absent.

GCyts are hypo- to isointense relative to cortex on T1WI and hyperintense on T2/FLAIR. Enhancement varies from none to striking homogeneous enhancement in the solid portions of the tumor **(21-30)**.

### Differential Diagnosis

The major differential diagnosis of a hemispheric GCyt is **ganglioglioma**. Gangliogliomas are far more common and may be indistinguishable from GCyt on imaging studies. **DNETs** have a bubbly appearance and often have a FLAIR-hyperintense rim. **Multinodular and vacuolating neuronal tumors (MVNTs)** are collections of multiple T2-/FLAIR-hyperintense nodules along the undersurface of the cerebral cortex and do not cause mass effect. The

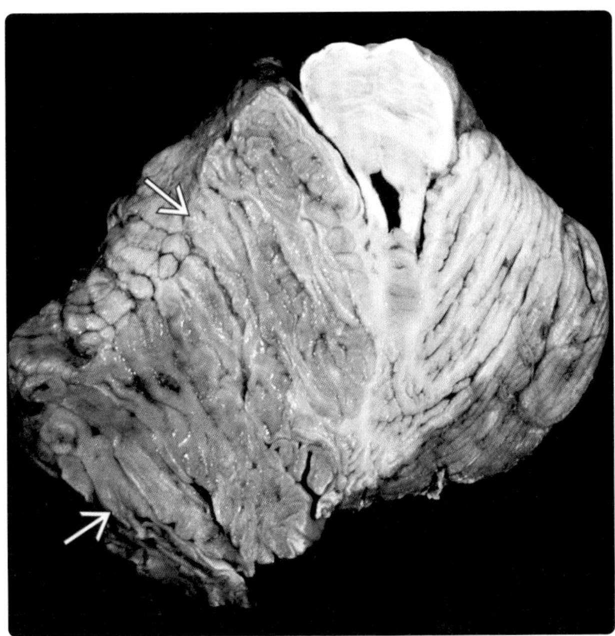

*(21-31) Cut section through a dysplastic cerebellar gangliocytoma shows grossly thickened cerebellar folia ➡ expanding the cerebellar hemisphere. (Courtesy AFIP Archives.)*

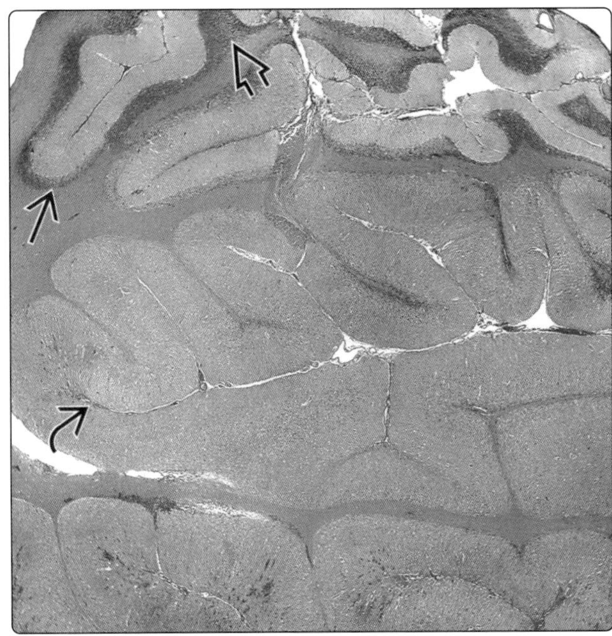

*(21-32) Folia expansion in Lhermitte-Duclos disease (LDD) is shown. Contrast normal cerebellum ➡ with expanded cerebellar cortex ➡. Compare normal dark-staining internal granule cells ➡ with absence in LDD. (Courtesy F. J. Rodriguez, MD.)*

multinodular configuration of MVNT on histopathology distinguishes this lesion from GCyt.

**Focal cortical dysplasia** (FCD), primarily FCD type 2a, is another common cause of refractory epilepsy in young patients and is in the neuropathologic differential diagnosis. FCD follows gray matter on all imaging sequences and does not enhance. In the suprasellar region, GCyt should be distinguished from **hypothalamic ("tuber cinereum") hamartoma**.

# Dysplastic Cerebellar Gangliocytoma

## Terminology

Dysplastic cerebellar gangliocytoma is a rare benign cerebellar mass composed of dysplastic ganglion cells that is better known as **Lhermitte-Duclos disease** (LDD).

LDD may occur as part of the multiple hamartoma syndrome called **Cowden syndrome** (CS). When LDD and CS occur together, they are sometimes called Cowden-Lhermitte-Duclos or **COLD syndrome**. CS is also known as **multiple hamartoma-neoplasia syndrome** or **PTEN hamartoma tumor syndrome (PHTS)**.

CS is an autosomal dominant phacomatosis. The vast majority of patients have hamartomatous neoplasms of the skin combined with neoplasms and hamartomas of multiple other organs. Breast, thyroid, endometrium, and gastrointestinal cancers are the most prevalent other neoplasms in CS.

## Etiology

Whether LDD constitutes a neoplastic, malformative, or hamartomatous lesion is debated. The majority of cases are sporadic, but the association of LDD with CS favors a hamartomatous origin.

Approximately 40% of dysplastic cerebellar gangliocytomas occur as part of CS. Approximately 85% of patients with CS have a *PTEN* germline mutation that results in uncontrolled cell proliferation. Multisystem hamartomas derived from all three germ cell layers and malignant neoplasms are characteristic.

## Pathology

LDD is always infratentorial, usually involving the cerebellar hemisphere or the vermis. Dysplastic cerebellar gangliocytomas often become very large, displacing the fourth ventricle and causing obstructive hydrocephalus.

The gross appearance of LDD is a tumor-like mass that expands and replaces the normal cerebellar architecture. On cut section, the cerebellar folia are markedly enlarged and distorted but not obliterated, leading to a grossly gyriform appearance **(21-31)** **(21-33)**.

Microscopically, LDD is characterized by marked disruption of the normal cerebellar cortical layers. Diffuse hypertrophy of the granular cell layer with absence of the Purkinje layer of the cerebellum is typical **(21-32)**. Mitoses and necrosis are absent.

Dysplastic cerebellar gangliocytoma (LDD) is designated as a CNS WHO grade 1 lesion in the 5th edition WHO.

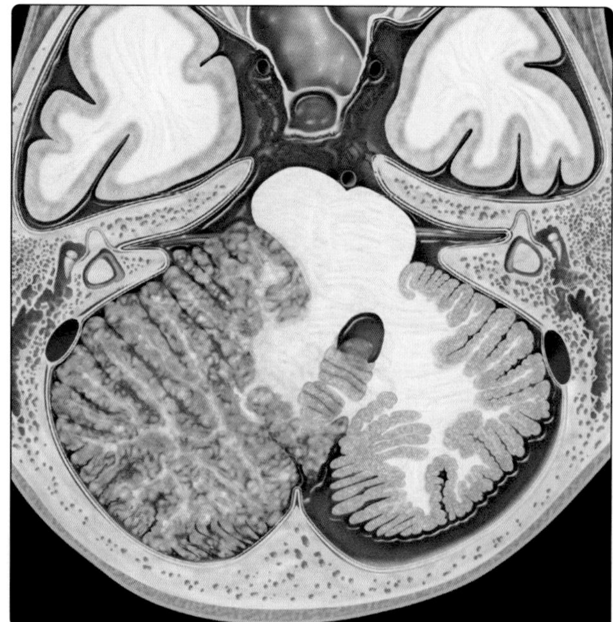

***(21-33) Graphic depicts dysplastic cerebellar gangliocytoma (LDD).***

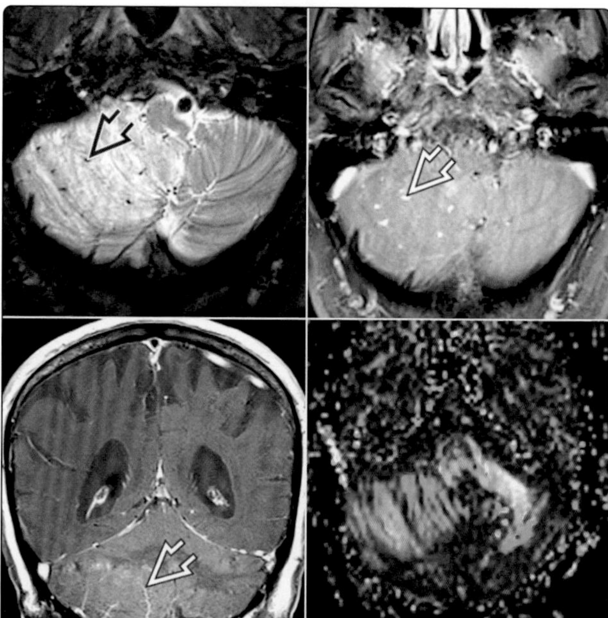

***(21-34) Tiger stripe configuration of thickened cerebellar folia and mass effect in LDD is best appreciated on T2 MR (upper left) and DTI (lower right). The "flow voids" ⇨ are prominent vessels ➡.***

## Clinical Issues

LDD occurs in all age groups, but most cases occur in adults between 20-40 years. The average age at diagnosis is 34 years. Patients may be asymptomatic or present with symptoms of increased intracranial pressure, such as headache, nausea, and vomiting. Cranial nerve palsies, gait disturbance, and visual abnormalities are also common.

LDD enlarges very slowly over many years. No cases of metastatic spread or CSF dissemination have been reported. Shunting or surgical debulking are options for symptomatic patients with hydrocephalus.

## Imaging

**General Features.** A nonenhancing, unilateral, cerebellar mass in a middle-aged patient that demonstrates a prominent tiger stripe pattern on MR is typical of LDD.

**CT Findings.** Most cases of LDD are hypodense on NECT. Mass effect with compression of the fourth ventricle, effacement of the cerebellopontine angle cisterns, and obstructive hydrocephalus is common. Calcification is rare. CECT generally shows no appreciable enhancement.

**MR Findings.** An expansile cerebellar mass with linear hypointense bands on T1WI is typical. T2WI shows the nearly pathognomonic tiger stripe pattern of alternating inner hyperintense and outer hypointense layers in enlarged cerebellar folia **(21-34)** **(21-35)**.

T2* (GRE, SWI) demonstrates prominent venous channels surrounding the grossly thickened folia. T1 C+ shows striking linear enhancement of these abnormal veins in between the folia **(21-34)**.

DWI may show restricted diffusion, probably reflecting the hypercellularity and increased axonal density characteristic of LDD. PWI shows increased relative cerebral blood volume, reflecting the prominent enlarged interfolial veins, not malignancy. MRS shows normal or slightly reduced NAA and normal Cho:Cr ratios. A lactate doublet may be present.

## Differential Diagnosis

Imaging findings of LDD are so characteristic that the diagnosis can usually be established without biopsy confirmation.

**Medulloblastoma**, especially the SHH-activated desmoplastic variant, may present as a lateral cerebellar mass but usually occurs in younger patients and rarely displays the "tiger stripes" that are so characteristic of LDD. **Cerebellar infarction** is confined to a specific vascular territory, and symptom onset is acute or subacute rather than chronic. Occasionally, **ganglioglioma** occurs in the posterior fossa and may mimic LDD. Gangliogliomas typically enhance and, although sometimes bizarre-appearing, rarely demonstrate prominent "tiger stripes."

A few rare **cerebellar cortical dysplasias** can mimic LDD. However, these malformations do not demonstrate progressive enlargement and rarely cause mass effect with hydrocephalus.

A few cases of posterior fossa **tuberous sclerosis complex** (TSC) that mimic LDD have been reported. However, these patients are generally younger and have other stigmata of TSC.

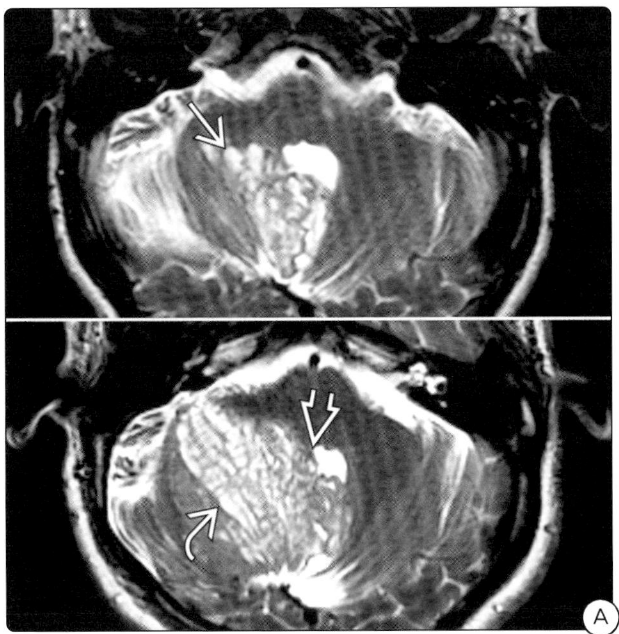

(21-35A) (Top) T2 MR in a 16-yo girl shows the typical tiger stripe pattern ➡ of LDD. (Bottom) T2 MR obtained 16 years later shows the lesion ➡ has increased in the interval as has the mass effect on the 4th ventricle ➡.

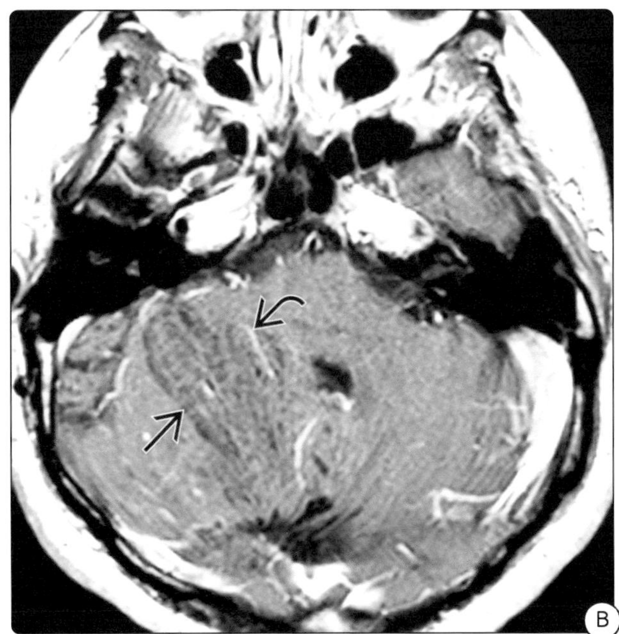

(21-35B) T1 C+ MR in the same patient shows the bubbly, laminated appearance of the mass ➡ with prominent vessels ➡ coursing between the expanded cerebellar folia. Surgical resection confirmed LDD.

**CEREBRAL GANGLIOCYTOMAS**

**Gangliocytoma**

- Pathology
  - Rare (< 1%) tumor
  - Mature but dysplastic ganglion cells
  - Temporal lobe (75%)
  - CNS WHO grade 1
- Clinical issues
  - Most patients < 30 years
  - Epilepsy
- Imaging findings
  - Mixed density on NECT (1/3 have $Ca^{++}$)
  - "Cyst + nodule" or solid
  - No hemorrhage, necrosis
  - T2/FLAIR hyperintense
  - Variable enhancement (none to striking)

**Dysplastic Cerebellar Gangliocytoma**

- Terminology
  - Lhermitte-Duclos disease (LDD)
  - LDD + multiple hamartomas = Cowden-Lhermitte-Duclos (COLD)
- Pathology
  - Enlarged, thick, "gyriform" cerebellar folia
  - Hypertrophied granular layer, absent Purkinje
  - CNS WHO grade 1
- Imaging findings
  - Mass with laminated, tiger stripe appearance
  - Linear enhancement of veins around thickened folia

# Central Neurocytoma

## Terminology

Central neurocytoma (CNC) is a well-differentiated neuroepithelial tumor with mature neurocytic elements. Most CNCs are located in the lateral ventricle(s) &/or the third ventricle.

## Pathology

CNCs are tumors of the lateral ventricle body, usually attached to the septi pellucidi and arising near the foramen of Monro **(21-36)**. They vary in size from small to huge lesions that extend through the foramen of Monro to involve the contralateral ventricle **(21-37)** and occasionally the third ventricle.

The gross appearance of CNC is that of a well-defined, lobulated, moderately vascular friable intraventricular mass arising from the septum pellucidum or lateral ventricular wall. Calcifications are present in 50% of cases, and intratumoral cysts and hemorrhage are common. CNCs rarely invade the adjacent brain parenchyma.

Microscopically, CNCs are neuroepithelial tumors composed of uniform round cells and often exhibit an oligodendroglioma-like monomorphic cells with honeycomb architecture. Mitotic activity is low with a Ki-67 (MIB-1) usually < 2-3%. In rare instances, brisk mitotic activity, microvascular proliferation, and necrosis may occur ("atypical" CNC).

Immunohistochemistry is positive for synaptophysin and generally negative for OLIG2. The methylation class (MC) of

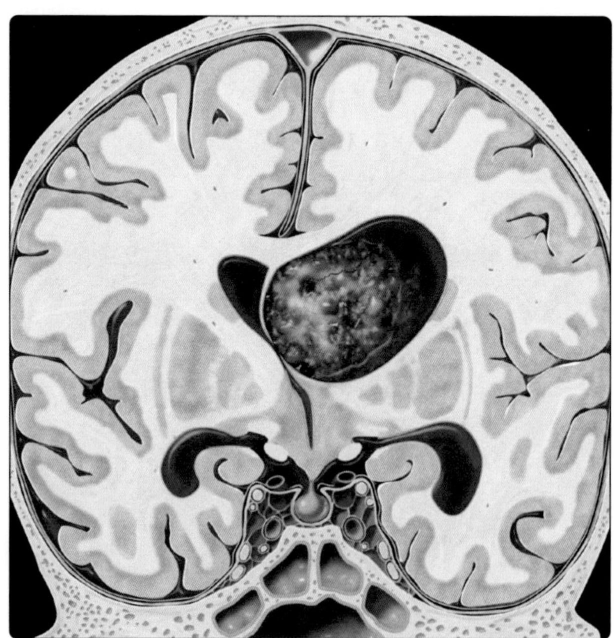

***(21-36) Coronal graphic depicts central neurocytoma as a multicystic, relatively vascular, occasionally hemorrhagic mass in the body of the lateral ventricle.***

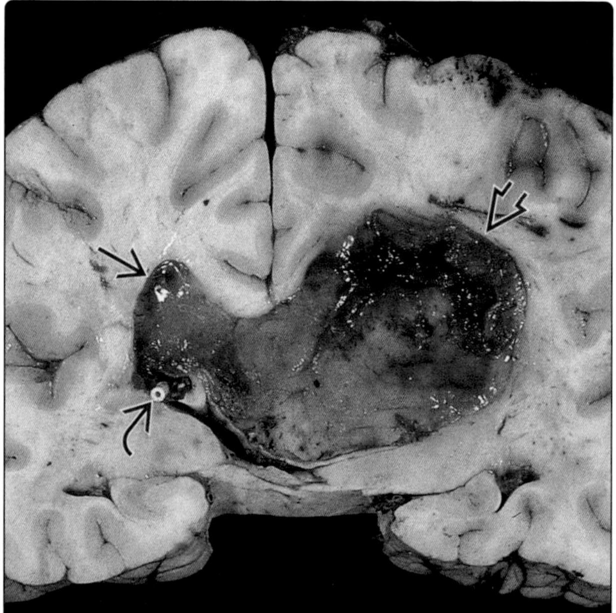

***(21-37) Autopsy shows a central neurocytoma expanding the left lateral ventricle ➡, crossing through the foramen of Monro to fill the right lateral ventricle ➡. Note ventricular shunt ➡. (From D. Ellison et al: Neuropathology, 2013.)***

CNC exclusively comprises tumors with the histologic diagnosis of CNC.

CNCs are CNS WHO grade 2 neoplasms. Distinguishing between CNC and atypical CNC is not possible based on current methylation clustering.

## Clinical Issues

**Epidemiology.** CNC is the most common primary intraventricular neoplasm of young and middle-aged adults between 20 and 40 years of age, accounting for nearly 1/2 of all cases. CNCs are rarely diagnosed in children or older adults. Overall, they are rare neoplasms that represent between 0.25-0.50% of intracranial neoplasms and 10% of all intraventricular tumors.

**Presentation.** Symptoms are usually those of increased intracranial pressure. Headache, mental status changes, and visual disturbances are common while focal neurologic deficits are rare. Sudden ventricular obstruction or acute intratumoral hemorrhage may cause abrupt clinical deterioration and even death.

**Natural History.** CNCs are slow-growing neoplasms that rarely recur following complete surgical resection. Five-year survival rate in tumors with gross total resection is 90-95%. Adjuvant radiotherapy may improve progression-free survival in patients with subtotal resection. Malignant behavior with craniospinal dissemination has been reported but is rare.

## Imaging

**General Features.** A "bubbly" mass in the body or frontal horn of the lateral ventricle is classic for CNC.

**CT Findings.** NECT shows a mixed-density solid and cystic intraventricular neoplasm attached to the septum pellucidum **(21-38A)**. Obstructive hydrocephalus is common. Calcification is present in 50-70% of cases. Gross intratumoral hemorrhage occurs but is rare. CNCs show moderately strong but heterogeneous enhancement on CECT.

**MR Findings.** CNCs are heterogeneous masses that are mostly isodense with gray matter on T1WI. Intratumoral cysts and prominent vascular "flow voids" are common. A soap-bubble appearance on T2WI is typical **(21-38C)**. CNCs are heterogeneously hyperintense on FLAIR **(21-38D)** and demonstrate moderate to strong but heterogeneous enhancement following contrast administration **(21-38F)**.

Decreased NAA and modestly elevated Cho are present on MRS. The presence of some NAA and glycine along with an inverted alanine peak at 1.5 ppm with a TE of 135 ms is highly suggestive of neurocytoma.

## Differential Diagnosis

The major differential diagnosis of CNC is **subependymoma**. Supratentorial subependymomas are typically located in the frontal horn adjacent to the foramen of Monro and may appear very similar. CNCs are tumors of younger adults, whereas subependymoma is more common in older adults. **Subependymal giant cell astrocytoma** also occurs in a similar location. Clinical and imaging stigmata of tuberous sclerosis (i.e., subependymal nodules and cortical tubers) are usually present.

**Myxoid glioneuronal tumor (MGNT)** is classically located in the septum pellucidum but may extend into/around the lateral ventricles. MGNTs are typically very hyperintense on

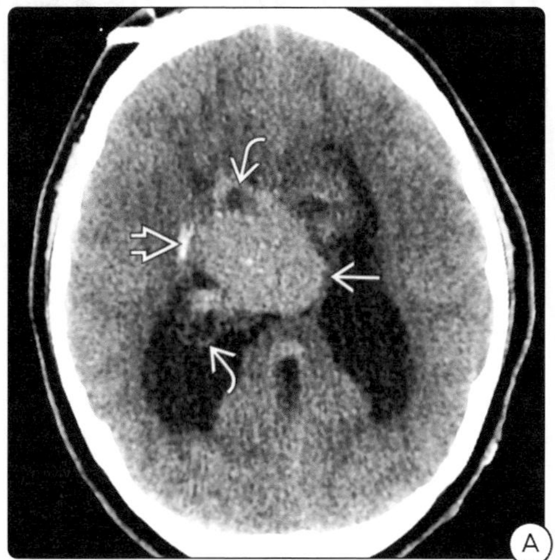


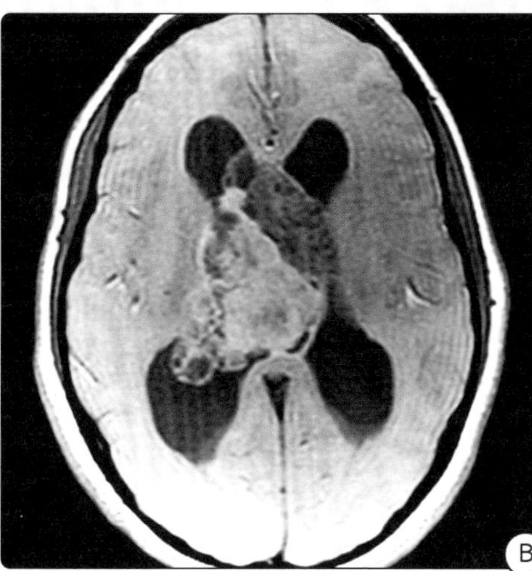


***(21-38A)*** *NECT in an 18-yo woman in the ER with 1 month of increasingly severe headaches shows a biventricular mass with hyperdense and hypodense components with focal calcifications.* ***(21-38B)*** *T1 MR in the same patient shows a very heterogeneous, mixed cystic/solid mass involving the bodies of both lateral ventricles. The mass appears confined to the ventricles without extension into the adjacent brain.*

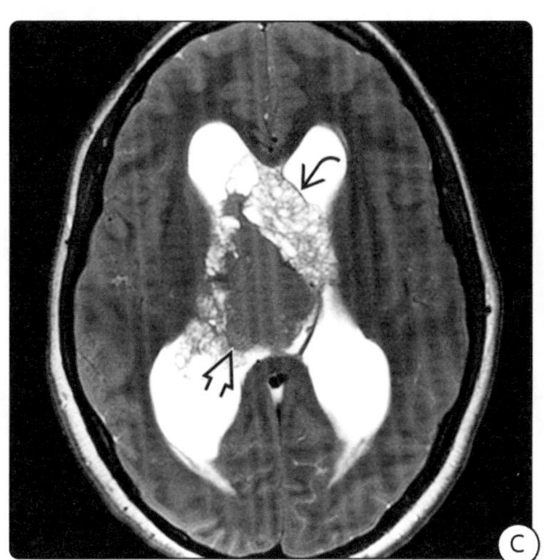


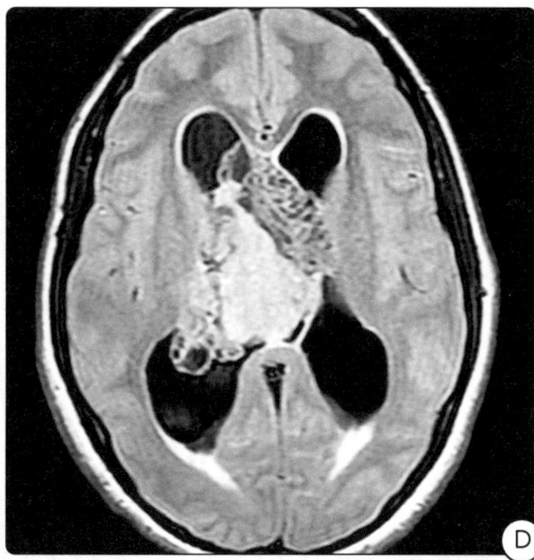


***(21-38C)*** *T2 MR in the same patient shows a solid portion of the mass is nearly isointense with cortex. Multiple tiny, hyperintense cysts with a distinct soap bubble appearance are present. The lateral ventricles are enlarged, but there is minimal periventricular fluid accumulation.* ***(21-38D)*** *The mixed cystic/solid mass is well delineated on FLAIR.*

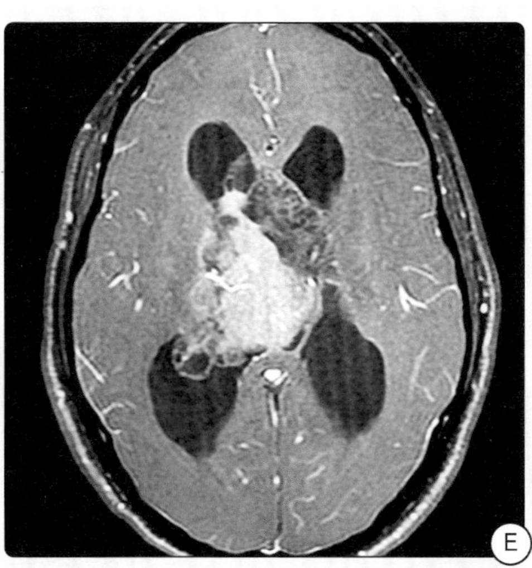


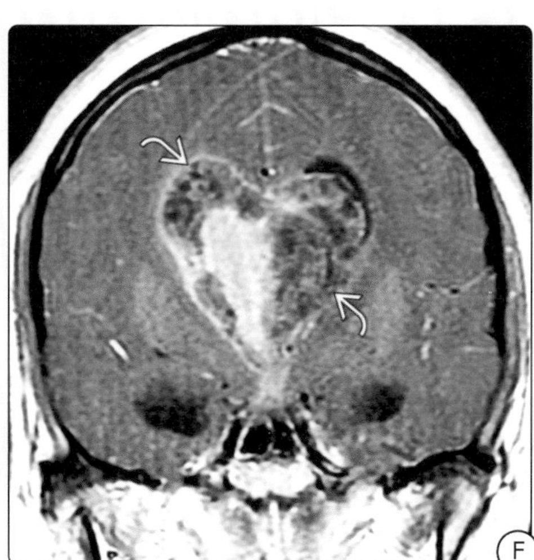


***(21-38E)*** *T1 C+ FS MR shows the solid portion enhances intensely and relatively uniformly. The walls of the cystic portion also enhance.* ***(21-38F)*** *Coronal T1 C+ MR shows the typical soap bubble appearance of central neurocytoma. Central neurocytoma, CNS WHO grade 2 was found at surgery.*

*__(21-39A)__ NECT in an 8-yo patient shows a partially calcified, partially cystic right frontal lobe mass. __(21-39B)__ Bone CT in the same patient shows the mass is extensively and densely calcified. Note focal thinning and remodeling of the overlying calvarium, suggesting the mass is likely a longstanding lesion.*

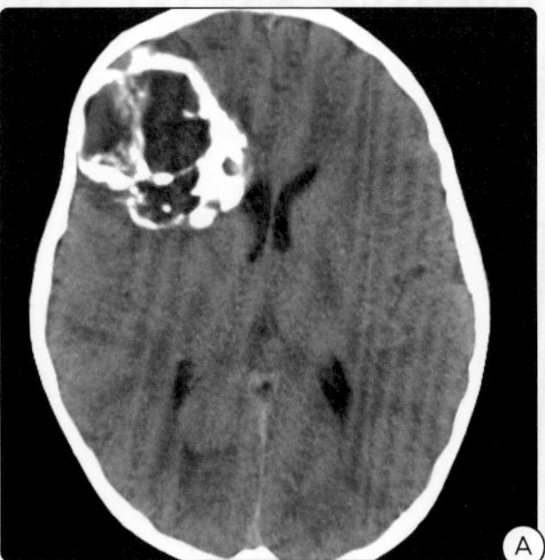

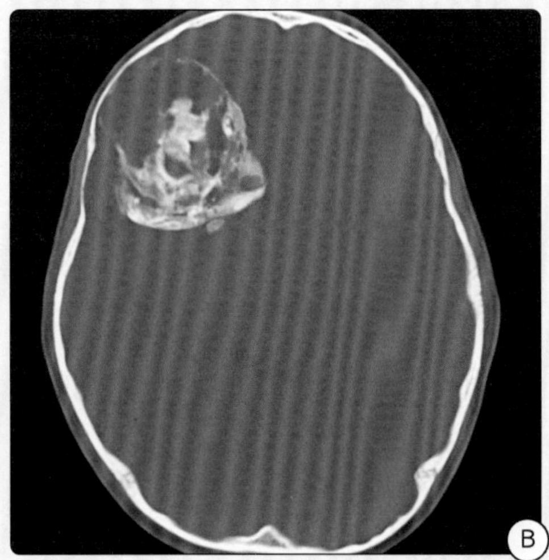

*__(21-39C)__ Axial T1 MR shows the mass is slightly hypointense compared to the cortex with some T1 shortening in the rim of the mass. __(21-39D)__ The mass is very heterogeneous on T2 MR with multiple hyperintense cysts and low signal intensity foci corresponding to the tumor calcifications. Note the minimal peripheral edema associated with the mass. Minimal mass effect on the adjacent frontal horn is present.*

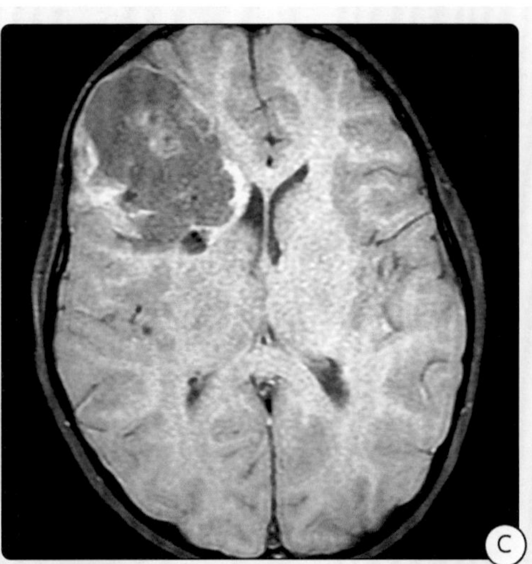

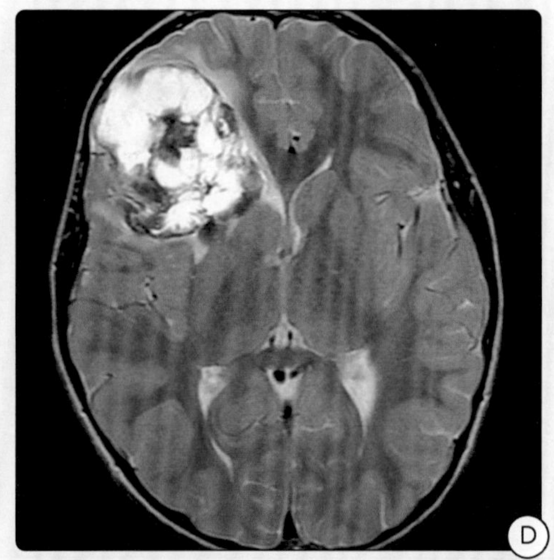

*__(21-39E)__ FLAIR shows fluid in the cysts does not completely suppress. Note remodeling of the adjacent calvarium and minimal edema relative to the overall size of the mass. __(21-39F)__ T1 C+ FS MR shows minimal internal enhancement of the mass. Extraventricular neurocytoma, CNS WHO grade 2 was found at surgery.*

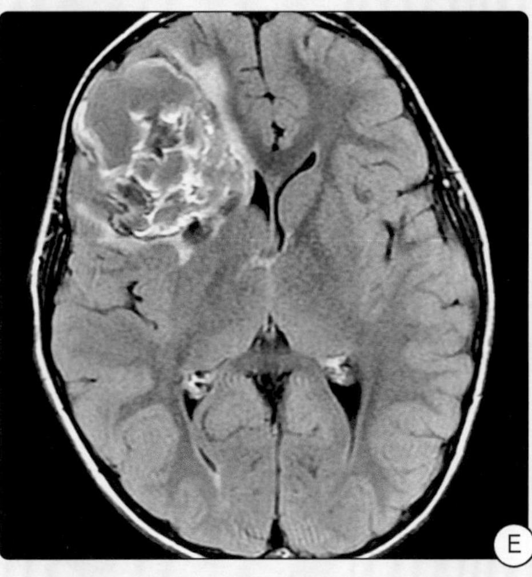

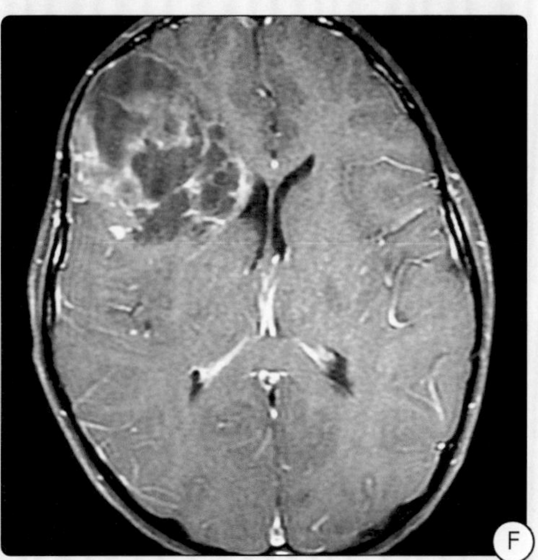

T2WI and exhibit a hyperintense rim around a central isointense area on FLAIR.

True intraventricular **oligodendroglioma** does occur but is rare. As the imaging appearance is indistinguishable from CNC, the diagnosis of intraventricular oligodendroglioma is established on the basis of immunohistochemistry and methylation profiling. Oligodendrogliomas are synaptophysin negative and often show mutations of *OLIG2*, and 1p,19q are co-deleted.

## Extraventricular Neurocytoma

**Extraventricular** neurocytomas (EVNs) are rare, well-circumscribed neurocytic neoplasms that occur throughout the CNS parenchyma but, by definition, do not contact the ventricular system. EVNs have been reported in patients of all ages but have a predilection for young adults. The most common locations are the frontal lobe and cerebellum followed by the temporal and occipital lobes.

Pathologically, EVNs are typically well-circumscribed lesions, often with a cyst + nodule configuration, although rare infiltrating tumors have been reported. Most EVNs correspond to CNS WHO grade 2 lesions. Some cases with anaplasia, increased mitoses, microvascular proliferation, &/or necrosis have been reported to follow a more aggressive clinical course.

EVNs have a widely varied imaging appearance. The most common finding is a large, relatively well-demarcated, cystic/solid mass that is frequently calcified on NECT scans **(21-39A)**. The solid portion is iso- to hypointense on T1WI and heterogeneously hyperintense on T2WI and FLAIR **(21-39)**. Heterogeneous enhancement after contrast administration is typical.

The differential diagnosis varies with age. In children, pediatric-type low-grade gliomas, such as **diffuse low-grade glioma, MAPK pathway altered**, should be considered. Smaller EVNs can mimic other cyst + nodule-type tumors in young adults, such as **ganglioglioma**, **polymorphous low-grade neuroepithelial tumor of the young**, **and pilocytic astrocytoma**.

## Cerebellar Liponeurocytoma

Cerebellar liponeurocytoma (CL) is a rare, molecularly distinct adult tumor of the cerebellar hemispheres characterized by lipid accumulation in oligodendroglioma-like neuroepithelial tumor cells **(21-40)**. The lipidized component can be prominent, reduced, or even largely absent. CLs are CNS WHO grade 2 neoplasms.

The most characteristic radiologic finding of CL is a relatively well-circumscribed mass in the cerebellar hemisphere with scattered, fatty, T1-hyperintense inclusions in the tumor **(21-41)**. CLs are T2/FLAIR heterogeneously hyperintense lesions. Enhancement is variable.

The major imaging differential diagnosis is **medulloblastoma. Central neurocytoma with lipomatous changes** have been reported but do not exhibit the methylation profile of CL.

*Selected References: The complete reference list is available on the eBooks+ version included with purchase.*

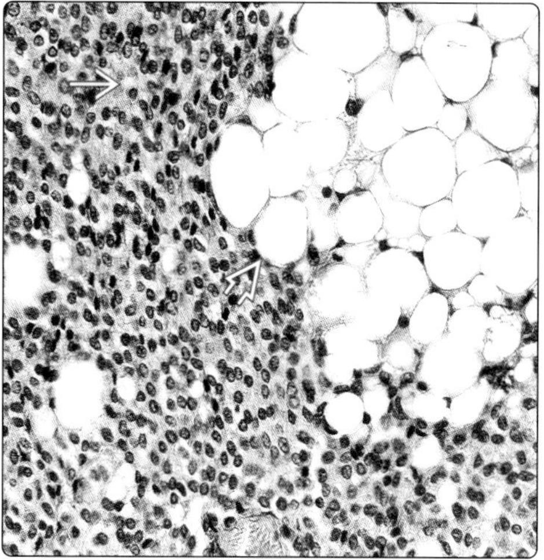

***(21-40)** Photomicrograph of classic cerebellar liponeurocytoma shows neurocytes ➡ and lipidized cells ➡. (From DP: Neuro.)*

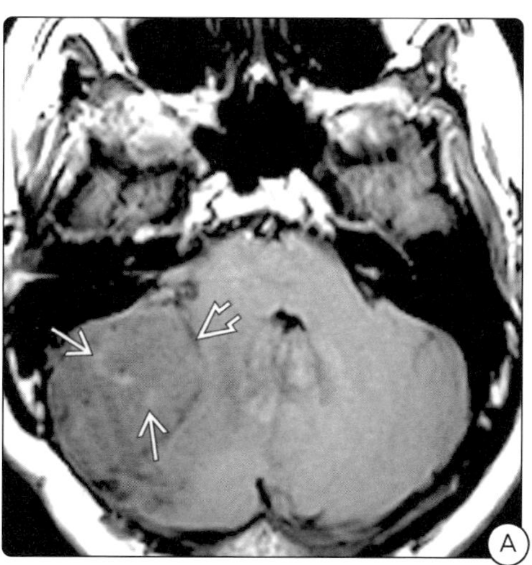

***(21-41A)** T1 MR of cerebellar liponeurocytoma shows a well-demarcated mass ➡ with T1-hyperintense foci ➡ representing lipid content.*

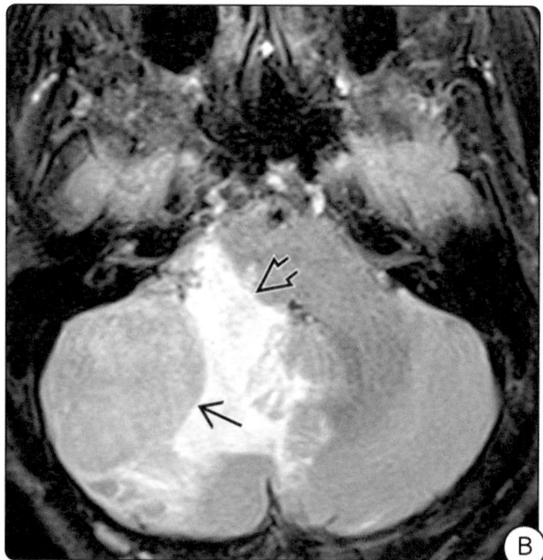

***(21-41B)** T2 FS MR shows the well-demarcated mass ➡ and edema ➡. Fatty streaks are suppressed.*

# Ependymal Tumors

*Overall, ependymomas represent 2-3% of all primary CNS neoplasms. Approximately 30% affect children and adolescents, although ependymal neoplasms occur at all ages, encompass multiple tumor types and subtypes, and can develop along the entire neuraxis. Clinically, ependymomas are a heterogeneous group ranging from relatively benign subependymomas to the deadly early childhood ependymomas of the posterior fossa.*



The 5th edition WHO recognizes ependymomas as a distinct family of tumors that are now classified according to a combination of (1) histopathologic features, (2) molecular features, and (3) anatomic site.

Ependymomas are divided into specific molecular groups in each of three anatomic sites, viz., the supratentorial, posterior fossa, and spinal compartments (SC). DNA methylation profiling results in distinct ependymoma subgroups divided among these three sites. Each molecular subgroup is genetically, transcriptionally, demographically, and clinically distinct.

In this chapter, we group and discuss CNS ependymomas by their respective anatomic compartments **(22-1)**. Two additional tumors—subependymoma (SE) and myxopapillary ependymoma (MPE)—are not restricted to a specific anatomic location (e.g., SEs can occur in all three anatomic compartments) and are discussed separately at the end of this chapter.

## Supratentorial Ependymomas

Supratentorial ependymomas (ST-EPNs) represent 30% of all ependymomas. The 5th edition WHO includes two molecularly defined types of ST-EPN: One with *ZFTA* fusion and the other with *YAP1* fusion. If no pathogenic gene fusion of *ZFTA* (formerly known as C11orf95) or *YAP1* can be detected, the diagnosis ST-EPN, not elsewhere classified (NEC) is used.

### Supratentorial Ependymoma, *ZFTA* Fusion-Positive

#### Terminology

*ZFTA* fusion-positive ependymoma is a circumscribed supratentorial neoplasm with *ZFTA* gene fusions with partner genes, mainly *RELA*. *ZFTA* fusion-positive is the new, updated designation for C11orf95, because fusion partners other than *RELA* (e.g., *MAML2*/*MAML3*, *NCOA1*/*NCOA2*, *MN1*, or *CTNNA2*) may also occur.

*(22-1) Graphic shows ependymoma subtype and correlation with geographic localization. Subependymomas are found in the frontal horn of the lateral ventricle (supratentorial subependymoma) and obex (posterior fossa subependymoma) ➡. Supratentorial ependymomas ➡ are most often RELA- or YAP-fusion tumors. Posterior fossa ependymomas ➡ are group A (PFA) or B (PFB). Spinal ependymomas can be myxopapillary ➡, which occur almost exclusively in the conus/filum terminale, or cellular/anaplastic ependymomas ➡ (spinal ependymomas), which occur in the central canal of the spinal cord and are intramedullary neoplasms.*

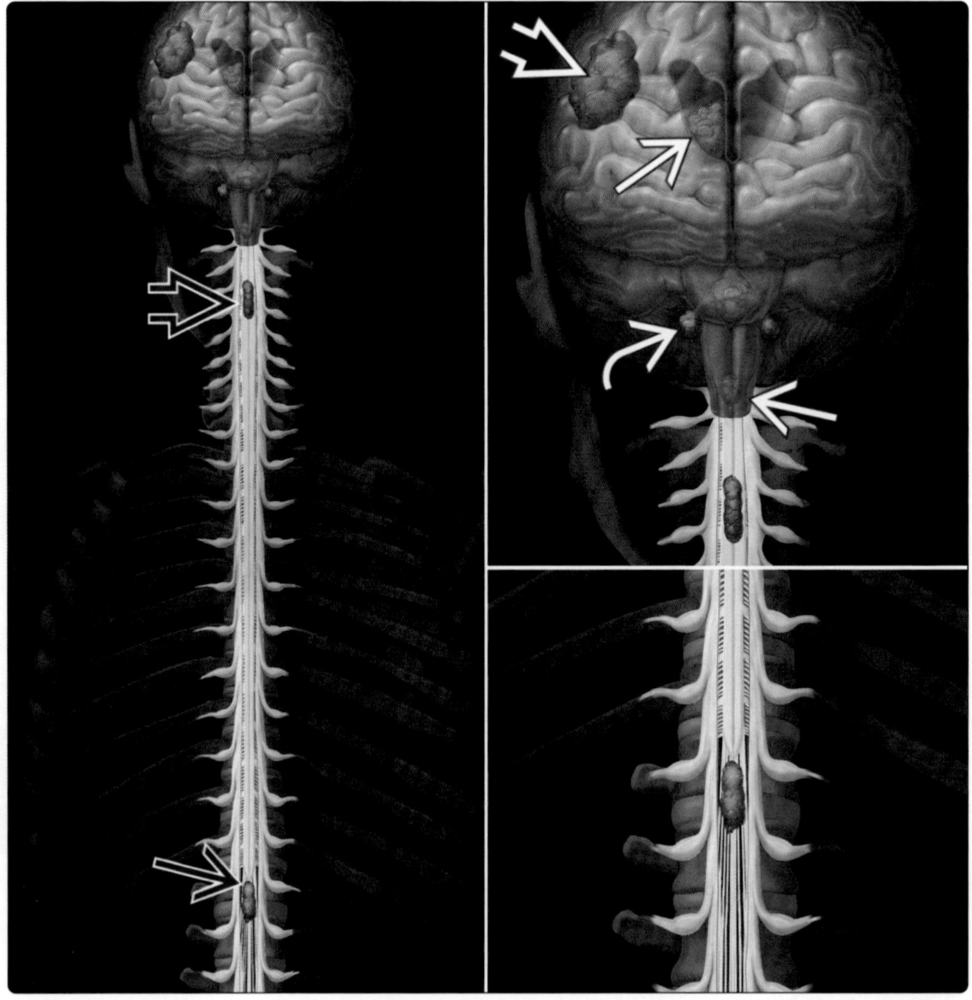

## Etiology

*ZFTA* fusion-positive ST-EPNs probably arise from radial glia stem cells. Fusion of the *ZFTA* gene with a partner gene—usually *RELA*—is the principal oncogenic driver of the neoplasm.

## Pathology

Grossly, *ZFTA* fusion-positive ependymomas are sharply demarcated extraventricular masses arising in the cerebral hemispheres, most commonly the frontal and parietal lobes. Less common reported sites include the thalamus and hypothalamus/third ventricle.

Perivascular pseudorosettes are a cornerstone histologic marker of *ZFTA* fusion-positive ependymomas. True ependymal rosettes are rare.

*ZFTA* fusion-positive ependymomas are usually positive for L1CAM immunostaining. *ZFTA* fusions with partners other than *RELA* are uncommon; these rare tumors have a highly variable morphologic spectrum, exhibiting features that can resemble pleomorphic xanthoastrocytoma or astroblastoma.

*ZFTA* fusion-positive ependymomas exhibit varying degrees of anaplasia and are designated CNS WHO grade 2 or 3.

## Clinical Issues

*ZFTA* fusion-positive ependymomas account for nearly 70% of ST-EPNs in children and most of the hemispheric ependymomas in adults. The five-year survival is 50%. Notably, recent evidence suggests progression-free survival in non-*ZFTA*::*RELA*-fused ependymomas is worse.

## Imaging

*ZFTA* fusion-positive ependymomas appear as large, bulky, heterogeneous-appearing para- or extraventricular hemispheric masses. Completely intraventricular ST-EPNs are rare. In many cases, no direct connection to the lateral ventricles can be identified.

NECT shows a mixed-density mass with solid and cystic components and peritumoral edema **(22-2A)** **(22-3A)**. Intratumoral hemorrhage and calcification are common. Heterogeneous enhancement on CECT is present in nearly all cases.

MR findings vary widely. Mixed solid with variable cystic components are typical. Signal intensity is quite variable with hypo- and isointense foci on T1WI and variably iso- to hyperintense foci on T2WI **(22-2)**. Cyst fluid does not suppress on FLAIR. "Blooming" hemorrhagic foci on T2* sequences are common **(22-3)**. Moderately cellular tumors may exhibit some restricted diffusion.

Over 85% exhibit strong, thick but inhomogeneous enhancement on T1 C+ **(22-3F)**. Cystic components usually exhibit an enhancing rim. Most *ZFTA* fusion-positive ependymomas show moderate restricted diffusion on DWI and elevated rCBV on pMR **(22-5)**.

## Differential Diagnosis

The main differential diagnosis includes **MN1-altered astroblastoma** and neoplasms with **BCOR internal tandem duplication**. In adults, **glioblastoma** and **pleomorphic xanthoastrocytoma** can mimic hemispheric ependymomas. Rare neoplasms, such as **extraventricular neurocytoma**, can be indistinguishable on imaging studies.

## Supratentorial Ependymoma, *YAP1* Fusion-Positive

The second subgroup of ST-EPNs is characterized by the absence of *ZFTA* alterations and presence of *YAP1* gene fusions. The most frequent rearrangement is with the *MAMLD1* gene, but other fusion partners occur.

These tumors are uncommon. Most occur in infants and young children, where they represent just 6-7% of pediatric ST-EPNs. Immunoreactivity for L1CAM is absent. *YAP1*-fused ST-EPNs are associated with a more favorable prognosis than *ZFTA*-fused ependymomas.

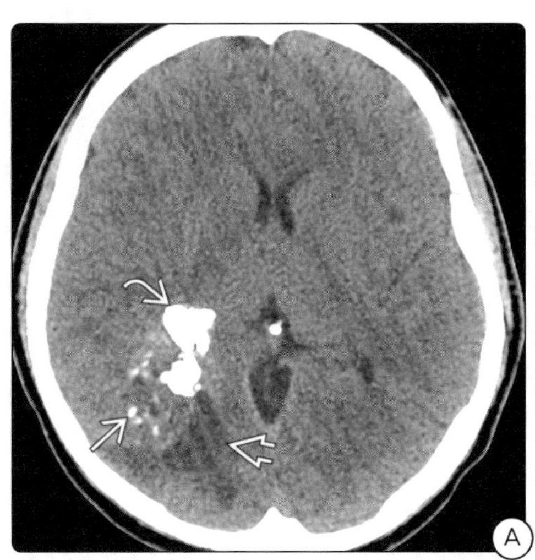


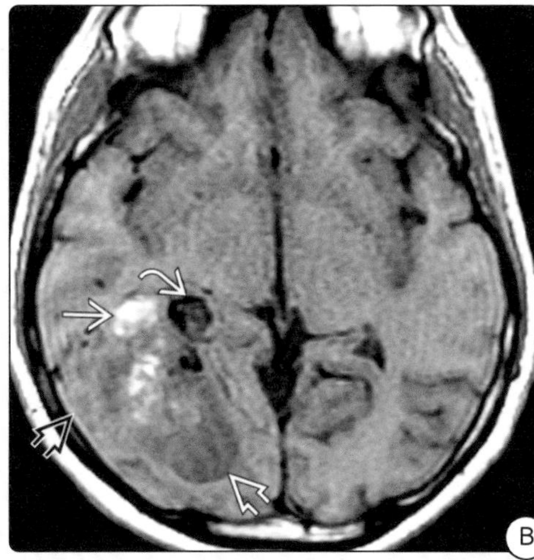


***(22-2A)** Axial NECT in a 25-yo man shows a very heterogeneous mass adjacent to the atrium of the right lateral ventricle. Note clumped ➔ and scattered punctate ➔ calcifications. A hypodense cystic-appearing component adjacent to the mass ➔ is visible. **(22-2B)** T1WI shows a heterogeneous mass with focal hypodensities from the calcifications ➔ and intermixed hyper- ➔, iso- ➔, and hypointense ➔ components.*

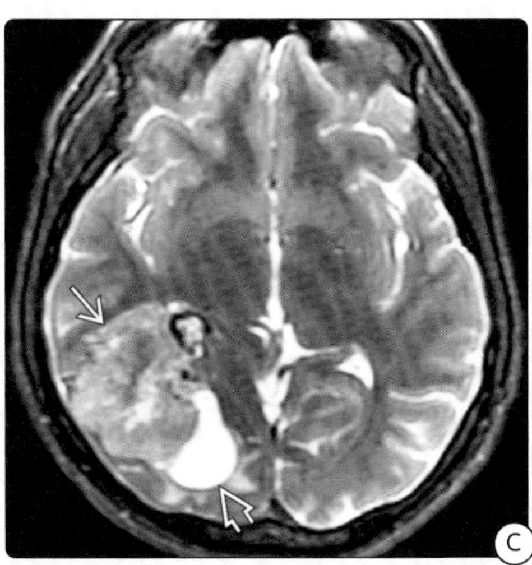


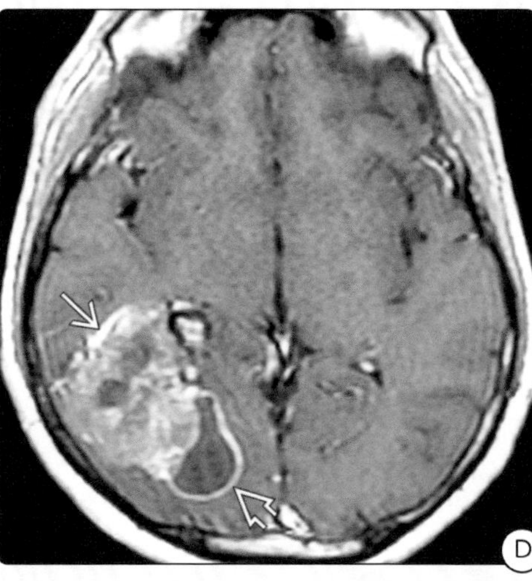


***(22-2C)** T2 FS shows the mass has heterogeneous solid ➔ and homogeneously hyperintense cystic ➔ areas. **(22-2D)** T1 C+ MR shows the solid portion of the mass enhances heterogeneously ➔. The adjacent cystic component exhibits rim enhancement ➔. This is ZFTA fusion-positive supratentorial ependymoma, CNS WHO grade 3.*

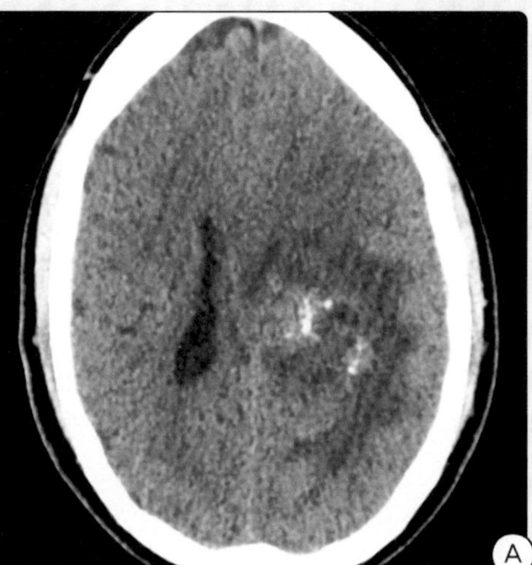

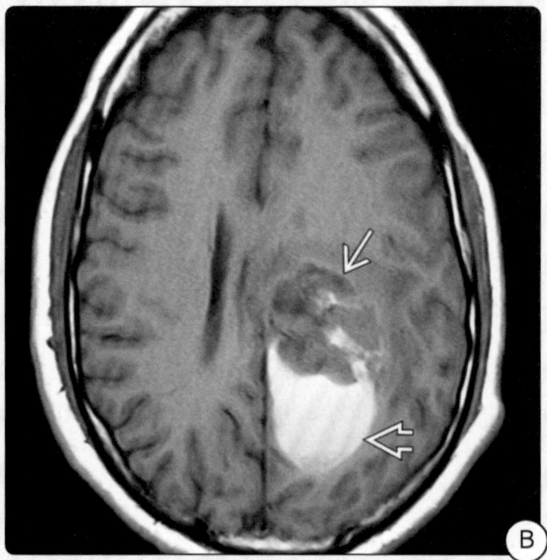

***(22-3A)** NECT in a 39-yo man with right-sided upper and lower extremity weakness shows a mixed-density left parietal mass with calcifications and surrounding edema. **(22-3B)** Axial T1WI in the same case shows a mixed signal intensity left hemispheric mass ➡ with an associated proteinaceous cyst that has a subtle internal signal gradient ➡.*

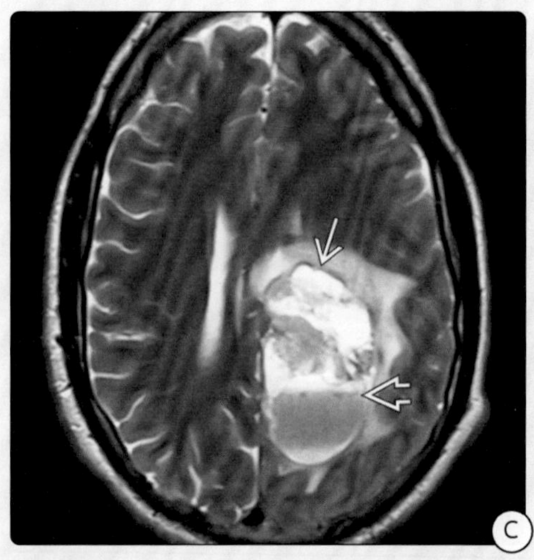

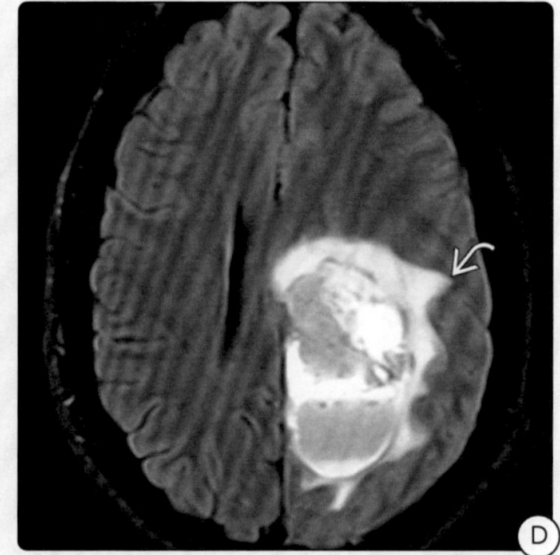

***(22-3C)** T2WI shows the mass ➡ is heterogeneously hyper- and isointense. Note fluid-fluid layering in the posterior cystic cavity ➡. **(22-3D)** The mass is extremely heterogeneous on FLAIR. Moderate peritumoral edema ➡ is present.*

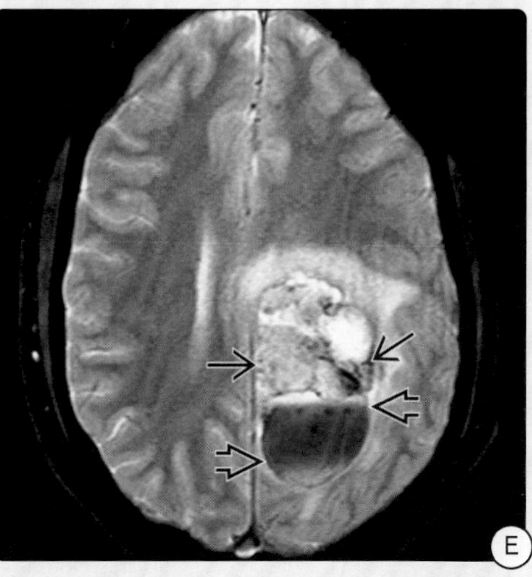

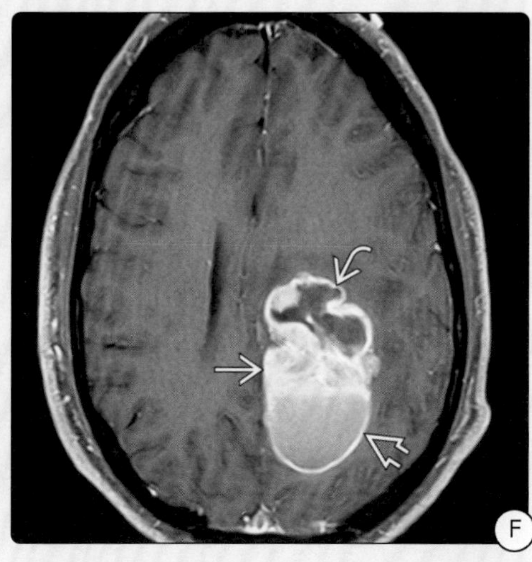

***(22-3E)** T2* GRE shows punctate linear hypointensities in the solid portion of the tumor ➡ and 3 distinct fluid-fluid levels in the dependent part of the lesion ➡. **(22-3F)** T1 C+ FS shows strong but heterogeneous enhancement in the solid portion of the tumor ➡ with enhancement around the necrotic superior portion ➡ and rim of the dependent cyst ➡. CNS WHO grade 3 ZFTA fusion-positive ependymoma with ZFTA::RELA fusion.*

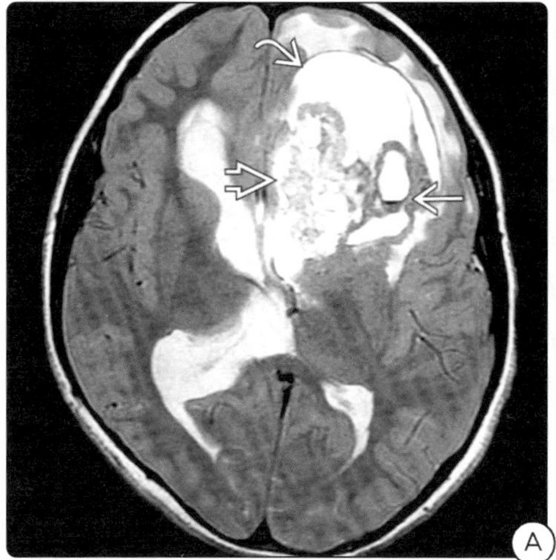

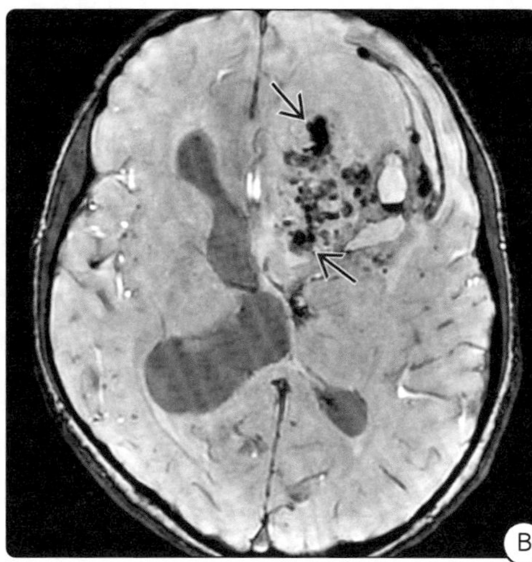

***(22-4A)** Axial T2WI in an 11-yo girl with 6 weeks of nausea and vomiting shows a large mixed cystic ➩ and solid ➩ mass occupying almost the entire left frontal lobe. Note hemorrhage with blood-fluid levels ➩ in several of the cysts. **(22-4B)** T2* SWI shows multiple hemorrhagic foci ➩ in the mass.*

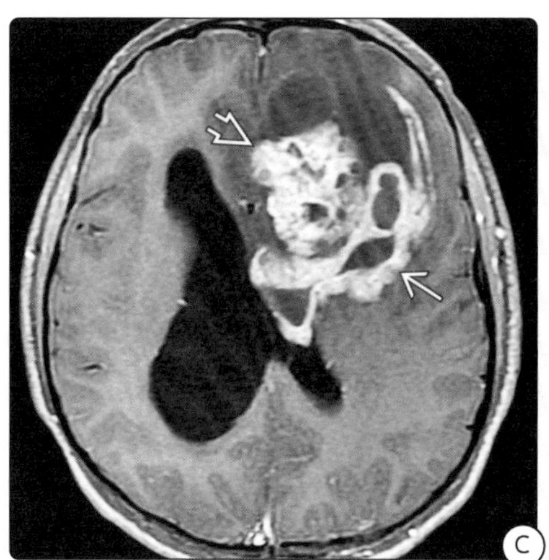

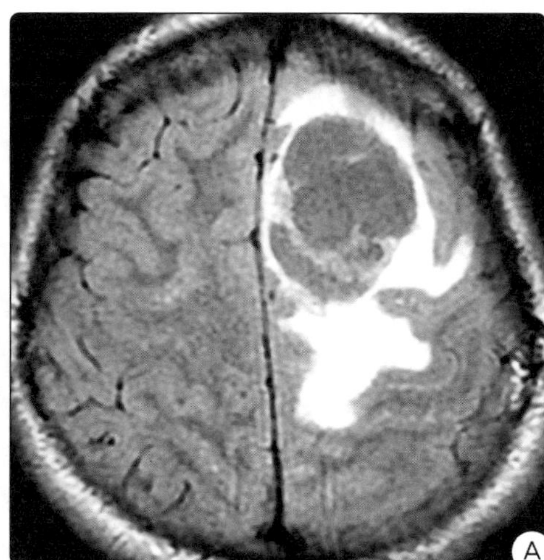

***(22-4C)** T1 C+ FS in the same case shows thick, irregular rinds of enhancing tumor ➩ around the cystic portions of the mass. The solid portion ➩ enhances heterogeneously. **(22-5A)** Axial FLAIR in a 19-yo man with 2 weeks of headache, nausea, and vomiting shows a left frontal mass with striking peritumoral edema.*

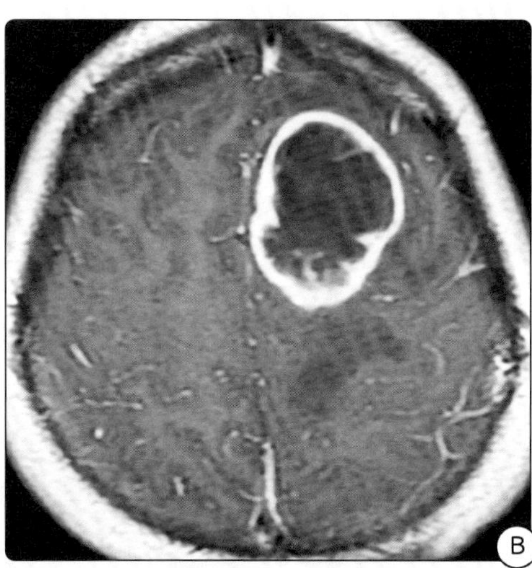

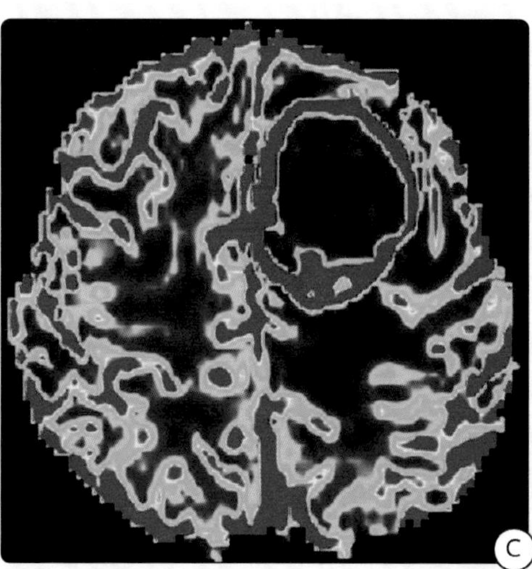

***(22-5B)** T1 C+ in the same case shows ring enhancement. **(22-5C)** pMR in the same case shows elevated rCBV in the enhancing tumor rind. Original diagnosis was astroblastoma. Diagnostic molecular pathology revealed the tumor was ZFTA::RELA fusion positive.*

# Posterior Fossa Ependymomas

Approximately 60% of all ependymomas are *infratentorial*. Of these, 95% are found in the fourth ventricle. The remainder occur as cerebellopontine angle (CPA) lesions.

Posterior fossa ependymomas have morphologic and immunohistochemical features of ependymoma. Two subtypes are defined: Posterior fossa group A (PFA) ependymoma and posterior fossa group B (PFB) ependymoma. Although they appear similar at gross pathology and on imaging studies, they differ in both age at onset and biologic behavior and so are discussed separately.

## Posterior Fossa Group A Ependymoma

### Terminology

PFA ependymoma is sometimes referred to as infantile posterior fossa ependymoma.

### Pathology

**Gross Pathology.** In general, posterior fossa ependymomas are reddish-tan or gray in color and form relatively well-demarcated, lobulated masses. They have a plastic appearance, extruding from the fourth ventricle through the foramina of Luschka and Magendie to fill the cisterns and encase cranial nerves and blood vessels **(22-6)** **(22-7)**.

Calcification, cyst formation, and hemorrhage are common **(22-11)**.

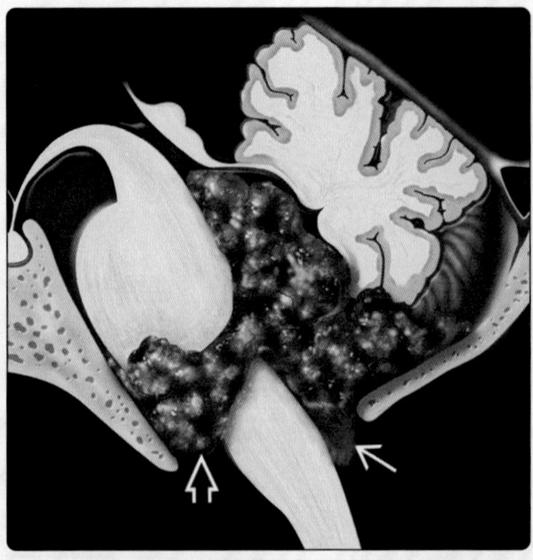

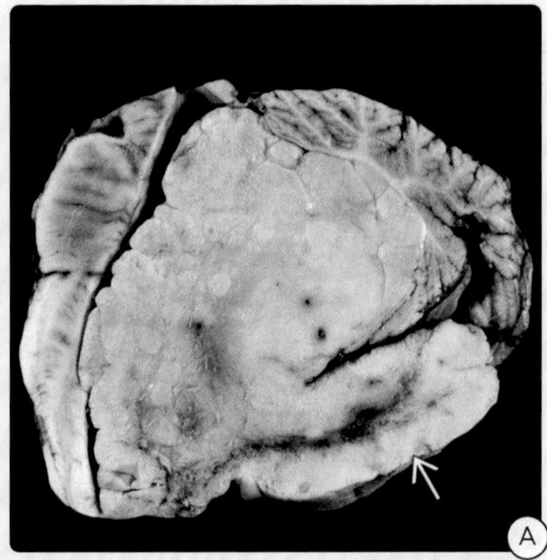

***(22-6)** Graphic depicts "classic" cellular ependymoma of the 4th ventricle extending through the foramen of Magendie into the cisterna magna ➡, around the pons, under the brachium pontis, and through the lateral recesses into the cerebellopontine angle (CPA) cisterns ➡. **(22-7A)** Sagittal autopsy case shows ependymoma filling the 4th ventricle, elevating the vermis, extending posteroinferiorly to fill the cisterna magna ➡.*

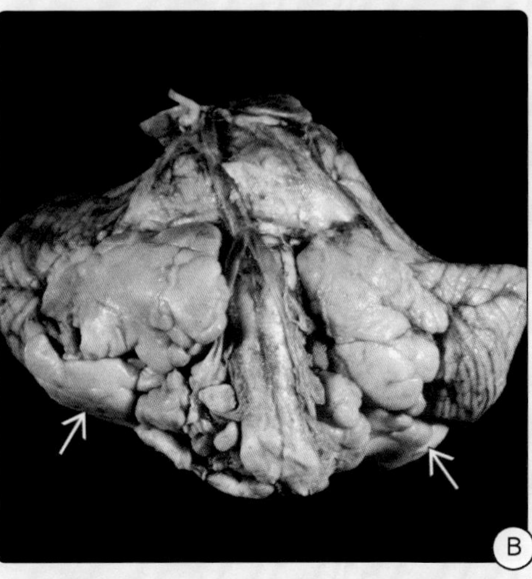

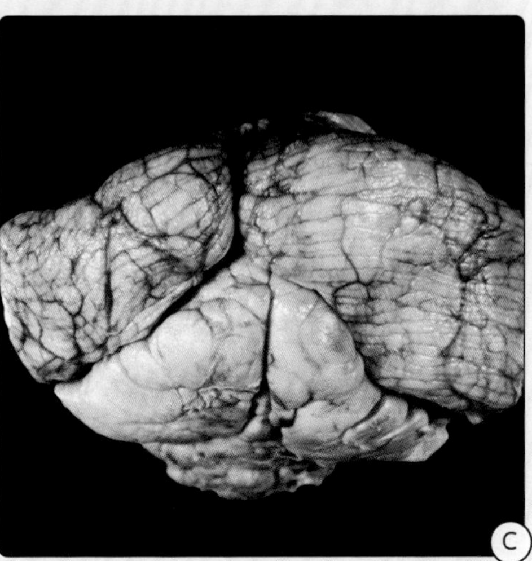

***(22-7B)** Coronal view in the same case shows massive tumor extension through both foramina of Luschka into the CPA cisterns ➡. **(22-7C)** Posterior view shows tumor bulging through the foramen of Magendie, completely filling the cisterna magna. Posterior fossa ependymomas squeeze out the foramina of the 4th ventricle, oozing like toothpaste into the surrounding CSF spaces. (Courtesy E. Ross, MD.)*

**Microscopic Features.** The most characteristic microarchitectural feature of ependymomas is the presence of perivascular pseudorosettes, in which tumor cells are arranged radially around blood vessels.

PFA ependymomas exhibit varying degrees of anaplasia. Nearly 2/3 exhibit high-grade features, including prominent mitotic activity and microvascular proliferation. Nuclear pleomorphism and necrosis have lesser prognostic significance.

PFA ependymomas are designated as CNS WHO grade 2 or 3 depending on the degree of anaplasia.

**Diagnostic Molecular Pathology.** Molecular characterization of posterior fossa ependymomas has a greater impact on risk stratification than histopathologic grading criteria. Therefore, posterior fossa ependymomas should be assigned to a specific molecular group (i.e., PFA, PFB, or SE). PFA is defined by its unique DNA methylation profile *or* reduced H3p.K28me3 in tumor cell nuclei.

## Clinical Issues

**Epidemiology.** Overall, ependymoma is the third most common posterior fossa tumor of childhood (after medulloblastoma and astrocytoma). PFA ependymoma accounts for nearly 30% of all brain tumors in children under the age of three years.

**Demographics.** PFA ependymomas are almost exclusively found in young children (median age = three years), and male patients predominate, nearly 2:1.

**Presentation.** Fourth ventricle ependymomas—both PFA and PFB—commonly cause intraventricular obstructive hydrocephalus. Infants with PFA ependymomas can present with a rapidly growing head circumference. Older children

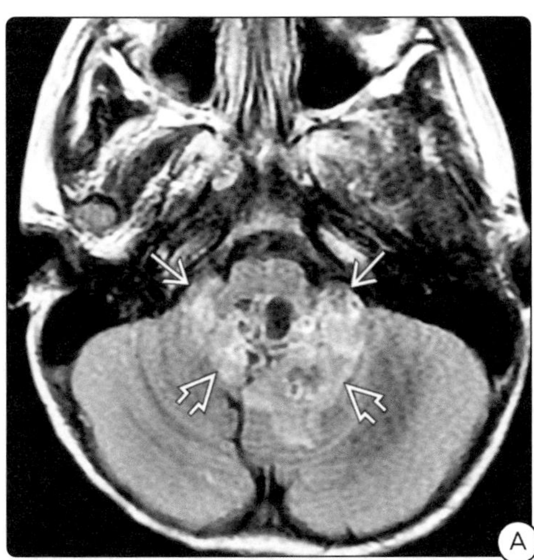


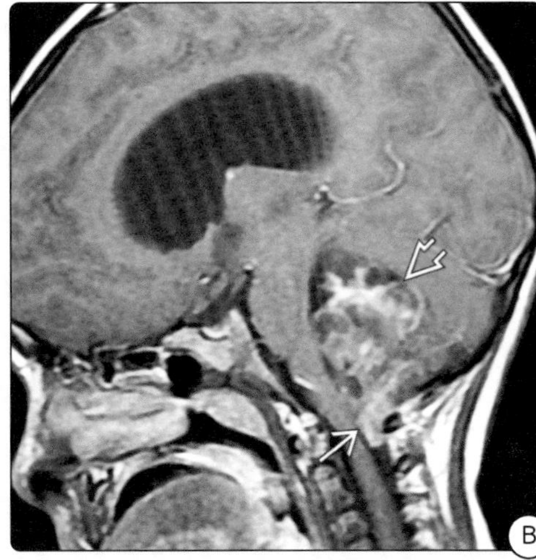


***(22-8A)** Axial FLAIR in a 3-yo boy shows a mixed signal intensity mass in the inferior 4th ventricle that extends anterolaterally through both foramina of Luschka into the CPA cisterns. **(22-8B)** Sagittal T1 C+ shows the heterogeneously enhancing 4th ventricle mass extrudes posteroinferiorly through the foramen of Magendie into the cisterna magna and upper cervical canal.*

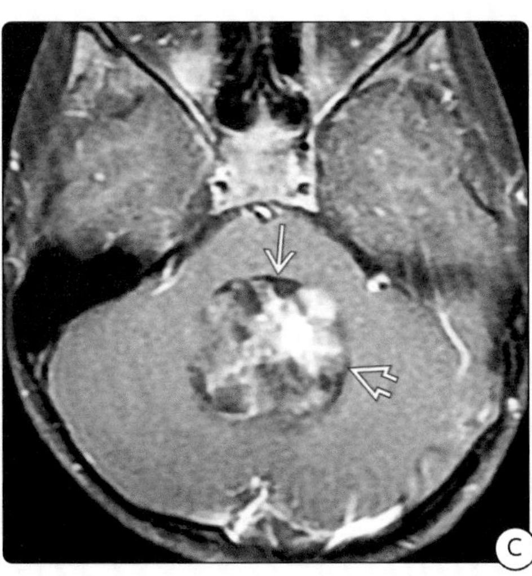


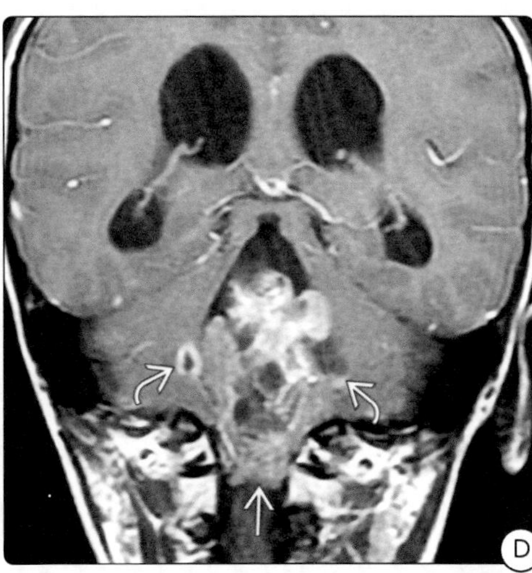


***(22-8C)** T1 C+ FS shows the mixed solid/cystic tumor enhances heterogeneously, expands and almost completely fills the 4th ventricle. **(22-8D)** Coronal T1 C+ shows tumor extends inferiorly into the cisterna magna, laterally into both foramina of Luschka. This is PFA ependymoma. The child survived 2 years.*

present with nonspecific symptoms (headache, vomiting, and lethargy).

**Natural History.** PFA ependymomas are associated with a high recurrence rate and poor clinical outcome. Overall five-year survival for this subgroup is ~ 50%, whereas it approaches 85-90% for the PFB ependymoma subgroup.

**Treatment Options.** Maximum cytoreduction surgery followed by conformal radiotherapy—not cranial spinal irradiation—is the standard treatment. Adjuvant therapy is generally reserved for recurrent tumor.

## Imaging

**General Features.** *Infratentorial* ependymomas (both PFA and PFB) are relatively well-delineated, "plastic" tumors that typically arise from the floor of the fourth ventricle and extrude through the outlet foramina. They extend laterally through the foramina of Luschka toward the CPA cistern **(22-8)** and posteroinferiorly through the foramen of Magendie into the cisterna magna **(22-9)**.

Sagittal images disclose a mass that fills most of the fourth ventricle and extrudes inferiorly into the cisterna magna **(22-10C)**. Axial and coronal images show lateral extension toward or into the CPA cisterns **(22-9)**.

Obstructive hydrocephalus is a frequent accompanying feature of infratentorial ependymomas. Extracellular fluid often accumulates around the ventricles, giving the appearance of "blurred" margins.

CSF dissemination is a key factor in staging, prognosis, and treatment of ependymoma. The only statistically significant preoperative imaging predictor of patient outcome is evidence of tumor spread. Therefore, *preoperative imaging of the entire cranial-spinal axis should be performed in any child with a posterior fossa neoplasm*, especially if medulloblastoma or ependymoma is suspected.

***(22-9A)** Axial T2 FS in a 3-yo boy shows a heterogeneously hyperintense mass ➡ centered in the 4th ventricle. Note anterolateral extension through the lateral recess into the left CPA cistern ➡. Posteroinferior extension into the cisterna magna ➡ is also present. **(22-9B)** Sagittal T2 FS shows the mass expands the 4th ventricle ➡, displaces the pons anteriorly ➡, extends into the cisterna magna and upper cervical spine ➡.*

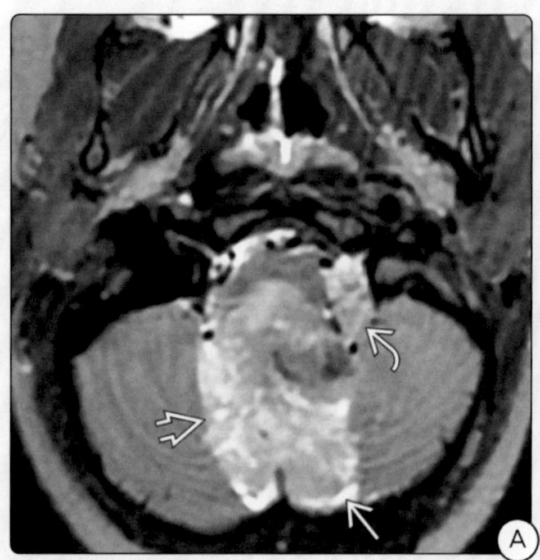


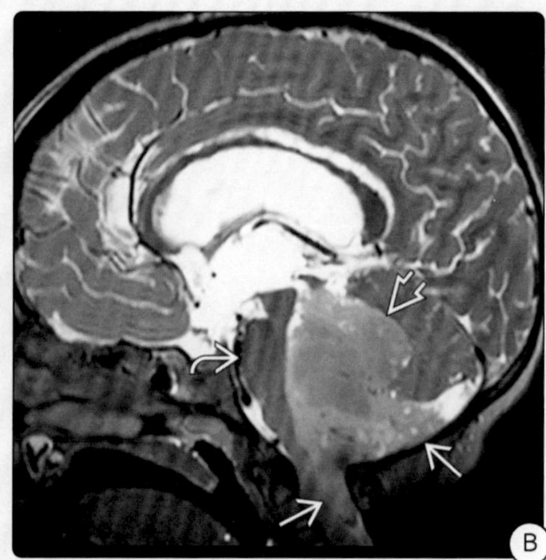


***(22-9C)** Axial T1 C+ SPGR shows almost no enhancement in the mass. **(22-9D)** Sagittal T1 C+ SPGR shows a few scattered enhancing foci ➡ in the mostly nonenhancing mass. This is PFA ependymoma. The child survived 18 months.*

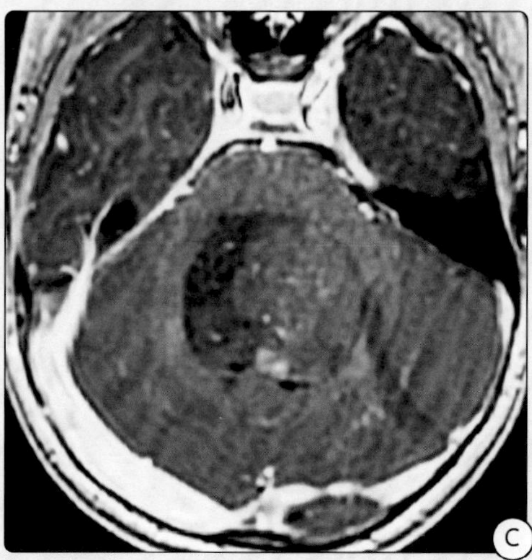


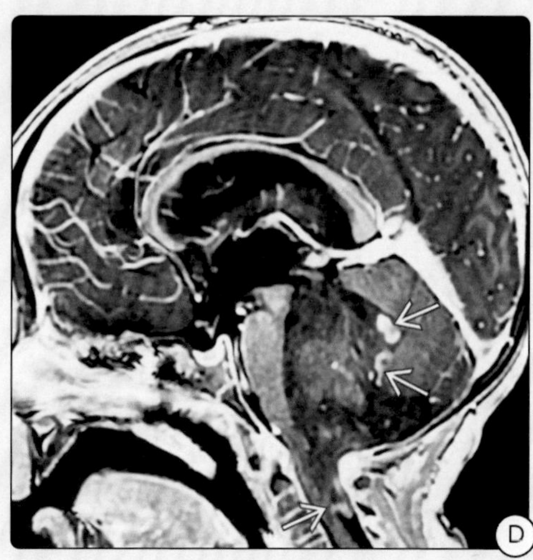

**CT Findings.** Ependymomas are generally mixed density on NECT scans with hypodense intratumoral cysts intermixed with iso- and hyperdense soft tissue portions. Coarse calcification occurs in ~ 1/2 of all ependymomas **(22-12A)**. Macroscopic hemorrhage can be identified in ~ 10% of cases.

Most ependymomas show mild to moderate heterogeneous enhancement.

**MR Findings.** Ependymomas are generally heterogeneously hypointense relative to brain parenchyma on T1WI and hyperintense on T2/FLAIR **(22-9)**. Following contrast administration, most ependymomas enhance. Areas of strong, relatively homogeneous enhancement are intermixed with foci of minimal or even no enhancement **(22-9D)**.

T2* imaging (GRE, SWI) commonly demonstrates "blooming" foci that can be caused by calcification **(22-12B)** &/or old hemorrhage. An ependymoma may bleed, causing nonaneurysmal subarachnoid hemorrhage and siderosis around the tumor and along the pial surfaces of the cerebellum.

Most ependymomas do not restrict on DWI, although foci of restricted diffusion can be identified in some cases.

General MRS metabolite ratios are nonspecific. Elevated choline and reduced NAA are common in ependymoma, as in many other brain tumors. pMR generally demonstrates markedly elevated CBV with poor return to baseline.

## Differential Diagnosis

Differential diagnosis of ependymoma is location dependent.

The major differential diagnosis of *infratentorial* ependymoma is **medulloblastoma**. Medulloblastomas are more common and typically arise from the roof of the fourth ventricle (not from the floor, as is typical of ependymoma). Medulloblastomas are hyperdense on NECT, often

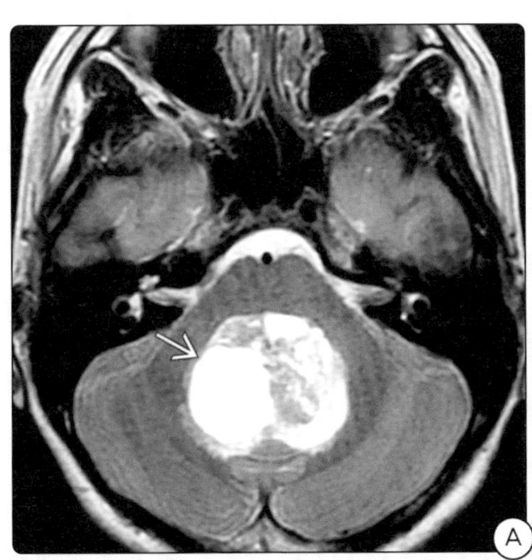

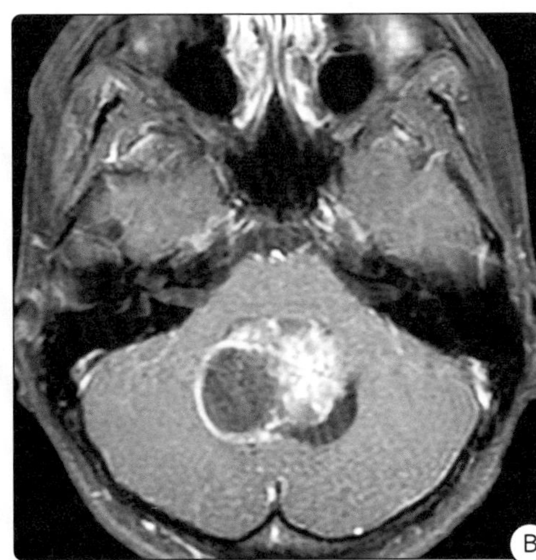

***(22-10A)** T2WI in a 12-yo girl with headaches shows a heterogeneously hyperintense mass ➡ filling a massively enlarged 4th ventricle. **(22-10B)** T1 C+ FS shows the solid portion of the mass enhances heterogeneously. An enhancing rim is present around the cystic component of the tumor.*

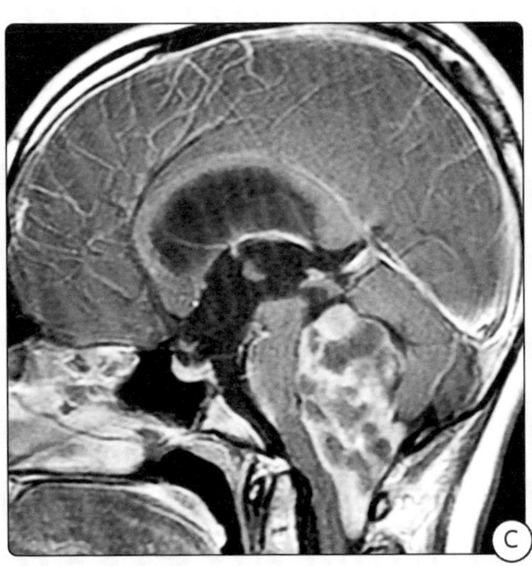

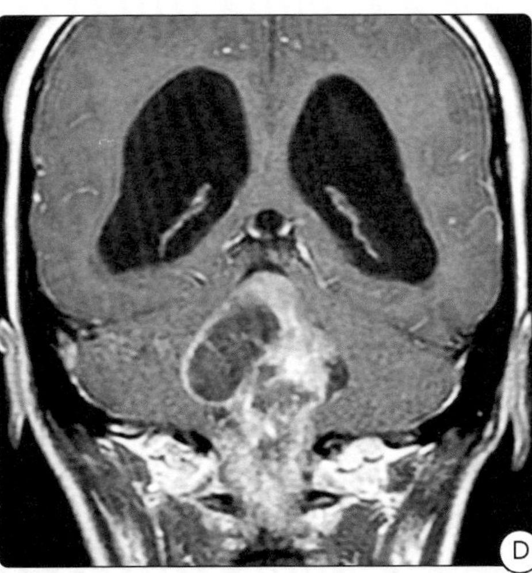

***(22-10C)** Sagittal T1 C+ shows the heterogeneously enhancing mass fills the 4th ventricle and extends posteroinferiorly into the cisterna magna and upper spinal cord. **(22-10D)** Coronal T1 C+ shows the mass expands the 4th ventricle, extends into the upper cervical canal. This is PFB ependymoma. Imaging resembles PFA (Fig. 22-8), but the patient is alive without evidence for disease 7 years following resection and chemotherapy.*

demonstrate diffusion restriction, and more frequently show evidence of CSF dissemination at the time of initial diagnosis. Cysts, hemorrhage, and calcification are less common in medulloblastoma compared with ependymoma.

## Posterior Fossa Group B Ependymoma

### Terminology

PFB ependymomas are identified as such by DNA methylation profiling.

### Pathology

Both the general macro- and microscopic features of PFB ependymomas are similar to PFA ependymomas. While PFB ependymomas can arise anywhere in the fourth ventricle, they more frequently arise from the floor rather than the roof or lateral recesses **(22-11)**.

In contrast to PFA ependymomas, almost all PFB ependymomas retain nuclear expression of H3p.K28me3, which can be readily assessed by immunohistochemistry.

Similar to the PFA ependymomas, PFB ependymomas can be CNS WHO grade 2 or 3 tumors depending on the degree of anaplasia and other high-grade features, such as prominent mitotic activity and microvascular proliferation.

### Clinical Issues

Frequency of PFB ependymomas compared to PFA ependymomas is highly age dependent. Median age at presentation is 30 years. Over 90% occur in adults or adolescents; < 5% occur in infants and children under five years.

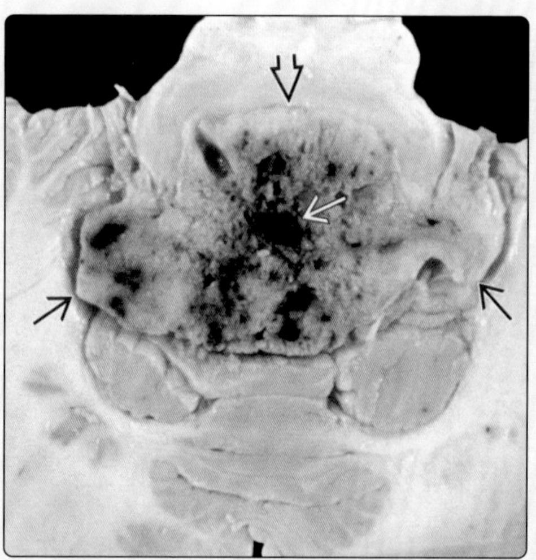

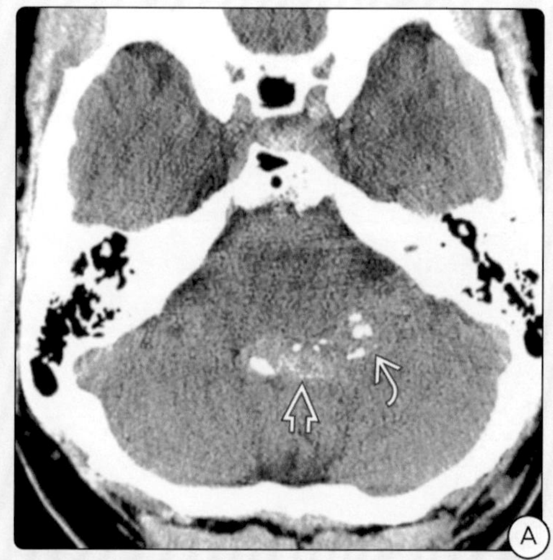

*(22-11) Axial gross pathology shows ependymoma filling the 4th ventricle ⇨ and extending anterolaterally through the lateral recesses towards the foramina of Luschka ⇨. Note patchy hemorrhagic foci ➡. (Courtesy E. Ross, MD.) (22-12A) NECT shows a partially calcified mass in the 4th ventricle ➡ extending through the lateral recess ➡ towards the CPA cistern.*

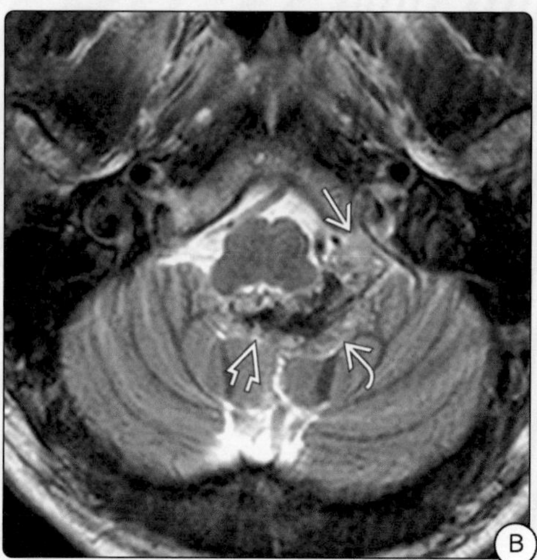

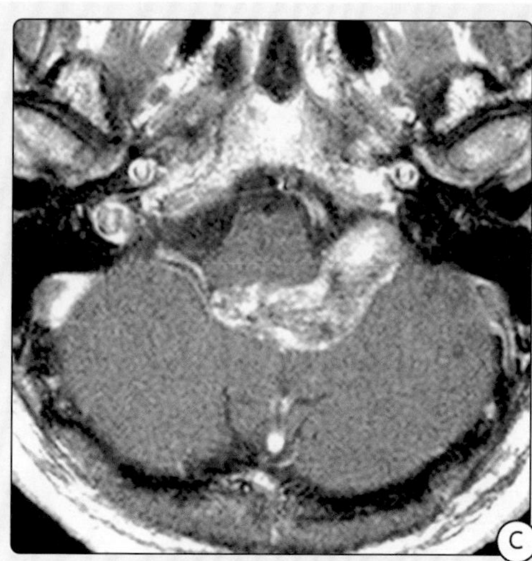

*(22-12B) T2WI shows the "plastic" nature of the partially calcified mass ➡ as it extrudes through the lateral recess ➡ into the adjacent CPA cistern ➡. (22-12C) T1 C+ shows the mass enhances heterogeneously. This is ependymoma (no methylation class specified), CNS WHO grade 2.*

DNA methylation profiling has identified five distinct PFB subtypes. PFB-1, PFB-2, and PFB-3 tumors tend to occur in patients aged 25-30 years, whereas the median age of PFB-4 tumors is 15 years. PFB-5 tumors occur in older adults where the median age at diagnosis is 40 years.

### Imaging

Imaging findings in PFB ependymomas **(22-10)** **(22-12)** are identical to PFA ependymomas.

### Differential Diagnosis

A posterior fossa ependymoma in an adult or adolescent older than eight years is either a **PFB ependymoma** or **subependymoma (SE)** **(22-17)**.

The other main differential diagnosis of PFB ependymoma is **medulloblastoma**, which can also occur in adolescents and adults. **Pilocytic astrocytoma** also occurs in the fourth ventricle but is more common in the cerebellar hemispheres. **High-grade astrocytoma with pilocytic features (HGAP)** is in the differential diagnosis, especially in patients with neurofibromatosis type 1. HGAPs are more common in the cerebellar hemispheres and brainstem.

## Subependymoma

### Terminology

Subependymomas (SEs) are rare, benign, slow-growing, noninvasive tumors that are often found incidentally at imaging or autopsy. SE is a well-circumscribed glial tumor with small, uniform, cytologically bland nuclei.

### Etiology

The origin of SEs is unclear. They may arise from pluripotential ependymal-glial precursor cells, astrocytes in the subependymal plate, or a preexisting hamartomatous lesion.

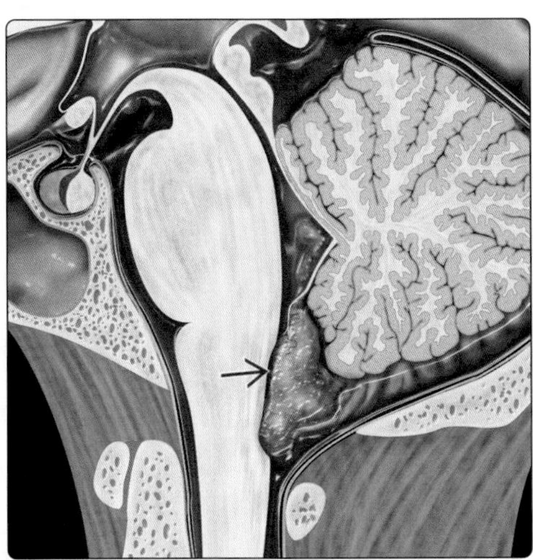

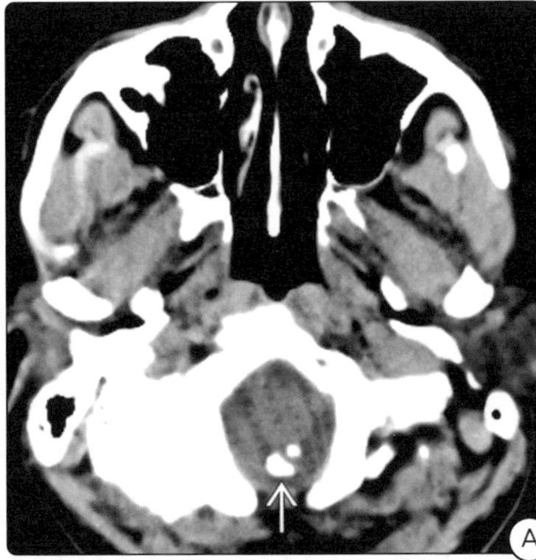


***(22-13)** Graphic depicts subependymoma ⇨ of the inferior 4th ventricle at the level of the obex. **(22-14A)** NECT in a 56-yo man in the ER with severe "thunderclap" headache and suspected subarachnoid hemorrhage shows chunky calcifications ➡ in the lower cisterna magna. No subarachnoid hemorrhage was found.*

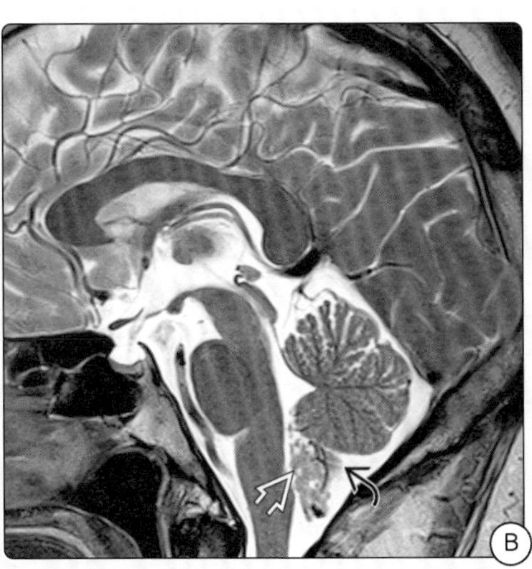


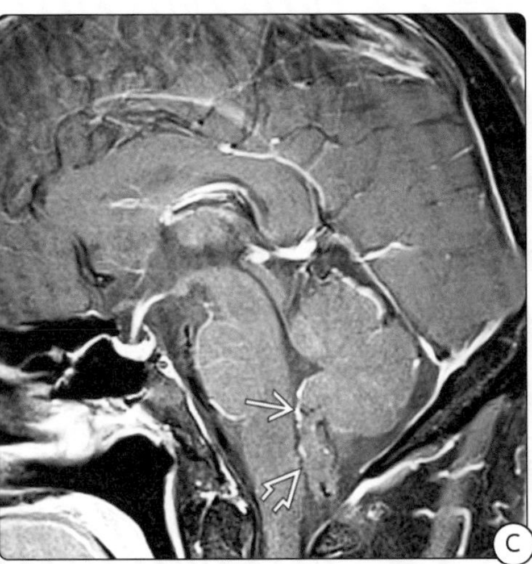


***(22-14B)** Sagittal T2WI shows a heterogeneous mass in the inferior 4th ventricle ➡ that extends into the cisterna magna. The cerebellar tonsil is displaced posteriorly ⇨. Compare to Fig. 22-13. **(22-14C)** T1 C+ FS in the same case shows the mass ➡ does not enhance, although the choroid plexus in the inferior 4th ventricle enhances intensely ➡. Subependymoma, CNS WHO grade 1. This was probably an incidental finding.*

A specific mutation on the *TRPS1* gene may play a role in at least some cases.

## Pathology

**Location.** While SEs can arise along the whole neuraxis, they are usually located within or adjacent to an ependyma-lined space. They occur in all three anatomic compartments (supratentorial, posterior fossa, and spinal).

The fourth ventricle is the most common site (50-60% of cases) **(22-13)** **(22-15)**. The lateral ventricles account for ~ 1/3 of all cases. Most of these occur in the frontal horn of the lateral ventricle, near the foramen of Monro, where they are often attached to the septi pellucidi **(22-18)**. SEs in the third ventricle and occipital horn of the lateral ventricle are rare. Parenchymal and intramedullary intraspinal SEs occur but are uncommon.

**Size and Number.** SEs are solitary tumors. Most are < 2 cm **(22-14)**, although some tumors may reach several centimeters in diameter **(22-16)**. A few cases of very large biventricular SEs that fill both lateral ventricles have been reported. Because the posterior fossa is more anatomically constrained, infratentorial tumors are generally smaller than their supratentorial counterparts.

**Gross Pathology.** SEs are solid, round to somewhat lobulated, well-delineated, gray-tan masses. Calcification, cysts, and hemorrhage are common in larger lesions.

**Microscopic Features.** Bland nuclei in a dense fibrillary stroma with variable microcystic degeneration is typical. Nuclear pleomorphism and nonpalisading necrosis are rare but may occur. Mitotic activity is absent or low level.

**Diagnostic Molecular Pathology.** Although SEs in the three anatomic compartments have distinct, site-specific epigenetic

*(22-15) Subependymomas can vary widely in size. This sagittal autopsy section shows a small 4th ventricle subependymoma ⇨ that was found incidentally at autopsy. Location in the inferior 4th ventricle near the obex is typical. (Courtesy P. Burger, MD.) (22-16A) Sagittal T1WI in a 63-yo man with a 10-year history of vertigo shows a very large, quite heterogeneous-appearing mass in the inferior 4th ventricle ➡.*

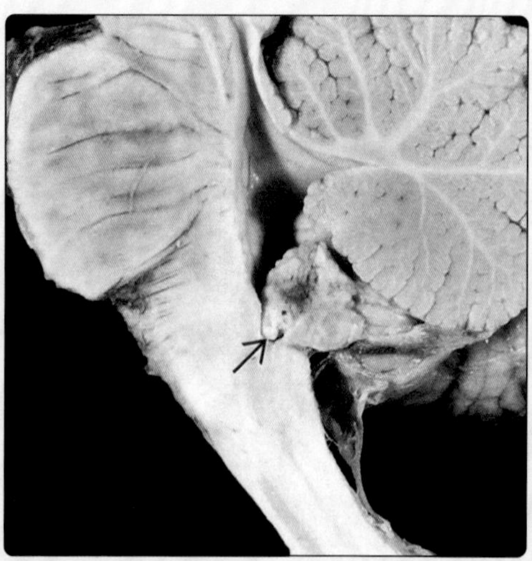

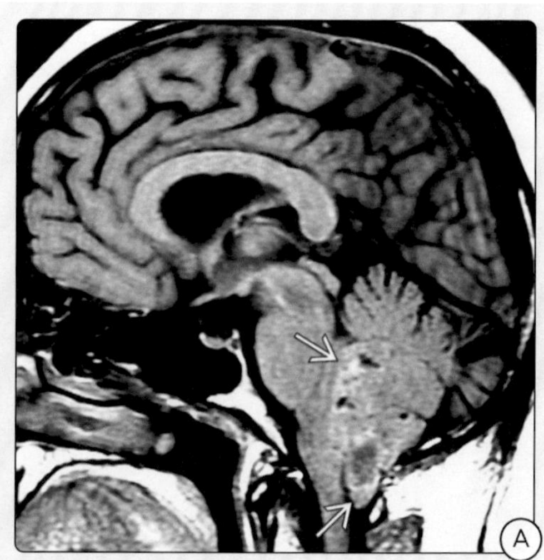

*(22-16B) Axial T2WI shows the mass ➡ is well demarcated but exhibits very heterogeneous signal intensity. Note posteroinferior extension into the cisterna magna ➡. (22-16C) The mass ➡ exhibits mild, heterogeneous enhancement on T1 C+ FS. This is subependymoma, CNS WHO grade 1.*

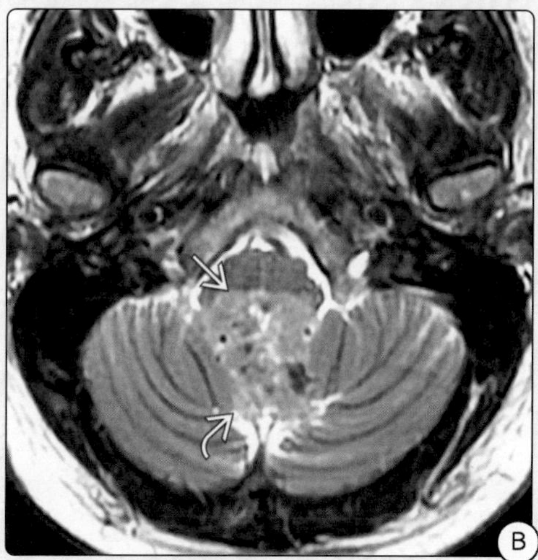

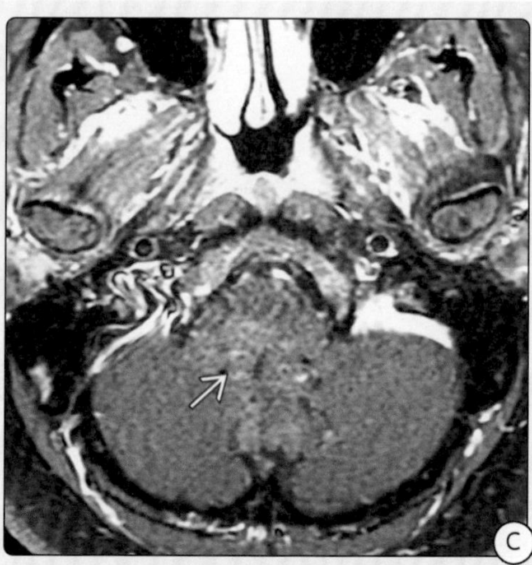

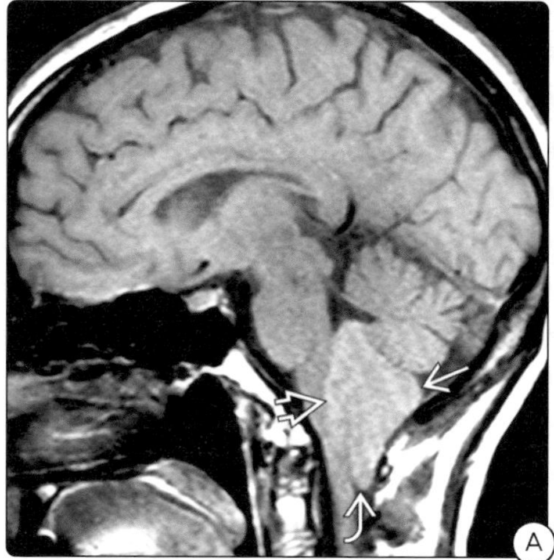

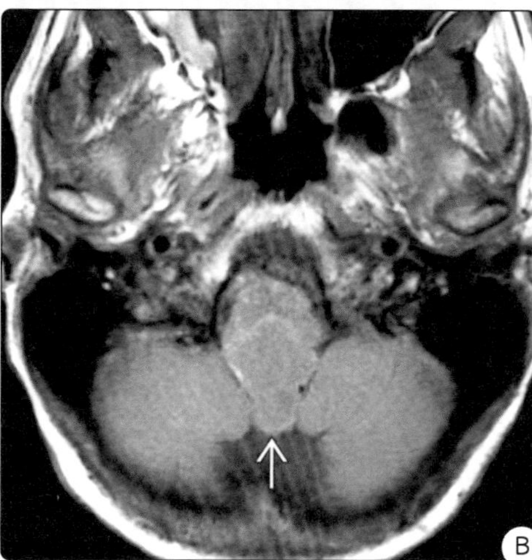

***(22-17A)*** *Sagittal T1WI in a 33-yo woman with suboccipital headaches shows a slightly hyperintense mass in the 4th ventricle ➡ that extends into the cisterna magna ➡ and upper cervical spine ➡.* ***(22-17B)*** *Axial T1WI in the same case shows the mass is well delineated, somewhat lobulated, and slightly hyperintense compared to adjacent brain. Posterior extension into the cisterna magna ➡ is well seen here.*

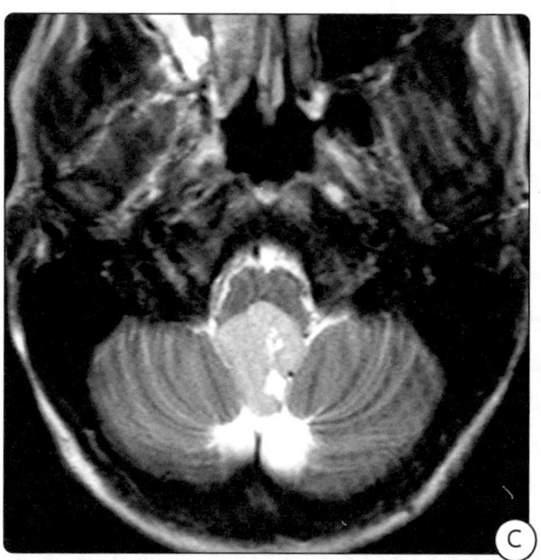

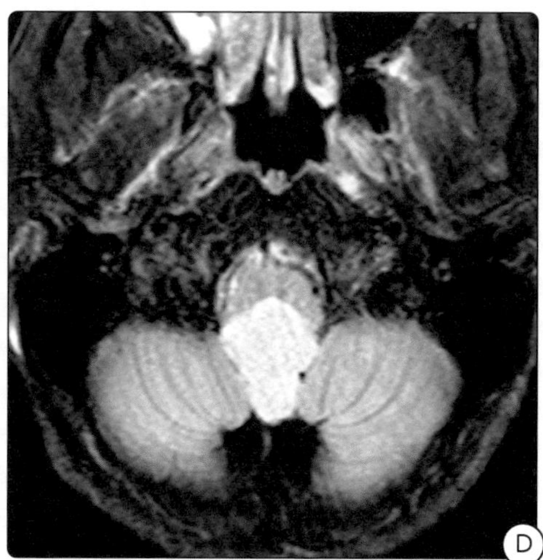

***(22-17C)*** *T2WI shows the mass is hyperintense and contains some even more hyperintense foci.* ***(22-17D)*** *The lobulated, well-delineated mass is uniformly hyperintense to brain on FLAIR.*

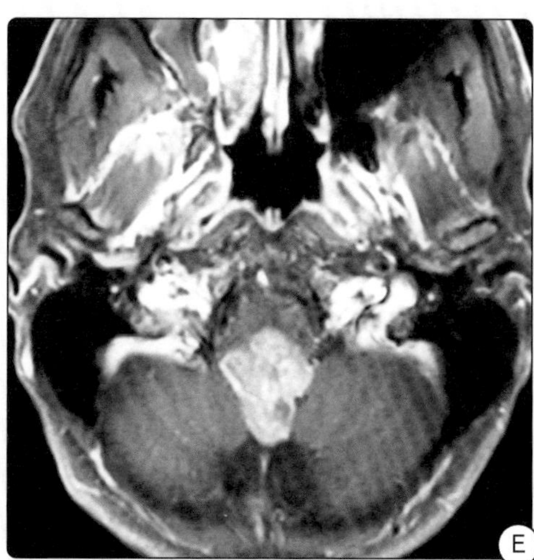

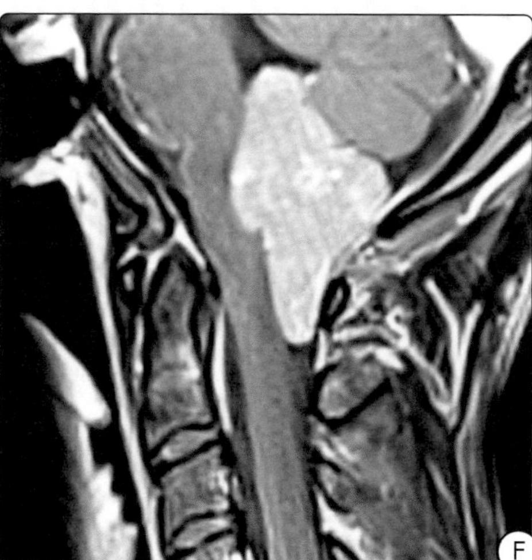

***(22-17E)*** *T1 C+ FS shows the mass enhances intensely but slightly heterogeneously.* ***(22-17F)*** *Sagittal T1 C+ FS from the cervical spine MR in the same case shows the lobulated mass begins at the midlevel of the 4th ventricle and extends intradurally to C2. Preoperative diagnosis was subependymoma but pathology disclosed PFB ependymoma by methylation profiling.*

methylation profiles, they all cluster together and are not placed in separate molecular groups.

**Staging, Grading, and Classification.** SEs are designated as CNS WHO grade 1 neoplasms even if rare pleomorphic features are present. Anaplastic transformation is exceptionally rare.

## Clinical Issues

**Epidemiology.** SEs are often clinically silent, so reliable incidence figures are lacking. SEs are found in 0.5-1.0% of autopsies. They account for 8% of all ependymomas and < 1% of intracranial neoplasms.

**Demographics.** SEs are tumors of middle-aged and older adults. They are very rare in children. There is a moderate male predominance.

**Presentation.** The majority of SEs are asymptomatic and discovered incidentally. Approximately 40% cause symptoms, mostly related to CSF obstruction or mass effect.

**Natural History.** SEs exhibit an indolent growth pattern, expanding slowly into a ventricular space. Larger tumors may cause obstructive hydrocephalus, but they rarely invade adjacent brain. Recurrence is rare even after subtotal resection. Cytologic pleomorphism, occasional mitoses, and even necrosis have not proved prognostically significant.

**Treatment Options.** "Watchful waiting" with serial imaging is appropriate in asymptomatic patients. Complete surgical resection of symptomatic SEs is the procedure of choice.

## Imaging

**General Features.** SEs are well-demarcated nodular masses that may expand the ventricle but usually cause little mass effect. Almost all fourth ventricle SEs are centered below the

*(22-18) Coronal autopsy shows frontal horn mass ➡ attached to the septum pellucidum ➡. This is subependymoma. This was an incidental finding. (22-19A) Axial T2WI shows a well-demarcated, hyperintense frontal horn mass ➡ that seems to be attached to the septum pellucidum ➡.*

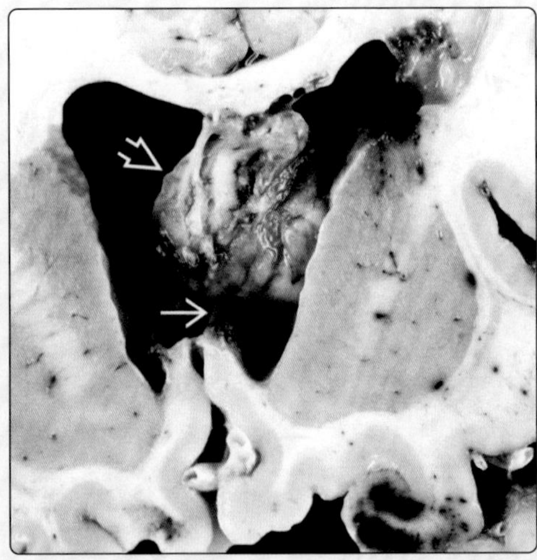

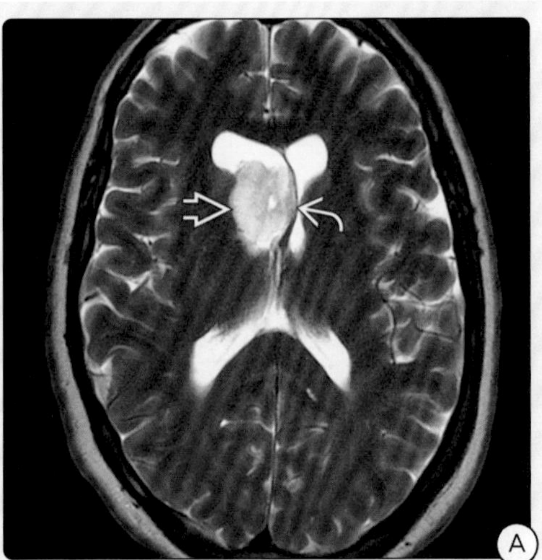

*(22-19B) FLAIR shows the mass is very hyperintense. There is no evidence for hydrocephalus or periventricular fluid accumulation. (22-19C) Sagittal T1 C+ shows the lobulated mass enhances intensely but heterogeneously and appears confined to the frontal horn of the lateral ventricle. This is subependymoma, CNS WHO grade 1.*

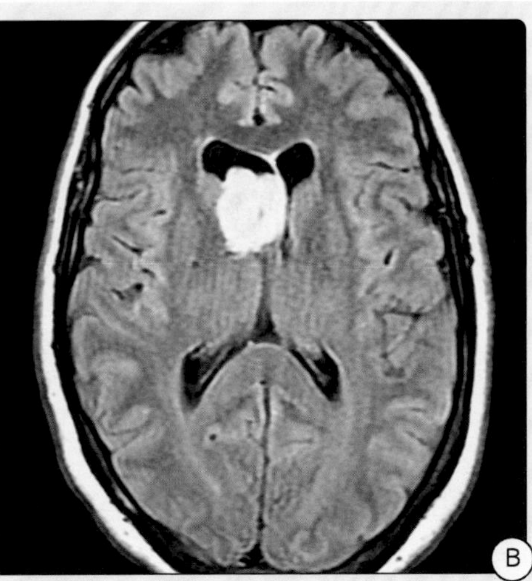

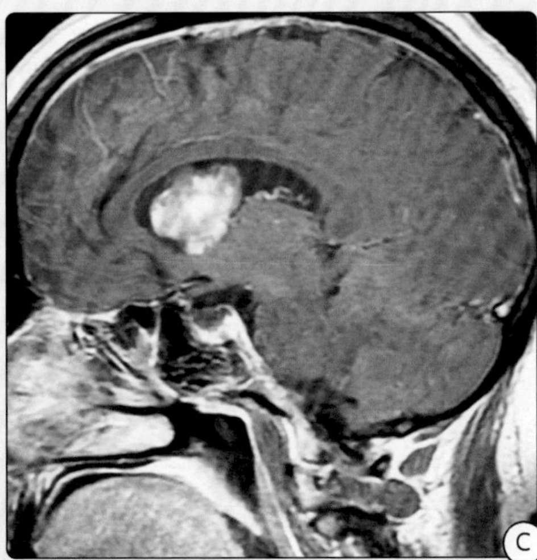

body of the fourth ventricle and above the obex **(22-14)**. Nearly 1/2 of these exhibit tumor extension into the foramen of Magendie or Luschka **(22-16)**.

**CT Findings.** SEs are iso- to slightly hypodense compared with brain on NECT scans. Calcification and intratumoral cysts may be present **(22-14A)**, especially in larger lesions. Hydrocephalus is variable, and hemorrhage is rare. Little or no enhancement is seen on CECT.

**MR Findings.** Most SEs are isointense or slightly hyperintense compared with brain on T1WI **(22-16A)**. Intratumoral cysts are common in larger lesions. SEs are heterogeneously hyperintense on T2 **(22-19A)** and hyperintense on FLAIR **(22-19B)**. Peritumoral edema is usually absent. T2* (GRE, SWI) shows "blooming" foci, probably secondary to calcification. Hemorrhage is seen in 10-12%.

The majority of SEs exhibit some degree of enhancement on T1 C+ that varies from none or mild **(22-16C)** to moderate **(22-19C)**. Typically only part of the tumor enhances. Avid enhancement is rare.

SEs do not restrict on DWI. MRS shows normal choline with mildly decreased NAA.

## Differential Diagnosis

The differential diagnosis of SE varies with age and anatomic location. In older patients, the major differential is intraventricular **metastasis**. Most intraventricular metastases arise in the choroid plexus. In young to middle-aged adults, **ST-EPNs** and **PFB ependymomas** **(22-17)** as well as **central neurocytoma** might considered **(22-20)**. Central neurocytoma is typically found in the body of the lateral ventricle, not the frontal horn or inferior fourth ventricle, and has a characteristic bubbly appearance.

In children, depending on age, **PFA and PFB ependymomas** and (in patients with tuberous sclerosis) **subependymal giant**

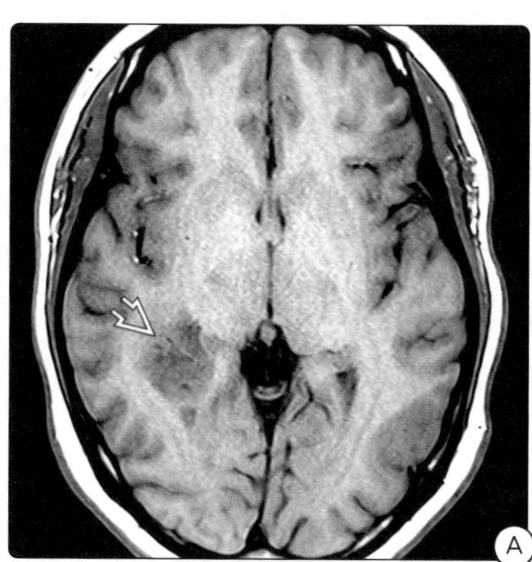

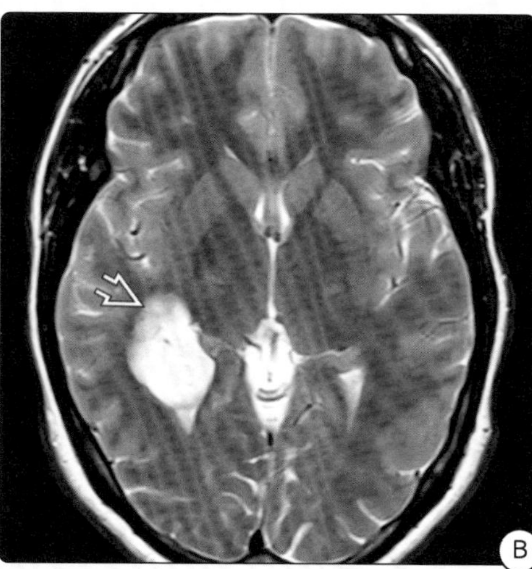

***(22-20A)*** *Axial T1WI in a 24-yo woman with left-sided paresthesias shows a mass in the atrium of the right lateral ventricle ➯ that is mostly isointense with cortex.* ***(22-20B)*** *The mass ➯ is well delineated, without surrounding edema, and is hyperintense compared to CSF in the adjacent occipital horn.*

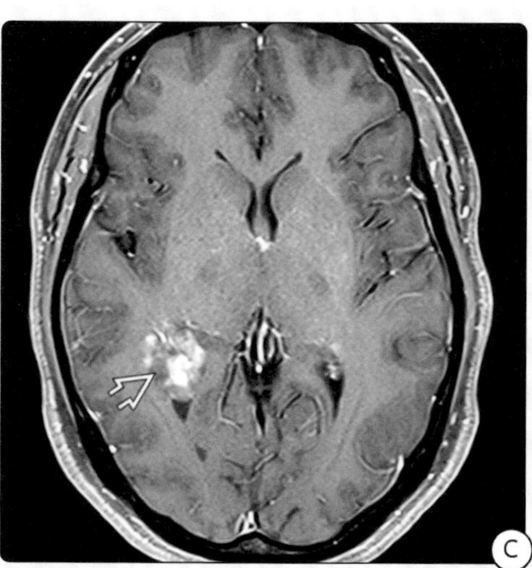

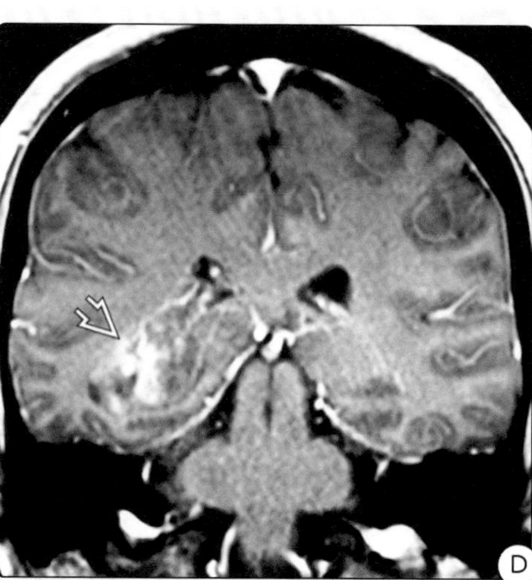

***(22-20C)*** *The mass ➯ is well demarcated and exhibits heterogeneous enhancement on T1 C+ FS.* ***(22-20D)*** *Coronal T1 C+ shows the mass ➯ appears to be completely contained within the lateral ventricle. Histology disclosed mixed features of ependymoma and subependymoma. DNA methylation class was supratentorial ependymoma.*

**cell astrocytoma** are considerations. **Choroid plexus papillomas** in children are usually in the atrium of the lateral ventricle. Choroid plexus papilloma also has a frond-like appearance and typically shows intense uniform enhancement.

# Spinal Ependymomas

Ependymal tumors of the spinal cord are relatively uncommon, accounting for 2-6% of all CNS tumors. Spinal ependymomas (SP-EPNs) primarily affect adults between the ages of 20-40 years.

Four distinct spinal ependymal tumor types are recognized: SP-EPN, SP-EPN with *MYCN* amplification (SP-MYCN), myxopapillary ependymoma (MPE), and SE. We discuss two of these—MPE and SP-MYCN—in this closing section, as the 5th edition WHO made some significant changes in these entities.

## Spinal Ependymoma, *MYCN*-Amplified

SP-MYCN was recognized in the 5th edition WHO as a novel, clinically aggressive type of ependymoma characterized by early metastases, rapid progression, leptomeningeal dissemination, and poor response to multimodal treatment strategies. In the most recent classification, *MYCN*-amplified high-grade glioma is one of the recognized subtypes of IDH- and H3-wildtype pediatric-type high-grade gliomas.

SP-MYCN is rare, accounting for 5% of all SP-EPNs. It has a distinct methylation profile that differs from all other ependymal tumor types. Practically all SP-MYCNs display microvascular proliferation, necrosis, and a high mitotic count. To date, no CNS WHO grade has been assigned, but investigators report these tumors are characterized by grade 3 histopathology. Reported median overall survival is 14 months.

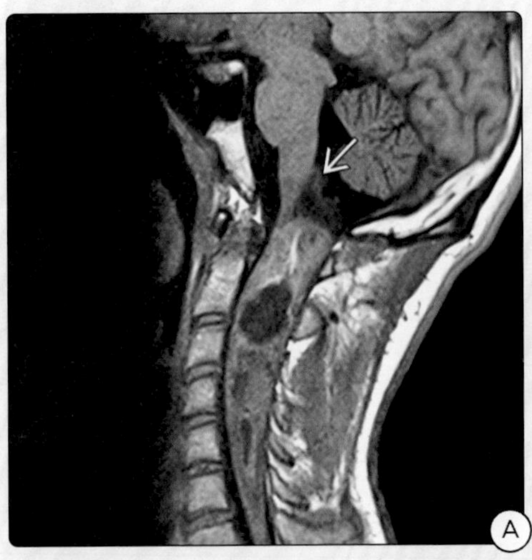


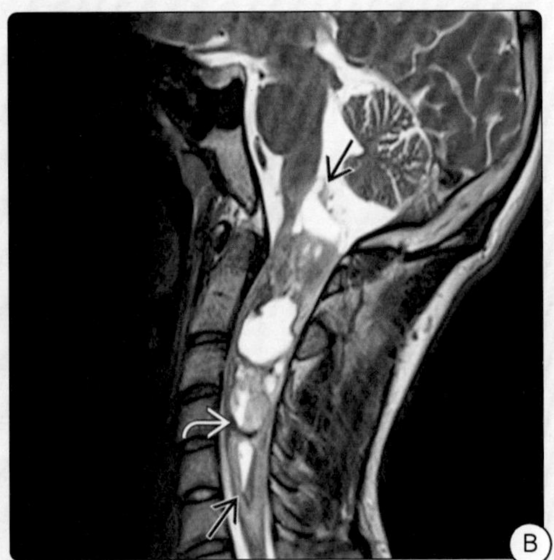


***(22-21A)** Sagittal T1WI in 21-yo man shows a heterogeneous intramedullary mass extending from the lower posterior fossa to C6-C7. **(22-21B)** T2WI shows a heterogenous cystic/solid mass with cap sign, suggesting intratumoral hemorrhage.*

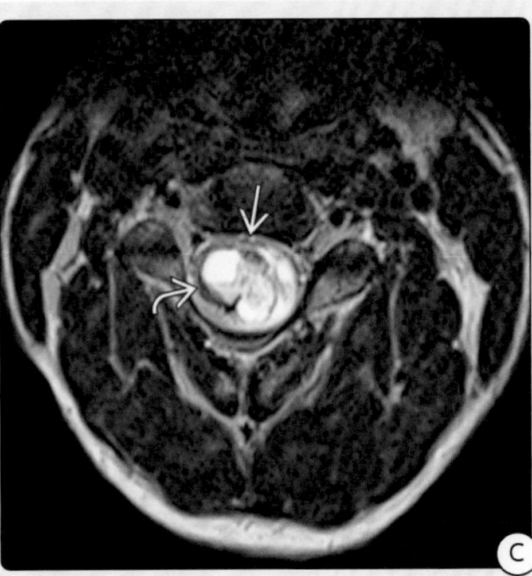


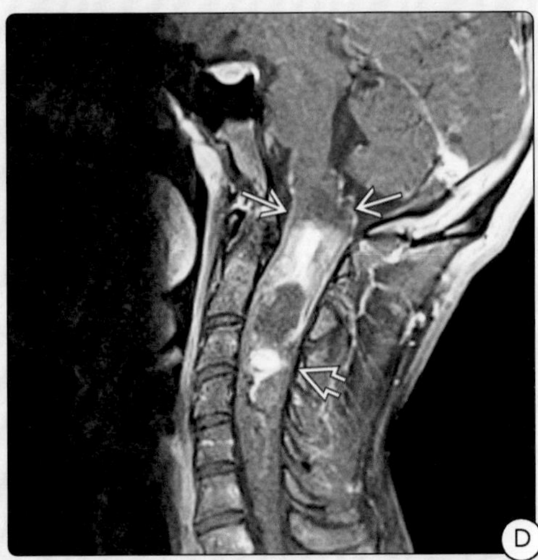


***(22-21C)** Axial T2WI shows the mixed solid/cystic mass occupies nearly the entire width of the cervical cord. Note intratumoral hemorrhage. **(22-21D)** T1 C+ shows the mass enhances heterogeneously. Note leptomeningeal tumor spread. Histopathology disclosed microvascular proliferation, necrosis, and brisk mitotic activity was consistent with a CNS WHO grade 3 tumor. Spinal ependymoma, MYCN-amplified.*

More than 80% are found in the cervical or thoracic spinal cord. Unlike classic spinal cord ependymomas, MYCN-amplified tumors appear diffusely infiltrative on MR. Imaging shows extremely heterogeneous signal intensity on T1- and T2WIs with intermixed cystic and solid components **(22-21)**. Hemorrhage with a hypointense cap sign is common. Enhancement is variable and leptomeningeal dissemination is frequent, so imaging the entire neuraxis is recommended prior to surgical intervention.

## Myxopapillary Ependymoma

MPE is a very slow-growing type of ependymoma that occurs at all ages but mostly affects young adults. MPEs are almost exclusively tumors of the conus medullaris, cauda equina, and filum terminale **(22-22)**.

Progressive lower back pain is the most common clinical presentation. Although disseminated tumor and recurrent or progressive disease after surgery are common, 10-year survival is > 90%.

In the typical MPE, MIB-1 labeling index is low (generally < 1%). MPEs are **CNS WHO grade 2 tumors**, a change from the 2016 edition.

MPEs are generally hypo- to isointense on T1WIs and hyperintense on T2WIs. Enhancement is typically strong and homogeneous **(22-23)**. Although adults rarely have multiple lesions, nearly 1/2 of MPEs in children and adolescents have leptomeningeal disease on initial presentation, so complete neuraxis imaging should be performed prior to surgery **(22-24)**.

**IMAGING FEATURES OF EPENDYMOMAS BY ANATOMIC COMPARTMENT**

Supratentorial Ependymomas
- Hemispheres (not ventricles)
  - Bulky, mixed cystic-solid

Posterior Fossa Ependymomas (Defined by Molecular Group)
- PFA = infants, very young children (adults rare)
  - Bulky, heterogeneous 4th ventricle mass
  - Extends into lateral recesses, cisterna magna
  - Poor prognosis
- PFB = adolescents or adults (infants very rare)
  - Imaging identical to PFA
  - Better prognosis
- SE (occurs in all 3 compartments)
  - 4th ventricle (centered below body, above obex)
  - Lateral ventricle (frontal horn) > temporal > occipital

Spinal Ependymomas
- *MYCN* amplified (cord)
  - Highly malignant, diffusely infiltrative
  - No formal grade but behaves like CNS WHO grade 3
  - Hemorrhage, cysts, leptomeningeal dissemination common
  - Strong but heterogeneous enhancement
- MPE
  - Slow growing but now CNS WHO grade 2!
  - Intradural, extramedullary
  - Cauda equina ± uphill "drop" metastases
  - Scan entire spine + brain before surgery!

*Selected References: The complete reference list is available on the eBooks+ version included with purchase.*

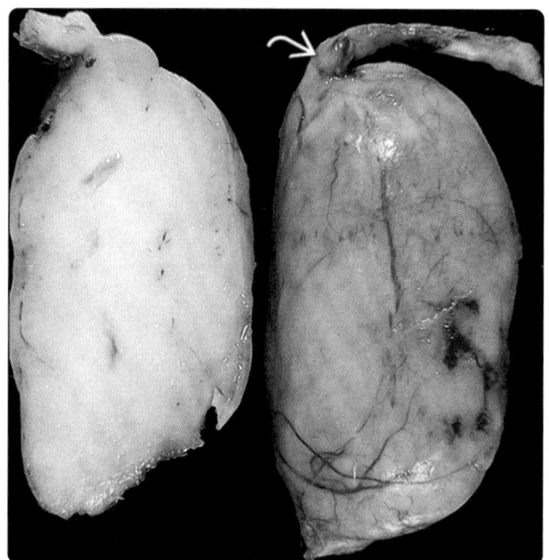

***(22-22)** Well-defined intradural extramedullary mass attached to the cauda equina ➲. Myxopapillary ependymoma, CNS WHO grade 2.*

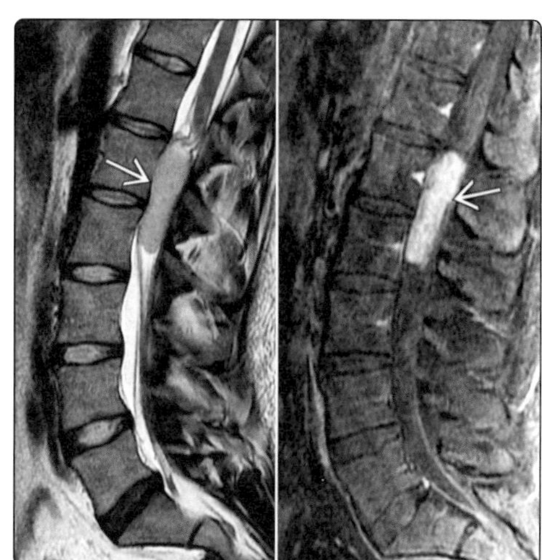

***(22-23)** Sagittal T2WI (L), T1 C+ FS (R) show classic myxopapillary ependymoma of the cauda equina ➲.*

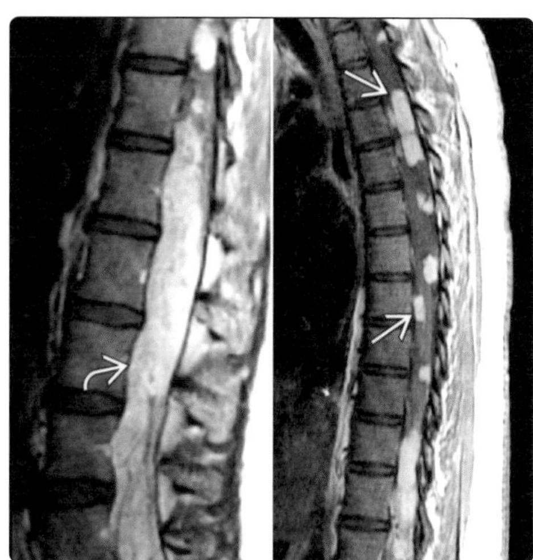

***(22-24)** (L) T1 C+ in 16-yo girl shows enhancing lumbar intradural mass ➲, (R) metastases ➲. Myxopapillary ependymoma, CNS WHO grade 2.*

# Choroid Plexus Tumors

*The 5th edition WHO separates choroid plexus tumors from gliomas, glioneuronal tumors, and neuronal tumors. Choroid plexus neoplasms are now considered as their own distinct category of tumors.*



## Choroid Plexus Tumors

The 5th edition WHO recognizes three *histologic* subtypes of choroid plexus tumors (CPTs): Choroid plexus papilloma (CPP), atypical CPP (APP), and choroid plexus carcinoma (CPC).

Recent DNA methylation profiling studies suggest further segregating CPTs into three *clinically/molecularly* relevant subclasses: (1) Pediatric low-risk CPT (CPP/APP) = "pediatric A" CPT; (2) infratentorial adult low-risk CPT (CPP/APP) = "adult" CPT; and (3) supratentorial pediatric high-risk CPT (all CPCs, very few APP/CPPs) = "pediatric B."

In this section, we discuss each of the three *histopathologic* types of choroid plexus neoplasms with the major focus on CPP—the most common primary CPT.

### Choroid Plexus Papilloma

#### Terminology

CPP is, by far, the most common, as well as the most benign, of the choroid plexus neoplasms. Both pediatric A and most adult low-risk infratentorial CPTs are CPPs.

#### Etiology

**Genetics.** Genomic analysis of CPPs suggests a role of genes involved in the development and biology of plexus epithelium (i.e., *OTX2* and *TRPM3*).

*SMARCB1* mutations with INI1 protein alterations and CPPs have been described in the **rhabdoid predisposition syndrome**. Both mutations are very rarely identified in sporadic CPPs.

CPPs also occur as part of **Aicardi syndrome**, an X-linked dominant syndrome that occurs almost exclusively in female patients. Aicardi syndrome is defined by the triad of infantile spasms, corpus callosum agenesis, and pathognomonic chorioretinal abnormalities (lacunae). Since it was first described in 1965, new features, such as cortical malformations, gray matter heterotopias, CPPs, and choroid plexus cysts, have been identified and added to the Aicardi spectrum. The prevalence of CPPs in Aicardi syndrome is estimated at 3-5%. Bilateral and triventricular CPPs occur in 1% of cases.

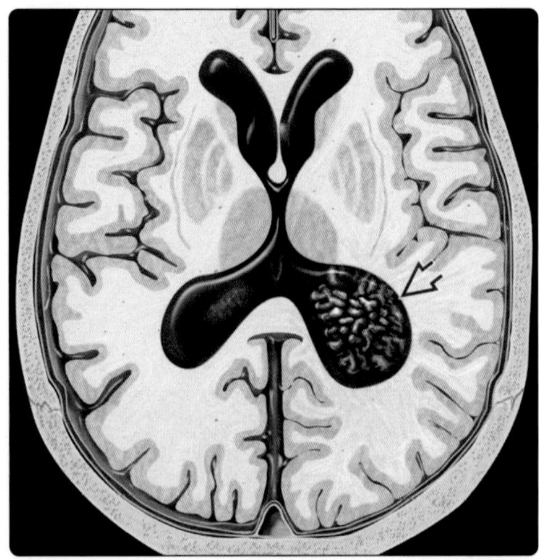

*(23-1) Graphic shows choroid plexus papilloma (CPP) ➾ in the left lateral ventricle atrium and enlarged ventricles from CSF overproduction.*

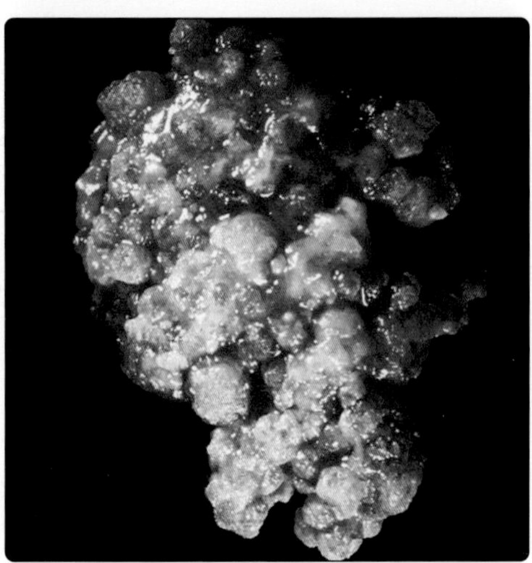

*(23-2) Resected CPP is shown. (From Fuller et al: Practical Surgical Neuropathology: A Diagnostic Approach, 6th ed.)*

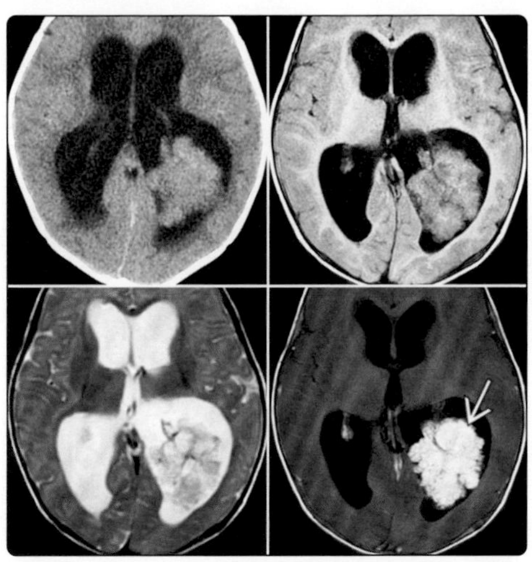

*(23-3) CPP in a child enhances strongly ➡. Note hydrocephalus caused by overproduction of CSF.*

## Pathology

**Location.** CPPs can arise wherever choroid plexus is normally found, in proportion to the amount of choroid plexus normally present in each location. Therefore, the vast majority arise in the lateral (50%) and fourth (40%) ventricles. The trigone is the most common overall site in the lateral ventricles **(23-1)** followed by the temporal horn. The body of the fourth ventricle is its most common site **(23-17)**. Tufts of normal choroid plexus extrude through the foramina of Luschka into the adjacent cerebellopontine angle (CPA) cisterns so CPPs within the lateral recesses or CPA also sometimes occur **(23-13)**.

Only 5-10% of all CPPs occur in locations other than the lateral and fourth ventricles. Just 5% are found in the third ventricle **(23-19)** **(23-20)**. Extraventricular CPPs are extremely rare. They have been reported in the brainstem, cerebellum, pituitary fossa, and septi pellucidi.

A few large CPPs involve multiple locations. Triventricular CPP is seen in 5% of cases and originates in the third ventricle, extending cephalad through the foramen of Monro into both lateral ventricles.

There is a strong effect of age on CPP location. More than 80% of all CPPs in infants arise in the atrium of the lateral ventricle. The fourth ventricle and CPA cisterns are more typical locations in adults. The lateral ventricles are an exceptionally rare site of CPP in older patients **(23-15)**.

**Size and Number.** CPPs are usually solitary tumors, varying in size from small to huge masses. Occasionally, multiple noncontiguous lesions are seen, but most represent CSF dissemination from the primary tumor site. Multiple CPPs arise independently as synchronous tumors are rarely seen.

**Gross Pathology.** CPPs are well-circumscribed papillary or cauliflower-like masses that may adhere to—but usually do not invade through—the ventricular wall **(23-2)**. Cysts and hemorrhage are common.

**Microscopic Features.** Histologically, the architecture of CPPs closely resembles that of normal nonneoplastic choroid plexus. A core of fibrovascular connective tissue covered by a single layer of uniform benign-appearing epithelial cells is typical. Cells tend to be more crowded and elongated or stratified. Cytokeratins, vimentin, and podoplanin are expressed by virtually all CPPs.

Mitotic activity is very low with MIB-1 < 1%. High cellularity, necrosis, nuclear pleomorphism, and focal blurring of the papillary pattern are unusual but may occur. CPPs are generally confined to the ventricle of origin and rarely exhibit an infiltrative growth pattern.

**Staging, Grading, and Classification.** CPPs are CNS WHO grade 1 neoplasms.

## Clinical Issues

**Epidemiology.** CPPs are rare lesions, accounting for < 1% of all primary intracranial neoplasms. However, CPPs represent 10-20% of brain tumors occurring in the first year of life.

**Demographics.** Median age at presentation is 1.5 years for lateral and third ventricular CPPs, 22.5 years for fourth ventricle CPPs, and 35.5 years for CPA CPPs. There is a very slight male predominance. About 80% of all lateral ventricle CPPs occur in patients < 20 years while fourth ventricle tumors are evenly distributed across all age groups.

**Presentation.** CPPs tend to obstruct normal CSF pathways. Infants present with increased head size and raised intracranial pressure. Children and adults may experience headache, nausea, and vomiting.

CPP can also present as a fetal brain tumor and is the fifth most common congenital brain neoplasm (after teratoma, astrocytoma, craniopharyngioma, and primitive neuroectodermal tumor). Macrocephaly with a large intracranial mass and hydrocephalus is the most common presentation.

**Natural History.** Surgical resection is often curative. The recurrence rate following gross total resection is low, only about 5-6%. Malignant progression of CPP to CPC has been reported but is very rare.

**CHOROID PLEXUS PAPILLOMA**

**Gross Pathology**
- Lateral ventricle trigone
    - 50%
    - Usually children
- Temporal horn
    - < 5%
    - Usually adults
- 4th ventricle/CPA cistern
    - 40%
    - Usually adults
- 3rd ventricle
    - 5-10%
    - Usually children
- Lobulated, frond-like configuration

**Microscopic Features**
- Well-developed papillary pattern
- Single layer of cuboidal/columnar epithelial cells
- Absent/low mitotic activity (< 2 mitoses/10 HPF)
- CNS WHO grade 1

**Clinical Issues**
- 13% of brain tumors in first year of life
- Mean age: 1.5 years for CPPs in lateral, 3rd ventricle
- Symptoms of obstructive hydrocephalus common
- Occurs with Aicardi, Li-Fraumeni, rhabdoid predisposition syndromes

**Imaging Findings**
- CT
    - Iso-/hyperdense, lobulated mass
    - Hydrocephalus common
    - Ca++ (25%)
    - CECT shows intense enhancement
- MR
    - Iso-/hypointense on T1
    - Iso-/hyperintense on T2/FLAIR
    - "Flow voids" common
    - May show "blooming" foci on T2*
    - Intense enhancement, no restriction
    - Occasionally demonstrates CSF dissemination (image entire neuraxis preoperatively!)

## Imaging

**General Features.** A well-delineated, lobulated intraventricular mass with frond-like papillary excrescences is typical (**23-3**). *Diffuse leptomeningeal dissemination is uncommon but does occur with histologically benign CPPs, so preoperative imaging of the entire neuraxis is recommended!*

**CT Findings.** The majority of CPPs are iso- to hyperdense compared with brain on NECT scans (**23-3**). Calcification is seen in 25% of cases (**23-16A**). Hydrocephalus—either obstructive or caused by CSF overproduction—is

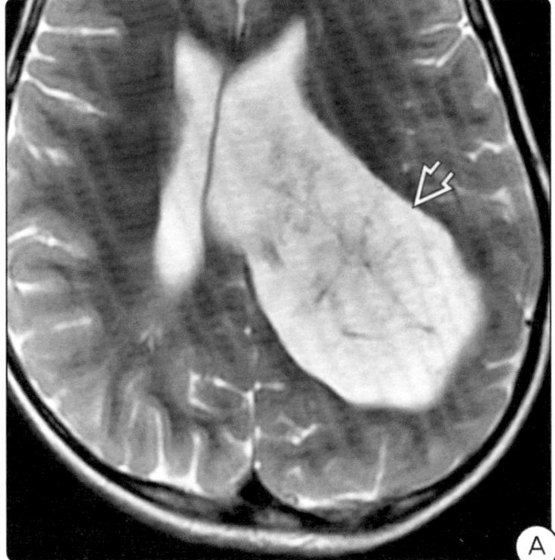

***(23-4A)** T2 MR in a 3-yo shows a heterogeneous, very hyperintense mass ➡ in the left lateral ventricle, which appears grossly enlarged.*

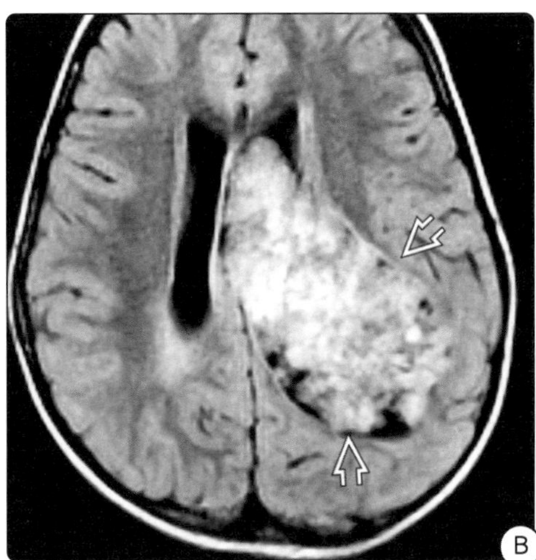

***(23-4B)** FLAIR MR shows the lobulated, hyperintense mass ➡ is contained within the grossly expanded left lateral ventricle.*

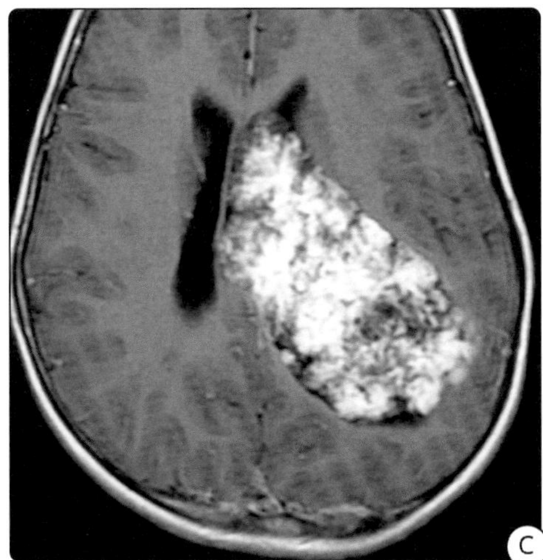

***(23-4C)** T1 C+ MR shows the cauliflower-like fronds of the mass enhance intensely. This is classic CPP, CNS WHO grade 1.*

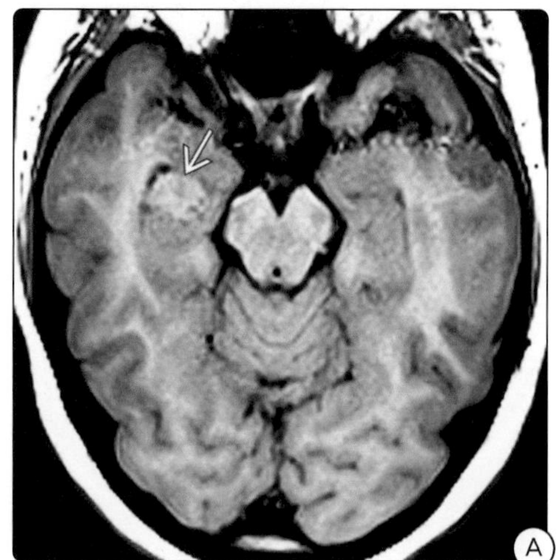


*(23-6A) T1 MR in a 19-yo asymptomatic woman shows a well-demarcated isointense mass in the right temporal horn ➡.*

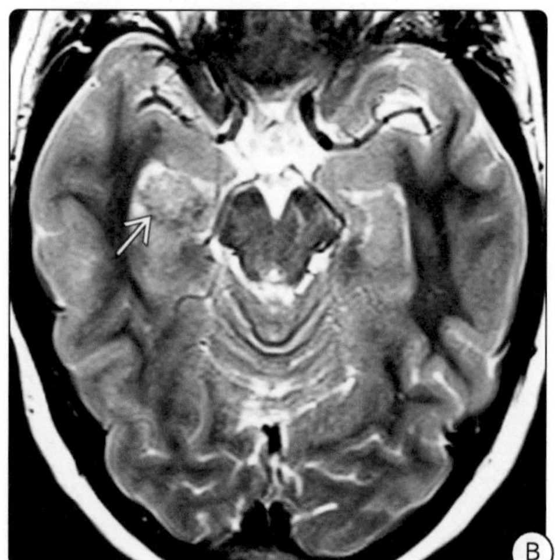


*(23-6B) T2 MR shows that the mass has a slightly lobulated appearance with peripheral hypointensity along its surface ➡.*

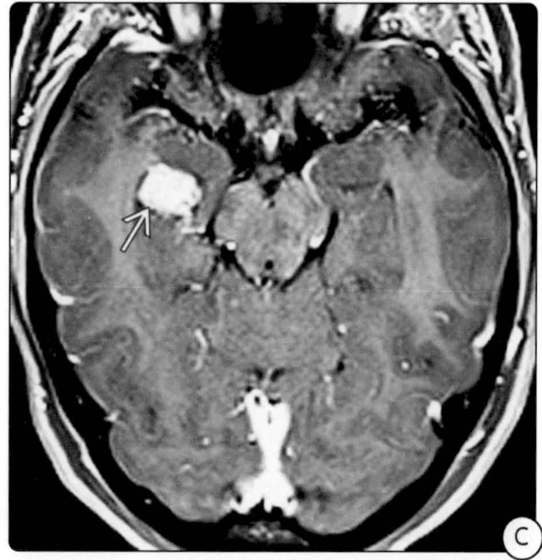


*(23-6C) T1 C+ FS MR shows the mass ➡ enhances intensely. Pathology proved CPP (WHO grade 1).*

common **(23-3)**. CECT scans show intense homogeneous enhancement **(23-10B)**.

**MR Findings.** A sharply marginated lobular mass that is iso- to slightly hypointense relative to brain is seen on T1WI. CPPs are iso- to hyperintense on T2WI and FLAIR **(23-4)**. Linear and branching internal "flow voids" reflect the increased vascularity common in CPPs. T2/T2* (GRE, SWI) may show hypointense foci secondary to calcification or intratumoral hemorrhage **(23-11)**.

Intense homogeneous enhancement is seen following contrast administration **(23-7) (23-10C) (23-18)**. CPPs generally do not restrict on DWI. MRS may show elevated myoinositol (mI).

Rare CPP variants include cystic extraaxial metastases from an intraventricular CPP. Cystic extraaxial metastases from CPP are seen as nonenhancing cisternal CSF-like cysts that resemble multiple parasitic cysts, such as neurocysticercosis **(23-31)**.

**Ultrasound.** CPPs appear as well-defined, lobular, hyperechoic intraventricular masses on transcranial US.

## Differential Diagnosis

The major differential diagnoses of CPP are **atypical CPP** (APP) and **choroid plexus carcinoma** (CPC). Both share similar imaging features on standard MR sequences. CPC is also far more likely to invade brain parenchyma than CPP. CSF dissemination occurs with all three histologic types of CPTs and is therefore neither a distinguishing feature nor a reliable predictor of malignancy.

**Choroid plexus hyperplasia**, also called **villous hypertrophy of the choroid plexus**, is a very rare cause of CSF overproduction and shunt-resistant hydrocephalus. Diffuse villous hyperplasia may result in CSF production exceeding three liters per day. Unlike CPP, most cases of choroid plexus hyperplasia are bilateral and diffusely enlarge the entire length of the choroid plexus.

**Choroid plexus xanthogranulomas** are benign incidental lesions that occur commonly in the lateral ventricular choroid plexus. They consist of desquamated epithelial cells with accumulated lipid together with macrophages and multinucleated foreign body giant cells. In contrast to most CPPs, they are found primarily in middle-aged and older patients. On imaging, they appear as bilateral multiloculated cysts within the enhancing choroid plexus glomus. **Choroid plexus metastasis** occurs in middle-aged and older adults and is not in the differential diagnosis of a pediatric CPP. **Subependymoma** is in the differential diagnosis of an adult fourth ventricular CPP.

### CHOROID PLEXUS PAPILLOMA: DIFFERENTIAL DIAGNOSIS

**Children**
- Atypical choroid plexus papilloma
- Choroid plexus carcinoma
- Villous hyperplasia

**Adults**
- Lateral ventricles
  - Choroid plexus xanthogranulomas
  - Metastases
- 4th ventricle
  - Subependymoma

## Atypical Choroid Plexus Papilloma

Atypical CPP (APP) has intermediate pathologic features, prognosis, and outcomes between CPP (a WHO grade 1 neoplasm) and CPC (a WHO grade 3 neoplasm). APPs represent ~ 15% of all CPTs. Although they can occur at all ages, APPs are more common in children compared with adults and are usually located in the lateral ventricles.

The main distinguishing histopathologic feature of APP is increased mitotic activity (≥ 2 mitoses/10 HPF) with elevated MIB-1 labeling **(23-23)**. One or two of the following four features may be present: Increased cellularity, nuclear pleomorphism, solid (not papillary) growth, and areas of necrosis.

Only a few imaging cases of APP have been reported. Most have the lobulated papillary appearance with strong uniform enhancement that also characterizes CPPs **(23-21)**. Cysts, necrosis, peritumoral edema, larger tumor volume, blurred borders, and CSF dissemination are more common in APPs compared to CPPs **(23-25)**. *However, imaging findings do not reliably discriminate between APP and CPP, so the definitive diagnosis depends on histopathology.*

## Choroid Plexus Carcinoma

### Terminology

CPC is a rare malignant tumor that occurs almost exclusively in young children.

### Etiology

**Genetics.** Nearly 1/2 of all CPCs harbor *TP53* mutations. The *TP53*-mutated tumor genome is associated with significant risk of progression and poor outcome. CPCs also occur in patients with **Li-Fraumeni syndrome**, a cancer predisposition syndrome caused by *TP53* germline mutation.

Recent data suggest that abnormalities in regulation of ventricular ependymal cell multiciliogenesis directed by the GMNC-MCIDAS transcriptional network may also be involved in the development of CPCs.

All CPCs fall into the supratentorial pediatric B, high-risk group and are associated with a mean progression-free survival of 55 months.

### Pathology

**Gross Pathology.** The vast majority of CPCs in children arise in the lateral ventricle. This heterogeneous, bulky intraventricular tumor often displays gross hemorrhage and necrotic foci. Invasion into adjacent brain parenchyma is common **(23-26)**. Adult CPCs are rare; when they occur, the fourth ventricle is the most common location.

**Microscopic Features.** Frank cytologic features of malignancy are seen. CPCs demonstrate at least four of five histologic features: Increased cellular density, nuclear pleomorphism, loss of papillary architecture with poorly structured sheets of tumor cells, foci of necrosis, and frequent mitoses (> 2.5/mm³ equating to > 5 mitoses/10 HPF). MIB-1 is elevated, ranging from 15% to 20%.

The presence of *TP53* mutation and a methylation profile of CPC also support the diagnosis.

**Staging, Grading, and Classification.** CPC is a CNS WHO grade 3 neoplasm. Malignant progression from CPPs to CPCs is exceedingly rare with only a handful of reported cases, mostly occurring with germline *TP53* mutation.

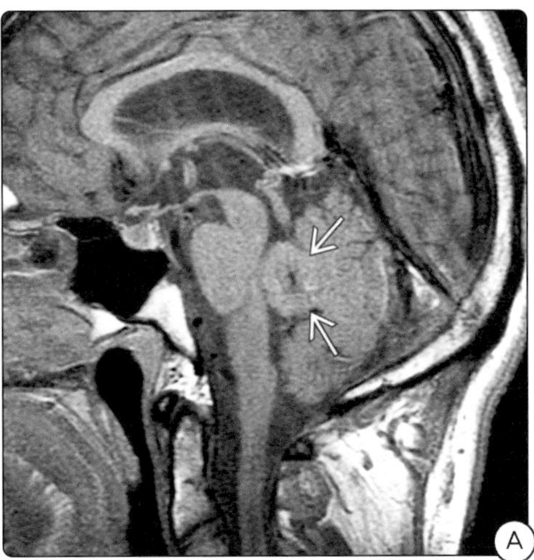

***(23-8A)** Sagittal T1 MR in a 28-yo man shows a well-demarcated 4th ventricle mass ➡.*

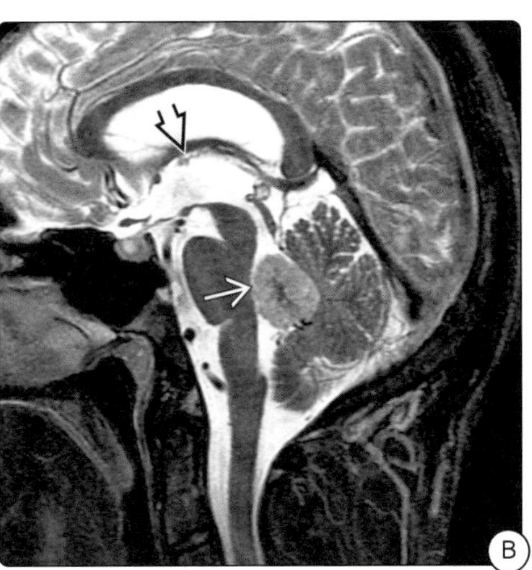

***(23-8B)** The mass ➡ is slightly hyperintense on T2 MR. Note hypoplastic choroid plexus in the roof of the 3rd ventricle ⇨.*

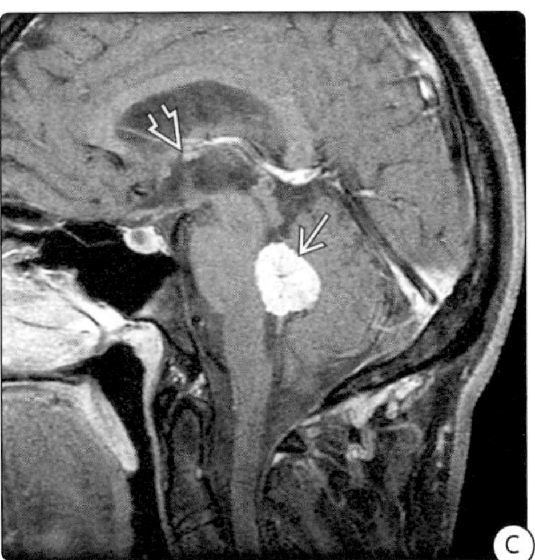

***(23-8C)** T1 C+ shows intensely enhancing mass ➡. Hypoplastic choroid plexus in 3rd ventricle enhances normally ➡. CPP, CNS WHO grade 1.*

*(23-10A) NECT in a 42-yo man with headaches and papilledema shows an isodense 4th ventricle mass ⮚ and dilated temporal horns ⮚. (23-10B) CECT shows the mass ⮚ enhances intensely and uniformly.*

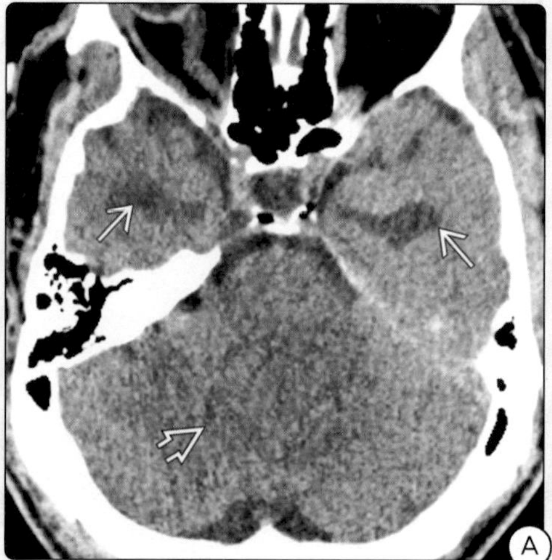

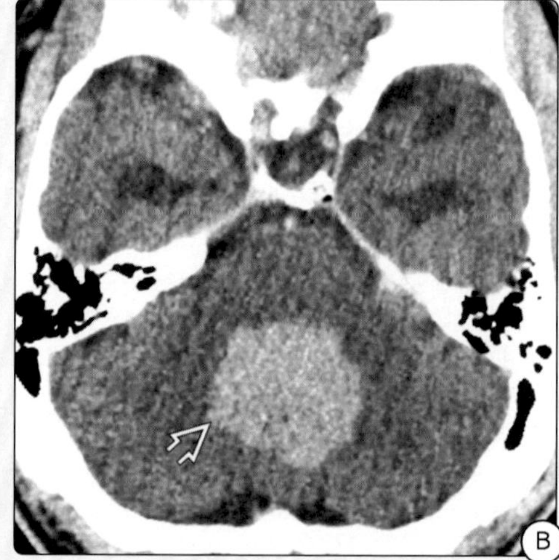

*(23-10C) The mass ⮚ enhances intensely on T1 C+ FS MR. Typical CPP, CNS WHO grade 1 was found at surgery. (23-12A) T1 MR in a 41-yo man with headache, nausea, vomiting, and ataxia shows a mixed cystic ⮚ and solid ⮚ intraaxial posterior fossa mass.*

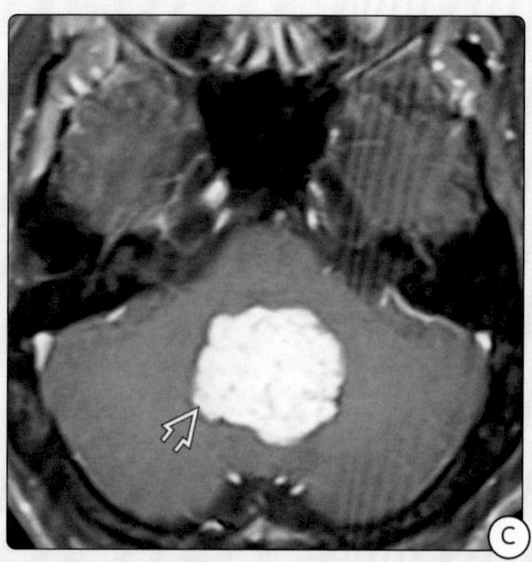

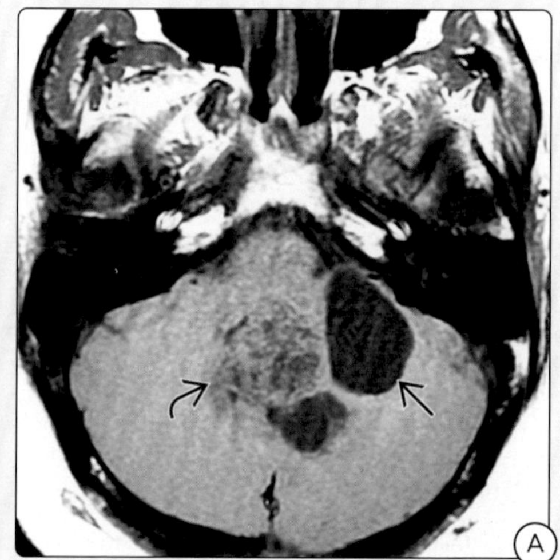

*(23-12B) T2 MR shows the solid ⮚ and cystic ⮚ portions of the mass. Note hyperintensity in displaced medulla ⮚ and cerebellum ⮚ surrounding the mass. (23-12C) T1 C+ MR shows the solid portion of the mass enhances strongly but heterogeneously ⮚. CPP, CNS WHO grade 1 was found at surgery.*

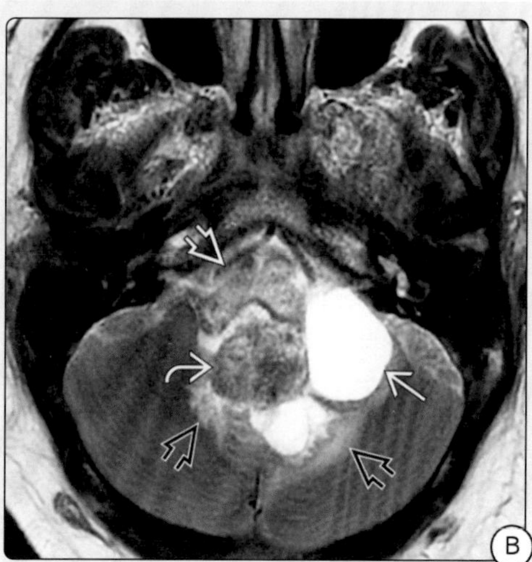

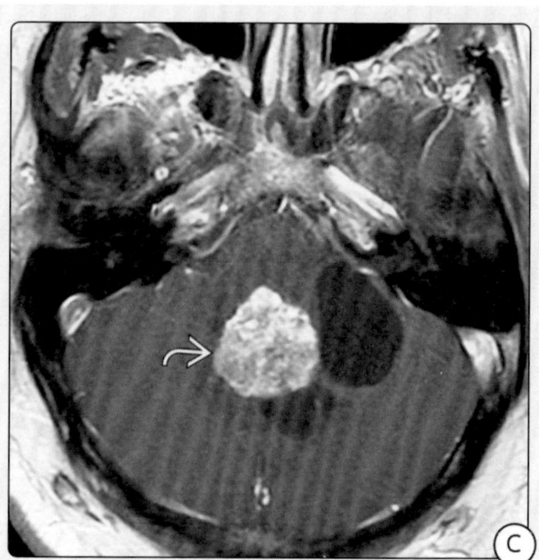

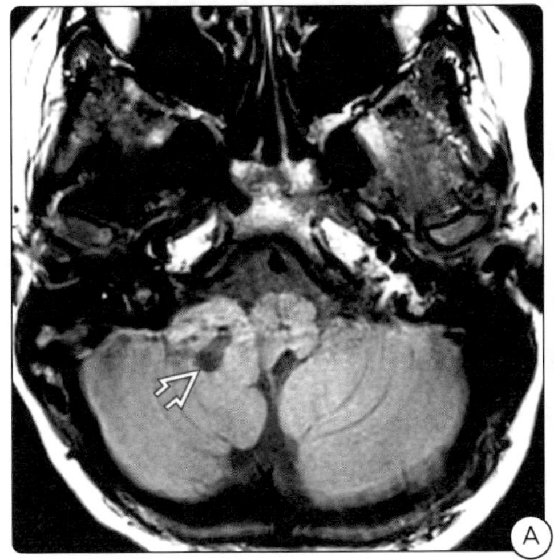

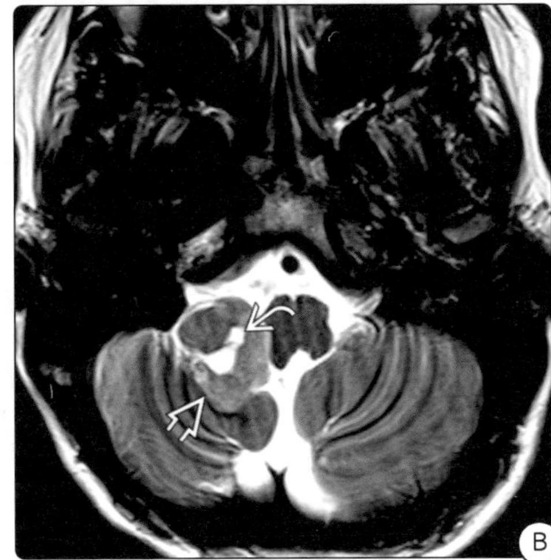

***(23-14A)** T1 MR in a 16-yo girl with headaches shows a mostly isointense, partially cystic mass in the right foramen of Luschka ➡. **(23-14B)** T2 MR shows the solid portion of the mass ➡ is isointense with the cerebellum and contains a focus of cystic degeneration ↪.*

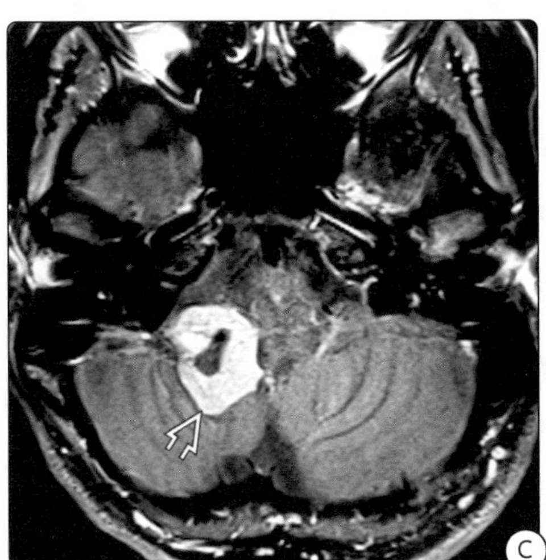

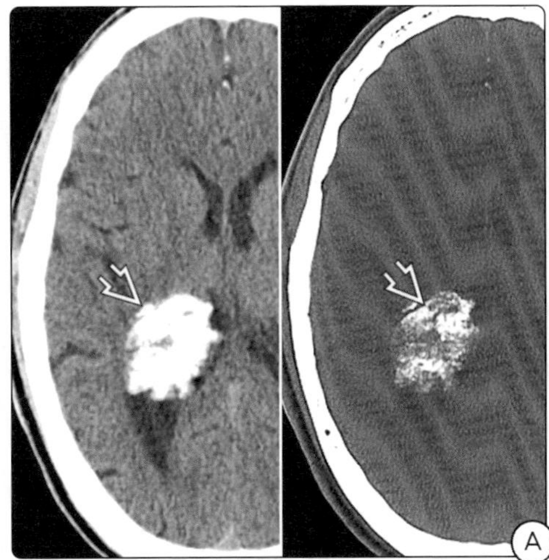

***(23-14C)** T1 C+ FS MR shows the solid portion of the mass ➡ enhances intensely. CPP, CNS WHO grade 1 was found at surgery. **(23-16A)** A 22-yo man presented with headaches. (L) NECT and (R) bone window show a densely calcified mass in the atrium of the right lateral ventricle ➡.*

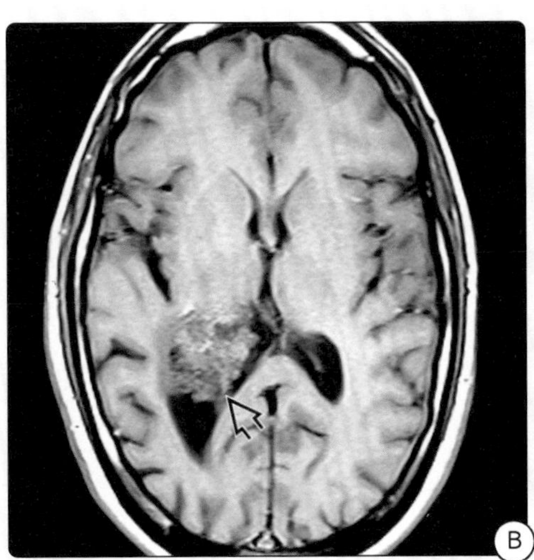

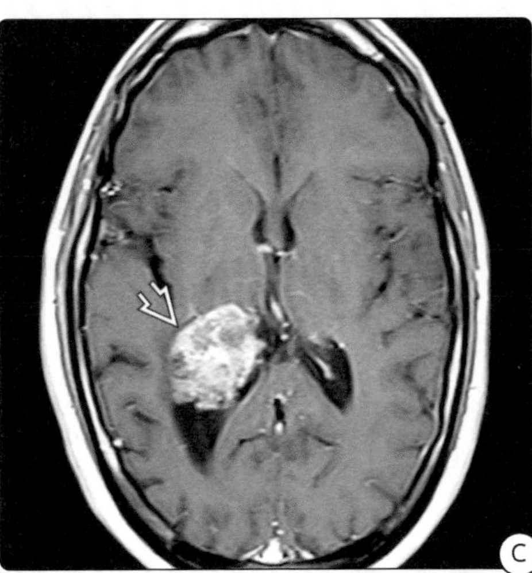

***(23-16B)** T1 MR in the same case shows a heterogeneous, lobulated mass ➡ in the atrium of the right lateral ventricle. **(23-16C)** T1 C+ FS MR shows the lesion ➡ exhibits strong but heterogeneous enhancement. CPP, CNS WHO grade 1 was found at surgery. CPPs in this location and in this age do occur but are unusual.*

*(23-18A) Sagittal T1 MR in a 23-yo woman with headaches and papilledema shows a large, lobulated, isointense mass ➡ in the body of the 4th ventricle causing obstructive hydrocephalus. (23-18B) Axial high-resolution T2 SPACE in the same case shows the mass is mostly isointense with the adjacent cerebellum. Note multiple hyperintense foci ➡ that likely represent CSF trapped between tumor fronds.*

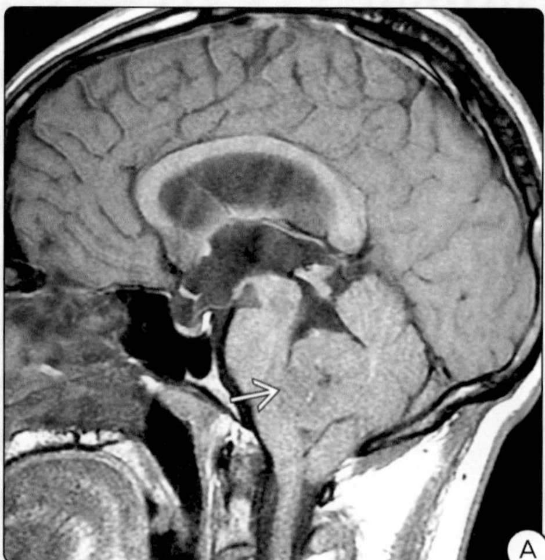

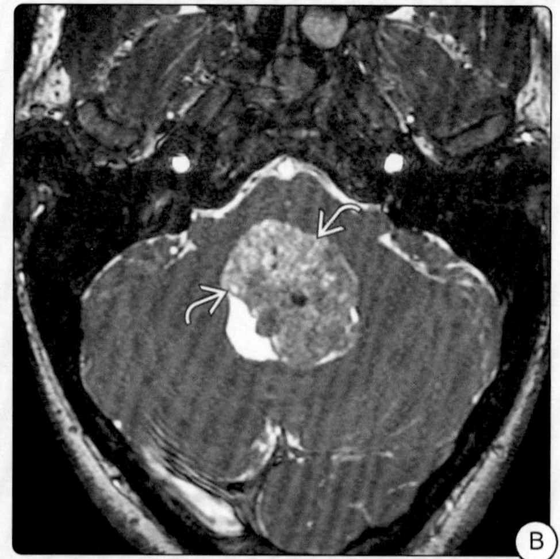

*(23-18C) Sagittal T1 C+ MR shows the mass enhances intensely but heterogeneously. (23-18D) Axial T1 C+ MR shows solid portions of the mass enhance. Note expanded, dilated 4th ventricle ➡ surrounding and containing the mass. This is CPP, CNS WHO grade 1.*

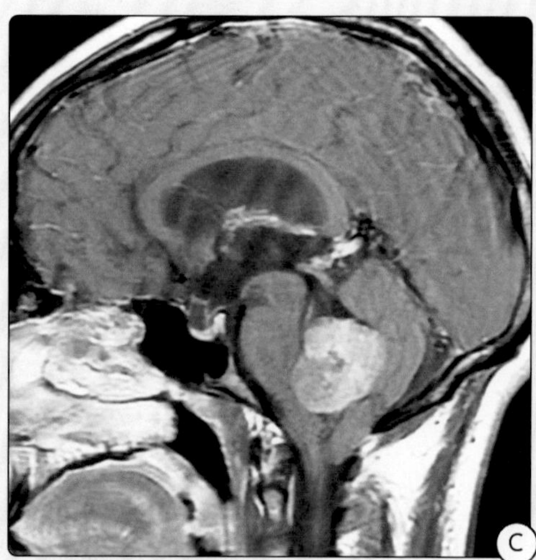

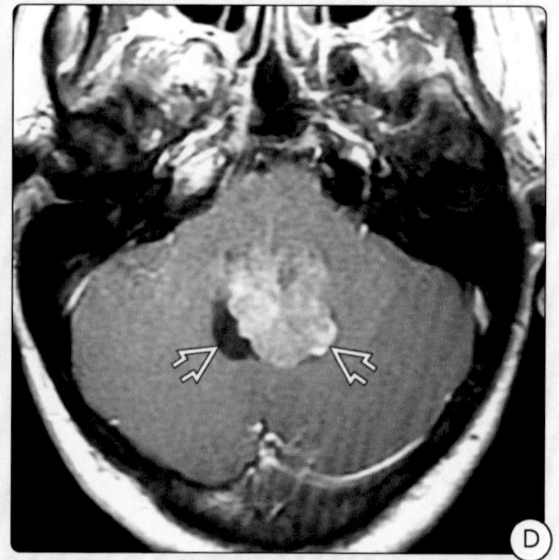

*(23-19) Axial T1 C+ FS MR in a 36-yo female patient with headaches and papilledema shows a well-demarcated enhancing mass in the posterior 3rd ventricle ➡. CPP, CNS WHO grade 1 was found at surgery. (23-20) T2 MR in an infant with macrocrania shows a heterogeneously hyperintense 3rd ventricle mass ➡. This is atypical CPP (APP), CNS WHO grade 2. (Courtesy M. Castillo, MD.)*

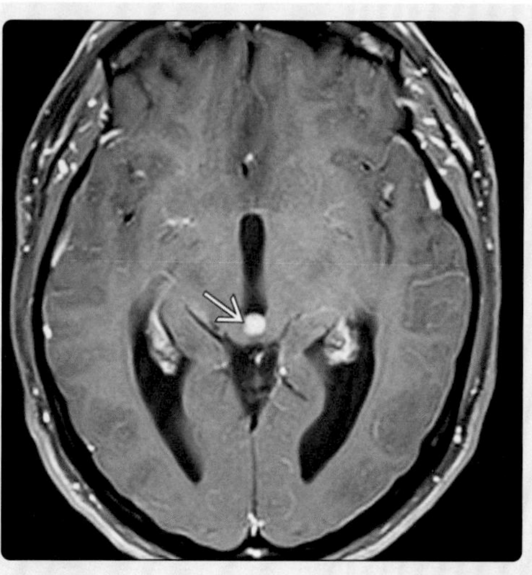

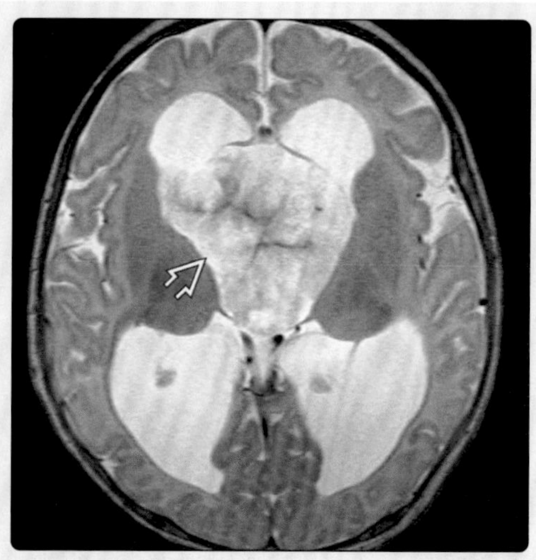

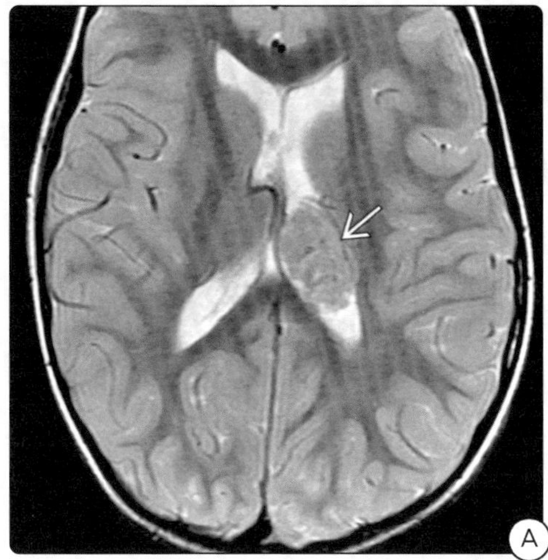

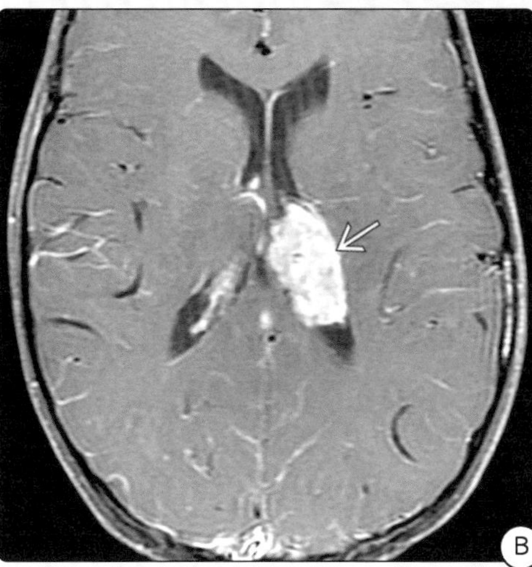

***(23-22A)** Axial T2 MR in a patient with headaches shows a mass ➡ in the left lateral ventricle that is isointense with gray matter. **(23-22B)** The mass ➡ enhances intensely on T1 C+ FS MR. APP (WHO grade 2) was histopathologically identified.*

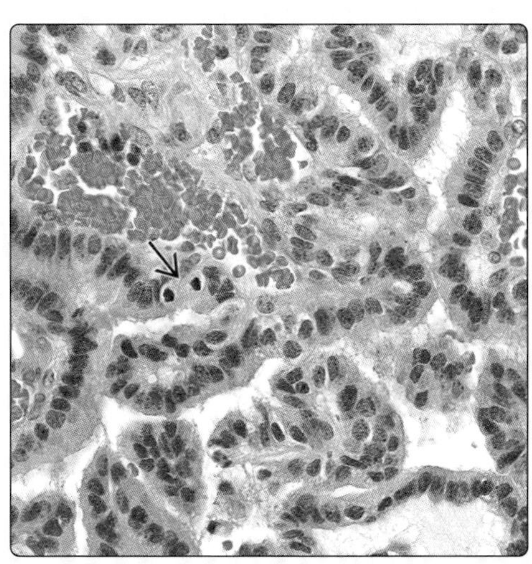

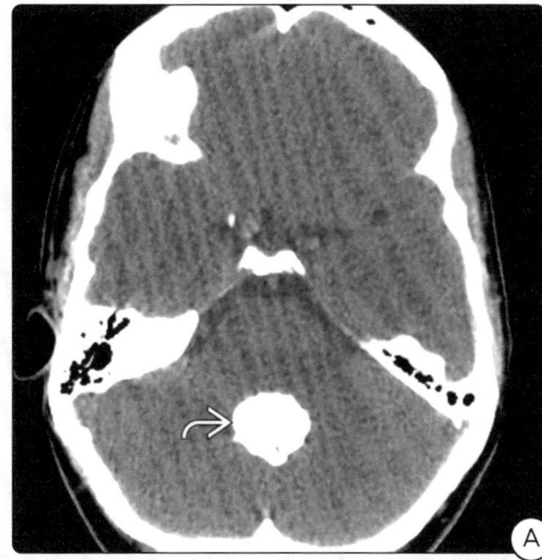

***(23-23)** CPPs are atypical based on ↑ mitotic activity ➡ (> WHO grade 1 CPPs). 2+ mitoses/10 HPF is the threshold and was met here. (Courtesy P. Burger, MD.) **(23-25A)** NECT in a 27-yo woman shows a densely calcified, well-demarcated mass ➡ in the 4th ventricle.*

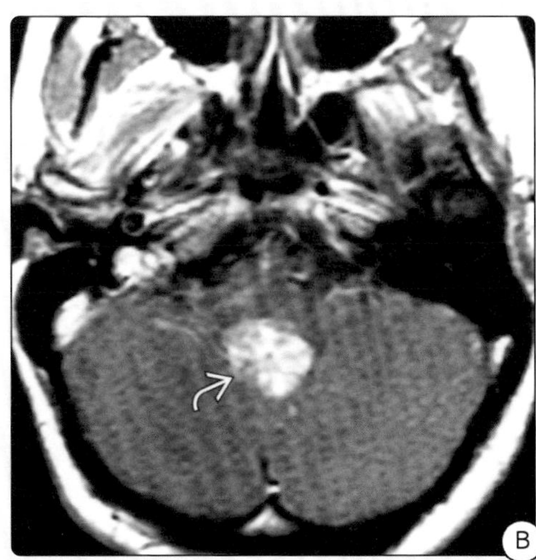

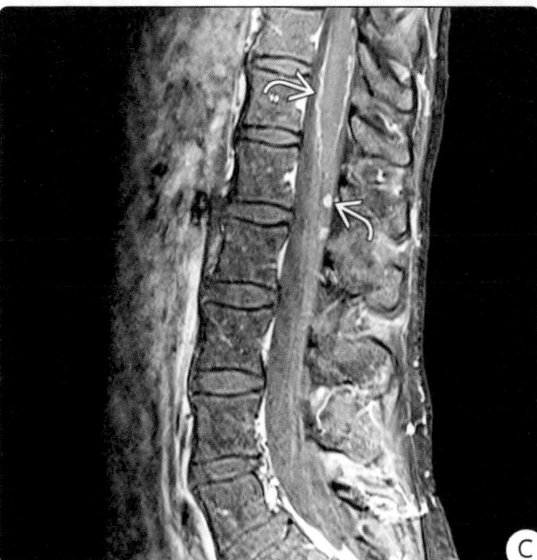

***(23-25B)** Axial T1 C+ MR shows the mass ➡ enhances intensely. No other intracranial lesions were identified. **(23-25C)** Complete spine imaging done at the time of initial diagnosis shows CSF dissemination ➡. This is APP, CNS WHO grade 2. Imaging findings, even with CSF dissemination, can be indistinguishable from grade 1 choroid plexus tumors.*

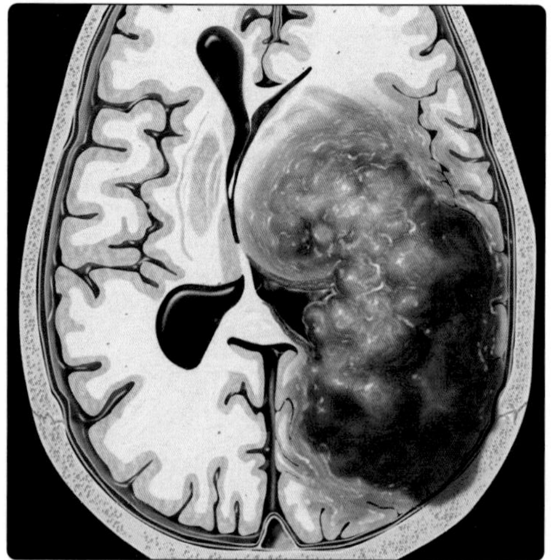

*(23-26) Choroid plexus carcinoma, seen here as a hemorrhagic, highly vascular mass that fills atrium of lateral ventricle, invades parenchyma.*

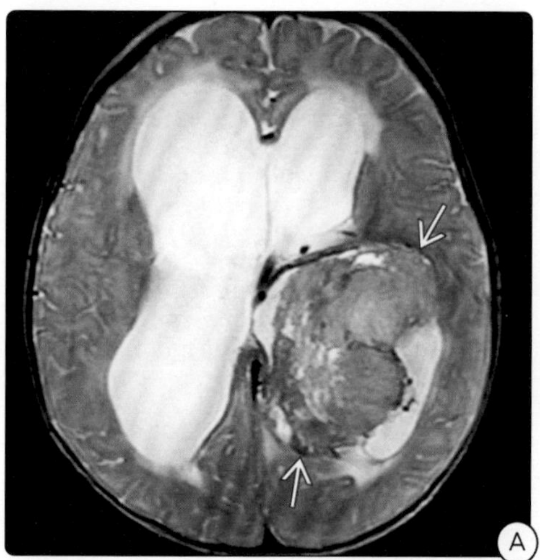

*(23-28A) T2 MR in an 8-mo girl with macrocrania, vomiting shows severe hydrocephalus, large mass ➡ in the atrium of the left lateral ventricle.*

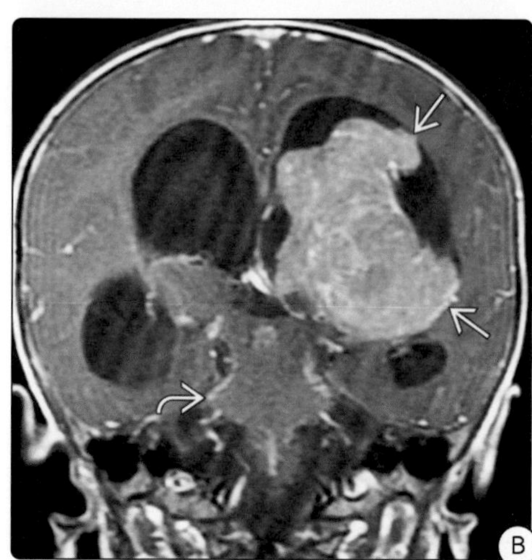

*(23-28B) T1 C+ shows intense but heterogeneous enhancement in the mass ➡. Note diffuse CSF spread ➡. This is choroid plexus carcinoma.*

## Clinical Issues

**Epidemiology.** Although CPC is uncommon, representing < 1% of all pediatric brain tumors, it accounts for 5% of supratentorial neoplasms. CPC represents 20-40% of all primary choroid plexus neoplasms.

**Demographics.** Between 70-80% of CPCs arise in children younger than three years. Median age at diagnosis is 18 months. CPCs in adults have been reported but are very rare.

**Natural History.** Prognosis in patients with these aggressive tumors is generally dismal, especially those with incomplete resection of a *TP53*-mutated genotype. Approximately 20% of patients with CPCs have metastases at initial diagnosis. Five-year overall survival is ~ 65%.

## Imaging

CPC often invades through the ventricular ependyma into adjacent brain. Edema, necrosis, intratumoral cysts, and hemorrhage are common **(23-29)**. Enhancement is typically strong but heterogeneous. CSF dissemination is common **(23-27)**.

## Differential Diagnosis

The major differential diagnoses are **CPP** and **APP**. Imaging features of all three tumors overlap. *CSF spread can occur with both benign and malignant CPTs*. The presence of frank parenchymal invasion and accompanying edema suggests CPC.

**OTHER CHOROID PLEXUS NEOPLASMS**

**Atypical Choroid Plexus Papilloma**
- WHO grade 2
- Imaging findings similar to those of choroid plexus papilloma

**Choroid Plexus Carcinoma**
- Rare
- Children < 3 years (70-80%)
- WHO grade 3
- Imaging
  - Invades through ependyma
  - Edema, necrosis, cysts, hemorrhage common
  - Strong, heterogeneous enhancement
  - CSF dissemination common

# Cystic Dissemination of Choroid Plexus Papillomas

Metastasis of both benign and malignant choroid plexus neoplasms may occur throughout the neuraxis. Although the majority of metastatic lesions are solid, enhancing lesions appearing similar to the primary tumor, widely disseminated cystic, nonenhancing leptomeningeal metastases may occur with CNS WHO grade 1 CPPs. In this rare presentation, numerous widely disseminated cysts are present within the cranial and spinal CSF spaces **(23-31)**. The natural history of such lesions is mostly benign with cysts exhibiting remarkably slow or no growth over time.

*Selected References: The complete reference list is available on the eBooks+ version included with purchase.*

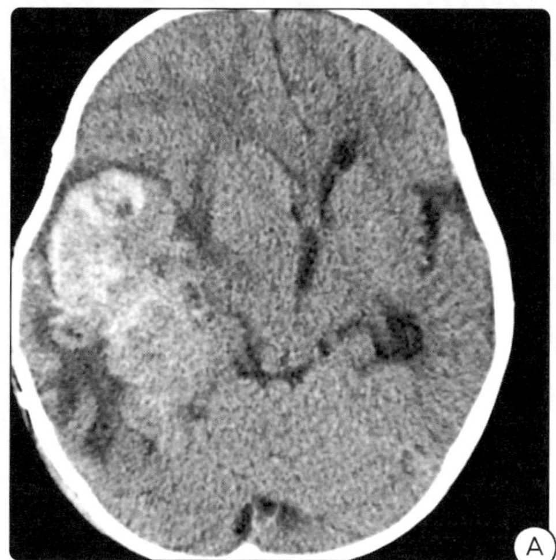

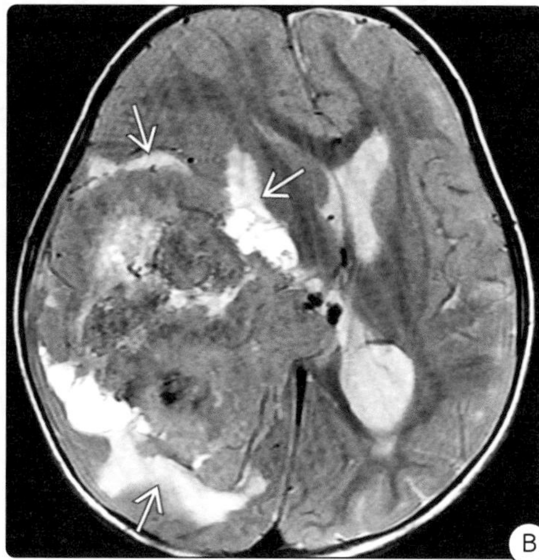

***(23-30A)** NECT in a 2-yo girl with a large head and papilledema shows a predominantly hyperdense, lobulated mass in the right lateral ventricle invading adjacent brain. **(23-30B)** T2 MR shows the extremely heterogeneous nature of the mass. Gross tumor invasion of the brain parenchyma with surrounding edema ➡ is present.*

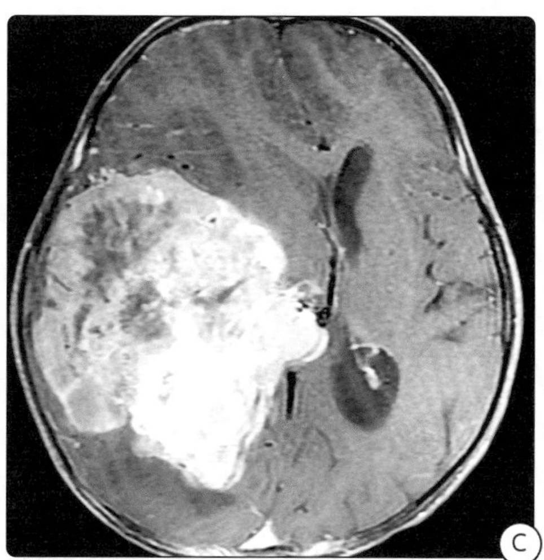

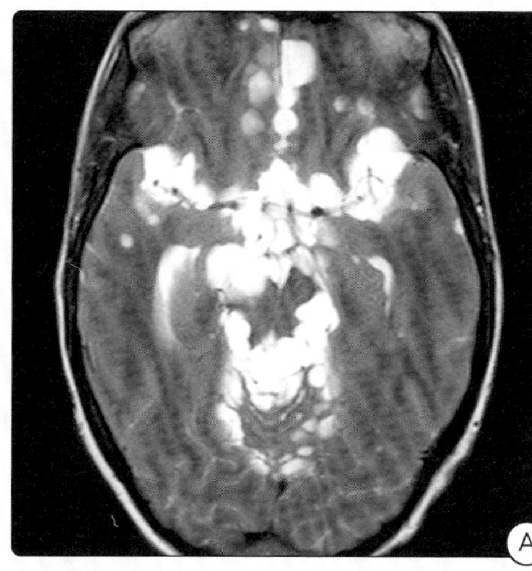

***(23-30C)** T1 C+ FS MR shows that the mass enhances intensely but heterogeneously. This is choroid plexus carcinoma, CNS WHO grade 3. **(23-32A)** T2 MR 10 years after resection of a 4th ventricle CPP, CNS WHO grade 1 shows disseminated T2-hyperintense cysts in the subarachnoid cisterns.*

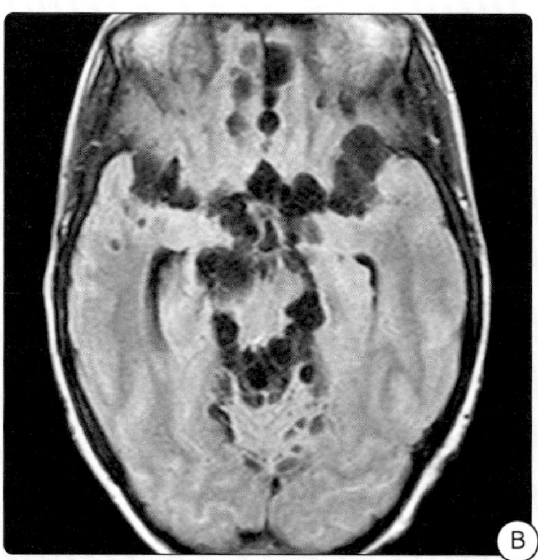

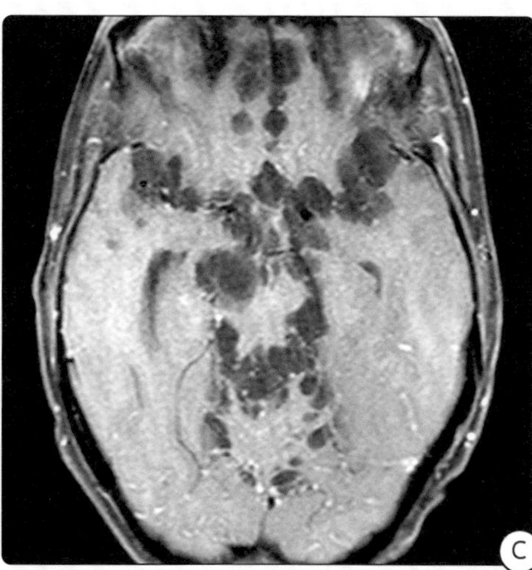

***(23-32B)** The subarachnoid cysts suppress completely on FLAIR MR. **(23-32C)** T1 C+ FS shows cysts do not enhance. Infection work-up was negative. Biopsy disclosed benign-appearing cysts without definite histologic evidence for metastases.*

# Embryonal Tumors

*The rapidly evolving molecular classification of brain tumors has fundamentally changed the understanding of embryonal neoplasms. In the 2021 WHO schema, the classification of the largest group of embryonal neoplasms—medulloblastoma—was revised to reflect clinically relevant molecular subgroups.*



The 2021 WHO classification recognizes two general categories of embryonal tumors: (1) Medulloblastoma (MB) (relatively common) and (2) other CNS embryonal tumors (rare). The term primitive neuroectodermal tumor (PNET) was previously removed from the diagnostic lexicon in the 2016 classification scheme. The tumors formerly included in this now-obsolete category have recently been redefined using molecular data and are now included in the "other CNS embryonal tumors."

We begin this chapter with an in-depth discussion of MB that follows the 2021 WHO, 5th edition presentation of this biologically heterogeneous neoplasm. We conclude the chapter with a brief discussion of the less common embryonal tumors.

## Medulloblastoma

### Histology and Genetics

MB is the most common malignant CNS neoplasm of childhood and the second most common overall pediatric brain tumor (after astrocytoma). As a group, MBs account for ~ 20% of childhood CNS neoplasms.

MB is not a single tumor entity but a heterogeneous cluster of multiple distinct, clinically relevant molecular subgroups. International consensus now recognizes five molecular subgroups, each differing in its demographics, recommended treatments, and clinical outcomes.

All MBs are designated CNS WHO grade 4 even though certain molecular groups and subgroups (e.g., WNT-activated tumors) have a good therapeutic response and cure is possible in some cases.

#### Medulloblastoma, Histologically Defined

MBs consist of densely packed small round poorly differentiated ("blue") cells. Moderate nuclear pleomorphism and a high mitotic index (MIB-1 or Ki-67) are characteristic.

The 2021 WHO classification recognizes four morphologic subtypes of medulloblastoma: (1) **Classic MB**, (2) **desmoplastic/nodular (D/N) MB**, (3) **MB with extensive nodularity (MBEN)**, (4) **large cell/anaplastic (LC/A) MB**.

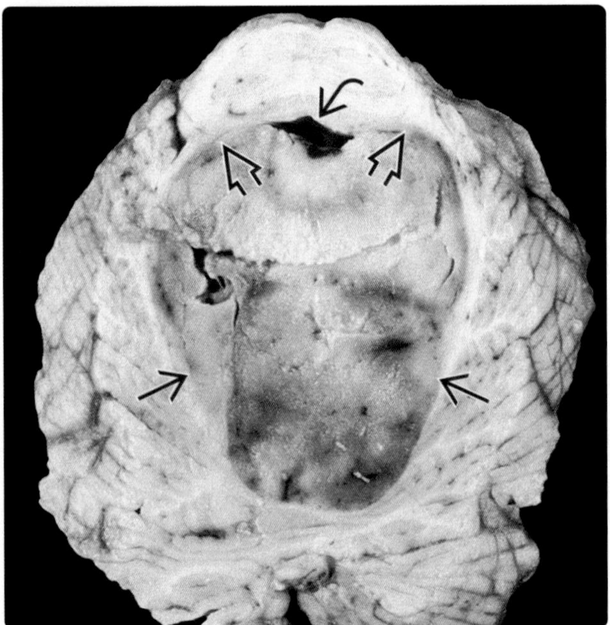

***(24-1)*** *Autopsy specimen demonstrates a large medulloblastoma (MB) ➡ nearly filling the 4th ventricle with some sparing of the uppermost aspect of the ventricle ⬀. Pons is compressed anteriorly ➡. (Courtesy R. Hewlett, MD.)*

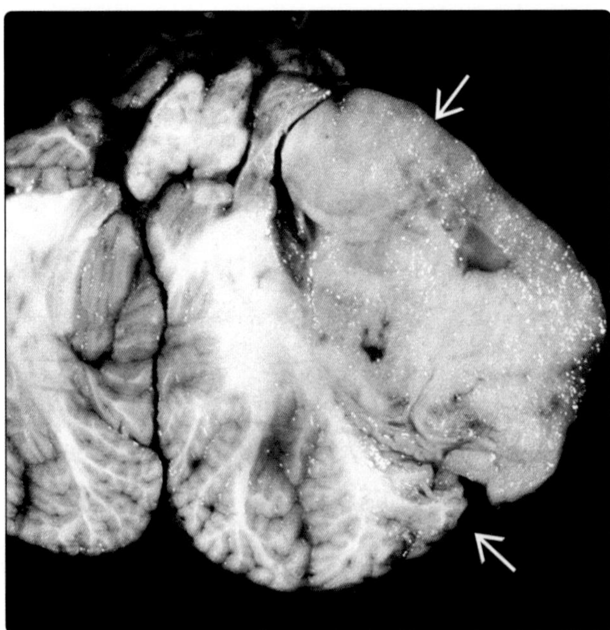

***(24-2)*** *Cut section shows the classic desmoplastic MB located in the lateral cerebellar hemisphere ➡. Most tumors in this location are SHH-activated. (Courtesy R. Hewlett, MD.)*

All MBs are currently designated as CNS WHO grade 4 neoplasms.

Classic MBs are typically located in the cerebellar midline and involve the fourth ventricle **(24-1)**. D/N MBs may arise both in the cerebellar hemisphere and vermis. D/N MBs in adults often arise in the lateral cerebellum **(24-2)**. MBENs are typically located in the vermis and frequently involve both cerebellar hemispheres **(24-9)**. LC/A MBs usually involve the fourth ventricle, brainstem, and adjacent cerebellum **(24-3)**.

## Medulloblastoma, Genetically Defined

MB is a genetically heterogeneous disease with five main molecular subgroups: (1) **WNT-activated**, (2) **SHH-activated and TP53-wildtype**, (3) **SHH-activated and TP53-mutant**, (4) **non-WNT/non-SHH, group 3** and (5) **non-WNT/non-SHH, group 4**. Groups 3 and 4—the non-WNT/non-SHH MBs—are further divided by DNA methylation profiling into eight subgroups.

All MB subtypes have different origins, preferred anatomic locations, and demographics, as well as different prognosis and therapeutic implications. Each of these subtypes has been further subdivided into distinctive molecular subgroups, adding more precision to patient-based risk stratification.

**WNT-Activated Medulloblastomas.** WNT-activated MB (WNT-MB) is the smallest molecular subgroup (10%) and appears strikingly different from the other MBs in origin, appearance, and prognosis. WNT-MBs are lateralized tumors that arise from the lower rhombic lip in the dorsolateral primitive brainstem around the foramen of Luschka and cerebellar peduncle **(24-3)**.

WNT-MBs are very rare in infants and usually affect older children and young adults. They almost always exhibit classic histology. Childhood patients with WNT-MBs have a favorable prognosis (five-year survival > 90%) and reduced intensity; risk-adapted therapies are often utilized.

Germline mutations in the WNT pathway inhibitor, *APC*, predispose individuals to develop MB in the setting of **Turcot syndrome**.

**SHH-Activated and TP53-Wildtype Medulloblastomas.** Overall, the two SHH-activated subgroups (distinguished by mutant or wildtype *TP53*) account for 25-30% of MBs. Both subgroups of SHH-activated MBs (SHH MBs) arise from granule neuron precursor cells, which are found in the external granular layer of the cerebellum. SHH MBs (both *TP53*-wildtype and *TP53*-mutant) comprise four provisional molecular subgroups (designated SHH-1 through 4) that can be demonstrated by DNA methylation or transcriptome profiling.

SHH MBs in infants frequently involve the vermis. In older children and young adults, SHH MBs are most often located laterally within the cerebellar hemispheres **(24-2)**.

The majority of SHH MBs are *TP53*-wildtype. There is a high incidence of germline mutations (~ 40%) in SHH MBs, including basal cell nevus (Gorlin) syndrome.

Compared with other subgroups, SHH-activated *TP53*-wildtype MBs are more likely to have desmoplastic or nodular pathology.

All four clinical subtypes of SHH MB may have *TP53*-wildtype status. *TP53*-wildtype SHH MBs have an intermediate prognosis that is generally better than those with *TP53*

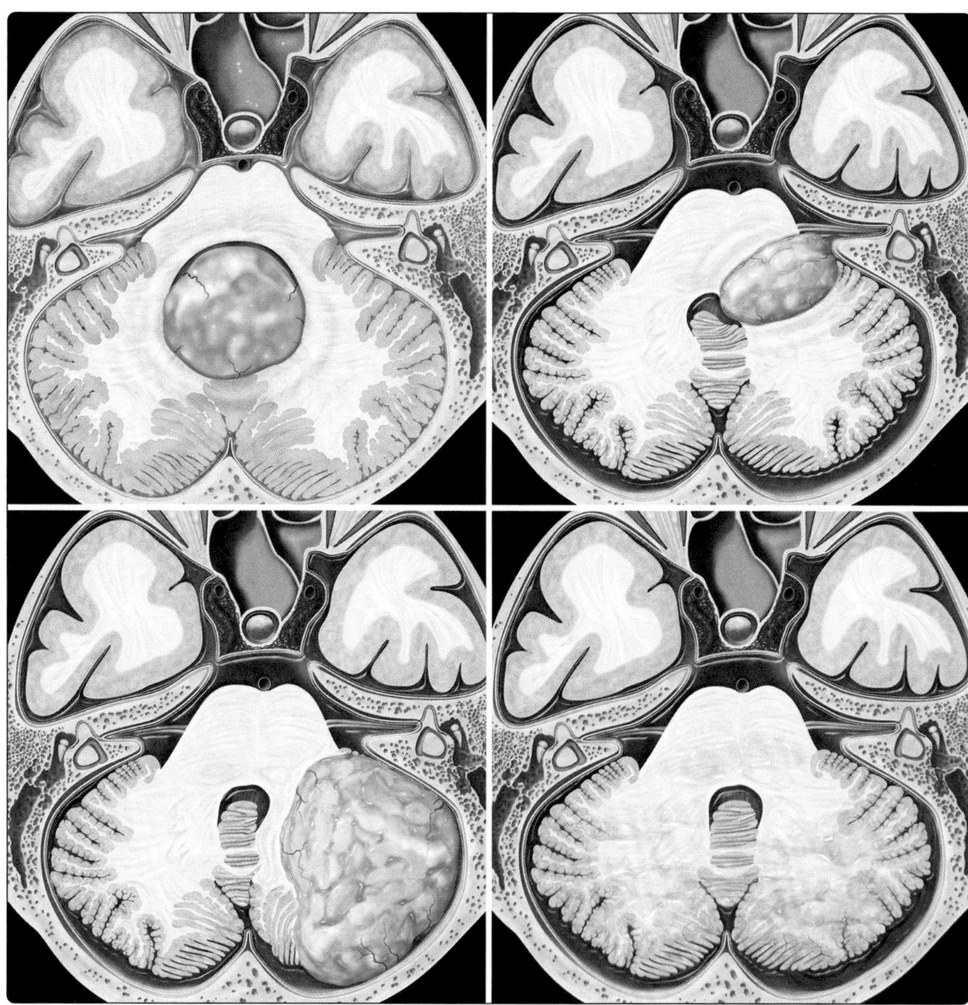

*(24-3) (Upper left) Graphic depicts classic MB in the midline 4th ventricle with CSF spread. All molecular subgroups and all histologies can be located here, but the most common subtypes are groups 3 and 4 (see Fig. 24-5). (Upper right) Graphic depicts an MB in the cerebellar peduncle/cerebellopontine angle (CPA) cistern. This location is classic for WNT-activated MB (compare to Fig. 24-7). (Lower left) Graphic depicts an MB in the lateral cerebellar hemisphere. This is the classic location for desmoplastic MB, SHH-activated and TP53-wildtype (compare to Fig. 24-6). (Lower right) Graphic depicts a nonfocal, diffusely infiltrating MB. Groups 3 and 4 can occasionally be diffusely infiltrating with no dominant mass. Group 4 MBs are sometimes characterized by exhibiting mild to minimal or no enhancement on T1 C+ FS (see Fig. 24-5C).*

mutations. However, specific gene alterations may alter the prognosis of patients within this subgroup.

#### SHH-Activated and TP53-Mutant Medulloblastomas

SHH-activated *TP53*-mutant MBs usually demonstrate LC/A histology. Compared to those SHH-activated tumors without a *TP53* mutation, this group has a generally worse prognosis. SHH-activated and *TP53*-mutant MBs almost always belong to subgroup SHH-3.

*TP53*-mutant MBs tend to occur in children 5-14 years. Most are found in the cerebellar hemispheres but can also involve midline structures. Leptomeningeal spread is often a presenting feature of this MB subgroup.

**Non-WNT/Non-SHH Medulloblastoma.** By definition, non-WNT/non-SHH MBs lack activation of the WNT and SHH signaling pathways.

Non-WNT/non-SHH MBs cluster into two groups (group 3 and group 4) and comprise eight molecular subgroups, as demonstrated by DNA methylation profiling. These MBs arise almost exclusively in the cerebellum, usually in the midline. Most exhibit classic histopathology. LC/A tumors can belong to either group.

Group 3 is the third largest MB subgroup (20-25%) and has the worst outcome. Group 3 tumors are common in infants but exceedingly rare in adults. *MYC* amplification is common, and ~ 50% of patients present with metastases at initial diagnosis **(24-8)**. *NOTCH1* has been identified as a pivotal driver of group 3 MB metastasis and self-renewal.

Group 4 is the largest (~ 35%) of the four molecular MB subgroups. Most group 4 MBs exhibit classic histology. Group 4 MBs affect all ages but are most common in children. The M:F ratio is 2:1. A minority of group 4 MBs present with metastasis. Overall prognosis is intermediate but poor in adults.

In both groups 3 and 4, *MYC* amplification plays an important role in prognosis, with those tumors expressing increasing *MYC* having a poorer prognosis.

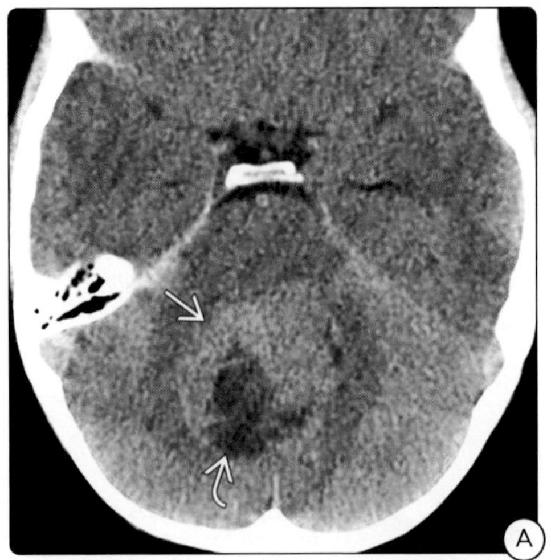


*(24-4A) NECT of MB shows mixed hyper-/hypodense midline posterior fossa mass ➡ with intratumoral cysts ➡.*

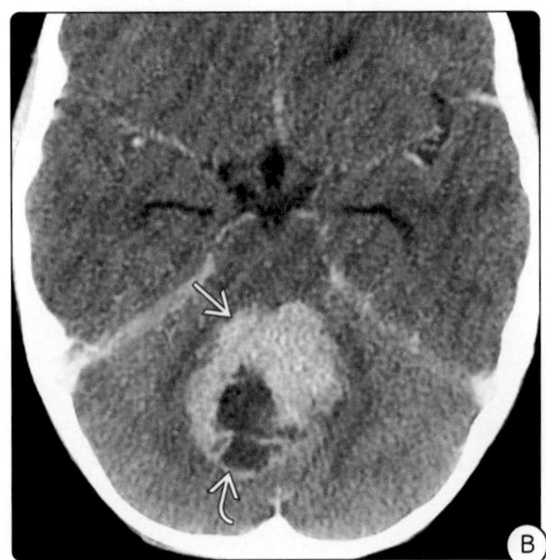


*(24-4B) CECT shows the solid portion of the 4th ventricle mass enhances ➡ while the cyst ➡ does not.*

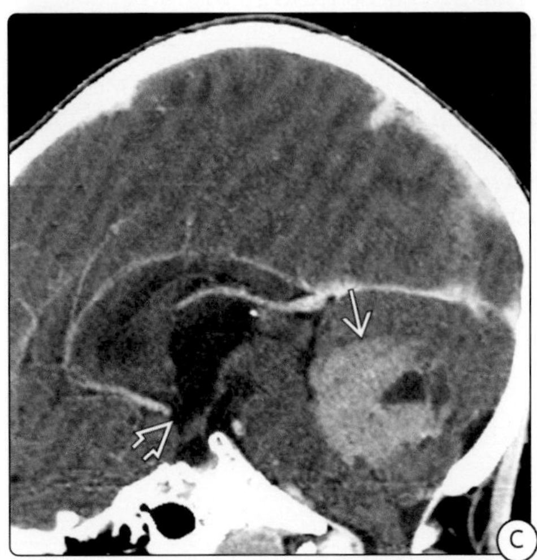


*(24-4C) Sagittal CECT shows 4th ventricle mass ➡ causes moderate hydrocephalus ➡. Classic MB, CNS WHO grade 4.*

**MEDULLOBLASTOMA CLASSIFICATION WITH RELATIVE FREQUENCIES**

**Histologically Defined Medulloblastomas**
- Medulloblastoma, histologically defined
- Desmoplastic/nodular medulloblastoma
- Medulloblastoma with extensive nodularity
- Large cell medulloblastoma
- Anaplastic medulloblastoma

**Genetically Defined Medulloblastomas**
- Medulloblastoma, WNT-activated (10%)
- Medulloblastoma, SHH-activated and *TP53*-wildtype (20%)
- Medulloblastoma, SHH-activated and *TP53*-mutant (10%)
- Medulloblastoma, non-WNT/non-SHH
  - Group 3 medulloblastoma (25%)
  - Group 4 medulloblastoma (35%)

## Pathology, Clinical, and Imaging Features

### Pathology

**Location.** While any histologic type can be found in any location, > 85% of classic, group 3, and group 4 MBs arise in the midline. They typically fill the fourth ventricle, displacing and compressing the pons anteriorly **(24-1)**. Posteroinferior extension into the cisterna magna is common. Unlike ependymoma, lateral extension into the cerebellopontine angle is uncommon.

WNT-MBs are also found at the cerebellopontine angle and along the lateral recess of the fourth ventricle. SHH MBs are most often located in the cerebellar hemispheres. Occasionally, MB occurs as a diffusely infiltrating lesion without a focal dominant mass **(24-3)**.

**Microscopic Features.** MBs are highly cellular tumors (small round blue cell tumor). Neuroblastic (Homer Wright) rosettes—radial arrangements of tumor cells around fibrillary processes—are found in 40% of cases.

### Clinical Issues

**Epidemiology and Demographics.** Most MBs occur before the age of 10 years old; median patient age at diagnosis is nine years. There is a second, smaller peak in adults aged 20-40 years with up to 25% of MBs occurring in adults.

MBs occur in the setting of several inherited cancer syndromes, including nevoid basal cell carcinoma (Gorlin) syndrome with *SUFU* and *PTCH1* mutations, *TP53* mutations (Li-Fraumeni syndrome), and *APC* (familial adenomatous polyposis), among others.

**Presentation.** The most common clinical manifestations of MB are vomiting (90%) and headache (80%). Because of their location, MBs tend to compress the fourth ventricle and cause obstructive hydrocephalus.

**Natural History.** Risk varies with the molecular subgroup. For example, almost all WNT-MBs exhibit classic histology and are considered low-risk neoplasms.

Poor prognostic factors include metastatic disease at time of diagnosis, *TP53* mutation, *MYC* amplification, non-WNT/non-SHH and LC/A histologies.

MEDULLOBLASTOMA: PATHOLOGY AND CLINICAL

**Etiology**

- All 5 molecular groups represented
- Many subgroups of diagnostic or prognostic or therapeutic value
  - 4 subgroups of SHH medulloblastomas
  - 8 subgroups of non-WNT/non-SHH medulloblastomas

**Pathology**

- Most common = midline (4th ventricle, vermis)
  - WNT-activated near foramen of Luschka/cerebellar peduncle, cerebellopontine angle cistern
  - SHH-activated in lateral cerebellar hemispheres
  - Non-WNT/non-SHH midline inferior cerebellum
- Small round blue cell tumor
- Neuroblastic (Homer Wright) rosettes
- All medulloblastomas are CNS WHO grade 4
  - Some groups/subgroups (e.g., WNT-activated) have good therapeutic response

**Clinical Features**

- Medulloblastoma = 20% of all pediatric brain tumors
- Most common malignant posterior fossa childhood neoplasm
- Most medulloblastomas in patients < 10 years
  - 2nd peak in patients 20-40 years
  - Up to 25% of medulloblastomas occur in adults!

## Imaging

The three main standard imaging phenotypes that can help predict MB molecular subgroups are (1) anatomic location **(24-3)**, (2) enhancement pattern, and (3) metastasis. Radiomics and machine learning approaches have recently been reported as significantly improving the prediction of the MB subgroup in individual cases.

As 40-50% of MBs have CSF dissemination at the time of initial diagnosis, preoperative contrast-enhanced MR of the entire neuraxis is recommended.

**CT Findings.** NECT scans show a moderately hyperdense, relatively well-defined mass in the midline posterior fossa (classic MB) **(24-4A)**, around the foramen of Luschka (WNT-subgroup MB) **(24-7)** or lateral cerebellum (SHH). Cyst formation (40%) and calcification (20-25%) are common **(24-4B) (24-5A)**. Gross hemorrhage is uncommon. Enhancement patterns are variable.

If dense tentorial or falcine calcifications are present, the patient should be evaluated for basal cell nevus (Gorlin) syndrome.

**MR Findings.** Almost all MBs are hypointense relative to gray matter on T1WI **(24-8A)** and hyperintense on T2WI **(24-5B)**. Peritumoral edema is present in 1/3 of cases. Obstructive hydrocephalus with periventricular accumulation of CSF is common and best delineated on FLAIR.

Because of their dense cellularity, MBs often show moderate restriction on DWI **(24-6B)**, helping distinguish them from other posterior fossa tumors. pMR shows low rCBV and increased permeability. MRS typically reveals a small taurine peak, high Cho peak, decreased NAA peak, and increased Cho:Cr and Cho:NAA ratios.

Enhancement patterns show striking variation. 2/3 of MBs show marked enhancement, whereas 1/3 show only subtle **(24-7B)**, marginal, or linear enhancement **(24-5C)**. Multinodular and gyriform tumor masses that enhance strongly and uniformly can be seen in MBs with extensive nodularity **(24-10B) (24-11)**.

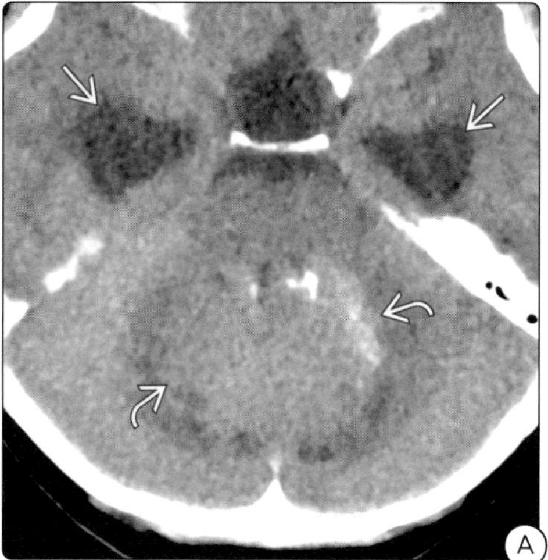

***(24-5A)** Axial NECT in a 7-yo shows a slightly hyperdense, partially calcified mass ➡ in the 4th ventricle. Note hydrocephalus ➡.*

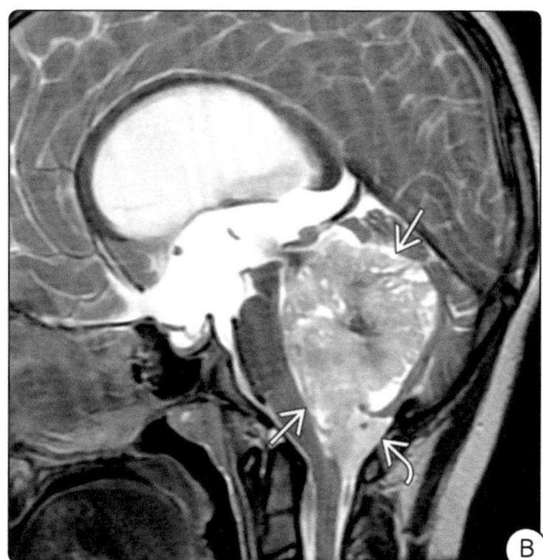

***(24-5B)** The 4th ventricle mass ➡ is hyperintense, extends posteroinferiorly through foramen of Magendie ➡ on this sagittal T2WI.*

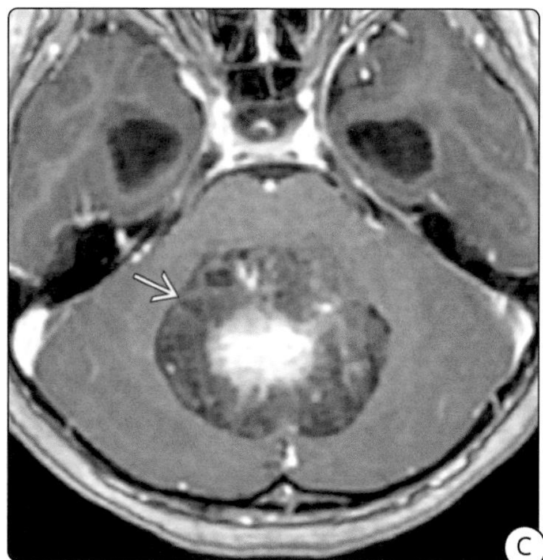

***(24-5C)** Mass ➡ enhances heterogeneously. MB, non-WNT/non-SHH, group 4 by DNA methylation profiling.*

***(24-6A)*** *Axial T2WI in a 14-yo boy shows a heterogeneously hyperintense mass ➡ in the left cerebellar hemisphere.* ***(24-6B)*** *The cerebellar mass ➡ restricts strongly on DWI.*

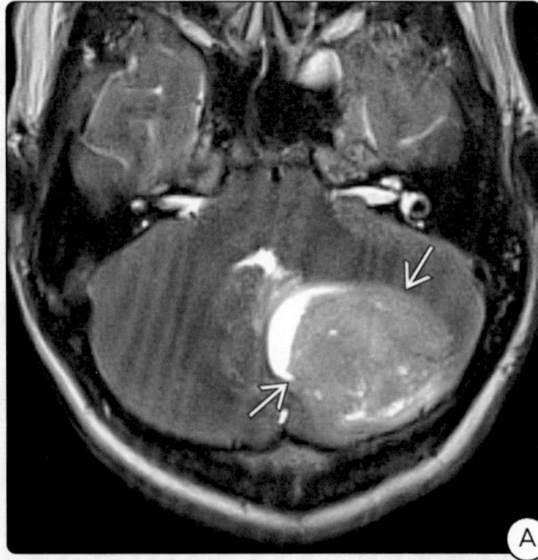


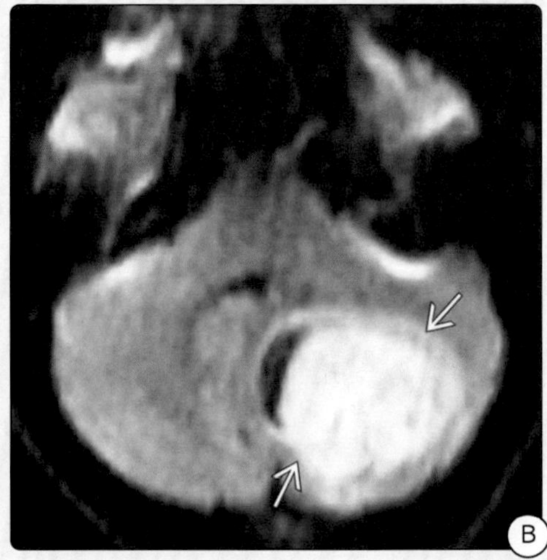


***(24-6C)*** *Axial T1 C+ in the same case shows the mass ➡ enhances only moderately and quite heterogeneously. MB, SHH-activated and TP53-mutant.* ***(24-7A)*** *T2WI in a 22-yo woman shows a heterogeneously hyperintense mass in the left cerebellar peduncle ➡.*

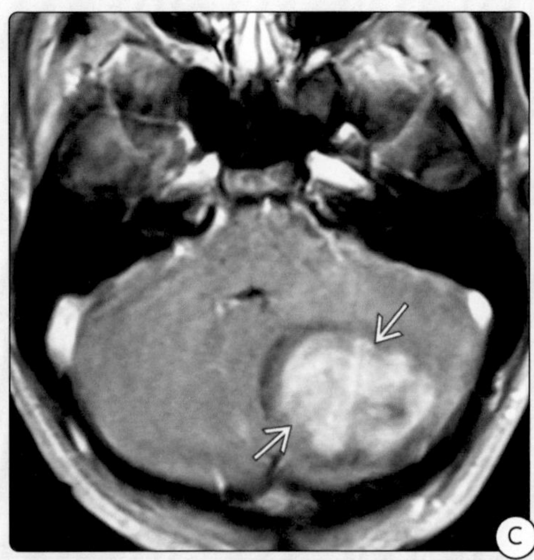


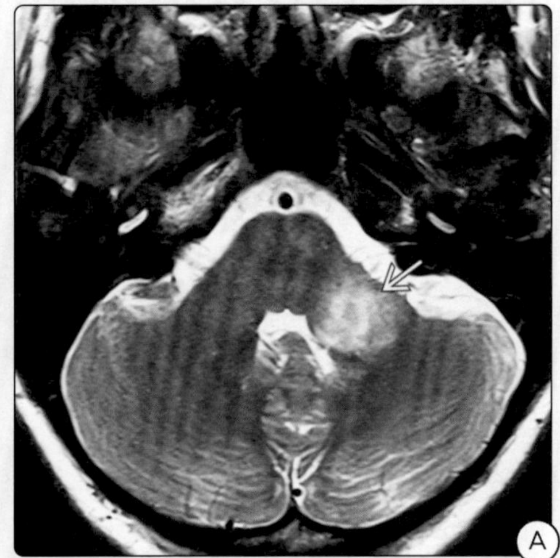


***(24-7B)*** *Axial T1 C+ FS MR shows mild enhancement in the brachium pontis mass ➡.* ***(24-7C)*** *DWI shows the mass ➡ restricts strongly. MB, WNT-activated. WNT-activated MBs account for 15-20% of MBs in adults.*

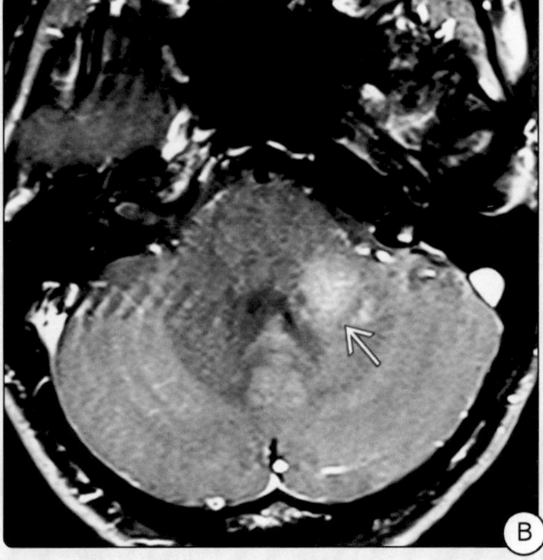


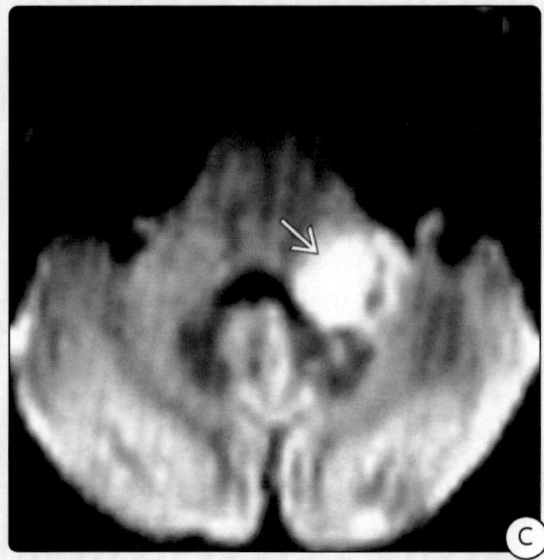

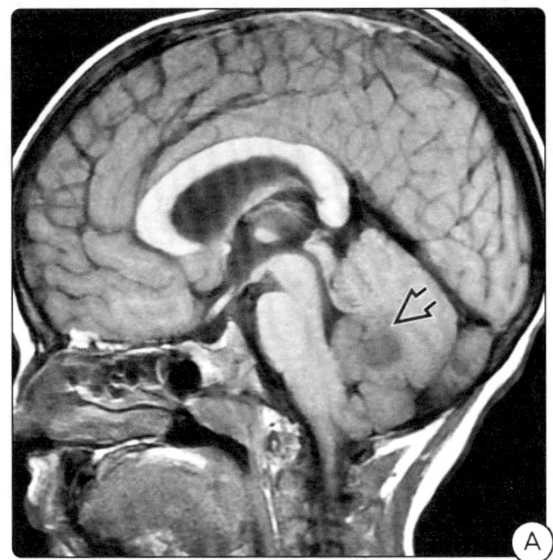

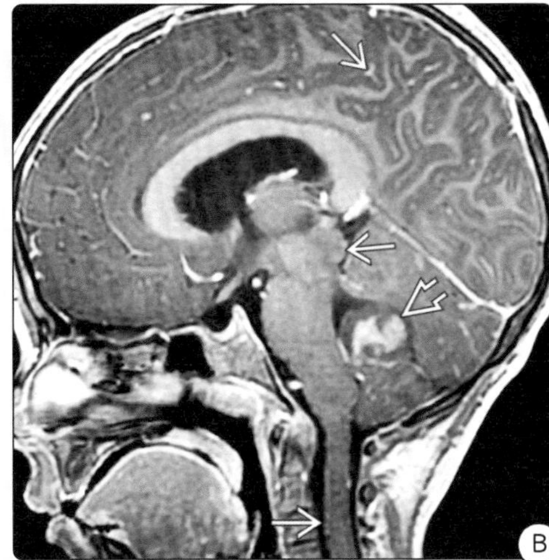

***(24-8A)** T1WI in a 4-yo boy with vomiting, bulging fontanelles shows a mixed iso- and hypointense mass ➩ in the midline posterior fossa. **(24-8B)** T1 C+ shows strong but patchy enhancement ➩ in the mass. Note subtle pial enhancement ➡.*

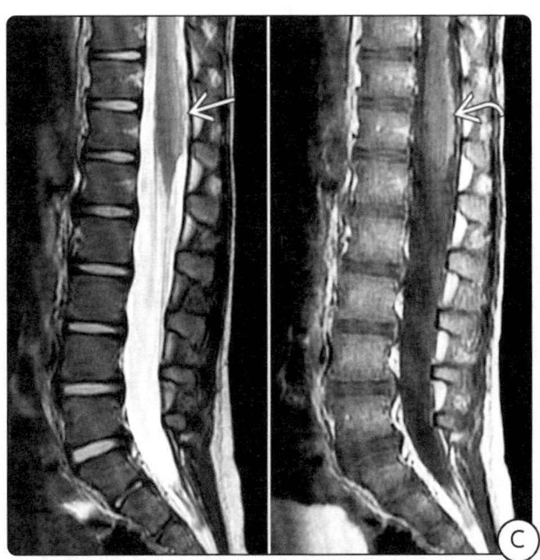

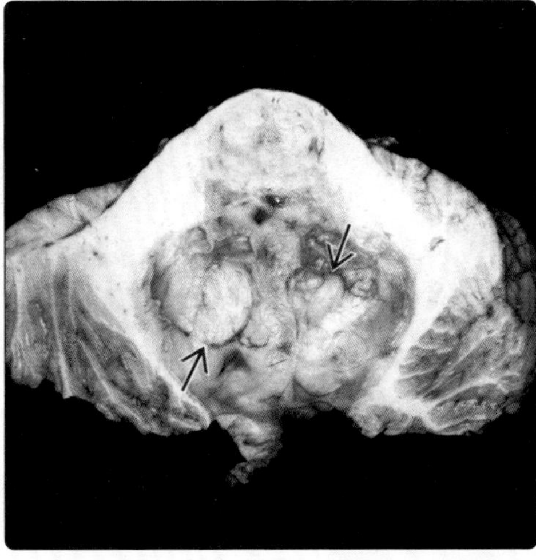

***(24-8C)** T2 (L), T1 C+ (R) show hyperintensity ➡, enhancement ➦ along distal cord. Group 3 MB with CSF dissemination at initial presentation. **(24-9)** Autopsied MB shows heterogeneous mass filling 4th ventricle, displacing and compressing the pons. Distinct nodules ➙ within the tumor mass suggest this could be a desmoplastic/nodular MB. Most of these are SHH-activated, TP53-wildtype.*

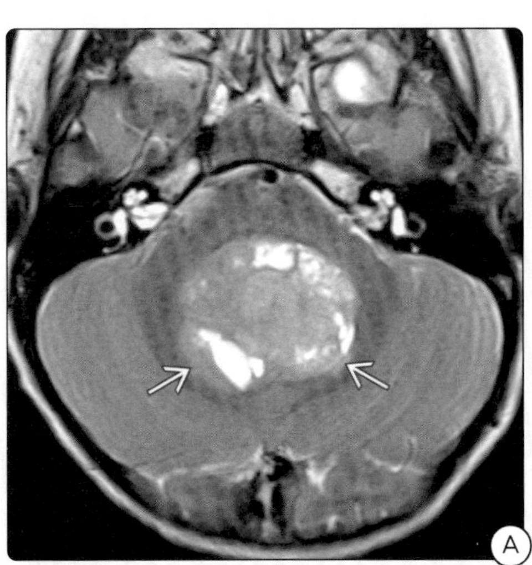

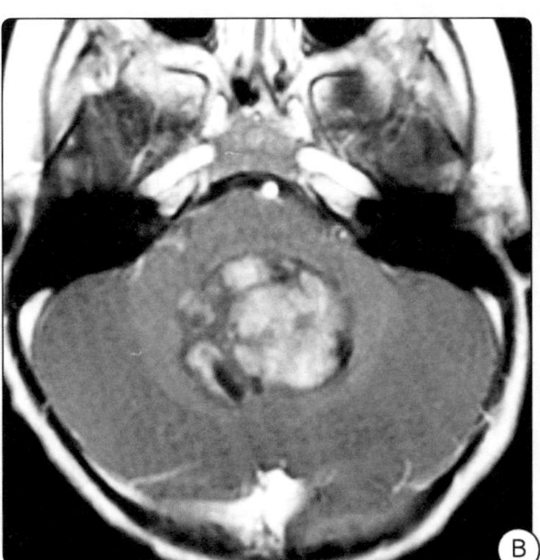

***(24-10A)** Axial T2WI in a 4-yo shows a heterogeneous mass ➡ filling the 4th ventricle. **(24-10B)** Axial T1 C+ in the same case shows the mass enhances heterogeneously in a nodular-appearing fashion. Non-WNT/non-SHH group 3 MB with desmoplastic/nodular histopathology.*

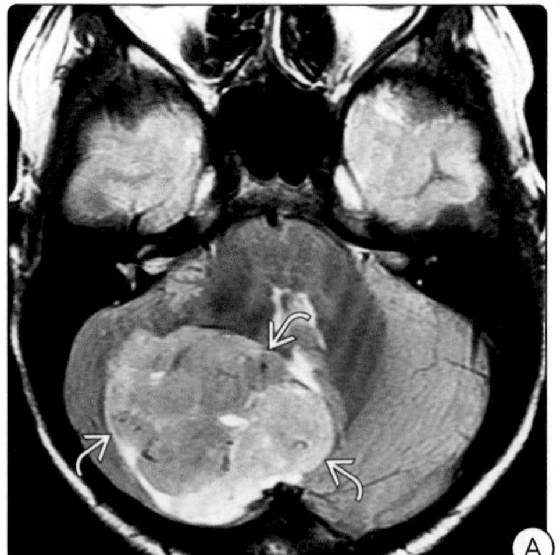


***(24-11A)** T2WI in a 10-yo boy shows a well-delineated multinodular ➔ heterogeneously hyperintense mass in right cerebellum, vermis.*

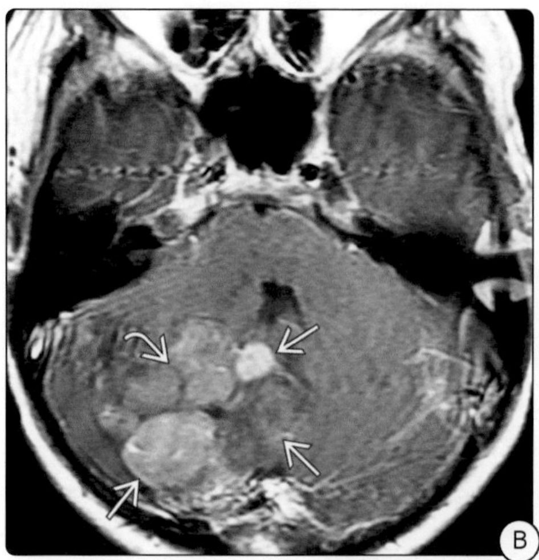


***(24-11B)** T1 C+ MR shows the distinct variably enhancing tumor nodules ➔ appear to be separated by nonenhancing septa ➔.*

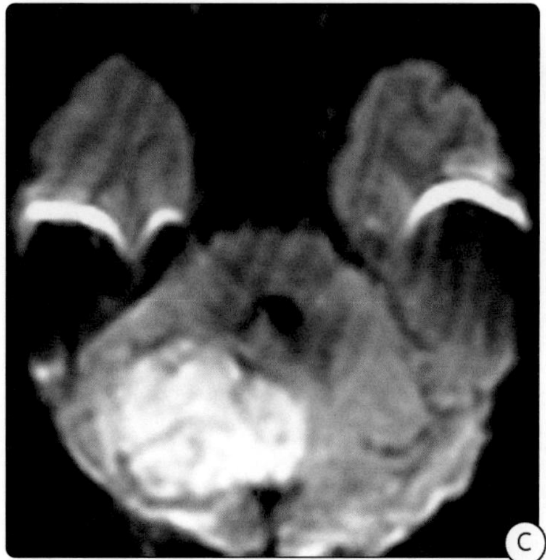


***(24-11C)** The tumor restricts strongly. Desmoplastic/nodular SHH-activated TP53-wildtype MB with extensive nodularity (MBEN).*

Group 4 MBs often exhibit minimal or no enhancement. Enhancing leptomeningeal metastases at initial diagnosis are common ("sugar icing") **(24-12)** and typically occur with groups 3 **(24-8)** and 4 **(24-13)**.

**MEDULLOBLASTOMA: IMAGING**

**CT**
- Hyperdense on NECT
- Cysts (40%)
- Calcification (20-25%)
- Hemorrhage rare

**MR**
- Hypointense on T1, iso- to hyperintense on T2
- Restricted diffusion on DWI
- Enhancement: None to strong
  - Strong but heterogeneous common
  - Little/no enhancement often seen in group 4

**Differential Diagnosis**
- Children
  - Atypical teratoid/rhabdoid tumor
  - Posterior fossa ependymoma (PFA, PFB)
  - Pilocytic astrocytoma
- Adults
  - Metastasis
  - High-grade astrocytoma with piloid features

## Differential Diagnosis

The main differential diagnoses in children are **atypical teratoid/rhabdoid tumor (AT/RT), ependymoma**, and **pilocytic astrocytoma**. AT/RT is a cellular rhabdoid tumor and is often indistinguishable from MB on imaging studies.

**Ependymoma** is also typically centered in the fourth ventricle but more often demonstrates lateral extension through the foramina of Luschka into the adjacent cisterns, sometimes described as a plastic appearance. The majority of ependymomas do not exhibit restricted diffusion.

The vast majority of **pilocytic astrocytomas** arise in the cerebellar hemispheres. The main differentiating factor from MB is the hypocellularity of the solid pilocytic tumor components, which are typically very bright on T2 and ADC.

The differential diagnosis of MB in adults differs. The most common parenchymal posterior fossa mass in adults is **metastasis**. A newly described neoplasm, **high-grade astrocytoma with piloid features (HGAP)**, occurs throughout the neuraxis but is most common in the cerebellum (75% of cases). Unlike pilocytic astrocytomas, HGAPs are more common in young and middle-aged adults but rare in the pediatric population.

# Other CNS Embryonal Tumors

CNS embryonal neoplasms other than medulloblastoma (MB) are a rare, aggressive and heterogeneous group of poorly differentiated tumors composed of immature cells that resemble neural progenitors. They are mostly—but not exclusively—neoplasms of childhood. In contrast to MBs (which arise in the posterior fossa), these embryonal tumors may arise throughout the neuraxis.

This group now consists of five specific pathologic entities: **Embryonal tumor with multilayered rosettes (ETMR), AT/RT, cribriform neuroepithelial tumor (CRINET), CNS neuroblastoma, FOXR2-activated, CNS tumor with BCOR internal tandem duplication**, and **CNS embryonal tumor, not elsewhere classified/not otherwise classified (NEC/NOS)**. DNA methylation profiling provides an indispensable tool in distinguishing these rare neoplasms.

## Embryonal Tumor With Multilayered Rosettes

### Terminology

ETMRs are aggressive CNS embryonal tumors that are characterized histologically by multilayered rosettes. ETMRs have three morphologic patterns: (1) Embryonal tumor with abundant neuropil and true rosettes, (2) ependymoblastoma, and (3) medulloepithelioma. Once considered separate entities, they now comprise a single clinicopathologic entity based on common molecular alterations.

### Pathology

Approximately 70% of ETMRs are supratentorial masses that appear relatively well demarcated with little surrounding edema. Tumors are highly variable in size but often reach > 5 cm in diameter when located in the cerebral hemispheres **(24-14)**. The cerebellum and brainstem are the primary site in 30% of cases.

Microscopically, ETMRs contain abundant neuropil and true rosettes with a pseudostratified neuroepithelium surrounding a central round or slit-like lumen. Mitoses are frequent, and CSF dissemination is common.

ETMRs harbor either C19MC alterations (most common) or *DICER1* mutation (rare). ETMR corresponds histologically to CNS WHO grade 4.

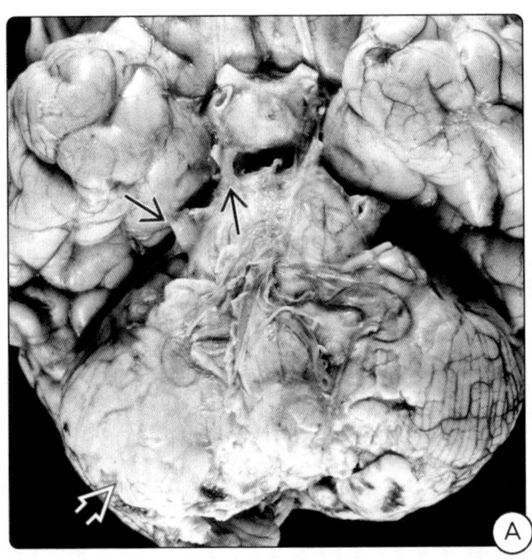


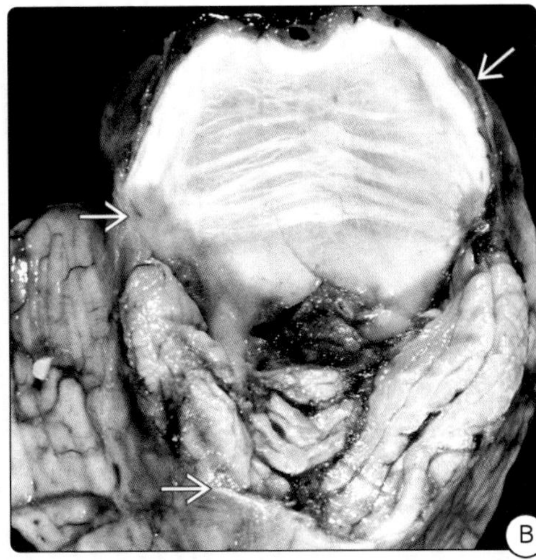


***(24-12A)** Gross pathology of metastatic MB shows diffuse "sugar icing" coating of the brain surfaces ➡ and cranial nerves ➡ by disseminated tumor. **(24-12B)** Gross pathology of the same case sectioned axially through the pons shows the diffuse coating of brain surfaces by disseminated MB ➡.*

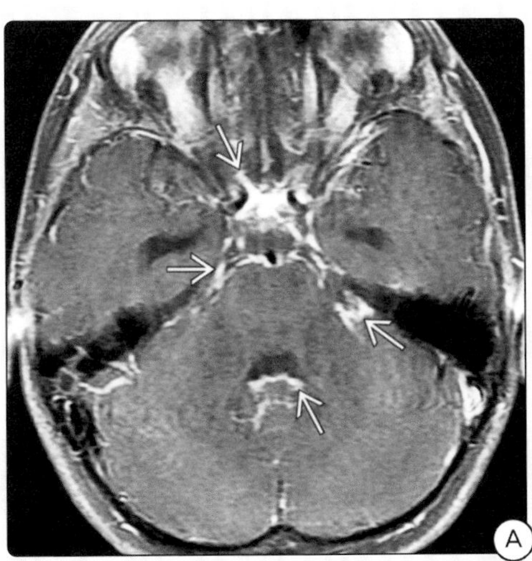


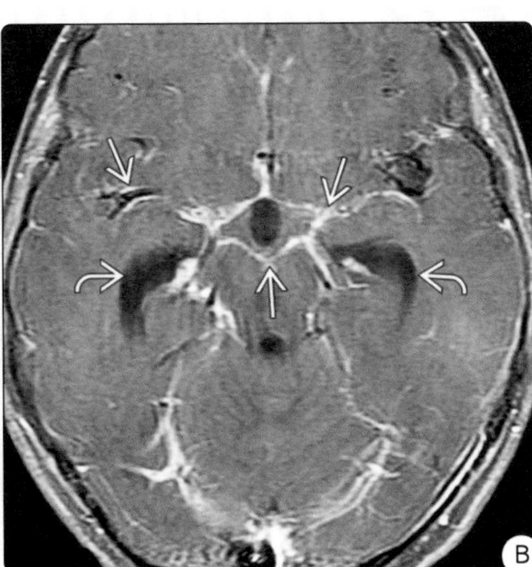


***(24-13A)** T1 C+ FS shows diffuse leptomeningeal metastases from MB coating pial surfaces of the pons, trigeminal nerves, optic chiasm, 4th ventricle, and CPA cisterns ➡. **(24-13B)** More cephalad T1 C+ FS shows metastatic MB causes obstructive hydrocephalus ➡, coats midbrain and sylvian fissures ➡.*

## Clinical Issues

Almost all ETMRs occur under the age of four years with the majority occurring in the first two years of life. Increasing head circumference and signs of elevated intracranial pressure are common. ETMRs are extremely aggressive neoplasms, and the clinical prognosis is dismal with poor overall survival.

## Imaging

**General Features.** ETMRs grow rapidly and are often very large, heterogeneous-appearing masses that cause gross distortion and effacement of the underlying brain architecture **(24-15)**.

**CT Findings.** A complex, heterogeneously iso- to hyperdense mass is typical on NECT. When large, they often become more heterogeneous and frequently develop cystic components. Hemorrhage and dystrophic calcifications may occur, especially in larger lesions.

**MR Findings.** Conventional sequences show T2/FLAIR iso-/hyperintensity of solid components **(24-16)**. With increasing size of tumor, signal characteristics typically become more heterogeneous, and T2-hyperintense cystic areas and areas of T1 hyperintensity and T2*/SWI signal loss consistent with hemorrhage are often seen. T2/FLAIR hyperintensity in cystic or necrotic segments and isointensity in the solid portions of the mass are typical. Peritumoral edema is typically minimal or absent **(24-15B)**.

Because of their relatively dense cellularity, C19MC-altered ETMRs solid components typically show moderately restricted diffusion **(24-15C)** **(24-16E)**. pMR shows areas of elevated rCBV and vascular permeability.

Enhancement varies from none **(24-16F)** to solid or rim enhancement.

*(24-14) Autopsy (L) and antemortem FLAIR scan (R) in an 8-mo infant with a supratentorial embryonal neoplasm show a large, aggressive-looking hemispheric mass with confluent areas of necrosis and hemorrhage. There is relatively little peritumoral edema. (Courtesy R. Hewlett, MD.) (24-15A) Axial T1 MR in an infant with macrocephaly shows a very large right frontal mass ➡ with areas of necrosis ➡ and hemorrhage ➡.*

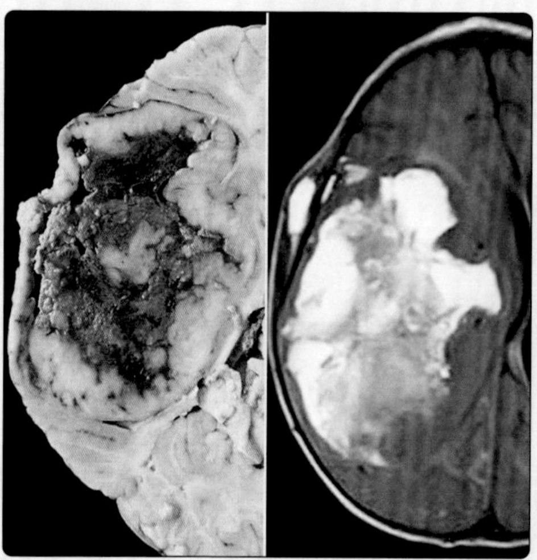

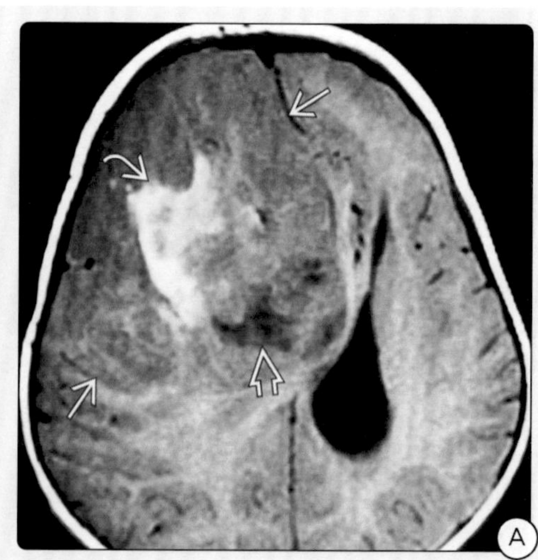


*(24-15B) T2 MR in the same patient shows that the mass is relatively well demarcated ➡ and mostly hyperintense with heterogeneously hypointense foci of hemorrhage ➡. (24-15C) The lesion restricts on DWI ➡. This is a supratentorial embryonal neoplasm [formerly designated as primitive neuroectodermal tumor and reclassified as embryonal tumor with multilayered rosettes (ETMR)].*

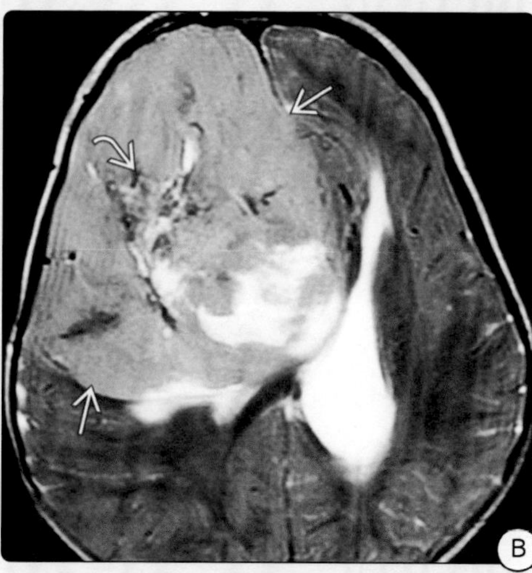


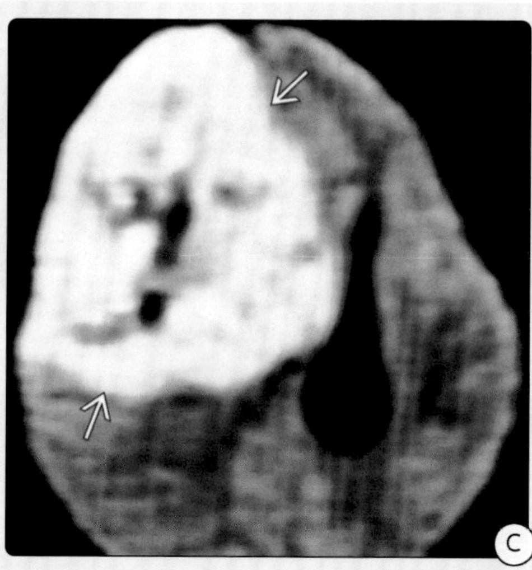

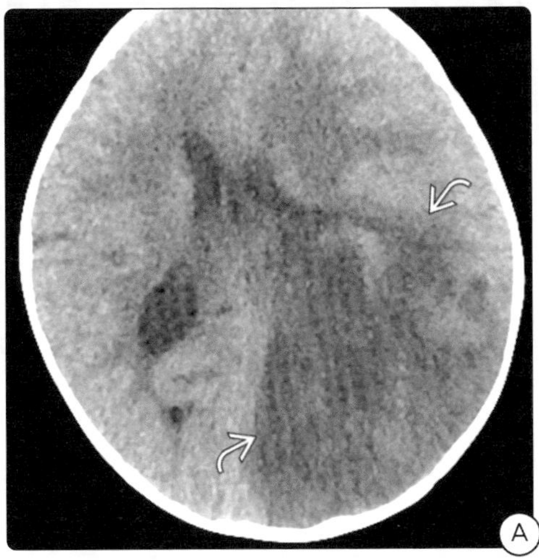

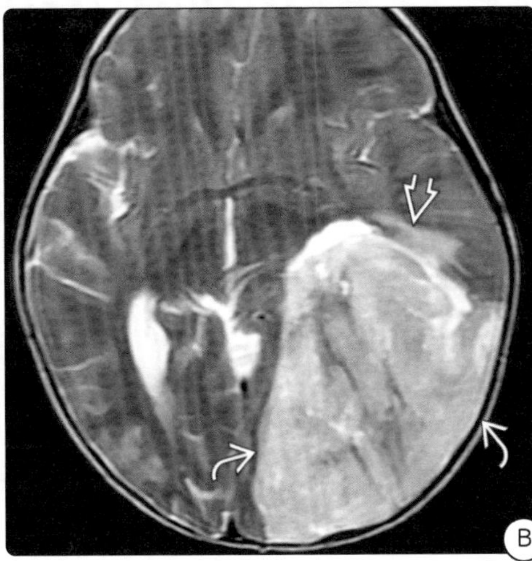

*(24-16A) Axial NECT in a 23-mo infant shows a large hypodense supratentorial mass ➔. (24-16B) The mass ➔ is heterogeneously hyperintense on T2WI. Note that, for the size of the mass, peritumoral edema ➔ is minimal.*

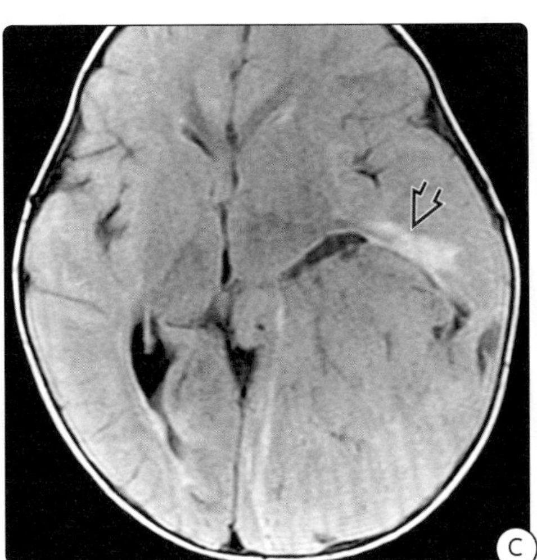

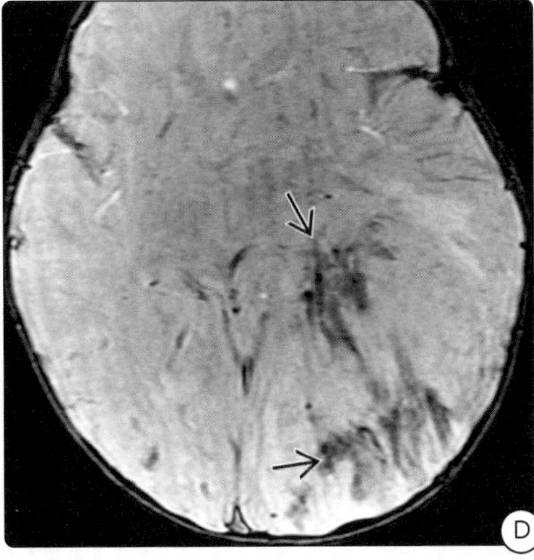

*(24-16C) The mass is mostly isointense on FLAIR with minimal peripheral edema ➔. (24-16D) T2* imaging shows foci of gradient susceptibility ➔, suggesting intratumoral hemorrhage.*

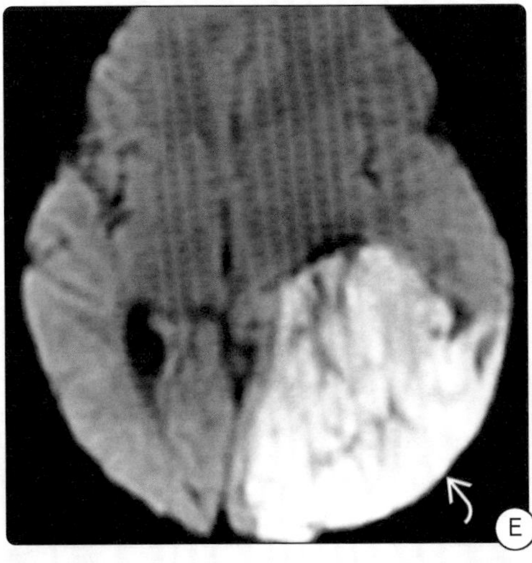

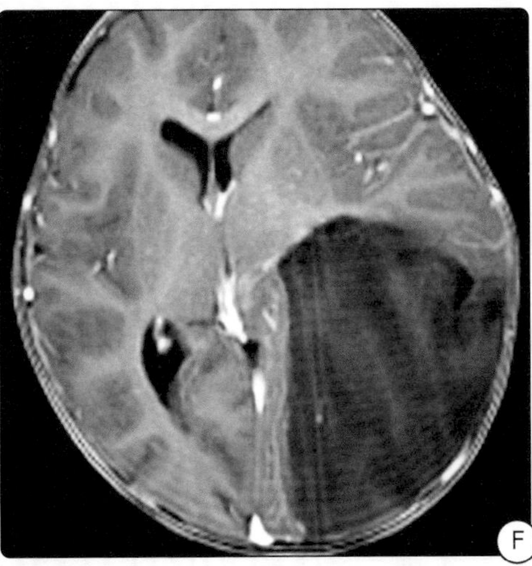

*(24-16E) The mass restricted strongly on DWI ➔ and was hypointense on ADC (not shown). (24-16F) T1 C+ shows no enhancement in the mass. ETMR, C19MC-altered.*

## Differential Diagnosis

The differential diagnosis of C19MC-altered ETMR in infants and children includes other bulky hemispheric masses, including **AT/RT, supratentorial ependymoma** (*ZFTA* or *YAP1* fusion-positive), **astroblastoma** (*MN1*-altered), **pediatric-type diffuse high-grade gliomas**, such as infant-type hemispheric glioma, **CNS neuroblastoma** (*FOXR2*-altered), and **CNS tumor with internal tandem duplication** (*BCOR*).

# Atypical Teratoid/Rhabdoid Tumor

Atypical teratoid/rhabdoid tumor (AT/RT) occurs at a younger age and is associated with a worse prognosis than MB. Although it accounts for just 1-2% of pediatric CNS tumors, it is the most common of the "other CNS embryonal neoplasms." AT/RTs occur at a younger age than MB.

## Terminology

AT/RT is a rare, highly malignant CNS embryonal tumor composed of poorly differentiated elements and a variable number of malignant rhabdoid cells.

## Etiology

AT/RT is a genetically defined tumor characterized by deletions and biallelic inactivating mutations of the *SMARCB1* (a.k.a. hSNF5 or INI1) gene. Loss of the SMARCB1 protein in AT/RT results in unopposed expression of *LIN28B* (a key gene in embryonic development and for maintaining pluripotency in stem cells).

Molecular profiling has identified three molecularly and clinically distinct AT/RT subgroups, currently designated as ATRT-TYR, ATRT-SHH, and ATRT-MYC.

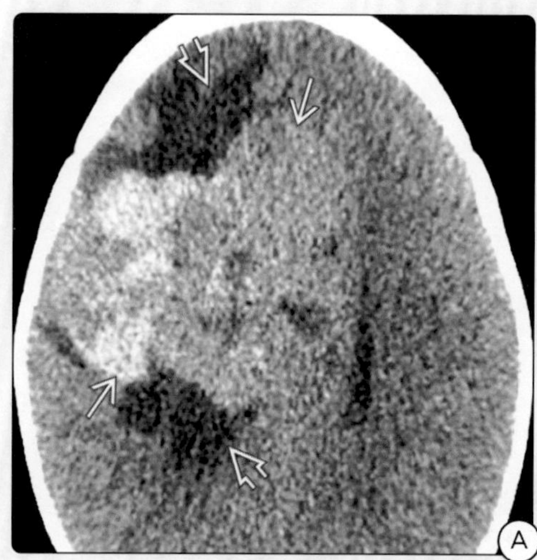


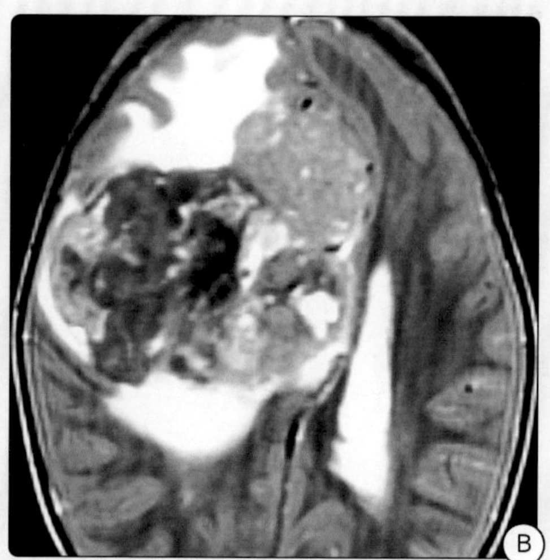


***(24-17A)** NECT in an 18-mo girl with vomiting for 1-2 weeks shows a mixed, mostly hyperdense right frontal mass ➡ with marked vasogenic edema ⮕. **(24-17B)** T2 MR shows that the mass has mixed, mostly hypo- and isointense signal intensity.*

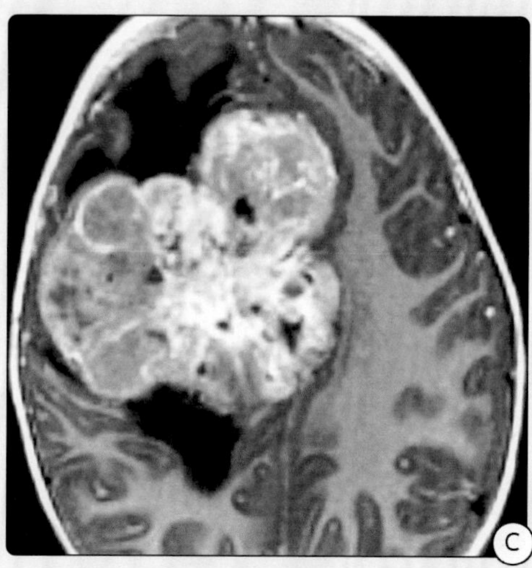


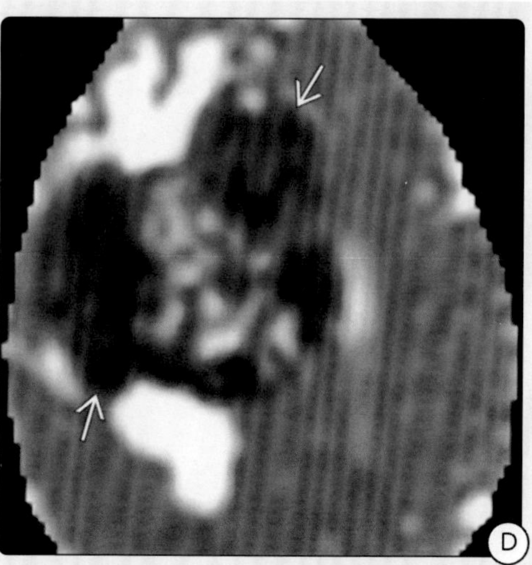


***(24-17C)** T1 C+ MR shows diffuse but very heterogeneous enhancement. **(24-17D)** ADC map shows marked diffuse restriction ➡ due to the high cellularity of the tumor. MRS (not shown) demonstrated elevated Cho and lactate. Histologic diagnosis was atypical teratoid/rhabdoid tumor (AT/RT). (Courtesy B. Jones, MD.)*

## Pathology

**Location.** AT/RTs occur throughout the neuraxis, in both the supra- **(24-17)** and infratentorial compartments **(24-18)**. Spinal cord AT/RTs are rare. Location is strongly correlated with molecular subgroup.

Slightly more than 1/2 of all AT/RTs are supratentorial, usually occurring in the cerebral hemispheres **(24-17)**, although cases in other sites (including the suprasellar cistern, ventricles, and pineal gland) have been reported. Most supratentorial AT/RTs are ATRT-MYC or ATRT-SHH subtypes.

Posterior fossa AT/RTs preferentially occur in the cerebellar hemispheres **(24-18A)**, although they can occur in the fourth ventricle, where they mimic MB. Although ATRT-MYC and ATRT-SHH subtypes occasionally occur here, the posterior fossa is the site of ~ 75% of ATRT-TYR neoplasms.

### ATYPICAL TERATOID/RHABDOID TUMOR: ETIOLOGY AND PATHOLOGY

**Etiology**

- Loss *SMARCB1* or *SMARCA4* expression required for diagnosis
- 3 distinct atypical teratoid/rhabdoid tumor molecular subgroups
    - ATRT-TYR, ATRT-SHH, ATRT-MYC

**Pathology**

- Supratentorial: ~ 50%
    - Most are ATRT-MYC or ATRT-SHH
- Infratentorial: ~ 50%
    - All 3 subgroups (75% of ATRT-TYR)
- Poorly differentiated neuroepithelial elements + rhabdoid cells
- CNS WHO grade 4

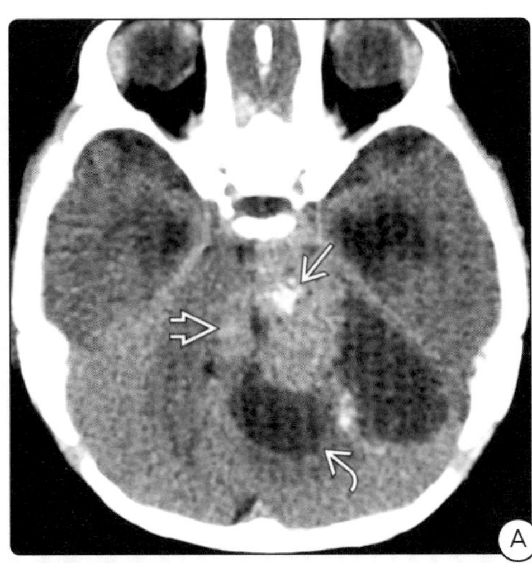


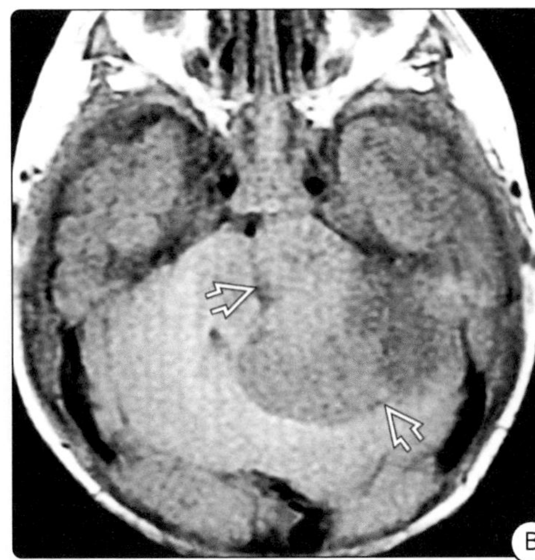


***(24-18A)** NECT in a 4-mo boy with vomiting, head tilt, and bulging fontanelle shows a partially solid ➡, partially cystic-appearing ➡ posterior fossa mass that exhibits focal calcifications ➡. **(24-18B)** Axial T1 MR in the same case shows that the mass ➡ is mixed iso-/hypointense compared with gray matter.*

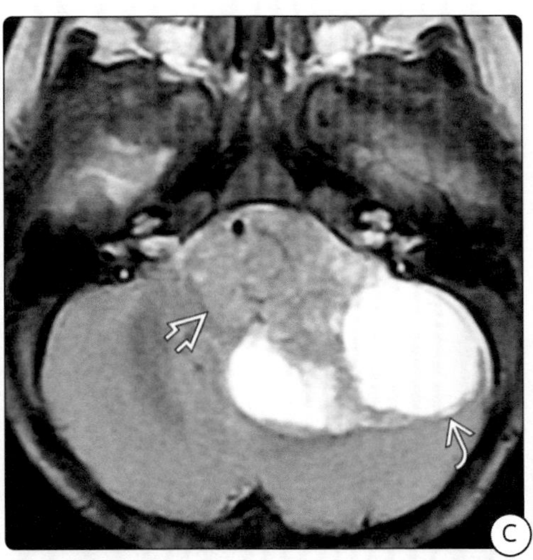


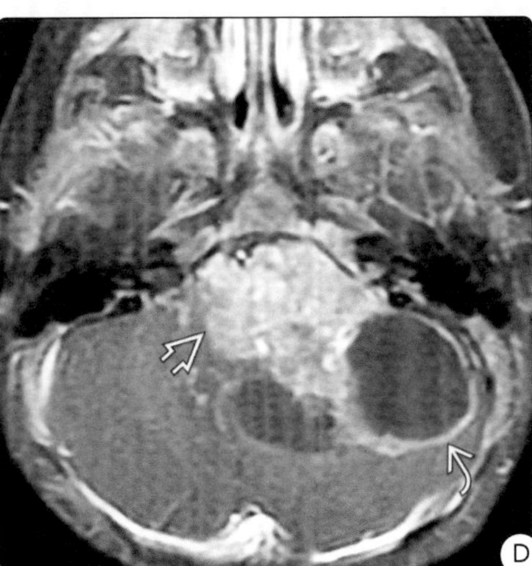


***(24-18C)** Axial T2 MR in the same case shows the mixed solid ➡, cystic ➡ mass. **(24-18D)** Axial T1 C+ FS MR shows the solid components ➡ of the mass enhancing strongly but heterogeneously. The cysts exhibit rim enhancement ➡. This is AT/RT, CNS WHO grade 4.*

**Gross Pathology.** The gross appearance—a large, soft, fleshy, hemorrhagic, necrotic mass—is similar to that of other CNS embryonal neoplasms.

**Microscopic Features.** AT/RTs are composed of poorly differentiated neural, epithelial, and mesenchymal elements together with prominent rhabdoid cells. Nuclear loss of SMARCB1 (INI1) protein expression is a highly sensitive marker for the diagnosis of AT/RT.

## Clinical Issues

**Epidemiology.** AT/RT accounts for just 1-2% of all pediatric brain tumors but up to 20% of patients under three years of age. AT/RT does occur in adults but is rare. There is a moderate male predominance.

AT/RT can occur sporadically or in **rhabdoid tumor predisposition syndrome** (RTPS). RTPS is a familial cancer syndrome characterized by a markedly increased risk of developing malignant rhabdoid tumors—including AT/RT—caused by loss or inactivation of the *SMARCB1* gene (less commonly, the mutation involves the *SMARCA4* gene).

Children with RTPS and AT/RT are even younger, have more extensive disease, and experience more rapid progression compared to sporadic tumors. Other CNS tumors associated with RTPS include choroid plexus carcinoma and rhabdoid meningioma.

**Natural History.** AT/RT is a highly malignant tumor with generally poor prognosis. Median survival is around 17 months. Most children die within 6-8 months despite aggressive therapy. Survival in adults is somewhat better, averaging two years.

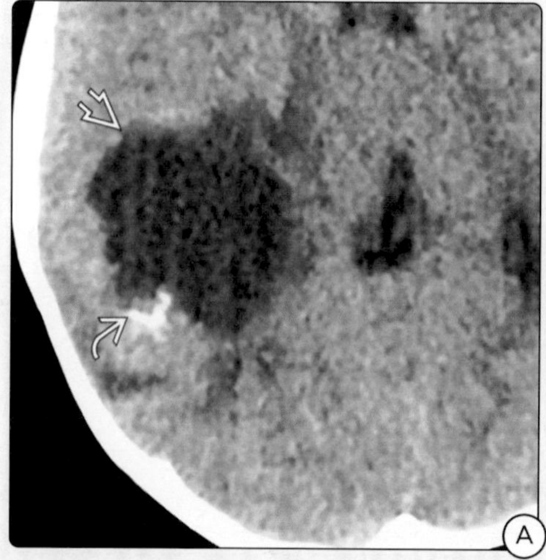


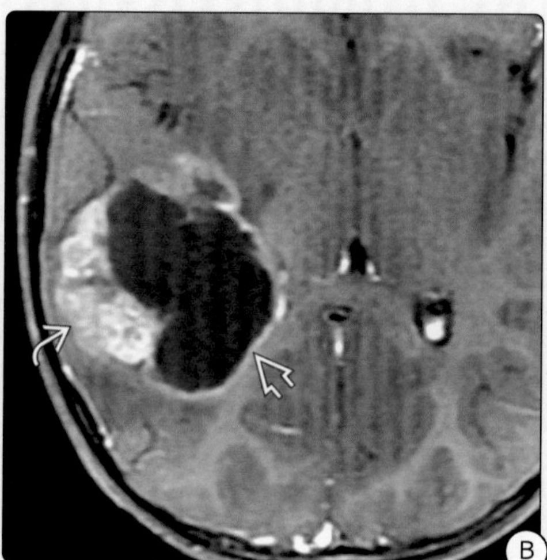


***(24-19A)** Axial NECT in a 2-yo shows a partially cystic, partially solid right parietal mass. A small focus of calcification is present in the solid portion of the mass. **(24-19B)** T1 C+ in the same case shows the rim of the partially cystic mass enhances. The solid portion of the mass enhances strongly but heterogeneously.*

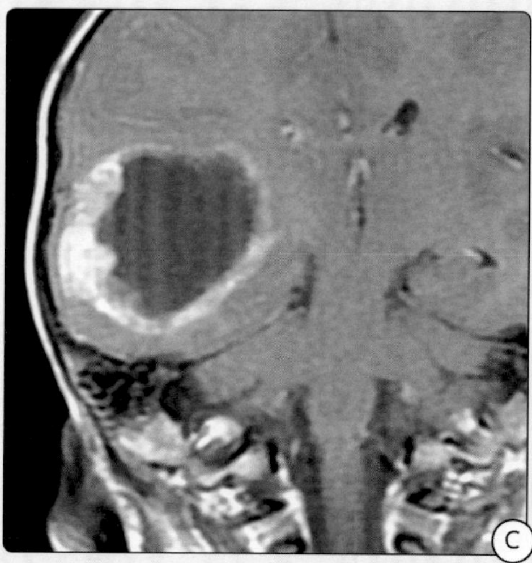


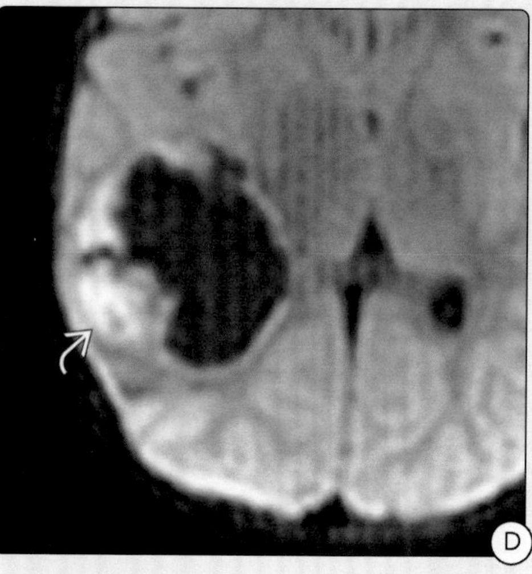


***(24-19C)** Coronal T1 C+ shows the hemispheric mass has irregular rim enhancement. **(24-19D)** The solid portion of the mass shows moderate restricted diffusion indicating cellularity. This is AT/RT.*

ATYPICAL TERATOID/RHABDOID TUMOR: CLINICAL ISSUES

**Epidemiology**
- 1-2% of pediatric brain tumors
  - Children < 5 years, most < 2 years
  - 10% of CNS neoplasms in infants
  - Occasionally occur in adults (rare)

**Rhabdoid Tumor Predisposition Syndrome**
- Malignant rhabdoid tumors
- Choroid plexus carcinoma

## Imaging

**General Features.** AT/RT shares many imaging features with other embryonal tumors, i.e., they are densely cellular neoplasms that frequently contain hemorrhage, necrosis, cysts, and calcifications **(24-17A)**. A moderately large, bulky tumor with mixed solid and cystic components and heterogeneous density/signal intensity is typical **(24-18A)**.

CSF dissemination is common, so the entire neuraxis should be imaged prior to surgical intervention.

**CT Findings.** NECT scan shows a mildly to moderately hyperdense mass with cysts and hemorrhagic foci **(24-17A)**. Peripheral cysts can be found in all molecular subgroups independent of location but occur most frequently in ATRT-TYR. Calcification **(24-19A)** and obstructive hydrocephalus—especially with posterior fossa AT/RT—are common. Enhancement is typically strong but heterogeneous.

**MR Findings.** AT/RTs are heterogeneously hypo- to isointense to brain on T1WI **(24-18B)** and iso- to hyperintense on T2WI **(24-18C)**. "Blooming" foci on T2* (GRE, SWI) from intratumoral hemorrhage are common. Mild to moderate diffusion restriction is seen in the majority of cases **(24-17D)** **(24-19)**. MRS shows elevated Cho and decreased or absent NAA.

Enhancement on T1 C+ is strong but heterogeneous, especially in ATRT-TYR and ATRT-MYC tumors **(24-18D)**. Although not present in the majority of AT/RTs, a distinct and unusual pattern of a "wavy" band-like enhancement surrounding a central hypointensity has been described in 38% of AT/RTs and is found throughout all molecular subgroups **(24-17C)**. Leptomeningeal spread at initial imaging is present in 15% of cases and occurs equally across all subgroups, so imaging the entire neuraxis prior to surgery is mandatory.

## Differential Diagnosis

The major differential diagnosis for *supratentorial* AT/RT includes **ETMR, supratentorial ependymoma, ZFTA fusion-positive** as well as **teratoma** and **pediatric-type diffuse high-grade gliomas** (such as infant-type hemispheric glioma). As all of these may be bulky—even massive—tumors with very heterogeneous imaging appearance, definitive diagnosis requires biopsy and loss of *SMARCB1* or *SMARCA4* immunostaining.

The major differential diagnosis for *infratentorial* (posterior fossa) AT/RT is **MB**. These tumors can look virtually identical on imaging studies. The rare spinal cord AT/RT can resemble an **MYCN-amplified spinal ependymoma**, but the latter occur in adolescents and young adults, not infants.

ATYPICAL TERATOID/RHABDOID TUMOR: IMAGING AND DIFFERENTIAL DIAGNOSIS

**Imaging**
- Heterogeneous, hyperdense on NECT
- Heterogeneous on both T1, T2
- Enhances strongly but heterogeneously
- CSF spread in 15-20% at diagnosis
- Restricts on DWI

**Differential Diagnosis**
- Of *supratentorial* atypical teratoid/rhabdoid tumor
  - Embryonal tumor with multilayered rosettes
  - Supratentorial ependymoma, *ZFTA* fusion-positive
  - Pediatric-type diffuse high-grade glioma (e.g., infant-type hemispheric glioma)
- Of *posterior fossa* atypical teratoid/rhabdoid tumor
  - Medulloblastoma (midline atypical teratoid/rhabdoid tumor may be indistinguishable)

# Cribriform Neuroepithelial Tumor

CRINET is a newly recognized benign tumor provisionally defined as a nonrhabdoid neuroectodermal tumor characterized by a large, heterozygous deletion in *SMARCB1*. CRINET shares molecular similarities with the TYR subgroup of AT/RT but has distinct histologic features and favorable long-term outcome.

Key histologic features of CRINET are a cribriform growth pattern with strands, ribbons, and loss of nuclear *SMARCB1* expression in tumor cells. CRINET is an intra- or paraventricular tumor with reported median age at diagnosis of 1.7 years. CRINETs generally have a benign clinical course with estimated mean overall survival of 10.4 years. No WHO grade has been defined.

Reported imaging findings are nonspecific with a large bulky mass that is T1 hypointense, T2/FLAIR hyperintense, and exhibits restricted diffusion and heterogeneous enhancement.

# CNS Neuroblastoma, *FOXR2*-Activated

*FOXR2*-activated neuroblastoma is a rare, highly malignant embryonal neoplasm that exhibits varying degrees of neuroblastic &/or neuronal differentiation. It is characterized by activation of, and complex inter- and intrachromosomal rearrangements in, the *FOXR2* gene. Stabilization and amplification of *MYCN* induced by activated FOXR2 are thought to play a pivotal role in tumorigenesis.

This embryonal tumor presents as a supratentorial hemispheric mass in a child between 2-6 years (median age =

4.2 years). Headache, vomiting, seizure, and focal neurologic deficits are the common presenting symptoms.

*FOXR2*-activated neuroblastomas are composed of uniform round, poorly differentiated cells with a high nuclear:cytoplasmic ratio and elevated mitotic count. Necrosis and intratumoral hemorrhage are common.

A large, lobulated mixed hyper- and isodense mixed solid/cystic mass with spotty calcification along the solid inner rim can be seen on NECT in 80% of cases **(24-20A)**. Peritumoral edema is minimal or absent. Tumors are generally heterogeneously hyperintense on T2WI and FLAIR **(24-20B)** and show variable enhancement in the solid portion of the tumor **(24-20D)**. Susceptibility artifacts are common and caused by calcification &/or hemorrhage **(24-20C)**.

Because of their cellularity, *FOXR2*-activated neuroblastomas restrict on DWI. pMR may show elevated rCBV and rCBF. As CSF spread can occur, imaging the entire neuraxis prior to surgery is a necessity.

The differential diagnosis for this rare tumor is broad and includes **AT/RT** as well as all the pediatric-type diffuse high-grade gliomas, including **diffuse hemispheric glioma, H3 G34-mutant, diffuse pediatric-type high-grade glioma, H3- and IDH-wildtype**, and **infant-type hemispheric glioma**. Intratumor calcification is rare in all of these high-grade pediatric-type gliomas, which may help in distinguishing them from *FOXR2*-activated neuroblastomas.

## CNS Tumor With *BCOR* Internal Tandem Duplication

CNS tumor with *BCOR* internal tandem duplication is a high-grade neuroepithelial tumor characterized by a predominately solid, compact growth pattern, ependymoma-like perivascular pseudorosettes, and immature neuronal-like areas.

*(24-20A) NECT in a 7-yo shows a large mixed hyper- and hypodense right hemispheric mass ➡ with foci of intratumoral calcifications ➡. (24-20B) Axial T2 FS in the same case shows numerous flow voids ➡ in this highly vascularized, very heterogeneous-appearing tumor.*

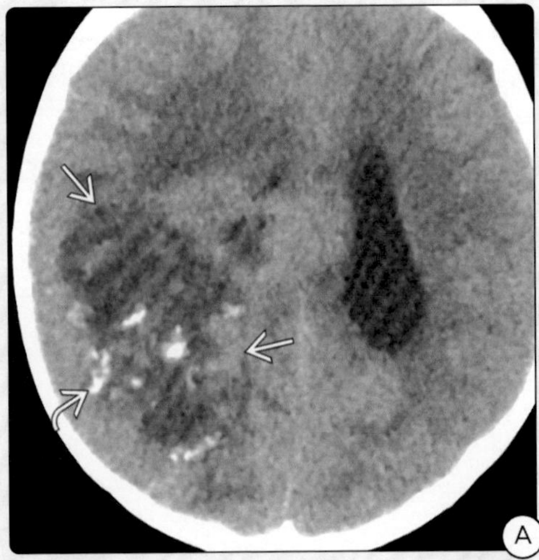


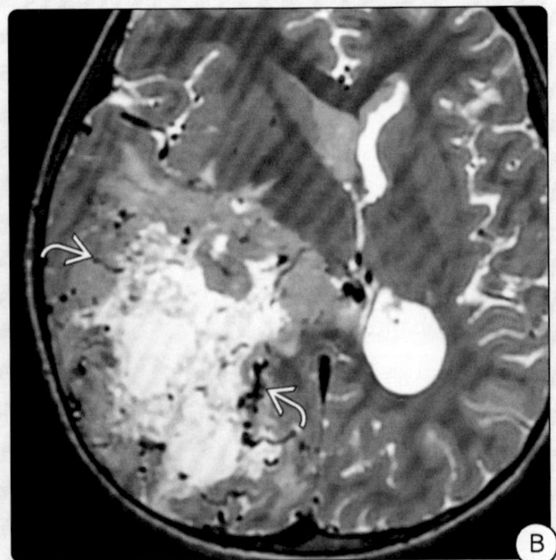


*(24-20C) T2* SWI shows multiple "blooming" foci within the mass ➡, representing a combination of calcifications and hemorrhage. (24-20D) T1 C+ FS shows thick, rind-like enhancement around the necrotic tumor core ➡. Note the diffuse "sugar icing" leptomeningeal metastatic disease ➡ in the frontal and temporal lobe sulci, as well as ependymal spread around the ventricles ➡. CNS neuroblastoma, FOXR2-activated.*

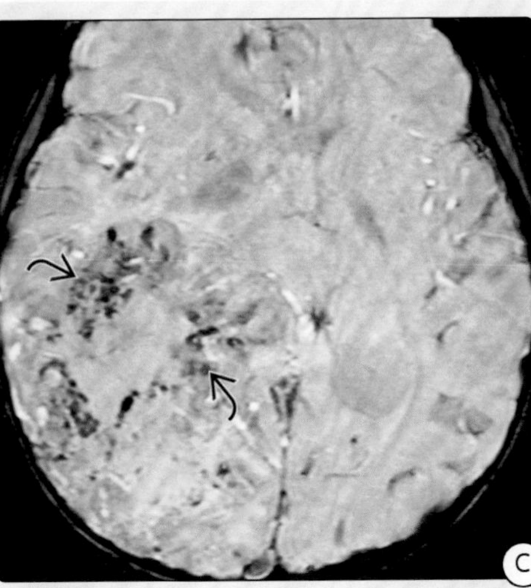


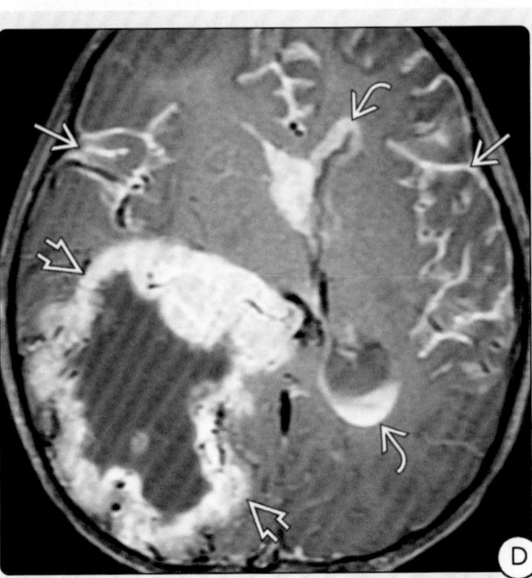

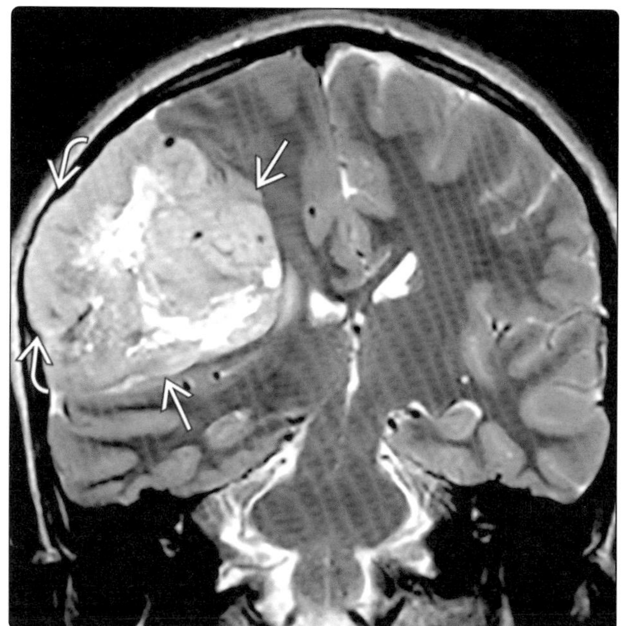

***(24-21)** Coronal T2WI in a 12-yo girl shows a well-demarcated, heterogeneously hyperintense hemispheric mass ➡. Note thinning, remodeling of the adjacent calvarium ➡. CNS tumor with BCOR internal tandem duplication. (From DP: Neuro.)*

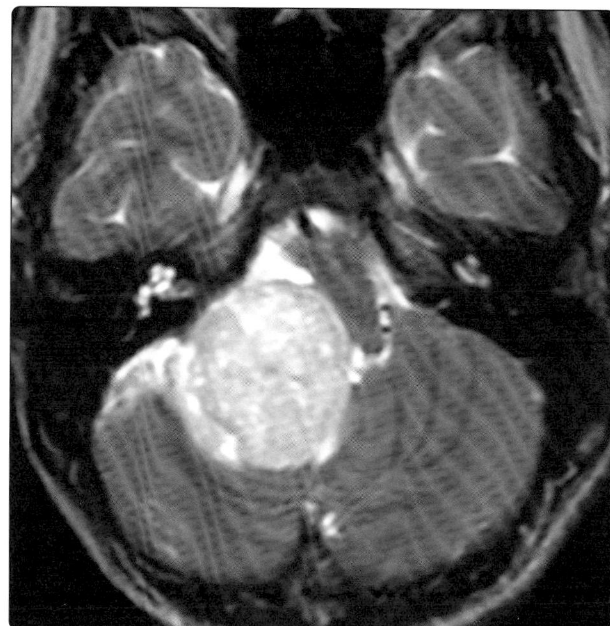

***(24-22)** Axial T2WI shows an infratentorial CNS tumor with BCOR internal tandem duplication as a heterogeneously hyperintense cerebellar mass. (From DP: Neuro.)*

*BCOR* internal tandem duplication tumors primarily affect infants. Tumors can be supra- **(24-21)** or infratentorial **(24-22)**. Most are large, solid, well-circumscribed masses that often abut the dura **(24-21)**. The few reported cases are heterogeneous on T1- and T2WIs, predominately T1 hypo- and T2 hyperintense. Because of their high cellularity, most restrict on DWI. Enhancement varies but is generally mild to moderate.

The imaging differential is other high-grade neuroepithelial neoplasms of infancy, such as **AT/RT**, **ETMR**, and **CNS neuroblastoma, FOXR2-activated**. Pediatric-type diffuse high-grade gliomas, such as **infant-type hemispheric glioma** and **diffuse pediatric-type high-grade glioma, H3- and IDH-wildtype**, are also differential diagnostic considerations.

*Selected References: The complete reference list is available on the eBooks+ version included with purchase.*

# Pineal and Germ Cell Tumors

*The region in and around the pineal gland is one of the most anatomically complex intracranial sites. There are many critical structures that surround the small gland, which makes surgery of pineal region masses challenging for our neurosurgical colleagues. Accurate preoperative assessment of lesions of the pineal region is essential. A broad spectrum of both neoplasms and nonneoplastic entities can arise from the pineal gland itself or the surrounding structures.*



Overall, pineal region tumors are rare, accounting for 1-3% of all intracranial neoplasms. Neoplasms in this region can be grouped into three simple overarching categories. The two most important groups arise in the midline or from cells within the pineal gland itself: (1) Germ cell tumors (GCTs) and (2) tumors of pineal parenchymal cells. The third group includes tumors of "other cells," including metastases, rare glial tumors and other rare tumors. We begin our discussion with a brief review of anatomy and then focus on the two major types of pineal neoplasms. We then close with a brief discussion of "other cell" tumors in the pineal gland and pineal region.

## Pineal Region Anatomy

The pineal region is located under the falx cerebri, near its confluence within the tentorium cerebelli. The pineal region includes the pineal gland, adjacent CSF spaces, brain parenchyma (corpus callosum splenium, quadrigeminal plate and upper vermis), vascular structures, and meninges **(25-1)**.

### Gross Anatomy

#### Pineal Gland

The pineal gland is a small, rounded endocrine organ that is in the midline nestled between the superior colliculi in the quadrigeminal cistern **(25-1)** **(25-3)** **(25-4)**. It is attached to the diencephalon and posterior wall of the third ventricle by the pineal stalk. The pineal gland also connects with the habenular and posterior commissures. The pituitary gland is supplied primarily by the medial posterior choroidal artery from P2 branches of the posterior cerebral artery (PCA). The pineal gland is primarily composed of pineal parenchymal cells called **pinealocytes**. Other contents include neuroglial cells, predominately astrocytes. The pineal gland produces **melatonin**, which plays a role in regulating the sleep/wake cycle in humans. The pineal gland is also responsible for regulation of reproductive function, such as onset of puberty in humans.

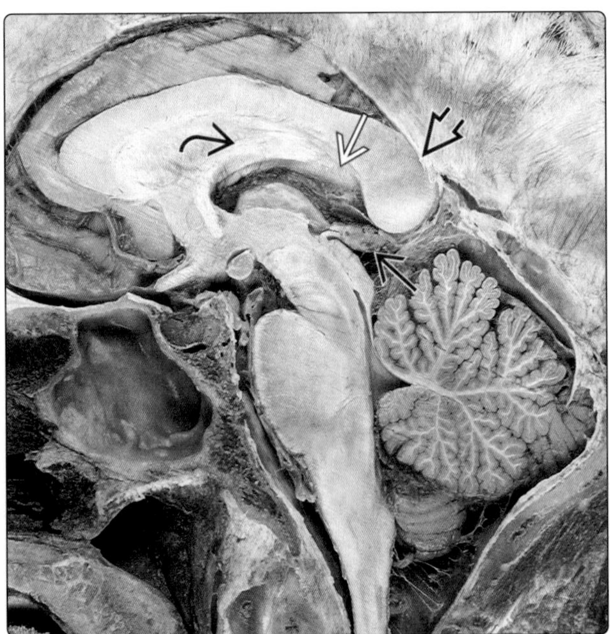

*(25-1) Sagittal midline autopsy section shows the pineal gland along the posterior 3rd ventricle within the quadrigeminal cistern under the corpus callosum splenium. The fornix is above the velum interpositum. (Courtesy M. Nielsen, MS.)*

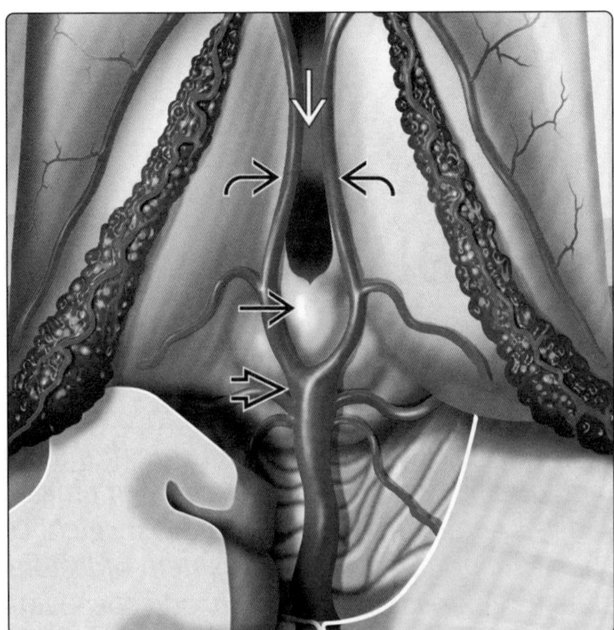

*(25-2) Axial graphic from above shows the pineal gland with corpus callosum and fornices removed. ICVs extend posteriorly from the foramen of Monro along the 3rd ventricle and unite posteriorly to form the vein of Galen.*

## Third Ventricle

The pineal gland is located at the posterior third ventricle and abuts the two posterior recesses. Just superior to the pineal gland is the **suprapineal recess** of the third ventricle, just below the splenium of the corpus callosum. There is a smaller **pineal recess** that points posteriorly, directly into the pineal gland.

There are two commissural fiber tracts that relate to the pineal gland. The habenular commissure lies just above the pineal gland, and the posterior commissure lies below the gland. The **habenular commissure** connects the habenular, amygdaloid nuclei, and hippocampi. The **posterior commissure** **(25-3)** has connections with the dorsal thalamus, superior colliculi, pretectal nuclei, and other nuclei. The medial longitudinal fasciculus fibers also cross at the posterior commissure.

## Fornix and Velum Interpositum

The **fornices** are part of the limbic system and provide primary efferent outputs from the hippocampus **(25-1)** **(25-4)**. The fornices are paired C-shaped nuclei that each has four parts. The fornix **crura** arch under the corpus callosum splenium and form part of the medial wall of the lateral ventricles. The **commissure** connects the two crura, which converge to form the body. The fornix **body** is attached to the inferior surface of septum pellucidum and is best seen on coronal imaging. The **columns** or "pillars" of the fornix extend to and terminate in the mammillary bodies.

The **velum interpositum** (VI) is formed by a double layer of pia known as the tela choroidea. The VI stretches between the bodies of the two fornices **(25-4)**. The VI forms the roof of the third ventricle and is closed anteriorly at the foramen of Monro. If the VI is open posteriorly, it may communicate posteriorly with quadrigeminal cistern, a normal variant called the cavum of the VI. The VI also covers the pineal gland and habenular commissure but is not attached to these structures.

## Vascular Structures

The **internal cerebral veins** (ICVs) are paired veins that course along the VI and terminate in the quadrigeminal cistern, where they unite. With the basal veins of Rosenthal, the ICVs form the great cerebral **vein of Galen** **(25-2)**. The ICVs lie above the pineal gland.

The **medial posterior choroidal arteries** arise from the P2 segments of the PCAs and provide the main arterial supply to the pineal gland **(25-3)**. The pineal gland lacks a blood-brain barrier and enhances avidly.

# Imaging

Physiologic pineal calcification is common and increases with age. Studies have shown that 40% of pineal glands are calcified in patients < 30 years of age. More than 1/2 of all adults have calcified pineal glands. Pineal glands are typically ≤ 10 mm but may be larger, up to 14-15 mm.

Thin-section, small FOV sagittal and coronal MR are the ideal planes to evaluate pineal region lesions. A simple way to recall the relationship of the pineal gland to its adjacent structures can be identified using sagittal sequences. From the top down, the mnemonic "**F**amous **V.I.P.**" identifies the **f**ornix, **V**I, **I**CVs, and the **p**ineal gland **(25-4)**. Lesions of the fornix, VI, and ICVs will displace the pineal gland inferiorly. Lesions that arise from the tectal plate displace the pineal gland anteriorly and

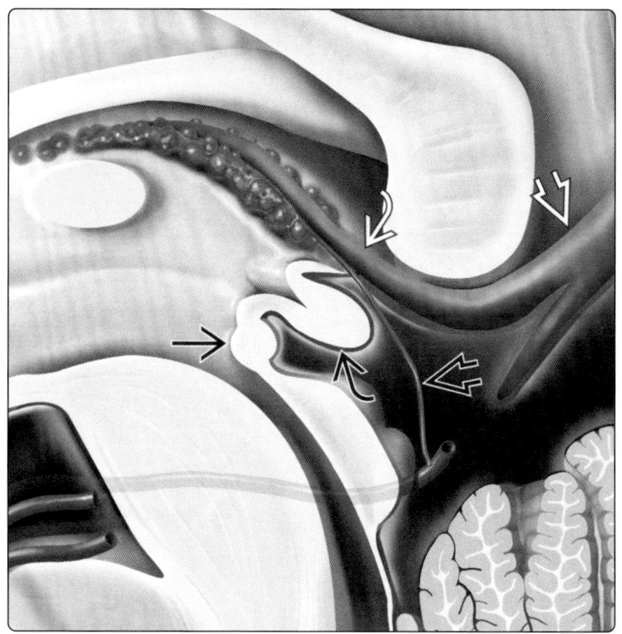

***(25-3) Sagittal graphic shows the pineal gland ➲ and posterior commissure ➲. The medial posterior choroidal artery ➲ from the PCA, P2 segment, provides the main vascular supply to the pineal gland. Vein of Galen ➲ and ICVs ➲.***

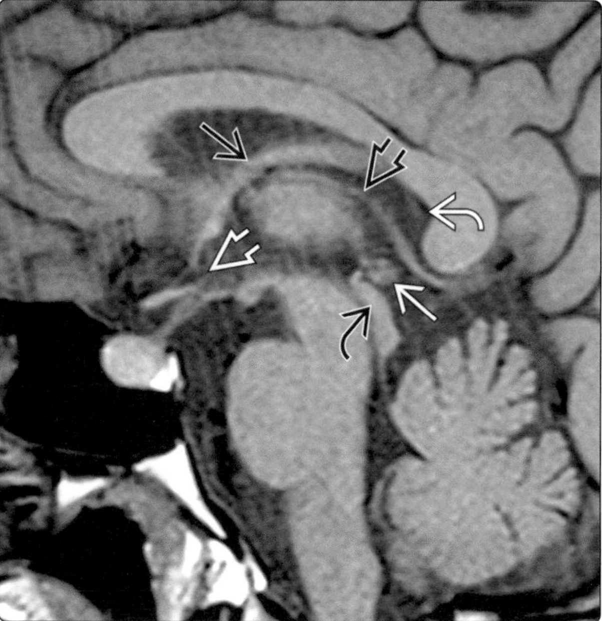

***(25-4) Sagittal T1 shows the pineal gland ➲ along posterior 3rd ventricle, below ICV ➲ and velum interpositum ➲, above superior colliculus ➲. The optic and infundibular recesses ➲ of the 3rd ventricle and fornix ➲ are seen.***

superiorly, while lesions of the third ventricle displace it posteriorly.

# Germ Cell Tumors

## Overview of Germ Cell Tumors

The most common pineal gland neoplasms are germ cell tumors (GCTs), accounting for ~ 40% of pineal neoplasm. GCTs are divided into two basic groups, **germinomas** and **nongerminomatous GCTs** (NGGCTs). CNS GCTs account for 2-3% of all primary intracranial neoplasms and 3-8% of pediatric brain neoplasms.

Germinomas represent ~ 2/3 of all GCTs. 1/3 are NGGCTs. NGGCTs include both teratomas and a heterogeneous group of miscellaneous nongerminomatous malignant germ cell neoplasms. According to the 2021 WHO classification of CNS tumors, NGGCT types are mature teratoma, immature teratoma, teratoma with somatic-type malignancy, embryonal carcinoma, yolk sac tumor, choriocarcinoma, and mixed GCTs.

## Germinoma

### Etiology

The normal mature pineal gland does not contain germ cells. Once thought to arise from "aberrant migration" of primordial germ cell layers, recent studies show that activation of the MAPK &/or PI3K-AKT signaling pathway is the genetic driver of pure GCTs as well as NGGCTs.

### Pathology

**Location.** Although GCTs may arise in many intracranial locations, they have a distinct predilection for midline structures **(25-5) (25-6)**. Between 80-90% "hug" the midline, extending along the midline axis from the pineal gland to the suprasellar region **(25-6) (25-7) (25-9)**. 1/2-2/3 are found in the pineal region with the suprasellar region, the second most frequent location, accounting for 1/4-1/3 of germinomas.

Off-midline germinomas occur in only 5-10% of cases **(25-10A)**. The basal ganglia and thalami are the most common off-midline sites. Periventricular lesions are an uncommon presentation.

**Size and Number.** Pineal germinomas that do not invade the tectum or cause hydrocephalus can be as large as several centimeters at the time of initial diagnosis. Infundibular stalk germinomas may become symptomatic (usually causing central diabetes insipidus) before they can be detected on high-resolution, contrast-enhanced MRs. Therefore, in young patients with diabetes insipidus, follow-up MR is recommended.

Approximately 20% of intracranial germinomas are multiple. The most frequent combination is a pineal + a suprasellar ("bifocal" or "double midline") germinoma **(25-5)**.

**Gross Pathology.** Germinomas are generally solid masses that often infiltrate adjacent structures. Intratumoral cysts, small hemorrhagic foci, and CSF dissemination are common.

**Microscopic Features.** A biphasic pattern of neoplastic germinoma cells mixed with benign lymphocytes is typical **(25-8)**. Some tumors exhibit such a florid immune cell infiltrate that it can obscure the neoplastic elements. Mitotic activity is common and may even be conspicuous, but frank necrosis is rare.

## Clinical Issues

**Demographics.** Germinoma is the most common intracranial GCT and accounts for 1-2% of all primary brain tumors. More than 90% of patients are younger than 20 years of age at initial diagnosis. Peak presentation is 10-14 years. The M:F ratio for pineal germinoma is 10:1. Suprasellar germinomas have no sex predilection.

**Presentation.** Pineal germinomas typically present with headache and Parinaud syndrome (paralysis of upward gaze) related to compression or invasion of the tectal plate. Ataxia and precocious puberty have also been described. The most common presentation for suprasellar germinoma is central diabetes insipidus. Hypothalamic-pituitary dysfunction and visual symptoms may also be present.

CSF cytology is rarely positive for tumor cells. Elevated serum or CSF markers (α-fetoprotein, β-hCG) are rare in pure germinomas but common with mixed GCTs.

**Natural History.** CSF dissemination and invasion are common, but pure germinomas have a very favorable response to radiation therapy. The five-year survival for treated patients with pure germinoma is > 90%.

**Treatment Options.** Histologic documentation followed by radiation therapy is the standard first-line treatment, as germinomas are extremely radiosensitive. Adjuvant chemotherapy is reserved for disseminated or recurrent tumors.

## Imaging

**General Features.** CSF dissemination is common, so MR imaging of the entire neuraxis should be performed in patients with suspected germinoma. Caution: Some

*(25-5) Pineal germinoma is shown with CSF dissemination to the 3rd, lateral, and 4th ventricles. Germinomas are the most common germ cell tumors (GCTs) and often have CSF spread. Imaging of entire neuraxis prior to surgery is key! (25-6) NECT shows a hyperdense mass "engulfing" the pineal calcification, typical of germinoma, with associated hydrocephalus. Note the subtle CSF dissemination along the anterior 3rd ventricle.*

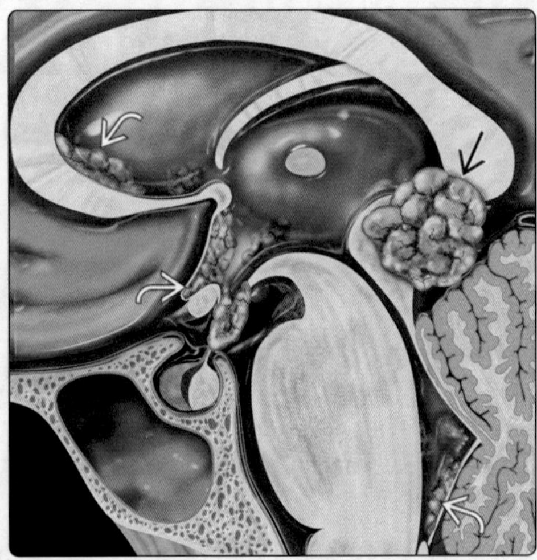

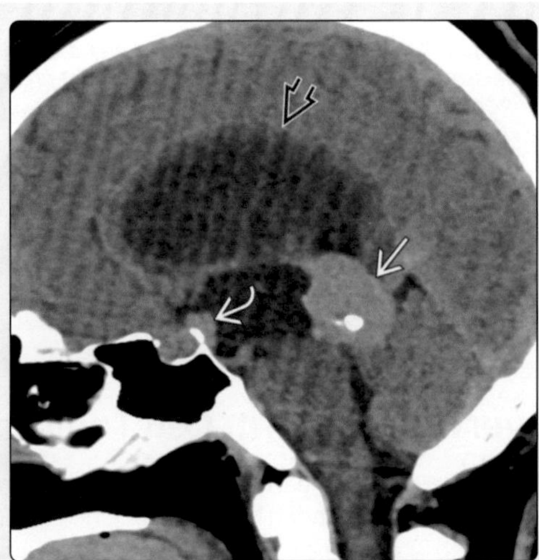

*(25-7A) Axial T2 MR in a 21-yo with headaches and Parinaud syndrome shows a homogeneous mass along the posterior 3rd ventricle with hydrocephalus. Small intraventricular air and blood products are related to recent ventriculostomy placement. (25-7B) Axial DTI trace image in the same patient shows hyperintensity (diffusion restriction) of the mass related to high cellularity, typical of germinoma.*

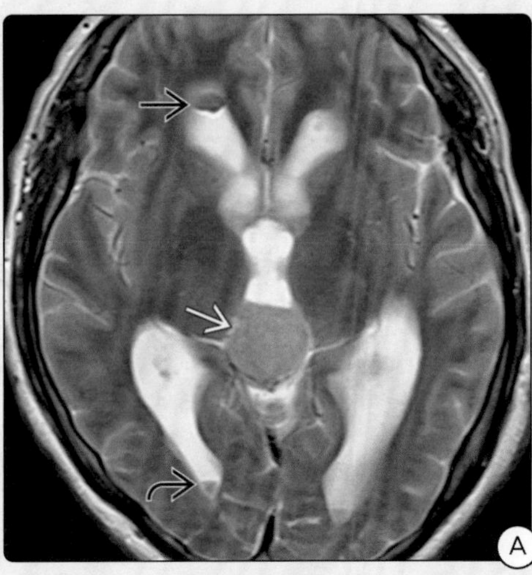


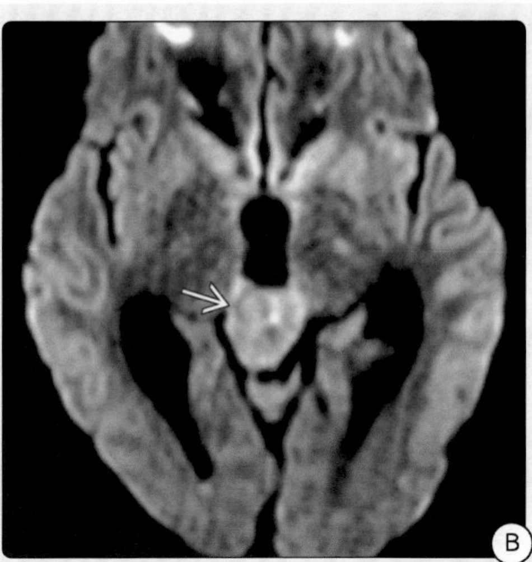

suprasellar germinomas may present with diabetes insipidus long before lesions are visible on MR. In such cases, serial imaging in 3-6 months should be performed.

**CT Findings.** Germinomas are typically hyperdense on NECT. Pineal calcifications can appear "engulfed" and surrounded by tumor **(25-6)**. Obstructive hydrocephalus is common. Strong uniform enhancement on CECT is typical.

**MR Findings.** Germinomas are iso- to slightly hyperintense to cortex on T1- and T2WI **(25-7A)**. Variably sized intratumoral cysts are common, especially in larger and "ectopic" lesions. Hemorrhage is generally uncommon except in basal ganglionic germinomas. T2* (GRE, SWI) may show "blooming" due to intratumoral calcification. Because of their high cellularity, germinomas may show restricted diffusion **(25-7B)**.

Enhancement is strong and usually homogeneous **(25-9)** **(25-11)**. Nearly 20% of germinomas are multiple, so look carefully for a second lesion in the suprasellar region (anterior third ventricle recesses, infundibular stalk) **(25-6)**! CSF spread is common, so imaging of the entire neuraxis prior to surgery is recommended.

"Inflammatory" germinomas may show extensive, nonenhancing peritumoral T2/FLAIR hyperintensity that extends into adjacent structures, such as the midbrain and thalami. In such cases, biopsies—especially small stereotaxic samples—may disclose only granulomatous reaction and be mistaken for tuberculosis or neurosarcoid.

## Differential Diagnosis

The major differential diagnosis of pineal germinoma is **mixed GCT** as well as **NGGCTs**. NGGCTs tend to be larger and more heterogeneous than germinomas. Bifocal lesions are almost always germinomas.

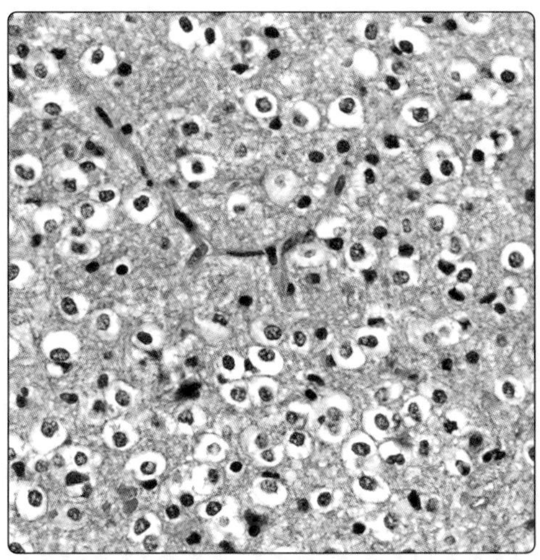

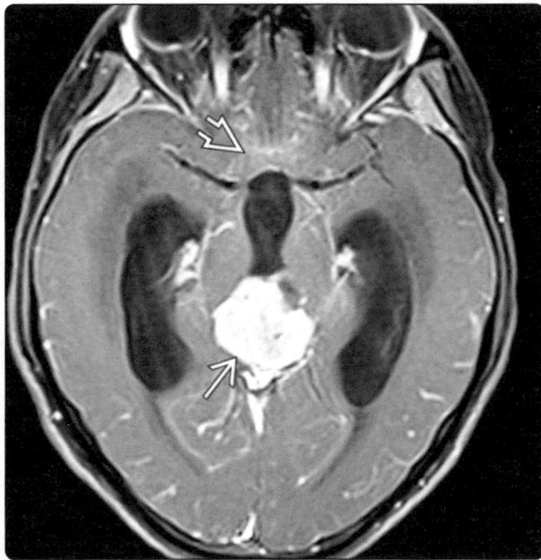

***(25-8)** Histologic image shows classic germinoma with large round cells with prominent nucleoli admixed with small lymphocytes. (Courtesy T. Tihan, MD.)* ***(25-9)** Axial T1 C+ FS MR shows an enhancing pineal mass ➔ and sulcal-cisternal enhancement ➔, suggesting CSF dissemination. Imaging the entire neuraxis is important, as CSF spread is common. Germinomas have a favorable response rate to radiation therapy.*

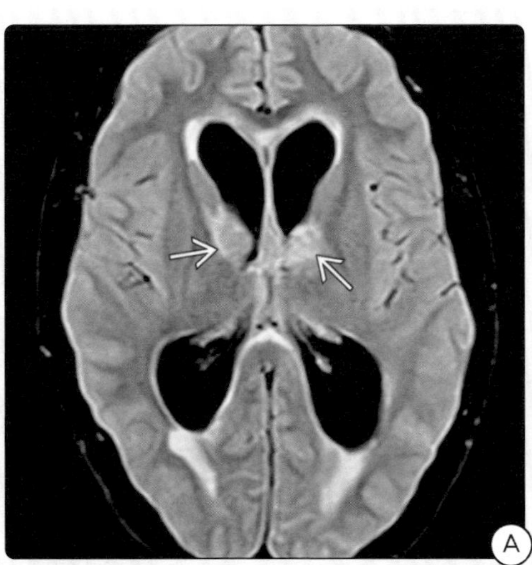


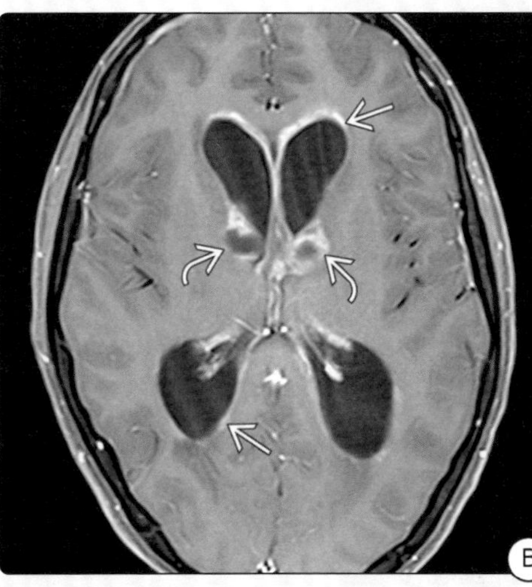


***(25-10A)** Axial FLAIR MR in an 18-yo with headaches shows bilateral anterior thalamic masses ➔ and acute hydrocephalus.* ***(25-10B)** Axial T1 C+ FS MR in the same patient shows enhancement along the ventricular margins ➔ related to subependymal tumor spread and enhancing masses along the thalami ➔. Germinomas typically involve the pineal or suprasellar regions but may present as basal ganglia, thalamic, or periventricular masses.*

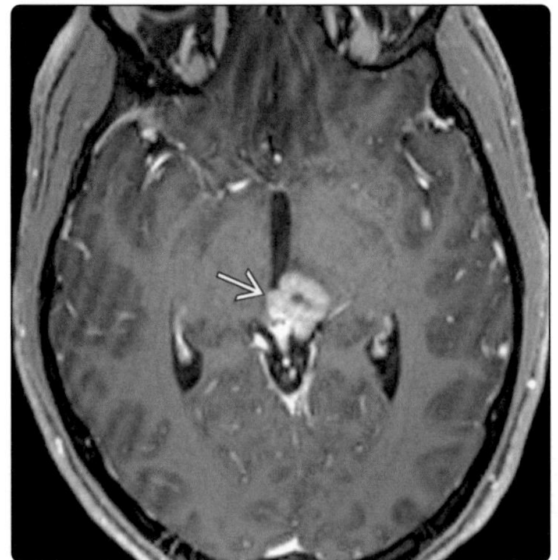

*(25-11) Axial T1 C+ FS MR shows a classic pineal germinoma ➡ with enhancement and mild mass effect on the posterior 3rd ventricle.*

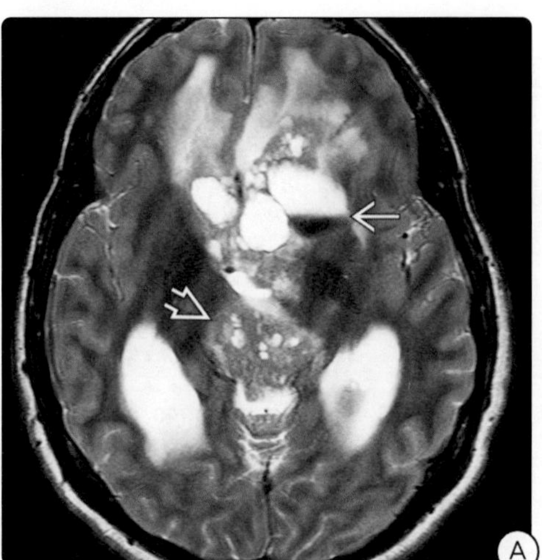

*(25-12A) Axial T2 MR in a 24-yo shows a heterogeneous pineal mass ➡, hydrocephalus, and frontal lobe cysts with blood-fluid levels ➡.*

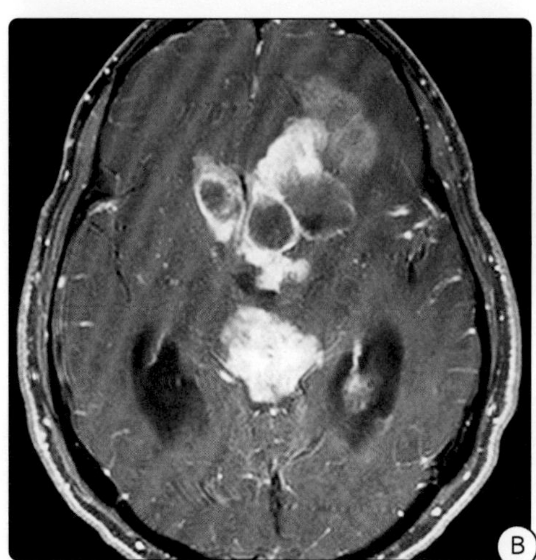

*(25-12B) Axial T1 C+ FS MR in the same patient shows intense enhancement of the pineal and frontal lobe masses. Germinoma at resection.*

Some **pineoblastomas** may appear similar to germinoma but "explode" rather than "engulf" pineal calcifications. **Pineal parenchymal tumor of intermediate differentiation** (PPTID) usually occurs in middle-aged and older adults.

The major differential diagnosis of suprasellar germinoma is **Langerhans cell histiocytosis** (LCH). Both are common in children, often cause diabetes insipidus, and may be indistinguishable on imaging studies alone. However, LCH does not produce oncoproteins. **Neurosarcoidosis** in an adult can cause a suprasellar mass that resembles germinoma.

### GERMINOMA: IMAGING AND DIFFERENTIAL DIAGNOSIS

**CT**

- NECT: Hyperdense, "engulfs" pineal calcifications
- CECT: Enhances strongly, uniformly

**MR**

- T1 iso-/hypointense, T2 iso-/hyperintense
- Inflammatory germinomas may have extensive peritumoral T2/FLAIR hyperintensity
- GRE may show calcification, hemorrhage
- Often restricts on DWI/DTI
- Enhances intensely, homogeneously
- CSF spread common (look for other lesions)
  - Anteroinferior 3rd ventricle, infundibular stalk
- Image entire neuraxis before surgery!

**Differential Diagnosis**

- Nongerminomatous germ cell tumor
- Pineal parenchymal tumors (pineoblastoma, pineal parenchymal tumor of intermediate differentiation)
- Histiocytosis (stalk lesion in child)
- Neurosarcoidosis (stalk lesion in adult)

## Teratoma

Teratomas are tridermic masses that originate from "misenfolded" or displaced embryonic stem cells. Teratomas recapitulate somatic development and differentiate along ectodermal, mesodermal, and endodermal cell types **(25-13)**.

There are three recognized types of teratoma. These range from a benign well-differentiated "mature" teratoma to an immature teratoma to a teratoma with somatic-type malignancy. All three share some imaging features, such as complex masses with striking heterogeneity in density &/or signal intensity. Cysts and hemorrhage are common.

Although they may originate anywhere in the body, teratomas are most commonly found in sacrococcygeal, gonadal, mediastinal, retroperitoneal, cervicofacial, and intracranial locations. Teratomas preferentially involve the midline; intracranial lesions most often arise in the pineal or suprasellar region.

Teratomas account for 2-4% of primary brain tumors in children and almost 1/2 of all congenital (perinatal) brain tumors. Teratomas are more common in Asian patients and male patients.

Imaging of mature teratomas shows a complex-appearing multiloculated lesion with fat, calcification, numerous cysts, and other tissues **(25-14)**. Hemorrhage is common. Enhancement is variable.

Immature teratomas contain a complex admixture of at least some fetal-type tissues from all three germ cell layers in combination with more mature tissue elements. It is common to have cartilage, bone, intestinal mucus, and smooth muscle intermixed with primitive neural ectodermal tissue. Hemorrhage and necrosis are common. CT or MR demonstrate almost complete replacement of brain tissue by a complex mixed-density or signal intensity mass.

Teratomas with somatic-type malignancy generally arise from immature teratomas and contain somatic-type cancers, such as sarcomas or carcinomas.

## Other Germ Cell Neoplasms

Germinomas are by far the most common of the germ cell neoplasms. Nongerminomatous malignant GCTs (NGMGCTs) are rare neoplasms that contain undifferentiated epithelial cells and are often mixed with other germ cell elements (most often germinoma). These include **yolk sac (formerly endodermal sinus) tumor, embryonal carcinoma, choriocarcinoma, and mixed GCT**.

NGMGCTs generally occur in adolescents with a peak incidence at 10-15 years of age. Prognosis is usually poor with overall survival of < 2 years.

Differentiating intracranial germ cell neoplasms on the basis of imaging studies alone is problematic. All intracranial GCTs—whether benign or malignant—tend to "hug" the midline.

Serum and CSF biomarkers can be helpful in the preoperative evaluation of a pineal mass. Embryonal carcinomas, immature teratomas, and yolk sac tumors can cause elevated α-fetoprotein. Choriocarcinomas and germinomas are associated with elevated β-hCG. Germinomas are also associated with elevated lactate dehydrogenase and placental alkaline phosphatase.

Many pineal neoplasms express different oncoproteins, so immunohistochemical profiling of biopsied tissue is an essential part of the diagnosis.

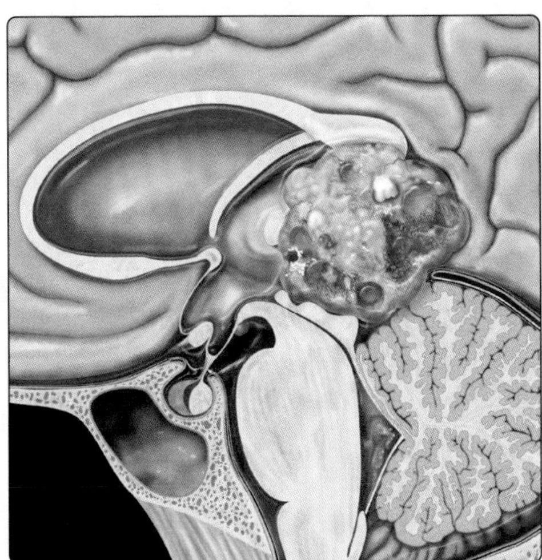

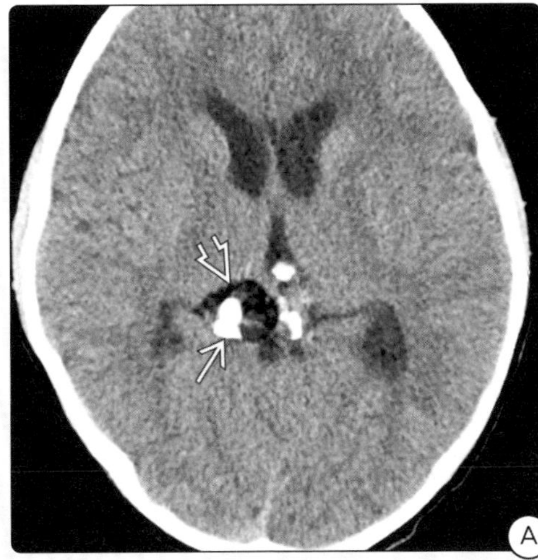


***(25-13)*** *Graphic showcases a pineal teratoma with the typical heterogeneous tissue components (cysts, solid tumor, calcifications, fat, etc.).* ***(25-14A)*** *Axial NECT in an 8-yo boy with headaches, nausea, and vomiting shows a very heterogeneous mass in the pineal region. Hypodense fat-attenuation tissue ➡ surrounds a densely calcified component ➡ that grossly resembles a tooth.*

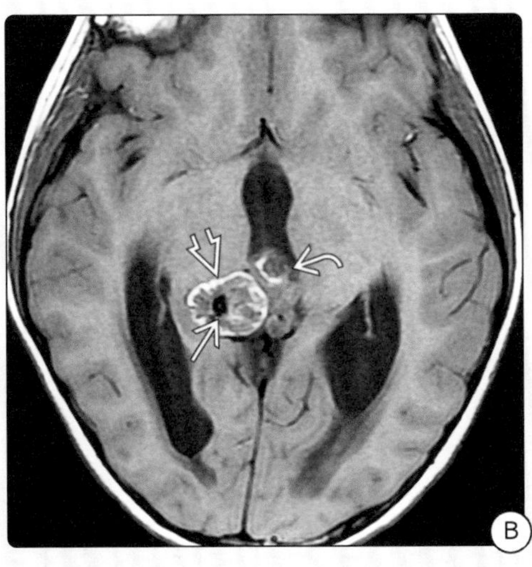


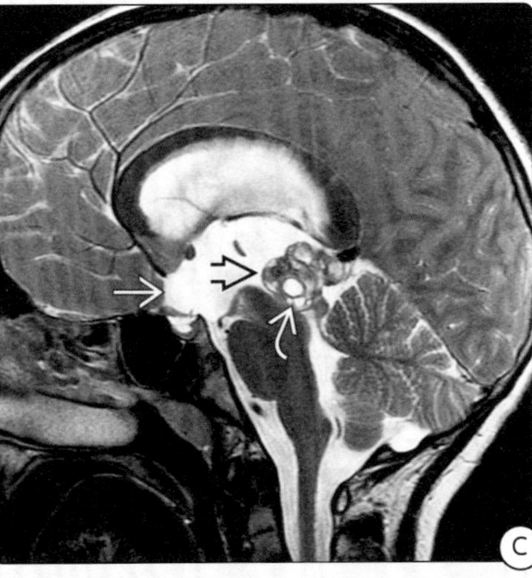


***(25-14B)*** *Axial T1 MR shows T1 shortening around the periphery of the mass ➡ consistent with fat. The internal signal void ➡ is caused by the densely calcified component. A lobulated mixed signal intensity component is present in the posterior 3rd ventricle ➡.* ***(25-14C)*** *Sagittal T2 MR shows that the heterogeneous-appearing mass ➡ also contains numerous cysts ➡. There is associated hydrocephalus with enlargement of the 3rd ➡ and lateral ventricles.*

Imaging of NGGCTs, including mixed GCTs, is nonspecific and may mimic the more common germinoma **(25-15)**. However, these GCTs may appear more heterogeneous with areas of calcification or cysts **(25-16)**. Choriocarcinomas have a tendency to hemorrhage.

# Pineal Parenchymal Tumors

**Pineal parenchymal tumors** (PPTs) are intrinsic primary tumors that arise from pinealocytes or their precursors. PPTs account for < 1% of all brain tumors but cause ~ 25-30% of pineal gland tumors.

Three grades are recognized: (1) **Pineocytoma** (WHO grade 1), (2) **PPTID** (WHO grades 2-3), and (3) **pineoblastoma** (WHO grade 4), the most malignant parenchymal cell tumors. The **papillary tumor of the pineal region** (PTPR) is a rare tumor that arises from the subcommissural organ. Lastly, the extremely rare desmoplastic myxoid tumor of the pineal region, *SMARCB1*-mutant, is a newly recognized tumor by the WHO classification of CNS tumors, 5th edition.

In the most recent epidemiologic studies, pineocytomas account for 20-25% of pineal parenchymal neoplasms (probably an underrepresentation, as many presumed cases are not resected or biopsied). PPTIDs represent nearly 45% of cases, and pineoblastomas account for ~ 35% of PPTs.

At present, the genetic alterations that drive PPTs are largely unknown, except for the subset of pineoblastomas that arise in patients with germline mutations in either *RB1* or as part of their eponymous tumor predisposition syndromes.

*(25-15A) Axial T2 MR in a 23-yo man shows a hyperintense pineal region mass ➡ with edema ➡ in the adjacent midbrain and hydrocephalus. (25-15B) Axial T1 C+ MR in the same patient shows avid enhancement ➡ of the mass. Imaging suggests a GCT or pineal parenchymal tumor. Yolk sac tumor was diagnosed at resection. Imaging of nongerminomatous GCTs is nonspecific and may resemble germinoma or have more heterogeneity.*

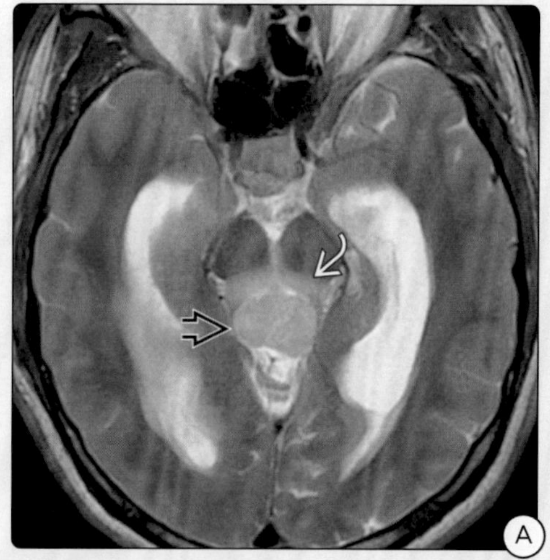


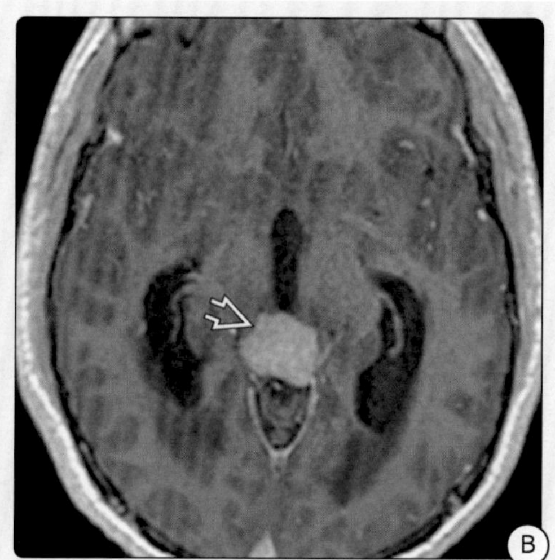


*(25-16A) Sagittal T2 MR in a 13-yo boy shows a heterogeneous pineal region mass ➡ with inferior displacement of the tectum ➡. (25-16B) Coronal T1 C+ MR in the same patient shows heterogeneous enhancement ➡ of the mass. A mixed GCT with both germinoma and teratomatous elements was diagnosed at resection.*

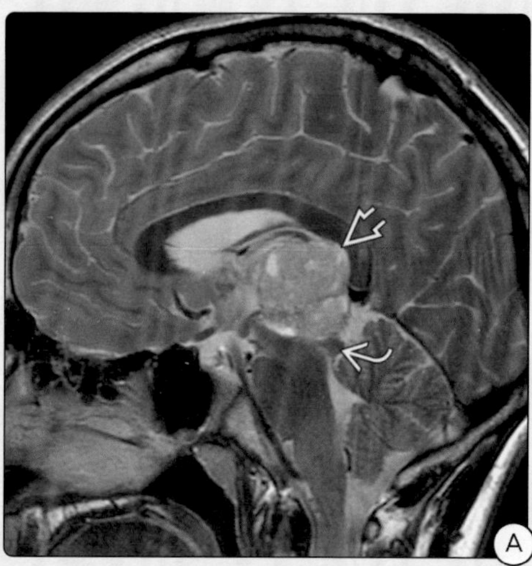


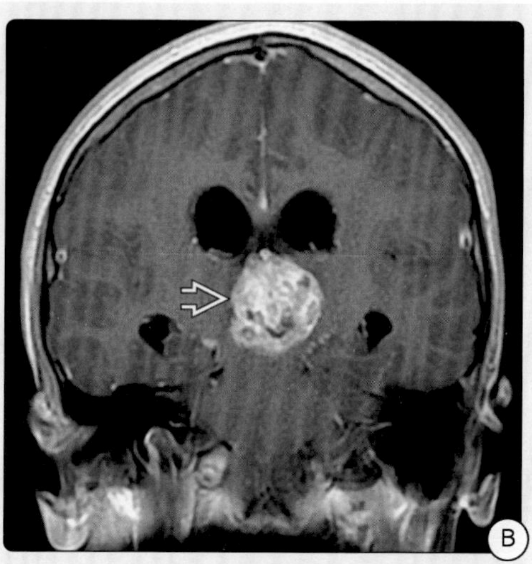

## Pineocytoma

These WHO grade 1 tumors may mimic benign pineal cysts or more aggressive PPTs. They are typically < 3 cm in size. In the most recent epidemiologic studies, pineocytomas account for ~ 20-25% of pineal parenchymal neoplasms.

### Pathology

Grossly, pineocytomas are well-circumscribed, round or lobular, gray-tan masses that are located behind the third ventricle and rarely invade adjacent structures. Although "giant" tumors have been reported, most are < 3 cm in diameter.

Pineocytomas are composed of small, uniform cells that resemble pinealocytes and are positive for both synaptophysin and neurofilament. Large "pineocytomatous rosettes" are the most characteristic feature. Mitoses are absent. Pineocytomas are designated as WHO grade 1 neoplasms. CSF dissemination has not been reported.

### Clinical Issues

Pineocytomas occur at all ages but are mostly tumors of adults. Mean age at diagnosis is 43 years. There is a slight female predominance (M:F = 0.6:1).

Many small pineocytomas are discovered incidentally on imaging studies. Larger lesions may compress adjacent structures or cause hydrocephalus. Headache and Parinaud syndrome (paralysis of upward gaze) are common in symptomatic patients.

Pineocytomas grow very slowly and often remain stable in size over many years. "Watchful waiting" is common with small lesions. Imaging is usually obtained only if the patient's symptoms change. Complete surgical resection is generally curative without recurrence or metastatic tumor spread.

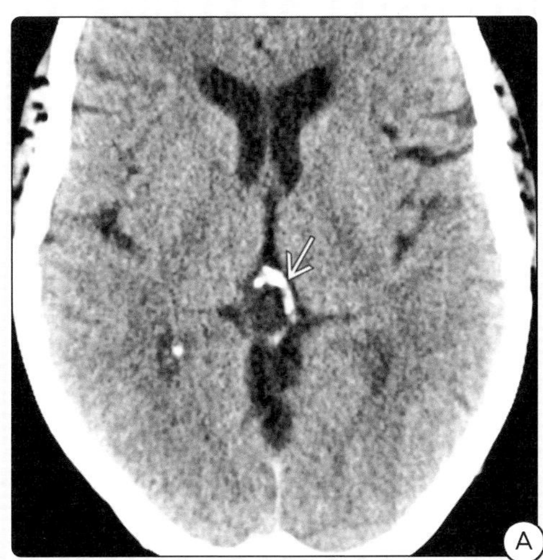


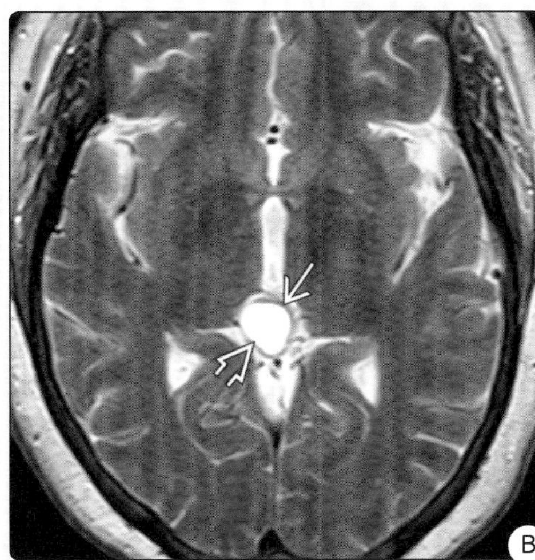


*(25-17A) NECT shows the typical findings of pineocytoma. The cystic-appearing pineal mass "explodes" calcifications toward the periphery of the lesion ➡. (25-17B) T2 MR in the same patient shows a cyst ➡ surrounded by a thin rim of solid tissue ➡. Note small size and lack of mass effect on the adjacent structures, typical of pineocytoma or pineal cyst.*

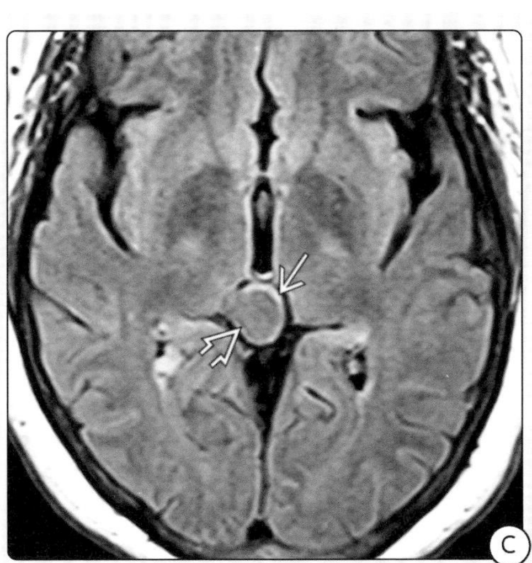


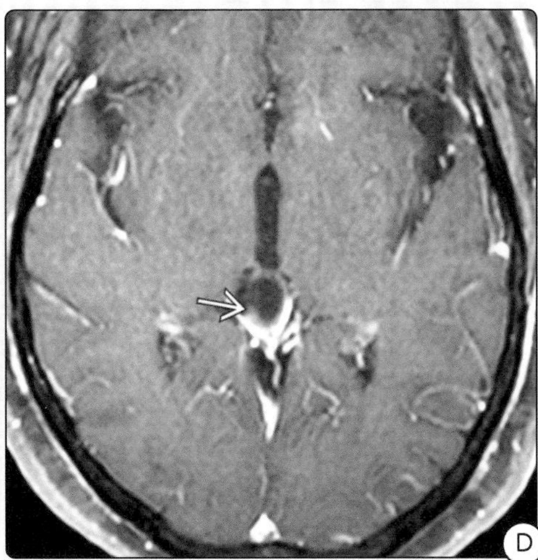


*(25-17C) FLAIR MR shows that the cyst wall ➡ is mildly hyperintense and that the cyst fluid ➡ does not suppress. (25-17D) T1 C+ FS MR demonstrates that the cyst wall enhances ➡. Imaging mimics a benign pineal cyst. These lesions may be followed conservatively or surgically resected. This is pathologically proven pineocytoma, WHO grade 1.*

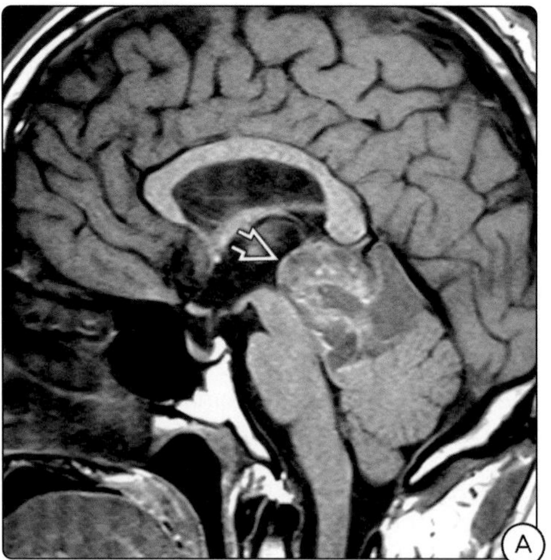

***(25-18A) Sagittal T1 MR in a 39-yo with headaches shows a large, heterogeneous pineal mass ➡ with areas of T1 hyperintensity.***

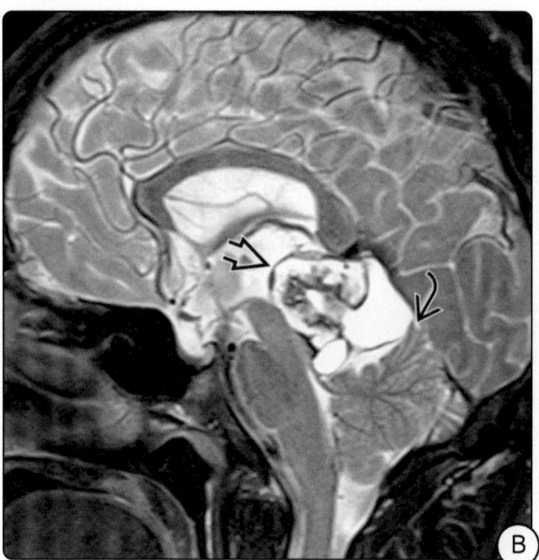

***(25-18B) Sagittal T2 MR in the same patient shows cystic and solid components within the mass ➡, inferior displacement of cerebellum ↷.***

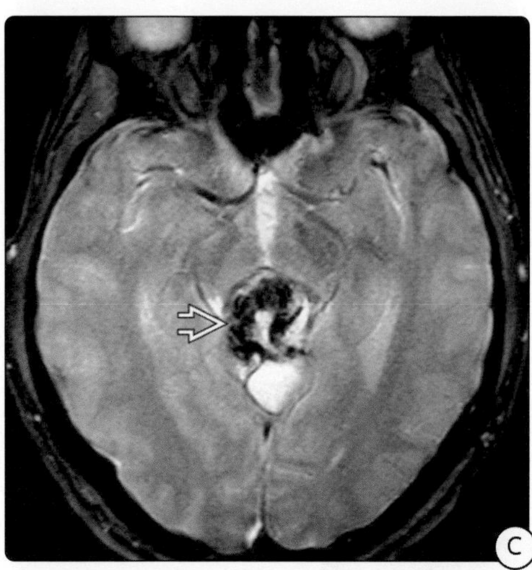

***(25-18C) Axial GRE in the same patient shows "blooming" related to blood products ➡ in the mass. PPTID grade 2 at resection.***

## Imaging

Pineocytomas are globular, well-delineated masses that are mixed iso- to hypodense on NECT scans. Calcifications typically appear "exploded" toward the periphery of the pineal gland **(25-17A)**.

Pineocytomas are well-demarcated, round or lobular masses that are iso- to hypointense on T1WI and hyperintense on T2WI and FLAIR **(25-17B)** **(25-17C)**. T2* GRE may show "blooming" foci secondary to calcification or hemorrhage. Pineocytomas typically enhance avidly with solid, rim, or even nodular patterns **(25-17D)**.

## Differential Diagnosis

The major differential diagnosis of pineocytoma is a benign, nonneoplastic **pineal cyst**. Pineal cysts may be indistinguishable from pineocytomas on imaging studies.

**Germinoma** typically "engulfs" rather than "explodes" the pineal calcifications, is most common in male adolescents, and enhances intensely and uniformly. **PPTID** is a tumor of middle-aged and older patients. The imaging appearance of PPTIDs is more "aggressive" than that of pineocytoma.

### PINEOCYTOMA

**Pathology**
- Most are 1-3 cm
- Well demarcated, round/lobulated
- WHO grade 1

**Clinical Issues**
- Adults (mean = 40 years)
- Grows very slowly, often stable for years

**Imaging**
- CT
  - Mixed iso-/hypodense
  - Pineal calcifications "exploded"
- MR
  - Iso-/hypointense on T1, hyperintense on T2
  - Cysts common, may hemorrhage
  - Variable enhancement (solid, rim, nodular)

**Differential Diagnosis**
- Benign pineal cyst (may be indistinguishable)
- Germinoma ("engulfs" calcifications; male adolescents)
- Pineal parenchymal tumor of intermediate differentiation (more aggressive-looking)

# Pineal Parenchymal Tumor of Intermediate Differentiation

Pineal parenchymal tumor of intermediate differentiation (PPTID) is intermediate in malignancy between pineocytoma and pineoblastoma. PPTID supersedes the terms "atypical" or "aggressive" pineocytoma.

## Pathology

Grossly, PPTID is a large, heterogeneous mass with peripheral calcification and variable cystic changes. Microscopically, PPTIDs are moderate to highly cellular tumors that exhibit dense lobular architecture. Two morphologic subtypes, small cell and large cell, have been recently described.

PPTIDs can be either WHO grade 2 or 3, although definite histologic grading criteria remain to be defined.

## Clinical Issues

PPTIDs are the most common PPT, representing ~ 45% of all cases. PPTIDs can occur at any age but are typically tumors of middle-aged adults. The medial patient age is 33 years.

Diplopia, Parinaud syndrome, and headache are the most common presenting symptoms. Biologic behavior is variable, and clinical progression can be seen in both grades 2 and 3 PPTIDs. Tumors tend to enlarge slowly and recur locally, although CSF dissemination may occur. Malignant degeneration into pineoblastoma has been reported in a few cases.

No serum or CSF biomarkers are currently available that inform the diagnosis or treatment of PPTIDs.

## Imaging

PPTIDs have a more "aggressive" imaging appearance than pineocytoma **(25-18)**. Extension into adjacent structures (e.g., the ventricles and thalami) is common. Size varies from < 1 cm to large masses that are 4-6 cm in diameter. CSF dissemination is uncommon but does occur, so imaging evaluation of the entire neuraxis should be performed prior to surgical intervention.

NECT scans show a heterogeneous mass centered in the pineal region that often have calcification "exploded" toward the periphery of the pineal gland **(25-19A)**. PPTIDs generally enhance strongly and uniformly.

PPTIDs are mixed iso- and hypointense on T1WI, isointense with gray matter on T2WI, and hyperintense on FLAIR. T2*

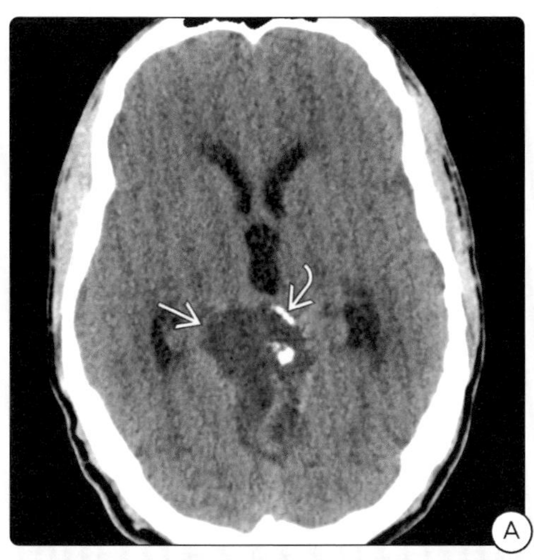


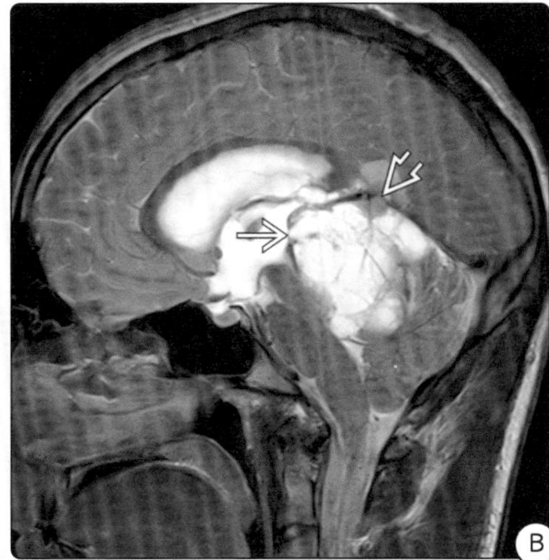


***(25-19A)** Axial CT in a 21-yo man with headaches and Parinaud syndrome shows a large, cystic pineal mass ➡ with areas of peripheral and central calcification ➡. Pineal parenchymal tumors classically "explode" the calcification. **(25-19B)** Sagittal T2 MR in the same patient shows a heterogeneous mass with large cysts ➡ and solid components ➡ centered in pineal region. There is associated hydrocephalus and mass effect on the tectum.*

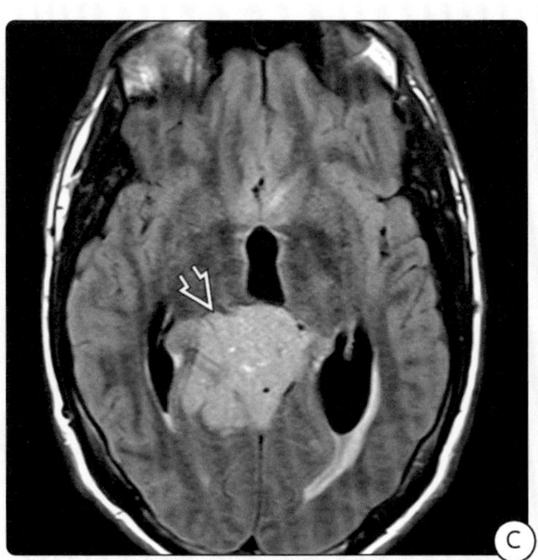


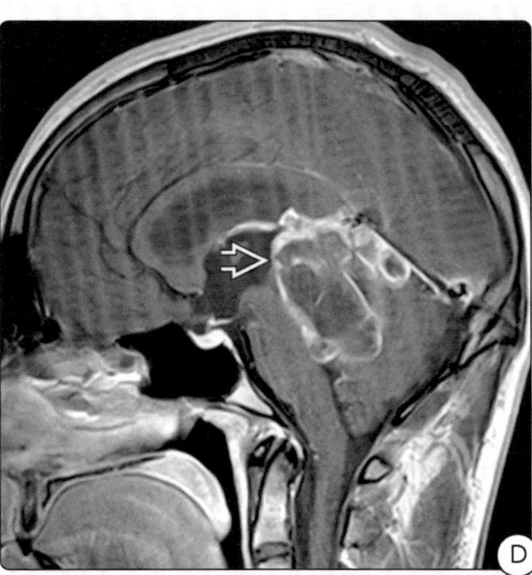


***(25-19C)** Axial FLAIR MR in the same patient shows a mildly heterogeneously hyperintense mass ➡ with hydrocephalus. **(25-19D)** Sagittal T1 C+ shows avid enhancement ➡ of the heterogeneous pineal mass. PPTID was found at resection. These tumors may be WHO grade 2 or 3 and represent the majority of pineal parenchymal tumors. There may be local invasion CSF dissemination of these tumors.*

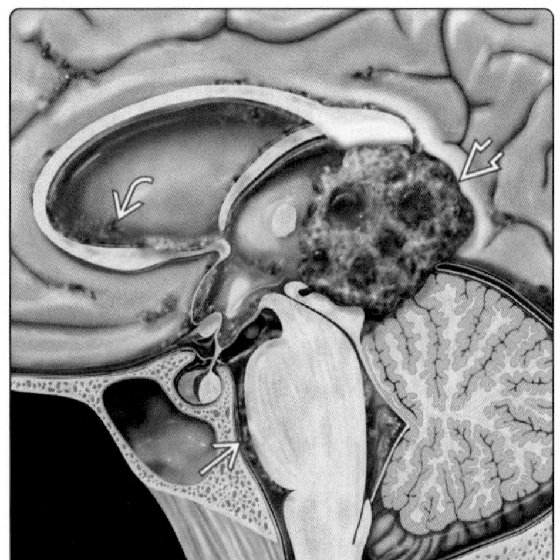

***(25-20)** Sagittal graphic depicts pineoblastoma ➡ with CSF dissemination into the ventricles and ➡ subarachnoid spaces ➡.*

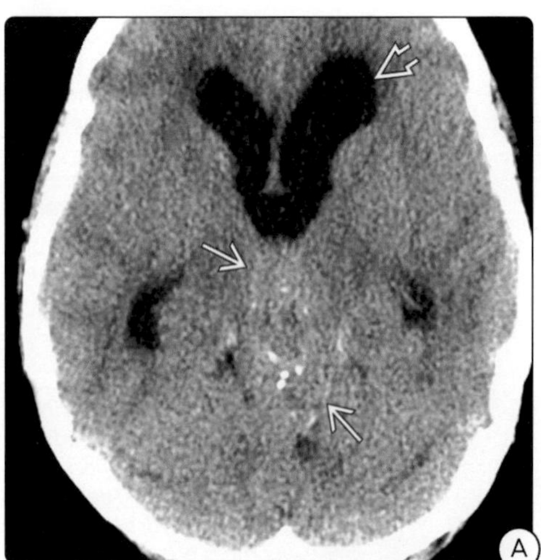

***(25-21A)** NECT of pineoblastoma shows a large, ill-defined, slightly hyperdense pineal region mass ➡ causing obstructive hydrocephalus ➡.*

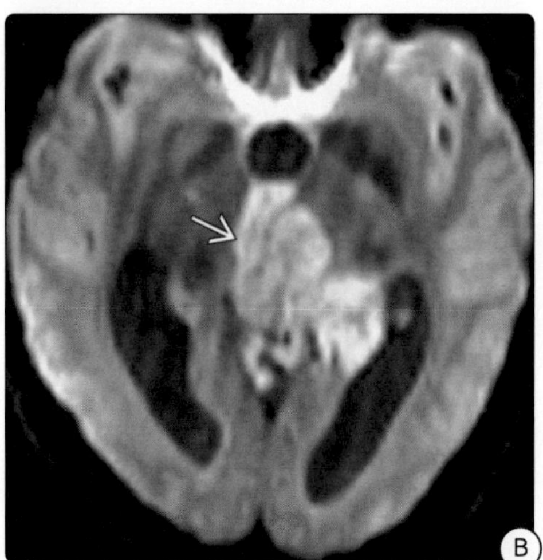

***(25-21B)** DWI in the same patient shows diffusion restriction ➡ related to high cellularity. This is pineoblastoma, WHO grade 4.*

(GRE, SWI) scans may show hypointense "blooming" foci **(25-18)**. Enhancement is generally strong but heterogeneous on T1 C+ **(25-18)** **(25-19)**.

## Differential Diagnosis

The major differential diagnosis of PPTID is **pineocytoma**. A more aggressive-appearing pineal mass in a middle-aged or older adult is most consistent with PPTID. **Pineoblastoma** is typically a tumor of younger patients but may occur at all ages. **Germinoma** is more common in male adolescents. **PTPR** can appear identical on imaging studies but is very rare.

### PINEAL PARENCHYMAL TUMOR OF INTERMEDIATE DIFFERENTIATION

**Pathology**
- 45% of pineal parenchymal tumors
- WHO grade 2 or 3

**Clinical Issues**
- Middle-aged adults

**Imaging**
- Appears more "aggressive" than pineocytoma
- Usually larger, more heterogeneous
- May disseminate via CSF

**Differential Diagnosis**
- Pineocytoma
- Pineoblastoma
- Germinoma

# Pineoblastoma

Pineoblastomas are the most primitive and biologically aggressive of all PPTs. They are poorly differentiated cellular embryonal tumors arising in the pineal parenchyma.

Pineoblastomas now have molecular profiling that may provide important prognostic information. There are four subtypes that have distinct clinical and molecular features: (1) **Pineoblastoma, miRNA processing altered_1** arises in children and is characterized by mutations of *DICER1*, *DROSHA*, or *DGCR8* and has an intermediate overall five-year survival of 67.5%; (2) **pineoblastoma, miRNA processing altered_2** arises in older children and is characterized by mutations of *DICER1*, *DROSHA*, or *DGCR8* and has an excellent overall five-year survival of 100%; (3) **pineoblastoma,** ***MYC/FOXR2*-activated** arises in infants and is characterized by *MYC* alteration and *FOXR2* overexpression and has a very poor prognosis with overall five-year survival of 20.5%; (4) **pineoblastoma,** ***RB1*-altered** arises in infants and has a very poor prognosis.

Pineoblastomas also occur in patients with familial (bilateral) retinoblastoma (the so-called trilateral retinoblastoma syndrome), and cases have been reported in familial adenomatous polyposis. Patients with **DICER1 syndrome** are at increased risk for developing pineoblastomas.

## Pathology

Grossly, a soft, friable, diffusely infiltrating tumor that invades adjacent brain and obstructs the cerebral aqueduct is typical. Necrosis and intratumoral hemorrhage are common, as is CSF dissemination with sheet-like coating of the brain and spinal cord **(25-20)**.

Microscopically, pineoblastomas are poorly differentiated, highly malignant tumors consisting of undifferentiated small round blue cells with hyperchromatic nuclei that exhibit a high nuclear:cytoplasmic ratio. Pineoblastomas are WHO grade 4 neoplasms.

## Clinical Issues

**Epidemiology.** Pineoblastomas account for 0.5-1.0% of primary brain tumors, 15% of pineal region neoplasms, and 30-35% of pineal parenchymal tumors. They can occur at any age, including adults, but pineoblastomas are decidedly more prevalent in children. The mean age at diagnosis in children is three years.

**Presentation and Natural History.** Symptoms of elevated intracranial pressure, such as headache, nausea, and vomiting, are typical. Parinaud syndrome is common.

Surgical debulking with adjuvant chemotherapy and craniospinal radiation compose the typical regimen. Prognosis is poor with a median survival of 16-25 months. CSF dissemination is frequent and the most common cause of death. Extracranial metastases are very rare.

## Imaging

Pineoblastomas are large, bulky, aggressive-looking pineal region masses that invade adjacent brain and usually cause obstructive hydrocephalus. CSF dissemination is common, so the entire neuraxis should be imaged prior to surgical intervention.

NECTs show a large, hyperdense, inhomogeneously enhancing mass with obstructive hydrocephalus **(25-21A)**. If pineal calcifications are present, they appear "exploded" toward the periphery of the tumor.

Pineoblastomas are heterogeneous tumors that frequently demonstrate necrosis and intratumoral hemorrhage on MR. They are usually mixed iso- to hypointense compared with brain on T1WI and mixed iso- to hyperintense on T2WI. They enhance strongly but heterogeneously **(25-22)**. Because they are densely cellular tumors, restriction on DWI is common **(25-21B)**.

## Differential Diagnosis

The major differential diagnosis of pineoblastoma is **PPTID**. Pineoblastomas tend to occur in children, and CSF dissemination at diagnosis is more common. **Germinoma** also frequently demonstrates CSF spread but is more common in adolescent and young adult males. **NGMGCTs** are a heterogeneous group of tumors that may be indistinguishable on imaging studies from pineoblastomas.

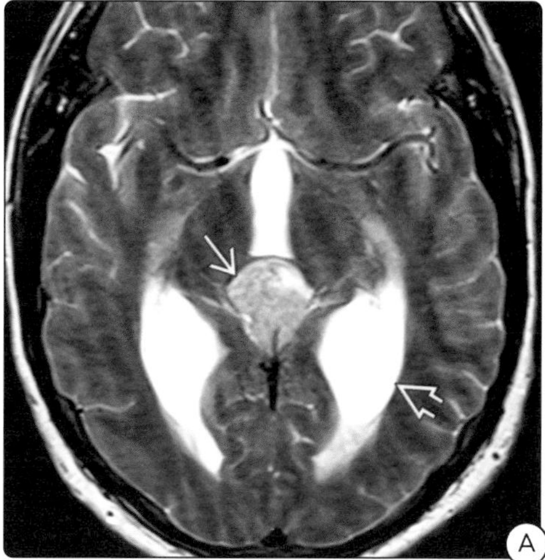

*(25-22A) T2 MR in 43-yo with headache, nausea, vomiting for 11 days shows hyperintense pineal mass ➡, acute obstructive hydrocephalus ➡.*

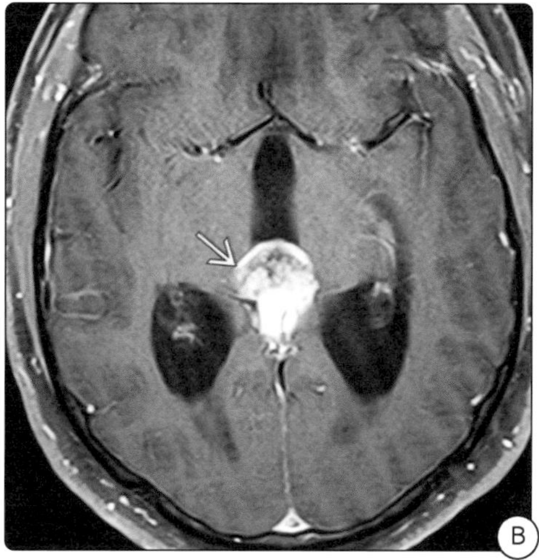

*(25-22B) T1 C+ FS MR shows mass ➡ enhancing intensely, heterogeneously with no evidence for CSF spread. Imaging diagnosis was PPTID.*

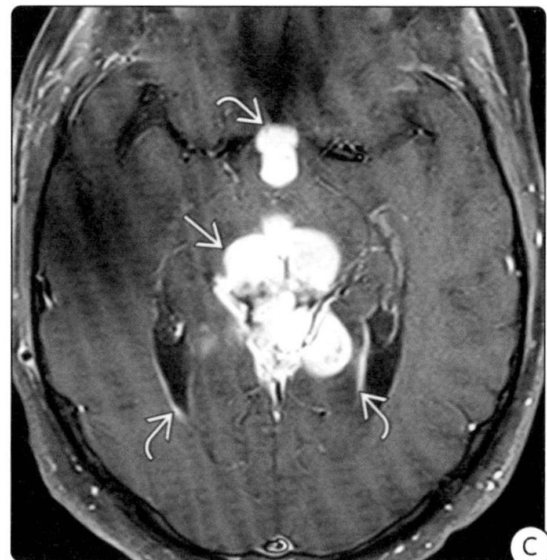

*(25-22C) T1 C+ FS MR 5 weeks later shows mass ➡ has increased significantly, and there is CSF dissemination ➡. Pineoblastoma, WHO grade 4.*

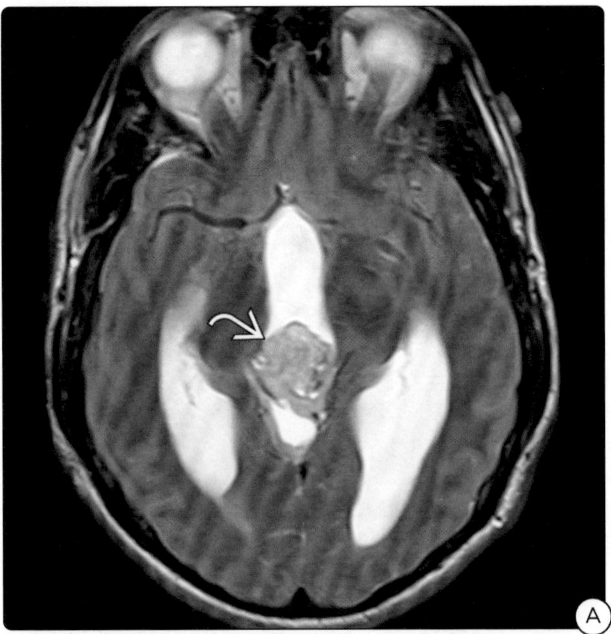

***(25-23A)** Axial T2 MR in a 40-yo with severe headaches shows a heterogeneous, hyperintense ➡ mass along the posterior 3rd ventricle with hydrocephalus. Pineoblastomas occur at all ages but most commonly in patients < 10 yo.*

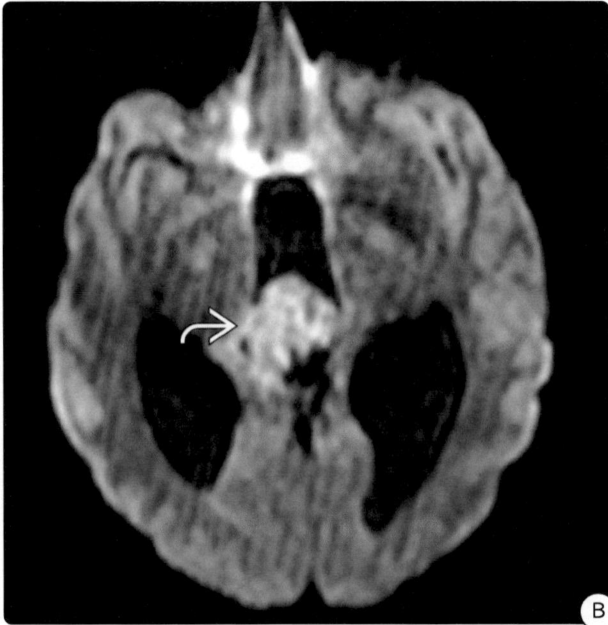

***(25-23B)** Axial DWI trace image in the same patient shows hyperintensity ➡ related to high cellularity of the tumor. CSF spread is common in these WHO grade 4 tumors.*

### PINEOBLASTOMA

**Pathology**
- Most primitive, malignant of all pineal parenchymal tumors
- Diffusely infiltrates adjacent structures
- Early, widespread CSF dissemination common
- WHO grade 4
- 4 subtypes with molecular profiles: Some with *RB1*, *DICER1* mutations
  - Pineoblastoma, miRNA processing altered_1
  - Pineoblastoma, miRNA processing altered_2
  - Pineoblastoma, *MYC/FOXR2*-activated
  - Pineoblastoma, *RB1*-altered

**Clinical Issues**
- 15% of pineal region tumors
- 30-35% of pineal parenchymal tumors
- All ages but primarily children (< 20 years old)
- Prognosis generally poor

**Imaging**
- CT
  - Heterogeneously hyperdense
  - Pineal calcifications "exploded"
- MR
  - Large, bulky, aggressive-looking
  - Necrosis, intratumoral hemorrhage common
  - Enhances strongly, heterogeneously
  - Restricts on DWI (densely cellular)
  - Look for CSF spread (image entire neuraxis)

## Papillary Tumor of the Pineal Region

Papillary tumors of the pineal region (PTPR) are neuroepithelial tumors with papillary and solid areas. They may be WHO grade 2 or 3. These tumors are rare and may occur in children and adults with a median age of 35 years.

### Clinical Issues

The clinical features are similar to other tumors of the pineal region. Patients often present with headaches, Parinaud syndrome, or diplopia. Hydrocephalus may be present in larger masses. There is no sex predilection for these tumors.

The clinical course of patients with PTPR is often complicated by local recurrence. CSF dissemination is rare in these tumors.

### Imaging

PTPR are well-circumscribed, heterogeneous masses with solid and cystic components **(25-24A)**. Aqueductal obstruction with hydrocephalus is common **(25-24B)**. Heterogeneous enhancement has been described **(25-24C)**. Imaging often mimics more common pineal region tumors. Recent reports suggest that proton MR spectroscopy may show extremely high myoinositol.

### Differential Diagnosis

The major differential diagnoses of PTPR are other pineal region neoplasms, including pineocytoma, PPTID, pineoblastoma, and GCTs.

# "Other Cell" Pineal and Pineal Region Neoplasms

## Miscellaneous Pineal Neoplasms

Rarely, tumors arising within the pineal gland are composed of neoplastic elements other than parenchymal or germ cells. Primary glial neoplasms, such as astrocytoma (including glioblastoma) and oligodendroglioma, can occur within the pineal gland itself as can melanoma arising from pineal melanocytes. Rosette-forming glioneuronal tumors are WHO grade 1 tumors that occur in the midline **(25-25)**. They may occur in the fourth ventricle, cerebellar vermis, pineal gland, or thalamus. They are slow growing and typically affect young adults. Metastases from extracranial sources also occasionally present as pineal masses **(25-26)**. Meningiomas may occur in the pineal region along the dura of the falx cerebri or tentorium cerebelli **(25-27)**.

In general, imaging findings with intrinsic pineal gland masses are nonspecific and often do not permit differentiation between the broad spectrum of histologic types. However, certain clinical and imaging features can help narrow down the differential diagnosis.

### APPROACH TO PINEAL MASSES

**Key Questions to Consider**

- Is mass in pineal gland or adjacent to it?
- What is patient's age, sex?
- Is there serum or CSF evidence for oncoproteins?
- Are additional lesions present?

**Pineal Gland Mass**

- Most common = benign, nonneoplastic cyst!
- Less common
  - Pineocytoma
  - Germinoma
  - Pineal parenchymal tumor of intermediate differentiation
- Rare but important
  - Pineoblastoma
  - Teratoma
  - Rare pineal tumors (e.g., papillary tumor of pineal region)
  - Rosette-forming glioneuronal tumor
  - Other (e.g., glioma, metastasis)

**Pineal Region Mass**

- Adjacent to, but not in, pineal gland
  - Arachnoid cyst
  - Dermoid or epidermoid cyst
  - Meningioma
  - Lipoma (quadrigeminal plate)
  - Astrocytoma (e.g., tectal glioma)
  - Metastasis
  - Aneurysm (basilar tip, PCA)
  - Vein of Galen malformation

*Selected References: The complete reference list is available on the eBooks+ version included with purchase.*

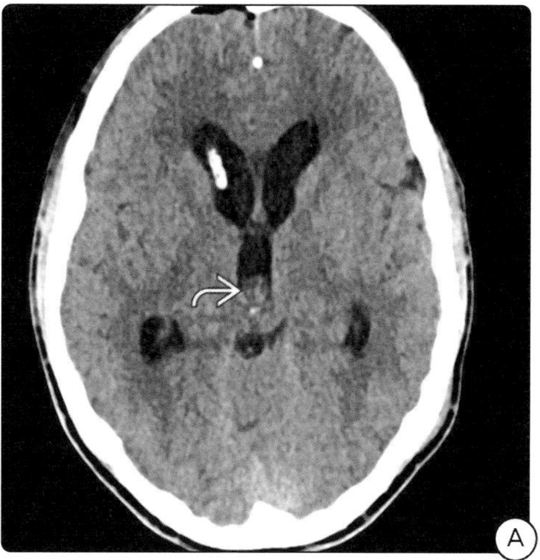


***(25-24A)** Axial CT in a 21-yo man with headaches shows a small mass in the pineal region ➡ along the posterior 3rd ventricle.*

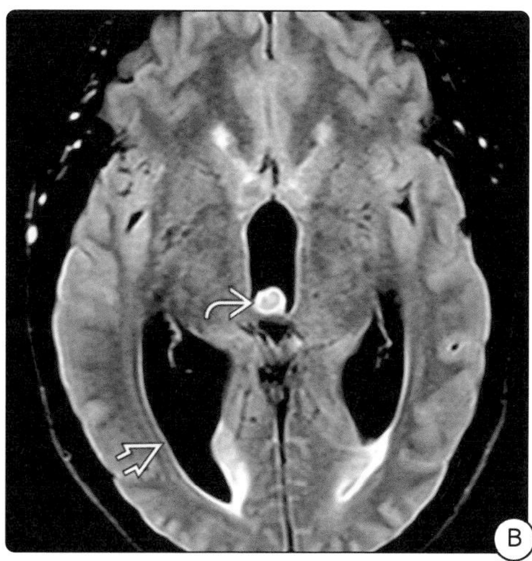


***(25-24B)** Axial FLAIR in the same patient shows the small mass ➡ along the posterior 3rd ventricle with associated hydrocephalus ➡.*

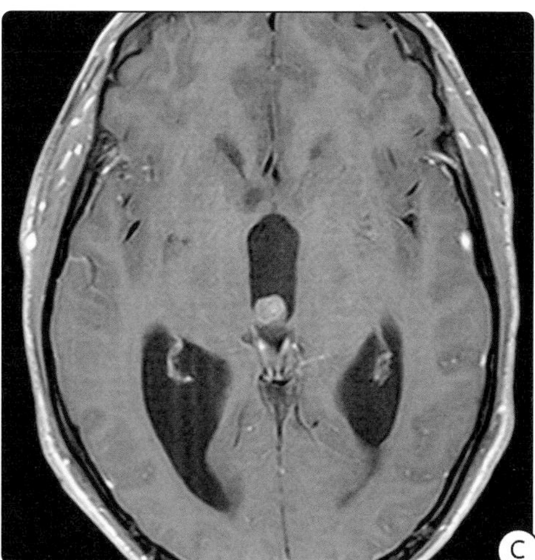


***(25-24C)** Axial T1 C+ MR shows enhancement of the mass. Differentials include GCTs and pineal parenchymal tumors. This was PTPR at resection.*

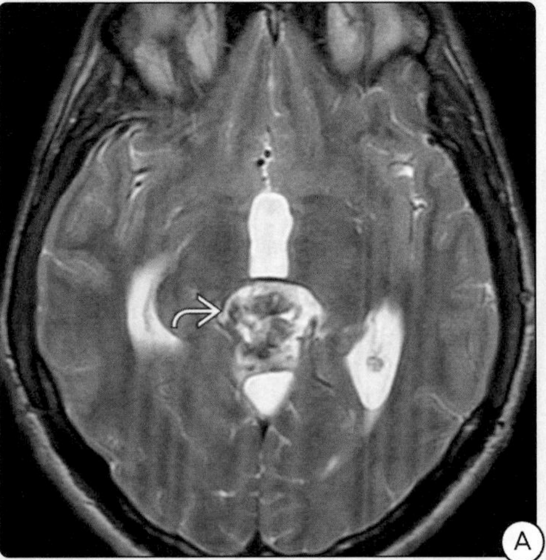
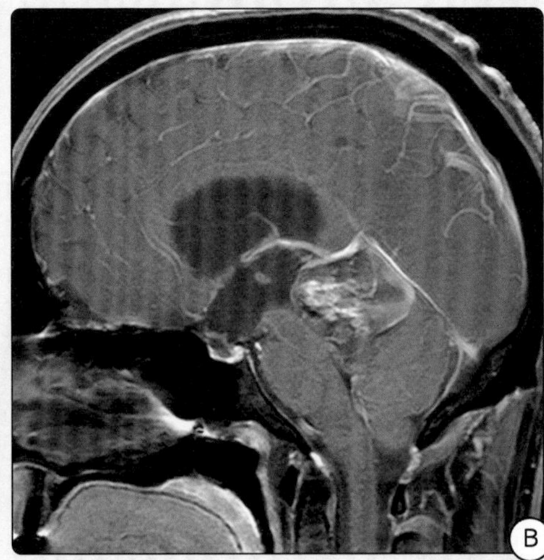

***(25-25A)*** *Axial T2 MR in a young adult with headaches shows heterogeneous pineal region mass ➡ along posterior 3rd ventricle. These tumors are often solid and cystic masses with variable calcification, hemorrhage.* ***(25-25B)*** *T1 C+ MR shows heterogenous enhancement of the mass. Rosette-forming glioneuronal tumors are rare, WHO grade 1, midline masses. They may occur in the 4th ventricle, cerebellar vermis, pineal gland, or thalamus.*

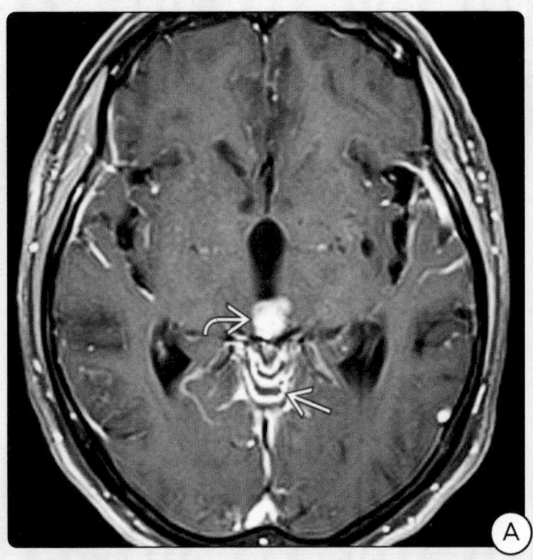
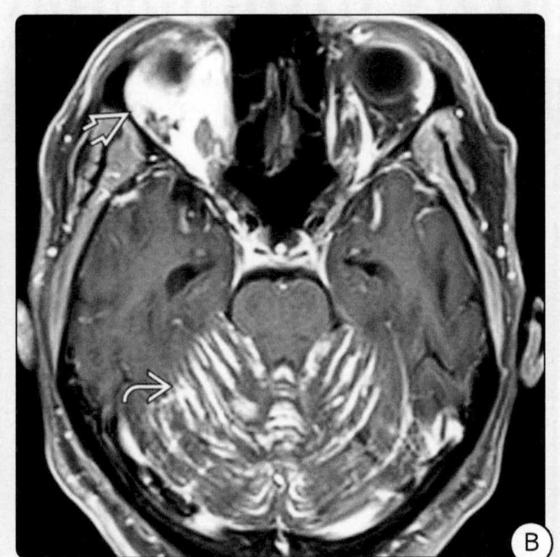

***(25-26A)*** *Axial T1 C+ MR in a woman with metastatic breast cancer, headaches, and Parinaud syndrome shows an avidly enhancing pineal region mass ➡ along the posterior 3rd ventricle. CSF dissemination of metastatic disease is noted in the folia ➡ of the superior cerebellar vermis.* ***(25-26B)*** *Axial T1 C+ MR shows extensive leptomeningeal enhancement in the cerebellar folia ➡. A right orbital metastatic lesion ➡ is also noted.*

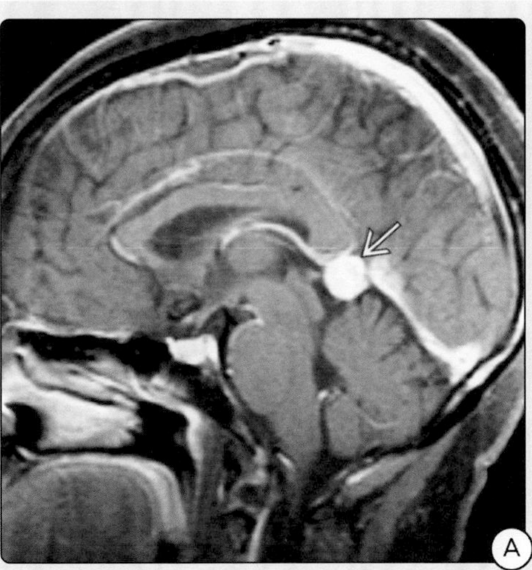
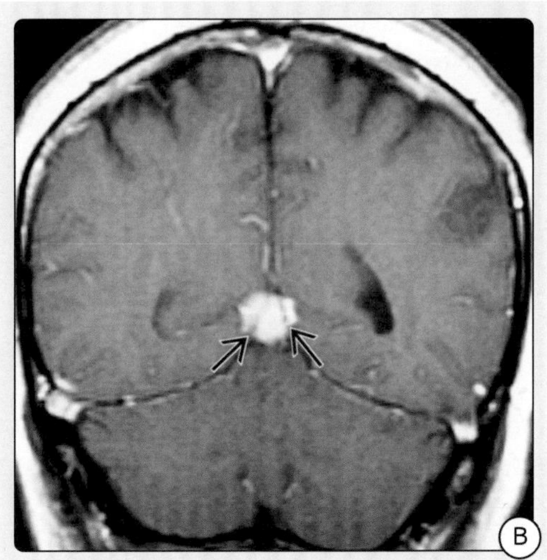

***(25-27A)*** *Sagittal T1 C+ MR shows a small, enhancing, dural-based mass in the pineal region ➡.* ***(25-27B)*** *Coronal T1 C+ MR shows the dural-based mass along the leaves of the tentorium cerebelli ➡. Meningiomas typically arise along the dura and may mimic a primary pineal parenchymal mass. These tumors are typically benign and may be treated conservatively or with surgery or radiation therapy.*

# Cranial Nerve Tumors

*Nerve sheath tumors occur throughout the CNS either sporadically (discussed here) or as part of tumor predisposition syndromes, such as neurofibromatosis types 1 and 2 (see Chapter 44).*



The 2021 WHO classification of CNS tumors made several changes in the way tumors of the cranial and paraspinal nerves are classified. The four basic categories of **schwannoma, neurofibroma, perineurioma**, and **malignant peripheral nerve sheath tumor** were retained. Newly recognized tumors include **hybrid nerve sheath tumor** and **malignant melanotic nerve sheath tumor**. Cauda equina "CNS paraganglioma" is now termed **cauda equina neuroendocrine tumor** and is considered biologically distinct from paragangliomas elsewhere in the body. Cauda equine neuroendocrine tumor is briefly discussed in this chapter even though it is an intradural-extramedullary spinal neoplasm.

With the exception of vestibular schwannoma (VS), all intracranial nerve sheath tumors are rare, and the vast majority are benign. The two major tumor types that are found intracranially and at or near the skull base are schwannomas and neurofibromas. Both are discussed here as are melanotic and malignant peripheral nerve sheath tumors. Intracranial hybrid nerve sheath tumors and perineuriomas are very rare and are not included in this chapter.

# Schwannomas

## Schwannoma Overview

### Terminology

Schwannomas are benign, slow-growing, encapsulated tumors of cranial and spinal nerves that are composed entirely of well-differentiated Schwann cells.

### Etiology

**General Concepts.** Schwannomas originate from Schwann cells, which are derived from the embryonic neural crest. Schwannomas may arise along the course of any peripheral nerve or cranial nerves (CNs) III-XII **(26-1)**. The olfactory and optic nerves do not contain Schwann cells so schwannomas do not arise from CNs I and II. "Olfactory groove schwannomas" are probably tumors that arise from olfactory ensheathing cells.

Schwann cells are also not a component of normal brain parenchyma. The exceptionally rare intraparenchymal schwannoma is thought to arise from neural crest remnants that later express aberrant Schwann cell differentiation.

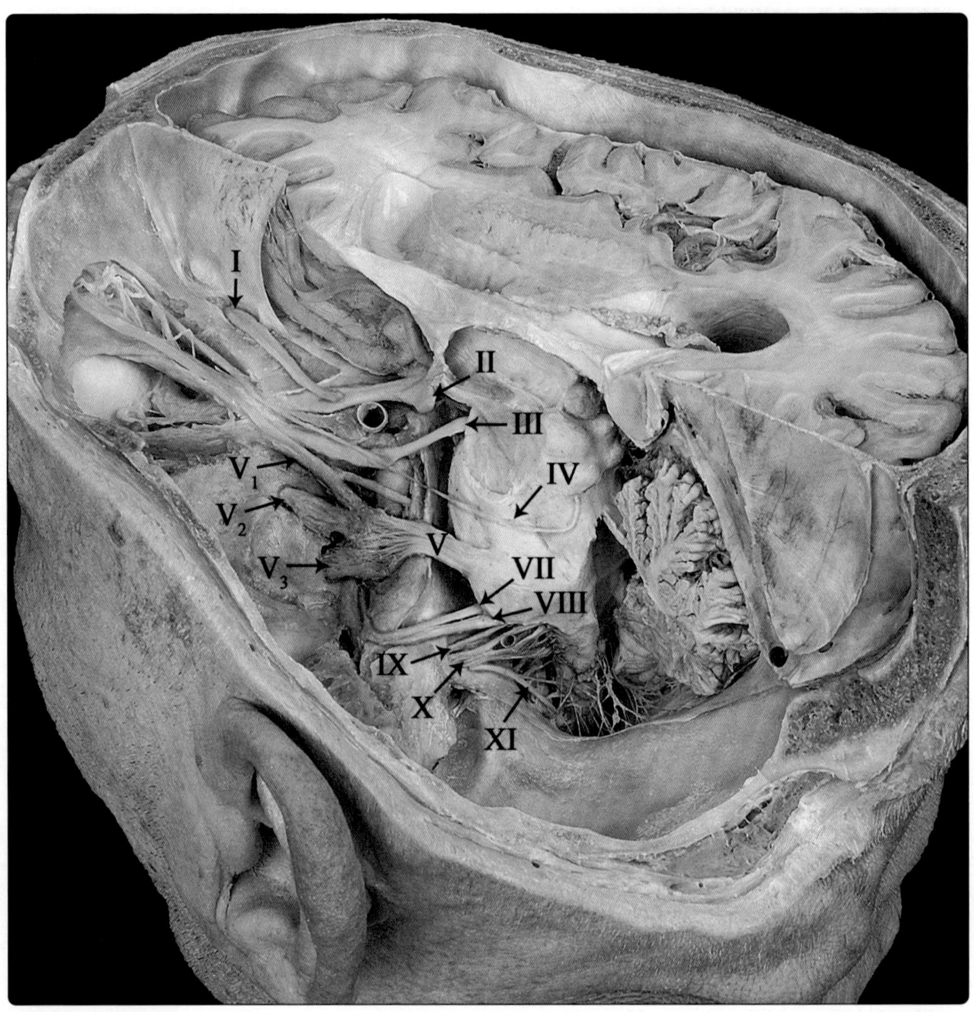


*(26-1) Olfactory nerve (I), optic chiasm (II), oculomotor nerve (III), trochlear nerve (IV) course anteriorly in the ambient cistern, and the trigeminal nerve (V) with its ophthalmic (V1), maxillary (V2), and mandibular (V3) branches are shown. Abducens (VI) and hypoglossal (XII) nerves are not visualized. Cerebellopontine angle (CPA) segments of the facial (VII) and vestibulocochlear (VIII) nerves are shown. Glossopharyngeal (IX), vagus (X), and spinal accessory (XI) nerves course toward the jugular foramen. (Courtesy M. Nielsen, MS.)*

**Genetics.** Inactivating mutations of the *NF2* gene are detected in 50-75% of sporadic schwannomas. The majority of VSs—the most common nerve sheath tumor—present sporadically without identification of germline pathogenic variants, although recent studies have identified a 9p21.3 hotspot associated with an increased risk of VS tumorigenesis.

Germline mutations of either the *SMARCB1* or *LZTR1* tumor suppressor gene are found in many patients with familial schwannomatosis (see Chapter 43).

## Pathology

**Location.** Schwannomas arise at the glial-Schwann cell junction of CNs III-XII **(26-1)**. The distance from the brain to the interface where the glial covering terminates and Schwann cell ensheathing begins varies with each CN. In some—such as the oculomotor nerve (CNIII)—the junction is in close proximity to the brain. Here, schwannomas arise close to the exit of the parent nerve from the brain. In others—such as the vestibulocochlear nerve (CNVIII)—the junction lies at some distance from the nerve exit or entrance into the brainstem.

Sensory nerves are much more commonly affected by schwannomas compared with pure motor CNs. The vestibulocochlear nerve is by far the most common intracranial site (90%). The second most common site is the trigeminal nerve (CNV) (2-4%). Schwannomas of CNs other than CNVIII and CNV (e.g., jugular foramen or hypoglossal tumors) are very rare, accounting for just 1-2% of cases.

**Size and Number.** Most intracranial schwannomas are small, globose tumors with nerve fascicles draped over the tumor capsule **(26-2)**. Some, especially trigeminal schwannomas, can attain huge size and involve both intra- and extracranial compartments.

Most schwannomas are "sporadic" or "solitary." The presence of multiple schwannomas in the same individual suggests an underlying tumor predisposition syndrome (see Chapter 43).

**Gross Pathology.** Schwannomas arise eccentrically from their parent nerves and are smooth or nodular well-encapsulated lesions **(26-3)**. Cystic change is common. Microhemorrhages occur, but gross macroscopic bleeds are rare **(26-4)**.

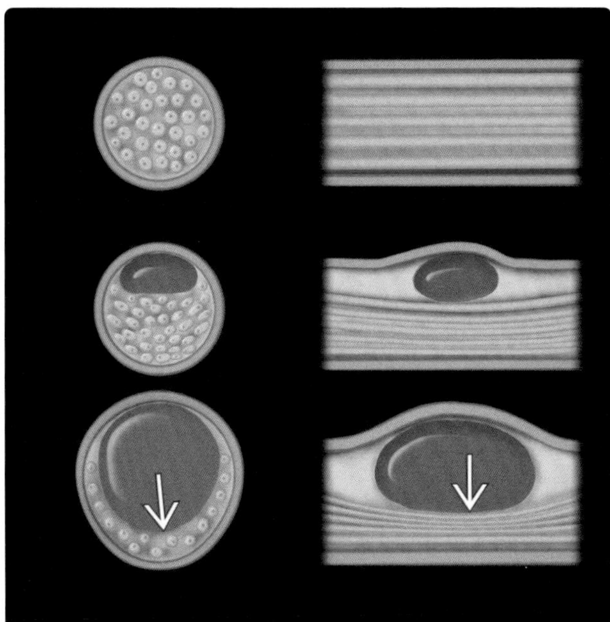

*(26-2) (L) Axial and (R) sagittal graphics show a schwannoma arising within a unifascicular nerve. The tumor displaces other nerve fibers peripherally ➡.*

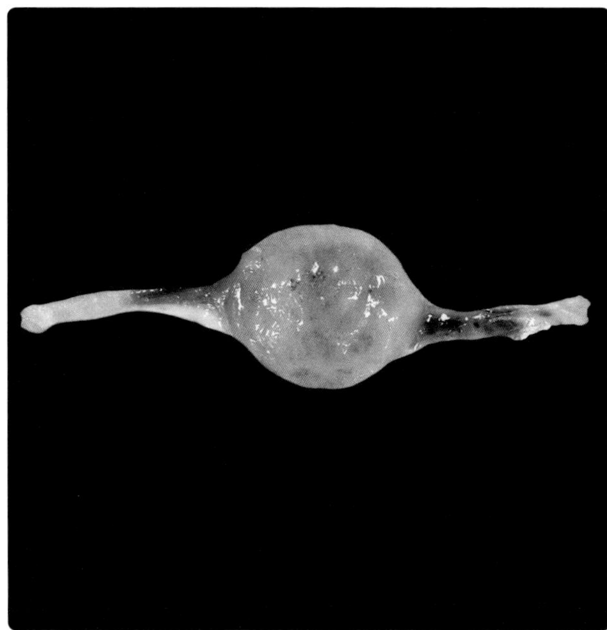

*(26-3) Schwannomas are encapsulated by perineurium and epineural collagen and grow eccentrically to the nerve of origin. (From DP: Neuro.)*

### INTRACRANIAL SCHWANNOMAS: PATHOLOGY

**Location**
- Vestibular (CNVIII): Most common (90-95%)
  - All other sites combined (1-5%)
- Trigeminal (CNV): 2nd most common
- Jugular foramen (CNs IX, X, XI): 3rd most common
- Solitary > > multiple (NF2, schwannomatosis)

**Pathology**
- Arise at glial-Schwann cell junction
  - Distance from brain varies according to CN
- Benign encapsulated nerve sheath tumor
  - CNS WHO grade 1
- Well-differentiated neoplastic Schwann cells
- Biphasic histology with 2 components
  - Compact, highly ordered cellularity ("Antoni A")
  - Less cellular, myxoid matrix ("Antoni B")

**Microscopic Features.** So-called conventional schwannomas are well-encapsulated spindle cell tumors composed of well-differentiated Schwann cells. The large majority exhibit a biphasic histopathology. The Antoni A pattern consists of compact fascicles of elongated spindle cells. A less cellular, loosely textured, more haphazard arrangement with lipid-laden cells is called the Antoni B pattern **(26-5)**. Schwannomas correspond to CNS WHO grade 1.

**Diagnostic Molecular Pathology.** Loss of chromosome 22q &/or mutation of *NF2* are frequent but nonspecific findings in sporadic schwannomas. Schwannomas exhibit a distinct DNA methylation pattern.

Syndrome-associated schwannomas [neurofibromatosis type 2 (NF2) or schwannomatosis] are often associated with *SMARCB1* or *LZTR1* germline mutations followed by a somatic *NF2* mutation on chromosome 22.

## Clinical Issues

Intracranial schwannomas are relatively uncommon, constituting ~ 7% of all primary neoplasms. All ages are affected, but the peak incidence is in the 4th-6th decades. Schwannomas do occur in children but are uncommon unless associated with NF2. Symptoms are location specific; tinnitus and hearing loss are the most common symptoms in VSs.

Schwannomas are benign tumors that tend to grow very slowly. VS growth can be episodic and nonlinear. Some small intracanalicular VSs are monitored with a "wait-and-scan" management. Between 10-13% may exhibit volumetric tumor regression. The exception is VSs in young patients with NF2. These tumors have higher MIB-1 indices and may grow more rapidly.

## Imaging

**General Features.** Neuroimaging findings reflect their slow growth and benign biologic behavior. A well-circumscribed extraaxial mass that originates within or near a CN and displaces but does not invade adjacent structures is typical **(26-6)**.

**CT Findings.** Most schwannomas exhibit low to intermediate attenuation on NECT scans and show smooth expansion/remodeling of osseous foramina on bone CT. Cystic change is common. Gross intratumoral hemorrhage is uncommon, and calcification is rare. Strong, moderately heterogeneous enhancement after contrast administration is typical.

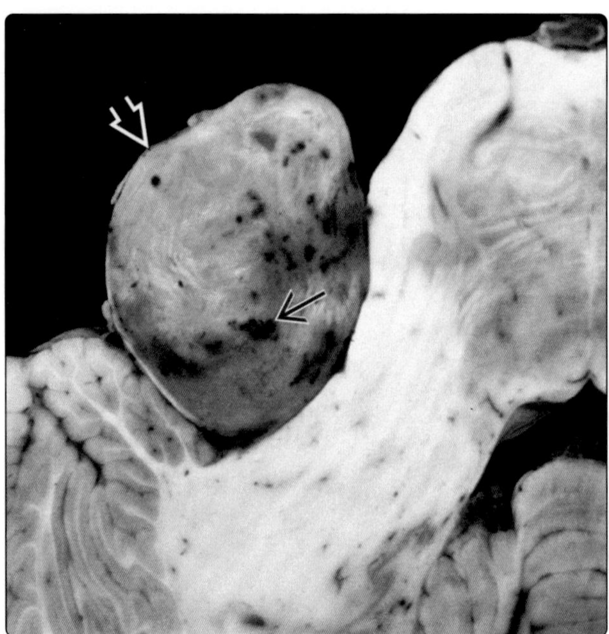

*(26-4) Gross pathology of vestibular schwannoma (VS) shows a large, well-demarcated, extraaxial mass ➡ in the CPA cistern. A few small hemorrhagic foci ➡ are present within the tumor. (Courtesy B. Horten, MD.)*

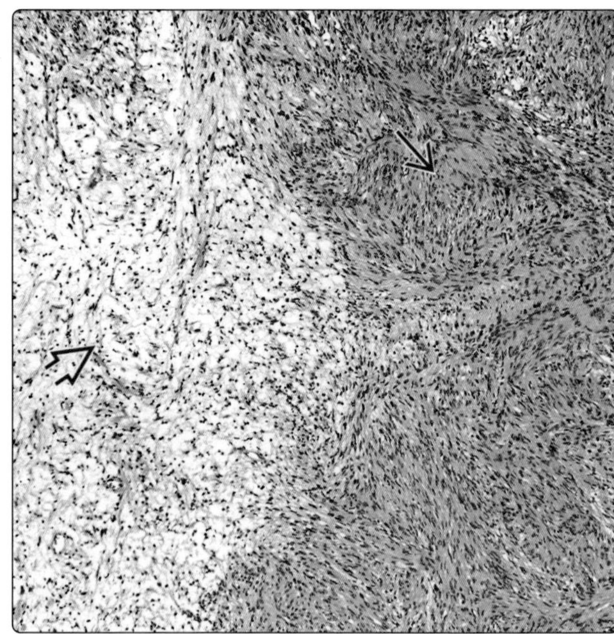

*(26-5) The juxtaposition of the cellular Antoni A ➡ and loose Antoni B ➡ patterns is classic for conventional schwannoma. (From DP: Neuro.)*

**MR Findings.** Schwannomas are generally isointense with cortex on T1WI **(26-8B)** and heterogeneously hyperintense on T2WI and FLAIR **(26-8A)**. Although macroscopic intratumoral hemorrhage is rare, T2* (GRE, SWI) scans often reveal "blooming" foci of microbleeds.

Secondary changes of muscle edema or denervation with atrophy and fatty infiltration can occur with motor nerve schwannomas. Vagal nerve schwannomas may cause vocal cord paralysis.

Virtually all schwannomas enhance intensely **(26-7)** **(26-8B)**. Approximately 15% have nonenhancing intratumoral cysts. Nonneoplastic peritumoral cysts occur in 5-10% of cases, especially with larger lesions **(26-11)**.

Dynamic susceptibility contrast perfusion sequences may be helpful in distinguishing sporadic schwannomas from other infratentorial tumors, such as paragangliomas.

## Differential Diagnosis

Cerebellopontine angle (CPA) masses that can mimic VS include **meningioma** and **paraganglioma**. Meningiomas often cap the internal auditory canal (IAC) like a mushroom and exhibit a dural tail sign. Paragangliomas of the jugular foramen have a salt and pepper enhancing pattern.

The differential diagnosis of a **solitary enlarged enhancing CN** includes schwannoma, multiple sclerosis, viral and postviral neuritis, Lyme disease, sarcoid, ischemia, and malignant neoplasms (metastases, lymphoma, and leukemia).

The most common cause of **multiple enhancing CNs** is metastasis. NF2, neuritis (especially Lyme disease), lymphoma, and leukemia are significantly less common than metastasis. Rare but important causes include multiple sclerosis and chronic inflammatory demyelinating polyneuropathy, a disorder that usually affects spinal nerves but may occasionally involve CNs.

# Vestibular Schwannoma

## Terminology

**Vestibular schwannoma** (VS) is the preferred term for a CNVIII schwannoma. VSs are also known as **acoustic schwannomas** and **acoustic neuromas**.

## Etiology

VSs arise from the vestibular portion of CNVIII at the glial-Schwann cell junction inside the IAC near the porus acusticus. Schwannomas rarely arise from the cochlear portion of CNVIII. The majority of sporadic VSs have inactivating mutations of *NF2*.

## Pathology

VSs may occur at any location along the course of the nerve. Small VSs are often completely intracanalicular. Larger lesions frequently protrude medially through the porus acusticus into the CPA cistern.

Small VSs are round or ovoid lesions that generally measure 2-10 mm in length. VSs that extend into the CPA cistern can become very large, up to 5 cm in diameter. Bilateral VSs are pathognomonic of NF2.

## Clinical Issues

VS is by far the most common intracranial schwannoma. VS is also the most common CPA cistern mass, accounting for 85-90% of lesions in this location.

Peak presentation is 40-60 years of age. The most common presentation is an adult with slowly progressive unilateral sensorineural hearing loss (SNHL). Small VSs may present initially with tinnitus. Large lesions often present with trigeminal &/or facial neuropathy.

The growth rate of VSs varies. On average, they tend to enlarge between 1 mm or 2 mm per year. Approximately 60% grow very slowly (< 1 mm per year), whereas 10% of patients experience rapid enlargement of their lesions (> 3 mm per year).

## Imaging

**General Features.** The classic imaging appearance of VS is an avidly enhancing mass that looks like ice cream on a cone **(26-7)**. Many VSs extend medially from their origin within the IAC. The intracanalicular part of the tumor represents the "cone." If a VS passes through the porus acusticus, it typically expands when it enters the CPA, forming the "ice cream" on the cone.

Precisely defining the size and extent of a VS is one of the most important goals of imaging. Some VSs remain as small, slow-growing lesions that are entirely intracanalicular **(26-9)** **(26-10)**. Many intracanalicular VSs have a distinctive fundal "cap" of CSF interposed between the lesion and the modiolus **(26-10)**. Others grow laterally, extending deep into the IAC fundus, and may eventually pass through the cochlear aperture into the modiolus.

**CT Findings.** CT is generally negative unless lesions are large enough to expand the IAC or protrude into the CPA cistern.

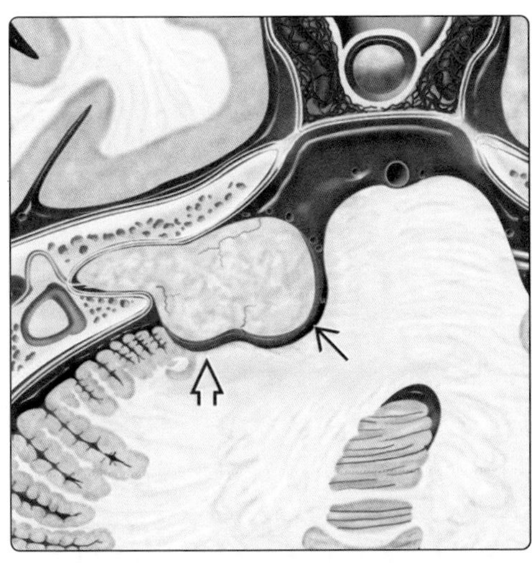

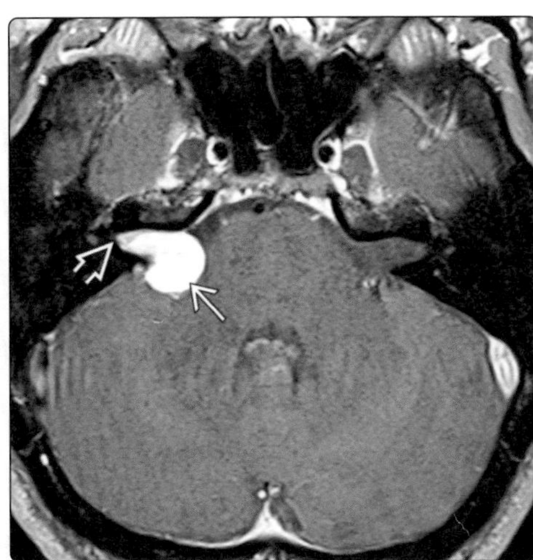

***(26-6)** Graphic of a large VS shows the typical ice cream on cone morphology. Note the prominent CSF-vascular "cleft" between the middle cerebellar peduncle ➩ and the cerebellar hemisphere ➩. **(26-7)** Classic ice cream on cone appearance of a VS is shown. Strong, relatively uniform enhancement ➡ is seen on T1 C+ FS MR. The tumor extends to the internal auditory canal (IAC) fundus ➡.*

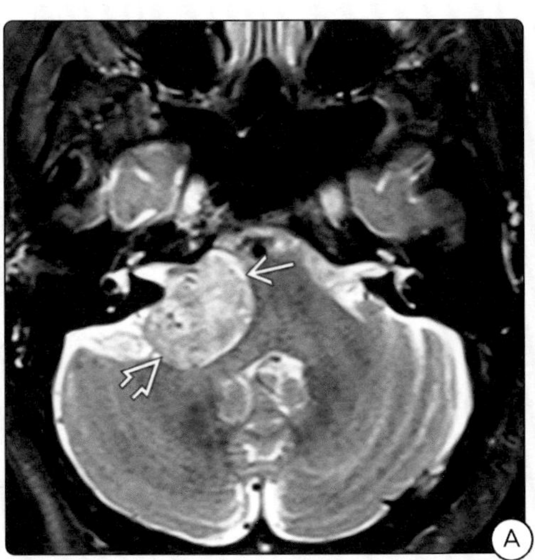

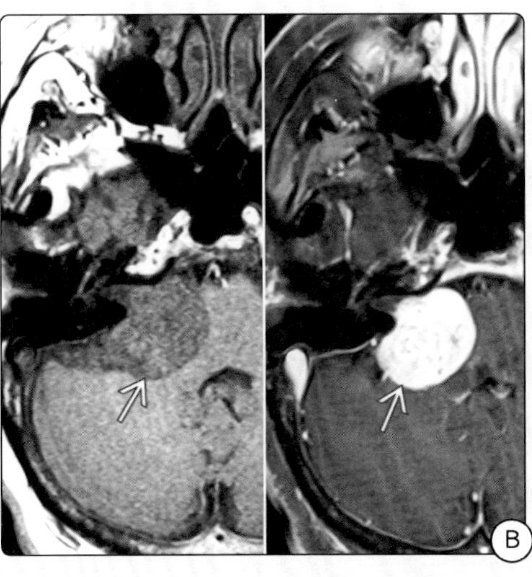

***(26-8A)** Axial T2 FS MR shows heterogeneously hyperintense signal of a typical large VS ➡. The tumor indents the pons and cerebellar peduncle, deforming the 4th ventricle. Note CSF "cleft" ➡ between the tumor and brainstem. **(26-8B)** (L) Precontrast T1 MR and (R) postcontrast T1 C+ FS MR (R) in the same patient show that the tumor ➡ enhances intensely but somewhat heterogeneously. This is a VS with conventional histology.*

**MR Findings.** VSs are generally iso-/hypointense with brain on T1WI **(26-8B)**. An intracanalicular VS appears as a hypointense filling defect within the bright CSF on CISS. Larger VSs are iso- to heterogeneously hyperintense on T2WI and may have associated cysts **(26-11)**. Microhemorrhage on T2* is common, although macroscopic hemorrhage is rare (0.4% of all newly diagnosed VSs but 5-6% of anticoagulated patients).

Virtually all VSs enhance strongly following contrast administration **(26-7)**. A schwannoma-associated dural tail sign occurs but is rare compared with CPA meningiomas.

### Differential Diagnosis

The major differential diagnosis of VS is **CPA meningioma**. Most meningiomas "cap" the IAC and do not extend deep to the porus. However, a reactive dural "tail" in the IAC may make distinction between VS and meningioma difficult unless other dural "tails" along the petrous ridge are also present.

A **facial nerve schwannoma** confined to the IAC may be difficult to distinguish from a VS. Facial nerve schwannomas are much less common and usually have a labyrinthine segment "tail." **Metastases** can coat the facial and vestibulocochlear nerves within the IAC. Metastases are usually bilateral with other lesions present.

Other CPA masses, such as **epidermoid cysts, arachnoid cysts, and aneurysms**, can usually be distinguished easily from VS. VSs occasionally have prominent intramural cysts, but a completely cystic schwannoma without an enhancing tumor rim is very rare.

## Trigeminal Schwannoma

Although trigeminal schwannomas are the second most common intracranial schwannoma, they are rare tumors. They may involve any part of the CNV complex, including extracranial peripheral divisions of the nerve. Nearly 2/3 of all Meckel cave tumors are schwannomas.

*(26-9) Graphic depicts an intracanalicular VS as round or fusiform enlargement of the nerve ➡. (26-10) (Top) Axial T1 C+ MR shows a small intracanalicular VS ➡. (Bottom) High-resolution axial T2 MR in the same patient nicely shows the VS as a round isointense mass in the IAC ➡. Note the fundal "cap" of CSF ➡.*

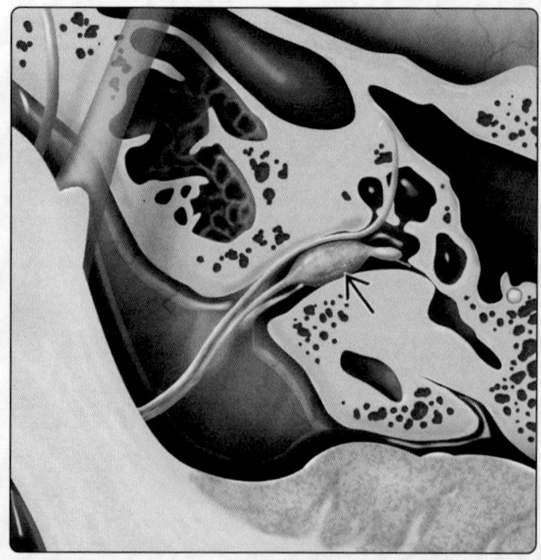

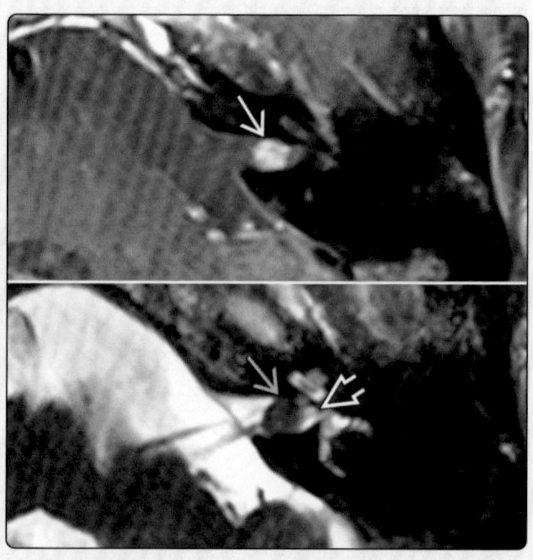

*(26-11A) Axial FIESTA MR in 31-yo man with headaches, left facial numbness shows large VS with intratumoral ➡, marginal cysts with fluid-fluid level suggesting hemorrhage ➡. Note peritumoral cysts ➡ exhibit different signal from normal CSF in CPA cistern ➡. (26-11B) T1 C+ FS MR shows nonenhancing intratumoral cysts ➡ and rim enhancement along marginal ➡, peritumoral cysts ➡. Cystic VS with intracystic hemorrhage.*

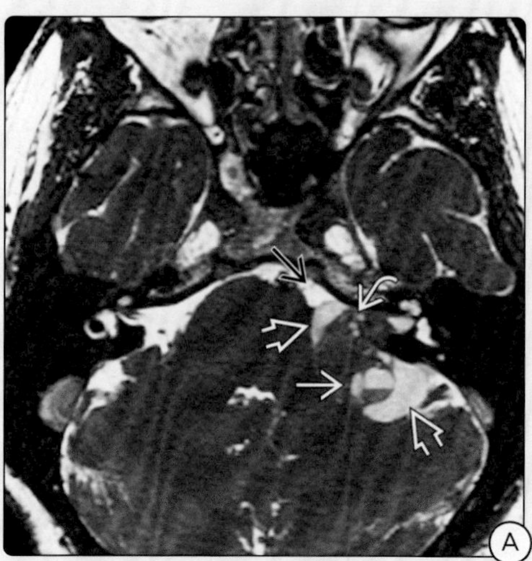


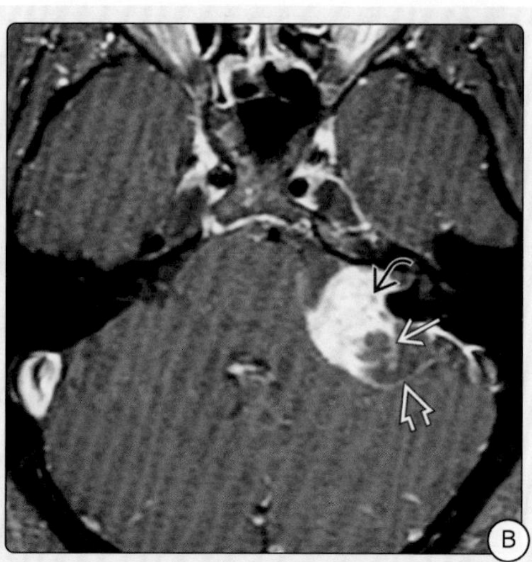

## Imaging

Trigeminal schwannomas arise from the junction of the gasserian ganglion and the trigeminal nerve root **(26-12)**. Small lesions may be confined to Meckel cave. They have a very characteristic appearance on coronal T2WI, the winking Meckel cave sign. Because at least 90% of each Meckel cave is normally filled with CSF, any lesion that fills the cave with soft tissue contrasts sharply with the bright signal on the opposite normal side **(26-13)**.

Bicompartmental tumors are common. Schwannomas that originate in Meckel cave can extend into the posterior fossa (through the porus trigeminus). These tumors have a characteristic dumbbell configuration **(26-14)**. Tumors that involve all three locations are uncommon and termed three-compartment trigeminal schwannomas **(26-15)**.

Schwannomas that involve the mandibular division (CNV3) may cause denervation atrophy of the muscles of mastication.

## Differential Diagnosis

The appearance of a bi- or tricompartmental CNV schwannoma is distinctive. The major differential diagnoses of a Meckel cave schwannoma are **meningioma** and **metastasis**.

# Jugular Foramen Schwannoma

Although schwannomas account for ~ 40% of all jugular foramen (JF) neoplasms, JF schwannomas constitute only 2-4% of all intracranial schwannomas.

**Glossopharyngeal schwannomas** are the most common JF schwannoma, but they are still rare. The vast majority present with vestibulocochlear symptoms secondary to compression and displacement, not CNIX symptoms. Glossopharyngeal schwannomas can occur anywhere along the course of CNIX, but the majority of symptomatic cases are intracranial/intraosseous.

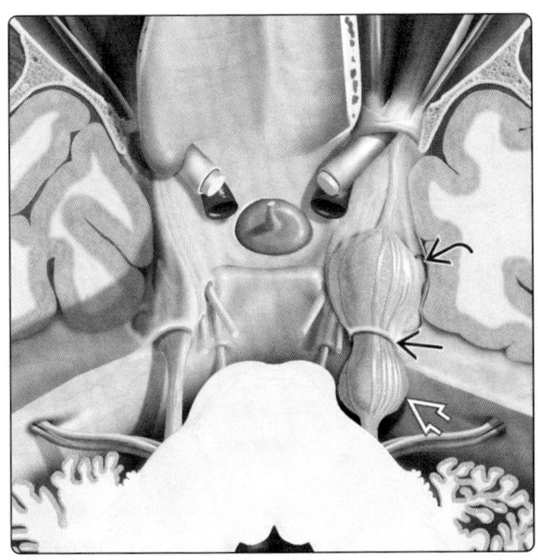

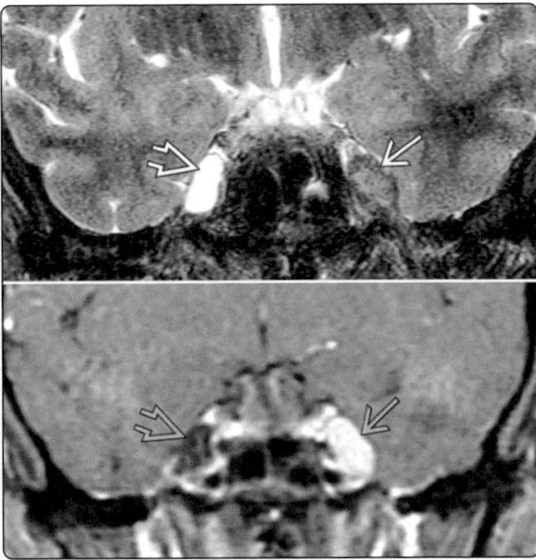

***(26-12)** "Dumbbell" trigeminal schwannoma shows that the cisternal tumor segment ➡ is constricted as it passes through porus trigeminus ➡. Schwannoma then expands again ➡ when it enters Meckel cave. **(26-13)** (Top) Coronal T2 MR of left CNV schwannoma shows winking Meckel cave sign. CSF-filled right side ➡ contrasts with tumor-filled left Meckel cave ➡. (Bottom) Schwannoma enhances ➡ while right side ➡ is normal.*

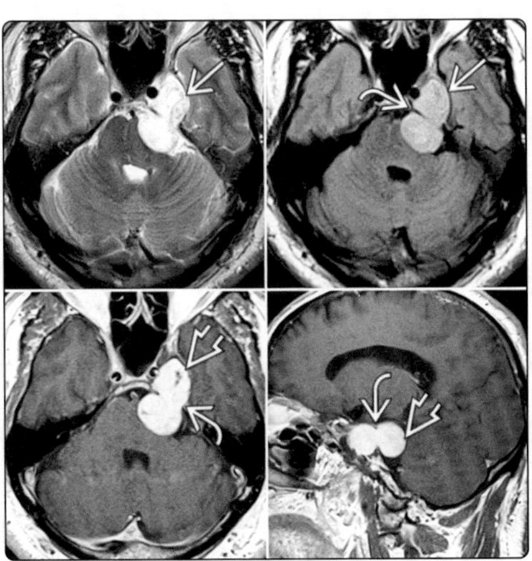

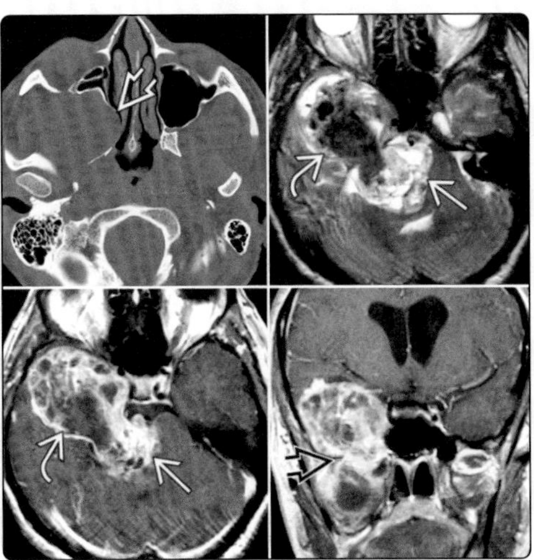

***(26-14)** This is a large "dumbbell" trigeminal schwannoma. Tumor is hyperintense on T2WI, and FLAIR ➡ enhances strongly on T1 C+ ➡. Note prominent constriction by dural ring of the porus trigeminus ➡. **(26-15)** Giant "tricompartmental" schwannoma of CNs V2 and V3 with cystic and hemorrhagic changes enlarges pterygopalatine fossa ➡, extends from posterior fossa ➡ into middle fossa ➡, through foramen ovale into masticator space ➡.*

Most **vagal schwannomas** are "dumbbell" lesions that extend from the basal cistern through the JF into the high, deep carotid space **(26-16)** **(26-17)**.

The major differential diagnoses of JF schwannoma include **meningioma, glomus jugulare tumor (paraganglioma)**, and **metastasis**. Only a JF schwannoma smoothly enlarges and remodels the jugular fossa. Paragangliomas exhibit a distinct salt and pepper appearance on contrast-enhanced sequences.

## Facial Nerve Schwannoma

Facial nerve schwannomas (FNSs) are rare lesions that can arise anywhere along the course of the facial nerve, from its origin in the CPA to its extracranial ramifications in the parotid space **(26-18)** **(26-19)**.

**CPA-IAC** FNSs are radiologically indistinguishable from vestibular schwannomas if they do not demonstrate extension into the labyrinthine segment of the facial nerve canal. Lesions that traverse the labyrinthine segment often have a dumbbell appearance.

Almost 90% of FNSs involve more than one facial nerve segment **(26-20)**. The **geniculate fossa** is the most common site, involved in > 80% of all FNSs **(26-21)**. The **labyrinthine** and **tympanic segments** are each involved in slightly over 1/2 of FNSs. **Tympanic segment** FNSs often pedunculate into the middle ear cavity, losing their tubular configuration.

## Schwannomas of Other Intracranial Nerves

Less than 1% of intracranial schwannomas arise from CNs other than VIII, V, VII, and IX/X. Most resemble their more common counterparts on imaging studies.

Olfactory nerve "schwannomas" actually arise from modified glial cells, not Schwann cells. Once termed "olfactory groove schwannoma" or "subfrontal schwannoma," these neoplasms

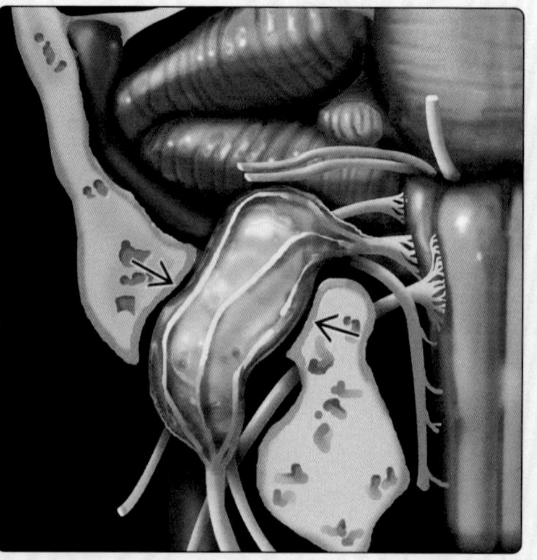

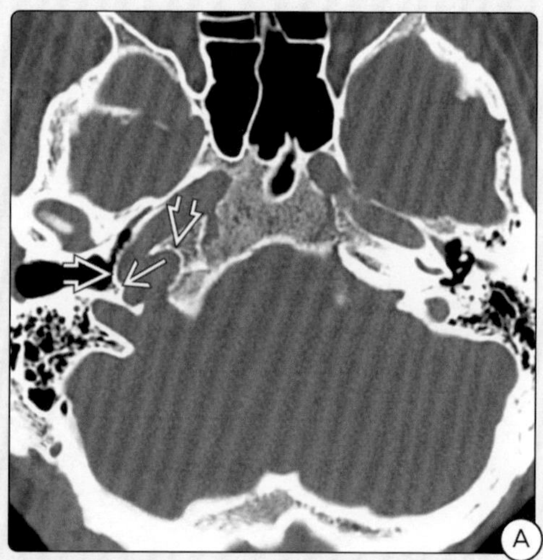


***(26-16)** Coronal graphic of a vagal schwannoma shows the tumor enlarging and remodeling the bony margins of the jugular foramen ➔. The "beak" of the "eagle" is eroded. **(26-17A)** NECT shows osseous remodeling of the right jugular foramen. The jugular spine ➔ is eroded, but the surrounding cortex ➔ appears intact.*

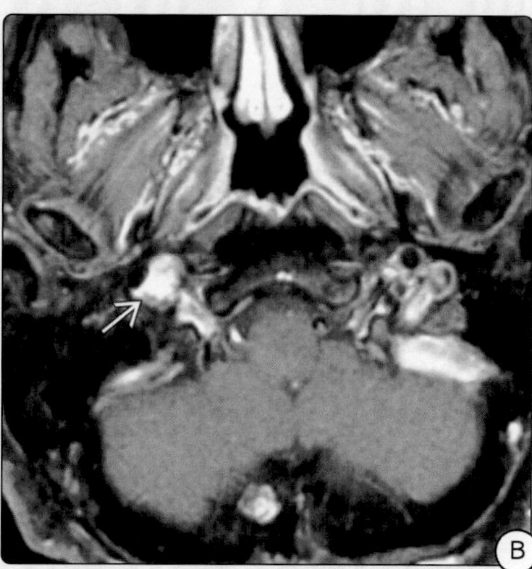


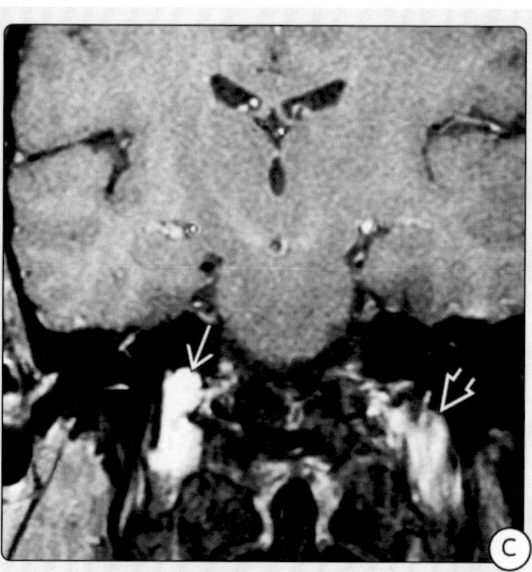


***(26-17B)** Axial T1 C+ FS MR shows an enhancing mass in the jugular foramen ➔. **(26-17C)** Coronal T1 C+ FS MR shows the intensely enhancing mass ➔. Contrast this with the normally enhancing left jugular bulb and vein ➔. At surgery, this jugular foramen schwannoma proved to be arising from the vagal nerve (CNX).*

are more accurately called **olfactory ensheathing cell (OEC) tumors**. Many reach a large size **(26-22)**, causing frontal lobe signs, such as emotional lability and complex partial seizures.

Neoplasms of the optic nerve (a brain tract) are astrocytomas, not schwannomas. Intraorbital schwannomas arise from peripheral branches of CNs IV, V1, or VI or from sympathetic or parasympathetic fibers (not the optic nerve).

**Oculomotor schwannomas** are the most common of all the pure motor nerve schwannomas **(26-23)**. The most frequent location of a CNIII schwannoma is in the interpeduncular cistern near the nerve exit from the midbrain **(26-24)**. **Trochlear schwannomas** are uncommon **(26-25)**. They cause diplopia (isolated unilateral superior oblique palsy) and compensatory head tilt that may be misdiagnosed clinically as "wry neck." Most CNIV schwannomas are small and either simply watched or treated with prism spectacles.

Hypoglossal tumors are the rarest of the "other" schwannomas, accounting for only 5% of all nonvestibular intracranial schwannomas **(26-26)**. Over 90% present with denervation hemiatrophy of the tongue. Most originate intracranially **(26-27)** but can also extend extracranially as a "dumbbell" tumor that expands and remodels the hypoglossal canal **(26-28)**.

## Parenchymal Schwannomas

Because the brain parenchyma does not normally contain Schwann cells, so-called ectopic schwannomas not associated with CNs are very rare (< 1% of cases). Most intraparenchymal schwannomas are solitary and nonsyndromic.

On imaging studies, most intracranial parenchymal schwannomas appear well demarcated. The most common imaging pattern is that of a cyst with a mural nodule and peripheral enhancement **(26-29)**. One-third are solid tumors

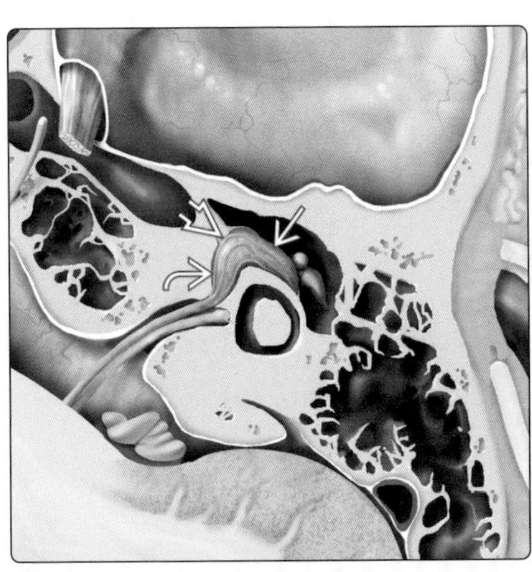

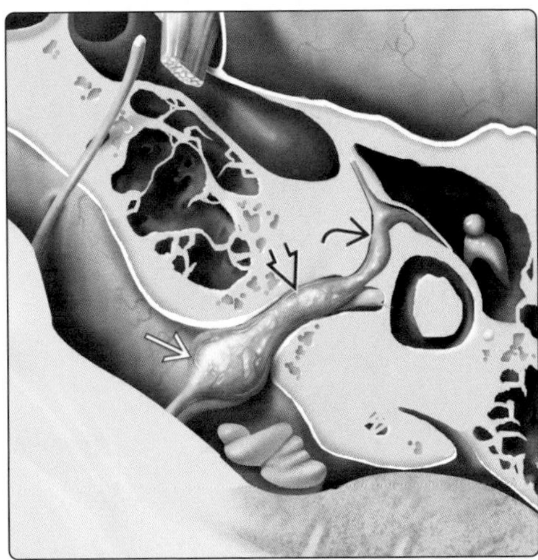

***(26-18)** Axial graphic depicts a small tubular facial nerve schwannoma involving the labyrinthine segment, geniculate ganglion, and anterior tympanic segment on CNVII. **(26-19)** Graphic depicts a larger facial nerve schwannoma with CPA and IAC segments. This can mimic a VS (ice cream on cone appearance) except for the "tail" of tumor extending into the labyrinthine segment.*

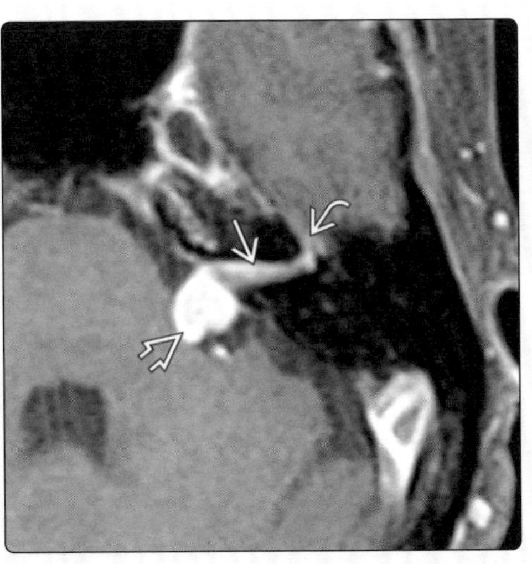

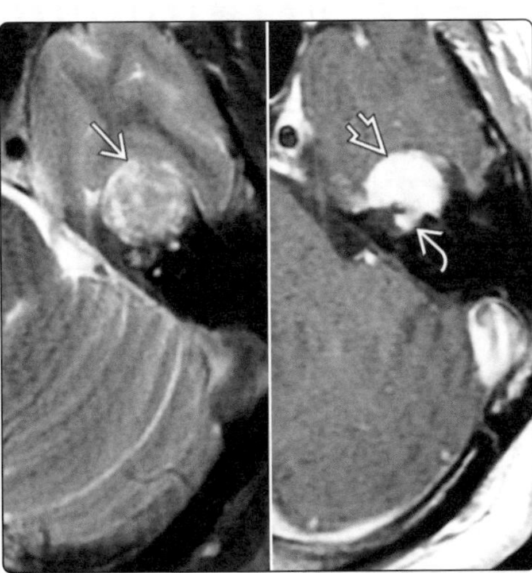

***(26-20)** Close-up view of T1 C+ FS MR shows a facial nerve schwannoma in the CPA extending into the IAC and geniculate ganglion. **(26-21)** Geniculate fossa VII schwannoma is shown. (L) T2 MR shows globular heterogeneously hyperintense mass tracking along the GSPN and extending extradurally into the middle cranial fossa. (R) The labyrinthine, geniculate ganglion segments enhance intensely. (Courtesy P. Hildenbrand, MD.)*

*(26-22A)* *Sagittal T1 C+ FS MR shows intensely enhancing, subfrontal, "dumbbell" mass ➡ extended through the eroded cribriform plate into the nasal cavity ➡.* *(26-22B)* *Axial T1 C+ MR in the same patient shows well-circumscribed, intensely enhancing mass centered on cribriform plate. Diagnosis was olfactory nerve schwannoma. Most similar-appearing cases are likely olfactory ensheathing cell tumors, not schwannomas. (Courtesy G. Parker, MD.)*

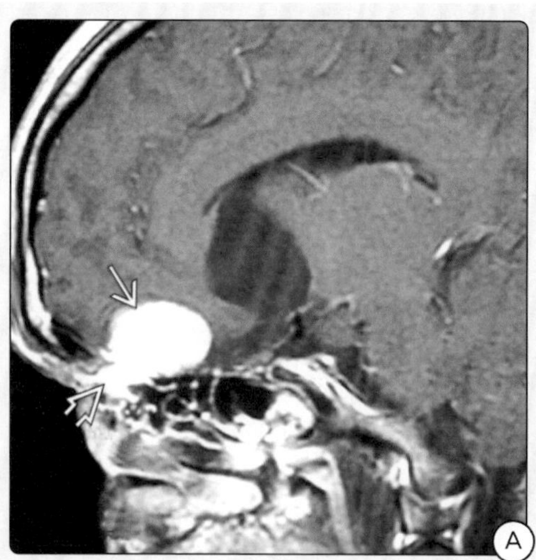

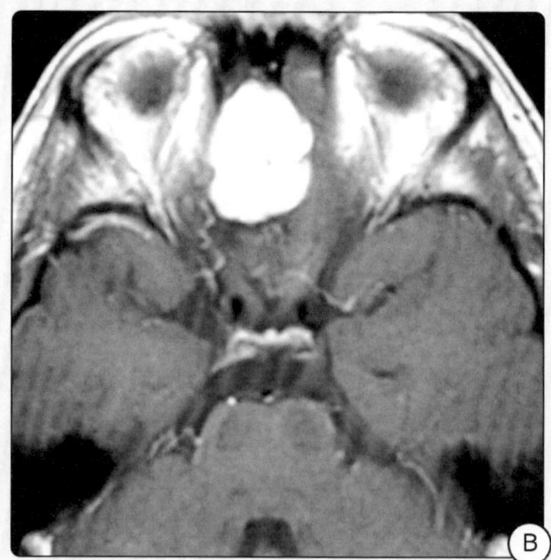

*(26-23)* *Coronal autopsy case shows an incidental left oculomotor schwannoma ➡ seen between the posterior cerebral artery above ➡ and the superior cerebellar artery below ➡. Contrast with the normal right CNIII ➡. (Courtesy E. T. Hedley-Whyte, MD.)* *(26-24A)* *Coronal T1 C+ MR demonstrates the enlarged, enhancing right oculomotor nerve ➡.*

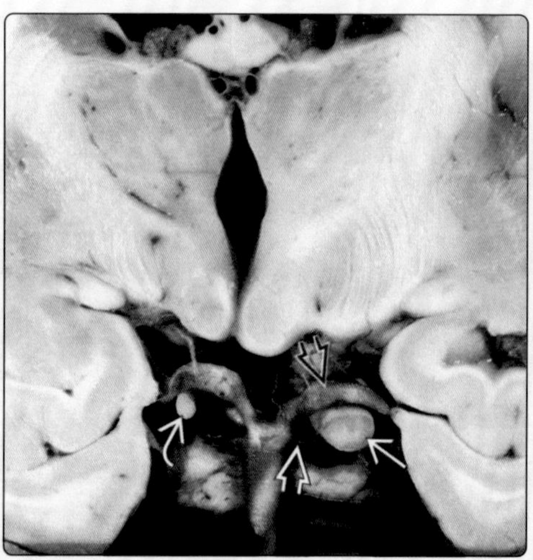

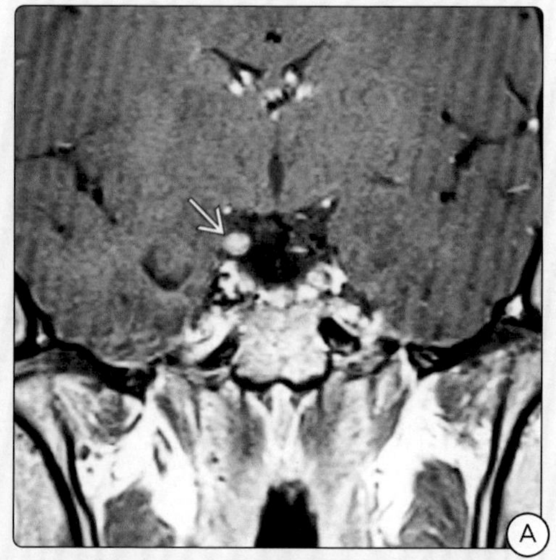

*(26-24B)* *Sagittal T1 C+ MR in the same patient shows tubular enlargement of the oculomotor nerve ➡ extending from its midbrain exit to the cavernous sinus.* *(26-24C)* *Axial T1 C+ MR in the same patient shows the enlarged, intensely enhancing, right oculomotor nerve ➡. The lesion was unchanged after 3 years. This was presumed schwannoma.*

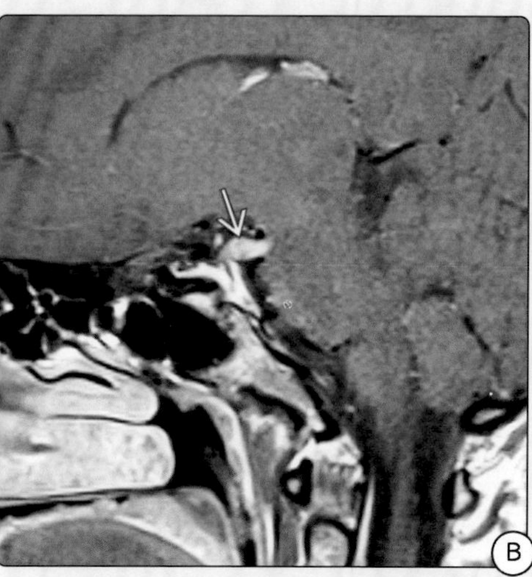

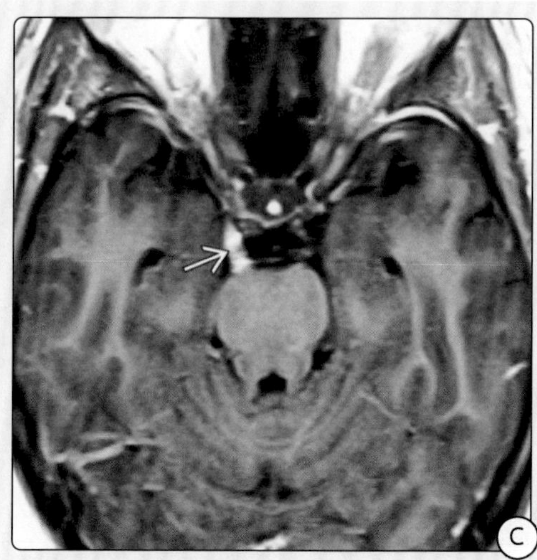

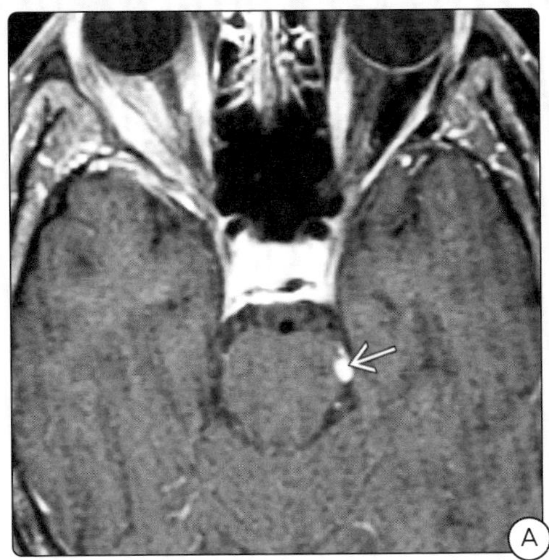

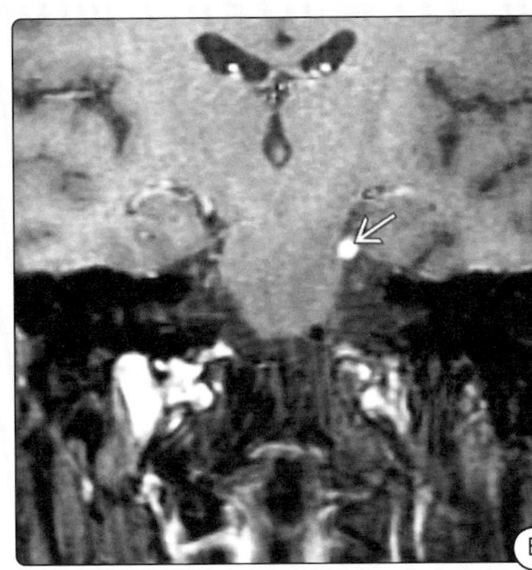

***(26-25A)** Axial T1 C+ FS MR shows a small enhancing tumor in the left ambient cistern ➡.* ***(26-25B)** Coronal T1 C+ FS MR in the same patient shows that the tumor ➡ lies along the expected course of CNIV. This was probable trochlear schwannoma.*

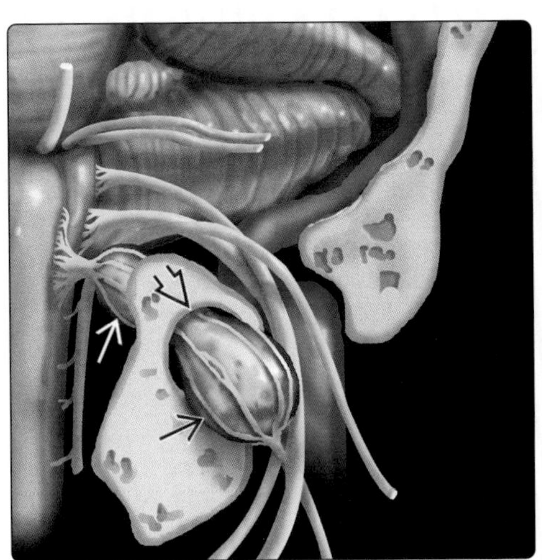

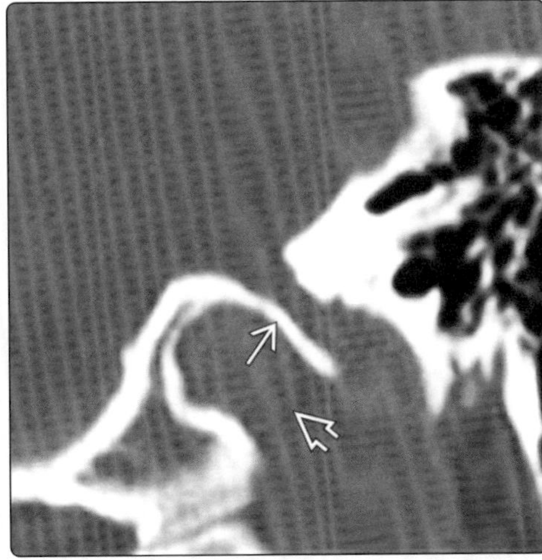

***(26-26)** Graphic depicts hypoglossal schwannoma. CNXII schwannomas have a dumbbell shape with a cisternal segment ➡, relative constriction in the bony hypoglossal canal ⇨, and a larger extracranial component ⇨.* ***(26-27)** Coronal bone CT with hypoglossal schwannoma shows enlarged hypoglossal canal ➡ with thinning and remodeling of the jugular tubercle ➡ ("head" and "beak" of the "eagle").*

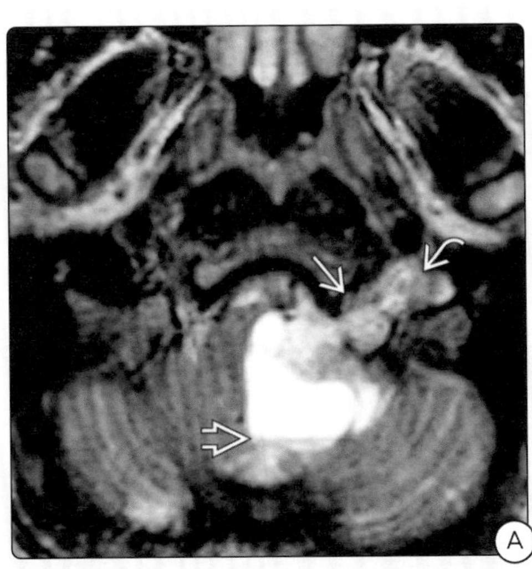

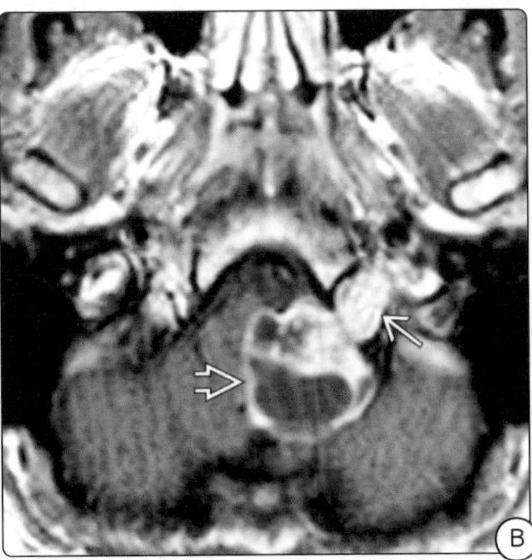

***(26-28A)** Axial T2 FS MR in a patient with excruciating left arm pain shows a heterogeneously hyperintense posterior fossa mass with a large, partially cystic intracranial component that exhibits a blood-fluid level ➡. Note extension through an enlarged hypoglossal canal ➡ into high deep carotid space ➡.* ***(26-28B)** T1 C+ MR shows the partially cystic ➡, partially solid ➡ enhancing mass. This is "dumbbell" hypoglossal schwannoma.*

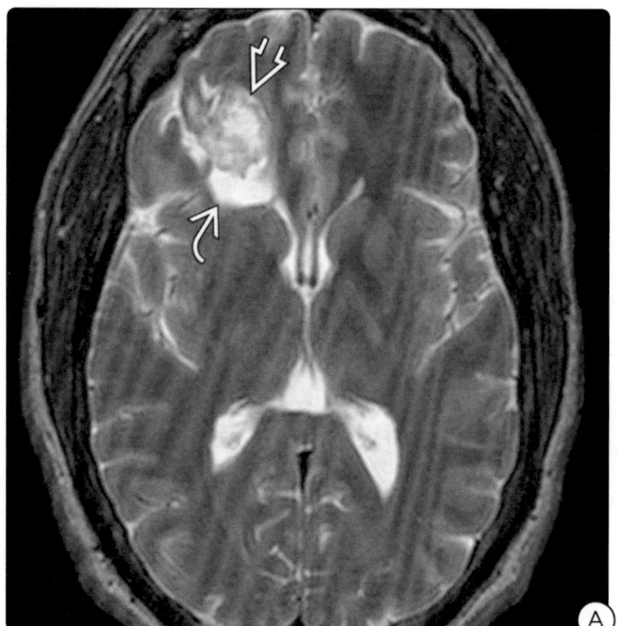


***(26-29A) Axial T2 MR shows a well-delineated mass in the right frontal lobe. Note hyperintense cyst ➢ with mixed-intensity solid nodule ➢.***

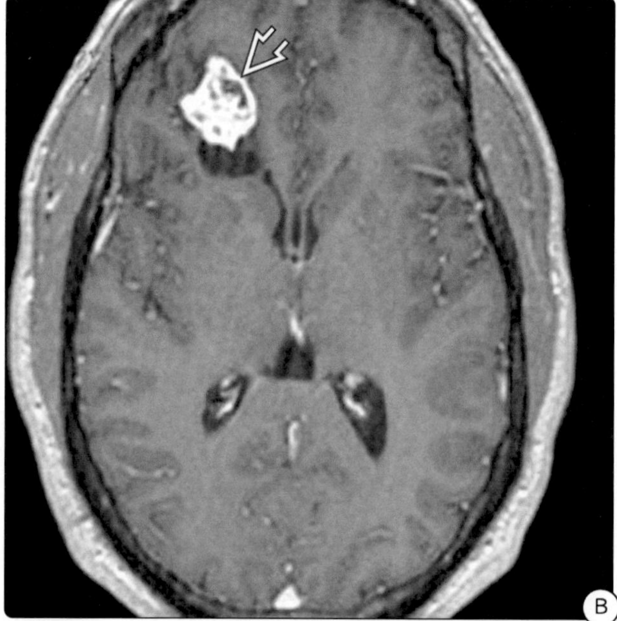


***(26-29B) T1 C+ MR shows the nodule ➢ enhancing strongly but heterogeneously. Intraparenchymal schwannoma was found at surgery. (Courtesy T. Hutchins, MD.)***

with strong homogeneous or heterogeneous enhancement. Peritumoral edema varies from none to moderate.

## Schwannomatosis

Nonsyndromic schwannomas are almost always solitary lesions. Multiple schwannomas occur in the setting of two familial tumor syndromes, **neurofibromatosis type 2** (NF2) and **schwannomatosis**. Bilateral vestibular schwannomas are pathognomonic of NF2. Multiple, mostly nonvestibular schwannomas in the absence of other NF2 features are characteristic of schwannomatosis. Both of these syndromes are discussed in Chapter 43.

# Neurofibromas

Neurofibromas (NFs) are much less common than schwannomas. In contrast to schwannomas, NFs consist of mature neoplastic Schwann cells intermixed with nonneoplastic cell types in a variable loose myxoid to collagenous stroma. NFs can affect the scalp, skull, some CNs (especially CNV1), or—rarely—the brain. They are found at all ages. Both sexes are affected equally.

NFs can be solitary or multiple. Multiple NFs and plexiform NFs occur only in connection with neurofibromatosis type 1 (NF1).

The gross appearance of NFs is different from that of schwannomas. Schwannomas are well-delineated encapsulated lesions that arise eccentrically from their parent nerve. Schwannomas typically displace elements of the normal parent nerve to one side **(26-2)**.

NFs generally present as more diffuse nerve expansions and tend to infiltrate adjacent soft tissues. They display single (localized) or multiple (plexiform) fascicles that enter and leave the affected nerve. Axons of the parent nerve pass through NFs and are intermixed with tumor cells **(26-30)**, distinguishing them from schwannoma.

NFs are all considered CNS WHO grade 1 neoplasms. Atypical histologic features, such as hypercellularity and mitoses, are rare. When present, these uncommon tumors are designated atypical neurofibromatous neoplasm of uncertain biological significance (ANNUBP) in the 2021 WHO.

## Solitary Neurofibroma

Solitary NFs are the most common subtype of NFs. Unlike the diffuse and plexiform NF subtypes, they are generally not associated with NF1.

A solitary NF in the head and neck rarely—if ever—involves CNs. Solitary NFs affect patients of all ages and are usually sporadic (nonsyndromic). Most occur in the absence of NF1 and present as a painless scalp or skin mass.

Scalp solitary NFs are usually well-defined lesions measuring < 5 cm in diameter. They abut but do not invade the calvarium. Solitary NFs are iso- to mildly hyperintense to muscle on T1WI and hyperintense on STIR and T2WI **(26-31)**. Strong but heterogeneous enhancement is typical. Solitary NFs do not undergo malignant degeneration.

## Plexiform Neurofibroma

Plexiform NF1 (PNF) is defined by its involvement of multiple nerve fascicles. PNFs demonstrate a predominant intrafascicular growth pattern with redundant loops of expanded nerve fascicles intermixed with collagen fibers and mucoid material. PNFs are infiltrative intra- and extraneural neoplasms with a ropy or bag of worms gross appearance **(26-32)**. PNFs are highly associated with NF1 and have an increased risk of transformation to malignant peripheral nerve sheath tumor (MPNST).

The most typical locations are the scalp, orbit, pterygopalatine fossa, and parotid gland.

PNFs are generally isodense with muscle on NECT. Calcification and hemorrhage are rare. CECT shows heterogeneous enhancement. Bone CT may show expansion of the superior orbital fissure and pterygopalatine fossa.

On MR, PNFs often appear as a bag of worms and are isointense on T1WI and hyperintense on T2WI. Strong, sometimes heterogeneous enhancement is common **(26-33)**. A target sign of hypointensity within an enhancing tumor fascicle is seen in some benign PNFs.

NEUROFIBROMAS

**Solitary Neurofibroma**
- Most are sporadic (nonsyndromic)
- All ages (children to adults)
- Scalp, skin
- Rarely (if ever) involves CNs

**Plexiform Neurofibroma**
- Pathology
  - Involves, expands multiple nerve fascicles
  - Composed of Schwann cells + fibroblasts, mucoid material
  - Fusiform, infiltrating
- Clinical
  - Usually diagnostic of NF1
  - Risk of malignant degeneration in PNF: 5%
- Imaging
  - Extensively infiltrating scalp; orbit lesions most common
  - Bag of worms appearance
  - May enlarge superior orbital fissure, extend into cavernous sinus
  - Intracranial involvement is rare unless malignant degeneration
  - Bone erosion should raise suspicion of MPNST

# Perineurioma and Hybrid Nerve Sheath Tumors

Benign peripheral nerve sheath tumors constitute 10-12% of benign soft tissue tumors. There are three common types: Schwannoma, neurofibroma, and perineurioma. The vast majority of peripheral nerve sheath tumors are schwannomas and neurofibromas.

**Perineurioma** is a rare, benign (CNS WHO grade 1) tumor of adolescents and young adults (mean age: 22 years). Perineuriomas are characterized histopathologically by concentric layers of perineurial cells around axons, forming a "pseudo-onion bulb" pattern in cross section. Most cases affect peripheral nerves, especially the sciatic and radial nerves. CN lesions are rare.

**Hybrid peripheral nerve sheath tumor** (HPNST) has at least two areas characteristic of perineurioma, schwannoma, or neurofibroma. HPNSTs tend to occur in mid-adulthood and present as slowly progressive, painless

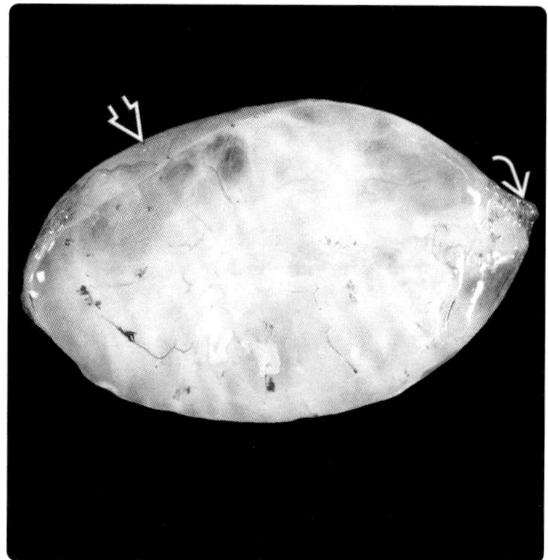

***(26-30)** Solitary neurofibroma ➡ has an almost translucent cut surface. The parent nerve is present at 1 end ➡. (From DP: Neuro.)*

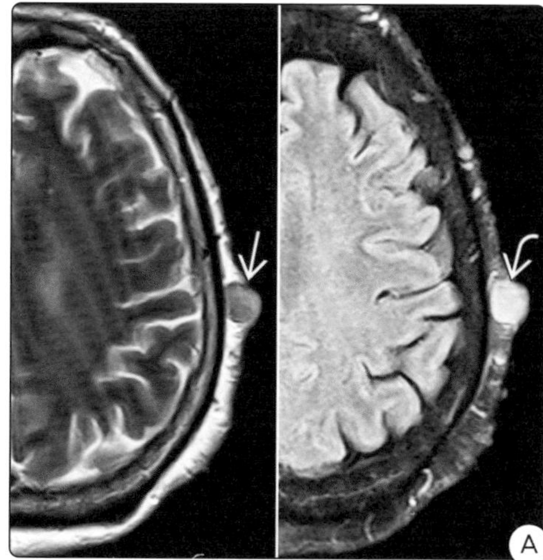


***(26-31A)** (L) T2 MR of solitary neurofibroma ➡ shows a well-demarcated, hypointense scalp mass that is (R) hyperintense on FLAIR ➡.*

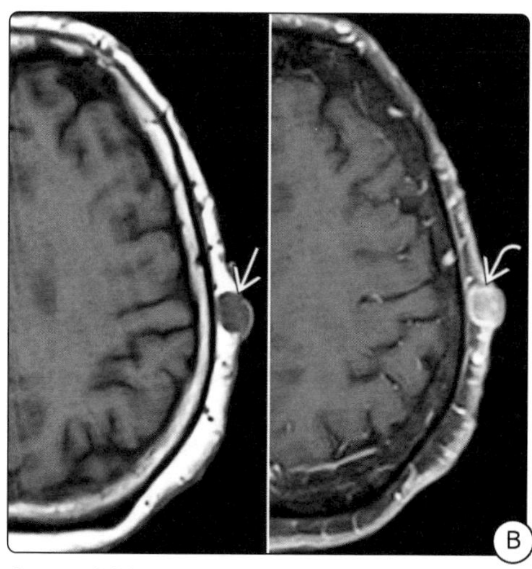


***(26-31B)** (L) T1 MR in same patient shows lesion is hypointense ➡ and (R) enhances strongly in a somewhat "target" fashion on T1 C+ FS MR ➡.*

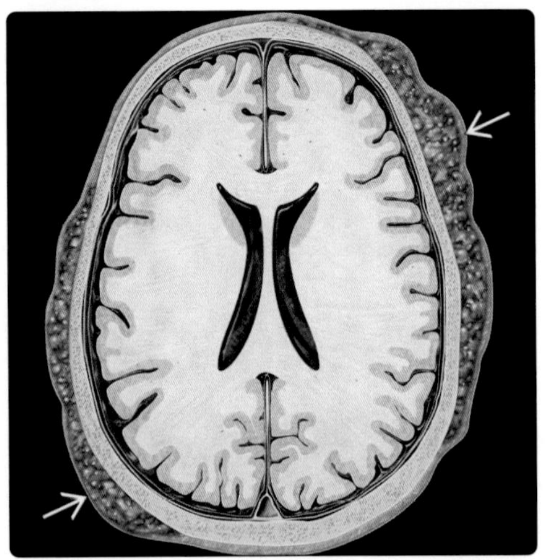

*(26-32) Graphic depicts plexiform neurofibromas (PNFs) diffusely infiltrating and deforming the scalp ➡.*

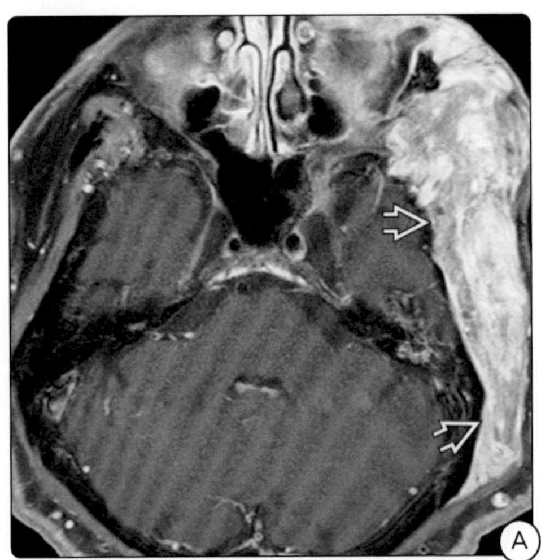

*(26-33A) T1 C+ FS MR shows extensively infiltrating PNF of the scalp ➡.*

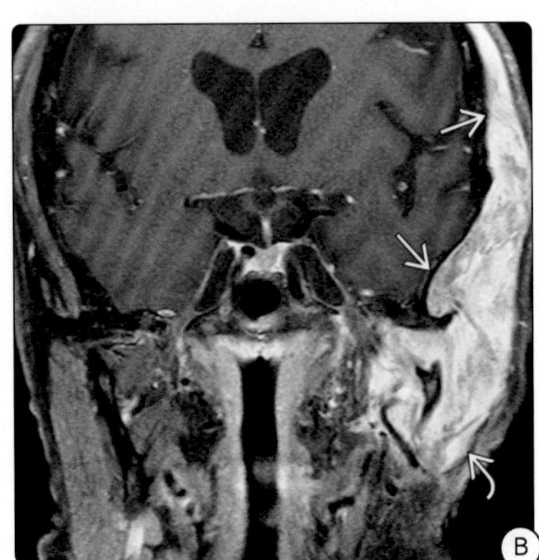

*(26-33B) Coronal T1 C+ FS MR shows that the extensive scalp PNF ➡ also extends into the masticator space ➡.*

superficial masses. Most involve cutaneous peripheral nerve but have been reported in the orbit.

# Malignant Peripheral Nerve Sheath Tumors

## Malignant Peripheral Nerve Sheath Tumor

A malignant peripheral nerve sheath tumor (MPNST) is any malignant tumor that arises from a peripheral nerve or shows nerve sheath differentiation. MPNSTs are relatively rare, accounting for 3-10% of soft tissue sarcomas.

MPNST is much more common in the peripheral or spinal nerves than in the CNs. The most commonly affected CNs are the vestibular, facial, and trigeminal nerves.

The 2021 WHO recognizes two histologic subtypes of MPNST: **Epithelioid MPNST** and **perineurial MPNST**. The pathogenesis of MPNST is complex and incompletely understood.

Approximately 1/2 of MPNSTs develop in patients with NF1. The overall lifetime risk of developing an MPNST at any location in patients with NF1 is estimated at 8-16%.

There is no clinically validated and reproducible grading system for MPNSTs, so tumors are generally grouped into low-grade and high-grade MPNSTs by mitotic count and presence or absence of necrosis.

On imaging studies, most MPNSTs are large (> 5 cm), heterogeneous enhancing lesions with infiltrative margins and central necrosis **(26-34)**. DWI/ADC mapping may help distinguish benign from MPNSTs. MRS may exhibit elevated choline.

## Malignant Melanotic Nerve Sheath Tumor

In the 2021 WHO classification, malignant melanotic nerve sheath tumor (MMNST) is now recognized as a highly distinct, frequently aggressive tumor with unique genetic alterations that distinguish it from all other nerve sheath tumors. The term melanotic schwannoma is no longer utilized.

MMNSTs exhibit features of both Schwann cell and melanocytic differentiation **(26-35)**. *PRKAR1A* mutations are present in almost all cases. Paraspinal and extraneural locations (e.g., skin, soft tissues, bone, and viscera) are the most common sites. Craniofacial and intracranial MMNSTs are very rare.

Peak age at diagnosis is about a decade younger compared with conventional schwannoma. MMNSTs can be sporadic or syndromic. Approximately 1/2 of all patients have **Carney complex**.

The biological behavior of MMNSTs is highly variable and unpredictable. Some lesions have a relatively indolent course, but metastases can occur in the absence of morphologically malignant features.

Most MMNSTs are relatively well-circumscribed lesions, although local bone invasion is present in 50% of cases. Because melanin causes T1 shortening, 90% of MMNSTs are hyperintense on T1WIs **(26-36B)**. Most are hypointense on T2WI **(26-36A)**. Enhancement varies from minimal to striking.

The main imaging differential diagnosis in MMNST is **metastatic melanoma** and **hemorrhagic conventional schwannoma**.

## Cauda Equina Neuroendocrine Tumor

The 2021 WHO Classification of CNS Neoplasms renamed the neoplasm formerly known as "paraganglioma" of the CNS as **cauda equina neuroendocrine tumor**.

Cauda equina neuroendocrine tumors are well-circumscribed, oval to sausage-shaped, intradural extramedullary masses that often hemorrhage **(26-37C)**. Neuroendocrine tumors of the cauda equina are CNS WHO grade 1 lesions.

Imaging studies show a hypervascular, intensely enhancing intradural extramedullary mass. Prominent flow voids and hemosiderin from prior hemorrhage may be present on MR **(26-37)**. Findings are indistinguishable from myxopapillary ependymoma. The differential diagnosis also includes schwannoma (rarely associated with dilated vessels) and hemangioblastoma of the filum terminale (rare).

## Nerve Sheath Tumor Mimics

Neoplastic and some nonneoplastic infiltrating disorders like **chronic interstitial demyelinating polyneuropathy (CIDP)** and **Charcot-Marie-Tooth (CMT) disease** occasionally affect CNs, causing enlargement and enhancement of one or more CNs.

**MULTIPLE ENLARGED, ENHANCING CRANIAL NERVES**

**Common**
- NF2
- Metastases
- Meningitis

**Less Common**
- Lyme disease
- Neurosarcoid
- Lymphoma/leukemia
- Viral, postviral neuritis

**Rare but Important**
- Guillain-Barré syndrome
- Chronic inflammatory demyelinating polyneuropathy
- Hereditary motor and sensory neuropathy (CMT, Dejerine-Sottas)

*Selected References: The complete reference list is available on the eBooks+ version included with purchase.*

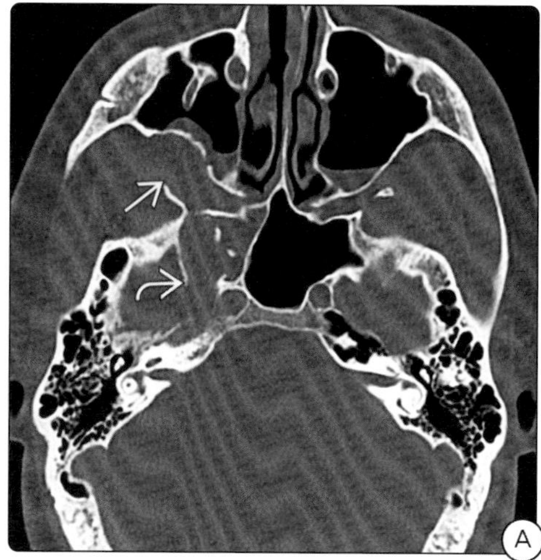


***(26-34A)** Bone CT shows destructive mass in the right cavernous sinus ➡ and pterygopalatine fossa ➡.*

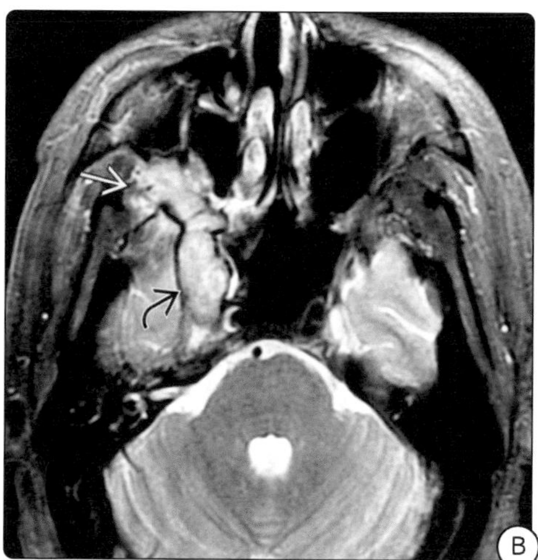


***(26-34B)** T2 MR shows hyperintense fusiform mass infiltrating and expanding the cavernous sinus ➡ and pterygopalatine fossa ➡.*

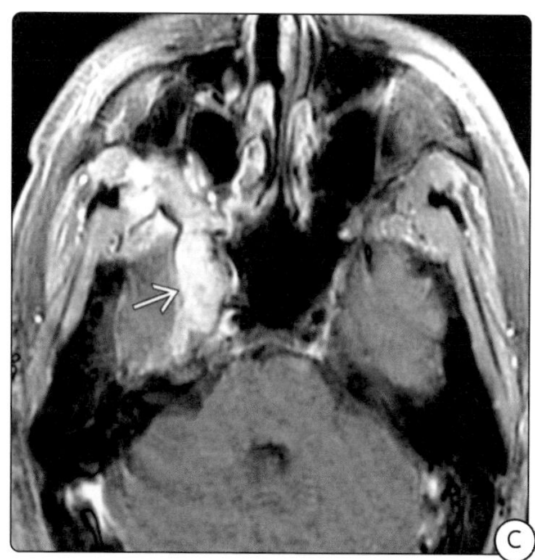


***(26-34C)** T1 C+ FS MR shows the mass ➡ enhancing strongly. Malignant peripheral nerve sheath tumor (MPNST) was found at surgery.*

*(26-35) Gross pathology shows a resected, heavily pigmented malignant melanotic nerve sheath tumor (MMNST). (From DP: Neuro.) (26-36A) T2 MR shows an "ice cream on cone" mass ➲ in the left CPA cistern that extends into the adjacent IAC ➲. The mass is very hypointense.*

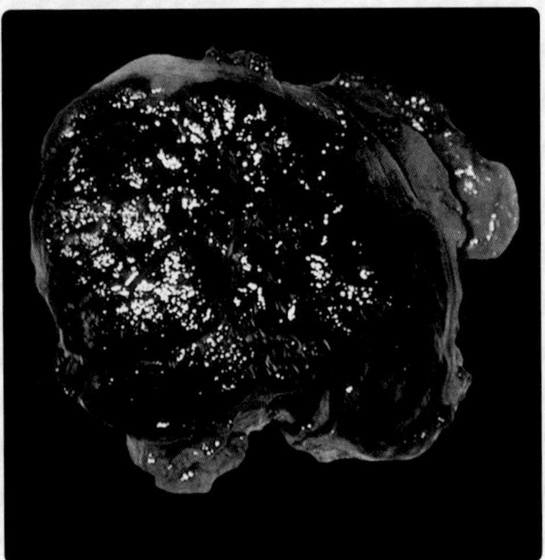

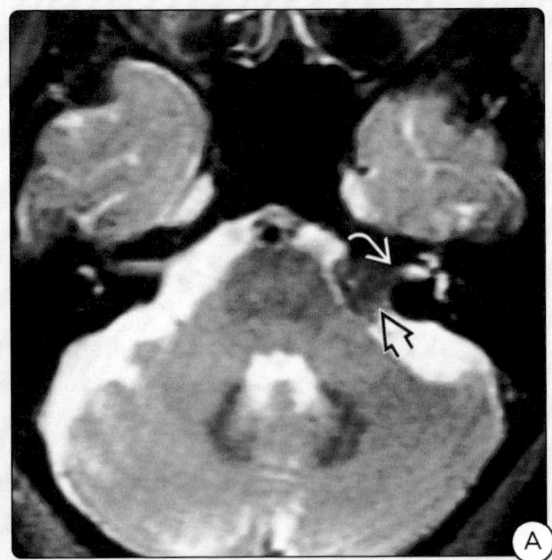

*(26-36B) (Top) T1 MR shows the CPA portion of the mass ➔ is heterogeneously hyperintense while the intracanalicular segment is homogeneously hyperintense ➔. MMNST was found at surgery. (Bottom) T1 C+ MR 6 months later shows tumor spread throughout the CPA ➔. Note brain invasion ➲. (26-37A) MR in a 61-yo woman with low back pain shows an intradural extramedullary mass ➔ that is isointense to the cord on both T1 (L) and T2 (R).*

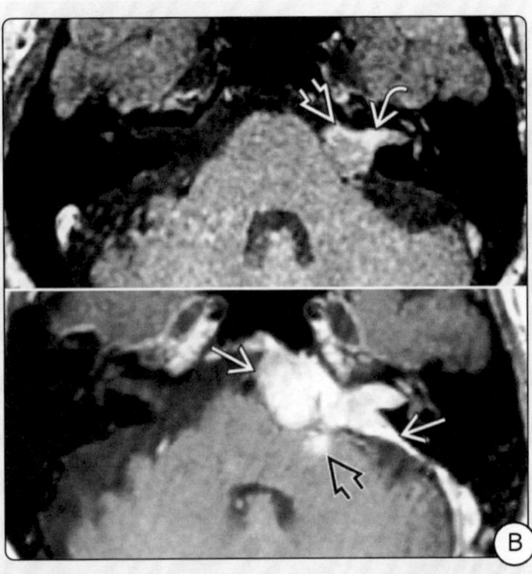

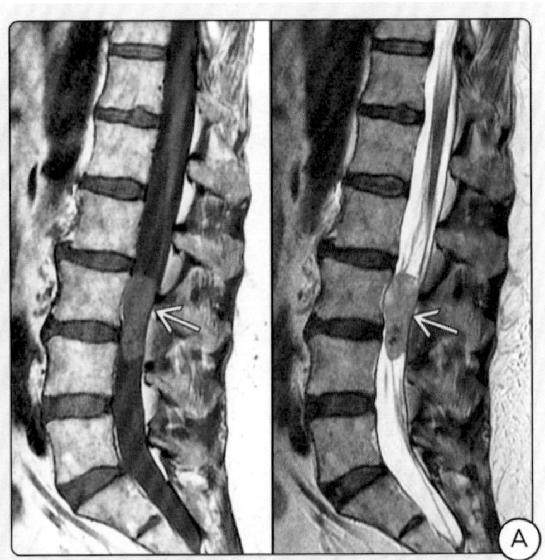

*(26-37B) Coronal T2 (L) and T1 C+ FS (R) MR images show the well-demarcated mass enhancing intensely ➔. Note enlarged vessels ➔ supplying the tumor. (26-37C) Gross pathology of a resected surgical specimen shows lobulated hypervascular mass. This is a cauda equina neuroendocrine tumor.*

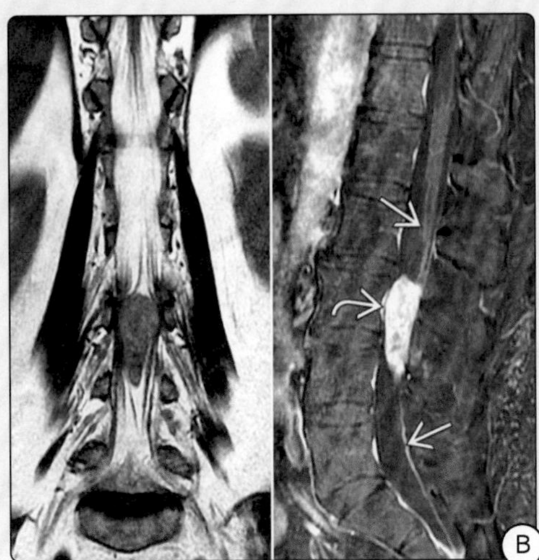

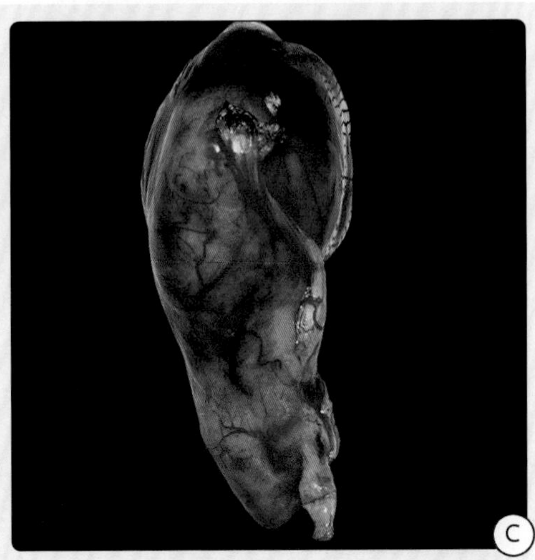

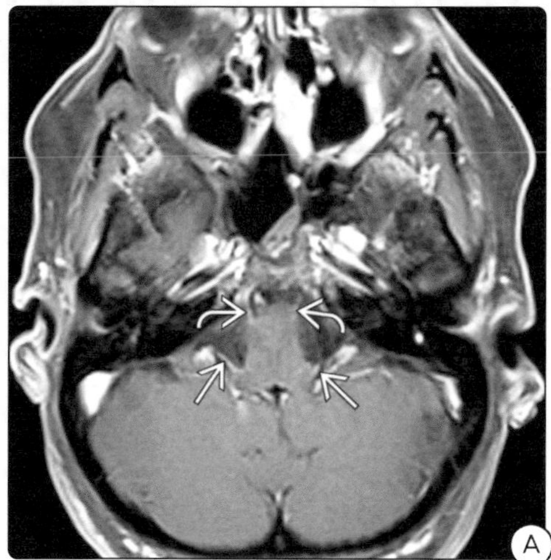

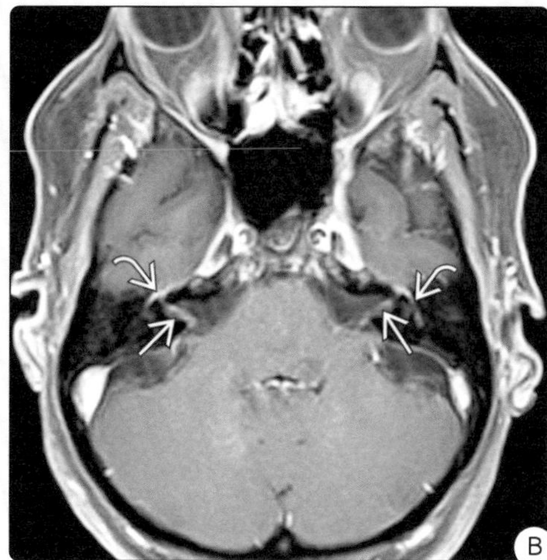

***(26-38A)*** *T1 C+ FS MR in a 47-yo woman with headaches, blurry vision, lower extremity weakness, and urinary incontinence shows bilateral enhancing CNs IX-XII ➡ and VI ➡.* ***(26-38B)*** *T1 C+ FS MR through the IACs shows enhancing CNVIII in the IACs ➡ and CNVII in the geniculate ganglions and facial nerve canals ➡.*

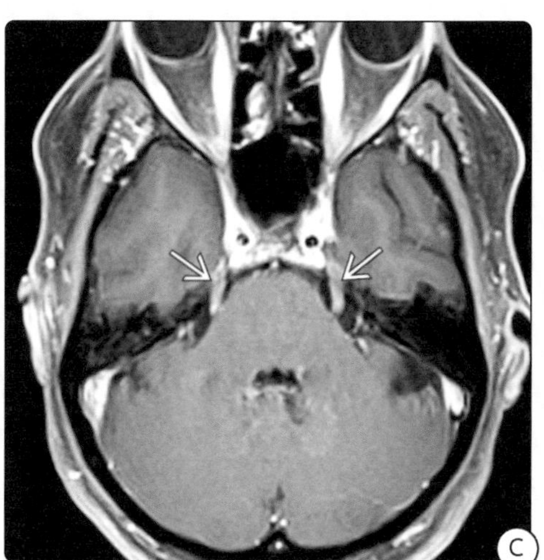

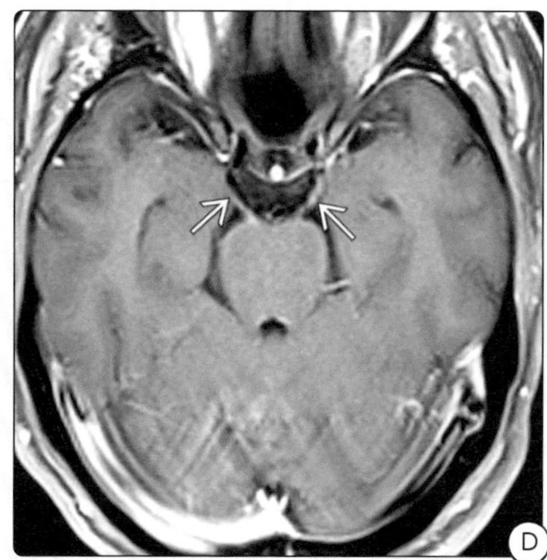

***(26-38C)*** *More cephalad T1 C+ FS MR in the same patient shows mildly enlarged but intensely enhancing trigeminal nerves ➡.* ***(26-38D)*** *T1 C+ FS MR through the midbrain shows enlarged, enhancing oculomotor nerves ➡.*

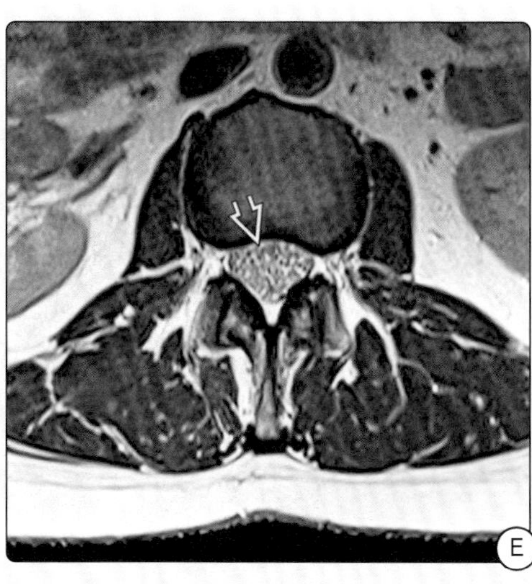

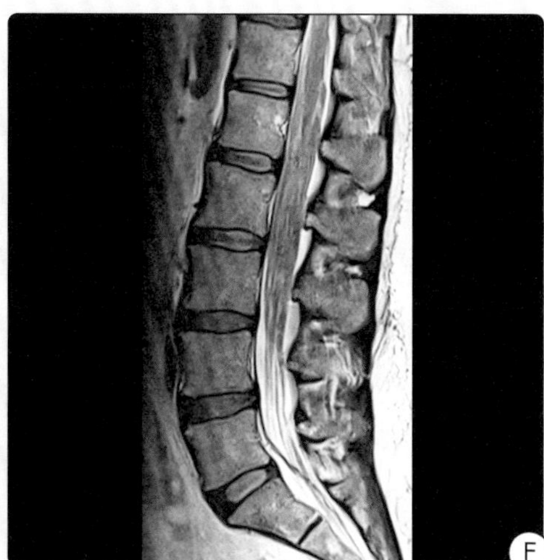

***(26-38E)*** *Axial T2 MR through the midlumbar spine shows multiple enlarged roots of the cauda equina ➡ filling and nearly effacing CSF in the canal.* ***(26-38F)*** *(L) Sagittal T2 MR shows that thickened cauda equina nerve roots fill the canal. (R) T1 C+ FS MR shows markedly thickened enhancing nerves. This is chronic interstitial demyelinating polyneuropathy (CIDP).*

# Chapter 27

# Meningiomas and Melanocytic Lesions

*Meningiomas are the most common of all brain tumors, accounting for > 1/3 of all primary intracranial neoplasms and nearly 40% of nonmalignant tumors. The 5th edition WHO separates meningiomas into a single family of neoplasms that are separated by grade into three groups: CNS WHO grades 1, 2, and 3 (formerly benign or typical meningioma, atypical meningioma, and anaplastic meningioma, respectively).*



In contrast to prior editions of the WHO classification of meningiomas, the 5th edition defines diagnostic criteria by tumor grade. Following a brief overview, we consider all three grades of meningioma in this chapter.

Following our focused and detailed discussion of meningiomas, we briefly discuss melanocytic tumors, which were assigned their own major tumor group in the 5th edition.

## Meningiomas

Meningiomas have a wide morphologic spectrum that includes numerous histopathologically defined subtypes. The 5th edition lists 15 subtypes of meningiomas (meningothelial, fibrous, transitional, psammomatous, angiomatous, microcystic, secretory, lymphoplasmacyte-rich, metaplastic, chordoid, clear cell, rhabdoid, and papillary meningiomas) plus atypical meningiomas (AMs) and anaplastic (malignant) meningiomas.

The WHO, 5th edition diagnostic criteria for meningioma include classic histopathologic features matching at least one of the meningioma subtypes, **or** suggestive histopathologic features combined with biallelic inactivation of *NF2* or other classic drivers of conventional meningioma (*TRAF7*, *AKT1*, *KLF4*, *SMO*, *PIK3CA*), clear cell meningioma (*SMARCE1*), or rhabdoid meningioma (*BAP1*), **or** (2) suggestive histopathologic features combined with a defined DNA methylation class of meningioma. The WHO, 5th edition also notes that the diagnosis of meningioma frequently requires matching of several of the above criteria.

Recent studies suggest dividing meningiomas into four consensus molecular groups: Two benign groups largely dichotomized by neurofibromatosis type 2 (NF2) status, and two clinically aggressive groups defined by their hypermetabolic transcriptome &/or their preponderance of proliferative, cell-cycling pathways.

In contrast to CNS WHO grade 1 meningiomas, CNS WHO grades 2 and 3 are associated with more aggressive clinical behavior and less favorable

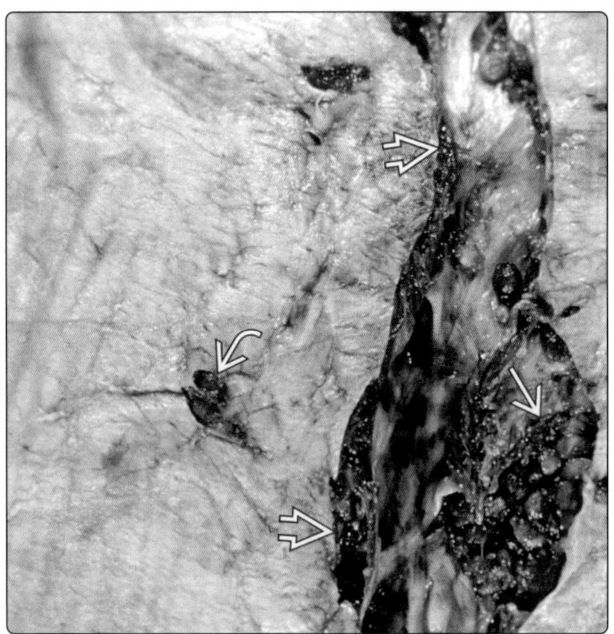

*(27-1) Close-up view of dura ➡, opened to show the superior sagittal sinus with numerous arachnoid granulations protruding into the sinus ➡, is shown. Note the small parasagittal venous lake with arachnoid granulation ➡. (Courtesy E. Ross, MD.)*

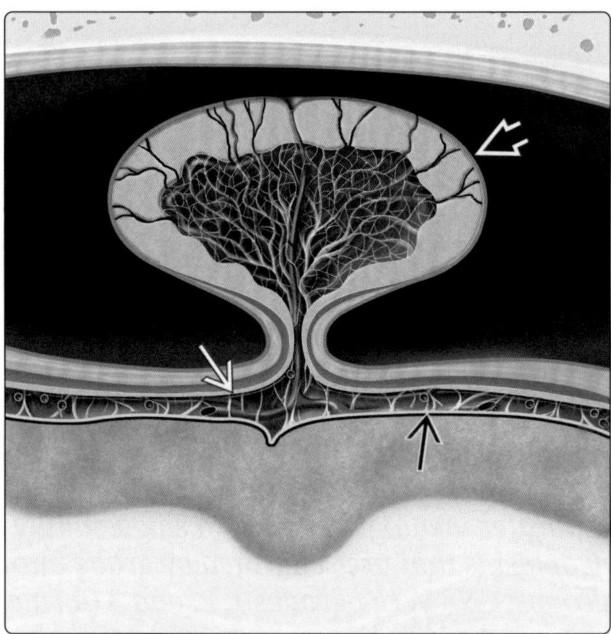

*(27-2) Graphic demonstrates pia ➡, arachnoid ➡, and arachnoid granulation projecting into venous sinus ➡. CSF from subarachnoid space is covered by a "cap" of arachnoid cells.*

outcomes. We discuss each of these three members of the meningioma family in sequence.

## Meningioma, CNS WHO Grade 1

Meningioma is a benign lesion with nonaggressive growth and a low recurrence risk. Histologically and biologically benign meningiomas correspond to WHO grade 1 and are by far the most common type, accounting for 70-80% of all meningiomas.

### Etiology

Meningiomas arise from progenitor cells that give rise to arachnoid meningothelial ("cap") cells positioned outside the thin arachnoid layer that covers the brain and spinal cord **(27-1) (27-2) (27-3)**.

Monosomy of chromosome 22, an early event in meningioma tumorigenesis, is the most frequent genetic abnormality. *NF2* mutations are detected in most meningiomas associated with NF2 and are found in 40-60% of sporadic meningiomas. *NF2* mutations occur in approximately equal frequency among all three WHO grades.

Mutations in non-*NF2* meningiomas include *TRAF7*, *KLF4*, *AKT1*, and *SMO* or *POLR2A*. These are found in ~ 1/4 of meningiomas. Most meningiomas with these non-*NF2* mutations are benign.

Higher grade meningiomas exhibit more complex genetic changes with losses on multiple chromosomes. Heterozygous or homozygous deletions of *CDKN2A* &/or *CDKN2B* and *TERT* promoter mutations are poor prognostic, grade 3-defining parameters.

### Pathology

**Location.** Tumor location is strongly associated with mutation spectrum. Although meningiomas can occur at virtually any site within the CNS, > 90% are supratentorial **(27-4)**. The most common location is parasagittal/convexity, accounting for ~ 1/2 of all meningiomas. The majority of these carry a 22q deletion &/or *NF2* mutations. Parasagittal/falx meningiomas also commonly exhibit *SMARCB1* mutations, while some convexity meningiomas have *BAP1* mutations.

Between 15-20% are located along the skull base, including the sphenoid ridge **(27-5)**. Most of these are non-*NF2* meningiomas. Non-*NF2* meningiomas have mutations in other "driver genes." Several mutations (*TRAF7*, *KLF4*, *AKT1*, *SMO*, &/or *PIK3CA*) have been identified. These non-*NF2* meningiomas are also usually benign and originate from the central or anterior skull base.

Less common supratentorial sites include the ventricles (usually in the choroid plexus glomus) and pineal region (tentorial apex).

Approximately 8-10% of intracranial meningiomas occur in the posterior fossa. Here, the cerebellopontine angle is by far the most common infratentorial site followed by the jugular foramen and foramen magnum, usually from the clivus or craniocervical junction. Meningiomas rarely arise from the squamous portion of the occipital bone.

Between 1-2% of meningiomas are entirely extracranial. Sites include the orbit (optic nerve sheath), paranasal sinuses, and nose. A few typical meningiomas (TMs) arise within the skull ("intradiploic" or "intraosseous" meningioma) and are most common where arachnoid granulations occur.

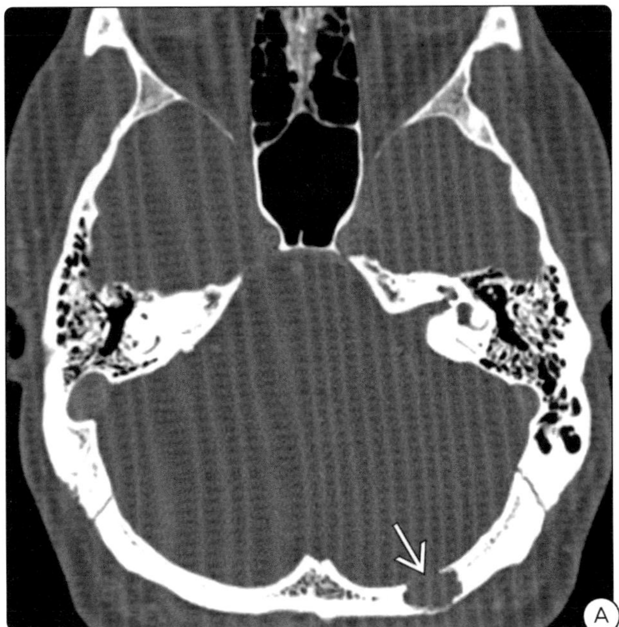

(27-3A) *A 34-yo man had a CT angiogram for trauma. A well-delineated scalloped lesion ➡ in the left occipital squama is likely an intraosseous arachnoid granulation.*

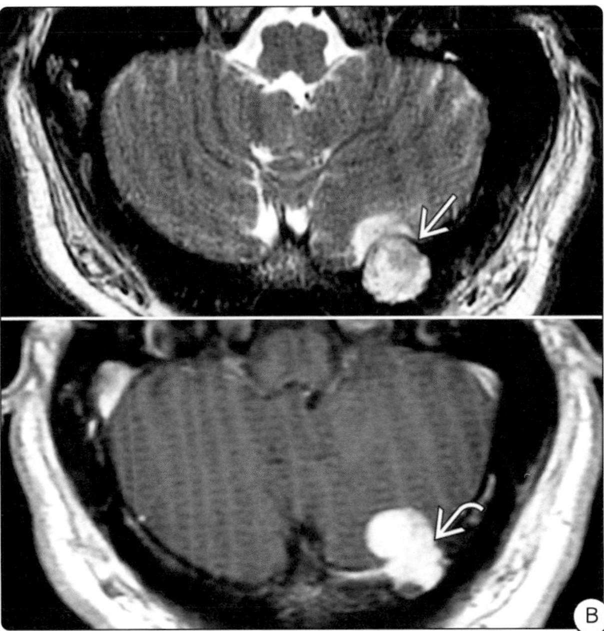

(27-3B) *14 years later, the patient was reimaged. Note occipital expansile, T2-hyperintense, dumbbell-shaped mass ➡ (top) that enhances intensely ➡ (bottom); this is meningioma originating from an intraosseous arachnoid granulation.*

**Size and Number.** Meningiomas vary widely in size. Most are small (< 1 cm) and found incidentally at imaging or autopsy. Some—especially those arising in the anterior fossa from the olfactory groove—may attain large size before causing symptoms.

Meningiomas can be solitary (90%) or multiple. Multiple meningiomas occur in **NF2** as well as in **multiple meningiomatosis syndrome**.

### MENINGIOMA: LOCATION

**General**

- Supratentorial (90%), infratentorial (8-10%)
- Multiple [10%; neurofibromatosis type 2 (NF2), meningiomatosis]

**Sites**

- Most common (60-70%)
  - Parasagittal (25%)
  - Convexity (20%)
  - Sphenoid ridge (15-20%)
- Less common (20-25%)
  - Posterior fossa (8-10%)
  - Olfactory groove (5-10%)
  - Parasellar (5-10%)
- Rare (2%)
  - Intraventricular
  - Pineal region/tentorial apex
  - Extracranial (optic nerve sheath, sinuses, nose)
  - Intraosseous (diploic space, often associated with arachnoid granulations)

**Gross Pathology.** Meningiomas have two general configurations: A round ("globose") **(27-5) (27-6) (27-7) (27-8)** and a flat, sheet-like or carpet-like ("en plaque") appearance **(27-16)**. Most meningiomas are well-demarcated, firm, rubbery, or gritty masses that have a broad base of dural attachment. As they grow, meningiomas typically invaginate toward adjacent brain. A CSF-vascular "cleft" is often present between the tumor and underlying cortex **(27-6) (27-7)**.

In contrast to higher grade meningiomas, most CNS WHO grade 1 meningiomas displace and compress, but do not invade, adjacent brain.

Meningiomas often cause reactive nonneoplastic thickening of the adjacent dura (dural tail sign on imaging) **(27-9) (27-10)**. They commonly invade dural venous sinuses and may extend through the dura to involve the skull, inducing calvarial hyperostosis **(27-17)**.

Although small intratumoral "microcysts" are not uncommon, gross cystic change is rare. Frank hemorrhage is uncommon, occurring in only 1-2% of cases **(27-20)**.

Rarely, metastasis from an extracranial primary to a meningioma occurs. Here, one primary tumor is the recipient and another tumor is the donor. Meningioma is the most common tumor to harbor metastases. Tumor-to-tumor metastasis, a.k.a. **"collision tumors,"** are typically lung or breast metastases to a histologically benign meningioma.

**Microscopic Features.** Meningiomas exhibit a wide spectrum of histologic appearances with 15 subtypes identified in the 2021 WHO classification. Of these subtypes, the most common are the **meningothelial, fibrous, and transitional** variants.

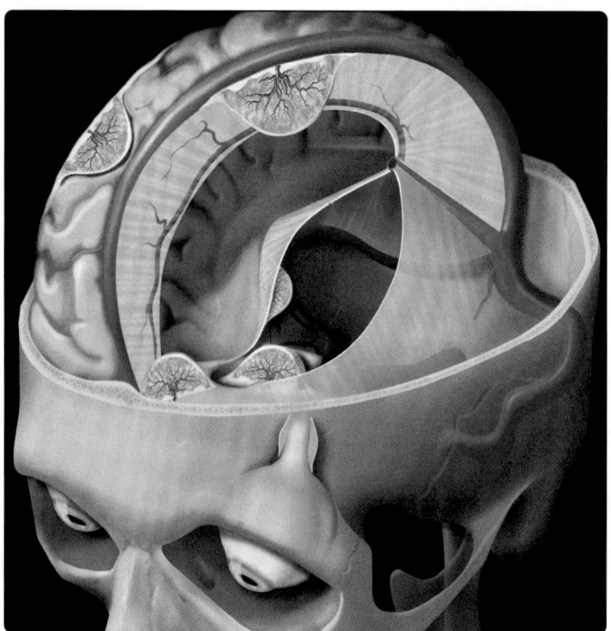

***(27-4) The most common meningioma sites are convexity, parafalcine, followed by sphenoid ridge, olfactory groove, sella/parasellar region. 8-10% are infratentorial. Extracranial sites include optic nerve sheath, nose, and paranasal sinuses.***

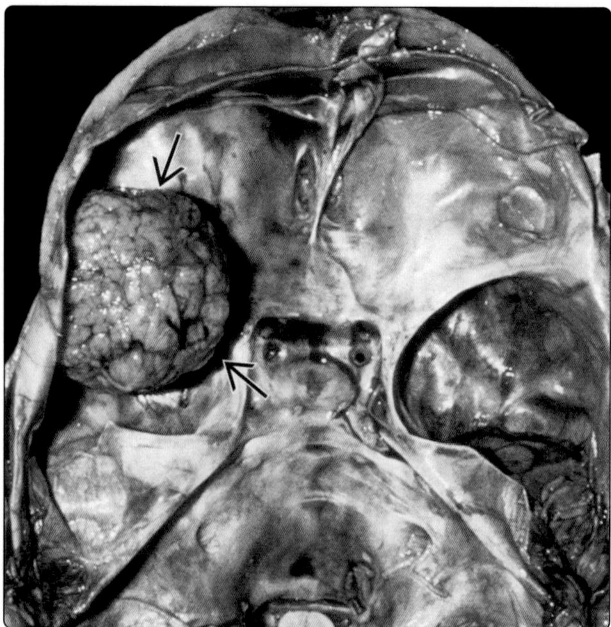

***(27-5) Autopsy specimen demonstrates classic globose meningioma ⇒ as a round, "bosselated" mass with a flat surface toward the dura. (Courtesy R. Hewlett, MD.)***

By definition, CNS WHO grade 1 meningiomas carry a low risk of recurrence &/or aggressive growth. Their mitotic index is low with MIB-1 usually < 1%. Brain invasion is absent.

Features of brain invasion &/or more aggressive growth can arise in any meningioma subtype. Histologically benign-appearing meningiomas that show *unequivocal* brain invasion (not isolated perivascular spread or indentation of the brain without pial breach) are designated as CNS WHO grade 2 neoplasms.

Because two specific histologic subtypes—chordoid and clear cell meningiomas—have a higher likelihood of recurrence, they are also assigned CNS WHO grade 2.

## Clinical Issues

**Epidemiology.** Recent epidemiologic data suggest that meningioma is the most frequently diagnosed primary brain tumor, accounting for > 1/3 of all reported CNS tumors. Grade 1 meningiomas account for 80-85% of these tumors.

Many meningiomas are small and discovered incidentally, often at imaging or autopsy. The lifetime risk of developing meningioma is ~ 1%; meningiomas are found in 1-3% of autopsies.

Multiple meningiomas are common in patients with NF2 and non-NF2 hereditary multiple meningioma syndromes **(27-8)**. Sporadic multiple (i.e., not syndromic) meningiomas occur in ~ 10% of cases.

**Demographics.** Meningiomas are classically tumors of middle-aged and older adults. Peak occurrence is in the sixth and seventh decades (mean = 65 years). Although meningioma accounts for slightly < 3% of primary brain tumors in children, meningioma still represents the most common dura-based neoplasm in this age group. Many (but by no means all) are related to NF2. NF2-related meningiomas occur at a significantly younger age compared with nonsyndromic meningiomas.

Meningioma is one of the few brain tumors that exhibits a female predominance. Women are almost twice as likely men to develop CNS WHO grade 1 meningiomas. The F:M ratio varies with age, peaking at 3.5-4:1 in premenopausal women in the 35- to 44-year age group.

**Presentation.** Symptoms relate to size and tumor location. Less than 10% of meningiomas become symptomatic.

**Natural History.** Longitudinal studies have demonstrated that most meningiomas < 2.5 cm grow very slowly—if at all—over five years. The majority of small, asymptomatic, incidentally discovered meningiomas show minimal growth and are usually followed with serial imaging.

Malignant degeneration of a CNS WHO grade 1 meningioma into an atypical or anaplastic variant is rare. Extracranial metastases are exceptionally rare, occurring in 1 in 1,000 cases. When they do occur, metastases are generally to the lung or axial skeleton. Metastases from both benign and atypical/malignant meningiomas have been reported.

**Treatment Options.** Stratified treatment risk:benefit ratios vary, not just with tumor type and grade, but also with size and location, vascular supply, and presence or absence of a brain/tumor cleavage plane.

Image-guided surgery with resection of symptomatic lesions can be curative. The major factor associated with meningioma recurrence is subtotal resection.

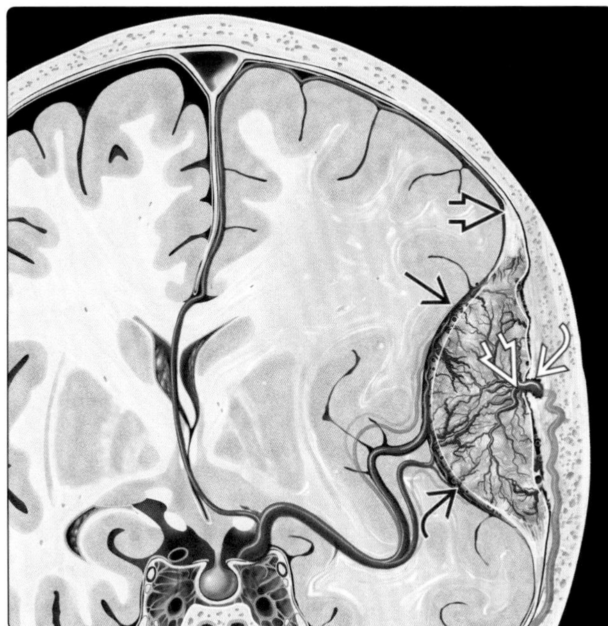

(27-6) *Classic meningioma has a broad base toward dura, reactive dural thickening (dural "tail") , enostotic "spur" , CSF-vascular "cleft" . MMA supplies tumor core in sunburst pattern ; pial vessels supply periphery .*

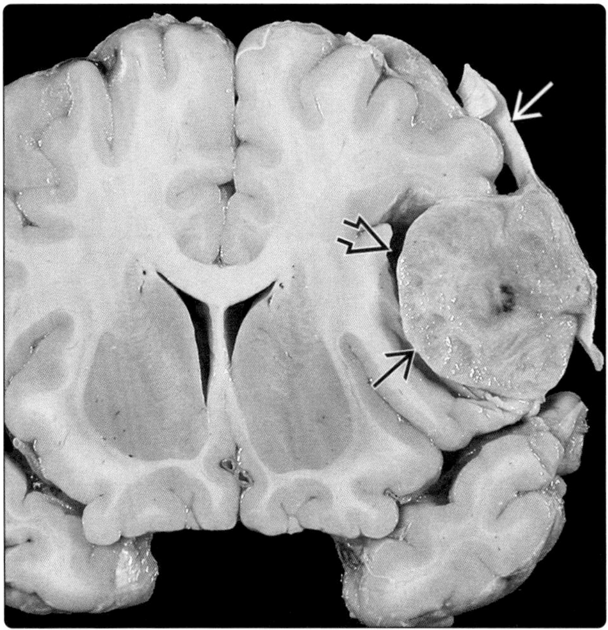

(27-7) *Autopsy specimen shows classic globose meningioma . Note prominent CSF-vascular "cleft"  and reactive dural thickening  (dural tail sign).*

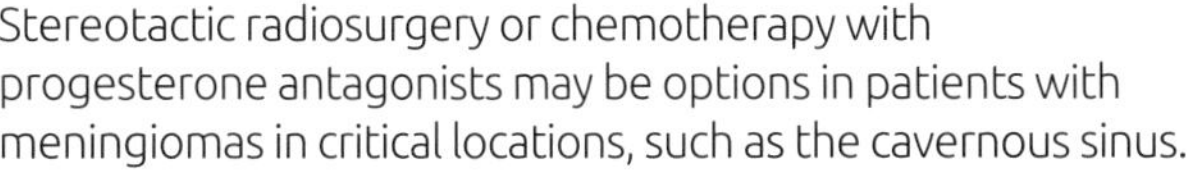

Stereotactic radiosurgery or chemotherapy with progesterone antagonists may be options in patients with meningiomas in critical locations, such as the cavernous sinus.

**MENINGIOMA: CLINICAL ISSUES**

**Epidemiology**
- Most common intracranial primary neoplasm
  - 36% of all primary CNS neoplasms
- Most are asymptomatic
  - Found incidentally at imaging/autopsy (1-3%)
- Solitary (> 90%)
  - Multiple in NF2, meningiomatosis

**Demographics**
- F:M = 2:1
  - Sex difference greatest prior to menopause
- Median age at diagnosis = 65 years
- Rare in children unless NF2

**Natural History**
- Grows slowly
- Rarely metastasizes

## Imaging

**General Features.** The general appearance of a CNS WHO grade 1 meningioma is a round or lobulated, sharply demarcated, extraaxial, dura-based mass that buckles the cortex inward. A discernible CSF-vascular "cleft" is often present, especially on MR.

Unequivocal parenchymal invasion—not just perivascular spread or indentation of the brain without breaching the pia—is uncommon. When present, it upgrades the tumor to atypical meningioma (AM), CNS WHO grade 2.

Meningioma-associated cysts are found in 4-7% of cases. These can be intra- or extratumoral. Occasionally, pools of CSF are trapped between the tumor and adjacent brain (creating the CSF-vascular "cleft"). Partially or almost completely cystic meningiomas occur but are rare.

### CT Findings

***NECT.*** Almost 3/4 of meningiomas are mildly to moderately hyperdense compared with cortex **(27-14A)**. About 1/4 are isodense **(27-12)** **(27-15A)**. Hypodense meningiomas occur but are uncommon **(27-19A)** **(27-13)**. Frank necrosis or hemorrhage is rare **(27-20A)**.

Peritumoral vasogenic edema, seen as confluent hypodensity in the adjacent brain, is present in ~ 60% of all cases.

Approximately 25% of TMs demonstrate calcification **(27-11)**. Focal globular or more diffuse, sand-like ("psammomatous") calcifications occur.

Bone CT may show hyperostosis that varies from minimal to striking **(27-17)**. Hyperostosis is often but not invariably associated with tumor invasion. Striking enlargement of an adjacent paranasal sinus may occur with skull base meningiomas **(27-18)**. Bone lysis or frank destruction can also occur. Bone involvement by meningioma occurs with both benign and malignant meningiomas and is not predictive of tumor grade.

***CECT.*** The vast majority of meningiomas enhance strongly and uniformly **(27-12)** **(27-14)**.

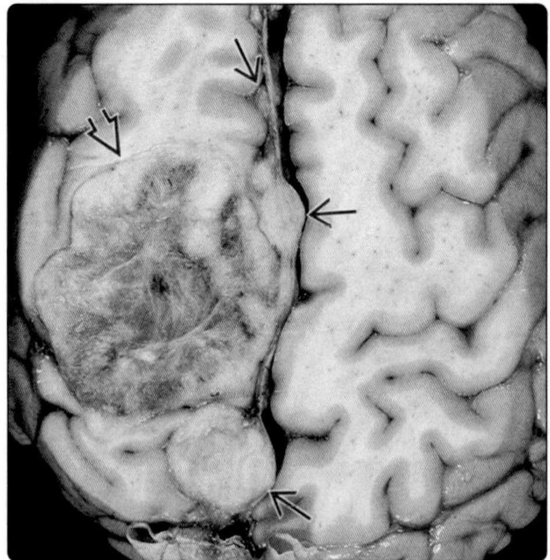

***(27-8) Autopsy specimen shows meningioma invaginating into brain ⮚, multiple falcine meningiomas ⮚. (Courtesy R. Hewlett, MD.)***

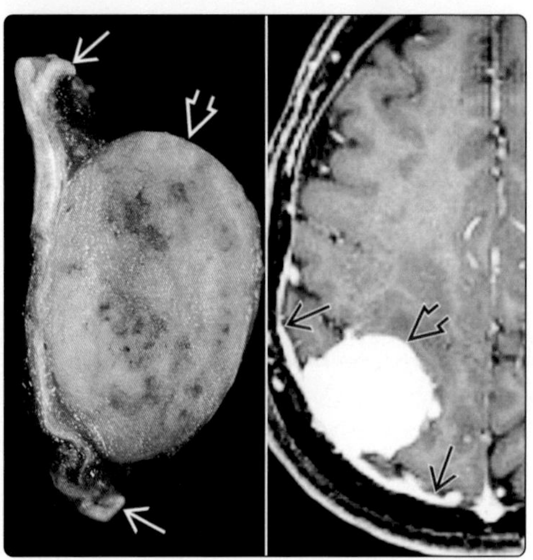

***(27-9) (L) Resected meningioma ⮚ with reactive dural thickening ⮚. (R) T1 C+ shows enhancing meningioma ⮚ with dural "tail" ⮚.***

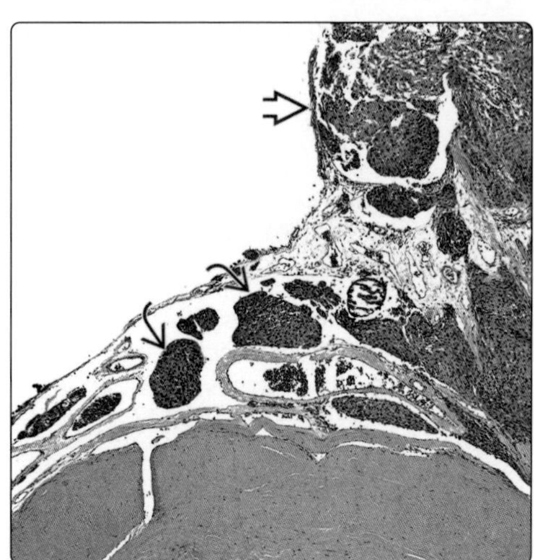

***(27-10) Micrograph of meningioma ⮚ with a tapering edge of tumor ⮚ ("tail") extending laterally at tumor edge. (From DP: Neuro.)***

### MR Findings

***General Features.*** The majority of meningiomas are isointense with cortex on all sequences **(27-14)**. Between 10-25% of cases demonstrate changes suggestive of cyst formation or necrosis **(27-13)**, although frank hemorrhage is uncommon.

***T1WI.*** Meningiomas are typically iso- to slightly hypointense compared with cortex. Predominant hypointensity on T1WI and hyperintensity on T2WI suggest the microcystic subtype of TM **(27-19)**.

***T2WI.*** Most meningiomas are iso- to moderately hyperintense compared with cortex **(27-23A)**. These are associated with a "soft" consistency at surgery, whereas T2-/FLAIR-hypointense tumors tend to be "hard" and somewhat gritty. Densely fibrotic and calcified meningiomas (appearing as "brain rocks" on NECT) can be very hypointense.

The CSF-vascular "cleft" **(27-6)** is especially well delineated on T2WI and is seen as a hyperintense rim interposed between the tumor and brain **(27-21D)** **(27-23A)**. A number of "flow voids" representing displaced vessels are often seen within the "cleft."

Sometimes, a sunburst pattern that represents the dural vascular supply to the tumor can be identified radiating toward the periphery of the mass **(27-22)**.

***FLAIR.*** Meningioma signal intensity varies from iso- to hyperintense relative to brain **(27-14E)**. FLAIR is very useful for depicting peritumoral edema, which is found with ~ 1/2 of all meningiomas **(27-21E)**. Peritumoral edema is related to the presence of pial blood supply and VEGF expression, not tumor size or grade. Some small meningiomas incite striking peritumoral edema, whereas some very large masses exhibit virtually none.

Pools of CSF trapped in the cleft between tumor and brain (nonneoplastic "peritumoral cysts") are usually proteinaceous and may not suppress completely on FLAIR.

***T2* (GRE, SWI).*** T2* sequences are helpful to depict intratumoral calcification. "Blooming" secondary to intratumoral hemorrhage is rare.

***T1 C+.*** Virtually all meningiomas, including densely calcified "brain rocks" and intraosseous tumors, demonstrate at least some enhancement following contrast administration. Over 95% enhance strongly and homogeneously **(27-15B)** **(27-14F)**.

A dural "tail" is seen in the majority of meningiomas and varies from a relatively focal area adjacent to the tumor **(27-9)** to dural thickening and enhancement that extends far beyond the site of tumor attachment. The dural "tail" often enhances more intensely and more uniformly than the tumor itself. A dural tail sign is not pathognomonic of meningioma, as it occasionally occurs with schwannomas or pituitary macroadenomas.

Most of the enhancing dural "tail" represents benign, reactive dural thickening, although small tumor foci can be seen adjacent to the main tumor mass **(27-10)**. Tumor extending 1 cm beyond the base of the tumor is rare.

Nonenhancing *intratumoral* cysts are seen in 5% of cases **(27-13)**. Nonneoplastic *peritumoral* cysts do not enhance. Enhancement around the rim of a cyst suggests the presence of marginal tumor in the cyst wall, so complete cyst resection is recommended if technically feasible.

***DWI.*** Most meningiomas do not restrict on DWI.

***Perfusion MR.*** Perfusion MR may be helpful in distinguishing CNS WHO grade 1 tumors from atypical/malignant meningiomas. High rCBV in the lesion or in the surrounding edema suggests a more aggressive tumor grade.

***MRS.*** Alanine (Ala; peak at 1.48 ppm) is often elevated in meningioma although glutamate-glutamine (Glx; peak at 2.1-2.6 ppm) and glutathione (GSH; peak at 2.95 ppm) may be more specific potential markers.

### Angiography

***CTA, MRA/MRV.*** CTA is very helpful in detecting dural venous sinus invasion or occlusion. Although it may be helpful in depicting the general status of the vascular supply to a meningioma **(27-21B)**, DSA is best for detailed delineation of tumor vascularity prior to embolization or surgery. Tumor invasion of major dural venous sinuses is especially well depicted on MRV.

***DSA.*** The classic angiographic appearance of a meningioma is a radial "sunburst" of vessels extending from the base of the tumor toward its periphery **(27-22)**. Dural vessels supply the core or center of the lesion, radiating outward from the vascular pedicle of the tumor **(27-24A)**. Pial vessels from internal carotid artery branches may become "parasitized" and supply the periphery of the mass **(27-24C)**.

A prolonged vascular "blush" that persists late into the venous phase is typical. In some cases, arteriovenous shunting with the appearance of "early draining" veins occurs **(27-24B)**. Careful examination of the venous phase should be conducted to detect dural sinus invasion or occlusion.

Preoperative embolization with tumor devascularization may substantially reduce operative time and blood loss. Careful delineation of tumor blood supply, including "dangerous" extra- to intracranial anastomoses, is essential to procedure success.

#### MENINGIOMA: IMAGING

**General**
- Round or flat ("en plaque"), dura based
- Extraaxial mass with "cleft" between tumor, brain

**CT**
- Hyperdense (70-75%)
- Calcified (20-25%)
- Cysts (peri- or intratumoral) (10-15%)
- Hemorrhage rare
- > 90% enhance

**MR**
- Usually isointense with gray matter
- CSF-vascular "cleft"
- ± vascular "flow voids"
- Strong, often heterogeneous, enhancement (> 98%)
- Dural "tail" (60%)

**Angiography**
- "Sunburst" vascularity
- Dural arteries to outside, pial to inside
- Prolonged, dense vascular "blush"

## Differential Diagnosis

The major differential diagnosis of TM is **AM** or **anaplastic (malignant) meningioma**. Although there are no pathognomonic imaging features that reliably distinguish grade 1 tumors from these more aggressive variants,

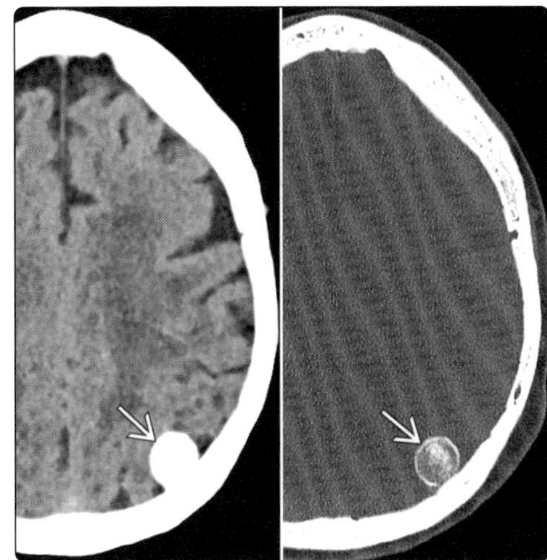

***(27-11)** NECT in 88-yo woman with soft tissue (L), bone algorithm (R) shows densely calcified meningioma ➡. This is an incidental finding.*

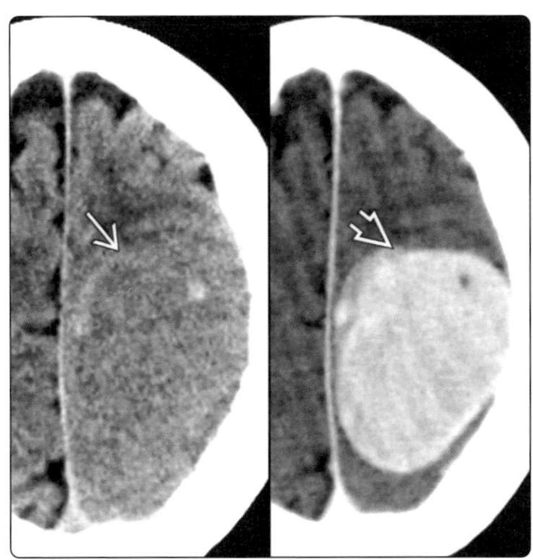

***(27-12)** NECT (L) and CECT (R) show isodense left convexity mass ➡ that enhances uniformly ➡. This is classic meningioma, WHO grade 1.*

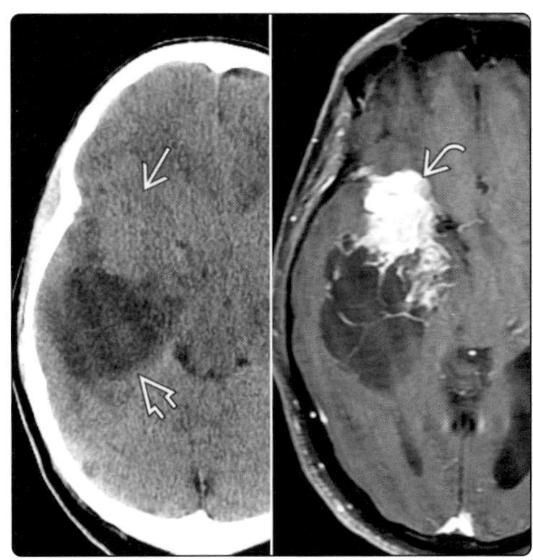

***(27-13)** (L) NECT shows mixed cystic ➡, solid ➡ mass. (R) T1 C+ shows enhancing solid ➡, cystic components of WHO grade 1 meningioma.*

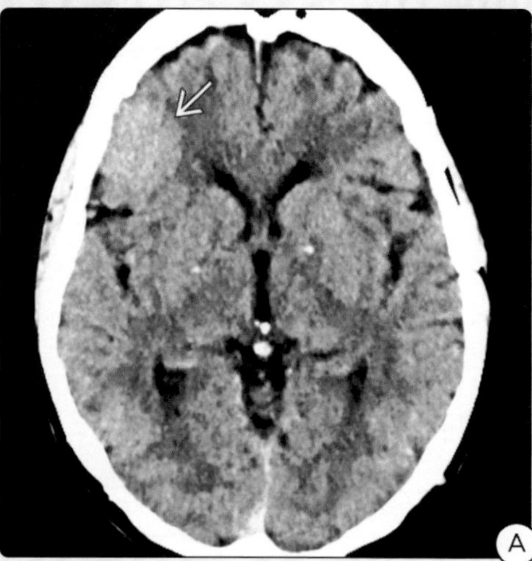

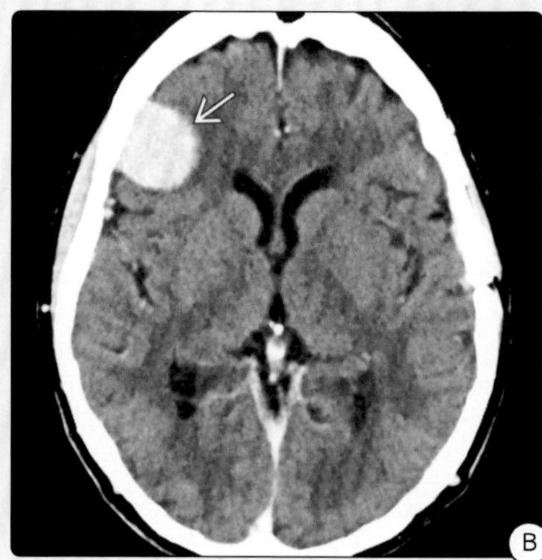

*(27-14A) Axial T1WI in a 69-yo woman shows a rounded, slightly hyperdense frontal lobe mass that abuts the inner table of the skull ➡. (27-14B) CECT in the same case shows the mass ➡ enhances intensely and uniformly with a broad base abutting the skull.*

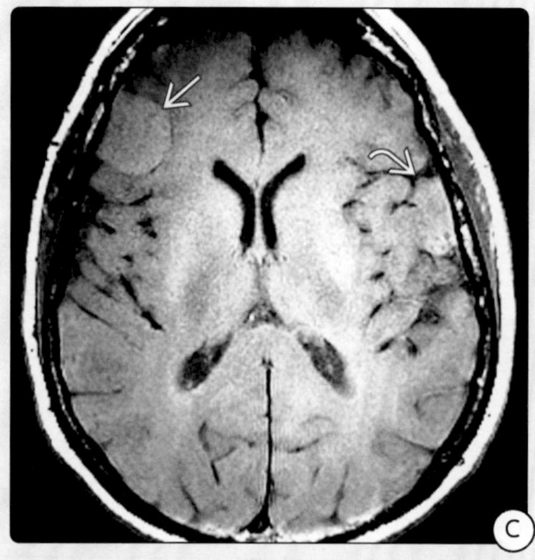

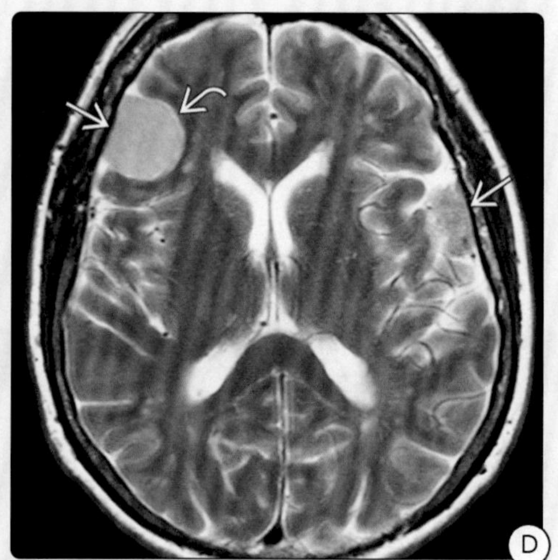

*(27-14C) T1WI in the same case shows the mass ➡ is isointense with the underlying brain. Note a 2nd, smaller isointense mass ➡ adjacent to the left sylvian fissure. (27-14D) Both masses ➡ are nearly isointense with cortex. The right frontal mass is extraaxial and indents the brain. Note thin rim of CSF and compressed cortex ➡ pushed medially by the invaginating mass.*

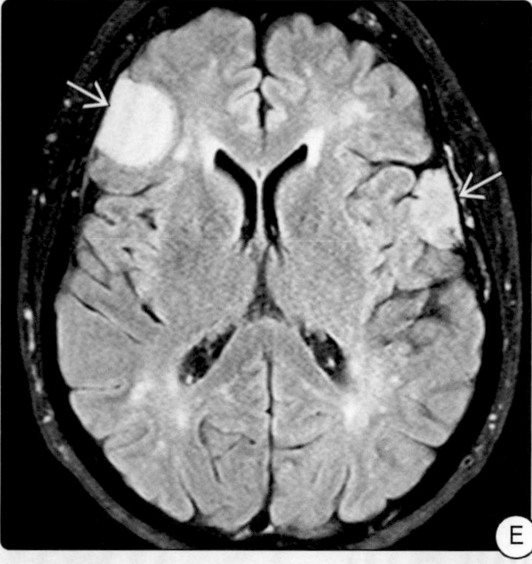

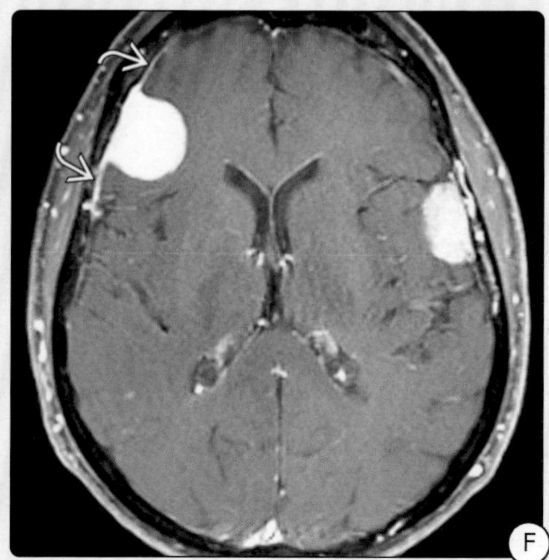

*(27-14E) Both masses ➡ are slightly hyperintense to brain on FLAIR. (27-14F) Both masses enhance intensely on T1 C+ FS. Note thickened, reactive dural "tail" ➡ adjacent to the right frontal mass. Classic meningioma, meningothelial subtype, CNS WHO grade 1.*

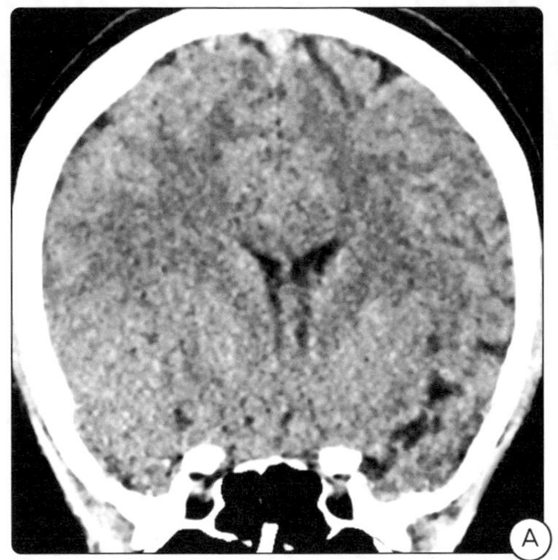


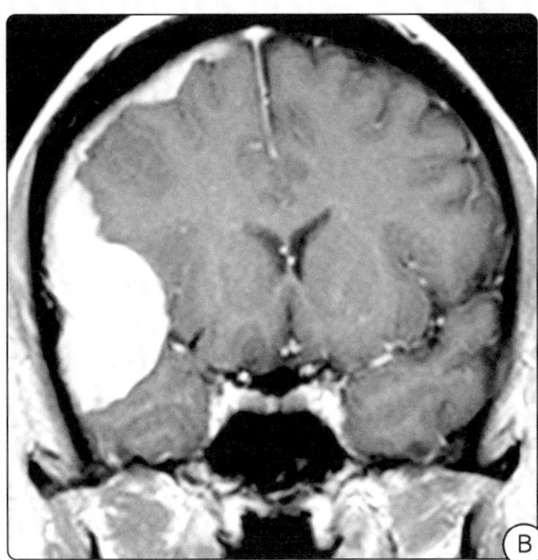


***(27-15A)*** *Coronal NECT in a 43-yo woman with headaches shows subtle effacement of the right sylvian fissure with slight left-to-right subfalcine herniation of the lateral ventricles.* ***(27-15B)*** *Coronal T1 C+ MR in the same case shows extensive "en plaque" meningioma. Because they are often isodense with cortex, noncalcified meningiomas can be difficult to detect on NECT scans.*

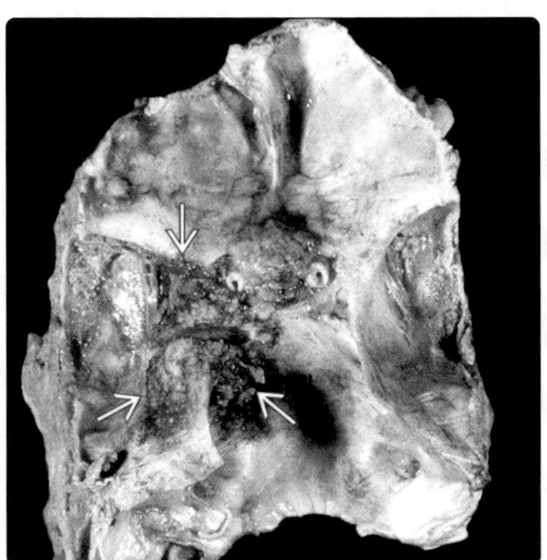

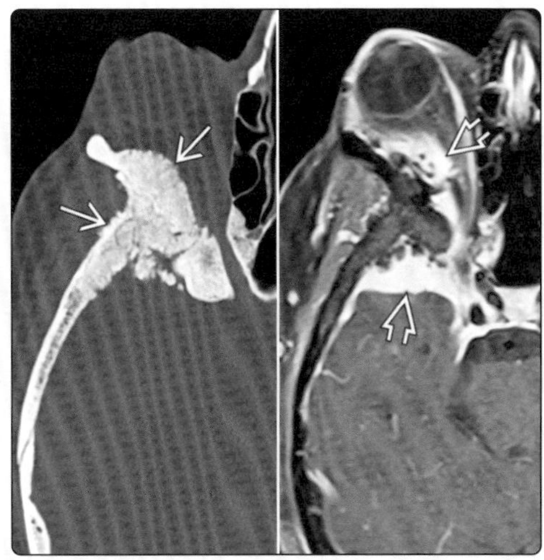

***(27-16)*** *Autopsy specimen shows an extensive skull base "en plaque" meningioma. Such tumors often affect > 1 compartment and infiltrate and thicken bone. The sphenoid wing and orbit are favored sites. (Courtesy R. Hewlett, MD.)* ***(27-17)*** *(L) Bone CT shows striking hyperostosis of the sphenoid wing in a middle-aged woman with proptosis. (R) T1 C+ FS shows enhancing "en plaque" meningioma.*

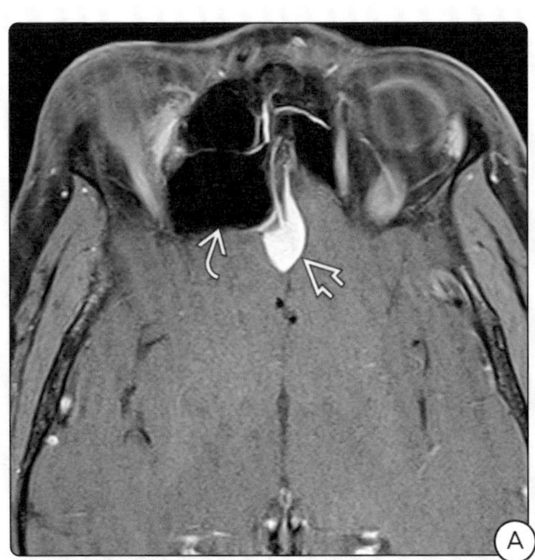


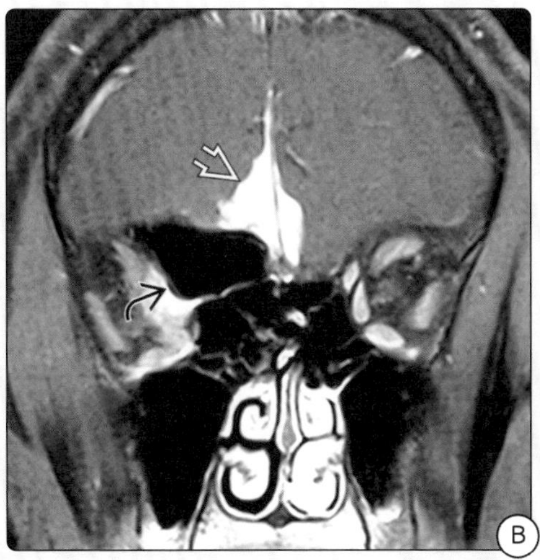


***(27-18A)*** *Occasionally, skull base meningiomas adjacent to a paranasal sinus cause massive enlargement of the sinus, a condition known as pneumosinus dilatans. This relatively small meningioma caused massive enlargement of the frontal sinus.* ***(27-18B)*** *Coronal T1 C+ FS in the same case shows the meningioma and markedly enlarged aerated orbital plate of the right frontal bone.*

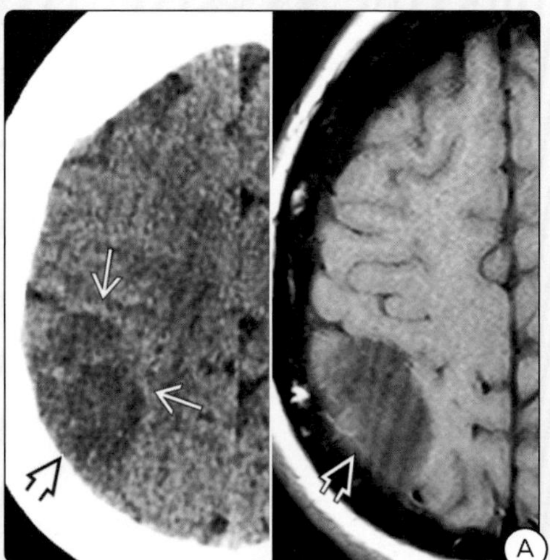


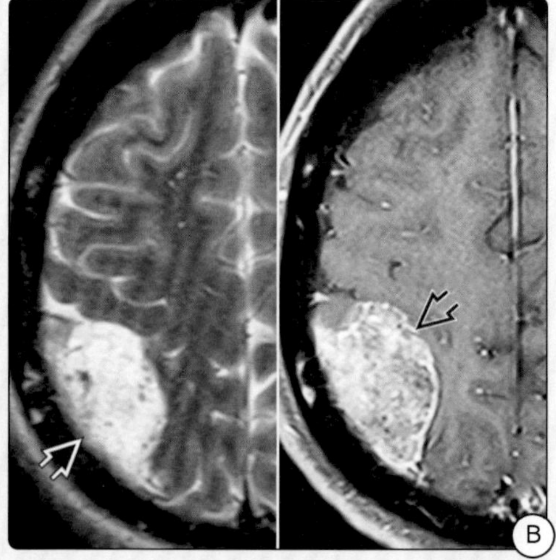


***(27-19A)** (L) NECT shows a hypodense right parietal mass. Note inward displacement of the adjacent cortex, suggesting that the mass is extraaxial. (R) The mass is well delineated, hypointense on T1WI. **(27-19B)** (L) The mass is very hyperintense on T2WI. (R) The mass enhances strongly but heterogeneously on T1 C+ FS. This is microcystic meningioma, CNS WHO grade 1.*

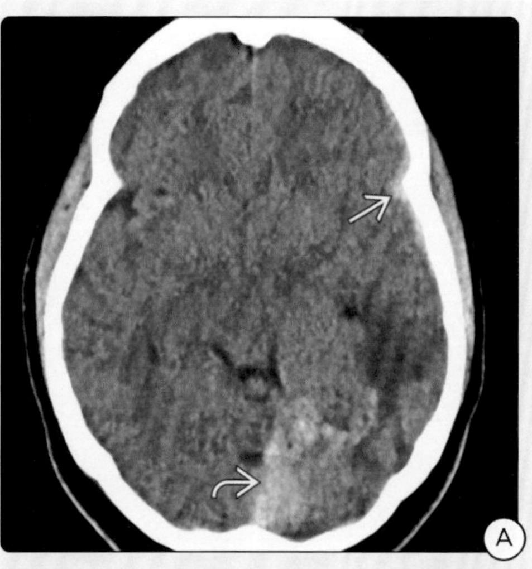


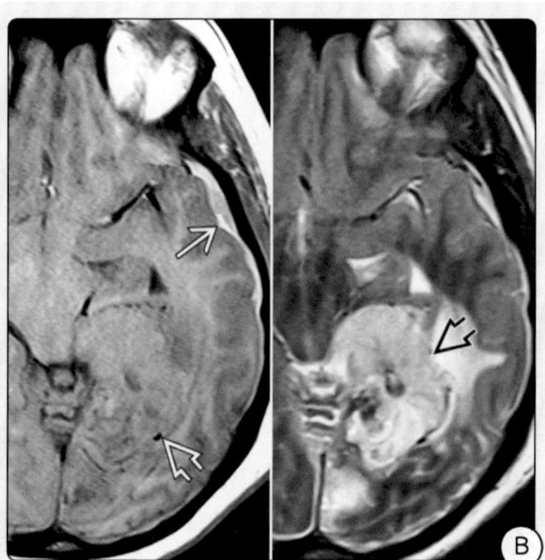


***(27-20A)** NECT in a 25-yo woman with worsening headache, nausea, and vomiting who presented with right-sided dysmetria shows a heterogeneously hyperdense left occipital mass and a thin ipsilateral subdural hematoma. **(27-20B)** (L) T1WI shows a heterogeneous, mostly isointense left occipital mass and subacute subdural hematoma. (R) The mass is heterogeneously hyperintense on T2WI.*

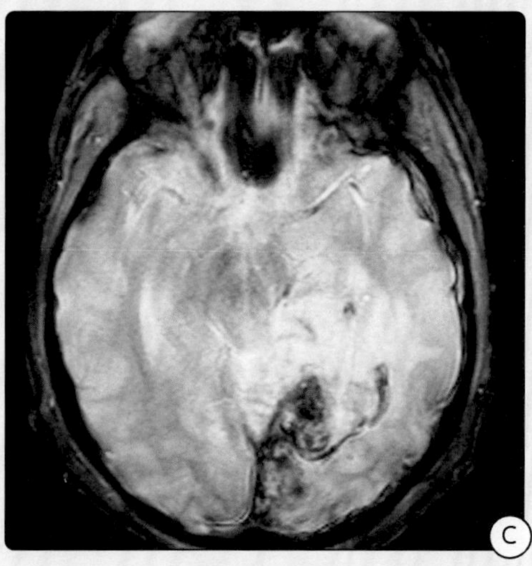


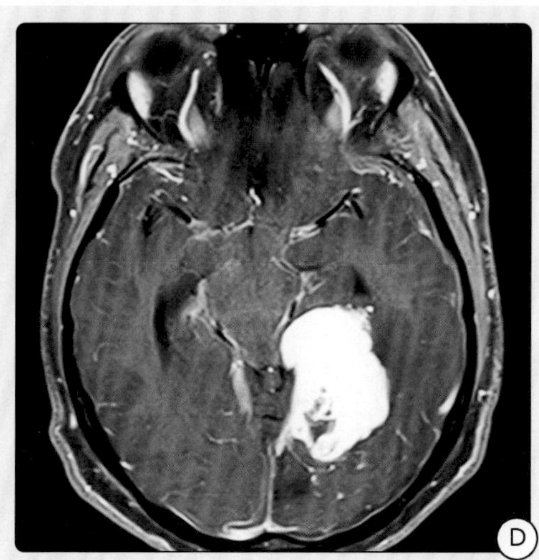


***(27-20C)** T2* GRE shows "blooming" hemorrhage within the mass, adjacent sulci, and the subdural hematoma. **(27-20D)** T1 C+ FS shows the mass enhances intensely and uniformly except for the intratumoral hemorrhage. Hemorrhagic meningioma, CNS WHO grade 1, was found at surgery.*

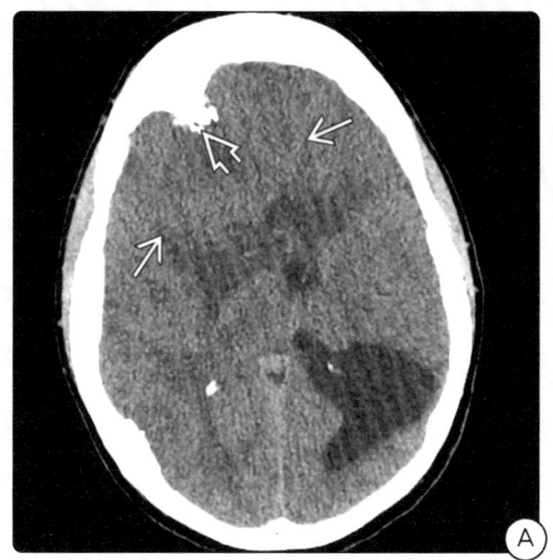

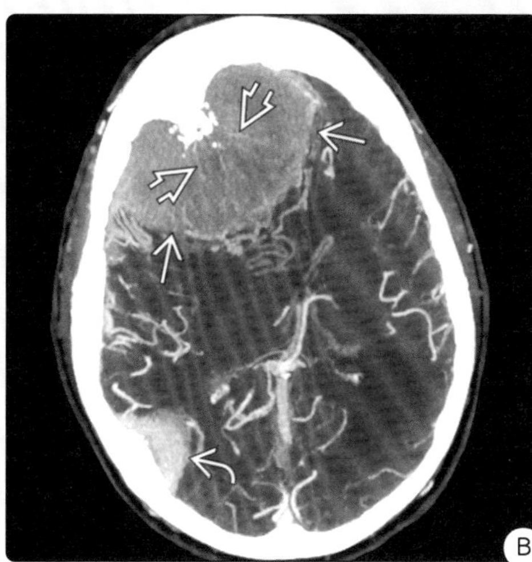

***(27-21A)*** *Axial NECT in a 48-yo woman with headaches shows a large isodense right frontal lobe mass ➡ adjacent to thickened calvarium with a prominent enostotic "spur" ➡.* ***(27-21B)*** *MIP of the CT angiogram in the same case shows intense, early enhancement in the mass ➡ with linear vessels ➡ radiating outwards from the enostotic "spur." A 2nd enhancing mass ➡ is present.*

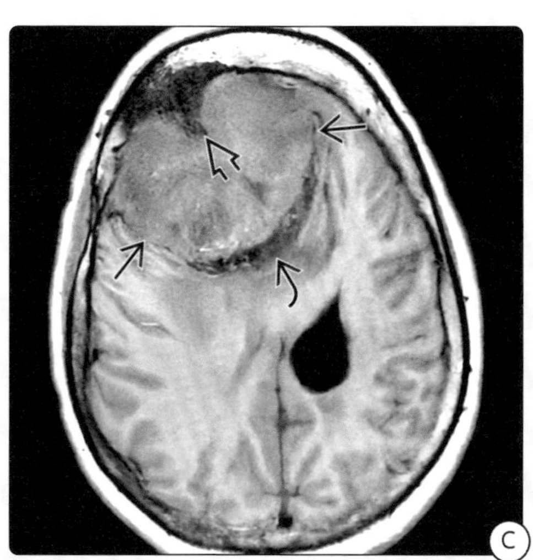

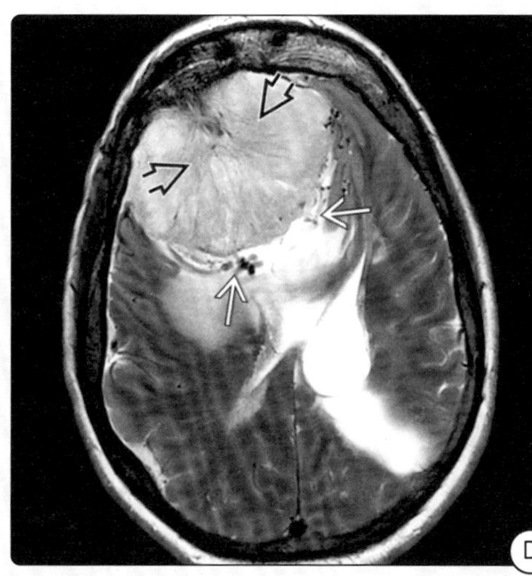

***(27-21C)*** *T1WI shows the huge right frontal mass ➡ is centered on a thick enostotic "spur" ➡ originating from the inner table of the calvarium. Hypointense cleft ➡ surrounding the mass is mostly CSF-like in signal intensity.* ***(27-21D)*** *The mass is hyperintense on T2WI. Prominent internal vasculature ➡ radiates outwards from the enostotic "spur" in a sunburst pattern. Note enlarged vessels ➡ in CSF "cleft" around the mass.*

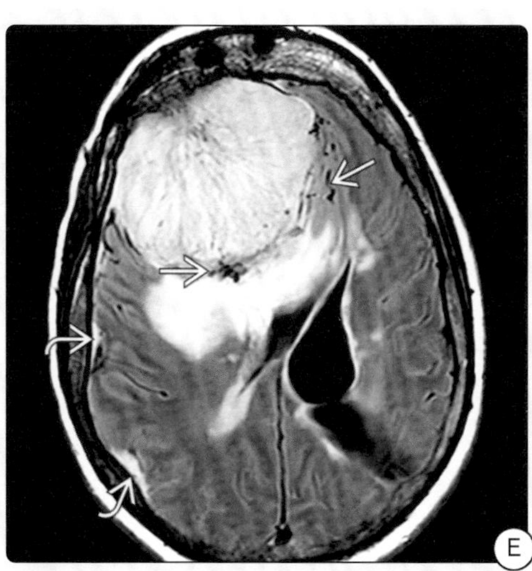

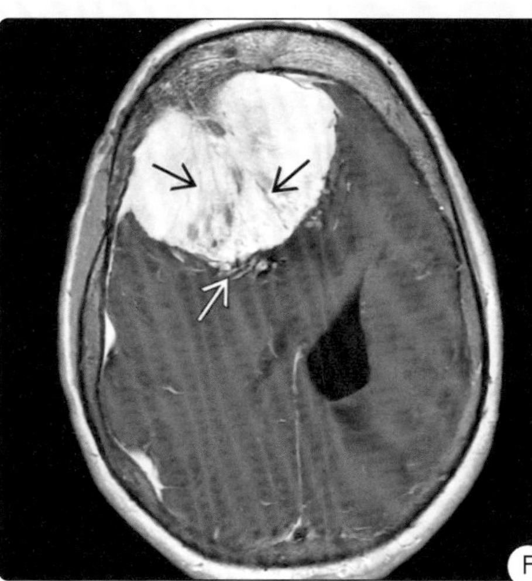

***(27-21E)*** *The mass is very hyperintense on FLAIR. Note prominent vascular "flow voids" ➡ surrounding the tumor. Two other small dural masses ➡ are present.* ***(27-21F)*** *The dural-based masses enhance intensely on T1 C+ FS. The linear hypointense "flow voids" ➡ within the mass are especially notable as are the enhancing vessels (probably draining veins) ➡ in the CSF-vascular "cleft." This is chordoid meningioma, CNS WHO grade 2.*

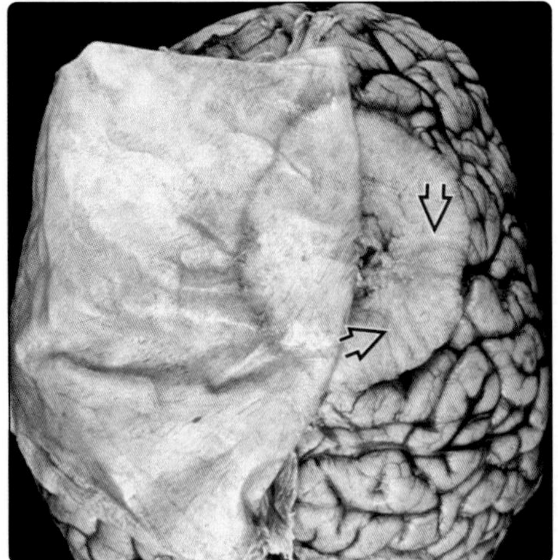

*(27-22) Autopsy shows convexity meningioma with dural attachment, "sunburst" of vessels radiating outward ⮚. (Courtesy AFIP Archives.)*

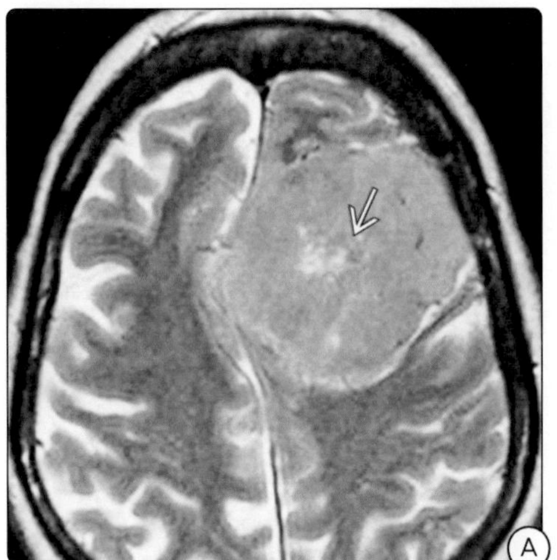


*(27-23A) T2WI shows an isointense convexity meningioma. Central hyperintensity ➡ is where dural vessels enter the mass (see Fig. 27-6).*

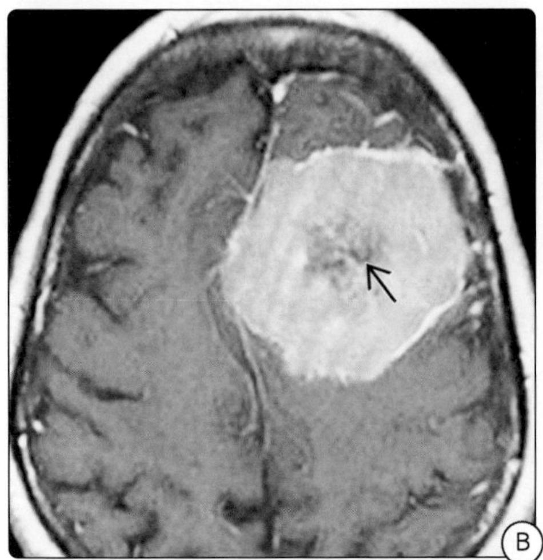


*(27-23B) T1 C+ shows that the mass enhances intensely. Note the "flow voids" in the vascular center of the mass ⮚.*

they are statistically far more common. Anaplastic meningiomas typically invade the brain and may exhibit a "mushrooming" configuration **(27-28)**.

**Dural metastasis**, usually from a breast or lung primary, may be virtually indistinguishable from meningioma on imaging studies.

Rare entities that can closely resemble meningioma include hemangioma and solitary fibrous tumor. A **hemangioma of the dura** or **venous sinuses** is a true vasoformative neoplasm that can resemble meningioma. Most hemangiomas are very hyperintense on T2WI, whereas most meningiomas are iso- to mildly hyperintense. Delayed slow centripetal "filling in" of the mass on dynamic contrast-enhanced MR is suggestive of hemangioma.

**Intracranial solitary fibrous tumor** is relatively rare. Most are found adjacent to the dura, venous sinuses, or choroid plexus. There are no specific imaging features that reliably distinguish solitary fibrous tumors from meningiomas.

Other meningioma mimics include **granuloma** (TB, sarcoid) and focal **idiopathic hypertrophic pachymeningitis**. Solitary dural granulomas are rare. Idiopathic hypertrophic pachymeningitis is uncommon. Most cases are found in or around the skull base, particularly the orbit, cavernous sinus, and posterior fossa (clivus/cerebellopontine angle). Idiopathic hypertrophic pachymeningitis can invade bone and may be virtually indistinguishable from "en plaque" meningioma.

**Intracranial mesenchymal tumor, FET::CREB fusion-positive** (sometimes called angiomatoid fibrous histiocytoma) is a rare extraaxial neoplasm attached to the meninges or dura that can exhibit a dural "tail," mimicking meningioma. Most occur in children or young adults, although cases in middle-aged adults have been reported.

**Extramedullary hematopoiesis** (EMH) can present as confluent or multifocal dura-based disease resembling "en plaque" solitary or multiple meningiomatosis. EMH occurs in the setting of chronic anemia or marrow depletion disorders.

### MENINGIOMA MIMICS

**Common**
- Metastasis
  - Most common = breast, lung, colon, prostate
- Lymphoma

**Less Common**
- Granuloma
  - TB, sarcoid most common
  - Other (less common) = plasma cell granuloma, Rosai-Dorfman disease

**Rare but Important**
- IgG4-related disease
- Dural/venous sinus hemangioma
- Solitary fibrous tumor
- Intracranial mesenchymal tumor, FET::CREB fusion-positive
- Extramedullary hematopoiesis

## Meningioma, CNS WHO Grade 2

While metastasis of meningiomas is extremely rare, tissue invasion is common and has wide implications for the treatment and clinical course of these tumors. In the 2016 WHO, 4th edition, breach of the "brain-meningioma interface" (i.e., brain invasion) led to acceptance of brain invasion as a standalone grading criterion for grade 2 meningioma. In the

2021 WHO, 5th edition, brain invasion must be unequivocal (i.e., not just perivascular spread or indentation of brain without pial breach) to establish the diagnosis of a CNS WHO grade 2 tumor.

## Terminology

Atypical meningioma (AM) is an intermediate-grade meningioma with specific diagnostic criteria that can be applied across all meningioma subtypes (see below).

## Etiology

There is a significant correlation between the number of inactivating *NF2* mutations and tumor grade. The rate of *NF2* mutations in high-grade meningiomas is 80%. Chromosomal abnormalities beyond chromosome 22 deletions are also much more common in high-grade meningiomas.

AMs demonstrate *NF2* loss, genomic instability, mutations in *SMARCB1*, and a hypermethylated subtype.

Biallelic *SMARCE1* inactivation and activating *TERT* promoter are rare mutations that are restricted to AM, CNS WHO grade 2 tumors. Most are clear cell subtypes.

## Pathology

**Location.** Most atypical and anaplastic (malignant) meningiomas arise from the calvaria. The skull base is a relatively uncommon location for these more aggressive lesions.

**Gross Pathology.** Approximately 1/2 of all AMs invade the adjacent brain. In such cases, there is no intervening layer of leptomeninges between the invading tumor and underlying parenchyma. Brain invasion is also strongly correlated with the presence of other histopathologic criteria of atypia or anaplasia (see below).

**Microscopic Features.** The 2021 WHO, 5th edition established specific criteria that must be met for a diagnosis of AM, CNS WHO grade 2. These include 4-19 mitoses in 10 consecutive HPF **or** unequivocal brain invasion (not only perivascular spread or indentation of brain without pial breach) **or** specific morphologic subtype (chordoid or clear cell). Extension along the perivascular spaces does not constitute brain invasion per se because the perivascular spaces are lined by pia.

A meningioma can be also designated as a grade 2 tumor with at least three of the following five features: Increased cellularity, small cells with high nuclear:cytoplasmic ratio, prominent nucleoli, sheeting (uninterrupted patternless or sheet-like growth), or foci of spontaneous (i.e., noniatrogenic) necrosis.

## Clinical Issues

**Epidemiology.** AMs represent 10-15% of all meningiomas.

**Demographics.** AMs tend to occur in slightly younger patients compared with grade 1 meningiomas and display a slight male predominance. Pediatric meningiomas also tend to be more aggressive.

Male patients with *SMARCE1*-inactivating mutations develop tumors in childhood, whereas carrier female patients develop tumors in adolescence or early adulthood.

**Natural History.** AMs are generally associated with a higher recurrence rate (25-30%) and shorter recurrence-free survival compared with TMs. The Simpson and modified Shinsu grading systems are the best predictors of

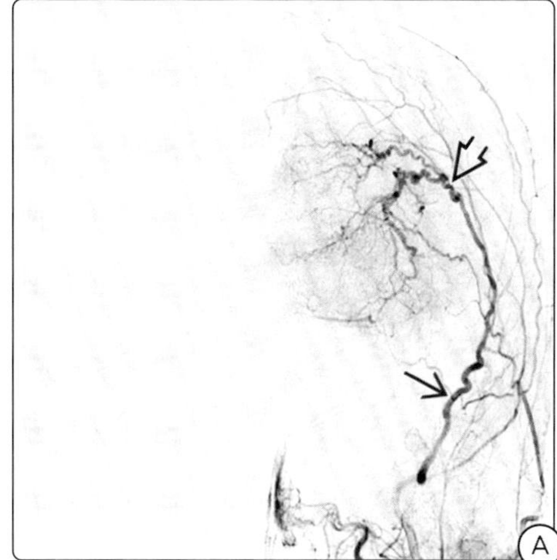

***(27-24A)** AP DSA of ECA shows enlarged MMA → with "sunburst" of vessels ⇨ supplying meningioma.*

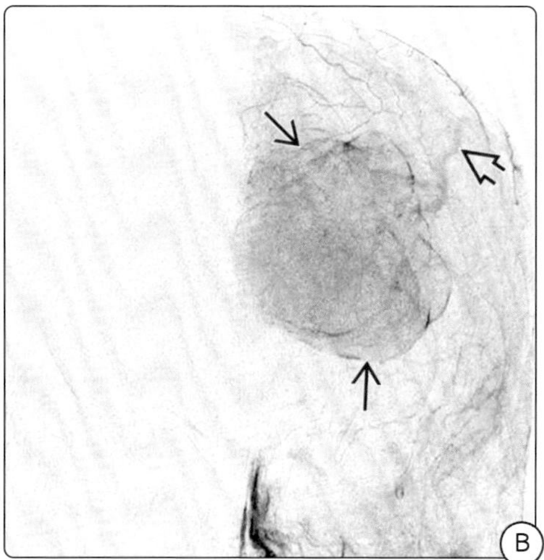

***(27-24B)** Later phase of ECA DSA shows prolonged vascular "blush" →, characteristic of meningioma. "Early draining" vein is seen ⇨.*

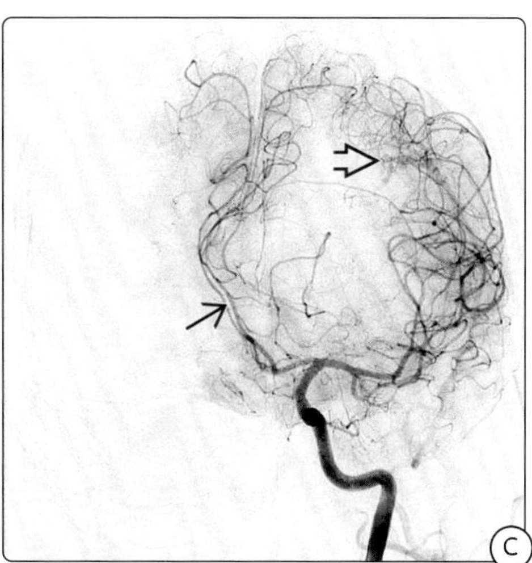

***(27-24C)** ICA DSA shows mass effect with the ACA shifted →. Only minimal supply to periphery of tumor ⇨ is coming from pial MCA branches.*

recurrence after resection. Grade I represents macroscopically complete tumor removal, including excision of its dural attachment and any abnormal bone. Grades II-IV represent progressively less complete resection, and grade V is simple decompression, with or without biopsy.

## Imaging

**General Features.** A good general rule is that it is difficult, if not impossible, to predict meningioma grade on the basis of imaging findings **(27-30)**. However, because brain invasion is a frequent (but not always visible) feature of AMs, the CSF-vascular "cleft" typically seen in CNS WHO grade 1 meningiomas **(27-23)** is often compromised or absent **(27-25)**.

**CT Findings.** AMs are usually hyperdense with irregular margins. Minimal or no calcification is seen, and frank bone invasion with osteolysis is common. Tumor may invade through the skull into the scalp.

**MR Findings.** Tumor margins are usually indistinct with no border between the tumor and the underlying cortex. A CSF-vascular "cleft" is often absent or partially effaced. Peritumoral edema and cyst formation are common but nonspecific findings **(27-25)**. Contrast enhancement is strong but often quite heterogeneous.

ADC is significantly lower in atypical and malignant meningiomas compared with grade 1 lesions. Perfusion MR may show elevated rCBV, especially in the peritumoral edema **(27-27)**. MRS often shows elevated choline **(27-27D)**.

## Differential Diagnosis

Because it is difficult to determine meningioma tumor grade on the basis of imaging findings alone, the major differential diagnosis of AM is **CNS WHO grade 1 meningioma**. **Dural metastasis** and **anaplastic (malignant) meningioma, CNS WHO grade 3**, can also be indistinguishable from AM. **Solitary**

*(27-25A) T2WI in a 74-yo man with seizures shows a lobulated, heterogeneously hyperintense mass in the right posterior frontal lobe. Note peritumoral edema and lack of a clear brain-tumor interface. (27-25B) FLAIR shows the mass is isointense with cortex, and the brain-tumor interface is indistinct.*

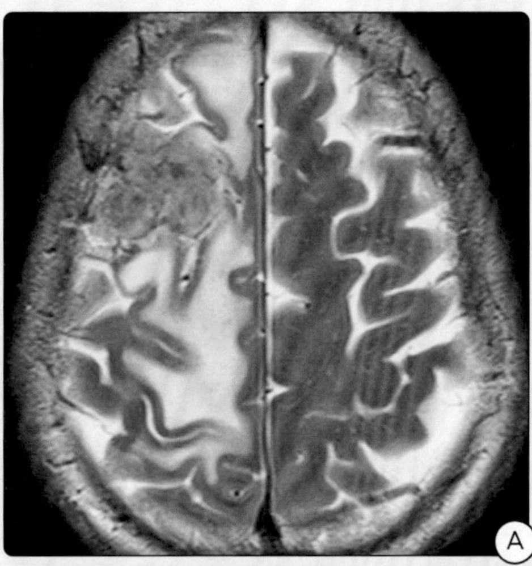


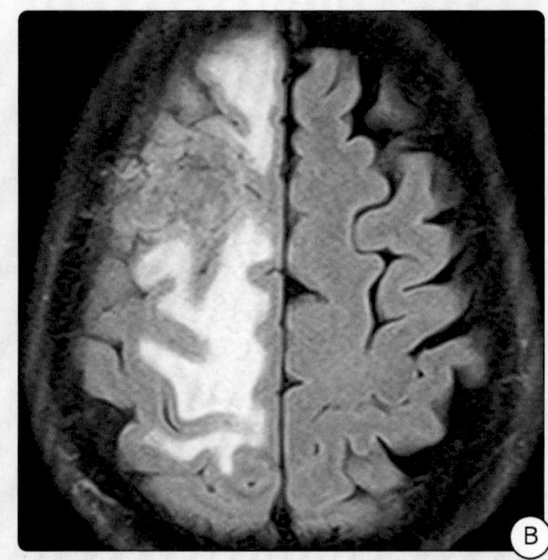


*(27-25C) The mass enhances intensely on T1 C+ FS. (27-25D) Coronal T1 C+ shows an indistinct brain-tumor interface with enhancing foci that appear to extend into the underlying parenchyma. Brain invasion was documented at surgery and histopathology. This is CNS WHO grade 2 meningioma.*

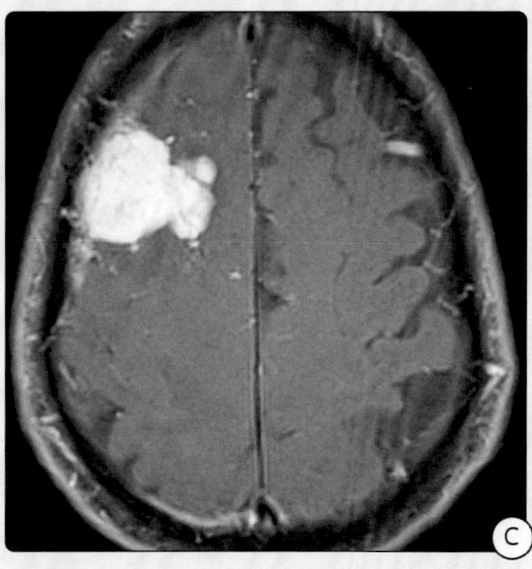


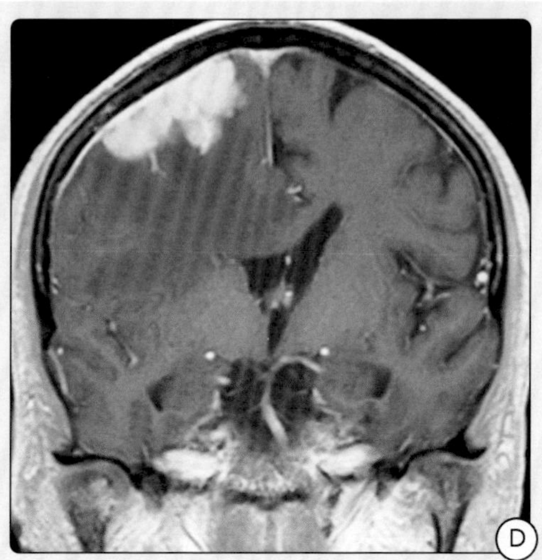

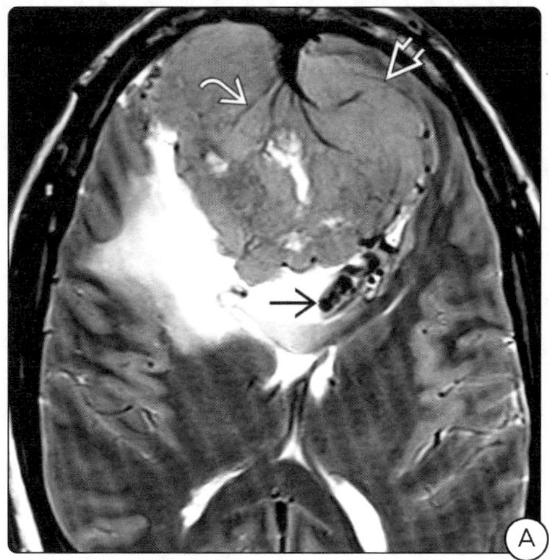


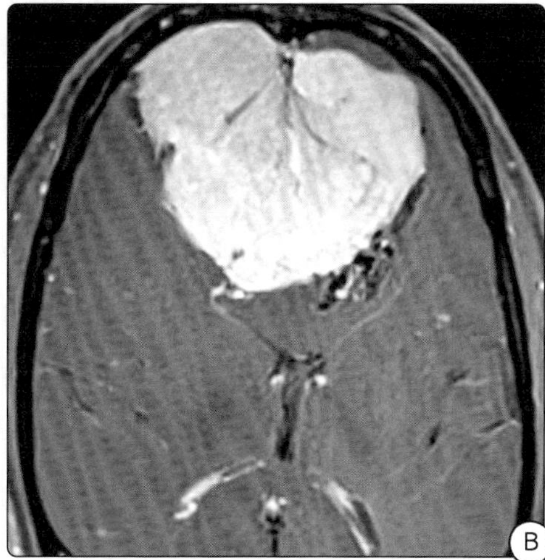


***(27-26A)** T2WI in a 43-yo man shows a lobulated bifrontal mass with prominent "sunburst" vessels within the mass as well as in the CSF-vascular "cleft" . **(27-26B)** The mass enhances intensely on T1 C+ FS. No definite brain invasion was seen at surgery or pathologic examination, but because this was a clear cell subtype meningioma, CNS WHO grade 2, was assigned to the tumor.*

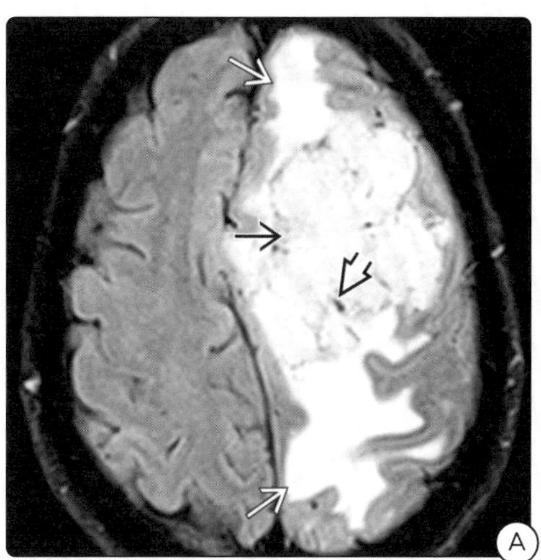


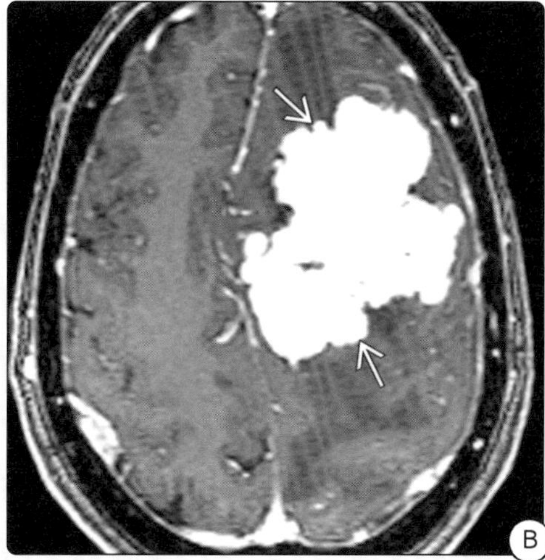


***(27-27A)** FLAIR scan in a 68-yo woman with right-sided weakness shows a hyperintense, lobulated convexity mass with numerous "flow voids" , edema . **(27-27B)** T1 C+ FS demonstrates that the mass enhances intensely and uniformly. Coronal T1 C+ (not shown) demonstrated that the mass was attached to the dura and exhibited a dural tail sign.*

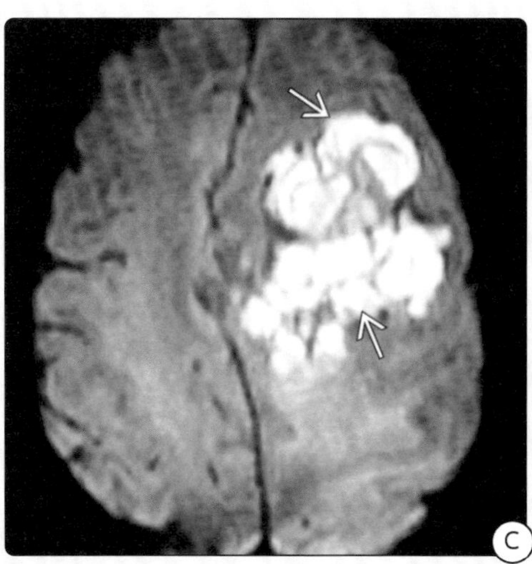


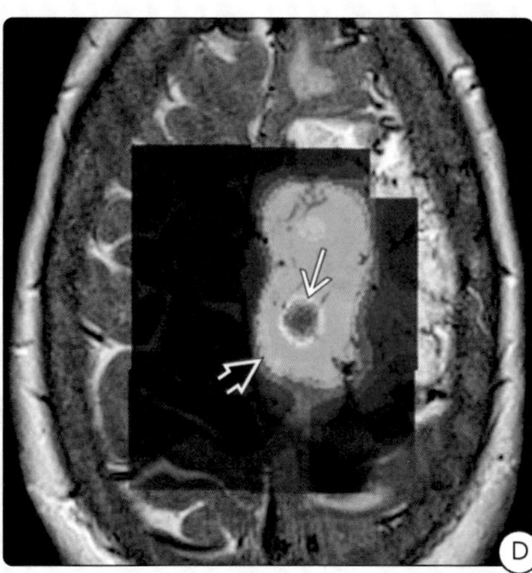


***(27-27C)** The mass shows restricted diffusion, consistent with high cellularity. **(27-27D)** MRS shows markedly elevated Cho, decreased NAA. Choline map shows the elevated Cho with the highest levels in the center of the lesion . This is atypical meningioma, clear cell type, CNS WHO grade 2. (Courtesy M. Thurnher, MD.)*

**fibrous tumor** can mimic meningiomas of all grades on imaging studies.

## Meningioma, CNS WHO Grade 3

### Terminology

Meningioma, CNS WHO grade 3, was formerly known as anaplastic or malignant meningioma. These uncommon tumors exhibit overtly malignant cytomorphology (anaplasia) &/or markedly elevated mitotic activity.

### Etiology

High-grade meningiomas often harbor a diverse and variable group of somatic mutations. Several genes have been associated with malignant progression in meningioma. Homozygous deletions or mutations of the tumor suppressor genes *CDKN2A* (ARF) and *CDKN2B* are found in most anaplastic meningiomas. A new meningioma-associated tumor suppressor gene, *NDRG2*, is downregulated in anaplastic meningioma and AMs with aggressive clinical behavior.

### Pathology

AM corresponds histologically to CNS WHO grade 3. Grossly, most AMs display extensive necrosis and often exhibit frank brain invasion **(27-28)**.

Either a markedly elevated mitotic index (≥ 20 mitoses/10 HPF) **or** histologic features of frank anaplasia (e.g., sarcoma-, carcinoma-, or melanoma-like appearance) is sufficient for the diagnosis of anaplastic meningioma. As the presence of *TERT* promoter mutation **or** homozygous deletion of *CDKN2A* &/or *CDKN2B* confers a high recurrence risk and short interval to progression, these molecular features designate a CNS WHO grade 3 tumor irrespective of other histologic features.

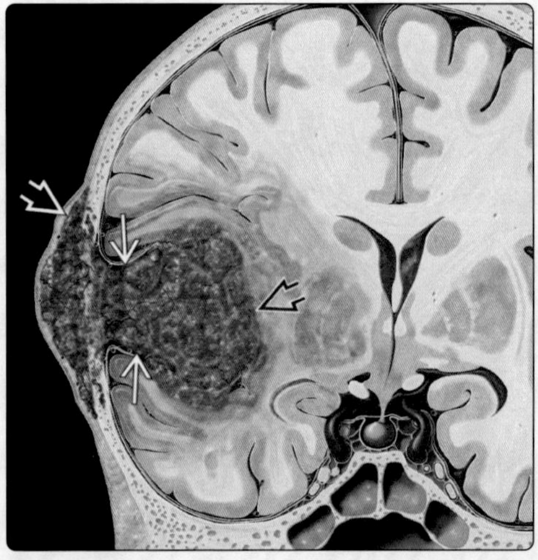

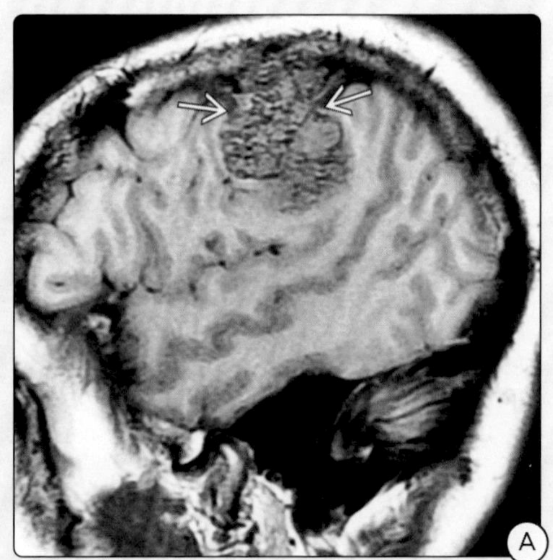


***(27-28)** Graphic shows malignant meningioma invading brain ➾ without CSF-vascular "cleft." The tumor also penetrates dura, invades calvarium, has a significant extracranial component ➾. Note "mushroom" configuration ➾, which may suggest more aggressive meningioma. **(27-29A)** Sagittal T1WI in a 50-yo man with left-sided weakness shows mixed iso-/hypointense extraaxial mass "mushrooming" ➾ into brain.*

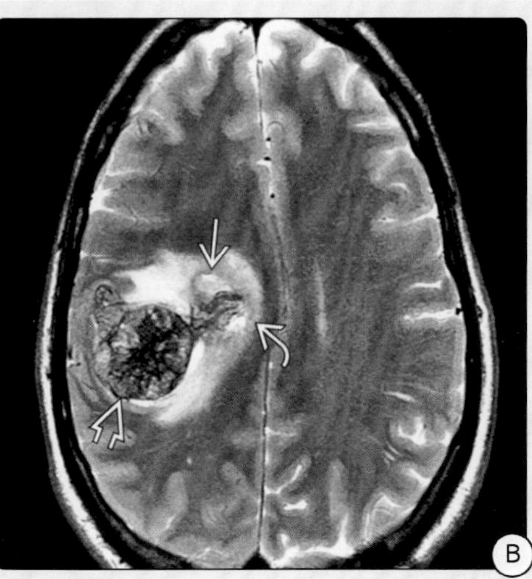


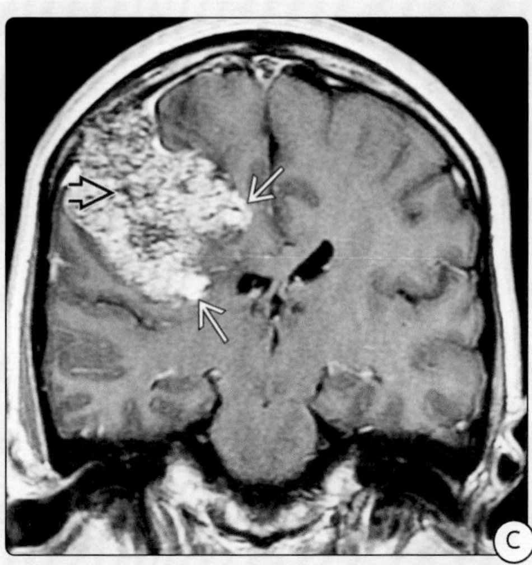


***(27-29B)** Axial T2WI shows the very heterogeneous signal of the lesion ➾, "mushroom" of focal brain invasion ➾ with adjacent edema ➾. **(27-29C)** Coronal T1 C+ MR shows that an intensely enhancing lesion contains numerous "flow voids" ➾ and invades adjacent brain ➾. This is papillary meningioma, CNS WHO grade 3.*

In the past, the rhabdoid meningioma subtype was designated a grade 3 anaplastic/malignant meningioma based on the presence of rhabdoid cells alone without fulfilling other criteria for a CNS WHO grade 3 designation. Recent studies have demonstrated that patient outcome is correlated with CNS WHO grade independent of rhabdoid features.

Similarly, focal papillary architecture—once considered indicative of an AM or anaplastic meningioma—does not itself suffice for designating tumors as CNS WHO grade 2 or 3. Therefore, histomorphologic features of a rhabdoid or papillary subtype alone do not designate a tumor as CNS WHO grade 2 or 3.

A subset of rhabdoid &/or papillary meningiomas arise in patients with BRCA (**br**east **ca**ncer gene)-associated protein 1 (*BAP1*) mutations and the *BAP1* tumor predisposition syndrome. Loss of *BAP1* expression is associated with aggressive clinical behavior consistent with CNS WHO grade 3 tumors.

## Clinical Issues

**Epidemiology.** Anaplastic (malignant) meningiomas are rare, representing only 1-3% of all meningiomas. Malignant meningiomas have a striking male predominance.

**Natural History.** Prognosis is poor. Recurrence rates following tumor resection range from 50-95%. Survival times range from 2-5 years and vary depending on resection extent.

## Imaging

**General Features.** The imaging triad of extracranial mass, osteolysis, and "mushrooming" intracranial tumor is present in most, but not all, cases of anaplastic meningioma **(27-28)** **(27-31)**. Calcification is rare, and contrast enhancement is typically heterogeneous **(27-29)**.

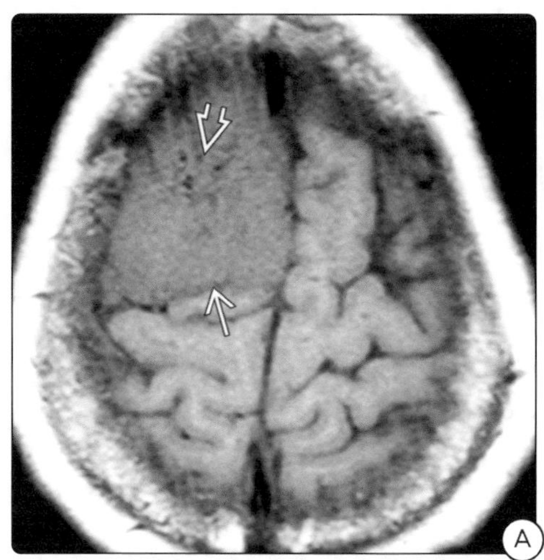


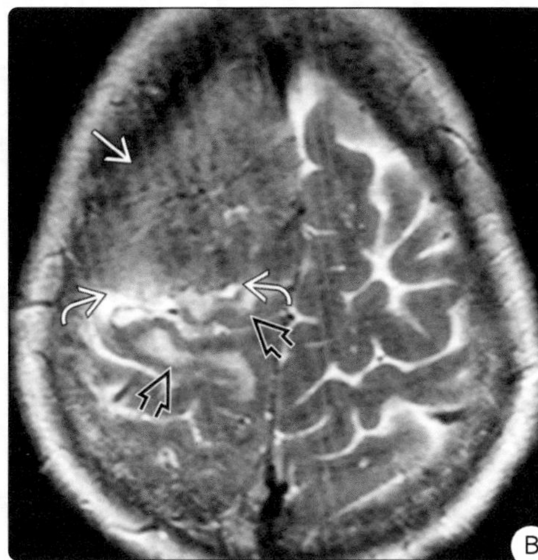


***(27-30A)** Axial T1WI in a 68-yo woman with headaches shows a right frontal mass that is isointense with cortex and exhibits a central cluster of "flow voids" . **(27-30B)** Axial T2WI in the same case shows that the mass appears mildly hypointense and has a relatively well-demarcated CSF-vascular "cleft" between the mass and adjacent brain. Mild edema is present in the white matter of the adjacent gyri .*

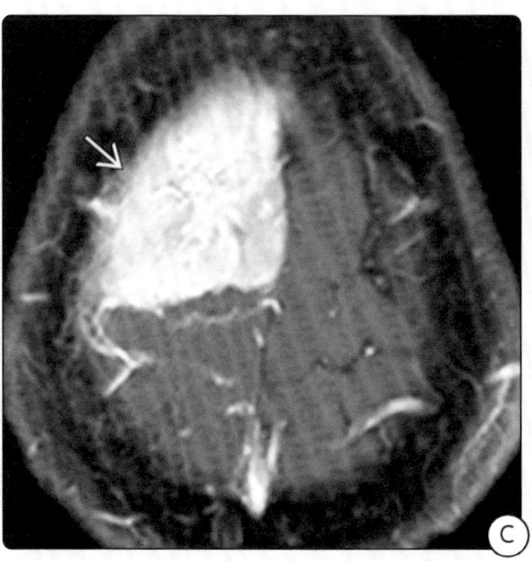


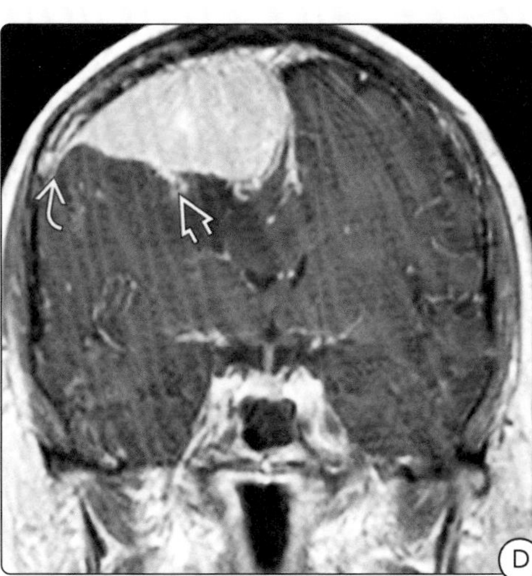


***(27-30C)** Axial T1 C+ FS shows that the mass enhances intensely, relatively uniformly. **(27-30D)** Coronal T1 C+ shows that the intensely enhancing mass has a relatively inconspicuous associated dural "tail" . There is a small area of enhancement in the adjacent brain , suggesting focal parenchymal invasion. This is CNS WHO grade 3 malignant meningioma.*

## Differential Diagnosis

The major differential diagnosis of anaplastic meningioma is **AM**. AMs can be indistinguishable from malignant meningiomas on imaging studies alone, as brain invasion may occur in both.

**Metastases, solitary fibrous tumors, and sarcomas**, such as meningeal fibrosarcoma, can all mimic anaplastic meningioma.

# Primary Melanocytic Lesions

By far the most frequent of all melanocytic CNS lesions are metastases from extracranial malignant melanomas (see Fig. 31-15). Primary melanocytic tumors of the CNS are a very rare, broad, and diverse group of entities with an estimated incidence of 0.9 per 10 million. These tumors can be circumscribed or diffuse and benign or malignant.

Primary CNS melanomas are thought to originate from leptomeningeal melanocytes, which are preferentially located at the base of the brain, ventral medulla, and along the upper cervical spinal cord. They can present as focal nodules or diffuse leptomeningeal infiltrates. Diffuse leptomeningeal melanotic infiltrates also occur in meningeal melanocytosis/melanomatosis [neurocutaneous melanosis (NCM)] **(27-32)** **(27-33)**.

Focal primary CNS melanotic masses span a morphologic spectrum from low-grade melanocytoma to the rare primary malignant melanoma. The 5th edition WHO specifies diagnostic criteria for circumscribed/localized primary melanocytic neoplasms in the meninges.

*Melanocytomas* have limited cytologic atypia, almost/no mitoses, no necrosis, and no CNS parenchymal invasion. For

***(27-31A)** Axial T2WI in a 50-yo man with seizures shows a heterogeneous extraaxial mass arising from the right sphenoid ala. **(27-31B)** T1 C+ shows the mass enhances intensely. The tumor-brain interface is poorly defined.*

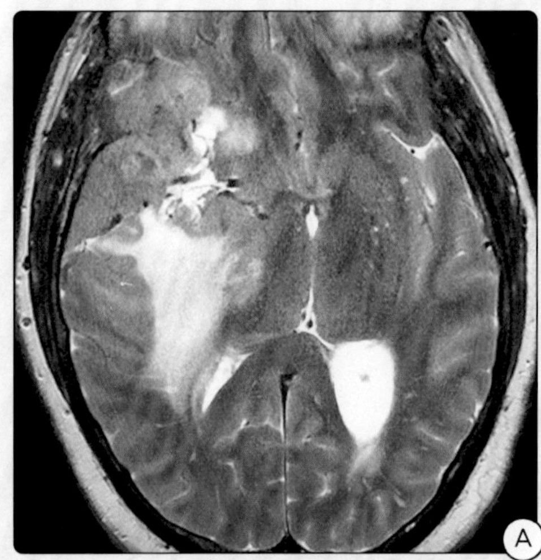


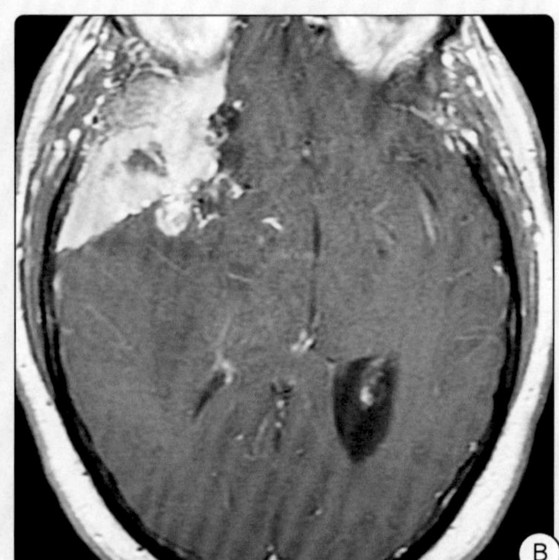


***(27-31C)** Coronal T1 C+ shows ill-defined tumor-brain interface. **(27-31D)** Sagittal T1 C+ shows poorly defined posterior tumor margins. Resection disclosed anaplastic (malignant) meningioma, CNS WHO grade 3. The patient expired from disseminated disease after multiple tumor recurrences.*

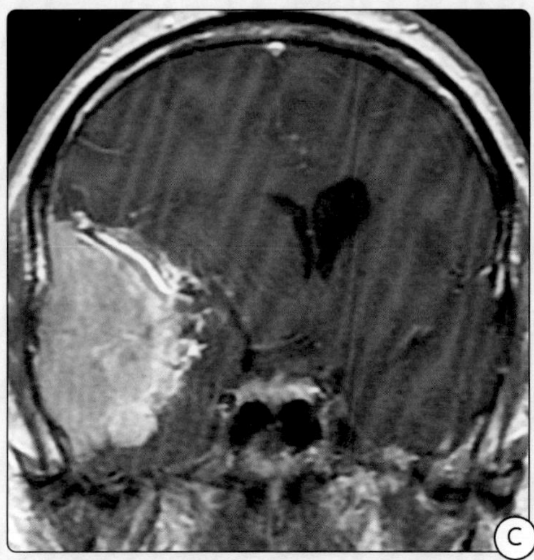


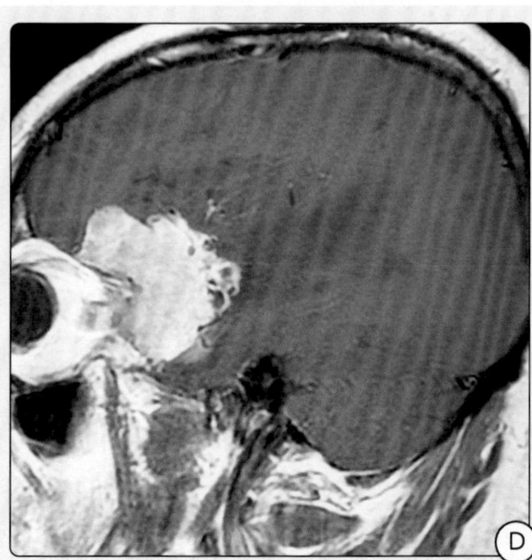

*intermediate-grade melanocytomas*, mitotic count of 0.5-1.5 mitoses/mm² (up to 5/HPF) &/or CNS invasion may be present, but cytologic atypia is limited and necrosis is absent. Melanomas should have > 5 mitoses/HPF &/or necrosis. Marked cytologic atypia is common.

## Melanocytoma and Melanoma

*Melanocytomas* account for < 0.1% of all CNS neoplasms. Molecular analyses have shown that melanocytomas carry *GNAQ/GNA11* mutations and present with copy number variants in chromosomes 3 and 6. Methylation profiling is especially useful in recognizing these neoplasms and distinguishing them from other pigmented CNS tumors.

Melanocytomas are solitary, darkly pigmented, low-grade tumors that do not invade adjacent brain. Preferred sites are the posterior fossa (skull base, cerebellopontine angle), temporal lobe, Meckel cave (with nevus of Ota), and spinal cord/nerve roots. Melanocytomas rarely undergo malignant transformation.

*Melanomas* frequently demonstrate *TERT* promoter mutations and frequently harbor additional oncogene mutations.

Prognosis is variable for melanocytic tumors of intermediate differentiation and poor for melanoma.

Imaging findings for melanocytic tumors depend largely on intrinsic melanin content and range from small, well-circumscribed focal lesions to diffuse meningeal involvement. Melanotic lesions are hyperdense on NECT and enhance strongly on CECT. The paramagnetic properties of melanin cause T1 shortening, so hyperintensity on T1WI and hypointensity on T2WI are characteristic **(27-35)** **(27-36)**.

The major differential diagnosis for primary melanocytic lesions of the brain is **metastatic malignant melanoma**.

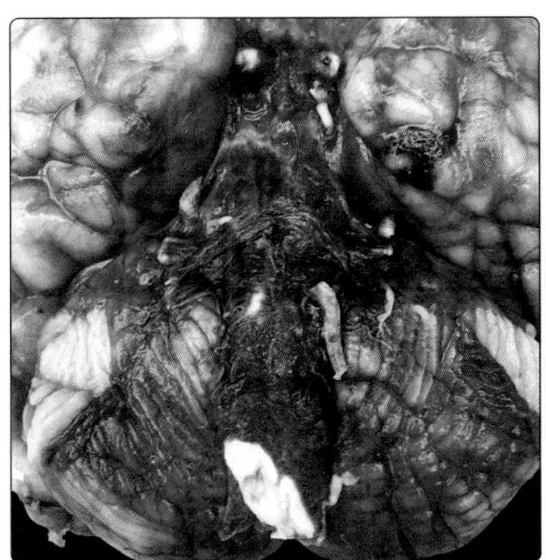

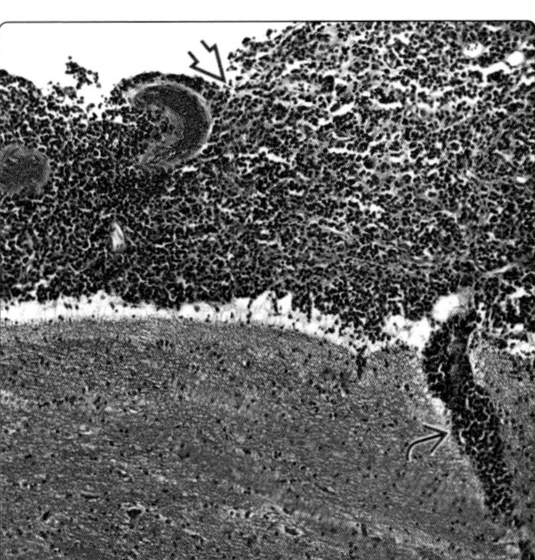

***(27-32)** Gross pathology in a patient with neurocutaneous melanosis shows diffuse black-brown infiltrates covering the basal leptomeninges. (From DP: Neuro.) **(27-33)** Diffuse leptomeningeal involvement ⇨ is one of the features of neurocutaneous melanosis. Spread into the perivascular (Virchow-Robin) spaces ⇨ from the leptomeninges may be present.*

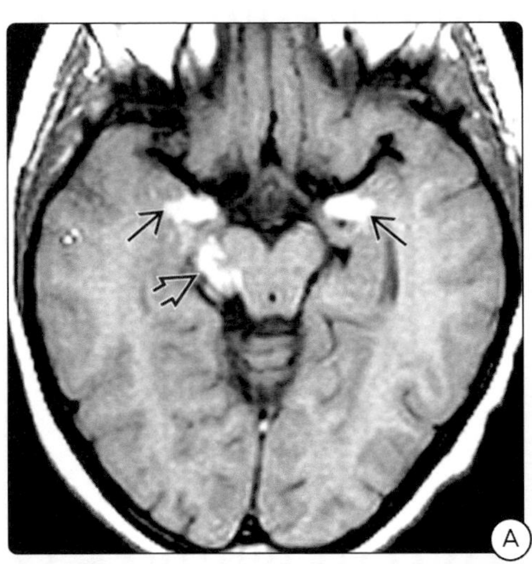


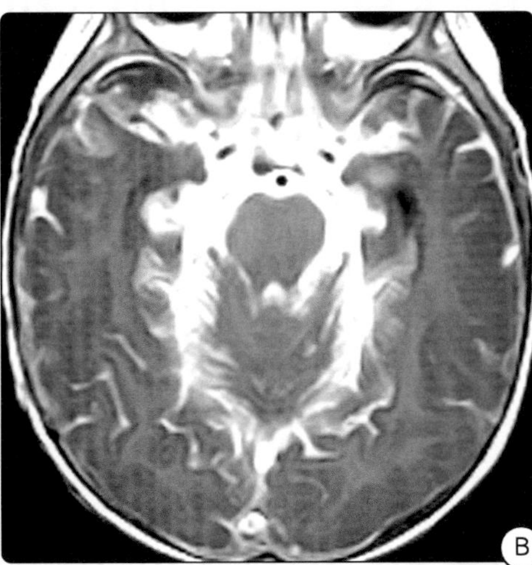


***(27-34A)** T1WI in a child with neurocutaneous melanosis shows characteristic ovoid hyperintensities in the amygdalae of both temporal lobes ⇨. Another focus of thick melanotic deposition with T1 shortening ⇨ is seen along the midbrain. **(27-34B)** T1 C+ MR in the same patient shows diffuse, thick meningeal enhancement. (Courtesy S. Blaser, MD.)*

## Diffuse Meningeal Melanocytosis/Melanomatosis

Diffuse leptomeningeal melanocytosis and melanomatosis are usually features of NCM, a rare neurocutaneous syndrome of childhood. Most patients present with numerous congenital melanotic nevi of the skin and neurologic dysfunction.

Diffuse melanocytic lesions appear as dense, thick, black confluent aggregates that fill the subarachnoid spaces and coat the pia **(27-32)** **(27-33)**. The amygdala, pons, and cerebellum are most commonly involved but melanosis can be seen anywhere in the CNS.

Bilateral T1-hyperintense foci in the amygdala is an early sign of NCM **(27-34A)**. Diffuse leptomeningeal enhancement **(27-34B)** and extension into the brain parenchyma via the perivascular spaces can occur and usually indicate malignant transformation with poor prognosis.

*Selected References: The complete reference list is available on the eBooks+ version included with purchase.*

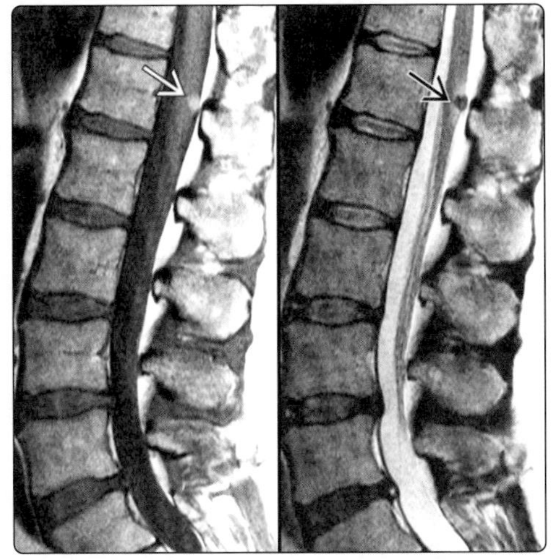

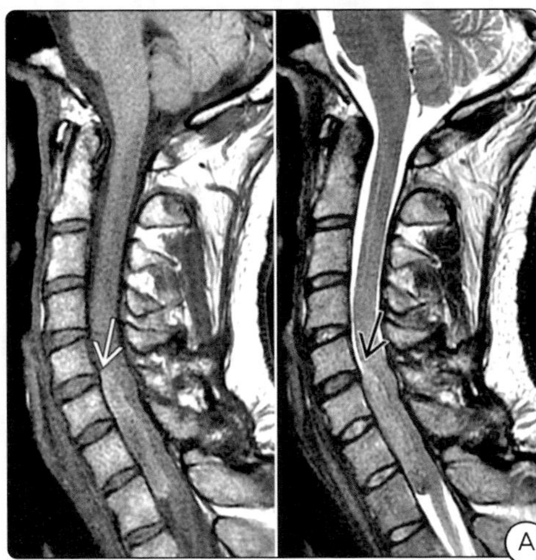

***(27-35)** (L) T1WI in a circumscribed low-grade primary meningeal melanocytoma of the spinal cord shows a well-demarcated hyperintense intramedullary lesion in the dorsal conus medullaris ➡. (R) The lesion is very hypointense on T2WI and is surrounded by hyperintense focal edema ➡. **(27-36A)** (L) T1WI shows a mildly hyperintense C5-C7 mass ➡ that is mildly hyperintense on T2WI ➡ (R).*

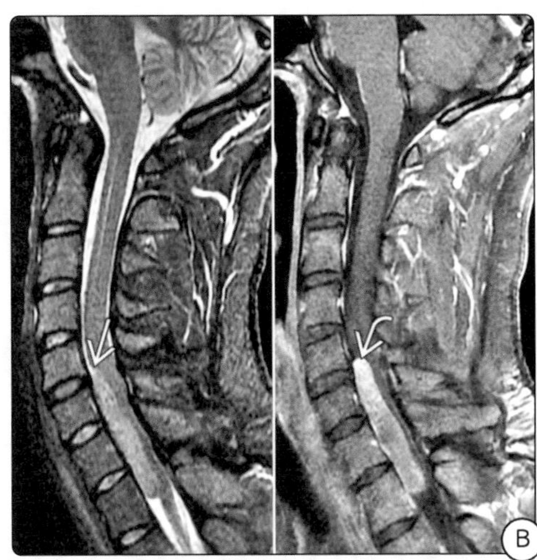

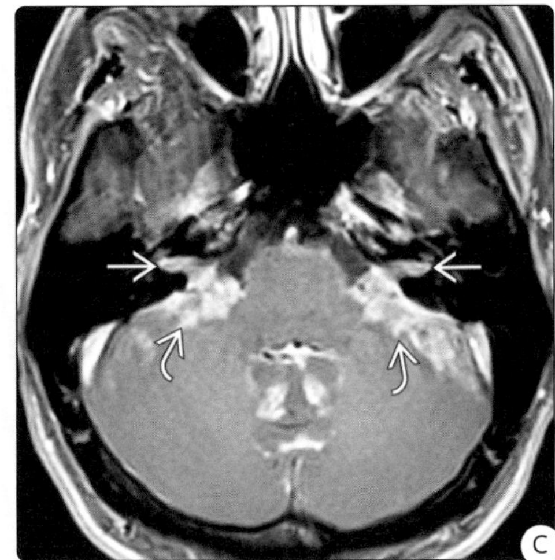

***(27-36B)** (L) The mass ➡ is hyperintense to cord on STIR and enhances strongly on T1 C+ FS ➡ (R). Meningeal melanocytoma of intermediate grade was found at histopathology. **(27-36C)** Two years later, the patient developed diffuse CSF metastases. This T1 C+ FS shows enhancing tumor in both IACs ➡ and CPA cisterns ➡.*

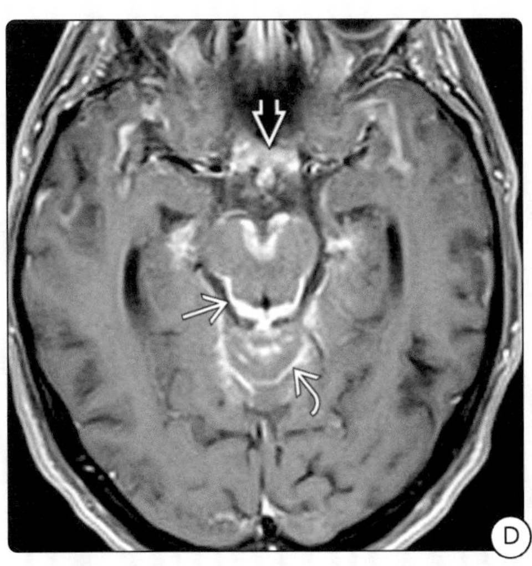

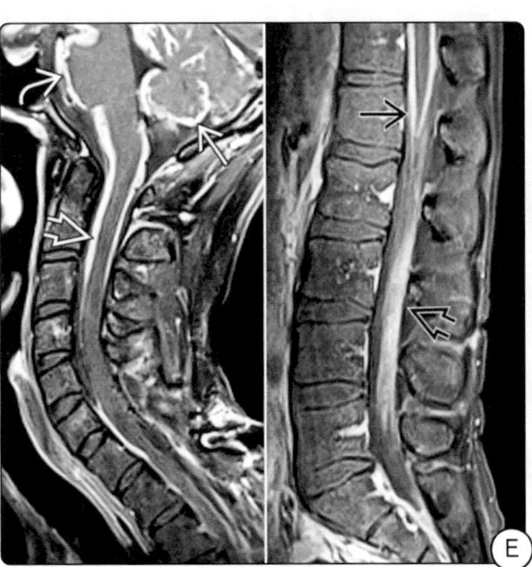

***(27-36D)** More cephalad T1 C+ FS shows thick pial enhancement around the midbrain ➡ and superior vermis ➡ as well as the optic chiasm ➡. **(27-36E)** Sagittal T1 C+ FS shows thick, enhancing leptomeningeal tumor spread around the pons ➡, vermis ➡, cervical cord ➡, conus ➡, and cauda equina ➡.*

# Mesenchymal, Nonmeningothelial Tumors

*The terminology and pathologic features of benign and malignant mesenchymal, nonmeningothelial neoplasms originating in the CNS correspond to soft tissue or bone tumors found elsewhere in the body.*



These unusual neoplasms can be tumors of adipose, fibrous, histiocytic, cartilaginous, or vascular tissues and can also arise from muscle or bone. Both benign and malignant varieties of each type occur, ranging from benign (CNS WHO grade 1) to highly malignant (grade 4) sarcomatous neoplasms.

Nonmeningothelial mesenchymal tumors rarely involve the CNS. When they do, they arise more commonly in the meninges than in the brain parenchyma or choroid plexus. They can occur in patients of any age.

The 2021 5th edition WHO divides these uncommon tumors into three groups: (1) Soft tissue tumors; (2) chondroosseous tumors, and (3) notochordal tumors. This chapter focuses on the most important of these rare neoplasms.

While the 2021 5th edition WHO does not include benign chondroosseous tumors, for the sake of completeness, we close this chapter with a fourth section that focuses briefly on these benign neoplasms.

## Soft Tissue Tumors

Soft tissue tumors involving the CNS usually originate from the meninges (typically the dura), choroid plexus, or skull base. The cranial meninges contain primitive pluripotential mesenchymal cells that can give rise to a broad spectrum of nonmeningothelial mesenchymal tumors. Most are supratentorial; the falx is the most common site.

Soft tissue tumors included in the 5th edition WHO include solitary fibrous tumor (SFT), hemangiomas, and vascular malformations (such as arteriovenous and cavernous malformations), hemangioblastoma, rhabdomyosarcoma, Ewing sarcoma, and a group of newly recognized but uncommon tumors, such as *DICER1*-mutant primary sarcoma and *CIC*-rearranged sarcoma. In this section, we focus on SFTs, hemangiomas, hemangioblastoma, and sarcomas. Vascular malformations are probably not neoplastic and were covered in Chapter 7.

### Solitary Fibrous Tumor

#### Terminology

Solitary fibrous tumor (SFT) represents a continuum of mesenchymal tumors with increasing cellularity. The term "hemangiopericytoma" (HPC) is no longer used.

Although relatively rare, SFT is the most common primary intracranial nonmeningothelial mesenchymal neoplasm. It is a very cellular, highly vascular neoplasm known for its aggressive clinical behavior, high recurrence rates, and distant metastases even after gross total surgical resection.

## Etiology

SFTs at all anatomic sites have a genomic inversion at 12q13, which leads to *NAB2::STAT6* gene fusion. Demonstration of this fusion is considered virtually pathognomonic of SFT.

## Pathology

**Location.** Most SFTs are dural based, usually arising from the falx or tentorium. The most common site is the occipital region, where they often straddle the transverse sinus. Intraparenchymal SFTs occur in the cerebrum and spinal cord, often without a discernible dural attachment. The cerebral ventricles are another common site.

**Size and Number.** SFTs are almost always solitary lesions. They are relatively large tumors, reaching up to 10 cm in diameter. Lesions more than 4-5 cm are not uncommon.

**Gross Pathology.** SFTs are solid, lobulated, relatively well-demarcated, dura-based neoplasms **(28-1)** that contain abundant vascular spaces. Myxoid change and intratumoral hemorrhage are common.

**Microscopic Features.** SFTs are variably cellular tumors composed of spindled to ovoid cells arranged around a branching and hyalinized vasculature. Necrosis is common. Nuclear atypia and mitotic activity vary.

**Diagnostic Molecular Pathology.** *STAT6* nuclear expression can be detected by sequencing techniques or RT-PCR and confirms the diagnosis of SFT. Immunohistochemical detection of strong nuclear STAT6 expression is also a sensitive and specific surrogate for all fusions.

*(28-1) Solitary fibrous tumors are firm, well-circumscribed masses that can appear identical to meningioma. (Courtesy E. Rushing, MD.) (28-3A) Sagittal T1 MR in a 42-yo man with headaches shows a well-delineated, mostly isointense frontal mass ➡ with prominent dural thickening ➡.*

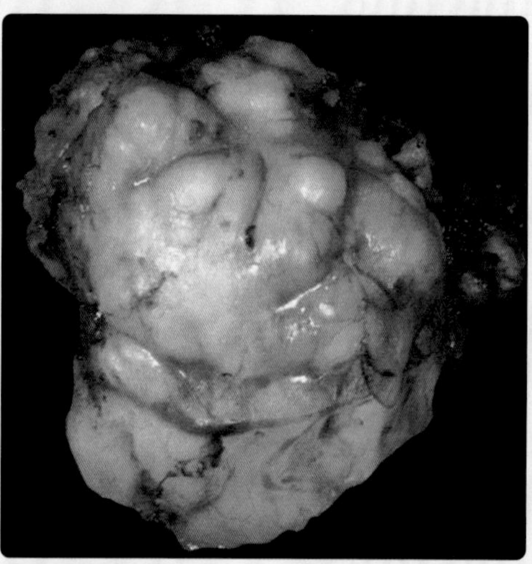

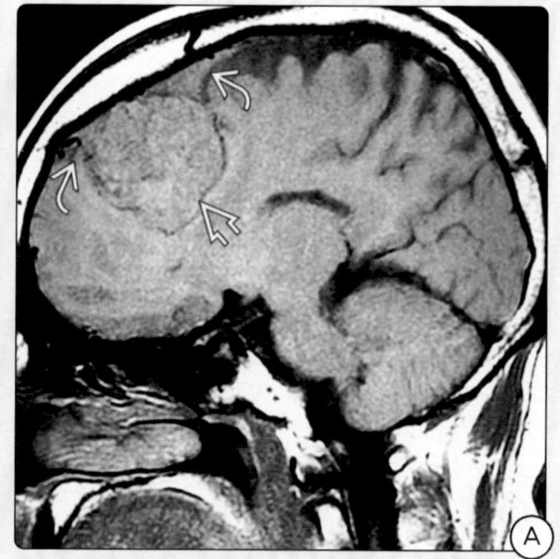


*(28-3B) Coronal T2 MR in the same patient shows that the mass ➡ is mostly isointense with cortex but contains numerous intratumoral cysts. Note a well-defined cleft ➡ between the mass and brain and edema ➡ in the corpus callosum. (28-3C) T1 C+ MR shows that the mass ➡ enhances strongly but heterogeneously. Note thickened, enhancing dural "tail" ➡ around the mass. This is solitary fibrous tumor, CNS WHO grade 2.*

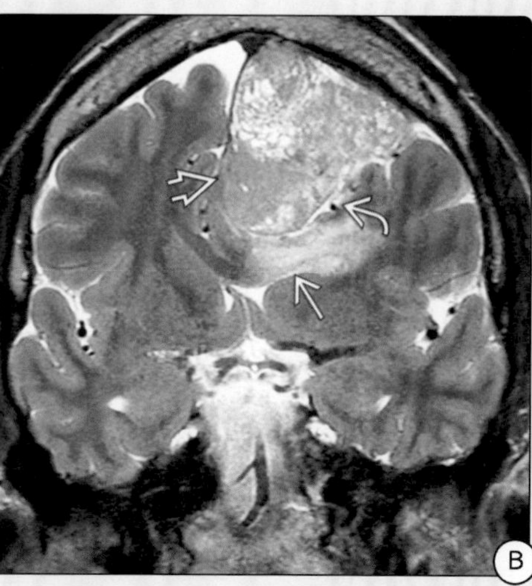


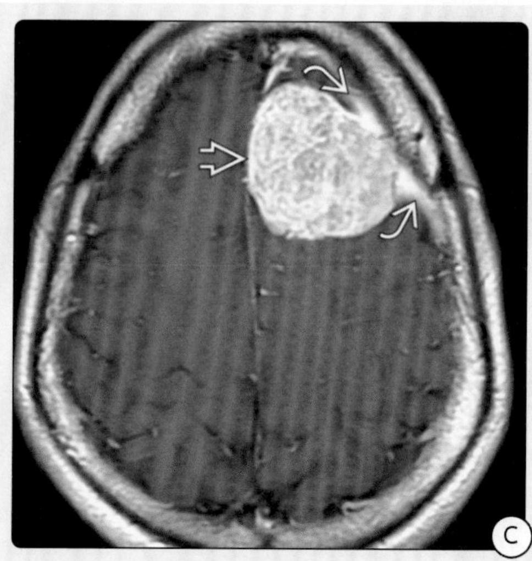

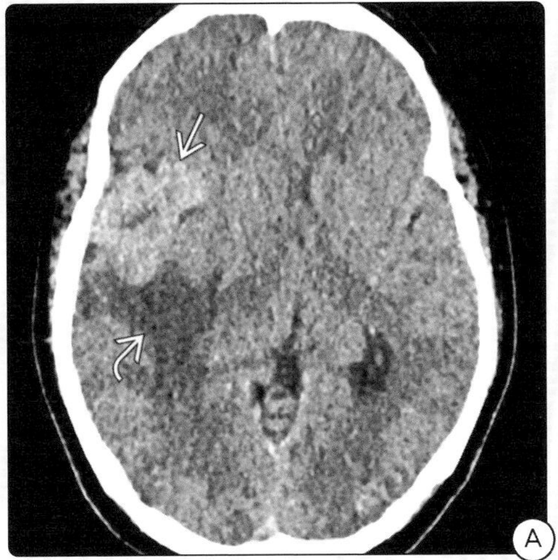


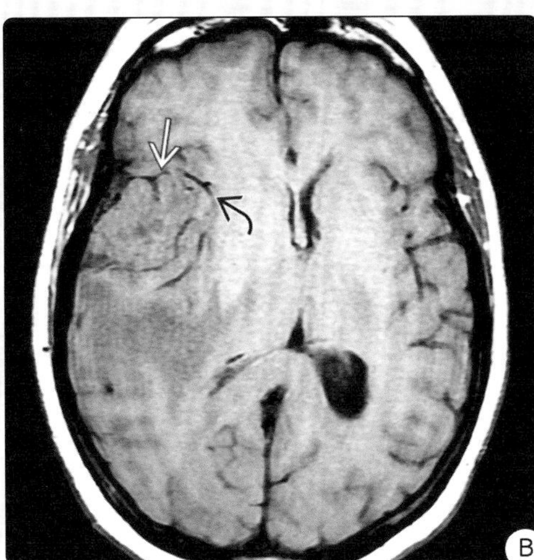


*(28-5A) NECT in a 55-yo woman with headaches shows a lobulated, hyperdense mass ➡ with adjacent edema ↷. (28-5B) Axial T1 MR in the same patient shows that the mass ➡ is mostly isointense with brain. Note prominent adjacent "flow voids" ↷ around the mass.*

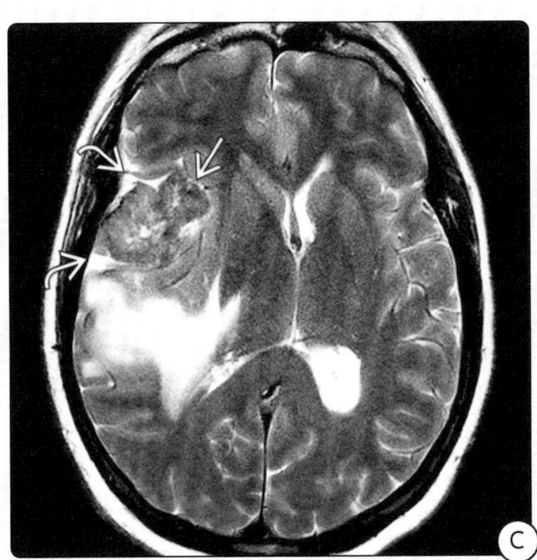


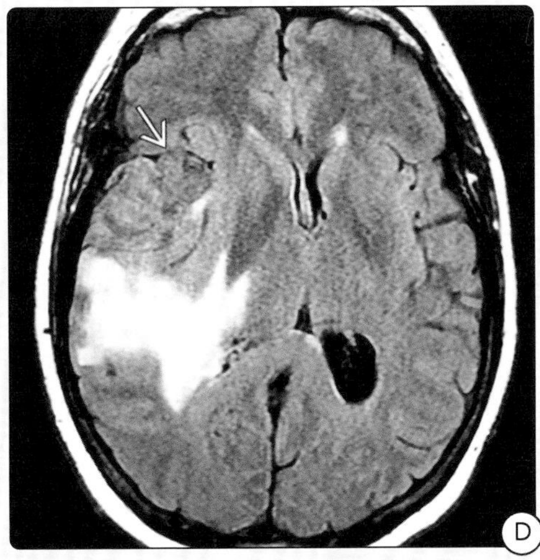


*(28-5C) The lobulated mass ➡ is quite hypointense and appears to be extraaxial, invaginating into the brain with an adjacent CSF "cleft" around the tumor ↷. (28-5D) The mass ➡ is mostly isointense with adjacent brain on FLAIR MR.*

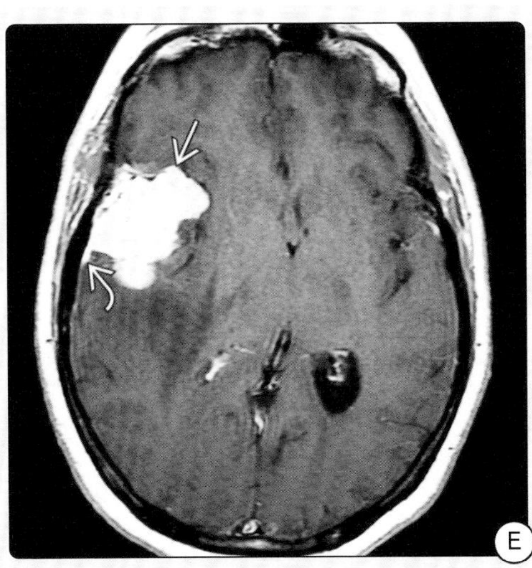


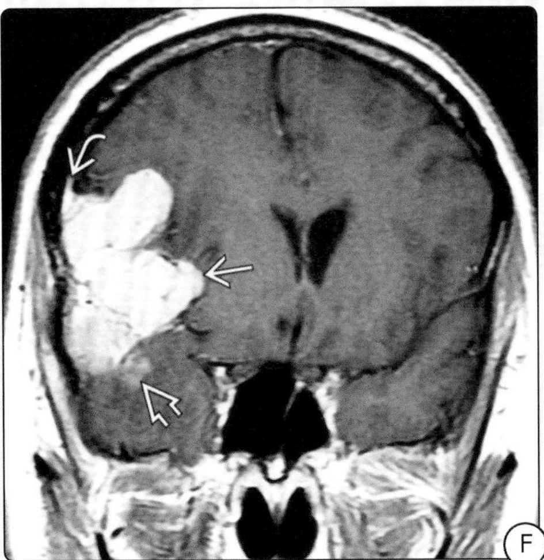


*(28-5E) The mass ➡ enhances intensely following contrast administration. Note a subtle dural "tail" ↷ associated with the mass. (28-5F) Coronal T1 C+ MR shows the lobulated mass ➡ with dural "tail" ↷. Note faint enhancement in the adjacent temporal lobe ⇨, suggesting brain invasion. Preoperative diagnosis was meningioma. Solitary fibrous tumor, CNS WHO grade 3 with STAT6 nuclear expression was found at pathology.*

**Staging, Grading, and Classification.** Three grades of SFT/HPC are recognized in the 2021 WHO. Grading is based on mitotic activity in 10 adjacent high-power fields (HPF). CNS WHO grade 1 tumors have ≤ 5 mitoses/10 HPF. Grade 2 tumors have ≥ 5 mitoses/10 HPF **without** necrosis. Grade 3 tumors have ≥ 5 mitoses/10 HPF **with** necrosis.

## Clinical Issues

**Epidemiology.** SFTs are rare, accounting for < 1% of all primary intracranial neoplasms and 2-4% of all meningeal tumors.

**Demographics.** Meningeal SFTs generally occur at a slightly younger age than meningiomas. Mean age at diagnosis is 43 years. There is a slight male predominance.

**Natural History.** Even with complete resection, local recurrence is the rule. The majority of meningeal SFTs eventually metastasize extracranially to bone, lung, and liver. There is no significant difference in survival between grade 2 and grade 3 SFTs.

**Treatment Options.** Surgical resection with radiation therapy or radiosurgery is the treatment of choice.

## Imaging

**CT Findings.** SFTs are hyperdense extraaxial masses **(28-5A)** that invade and destroy bone. Extracalvarial extension under the scalp is common. Calcification and reactive hyperostosis are absent. Strong but heterogeneous enhancement is typical.

**MR Findings.** Low-grade intracranial SFTs are circumscribed masses that are usually dura based and resemble meningioma. Lesions are isointense with gray matter on T1WI **(28-3A)** and have variable signal intensity on T2WI **(28-3B)**. A mixed hyper- and hypointense pattern is common. Collagen-rich areas can be very hypointense **(28-5C)**. Avid enhancement following contrast administration is typical **(28-5E)**.

Most SFTs demonstrate mixed signal intensity on all sequences **(28-5)**. They tend to be predominantly isointense to gray matter on T1 scans and iso- to hyperintense on T2 scans **(28-3B)**. Prominent "flow voids" are almost always present. Contrast enhancement is marked but heterogeneous. Nonenhancing necrotic foci are common. A dural tail sign is absent.

**Angiography.** SFTs may invade and occlude dural sinuses, so CTV or MRV are helpful noninvasive techniques for delineating patency.

DSA shows most SFTs as hypervascular masses with prominent vascularity, "early draining" veins, and intense prolonged tumor "staining." SFTs usually recruit blood supply from both dural and pial vessels.

## Differential Diagnosis

The major differential diagnosis of grade 1 SFT is CNS WHO grade 1 **meningioma**. Grades 2 and 3 SFTs may resemble higher grade (2, 3) meningiomas. Unlike meningiomas, SFTs rarely calcify or cause hyperostosis, and a dural tail sign is typically absent.

**Dural metastases** with skull invasion can be indistinguishable from SFTs. Rare neoplasms that can resemble SFTs include other sarcomas.

### SOLITARY FIBROUS TUMOR

**Terminology and Etiology**
- SFT
  - "Hemangiopericytoma" (HPC) is no longer used
  - Spectrum of tumors sharing common molecular features
  - *NAB2::STAT6* gene fusion

**Pathology**
- SFT CNS WHO grade 1
  - Collagenous, low-cellularity spindle cell lesion
  - ≤ 5 mitoses/10 HPF
- SFT CNS WHO grade 2
  - More cellular, "staghorn" vasculature
  - ≥ 5 mitoses/10 HPF, no necrosis
- SFT CNS WHO grade 3
  - ≥ 5 mitoses/10 HPF with necrosis

**Clinical Features**
- Rare (< 1% of CNS primary neoplasms)
  - However, most common CNS nonmeningothelial mesenchymal tumor
  - SFT/HPC grades 2, 3 recur, metastasize

**Imaging Findings**
- CT
  - Calcification absent
  - Hyperdense, lobulated dural-based mass
- MR
  - Isointense on T1WI
  - Hypointense on T2WI
  - Strong heterogeneous enhancement ± dural tail on T1 C+
  - May have prominent "flow voids"

**Differential Diagnosis**
- SFT grade 1 = meningioma
- SFT grades 2 and 3
  - Atypical/malignant meningioma
  - Dural metastases
  - Sarcomas
  - Malignant mesenchymal tumor

# Hemangioma

## Terminology

Hemangiomas are true benign mesenchymal nonmeningothelial tumors. They closely resemble normal vessels and are found in all organs of the body **(28-6)**. Hemangiomas are completely different from—and should not be confused with—cavernous or capillary malformations and arteriovenous malformations, which are all vascular malformations rather than true neoplasms. Vascular malformations were discussed in Chapter 7.

## Etiology

Hemangiomas probably arise by endothelial hyperplasia and hamartomatous-like proliferation.

## Pathology

**Location.** Hemangiomas arise preferentially in the spine. Intracranial hemangiomas can be located in different cranial compartments but are almost always extraaxial. They are found in the calvarium **(28-7)**, dural venous sinuses, and dura.

**Size and Number.** Hemangiomas vary in size from microscopic to massive. Transspatial extension across different anatomic compartments (e.g., scalp and skull, soft tissues, orbit, and cavernous sinus) is common. Multicentric lesions are uncommon in the CNS.

**Gross Pathology.** Hemangiomas are nonencapsulated, vascular-appearing, soft reddish-brown lesions. When they involve the calvaria, radiating spicules of lamellar bone are interspersed with vascular channels of varying sizes **(28-7)**. Hemangiomas of the venous sinuses and dura do not contain bone but otherwise resemble calvarial hemangiomas, consisting of large vascular channels in a soft, compressible mass.

**Microscopic Features.** Most intracranial hemangiomas consist of tightly packed, capillary-sized, and cavernous vessels with large, endothelium-lined spaces separated by fibrous septa.

**Staging, Grading, and Classification.** Hemangiomas are CNS WHO grade 1 neoplasms.

## Clinical Issues

**Demographics.** Hemangiomas represent only about 1% of all bone tumors. Most are found in the spine; the diploic space of the calvaria is the most common intracranial site. Dural and venous sinus hemangiomas are rare.

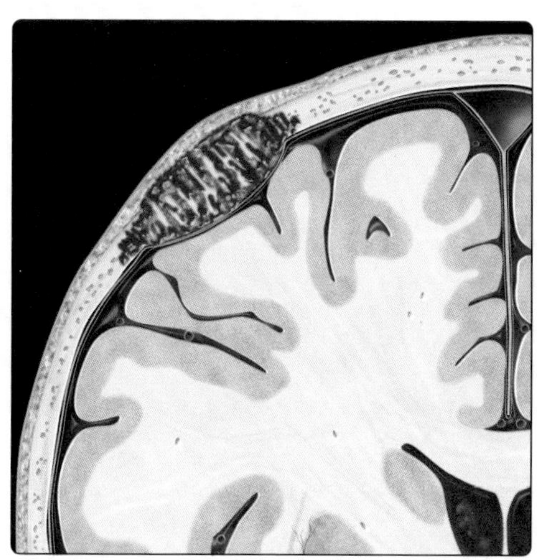

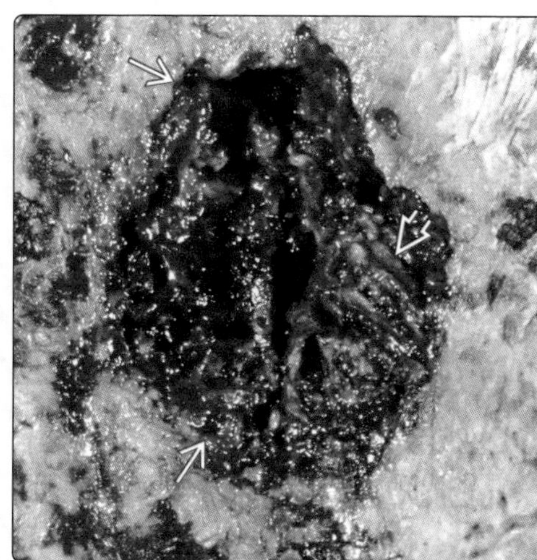

***(28-6)** Coronal graphic depicts a typical hemangioma of the calvaria as spicules of lamellar bone interspersed with vascular channels. **(28-7)** Photograph of a resected calvarial hemangioma shows an unencapsulated, very vascular-appearing mass ➡ with radiating spicules of bone ➡.*

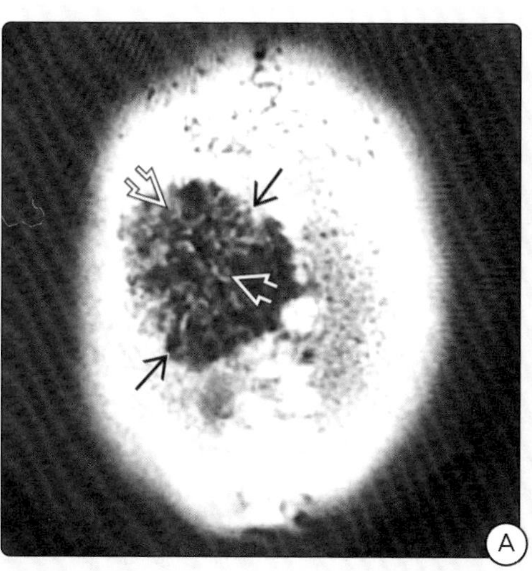


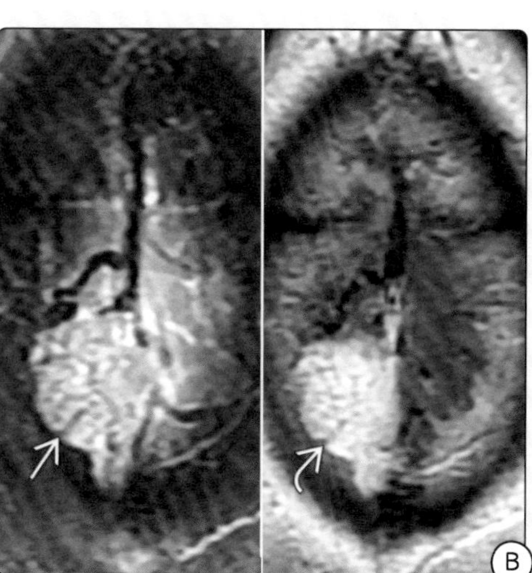


***(28-8A)** Bone CT show a well-defined lytic lesion ➡ at the vertex of the skull. Note spicules of preserved bone ➡ within the lesion. **(28-8B)** The lesion ➡ is extremely hyperintense on T2 MR (L) and enhances strongly on T1 C+ MR ➡ (R). This is calvarial hemangioma.*

Hemangiomas can occur at any age, although the peak presentation is between the fourth and fifth decades. The M:F ratio is 1:2-4.

**Presentation.** Most calvarial hemangiomas are asymptomatic, limited to the diploic space, and do not extend beyond the inner and outer tables of the skull **(28-10)**. Large lesions may present as painless firm masses. Scalp hemangiomas presenting with Kasabach-Merritt syndrome (consumptive coagulopathy due to sequestration and destruction of clotting factors within the lesion) have been reported.

Cavernous sinus hemangiomas can be asymptomatic but often present with headache, diplopia, or other cranial neuropathies, such as anisocoria.

Intracranial hemangiomas occasionally occur as part of **POEMS** syndrome, a rare, multisystem disease with typical features of **p**olyneuropathy, **o**rganomegaly, **e**ndocrinopathy, **m**onoclonal plasma-proliferative disorders, and **s**kin changes.

**Natural History.** Hemangiomas typically grow very slowly and do not undergo malignant degeneration. Pregnancy or hormone administration may trigger enlargement.

Capillary hemangiomas of infancy (usually in the skin, scalp, orbit, or oral mucosa and only rarely involving the brain) appear within a few months of birth, grow rapidly, plateau, and then involute.

**Treatment Options.** Calvarial hemangiomas are typically left alone unless tumor growth is demonstrated. The treatment of venous sinus hemangiomas is much more problematic. These highly vascular lesions bleed easily, and surgical mortality is high. Radiation (gamma knife surgery) has been used with some success in a few reported cases and may become the primary treatment choice for hemangiomas in critical locations, such as the cavernous sinus.

*(28-10A) Axial bone CT in a 32-yo woman with headaches shows an extensive salt and pepper lesion ➡ that causes slight expansion of the right parietal diploë. (28-10B) Axial T1 MR in the same patient shows that the extensive lesion ⇨ is slightly hyperintense compared with the normal diploic space. The cortex appears thinned in some areas ↪ but is largely intact.*

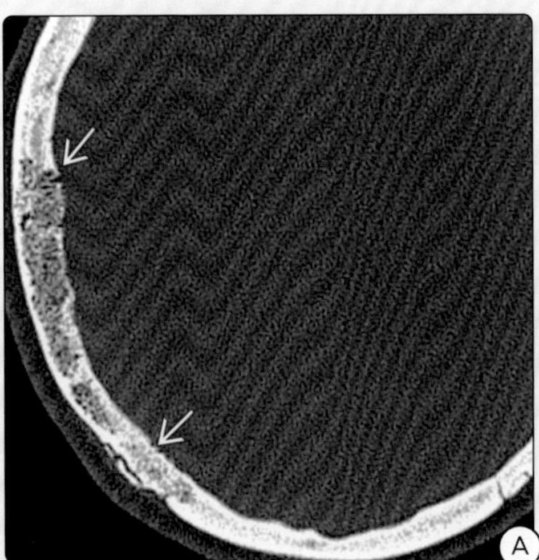

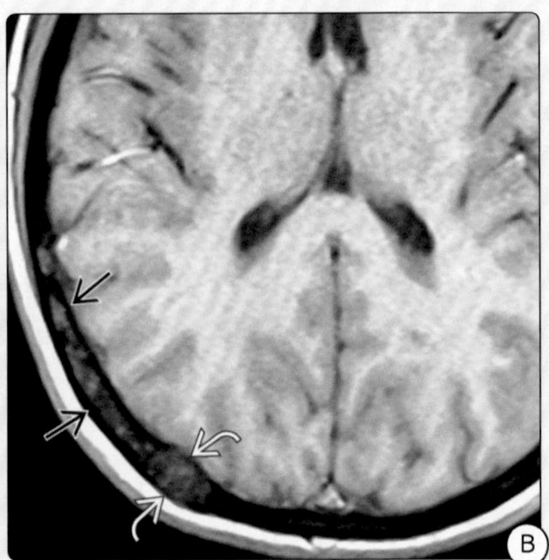

*(28-10C) Axial T2 MR in the same patient shows that the extensive diploic space lesion ➡ has a very hyperintense but speckled appearance and has focally thinned and broken through the cortex ↪. (28-10D) Axial T1 C+ FS MR shows that the lesion enhances intensely ➡ and has a striated or speckled appearance ↪. This is calvarial hemangioma.*

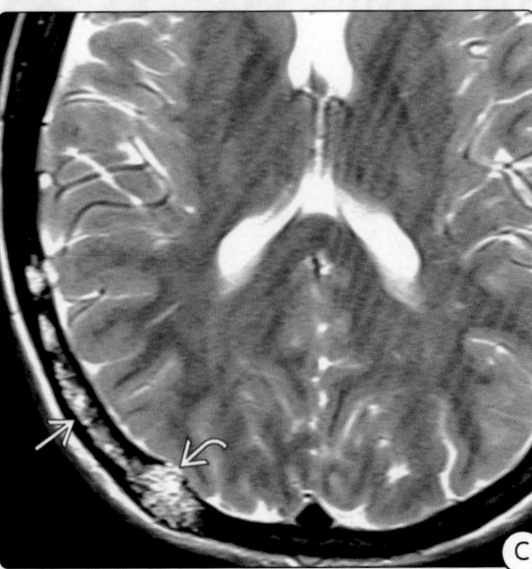

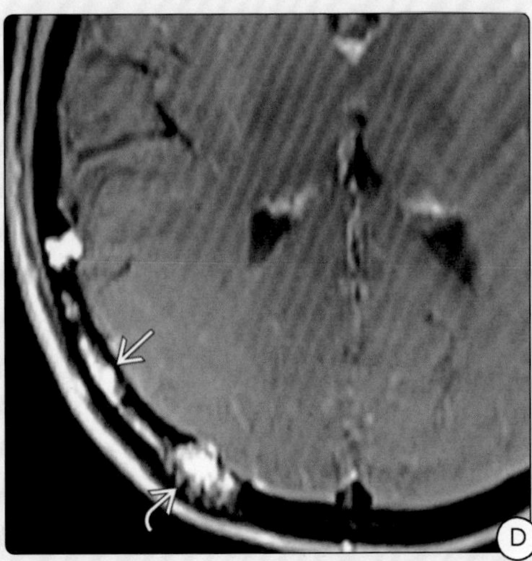

## Imaging

**CT Findings.** A calvarial hemangioma is seen as a sharply marginated, expansile diploic mass on NECT. Some lesions isolated to the scalp may have no underlying bony involvement.

Bone CT shows that the inner and outer tables are thinned but usually intact **(28-10A)**. A thin sclerotic margin may surround the lesion. "Spoke-wheel" or reticulated hyperdensities caused by fewer but thicker trabeculae are present within the hemangioma, giving it a honeycomb or jail bars appearance **(28-8A)**.

On CECT, foci of intense enhancement interspersed with focal hypodensities caused by the residual thickened trabeculae are typical.

**MR Findings.** Mixed hypo- to isointensity is the dominant pattern on T1WI. Scattered hyperintensities usually are caused by fat—not hemorrhage—within the lesion. Most hemangiomas are markedly hyperintense on T2WI **(28-10C)** **(28-12B)**.

Contrast-enhanced scans show diffuse intense enhancement **(28-8B)**. Dynamic scans show slow centripetal "filling in" of the lesion **(28-12C)**.

**Angiography.** Dural and venous sinus hemangiomas can closely resemble meningiomas with slow, persistent contrast accumulation in the capillary and venous phases of the angiogram.

## Differential Diagnosis

The differential diagnosis of calvarial hemangioma includes "holes in the skull" caused by venous lakes and arachnoid granulations, burr holes, dermoids, eosinophilic granuloma, and metastasis.

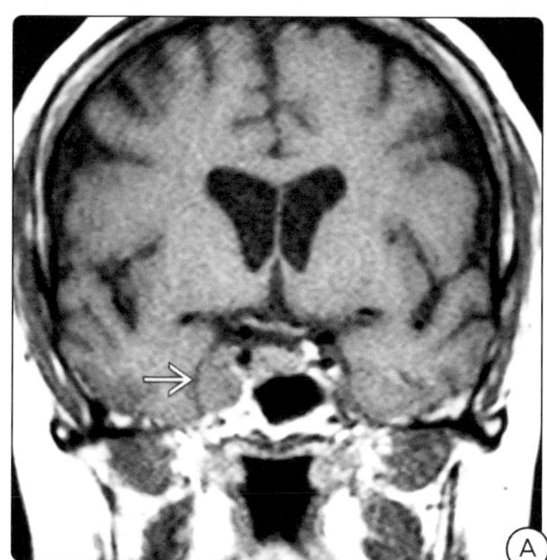


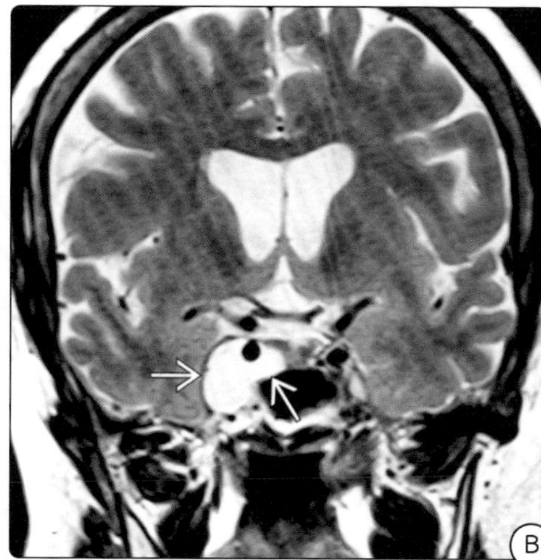


***(28-12A)** Coronal T1 MR in a 66-yo woman with a diagnosis of meningioma on outside MR shows a mass ➡ in the right cavernous sinus that is isointense with gray matter. **(28-12B)** Coronal T2 MR in the same patient shows that the mass ➡ is extremely and uniformly hyperintense.*

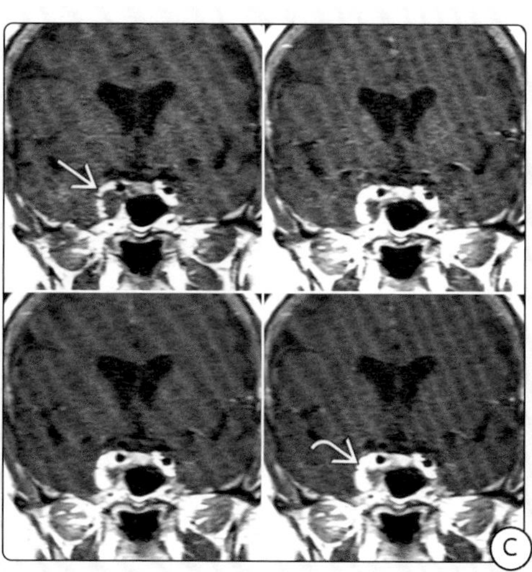


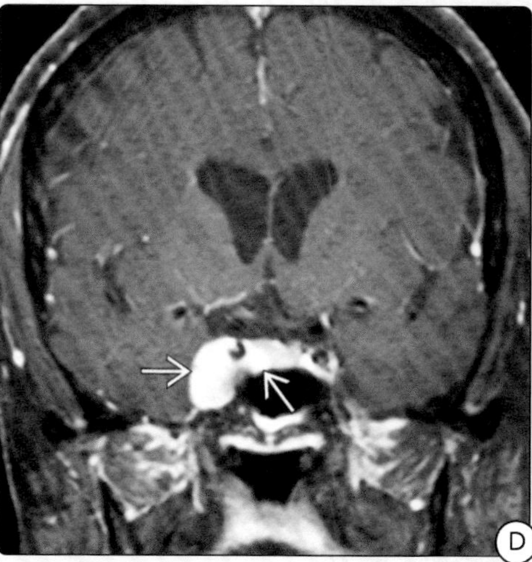


***(28-12C)** Dynamic C+ FS T1 MR images show progressive "filling in" of the mass by contrast with the periphery of the lesions filling first ➡, followed by centripetal (central) enhancement of the rest of the lesion with time ➥. **(28-12D)** T1 C+ FS MR 5 min after contrast injection for the dynamic sequence shows that the entire mass ➡ now enhances intensely and uniformly. This is cavernous sinus hemangioma. Surgery was canceled.*

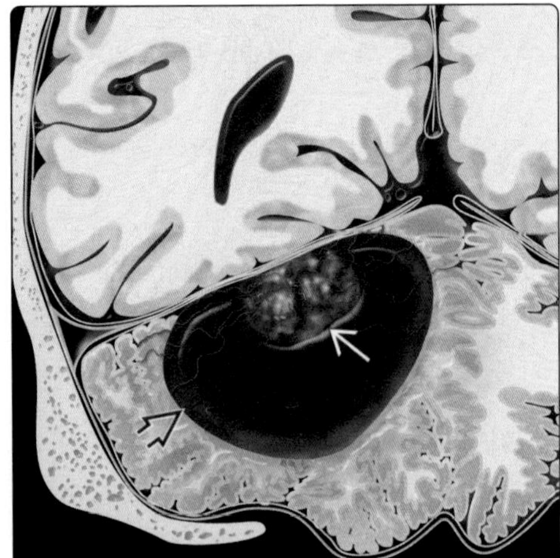

(28-13) Graphic depicts typical HGBL with cyst wall ⇨ composed of compressed cerebellum. Vascular tumor nodule ➡ abuts pial surface.

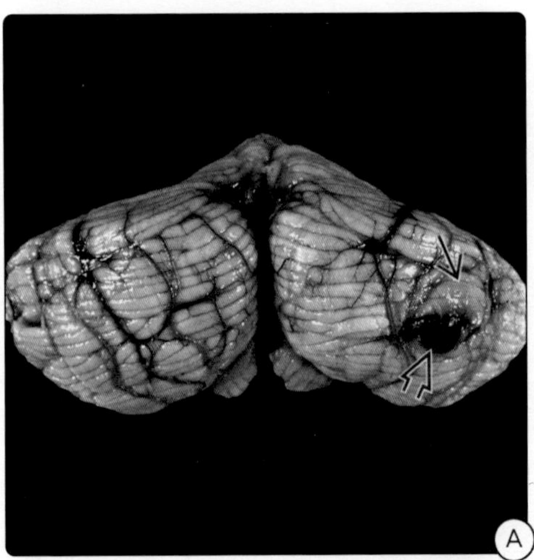

(28-15A) Autopsy specimen shows superficial nodule abutting the pia ⇨ and a hemorrhagic cyst ⇨ of a typical HGBL. (Courtesy E. Ross, MD.)

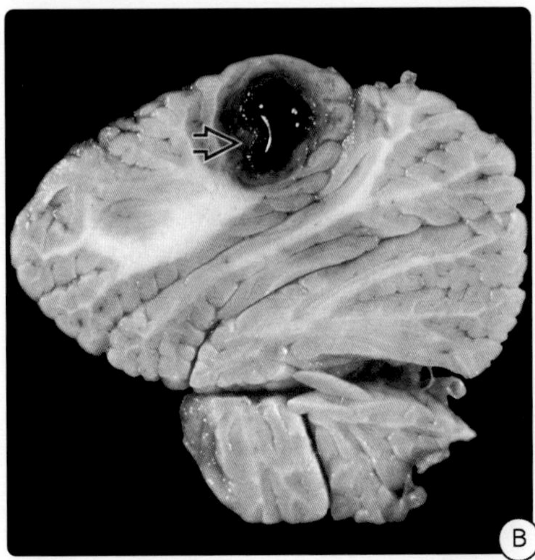

(28-15B) Sagittal section in the same patient shows the hemorrhagic cyst ⇨. The tumor nodule is not visible. (Courtesy E. Ross, MD.)

The major differential diagnosis for dural/venous sinus hemangioma is **meningioma**. Except for the microcystic variant, meningiomas do not display the marked hyperintensity on T2WI seen in most hemangiomas. Hemangiomas also exhibit the classic "filling in" from the periphery to the center of the lesion on rapid-sequence, dynamic contrast-enhanced T1WIs.

CALVARIAL AND DURAL HEMANGIOMAS

**Pathology**
- Benign vasoformative neoplasm with capillary-type growth pattern
- Calvarium (diploic space) more than dura, dural venous sinuses

**Clinical Features**
- Any age; mostly small/asymptomatic

**Imaging Findings**
- CT: Radiating "spoke-wheel" bone spicules
- MR: T2 "honeycomb" hyperintensities
  - Dynamic T1 C+ shows "filling in" of lesion

**Differential Diagnosis**
- Calvarial: Venous channels, arachnoid granulations, etc.
- Dura/venous sinus: Meningioma

# Hemangioblastoma

## Terminology

Hemangioblastoma (HGBL) is a benign, slow-growing, relatively indolent vascular neoplasm. HGBL occurs in both sporadic (70%) and multiple (30%) familial forms.

Multiple HGBLs are almost always associated with the autosomal-dominant inherited cancer syndrome **von Hippel-Lindau disease** (VHL). A rare non-VHL form of multiple disseminated HGBLs is termed **leptomeningeal hemangioblastomatosis**.

## Etiology

Allelic losses or mutations of the *VHL* gene at 3p25-26 are found in both sporadic HGBL and VHL. *VHL* gene mutations (losses or inactivations) are present in up to 80% of sporadic HGBLs. Multiple key angiogenic pathways, including VEGF-related angiogenesis, are massively activated in HGBL and contribute synergistically to the tumor's abundant vascularization.

## Pathology

**Location.** HGBLs can occur in any part of the CNS, although the vast majority (90-95%) of intracranial HGBLs are located in the posterior fossa **(28-15)**. The cerebellum is, by far, the most common site (80%) followed by the vermis (15%). Approximately 5% occur in the brainstem, usually the medulla. The nodule of an HGBL is superficially located and typically abuts a pial surface **(28-13)**.

Supratentorial tumors are rare, accounting for 5-10% of all HGBLs. Most are clustered around the optic pathways and occur in the setting of VHL.

**Size and Number.** HGBLs vary in size from tiny to large, especially when associated with a cyst. Unless they are syndromic, HGBLs are solitary lesions. If > one HGBL is present, the patient, by definition, has VHL. A positive family history or presence of other VHL markers (such as visceral cysts, retinal angioma, renal cell carcinoma) should prompt genetic screening.

**Gross Pathology.** The common appearance is that of a beefy red, vascular-appearing nodule that abuts a pial surface **(28-14)**. A variably sized cyst is present in 50-60% of cases **(28-15B)**. Cyst fluid is typically yellowish, and the cyst wall is usually smooth. Approximately 40% of HGBLs are solid tumors.

**Microscopic Features.** HGBLs contain two different cell types, stromal and vascular cells. Generally, it is the stromal (not the vascular) cells that are the neoplastic element of an HGBL.

The cyst wall of most HGBLs is nonneoplastic, composed of compressed brain with fibrillary neuroglia devoid of tumor cells. The intratumoral cyst fluid shares a proteomic fingerprint with normal serum and has no proteins in common with HGBL tumor tissue. Cyst formation in HGBLs is therefore a result of vascular leakage from tumor vessels, not tumor liquefaction or active secretion.

Mitoses in HGBLs are few or absent, so proliferation rates are low, too (usually MIB-1 < 1). HGBL is a CNS WHO grade 1 neoplasm. There is no recognized atypical or anaplastic variant.

#### HEMANGIOBLASTOMA: PATHOLOGY AND CLINICAL ISSUES

**Pathology**

- Posterior fossa (90-95%)
  - Cerebellum most common site
- Cyst + nodule (60%), solid (40%)

**Clinical Issues**

- Epidemiology/demographics
  - Uncommon (1.0-2.5% of primary brain tumors)
  - 7% of all adult primary posterior fossa tumors
  - Peak age: 30-65 years (younger with VHL), rare < 15 years
- Presentation/natural history
  - May cause hydrocephalus
  - Dysmetria, ataxia
  - 5% have secondary polycythemia
  - Slow, "stuttering" growth
  - Metastasis rare

## Clinical Issues

**Epidemiology.** HGBL accounts for 1.0-2.5% of primary CNS neoplasms and approximately 7% of all primary posterior fossa tumors in adults. It is the second most common infratentorial parenchymal mass in adults (after metastasis).

Between 25-40% of HGBLs are associated with VHL.

**Demographics.** HGBL is generally a tumor of adults between the ages of 30 and 65 years. Pediatric HGBLs are rare. VHL-associated HGBLs tend to present at a significantly younger age but are still relatively rare in children under the age of 15. There is a slight male predominance.

**Presentation.** Most symptoms in patients with the cystic form of HGBL are caused by the cyst, not the neoplastic nodule. Headache is the presenting symptom in 85% of cases. HGBLs produce erythropoietin, which causes secondary polycythemia in approximately 5% of patients.

**Natural History and Treatment Options.** Because HGBLs exhibit a stuttering growth pattern, they are frequently stable lesions that can remain asymptomatic for long intervals. Imaging progression alone is not an indication for treatment, although tumor/cyst growth rates can be used to predict symptom formation and future need for treatment.

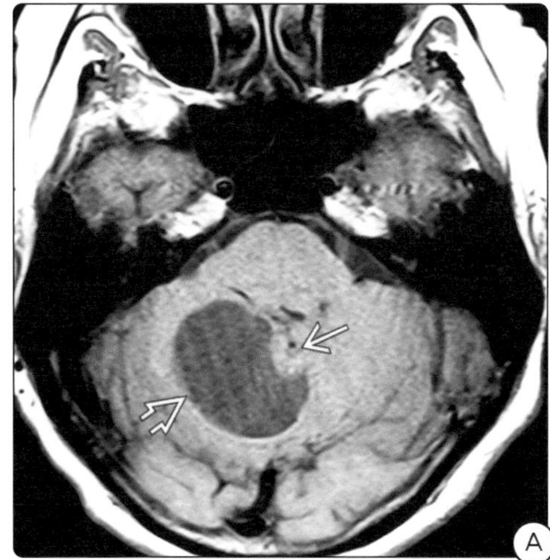


***(28-17A)** Axial T1 MR in a 70-yo woman with ataxia shows a cystic cerebellar mass ➲ with a mural nodule ➲.*

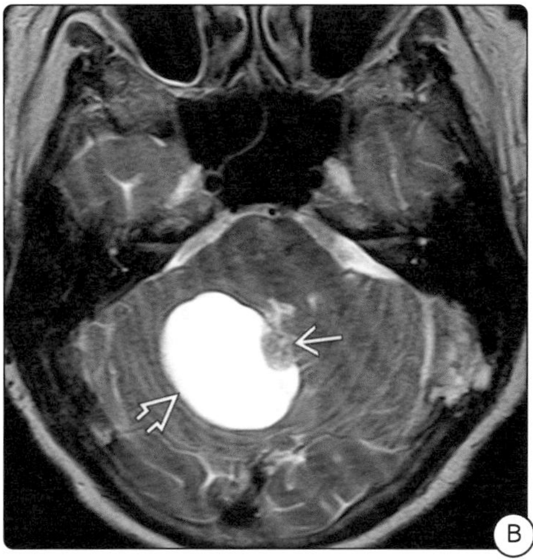


***(28-16B)** T2 FS MR shows that the cyst fluid ➲ is very hyperintense, while the nodule is mostly isointense ➲ with adjacent brain.*

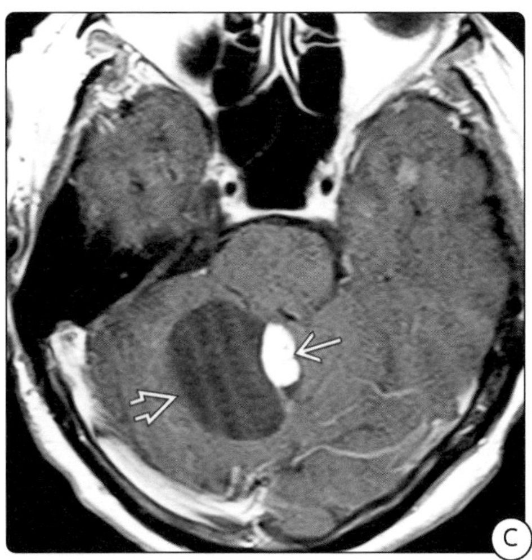


***(28-16C)** T1 C+ MR shows mural nodule enhancing intensely ➲ while the cyst wall does not ➲. This is solitary HGBL, WHO grade 1.*

Although HGBLs show no intrinsic tendency to metastasize, there are sporadic reports of intraspinal dissemination. Complete en bloc resection is the procedure of choice. Total resection eliminates tumor recurrence, although new HGBLs may develop in the setting of VHL.

## Imaging

**General Features.** HGBLs have four basic imaging patterns: (1) Solid HGBLs without associated cysts, (2) HGBLs with intratumoral cysts, (3) HGBLs with peritumoral cysts (nonneoplastic cyst with solid tumor nodule), and (4) HGBLs associated with both peri- and intratumoral cysts (nonneoplastic cyst with cysts in the tumor nodule). A nonneoplastic peritumoral cyst with solid nodule is the most common pattern, seen in 50-65% of cases. The second most common pattern is the solid form, seen in about 40% of cases.

### HEMANGIOBLASTOMA: IMAGING

**General Features**
- "Cyst + nodule" (60%)
  - Nodule abuts pial surface
- Solid (40%)

**CT**
- Low-density cyst
- Strongly enhancing nodule

**MR**
- Cyst
  - Fluid slightly hyperintense to CSF
  - Wall usually nonneoplastic
- Nodule
  - Isointense to brain
  - "Flow voids" common
  - Enhances intensely

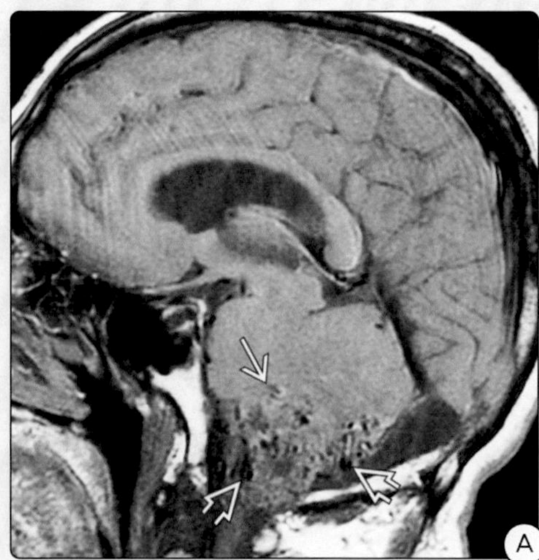


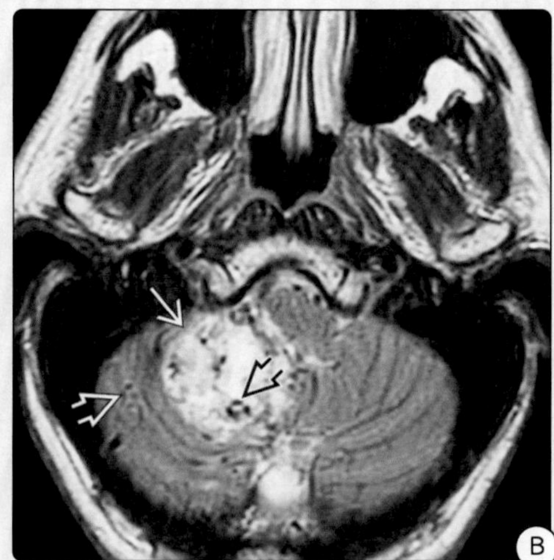


*(28-19A) Sagittal T1 MR in a 63-yo man with vertigo shows a posterior fossa mass ➡ with numerous prominent "flow voids" ➡. (28-19B) Axial T2 MR in the same patient shows that the mass ➡ is very hyperintense. Prominent "flow voids" are seen within the mass ➡ and adjacent cerebellum ➡.*

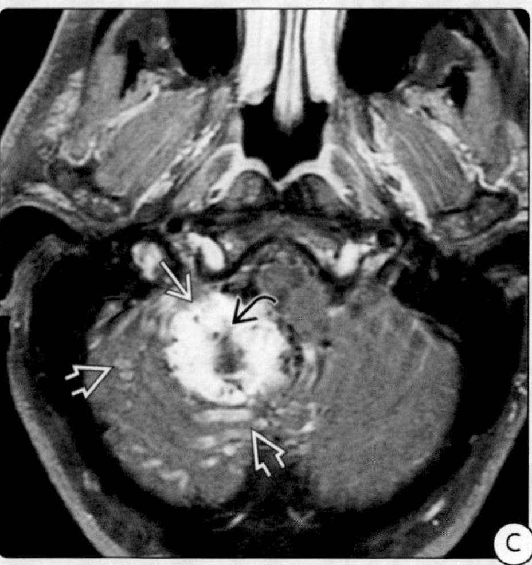


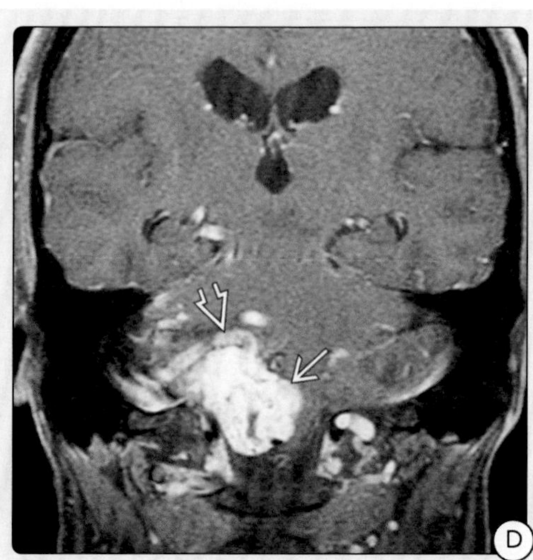


*(28-19C) Axial T1 C+ FS MR in the same patient shows that the mass ➡ enhances intensely and appears solid with an area of central necrosis ➡. Note numerous prominent serpentine enhancing vessels ➡ in the adjacent cerebellum. (28-19D) Coronal T1 C+ FS MR shows the solid mass ➡ and prominent draining vein ➡. This is HGBL, WHO grade 1.*

**CT Findings.** The most common appearance is a well-delineated iso- to slightly hyperdense nodule associated with a hypodense cyst. Calcification and gross hemorrhage are absent. The nodule enhances strongly and uniformly following contrast administration.

**MR Findings.** An isointense nodule with prominent "flow voids" is seen on T1WI. If an associated peritumoral cyst is present, it is typically hypointense to parenchyma on T1WI but hyperintense compared with CSF **(28-17)**.

Compared with brain parenchyma, the tumor nodule of an HGBL is moderately hyperintense on T2WI and FLAIR. Intratumoral cysts and prominent "flow voids" are common. The cyst fluid is very hyperintense on both T2WI and FLAIR **(28-17)**.

Occasionally, an HGBL hemorrhages. If present, blood products "bloom" on T2*.

Intense enhancement of the nodule—but not the cyst itself—is typical **(28-16C)**. Cyst wall enhancement should raise the possibility of tumor involvement, as compressed, nonneoplastic brain does not enhance.

Noncystic HGBLs enhance strongly but often heterogeneously **(28-18)**. Multiple HGBLs are seen in VHL and vary from tiny punctate to large solid tumors (see Chapter 43).

Supratentorial HGBLs are rare. Most occur around the optic nerves or chiasm. HGBL also sometimes occurs as a hemispheric mass with a cyst + nodule appearance.

**Angiography.** The most common appearance is that of an intensely vascular tumor nodule that shows a prolonged vascular "blush" **(28-21)**. "Early draining" veins are common. If a tumor-associated cyst is present, vessels appear displaced and "draped" around an avascular mass.

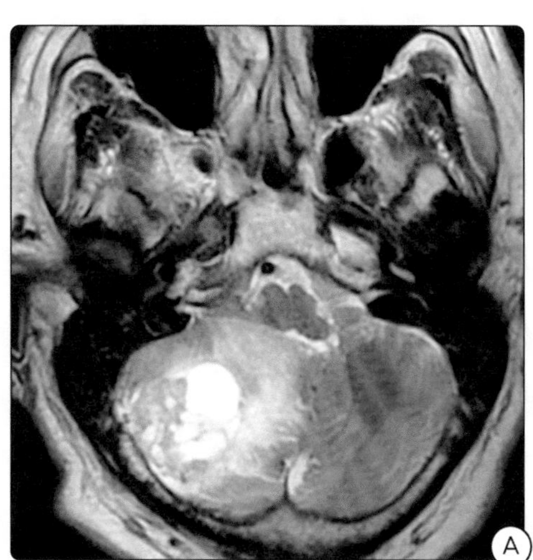


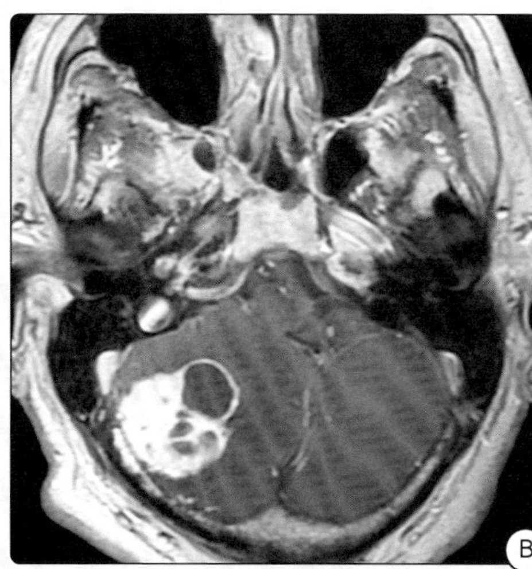


***(28-20A)** Axial T2 MR in a 62-yo man with a 2-month history of imbalance and vertigo shows a very heterogeneous iso- and hyperintense mass in the right cerebellar hemisphere with significant surrounding edema. **(28-20B)** T1 C+ MR in the same patient shows a mixed solid and cystic enhancing mass. HGBL, CNS WHO grade 1 was found at surgery.*

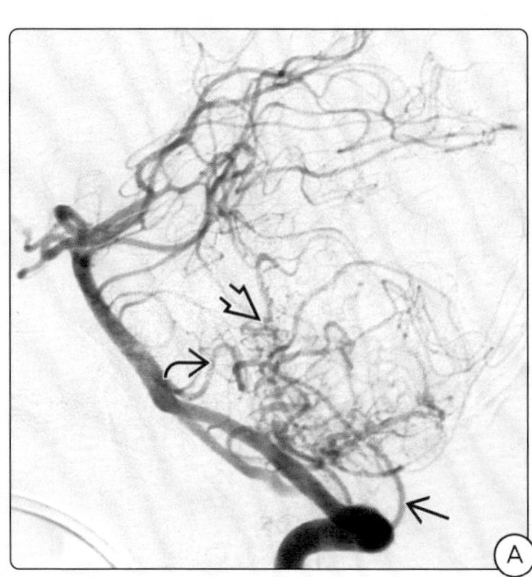


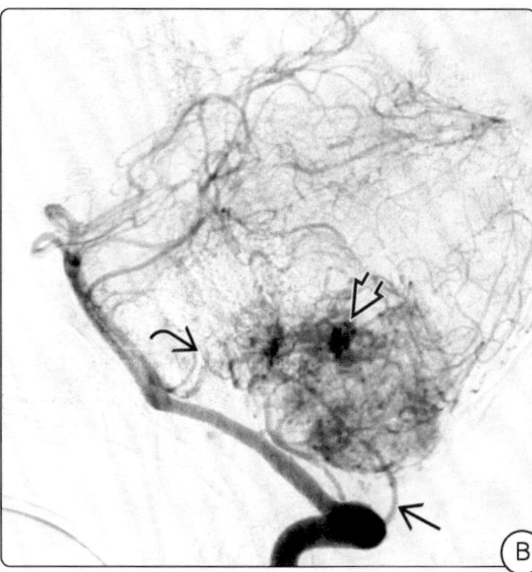


***(28-22A)** Early arterial phase, lateral view of a vertebrobasilar DSA shows a patient with cerebellar HGBL. Note a vascular tumor mass ➡ supplied primarily by enlarged branches of the anterior ➡ and posterior inferior cerebellar arteries ➡. **(28-22B)** Late arterial phase in the same patient shows the characteristic prolonged tumor "blush" ➡ coming from branches of enlarged posterior ➡ and anterior ➡ inferior cerebellar arteries.*

### Differential Diagnosis

The differential diagnosis of HGBL varies with age. In a middle-aged or older adult, the statistically most common cause of an enhancing posterior fossa intraaxial (parenchymal) mass is **metastasis**, not HGBL! DWI and DSC-PWI are helpful in the characterization and differentiation of HGBL from brain metastases. HGBL has higher minimum ADC values and relative ADC ratios compared with metastases.

A cerebellar mass with "cyst + nodule" in a child or young adult is most likely a **pilocytic astrocytoma**, not HGBL or metastasis. Occasionally, a **cavernous malformation** can mimic an HGBL with hemorrhage.

## Tumors of Uncertain Differentiation

The 2021 WHO groups a number of rare sarcomas together as "tumors of uncertain differentiation." These include intracranial mesenchymal tumor, *FET::CREB* fusion-positive, *CIC*-rearranged sarcoma, primary intracranial sarcoma *DICER1*-mutant, and Ewing sarcoma. Most of these appear as relatively circumscribed extraaxial tumors attached to the dura. Mixed solid and cystic components, variable edema, and avid enhancement are typical features on imaging studies. Many have an enhancing dural "tail" and mimic meningioma **(28-23)**.

# Chondroosseous Tumors

Chondroosseous tumors include mesenchymal chondrosarcoma and chondrosarcoma. Approximately 1% of all chondrosarcomas are intracranial.

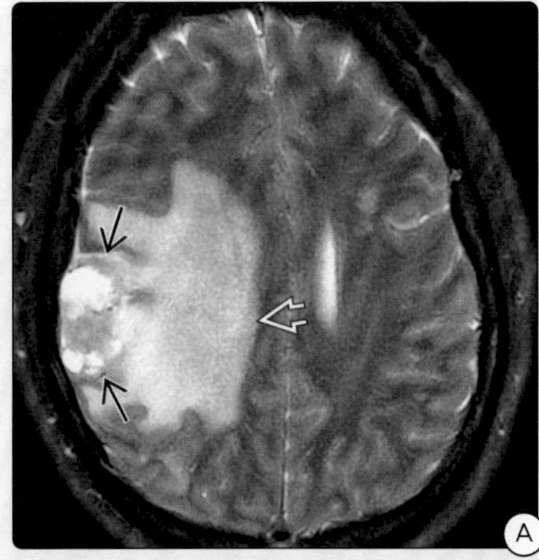
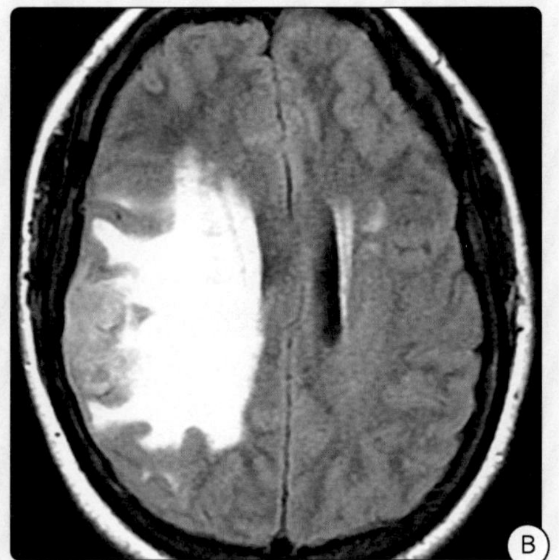

***(28-23A)** Axial T2 MR in a 37-yo woman shows a heterogeneous, mixed iso- and hyperintense lesion ⇨ in the right cerebral hemisphere with adjacent edema ⮕. **(28-23B)** The superficially located lesion is mostly isointense with gray matter on FLAIR MR.*

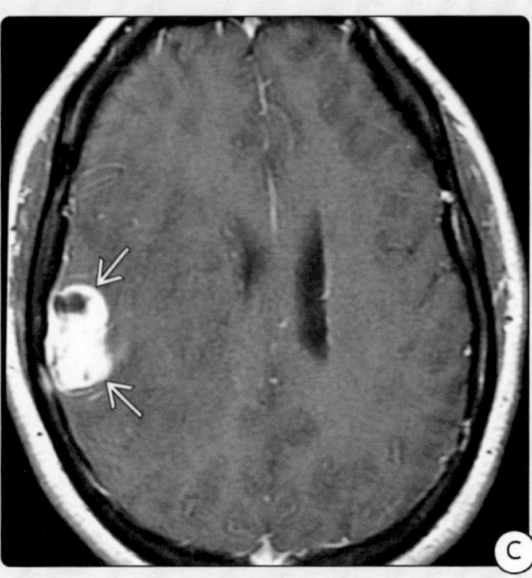
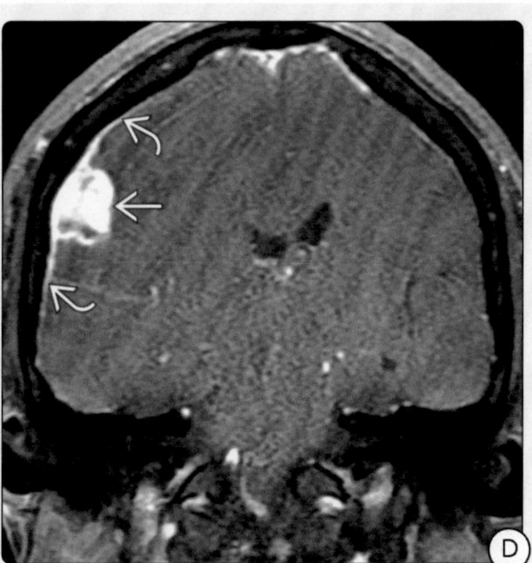

***(28-23C)** T1 C+ MR in the same patient shows the mass ⮕ enhancing strongly but somewhat heterogeneously. **(28-23D)** Coronal T1 C+ FS MR shows the heterogeneously enhancing mass ⮕ has an associated "dural tail" ⮫. Preoperative diagnosis was meningioma. Intracranial mesenchymal tumor with myxoid elements and EWSR1::CREB fusion was found at pathology.*

## Chondrosarcoma

### Terminology

Chondrosarcomas are a family of malignant mesenchymal tumors with cartilaginous differentiation.

### Etiology

Chondrosarcomas arise from remnants of embryonal cartilage, endochondral bone, or from primitive mesenchymal cells in the meninges. The majority of skull base chondrosarcomas harbor an *IDH1* or *IDH2* mutation.

Most chondrosarcomas are sporadic, but individuals with enchondromatosis (Ollier disease, Maffucci syndrome) have an increased risk of developing a chondrosarcoma.

### Pathology

**Location.** Most intracranial chondrosarcomas are located in the skull base, typically off-midline and centered on the petrooccipital fissure.

**Gross Pathology.** A smooth, lobulated, grayish-white mass arising from the petrooccipital fissure is the typical appearance.

**Microscopic Features.** Moderate hypercellularity with cartilaginous differentiation in a myxoid or hyaline matrix is typical. Chondrosarcomas are distinguished from chordoma by the absence of cohesive nests of cells. The neoplastic chondrocytes are negative for cytokeratin.

**Staging, Grading, and Classification.** CNS sarcomas are designated CNS WHO grade 1, 2, or 3 based on the degree of cellularity, cytologic atypia, and mitotic activity. Most skull base chondrosarcomas are grade 1 neoplasms.

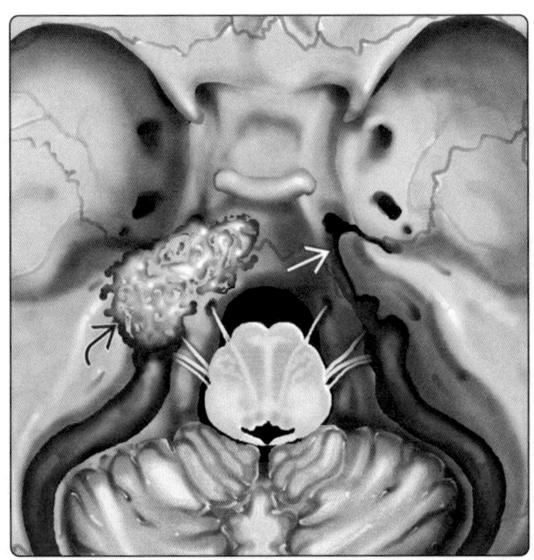

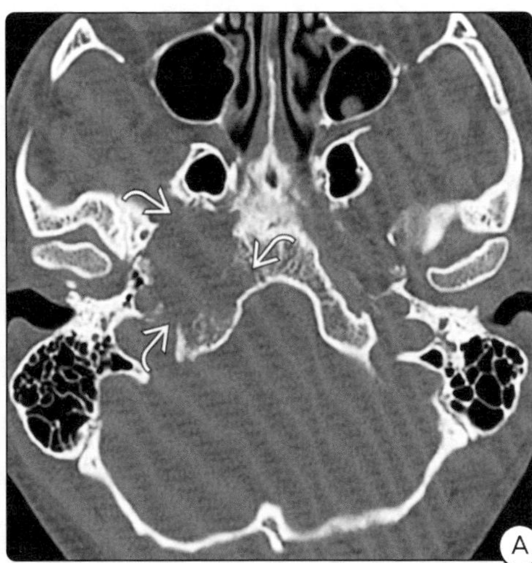

*(28-24) Axial graphic depicts the classic location of skull base chondrosarcoma centered at the petrooccipital fissure ➩. Note the normal contralateral petrooccipital fissure ➡. Chondroid calcifications are present within the lesion. (28-25A) Bone CT in a 29-yo man with right 6th cranial nerve palsy shows a destructive lesion centered in the right petrooccipital fissure ➡.*

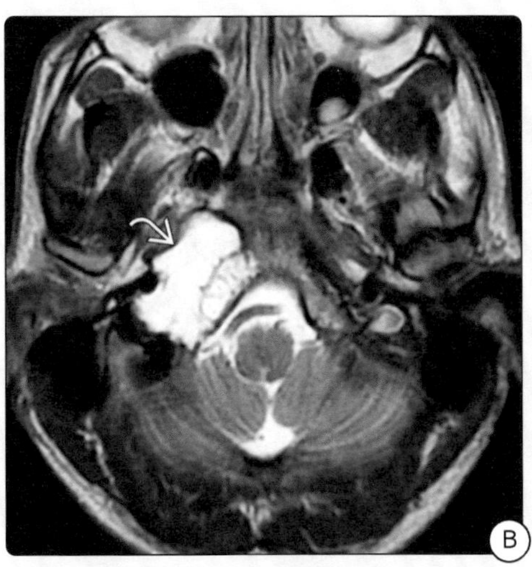

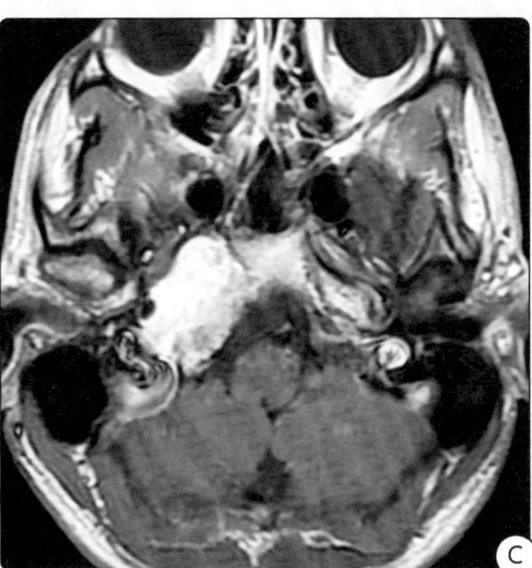

*(28-25B) T2 MR in the same patient shows the mass ➡ is extremely, almost uniformly hyperintense. (28-25C) T1 C+ MR shows the mass enhancing strongly and quite uniformly. CNS WHO grade 1 chondrosarcoma of the skull base centered at the petrooccipital fissure was found at surgery.*

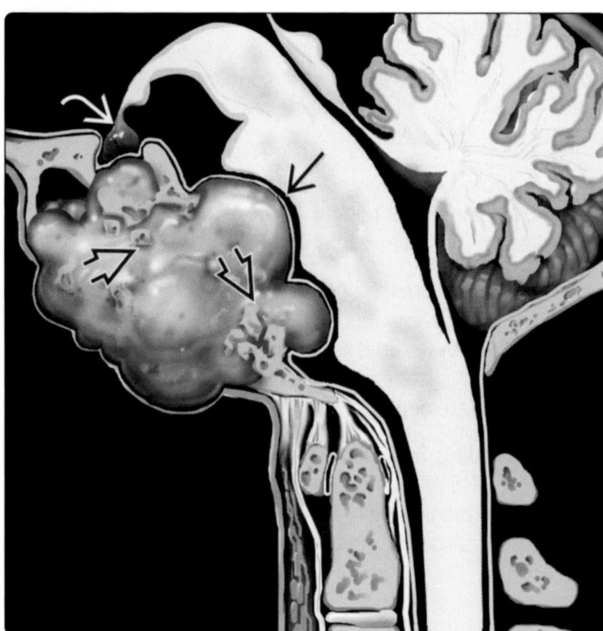

***(28-26)** Sagittal graphic shows an expansile, destructive, lobulated clival mass with a "thumb" of tumor ⇒ indenting the pons. The pituitary gland ➡ is elevated by the tumor. Note the bone fragments ⇒ "floating" in the chordoma.*

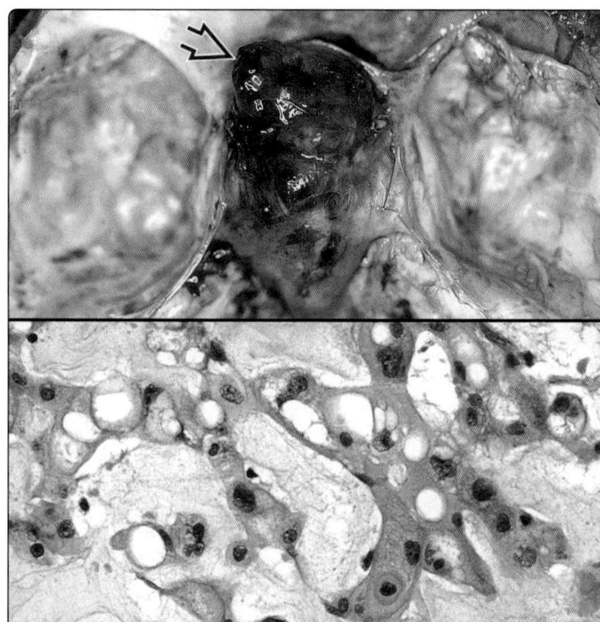

***(28-27)** (Top) Autopsy of clival chordoma shows a lobulated mass ⇒ invading the sella. (Bottom) Microscopy shows physaliphorous cells with vacuolated cytoplasm. (From Ellison: Neuropathology, 2013.)*

### Clinical Issues

Most patients are middle aged with headache and sometimes cranial nerve palsies.

### Imaging

CT shows an expansile mass at the petrooccipital fissure with erosive/destructive bone changes in the adjacent clivus and petrous apex **(28-25A)**. Approximately 50% of cases have a classic chondroid matrix with "rings and arcs" calcification.

Chondrosarcomas are low to intermediate signal intensity on T1WI and usually hyperintense on T2WI **(28-25B)**. Heterogeneous enhancement on T1 C+ is typical **(28-25C)**.

### Differential Diagnosis

The major differential diagnosis for chondrosarcoma is **chordoma**. Chordomas are more often midline, centered in the clivus. **Metastases** to the skull base are often multiple, hypointense on T2WI, and exhibit moderately strong enhancement. DWI and dynamic contrast-enhanced pMR can be helpful in differentiating these three common skull base tumors.

# Notochordal Tumors

There is only one notochordal neoplasm in the 2021 5th edition WHO classification of CNS tumors: Chordoma.

## Chordoma

### Terminology

Chordomas are rare, locally aggressive primary malignant bone neoplasms with a phenotype that demonstrates notochordal differentiation.

### Etiology

Skull base (clival) chordomas probably arise from the cranial end of primitive notochordal remnants. Subpopulations of cancer stem-like cells have been identified in some chordomas.

Signal transducer and activation of transcription (STAT) proteins regulate key cellular fates, including proliferation and apoptosis. *STAT3* is activated in chordoma.

### Pathology

Chordomas almost always arise within the axial skeleton, anywhere along the primitive notochord. The sacrum is the most common site (50% of all chordomas) followed by the sphenooccipital (clival) region (35%) **(28-26)** and spine (15%).

Most sphenooccipital chordomas are midline lesions. Occasionally, a chordoma is predominantly extraosseous and arises off-midline, usually in the nasopharynx or cavernous sinus.

Four major histologic forms of chordoma are recognized: Conventional ("classic"), chondroid, differentiated, and poorly differentiated *SMARCB1*-deficient types. Conventional chordoma is the most common type and consists of physaliphorous cells that contain mucin and glycogen vacuoles, giving this tumor a characteristic bubbly appearance to its cytoplasm.

Chondroid chordomas have stromal elements that resemble hyaline cartilage with neoplastic cells nestled within lacunae **(28-27)**. Dedifferentiated chordoma represents < 5% of chordomas and typically occurs in the sacrococcygeal region, not the clivus.

Both conventional and chondroid chordomas are strongly immunopositive for the epithelial markers cytokeratin (especially CK8) and epithelial membrane antigen (EMA). Dedifferentiated chordomas exhibit *SMARCB1*/INI1 loss and are associated with dismal prognosis.

## Clinical Issues

Chordomas account for 2-5% of all primary bone tumors but cause almost 40% of sacral tumors. Although chordomas may occur at any age, peak prevalence is between the fourth and sixth decades. *SMARCB1*-deficient chordomas are childhood tumors, presenting at a median age of seven years. There is a moderate male predominance.

Clival chordomas typically present with headaches and diplopia secondary to CNVI compression. Large chordomas may cause multiple cranial neuropathies, including visual loss and facial pain.

Although they grow slowly, chordomas are eventually lethal unless treated with aggressive resection and proton beam irradiation. Chondroid chordomas exhibit the most favorable outcomes, whereas dedifferentiated and poorly differentiated tumors are associated with the most rapid progression and worst overall survival.

## Imaging

NECT shows a relatively well-circumscribed, moderately hyperdense midline or paramedian clival mass with

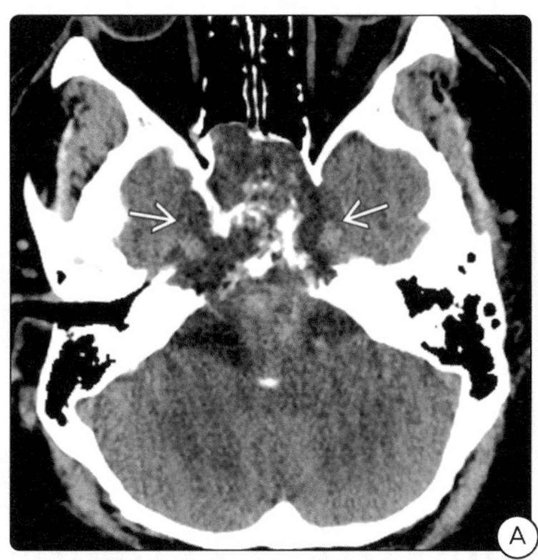


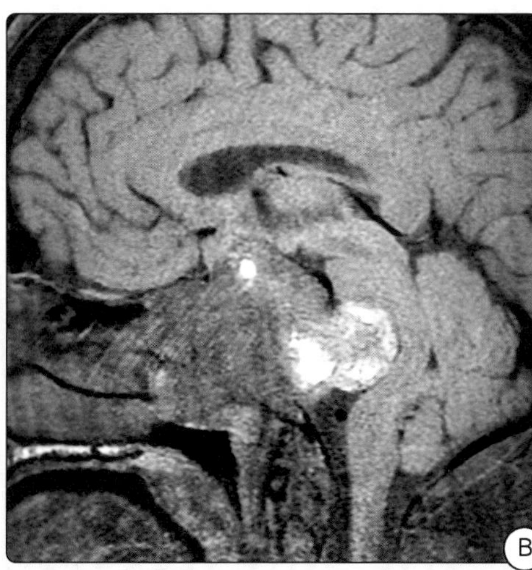


***(28-28A)** Axial NECT in a 39-yo man with multiple cranial nerve palsies shows a destructive, heterogeneous-appearing central skull base mass ➡. **(28-28B)** Sagittal T1 MR shows that the mass has destroyed almost the entire sphenoid bone with the "thumb" of tumor indenting the pons.*

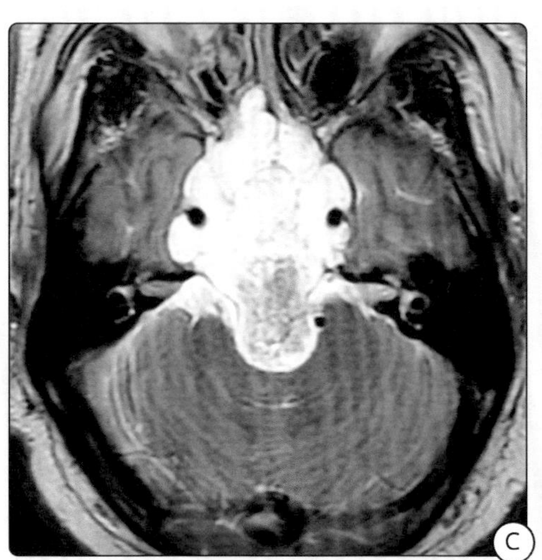


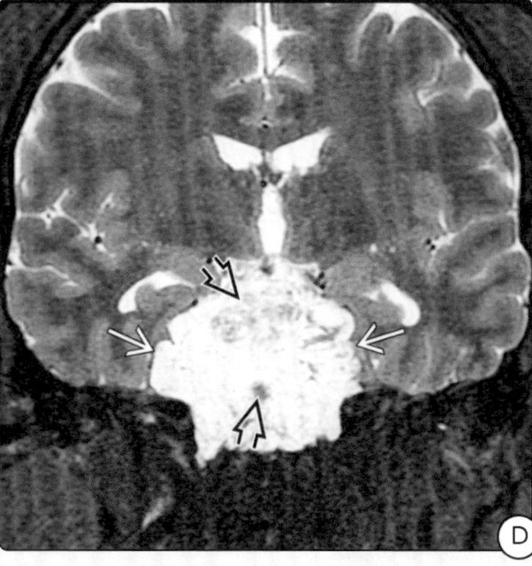


***(28-28C)** Axial T2 MR shows that the lobulated extradural mass is very hyperintense and displaces both carotid arteries laterally and the basilar artery posteriorly. **(28-28D)** T2 FS MR in the same patient shows that the destructive central skull base mass ➡ is exceptionally hyperintense. Iso-/hypointense foci within the mass ⇨ can represent calcifications or bone remnants. Conventional chordoma was found at surgery.*

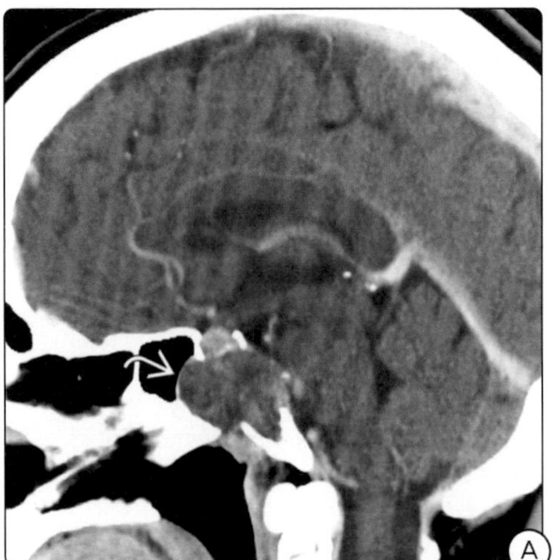


***(28-29A)** Sagittal CECT in a 54-yo woman with multiple cranial nerve palsies shows a destructive hypodense mass ➡ in the clivus.*

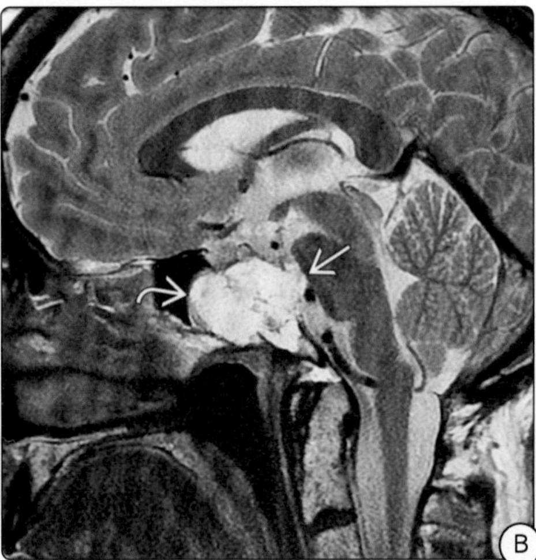


***(28-29B)** Sagittal T2 MR shows that the mass ➡ is extremely hyperintense and extends dorsally through the clivus ➡ to displace the pons.*

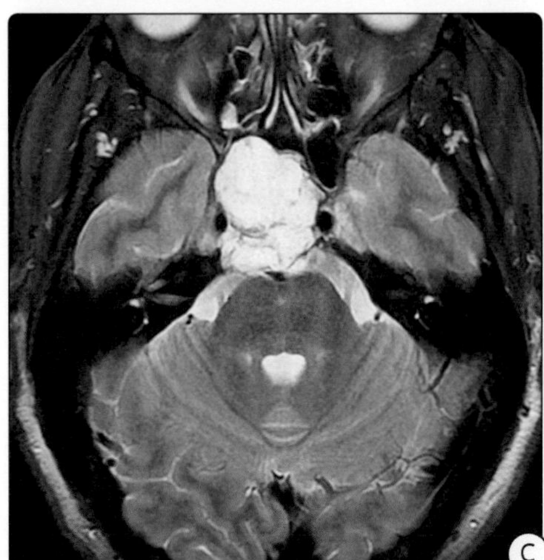


***(28-29C)** Axial T2 MR shows the hyperintense mass compresses and displaces the basilar artery. This is chordoma. (Courtesy A. Csillag, MD.)*

permeative lytic bony changes **(28-28A)** **(28-29A)**. Intratumoral calcifications generally represent sequestrations from destroyed bone.

Chordomas exhibit substantial heterogeneity on MR. Most conventional chordomas are typically intermediate to low signal intensity on T1WI. On sagittal images, a "thumb" of tumor tissue is often seen extending posteriorly through the cortex of the clivus and indenting the pons **(28-28B)**.

Conventional chordomas are very hyperintense on T2WI, reflecting high fluid content within the physaliphorous cells **(28-28C)** **(28-29B)**. Intratumoral calcifications and hemorrhage may cause foci of decreased signal within the overall hyperintense mass.

Enhancement is quite variable. Some cases demonstrate moderate heterogeneous enhancement, although many clival chordomas demonstrate minimal or no enhancement.

### CHORDOMA

**Etiology**
- Arises from cranial end of primitive notochordal remnants
- *STAT3* activation

**Pathology**
- Typically midline
  - 50% sacrum
  - 35% sphenooccipital (clivus)
  - 15% vertebral body
- 3 types
  - Typical ("classic") with physaliphorous cells
  - Chondroid
  - Dedifferentiated (< 5%, usually sacral)

**Clinical Features**
- Any age, but peak in 4th-6th decades
- Cranial neuropathies

**Imaging Findings**
- CT
  - Permeative destructive central skull base lesion
  - Often contains sequestered bony fragments
- MR
  - T1 hypointense, T2 hyperintense
  - "Thumb" of tumor extends posteriorly, indents pons
  - Variable, usually moderate enhancement

**Differential Diagnosis**
- Invasive pituitary macroadenoma
- Chondrosarcoma
- Ecchordosis physaliphora

## Differential Diagnosis

A large, **invasive pituitary macroadenoma** can mimic chordoma. Chordomas typically displace but do not invade the pituitary gland, whereas macroadenomas cannot be identified separate from the gland.

Signal intensity of a **skull base chondrosarcoma** is very similar to that of chordoma. Chondrosarcomas typically arise off-midline, along the petrooccipital fissure. **Ecchordosis physaliphora** is a rare nonneoplastic notochordal remnant that may arise anywhere from the skull base to the sacrum. Most are small and found incidentally at autopsy or imaging. They usually lie just in front of the pons and have a thin stalk-like connection to a smaller intraclival component.

Skull base **metastases** and **plasmacytoma** are destructive lesions that are usually isointense with brain on all sequences. Predominantly intraosseous **meningioma** is rare in the skull base. It usually causes sclerosis and hyperostosis rather than a permeative destructive pattern.

## Benign Chondroosseous Tumors

### Terminology

Benign chondroosseous tumors correspond in name and histology to their extracranial counterparts. Osteocartilaginous tumors, such as chondroma, osteochondroma, and osteoma, are the most common such tumors that occur within the CNS.

### Etiology

The skull base and clivus develop by enchondral ossification. **Chondromas** and **enchondromas** usually arise from cartilaginous synchondroses in the skull base. Therefore, the central skull base, especially the sella/parasellar region, is the most common site. Less commonly, chondromas can arise from the dura or falx. **Osteochondromas** also typically arise in or near the skull base.

In contrast to the skull base, the calvarial vault develops by membranous ossification. **Osteomas** are benign tumors that arise from membranous bone. In the head, the paranasal sinuses and calvaria are the most common sites.

### Pathology

Macro- and microscopic appearances depend on their cell type and are similar to their extracranial soft tissue counterparts, e.g., **chondromas** and **enchondromas** are sharply demarcated "bosselated" tumors that generally have a broad flat base and grossly resemble cartilage. **Osteochondromas** appear as a sessile or pedunculated cartilage-capped bony exostosis.

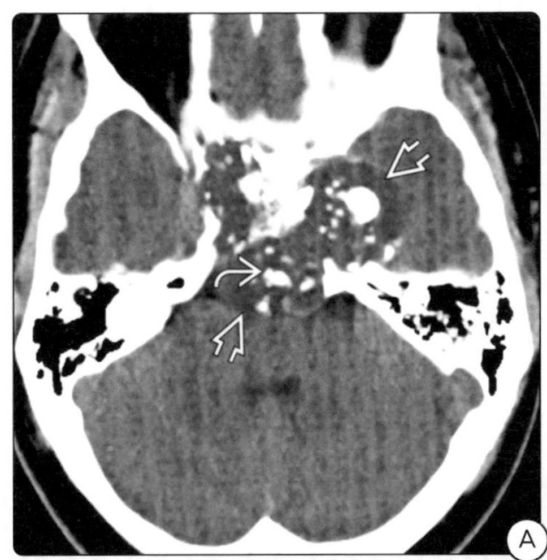


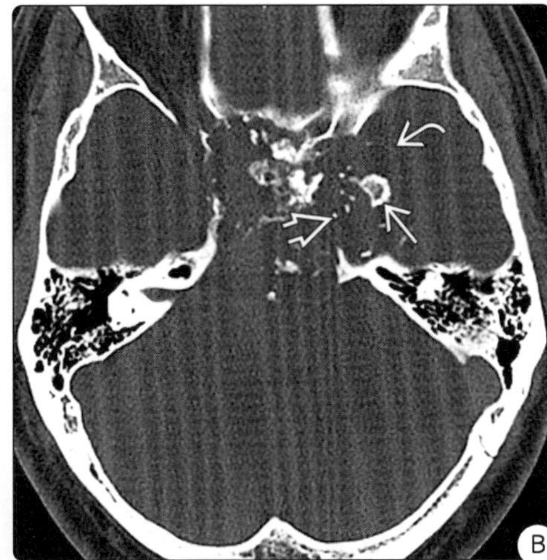


***(28-31A)** NECT in a 21-yo man with blurred vision shows a hypodense central skull base mass ➡ with numerous matrix calcifications ➡. **(28-30B)** Bone CT in the same patient shows erosion of the central skull base and anterior clinoid processes by the mass. Note matrix mineralization ➡, calcified arcs ➡, and dysplastic cortical bone ➡ within the mass.*

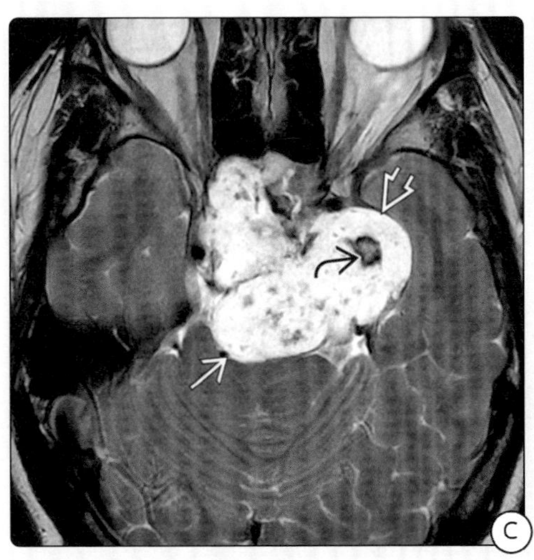


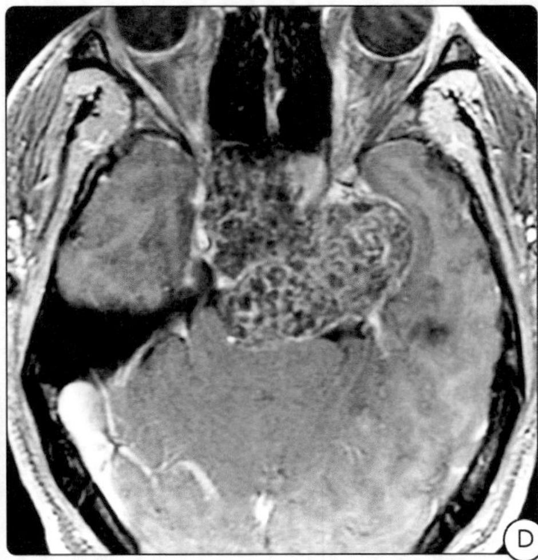


***(28-31C)** Axial T2 FS MR in the same patient shows that the lobulated mass ➡ is well delineated and extremely hyperintense and compresses/displaces the pons posteriorly ➡. Dysplastic cortical bone ➡ within the mass is well seen. **(28-30D)** T1 C+ FS MR shows a "bubbly" enhancement pattern within the mass. Pathology showed enchondroma with foci of chondrosarcoma arising within the mass.*

**Osteomas** resemble dense lamellar bone. Benign chondroosseous tumors are all CNS WHO grade 1 neoplasms.

## Clinical Issues

**Epidemiology.** Benign chondroosseous tumors account for < 1% of all intracranial neoplasms and can occur at any age. Overall, **chondroma/enchondroma** is the most common benign osteocartilaginous tumor of the skull base. **Osteoma** is the most common benign osseous tumor of the calvaria.

Most benign chondroosseous tumors occur as solitary nonsyndromic lesions. Multiple lesions generally occur as part of inherited tumor syndromes. Multiple osteomas occur as part of **Gardner syndrome** (together with skin tumors and colon polyps). Multiple enchondromas or "enchondromatosis" are part of **Ollier disease**. Enchondromas associated with soft tissue hemangiomas are found in **Maffucci syndrome**.

**Presentation.** Most benign chondroosseous tumors are asymptomatic and discovered incidentally. Others, such as osteomas, may present as a longstanding skull "bump." Occasionally, large tumors, especially those arising within or near the skull base, cause cranial nerve palsies.

**Natural History.** Most benign chondroosseous tumors can be completely resected and have a favorable prognosis. Malignant degeneration is generally rare. Multiple osteochondromas ("osteochondromatosis") have a higher propensity to undergo malignant transformation. The risk increases as the number and size of the lesions increase.

## Imaging

**General Features.** Imaging findings vary with tumor type. Most are benign-appearing nonaggressive masses of the scalp, skull, or dura that resemble their counterparts found elsewhere in the body.

**CT Findings. Chondroma/enchondromas** of the skull base are sessile, smoothly lobulated, expansile masses that contain curvilinear matrix calcifications and sometimes mature bone **(28-31)**. Slight enhancement on CECT may occur.

**Osteochondromas** are sessile or pedunculated bony masses that are contiguous with and project from their underlying bone of origin. Osteochondromas may exhibit a "cap" of matrix with speckled calcification that enhances mildly following contrast administration.

**Osteomas** are seen as dense masses of well-demarcated mature lamellar bone. They occur in paranasal sinuses—the most common site—or the calvarium **(28-32)**.

**MR Findings.** All benign chondroosseous tumors are typically well-delineated, noninvasive-appearing masses with variable signal intensity on both T1- and T2WI. A ring and arc pattern of contrast enhancement can be seen with chondromas. These tumors generally do not incite dural reaction, so a dural tail sign is absent.

*Selected References: The complete reference list is available on the eBooks+ version included with purchase.*

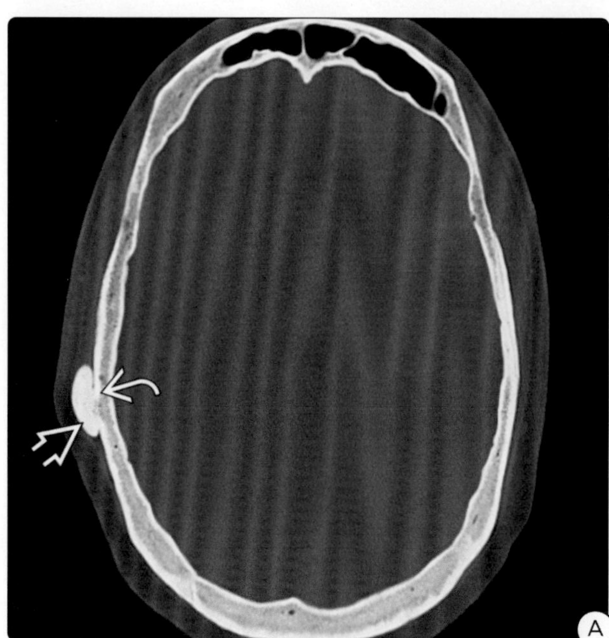


***(28-32A)** Axial bone CT of a 42-yo woman with a longstanding "lump" on her head shows a smooth, well-delineated, hyperdense mass ➡ that can clearly be seen to arise directly from the cortex of the calvarium ➡.*

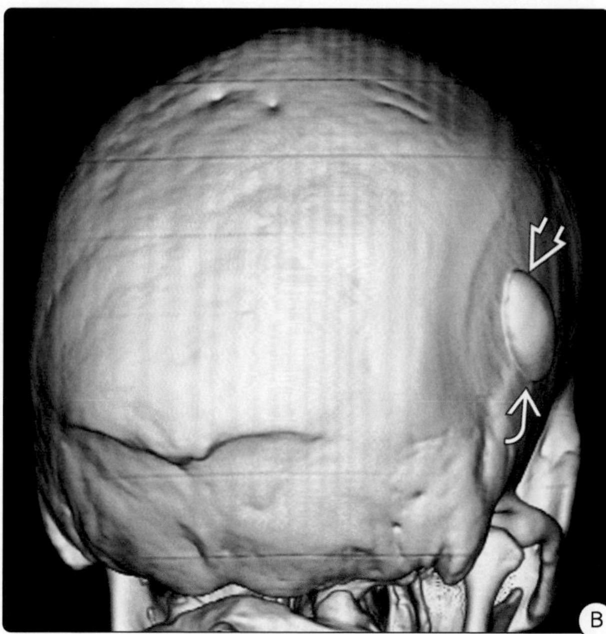


***(28-32B)** 3D shaded surface rendering shows that the bony mass ➡ arises from the outer table of the skull ➡. This is calvarial osteoma.*

# Hematolymphoid and Hematopoietic Tumors

*This chapter focuses on hematopoietic tumors and tumor-like conditions. We begin with an increasingly common group of neoplasms, **lymphomas and related disorders**, then turn our attention briefly to **histiocytic tumors**, such as Langerhans cell histiocytosis and Erdheim-Chester disease.*

**Plasma cell myeloma** and **solitary plasmacytoma** affecting the skull and brain are usually secondary to extracranial disease, but they are a form of mature B-cell neoplasms and hence are included here rather than in Chapter 31 on metastases. We conclude the chapter with a brief discussion of **extramedullary hematopoiesis**—benign, nonneoplastic proliferations of blood-forming elements—which can appear virtually identical to malignant hematopoietic neoplasms.



## Lymphomas and Related Disorders

The 2021 WHO divides primary CNS lymphoma (PCNSL) into **primary diffuse large B-cell lymphoma of the CNS** (CNS-DLBCL) (> 95% of lesions), immunodeficiency-associated CNS lymphomas, intravascular large B-cell lymphoma, anaplastic large cell lymphoma [ALK(+)/ALK(-)], T-cell and NK/T-cell lymphomas, and "other low-grade B-cell lymphomas of the CNS, which includes extranodal marginal zone lymphoma," as well as mucosa-associated lymphoid tissue (MALT) lymphoma of the dura.

We begin this chapter by focusing on CNS-DLBCL. We then consider the fascinating spectrum of **immunodeficiency-associated CNS lymphomas** and other lymphoproliferative disorders, including **lymphomatoid granulomatosis** (LG) and **posttransplant lymphoproliferative disorder** (PTLD).

We follow with a discussion of **intravascular large B-cell lymphoma**, an uncommon but increasingly well-recognized cause of unexplained cognitive decline in older adult patients. Uncommon PCNSLs, such as MALT lymphoma of the dura, are then briefly discussed. We close the section with a brief review of CNS metastatic lymphoma.

### Diffuse Large B-Cell Lymphoma of CNS

#### Terminology

CNS-DLBCL is an extranodal B-cell lymphoma that arises exclusively inside the CNS. The vast majority of PCNSLs are diffuse large B-cell lymphomas

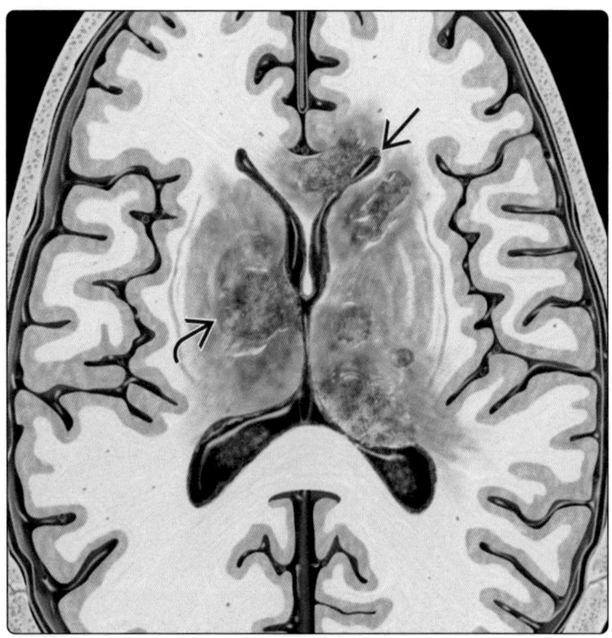

*(29-1) This is primary CNS lymphoma (PCNSL). Periventricular lesions ⮕ are in basal ganglia (BG), thalamus, corpus callosum with extensive subependymal spread of disease ⮕.*

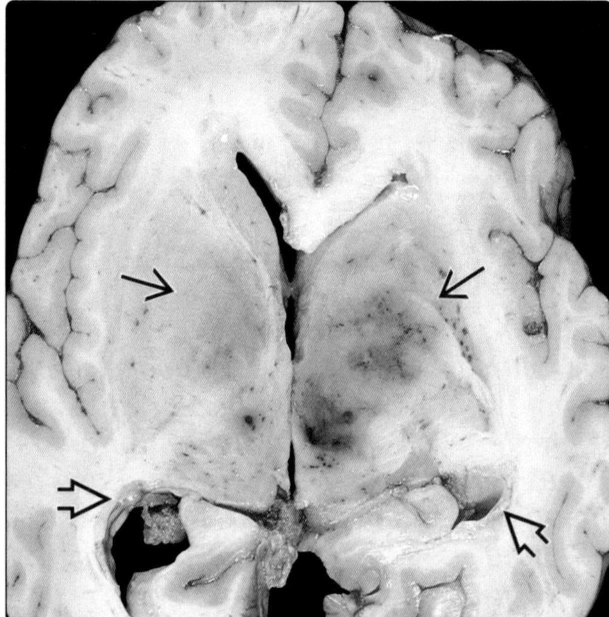

*(29-2) Autopsy shows PCNSL with bilateral deep basal ganglionic, thalamic masses ⮕, ependymal spread ⮕. (Courtesy R. Hewlett, MD.)*

(DLBCLs). For purposes of discussion, in this text, the terms PCNSL and DLBCL are used interchangeably.

### 2021 WHO CLASSIFICATION OF CNS LYMPHOMAS

**Primary Diffuse Large B-Cell Lymphoma of CNS**

**Immunodeficiency-Associated CNS Lymphomas**
- AIDS-related primary DLBCL
- EBV(+) DLBCL of older adults

**Lymphoproliferative Disorders**
- Lymphomatoid granulomatosis
- PTLD

**Intravascular Large B-Cell Lymphoma**

**Miscellaneous Rare CNS Lymphomas**
- Low-grade B-cell lymphomas
- T-cell and NK/T-cell lymphoma
- Anaplastic large cell lymphoma [ALK(+)/ALK(-)]

**MALT Lymphoma of Dura**

## Etiology

The brain parenchyma normally contains very few lymphocytes. So how and why lymphomas arise as primary CNS neoplasms in immunocompetent individuals is unknown. To date, no genetic predispositions to PCNSL have been identified. No viral associations have been identified.

What is clear is that lymphoma cells—regardless of whether they originate within or outside the brain—exhibit a distinct, highly selective neurotropism for the CNS microenvironment and its vasculature. Intra- and perivascular tumor spread is common.

## Pathology

**Location.** CNS-DLBCL can affect any part of the neuraxis. Up to 75% all PCNSLs contact a CSF surface, either the ventricular ependyma or pia **(29-1)**. Lesions are often deep seated with a predilection for the periventricular white matter, especially the corpus callosum **(29-5A)**. The basal ganglia and thalami are the next most common locations **(29-2)**.

The hypothalamus, infundibulum, and pituitary gland are less common sites. Primary DLBCL may also develop in the leptomeninges, calvarial vault, and central skull base, although these areas are more commonly involved by metastatic spread from extracranial primary tumors. Ocular manifestations may occur in ~ 20% of patients and spinal cord involvement is rare, < 1%.

**Gross Pathology.** DLBCL lesions vary in size from microscopic implants to large bulky masses. Up to 2/3 are solitary lesions.

Single or multiple hemispheric masses that appear relatively well demarcated rather than diffusely infiltrating lesions are typical. Large confluent areas of frank necrosis and gross intratumoral hemorrhage are more common in AIDS-related PCNSLs **(29-8)**.

Rarely, DLBCL diffusely infiltrates the brain, involving both gray and white matter structures. So-called lymphomatosis cerebri, like "gliomatosis cerebri," is an anatomic pattern, not a distinct disease entity. Lymphomatosis cerebri often presents as patchy or confluent T2/FLAIR hyperintensities in the deep white matter and basal ganglia with variable enhancement.

**Microscopic Features.** PCNSLs are highly cellular tumors. MIB-1 is high, often exceeding 50% (significantly higher than with glioblastoma). The WHO does not assign a grade to PCNSL.

PRIMARY CNS LYMPHOMA: ETIOLOGY AND PATHOLOGY

**Etiology**
- CNS lacks lymphatics, normally contains few lymphocytes
- Precise origin in immunocompetent individuals unknown

**Pathology**
- 3-6% of all primary CNS neoplasms
- Vast majority (90-95%) are DLBCLs
    - Large atypical cells
    - CD20(+), CD45(+)
    - MIB-1 > 50%
- Predilection for deep brain
    - Periventricular white matter, basal ganglia
    - Perivascular lymphoid clusters also common
- Solitary (2/3), multiple (1/3)
    - Multiple compartments may be involved
- Focal > > diffusely infiltrating lesions (lymphomatosis cerebri)
- Hemorrhage, necrosis rare in immunocompetent patients
- "Sentinel" demyelinating lesion indistinguishable from MS or ADEM can precede PCNSL!
- Corticosteroids → ↑ apoptosis, can obscure diagnosis of PCNSL!

## Clinical Issues

Lymphomas of the CNS are the second most frequent primary brain malignancy in adults after gliomas, accounting for 7% of all malignant tumors. Although PCNSLs account for only 3% of all malignant CNS neoplasms, worldwide prevalence is increasing as a result of the HIV/AIDS epidemic and the use of immunosuppressive therapies. PCNSLs are generally tumors of middle-aged and older adults. Peak age (in immunocompetent patients) is 60 years. CNS-DLBCL is typically EBV(-).

Most patients present with focal neurologic deficits, altered mental status, and neuropsychiatric disturbances. Seizures are less common than in patients with other primary brain tumors.

CNS-DLBCL is an aggressive tumor with a median survival of only a few months in untreated patients. In general, immunocompetent patients younger than 60 years fare slightly better than older patients and patients with acquired immunodeficiency syndromes.

Early diagnosis is crucial for proper management of PCNSLs. Stereotactic biopsy is typically performed for diagnostic confirmation and histologic tumor typing. Treatment options include corticosteroids, high-dose methotrexate-based polychemotherapy, and radiation. Newer therapies include consolidative high-dose chemotherapy and autologous stem cell transplantation after methotrexate-based chemotherapy with prolonged survival.

Approximately 70% of patients initially respond to treatment, but relapse is very common. Progression-free survival is approximately one year, and overall survival is approximately three years. Only 20-40% of patients experience prolonged progression-free survival.

## Imaging

**General Features.** Contrast-enhanced cranial MR is the modality of choice in evaluating patients with suspected PCNSL. CECT of the chest, abdomen, and pelvis or PET/CT is generally recommended in patients with suspected PCNSL to look for an extracranial source of disease. Occult systemic lymphomas are found in 5-8% of patients with putative PCNSL.

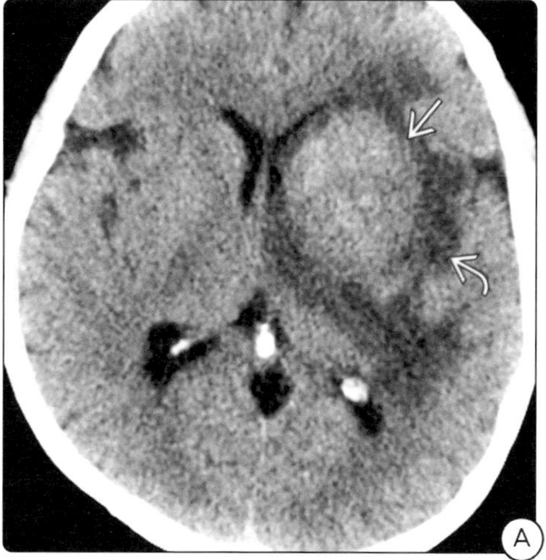


***(29-3A)** NECT in a 63-year-old woman with right-sided weakness shows a solitary hyperdense mass ➡ in the left BG with moderate edema ➡.*

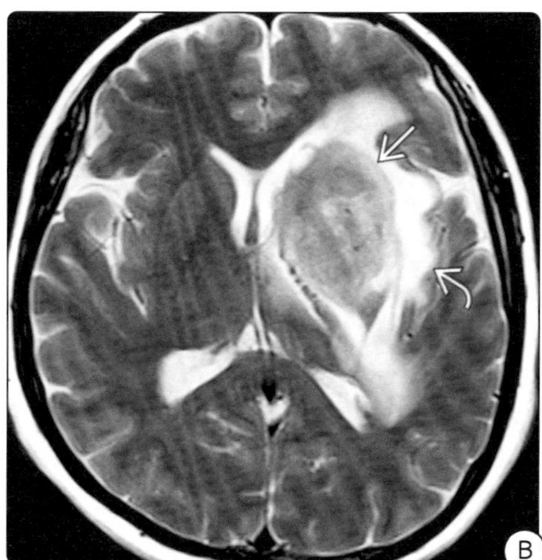


***(29-3B)** T2 MR shows mass ➡ is mixed iso- to hypointense relative to cortex. Moderate amount of hyperintense peripheral edema ➡ is present.*

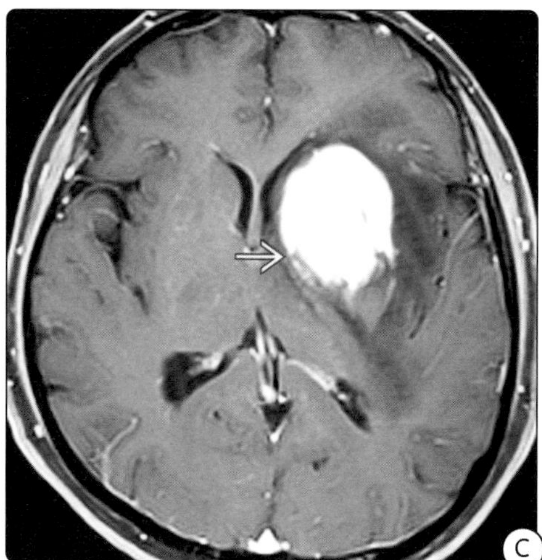


***(29-3C)** T1 C+ FS MR shows that the mass ➡ enhances intensely and uniformly. Diffuse large B-cell lymphoma (DLBCL) was found at surgery.*

**CT Findings.** All PCNSLs are highly cellular tumors. White matter or basal ganglia lesions in contact with a CSF surface are typical. Most lesions appear hyperdense compared with normal brain on NECT scans **(29-3A)** **(29-4)**. Marked peritumoral edema is common, but gross necrosis, hemorrhage, and calcification are rare (2-5%) unless the patient is immunocompromised **(29-9A)**.

DLBCLs in immunocompetent patients show mild to moderate, relatively homogeneous enhancement on CECT. Irregular ring enhancement is rare unless the patient is immunocompromised.

**MR Findings.** Over 3/4 of DLBCLs in **immunocompetent** patients are iso- or slightly hypointense compared with gray matter on T1WI and isointense on T2WI **(29-3B)** **(29-6A)**.

FLAIR signal is variable but usually iso- or hyperintense **(29-5A)**. Microhemorrhages with intratumoral "blooming" on T2* are present in 5-8% of cases, but gross hemorrhage is uncommon unless the patient is immunocompromised.

Nearly all PCNSLs in immunocompetent patients enhance **(29-3C)**. Solid homogeneous **(29-3C)** **(29-5C)** or mildly heterogeneous enhancement is common **(29-6B)**; ring enhancement is much less common (10-15%) **(29-7)**. MRS typically demonstrates elevated choline and high lipids.

Because of their high cellularity, > 95% of PCNSLs show mild to moderate diffusion restriction with low ADC values **(29-5B)**. MRS is nonspecific with elevated choline, reduced NAA and myoinositol, and prominent lipids. Tumor neovascularization is absent in PCNSLs; therefore, rCBV is relatively low, and permeability is not increased on DCE pMR even though the tumor is highly malignant.

Lymphomatosis cerebri mimics diffuse white matter disease with confluent T2/FLAIR hyperintensities. Enhancement can be subtle, patchy, or even absent.

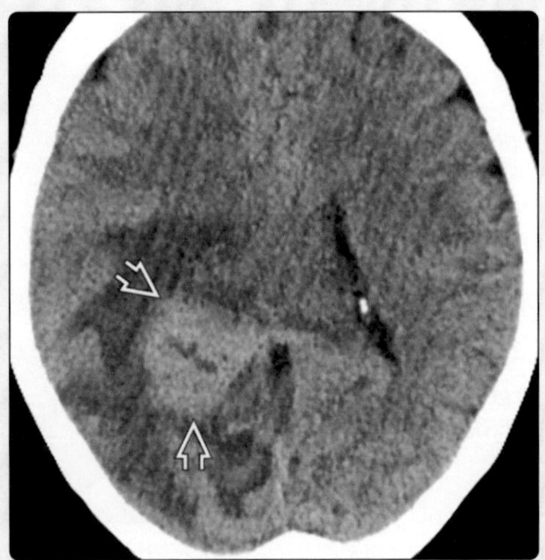

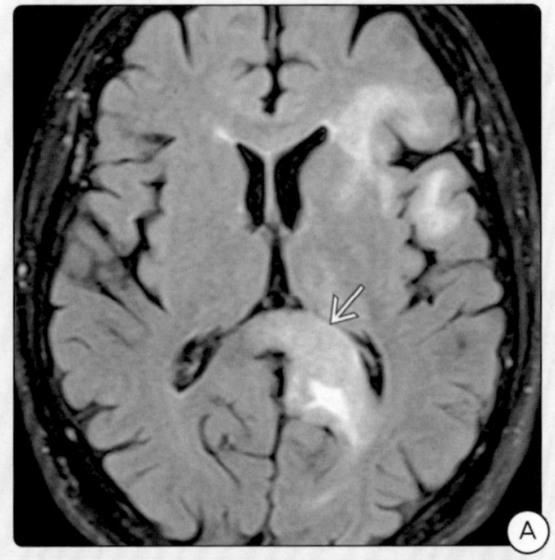


***(29-4)** Axial NECT shows a hyperdense mass ➔ along the corpus callosum with surrounding vasogenic edema. CT hyperdensity and diffusion restriction are typical of primary DLBCL related to high cellularity of the tumor. **(29-5A)** FLAIR MR in a patient with CNS-DLBCL shows a hyperintense mass in the corpus callosum splenium ➔ with mild expansion. The main imaging differential for a corpus callosum mass is GBM.*

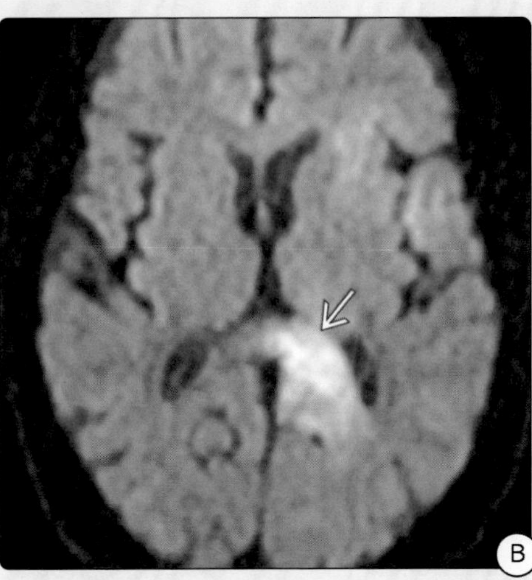


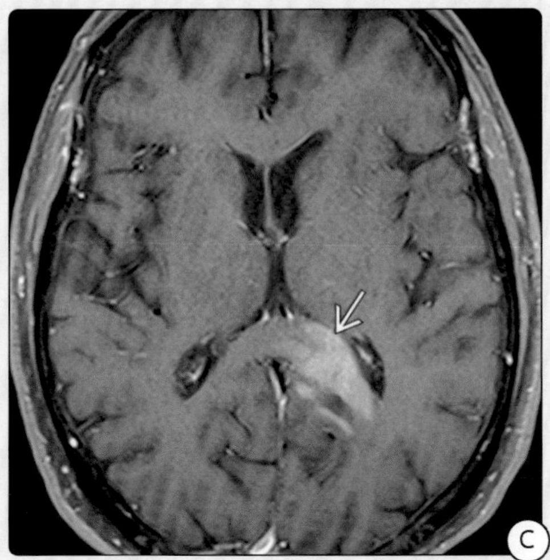


***(29-5B)** DWI trace MR in the same patient shows diffusion restriction ➔ (low ADC not shown) characteristic of a densely cellular mass, typical of DLBCL. **(29-5C)** T1 C+ FS MR in the same patient shows the mass ➔ enhances strongly and uniformly, typical for CNS-DLBCL. On occasion, heterogeneous or rim enhancement may be present, though it is more often seen in immunocompromised patients.*

Steroid administration significantly alters the imaging findings of PCNSLs. Cell lysis with tumor regression and normalization of the blood-brain barrier occurs in 40-85% of patients with **corticosteroid-treated PCNSLs**. Tumors typically diminish in size. Contrast enhancement also decreases or even disappears completely ("ghost tumor"), although some T2 and FLAIR signal abnormalities may persist.

## Differential Diagnosis

The major differential diagnosis of PCNSL is **glioblastoma** (GBM). Although both tumors often cross the corpus callosum, hemorrhage and necrosis are rare in PCNSL. Enhancement in immunocompetent patients with PCNSL is strong and relatively homogeneous, whereas a peripheral ring pattern is more typical of GBM. Advanced MR techniques, such as DWI, MRS, and DCE pMR are helpful in distinguishing PCNSLs from other highly aggressive primary brain tumors.

### PRIMARY CNS LYMPHOMA: IMAGING AND DIFFERENTIAL DIAGNOSIS IN IMMUNOCOMPETENT PATIENTS

**General Features**
- Periventricular white matter, basal ganglia common sites
  - 95% contact CSF surface
- Cautions
  - Findings vary with immune status
  - Steroids may mask/↓ imaging findings!

**CT**
- Hyperdense on NECT
- Hemorrhage, necrosis rare

**MR**
- Generally isointense with gray matter on T1-, T2WI
- Petechial hemorrhage in immunocompetent patients
- Gross hemorrhage, necrosis rare
- Strong, relatively uniform enhancement
- Often restricts on DWI/DTI
- Lymphomatosis cerebri
  - Mimics diffuse white matter disease with T2/FLAIR confluent hyperintensity
  - Enhancement can be subtle or patchy, occasionally absent

**Differential Diagnosis**
- Glioblastoma, metastasis
- Lymphomatosis cerebri
  - Microvascular disease
  - Encephalitis (infectious, inflammatory, autoimmune)
  - Toxic-metabolic disorders
  - Diffusely infiltrating glioma
  - Vasculitis

The second most common differential diagnosis of PCNSL is **metastasis**. Dura-based PCNSLs may resemble **meningioma** or—due to their hyperdensity—even look like an acute epi- or subdural hematoma.

In the setting of solid organ or hematopoietic stem cell transplants, **LG** and **PTLD** may closely resemble PCNSL. Biopsy is necessary for confirmation and patient management.

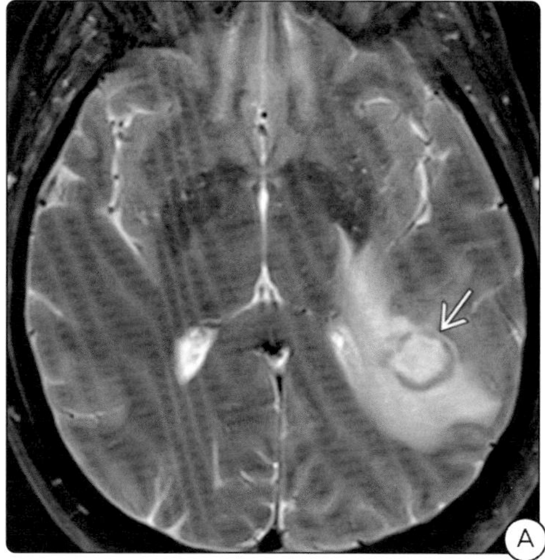


***(29-6A)** Axial T2 FS MR shows a mass with peripheral low signal ➡ and marked vasogenic edema. This is DLBCL.*

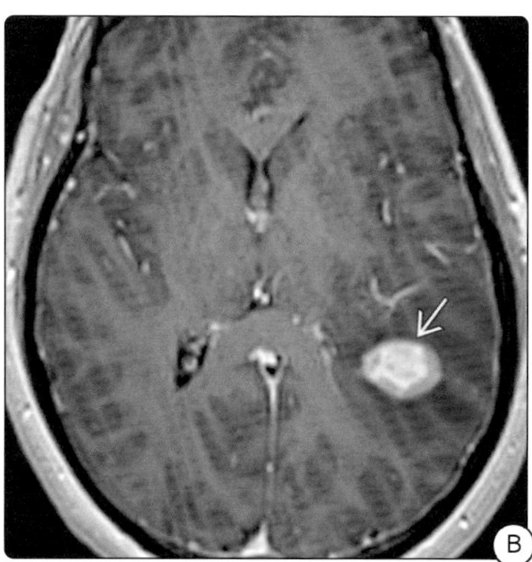


***(29-6B)** Axial T1 C+ FS MR in the same patient shows the mass ➡ enhances strongly with mild heterogeneity, CNS-DLBCL.*

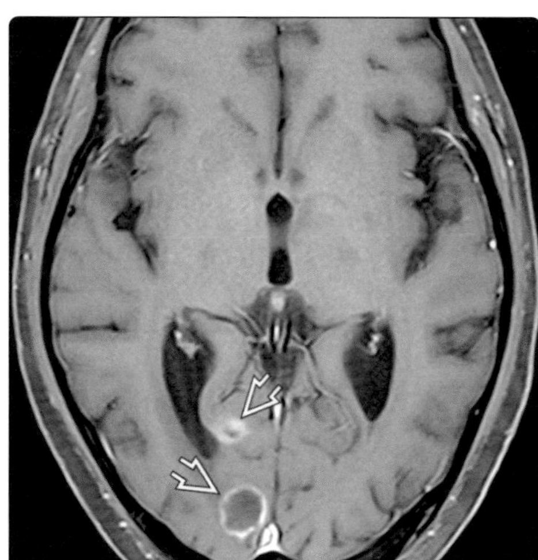

***(29-7)** T1 C+ FS MR in a patient with DLBCL shows the rare peripheral enhancement ➡ more typical in immunocompromised patients.*

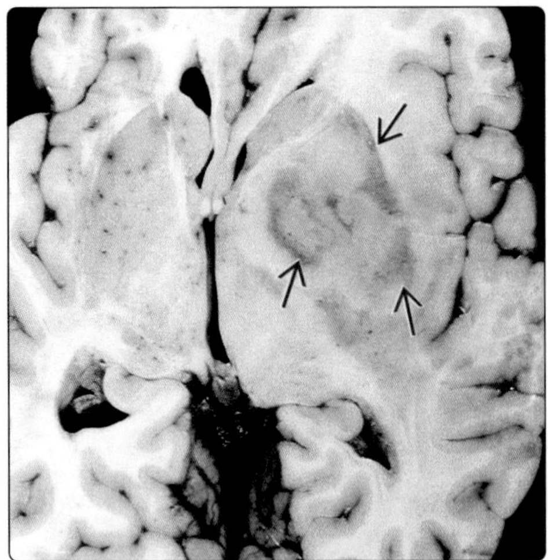

*(29-8) Autopsy of CNS-DLBCL in HIV/AIDS shows hemorrhagic, necrotic left BG masses ⇒. (Courtesy R. Hewlett, MD.)*

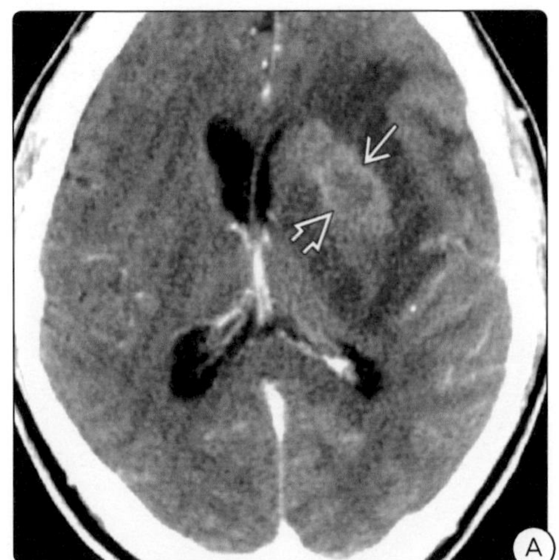

*(29-9A) CECT scan shows necrosis ⇒ and only faint rim enhancement ⇒ in this HIV(+) patient with primary DLBCL.*

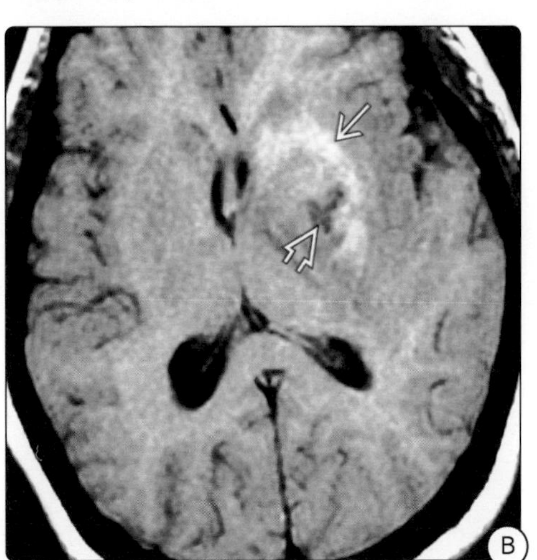

*(29-9B) T1 MR shows T1 shortening due to subacute hemorrhage ⇒ with more acute hemorrhage in the necrotic core of the lesion ⇒.*

## Immunodeficiency-Associated CNS Lymphomas

Lymphomas associated with either inherited or acquired immunodeficiency are grouped together as immunodeficiency-associated CNS lymphomas. The immunodeficiency-associated CNS lymphomas include **AIDS-related DLBCL and EBV(+) DLBCL** in older adult patients (> 50 years) with no known immunodeficiency.

PCNSLs associated with **EBV** account for 10-15% of all cases. Congenital immunodeficiency syndromes increase the risk of lymphoma, as do severe acquired immunosuppression and autoimmune diseases, such as Sjögren syndrome and systemic lupus erythematosus.

## AIDS-Related Diffuse Large B-Cell Lymphoma

Although HIV-associated PCNSL has become rarer with the introduction of highly active antiretroviral therapy (HAART), between 2-12% of HIV/AIDS patients eventually develop CNS lymphoma, generally during the later stages of their disease.

### Pathology

Multiple lesions are common, as are larger, more confluent necrotic areas and intratumoral hemorrhages **(29-8)**.

### Clinical Issues

Mean age at onset in HIV/AIDS patients is 40 years, two decades younger than immunocompetent patients. Lymphomas in transplant recipients occur even earlier, generally between 35-40 years of age. Mean age of onset in children with inherited immunodeficiencies is 10 years.

### Imaging

Multiple lesions are common, as are more frequent and larger confluent areas of necrosis **(29-9A)**. Intratumoral hemorrhage with T1 shortening **(29-9B)** and "blooming" on T2* scans is common. Enhancement is variable but often mild. Ring enhancement surrounding a nonenhancing core of necrotic tissue is typical.

### Differential Diagnosis

In immunocompromised patients, the major differential diagnosis of PCNSL is **toxoplasmosis**. *A solitary ring-enhancing lesion in an HIV/AIDS patient is most often lymphoma*, whereas multiple lesions are more characteristic of toxoplasmosis. An eccentric target sign is suggestive of toxoplasmosis, although necrotic lymphomas occasionally show an enhancing ring with a nodule pattern. Additional differential considerations for immunodeficiency-associated CNS lymphomas include **glioblastoma** or **metastases.** These two entities often present as ring-enhancing lesions with marked surrounding T2/FLAIR signal abnormality.

## Lymphomatoid Granulomatosis

LG is an angiocentric and angiodestructive lymphoproliferative disorder characterized by polymorphous lymphoid infiltrates with EBV(+) atypical B cells in a T-cell-rich inflammatory background.

## Etiology

LG is an EBV-driven disease and is present in the majority of cases. Immunodeficiency, such as HIV/AIDS and patients on immunosuppression for solid organ transplants, increases the risk of LG.

## Pathology

The lung is the most common location for LG followed by the skin. The CNS is involved in ~ 25% of cases. Macroscopically, the lesions may resemble tumor or infarct-like areas of necrosis.

LG is characterized histologically by polymorphous lymphoid infiltrates, primarily lymphocytes and plasma cells, angiitis and granulomatosis with central necrosis. LG may be graded as grade 1, grade 2, or grade 3 based on the proportion of EBV-expressing CD20(+) B cells. The majority of CNS LG is grade 2 or grade 3.

## Clinical Issues

LG is a rare disease that usually occurs in adults in the fifth and sixth decades with a male predilection. The typical patient is a middle-aged man with fever, dry cough, and weight loss. Patients with CNS LG often present with focal neurologic symptoms, headaches, &/or cognitive impairment. CNS LG is often aggressive and has similar treatment to DLBCL, including steroids, radiation, &/or chemotherapy.

## Imaging

LG may occur in the brain parenchyma, leptomeninges, or cranial nerves. Spinal cord involvement is rare. Imaging is often nonspecific with multifocal T2/FLAIR nodular hyperintensities as well as solid and ring-like enhancement patterns **(29-10)**.

Other imaging patterns described include multifocal punctate, nodular, linear enhancing foci. Leptomeningeal and cranial nerve enhancement has also been described. Dural-based enhancing masses and choroid plexus lesions have been reported.

## Differential Diagnosis

The major differential diagnosis of LG is **vasculitis** and lymphoma, particularly **intravascular lymphoma** (IVL). Vasculitis is typically characterized by multifocal T2 hyperintensities, often with restricted diffusion, and blood products on MR. IVL typically shows small ischemic foci with infarct-like lesions and microhemorrhages, as well as linear or punctate enhancement along perivascular spaces. Other imaging considerations include **CLIPPERS** (**c**hronic **l**ymphocytic **i**nflammation with **p**ontine **p**erivascular **e**nhancement **r**esponsive to **s**teroids), which often shows enhancing punctate or curvilinear lesions "peppering" the pons. Other regions of involvement in CLIPPERS include the cerebellar hemispheres, basal ganglia, and cerebral white matter.

# Posttransplant Lymphoproliferative Disorder

Posttransplant lymphoproliferative disorder (PTLD) is a potentially life-threatening complication of immunosuppressive therapy in patients with solid organ or hematopoietic cell transplantation.

The PTLD clinical spectrum can range from an infectious mononucleosis-like illness with reactive lymph node hyperplasia to malignant lymphoma. PTLD is related to EBV.

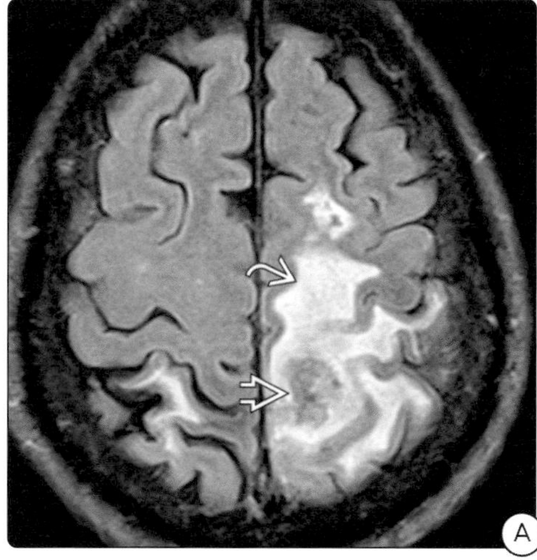


***(29-10A)** Axial FLAIR MR in a 63-year-old with sensory deficits shows a heterogeneous hypointense mass ➡ with vasogenic edema ➡.*

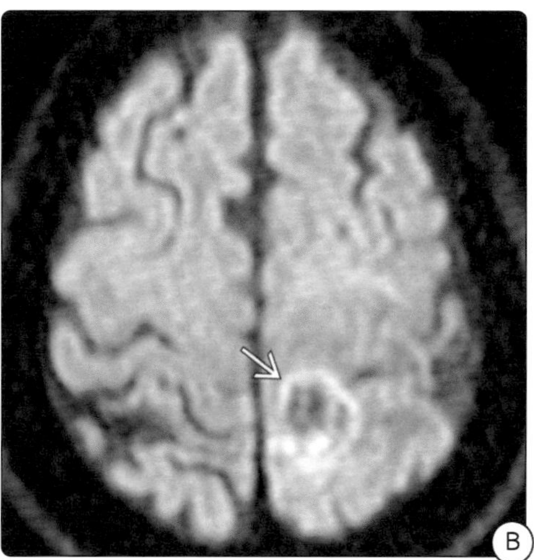


***(29-10B)** Axial DWI trace image shows a hyperintense rim ➡, which was hypointense on ADC map, with central low signal.*

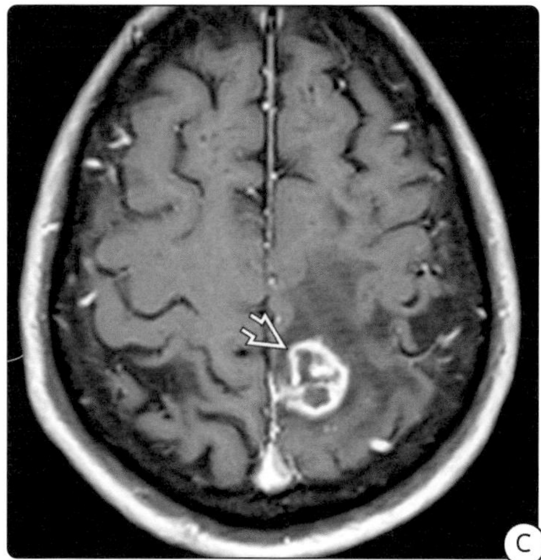


***(29-10C)** Axial T1 C+ MR shows strong peripheral and heterogeneous central enhancement ➡. Lymphomatoid granulomatosis at resection.*

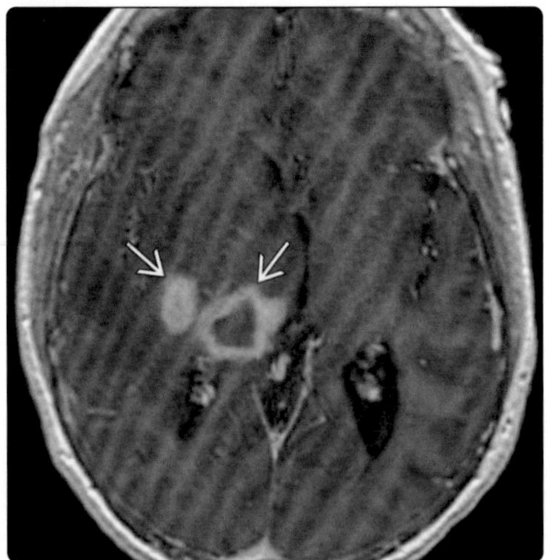

*(29-11) Axial T1 C+ MR in a liver transplant patient shows enhancing lesions ➡ in deep gray nuclei. Additional lesions were present. PTLD.*

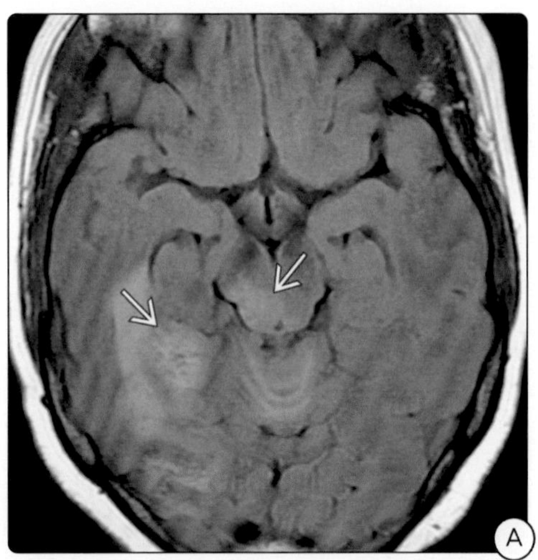

*(29-12A) Axial FLAIR MR in a 28-year-old on immunosuppression for rheumatoid arthritis shows hyperintense lesions ➡ with edema.*

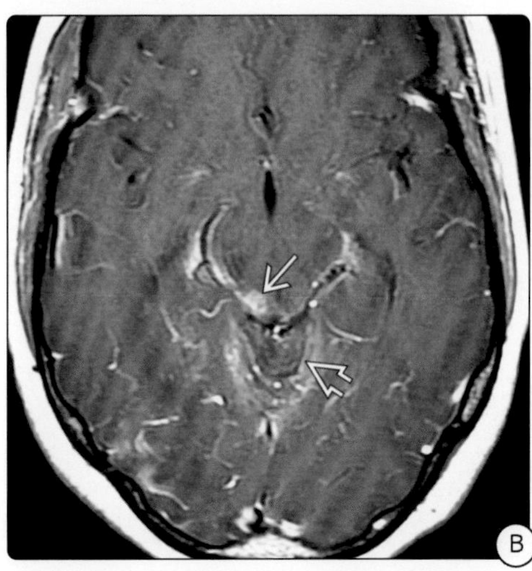

*(29-12B) Axial T1 C+ MR in the same patient shows leptomeningeal enhancement ➡ and enhancing parenchymal lesions ➡. PTLD.*

## Pathology

PTLD may be monomorphic or polymorphic. Monomorphic resembles aggressive DLBCL with a predisposition for growth in perivascular spaces. Polymorphic PTLD has a heterogeneous cell population.

## Clinical Issues

PTLD often presents several years following the transplant and symptoms vary with tumor location. Treatment is variable but often includes discontinuing immunosuppressive medications. Surgery, chemotherapy, and radiation therapy are sometimes required.

**Epidemiology.** The overall prevalence of PTLD following solid organ transplantation is 0.5-2.5%. Up to 15-20% of patients who develop PTLD have CNS involvement. Isolated CNS PTLD is rare, occurring in < 0.5% of transplant patients.

**Demographics.** Pediatric transplant patients develop PTLD more often than adult patients, as children are less likely to have EBV-specific immunity at the time of transplantation. The frequency varies with the type of transplant. The highest prevalence is seen with multiple organ transplant or intestinal (20%), lung or heart (8-20%), liver (4-15%), and kidney (1-8%). PTLD after bone marrow transplant is rare.

## Imaging

Imaging features of CNS PTLD often resemble those of AIDS-related lymphoma or metastatic disease **(29-11)**. Most lesions are single masses, hypointense to cortex on T1WI and heterogeneous on T2WI **(29-12A)**. Solid or ring enhancement is common following contrast administration **(29-12B)**. Moderate restriction is often present on DWI/DTI. Hemorrhage is not a typical feature of PTLD. Perfusion parameters, rCBV are lower than lymphoma or metastatic disease.

Extracranial head and neck PTLD results in a bilateral cervical lymphadenopathy in 75% of cases. Necrosis may be present. Other manifestations include orbital or sinonasal involvement.

## Differential Diagnosis

The major differential diagnosis of PTLD is **CNS-DLBCL**, especially AIDS-related lymphoma. Other considerations include opportunistic infections, such as **toxoplasmosis** and **metastatic disease.** Toxoplasmosis typically involves the basal ganglia and corticomedullary junctions. Multiple lesions are more common with toxoplasmosis. Toxoplasmosis often shows an eccentric target on postcontrast images. Metastatic disease often has multiple lesions and marked FLAIR hyperintensity related to vasogenic edema.

# Intravascular Large B-Cell Lymphoma

IVL is a distinctive type of aggressive B-cell lymphoma characterized by proliferating malignant cells within small and medium-sized vessels **(29-15)**. Although it can involve any organ, IVL typically affects the skin and the CNS. The brain is nearly always involved. Spinal cord involvement is rare.

## Terminology

IVL was formerly called angiocentric or angioendotheliotropic lymphoma, angiotropic large cell lymphoma, endovascular lymphoma, and malignant angioendotheliomatosis. The WHO 2021 term is **intravascular large B-cell lymphoma**.

## Etiology

IVL is an aggressive malignant lymphoma that usually arises from B cells. T cells or NK cells may occasionally be the cell of origin. A possible association of IVL (especially the NK type) with EBV has been reported.

## Pathology

The gross macroscopic appearance varies from normal to small multifocal infarcts of varying ages scattered throughout the cortex and subcortical white matter **(29-15)**. Focal cerebral masses are rare. Petechial microhemorrhages may be present and are more common than confluent macroscopic bleeds.

At histologic examination, markedly atypical cells with large round nuclei and prominent nucleoli are found in small and medium-sized vessels. Extension into the adjacent perivascular spaces is minimal or absent. CD20 staining is helpful in identifying tumor cells, especially when they are sparse and widely scattered.

## Clinical Issues

**Epidemiology.** IVL is rare. CNS involvement occurs in 75-85% of patients.

**Demographics.** IVL is typically a tumor of middle-aged and older adult patients. Mean age at presentation is 60-65 years.

**Presentation.** Sensory and motor deficits, neuropathies, and multiple stroke-like episodes are common symptoms. Some patients present with progressive neurologic deterioration and cognitive decline characterized by confusion and memory loss. Skin changes with elevated plaques or nodules are present in 1/2 of all cases.

**Natural History.** Outcome is generally poor. By the time of initial presentation, most patients have advanced

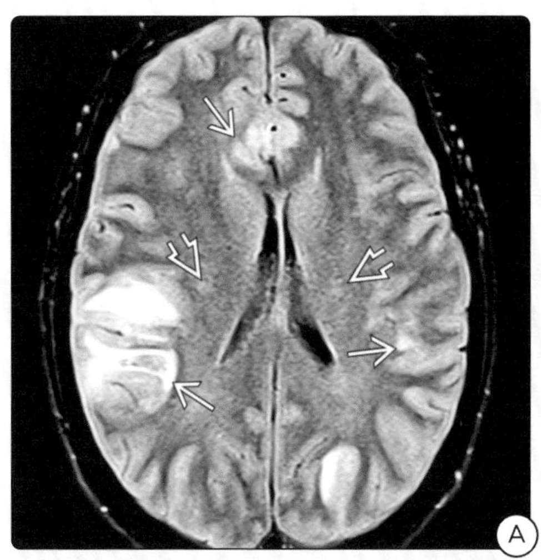


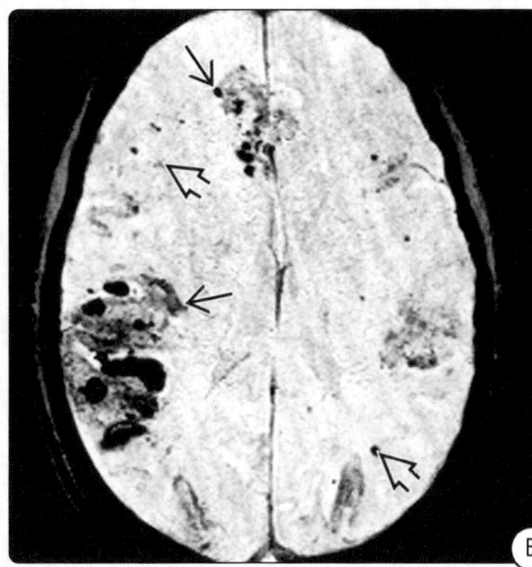


***(29-13A)** FLAIR MR in a 47-year-old patient with confusion and altered mental status shows multiple subcortical ➡, deep ➡, and white matter (WM) hyperintensities. **(29-13B)** T2* SWI MIP shows multifocal petechial WM ➡ and confluent cortical/subcortical hemorrhages ➡. Intravascular lymphoma (IVL) is rare, but characterized by WM lesions, blood products, and perivascular enhancement.*

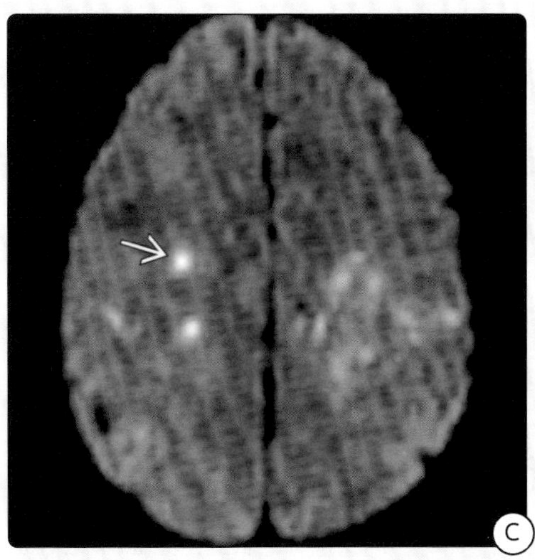


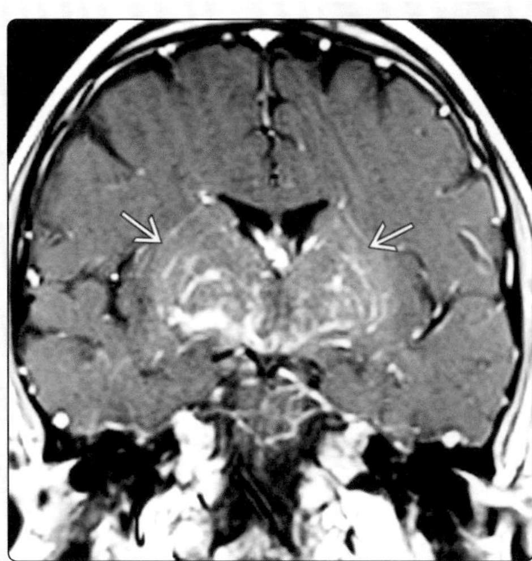

***(29-13C)** Axial DTI trace image in the same patient shows multiple foci of hyperintensity ➡ related to acute infarcts in this patient with intravascular large B-cell lymphoma. Imaging often mimics vasculitis. **(29-14)** Coronal T1 C+ MR shows prominent curvilinear enhancement following the penetrating arteries ➡ within the perivascular spaces. Intravascular large B-cell lymphoma was found at biopsy.*

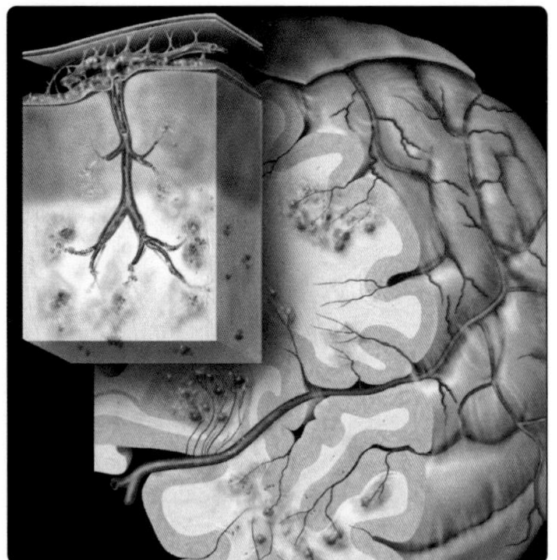

*(29-15) Graphic shows malignant cells filling the vessels, causing perivascular infiltrates and petechial hemorrhages. IVL.*

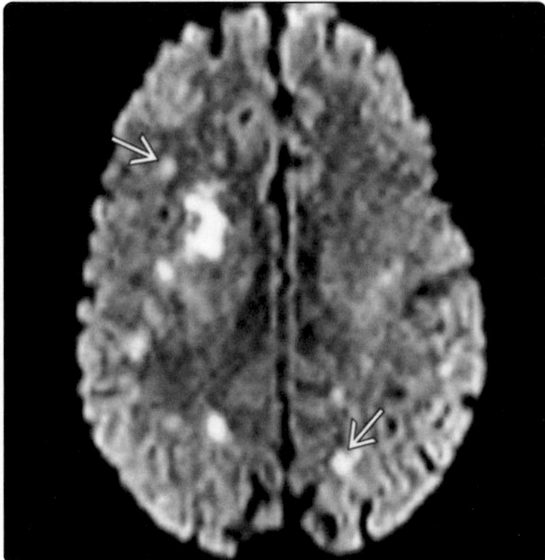

*(29-16) Axial DWI trace images shows multiple small infarcts ➡ related to IVL. Imaging and clinical features may mimic vasculitis.*

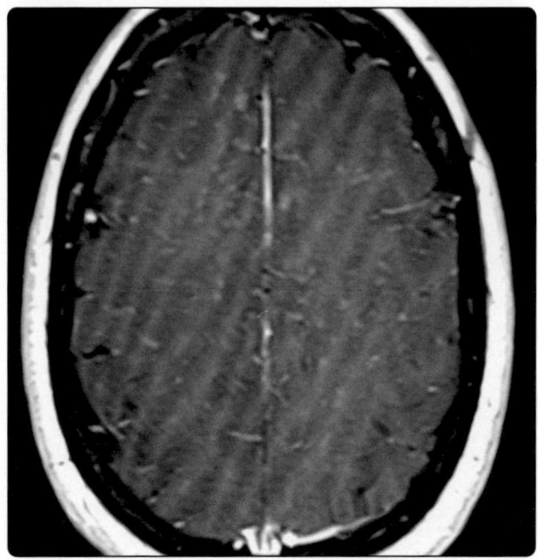

*(29-17) Axial T1 C+ MR shows prominent linear enhancement related to vasculitis. IVL often mimics vasculitis.*

disseminated disease. IVL is a relentless, rapidly progressive disease with a high mortality rate. Mean survival is 7-12 months.

**Treatment Options.** Because IVL is a widely disseminated disease, systemic chemotherapy is the recommended treatment. High-dose chemotherapy with autologous stem cell transplantation is often used in younger patients.

## Imaging

There are no pathognomonic neuroimaging findings for IVL. Ischemic foci with infarct-like lesions are the most common imaging finding **(29-13C)**. CT may be normal or nonspecific, demonstrating only scattered white matter hypodensities. MR shows multiple T2/FLAIR hyperintensities **(29-13A)**. Both macro- and microhemorrhages are common, so "blooming" foci on T2* (GRE, SWI) are often present **(29-13B)**. Linear/punctate enhancement oriented along penetrating arteries and perivascular spaces is suggestive of IVL **(29-14)**. Multifocal areas of diffusion restriction may be present **(29-16)**.

## Differential Diagnosis

IVL is a "great imitator," both clinically and on imaging studies. Stereotactic biopsy is thus necessary to establish the definitive diagnosis**. Vasculitis** with punctate and linear enhancing foci may be virtually indistinguishable from IVL on imaging studies alone **(29-17)**.

**PCNSL**, especially in the setting of immunodeficiency syndromes, may mimic IVL. IVL is most often multifocal, whereas 2/3 of PCNSLs are solitary lesions. Diffuse multifocal PCNSL, especially when it occurs in the form of **lymphomatosis cerebri**, may be difficult to distinguish from IVL. Lymphomatosis cerebri often shows little or no enhancement.

### INTRAVASCULAR LARGE B-CELL LYMPHOMA

**Pathology**
- Small/medium-sized vessels filled with tumor
- Little/no parenchymal tumor; focal masses rare
- Microhemorrhages common
- Multifocal infarcts

**Clinical Issues**
- Older patients with dementia, cognitive decline, transient ischemic attacks
- Skin lesions (50%)

**Imaging**
- Multifocal T2/FLAIR hyperintensities
- Punctate hemorrhages on T2* (SWI > GRE)
- Foci of restricted diffusion
- Linear/punctate enhancement

**Common Differential Diagnoses**
- PCNSL
- Vasculitis

Rapidly progressive leukoencephalopathy with confluent nonenhancing white matter lesions is a rare presentation of diffusely infiltrating CNS IVL and may mimic a cerebral **demyelinating disorder**.

Diffuse **subacute viral encephalitis** can likewise mimic IVL, especially on biopsy. Parenchymal **neurosarcoid** with perivascular nodular spread may also resemble IVL on imaging studies.

## Miscellaneous Rare CNS Lymphomas

Other than DLBCL, PCNSLs are rare. These lymphomas include anaplastic large cell lymphoma [ALK(+)/ALK(-)], T-cell and NK/T-cell lymphomas and "other low-grade B-cell lymphomas of the CNS," which includes extranodal marginal zone lymphoma.

**Low-grade lymphomas**, most of which are B cell, account for ~ 3% of all CNS lymphomas and almost exclusively affect immunocompetent adults. **Primary CNS T-cell lymphomas and NK/T-cell lymphomas** are very rare, accounting for ~ 2% of all PCNSLs **(29-18)**. Most reported cases are associated with prior EBV infection. Imaging findings are generally indistinguishable from parenchymal DLBCL.

## MALT Lymphoma of Dura

**Extranodal marginal zone lymphomas of mucosa-associated lymphoid tissue (MALT lymphomas)** in the head and neck are most often ocular adnexal tumors, occurring in the conjunctiva, lacrimal glands, orbit, and eyelids. The cranial meninges, especially the dura, are occasional intracranial sites. Diffuse dura-arachnoid thickening with one or more meningioma-like masses is the most typical imaging finding **(29-19)**. Parenchymal lesions are rare. Prognosis is excellent with a five-year survival rate of 85%.

## Metastatic Intracranial Lymphoma

Metastatic intracranial lymphoma is also called secondary CNS lymphoma (SCNSL). Between 5-10% of patients with diffuse large B-cell systemic lymphomas eventually develop CNS involvement.

Metastatic lymphoma rarely presents as a parenchymal mass. In contrast with PCNSL, skull and dural involvement is much more frequent. Both calvarial vault and skull base metastases are common. More recent studies suggest brain parenchymal

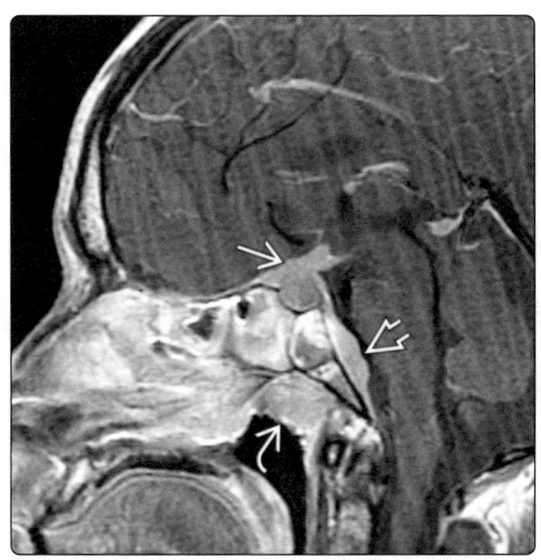

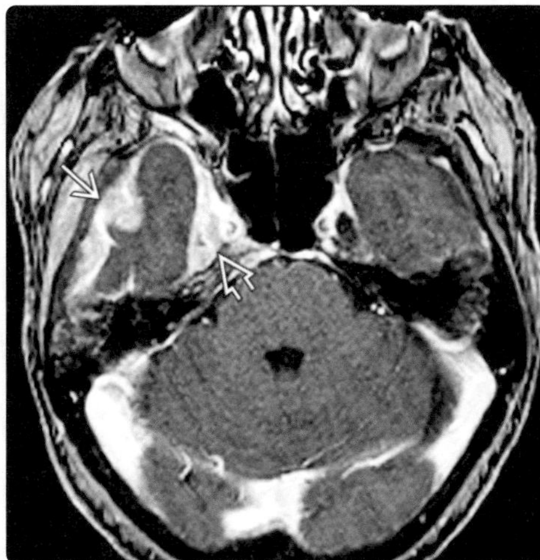

***(29-18)** T1 C+ MR of extranodal NK-/T-cell lymphoma shows an enhancing infiltrative mass involving the nasopharynx ➡, clivus, and adjacent dura ➡ with involvement of the pituitary gland and stalk ➡. These rare tumors are associated with prior EBV infection. **(29-19)** T1 C+ FS in 67-year-old woman with right CNVI palsy shows dural-based masses in right middle cranial fossa ➡ and cavernous sinus/Meckel cave ➡. MALT lymphoma.*

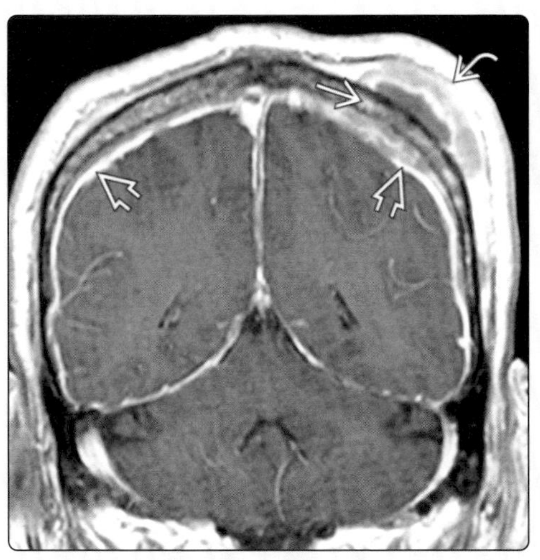

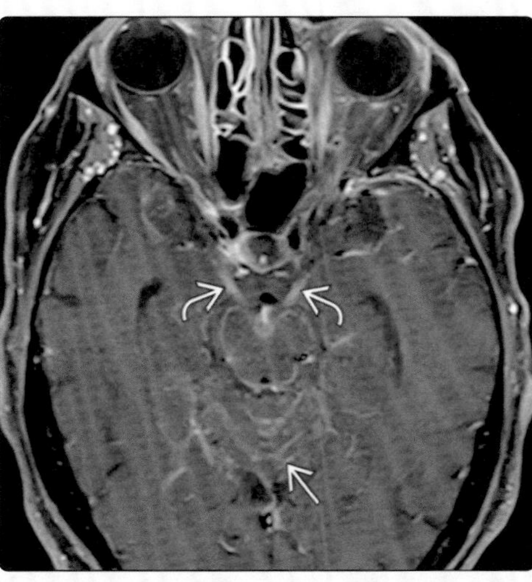

***(29-20)** Coronal T1 C+ MR shows systemic large B-cell lymphoma metastatic to the skull ➡, scalp ➡, and dura ➡. About 3-5% of systemic lymphomas develop CNS involvement. **(29-21)** Axial T1 C+ FS in a patient with cranial neuropathy and secondary DLBCL shows diffuse leptomeningeal involvement in the cerebellar folia ➡ and coating the midbrain. There is marked enlargement and enhancement along CNIII bilaterally ➡.*

involvement is more common than leptomeningeal disease and both are present in 10% of cases.

Calvarial lesions often involve the adjacent scalp and epidural space **(29-20)**. Dural "tails" are common. Involvement of the leptomeninges and underlying brain parenchyma may occur as late complications. Parenchymal lesions in the absence of skull and dural disease are uncommon. Leptomeningeal and CSF spread with cranial nerve, choroid plexus, and spine "drop" metastases occur but are rare **(29-21)**.

# Histiocytic Tumors

Histiocytic CNS neoplasms are a heterogeneous group of tumors that are histologically and immunologically identical to their extracranial counterparts. The 2021 WHO classification recognizes five histiocytic tumors that affect the CNS: **Langerhans cell histiocytosis (LCH), Erdheim-Chester disease (ECD), Rosai-Dorfman disease (RDD), juvenile xanthogranuloma**, and **histiocytic sarcoma**.

## Langerhans Cell Histiocytosis

LCH is a clonal neoplastic proliferation of immature, partially activated dendritic Langerhans cells. Between 50-60% of patients with LCH have *BRAF* V600E mutations, but the RAF-MEK-ERK pathway is activated in all patients. *MAP2K1*, which encodes MEK1, is mutated in 25% of cases.

LCH is now classified on the basis of disease extent as unifocal, multifocal (usually polyostotic), and disseminated disease. Most cases with isolated lesions present in young children under two years of age. Multifocal disease onset is generally between 2-5 years of age.

Geographic destructive bone lesions with "beveled edges" are the most common manifestation of LCH (80-95% of cases) **(29-22)**. The craniofacial bones and skull base are the most

***(29-22)** Graphic depicts the well-defined lytic skull lesions typical for LCH. There is lack of marginal sclerosis and classic "beveled" edges. Craniofacial and skull base bones are the most commonly affected sites in LCH. **(29-23A)** CECT in 15-month-old girl with mastoid region swelling, central diabetes insipidus (DI), and ataxia shows bilateral destructive temporal bone masses.*

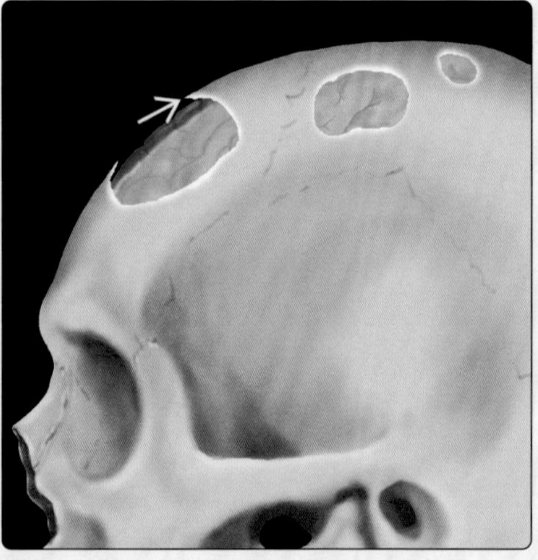

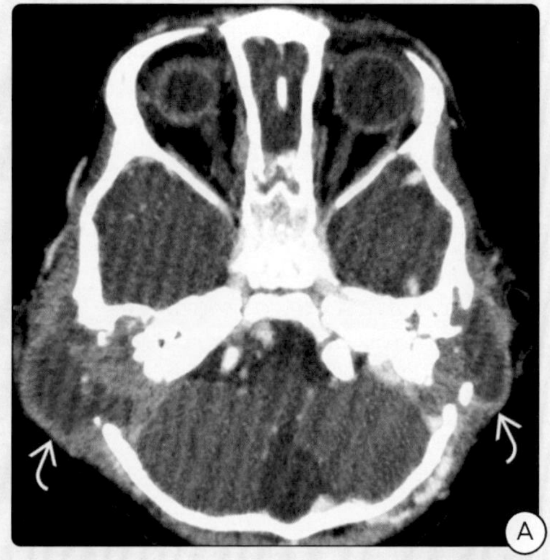


***(29-23B)** Axial T1 C+ FS MR shows a thickened, enhancing infundibular stalk. There was a lack of a normal "posterior bright spot" on precontrast T1 MR. **(29-23C)** T2 MR shows dentate hyperintensities representing autoimmune-mediated demyelination. About 1/3 of LCH patients have brain parenchymal lesions that present as a leukoencephalopathy-like pattern with dentate nuclei &/or BG involvement.*

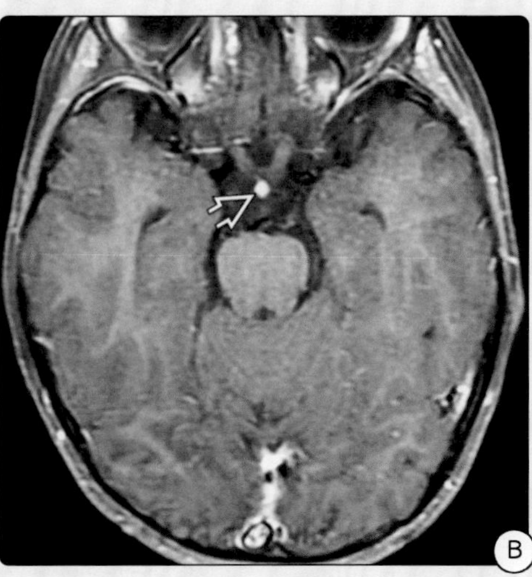


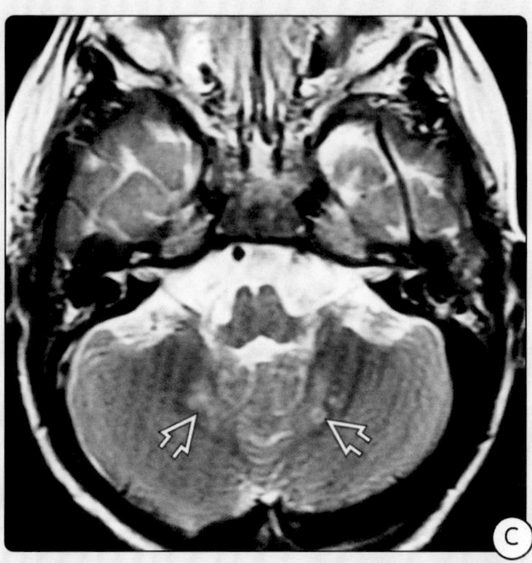

commonly affected sites (55%) **(29-23A)**. 1/2 of LCH cases affect the hypothalamic-pituitary region, often with absence of the posterior pituitary "bright spot" and a thickened, enhancing nontapering infundibular stalk **(29-23B)**. Nearly 1/3 of cases involve the cranial meninges.

Approximately 1/3 of patients exhibit parenchymal lesions. A leukoencephalopathy-like pattern, often with degenerative changes in the dentate nuclei &/or basal ganglia, occurs in nearly 1/3 of all LCH cases **(29-23C)**.

**LANGERHANS CELL HISTIOCYTOSIS: IMAGING**

CT
- > 50% have lytic craniofacial lesion(s)
- "Beveled" lesion > geographic destruction

MR
- Soft tissue mass adjacent to bone lesion
- Hypothalamus/pituitary stalk
  - Absent posterior pituitary "bright spot"
  - Thickened (> 3 mm), nontapering stalk
- Enhancing lesions
  - Dura-based mass(es)
  - Choroid plexus
  - Punctate/linear parenchymal enhancing foci
- Nontumorous degenerative changes
  - Symmetric T2/FLAIR hyperintensity in cerebellum/dentate nuclei, basal ganglia

## Rosai-Dorfman Disease

RDD, a.k.a. sinus histiocytosis with massive lymphadenopathy, is a rare benign histioproliferative disorder of unknown etiology. It is defined histopathologically by the accumulation of CD68(+), S100(+) proliferating histiocytes with intact, mature hematolymphoid cells floating freely within their cytoplasm ("emperipolesis"). A prominent lymphoplasmacytic infiltrate is also frequently present within the tumor mass.

RDD can occur at any age, but almost 80% of patients are younger than 20 years old at the time of initial diagnosis. Bilateral massive but painless cervical lymphadenopathy is the most common presentation. CNS involvement is rare and generally occurs *without* cervical adenopathy or other extranodal involvement. The mean age of patients with CNS RDD is 40 years.

RDD has a protean imaging appearance but most frequently presents as bilateral cervical lymphadenopathy. Extranodal involvement is seen in 50% of cases. The skin, nose, sinuses, and orbit (especially the eyelids and lacrimal glands) are often affected.

Intracranial RDD occurs in 5% of cases. Solitary or multiple dura-based masses that are isointense with gray matter on T1WI **(29-24A)** and slightly hypointense on T2WI **(29-24B)** are typical. Intense homogeneous enhancement occurs following contrast administration **(29-24C)**. Less commonly, multiple cranial and peripheral enhancing nerves can be identified. Sellar/suprasellar and intraspinal lesions are even less common. They can be isolated or occur in concert with more typical dura-based &/or orbital lesions.

The major imaging differential diagnosis of *intra*cranial RDD is **meningioma**. **Neurosarcoid** with dura-based and sellar/suprasellar involvement can mimic RDD, as can other dural-based masses, such as **metastasis, plasma cell**

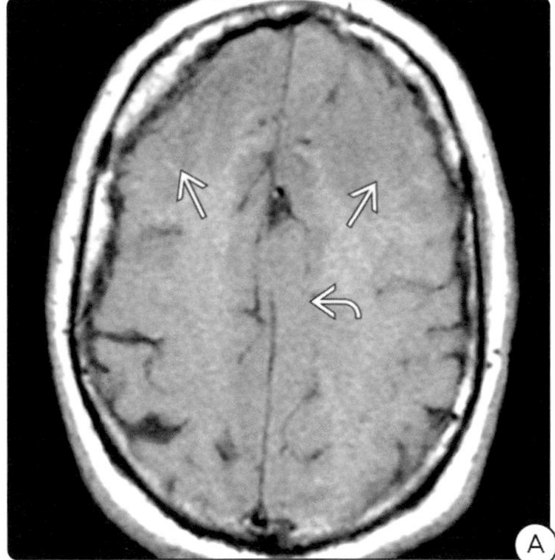


***(29-24A)** T1 MR shows effaced sulci and gray matter-WM interfaces in both frontal lobes ➡ and along the interhemispheric fissure ↪.*

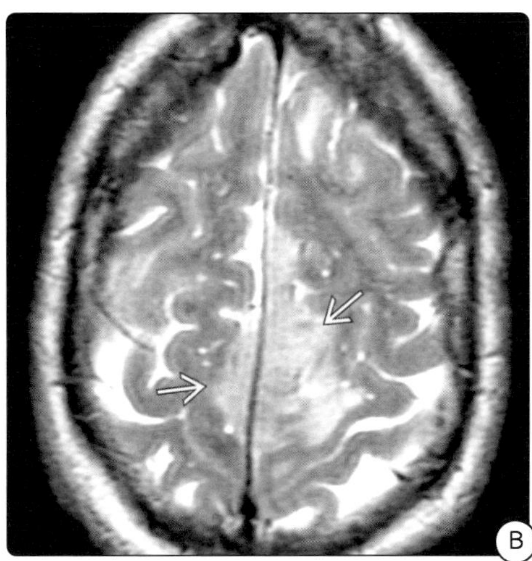


***(29-24B)** T2 MR shows lobulated parafalcine masses ➡ that are iso- to slightly hyperintense relative to cortex.*

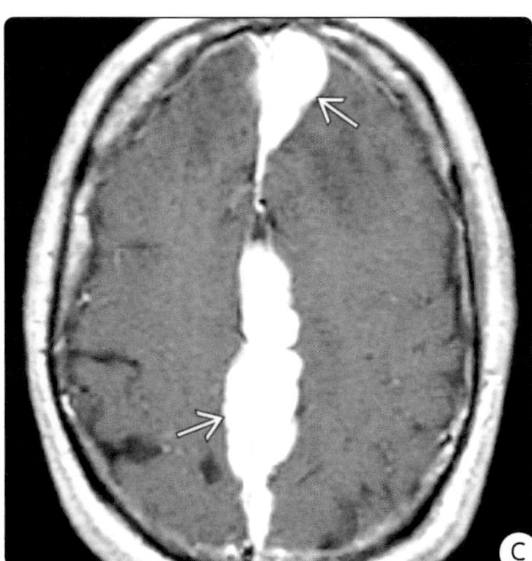


***(29-24C)** T1 C+ MR shows lobulated, intensely enhancing parafalcine masses ➡. Rosai-Dorfman disease diagnosed by cervical lymph node biopsy.*

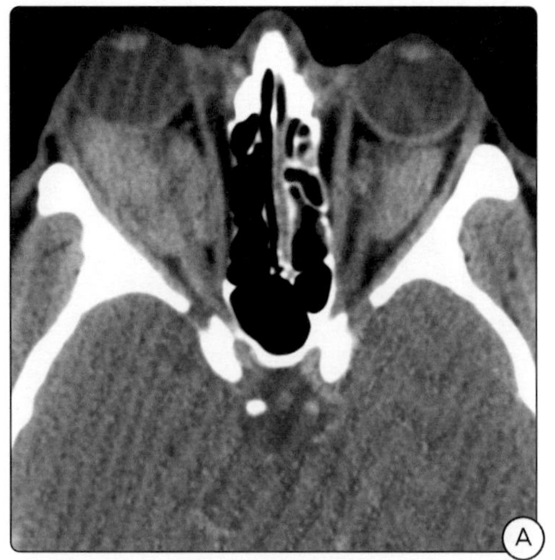

*(29-25A) Axial CECT of the orbits shows retrobulbar bilateral soft tissue masses in a 39-year-old man with proptosis. ECD.*

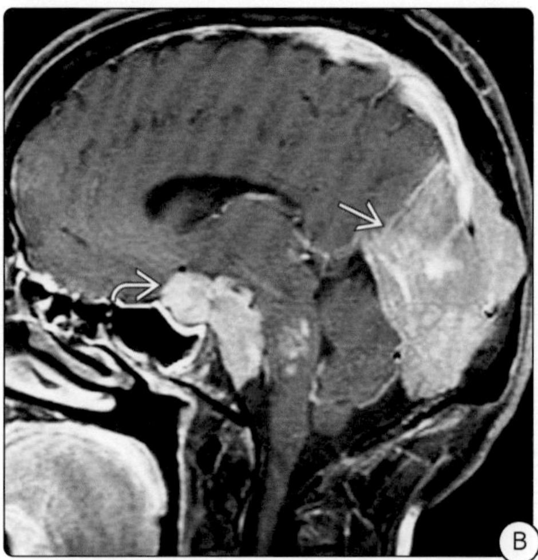

*(29-25B) Sagittal T1 C+ MR shows extensive dural-based masses along the falx ➡, pituitary region ➡ and within brainstem. ECD at biopsy.*

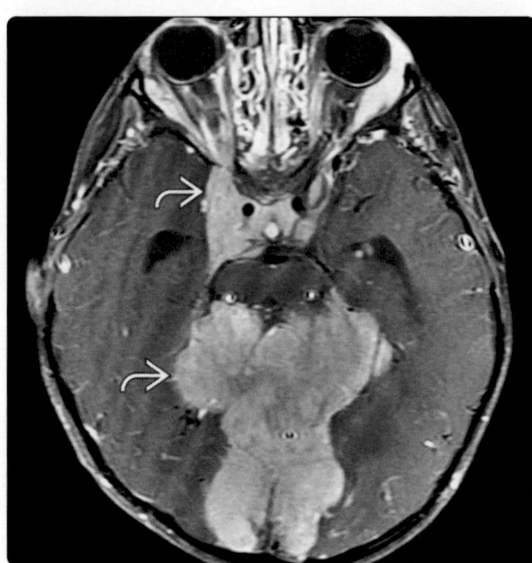

*(29-26) Axial T1 C+ in a 7-year-old shows extensive enhancing dural-based masses ➡ related to juvenile xanthogranuloma.*

**granuloma, infectious granuloma** (e.g., TB), **IgG4-related disease**, and **extramedullary hematopoiesis (29-28)**.

## Erdheim-Chester Disease

ECD of the CNS or the meninges is rare, non-LCH that affects multiple organs characterized by foamy histiocytes, occasional Touton giant cells, chronic inflammation, and variable fibrosis. CNS disease may occur with or without systemic lesions.

ECD is often seen in male patients ~ 50 years old. Neurologic complications occur in 30-50% of patients. ECD affects multiple organs, most often a disease of long bones. However, extraskeletal manifestations are present in ~ 50% of cases. Common genetic alterations include *BRAF* V600E mutations in ~ 50% of cases, *MAP2K1* mutations in up to 30% of cases. Patients may have both LCH and ECD.

ECD of the CNS may affect the brain parenchyma, hypothalamic-pituitary axis, orbits, dura, brainstem, and cerebellum **(29-25)**. Typical imaging appearance includes enhancing pontine and cerebellar lesions as well as dural-based masses **(29-25B)**. Some patients present with a thick enhancing pituitary infundibulum. Bony abnormalities, including symmetric bilateral osteosclerosis of the facial bones and calvarium, spine and long bones may be present.

In the brain parenchyma, FLAIR-hyperintense lesions with nodular enhancement is common. When affecting the dura, strong, homogeneous enhancement is typical, mimicking meningioma. A unique finding of ECD is perivascular disease. Periaortic fibrosis and perivascular infiltration along the carotid arteries may be seen as T2-hypointense lesions with strong enhancement.

The major imaging differential diagnosis of CNS ECD is **meningioma and neurosarcoid** with dura-based enhancing masses. Other differential considerations include **lymphoma** and **metastases**.

## Juvenile Xanthogranuloma

Juvenile xanthogranuloma is a rare non-LCH characterized by foamy histocytes, occasional Touton giant cells, and inflammation. Often, juvenile xanthogranuloma is a self-limited disorder of infancy or young children, often presenting as a solitary skin lesion. However, a small subset of patients present with systemic juvenile xanthogranuloma, which may include the CNS. CNS involvement is typically the brain, meninges, or spinal nerve roots.

Juvenile xanthogranuloma may present with T2- and FLAIR-hyperintense brain parenchymal lesions. Enhancement of the lesions is typically present. When affecting the dura, there is typically mild T2 hypointensity and homogeneous enhancement **(29-26)**.

The major imaging differential diagnosis of juvenile xanthogranuloma is similar to other histiocytoses and includes **meningioma, neurosarcoid, lymphoma**, and other **histiocytoses**, including **LCH**.

## Histiocytic Sarcoma

Histiocytic sarcoma is a malignant proliferation of cells showing morphologic and immunophenotypic features of tissue histiocytes. Rare cases of CNS histiocytic sarcoma have involved the brain parenchyma, meninges, and cavernous sinus.

These tumors have been reported primarily in adults. Presenting symptoms are related to tumor location. Imaging may mimic a primary malignant glioma or meningioma.

# Hematopoietic Tumors and Tumor-Like Lesions

## Leukemia

Leukemia is the most common form of childhood cancer, representing ~ 1/3 of all cases. Acute lymphoblastic leukemia (ALL) accounts for 80% and acute myeloid leukemia (AML) for most of the remaining 15-20%. Chronic myelocytic leukemia (CML) and lymphocytic leukemia are much more common in adults. Regardless of specific type, the general clinical features of leukemias are similar.

Leukemic masses were initially called **chloromas** (for the greenish discoloration caused by high levels of myeloperoxidase in immature cells). These tumors have been renamed **granulocytic sarcomas**.

Overt CNS leukemia presents in three forms: (1) Meningeal disease ("carcinomatous meningitis"), (2) intravascular tumor aggregates with diffuse brain disease ("carcinomatous encephalitis"), and (3) focal tumor masses (granulocytic sarcoma) **(29-27)**.

Most intracranial lesions are located adjacent to malignant deposits in the orbits, paranasal sinuses, skull base, or calvarium. Multifocal involvement is typical. Extraaxial lesions are generally large and seen as extensive bony infiltrates and dura-based masses **(29-28)**. Intraaxial granulocytic sarcomas occur but are less common and usually smaller, ranging from a few millimeters to 1 or 2 cm.

Imaging is key to the diagnosis of CNS involvement, as CSF studies may be negative.

Granulocytic sarcomas typically present as one or more iso- or hyperdense dura-based masses on NECT. Strong uniform enhancement is typical. Bone CT often shows infiltrating, permeative, destructive lucent lesions. An adjacent soft tissue mass may be present.

Nearly 75% of patients with leukemia and positive CSF cytology have abnormal findings on MR. Pachymeningeal (30%), leptomeningeal (25%), cranial nerve (30%), and spinal meningeal (70%) types of enhancement are typical. Parenchymal lesions ("chloroma") are much less common than meningeal disease. Chloromas are hypo- to isointense on T1WI and heterogeneously iso- to hypointense on T2/FLAIR. Enhancement of parenchymal and focal dural chloromas is typically strong and relatively homogeneous.

Differential diagnosis depends on location. Dura-based granulocytic sarcomas may resemble **extraaxial hematoma, lymphoma**, or **meningioma**. In younger children, **metastatic neuroblastoma** and **LCH** can mimic granulocytic sarcoma. **Extramedullary hematopoiesis** is a diagnostic consideration but is typically more hypointense than granulocytic sarcoma on T2WI.

## Plasma Cell Tumors

Three major forms of neoplastic plasma cell proliferations are recognized: (1) Solitary bone plasmacytoma (SBP), (2) solitary extramedullary plasmacytoma (EMP), and (3) multiple myeloma (MM).

**SBPs** are sometimes simply called plasmacytoma or solitary plasmacytoma. Solitary plasmacytomas are characterized by a mass of neoplastic monoclonal plasma cells in either bone or soft tissue without evidence of

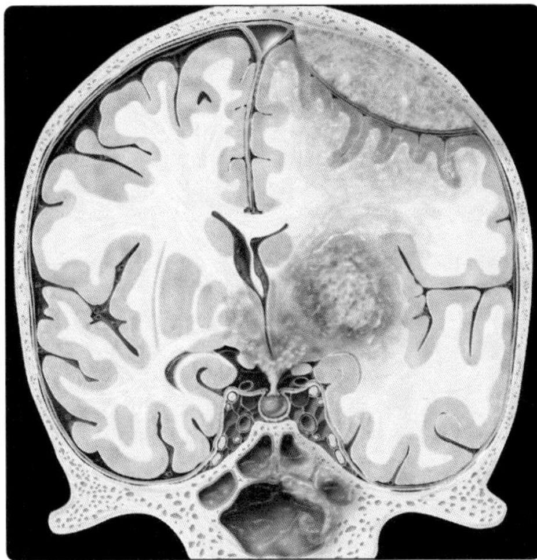

***(29-27)** Graphic depicts CNS leukemia with skull, dura, sinus, parenchymal, and juxtasellar disease.*

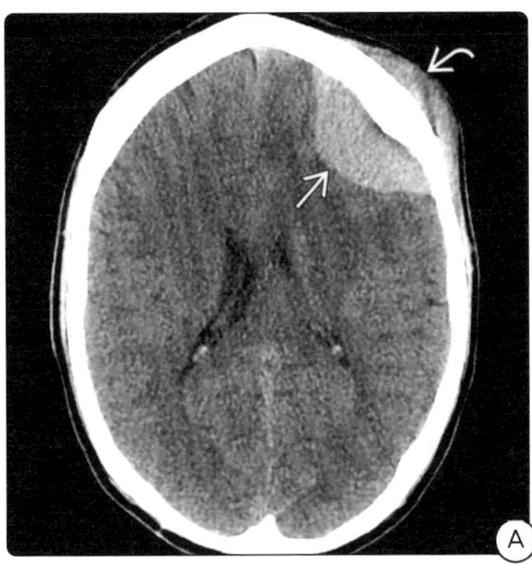


***(29-28A)** NECT in a 28-year-old man with AML and a scalp "lump" shows left frontal subgaleal ➡ and hyperdense extraaxial mass ➡.*

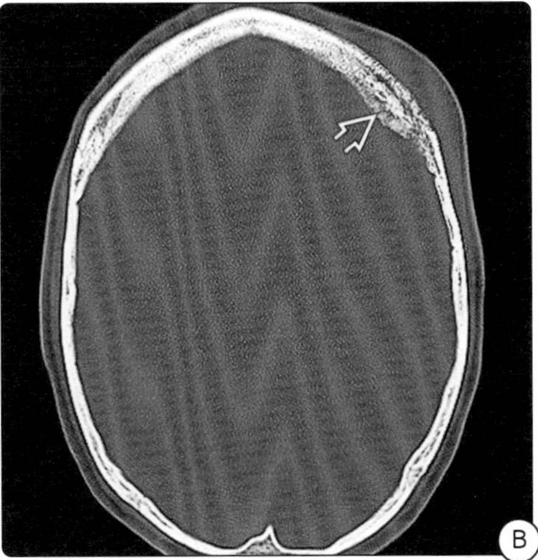


***(29-28B)** Bone CT with edge enhancement shows permeative, destructive changes in the adjacent calvarium ➡.*

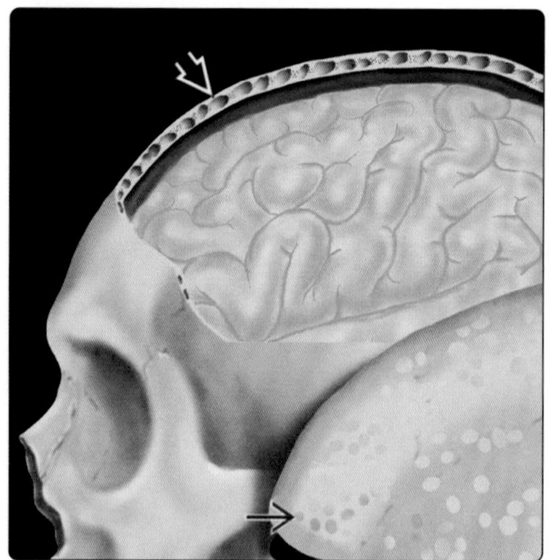

*(29-29) Graphic shows multiple lytic foci ⇒, characteristic of MM. Sagittal section shows the "punched-out" lesions in the diploic space ➡.*

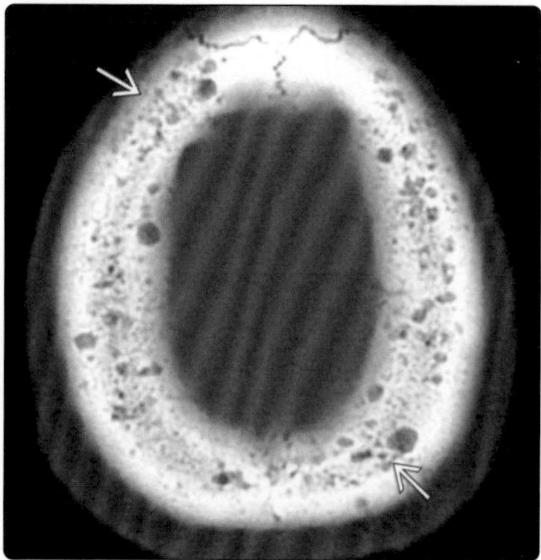

*(29-30) Bone CT shows MM. Innumerable lytic "punched-out" lesions ➡ give the calvarium the characteristic salt and pepper appearance.*

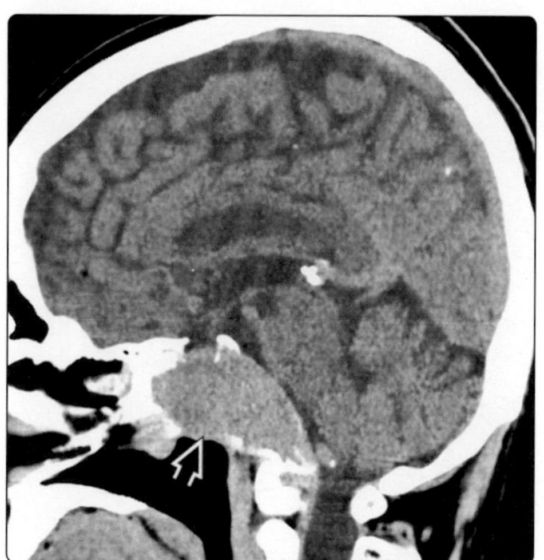

*(29-31) Sagittal NECT in a 67-year-old man with multiple cranial neuropathies shows hyperdense, destructive central skull base mass ➡.*

systemic disease. Solitary plasmacytomas are rare (5-10% of all plasma cell neoplasms) and are most commonly found in the red marrow of the spine vertebrae and skull.

**EMP** is usually seen in the head and neck, typically in the nasal cavity or nasopharynx.

Multifocal disease is **MM** **(29-29)**. **Plasmablastic lymphoma** is an uncommon, aggressive lymphoma that most frequently arises in the oral cavity of HIV-infected patients. Rarely, **atypical monoclonal plasma cell hyperplasia** occurs as an intracranial inflammatory pseudotumor (discussed in Chapter 15).

MM shows numerous lytic lesions on bone CT **(29-30)**, usually centered in the spine, skull base **(29-31)**, calvarial vault, or facial bones. A variegated salt and pepper pattern is typical.

Osseous lesions replace normal hyperintense fatty marrow and are typically hypointense on T1WI. T2 and fat-saturated sequences, such as T2-weighted STIR imaging, also highlight the extent of marrow infiltration. Focal and diffuse lesions appear hyperintense. Both SBPs and MM enhance strongly following contrast administration. Leptomeningeal and parenchymal disease occurs but is uncommon.

Multiple "punched-out" destructive myeloma lesions can appear virtually identical to lytic **metastases**. Spine and skull base MM can resemble **leukemia** or non-Hodgkin **lymphoma. Invasive pituitary macroadenoma** may be difficult to distinguish from MM, as both are isointense with gray matter. An elevated prolactin is often present with macroadenoma, and the pituitary gland cannot be separated from the mass.

## Extramedullary Hematopoiesis

Extramedullary hematopoiesis (EMH) is the compensatory formation of blood elements due to decreased medullary hematopoiesis. Various anemias (thalassemia, sickle cell disease, hereditary spherocytosis, etc.) are the most common etiologies, accounting for 45% of cases. Myelofibrosis/myelodysplastic syndromes (35%) are the next most common underlying causes associated with EMH.

Multiple smooth, juxtaosseous, circumscribed, hypercellular masses are typical **(29-32)**. The most common site is along the axial skeleton. The face and skull are the most common head and neck sites. The subdural space is the most common intracranial location.

EMH is hyperdense on NECT **(29-33A)**, enhances strongly and homogeneously on CECT, and may show findings of underlying disease on bone CT (e.g., hair on end pattern in thalassemia, dense bone obliterating the diploic space in osteopetrosis).

### EXTRAMEDULLARY HEMATOPOIESIS

**Etiology**
- ↓ medullary hematopoiesis
- Compensatory formation of blood elements
- Anemias (45%), myelofibrosis/myelodysplasia (35%)

**Imaging**
- Multiple smooth juxtaosseous masses
  - Spine, face, skull, dura
- Hyperdense on NECT
- T1 iso-/hypointense, T2 hypointense
- Enhances strongly

**Differential Diagnosis**
- Dural metastases
- Meningioma
- Neurosarcoid
- Lymphoma

Round or lobulated subdural masses that are iso- to slightly hyperintense relative to gray matter on T1WI and hypointense on T2WI are typical **(29-33B)**. EMH enhances strongly and uniformly on postcontrast T1WI **(29-33C)**.

The major differential diagnoses of intracranial EMH are **dural metastases** and **meningioma**. **Neurosarcoid** and **lymphoma** are other considerations. **RDD** and other histiocytoses can cause multiple dural-based masses.

*Selected References: The complete reference list is available on the eBooks+ version included with purchase.*

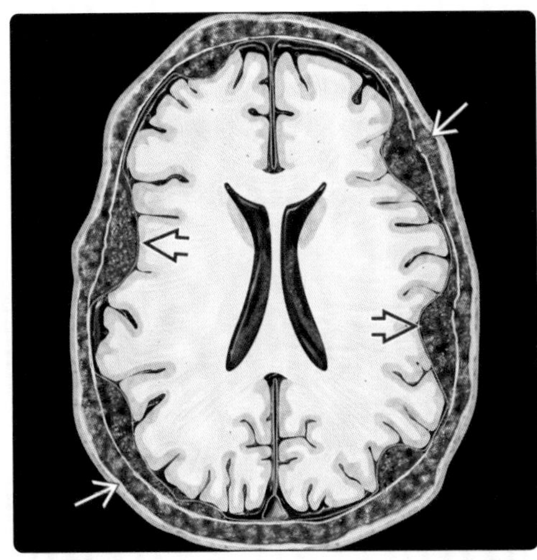

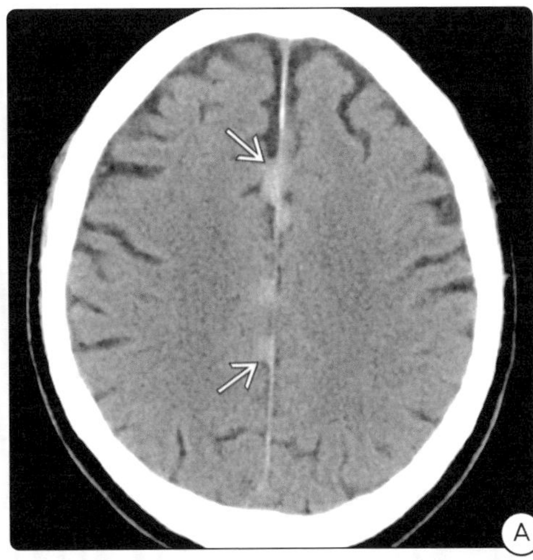


***(29-32)** Graphic shows extramedullary hematopoiesis (EMH), hematopoietic calvarial marrow ➡, and lobulated extraaxial masses ⇨. Various anemias (thalassemia, sickle cell disease, etc.) are the most common etiologies for EMH. **(29-33A)** NECT of EMH shows several hyperdense nodules ➡ along the falx cerebri. Imaging mimics the more common meningioma or dural metastatic disease.*

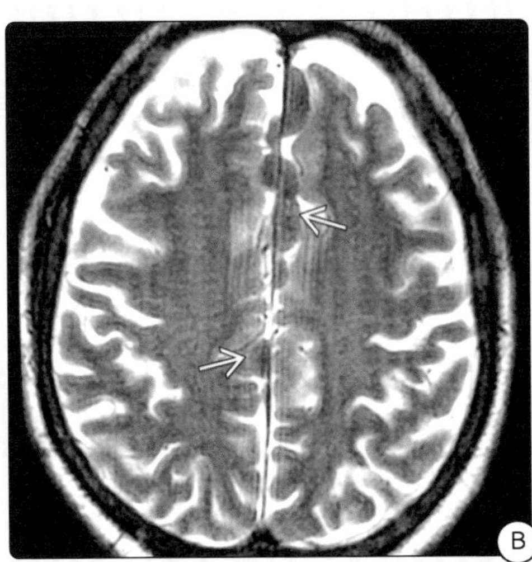


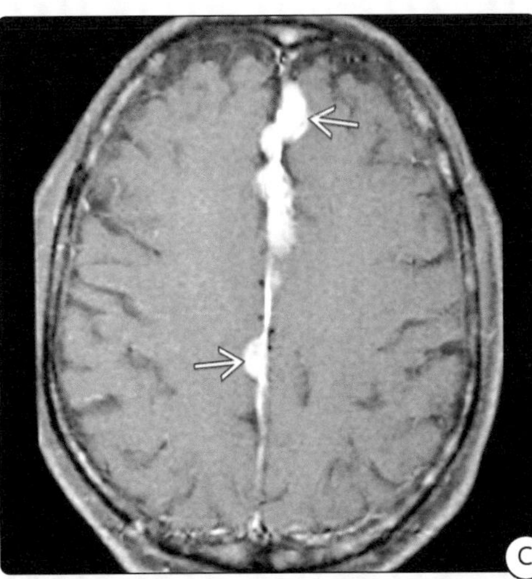


***(29-33B)** The lobulated lesions are very hypointense on T2WI ➡. **(29-33C)** EMH enhances strongly and uniformly ➡, as shown on this T1 C+ FS MR in the same patient. The main imaging differential considerations include meningioma, lymphoma, dural metastatic disease, and neurosarcoid.*

# Sellar Region Tumors and Tumor-Like Conditions

*The sellar region is one of the most anatomically complex areas in the brain. It encompasses the bony sella turcica and pituitary gland plus all the normal structures that surround it. Virtually any of these can give rise to pathology that ranges from incidental and innocuous to serious, potentially life-threatening, disease.*



At least 30 different lesions occur in or around the pituitary gland, arising from either the pituitary gland itself **(30-1)** or the structures that surround it **(30-2)**. These include the cavernous sinus and its contents, arteries (the circle of Willis), cranial nerves, meninges, CSF spaces (the suprasellar cistern and third ventricle), central skull base, and brain parenchyma (the hypothalamus).

Despite the overwhelming variety of lesions that can occur in this region, at least 75-80% of all sellar/juxtasellar masses are due to one of the **"Big Five": Macroadenoma, meningioma, aneurysm, craniopharyngioma (CP), and astrocytoma**. All other lesions combined account for < 1/4 of sellar region masses.

We begin the chapter with normal variants, such as physiologic hypertrophy, that can mimic pituitary pathology. Congenital lesions (such as tuber cinereum hamartoma) that can be mistaken for more ominous pathology are also delineated. Pituitary gland and infundibular stalk neoplasms are then discussed. A brief consideration of miscellaneous lesions, such as lymphocytic hypophysitis (LH), pituitary apoplexy (PAP), and the postoperative sella, follows.

The goal of imaging is to determine the precise location and characteristics of a sellar mass, delineate its relationship to—and involvement with—surrounding structures, and construct a reasonable, limited differential diagnosis to help direct patient management. We then conclude the chapter with a summary of—and approach to—a differential diagnosis of sellar masses.

## Diagnostic Considerations

**Anatomic sublocation** is the single most important key to establishing an appropriate differential diagnosis of a sellar region mass. The first step is assigning a lesion to one of three anatomic compartments, identifying it as an (1) intrasellar, (2) suprasellar, or (3) infundibular stalk lesion.

The key to determining anatomic sublocation accurately is the question, "can I find the pituitary gland separate from the mass?" If you cannot, and the gland *is* the mass, the most likely diagnosis is macroadenoma.

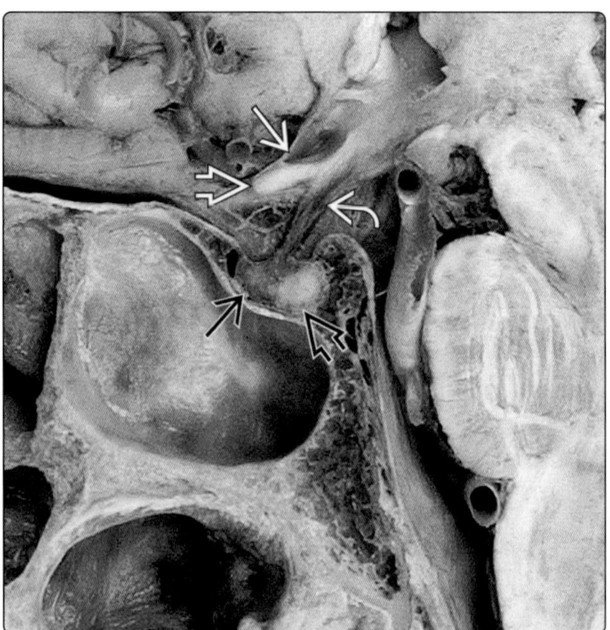

***(30-1) Midline anatomic section depicts sella and surrounding structures. Adenohypophysis ➲, neurohypophysis ➲ are shown, along with the optic chiasm ➲ and optic ➲ and infundibular ➲ recesses of the 3rd ventricle. (Courtesy M. Nielsen, MS.)***

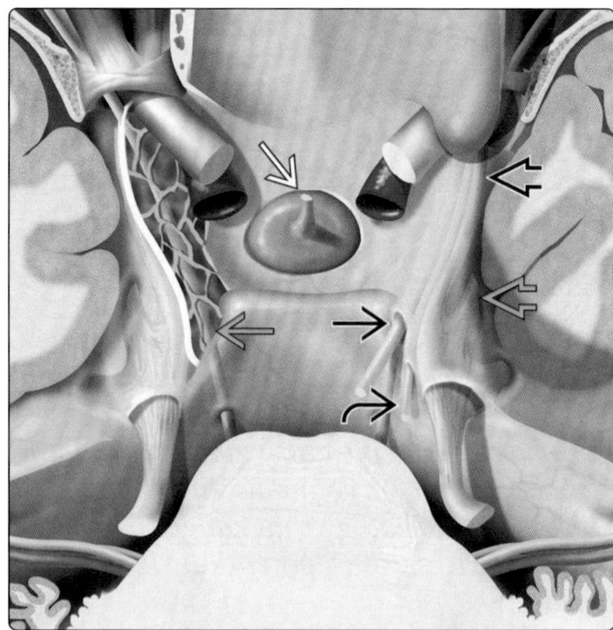

***(30-2) Graphic shows the pituitary gland and stalk ➲ from above. Note the cranial nerves in the lateral dural wall of the cavernous sinus: CNIII ➲, CNIV ➲, CNV1 ➲ and V2 ➲. CNVI ➲ is the most medial, located inside the cavernous sinus.***

If the mass is clearly *separate* from the pituitary gland, it is extrapituitary and therefore not a macroadenoma. Other pathologies, such as meningioma in an adult or CP in a child, should be considered in such cases.

## Clinical Considerations

The single most important clinical feature in establishing an appropriate differential diagnosis for a sellar region mass is **patient age**. Lesions that are common in adults (macroadenoma, meningioma, and aneurysm) are generally rare in children. A lesion in a prepubescent child—especially a boy—that looks like a macroadenoma is almost never a neoplasm. Nonneoplastic pituitary gland enlargement in children is much more common than tumors. Therefore, an enlarged pituitary gland in a child is almost always either normal physiologic hypertrophy or nonphysiologic nonneoplastic hyperplasia secondary to end-organ failure (most commonly hypothyroidism).

Some lesions that are common in children (e.g., opticochiasmatic/hypothalamic pilocytic astrocytoma and CP) are relatively uncommon in adults.

Sex is also important. Imaging studies of young menstruating female patients and postpartum women often demonstrate plump-appearing pituitary glands due to temporary physiologic hyperplasia.

## Imaging Considerations

Imaging appearance is very helpful in evaluating a lesion of the sellar region. After establishing the anatomic sublocation of a lesion, look for imaging clues. Are other lesions present? Is the lesion calcified? Does it appear cystic? Does it contain blood products? Is it focal or infiltrating? Does it enhance? Does it enlarge or invade the sella turcica?

# Normal Imaging Variants

A number of variants occur in the pituitary gland and around the sella turcica; these should not be mistaken for disease on imaging studies. Pituitary hyperplasia can be abnormal, but it can also be physiologic and normal. An ES is a common normal variant but can be a manifestation of idiopathic intracranial hypertension (IIH) (pseudotumor cerebri).

## Pituitary Hyperplasia

*Physiologic* increase in pituitary volume is common and normal in many circumstances **(30-3)**. Physiologic hypertrophy of puberty and enlarged pituitary glands in young menstruating female patients is very common **(30-4)**. Pituitary gland enlargement also occurs during pregnancy and lactation or in response to exogenous estrogen treatment.

*Pathologic* hyperplasia most commonly occurs in response to **end-organ failure**. Primary hypothyroidism, usually in the setting of longstanding primary hypothyroidism, is the most common cause of pathologic pituitary hyperplasia **(30-5)**. Other etiologies of pathologic pituitary hyperplasia include ectopic excess of releasing hormones that may occur with pancreas tumors, neuroendocrine tumors, pheochromocytomas as well as ACTH-dependent Cushing disease, and other less common conditions.

NECT scans of pituitary hyperplasia show that the superior margin of the gland is convex upward, measuring 10-15 mm in height. There is no evidence of erosion of the bony sella turcica. Enhancement is strong and generally uniform on CECT.

MR demonstrates an enlarged gland that bulges upward and may even contact the optic chiasm. The enlarged pituitary is isointense with cortex on both T1- and T2WI. Dynamic contrast-enhanced MR scans with 2- to 3-mm slice thickness and small FOV show that the gland enhances homogeneously.

Pituitary hyperplasia must be distinguished from **macroadenoma**. Age, sex, and endocrine status are helpful. Primary neoplasms of the pituitary gland are rare in children, whereas physiologic enlargement is common. Remember: **An enlarged pituitary gland in a prepubescent male patient is almost always hyperplasia, not adenoma!**

Other important causes of a diffusely enlarged pituitary gland include **LH**. LH is most common in pregnant and postpartum female patients and may be difficult to distinguish from physiologic hyperplasia on imaging studies alone. Other etiologies include granulomatous, IgG4-related, and drug-related hypophysitis. If stalk enlargement is present, hypophysitis is more likely than hyperplasia.

**Intracranial hypotension** results in pituitary enlargement above the sella turcica in 50% of patients. These patients typically present with headaches related to decreased intracranial CSF pressure. The classic imaging appearance of intracranial hypotension includes diffuse dural thickening and enhancement, downward displacement of the brain through the incisura ("slumping midbrain"), and distention of the venous structures and dural sinuses. Patients may also present with small subdural hygromas or, rarely, with subdural hematomas. Additional helpful features for diagnosis include a decreased pontomesencephalic angle between the pons and midbrain and a decreased vertical distance between the pons and mammillary bodies, the mamillopontine distance.

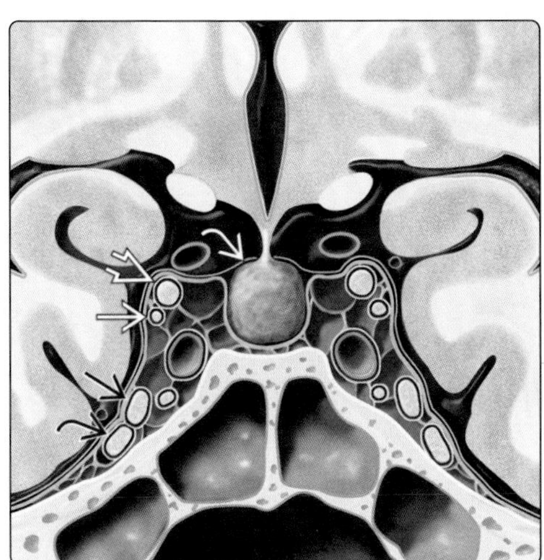

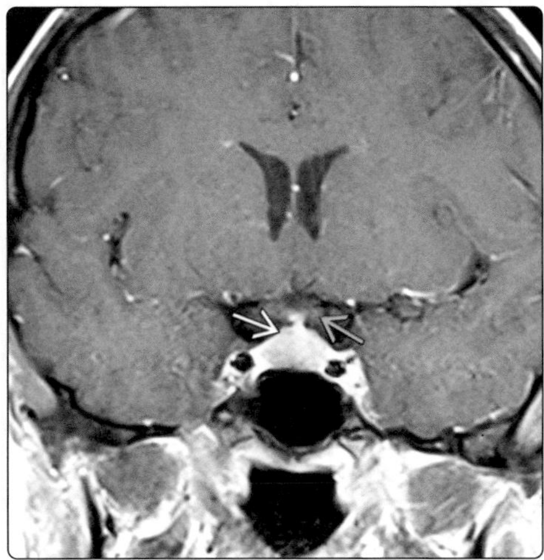

***(30-3)** Coronal graphic shows physiologic pituitary hyperplasia. The gland is uniformly enlarged and has a mildly convex superior margin ➡. Note cranial nerves in lateral dural wall of cavernous sinus: CNIII ➡, CNIV ➡, CNV1 ➡ and V2 ➡. **(30-4)** Coronal T1 C+ MR shows the upwardly convex gland ➡ almost touching the optic chiasm ➡. The overall volume of the pituitary gland is almost 2x the size of one in a postmenopausal woman.*

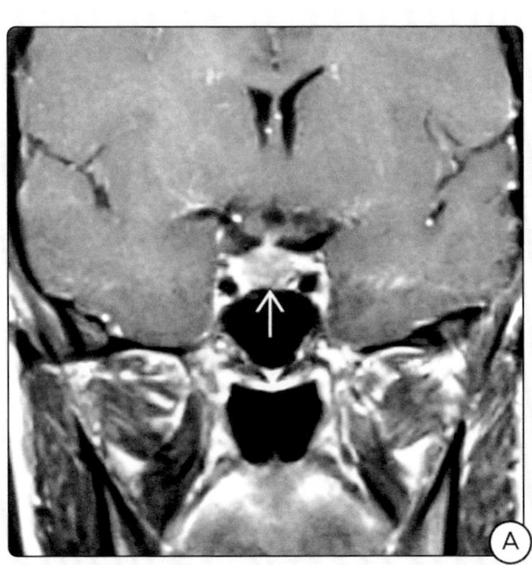



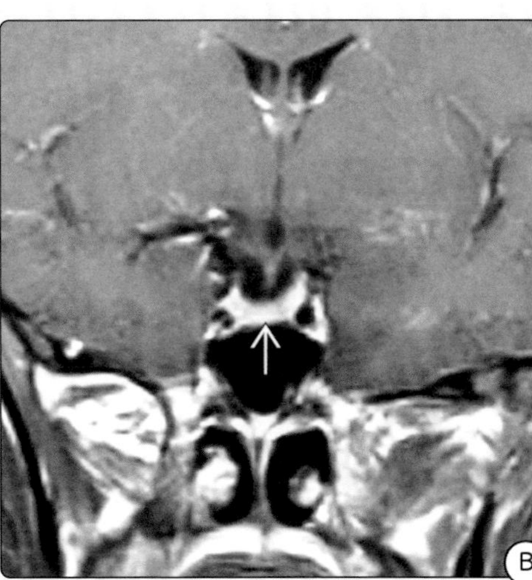



***(30-5A)** Coronal T1 C+ MR in a prepubescent male patient with hypothyroidism shows pituitary hyperplasia ➡ with an upwardly bulging gland that mimics macroadenoma. **(30-5B)** Repeat scan obtained a few weeks following initiation of thyroid hormone replacement therapy shows that the pituitary gland returned to a normal size ➡.*

## Empty Sella

An **empty sella (ES)** is an arachnoid-lined, CSF-filled protrusion that extends from the suprasellar cistern through the diaphragma sellae into the sella turcica **(30-6)**. An ES is rarely completely "empty"; a small remnant of flattened pituitary gland is almost always present at the bottom of the bony sella **(30-7)**, even if it is inapparent on imaging studies. An ES is identified in ~ 5-10% of cranial MR scans.

The major differential diagnosis of an ES is a **suprasellar arachnoid cyst** that may herniate into the sella turcica **(30-8)**. The bony sella is often not simply enlarged but eroded and flattened. Sagittal T2WI often shows an elevated, compressed third ventricle draped over the suprasellar arachnoid cyst. The optic chiasm is also typically elevated superiorly by the arachnoid cyst. Although often incidental, when they enlarge, arachnoid cysts may result in mass effect on the pituitary infundibulum and gland.

The other major consideration of patients with an ES is **IIH** a.k.a. "pseudotumor cerebri." Both incidental ES and patients with IIH have an increased prevalence in obese female patients. Imaging findings also show some overlap, as both conditions often demonstrate an ES. In IIH, the optic nerve sheaths are often dilated, and the ventricles and CSF cisterns often appear smaller than normal. Patients with IIH will also typically have papilledema, which can be seen on MR as protrusion of the optic nerve papilla into the posterior globes **(30-9)**.

**Increased intracranial pressure** (↑ ICP) caused by obstructive hydrocephalus usually results in displacement of the enlarged anterior third ventricle recesses—not the suprasellar cistern—toward or into the bony sella. Transependymal CSF migration is common in ↑ ICP but absent in ES.

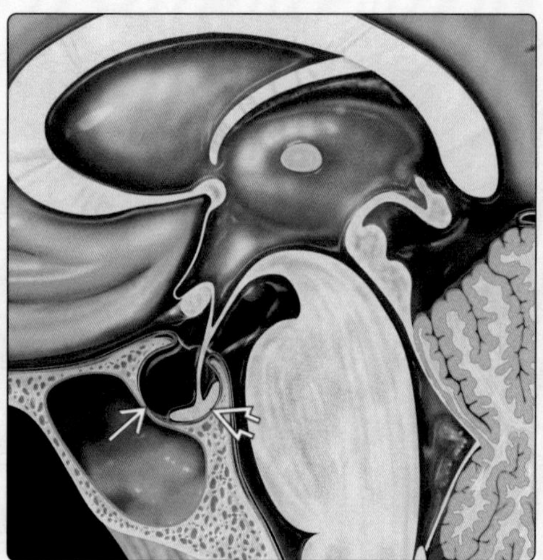

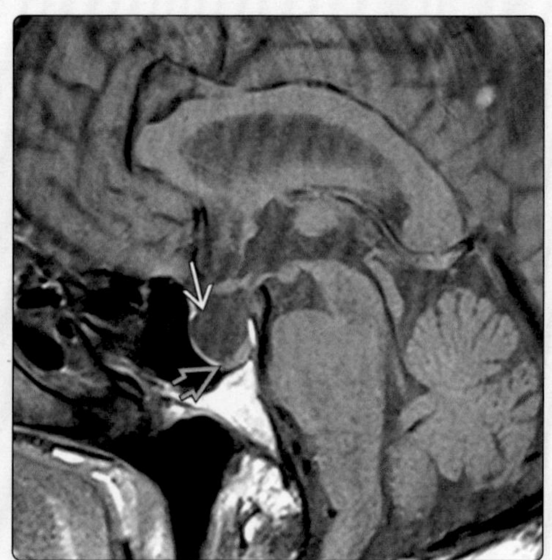

***(30-6)** Graphic depicts primary empty sella ➡ with CSF-filled arachnoid cistern protruding inferiorly into the enlarged sella turcica, flattening the pituitary gland posteroinferiorly against the sellar floor ➡. **(30-7)** Sagittal T1 MR shows a classic empty sella ➡ with an enlarged sella turcica in this 58-year-old woman with Cushing syndrome. The pituitary gland is thinned and flattened against the sellar floor ➡.*

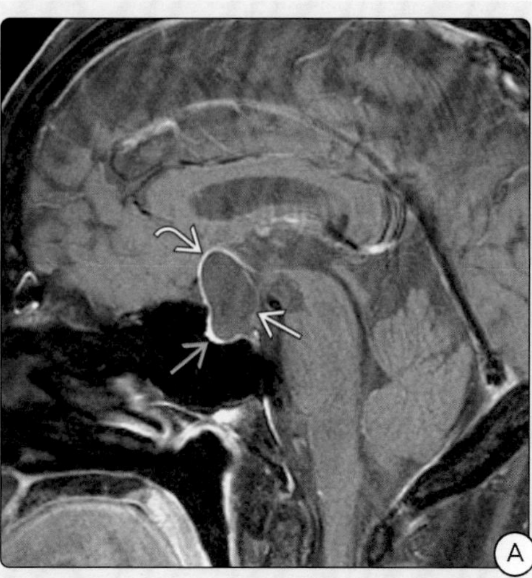

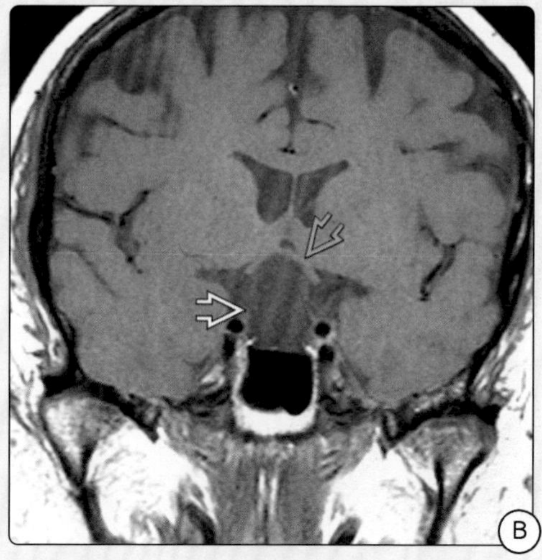

***(30-8A)** Sagittal T1 C+ MR in a 61-year-old woman with headaches shows an arachnoid cyst filling the sella and suprasellar regions ➡. Note the gland is flattened anteriorly within the sella ➡, and the infundibulum ➡ is displaced superiorly. **(30-8B)** Coronal T1 MR in the same patient shows the optic chiasm ➡ is displaced superiorly over the arachnoid cyst ➡. Arachnoid cysts follow CSF signal intensity on all MR sequences.*

# Congenital Lesions

## Pituitary Anomalies

A **hypoplastic pituitary gland** is the most frequent abnormality in children with *isolated* growth hormone deficiency, whereas **stalk abnormalities** are more common in children with *multiple* hormone deficiencies. Nearly 75% of children with hypopituitarism are male. Many affected have growth hormone deficiency and short stature.

Imaging abnormalities include a small sella and anterior pituitary lobe, hypoplasia or absence of the stalk, and an "ectopic" posterior pituitary "bright spot" (PPBS) seen as displacement of the T1-hyperintense posterior lobe into the infundibulum or median eminence of the hypothalamus **(30-10)**.

Pituitary duplication is a rare anomaly in which two pituitary stalks are present. The tuber cinereum of the hypothalamus and mammillary bodies are fused into a single thick mass. Associated craniofacial and craniocervical anomalies are common in these cases. Female patients are more commonly affected.

## Hypothalamic Hamartoma

Hypothalamic hamartoma (HH), a.k.a. diencephalic or **tuber cinereum hamartoma**, is a nonneoplastic congenital malformation associated with precocious puberty, behavioral disturbances, and gelastic seizures.

The majority of HHs are located in the tuber cinereum, i.e., between the infundibular stalk anteriorly and the mammillary bodies posteriorly. They can be pedunculated or sessile. Pedunculated lesions extend inferiorly from the hypothalamus into the suprasellar cistern, whereas sessile HHs project from the floor of the third ventricle into its lumen. HHs

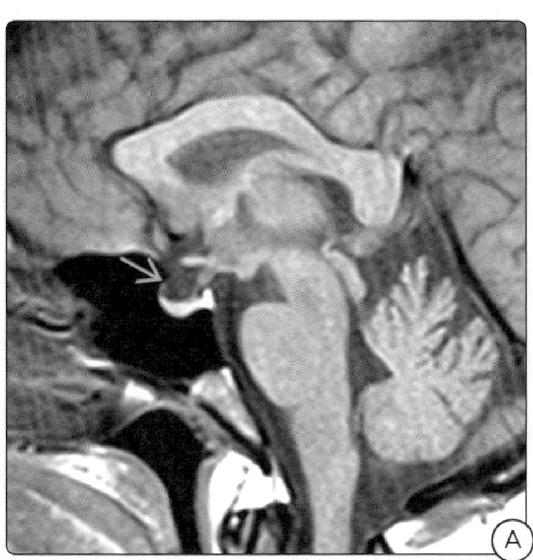

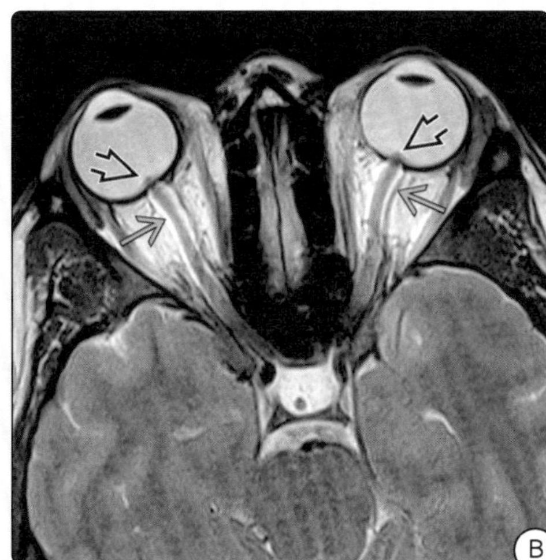

***(30-9A)** Sagittal T1 MR in a 24-year-old woman with headaches demonstrates a partially empty sella ⇨. A normal pituitary gland should have an upwardly convex margin. **(30-9B)** Axial T2 MR in the same patient with papilledema related to idiopathic intracranial hypertension shows dilated optic nerve sheaths ⇨ and protrusion of the optic nerve heads into the posterior globes ⇨.*

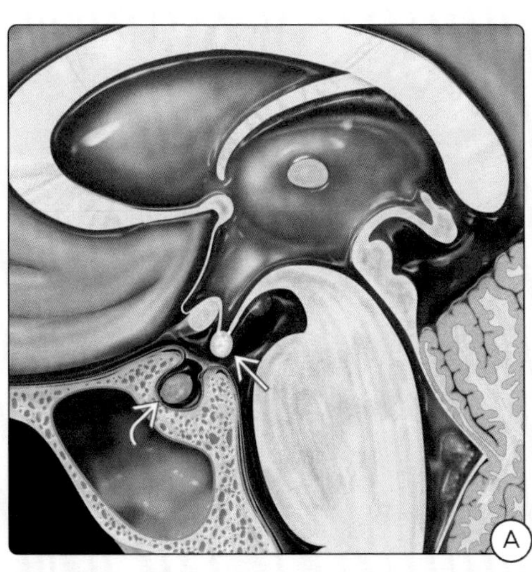

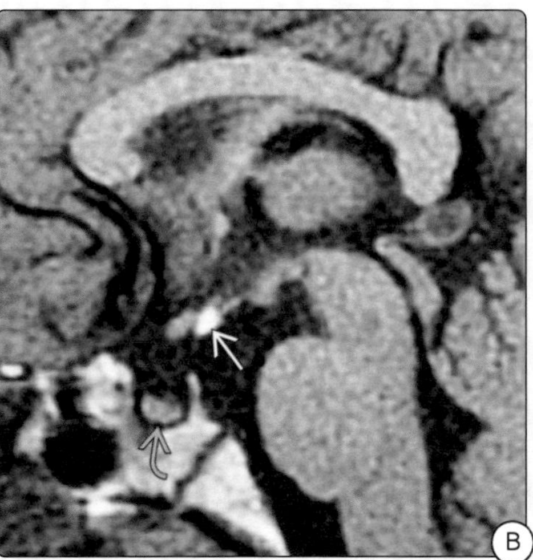

***(30-10A)** Sagittal graphic demonstrates ectopia of the posterior pituitary gland ➡, located at the distal end of a truncated pituitary stalk. The sella turcica and adenohypophysis ➡ are both small. **(30-10B)** Sagittal T1 MR shows an ectopic posterior pituitary gland at the hypothalamic median eminence ➡. The infundibulum is absent, and the anterior pituitary gland ⇨ is small. The normal posterior pituitary "bright spot" is not in its typical location.*

are solitary lesions that vary in size from a few millimeters to huge mixed solid/cystic lesions measuring several centimeters in diameter.

Most HHs present between 1-3 years of age. 3/4 of patients with histologically verified HHs have precocious puberty, and 50% have seizures, often "gelastic" (ictal laughing fits). Gelastic seizures are more common with sessile tumors, whereas precocious puberty is more often present in patients with small, pedunculated lesions.

NECT scan shows a homogeneous suprasellar mass that is isodense to slightly hypodense compared with brain. HHs do not enhance on CECT.

Pedunculated HHs are shaped like a collar button on sagittal T1WI, extending inferiorly into the suprasellar cistern. Signal intensity is usually isointense to normal gray matter on T1WI and iso- to slightly hyperintense on T2/FLAIR **(30-13A)**. Intralesional cysts may be present in larger HHs. HHs do not enhance with contrast **(30-13B)**. If contrast enhancement is present, a more aggressive neoplastic lesion should be considered.

The differential diagnoses of HH are CP and chiasmatic/hypothalamic astrocytoma. **CP** is the most common suprasellar mass in children. Over 90% of CPs are cystic, 90% calcify, and 90% show nodular and rim enhancement. **Optic pathway/hypothalamic pilocytic astrocytoma** is the second most common pediatric suprasellar mass. Astrocytomas are hyperintense on T2/FLAIR and often enhance on T1 C+.

## Rathke Cleft Cyst

Rathke cleft cyst (RCC) is a benign endodermal cyst of the sellar region, thought to arise from remnants of the fetal Rathke pouch. Approximately 40% are completely intrasellar and 60% are either suprasellar or combined intra- and suprasellar **(30-14)**.

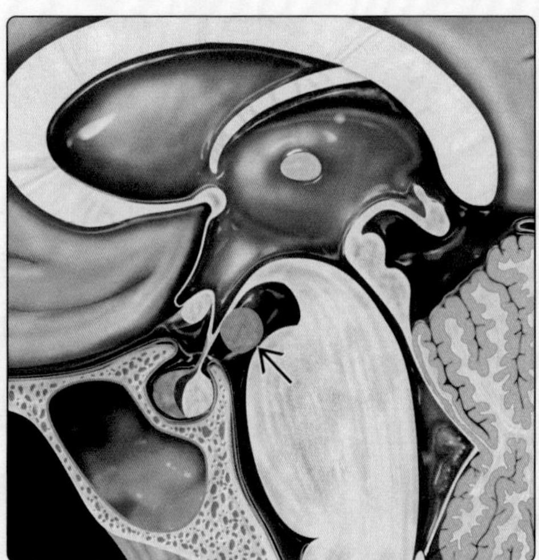

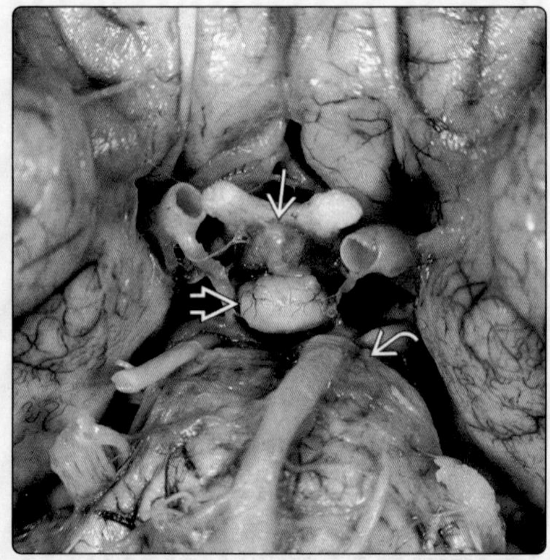

***(30-11)** Sagittal graphic shows a pedunculated hypothalamic hamartoma (HH) ➡ interposed between the infundibulum anteriorly and the mammillary bodies posteriorly. The mass resembles gray matter. **(30-12)** Submentovertex view shows a classic "collar button" pedunculated HH ➡ positioned between infundibular stalk ➡ in front, mammillary bodies (not visible), and pons ➡ behind. (Courtesy R. Hewlett, MD.)*

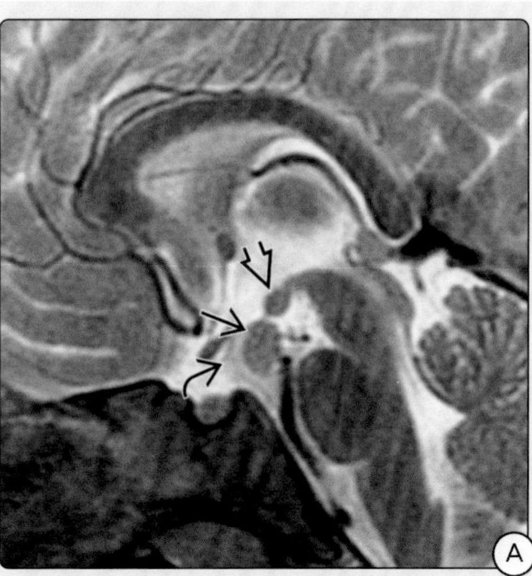


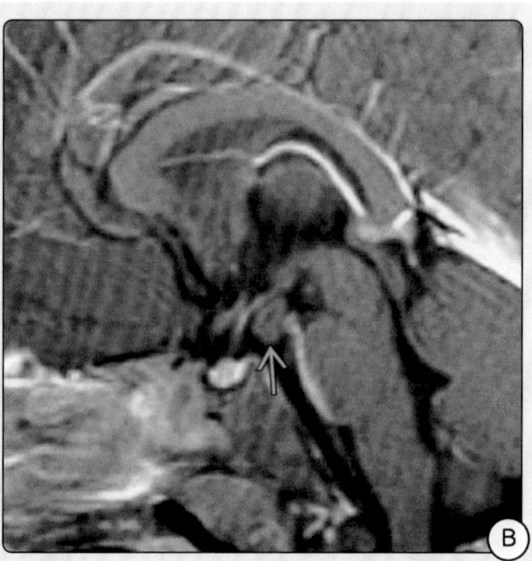


***(30-13A)** Sagittal T2 MR in a 12-month-old child with central precocious puberty shows a classic "collar button" HH ➡ between the infundibular stalk ➡ and the mammillary bodies ➡. The mass is isointense with gray matter. **(30-13B)** Sagittal T1 C+ MR in the same patient shows that the HH ➡ does not enhance. If the mass enhanced, a glioma should be considered.*

Most RCCs are asymptomatic and discovered incidentally at imaging. Symptomatic RCCs cause pituitary dysfunction, visual disturbances, and headache. Mean age at presentation is 45 years. Most RCCs remain stable and do not change in size or signal intensity. They do not undergo malignant degeneration.

NECT scans show a well-delineated round or ovoid mass within or just above the sella. 3/4 of RCCs are hypodense, 20% are of mixed density, and 5-10% are hyperdense. Calcification is rare. Lack of calcification helps differentiate an RCC from a CP.

Signal intensity varies with cyst contents; 1/2 of RCCs are hypointense on T1WI and 1/2 are hyperintense **(30-15)**. The majority are hyperintense on T2WI **(30-16)**, whereas 25-30% are iso- to hypointense. A hypointense intracystic nodule occurs in 40-75% of cases **(30-16)**. RCCs are almost always hyperintense on FLAIR. An enhancing rim (claw sign) of compressed pituitary gland can often be seen surrounding the nonenhancing cyst on T1 C+ **(30-17)**.

The major differential diagnosis of RCC is an **adamantinomatous CP**. Calcifications are common in CP. The rim or nodular enhancement in CP is generally thicker and more irregular than the "claw" of enhancing pituitary gland that surrounds the nonenhancing RCC. A cystic pituitary adenoma—especially a **nonfunctioning cystic microadenoma**—can be difficult to distinguish from a small intrasellar RCC.

**Other nonneoplastic cysts** that can occur in the sellar region are dermoid (fat, calcification common) and epidermoid cysts (ECs) (rarely midline, usually CSF-like, DWI hyperintense), arachnoid cysts (larger, CSF-like, lacking an intracystic nodule), and inflammatory cysts (e.g., neurocysticercosis; multiple far more prevalent than solitary cysts).

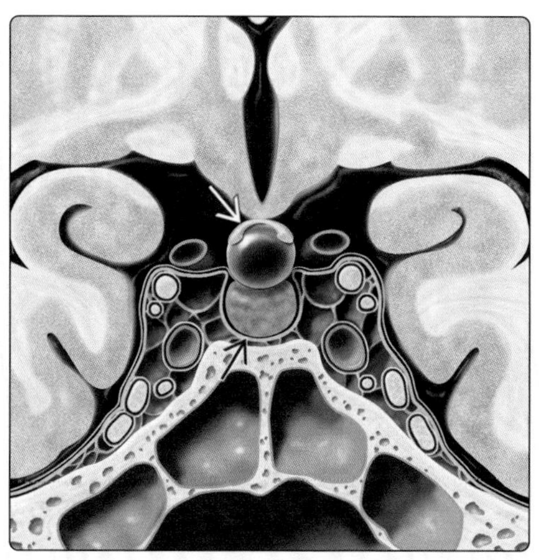

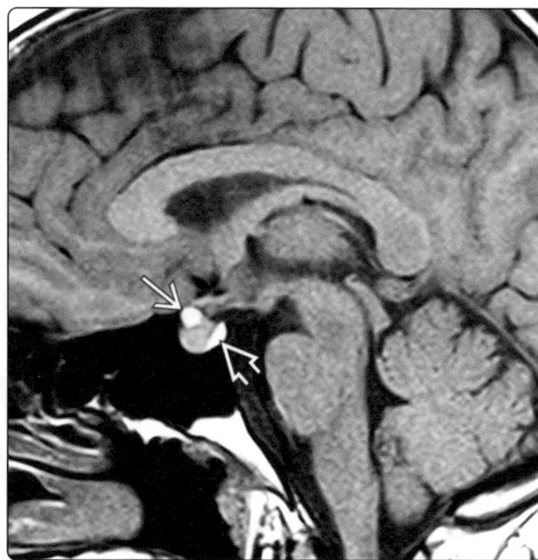

***(30-14)** Coronal graphic shows a typical suprasellar Rathke cleft cyst interposed between the pituitary gland ⇨ and the optic chiasm ➡. **(30-15)** Sagittal T1 MR in an asymptomatic patient shows a tiny hyperintense suprasellar mass ➡ that appears separate from the pituitary gland "bright spot" of the neurohypophysis ➡. This is presumed Rathke cleft cyst.*

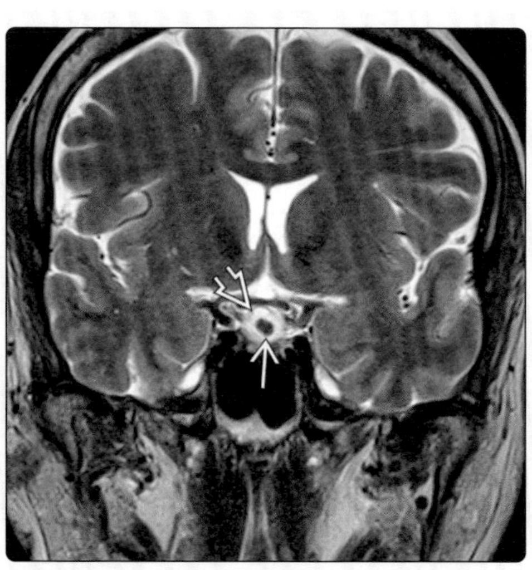

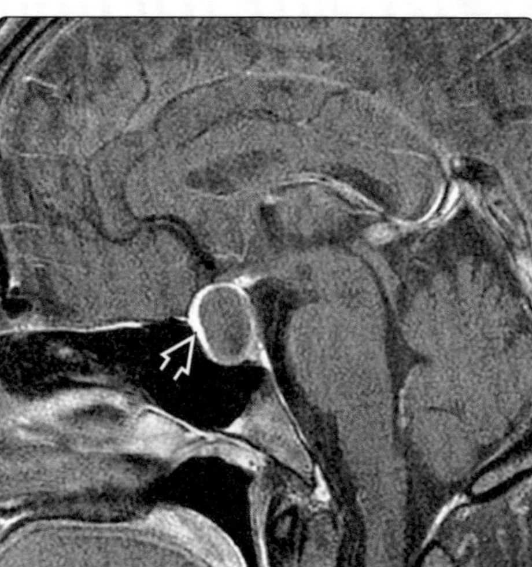

***(30-16)** Coronal T2 MR in a 62-year-old woman with headaches shows a hyperintense intra- and suprasellar cyst ➡ with a hypointense intracystic nodule ➡ related to a Rathke cleft cyst. These nodules do not enhance. **(30-17)** Sagittal T1 C+ MR in a 42-year-old patient with a Rathke cleft cyst shows the classic claw sign ➡ of compressed pituitary gland wrapping around the anterior aspect of the cyst.*

# Neoplasms

## Pituitary Adenomas

### Terminology

Pituitary adenomas, now a.k.a. pituitary neuroendocrine tumors (PitNET) according to the new 2021 WHO classification, are adenohypophysial tumors composed of secretory cells that produce pituitary hormones. **Microadenomas** are defined as tumors ≤ 10 mm in diameter, whereas larger adenomas are designated **macroadenomas (30-18) (30-19) (30-20)**.

### Pathology

**Location.** Adenomas/PitNETs arise from the adenohypophysis. Specific sublocation follows the normal distribution of peptide-containing cells. Prolactinomas and growth-hormone-secreting tumors—the two most common pituitary adenomas—tend to arise laterally within the adenohypophysis, whereas thyroid-stimulating hormone (TSH)- and ACTH-secreting tumors are more often midline.

**Size and Number.** These adenomas/PitNETs vary in size from microscopic lesions to giant tumors that invade the skull base and extend into multiple cranial fossae.

**Gross Pathology.** Macroadenomas/PitNETs are red-brown, lobulated masses that often bulge upward through the opening of diaphragma sella **(30-19)** or, less commonly, extend laterally toward the cavernous sinus. Approximately 1/2 of macroadenomas/PitNETs contain cysts &/or hemorrhagic foci. These are typically nonaggressive tumors with low recurrence rates. However, when there is craniospinal dissemination &/or systemic metastases, these are called pituitary carcinomas. These carcinomas are rare, representing < 0.5% of all pituitary adenomas/PitNETs.

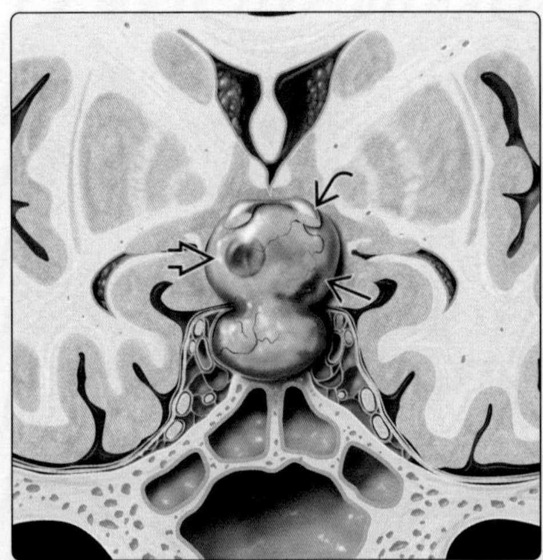

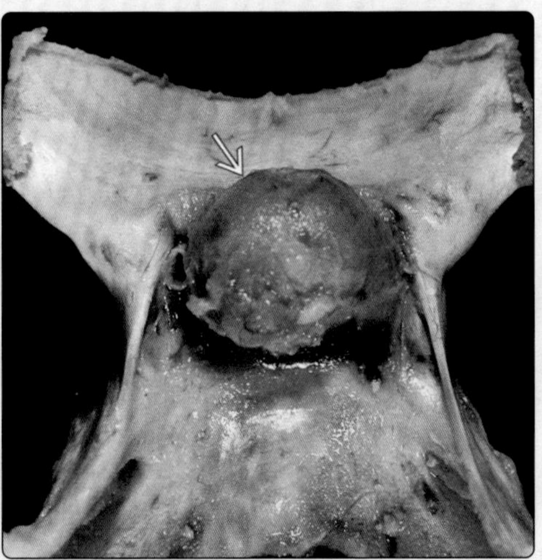

***(30-18)** Coronal graphic shows a snowman-shaped or "figure 8" sellar and suprasellar mass ➔. Small foci of hemorrhage ➔ and cystic change ➔ are present within the lesion. The pituitary gland cannot be identified separately from the mass; indeed, the gland is the mass. **(30-19)** Autopsy specimen shows a macroadenoma/PitNET ➔ protruding superiorly into the suprasellar cistern. (Courtesy R. Hewlett, MD.)*

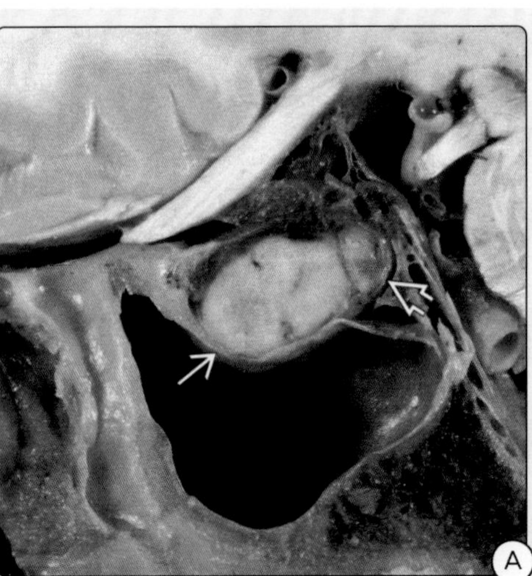



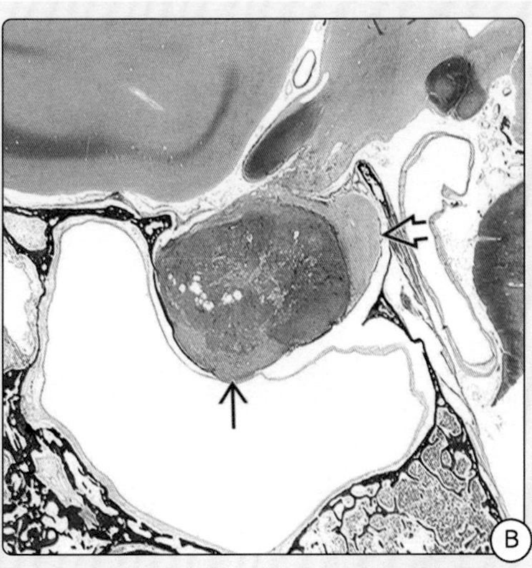



***(30-20A)** Pituitary adenomas/PitNETs ➔ are well-circumscribed masses that compress and displace the normal pituitary gland ➔. (Courtesy A. Ersen, MD; B. Scheithauer, MD.) **(30-20B)** Sagittal low-power photomicrograph shows a prolactinoma eroding the sellar floor ➔, compressing and displacing the normal pituitary gland posteriorly ➔. (Courtesy A. Ersen, MD; B. Scheithauer, MD.)*

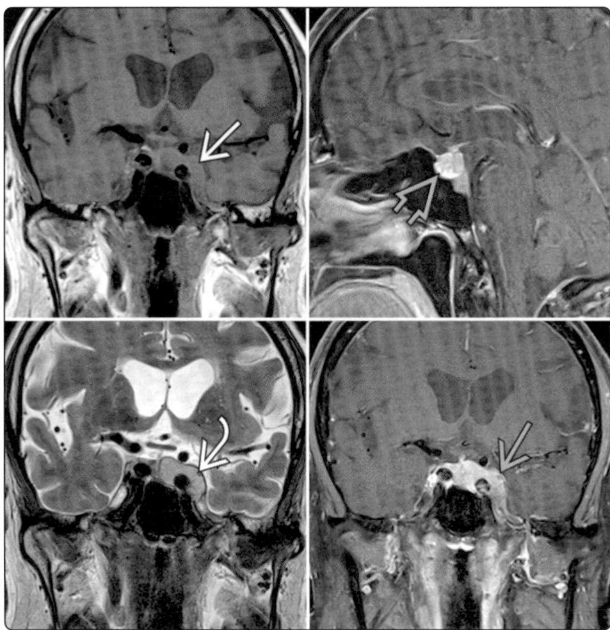

***(30-21)** Series of MR images shows an adenoma with cavernous sinus invasion seen as tumor between the cavernous ICA and the lateral dural wall. The mass is isointense with gray matter on T1- and T2WI and enhances strongly and uniformly.*

***(30-22)** Sagittal T1, T2, coronal FLAIR, and T1 C+ MR show a very large "snowman" or "figure 8" sellar and suprasellar mass typical of macroadenoma/PitNET. The pituitary gland cannot be identified as separate from the mass.*

## Clinical Issues

**Epidemiology.** Pituitary adenomas/PitNETs are among the most common of all CNS neoplasms, accounting for 10-15% of primary intracranial neoplasms. Microadenomas are much more common than macroadenomas; clinically silent incidental microadenomas are identified in 15-25% of autopsies.

Peak age of presentation is between 4th-7th decades. Only 2% of pituitary adenomas/PitNETs are found in children. Most of these occur in adolescent girls. Pituitary adenomas/PitNETs in prepubescent boys are very rare.

**Presentation.** Almost 2/3 of pituitary adenomas/PitNETs secrete a hormone (~ 40-50% prolactin, 10% growth hormone, 6% corticotropin, 1% thyrotropin) and cause typical hypersecretory syndromes. 1/3 do not produce hormones and are referred to as "nonfunctioning" or "null cell" adenomas/PitNETs.

Macroadenomas generally present with mass effect. Headache and visual disturbances are common. Diabetes insipidus is rarely associated with pituitary adenoma/PitNETs, so its presence should prompt consideration of an alternative diagnosis.

Although pituitary adenoma/PitNET growth rates are quite variable, most enlarge slowly over a period of years. Malignant degeneration into pituitary carcinoma is exceptionally rare and is diagnosed when craniospinal spread or distant metastases are identified. Treatment options are numerous and range from medical treatment to surgical resection and radiation therapy. Chemotherapy is reserved for pituitary carcinomas.

## Imaging

**General Features.** A sellar or combined intra- and suprasellar mass that cannot be identified separately from the pituitary gland (the mass *is* the gland) is the most characteristic imaging finding.

**CT Findings.** Pituitary adenomas/PitNETs demonstrate variable attenuation on NECT scans. Macroadenomas are usually isodense with gray matter, but cysts (15-20%) and hemorrhage (10%) may be seen. Calcification is rare (< 2%). Moderate but heterogeneous enhancement of macroadenomas/PitNETs is typical on CECT.

Bone CT may show an enlarged, remodeled sella turcica. "Giant" pituitary adenomas/PitNETs may erode and extensively invade the skull base **(30-24)**.

### MR Findings

***Macroadenomas.*** Macroadenomas are usually isointense with cortex on T1WIs **(30-22)**. Small cysts and hemorrhagic foci are common. Fluid-fluid levels can be present but are more common in patients with pituitary apoplexy (PAP).

Adenomas are generally isointense with gray matter on T2WI but can also demonstrate heterogeneous signal intensity **(30-23)**. Hemorrhagic adenomas "bloom" on T2* sequences.

Most macroadenomas enhance strongly but heterogeneously on T1 C+ **(30-22)**. Subtle dural thickening (a dural "tail") is present in 5-10% of cases.

Approximately 10% of pituitary adenomas invade the cavernous sinus, which often prevents complete surgical resection. There are several classification systems used to

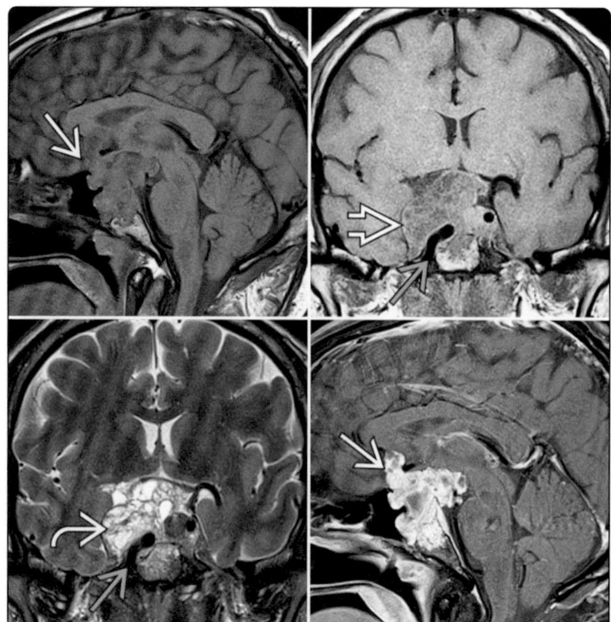

***(30-23)** Lobulated, invasive sellar/suprasellar mass ➡ has multiple medium/small-sized T2-hyperintense cysts ➡. Macroadenoma also invades the right cavernous sinus ➡ with tumor lateral to the cavernous carotid artery ➡.*

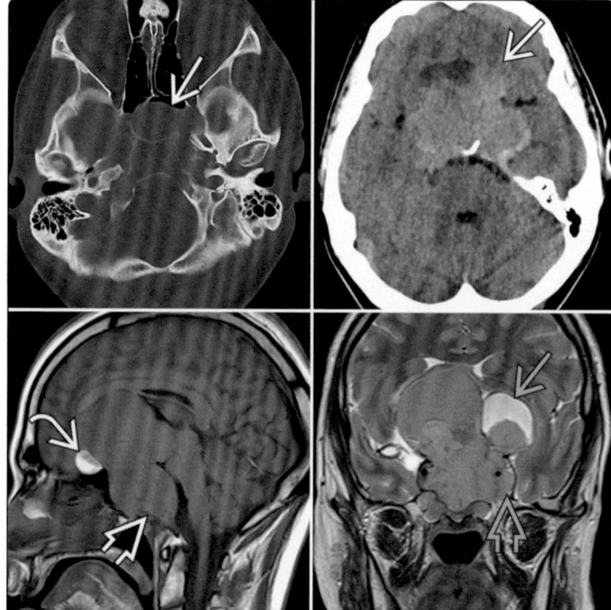

***(30-24)** Bone CT (top left), CECT (top right) show a very large, invasive macroadenoma ➡. Sagittal T1 shows invasion of the clivus ➡ and blood products ➡. Coronal T2 shows heterogeneous cysts ➡ and cavernous sinus invasion ➡.*

evaluate cavernous sinus invasion. The Knosp system assesses the impact of the tumor on the lateral cavernous sinus and encasement of the internal carotid artery (ICA), based on MR findings. The Knosp classification includes five grades: Grade 0 (normal) to grade 4 (complete encasement of cavernous ICA). A higher grade implies higher likelihood of cavernous sinus invasion, which translates into greater surgical risk and lower likelihood of gross total resection. MR imaging findings of tumor between the lateral cavernous carotid artery and the lateral dural sinus wall is a reliable feature of cavernous sinus invasion **(30-21) (30-23) (30-24)**.

***Microadenomas.*** Unless they hemorrhage, small microadenomas may be inapparent or mildly hypointense on standard nonenhanced sequences **(30-25)**. Many microadenomas appear slightly hypointense on T1 C+ **(30-26) (30-27)**, as they enhance less than the normal pituitary gland, which lacks a blood-brain barrier. Others enhance more strongly and may become isointense with the enhancing pituitary gland, rendering them virtually invisible on delayed postcontrast imaging.

Microadenomas enhance more slowly than the normal pituitary tissue. This discrepancy in enhancement timing can be exploited by using thin-section coronal dynamic contrast-enhanced scans. Fast image acquisition during contrast administration can often discriminate between the slowly enhancing microadenoma and rapidly enhancing normal gland. Between 10-30% of microadenomas are seen only on dynamic T1 C+ imaging.

## Differential Diagnosis

The major differential diagnosis of pituitary *macro*adenoma is **pituitary hyperplasia**. Tumors that can resemble pituitary adenoma/PitNETs include meningioma, metastasis, and CP. **Meningioma** of the diaphragma sellae can usually be identified as clearly separate from the pituitary gland below with different signal intensity and enhancement than the pituitary gland. Meningiomas also typically have an enhancing dural tail and avid homogeneous enhancement.

**Metastasis** to the stalk &/or pituitary gland from an extracranial primary neoplasm is uncommon. Lung, breast, and systemic **lymphoma** are the most common sources. Lymphoma involving the sellar region is often infiltrative and may show low T2 signal.

**Adamantinomatous CP** is the most common suprasellar tumor of childhood, whereas pituitary adenomas/PitNETs in children are rare. **Papillary CPs** in middle-aged adults are typically solid papillary tumors that infrequently calcify. In adults with CP, the pituitary gland can usually be identified as anatomically separate from the mass.

Nonneoplastic entities that can mimic macroadenoma include **hypophysitis** and, rarely, aneurysm. An aneurysm arises eccentrically from the circle of Willis and is usually not in the midline. Flow voids are typically present on MR.

Pituitary *micro*adenoma may be difficult to distinguish from incidental nonneoplastic intrapituitary cysts, such as **RCC** or **pars intermedia cyst**. Microadenomas enhance; cysts are seen as nonenhancing foci within the intensely enhancing pituitary gland. A cystic microadenoma cannot be reliably distinguished from other benign pituitary cysts.

**PITUITARY MACROADENOMA: IMAGING AND DIFFERENTIAL DIAGNOSIS**

**CT**
- Sella usually enlarged, remodeled; cortex intact
- Invasive adenomas erode, destroy bone
- Majority are isodense with brain
  - Cysts (15-20%), hemorrhage (10%)
  - Calcification rare (1-2%)

**MR**
- Usually isointense with cortex
- Heterogeneous signal intensity common (cysts, hemorrhage)
- Strong, heterogeneous enhancement
- Microadenomas sometimes seen only with dynamic T1 C+

**Differential Diagnosis**
- Pituitary hyperplasia (know patient age, sex, endocrine status!)
- Other tumors
  - Meningioma, craniopharyngioma, metastasis, lymphoma
  - Aggressive-looking adenoma is almost never malignant!
- Nonneoplastic lesions
  - Hypophysitis
  - Aneurysm (usually eccentric, "flow void")

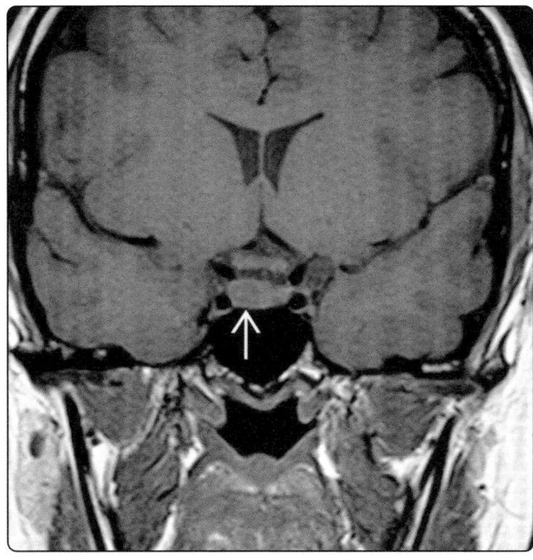

***(30-25)** T1WI in a 22-year-old with amenorrhea and elevated prolactin shows a hypointense mass ➡ in the right lateral pituitary gland.*

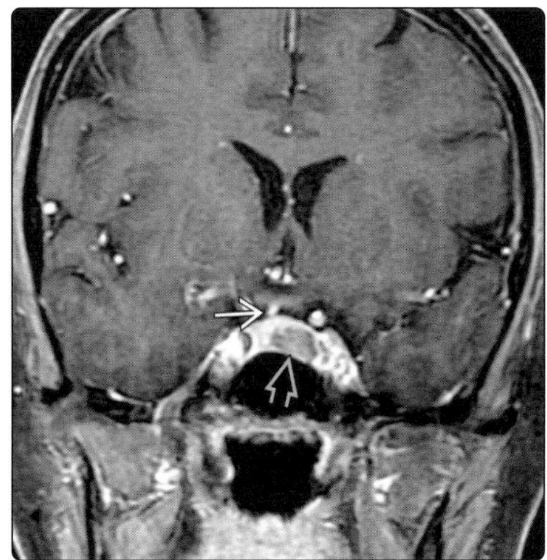

***(30-26)** T1 C+ MR shows a microadenoma ⇨ displacing the infundibulum ➡. Mass enhances more slowly than gland, appearing hypointense.*

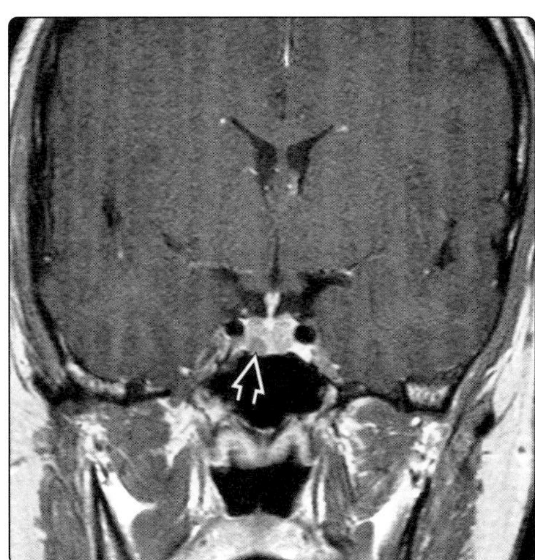

***(30-27)** T1 C+ shows a microadenoma ➡ in a Cushing syndrome patient. These tumors enhance less than intensely enhancing normal gland.*

## Pituitary Carcinoma

Pituitary carcinomas are rare and represent between 0.12-0.4% of all pituitary tumors. They are characterized by craniospinal dissemination &/or systemic metastases. Pituitary carcinomas do not have unique imaging features and may be indistinguishable from an invasive, but histologically typical, adenoma. Diagnosis is made at time of craniospinal metastases or systemic tumor spread.

## Pituitary Blastoma

Pituitary blastoma is a very rare tumor that usually occurs in children under two years of age. It is an embryonal neoplasm of the sellar region composed of three types of cells: Primitive blastema cells, neuroendocrine cells, and Rathke pouch epithelium. These tumors are located in the sellar and suprasellar regions, and cavernous sinus invasion is common. Cushing syndrome is one of the most common presenting symptoms.

## Germinoma

Germinomas are discussed in detail in Chapter 25. Germinomas of the suprasellar region are classically hyperdense on CT, similar to lymphoma. When involving the pituitary axis, a germinoma involves the infundibulum &/or neurohypophysis and often presents in a child with an absent PPBS. T2 hypointensity and diffuse enhancement of an enlarged infundibulum/anterior third ventricle is the typical MR appearance. Diffusion restriction on DWI is typical.

## Craniopharyngioma

### Terminology and Etiology

Craniopharyngioma (CP) is a benign, often partly cystic sellar/suprasellar mass that probably arises from epithelial remnants of Rathke pouch.

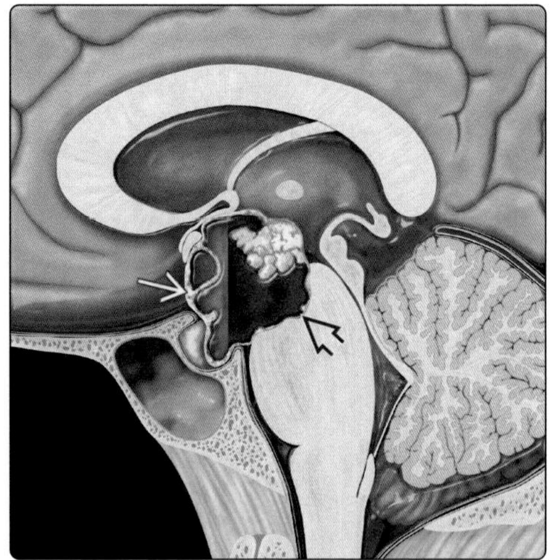

*(30-28) Graphic shows adamantinomatous craniopharyngioma as a cystic/solid suprasellar mass with rim Ca++ ➡, dark, viscous fluid ⇨.*

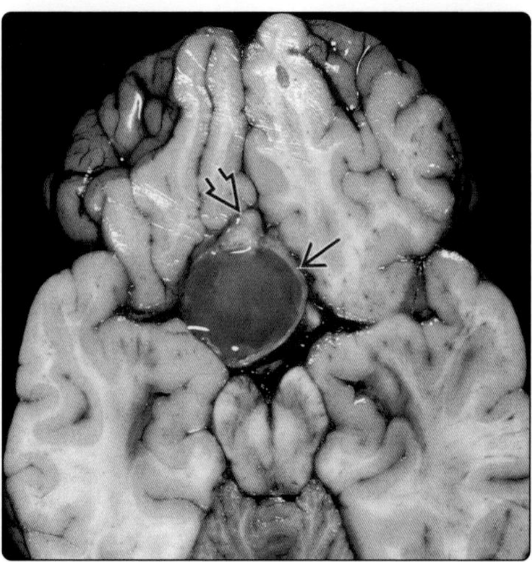

*(30-29) Specimen shows mostly cystic craniopharyngioma ⇨ with small tumor nodule present ⇨. (Courtesy R. Hewlett, MD.)*

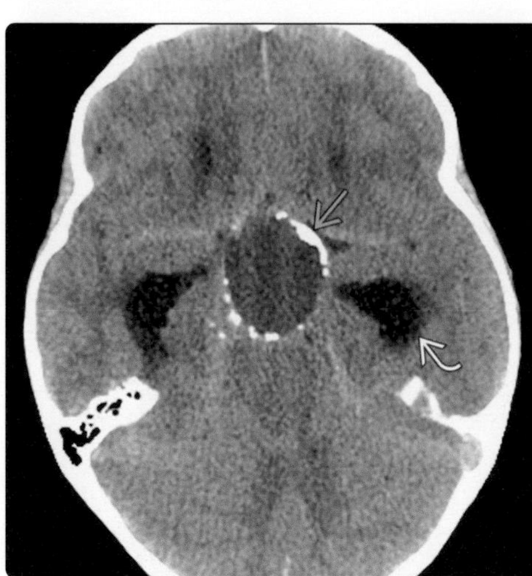

*(30-30) NECT shows a cystic suprasellar adamantinomatous craniopharyngioma with rim Ca++ ⇨. Note associated hydrocephalus ➡.*

## Pathology

Completely intrasellar CPs are rare. CPs are primarily suprasellar tumors (75%). A small intrasellar component is present in 20-25% of cases. Occasionally, CPs (especially the papillary type) arise mostly or entirely within the third ventricle.

Lesions > 5 cm are common. Giant CPs may extend into both anterior and middle cranial fossae. Posteroinferior extension between the clivus and pons down to the foramen magnum can be seen in exceptionally large lesions.

Two types of CPs are recognized: Adamantinomatous (90%) and papillary (10%). The typical gross appearance of an **adamantinomatous CP** is that of a multilobulated, partially solid, but mostly cystic, suprasellar mass **(30-28)**. Multiple loculated cysts are common. The cysts often contain dark, viscous, "machinery oil" fluid rich in cholesterol crystals **(30-29)**. Adamantinomatous CPs often adhere to adjacent structures, such as the hypothalamus.

**Papillary CP** is usually a discrete encapsulated mass with a smooth surface that does not adhere to adjacent brain. Papillary CPs are often solid with a cauliflower-like configuration **(30-34)**. When they contain cysts, the fluid is clear (unlike the "machinery oil" cholesterol-rich contents of adamantinomatous CPs).

Both adamantinomatous and papillary CPs are WHO grade 1 neoplasms. MIB-1 is low.

### CRANIOPHARYNGIOMA: ETIOLOGY AND PATHOLOGY

**Etiology**
- Epithelial remnants of Rathke pouch

**Pathology**
- 2 types
  - Adamantinomatous (90%)
  - Papillary (10%)
  - Both are WHO grade 1
- Adamantinomatous
  - Multiple cysts
  - Squamous epithelium, "wet" keratin
  - Cholesterol-rich "machinery oil" fluid
- Papillary
  - Solid > > cystic (clear fluid)
  - Almost always adults (30-59 years old)

## Clinical Issues

CP is the most common nonglial neoplasm in children, accounting for 6-10% of all pediatric brain tumors and slightly > 1/2 of suprasellar neoplasms.

CPs occur nearly equally in children and adults. Adamantinomatous CPs have a bimodal age distribution with a large peak at 5-15 years and a second, smaller peak at 45-60 years. CPs are rare in newborns and infants; only 5% arise in patients between birth and five years of age. Papillary CPs almost always occur in adults with a peak incidence at 30-59 years.

Patients most commonly present with visual disturbances, either with or without accompanying headache. Endocrine deficiencies, including growth failure, delayed puberty, and diabetes insipidus, are common.

CPs are slow-growing neoplasms with a propensity to recur following surgery. More than 85% of patients survive at least three years following diagnosis. However, the recurrence rate at 10 years approaches 20-30%, even in patients with gross total resection.

## Imaging

**General Features.** A partially calcified, mixed solid/cystic extraaxial suprasellar mass in a child is the classic appearance of adamantinomatous CP. A compressed, displaced pituitary gland can sometimes be identified as separate from the mass. If the mass is large, associated hydrocephalus may be present.

**CT Findings.** Adamantinomatous CPs follow a "rule of 90," i.e., 90% are mixed cystic/solid, 90% are calcified, and 90% enhance **(30-30)**. Papillary CPs rarely calcify. They are often solid or mostly solid **(30-35)**.

**MR Findings.** Signal intensity varies with cyst contents **(30-31)**. Multiple cysts are common, and intracystic fluid within each cyst varies from hypo- to hyperintense compared with brain on T1WI **(30-33)**.

CP cysts are variably hyperintense on T2WI and FLAIR. The solid nodule is often calcified and moderately hypointense. Hyperintensity extending along the optic tracts is common and usually represents edema, not tumor invasion. Cyst walls and solid nodules typically enhance following contrast administration **(30-31C)**.

MRS shows a large lipid-lactate peak, characteristic of the cholesterol and lipid constituents of a CP. pMR shows low rCBV.

### CRANIOPHARYNGIOMA: CLINICAL ISSUES, IMAGING, AND DIFFERENTIAL DIAGNOSIS

**Clinical Issues**
- Occurs equally in children, adults
  - Peak in children = 5-15 years (usually adamantinomatous)
  - Peak in adults = 40-55 years (papillary more common)

**Imaging**
- CT
  - Adamantinomatous: 90% cystic, 90% calcify, 90% enhance
  - Papillary: Solid > cystic
- MR
  - Variable signal on T1WI
  - Usually hyperintense on T2/FLAIR
  - Enhancement (nodular or rim) 90%
  - MRS: Large lipid-lactate peak
  - Main differential diagnosis = Rathke cleft cyst

## Differential Diagnosis

The major differential diagnosis of CP is **Rathke cleft cyst** (RCC). RCCs do not calcify, appear to be much less heterogeneous, and do not show nodular enhancement. RCCs often have an intracystic nodule. The ADC of RCC is significantly increased compared with that of cystic CPs. Immunohistochemistry is helpful, as RCCs express specific cytokeratins that CPs do not.

**Hypothalamic/chiasmatic astrocytoma** is usually a solid suprasellar mass that is clearly intraparenchymal. Calcifications and cysts are uncommon. These tumors are T2 hyperintense and have variable enhancement.

**Pituitary adenoma** is rare in prepubescent children (peak age period for CP). A **dermoid cyst** can be hyperintense on T1WI related to lipid contents and may demonstrate calcification. Dermoid cysts may present with rupture into the subarachnoid spaces. An **epidermoid cyst** (EC) is usually off-midline with DWI restriction. Suprasellar ECs are uncommon. Neither dermoid cysts nor ECs enhance.

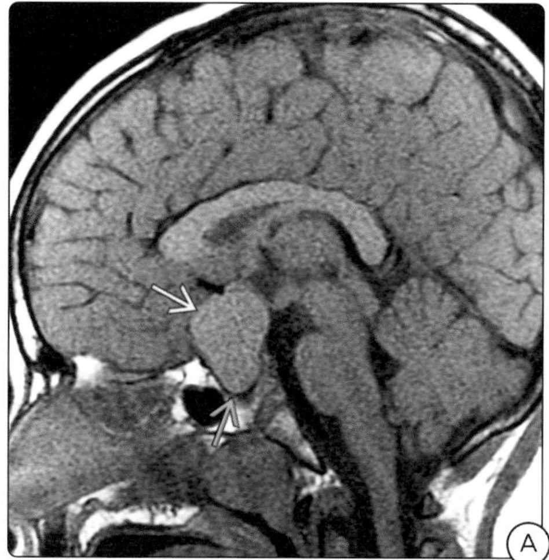


***(30-31A)** Sagittal T1 MR in a 7-year-old with vision change shows a lobular sellar/suprasellar mass ➡ with sella turcica expansion ⇨.*

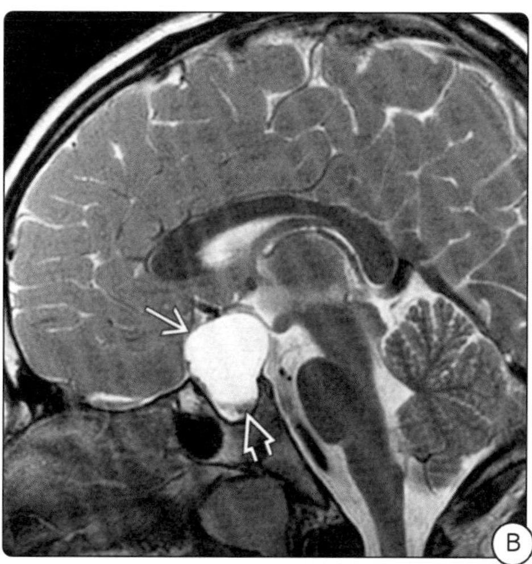


***(30-31B)** Sagittal T2 MR shows a hyperintense mass ➡ with hypointense debris ➡. Remember 90% rule: 90% $Ca^{++}$, 90% cystic, 90% enhance.*

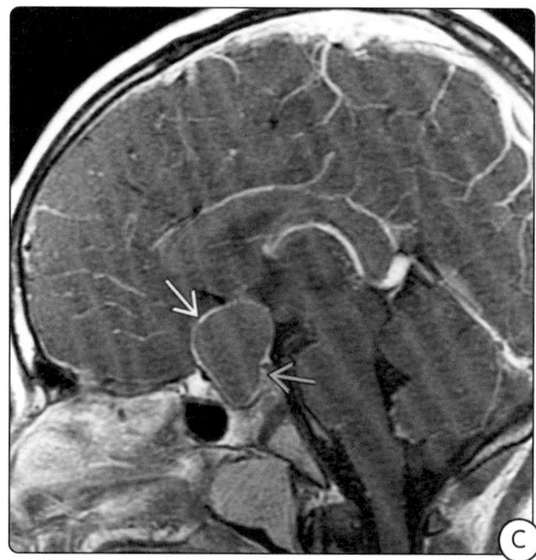


***(30-31C)** Sagittal T1 C+ MR shows thin rim enhancement of the mass ➡ with focal nodular enhancement ⇨, typical of craniopharyngioma.*

## Nonadenomatous Pituitary Tumors

The 2021 WHO recognizes three rare, histologically distinct pituitary region neoplasms: Pituicytoma, spindle cell oncocytoma (SCO), and granular cell tumor of the sellar region. These three tumors constitute a distinct family of low-grade neoplasms that arise from pituicytes, modified glial cells that reside in the posterior pituitary or infundibulum **(30-36)**. They all show expression of thyroid transcription factor 1 (TTF-1). These tumors likely represent a spectrum of a single nosologic entity. All are WHO grade 1 tumors. These tumors arise in adults in the fifth and sixth decades of life. Most patients present with headaches, visual disturbances, or panhypopituitarism and rarely present with diabetes insipidus. These tumors are slow growing and typically curable by surgical resection.

**Pituicytoma** arises from modified glial cells ("pituicytes") that reside in the infundibular stalk and neurohypophysis. The majority of pituicytomas are isointense with brain on T1WI and hyperintense on T2WI. They usually arise along the infundibulum or neurohypophysis and enhance homogeneously following contrast enhancement **(30-36A)**. Imaging may mimic an adenoma.

Like pituicytoma, **granular cell tumor** is a tumor of the neurohypophysis and may be asymptomatic. Granular cell tumors are typically suprasellar masses. They are hyperdense on NECT and isointense with brain on both T1- and T2WI. Granular cell tumors enhance strongly and homogeneously following contrast administration **(30-36B)**.

**SCO** has imaging findings that are similar to—and cannot be distinguished from—those of pituitary adenoma/PitNET, pituicytoma, or LH. These tumors are typically sellar and suprasellar **(30-36C)**. They are reportedly highly vascular.

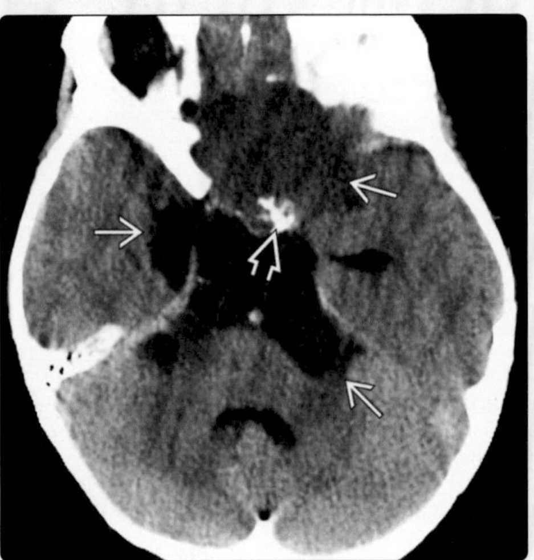

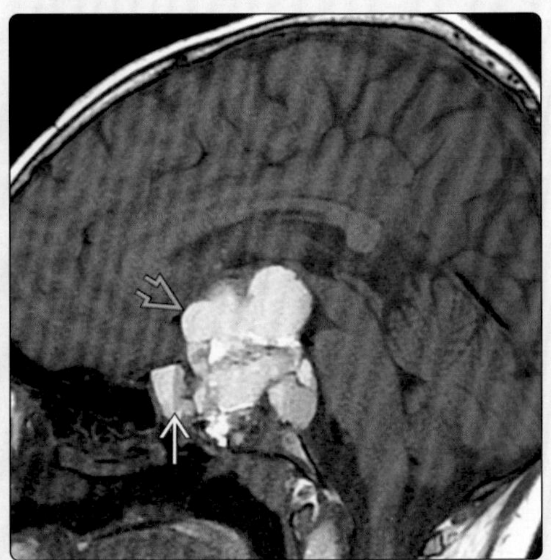

***(30-32)** Axial NECT in a 9-year-old shows a large cystic mass involving the anterior, middle, and posterior cranial fossae ➡. A small focus of Ca⁺⁺ ➡ is present in the mass, typical of adamantinomatous craniopharyngioma. **(30-33)** Sagittal T1 MR in a 10-year-old shows a large sellar and suprasellar mass ➡ with multiple cysts of variable signal intensity. Small fluid levels are present ➡ in this adamantinomatous craniopharyngioma.*

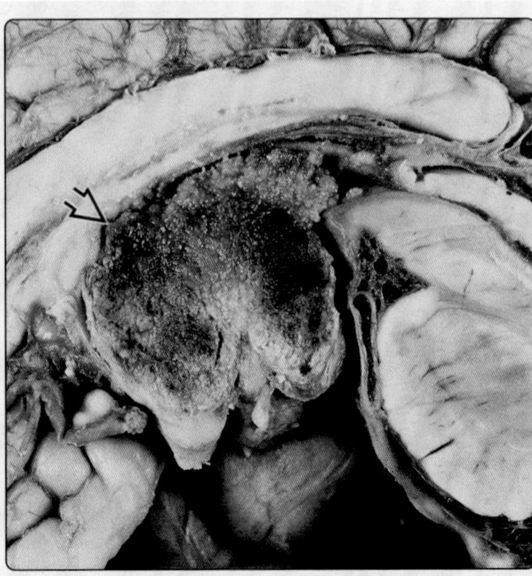

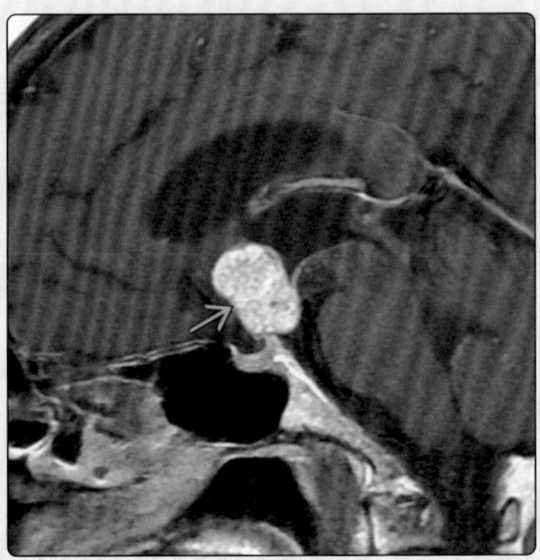

***(30-34)** Midline sagittal autopsy section shows a solid mass filling the 3rd ventricle ➡. This was papillary craniopharyngioma. (Courtesy B. Scheithauer, MD.) **(30-35)** Sagittal T1 C+ MR in a 60-year-old man shows a solidly enhancing mass in the anterior 3rd ventricle ➡. Note that the pituitary gland is separate from the mass. Imaging is typical of a papillary craniopharyngioma.*

# Miscellaneous Lesions

## Hypophysitis

Hypophysitis is an inflammation of the pituitary gland. There are two main histologic forms of hypophysitis: Lymphocytic hypophysitis (LH) **(30-37)** and non-LH. We focus on LH, the most common form. We then briefly discuss non-LH, including granulomatous hypophysitis, and some of the newly described entities that are often characterized by plasma cell infiltrates.

### Lymphocytic Hypophysitis

LH is also called lymphocytic adenohypophysitis, primary hypophysitis, and stalkitis. LH is an uncommon autoimmune inflammatory disorder of the pituitary gland **(30-37)**. Between 80-90% of patients with LH are female; 30-60% of cases occur in the peripartum period.

The most common presenting symptoms are headache and multiple endocrine deficiencies with partial or total hypopituitarism. Diabetes insipidus is common. ACTH deficits often appear first. Hyperprolactinemia occurs in 1/3 of all patients, probably secondary to stalk compression known as "stalk effect."

Imaging shows a combined intra- and suprasellar mass with a thickened, nontapering infundibular stalk **(30-37)** **(30-39)**. A rounded, symmetrically enlarged pituitary gland is common. The sellar floor is intact, not expanded or eroded. The posterior pituitary "bright spot" (PPBS) is absent in 75% of cases. LH enhances intensely and uniformly.

The major differential diagnosis for LH is nonsecreting **pituitary macroadenoma**. The distinction is important, as treatment differs significantly. LH is often treated medically, unless there is significant potential for vision loss, whereas surgical resection is the primary treatment for pituitary macroadenoma. Macroadenomas can be giant, but LH only occasionally exceeds 3 cm in diameter. Clinical findings are also helpful, as LH commonly presents with diabetes insipidus.

The stalk is usually normal in **pituitary hyperplasia**, although patient age and sex are similar. **Metastasis** usually occurs in older patients with known systemic primary tumor.

**Granulomatous hypophysitis** may occur secondary to infection, sarcoidosis, or Langerhans cell histiocytosis. Granulomatous hypophysitis is less common than LH, has a different epidemiologic profile, and tends to enhance more heterogeneously. **IgG4-** and **drug-related hypophysitis** are very rare. Imaging features are similar to classic hypophysitis **(30-38)**.

### Granulomatous Hypophysitis

Granulomatous hypophysitis has different epidemiologic characteristics than LH does. Granulomatous hypophysitis is equally common in both sexes, and there is no association with pregnancy.

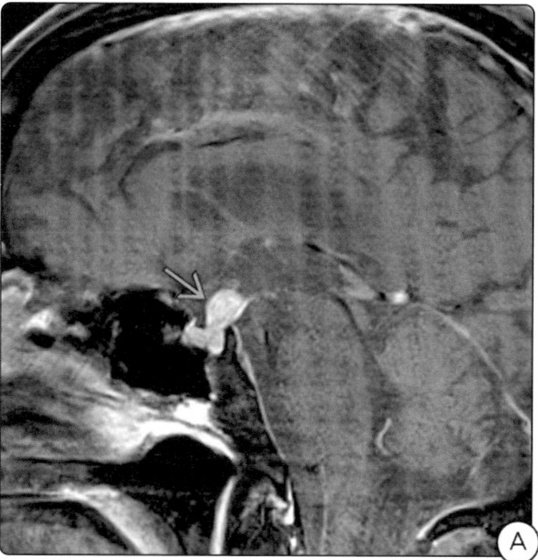


***(30-36A)** Sagittal T1 C+ MR shows an enhancing mass in the pituitary infundibulum ➡ typical of a pituicytoma, which arises from pituicytes.*

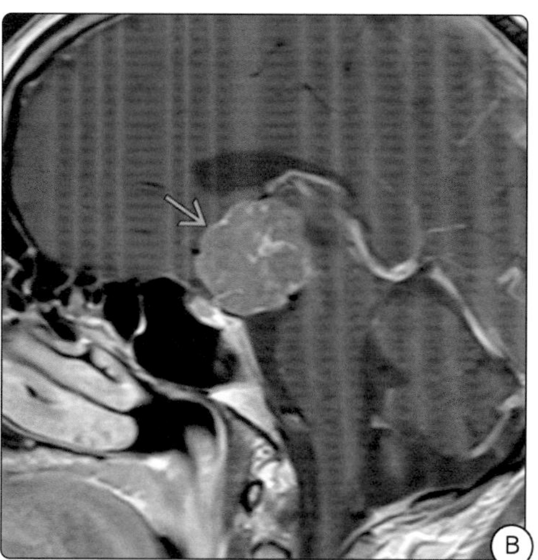


***(30-36B)** Sagittal T1 C+ MR shows an enhancing suprasellar mass ➡ in the pituitary infundibulum related to a granular cell tumor.*

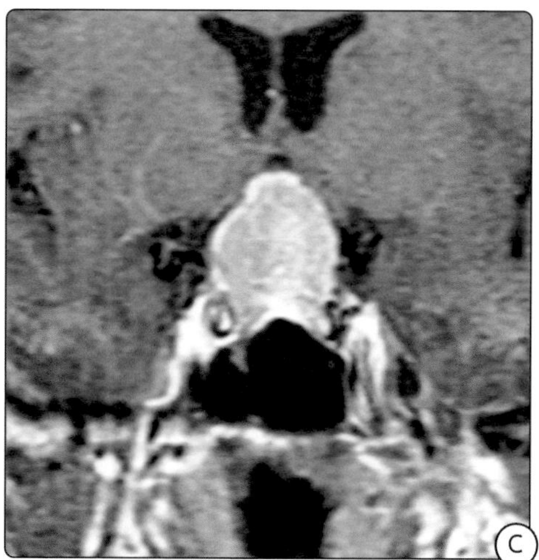


***(30-36C)** Coronal T1 C+ MR shows an enhancing sellar/suprasellar mass that mimics the more common adenoma. Spindle cell oncocytoma.*

Granulomatous hypophysitis can be primary (idiopathic) or secondary. **Secondary granulomatous hypophysitis** is far more common than primary granulomatous hypophysitis and typically results from necrotizing granulomatous inflammation. Infectious/inflammatory secondary granulomatous hypophysitis can be caused by TB, sarcoid, fungal infection, syphilis, Langerhans cell histiocytosis, Wegener granulomatosis, Erdheim-Chester disease, granulomatous autoimmune hypophysitis, ruptured RCC, or CP. Secondary granulomatous hypophysitis may also occur as a reaction to systemic inflammatory disorders, such as Crohn disease. Imaging findings are nonspecific, resembling those of LH or pituitary adenoma.

**Primary granulomatous hypophysitis** is a rare inflammatory disease without identifiable infectious organisms. The precise etiology of primary granulomatous hypophysitis is unknown. Nonnecrotizing granulomas with multinucleated giant cells, histiocytes, and various numbers of plasma cells and lymphocytes are typical. Primary granulomatous hypophysitis usually presents with diabetes insipidus. A symmetric sellar mass that enhances strongly but heterogeneously is seen on imaging studies.

## Other Hypophysitis Variants

A number of new hypophysitis variants have been recently described. **IgG4-related hypophysitis** has a marked mononuclear infiltrate mainly characterized by increased numbers of IgG4-positive plasma cells. Imaging findings resemble those of lymphocytic infundibuloneurohypophysitis. The pituitary stalk and posterior pituitary lobe are enlarged and enhance intensely following contrast administration.

**Drug-related hypophysitis** has been reported in cases of cancer immunotherapy with antibodies that stimulate T-cell responses (e.g., ipilimumab) **(30-38)**. Clinicians and radiologists should be aware of autoimmune-induced hypophysitis as a complication of new treatments. Imaging of

*(30-37) Sagittal graphic shows lymphocytic hypophysitis. Note thickening of the infundibulum ➡ and infiltration into the anterior lobe of the pituitary gland ➡. (30-38) Patient on ipilimumab for metastatic melanoma developed drug-induced hypophysitis with infiltration of the stalk and pituitary gland ➡.*

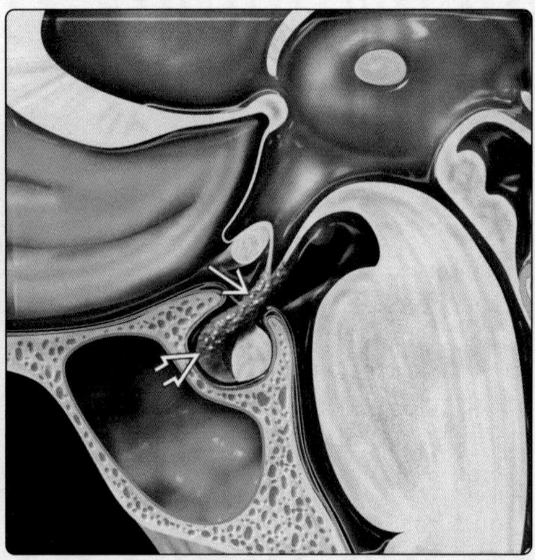

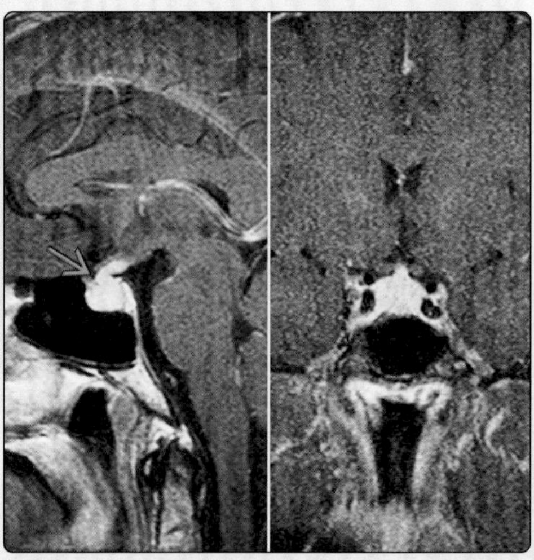

*(30-39A) Coronal T1WI in a 19-year-old pregnant woman with acute vision changes shows a sellar and suprasellar snowman-shaped mass ➡ with superior displacement of the optic chiasm ➡. (30-39B) Coronal T2 in the same patient shows the mass is hyperintense ➡. Superior displacement and draping of the optic chiasm ➡ over the mass is well visualized. Lymphocytic hypophysitis may mimic an adenoma, as in this patient.*

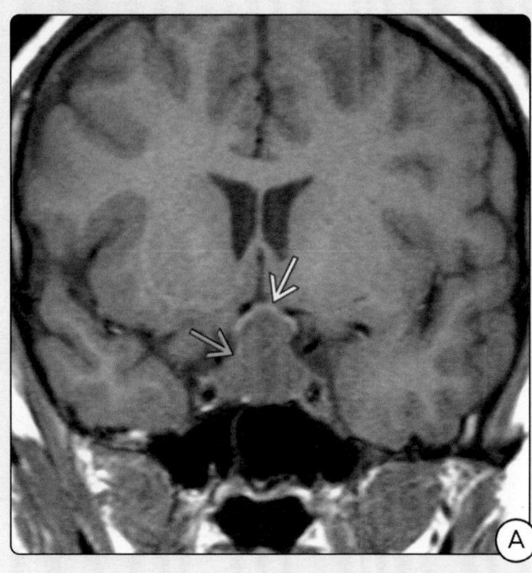


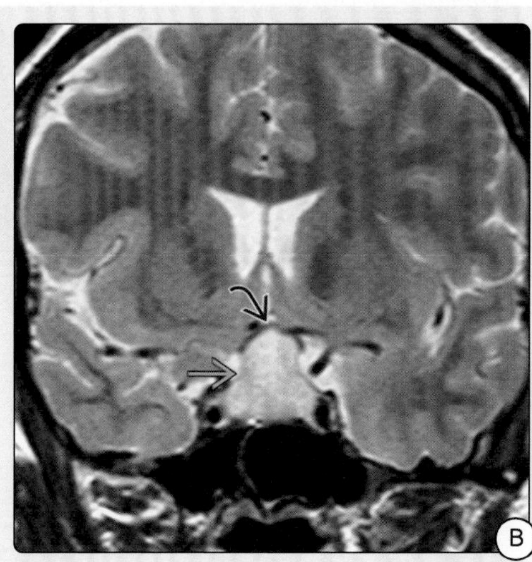

drug-related hypophysitis usually shows enlargement of the pituitary gland with or without infundibulum.

## Langerhans Cell Histiocytosis

Langerhans cell histiocytosis is discussed in detail in Chapter 29. Langerhans cell histiocytosis typically presents with diabetes insipidus. The typical patient is under two years of age.

The classic imaging of Langerhans cell histiocytosis of the pituitary axis is an absent PPBS with a thickened, enhancing pituitary infundibulum **(30-40)**. Langerhans cell histiocytosis may also present as a sellar and suprasellar mass. The major differential diagnosis of Langerhans cell histiocytosis in a child is **germinoma**. In an adult, the major differential diagnosis of Langerhans cell histiocytosis affecting the pituitary axis is **neurosarcoid** or **hypophysitis**.

## Neurosarcoid

Neurosarcoid is a multisystem inflammatory disease characterized by noncaseating epithelioid cell granulomas. Neurosarcoid is discussed in more detail in Chapter 15. Neurosarcoid may present as diffuse or focal dural (pachymeningeal) &/or leptomeningeal thickening and enhancement, pituitary infundibulum &/or hypothalamic thickening and enhancement, cranial nerve enhancement, brain parenchymal lesions, or, less commonly, choroid plexus lesions.

The main differential diagnoses for pituitary axis neurosarcoid are LH, lymphoma, and metastatic disease.

### INFUNDIBULAR STALK MASSES

**Adults**
- Neurosarcoid (isolated stalk lesion rare)
- Hypophysitis ("stalkitis")
- Metastasis
- Lymphoma
- Pituicytoma
- IgG4-related disease

**Children**
- Germinoma
- Langerhans cell histiocytosis (look for other lesions)
- Ectopic neurohypophysis (displaced posterior pituitary "bright spot")
- Leukemia

## Pituitary Apoplexy

Pituitary apoplexy (PAP) is a well-described acute clinical syndrome with headache, visual defects, and variable endocrine deficiencies. In some cases, profound pituitary insufficiency develops and may become life threatening.

### Etiology

PAP is caused by hemorrhage into—or ischemic necrosis of—the pituitary gland **(30-41)**. A preexisting macroadenoma is present in 65-90% of cases **(30-42)**, but PAP can also occur in microadenomas or histologically normal pituitary glands. What precipitates the hemorrhage or necrosis is unknown.

In rare cases, patients undergoing treatment with bromocriptine or cabergoline for pituitary adenoma have developed life-threatening PAP. More often, this medical therapy results in a subclinical hemorrhage into the adenoma.

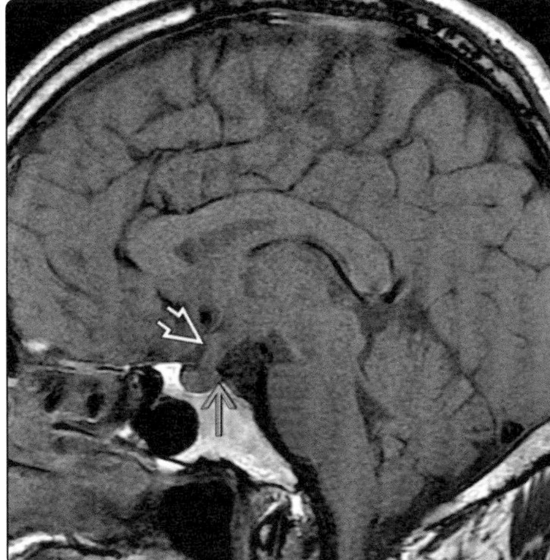

***(30-40)** Sagittal T1 MR shows a thickened pituitary infundibulum ➡ and lack of a posterior "bright spot" ⇨, typical of LCH.*

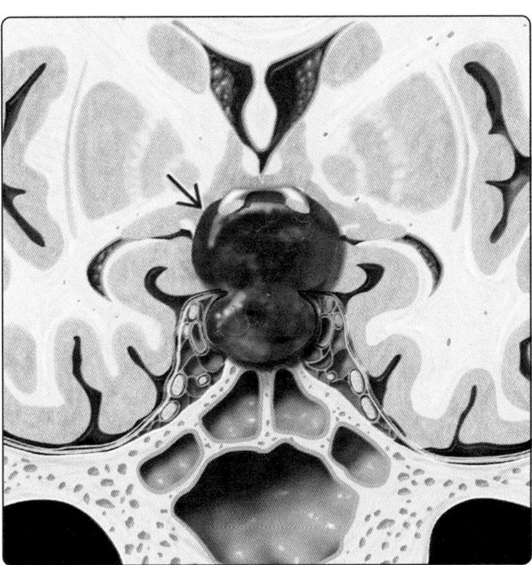

***(30-41)** Coronal graphic shows a macroadenoma with acute hemorrhage ⇨ causing pituitary apoplexy.*

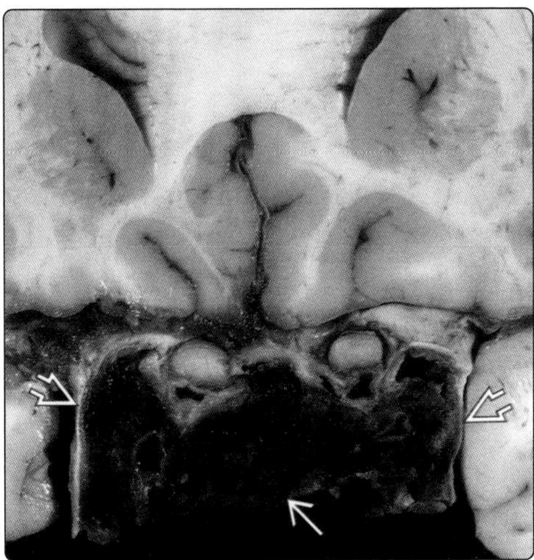

***(30-42)** Autopsy specimen of pituitary apoplexy shows hemorrhagic mass ➡ extending into the cavernous sinuses ➡. (Courtesy R. Hewlett, MD.)*

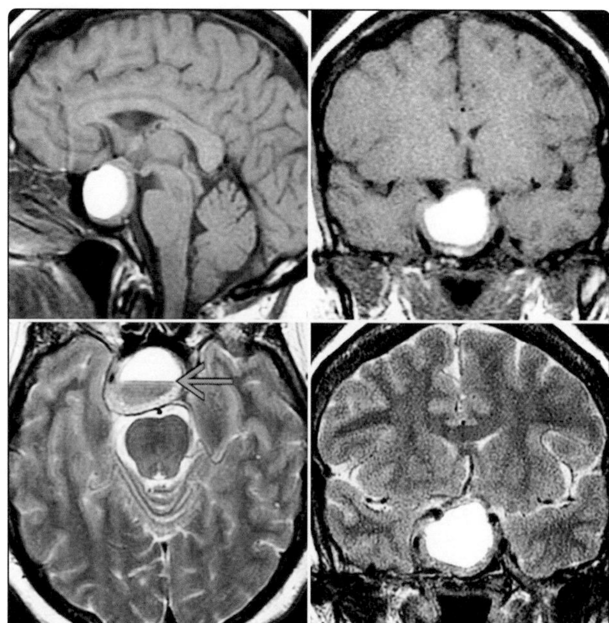

***(30-43) Pituitary apoplexy in a 50-year-old woman with 4 days of visual changes shows subacute hemorrhage in a macroadenoma with a blood-fluid level ⇒.***

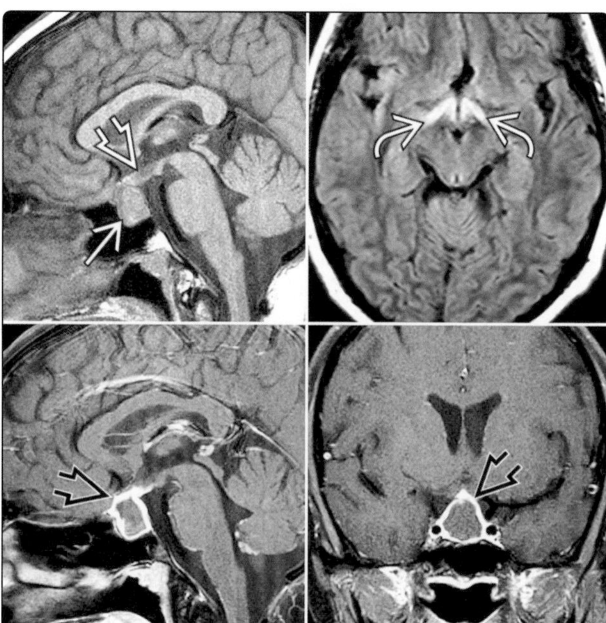

***(30-44) T1WI shows an enlarged pituitary gland ➡, thick hypothalamus ➡. FLAIR hyperintensity is along both optic tracts ➡. Rim enhancement ⇒ is shown. This is nonhemorrhagic pituitary apoplexy.***

## Pathology

The most common gross appearance of PAP is that of a large intrasellar or combined intra- and suprasellar mass **(30-41)**. Between 85-90% of cases demonstrate gross hemorrhagic infarction **(30-42)**. Nonhemorrhagic ("bland") pituitary infarction causes an enlarged, edematous-appearing pituitary gland. Microscopic features are nonspecific and generally unremarkable.

## Clinical Issues

PAP is rare, occurring in ~ 1% of all patients with pituitary macroadenomas. Peak age is 55-60 years. PAP is rare in patients under the age of 15 years. The M:F ratio is 2:1.

Headache is almost universal in patients with PAP and is the most common presenting symptom followed by nausea (80%) and visual field disturbance (70%). Hemorrhagic tumors that extend into the cavernous sinus may compress CNIII, IV, V, and VI. Almost 80% of patients with PAP have panhypopituitarism.

PAP varies from a clinically benign event to catastrophic presentation with permanent neurologic deficits. Coma or even death may ensue in severe cases.

## Imaging

An enlarged pituitary gland with peripheral rim enhancement is typical of PAP. Gross intraglandular hemorrhage is common but not invariably present.

NECT scans are often normal. Hemorrhage into the pituitary gland with a hyperdense sellar/suprasellar mass can be identified in 20-25% of cases.

MR is the procedure of choice to evaluate suspected PAP. Signal intensity depends on whether the PAP is hemorrhagic or nonhemorrhagic. Hemorrhage can be identified in 85-90% of cases **(30-43)**.

Signal intensity depends on clot age. Acute PAP is heterogeneously iso- to hypointense to brain on T1WI. Initially iso- to mildly hyperintense on T2WI, PAP rapidly becomes hypointense on T2WI. Acute compression of the hypothalamus and optic chiasm may cause visible edema along the optic tracts on T2/FLAIR scans.

"Blooming"/susceptibility artifact on T2* is common if blood products are present but may be obscured by artifact from the adjacent paranasal sinuses. T1 C+ shows rim enhancement **(30-44)**. Dural thickening and enhancement is seen in 50%, and mucosal thickening in the adjacent sphenoid sinus occurs in 80% of all patients. PAP usually restricts on DWI. Associated subarachnoid hemorrhage is rare.

## Differential Diagnosis

The major differential diagnosis of PAP is **hemorrhagic macroadenoma**. Focal hemorrhages in adenomas are common, but, in contrast to PAP, the clinical course is typically subacute or chronic. Most adenomas enhance strongly but heterogeneously, whereas PAP demonstrates rim enhancement around a predominantly nonenhancing, expanded pituitary gland.

Other differential considerations would include a CP or an unusual RCC. Rarely, an RCC may have apoplexy where there is acute hemorrhage. Less likely considerations would include a giant aneurysm.

## PITUITARY APOPLEXY

**Etiology**
- Hemorrhagic or nonhemorrhagic pituitary necrosis
- Preexisting macroadenoma (65-90%)

**Clinical Issues**
- Sudden onset
- Headache, visual defects, cranial neuropathies
- Hypopituitarism (80%)
- Can be life threatening
- Can result in permanent pituitary insufficiency
- Sheehan syndrome = postpartum pituitary necrosis

**Imaging**
- Enlarged pituitary
  - ± hemorrhage (85-90%)
- Rim enhancement around nonenhancing gland
- May cause hypothalamic, optic tract edema

**Differential Diagnosis**
- Hemorrhagic macroadenoma without apoplexy
- Rathke cleft cyst apoplexy
- Pituitary abscess
- Acute thrombosed aneurysm

# Pre- and Postoperative Sella

## Preoperative Evaluation

Most surgical approaches (transethmoid, transnasal, or transseptal) pass through the sphenoid sinus to reach the sella. Regardless of which operative technique—microscopic or endoscopic—is used, delineating sphenoid sinus anatomy and identifying anatomic variants that might impact surgery are important to successful patient outcome.

CT and MR each has a unique contribution to the full preoperative evaluation of sellar lesions. Multiplanar MR is the procedure of choice to characterize the lesion and define its extent. In concert with MR, preoperative CT helps define relevant bony anatomy.

Location and extent of sphenoid sinus pneumatization as well as the presence and location of bony septa are the major concern. Pneumatization of the planum sphenoidale and dorsum sellae should also be noted. The specific type of pneumatization is generally determined from sagittal MRs.

## Postoperative Evaluation

To evaluate the postoperative sella, thin-section, small FOV imaging in both the sagittal and coronal planes is mandatory. Precontrast T1- and T2WI images + postcontrast fat-saturated sequences are standard.

The appearance on postoperative MR scans is complicated by hemorrhage, use of hemostatic agents, packing materials (muscle, fat, fascia lata), and residual tumor. Typical findings include a bony defect in the anterior sphenoid sinus wall, fluid and mucosal thickening in the sinus, fat packing within the sella turcica, hemorrhage, and varying amounts of residual mass effect **(30-45)**.

The first postoperative scan provides the baseline against with which subsequent imaging is compared. With time, hemorrhage evolves and resorbs, fat packing fibroses and retracts, and mass effect decreases. A partially ES with or without traction on the infundibular stalk and optic chiasm is typical in the months and years following the initial surgery.

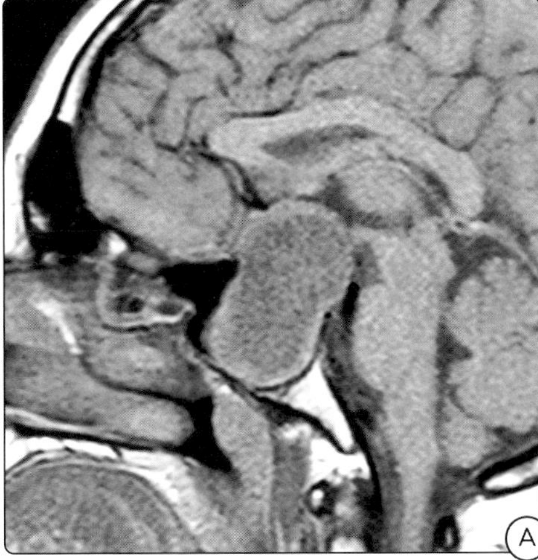


***(30-45A)** Preoperative sagittal T1 MR shows a large sellar/suprasellar solid and cystic mass that expands, erodes, and deepens the sella turcica.*

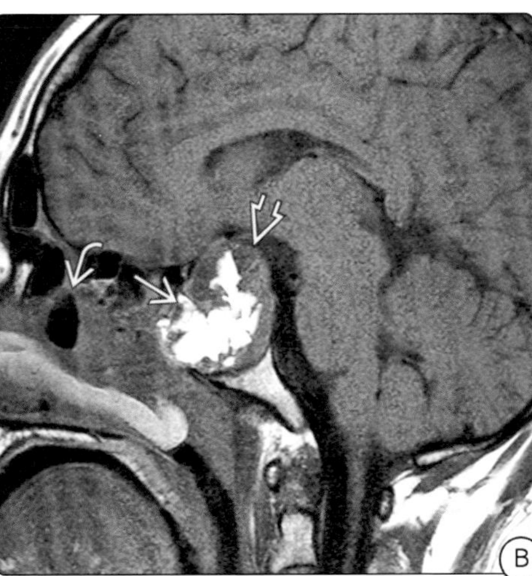


***(30-45B)** Postoperative T1 C+ MR after tumor debulking shows fat packing ➡, residual tumor ➡, and sphenoid air-fluid level ➡.*

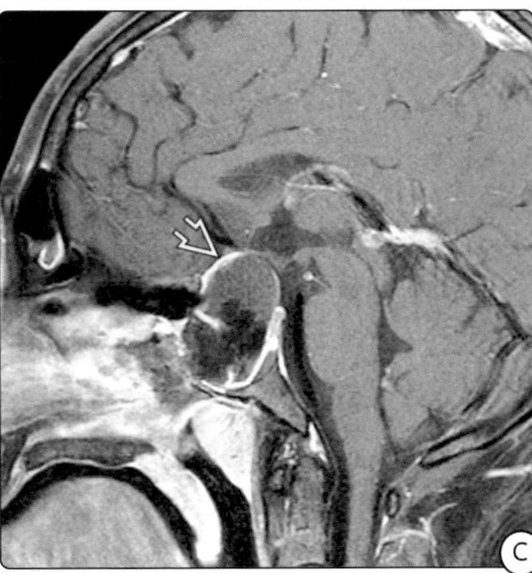


***(30-45C)** T1 C+ FS MR shows suppressed fat and a thin rim of enhancing tissue ➡.*

Complications, such as diabetes insipidus, stalk transection, and electrolyte disturbances, are usually temporary. Long-term complications include CSF leaks and cranial neuropathy.

# Differential Diagnosis of Sellar Region Mass

In establishing a helpful differential diagnosis of a sellar mass, determining anatomic sublocation is the first, most important step. Is the lesion (1) intrasellar, (2) suprasellar, or (3) in the infundibular stalk? Or is it a combination of these locations?

Whether a sellar/suprasellar mass *is* the pituitary gland itself or is separate from the mass is the most important imaging task and the most helpful finding **(30-46)** **(30-47)**. Masses that can be clearly distinguished as separate from the pituitary gland are rarely, if ever, macroadenomas.

The most helpful clinical feature is patient age. Some lesions are common in adults but rarely occur in children. Sex and endocrine status are helpful ancillary clues. For example, pituitary macroadenomas rarely cause diabetes insipidus, but it is one of the most common presenting symptoms of hypophysitis.

Lastly, consider some specific imaging findings. Is the mass cystic? Is it calcified? What is the MR signal intensity? Does the lesion enhance?

## Intrasellar Lesions

Intrasellar lesions can be mass-like or non-mass-like. Keep two concepts in mind: (1) Not all "enlarged pituitary glands" are abnormal. Pituitary size and height vary with sex and age. A "fat" pituitary can also occur with intracranial hypotension **(30-50)**. (2) Pituitary "incidentalomas" are common (identified in 15-20% of normal MR scans); often cystic microadenomas or RCCs **(30-49)**.

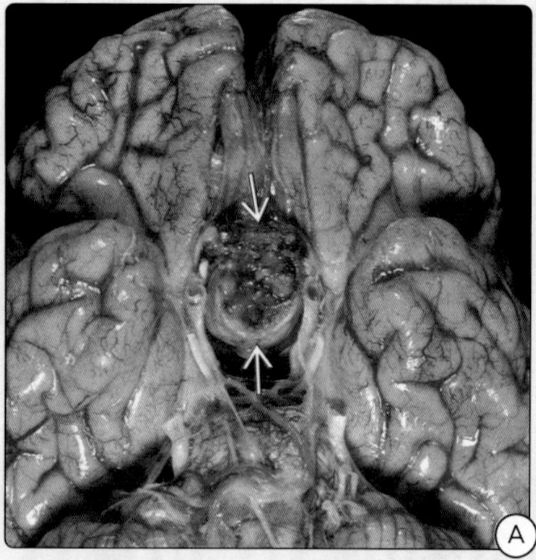

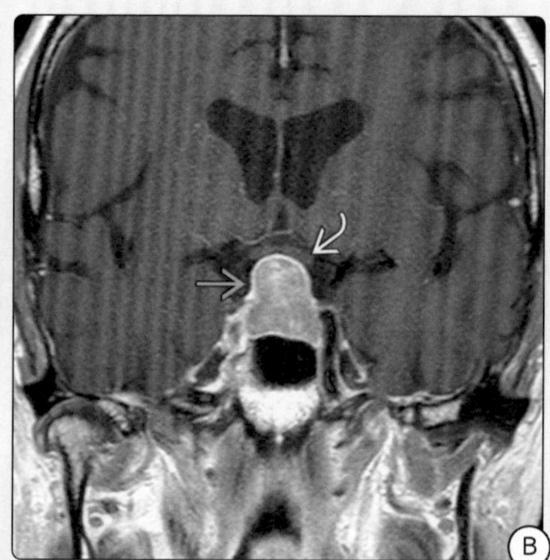

***(30-46A)** Submentovertex view of autopsied brain shows large intra- and suprasellar mass ➡. The pituitary gland cannot be separated from the mass and indeed is the mass. (Courtesy R. Hewlett, MD.) **(30-46B)** Coronal T1 C+ MR shows the classic snowman or figure 8 shape of a macroadenoma ➡ with mild superior displacement of the optic chiasm ➡. The mass and pituitary gland are indistinguishable from each other.*

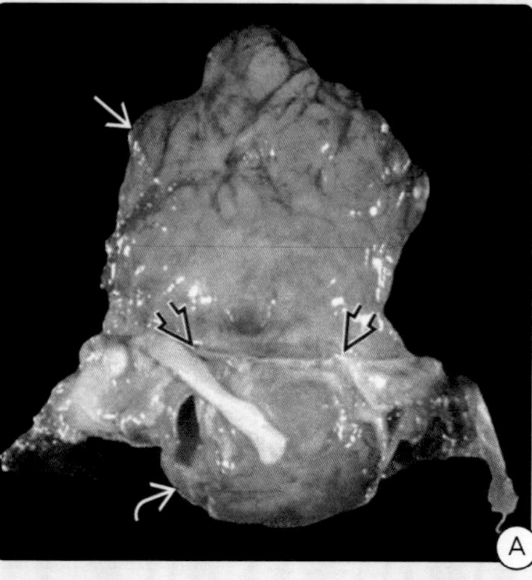

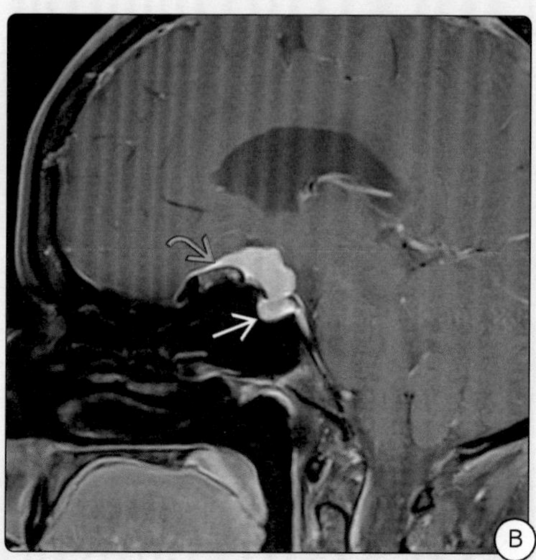

***(30-47A)** Autopsy coronal view shows a suprasellar meningioma. Tumor ➡ is separated from the pituitary gland below ➡ by the diaphragma sellae ➡ from which the meningioma arose. (Courtesy J. Paltan, MD.) **(30-47B)** Sagittal T1 C+ MR shows an enhancing suprasellar mass ➡ with a dural tail along the planum sphenoidale, classic location for meningioma. Meningiomas often have different enhancement characteristics than the pituitary gland ➡.*

## WHEN MASS *CANNOT* BE SEPARATED FROM PITUITARY GLAND

**Common**
- Pituitary macroadenoma
- Pituitary hyperplasia (physiologic, pathologic)

**Less Common**
- Neurosarcoid
- Langerhans cell histiocytosis
- Hypophysitis

**Rare but Important**
- Metastasis
- Lymphoma
- Germinoma

## INTRASELLAR LESION

**Common**
- Pituitary hyperplasia (physiologic, pathologic), pituitary microadenoma, empty sella

**Less Common**
- Pituitary macroadenoma, Rathke cleft (or other) cyst, craniopharyngioma, neurosarcoid

**Rare but Important**
- Lymphocytic hypophysitis, intracranial hypotension (venous congestion), vascular ("kissing" carotids, aneurysm), meningioma, metastasis, lymphoma

## Common Suprasellar Masses

The five most common overall suprasellar masses, i.e., the "Big Five," are pituitary macroadenoma, meningioma, aneurysm,

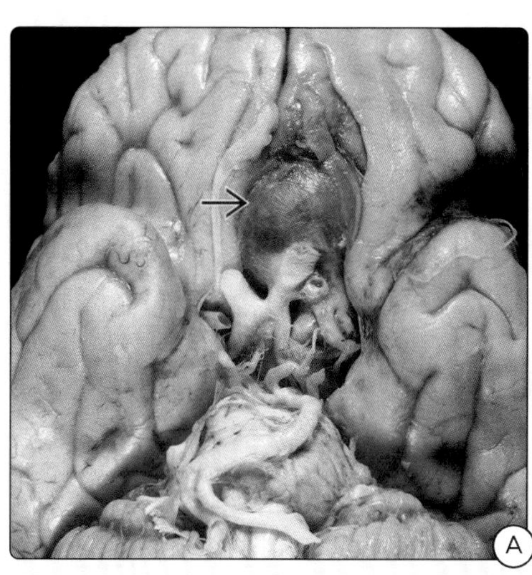


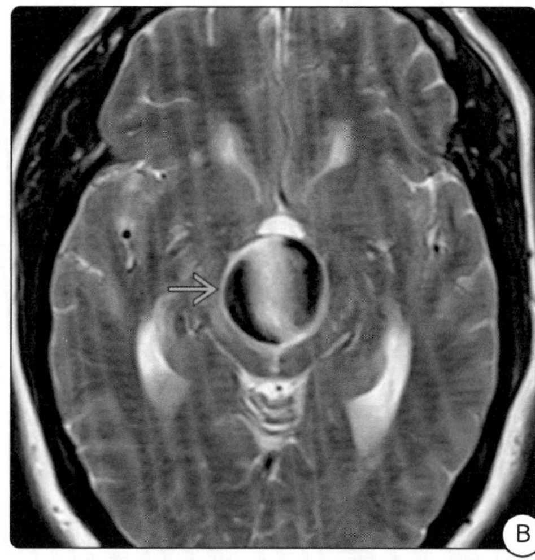


***(30-48A)** Autopsy specimen demonstrates an unruptured suprasellar aneurysm ➙. (Courtesy R. Hewlett, MD.)* ***(30-48B)** Axial T2 MR in a patient with headaches shows a heterogeneous mass ➙ in the suprasellar cistern. Considerations in an adult include macroadenoma, meningioma, and aneurysm. This is a giant basilar tip aneurysm. Flow voids, pulsation artifact, and a laminated appearance may be seen with aneurysms.*

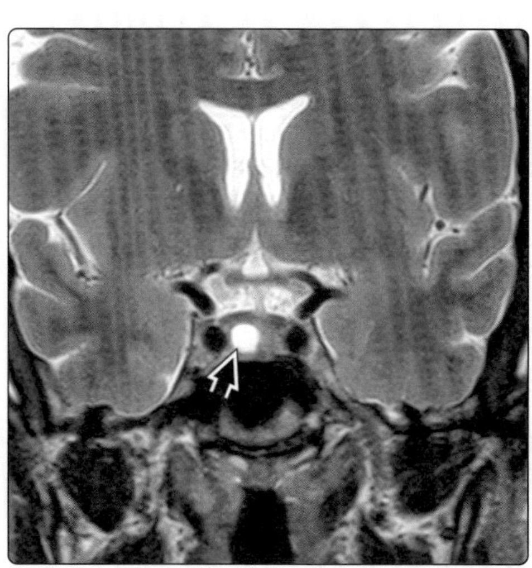

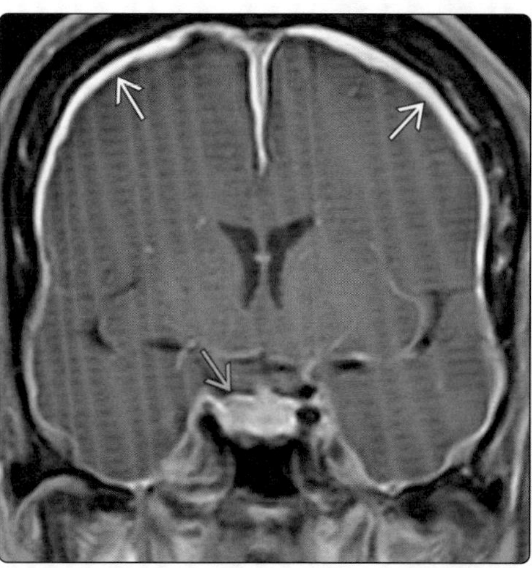

***(30-49)** Coronal T2 MR shows a cystic intrasellar mass ➙ in a young adult with elevated prolactin. Cystic microadenoma was found at resection. Imaging mimics a Rathke cleft cyst.* ***(30-50)** Coronal T1 C+ MR in a headache patient shows an enlarged pituitary gland ➙ and diffuse dural enhancement ➙, a classic feature of intracranial hypotension. Other features include "sagging midbrain," engorged veins, and subdural collections.*

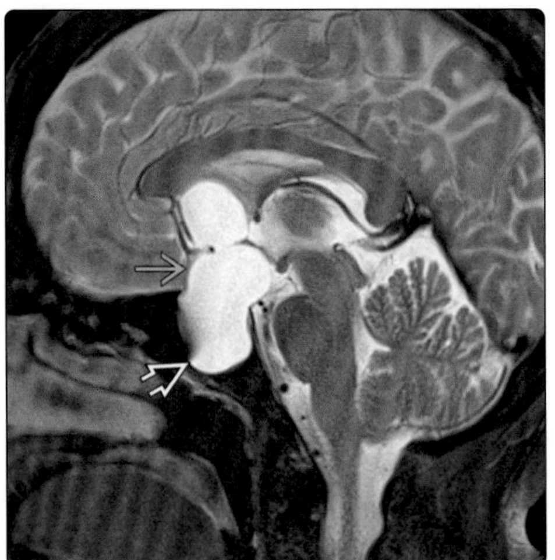

***(30-51)** Sagittal T2 MR shows a cystic sellar and suprasellar mass ⇒ related to an arachnoid cyst. There is enlargement of the sella turcica ⇒.*

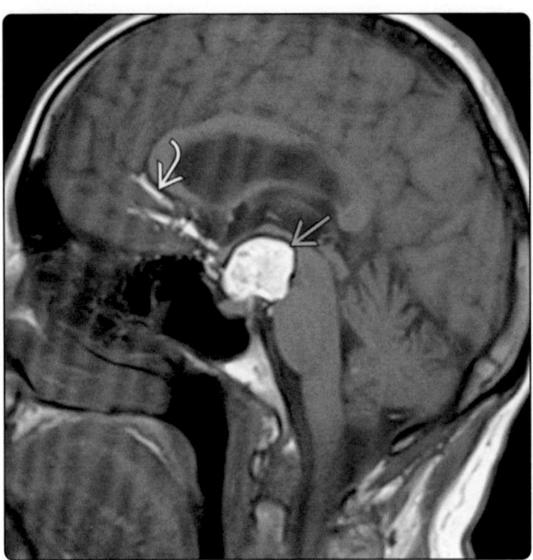

***(30-52)** Sagittal T1 MR shows a hyperintense mass ⇒ with subarachnoid space linear T1 hyperintensity ⇒ related to a ruptured dermoid.*

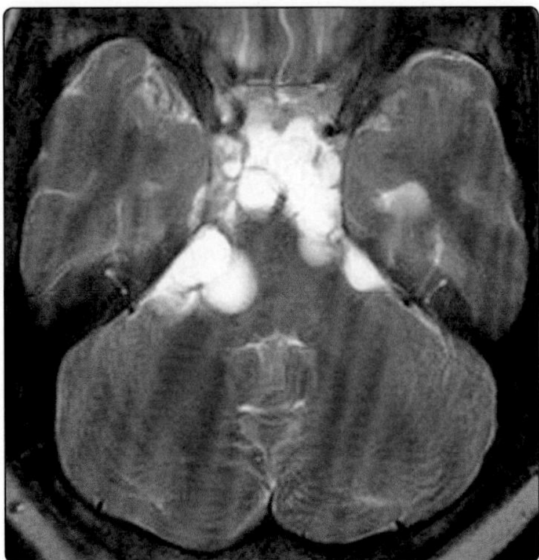

***(30-53)** Axial T2 MR shows multiple hyperintense cysts related to neurocysticercosis in the suprasellar region and along the pons.*

CP, and astrocytoma. Together, they account for 75-80% of all sellar region masses. Three of the "Big Five" (the "Big Three")—adenoma, meningioma, aneurysm—are common in adults but rare in children **(30-46)** **(30-47)** **(30-48)**.

**COMMON SUPRASELLAR MASSES**

**Adults**
- Pituitary adenoma (mass = gland)
- Meningioma (mass separate from gland)
- Aneurysm ("flow void," pulsation artifact)

**Children**
- Craniopharyngioma (90% cystic, 90% calcify, 90% enhance)
- Hypothalamic/optic chiasm astrocytoma (solid, no calcification)
- Germ cell tumor (germinoma most common)

## Less Common Suprasellar Masses

The presence of some less common lesions can often be inferred from imaging studies. The typical MR signal intensity of the lesion is often key to the diagnosis. Arachnoid cysts follow CSF signal intensity on all sequences and do not enhance **(30-51)**. Dermoid cysts have T1-hyperintense fat that will suppress on fat-saturated MR sequences **(30-52)**. Neurocysticercosis (NCC) is an intracranial parasitic infection caused by the pork tapeworm *Taenia solium* and may present as multiple T2-hyperintense racemose cysts in the basal cisterns **(30-53)**.

**LESS COMMON SUPRASELLAR MASSES**

- Rathke cleft cyst (well delineated, separate from pituitary)
- Arachnoid cyst (behaves just like CSF)
- Dermoid cyst (looks like fat)
- Neurocysticercosis (usually multiple)

## Rare Suprasellar Masses

Keep these lesions in mind—they can mimic more common lesions, but the appropriate treatment differs sharply. Hypophysitis may affect the gland or the infundibulum or both. It may be autoimmune, granulomatous, IgG4 related to drug related. Germinomas are classically CT hyperdense and enhance diffusely. They may occur in the suprasellar or pineal region **(30-56)**.

**RARE BUT IMPORTANT SUPRASELLAR MASSES**

- Hypophysitis (may look like adenoma)
- Hypothalamic hamartoma ("collar button" between stalk, mammillary bodies)
- Germinoma (or other germ cell tumor)
- Metastasis (systemic cancer; look for other lesions)
- Lymphoma (often infiltrates adjacent structures)

## Cystic Intra-/Suprasellar Mass

If an intra- or suprasellar mass is primarily or exclusively cystic, the differential diagnosis considerations change. The key issue is to distinguish a cystic mass that originates *within* the sella vs. intrasellar extension *from* a suprasellar lesion **(30-49)**. Other than RCC, completely intrasellar nonneoplastic cysts are rare, as is a totally intrasellar CP without suprasellar extension.

In a **child** with a suprasellar cystic mass, consider an enlarged third ventricle, CP, NCC, and astrocytoma. In an **adult**, consider arachnoid cyst, NCC, RCC, adenoma, and aneurysm **(30-51)**.

## CYSTIC *INTRA*SELLAR MASS

**Common**
- Empty sella
- Idiopathic intracranial hypertension

**Less Common**
- Cystic pituitary adenoma
- Rathke cleft cyst
- Neurocysticercosis cyst

**Rare but Important**
- Craniopharyngioma
- Epidermoid cyst, arachnoid cyst
- Pituitary apoplexy
- Thrombosed aneurysm

## CYSTIC *SUPRA*SELLAR MASS

**Common**
- Enlarged 3rd ventricle
- Arachnoid cyst
- Craniopharyngioma
- Neurocysticercosis cyst

**Less Common**
- Rathke cleft cyst
- Dermoid cyst
- Epidermoid cyst

**Rare but Important**
- Pituitary macroadenoma, apoplexy
- Astrocytoma (usually solid)
- Ependymal cyst
- Aneurysm (patent or thrombosed)

*Selected References: The complete reference list is available on the eBooks+ version included with purchase.*

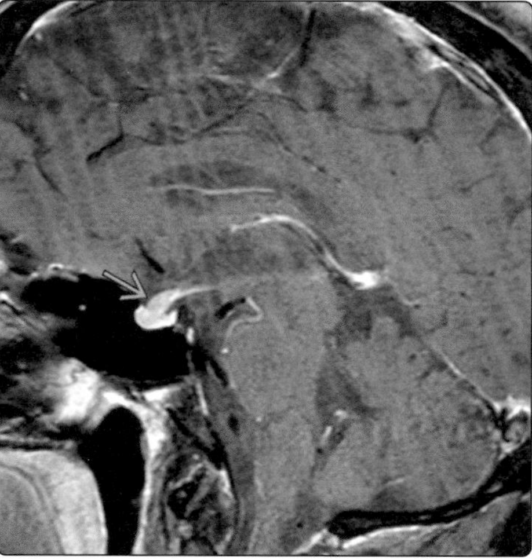

***(30-54)** Sagittal T1 C+ MR shows a thickened pituitary infundibulum related to autoimmune lymphocytic hypophysitis ⇒.*

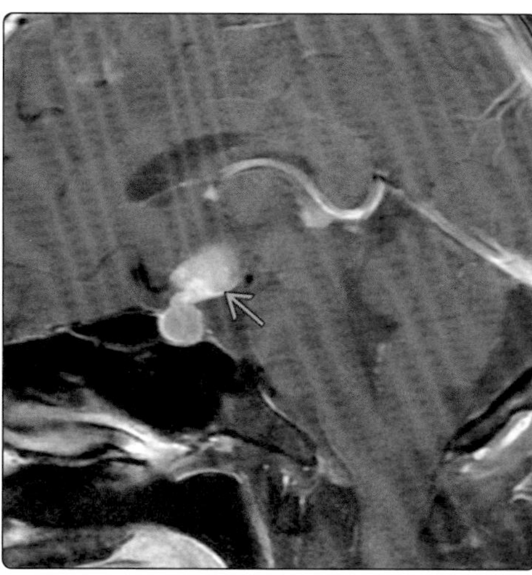

***(30-55)** Sagittal T1 C+ MR shows avid enhancement along the infundibulum and hypothalamus ⇒ related to B-cell lymphoma.*

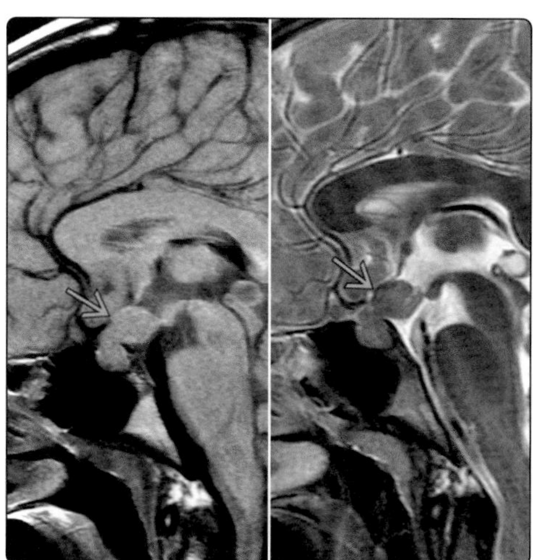

***(30-56)** Sagittal T1 and T2 MR in a teenager with abnormal menses shows an infundibular and suprasellar mass ⇒. Biopsy-proven germinoma.*

# Metastases and Paraneoplastic Syndromes

*Brain metastases are the most common type of intracranial neoplasm in adults. Between 20-45% of all patients with advanced cancers (particularly lung and breast) will eventually develop CNS involvement. Brain metastases are often ultimately responsible for patient mortality, even in the face of controlled systemic disease.*



We begin this chapter with a brief overview of CNS metastases, then follow with a discussion of cranial metastases by anatomic location, beginning with the brain parenchyma (the most common overall CNS location). We conclude with remote effects of cancer on the CNS, so-called paraneoplastic syndromes.

## Metastatic Lesions

Metastases are secondary tumors that arise from primary neoplasms at another site. As a group, metastases are now the most common CNS neoplasm in adults.

### Overview

#### Etiology

**Routes of Spread.** CNS metastases can arise from both extra- and intracranial primary tumors. Metastases from **extracranial primary neoplasms** ("body-to-brain metastases") most commonly spread via **hematogenous dissemination**.

**Direct geographic extension** from a lesion in an adjacent structure (such as squamous cell carcinoma in the nasopharynx) also occurs but is much less common than hematogenous spread. Invasion is usually through natural foramina and fissures where bone is thin or absent. **Perineural** and **perivascular spread** are less common but important direct geographic routes by which head and neck tumors gain access to the CNS.

**Primary intracranial neoplasms** sometimes spread from one CNS site to another, causing brain-to-brain or brain-to-spine metastases. Spread occurs preferentially along compact white matter tracts, such as the corpus callosum and internal capsule, but can also involve the ventricular ependyma, pia, and perivascular spaces.

**CSF dissemination** with "carcinomatous meningitis" occurs with both extra- and intracranial primary neoplasms.

**Origin of CNS Metastases.** Both the source and location of metastases vary significantly with patient age. Approximately 10% of all brain metastases

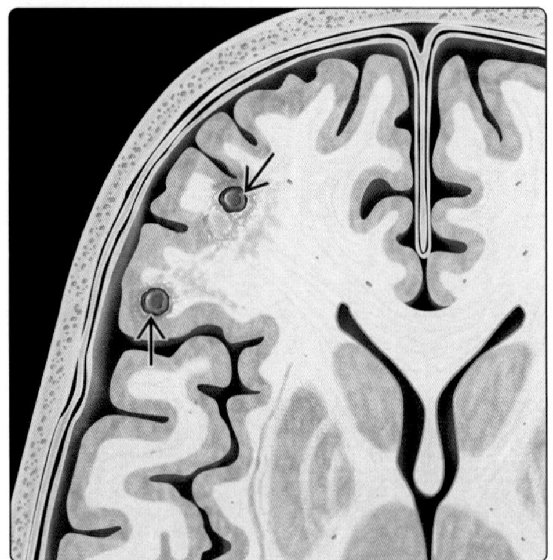

***(31-1)** Graphic shows parenchymal metastases ➡ at the GM-WM junction, the most common site. Most metastases are round, not infiltrating.*

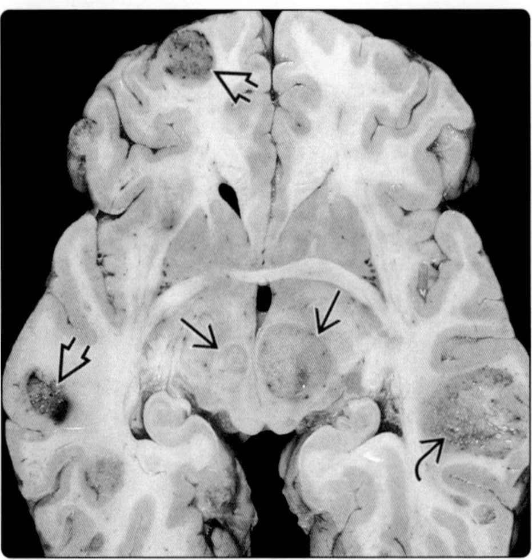

***(31-2)** Multiple metastases shown, some with hemorrhage ➡ or necrosis ➡. Midbrain lesions are gray-tan ➡. (Courtesy R. Hewlett, MD.)*

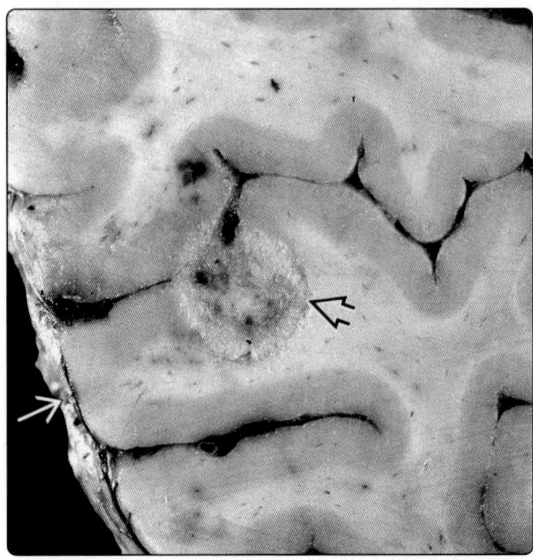

***(31-3)** Metastases are often at the depths of sulci ➡. This specimen also has pial metastases ➡.*

(BMs) originate from an unknown primary neoplasm at the time of initial diagnosis.

***Children.*** Metastases are rare in children, accounting for only 2% of all pediatric CNS tumors. The most common sources of cranial metastases in children are hematologic malignancies, such as leukemia and lymphoma. The preferential locations are the skull and dura. Parenchymal metastases are much less common in children compared with adults.

***Adults.*** Lung, breast, and melanoma account for at least 2/3 of all BMs in adults. The most common primary tumor that metastasizes to the brain is lung cancer. Breast is the second most common primary tumor source followed by melanoma, renal carcinoma, and colorectal cancer. In ~ 10% of cases, no primary tumor is found at initial presentation.

Skull, dura, and spine metastases are typically caused by prostate, breast, or lung cancer followed by renal cancers and hematologic malignancies, such as non-Hodgkin lymphoma and multiple myeloma.

### CNS METASTASES: EPIDEMIOLOGY AND ETIOLOGY

**Epidemiology**

- Adults > > children
  - Metastases: Most common CNS neoplasm in adults
  - 5x increase in past 50 years
  - BMs occur in > 30-40% of cancer patients

**Routes of Spread**

- Most common: Extracranial primary to CNS via
  - Hematogenous dissemination
  - CSF, leptomeninges (pia)
  - Direct geographic extension (nasopharynx, sinuses)
  - Perineural, perivascular spread
- Less common
  - Brain to brain from CNS primary
  - Brain to CSF from CNS primary
- Least common
  - Tumor-to-tumor metastasis
  - Sometimes called collision tumor
  - Most common "donor" tumor: Breast, lung
  - Most common "recipient" tumor: Meningioma

**Origin**

- 10% unknown primary at initial diagnosis
  - Children: Leukemia, lymphoma, sarcoma
  - Adults: Lung, breast cancer, melanoma, renal carcinoma, colorectal cancer

## Pathology

**Location.** The brain parenchyma is the most common site (80%) followed by the skull and dura (15%) and leptomeninges (pia)/subarachnoid space (5%).

The vast majority of parenchymal metastases are located in the cerebral hemispheres, especially at the junction between the cortex and subcortical white matter **(31-1)** **(31-2)**. While only 15% of metastases are found in the cerebellum, *a solitary cerebellar mass in a middle-aged or older adult is more likely to be metastasis than a primary neoplasm!*

Uncommon sites include the pons and midbrain, choroid plexus, ventricular ependyma, pituitary gland/stalk, and retinal choroid. Rarely, tumor cells diffusely infiltrate the brain perivascular spaces, a process termed carcinomatous encephalitis.

**Size and Number.** Most parenchymal metastases are between a few millimeters and 1.5 cm **(31-3)**. Large hemispheric metastases are rare. In contrast, skull and dural metastases can become very large.

Approximately 50% of metastases are solitary while 50% are multiple. About 20% of patients have two lesions, 30% have three or more, and only 5% have more than five lesions.

### Gross Pathology

***Parenchymal Metastases.*** Parenchymal metastases are focal, round, relatively circumscribed, grayish-white or tan lesions that exhibit sharp borders with the adjacent brain **(31-3)**. Melanoma metastases are often brown to black in color. Peritumoral edema, necrosis, hemorrhage, and mass effect range from none to striking.

Diffusely infiltrating parenchymal metastases are rare, and when they do occur, they typically extend along perivascular spaces.

***Skull/Dural Metastases.*** Calvarial and skull base metastases are typically destructive, poorly marginated lesions **(31-4)** **(31-5)**.

Dural metastases usually occur in combination with adjacent skull lesions, appearing as focal nodules **(31-6)** or more diffuse, plaque-like sheets of tumor. Dural metastasis without skull involvement is much less common.

***Leptomeningeal Metastases.*** The term leptomeningeal metastases actually describes metastases to the subarachnoid spaces and pia **(31-7)**. Diffuse sugar-like coating of the pia is typical **(31-8)**. Multiple nodular deposits and infiltration of the perivascular (Virchow-Robin) spaces with extension into the adjacent cortex may occur **(31-9)** **(31-20)**.

**Microscopic Features.** Although metastases may display more marked mitoses and elevated labeling indices compared with their primary systemic source, they generally preserve the same cellular features.

#### CNS METASTASES: PATHOLOGY

**Location**
- Adults
  - Brain (80%, cerebral hemispheres > > cerebellum)
  - Skull/dura (15%)
  - Pia ("leptomeningeal"), CSF (5%), perivascular spaces
  - Other (1%): Choroid plexus, ventricular ependyma, pituitary
- Children
  - Skull/dura > > brain parenchyma

**Number**
- Solitary (50%)
- 2 lesions (20%)
- ≥ 3 lesions (30%)
  - Only 5% have > 5 lesions

**Gross Pathology**
- Round, well circumscribed
  - Less common: Infiltrating, poorly delineated
- Variable edema, necrosis, hemorrhage

**Microscopic Features**
- Preserves general features of primary tumor
- May have more mitoses, elevated labeling indices

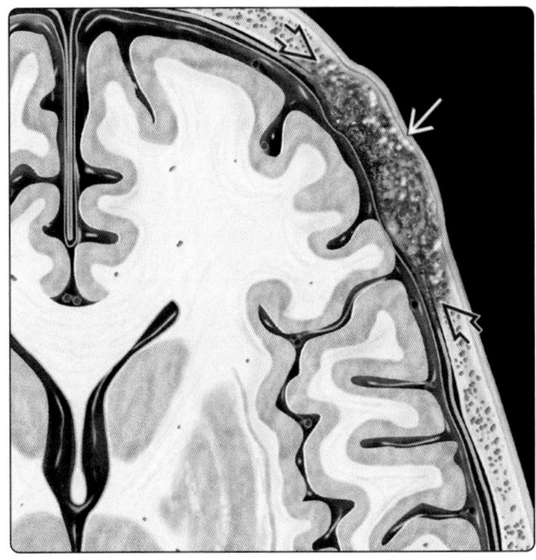

***(31-4)** Graphic shows skull metastasis ➡ expanding diploic space, invading/thickening the underlying dura (light blue linear structure) ⇨.*

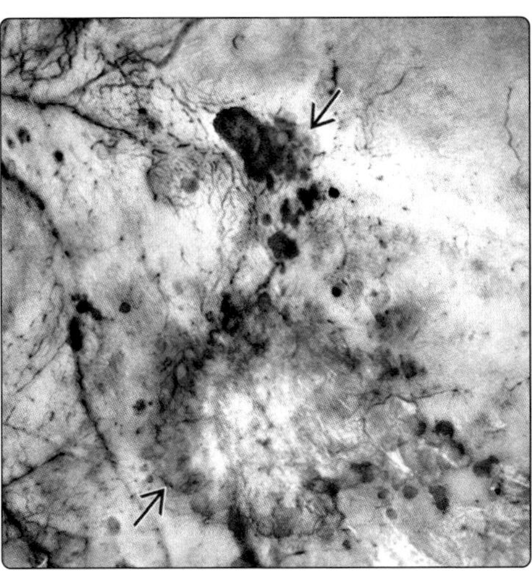

***(31-5)** Skull metastases are seen here as permeative, lytic, and destructive lesions ⇨.*

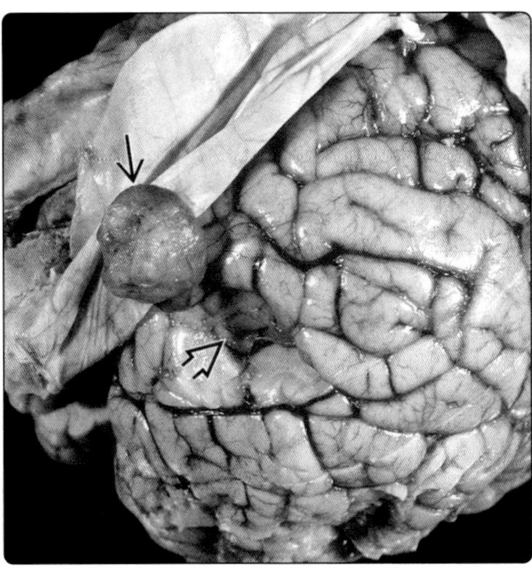

***(31-6)** Solitary dural metastasis ⇨ indents the brain ⇨ and appears identical to a meningioma. (Courtesy R. Hewlett, MD.)*

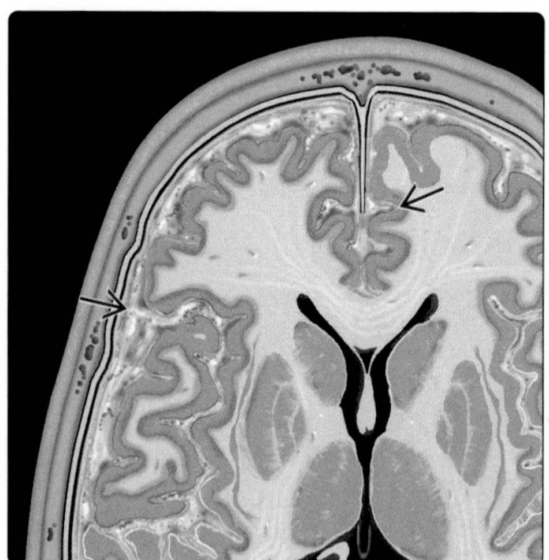

*(31-7) Graphic depicts a sugar icing appearance of leptomeningeal metastases ➡ covering the brain and extending into the sulci.*

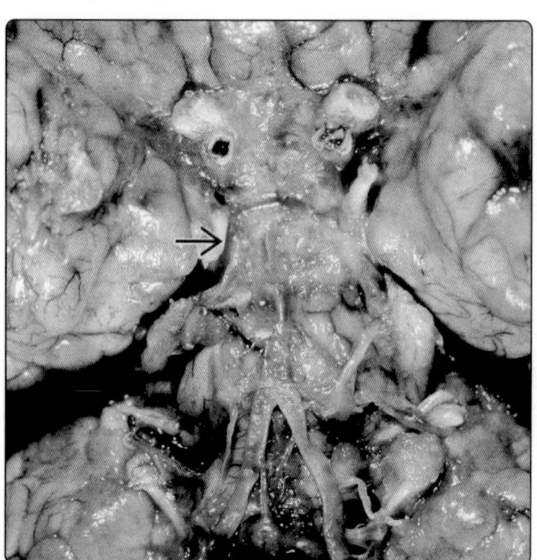

*(31-8) Pia-subarachnoid ("leptomeningeal") metastases coat the brain, fill the subarachnoid cisterns ➡. (Courtesy R. Hewlett, MD.)*

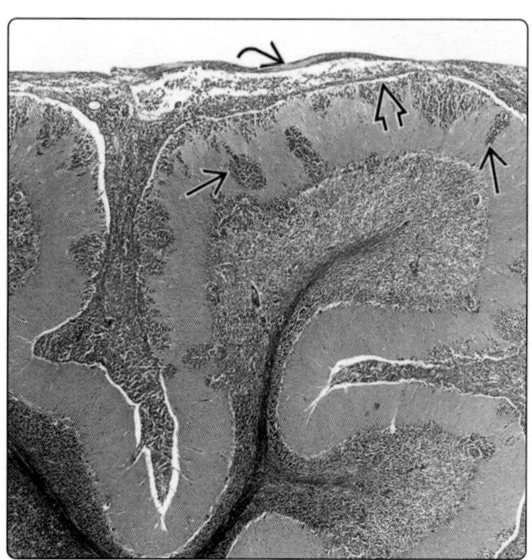

*(31-9) Mets fill space between the arachnoid ➡ and pia ➡ and extend along PVSs into cortex ➡. (Courtesy P. Burger, MD.)*

## Clinical Issues

**Demographics.** Up to 40% of patients with treated systemic cancers eventually develop BMs. Peak prevalence is in patients older than 65 years of age. Only 6-10% of children with extracranial malignancies develop BMs.

**Presentation.** Seizure and focal neurologic deficit are the most common presenting symptoms of parenchymal metastases. 1/2 of all patients with skull/dural metastases present with headache. Seizure, sensory or motor deficit, cranial neuropathy, or a palpable mass under the scalp are other common symptoms.

**Natural History.** Although gross total resection of BMs improves symptoms and survival in selected patients, the natural history of parenchymal metastases is grim. Relentless, progressive increase in both number and size of metastases is typical. Median survival after diagnosis is short, generally averaging between 3 and 6 months, although in patients with gross total resection of a solitary metastasis, survival averages 13 months.

## Imaging

Imaging findings and differential diagnosis vary with metastasis location. Each anatomic site has special features; each is discussed separately in this chapter.

# Parenchymal Metastases

## Imaging

Recent analyses indicate nearly 1/2 of systemic cancer therapy trials do not require mandatory cerebral imaging at baseline and only rare trials require continued surveillance imaging for patients without BMs at baseline. Despite this, there is increasing evidence supporting screening for BMs in many common cancers, such as advanced breast cancer, melanoma, and non-small cell lung cancer (NSCLC), both at diagnosis and after initiation of palliative systemic therapy.

Early detection of metastases improves the impact of treatments and increases patient survival rates. Contrast-enhanced MR is the preferred modality for diagnosing BMs and is more sensitive than either CT or nonenhanced MR. Because manual detection and delineation of BMs is time consuming, a variety of artificial intelligence (AI) methods have been utilized to detect brain tumors in their initial stages. Computer-aided deep learning using MR may be increasingly utilized in the future to detect BMs in patients with systemic cancers.

In this section, we review the findings of parenchymal BMs on standard imaging studies used in typical clinical practices.

**CT Findings.** Parenchymal metastases can be iso-, hypo- or hyperdense on NECT with variable surrounding hypodense vasogenic edema **(31-11A) (31-12)**. With the exception of treated metastases, calcification is rare. Occasionally, the first manifestation of an intracranial metastasis is a brain bleed.

The vast majority of parenchymal metastases enhance strongly following contrast administration **(31-11B)**. Double-dose delayed scans may increase lesion conspicuity. Solid, punctate, nodular, or ring patterns can be seen.

### MR Findings

***T1WI.*** Most metastases are iso- to mildly hypointense on T1WI. The exception is melanoma metastasis, which has intrinsic T1 shortening and thus appears moderately hyperintense **(31-15)**. Subacute hemorrhagic metastases show disordered, heterogeneous signal intensity, often with bizarre-appearing intermixed foci of T1 hyper- and hypointensities **(31-31)**.

***T2/FLAIR.*** Signal intensity on T2WI varies widely depending on tumor type, lesion cellularity, presence of hemorrhagic residua, and amount of peritumoral edema. In contrast to high-grade gliomas, peritumoral hyperintense T2/FLAIR signal in metastases generally represents pure vasogenic edema, not tumor infiltration **(31-14A)**. Many metastases are hypointense on T2WI and FLAIR. Exceptions are mucinous tumors, cystic metastases, and tumors with large amounts of central necrosis, all of which can appear moderately hyperintense.

Some hyperintense metastases show little or no surrounding edema. Multiple small hyperintense metastases ("miliary metastases") can be mistaken for small vessel vascular disease unless contrast is administered.

***T2*.*** Both subacute hemorrhage and melanin cause prominent signal intensity loss ("blooming") on T2* (GRE, SWI) images **(31-31A)**.

***T1 C+.*** Virtually all nonhemorrhagic metastases enhance following contrast administration **(31-14B)**. Patterns vary from solid, uniform enhancement to nodular, "cyst + nodule," and ring-like lesions. Multiple metastases in the same patient may exhibit different patterns.

***DWI, MRS.*** DWI is variable, but metastases generally do not exhibit restricted diffusion. Some highly cellular tumors show low ADC values. MRS may show a prominent lipid peak.

**PARENCHYMAL METASTASES: IMAGING**

CT
- Variable density (most iso-, hypodense)
- Most enhance on CECT
- Perform bone CT for calvarial, skull base metastases

T1WI
- Most metastases: Iso- to slightly hypointense
- Melanoma metastases: Hyperintense
- Hemorrhagic metastases: Heterogeneously hyperintense

T2/FLAIR
- Varies with tumor type, cellularity, hemorrhage
- Most common: Iso- to mildly hyperintense
- Can resemble small vessel vascular disease

T2*
- Subacute blood, melanin "bloom"

T1 C+
- Almost all nonhemorrhagic metastases enhance strongly
- Solid, punctate, ring, "cyst + nodule"

DWI
- Variable; most common: No restriction
- Highly cellular metastases may restrict

MRS
- Most prominent feature: Lipid peak
- Elevated Cho, depressed/absent Cr

## Differential Diagnosis

The major differential diagnosis for punctate and ring-enhancing metastases is abscess. **Abscesses** and **septic emboli** typically restrict on DWI. Primary neoplasms like **glioblastoma** tend to be infiltrating, whereas metastases are almost always round and relatively well demarcated.

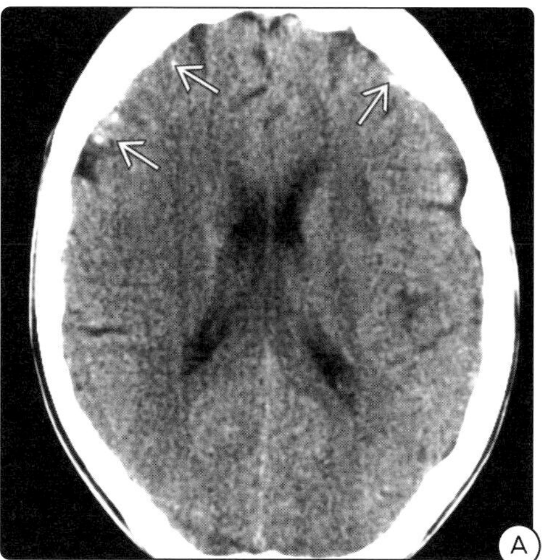


***(31-11A)** Axial NECT in a 63-year-old woman with known breast carcinoma shows a few scattered, bifrontal hyperdensities ➔.*

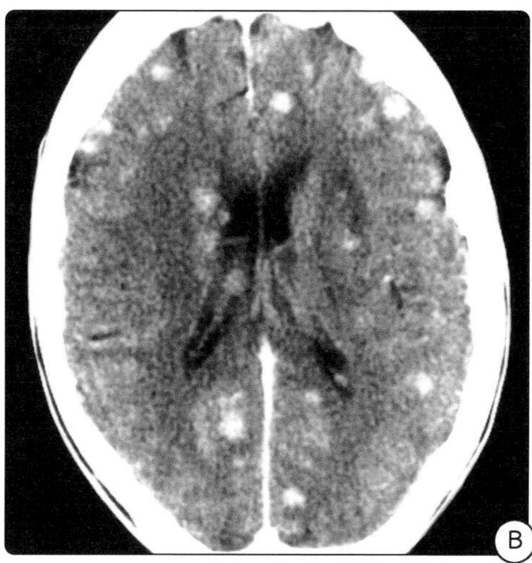


***(31-11B)** CECT shows "too numerous to count" enhancing metastases, most of which were invisible on the precontrast study.*

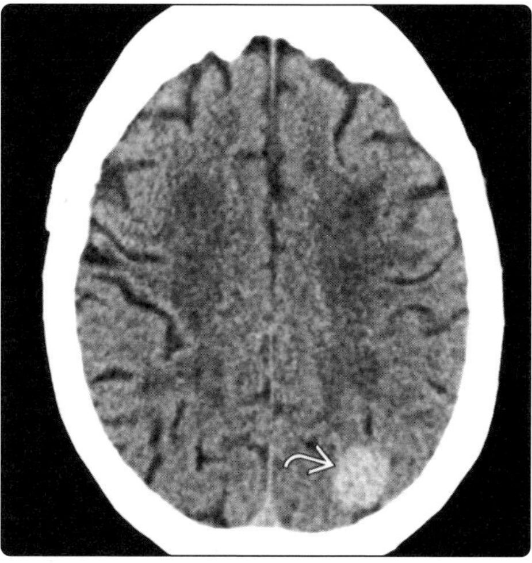

***(31-12)** Axial NECT shows a solitary hyperdense parenchymal mass ➔. This is metastatic thyroid carcinoma.*

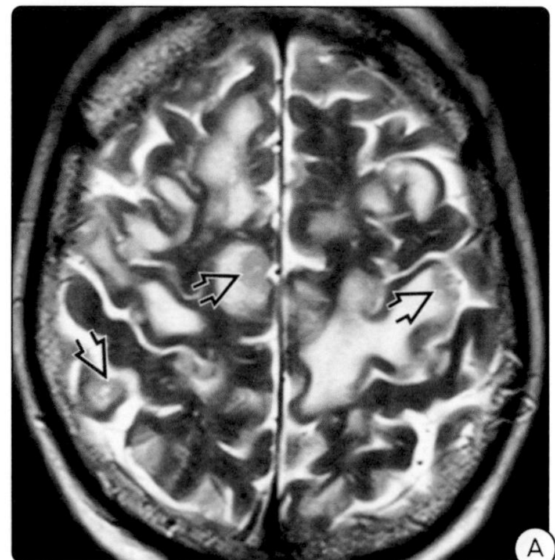

***(31-14A)*** *T2 MR shows multiple iso- to slightly hyperintense nodules at the GM-WM interfaces ➱ surrounded by edema.*

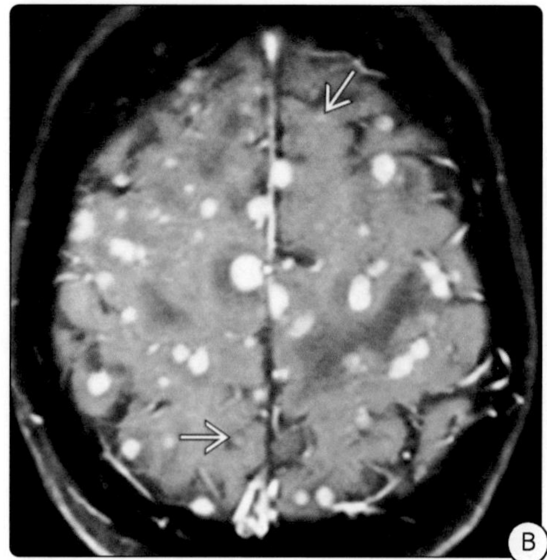

***(31-14B)*** ***Lesions enhance on T1 C+ FS MR. Tiny enhancing foci ➡ not seen on T2 or FLAIR are identified. This is metastatic renal cell carcinoma.***

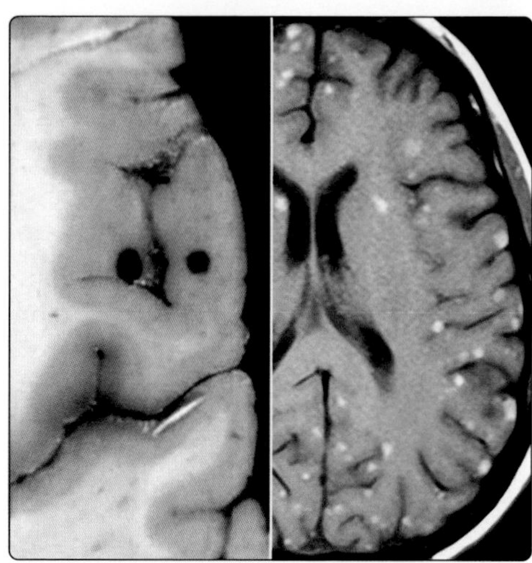

***(31-15)*** ***(L) Autopsy shows melanoma metastases at GM-WM interfaces. (R) T1WI shows innumerable hyperintense melanoma metastases.***

Both metastases and **multiple embolic infarcts** share a predilection for arterial "border zones" and the gray matter-white matter interfaces. Most acute infarcts restrict strongly on DWI and rarely demonstrate a ring-enhancing pattern on T1 C+ scans. Chronic infarcts and age-related microvascular disease are hyperintense on T2WI and do not enhance following contrast administration.

**Multiple cavernous malformations** can mimic hemorrhagic metastases but are typically surrounded by a complete hemosiderin rim. **Multiple sclerosis** occurs in younger patients and is preferentially located in the deep periventricular white matter, not the gray matter-white matter interface.

Primary infratentorial parenchymal brain tumors in adults are rare. No matter what the imaging findings are, *a solitary cerebellar mass in a middle-aged or older adult should be considered a metastasis until proven otherwise!*

## Skull and Dural Metastases

### Terminology

The term "skull" refers both to the calvarium and to the skull base. As one cannot distinguish neoplastic involvement of the periosteal vs. meningeal dural layers, we refer to these layers collectively as the "dura." In actuality, the arachnoid—the outermost layer of the leptomeninges—adheres to the dura, so it, too, is almost always involved any time tumor invades the dura.

### Overview

The skull and dura are the second most common sites of CNS metastases from extracranial primary tumors. Calvarial and skull base metastases can occur either with or without dural involvement.

In contrast, dural metastases without coexisting calvarial lesions are less common. Between 8-10% of patients with advanced systemic cancer have dural metastases. Breast (35%) and prostate (15-20%) cancers are the most frequent sources. Single lesions are slightly more common than multiple dural metastases.

### Imaging

**General Features.** Solitary or multiple focal lesions involve the skull, dura (and underlying arachnoid), or both. A less common pattern is diffuse neoplastic dura-arachnoid thickening, seen as a curvilinear layer of tumor that follows the inner table of the calvarium.

**CT Findings.** Complete evaluation requires **both** soft tissue and bone algorithm reconstructions of the imaging data **(31-16)**. The most common finding on NECT is a focal soft tissue mass centered on the diploic space. A biconvex shape with both subgaleal and dural extension is typical. Most dural metastases enhance strongly on CECT.

Bone CT usually demonstrates one or more relatively circumscribed intraosseous lesions **(31-19)**. Permeative, diffusely destructive lesions are the second most common pattern **(31-16)**. A few osseous metastases—mostly those from prostate and treated breast cancer—can be blastic and sclerotic.

Large dural metastases displace the brain inward, buckling the gray matter-white matter interface medially **(31-17)**. Hypodensities in the underlying brain suggest parenchymal invasion or venous ischemia.

**MR Findings.** Hyperintense fat in the diploic space provides excellent, naturally occurring demarcation from skull metastases on T1WIs. Metastases replace hyperintense yellow marrow and appear as hypointense infiltrating foci. Dural metastases thicken the dura-arachnoid and are typically iso- or hypointense to underlying cortex.

Most skull metastases are hyperintense to marrow on T2WI, but the signal intensity of dural metastases varies. FLAIR hyperintensity in the underlying sulci suggests pia-subarachnoid tumor spread. Hyperintensity in the underlying brain is present in 1/2 of all cases and suggests either tumor invasion along the perivascular spaces or compromise of venous drainage.

Nearly 70% of dural metastases are accompanied by metastases in the overlying skull. Involvement of the adjacent scalp is also common. Contrast-enhanced T1WI should be performed with fat saturation (T1 C+ FS) for optimal delineation, as some calvarial lesions may enhance just enough to become isointense with fat.

Most dural metastases enhance strongly, appearing as biconvex masses centered along the adjacent diploic space. Dural "tails" are present in ~ 1/2 of all cases. Frank tumor invasion into the underlying brain is seen in 1/3 of cases. Dural thickening can be smooth and diffuse or nodular and mass-like.

Hypercellular metastases with enlarged nuclei and reduced extracellular matrix may show diffusion restriction (hyperintense) and decreased ADC values (hypointense) on diffusion-weighted sequences.

## SKULL/DURA METASTASES

**General Features**
- 2nd most common site of CNS metastases
- Skull alone or skull + dura > > isolated dural metastases
- "Dural" metastases: Usually dura **plus** arachnoid!

**CT**
- Use both soft tissue, bone reconstructions
- Skull: Permeative lytic lesion(s)
- Scalp, dura: Biconvex mass centered on skull

**MR**
- T1WI: Metastases replace hyperintense fat
- T2WI: Most skull metastases are hyperintense
- FLAIR: Look for
    - Underlying sulcal hyperintensity (suggests pia-subarachnoid space tumor)
    - Parenchymal hyperintensity (suggests brain invasion along perivascular spaces)
- T1 C+
    - Use fat-saturation sequence
    - Skull/scalp/dural lesion(s) can be focal or diffuse, enhance strongly
    - Dural tail sign (50%)
    - Less common: Diffuse dura-arachnoid thickening ("lumpy-bumpy" or smooth)
- DWI: Hypercellular metastases may restrict

**Differential Diagnosis**
- Skull metastases
    - Surgical defect, venous lakes/arachnoid granulations
    - Myeloma
    - Osteomyelitis
- Dural metastases
    - Meningioma (solitary or multiple)

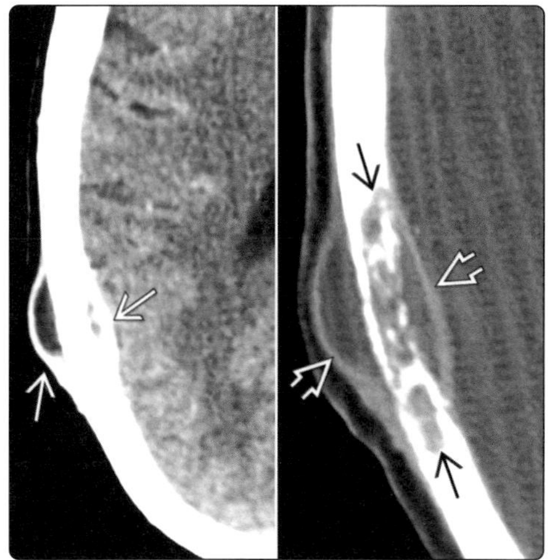

*(31-16) (L) CECT shows lesion ➡ centered on diploic space. (R) Bone window shows subgaleal, extradural components ➡ of lesion ➡.*

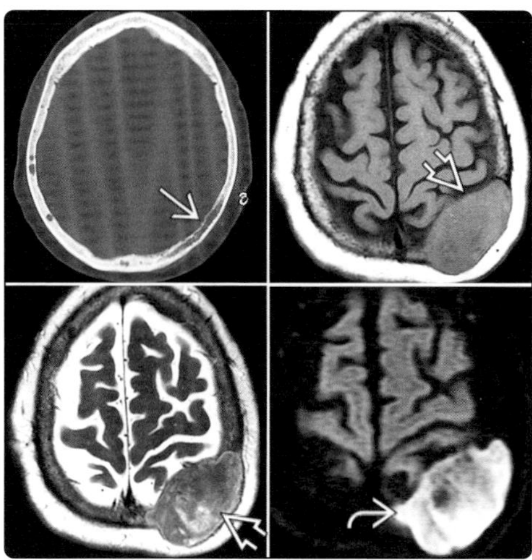

*(31-17) Metastatic breast carcinoma is seen as permeative ➡. Lesion is mostly isointense to brain on T1 and T2 ➡ and restricts on DWI ➡.*

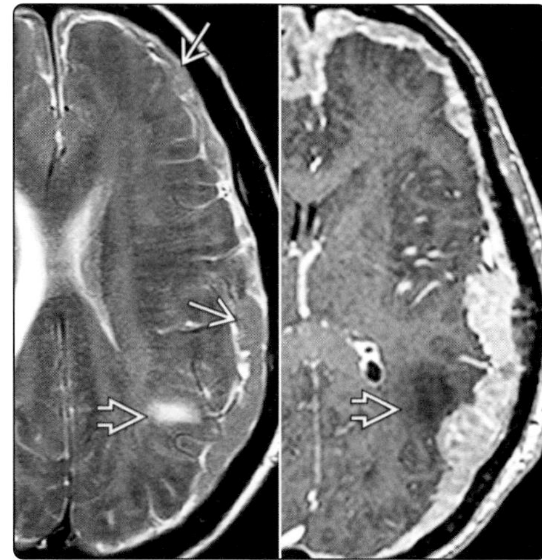

*(31-18) Metastases thicken the dura, fill the subarachnoid space ➡, and infiltrate via PVSs into brain ➡. (Courtesy N. Agarwal, MD.)*

*(31-19A) CECT in a 49-year-old man with a lump on his head shows a lytic, destructive mass centered on the diploic space. (31-19B) Coronal CECT shows subgaleal ➢, intraosseous ➩, and bilateral epidural tumor masses ➢.*

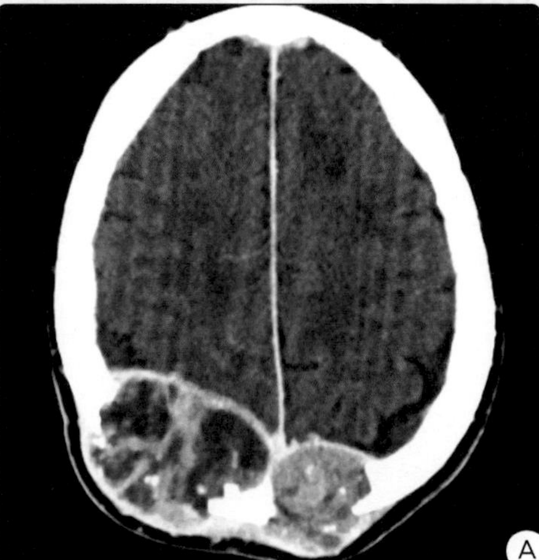

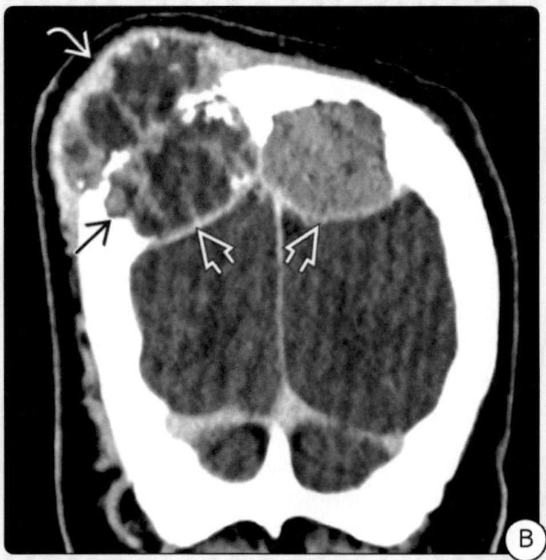

*(31-19C) T1 MR shows the lesions are mixed iso- and hyperintense compared to brain. (31-19D) The lesions are very heterogeneous on T2 MR, ranging from hypo- to iso- to hyperintense compared to cortex.*

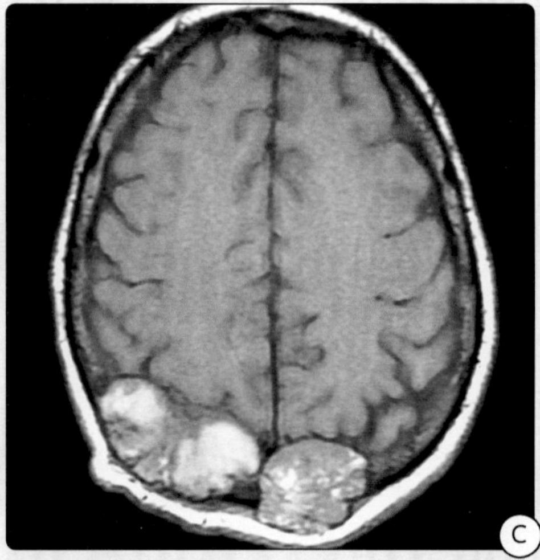

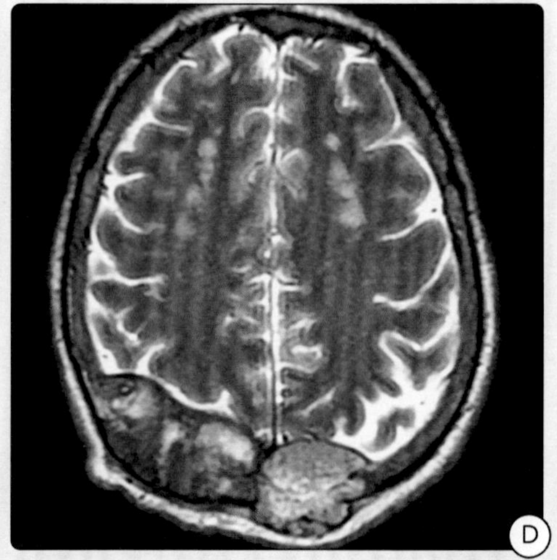

*(31-19E) T1 C+ FS MR shows the lesions enhancing heterogeneously. (31-19F) T2* GRE MR shows some susceptibility in the masses, suggesting intratumoral hemorrhage. Preoperative diagnosis was anaplastic meningioma or solitary fibrous tumor. Pathology disclosed occult metastatic thyroid carcinoma.*

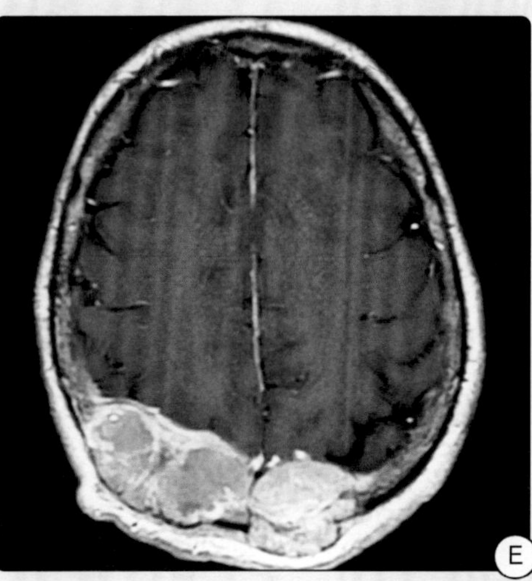

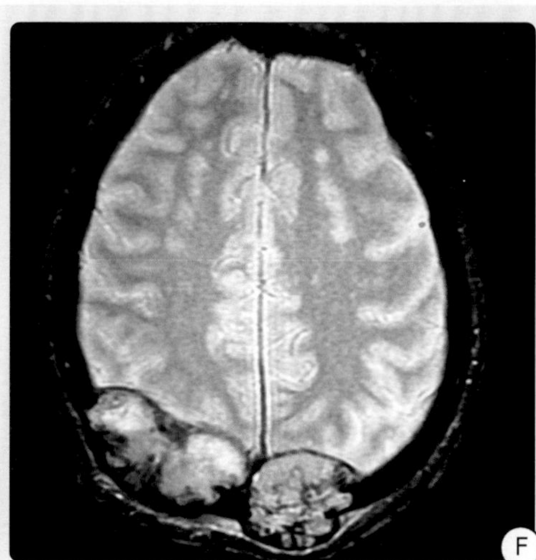

## Differential Diagnosis

The major differential diagnoses for skull metastases are surgical defects and normal structures. A **surgical defect**, such as a burr hole or craniotomy, can be distinguished from a metastasis by clinical history and the presence of defects in the overlying scalp. **Venous lakes, vascular grooves, arachnoid granulations**, and sometimes even **sutures** can mimic calvarial metastases. Normal structures are typically well corticated, and the underlying dura is normal.

**Myeloma** can be indistinguishable from multiple lytic skull metastases. Skull base **osteomyelitis** is a rare but life-threatening infection that can resemble diffuse skull base metastases. ADC values are generally higher in infection than in malignant neoplasms.

The major differential diagnosis for solitary or multifocal dura-arachnoid metastases is **meningioma**. Metastases, especially from breast cancer, can be virtually indistinguishable from solitary or multiple meningiomas on the basis of imaging studies alone.

The differential diagnosis of diffuse dura-arachnoid thickening is much broader. Nonneoplastic pachymeningopathies, such as meningitis, chronic subdural hematoma, and intracranial hypotension, can all cause diffuse dura-arachnoid thickening. Metastatic dural thickening is generally—although not invariably—more "lumpy-bumpy" **(31-18)**.

# Leptomeningeal Metastases

## Terminology

The anatomic term **leptomeninges** refers to both the arachnoid **and** the pia. The widely used term **leptomeningeal metastases** (LMs) is technically incorrect, as it is employed to designate the imaging pattern seen when tumor involves the subarachnoid spaces and pia **(31-9)**.

Synonyms for LMs include meningeal carcinomatosis, neoplastic meningitis, and carcinomatous meningitis.

## Epidemiology and Etiology

LMs from **systemic cancers (31-8)** are rare, occurring in 5% of cases. The most common sources are breast and small cell lung cancers.

**Intracranial primary tumors** more commonly cause LM. In adults, the two most common are glioblastoma and lymphoma. The most common intracranial sources of childhood LM are medulloblastoma and other embryonal tumors, such as embryonal tumors with multilayered rosettes C19MC-altered, ependymoma, and germinoma.

## Imaging

**General Features.** LMs follow the brain surfaces, curving along gyri and dipping into the sulci. The general appearance on contrast-enhanced scans is as though the CSF "turns white" **(31-7)**.

**CT Findings.** NECT scans may be normal or show only mild hydrocephalus. Sulcal-cisternal enhancement, especially at the base of the brain, can sometimes be seen on CECT.

CECT scans may also be normal.

**MR Findings.** T1 scans may be normal or show only "dirty" CSF. Most LMs are hyperintense on T2WI and may be indistinguishable from normal CSF. Sulcal-cisternal hyperintensity on FLAIR is common **(31-24A) (31-26A)**. If tumor

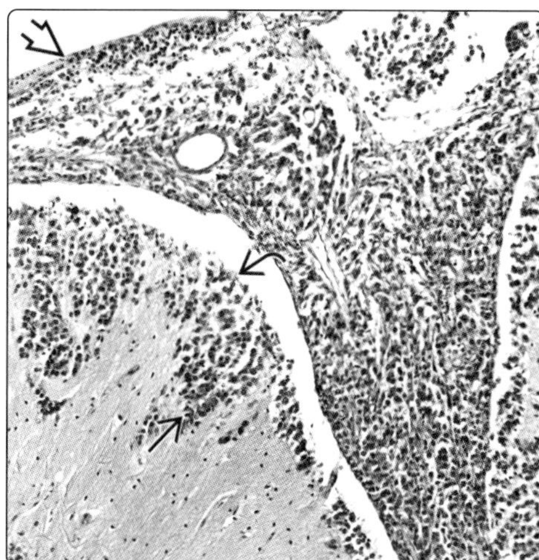

***(31-20)** Micrograph shows metastatic tumor in subarachnoid space ➮ infiltrating pia ➮ and extending into the cortex ➙. (From DP: Neuro.)*

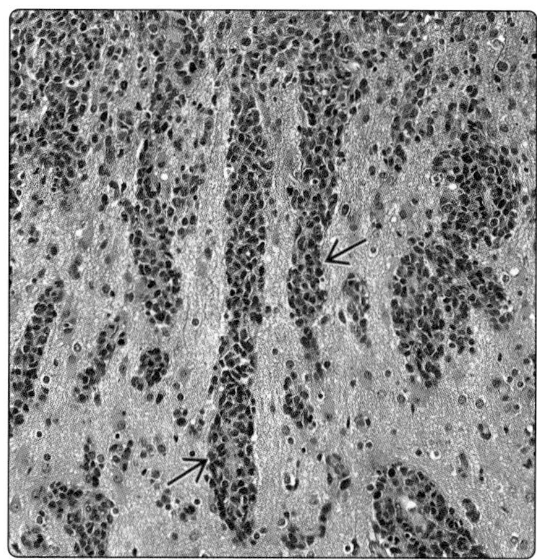

***(31-21)** Metastatic disease to the brain is shown with tumor cells infiltrating the parenchyma along the PVSs ➙. (From DP: Neuro.)*

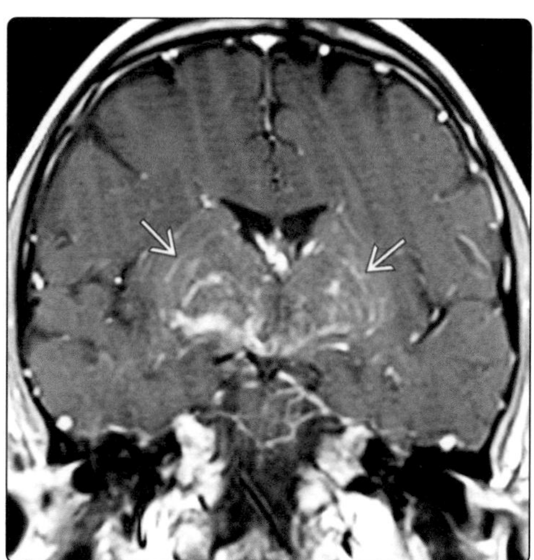

***(31-22)** Coronal T1 C+ MR in large B-cell lymphoma shows a tumor infiltrating along enlarged, enhancing PVSs ➡ in the basal ganglia.*

*(31-23) Graphic of CNS metastases from systemic cancers shows tumor in thickened dura-arachnoid ➡, sulci, and cisterns ➡. (31-24A) FLAIR MR in a patient with metastatic breast cancer shows hyperintensity in the sulci ➡ and pia around the sylvian fissures ➡.*

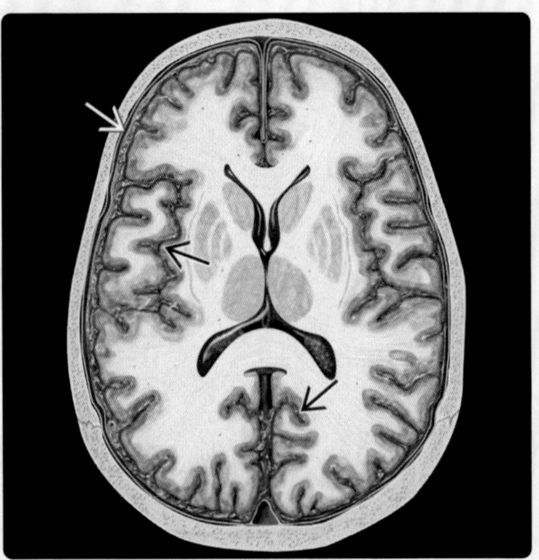

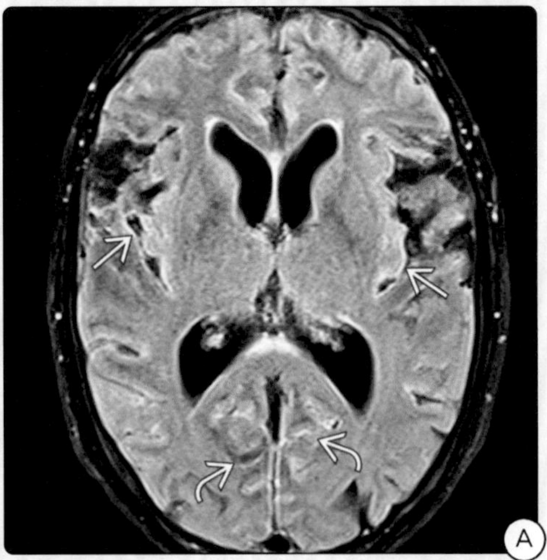

*(31-24B) T1 C+ FS MR in the same patient shows enhancing tumor coating the medulla ➡, cerebellar vermis ➡, and cranial nerves (CNs) IX-XI ➡. (31-24C) More cephalad T1 C+ MR shows enhancing metastases coating the midbrain ➡, vermis ➡, and filling the superficial sulci ➡.*

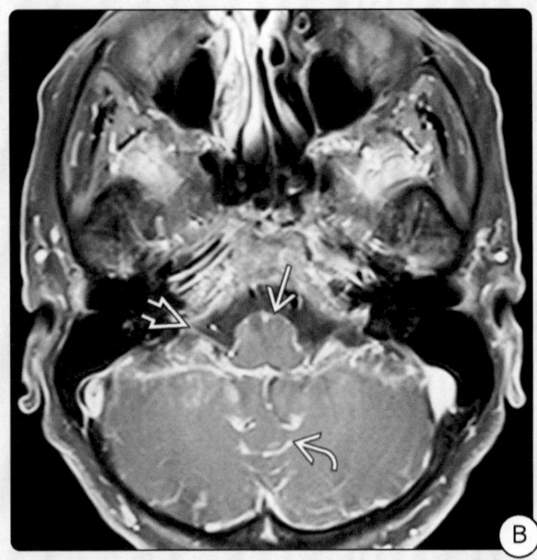

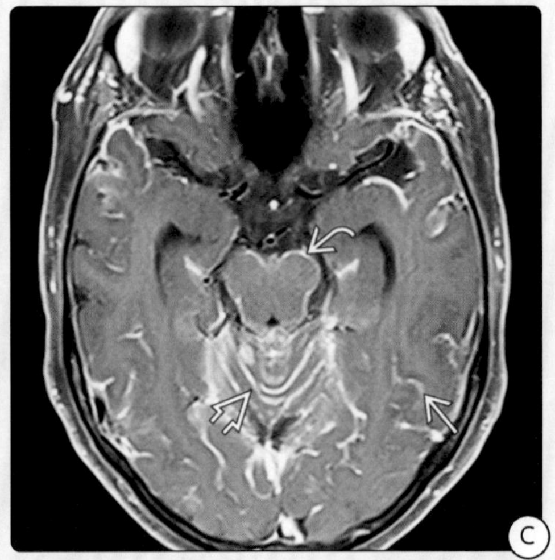

*(31-24D) T1 C+ FS MR shows the extensive nature of the pial metastases. (31-24E) T1 C+ FS MR through the ventricles shows the tumor coating the brain along the sylvian fissures and filling in numerous superficial sulci ➡. Note subtle dura-arachnid thickening over the left frontal lobe ➡.*

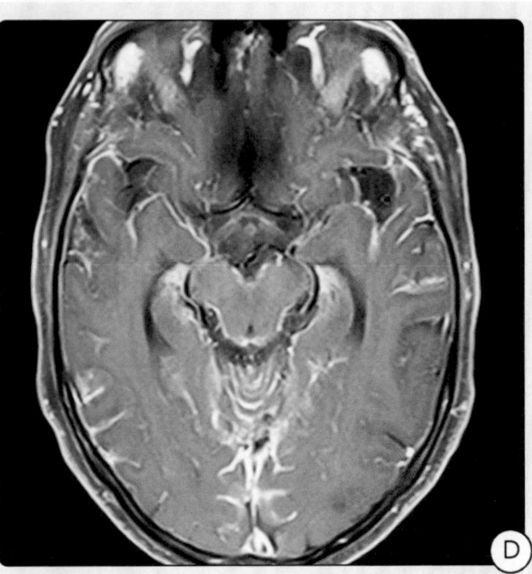

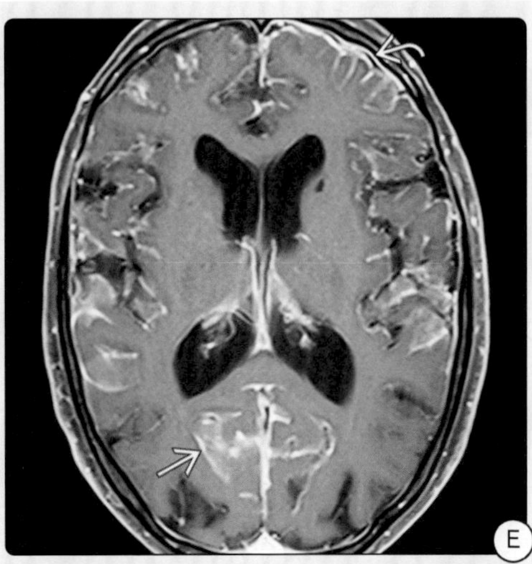

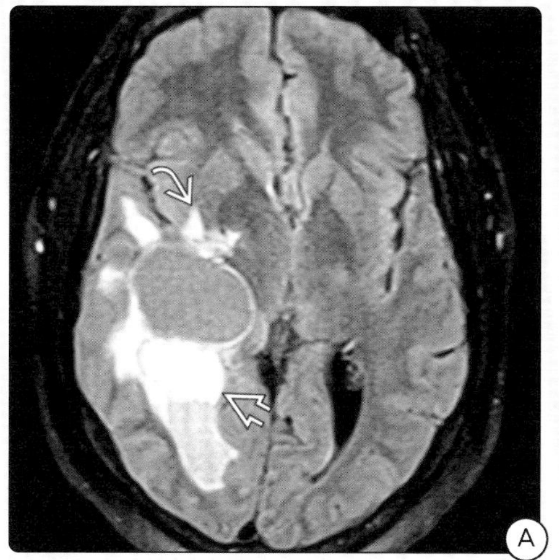

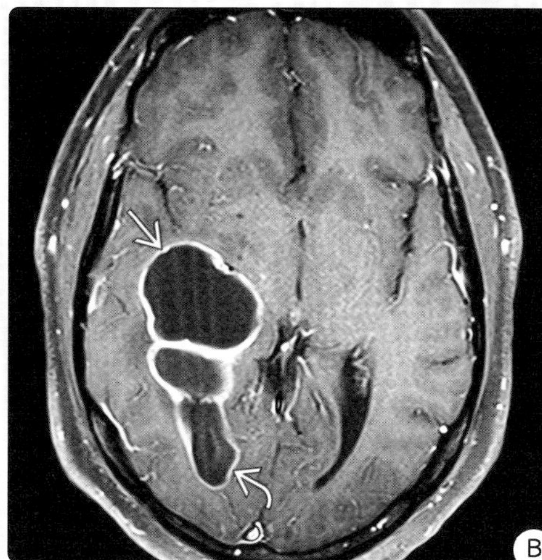

***(31-25A)** Axial FLAIR MR in a 39-year-old man with metastatic adnexal skin cancer shows an unusual multicystic, iso- and hyperintense mass ➡ in the right lateral ventricle with surrounding vasogenic edema ➡. **(31-25B)** T1 C+ FS MR in the same patient shows the walls of the cystic intraventricular metastasis enhancing strongly ➡. Note entrapment and enlargement of the right atrium with ependymal enhancement ➡.*

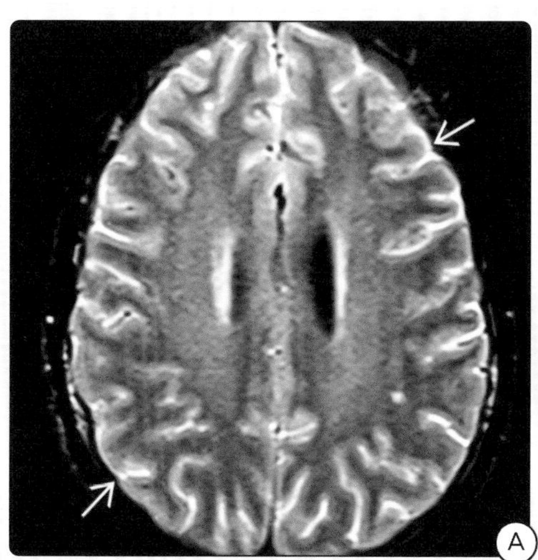

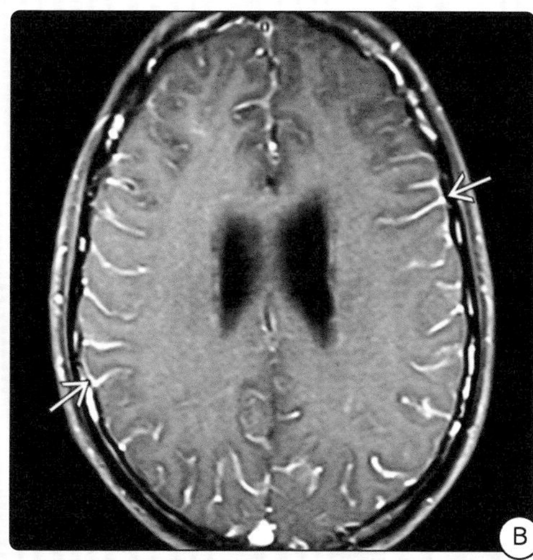

***(31-26A)** Axial FLAIR MR in a patient with metastatic melanoma shows diffuse hyperintensity in all the visible sulci ➡. **(31-26B)** T1 C+ FS MR shows widespread sulcal enhancement ➡ from leptomeningeal carcinomatosis.*

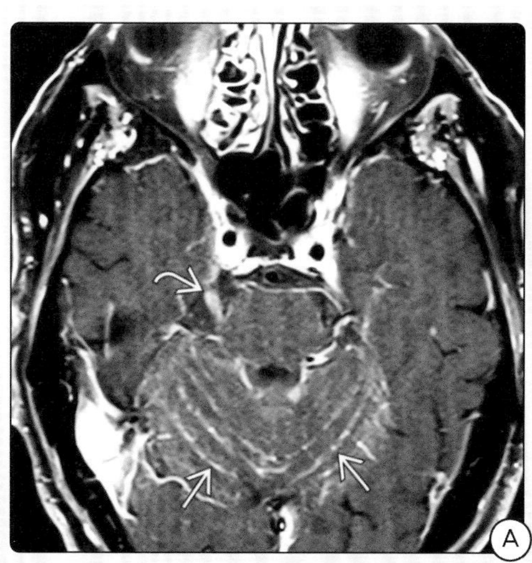

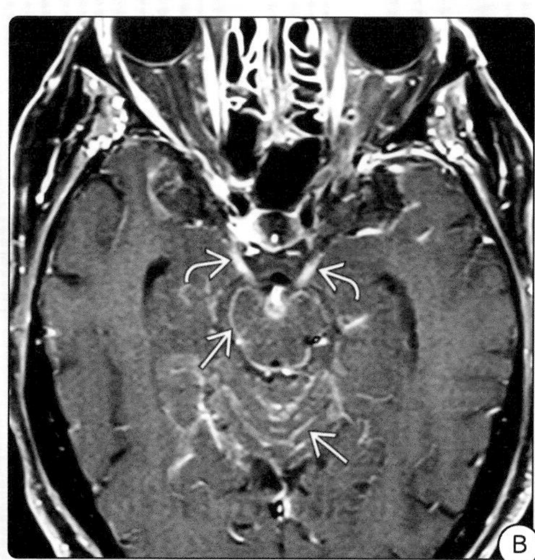

***(31-27A)** Axial T1 C+ FS MR in a patient with a known primary large B-cell lymphoma and multiple CN palsies shows diffuse sulcal-cisternal enhancement along the cerebellar hemispheres ➡. The right trigeminal nerve is thickened and enhancing ➡. **(31-27B)** More cephalad T1 C+ FS MR shows diffuse leptomeningeal/pial enhancement ➡ and thickening and enhancement of both oculomotor nerves ➡.*

has extended from the pia into the perivascular spaces, underlying brain parenchyma may show hyperintense vasogenic edema **(31-18)**.

Postcontrast T1 scans show meningitis-like findings. Smooth or nodular enhancement seems to coat the brain surface, filling the sulci **(31-26B)** and sometimes almost the entire subarachnoid space, including the thecal sac **(31-24)**. Cranial nerve thickening with linear, nodular, or focal mass-like enhancement may occur with or without disseminated disease **(31-27)**.

Tiny enhancing miliary nodules or linear enhancing foci in the cortex and subcortical white matter indicate extension along the penetrating perivascular spaces **(31-22)**.

### Differential Diagnosis

The major differential diagnosis of LMs is **infectious meningitis**. It may be difficult or impossible to distinguish between carcinomatous and infectious meningitis on the basis of imaging findings alone. Other diagnostic considerations include **neurosarcoid**. Clinical history and laboratory features are essential elements in establishing the correct diagnosis.

**LEPTOMENINGEAL METASTASES**

**General Features**
- Pia + subarachnoid space metastases
- Uncommon
  - 5% of systemic cancers
  - More common with primary tumors (e.g., glioblastoma, medulloblastoma, germinoma)

**CT**
- NECT: May be normal ± mild hydrocephalus
- CECT: Sulcal-cisternal enhancement (looks like pyogenic meningitis)

**MR**
- T1WI: Normal or "dirty" CSF
- T2WI: Usually normal
- FLAIR: Sulcal-cisternal hyperintensity (nonspecific)
- T1 C+: Sulcal-cisternal enhancement (nonspecific)

**Differential Diagnosis**
- Meningitis
- Neurosarcoid

## Miscellaneous Metastases

Several "secret" sites may also harbor metastases. The ventricles and choroid plexus, pituitary gland/infundibular stalk, pineal gland, and eye are less obvious places where intracranial metastases occur and may escape detection.

### CSF Metastases

Both extra- and intracranial metastases can seed the CSF. Intracranial CSF metastases are usually seen as "dirty" CSF on T1WI and FLAIR **(31-26)**, often occurring together with diffuse pial spread. "Drop metastases" into the spinal subarachnoid space are a manifestation of generalized CSF spread.

Ependymal spread around the ventricular walls occurs with primary CNS tumors much more often than with extracranial sources **(31-25)**.

### Ventricles/Choroid Plexus Metastases

The lateral ventricle choroid plexus is the most common site for ventricular metastases followed by the third ventricle **(31-32)**. Only 0.5% of ventricular metastases occur in the fourth ventricle. Solitary choroid plexus metastases **(31-30)** are more common than multiple lesions.

Choroid plexus metastases enlarge the choroid plexus and are iso- to hyperdense compared with normal choroid plexus on NECT scans. They enhance strongly but heterogeneously on CECT and T1 C+ **(31-28)**.

Most nonhemorrhagic choroid plexus metastases are hypointense to brain on T1WI and hyperintense on T2/FLAIR. Intense enhancement following contrast administration is typical.

In an older patient (especially one with known systemic cancer, such as renal cell carcinoma), the differential diagnosis of a choroid plexus mass should always include metastasis. Other common choroid plexus lesions in older patients are **meningioma** and **choroid plexus xanthogranuloma**. Choroid plexus meningiomas enhance strongly and generally uniformly. Choroid plexus cysts (xanthogranulomas) are usually bilateral, multicystic-appearing lesions.

### Pituitary Gland/Infundibular Stalk Metastases

Metastasis causes ~ 1% of all pituitary tumors and is found in 1-2% of autopsies. Breast and lung primaries account for 2/3 of cases.

Most pituitary metastases involve the posterior lobe, probably because of its direct systemic arterial supply via the hypophyseal arteries. Coexisting BMs are common, but solitary lesions do occur.

A sellar mass with or without bone erosion, stalk thickening, loss of posterior pituitary "bright spot," and cavernous sinus invasion is typical but nonspecific. An infiltrating, enhancing pituitary &/or stalk mass is the most common finding **(31-28)**.

The major differential diagnosis of pituitary metastasis is **macroadenoma**. Macroadenomas rarely present with diabetes insipidus. In the setting of a known systemic cancer, rapid growth of a pituitary mass with onset of clinical diabetes insipidus is highly suggestive but certainly not diagnostic of metastasis. **Lymphocytic hypophysitis** can also resemble pituitary metastasis on imaging studies.

### Pineal Gland Metastases

Although the pineal gland is a relatively common source of primary CNS tumors that seed the CSF, it is one of the rarest sites to harbor a metastasis. Only 0.3% of intracranial metastases involve the pineal gland. Lung, breast, skin (melanoma), and kidney are the most frequent sources. When pineal metastases do occur, they are usually solitary lesions

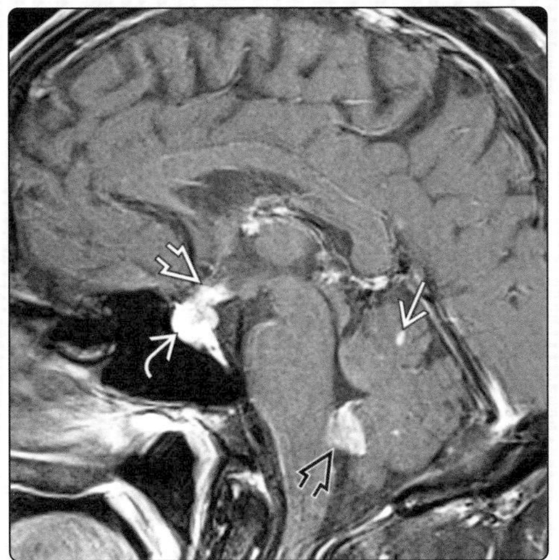

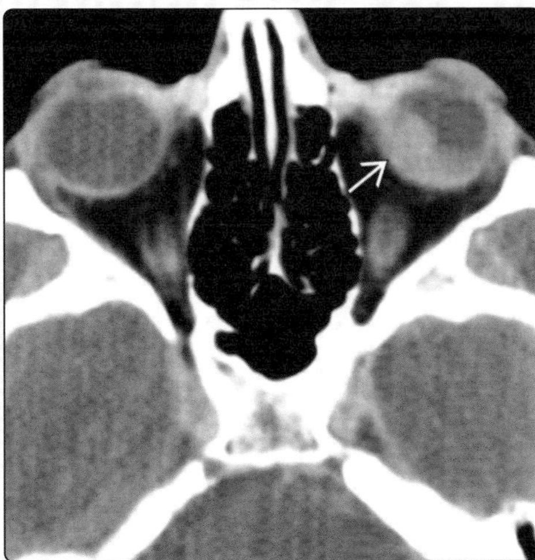

*(31-28) T1 C+ FS MR shows metastases to pituitary gland/stalk ➩, 3rd ventricle ➩, 4th ventricle choroid plexus ➩, and vermian folia ➩. (31-29) CECT shows a lobulated enhancing mass in the posterior segment of the left globe ➩. This is metastatic breast carcinoma.*

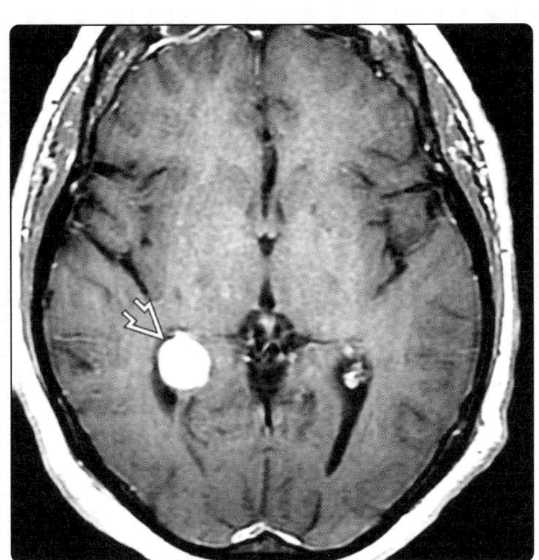

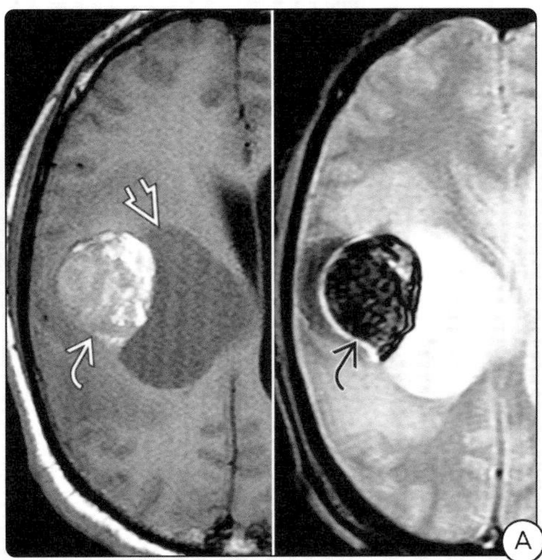

*(31-30) T1 C+ FS MR in a patient with headaches shows an enhancing mass ➩ in the atrium of the right lateral ventricle. Preoperative diagnosis was meningioma. Solitary metastasis from an unsuspected lung carcinoma. (31-31A) (L) T1WI in a patient with melanoma and left hemiplegia shows a cystic mass ➩ with a mixed hyper- and isointense mural nodule ➩. (R) T2* GRE shows striking gradient blooming ➩, consistent with hemorrhage.*

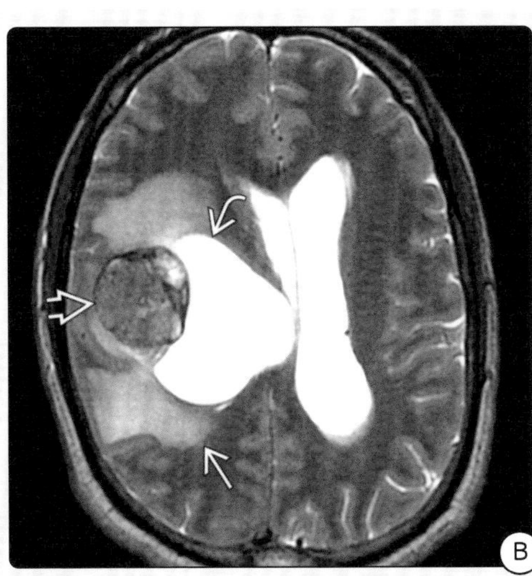

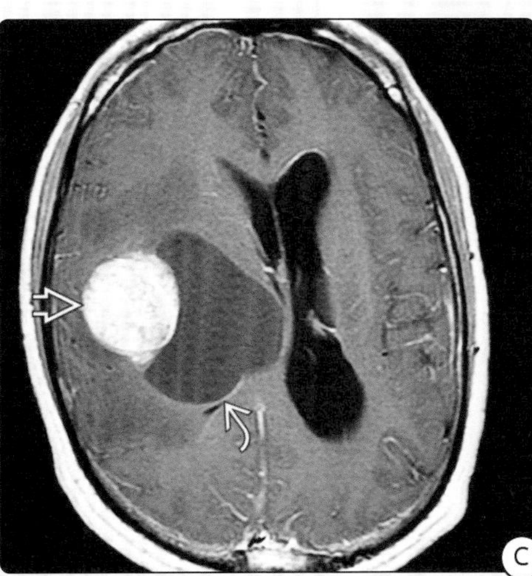

*(31-31B) T2 FS MR in the same patient shows a cystic mass in the right hemisphere ➩ with a mixed iso- and very hypointense nodule ➩ and moderate parenchymal edema ➩. (31-31C) T1 C+ FS MR shows the nodule of the cyst enhances intensely ➩. Note subtle enhancement of the associated cyst wall ➩. No other lesions were identified. This is cystic melanoma metastasis.*

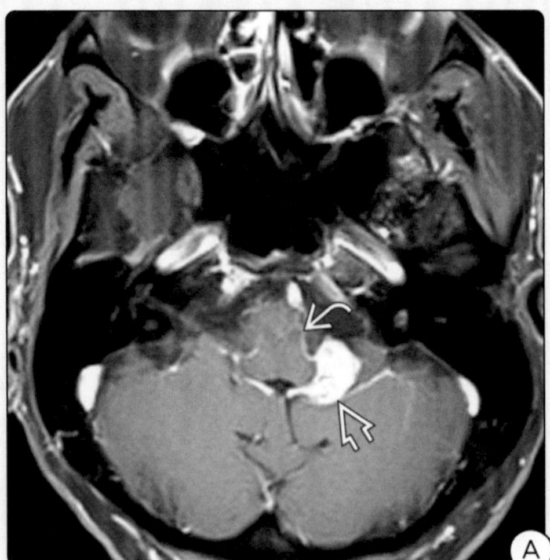

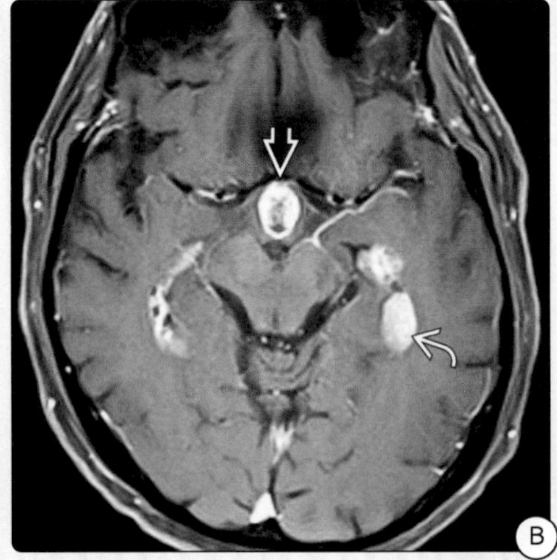

***(31-32A)*** *Axial T1 C+ FS MR in a patient with melanoma shows metastasis to the choroid plexus in the left lateral recess of the 4th ventricle ➡ and pial surface of the medulla ➡.* ***(31-32B)*** *More cephalad T1 C+ FS MR shows metastasis to the pituitary stalk, infundibulum, and hypothalamus ➡ as well as the choroid plexus ➡ of the left lateral ventricle.*

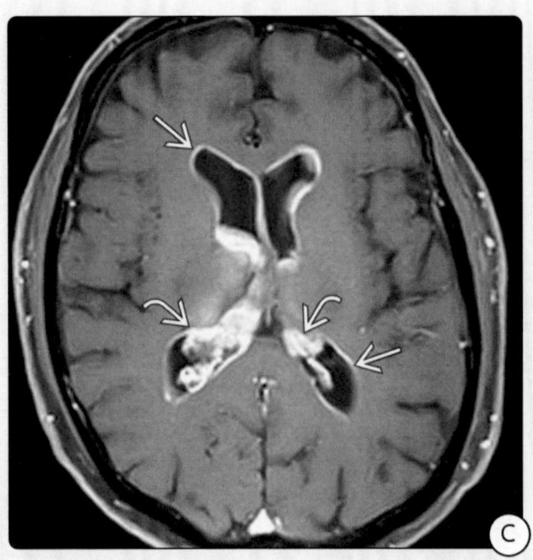

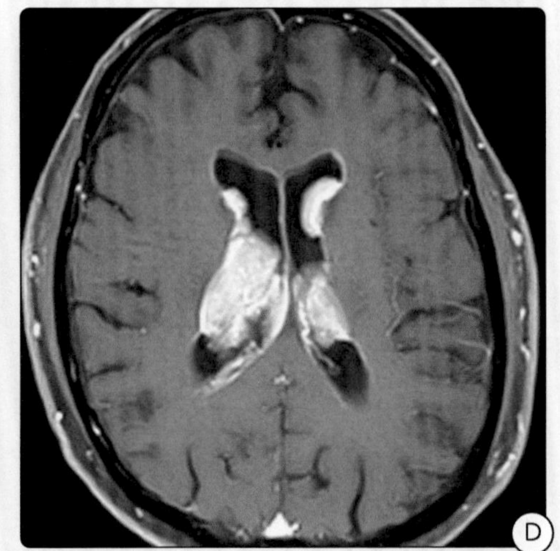

***(31-32C)*** *More cephalad T1 C+ MR shows extensive metastases to the choroid plexi ➡ and ventricular ependyma ➡.* ***(31-32D)*** *T1 C+ FS MR through the bodies of the lateral ventricle shows extensive ependymal, choroid plexus metastases from the patient's known melanoma.*

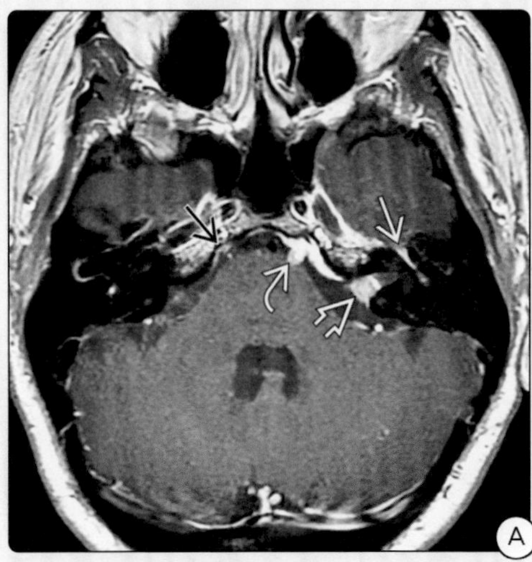

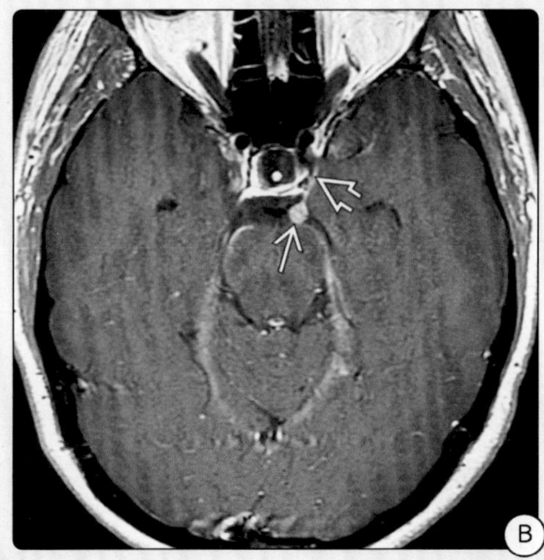

***(31-33A)*** *Axial T1 C+ FS MR with known invasive squamous cell carcinoma and multiple CN palsies shows dural metastasis with involvement of the left CNVI ➡. Very subtle enhancement of the right CNVI and Dorello canal is present ➡. Note metastasis to the left IAC ➡ and facial nerve ➡.* ***(31-33B)*** *More cephalad T1 C+ FS MR shows focal metastasis to the left CNIII ➡. Note diffuse enhancement of CNIII in the oculomotor cistern ➡.*

without evidence of metastatic deposits elsewhere and are indistinguishable on imaging studies from primary pineal neoplasms.

## Ocular Metastases

Metastases to the eye are rare. The highly vascular choroid is, by far, the most commonly affected site, accounting for nearly 90% of all ocular metastases. Breast cancer is the most common cause of ocular metastases followed by lung cancer.

CT and MR findings are nonspecific, demonstrating a posterior segment mass that often enhances strongly after contrast administration **(31-29)**. Whole-brain imaging is recommended, as 20-25% of patients with choroidal metastases have concurrent CNS lesions.

The differential diagnosis of choroidal metastasis includes other hyperdense posterior segment masses. Primary **choroidal melanoma** and **hemangioma** may appear similar on both CT and MR. Melanoma and metastases may also incite **hemorrhagic choroidal** or **retinal detachment**.

## Perineural Metastases

Perineural tumor (PNT) spread is defined as the extension of malignant tumor along neural sheaths. Squamous cell carcinoma (SCCa) and major/minor salivary gland malignancies, such as adenoid cystic carcinoma, are all prone to PNT spread **(31-33)**. Other tumors, such as non-Hodgkin lymphoma, also frequently spread along major nerve sheaths. Perineural invasion occurs in 2-6% of cutaneous head and neck basal carcinomas and SCCas.

The most common nerves to be affected by PNT are the maxillary division of the trigeminal nerve (CNV2) **(31-27A)** and the facial nerve (CNVII) **(31-33A)**.

Tubular enlargement and enhancement of the affected nerve together with widening of its bony canal or foramen is typical.

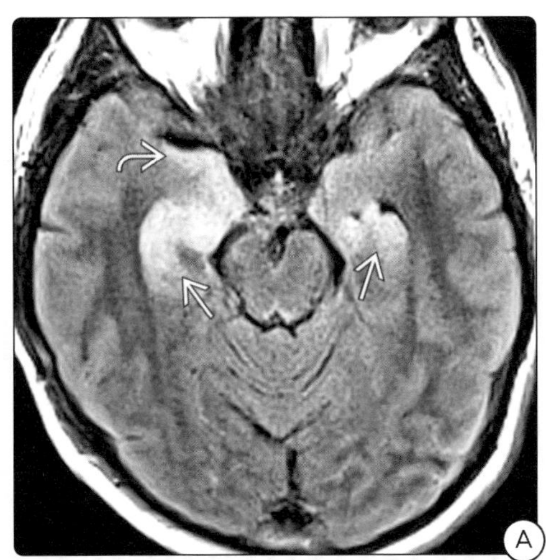


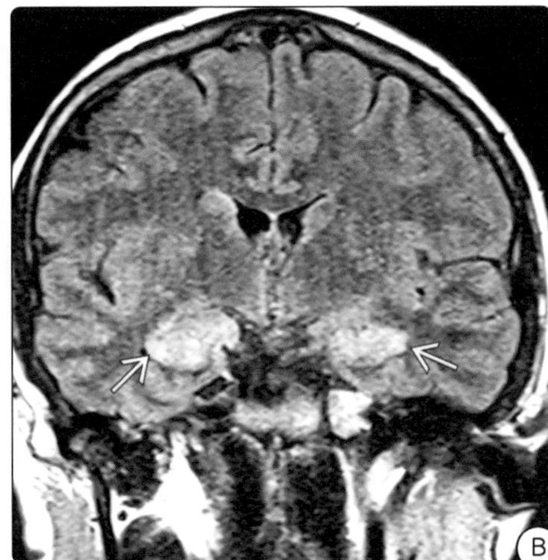


***(31-34A)** FLAIR MR in a 24-year-old man with progressive behavioral changes, altered mental status, and then seizure shows hyperintensity in the right medial temporal lobe cortex ↷ as well as both hippocampi ➔. **(31-34B)** Coronal FLAIR MR in the same patient shows that both hippocampi are swollen and hyperintense ➔.*

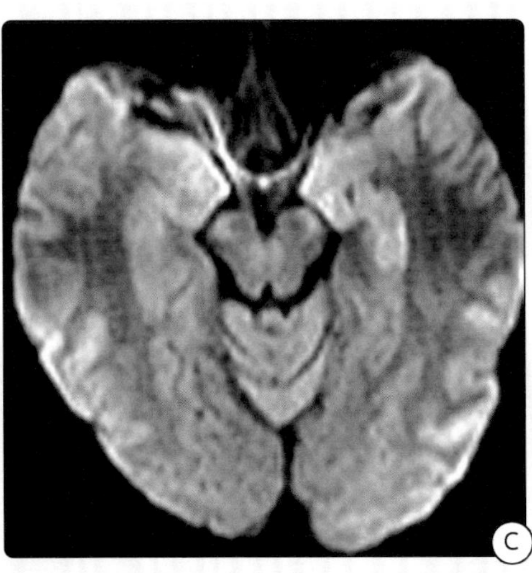


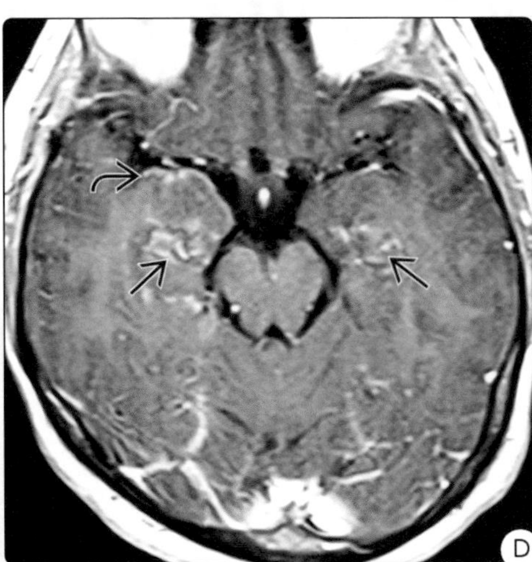


***(31-34C)** DWI MR shows no evidence for restricted diffusion to suggest herpes encephalitis or seizure. **(31-34D)** T1 C+ MR shows patchy enhancement in both hippocampi ➔ and the right temporal lobe cortex ↷. Chest x-ray disclosed an anterior mediastinal mass. Biopsy showed Hodgkin lymphoma. This is paraneoplastic limbic encephalitis.*

If the nerve passes through a structure, such as the pterygopalatine fossa that is normally filled with fat, the fat becomes "dirty" or effaced. *Look for denervation atrophy*—common with CNV3 lesions—seen as small, shrunken muscles of mastication with fatty infiltration.

# Paraneoplastic Syndromes

We close this chapter with a brief discussion of remote effects of cancer with an immune-mediated pathogenesis. These cancer-induced remote neurologic effects are collectively called **paraneoplastic neurologic syndromes** (PNSs). Here, neurologic signs and symptoms are associated with malignancy **but** are neither explained by nor related to direct (local or metastatic) tumor invasion, adverse effects of chemotherapy, malnutrition, or infection. Instead, PNSs are secondary to an immune response triggered by the underlying tumor, which affects the central or peripheral nervous system.

PNSs are defined as neurologic disorders that (1) can affect any part of the nervous system (often with stereotyped clinical manifestations), (2) occur in association with cancer, and (3) have an immune-mediated pathogenesis supported by the frequent presence of specific neuronal antibodies.

In paraneoplastic syndromes, extra-CNS tumors exert their adverse influence on the brain, not via metastasis but indirectly. Neural antigens are ectopically expressed by tumor, and the immune attack is directed at the CNS or PNS.

PNSs are rare, affecting < 1% of all patients with systemic cancer. In most cases, a paraneoplastic syndrome is diagnosed only after other etiologies—primarily metastatic disease—have been excluded. However, in 70% of patients with PNSs, neurologic symptoms are the **first** manifestation of a tumor.

PNSs may involve any part of the CNS (brain, spinal cord) or peripheral nervous system, although the temporal lobes seem

***(31-35A)** Baseline sagittal T1 MP-RAGE in a 53-year-old woman with breast cancer is normal. **(31-35B)** Five months later, the patient developed progressive ataxia. Sagittal MP-RAGE shows interval development of gross cerebellar atrophy ➲.*

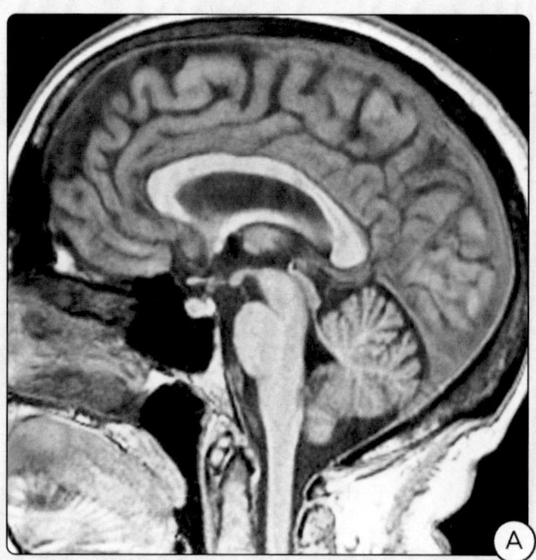


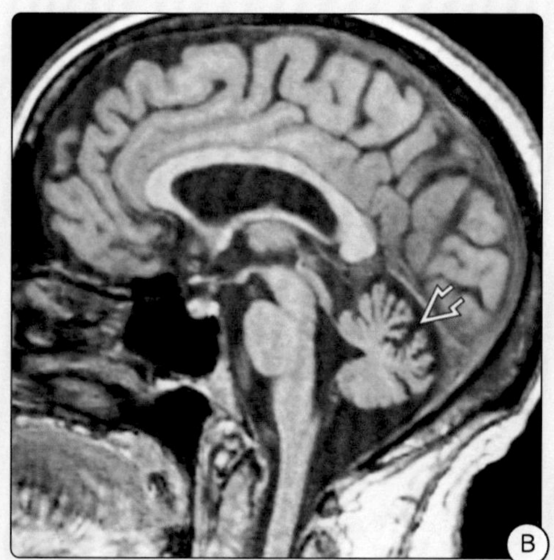


***(31-35C)** Axial T2 MR shows marked enlargement of the 4th ventricle ➲ together with gross atrophy of the cerebellar hemispheres ➲. The pons appears normal. **(31-35D)** Coronal T1 C+ MR shows the grossly enlarged 4th ventricle ➲ and cerebellar atrophy ➲. No metastases were identified. This is paraneoplastic cerebellar degeneration/encephalitis (a.k.a. cerebellar paraneoplastic disease).*

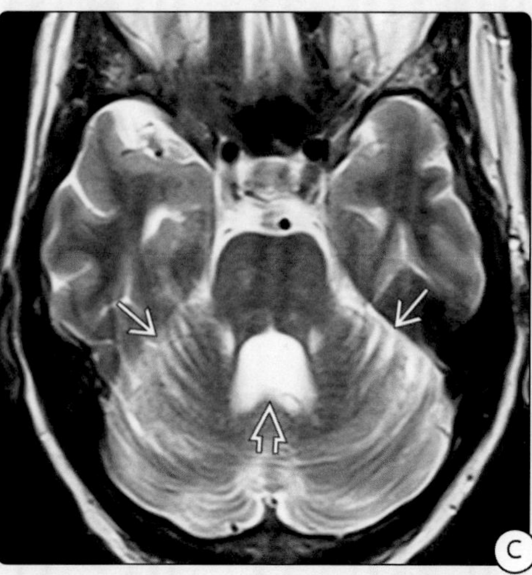


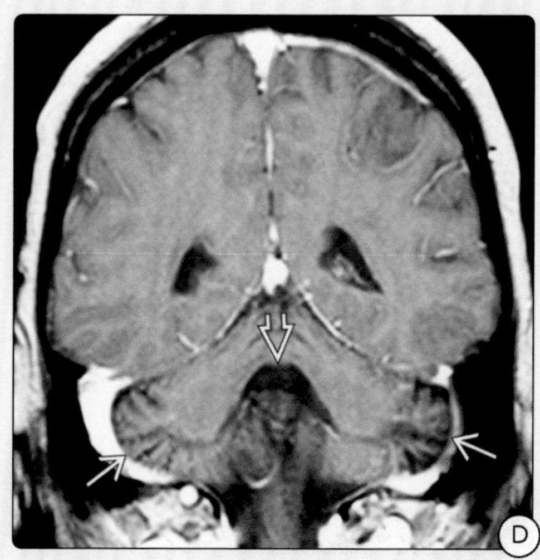

to be the most favored site, and paraneoplastic limbic encephalitis is the most common PNS. **Keep in mind that the major clinical and imaging findings in all the autoimmune encephalitides—including PNSs—are often nonspecific and demonstrate considerable overlap between the different subtypes as well as various other infectious, inflammatory, or toxic-metabolic encephalitides.**

In 2020, an imaging-based review of PNSs classified them by anatomic location: Limbic encephalitis, paraneoplastic cerebellar degeneration, brainstem encephalitis, cranial neuropathy, myelitis, and polyneuropathy.

In 2021, a group of international experts revised the diagnostic criteria of PNSs, identifying seven phenotypes with the presence of "high-risk" antibodies (i.e., > 70% are associated with cancer): Encephalomyelitis, limbic encephalitis, rapidly progressive cerebellar syndrome, opsoclonus-myoclonus, sensory neuropathy, gastrointestinal pseudoobstruction (enteric neuropathy), and Lambert-Eaton myasthenic syndrome.

We will briefly discuss the most common of these "high-risk" disorders in which imaging may play a central role in diagnosis and conclude the chapter with a brief synopsis of conditions with well-defined diagnostic criteria that are less frequently associated with systemic cancers (so-called **intermediate-risk** phenotypes).

## Encephalomyelitis

The term **encephalomyelitis** (EM) is used only in patients with clinical manifestations at multiple sites, including peripheral involvement, such as dorsal root ganglia, peripheral nerve/nerve roots. EM is almost always associated with small cell lung cancer with anti-Hu or CV2 antibodies.

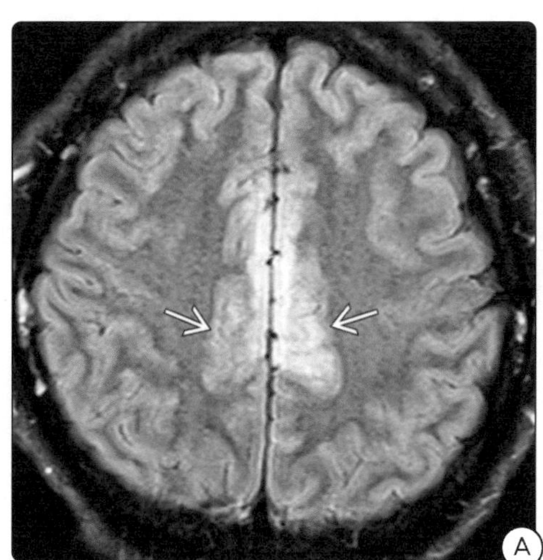


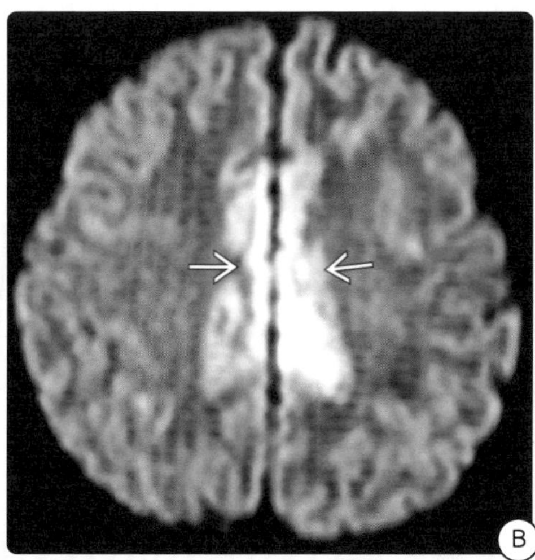


***(31-36A)** A 25-year-old man presented to the ED with altered mental status. Head CT was normal. Axial FLAIR MR shows hyperintensity in both cingulate gyri ➡. **(31-36B)** The cingulate gyri show restricted diffusion ➡ on DWI MR.*

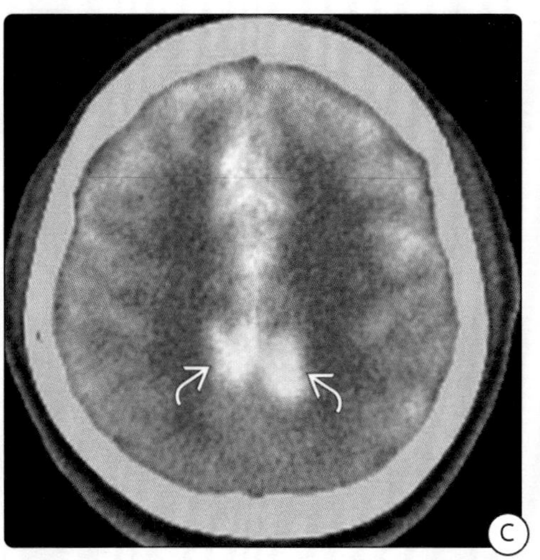


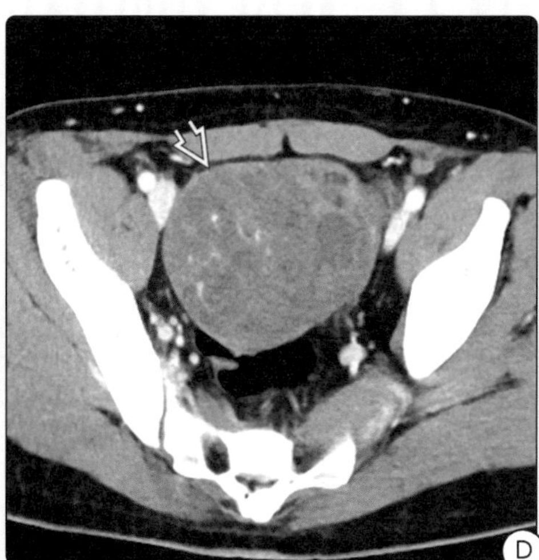


***(31-36C)** Axial PET/CT shows striking hypermetabolism in the cingulate gyri ➡. A pelvic mass was also identified on the study. **(31-36D)** CT shows a mixed-density mass ➡ in the pelvis. Surgery disclosed carcinoma in an undescended testicle. Paraneoplastic encephalitis in the cingulate gyri, part of the limbic system, was confirmed by finding anti-Ma autoantibodies in the CSF.*

## Limbic Encephalitis

One of the most common PNSs is limbic encephalitis (LE). There are multiple variants of LE. LE is a heterogeneous group of immune-mediated disorders that also includes **non**paraneoplastic autoimmune encephalitides, such as anti-GAD and LGI1 encephalitis. The neurologic presentation of paraneoplastic and nonparaneoplastic cases can be clinically indistinguishable. Nonparaneoplastic autoimmune encephalitides were discussed in Chapter 15.

### Terminology

By definition, paraneoplastic LE (PLE) is a limbic system disorder. The medial temporal lobes are preferentially involved, but the inferior frontal region, insular cortex, and cingulate gyrus can also be affected.

### Etiology

The most frequent neoplasm associated with PLE is small cell lung cancer identified in ~ 1/2 of all cases. Other associated tumors include testicular neoplasms (20%) **(31-36)**, breast carcinoma (8%), thymoma, and lymphoma.

Antineuronal antibodies are frequently but not invariably found in the CSF or serum of patients with PLE. The most common is the anti-Hu antibody, which is present in ~ 1/2 of the patients with small cell lung cancer-associated PLE. Anti-Ma2 PLE is associated with testicular germ cell tumors. Keep in mind that multiple autoantibodies may be produced in response to malignancy, and overlapping of clinical presentations may occur.

Other neuronal autoantibodies include anti-Ri (breast, small cell lung cancer), anti-Yo (ovarian, breast), and anti-Ma2 (testicular germ cell cancer). These often affect the brainstem (midbrain, pons, medulla) either in isolation or as part of a more widespread autoantibody-mediated encephalitis.

### Clinical Issues

The presence of onconeuronal antibodies, such as anti-Hu and anti-Ma2, almost always occurs in adults. Neurologic symptoms often precede identification of the inciting tumor by weeks or months. Confusion and short-term memory loss with relative preservation of other cognitive functions—with or without mood and behavioral changes—are typical. Complex partial seizures are common.

Misdiagnoses are common, so CSF and serum testing for autoantibodies should be performed. A positive serum result for antibodies against neuronal surface proteins mandates the confirmation of antibodies in the CSF, as the risk for clinical misdiagnosis of autoimmune encephalitis dramatically increases if the CSF status is negative or unknown.

### Imaging

MR is the procedure of choice in diagnosing PLE. T2/FLAIR shows hyperintensity in one or both medial temporal lobes. Enhancement is variable **(31-34)**.

### Differential Diagnosis

The major differential diagnosis of PLE is **herpes encephalitis**. Other causes of LE that can mimic PLE include **glutamic acid decarboxylase 65 (GAD65) autoantibody-associated LE**, **posttransplant acute LE** (PALE) syndrome, and **human herpesvirus 6 (HHV-6) encephalitis**.

HHV-6 encephalitis is associated with hematologic malignancies, such as Hodgkin and angioimmunoblastic T-cell lymphoma and leukemia.

## Rapidly Progressive Cerebellar Syndrome

This disorder, previously known as subacute cerebellar degeneration, is characterized by a rapidly progressive cerebellar syndrome without substantial cerebellar atrophy at early stages of the disease. Most patients rapidly develop a severe, bilateral cerebellar syndrome with gait ataxia, with or without truncal and limb involvement later. Unlike LE, specific antibodies suggestive of the diagnosis (e.g., anti-Yo) are often not identified.

Initial imaging early in the disease may be normal followed by rapid onset of cerebellar atrophy **(31-35)**. Rare cases with a hot cross bun sign (erroneously considered specific for multiple system atrophy with cerebellar features) causing paraneoplastic cerebellar ataxia have been reported.

## Miscellaneous Phenotypes

"Intermediate-risk" antibody-related phenotypes are neurologic disorders that can occur with or without cancer (30-70% associated with cancer). Conditions with well-defined diagnostic criteria but rare/unusual oncologic associations include anti-NMDAR encephalitis (ovarian teratomas), anti-GABA R encephalitis (older male smokers), and brainstem encephalitis with anti-Ma2 antibodies (testicular tumors or NSCLC).

Lower risk antibodies (< 30% associated with cancer) can cause phenotypes, such as stiff-person syndrome (anti-GAD65) and Morvan syndrome (malignant thymoma with LGI1 and CASPR2 antibodies).

*Selected References: The complete reference list is available on the eBooks+ version included with purchase.*

# Nonneoplastic Cysts

*There are many types of intracranial cysts. Some are incidental and of no significance. Others may cause serious—even life-threatening—symptoms.*



In this chapter, we consider a number of different intracranial cysts: Cystic-appearing anatomic variants that can be mistaken for disease, congenital/developmental cysts, and a variety of miscellaneous cysts. Parasitic cysts, cystic brain malformations, and cystic neoplasms are excluded as they are discussed in their respective chapters.

While there are many different ways to classify cysts, an **imaging-based** approach to classification of intracranial cysts is the most practical, as most of these lesions are discovered on CT or MR examination.

An imaging-based approach takes into account three easily defined features: (1) Anatomic location, (2) imaging characteristics (i.e., density/signal intensity of the contents, presence/absence of calcification &/or enhancement), and (3) patient age. Of these three, anatomic location is the most helpful.

While many types of intracranial cysts occur in more than one location, some sites are "preferred" by certain cysts. In this chapter, we discuss cysts by location from the outside in, beginning with scalp and intracranial extraaxial cysts before turning our attention to intraaxial (parenchymal and intraventricular) cysts.

The following are four key anatomy-based questions to consider about a cystic-appearing intracranial lesion. A summary chart based on these simple questions, together with the cysts discussed throughout the text, is also included **(Table 32-1)**.

**4 KEY ANATOMY-BASED QUESTIONS**

- Is the cyst extra- or intraaxial?
- Is the cyst supra- or infratentorial?
- If the cyst is extraaxial, is it midline or off-midline?
- If the cyst is intraaxial, is it in the brain parenchyma or inside the ventricles?

# Scalp Cysts

Nonneoplastic scalp cysts are sometimes identified on imaging studies intended to visualize intracranial structures. The most common incidental scalp masses in adults are epidermoid cysts (50%), trichilemmal ("sebaceous") cysts (40%), and dermoid cysts (10-20%). Epidermoid and dermoid cysts are discussed later in this chapter. We discuss trichilemmal (pilar or "sebaceous") cysts of the scalp here.

## Intracranial Cystic-Appearing Lesions

| | Supratentorial | Infratentorial |
|---|---|---|
| **Extraaxial** | | |
| Midline | Pineal cyst<br>Dermoid cyst<br>Rathke cleft cyst<br>Arachnoid cyst (suprasellar) | Neurenteric cyst<br>Arachnoid cyst (retrocerebellar) |
| Off-midline | Arachnoid cyst (middle cranial fossa, convexity)<br>Epidermoid cyst<br>Tumor-associated cyst<br>Trichilemmal ("sebaceous") cyst (scalp)<br>Leptomeningeal cyst ("growing fracture") | Epidermoid cyst (CPA)<br>Arachnoid cyst (CPA)<br>Tumor-associated cyst |
| **Intraaxial** | | |
| Parenchymal | Enlarged perivascular spaces<br>Neuroglial cyst<br>Porencephalic cyst<br>Hippocampal sulcus remnants | Enlarged perivascular spaces (dentate nuclei) |
| Intraventricular | Choroid plexus cyst<br>Colloid cyst<br>Choroid fissure cyst<br>Ependymal cyst | Epidermoid cyst (4th ventricle, cisterna magna)<br>Cystic ("trapped") 4th ventricle |

***(Table 32-1)*** *CPA = cerebellopontine angle. Rathke cleft cyst and cystic/trapped 4th ventricle are discussed in chapters 30, and 38, respectively. Other entities listed in the table are considered here.*

# Trichilemmal ("Sebaceous") Cyst

## Terminology

Although the term "sebaceous cyst" is commonly used by radiologists, this type of cyst does not actually contain sebaceous material. These cysts are more accurately called **trichilemmal cysts** (TCs) or pilar cysts.

## Etiology

TCs are derived from the outer root sheath of hair follicles, not sebaceous glands.

## Pathology

**Location, Size, and Number.** Most TCs are found within the dermis or subcutaneous tissue. TCs can be single or multiple and vary in size from a few millimeters to several centimeters in diameter.

**Gross and Microscopic Features.** TCs are oval/round (75%) or lobulated (25%) and consist of a fibrous capsule lined by stratified squamous epithelium. Cyst contents consist of waxy desquamated keratin without a granular layer.

## Clinical Issues

**Demographics.** TCs affect 5-10% of the population. Although they can occur at any age, most are found in middle-aged and older women.

**Presentation and Natural History.** TCs generally appear as hairless, mobile, slightly compressible subcutaneous scalp masses.

TCs grow slowly and have often been present for years. Up to 2% of TCs give rise to a proliferating trichilemmal tumor known as pilar or "turban" tumors. Rarely, TCs can become locally aggressive and even invade bone. Malignant degeneration ("proliferating trichilemmal cystic carcinoma") is extremely rare.

## Imaging

**CT Findings.** TCs are generally sharply delineated solid, cystic, or mixed solid/cystic masses that are heterogeneously hyperdense compared with subcutaneous fat. Calcification is seen in 80% of cases and can appear as punctate, curvilinear, or coarsely clumped aggregations **(32-1A)**.

Soft tissue density and hyperdense foci are common. Typical TCs do not enhance. Calvarial remodeling or invasion is absent.

**MR Findings.** TCs are well-circumscribed scalp masses that appear incompletely surrounded by fat. They are generally homogeneously iso- to mildly hyperintense relative to brain on T1WI and inhomogeneously hypointense on T2WI and FLAIR **(32-1)**. TCs do not suppress on FLAIR.

"Blooming" foci on T2* (GRE, SWI) are caused by calcifications, not hemorrhage. Simple, uncomplicated TCs do not enhance, although the proliferating variant may show significant enhancement with solid lobules interspersed with nonenhancing cystic foci.

## Differential Diagnosis

In adults, the imaging differential diagnoses are benign and malignant scalp tumors. **Basal cell carcinomas** and **scalp metastases** are ill-defined, poorly delineated scalp masses that invade the subcutaneous soft tissues and may erode bone. Superficial ulceration is common. **Dermoid** and **epidermoid cysts** as well as **hemangiomas** are all much more common in the skull than in the scalp.

# Extraaxial Cysts

Extraaxial cysts lie between the skull and brain. With few exceptions, most are contained within the arachnoid membrane or in the subarachnoid space.

Determining sublocation of an extraaxial cyst (supra- vs. infratentorial, midline vs. off-midline) is helpful in establishing a meaningful differential diagnosis **(Table 32-1)**. For example, an arachnoid cyst is the only type that commonly occurs in the posterior fossa. Some extraaxial cysts are usually (although not invariably) off-midline. Others—pineal and Rathke cleft cysts—occur only in the midline.

## Arachnoid Cyst

### Terminology and Etiology

Arachnoid cyst (AC) is also known as a meningeal cyst. ACs are CSF-containing cysts that arise as an anomaly of meningeal development. The embryonic endomeninges fail to merge and remain separated, forming a "duplicated" arachnoid. CSF is secreted by cells in the cyst wall and accumulates between the layers.

Most ACs are solitary, isolated sporadic, nonsyndromic lesions. Syndromic ACs have been reported in association with acrocallosal, Aicardi, and Pallister-Hall syndromes. A rare familial form of ACs with *FOXC2* and *RERE* mutations has been reported.

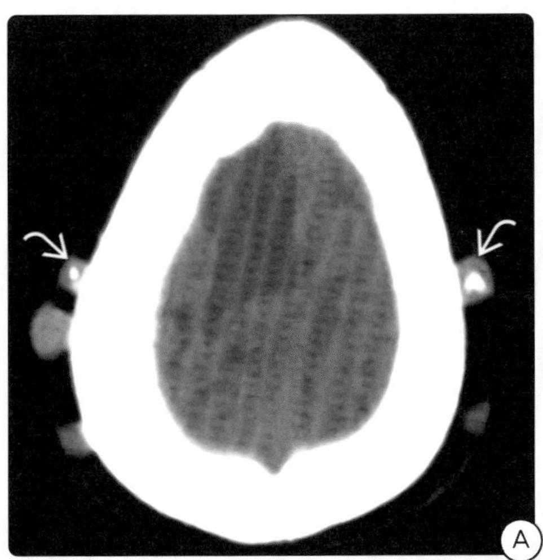

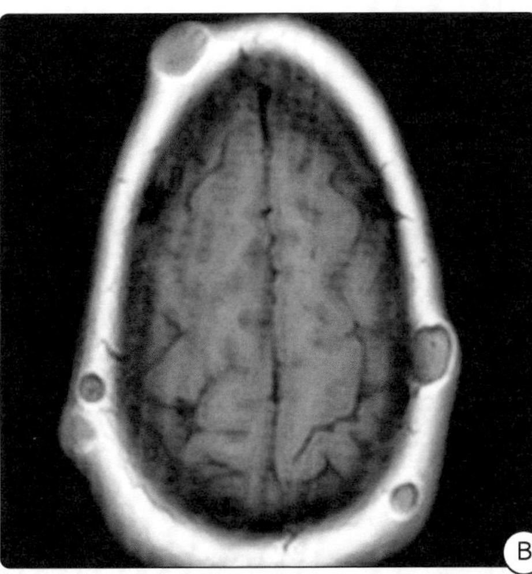

***(32-1A)** NECT in a patient imaged for acute stroke symptoms shows an incidental finding of 5 hyperdense trichilemmal scalp cysts, 2 of which contain calcification ➡ while the other 3 do not.* ***(32-1B)** T1 MR in the same patient shows that the well-delineated scalp cysts are hypointense relative to fat and isointense compared to brain.*

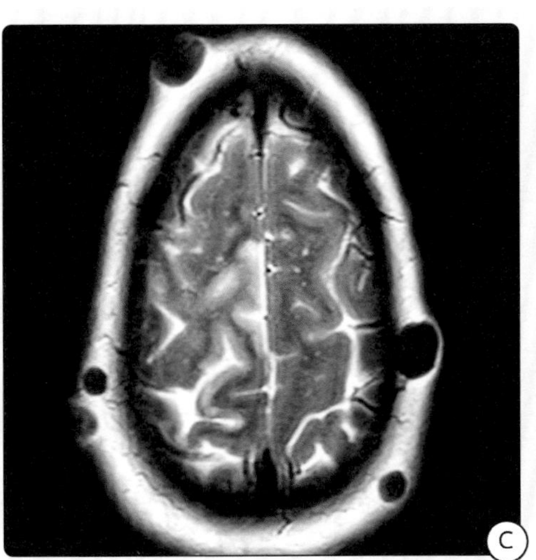

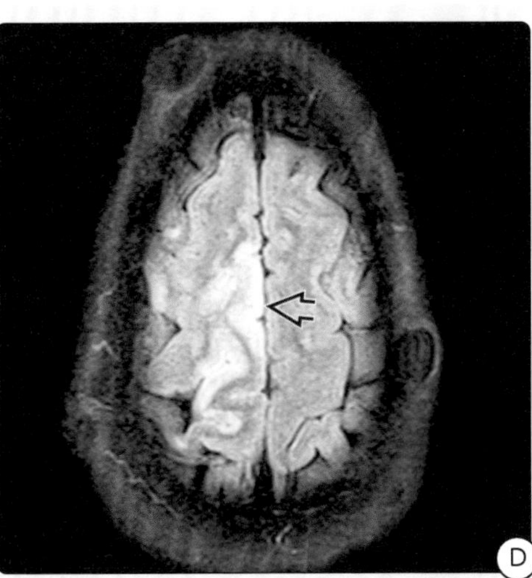

***(32-1C)** Most of the large cysts appear quite hypointense on T2 MR.* ***(32-1D)** On FLAIR MR, the scalp cysts are hypointense relative to brain. The patient's acute infarct is seen as cortical hyperintensity ➡.*

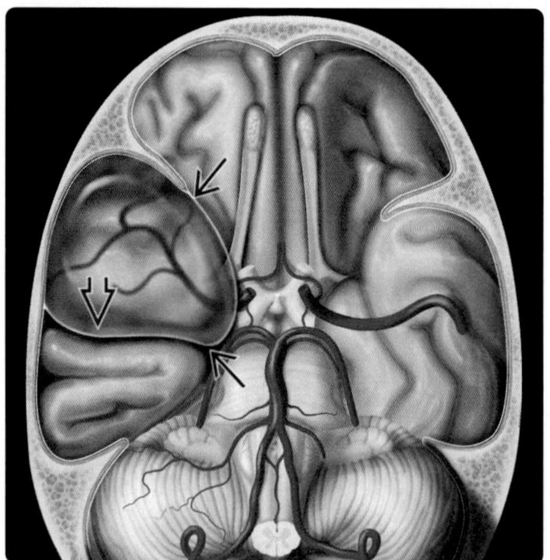

(32-2) Graphic shows the arachnoid ➡ splitting, enclosing CSF. Middle fossa is expanded; temporal lobe ➡ is displaced posteriorly.

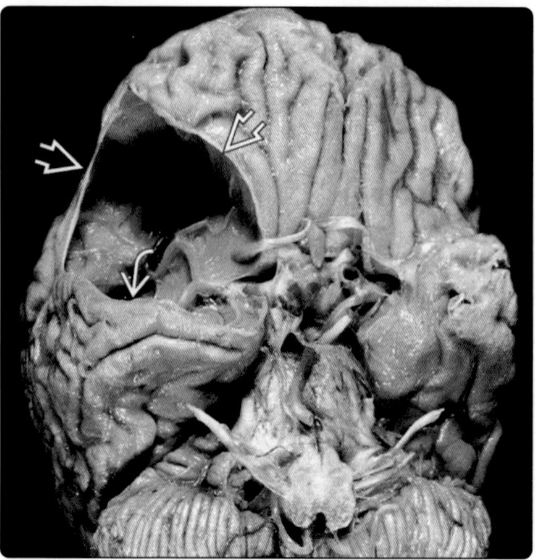

(32-3) Middle fossa AC is contained between layers of "duplicated" arachnoid ➡. Temporal lobe ➡ is displaced. (Courtesy J. Townsend, MD.)

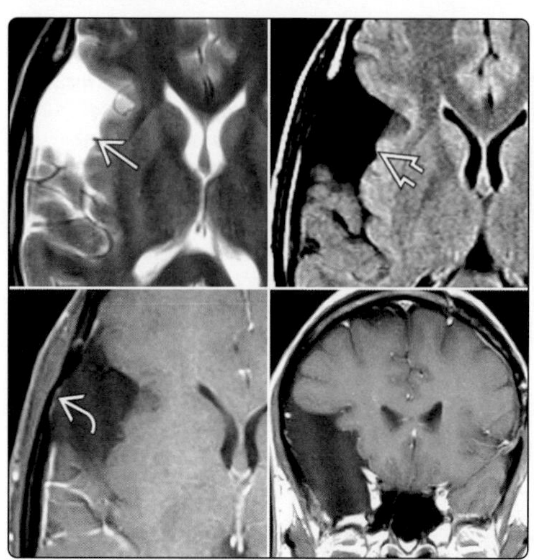

(32-4) ACs often have scalloped margins and are CSF-like on T2 ➡. They suppress on FLAIR ➡, remodel the skull ➡, and do not enhance.

## Pathology

**Location.** Most ACs are supratentorial. They are usually off-midline and are the most common off-midline, extraaxial, supratentorial cyst. Nearly 2/3 are found in the middle cranial fossa, anteromedial to the temporal lobe **(32-2)**. 15% of ACs are found over the cerebral convexities, predominantly over the frontal lobes. Between 10-15% of ACs are found in the posterior fossa, predominately the cerebellopontine angle (CPA) cistern.

**Size and Number.** ACs are almost always solitary. Size ranges from small incidental cysts to large space-occupying lesions.

**Pathology.** ACs are well-marginated cysts filled with clear, colorless fluid that resembles CSF. They are devoid of internal septations and are completely encased by a delicate translucent membrane lined by a single layer of mature, histologically normal arachnoid cells **(32-3)**. Focal inflammatory infiltrates may occur but are rare.

### ARACHNOID CYST: PATHOLOGY

**Location**

- Supratentorial (90%)
  - Middle fossa (67%)
  - Convexities (15%)
  - Other (5-10%): Suprasellar, quadrigeminal cisterns
- Infratentorial (10-12%)
  - Mostly CPA cistern (2nd most common cystic CPA mass)
  - Less common: Cisterna magna

**Gross Pathology**

- Thin, translucent cyst wall bulging with clear fluid
- Lined by mature arachnoid cells

## Clinical Issues

ACs are the most common of all congenital intracranial cysts. They account for ~ 1% of all space-occupying intracranial lesions and are identified on imaging studies in 1-2% of patients. ACs can be seen at any age. Most (nearly 75%) are found in children and young adults. There is no significant sex predilection.

More than 94% of ACs are asymptomatic and found incidentally, remaining stable over many years. Enlargement—if any—is very gradual. Some ACs—especially in the sylvian fissure—often reach a large size without causing symptoms. Large cysts in locations compressing CSF pathways (e.g., suprasellar ACs) may be candidates for surgical fenestration.

Hemorrhage—either traumatic or spontaneous—into an intracranial AC is rare but may cause sudden enlargement. ACs carry a slightly increased risk of subdural hematoma (SDH) **(32-6)**.

Reduction or disappearance of an AC is rare. Some cases occur spontaneously while others have been reported following inciting events, such as trauma. Cyst wall rupture with CSF flow perturbation seems to be the most applicable pathophysiologic mechanism in so-called triggered spontaneous AC resolution.

## Imaging

ACs vary in size, ranging from small incidental cysts to large space-occupying lesions. Uncomplicated ACs behave **exactly** like CSF on CT and MR **(32-4)**. FLAIR and DWI are the best sequences to distinguish cystic-appearing intracranial masses from one another.

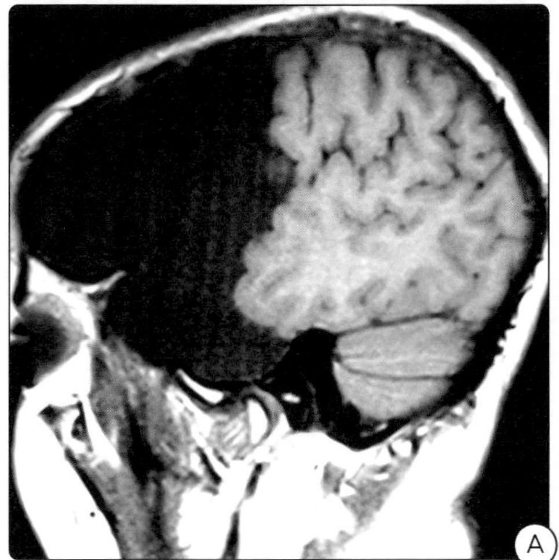

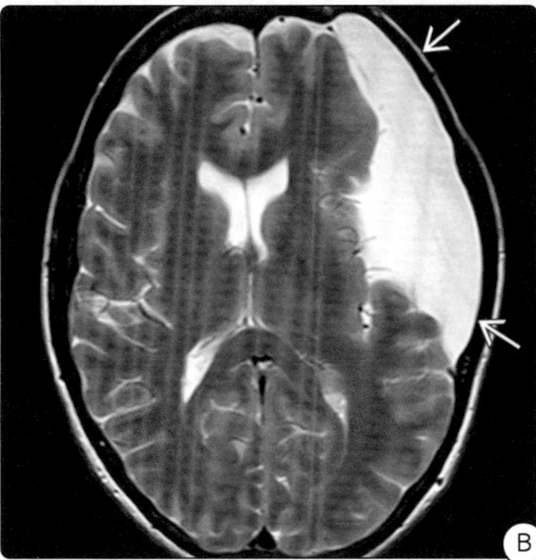

***(32-5A)** Sagittal T1 MR in a 53-yo woman with nonspecific headaches shows a large CSF collection in the anterior and middle cranial fossae that displaces the parietal and temporal lobes posteriorly. **(32-5B)** T2 MR shows the fluid collection has expanded and thinned the overlying calvarium ➡. Signal intensity of the fluid collection is exactly like CSF in the lateral ventricles.*

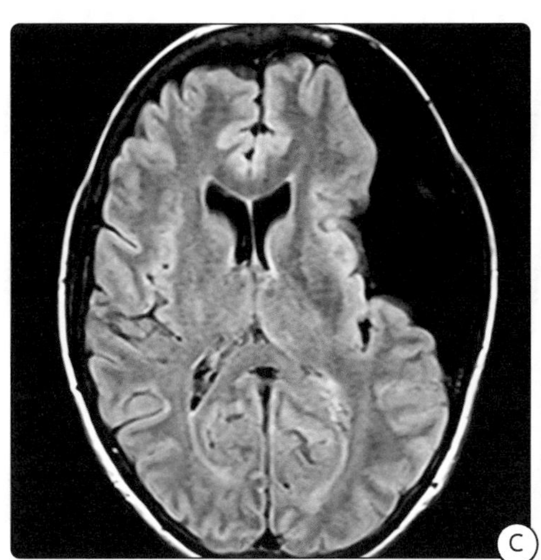

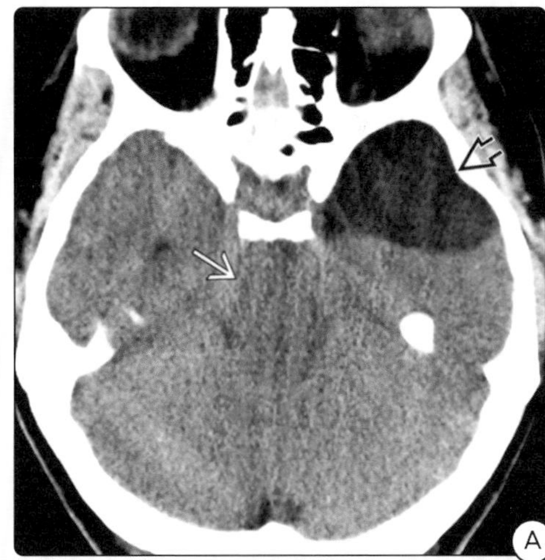

***(32-5C)** FLAIR MR in the same patient shows fluid in the cyst suppresses completely. The underlying brain shows no evidence for malformation or other abnormalities. This is an incidental AC. **(32-6A)** NECT in a 59-yo woman with severe headaches and confusion shows a CSF-density fluid collection in the left anterior middle cranial fossa ➲. Note tight appearance of brain with basilar cistern effacement and midbrain compression ➡.*

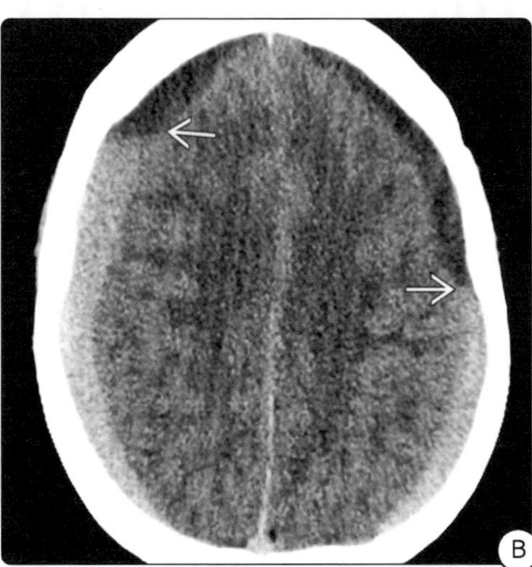

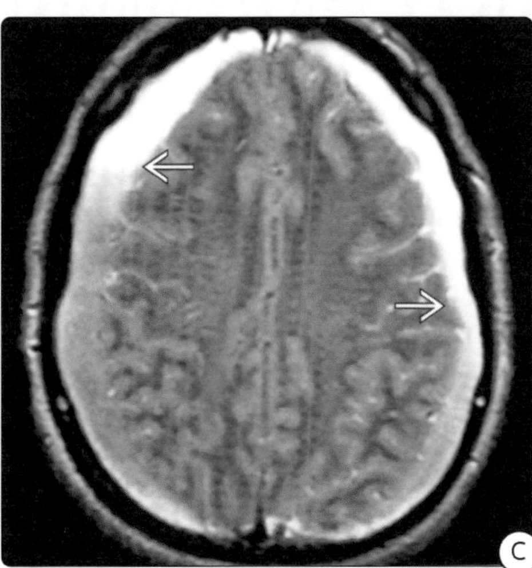

***(32-6B)** More cephalad NECT in the same patient shows mixed-density, acute-on-chronic, bilateral subdural hematomas (SDHs) with blood-fluid levels ➡. **(32-6C)** T2 MR shows mixed-age SDHs with fluid-fluid levels ➡ between the chronic SDH above and the more acute component below. This is an AC with associated bilateral SDHs.*

There is a relationship between SDHs and ACs, although whether this is causative or coincidental is unclear. Traumatic SDHs can rupture into ACs. The converse—AC rupture causing a spontaneous SDH—occurs but is rare.

**CT Findings.** Uncomplicated ACs are CSF density **(32-6A)**. If intracystic hemorrhage has occurred, the cyst fluid may be moderately hyperdense compared with CSF **(32-6B)**. Large middle cranial fossa ACs expand the fossa and cause temporal lobe hypoplasia or displacement **(32-3)**.

With moderately large ACs, bone CT may show pressure remodeling of the adjacent calvarium. ACs do not cause frank bone invasion. ACs do not enhance.

**MR Findings.** ACs are sharply marginated, somewhat scalloped-appearing lesions that parallel CSF signal intensity on all sequences. They are therefore isointense with CSF on T1- and T2-weighted images. ACs cause moderate focal mass effect, **displacing but not engulfing adjacent brain, vessels, and cranial nerves (32-7)**.

The internal appearance of an AC is intrinsically featureless, containing neither septations, vessels, nor cranial nerves **(32-8)**.

ACs suppress completely with FLAIR **(32-9)**. Occasionally, CSF pulsations within large lesions may cause spin dephasing, producing heterogeneous signal intensity and significant propagation of phase artifact across the scan **(32-10)**. ACs do not restrict on DWI and do not enhance.

## Differential Diagnosis

The major differential diagnosis of AC is **epidermoid cyst** (EC). ECs are often almost—but not quite—exactly like CSF. They have a cauliflower-like, lobulated configuration instead of the sharply marginated borders of an AC. ECs engulf vessels and nerves, insinuating themselves along CSF cisterns. ECs do not

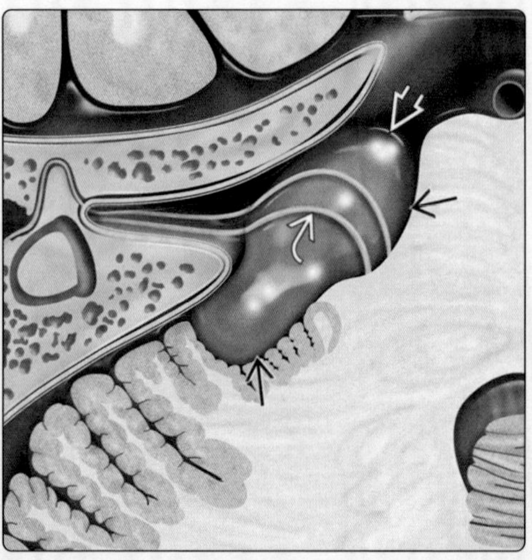

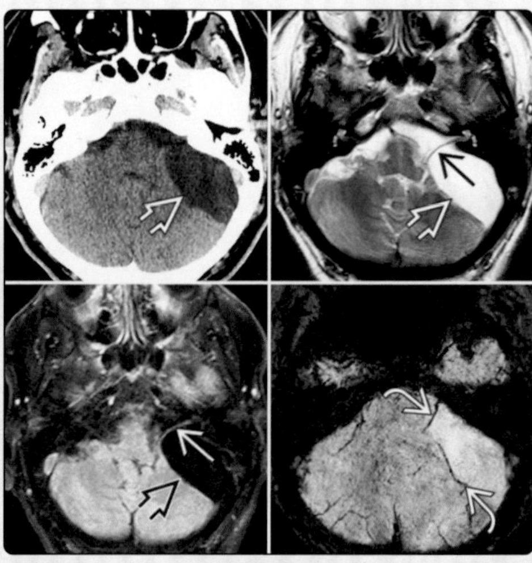

*(32-7) Graphic shows cerebellopontine angle (CPA) AC. Cyst ➡ causes mild mass effect on the adjacent brain ➡. Note CNVII-VIII ➡ are displaced over the translucent, glistening cyst. (32-8) (Upper L) AC ➡ is CSF-like on NECT and hyperintense-like on T2 (upper R). CNVII-VIII are displaced over/around ➡ the AC. (Lower L) Cyst ➡ suppresses completely on FLAIR MR and displaces nerves ➡. (Lower R) T2* SWI shows vessels ➡ displaced around AC.*

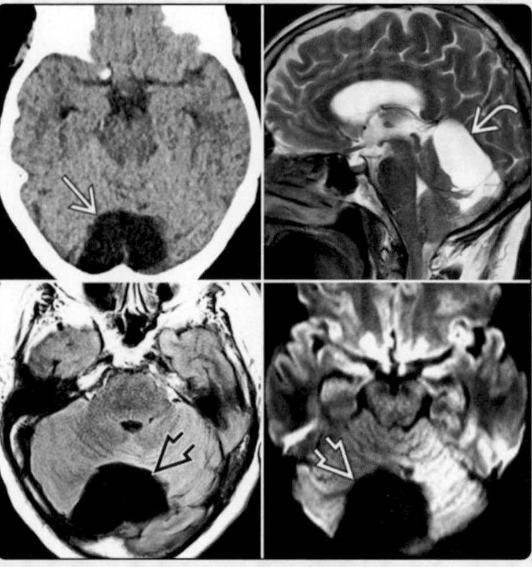

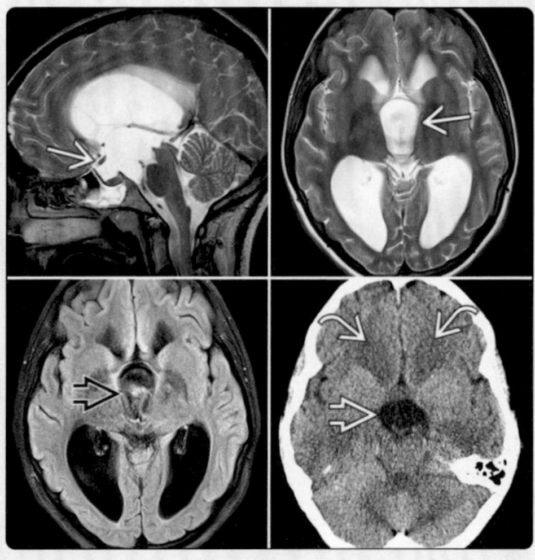

*(32-9) Large midline posterior fossa AC is isodense with CSF on NECT ➡. AC ➡ compresses, displaces vermis and brainstem anteriorly, suppresses on FLAIR ➡, and does not restrict on DWI ➡. (32-10) CSF-filled suprasellar AC is shown on T2 MR ➡. CSF pulsations in cyst do not suppress completely on FLAIR ➡. CT ventriculogram shows dilute contrast in lateral ventricles ➡. Noncommunicating cyst ➡ does not opacity.*

suppress completely on FLAIR and typically show moderate to marked hyperintensity on DWI.

**Enlarged subarachnoid spaces** caused by brain volume loss are usually more diffuse CSF collections and do not cause mass effect on adjacent structures.

A **subdural hygroma** or **chronic SDH** (cSDH) is not precisely like CSF and is usually crescentic, not round or scalloped. cSDHs usually show evidence of prior hemorrhage, especially on T2* sequences, and may have enhancing encasing membranes.

A **porencephalic cyst** looks just like CSF, but it is intraaxial and lined by gliotic white matter that is often hyperintense on FLAIR.

## ARACHNOID CYST: CLINICAL ISSUES, IMAGING

**Clinical Issues**

- Most common nonneoplastic intracranial cyst
  - All ages; children + young adults (75%)
  - Prevalence: 1-2% on imaging studies

**Imaging**

- Behaves **exactly** like CSF
- FLAIR/DWI best to distinguish from other cysts

**Differential Diagnosis**

- Most common: EC
- Less common
  - Enlarged subarachnoid spaces
  - Loculated subdural hygroma/hematoma
  - Porencephalic cyst
- Rare: Neurenteric cyst

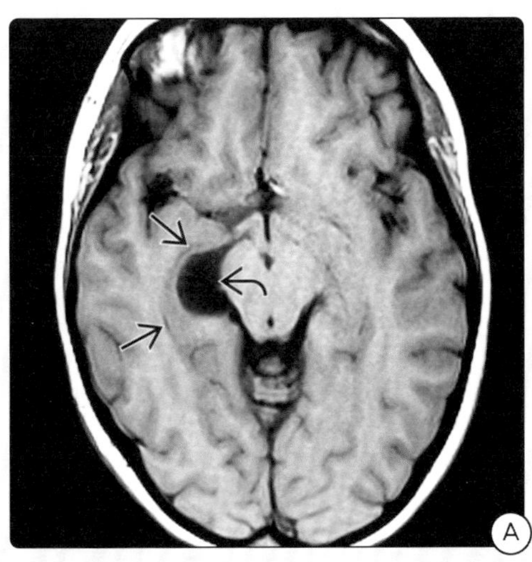

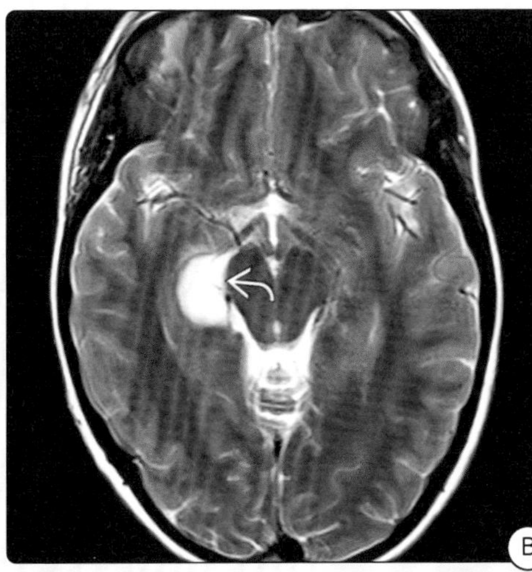

***(32-11A)** Axial T1 MR in a 21-yo woman with headaches and normal neurologic examination shows a sharply demarcated CSF-like collection ➩ just medial to the right temporal horn of the lateral ventricle ➩. **(32-11B)** T2 MR shows the fluid collection ➩ is exactly like CSF.*

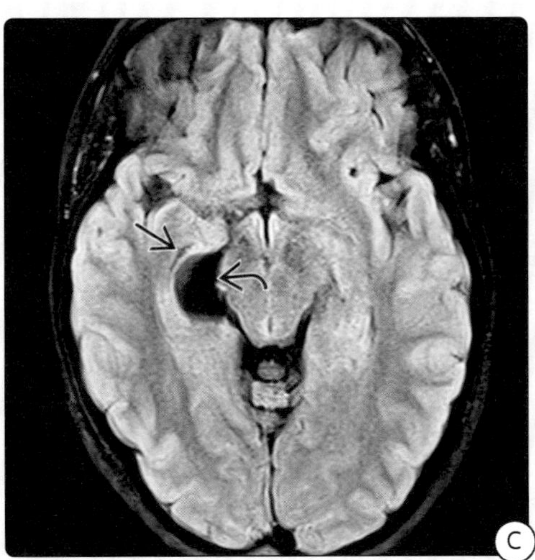

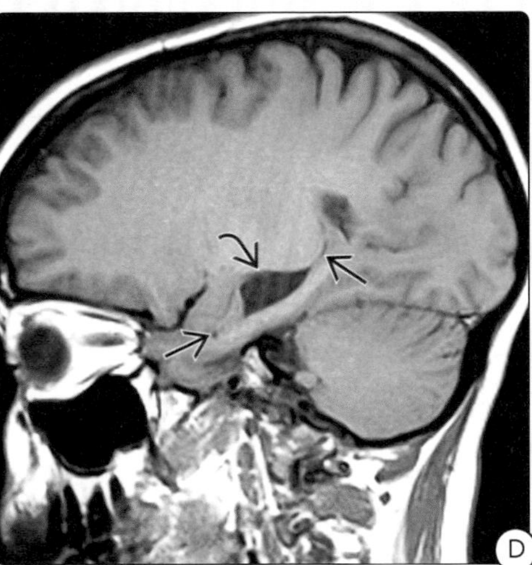

***(32-11C)** The well-demarcated collection ➩ suppresses completely on FLAIR MR, as does CSF in the adjacent temporal horn ➩. **(32-11D)** Sagittal T1 MR shows the classic spindle shape ➩ of a choroid fissure cyst. Note CSF in the adjacent temporal horn ➩.*

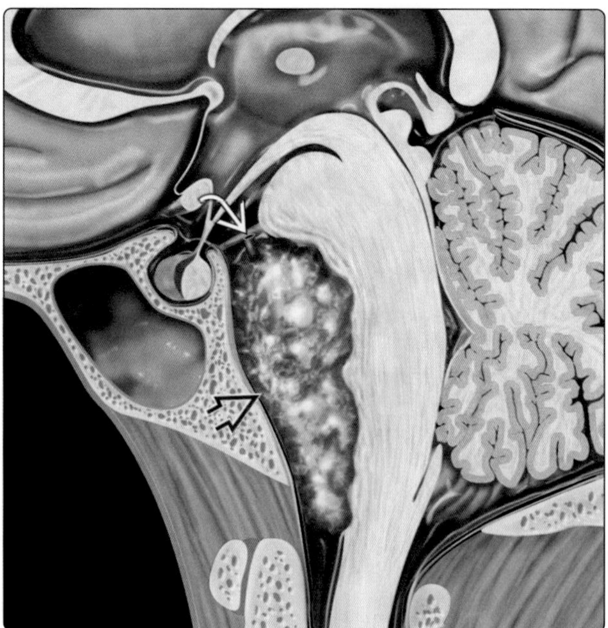

*(32-12) Graphic shows a multilobulated epidermoid cyst (EC) ⇒ within the prepontine cistern encasing the basilar artery ➡ and displacing the pons.*

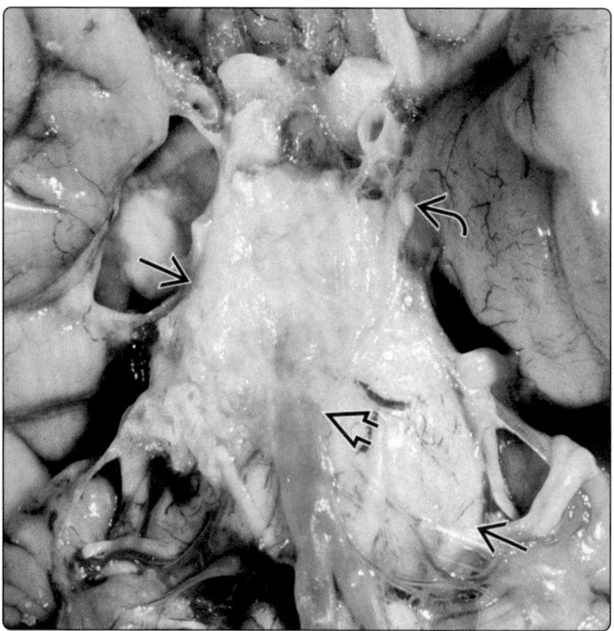

*(32-13) Autopsy shows EC as a whitish, pearly tumor ⇒. Note the encased basilar artery ⇒ and oculomotor nerves ⇒.*

## Choroid Fissure Cyst

The C-shaped choroid fissure is an infolding of CSF positioned centrally between the fornix and thalamus with the former forming its outer margin and the latter forming its inner margin.

The choroid fissure is normally a shallow, inconspicuous, C-shaped cleft that curves posterosuperiorly from the anterior temporal lobe all the way to the atrium of the lateral ventricle. The choroidal arteries and choroid plexus lie just medial to the choroid fissure.

A CSF-containing cyst can form anywhere in the plane of the choroidal fissure. These "choroid fissure cysts" (CFCs) are probably caused by maldevelopment of the embryonic tela choroidea, a double layer of pia that invaginates through the choroid fissure to reach the lateral ventricles. CFCs may thus have a neuroglial, neuroepithelial, or arachnoidal origin.

### Imaging

Most CFCs are discovered incidentally on imaging studies. They lie just medial to the temporal horn of the lateral ventricle between the hippocampus and diencephalon and thus will shift the lateral ventricle and its choroid plexus laterally. Patients are usually asymptomatic or exhibit symptoms that do not correlate with the anatomic location of the cyst.

CT scans show a well-delineated, homogeneously hypodense mass with CSF-like attenuation. Calcification and contrast enhancement are absent. CFCs follow CSF signal intensity on all MR sequences, suppressing completely on FLAIR **(32-11)**.

On axial and coronal images, CFCs are round to ovoid in shape, but on sagittal images, they have a distinctive, pathognomonic, elongated spindle configuration **(32-11D)**.

## Epidermoid Cyst

Both congenital and acquired epidermoid cysts (ECs) are found in the CNS. Although spinal ECs are often acquired lesions, intracranial ECs are always congenital in origin.

### Terminology

An intracranial EC is a congenital, developmental, nonneoplastic inclusion cyst. ECs arise when the embryonic neural and cutaneous ectoderm fail to separate completely during neural tube closure, resulting in transplantation of epithelial cell rests into the developing neural tube.

ECs have incorrectly been called "tumors," but they are not neoplastic. The term "cholesteatoma" should be reserved for an acquired lesion arising as a complication of chronic otitis media.

### Pathology

**Location. Extracranial** ECs commonly involve the scalp, face, and neck. Over 90% of **intracranial** ECs are intradural and are almost always extraaxial. They have a distinct predilection for the basilar cisterns and are usually off- or paramidline. ECs insinuate themselves around cranial nerves and vessels **(32-12)**.

The CPA cistern is the single most common site, accounting for 50% of all intracranial ECs. ECs are the third most common CPA mass (after vestibular schwannoma and meningioma).

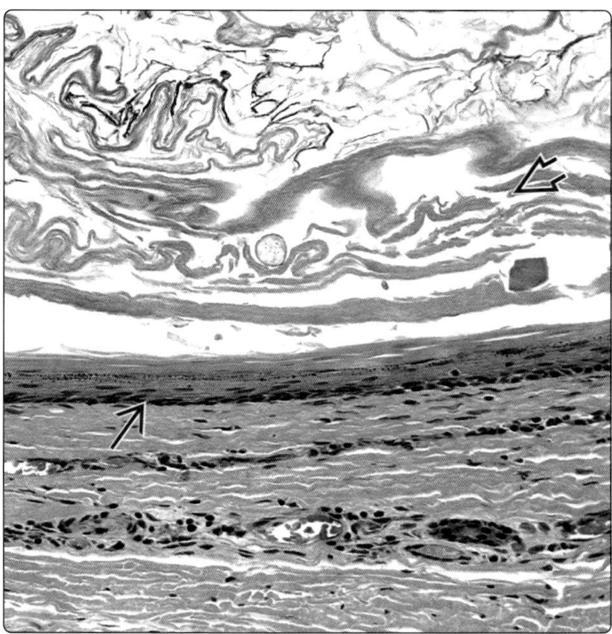

*(32-14) ECs contain anuclear laminate keratin ⇨ and are lined by cytologically benign squamous epithelium ➡. Note absence of adnexal glands. (From DP: Neuro.)*

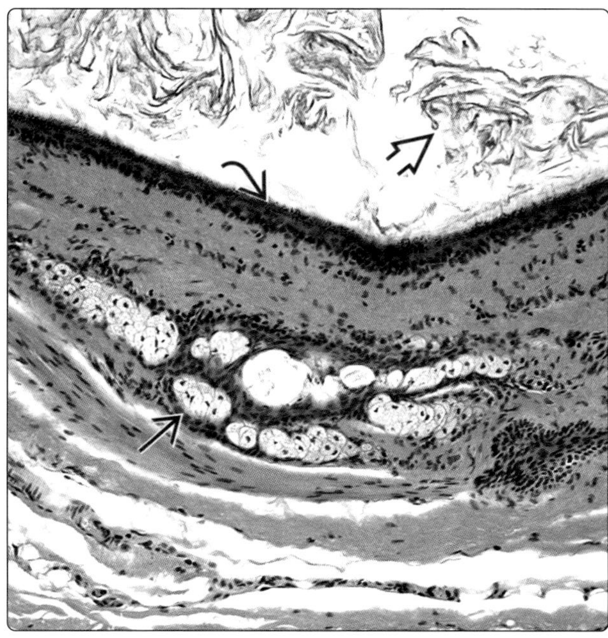

*(32-15) Dermoid cyst (DC) wall shows the presence of adnexal glands ➡. Like ECs, DCs also contain benign squamous epithelium ➡ and desquamated keratinaceous debris ⇨.*

The middle cranial fossa (sylvian fissure) and parasellar region together account for 10-15% of ECs. Less common locations are the cerebral ventricles, most commonly the fourth ventricle. Intradiploic ECs account for 5-10% of cases.

**Gross Pathology.** The outer surface of an EC is often shiny, resembling mother of pearl **(32-13)**. Multiple "cauliflower" excrescences are typical. The cyst wall consists of an outer fibrous capsule lined by stratified squamous epithelium. The cyst itself is filled with soft, waxy, creamy, or flaky material with keratinaceous debris and solid crystalline cholesterol **(32-14)**. **Dermal appendages, such as hair follicles (a characteristic of dermoid cysts), are absent.**

## Clinical Issues

**Epidemiology.** ECs are the most common intracranial developmental cyst and are 4-9x more common than dermoid cysts. Peak age of presentation is 20-50 years. Symptomatic ECs are rare in children.

**Natural History.** ECs may remain clinically silent for many years. They grow very slowly via progressive accumulation of epidermal cells and accretions of desquamated keratin. ECs often reach considerable size before becoming symptomatic. Headache and cranial neuropathy are common features.

In contrast to dermoid cysts, rupture of an EC is rare. Malignant transformation occurs but is very rare.

### EPIDERMOID CYST: PATHOLOGY AND EPIDEMIOLOGY

**Pathology**
- Gross pathology
  - Congenital inclusion cyst
  - Insinuates in/around CSF cisterns
  - Encases vessels/cranial nerves
  - Cauliflower-like excrescences
  - Pearly whitish surface
  - Waxy, creamy, or flaky contents
- Microscopic pathology
  - Squamous epithelium + keratin debris, solid cholesterol
  - **No** dermal appendages!

**Epidemiology**
- 4-9x more common than dermoid cysts
- Peak age: 20-60 years (rare in children)

## Imaging

ECs resemble CSF on imaging. Irregular frond-like excrescences and an insinuating growth pattern within CSF cisterns are characteristic.

**CT Findings.** The vast majority (> 95%) of ECs are hypodense ("black epidermoids") and appear almost identical to CSF on NECT scans **(32-16A)**. Calcification is present in 10-25%. Hemorrhage is very rare as is enhancement on CECT sequences.

An atypical hyperdense variant, the so-called **white epidermoid**, is uncommon, representing between 1.5 and 5.6% of all intracranial ECs. The hyperdensity of white epidermoids **(32-19A)** has been variously attributed to hemorrhage, formation of calcium soaps, or high protein content.

**MR Findings.** Classic ("black") ECs are iso- or slightly hyperintense compared with CSF on both T1- **(32-17A)** and T2-weighted **(32-17B)** sequences. Slight heterogeneity in signal intensity is often present.

Typical ECs either do not suppress at all or suppress incompletely on FLAIR **(32-17C)**. They restrict on DWI **(32-17D)** and are therefore moderately to strikingly hyperintense. Enhancement is generally absent, although mild peripheral enhancement can be seen in 25% of cases **(32-18)**.

"White" ECs generally display reversed MR signal intensities (i.e., hyperintense on T1WI, hypointense on T2WI) **(32-19)**. Most articles attribute the T2 hypointensity to high protein level and high viscosity of the cystic content, not intracystic hemorrhage. Partial FLAIR suppression may be present and has been termed the shading sign. DWI hypointensity is common and may be due to a T2 "blackout" effect.

## Differential Diagnosis

The major differential diagnosis is **arachnoid cyst (AC)**. ACs are smoothly marginated, behave **exactly** like CSF on all sequences, suppress completely on FLAIR, and do not restrict on DWI. ACs displace nerves and vessels while ECs surround and engulf them. **Dermoid cysts** should not be confused with ECs. Dermoid cysts contain fat and dermal appendages and do not resemble CSF on imaging studies. **Neurenteric (endodermal) cysts** are rare; the most common intracranial site is the prepontine medullary cistern.

**Parasitic cysts**, such as neurocysticercosis (NCC), are usually multiple and comparatively small. NCC cysts often contain a discernible scolex. **Cystic neoplasms** are rarely mistaken for ECs, as the cyst wall &/or nodule typically enhances.

*(32-16A) NECT in a 34-yo woman shows a hypodense extraaxial mass ➡ in the left CPA cistern that extends anteromedially in front of the pons. (32-16B) T1 MR in the same patient shows the mass ➡ is heterogeneously hypointense relative to brain but slightly hyperintense compared to CSF in the 4th ventricle.*

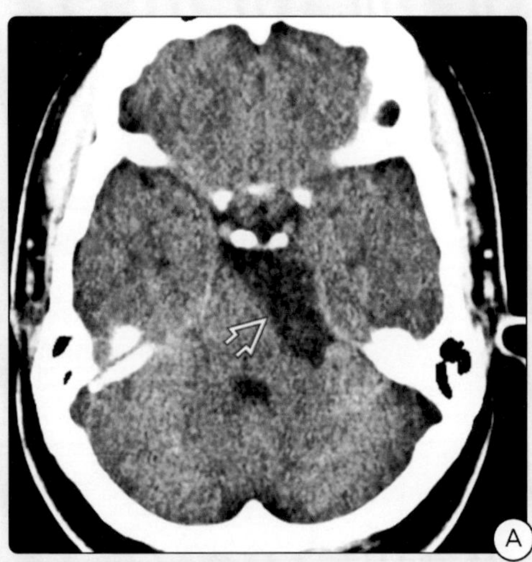


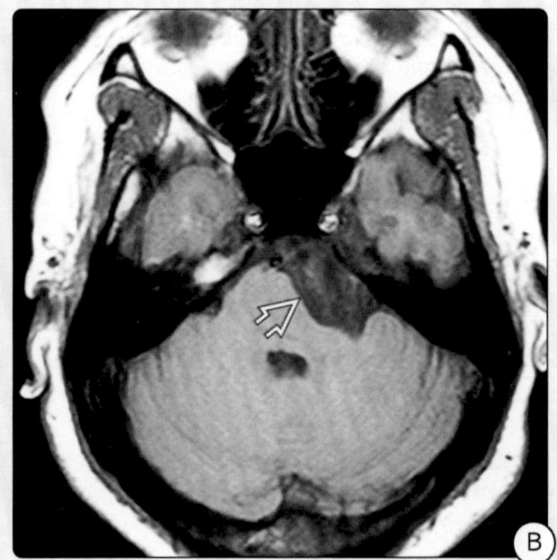


*(32-16C) T2 MR shows the mass ➡ is very hyperintense and surrounds, encases, and narrows the basilar artery ➡. (32-16D) The mass ➡ restricts on DWI MR. EC was found at surgery.*

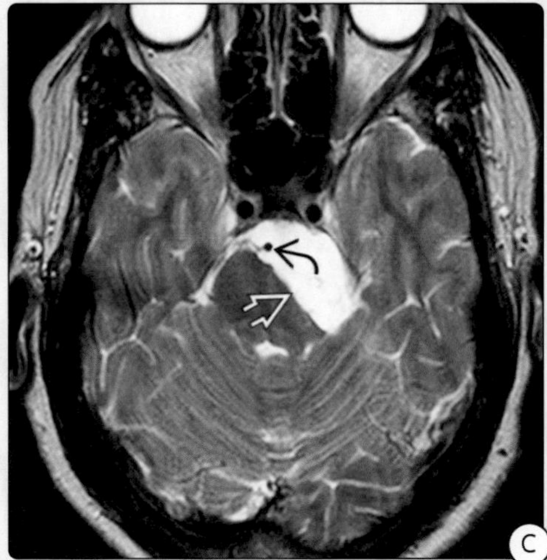


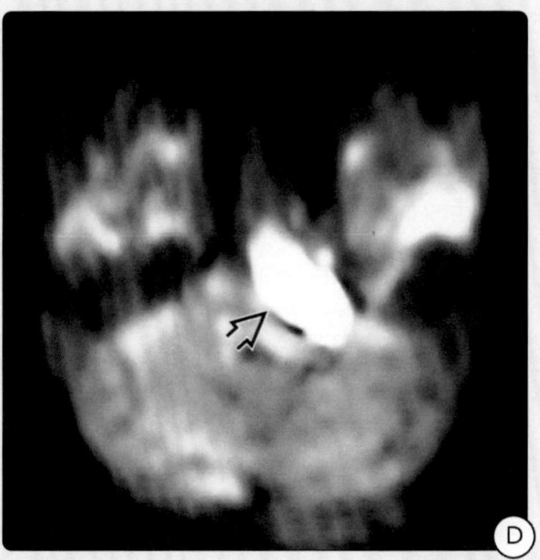

**EPIDERMOID CYST: IMAGING FEATURES**

**General Features**
- Resembles CSF (vs. fat-like dermoid)
- Insinuates around/along CSF cisterns
- Encases, displaces vessels and cranial nerves

**Imaging**
- Hypodense (> 95%)
- Slightly hyperintense to CSF on T1WI
- Does not suppress on FLAIR
- Restricts ("bright") on DWI

**Differential Diagnosis**
- AC (suppresses on FLAIR, restricts)
- Parasitic cyst (neurocysticercosis)
- Endodermal cyst (pontomedullary junction)

# Dermoid Cyst

## Pathology

Dermoid cysts (DCs) are congenital inclusion cysts. The cyst wall contains mature squamous epithelium, keratinous material, and adnexal structures (hair follicles and sebaceous and sweat glands). DCs typically contain a thick, greasy sebaceous material with lipid and cholesterol elements **(32-21)**.

DCs are usually extraaxial lesions that are most often found in the midline. The suprasellar cistern is the most common site **(32-20)** followed by the posterior fossa and frontonasal region.

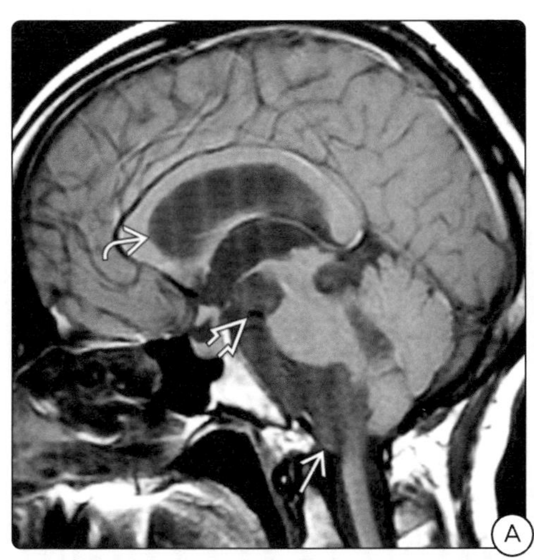


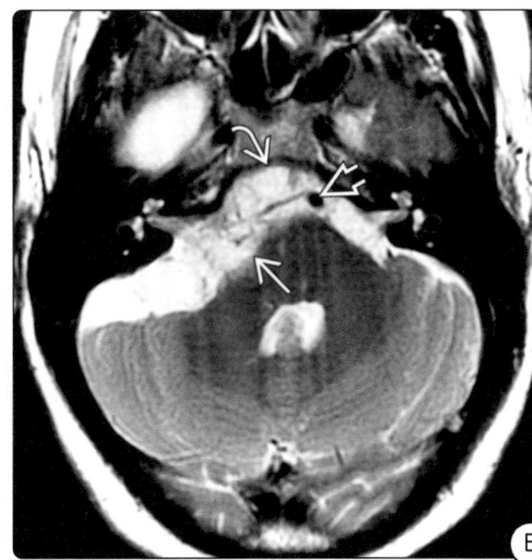


***(32-17A)** Sagittal T1 MR shows a scalloped posterior fossa mass ➡ that encases the basilar artery ➡, wraps around the midbrain, elevates the 3rd ventricle, and deforms the pons. Mass is slightly hyperintense compared to CSF in the 3rd ventricle ➡. **(32-17B)** T2 MR in the same patient shows a lobulated, irregular hyperintense mass in the right CPA ➡ and basilar ➡ cisterns encasing the basilar artery ➡. The CSF looks "dirty."*

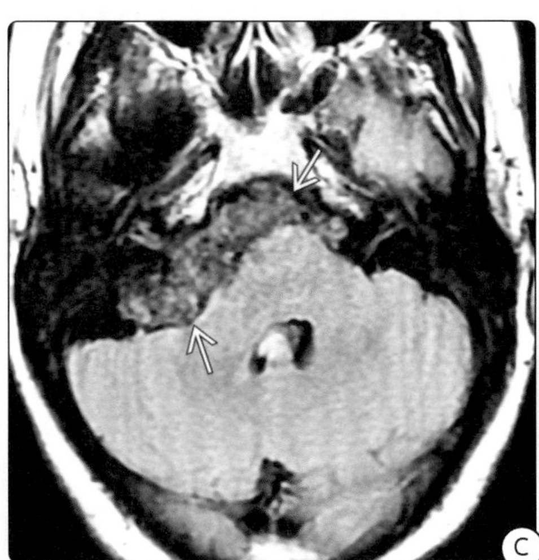


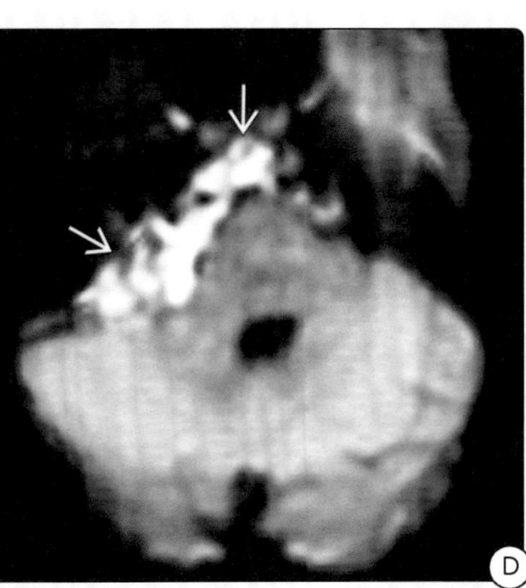


***(32-17C)** FLAIR MR demonstrates that the lobulated, cauliflower-like mass ➡ does not suppress. **(32-17D)** The mass ➡ restricts on DWI MR. This is a classic EC.*

*(**32-18A**) NECT in a 48-yo woman with headaches shows a well-delineated, hypodense mass ➡ eroding the right orbital roof and greater sphenoid wing. (**32-18B**) T1 MR in the same patient shows a well-demarcated, extraaxial mass ➡ that is mixed hypo- and isointense relative to brain. Note smooth remodeling of the adjacent frontal bone ➡.*

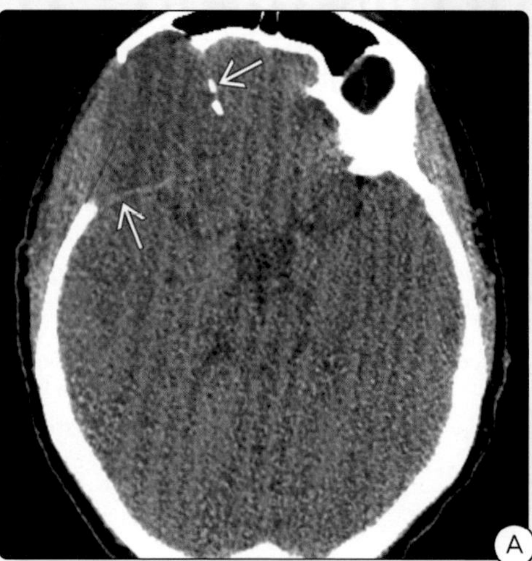

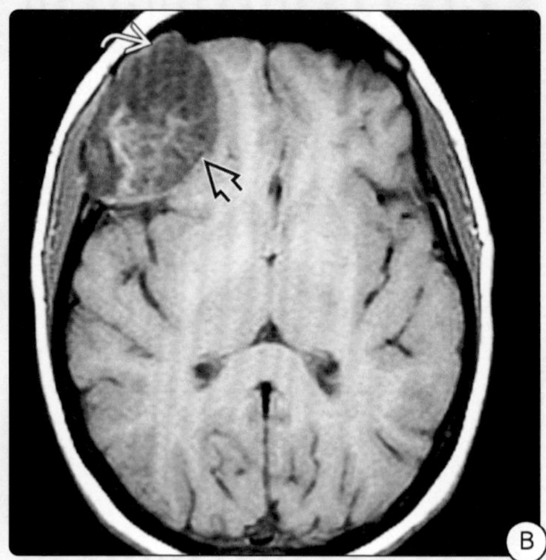

*(**32-18C**) The mass is very hyperintense relative to brain and even hyperintense compared to CSF on this T2 MR. Note the displaced dura, seen here as a thin, linear hypointensity ➡ adjacent to the mass. (**32-18D**) The mass does not suppress on FLAIR MR and is heterogeneously hyper- to isointense relative to the cortex.*

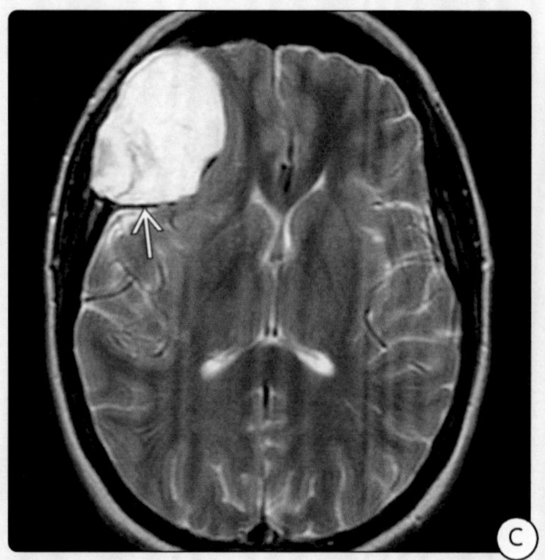

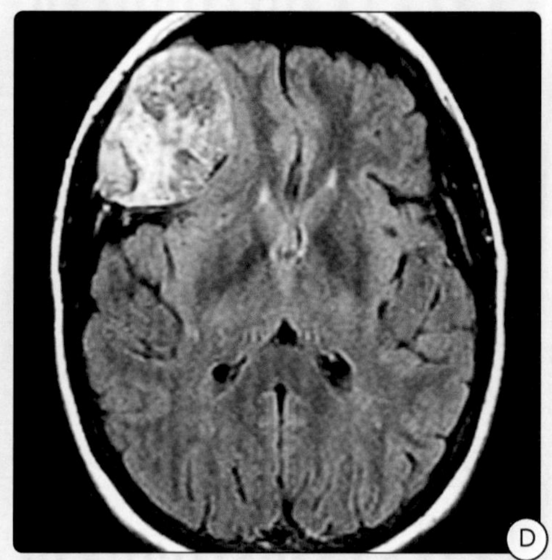

*(**32-18E**) T1 C+ FS MR shows the mass does not enhance, but the displaced, enhancing, slightly thickened dura ➡ is well seen. (**32-18F**) Coronal T1 C+ MR shows the mass is centered on the skull and orbital roof. Preoperative diagnosis of intradiploid EC was confirmed at surgery.*

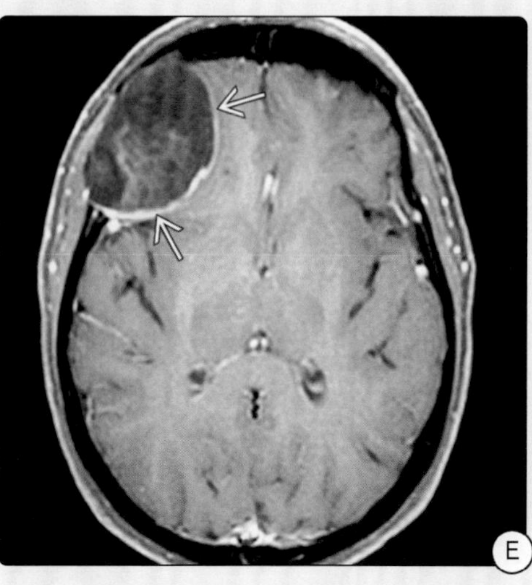

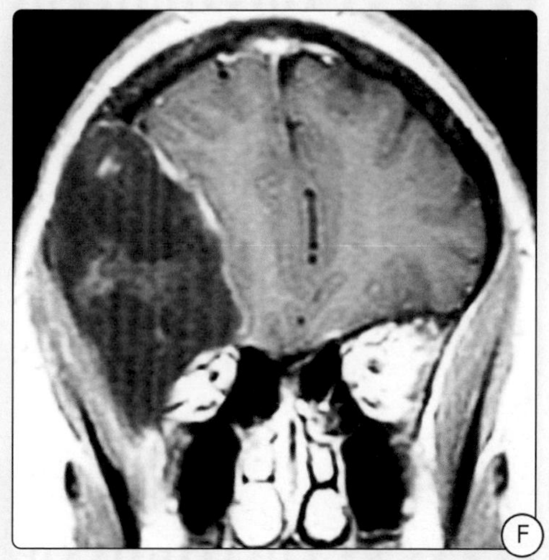

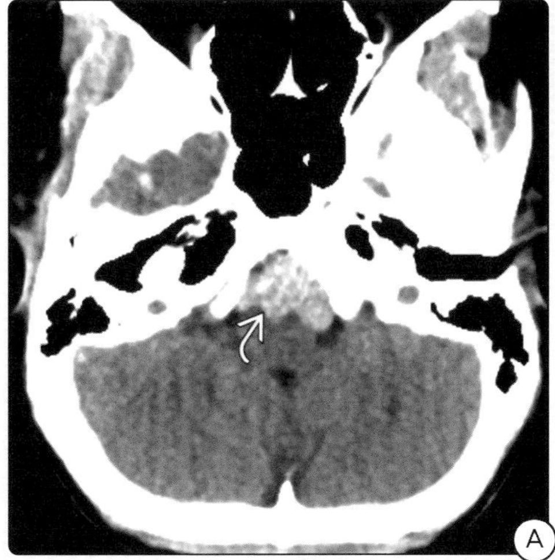

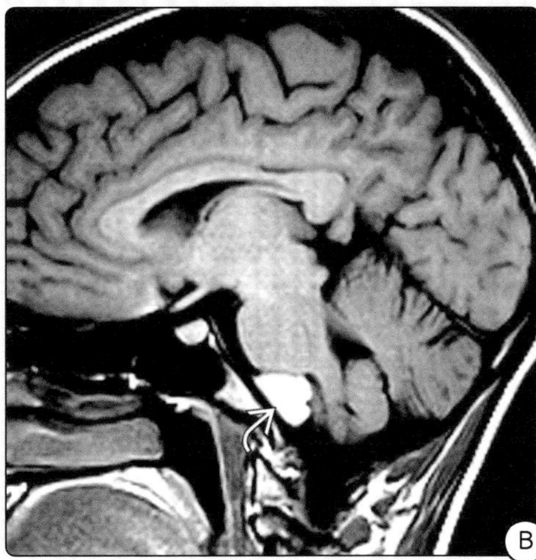

***(32-19A)** Axial NECT in a 22-yo woman shows a heterogeneously hyperdense extraaxial mass ➡ anterior to the medulla. The adjacent skull was normal on bone CT (not shown). **(32-19B)** Sagittal T1 MR shows the extraaxial mass ➡ is very hyperintense.*

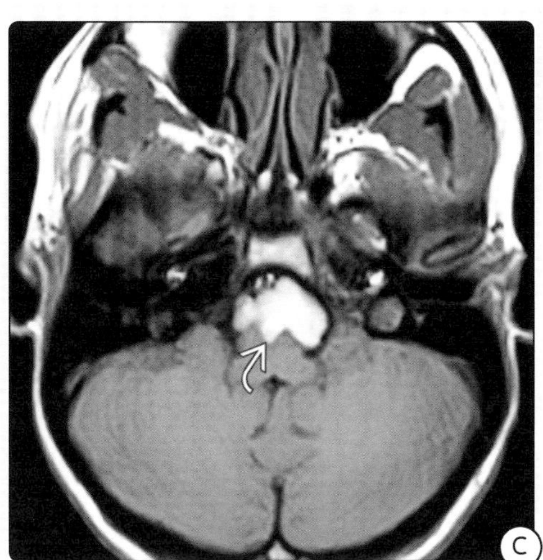

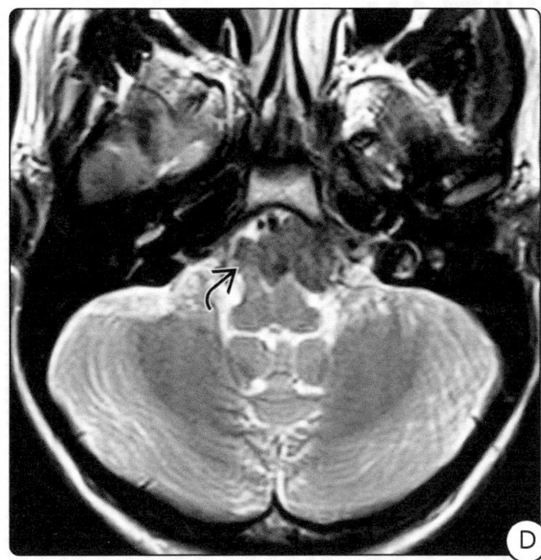

***(32-19C)** The mass ➡ is very hyperintense on axial T1 MR. **(32-19D)** The mass ➡ is quite hypointense relative to the adjacent brain on T2 MR.*

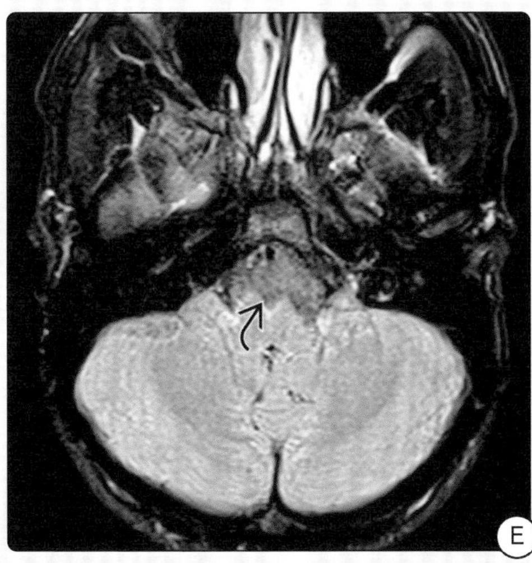

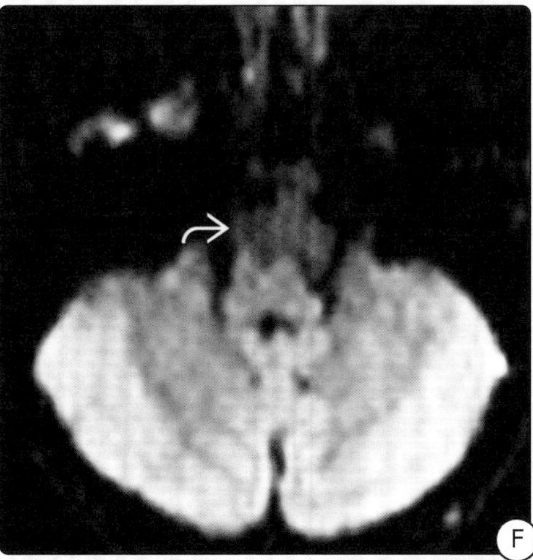

***(32-19E)** The mass ➡ does not suppress on FLAIR MR. **(32-19F)** The mass ➡ does not restrict on DWI MR. Preoperative diagnosis was neurenteric cyst. "White" epidermoid was found at surgery.*

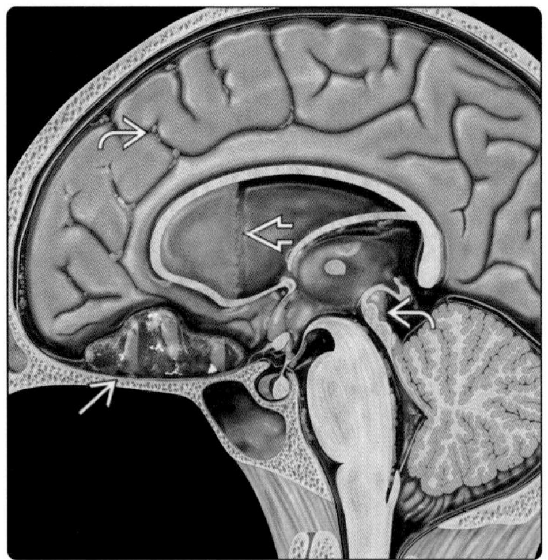

*(32-20) Ruptured DC ➡ is a heterogeneous, fat-containing midline mass with ventricular fat-fluid level ➡ and fat droplets in SASs ➡.*

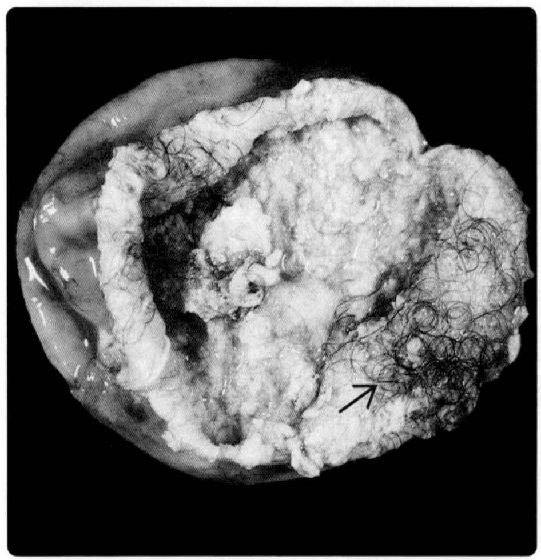

*(32-21) DC contains thick, greasy sebaceous material, keratin debris, and hair ➡.*

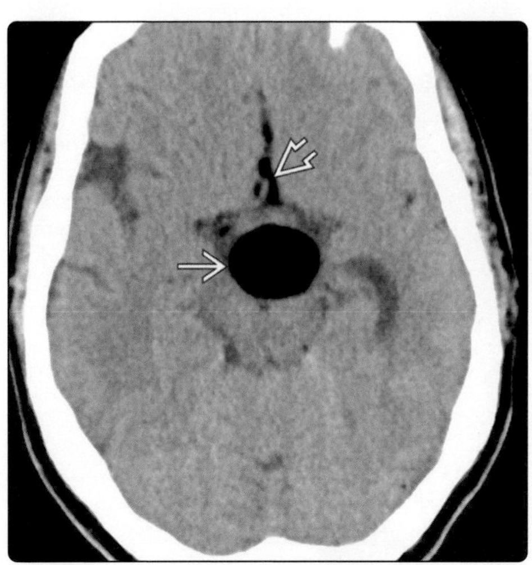

*(32-22) Axial NECT of a ruptured DC shows a hypodense suprasellar mass ➡ and fat droplets in the interhemispheric fissure ➡.*

## Clinical Issues

DCs are much less common than epidermoid cysts (ECs) (ECs are 4-10x more common). DCs grow slowly secondary to the production of hair and oils from the internal dermal elements.

Presentation occurs at significantly younger ages compared with epidermoids, peaking in the second to third decades. DCs often remain asymptomatic until they rupture. Chemical meningitis with seizure, coma, vasospasm, infarction, and even death may ensue as a consequence.

Malignant transformation of intracranial DCs into squamous cell carcinoma is extremely rare.

## Imaging

**CT Findings.** DCs are quite hypodense on NECT scans. With rupture, hypodense fatty "droplets" disseminate in the CSF cisterns and may cause discernible fat-fluid levels in the ventricles **(32-23A)**.

**MR Findings.** Signal intensity varies with fat content in the cyst. Most DCs are heterogeneously hyperintense on T1WI. T1WI is also the most sensitive sequence to detect disseminated fat "droplets" in the subarachnoid space, diagnostic of ruptured dermoid **(32-23C)**. Fat suppression is helpful to confirm the presence of lipid elements.

Standard PD and T2 scans show increasingly more pronounced "chemical shift" artifact in the frequency-encoding direction as the time of repetition is lengthened. Fat is very hypointense on standard T2WI **(32-23D)** but is "bright" (hyperintense) on fast spin-echo T2-weighted sequences. DCs demonstrate heterogeneous hyperintensity with linear or striated laminations if hair is present within the cyst.

Uncomplicated DCs are heterogeneously hyperintense on FLAIR. Ruptured DCs demonstrate subtle FLAIR sulcal hyperintensity **(32-23E)** and "bloom" on T2* GRE or SWI **(32-23F)**.

Most DCs do not enhance, although ruptured DCs may cause significant chemical meningitis with extensive leptomeningeal reaction and enhancement.

Spectroscopy may show an elevated lipid peak at 0.9-1.3 ppm.

### DERMOID CYST

**Pathology**
- Location
  - Extraaxial; midline > off-midline
  - Suprasellar > posterior fossa > frontonasal
- Wall of squamous epithelium
  - Cyst contains fatty sebaceous material, keratin, adnexa

**Clinical Findings**
- Grow slowly
- Usually asymptomatic until rupture

**Imaging**
- NECT
  - Hypodense, $Ca^{++}$ in 20%
  - "Fatty" droplets in cisterns if ruptured
- MR
  - Heterogeneously hyperintense on T1WI/FSE T2
  - Heterogeneously hyperintense on FLAIR
  - Ruptured DCs "bloom" on T2* GRE

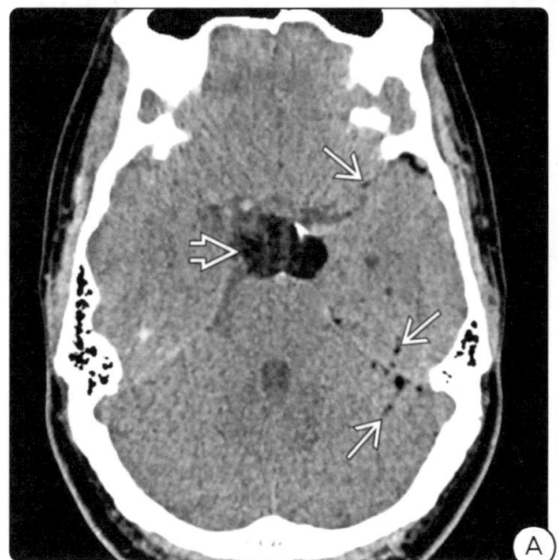

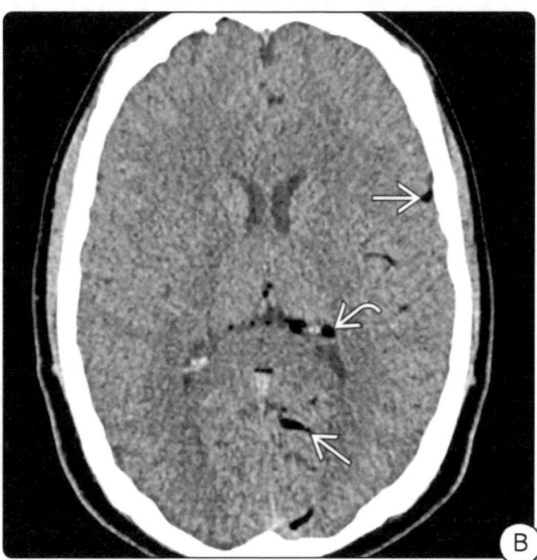

*(32-23A) Axial NECT in a 24-yo man with sudden onset of severe headaches shows a well-delineated, lobulated hypodense mass ➡ in the suprasellar cistern. Note multiple scattered hypodense droplets ➡ in the SASs. (32-23B) More cephalad NECT shows additional low-attenuation droplets in the ventricles ➡ and SASs ➡. Droplets measured -50 HU (consistent with fat, not air).*

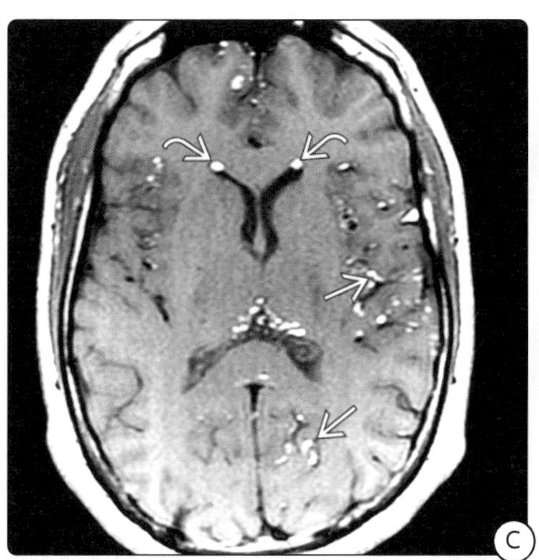

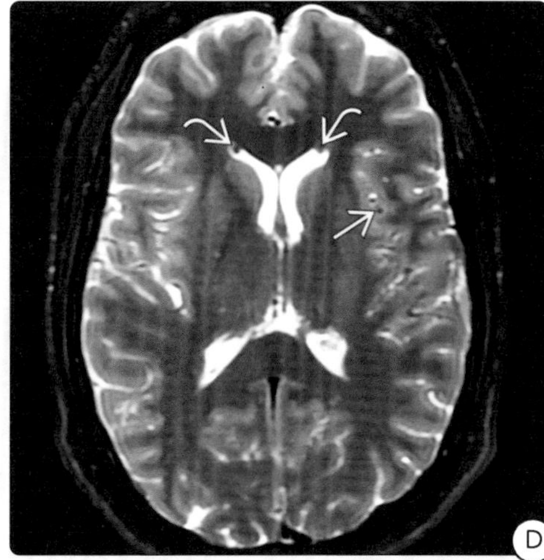

*(32-23C) T1 MR in the same patient shows hyperintense droplets ➡ floating on top of CSF in the frontal horns. Additional fatty droplets are scattered throughout the SASs ➡. (32-23D) T2 FS MR shows that the T1-hyperintense droplets of ruptured dermoid in the frontal horns of the lateral ventricle ➡ and sylvian fissure ➡ now appear hypointense (fat-saturated sequence).*

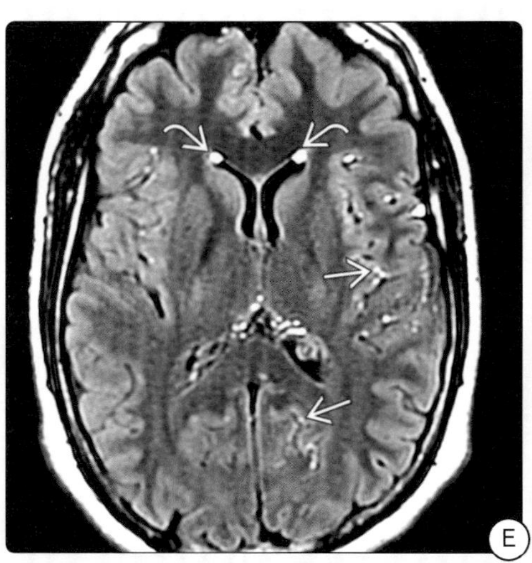

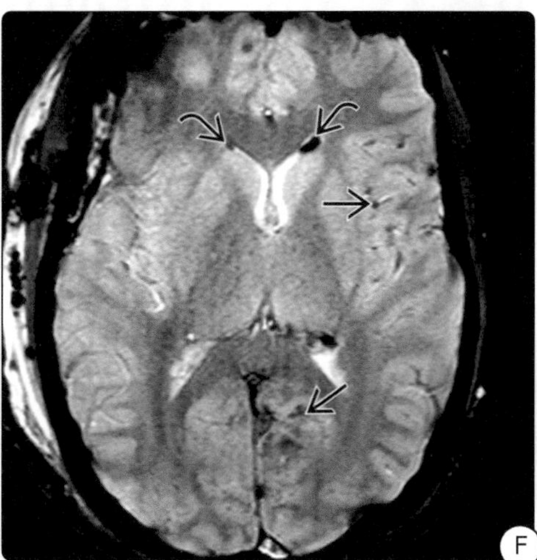

*(32-23E) Fatty droplets ➡ from the ruptured DC float on top of CSF in the frontal horns of the lateral ventricles and are hyperintense on FLAIR MR. Numerous small, hyperintense droplets are scattered throughout the SASs ➡. (32-23F) Postoperative T2* GRE MR shows the fatty droplets in the frontal horns ➡ and SASs ➡ have "blooming" hypointensity. This is classic imaging of a ruptured DC.*

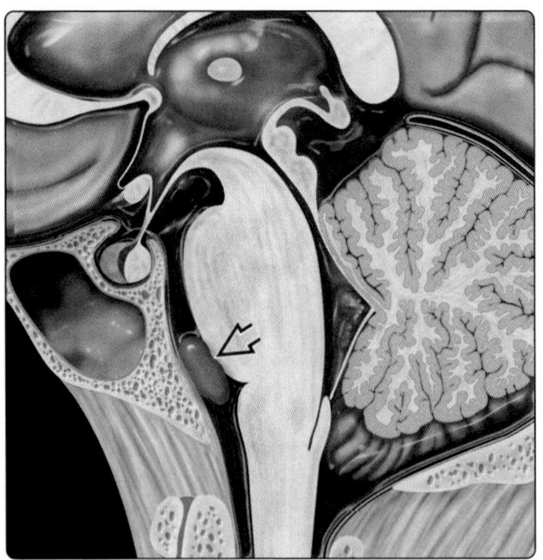

*(32-24) Sagittal graphic shows a neurenteric cyst ➲ anterior to the pontomedullary junction.*

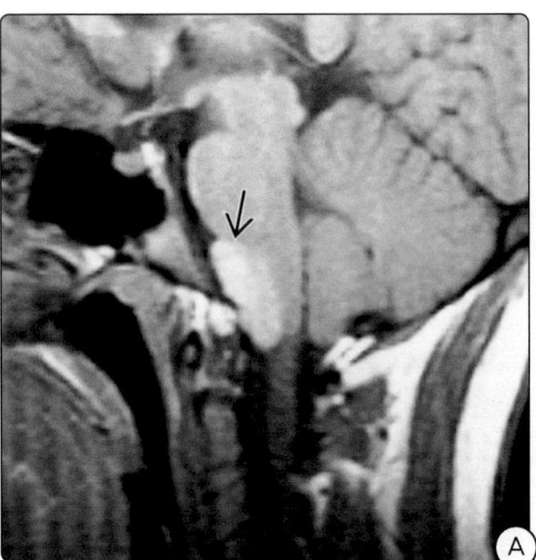

*(32-25A) Sagittal T1 MR shows hyperintense, lobulated, midline extraaxial mass ➲ anterior to the pontomedullary junction.*

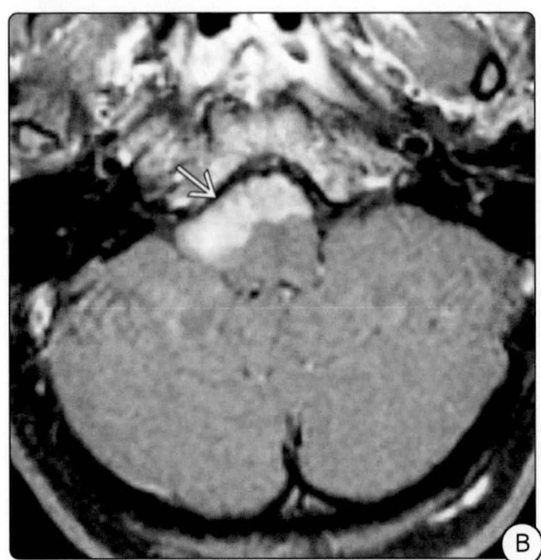

*(32-25B) Axial T1 MR shows mass ➡ anterior to medulla and extends laterally into CPA cistern. Neurenteric (endodermal) cyst found at surgery.*

## Differential Diagnosis

The major differential diagnosis of DC is **EC**. ECs behave more like CSF on both CT and MR imaging, whereas DCs resemble fat. **Lipoma** may resemble a DC, but it is generally much more homogeneous on MR imaging, and it is often associated with other congenital malformations, such as callosal dysgenesis.

**Craniopharyngioma** is often multicystic, extends into the sella, calcifies, and enhances. **Teratoma** may resemble a DC but most commonly occurs in the pineal gland and is much more heterogeneous on imaging than the typical DC.

### DERMOID vs. EPIDERMOID CYST

**Pathology**
- **Both** dermoid, epidermoid contain squamous epithelium + keratin debris
- **Only** dermoid also contains fat, dermal appendages

**Clinical Issues**
- DCs **less** common than epidermoids
- DCs more common in children/young adults
- DCs commonly rupture

**Imaging**
- DC behaves mostly like fat
  - Most often midline, supra- or juxtasellar
- EC more like CSF
  - Most often midline
  - Most common site: Posterior fossa (CPA cistern)

# Endodermal (Neurenteric) Cyst

Endodermal/neurenteric (NE) cysts are rare endodermal-derived developmental CNS lesions. Spinal NE cysts are significantly more common than their intracranial counterparts.

## Terminology

Endodermal cysts are also called enterogenous cyst, enteric cyst, NE cyst, and neuroendodermal cyst **(32-26)**. Similar lesions can occur in the bronchi and foregut.

## Etiology

NE cysts, along with Rathke cleft and colloid cysts, are endodermally derived developmental lesions of the CNS. Embryonic multipotent endodermal cells freely migrate along the embryonic neuroectoderm, which lies just dorsal to the developing notochord. If the neuroectoderm fails to separate from the notochord, displaced nests of respiratory or alimentary tissue may ultimately form an NE cyst.

## Pathology

**Location.** The most common CNS site is the spine; intracranial NE cysts are rare, accounting for 25% of all cases. The majority of these occur as extraaxial lesions in the posterior fossa, most commonly in/near the midline at the pontomedullary junction or the CPA cistern **(32-24)**. Between 15-20% of intracranial cysts are supratentorial.

**Size and Number.** NE cysts vary widely in size. Most are relatively small, but occasionally, these cysts can become very large. NE cysts are almost always solitary lesions. Rare cases of intracranial cyst dissemination following surgical excision have been reported.

**Gross Pathology.** NE cysts are typically well delineated with a thin, translucent wall. Contents vary from clear colorless fluid that resembles CSF to thick viscous mucoid secretions.

**Microscopic Features.** NE cysts are lined with pseudostratified columnar epithelium with ciliated cells and mucous-secreting goblet cells. Neoplastic metaplasia is rare.

## Clinical Issues

NE cysts occur in patients of all ages. Posterior fossa NE cysts typically present with waxing and waning neck pain, occipital headaches, and gait disturbance. NE cysts grow very slowly and are often stable for years.

## Imaging

**General Features.** NE cysts are all well-circumscribed round to ovoid masses. Imaging characteristics—density and signal intensity—vary according to protein content of the cyst fluid and do not exactly follow CSF characteristics.

**CT Findings.** Most NE cysts are iso- to slightly hyperdense compared with CSF. Calcification and intracystic hemorrhage are absent. Bony anomalies are rare.

**MR Findings.** Signal intensity varies. Cyst contents are usually iso- to hyperintense compared to CSF on T1WIs **(32-25)**. Most are hyperintense on T2WI and do not suppress on FLAIR. NE cysts with inspissated cyst contents may appear hypointense on T2WI. Most do not exhibit enhancement on T1 C+ sequences and do not restrict on DWI.

## Differential Diagnosis

The major differential diagnosis of NE is **epidermoid cyst** (EC). ECs are insinuating lesions with lobulated, frond-like surfaces and are usually off-midline in the cerebellopontine angle cistern. Most ECs restrict strongly on DWI. **A "white" epidermoid (32-19) (32-19) (hyperdense on NECT and hyperintense on T1WI) may be indistinguishable from EC.**

**Arachnoid cyst** follows CSF signal intensity on all sequences. **Ecchordosis physaliphora** is a gelatinous-appearing notochordal remnant that typically occurs in the prepontine cistern and is attached to a visible defect in the dorsal clivus by a thin, stalk-like pedicle.

# Pineal Cyst

Cystic-appearing lesions in the pineal gland are common incidental findings on MR scans, seen in 1.5-11% of cases.

## Terminology and Etiology

A pineal cyst (PC) is a benign glia-lined, fluid-containing cyst within the pineal gland parenchyma. The precise etiology of PCs is unknown. Persistent coalescing embryonic pineal cavities and glial degeneration with cavitation have been cited as possible etiologies.

## Pathology

Up to 40% of autopsied pineal glands in the general population contain cysts. PCs are well-demarcated, round or ovoid expansions within an otherwise normal-appearing pineal gland **(32-29)**. Most are < 10 mm in

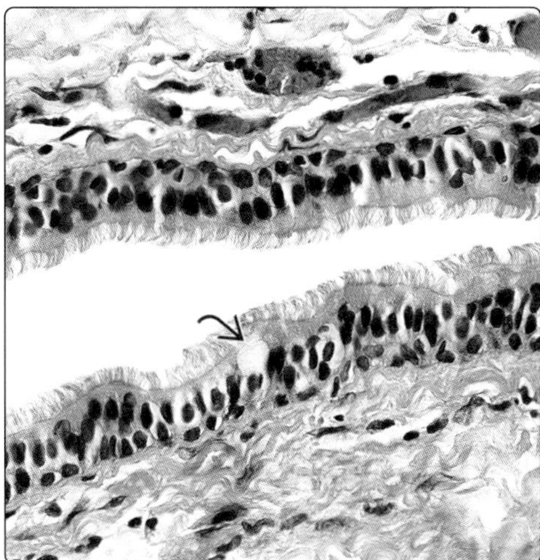

*(32-26) Neurenteric cyst has pseudostratified ciliated epithelium and occasional goblet cells ➲.*

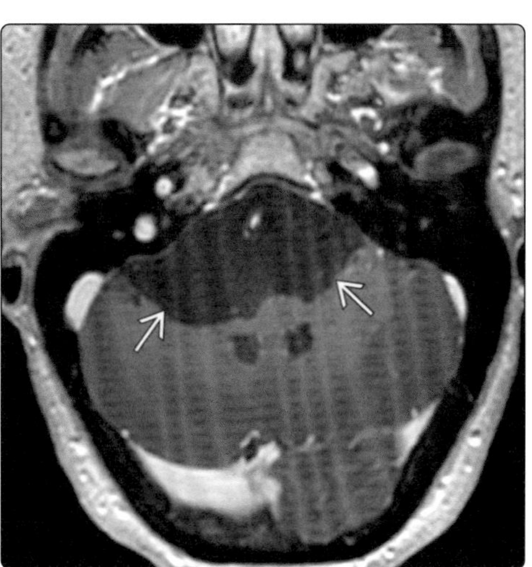

*(32-27) T1 C+ FS MR shows a nonenhancing extraaxial cyst ➡ anterior to the pontomedullary junction (endodermal cyst). (From DP: Neuro.)*

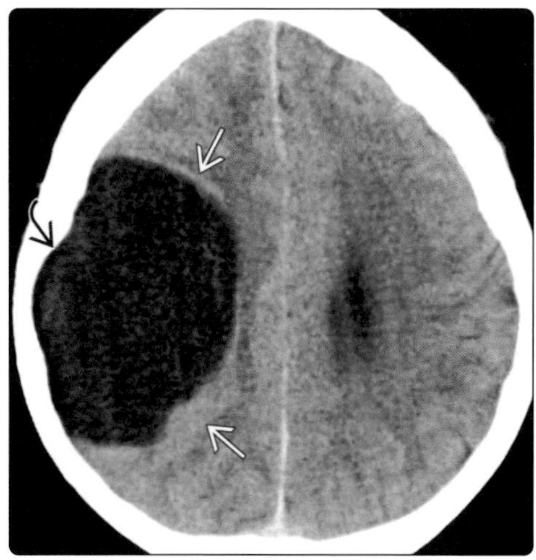

*(32-28) NECT shows a large, CSF-like, extraaxial cyst displacing the cortex ➡ and remodeling the skull ➲ [endodermal (neurenteric) cyst].*

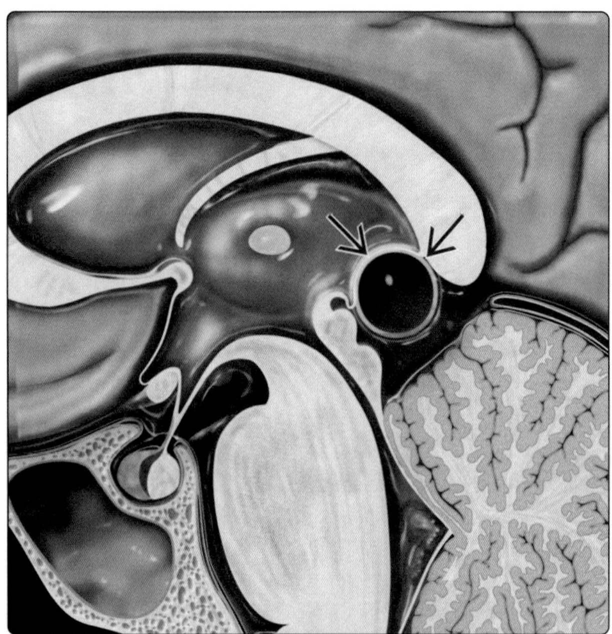

*(32-29) Sagittal graphic shows a small cystic lesion within the pineal gland ⇒. Small, benign pineal cysts are often found incidentally at autopsy or imaging.*

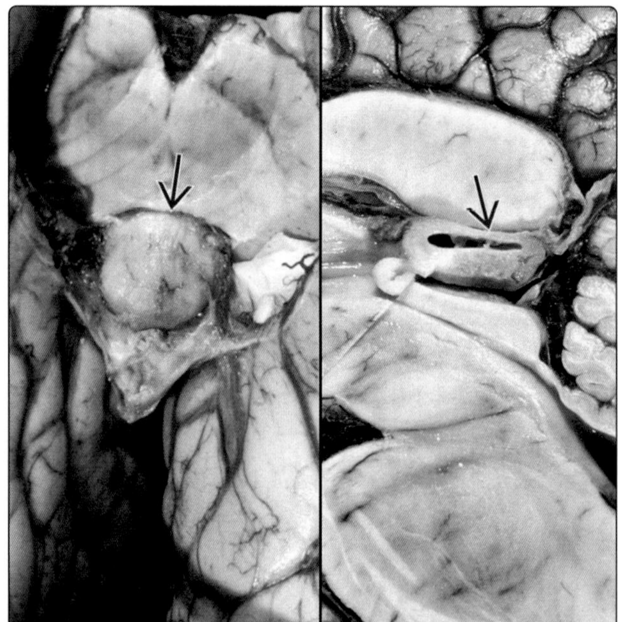

*(32-30) Axial (L) and sagittal (R) autopsy views of a pineal cyst ⇒ show the typical location behind the tectal plate. (Courtesy E. T. Hedley-Whyte, MD.)*

diameter. The largest reported PC is 4.5 cm. PCs are usually unilocular, but lesions containing multiple smaller cysts do occur.

**Gross Pathology.** The general appearance is that of a smooth, soft, tan-yellow pineal gland that contains a uni- or multilocular cyst **(32-30)**. PCs do not have ependymal or epithelial lining, so the cyst "wall" is actually compressed pineal parenchyma. The inner surface of the cyst cavity is often hemosiderin stained as the result of intralesional hemorrhage. Cyst fluid is clear to yellowish.

There are no gross pathologic or histologic features that distinguish symptomatic from asymptomatic PCs.

## Clinical Issues

**Demographics.** PCs can occur at **any** age, although they are more often discovered in middle-aged and older adults.

The overall F:M ratio is 2:1. The incidence among women ages 21-30 years is significantly higher than in any other group.

**Presentation.** PCs rarely cause symptoms. Most are clinically benign and discovered incidentally at imaging or autopsy. Large PCs may compress or obstruct the cerebral aqueduct, resulting in hydrocephalus and headache. Parinaud syndrome (tectal compression) is less common.

Pineal "apoplexy" occurs with sudden intracystic hemorrhage. Acute worsening of headaches combined with visual symptoms can occur. A "thunderclap" headache may mimic symptoms of aneurysmal subarachnoid hemorrhage. Pineal "apoplexy" can result in acute intraventricular obstructive hydrocephalus.

**Natural History.** Only 5% of PCs (mainly in patients younger than 50 years of age) grow; cyst stability or shrinkage is more likely across all age groups. Routine follow-up of PCs is unnecessary in the absence of unusual radiologic characteristics or related clinical symptoms. Surgery is rarely needed or indicated for PCs.

Follow-up of indeterminate cystic lesions of the pineal region usually shows no significant change over time intervals varying from months to years. Patients with growing lesions, atypical contrast enhancement, or hemorrhage on MR are more likely to develop hydrocephalus or exhibit malignant pathology, so follow-up serial MRs are recommended.

## Imaging

**CT Findings.** At least 25% of PCs show calcification within the cyst wall **(32-31A)**. The cyst fluid is iso- to slightly hyperdense compared with CSF **(32-35)**. A very hyperdense PC in a patient with severe headache should raise suspicion of hemorrhage with cyst "apoplexy." Rim, crescentic, or nodular enhancement patterns have all been described with PCs.

The ventricles are usually normal. Large ventricles with "blurred" margins indicate acute obstructive hydrocephalus.

**MR Findings.** As with other cysts, PC signal intensity varies with imaging sequence and cyst contents. Between 50% and 60% of PCs are slightly hyperintense compared with CSF on T1WI **(32-31B)**. Approximately 40% are isointense with CSF. Approximately 1-2% are very hyperintense, which may indicate intracystic hemorrhage. A blood-fluid level may be present **(32-36)**.

Most PCs are small and cause minimal or no mass effect. Large cysts may cause obstructive hydrocephalus. In such cases,

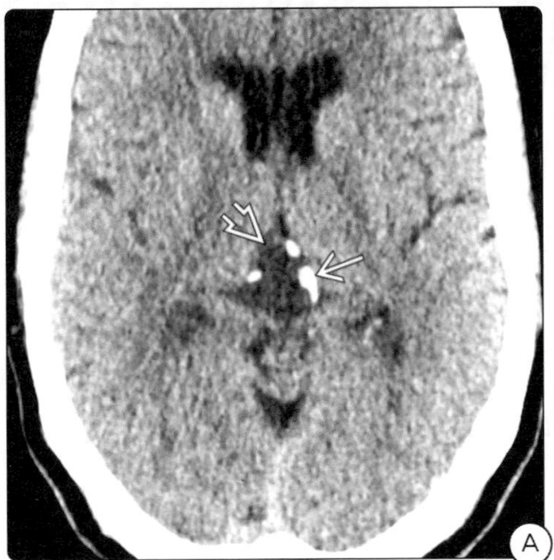

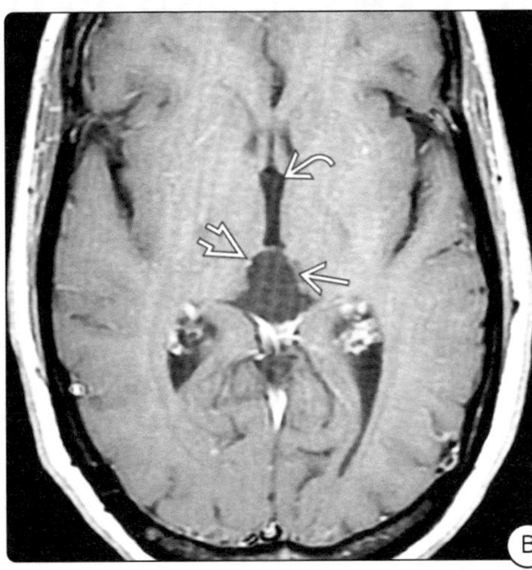

*(**32-31A**) Axial NECT in a 49-yo woman with chronic headaches shows a large, cystic pineal gland ➡ with thick rim calcifications ➡. The cyst appears slightly hyperdense compared to CSF in the frontal horns. (**32-31B**) T1 C+ MR shows that the cyst fluid ➡ is slightly hyperintense compared with CSF in the adjacent 3rd ventricle ➡. Minimal enhancement of the cyst wall ➡ is present. This is a nonneoplastic pineal cyst.*

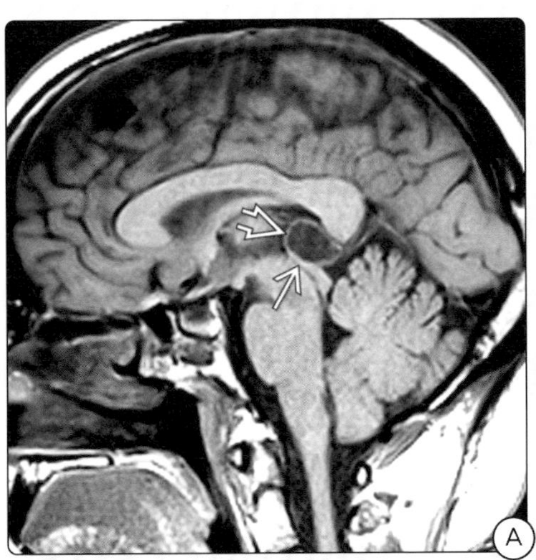

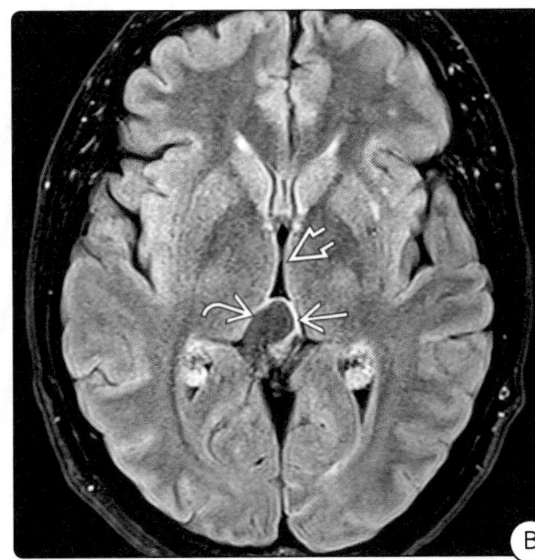

*(**32-32A**) Sagittal T1 MR in a 39-yo woman with headaches, normal neurologic examination shows a nearly 2-cm pineal cyst ➡ that is compressing the tectal plate ➡. (**32-32B**) Axial FLAIR MR in the same patient shows the cyst fluid ➡ is hyperintense relative to CSF in the adjacent 3rd ventricle ➡. The hyperintense cyst rim ➡ enhanced on T1 C+ (not shown). This is surgically proven nonneoplastic benign pineal cyst.*

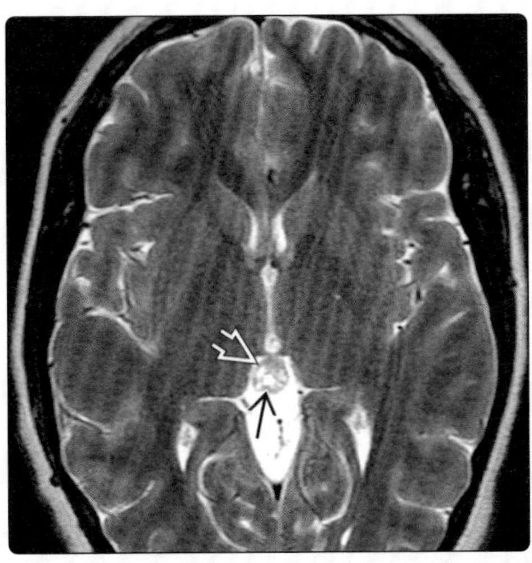

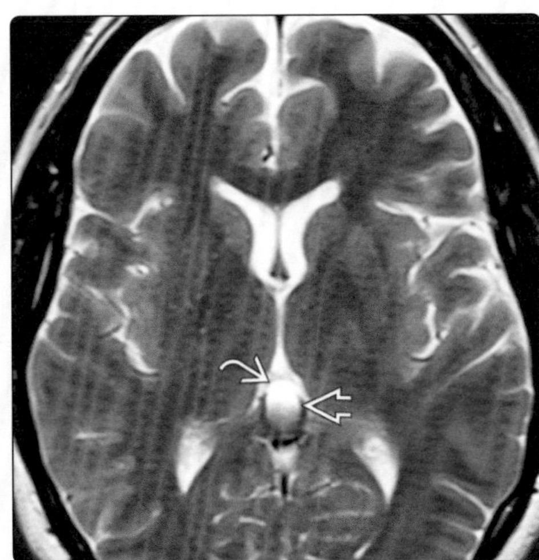

*(**32-33**) Axial T2 MR shows a normal-sized pineal gland ➡ that is isointense with brain. The gland contains multiple small, hyperintense cysts ➡. (**32-34**) T2 MR in a 30-yo woman with 1 week of severe headaches shows a 1.5-cm pineal cyst ➡ with blood-fluid level ➡. This is pineal cyst apoplexy.*

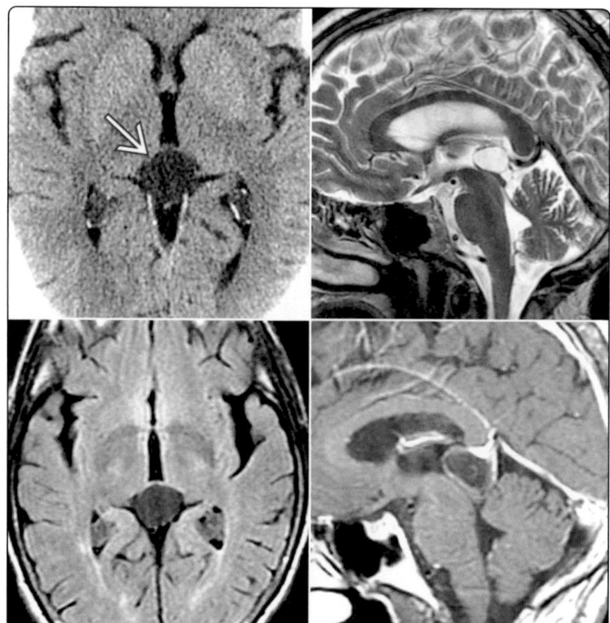

*(32-35) NECT (upper L) demonstrates a large, surgically proven, benign pineal cyst ➡ that is slightly hyperdense compared to CSF. Sagittal T2 (upper R), axial FLAIR (lower L), and sagittal T1 C+ (lower R) MR images show the cyst is not exactly like CSF.*

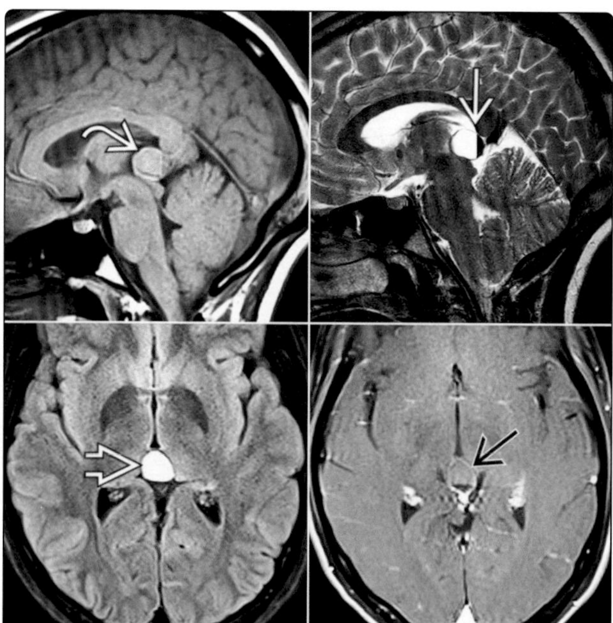

*(32-36) Sagittal T1 MR shows a large pineal cyst ➡ that exhibits a blood-fluid level ➡ on the sagittal T2 MR and does not suppress ➡ on FLAIR MR. Some rim enhancement ➡ is present on T1 C+ FS MR. This is pineal cyst "apoplexy."*

T2/FLAIR scans show "fingers" of hyperintensity extending into the periventricular white matter due to subependymal accumulation of brain interstitial fluid. These are especially well demonstrated on sagittal scans.

The vast majority of PCs are iso- to slightly hyperintense on T2WI **(32-35)** and do not suppress completely on FLAIR **(32-32)**. Internal septations are visible in 20-25% of cases, and up to 60% are multicystic on CISS or FIESTA sequences. If acute hemorrhage has occurred, intracystic blood may appear very hypointense on T2WIs and "bloom" on T2* (GRE, SWI). PCs typically do not restrict on DWI.

Between 1/3 and 2/3 of PCs enhance. The most common pattern is a thin (< 2-mm), circumferential rim of enhancement **(32-31B)**. Less common patterns include nodular or crescentic enhancement. Enhancing internal septa, rim thickness > 2 mm, or irregular enhancing nodules can be seen in 15-20% of PCs and may make differentiation between a nontumoral PC and cystic pineal neoplasm challenging.

On delayed imaging, contrast may accumulate within the cystic component and can be confused with a solid lesion.

## Differential Diagnosis

The most common differential diagnosis is **normal pineal gland**. Normal pineal glands often contain one or more small cysts **(32-33)** and can have nodular, crescentic, or ring-like enhancement. Quadrigeminal cistern **arachnoid cysts** occur dorsal to the pineal gland and follow CSF signal intensity on all sequences.

The most important pathologic entity to be differentiated from a PC is **pineocytoma**. Pineocytoma is a CNS WHO grade 1 pineal parenchymal tumor that is usually solid or at least partially solid/cystic. Purely cystic pineocytomas are much less common and can be indistinguishable from PCs on imaging. Pineocytomas can remain stable for many years without significant change on serial imaging.

Atypical imaging findings, focal invasion, or significant interval change in a presumed PC or pineocytoma should raise suspicion for the more aggressive **pineal parenchymal tumor of intermediate differentiation** (PPTID), which is a CNS WHO grade 2 or 3 lesion.

### PINEAL CYST

**Pathology**
- Usually < 1 cm
- Unilocular > multicystic
- Wall consists of compressed pineal parenchyma
- Fluid clear to yellowish

**Clinical Issues**
- Common
  - 23% of normal MRs
  - 25-40% of autopsies
- Occurs at any age
  - More common in adults
- Usually asymptomatic; found incidentally

**Imaging**
- $Ca^{++}$ (25%)
- Fluid slightly hyperintense to CSF on MR
- Rim, nodular, or crescentic enhancement
- Blood-fluid level = PC "apoplexy"

**Differential Diagnosis**
- Normal pineal gland
- Pineocytoma

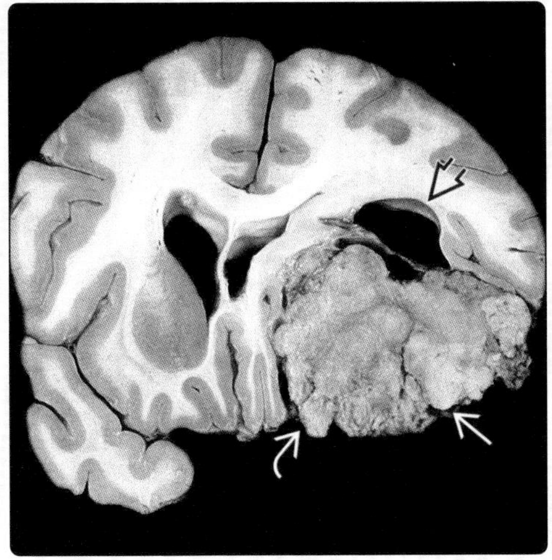

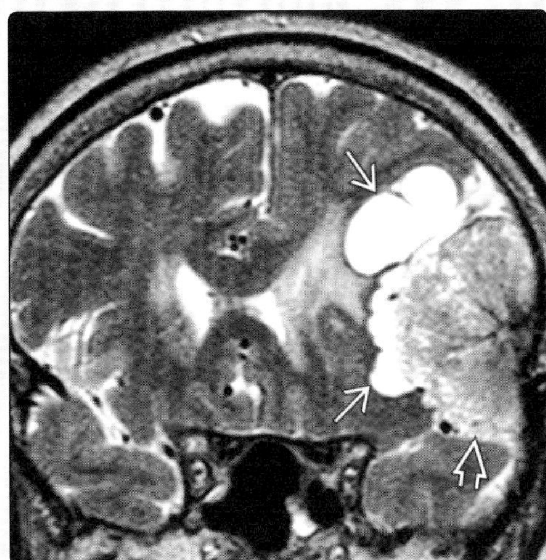

***(32-37)** Coronal autopsy shows a lobulated dural-based meningioma ➡ with CSF-vascular "cleft" ➦ and a large tumor-associated cyst ⇨. **(32-38)** Coronal T2 MR shows a typical sphenoid wing meningioma ➡ with hyperintense pools of trapped fluid ➡ between the tumor and brain. (Courtesy M. Thurnher, MD.)*

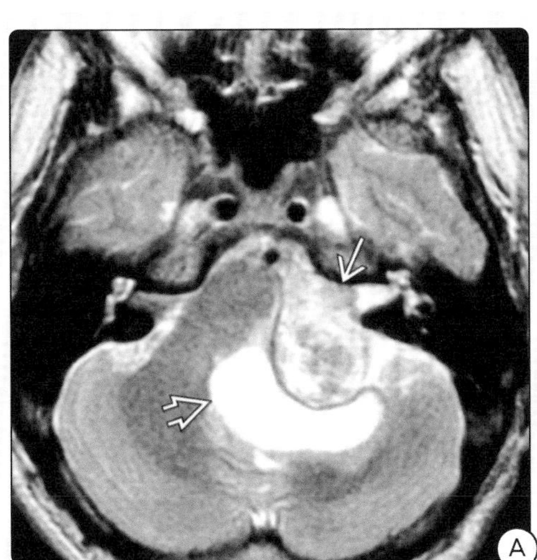

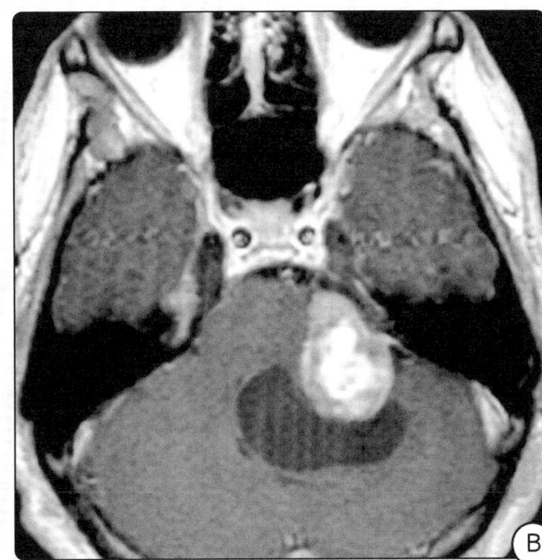

***(32-39A)** Axial T2 MR shows a mixed iso- and hyperintense dumbbell-shaped mass ➡ in the left internal auditory canal (IAC) and CPA cistern. Note the large tumor-associated cyst ➡. **(32-39B)** T1 C+ MR in the same patient shows the cyst wall does not enhance. Vestibular schwannoma with adjacent nonneoplastic peritumoral cyst was found at surgery.*

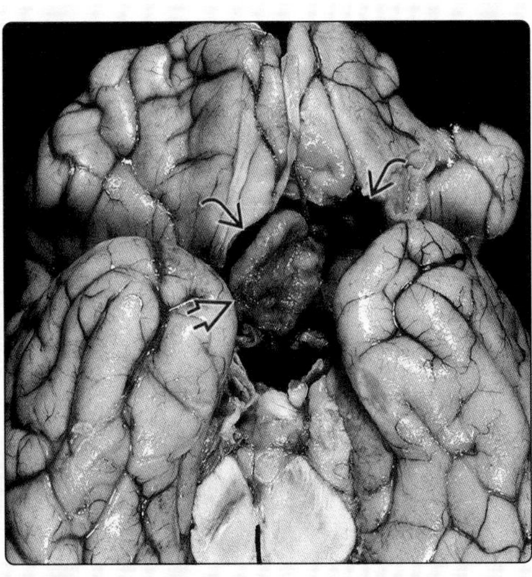

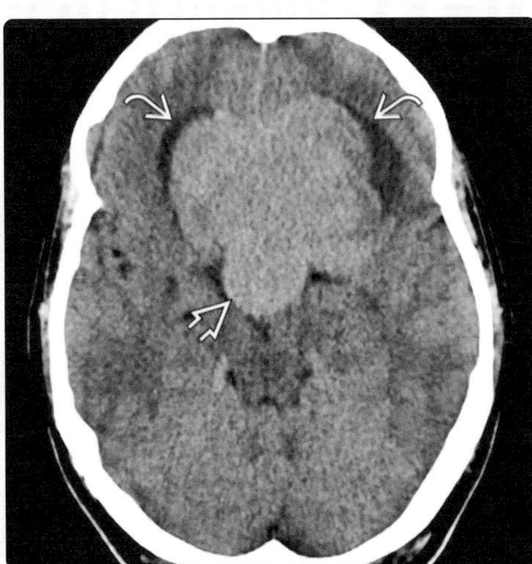

***(32-40)** Autopsied brain, submentovertex view, shows an enormous macroadenoma ⇨ with invagination into the brain and large peritumoral cysts ➦. **(32-41)** NECT shows a huge, lobulated pituitary macroadenoma ➡ with peritumoral cysts ➦.*

## Nonneoplastic Tumor-Associated Cysts

Tumor-associated cysts (TACs)—also referred to as peritumoral cysts—are rare, benign cysts that are adjacent to, but not contained within, a neoplasm.

Most TACs represent trapped, encysted "pools" of CSF adjacent to a large benign extraaxial tumor, such as meningioma **(32-37)**, schwannoma **(32-39)**, pituitary macroadenoma **(32-40)**, and craniopharyngioma. These trapped, encysted "pools" of CSF vary from clear, CSF-like liquid to turbid proteinaceous fluid. TACs are usually positioned at the tumor-brain interface between the extraaxial mass and adjacent cortex **(32-41)**. Size varies from small insignificant collections to very large cysts.

Imaging findings vary with cyst content. Most are hypointense relative to brain on T1WIs and are very hyperintense on T2WI and FLAIR **(32-39A)**. Enhancement is minimal or absent **(32-39B)**.

TACs must be distinguished from **cystic neoplasms** (cysts are contained within the tumor), **arachnoid cysts** (not tumor associated), and **enlarged perivascular (Virchow-Robin) spaces**. The latter two behave like CSF on imaging studies.

# Parenchymal Cysts

Parenchymal (intraaxial) cysts are much more common than either their extraaxial or intraventricular counterparts. Once a cyst has been identified as lying within the brain itself, the differential diagnosis is limited. The most common parenchymal cysts—prominent perivascular spaces and hippocampal sulcus remnants—are anatomic variants.

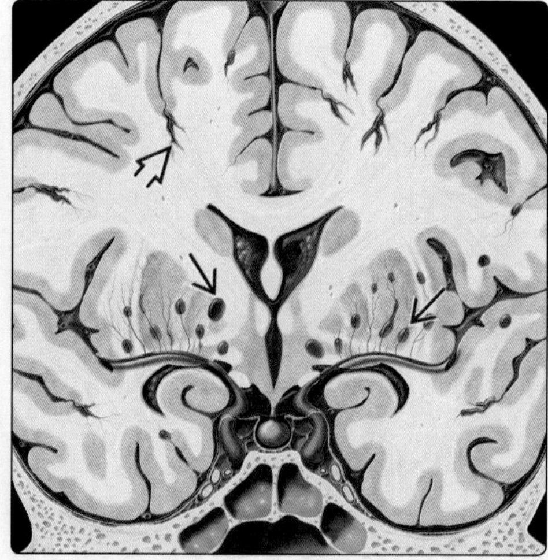

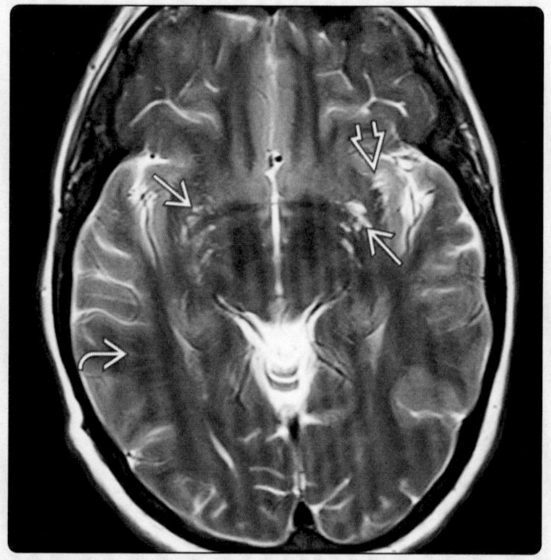

***(32-42)** Graphic shows normal perivascular spaces (PVSs) along penetrating arteries in the basal ganglia and subcortical white matter. **(32-43)** 3T T2 MR shows normal PVSs in the inferior basal ganglia, extreme capsule, and subcortical white matter.*

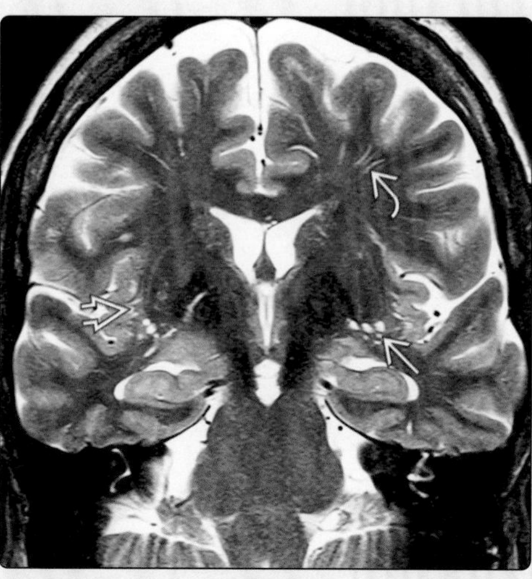

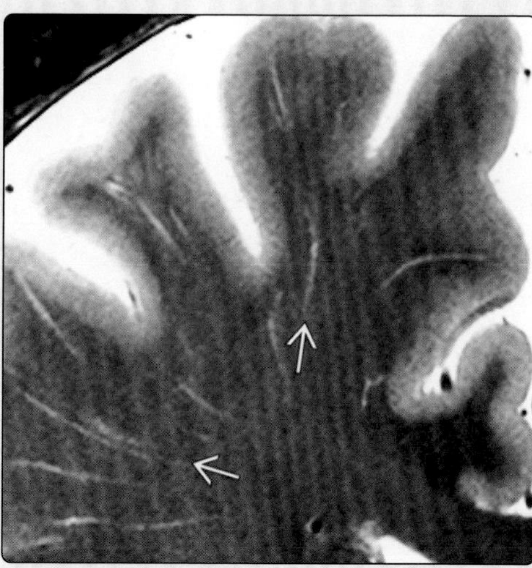

***(32-44)** Coronal T2 MR shows normal PVSs in inferior basal ganglia, external capsule, and corona radiata. **(32-45)** Close-up view of coronal 7T T2 MR shows normal PVSs can be seen throughout the subcortical white matter. Note that even at 7T, PVSs are not seen as they pass through the cortex. (Courtesy M. Law, MD.)*

Neuroglial cysts and porencephalic cysts are relatively uncommon. All other nonneoplastic, noninfectious brain cysts are rare.

## Enlarged Perivascular Spaces

By far, the most common parenchymal brain "cysts" are enlarged perivascular spaces (PVSs). They vary from solitary, small, inconspicuous, and unremarkable to multiple, large, bizarre, alarming-looking collections of CSF-like fluid. They are often asymmetric, may cause mass effect, and have frequently been mistaken for multicystic brain tumors.

### Terminology

PVSs are also known as Virchow-Robin spaces (VRSs). PVSs are pia-lined spaces that accompany penetrating arteries and arterioles into the brain parenchyma **(32-42)**. The PVSs do not communicate directly with the subarachnoid space.

The PVSs form an essential part of the brain's "glymphatic system." This system allows for dynamic exchange of interstitial fluid (ISF) and CSF along paravascular channels of the penetrating arteries and draining veins. The glymphatic system is essential in the clearance of neurotoxic solutes (such as amyloid) from the brain interstitium to the CSF efflux pathways.

### Etiology

**General Concepts.** The brain PVSs are distributed throughout the cerebral hemispheres, midbrain, and cerebellum. The PVSs are filled with ISF, not CSF. In addition to clearing neurotoxic solutes, recent evidence suggests the PVSs also perform an essential role in maintaining brain fluid and intracranial pressure homeostasis.

Precisely why some PVSs become enlarged is unknown. Most investigators believe ISF egress is blocked, causing cystic enlargement of the PVSs. Extreme enlargement of the PVSs is unusual and sometimes referred to as tumefactive VRSs.

### Pathology

**Location.** Although PVSs can be found virtually anywhere in the brain, they have a striking predilection for the inferior 1/3 of the basal ganglia, especially near the anterior commissure **(32-42)**. They are also common in the subcortical and deep white matter as well as the midbrain and dentate nuclei of the cerebellum.

**Size and Number.** Enlarged PVSs tend to occur in clusters. Collections of multiple variably sized PVSs are much more common than solitary unilocular lesions.

Most PVSs are smaller than 2 mm. PVSs increase in size and prevalence with age. Giant so-called tumefactive PVSs measuring up to 9 cm in diameter have been reported.

**Microscopic Features.** Enlarged PVSs appear as collections of smoothly demarcated cysts filled with clear colorless fluid.

PVSs are bounded by a single or double layer of invaginated pia. Cortical PVSs are lined by a single layer of pia, whereas two layers accompany lenticulostriate and midbrain arteries.

As a PVS penetrates into the subcortical white matter, it becomes fenestrated and discontinuous. The pial layer disappears completely at the capillary level.

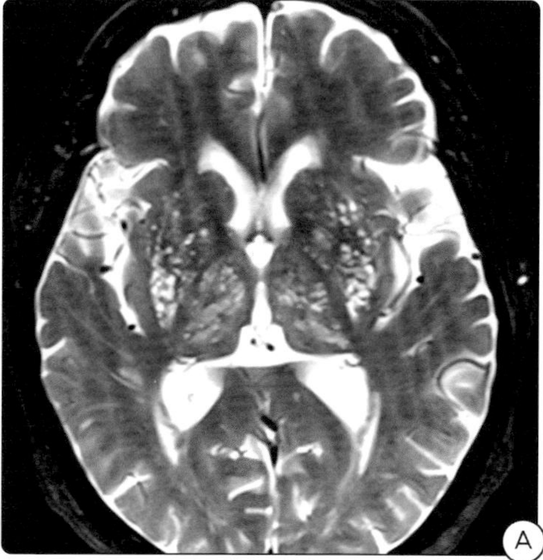

***(32-46A)** T2 MR in an intellectually normal 92-yo woman shows innumerable hyperintense PVSs scattered throughout the basal ganglia, thalami.*

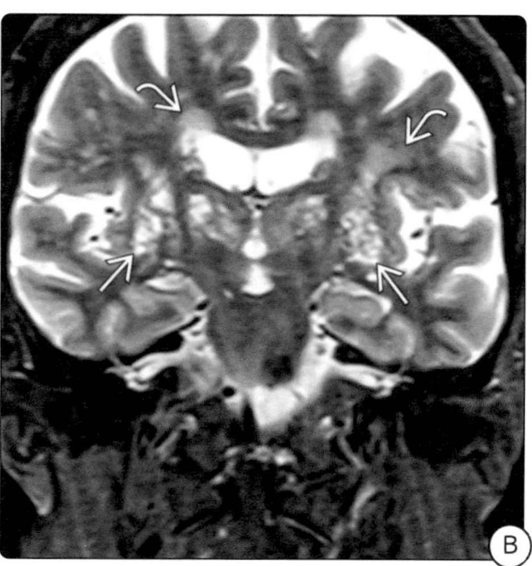

***(32-46B)** Coronal T2 MR shows the PVSs ➡ are distinct from more ill-defined, less hyperintense confluent white matter ➡.*

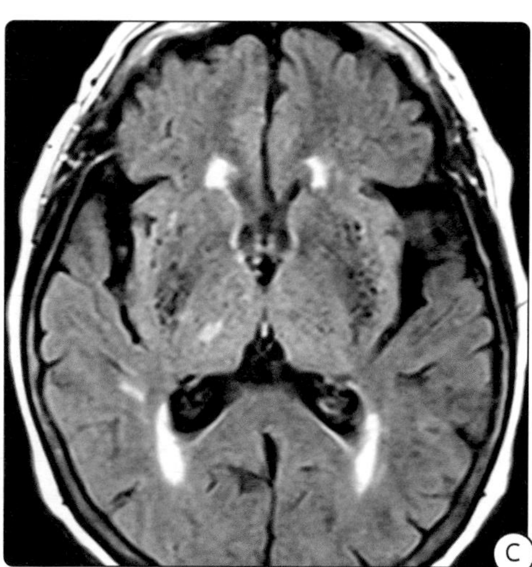

***(32-46C)** The basal ganglia PVSs suppress on FLAIR MR while the periventricular white matter hyperintensity does not (état criblé).*

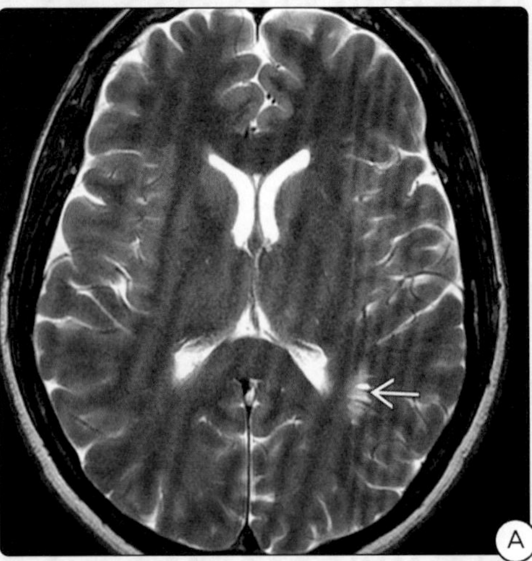

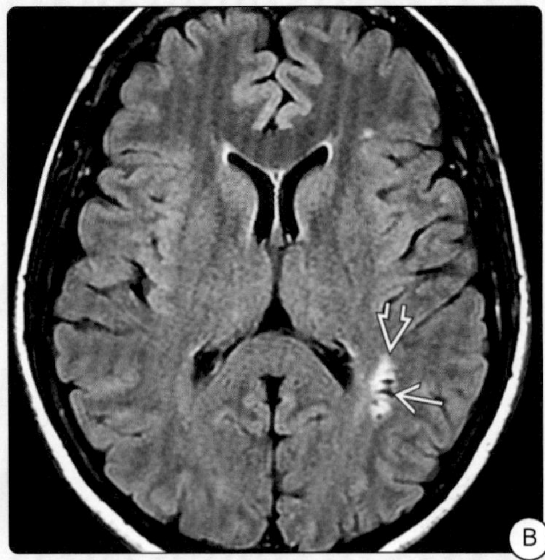

*(32-47A) T2 MR in a patient with headaches and normal neurologic examination shows a collection of hyperintense, ovoid-shaped, cystic-appearing structures ➡ in the left parietal white matter. (32-47B) FLAIR MR shows a collection of ovoid cyst-like structures suppresses completely ➡ and is surrounded by hyperintense white matter ➡. Approximately 25% of enlarged PVSs have FLAIR hyperintensity in the adjacent brain.*

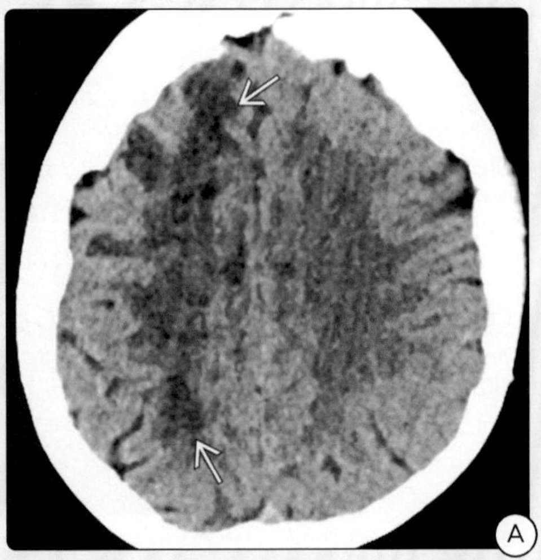

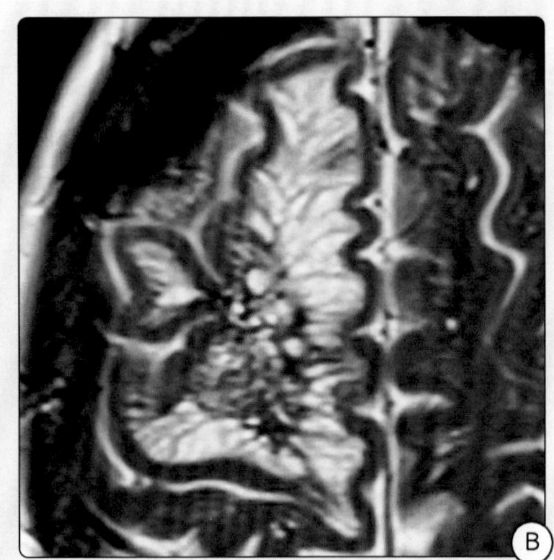

*(32-48A) NECT shows confluent hypodensity ➡ in the subcortical white matter of the right cerebral hemisphere (compare to the normal-appearing left hemisphere). (32-48B) Close-up view of T2 MR in the same patient shows multiple enlarged, confluent PVSs in the subcortical white matter. Gyri overlying over the tumefactive PVS are expanded. Note enlarged PVSs are not visible in the cortex.*

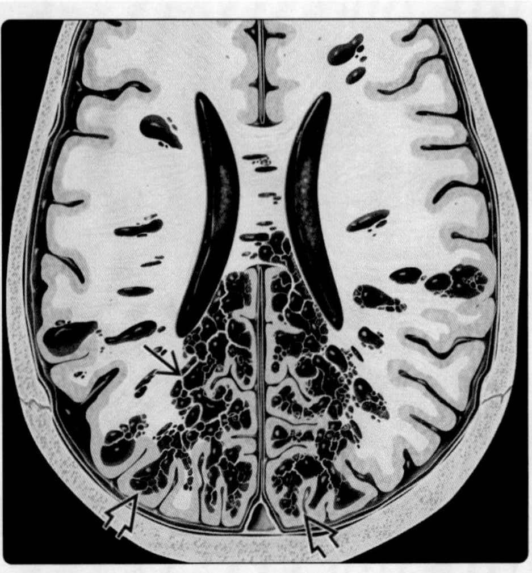

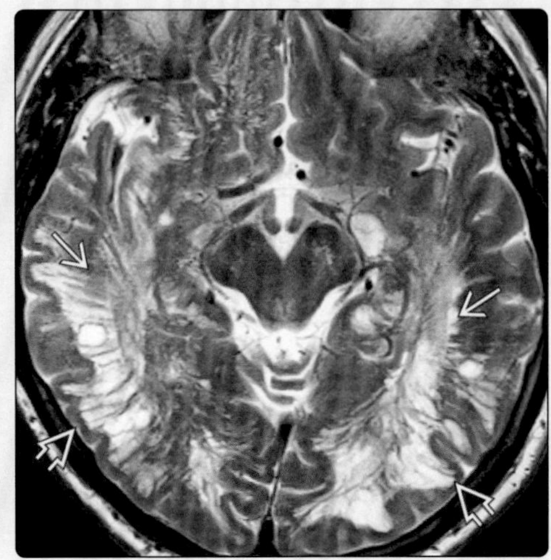

*(32-49) Graphic depicts innumerable hemispheric enlarged PVSs ➡ in the subcortical, deep white matter. Note that the overlying gyri ➡ are expanded but otherwise normal. (32-50) Axial T2 MR in a 69-yo moderately demented man shows innumerable enlarged PVSs ➡. Note sparing of overlying cortex, which appears expanded ➡. (Courtesy M. Warmuth-Metz, MD.)*

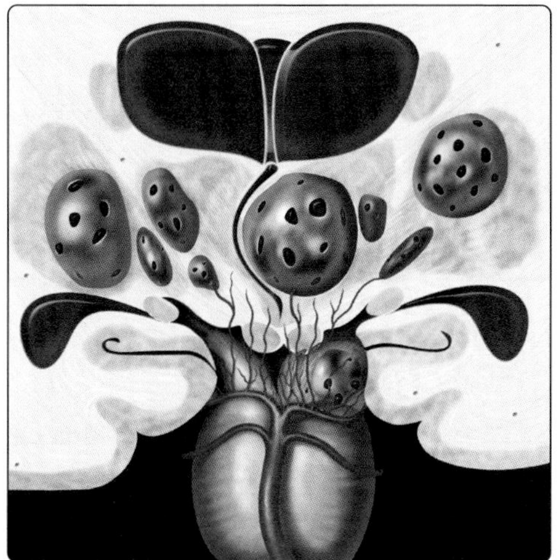

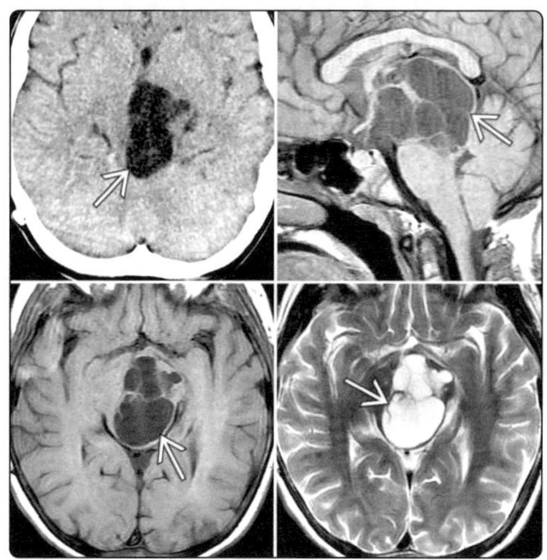

***(32-51)** Graphic shows tumefactive PVSs in the midbrain/thalami causing aqueduct obstruction and hydrocephalus.* ***(32-52)** Cluster of variably sized, CSF-like cysts → grossly expands the midbrain. These are giant tumefactive PVSs.*

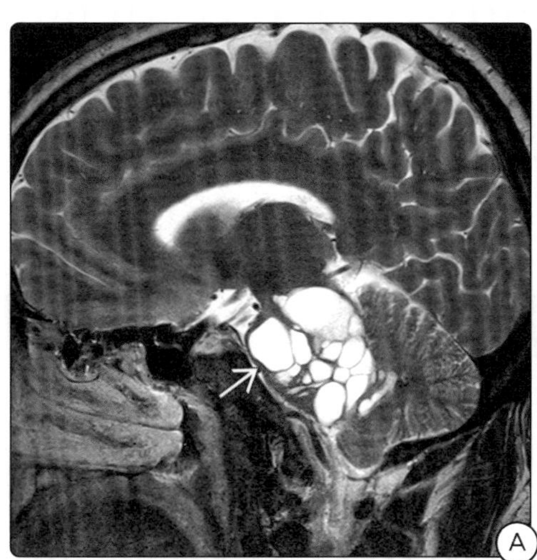

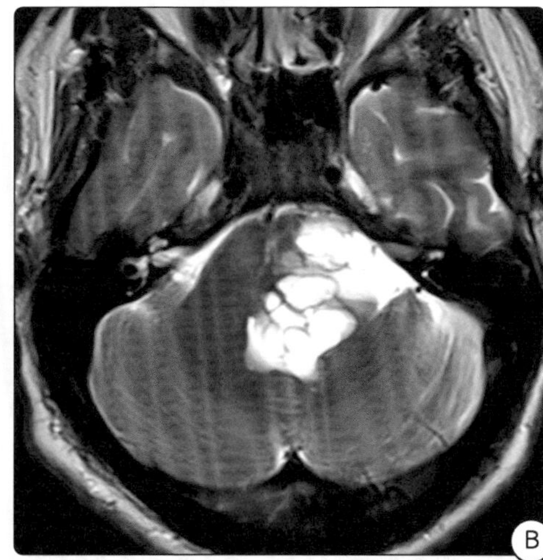

***(32-53A)** Sagittal T2 MR in a 41-yo man with facial numbness, ataxia, and double vision shows a collection of various-sized hyperintense cysts expanding the pons →.* ***(32-53B)** Axial T2 MR in the same patient shows the collection of CSF-like cysts extends from the pons into the dentate nuclei.*

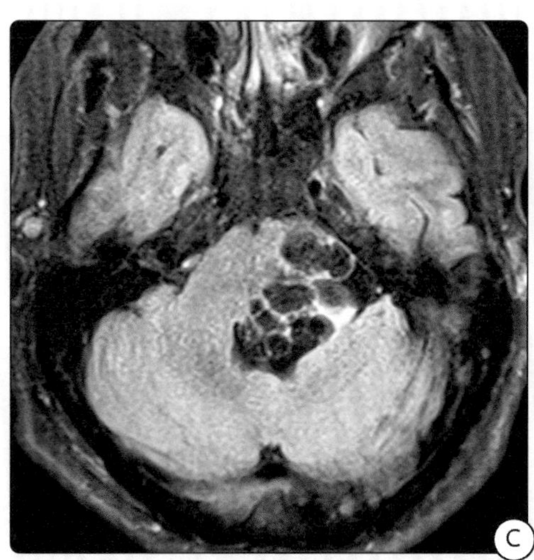

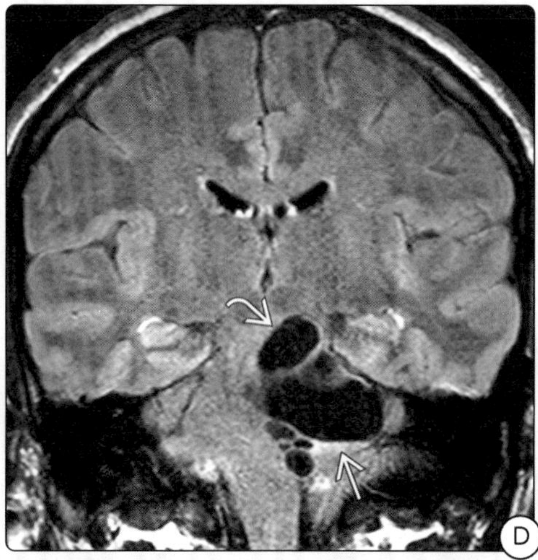

***(32-53C)** The cysts suppress on FLAIR MR and can be seen extending through the brachium pontis to the 4th ventricle.* ***(32-53D)** Coronal FLAIR MR shows the cysts → vary in size from extremely large to tiny. A small amount of gliosis in the adjacent brain is present →. Pial-lined cysts consistent with PVSs were found at surgery.*

The brain parenchyma surrounding enlarged PVSs is typically normal without gliosis, inflammation, hemorrhage, or discernible amyloid deposition.

## Clinical Issues

**Epidemiology.** PVSs are the most common nonneoplastic parenchymal brain "cysts" **(32-43)**. With high-resolution 3T or 7T MR **(32-45)**, small PVSs are seen in nearly all patients **(32-44)**, in virtually every location, and at all ages. Between 25-30% of children have identifiable PVSs on high-resolution MR scans.

**Demographics.** Enlarged PVSs are more common in middle-aged and older patients and increase in both size and number with age. Recent studies have linked enlarged PVSs with age, lacunar stroke subtype, and white matter lesions and consider them as an MR marker of cerebral small vessel disease.

**Presentation.** Most enlarged PVSs do not cause symptoms and are discovered incidentally on imaging studies or at autopsy. Neuropsychological evaluation is typically normal. Nonspecific symptoms, such as headache, dizziness, memory impairment, and Parkinson-like symptoms, have been reported in some cases, but their relationship to enlarged PVSs is unclear. Large PVSs in the midbrain may cause obstructive hydrocephalus and present with headache.

**Natural History.** Enlarged PVSs tend to be stable in size and remain unchanged over many years, although a few cases of progressively enlarging PVSs have been reported.

**Treatment Options.** Enlarged PVSs are "leave me alone" lesions that should not be mistaken for serious disease. If midbrain PVSs cause obstructive hydrocephalus, the generally accepted treatment is to shunt the ventricles, not the cysts.

## Imaging

**General Features.** The common pattern of enlarged PVSs is one or more clusters of variably sized CSF-like cysts. They commonly cause focal mass effect. For example, if they occur in the subcortical white matter, the overlying gyri are enlarged with concomitant compression of adjacent sulci **(32-49)**.

The clinical significance and MR appearance of tumefactive VRSs depends on their anatomic location. Type 1 tumefactive VRSs are located in the basal ganglia along the lenticulostriate arteries. Type 2 lesions are found in the subcortical white matter along perforating cortical arteries. Type 3 tumefactive PVSs occur in the mesencephalothalamic region **(32-52)**. Recently, a fourth type (type 4) has been described in the subcortical white matter of the anterior temporal lobe adjacent to the middle cerebral artery.

**CT Findings.** Enlarged PVSs are groups of round/ovoid/linear/punctate CSF-like lesions that do not demonstrate calcification or hemorrhage **(32-48A)**. PVSs do not enhance following contrast administration.

**MR Findings.** Even though they are filled with ISF, PVSs closely parallel CSF signal intensity on all imaging sequences. Focal mass effect is common. Enlarged PVSs in the subcortical white matter expand overlying gyri **(32-48B)**. Enlarged tumefactive PVSs in the midbrain may compress the aqueduct and third ventricle, resulting in intraventricular obstructive hydrocephalus **(32-51)**.

PVSs are isointense with CSF on T1-, PD, and T2WI **(32-50)**. They suppress completely on FLAIR. Edema in the adjacent brain is absent, although 25% of tumefactive PVSs have minimal increased signal intensity around the cysts **(32-47)**.

PVSs do not hemorrhage, enhance, or demonstrate restricted diffusion.

## Differential Diagnosis

The major differential diagnosis is chronic **lacunar infarction**. Although they often affect the basal ganglia and suppress on FLAIR, lacunar infarcts do not cluster around the anterior commissure, are often irregular in shape, and frequently exhibit hyperintensity in the adjacent brain.

In some older patients, very prominent PVSs in the basal ganglia are present **(32-46)**. This condition, called **"état criblé"** (cribriform state), should not be mistaken for multiple lacunar infarcts. PVSs are round/ovoid and regular in configuration, and the adjacent brain parenchyma is usually normal without gliosis or edema.

**Infectious cysts** (especially parenchymal neurocysticercosis cysts) are usually small. Although often multiple or multilocular, they typically do not occur in clusters of variably sized cysts as is typical for enlarged PVSs.

### ENLARGED PERIVASCULAR SPACES

**Terminology**

- a.k.a. VRSs
- Found around penetrating blood vessels
- Lined by pia
- Filled with ISF
- Do not communicate directly with subarachnoid space

**Pathology**

- Normal PVSs common, seen on 3T and 7T
  - Most are tiny, < 2 mm
  - Tend to occur in clusters
  - Inferior 1/3 of basal ganglia around anterior commissure
  - Also extreme capsule, anterior temporal lobes, dentate nuclei
  - Not visualized as they pass through cortex, even at 7T
- Giant tumefactive PVSs up to 9 cm reported

**Imaging**

- Often bizarre-looking
- Occur in clusters
- Variably sized cysts
- Follow CSF density/signal intensity
  - 25-40% have FLAIR hyperintensity in surrounding brain
- Tumefactive PVSs
  - Midbrain lesions may cause hydrocephalus
  - Subcortical lesions may expand gyri

## Hippocampal Sulcus Remnants

### Etiology

At 15 fetal weeks, the hippocampus normally surrounds an "open" shallow fissure—the hippocampal sulcus—along the medial surface of the temporal lobe. The walls of the hippocampal sulcus gradually fuse, and the sulcus is eventually obliterated. One or more residual cystic cavities may remain and persist into adult life **(32-54)**. These remnant cavities—hippocampal remnant cysts—are normal anatomic variants and are of no clinical significance.

### Imaging

Hippocampal sulcus remnants (HCSRs) are seen in 10-15% of normal high-resolution MR scans. They appear as a string of beads with multiple small round or ovoid cysts curving along the hippocampus between the dentate gyrus and subiculum, just medial to the temporal horn of the lateral ventricle. HCSRs follow CSF in signal intensity on all sequences **(32-55)**. They suppress completely on FLAIR, do not enhance, and do not restrict on DWI.

### Differential Diagnosis

The major differential diagnosis is **enlarged perivascular spaces**. When they occur in the temporal lobe, enlarged perivascular spaces are found in the subcortical white matter of the insula and anterior tip of the temporal lobe, not medial to the temporal horn of the lateral ventricle.

A **choroid fissure cyst** forms along the choroid fissure and lies medial to the hippocampus. It is a large, solitary CSF collection in contiguity with the subarachnoid space and has a characteristic spindle shape configuration on sagittal images.

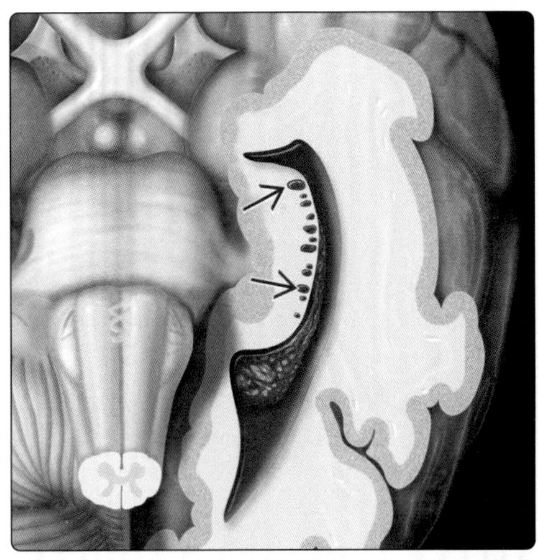

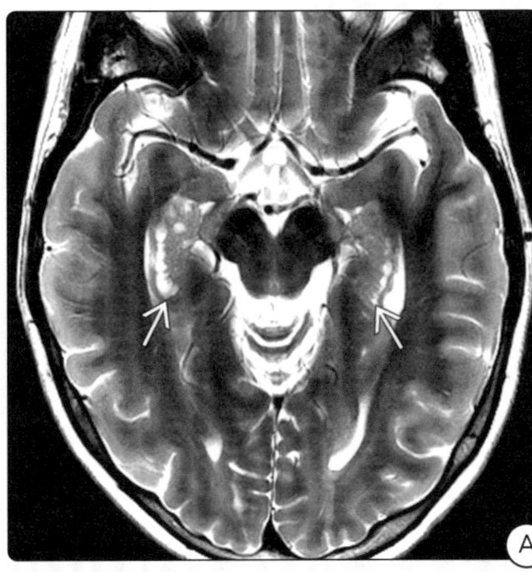

***(32-54)** Graphic of a normal temporal lobe shows a string of cysts within the lateral hippocampus, along the residual cavity of the primitive hippocampal sulcus ➡. Hippocampal sulcus remnant cysts are incidental, a normal finding. **(32-55A)** Axial T2 MR in a 51-yo woman shows a collection of CSF-like cysts ➡ in both hippocampi just medial to the temporal horns of the lateral ventricles.*

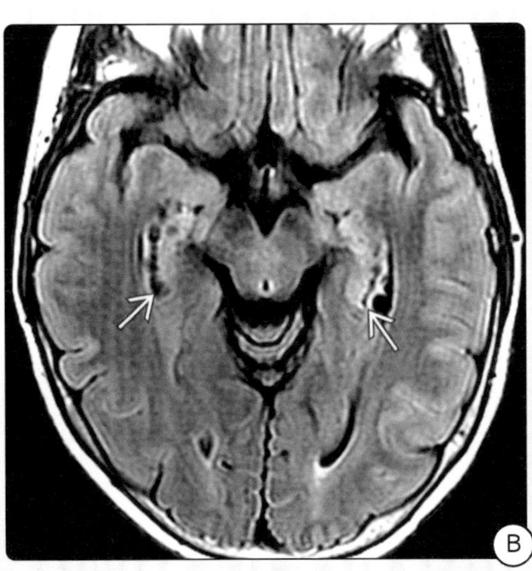

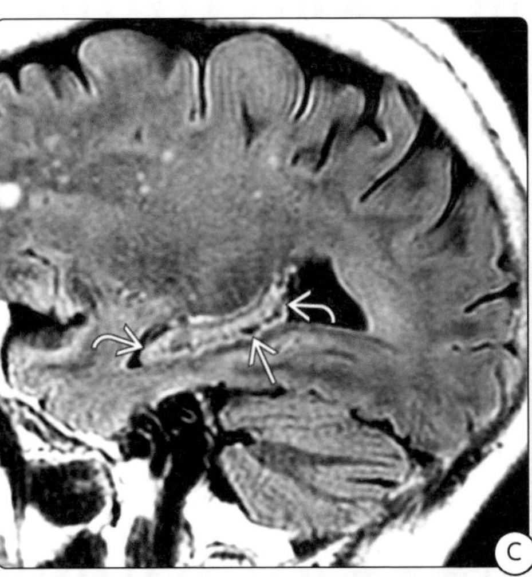

***(32-55B)** The cysts ➡ suppress on FLAIR and are identical in signal intensity compared to CSF in the temporal horns and suprasellar cistern, sylvian fissures. **(32-55C)** Sagittal FLAIR MR through the right temporal horn of the lateral ventricle nicely demonstrates the hippocampus ➡. The CSF-like cysts ➡ are remnants of the embryonic hippocampal sulci that did not fuse completely. This is a benign, incidental finding.*

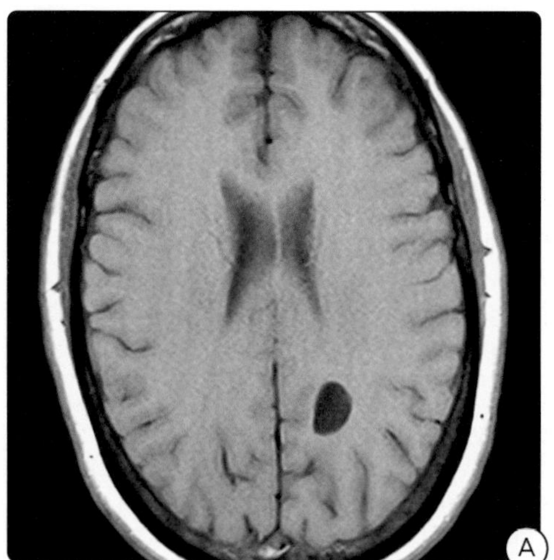


***(32-56A)** Axial T1 MR in a 63-yo woman with headaches shows a sharply demarcated CSF collection in the left parietal white matter.*

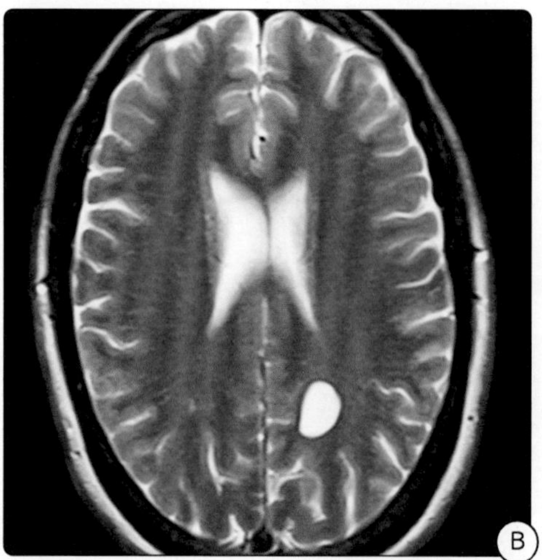


***(32-56B)** The cyst follows CSF on T2 MR.*

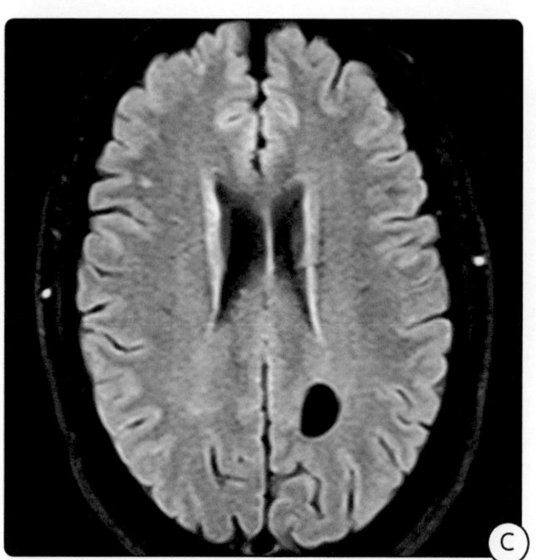


***(32-56C)** The cyst suppresses completely on FLAIR MR, and there is no surrounding signal abnormality. This is probable neuroglial cyst.*

## Neuroglial Cyst

### Terminology

Neuroglial cysts (NGCs) are sometimes called **glioependymal cysts** or **neuroepithelial cysts**. They are benign, fluid-containing cavities buried within the cerebral white matter.

### Pathology

The frontal lobe is the most common site. NGCs often lie adjacent to—but do not communicate directly with—the cerebral ventricles. Most are solitary, unilocular cysts that vary in size from a few millimeters up to several centimeters in diameter.

Grossly, NGCs are rounded, smooth, unilocular cysts that contain clear CSF-like fluid. Most NGCs are lined with a simple, nonstratified, low columnar/cuboidal epithelium.

### Clinical Issues

Parenchymal NGCs are uncommon, representing < 1% of all intracranial cysts. NGCs occur in all age groups but are generally more common in adults. There is no sex predilection.

NGCs are often asymptomatic and found incidentally at imaging or autopsy. Many—if not most—NGCs remain stable over many years. Serial observation with imaging studies is the usual course, although some large NGCs have been fenestrated or drained.

### Imaging

NGCs are fluid density, typically resemble CSF on NECT, do not contain calcifications, and do not hemorrhage.

MR signal intensity varies with cyst content. Most NGCs are iso- or slightly hyperintense to CSF. They usually suppress on FLAIR, do not restrict, and do not enhance **(32-56)**. The parenchyma surrounding an NGC is usually normal or may show minimal gliosis.

### Differential Diagnosis

The diagnosis of NGC is mostly a process of elimination, excluding other, sometimes more ominous possibilities.

The major differential diagnosis of NGC is a solitary **enlarged perivascular space**. Most enlarged PVSs are multiple (not solitary) and occur as clusters of variably sized cysts. A **porencephalic cyst** is a result of an insult to the brain parenchyma. Porencephalic cysts communicate with the ventricle and are lined by gliotic or spongiotic white matter.

**Arachnoid cysts** are extraaxial, not intraaxial, and lined with flattened arachnoid cells. **Epidermoid cysts** are almost always extraaxial, do not suppress on FLAIR, and restrict on DWI. **Ependymal cysts** are intraventricular. **Neoplastic** and **inflammatory cysts** generally do not follow CSF, often demonstrate wall enhancement or calcification, and are frequently surrounded by edema.

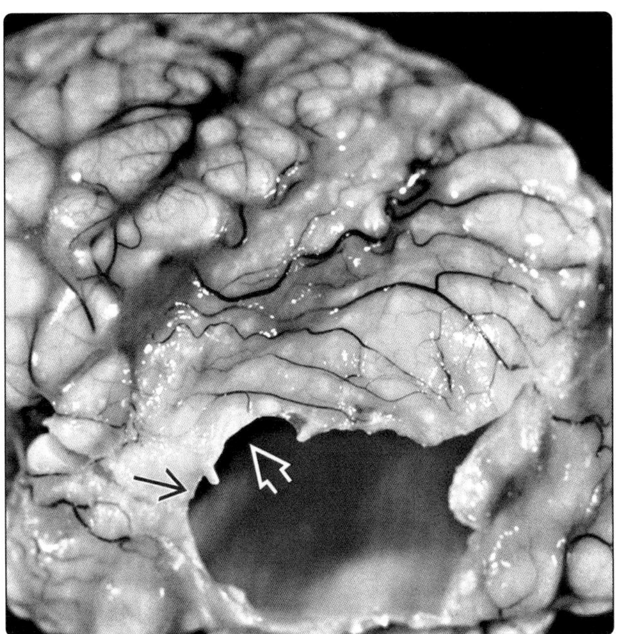

*(32-57) Autopsy specimen shows a typical porencephalic cyst as a CSF-filled cavity that extends from the brain surface ⇒ to the ventricular ependyma ➡. (Courtesy J. Townsend, MD.)*

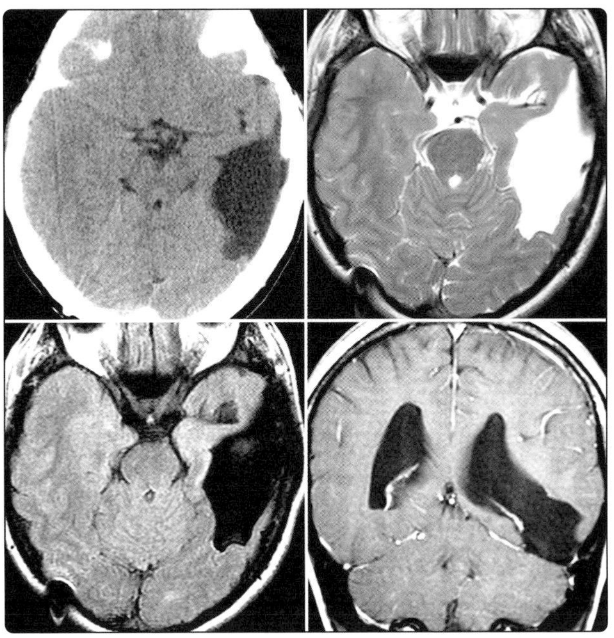

*(32-58) NECT, MR scans show a posttraumatic porencephalic cyst extending from the surface of the temporal lobe to the temporal horn of the lateral ventricle. The cyst contains CSF.*

## Porencephalic Cyst

### Terminology

"Porencephaly" literally means a hole in the brain. Porencephalic cysts are congenital or acquired CSF-filled parenchymal cavities that usually—but not invariably—communicate with the ventricular system.

### Pathology

Porencephalic cysts are the end result of a destructive process (e.g., trauma, infection, vascular insult, surgery) that compromises brain parenchyma. They range in size from a few centimeters to cysts that involve virtually an entire cerebral hemisphere.

Porencephalic cysts are typically deep, uni- or bilateral, smooth-walled cavities, or excavations within the brain parenchyma. They are often full-thickness lesions, extending from the ventricle to the cortex **(32-57)**.

### Clinical Issues

Porencephalic cysts are relatively common, especially in children in whom they represent 2.5% of congenital brain lesions. Spastic hemiplegia, medically refractory epilepsy, and psychomotor retardation are the most common symptoms.

Most porencephalic cysts remain stable for many years. Occasionally, a porencephalic cyst will continue to sequester fluid and expand, causing mass effect.

### Imaging

**CT Findings.** Porencephalic cysts are sharply marginated, smooth-walled, CSF-filled cavities that usually communicate directly with an adjacent ventricle **(32-58)**. The ipsilateral ventricle is often enlarged secondary to volume loss in the adjacent parenchyma. Bone CT may show skull thinning and remodeling caused by chronic CSF pulsations. Porencephalic cysts do not enhance.

**MR Findings.** Porencephalic cysts follow CSF signal intensity on all sequences **(32-58)**. Large cysts may show internal inhomogeneities secondary to spin dephasing. These cysts suppress completely on FLAIR, although there is often a rim of hyperintense gliotic or spongiotic white matter around the cyst.

### Differential Diagnosis

The major differential diagnosis is **cystic encephalomalacia**. An encephalomalacic cavity is often more irregular and does not communicate with the adjacent ventricle.

An **arachnoid cyst** is extraaxial and does not communicate with the ventricle. **Schizencephaly** (literally "split brain") is a congenital lesion that can be either "open lip" or "closed lip." An "open-lip" schizencephalic cleft can look very much like a porencephalic cyst but is lined with dysplastic gray matter, not gliotic white matter.

A **neuroglial cyst** does not communicate with the ventricles nor the brain surface, is typically round or ovoid, and is not surrounded by gliotic or spongiotic white matter.

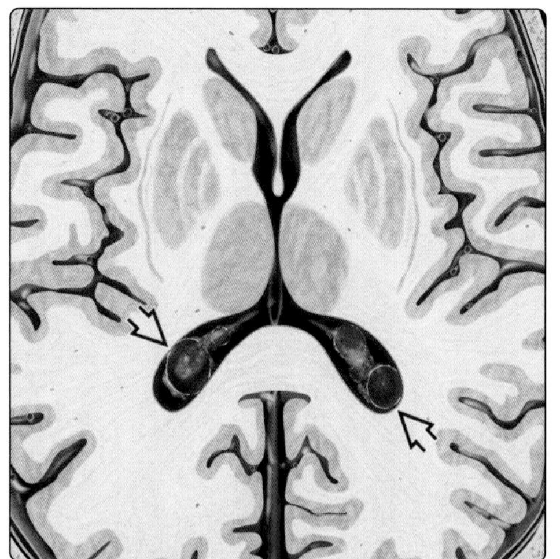

*(32-59) Multiple cystic masses are in the choroid plexus glomi ➡; in adults, it increases with age. Most are degenerative xanthogranulomas.*

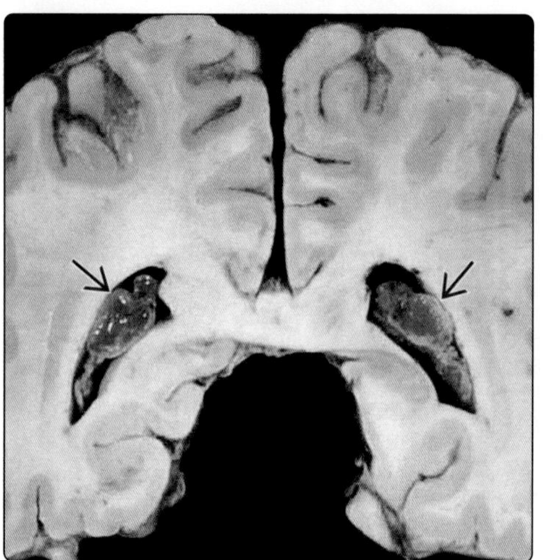

*(32-60) Autopsy specimen shows multiple cysts in the choroid plexus glomi of both lateral ventricles ➡. (Courtesy N. Nakase, MD.)*

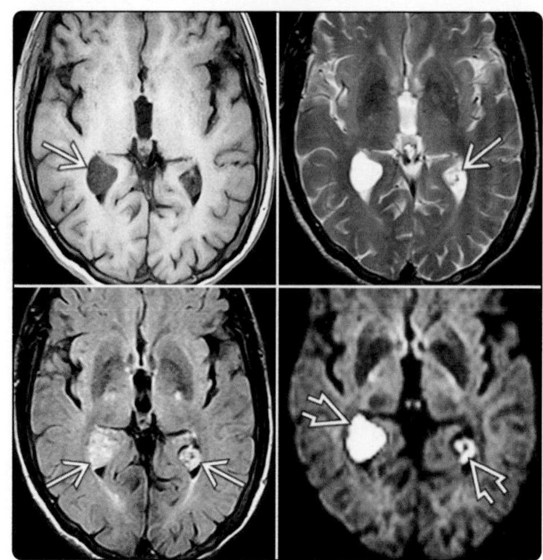

*(32-61) Choroid plexus cysts are usually bilateral and hyperintense compared with CSF ➡ and are often very bright on DWI ➡.*

# Intraventricular Cysts

Intraventricular cysts include choroid plexus cysts, colloid cysts, and ependymal cysts.

## Choroid Plexus Cysts

Choroid plexus cysts (CPCs), also called choroid plexus xanthogranulomas, are one of the most common types of intracranial cyst. Most are small and unremarkable. Occasionally, large cysts may appear somewhat atypical and cause diagnostic concern.

### Terminology

A CPC is also often called a choroid plexus xanthogranuloma. CPCs are nonneoplastic noninflammatory cysts of the choroid plexus **(32-59)**.

### Etiology

**General Concepts.** CPCs can be either congenital or acquired. Acquired lesions are much more common; lipid that accumulates from desquamating, degenerating choroid plexus epithelium coalesces into macrocysts and provokes a xanthomatous response.

**Genetics.** Large (> 10 mm), congenital CPCs can be associated with aneuploidy, particularly trisomy 18. CPCs, together with choroid plexus papillomas, also occur as part of Aicardi syndrome.

### Pathology

Most CPCs are found in the atrium of the lateral ventricle, within the choroid plexus glomus **(32-60)**. Most are small, ranging from a few millimeters up to 1 cm, although occasionally larger cysts exceed 2 cm in diameter. Multiple bilateral lesions are significantly more common than solitary unilateral CPCs.

CPCs are nodular, partly cystic, yellowish gray masses that are most often found in the choroid plexus glomus. They are highly proteinaceous and often gelatinous. Gross hemorrhage is rare.

**CHOROID PLEXUS CYSTS: ETIOLOGY, PATHOLOGY, AND CLINICAL ISSUES**

**Etiology**
- Congenital
  - Aicardi syndrome
  - Trisomy 18
- Acquired
  - Desquamated, degenerated epithelium
  - Xanthomatous response

**Pathology**
- Bilateral, usually multiloculated
- Most common in glomi of choroid plexus
- Proteinaceous, gelatinous contents

**Clinical Issues**
- Most common intracranial cyst
- Most found incidentally
- Most common in fetus/infants, older adults

## Clinical Issues

CPCs are the most common of all intracranial cysts, occurring in up to 50% of autopsies. CPCs are found at both ends of the age spectrum. In adults, their prevalence increases with age, whereas fetal CPCs decrease with gestational age. There is no sex predilection.

Most adult CPCs are found incidentally and are asymptomatic, remaining stable for many years. Congenital CPCs are detected on prenatal ultrasound in 1% of fetuses during the second trimester and generally resolve during the third trimester. When detected postnatally, CPCs are of no clinical significance in otherwise normal neonates.

## Imaging

**CT Findings.** CPCs are iso- to slightly hyperdense compared with intraventricular CSF. Irregular clumps of calcification around the margins are common findings. Enhancement varies from none to a complete rim surrounding each cyst.

**MR Findings.** CPCs do not precisely follow CSF signal intensity. They are iso- to slightly hyperintense compared with CSF on T1WI and are hyperintense on PD and T2WI. FLAIR signal is variable **(32-61)**.

Enhancement following contrast administration varies from none to striking. Solid, ring, and nodular patterns occur **(32-62)**.

Because of T2 "shine through," between 60-80% of CPCs appear quite bright on DWI but often remain isointense with parenchyma on ADC. This therefore represents "pseudorestriction" rather than true restricted diffusion.

## Differential Diagnosis

The major differential diagnosis of a CPC is an **ependymal cyst**. Ependymal cysts generally displace and compress the choroid plexus rather than arise from it. Ependymal cysts usually behave much more like CSF than CPCs do. **Neurocysticercosis cysts** are relatively uncommon and are not associated with the choroid plexus.

**Choroid plexus papilloma** of the lateral ventricle is a tumor of children younger than five years old. An enhancing, enlarged choroid plexus without frank cyst formation can also be seen with **Sturge-Weber malformation, collateral venous drainage**, and **diffuse villous hyperplasia**.

### CHOROID PLEXUS CYST: IMAGING AND DDx

CT
- Iso-/mildly hyperdense
- $Ca^{++}$ common

MR
- Iso-/mildly hyperintense to CSF on T1WI
- Hyperintense on PD/T2WI, FLAIR variable
- Variable enhancement (usually thin rim)
- Bright on DWI but isointense on ADC

**Differential Diagnosis**
- Most common: Ependymal cyst
- Uncommon/rare
  - Epidermoid cyst (rarely intraventricular)
  - Cystic metastasis

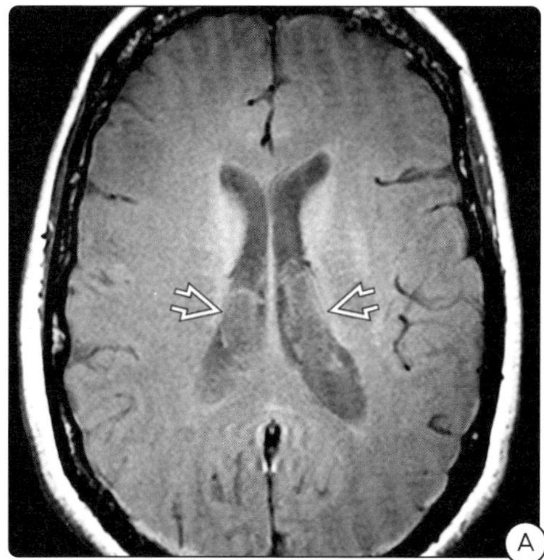


***(32-62A)** Variant choroid plexus cysts are in the body of the lateral ventricle. Cyst contents ➡ are slightly hyperintense compared with CSF.*

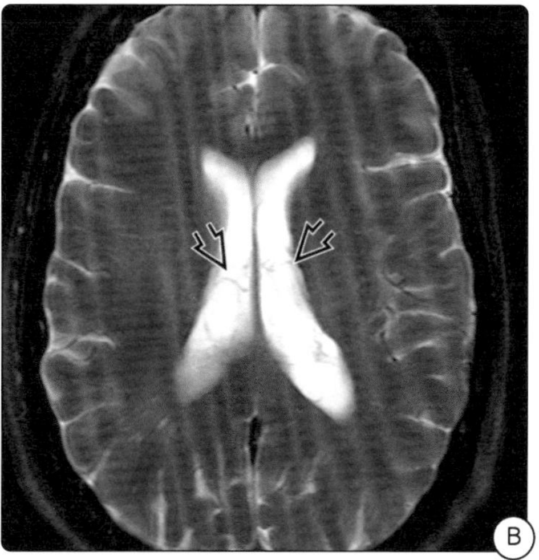


***(32-62B)** The cysts are so hyperintense on T2 MR that the thin cyst walls are barely visible ➡.*

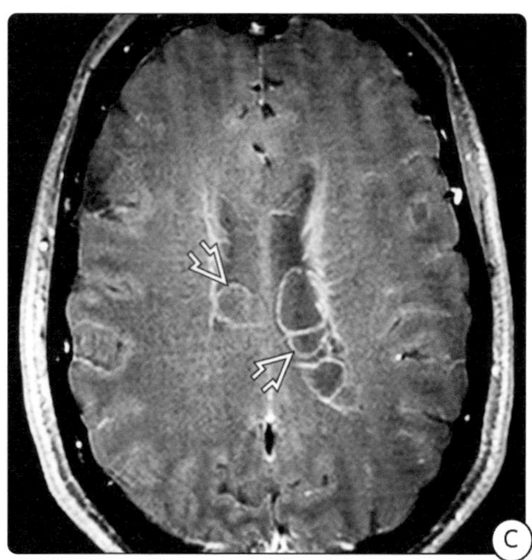


***(32-62C)** T1 C+ FS MR shows that the thin walls of these multiloculated choroid plexus cysts enhance moderately ➡.*

## Colloid Cyst

### Terminology

Colloid cysts (CCs) are unilocular, mucin-containing endodermal cysts. They are almost always found wedged into the top of the third ventricle at the foramen of Monro **(32-63)**. Rare reported locations include the velum interpositum and lateral ventricles.

### Pathology

CCs are virtually always solitary lesions. Size varies from tiny (a few millimeters) up to 3 cm. Mean diameter is 1.5 cm. CCs are smooth-walled, well-demarcated, spherical or ovoid cysts that have a thin fibrous capsule and gelatinous center of variable viscosity **(32-67)**. They are lined with simple or pseudostratified columnar epithelium with variable mucin-secreting goblet cells interspersed throughout the cyst lining.

### Clinical Issues

CCs represent ~ 1% of all intracranial tumors but 15-20% of all intraventricular tumors. They occur with equal frequency in men and women.

Most symptomatic CCs present between the third and fifth decades. The peak age is 40 years. Although CCs are congenital lesions, < 8% of all patients are younger than 15 years old at the time of initial diagnosis. Familial CCs do occur but are rare, representing < 5% of cases.

The clinical presentation of CCs is diverse. Many cases (50-75%) of CCs are asymptomatic and discovered incidentally on imaging studies. When CCs obstruct CSF flow at the foramina of Monro, symptoms range from headache to sudden neurologic deterioration and even death.

There are no standardized guidelines recommending observation vs. intervention. Over 90% of CCs—especially

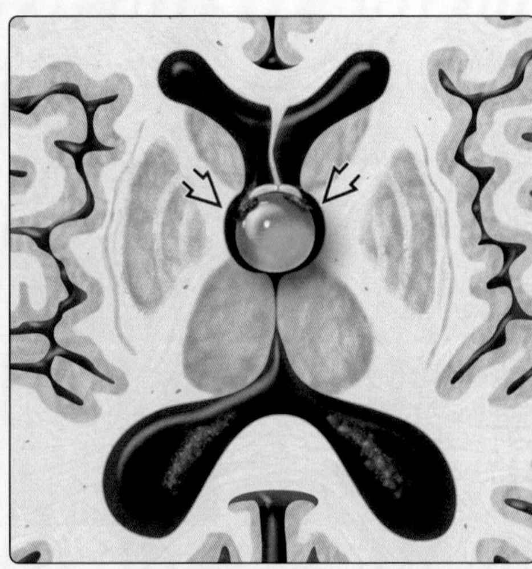

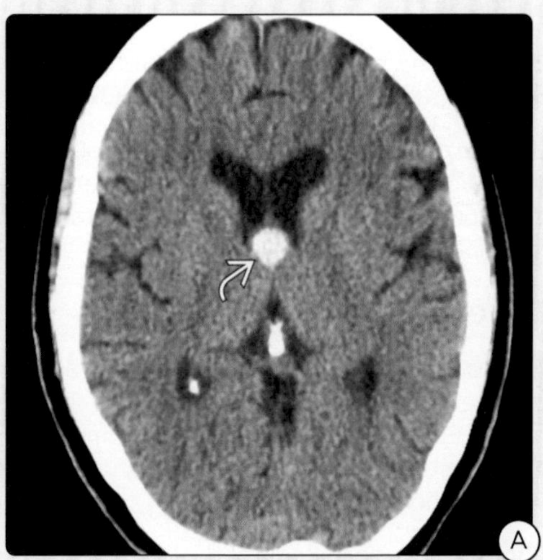


***(32-63)** Graphic shows a colloid cyst ⇨ at the foramen of Monro causing mild/moderate obstructive hydrocephalus. **(32-64A)** Axial NECT in a 65-yo woman with headaches shows an 8-mm round hyperdense mass ➡ in the foramen of Monro.*

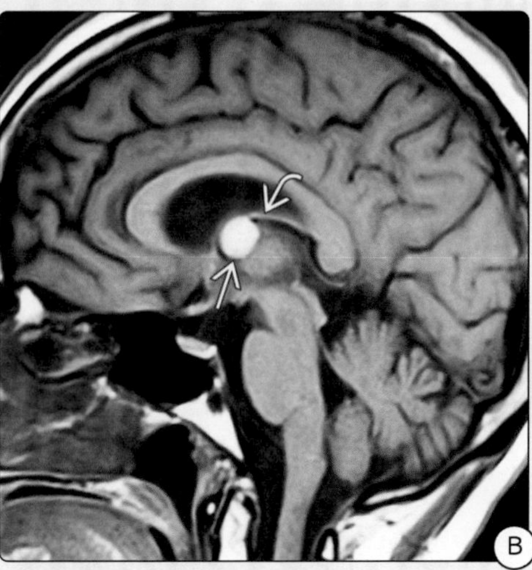


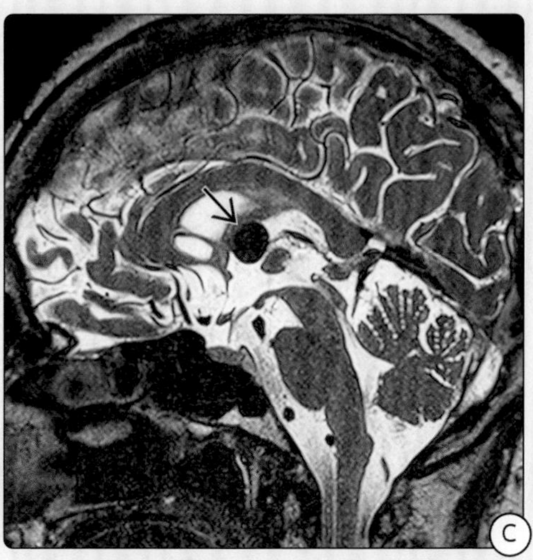


***(32-64B)** Sagittal T1 MR shows the mass ➡ is well delineated and uniformly hyperintense. Location is in the roof of the 3rd ventricle at the foramen of Monro. Note internal cerebral veins and fornix ➡ are draped over the mass. **(32-64C)** Sagittal T2 SPACE shows the mass ⇨ is uniformly hypointense. This is a colloid cyst.*

small cysts found in older patients—are stable and do not enlarge over time. Recent data suggest that only a few asymptomatic CCs demonstrate progression requiring surgery, whereas the vast majority remain stable over time, perhaps supporting a more conservative approach for this group of patients.

The roughly 10% that **do** enlarge tend to be larger lesions. Higher risk for developing symptomatic CC has recently been defined by a risk score that includes hyperintensity or heterogeneous appearance on T1WI, location in a "high risk" zone within the third ventricle (i.e., between the lamina terminalis and a vertical line drawn from the mammillary body tangential to the massa intermedia), and cyst volume ≥ 236.49 mm³.

CC "apoplexy" with intracystic hemorrhage and sudden enlargement occurs but is rare.

**Treatment Options.** Small, asymptomatic CCs that are discovered incidentally and followed with serial imaging rarely grow or cause obstructive hydrocephalus. However, their treatment is debated. Neuroendoscopic management has emerged as a safe, effective alternative.

## Imaging

CCs are well-delineated round or ovoid masses. Imaging appearance depends on their viscosity &/or cholesterol content. The relative amounts of mucous material, cholesterol, protein, and water content all affect density/signal intensity. Desiccated, inspissated cysts appear very different from water-rich lesions.

**CT Findings.** Density on NECT correlates directly with the hydration state of the cyst contents. Approximately 80% of all CCs are hyperdense compared with brain **(32-64A)**, whereas 20% are iso- to hypodense. Hydrocephalus is variable. Intracystic hemorrhage is rare, and calcification is very rare.

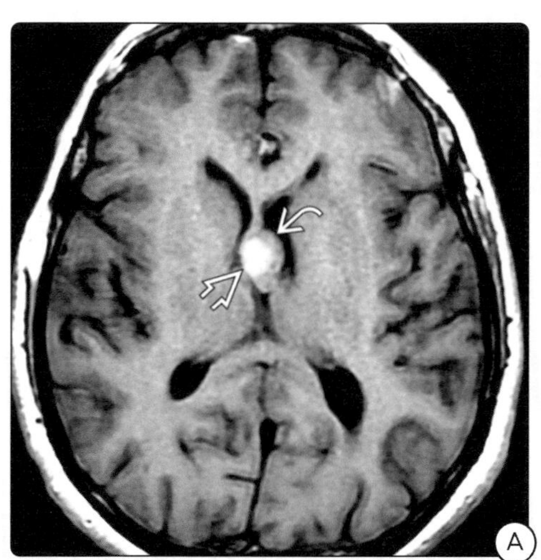


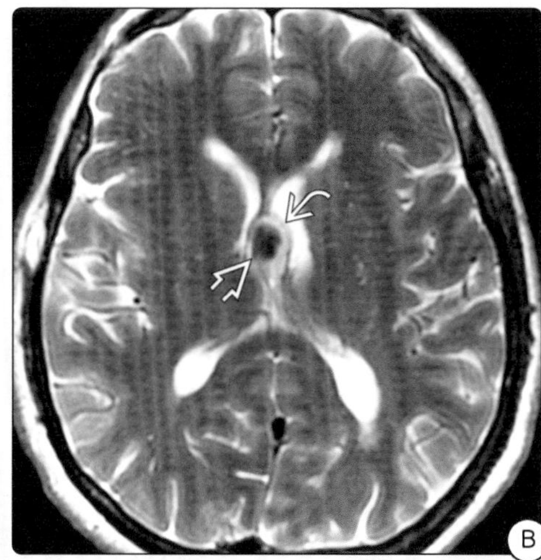


***(32-65A)** Axial T1 MR in a 55-yo woman with headaches shows a well-demarcated mass at the foramen of Monro. The majority of the mass is isointense with brain but has a distinctly hyperintense center. **(32-65B)** T2 MR in the same patient shows the periphery of the mass is relatively hyperintense, but the center is profoundly hypointense. Inspissated colloid cyst was found at surgery.*

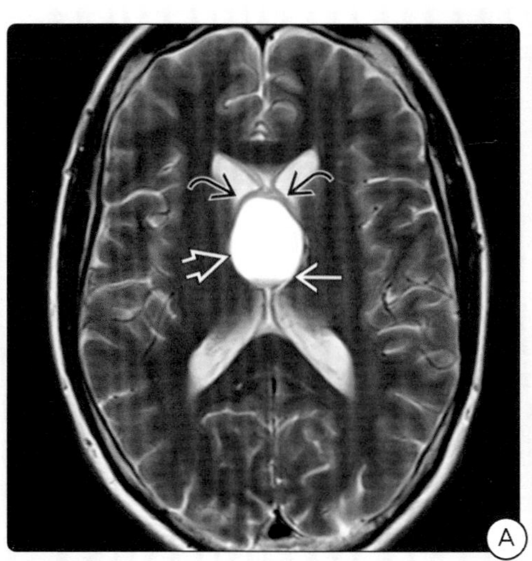


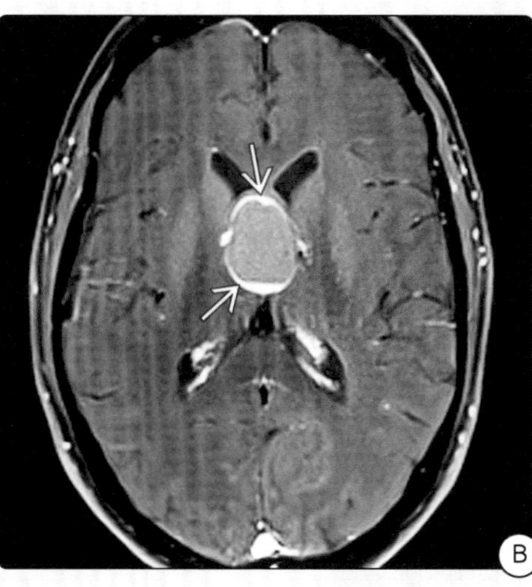


***(32-66A)** Axial T2 MR in a 52-yo man with severe headaches shows a large, very hyperintense mass that is splaying the fornices apart. A subtle fluid-fluid level is present in the dependent portion of the mass. **(32-66B)** T1 C+ FS MR in the same patient shows rim enhancement. A colloid cyst with xanthomatous and inflammatory changes was found at histopathology.*

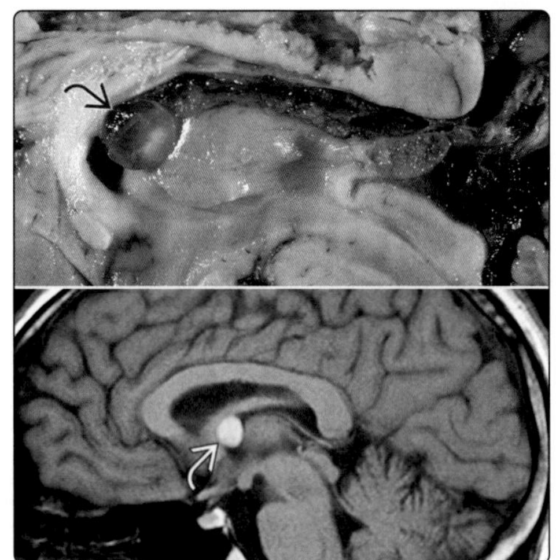

*(32-67) (Top) Sagittal close-up view of autopsy shows a colloid cyst ➩. (Bottom) Sagittal T1 MR shows a classic hyperintense colloid cyst ➩.*

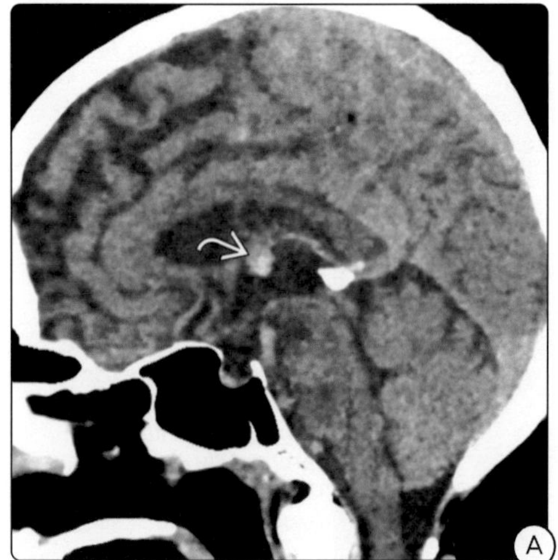

*(32-68A) Sagittal reformatted NECT in a 69-yo woman with headaches shows hyperdense mass at the foramen of Monro ➩.*

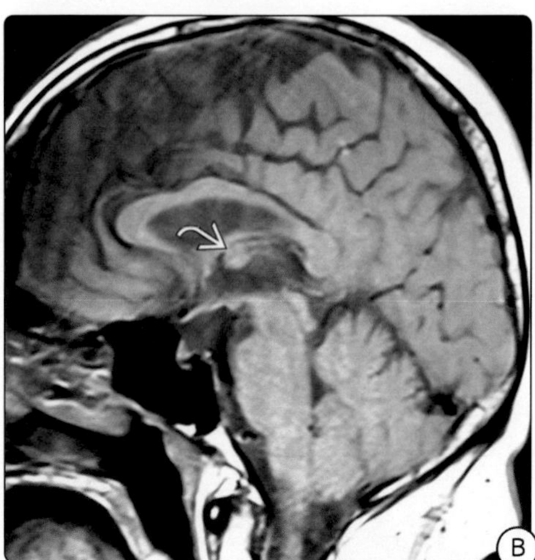

*(32-68B) Sagittal T1 MR in the same patient illustrates how difficult it may be to recognize a colloid cyst ➩ when it is isointense with brain.*

Most CCs show no enhancement. Occasionally, a thin enhancing rim surrounds the cyst. Solid or nodular enhancement almost never occurs.

**MR Findings.** Signal intensity varies with cyst content.

Signal intensity on T1WI reflects cholesterol concentration. Approximately 50% of CCs are hyperintense compared with brain **(32-64B)**, and 50% are isointense. Small, isointense CCs may be very difficult to identify on T1WI **(32-68B)**.

Signal intensity on T2/FLAIR is variable. Approximately 60% are hyperintense and exhibit three different patterns: Homogeneously hyperintense, cysts with rim (hyperintense rim, iso- to hypointense central core), and cysts with a dot sign (hyperintense with a small internal hypointense nodule) **(32-65)**. Approximately 40% are hypointense **(32-64C)**. Some cysts exhibit a hyperintense rim and an iso- to hypointense center.

CCs generally do not enhance. A thin peripheral rim of enhancement can be seen in some cases **(32-66)**. Susceptibility artifact on SWI is typically absent, although a thin black rim of susceptibility has been described in a few cases. CCs do not restrict on DWI.

## Differential Diagnosis

A well-delineated focal hyperdense lesion at the foramen of Monro on NECT scan is virtually pathognomonic of a CC. On MR, the most common "lesion" that mimics a CC is artifact caused by **pulsatile CSF flow**.

Neoplasms, such as **metastasis** and **subependymoma** (usually in the frontal horn or foramen of Monro, not anterosuperior third ventricle), can be hyperdense on NECT scans. Large **craniopharyngiomas** and pituitary **macroadenomas** occasionally extend superiorly almost to the foramen of Monro.

### COLLOID CYST: IMAGING AND DDx

**Imaging**
- CT
  - 2/3 hyperdense
  - 1/3 iso- to hypodense
- MR
  - Signal intensity varies with sequence, cyst contents
  - 50% T1 hyper-, 50% iso-/hypointense relative to brain
  - T2/FLAIR variable; 60% mixed, 40% hypointense
  - Generally do not enhance
  - Thin peripheral rim enhancement may occur
  - No restriction on DWI

**Differential Diagnosis**
- Most common
  - CSF flow artifact (MR)
  - Blood (trauma, surgery)
- Less common
  - Metastasis
  - Subependymoma
  - Pituitary macroadenoma
  - Craniopharyngioma
- Rare but important
  - Pilocytic astrocytoma
  - Lymphoma
  - Choroid plexus papilloma
  - Myxoid glioneuronal tumor

## Ependymal Cyst

Ependymal cysts are also called glioependymal cysts.

### Pathology

Ependymal cysts are solitary, thin-walled, usually unilocular cysts that are filled with clear, CSF-like liquid and lined with low columnar/cuboidal epithelium **(32-69)**. No glial capsule is present. They are most often found in the atrium of the lateral ventricles or the CPA cistern, where they may cause significant ventricular asymmetry.

### Clinical Issues

Ependymal cysts are typically asymptomatic and discovered incidentally at imaging or autopsy.

### Imaging

Intraventricular ependymal cysts can be rounded, ovoid, or multiseptated. They displace the choroid plexus and exhibit CSF-like density/signal intensity **(32-70)**. They suppress completely on FLAIR, do not enhance, and do not demonstrate diffusion restriction. Thin-section, heavily T2-weighted sequences, such as CISS, may be necessary to delineate the cyst wall **(32-70B)**.

### Differential Diagnosis

The major intraventricular mass that can mimic ependymal cyst is a **choroid plexus cyst**. Choroid plexus cysts are typically bilateral, often multilocular, and located **within** the choroid plexus glomi. Ependymal cysts arise **outside** the choroid plexus and usually displace it superolaterally.

**Epidermoid cysts** are rare in the lateral ventricle. They do not suppress completely on FLAIR and demonstrate diffusion restriction on DWI. **Arachnoid cysts** are identical to ependymal cysts in density and signal intensity but are extraaxial, not intraventricular. **Cystic metastases** to the choroid plexus are rare; nodular or irregular rim enhancement is typical.

**EPENDYMAL CYST**

**Terminology**
- Also called glioependymal or neuroepithelial cyst

**Pathology**
- 1% of intracranial cysts
- Solitary, usually unilocular intraventricular cyst
- Lined by columnar epithelium, contain CSF

**Clinical Issues**
- Most are asymptomatic, discovered incidentally
- All ages, but usually < 40 years

**Imaging**
- Density, signal intensity = CSF
- No enhancement, no restriction

**Differential Diagnosis**
- Most common: Choroid plexus cyst
- Uncommon/rare
  - Epidermoid cyst
  - Arachnoid cyst

*Selected References: The complete reference list is available on the eBooks+ version included with purchase.*

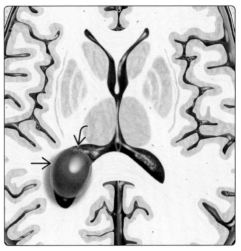

***(32-69)** Graphic depicts ependymal cyst of the lateral ventricle as CSF-containing simple cyst that displaces the choroid plexus around it.*

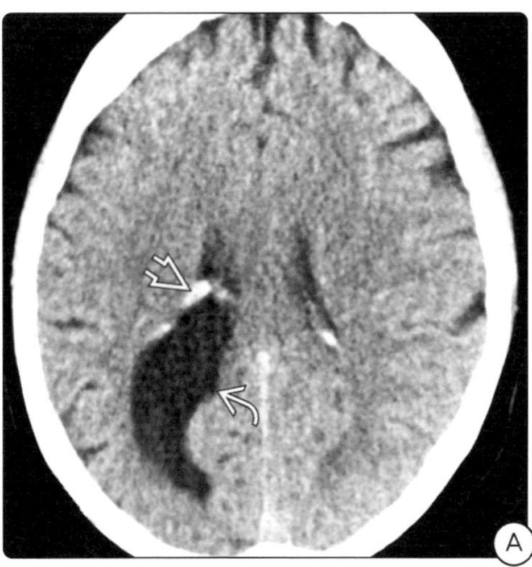

***(32-70A)** Axial NECT of an ependymal cyst shows a CSF-containing mass displacing the calcified choroid plexus around it.*

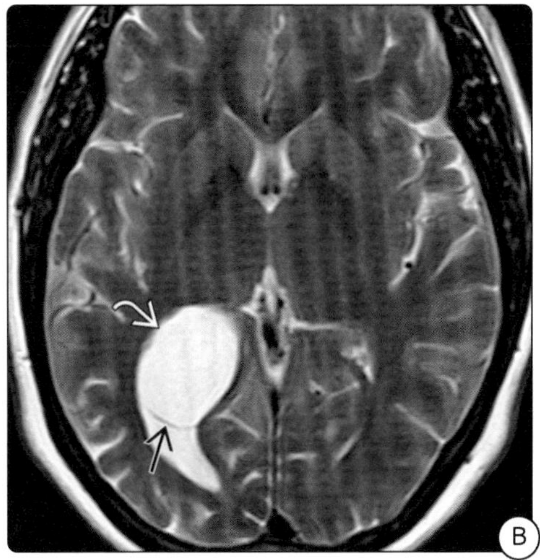

***(32-70B)** T2 MR in the same patient shows that the unilocular ependymal cyst is exactly like CSF. Note the distinct cyst wall.*

# Miscellaneous Tumors and Tumor-Like Conditions

*Some important neoplasms that affect the calvaria, skull base, and cranial meninges are not included in the 2021 5th edition WHO classification of CNS tumors. This chapter covers several of these intriguing tumors as well as tumor-like lesions that do not easily fit into other sections. Although infections, granulomatous disease, demyelinating disorders, and vascular diseases (among others) may sometimes mimic CNS neoplasms, they are treated separately in their own respective chapters.*



We begin with *extra*cranial tumors and tumor-like conditions. These lesions mostly arise within the calvaria or skull base. We then turn our attention to an interesting group of *intra*cranial lesions that all mimic neoplasms, i.e., they are pseudotumors. These tumor-like lesions may arise within the meninges, CSF cisterns, or brain parenchyma. Some lesions may involve multiple compartments and can be intracranial, extracranial, or a combination of both.

## Extracranial Tumors and Tumor-Like Conditions

### Fibrous Dysplasia

Benign fibroosseous lesions of the craniofacial complex are represented by a variety of intraosseous disease processes. These include bone dysplasias, the most common of which is fibrous dysplasia (FD).

#### Terminology

FD is a benign, dysplastic fibroosseous lesion that is also known as fibrocartilaginous dysplasia, osteitis fibrosa, and generalized fibrocystic disease of bone. FD can occur in one (monostotic FD) or multiple bones (polyostotic FD).

#### Etiology

**General Concepts.** FD is a developmental lesion with local arrest of normal structural/architectural development. Abnormal differentiation of osteoblasts results in replacement of normal marrow and cancellous bone by immature "woven" bone and fibrous stroma.

**Genetics.** Recent studies have demonstrated that FD is a neoplastic—not dysplastic—lesion. Activating mutations of the *GNAS* gene result in

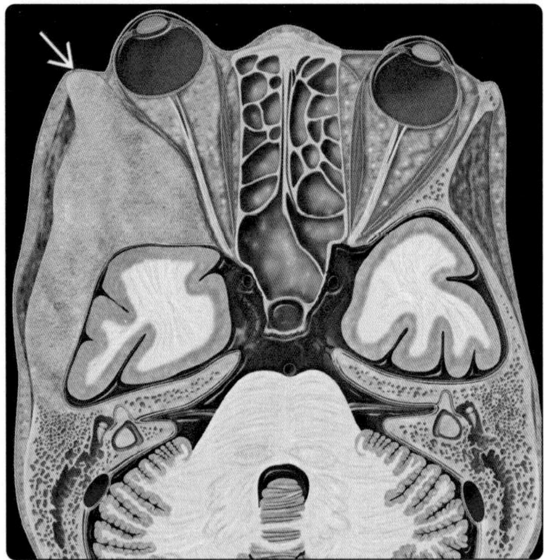

*(33-1) FD is with expansion of lateral orbital rim ➡, sphenoid wing, temporal squamosa. Note exophthalmos and stretching of optic nerve.*

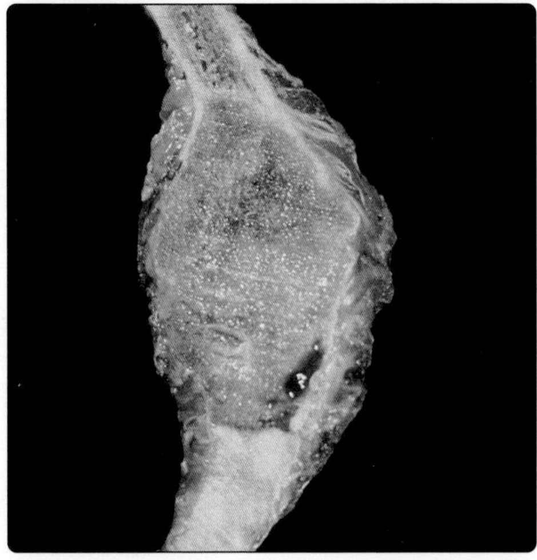

*(33-2) FD in a rib is a solid tan tumor that expands bone and has ground-glass appearance. (Courtesy A. Rosenberg, MD, G. P. Nielsen, MD.)*

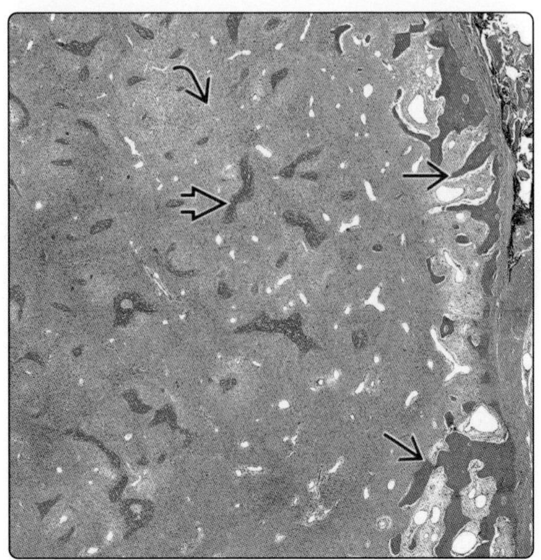

*(33-3) FD shows "woven" bony trabeculae ➡, fibrous stroma ➡, reactive subperiosteal new bone ➡. (A. Rosenberg, MD, G. P. Nielsen, MD.)*

overexpression of the c-Fos protooncogene, which contributes to the initiation and progression of FD.

## Pathology

**Location.** Although FD occurs throughout the skeleton, it is most commonly found in craniofacial bones, long bones, and spine.

Virtually any bone in the head and neck can be affected by FD. The skull and facial bones are the location of 10-25% of all monostotic FD lesions. The frontal bone is the most common calvarial site, followed by the temporal bone, sphenoid, and parietal bones. Involvement of the clivus is rare. The orbit, zygoma, maxilla, and mandible are the most frequent sites in the face **(33-1)**.

**Size and Number.** FD lesions range in size from relatively small (< 1 cm) to massive lesions that involve virtually an entire bone. Altered osteogenesis may occur within a single bone ("monostotic FD") or multiple bones ("polyostotic FD"). **Monostotic FD** accounts for ~ 60-80% of all lesions; **polyostotic FD** occurs in 20-40% of cases.

Polyostotic FD with endocrinopathy is known as **McCune-Albright syndrome** (MAS) and occurs in 3-5% of cases. The classic MAS triad consists of multiple FD lesions, endocrine dysfunction (typically precocious puberty), and cutaneous hyperpigmentation ("café au lait" spots).

**Gross Pathology.** FD is a well-defined, tan to whitish gray mass **(33-2)**. Depending on the relative amount of fibrous vs. osseous content, texture varies from firm and rubbery to "gritty." Prominent cyst formation can be present in older lesions.

**Microscopic Features.** Fibrous and osseous tissues are admixed in varying proportions **(33-3)**. In the early stages, pronounced osteogenesis with thin osteoid anastomosing trabeculae rimmed with osteoblasts is seen. A stromal fibroblastic element with variable vascularity is interspersed between irregular, curvilinear trabeculae of immature "woven" bone that resembles Chinese letters.

Almost 60% of cases demonstrate different stromal patterns admixed with the usual fibroblastic elements. These include focal fatty metamorphosis (20-25%), myxoid stroma (15%), and calcifications (12%). Cystic degeneration occurs but is uncommon.

## Clinical Issues

**Epidemiology.** FD is rare, representing ~ 5-7% of all benign bone tumors. It is the second most common pediatric primary skull lesion (after dermoid cysts).

**Demographics.** Although FD can present at virtually any age, most patients are younger than 30 years at the time of initial diagnosis. Polyostotic FD presents earlier; the mean age is eight years. With the exception of FD as part of MAS, which affects female patients more than male patients, there is no sex predilection.

**Presentation.** Symptoms of craniofacial FD depend on lesion location. Painless osseous expansion with calvarial or facial asymmetry is common. Proptosis and optic neuropathy are common in patients with orbital disease. Conductive hearing loss and facial weakness are typical in patients with temporal bone FD. Mandibular FD typically presents with "cherubism."

Polyostotic FD may cause "leontiasis ossea" (lion-like physiognomy) or complex cranial neuropathies (secondary to severe narrowing of the neural foramina).

**Natural History.** Disease course varies. Monostotic lesions do not regress or disappear, but they generally stabilize at puberty. In contrast, polyostotic FD generally becomes less active after puberty, although long bone deformities may progress, and microfractures may develop.

Patients with MAS are more likely to have pain, pathologic fractures, more bones involved, more aggressive disease, and more complications than those with polyostotic or monostotic FD.

Malignant sarcomatous transformation is a rare and challenging complication of craniofacial FD, occurring in < 1-9% of all FD cases, and has been described in both the monostotic and polyostotic forms.

Treatment options for FD are limited. Recurrence is very high following curettage and bone grafting. Radiation therapy is generally avoided, as it may induce malignant transformation. Intravenous bisphosphonate therapy has been used to ameliorate the disease course with some reported success.

**FIBROUS DYSPLASIA: PATHOLOGY AND CLINICAL ISSUES**

**Pathology**
- Location, number
  - Any bone
  - Craniofacial (10-25%)
  - Solitary (60-80%) or polyostotic (20-40%)
- Gross pathology: "Woven" bone
- Microscopic pathology
  - Variable admixture of fibrous, osseous components
  - Less common: Fat, myxoid tissue, $Ca^{++}$, cysts

**Clinical Issues**
- Rare (< 1% of biopsied bone tumors)
  - One of the most common fibroosseous lesions
- Monostotic patients < 30 years
- Polyostotic FD
  - Younger (mean age: 8 years)
  - McCune-Albright (3-5%)
  - Craniofacial > calvarial involvement

## Imaging

**General Features.** Most craniofacial lesions are monostotic. However, skeletal survey or whole-body MR is recommended to detect asymptomatic lesions in other bones that would indicate polyostotic disease or MAS.

Imaging findings depend on disease stage. In general, very early lesions are radiolucent and then undergo progressive calcification, resulting in a ground-glass appearance. Mixed patterns are common.

**CT Findings.** Nonaggressive osseous remodeling and thickening of the affected bone are typical. NECT shows a geographic expansile lesion centered in the medullary cavity. Abrupt transition between the lesion and adjacent normal bone is typical.

Bone CT appearance varies with the relative content of fibrous vs. osseous tissue. FD can be sclerotic, cystic, or mixed (sometimes called pagetoid). A pattern with mixed areas of radiopacity and radiolucency is found in almost 1/2 of all cases **(33-4A)** **(33-5)**. The classic, relatively homogeneous ground-glass appearance occurs in 25%. Densely sclerotic lesions are common in the skull base. Almost 1/4 of all FD cases have some cystic changes, seen as central lucent areas with thinned but sclerotic borders.

**MR Findings.** Signal intensity on MR is quite variable, and the diagnosis of FD should not be based on MR alone. FD lesions may show evidence of cortical

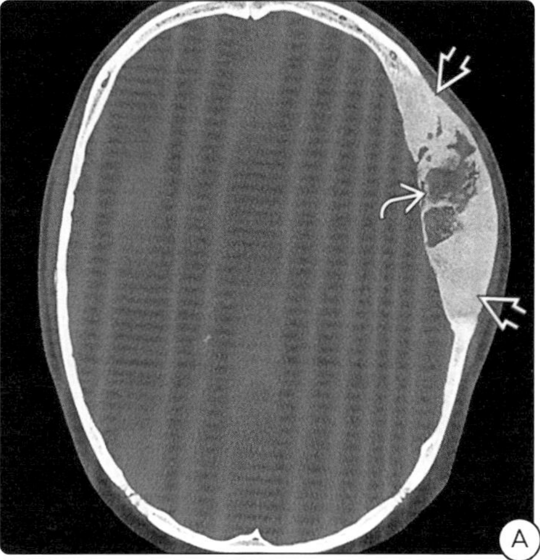


***(33-4A)** Bone CT in a 26-yo woman shows classic monostotic FD with ground-glass appearance ➡, central noncalcified fibrous stroma ➡.*

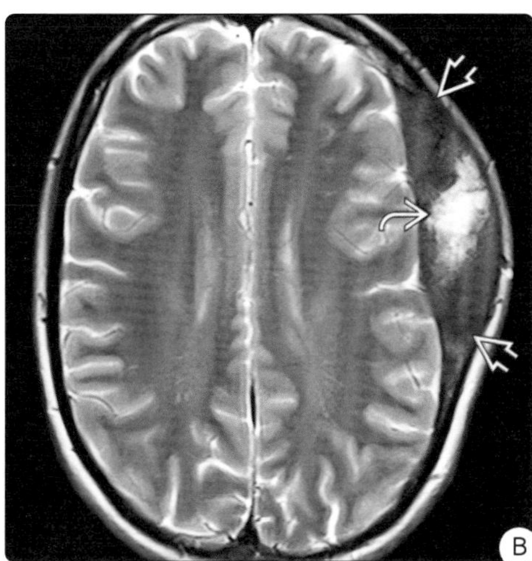


***(33-4B)** T2 MR shows that dense, ossified bone is hypointense ➡, but a central area of active disease is hyperintense ➡.*

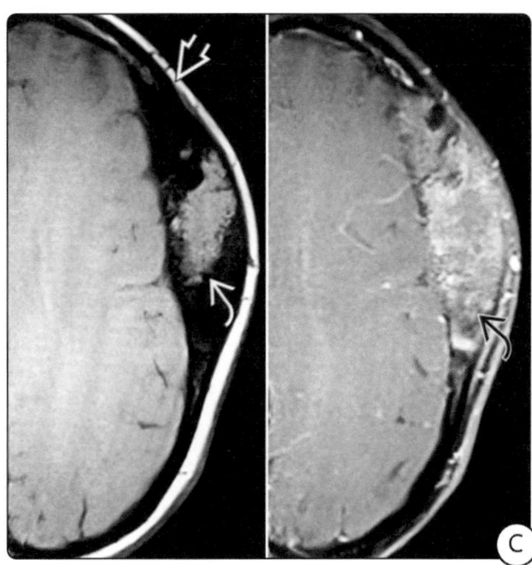


***(33-4C)** (L) T1 MR in the same patient shows hypointense periphery ➡, isointense center ➡. (R) T1 C+ FS shows most of mass ➡ enhances.*

destruction &/or soft tissue extension and still be benign. Recent studies have shown FD is homogeneously hypointense on T1WI in 60% of cases, although almost 20% have some hyperintense foci.

Signal intensity on T2WI is also quite variable. Moderate hypointensity is characteristic of ossified &/or fibrous portions of the lesion **(33-4B)**. Active lesions may be heterogeneous and may have hyperintense areas on T2 or FLAIR **(33-5D)**. Cysts appear as rounded high-signal foci.

Enhancement following contrast administration varies depending on the lesion stage and ranges from no enhancement to diffuse, avid enhancement in active lesions **(33-4C)**. Slightly over 50% of cases exhibit at least some enhancement.

Secondary aneurysmal bone cyst-like changes are relatively common, seen in 5-6% of cases. In these cases, fluid-fluid levels are present in 50%.

**Nuclear Medicine.** FDG PET and Ga-68 PET/CT show increased metabolic activity in one or more sites and can mimic metastatic disease.

## Differential Diagnosis

The major differential diagnoses for craniofacial FD are Paget disease and ossifying fibroma (OF).

**Paget disease** typically occurs in older adult patients and usually involves the calvaria and temporal bone. A cotton wool appearance is typical on digital skull radiographs and bone CT.

**OF** may mimic the cystic monostotic form of FD. OF has a thick, bony rim with a lower density center on bone CT and generally appears more mass-like and localized. Diffuse **sclerosing osteomyelitis** of the mandible may also resemble FD.

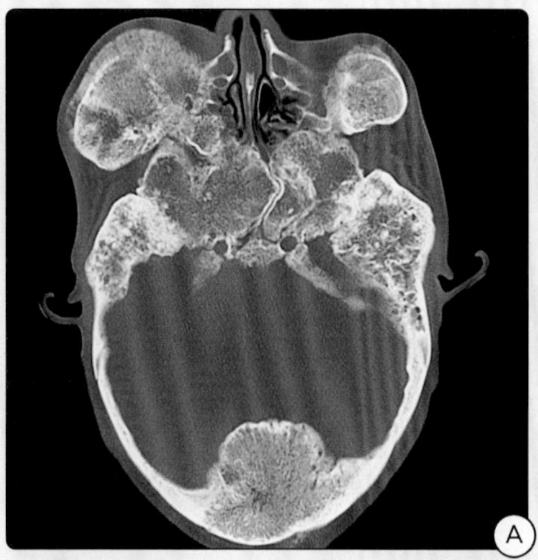


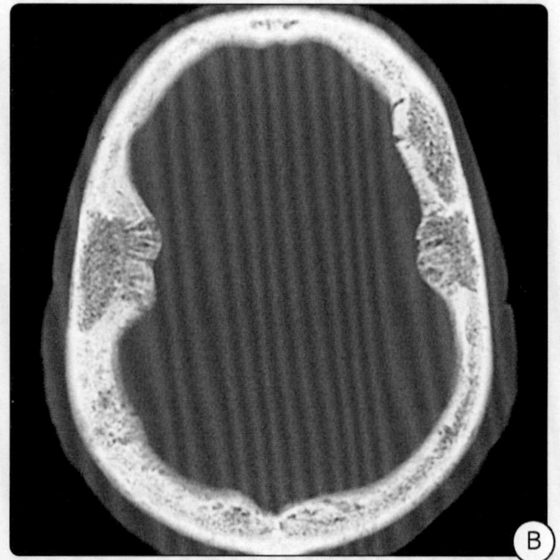


***(33-5A)** Bone CT in a 19-yo man with polyostotic FD and cranial nerve palsies shows multiple lesions in the facial bones and calvarium. **(33-5B)** More cephalad bone CT shows several lesions expanding the calvarium.*

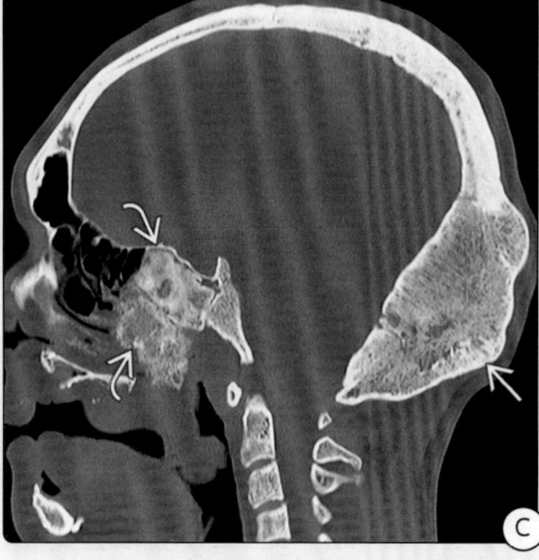


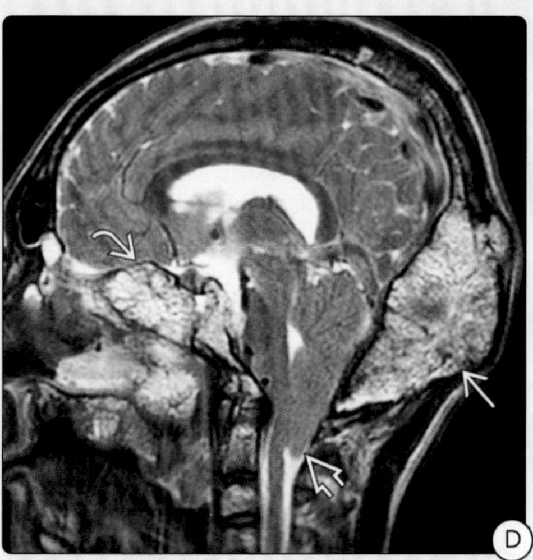


***(33-5C)** Sagittal reformatted bone CT shows the expansile, ground-glass appearance of the skull base ➡ and calvarial lesions ➡. **(33-5D)** Sagittal T2 MR shows that the expansile skull base ➡ and calvarial ➡ lesions are heterogeneously hyperintense. Note severe posterior fossa crowding with acquired tonsillar herniation ➡.*

**Intraosseous meningioma** is another differential consideration. Intraosseous meningiomas are more common in the calvaria than in the skull base and facial bones. A strongly enhancing en plaque soft tissue mass is often associated with the bony lesion. A mixed sclerotic-destructive skull base **metastasis** may mimic FD. In most cases, an extracranial primary site is known.

The DDx of FD includes rare fibroosseous disorders that can affect the craniofacial bones. These include **osteitis deformans, florid osseous dysplasia, focal cementoosseous dysplasia,** and **periapical cemental dysplasia**.

Facial bone changes associated with hyperparathyroidism and **renal osteodystrophy** may present with a classic ground-glass appearance on both conventional radiography and CT. However, in contrast to FD, these changes are generalized and diffuse.

### FIBROUS DYSPLASIA: IMAGING AND DDx

**Imaging**

- CT
  - Bone remodeled, expanded
  - Ground-glass appearance classic
  - Sclerotic, cystic, mixed ("pagetoid") changes
- MR
  - T1 hypointense, T2 variable (usually hypointense)
  - Enhancement varies from none to intense

**Differential Diagnosis**

- Paget disease (older patients)
- Ossifying fibroma, other benign fibroosseous lesions
- Intraosseous meningioma
- Renal osteodystrophy

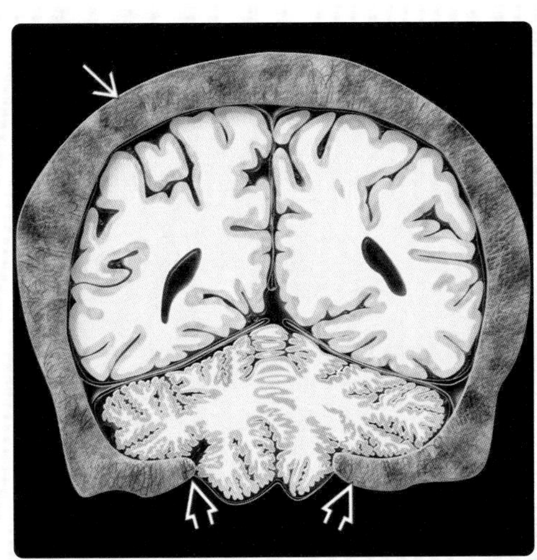

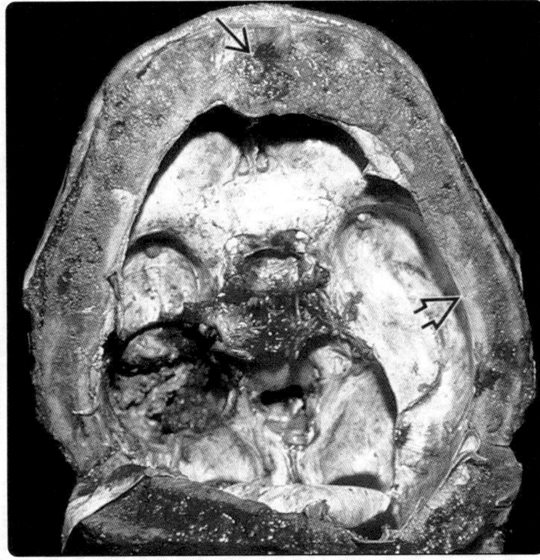

*(33-6) Graphic shows diffuse Paget disease of the skull with severe diploic widening ➡ and basilar invagination ⇨. (33-7) Autopsied Paget disease shows calvarial thickening with sclerotic bone ➡ and patches of fibrovascular tissue ⇨. (From Dorfman, 2016.)*

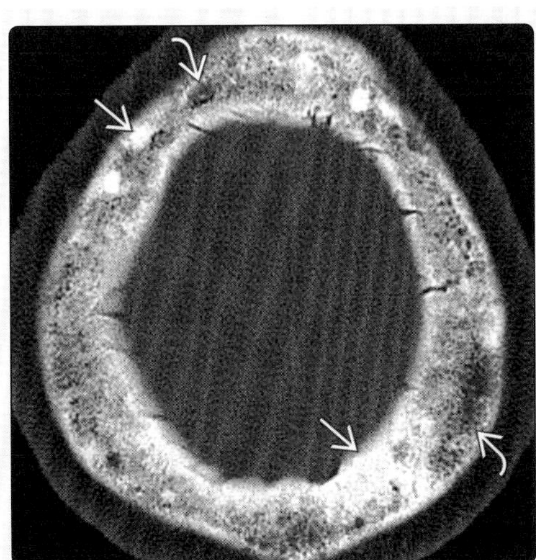

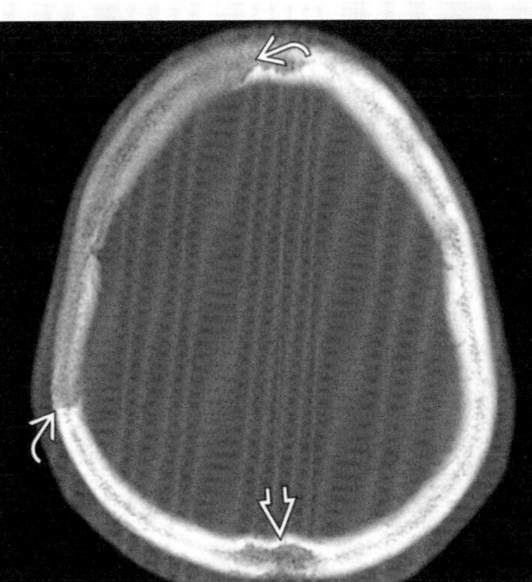

*(33-8) Bone CT in a 63-yo woman with Paget disease shows a thick calvarium with mixed sclerotic ➡ and lucent areas ↪. (33-9) Axial bone CT shows classic osteoporosis circumscripta ↪ in Paget disease. A smaller focal calvarial lesion ⇨ is also present. (Courtesy M. Jhaveri, MD.)*

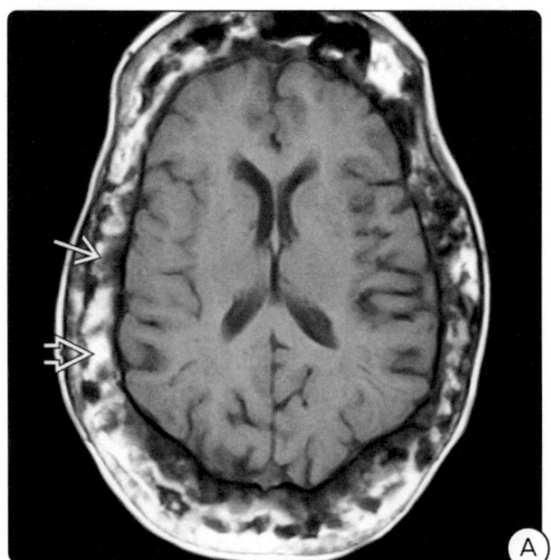

**(33-10A)** *T1 MR shows mixed hyper- ➡ and hypointense ➡ diploic lesions in a calvarium massively expanded by Paget disease.*

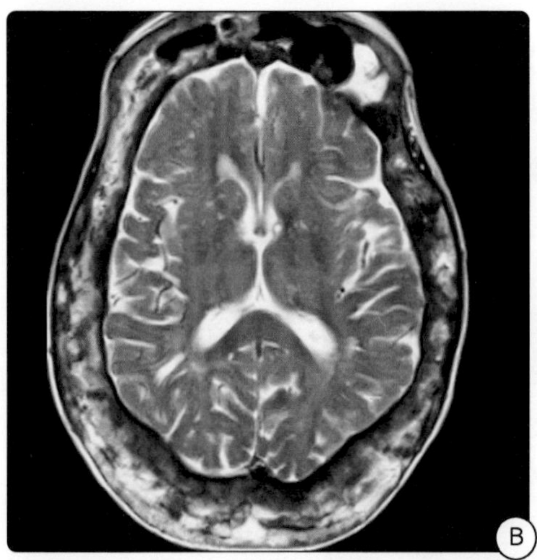

**(33-10B)** *T2 MR in the same patient shows the extremely mottled heterogeneous appearance of calvarial Paget disease.*

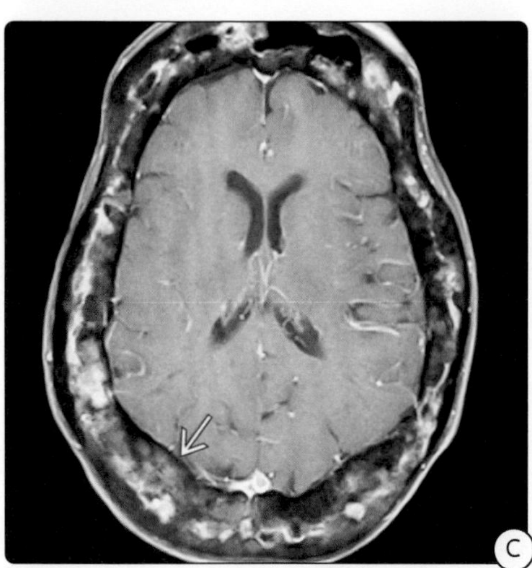

**(33-10C)** *Patchy enhancement ➡ is seen on T1 C+ FS MR, indicating that some active disease is present in this longstanding case.*

# Paget Disease

## Terminology

Paget disease (PaD) of bone is a metabolic bone disorder characterized by bone resorption followed by compensatory bone formation.

## Etiology

The initial abnormality is an increase in osteoclast activity followed by rapid compensatory bone formation. Lamellar bone is replaced by weak "woven bone" that is more susceptible to fractures and deformities.

Genetic alterations occur in both classic PaD of older adults and the uncommon familial Paget-like bone dysplasias that arise during childhood. Mutations involved in osteoclast differentiation affect function of the RANKL molecular pathway, a membrane protein on osteoblasts that induces differentiation and activation.

## Pathology

PaD follows a well-established sequence of events. First, osteoclast expansion generates lytic lesions. A combination of bone resorption with new disorganized bone formation then ensues. In the final phase, bone formation predominates, leading to bone enlargement and sclerosis.

**Location, Size, and Number.** The skull (both calvaria and skull base) is affected in 25-65% of patients and is often asymptomatic **(33-6)**. In contrast to FD, PaD is more commonly polyostotic (65-90% of cases).

**Gross Pathology.** The pagetoid skull shows diffuse thickening **(33-7)**. Patches of fibrovascular tissue initially replace fatty marrow.

**Microscopic Features.** In the early lytic stage, active PaD is characterized by cellular fibroosseous lesions with minimally calcified osteoid trabeculae. Increased vascularity is common. Osteoblastic rimming is present together with osteoclastic resorptive lacunae. Osteoclasts are numerous and larger than normal; they also have increased numbers of nuclei.

In the inactive stage, bone turnover and excessive vascularity decrease and the trabeculae coarsen.

## Clinical Issues

**Epidemiology.** PaD is common, affecting up to 10% of individuals over the age of 80 years. It is especially prevalent in the United States, the British Isles, Canada, Australia, and some parts of Western Europe. PaD is rare in Asia and Africa.

**Demographics.** Classic PaD is a disease of older adults. Most patients are 55-85 years of age with < 5% of cases occurring in patients under the age of 40 years. There is a moderate male predominance.

Juvenile PaD, a.k.a. idiopathic hyperphosphatasia, is an autosomal-recessive bone dysplasia. It begins in infancy or early childhood and is characterized by long bone widening, acetabular protrusion, pathologic fractures, and skull thickening.

**Presentation.** Presentation varies with location, and all bones of the craniofacial complex can be affected. Patients with calvarial PaD may experience increasing hat size. Cranial neuropathy is common with skull base lesions, most commonly affecting CNVIII. Patients may present with either conductive (ossicular involvement) or sensorineural hearing loss (cochlear involvement or bony compression).

Markedly elevated serum alkaline phosphatase is a constant feature, whereas calcium and phosphate levels remain within normal range.

**Natural History.** In the extracranial skeleton, osseous expansion with progressive skeletal deformity is typical. Osseous weakening leads to long bone deformities and fractures. In comparison, craniofacial PaD generally has a more benign course and may remain asymptomatic for many years.

Two neoplastic processes are associated with PaD: Giant cell tumor (benign) and sarcoma (malignant). **Giant cell tumor** is an expansile intraosseous mass that usually occurs in the epiphyses and metaphyses of long bones in patients with longstanding polyostotic PaD. Giant cell tumors that arise secondarily in pagetoid bone are rare. Just 2% occur in the skull, where the most common site is the sphenoid bone. Involvement of the calvarial vault is rare.

The most feared complication in PD is sarcomatous transformation. Malignant transformation to **osteosarcoma** occurs in 0.5-1.0% of cases and is generally seen in patients with widespread disease. The humerus, femur, and pelvis are the most common sites; sarcomatous transformation in the craniofacial bones is rare.

Most pagetic osteosarcomas are high grade and have already metastasized at the time of diagnosis. Only 15% of patients survive beyond two or three years.

**Treatment Options.** Bisphosphonates reduce bone turnover and have been effective in many cases of PaD.

## Imaging

**General Features.** Imaging findings in PaD vary with disease stage. In the early active "lytic" phase, radiolucent lesions develop in one or multiple bones. In the calvaria, this condition is termed **osteoporosis circumscripta** and is characterized by round osteolysis that may cross suture lines.

In the "mixed" phase, enlarged bone with mixed lytic and sclerotic foci and confluent nodular calcifications follows (the **cotton wool** appearance). The final inactive or quiescent stage is seen as **dense bony sclerosis**.

**CT Findings.** In early PaD, bone CT shows well-defined lytic foci (osteoporosis circumscripta) **(33-9)**. Mixed areas of bony lysis and sclerosis then develop, producing the cotton wool appearance **(33-8)**. Varying degrees of dense bony sclerosis eventually develop **(33-11)**.

In severe cases, the softened expanded skull base can produce basilar invagination.

**MR Findings.** The MR features of PaD depend on the phase of the disorder. Multifocal T1-hypointense lesions are intermixed with foci of residual yellow fatty marrow **(33-10A)**. Signal intensity on T2WI is often heterogeneous **(33-10B)**. Patchy enhancement on T1 C+ can occur in the advancing hypervascular zone of active PaD **(33-10C)**.

**Nuclear Medicine.** Bone scans detect the reaction of bone to the disease and not the destruction of bone. The active stage of PaD shows markedly increased uptake on Tc-99m bone scans with well-delineated margins between the affected and normal regions of bone. Nonactive pagetic lesions in the late "burnt-out" disease stage may not be detected.

18F-NaF PET/CT can also demonstrate high uptake in PD, mimicking metastatic disease.

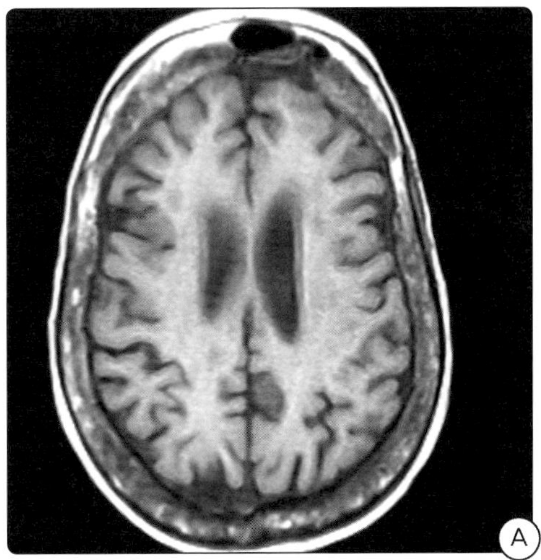


***(33-11A)** T1 MR in a 75-yo woman shows diffuse calvarial thickening with mottled hyper- and isointense foci.*

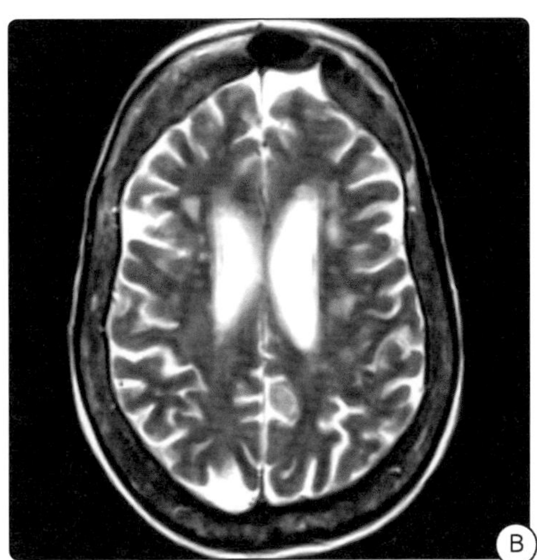


***(33-11B)** The thickened calvarium is heterogeneously hypointense on T2 MR.*

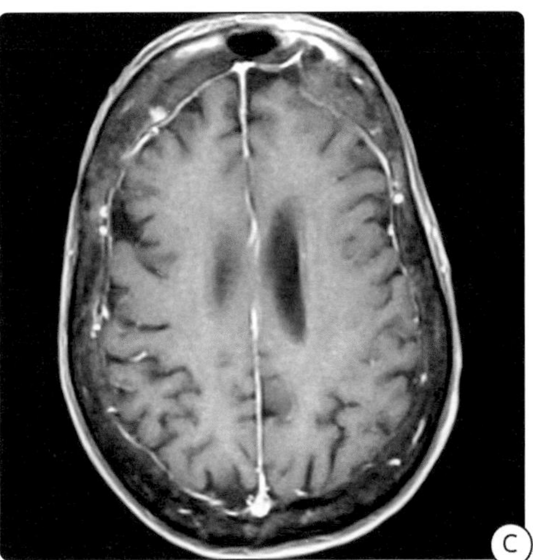


***(33-11C)** T1 C+ FS shows suppression of fatty foci without enhancement. Dense bony sclerosis is the final inactive (quiescent) stage of Paget disease.*

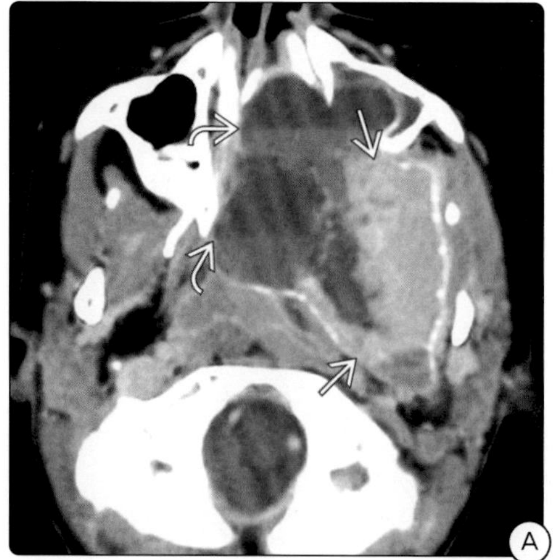

**(33-12A)** *CECT shows an expansile mass with cysts and fluid-fluid levels ➡, solid portion exhibiting relatively uniform enhancement ➡.*

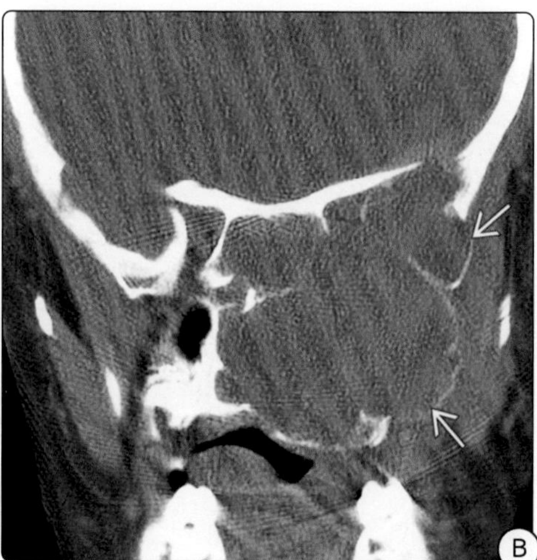

**(33-12B)** *Coronal bone CT demonstrates a thin "eggshell" rim of expanded bone around the lesion ➡.*

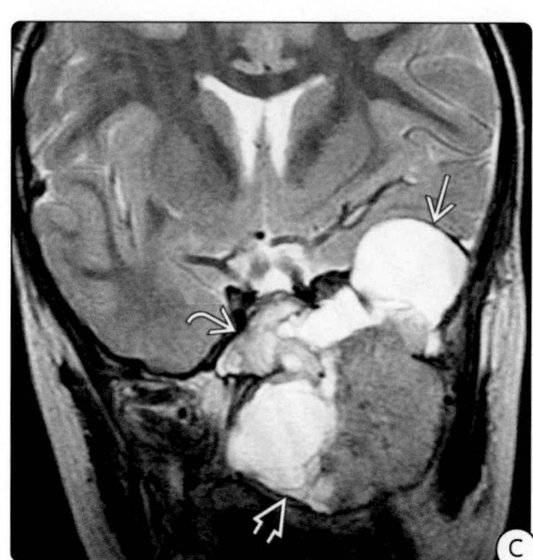

**(33-12C)** *T2 MR of aneurysmal bone cyst shows the lesion ➡ expands intracranially ➡, extends into sphenoid sinus ➡. (Courtesy A. Illner, MD.)*

## Differential Diagnosis

**FD** may appear very similar to craniofacial PaD. However, PaD occurs mostly in older adults and does not have the typical ground-glass appearance that often characterizes FD.

**Sclerotic metastases** may resemble PaD, but no trabecular coarsening or bony enlargement is present. The early lytic phase of PaD may resemble lytic metastases or multiple myeloma; neither enlarges the affected bone.

**PAGET DISEASE**

**Pathology**

- Monostotic (65-90%)
- Calvaria, skull base affected (25-60%)
- Fibroosseous tissue replaces fatty marrow

**Clinical Issues**

- Affects up to 10% of patients > 80 years
- Enlarging skull, CNVIII neuropathy common
- Malignant transformation (0.5-1.0%)
  - Sarcoma > giant cell tumor

**Imaging**

- Early: Lytic ("osteoporosis circumscripta")
- Mid: Mixed lytic, sclerotic ("cotton wool")
- Late: Dense bony sclerosis

**Differential Diagnosis**

- Fibrous dysplasia (younger patients)
- Metastases, myeloma

# Aneurysmal Bone Cyst

## Terminology

Aneurysmal bone cysts (ABCs) are benign, expansile, multicystic lesions that typically develop in childhood or early adulthood. At least 70% of ABCs are primary lesions; the rest arise secondarily within a preexisting benign tumor, such as giant cell tumor or osteoblastoma.

## Pathology

The most common overall ABC location is the metaphysis of long bones (70-80% of cases) with the vertebrae (generally the posterior elements) being the site of 15% of lesions.

The craniofacial bones are a relatively uncommon location. Lesions can occur in the jaws (maxilla, mandible), petrous temporal bone, basisphenoid, and paranasal sinuses. ABCs of the skull and orbit are rare, accounting for < 1% of all cases.

ABCs consist of blood-filled cavernous spaces with intracystic hemorrhages of variable ages. Multiple variably sized cysts are separated by septa lined by endothelium, spindle-shaped fibroblasts, and scattered multinucleated giant cells.

## Clinical Issues

ABCs represent 5% of all primary bone tumors and are the second most common pathologically proven bone tumor of childhood. About 70% occur in the first two decades with a slight male predominance. Symptoms vary with location. Many lesions are asymptomatic or present with slowly progressive swelling.

Treatments for symptomatic ABC are curettage, cryosurgery, and bone graft. Recurrence rates are high, varying from 20-50%. Preoperative embolization may be helpful in selected cases.

## Imaging

NECT scans show an eccentric lesion with expanded, remodeled, ballooned ("aneurysmally dilated") bone surrounded by a thin sclerotic rim **(33-12)**. Multiple cystic spaces with fluid-fluid levels are present **(33-13)**.

MR shows a multicystic lesion with a hypointense rim surrounding multiple fluid-filled spaces. Hemorrhages of varying ages with fluid-fluid levels are a prominent imaging feature, as are smaller cysts ("diverticula") that project from larger lesions. The surrounding rim and fibrous septa enhance following contrast administration **(33-13)**.

A rare manifestation is so-called solid variant ABCs. These typically lack the characteristic radiographic features and have a wide differential diagnosis, including Ewing sarcoma, Langerhans cell histiocytosis, osteosarcoma (OS), metastasis, and giant cell tumor.

## Differential Diagnosis

Some ABCs may have a phase of relatively rapid growth and can be mistaken clinically for a more aggressive lesion. The most important imaging differential diagnosis of ABC is **telangiectatic OS**, which may have fluid-fluid levels that resemble those of ABC. Incomplete margination, soft tissue mass, cortical destruction, and significant solid portions should suggest telangiectatic OS instead.

**Giant cell tumor** and **osteoblastoma** are associated with secondary ABC, and both show significant solid components.

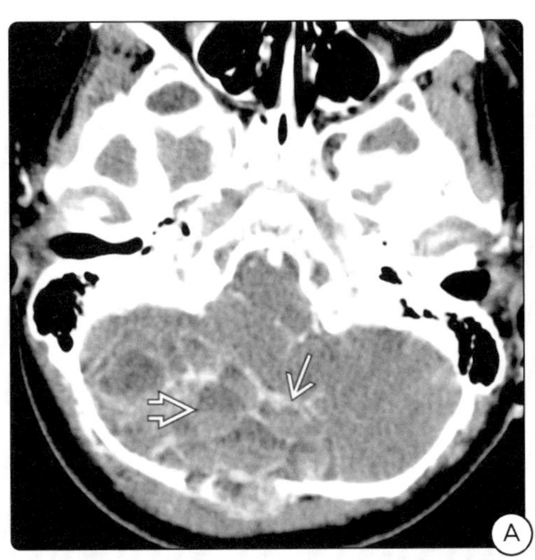


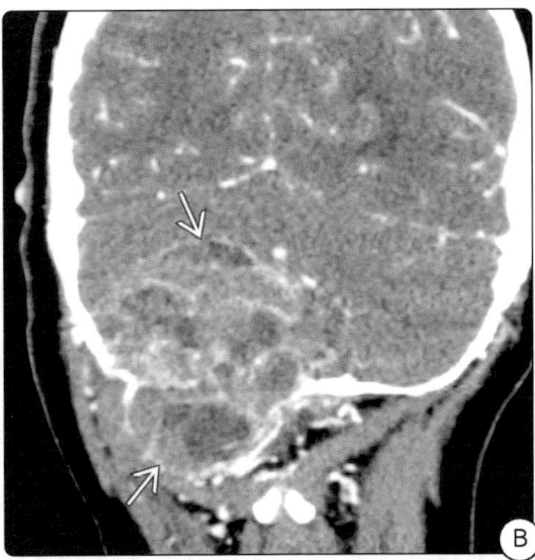


***(33-13A)** Axial CECT of an aneurysmal bone cyst demonstrates multiple cysts with fluid-fluid levels ➡ and enhancing rims ➡. **(33-13B)** Coronal CECT shows that the mass ➡ is both intra- and extracranial. The dependent blood-fluid levels in the cysts are better appreciated on the axial scan.*

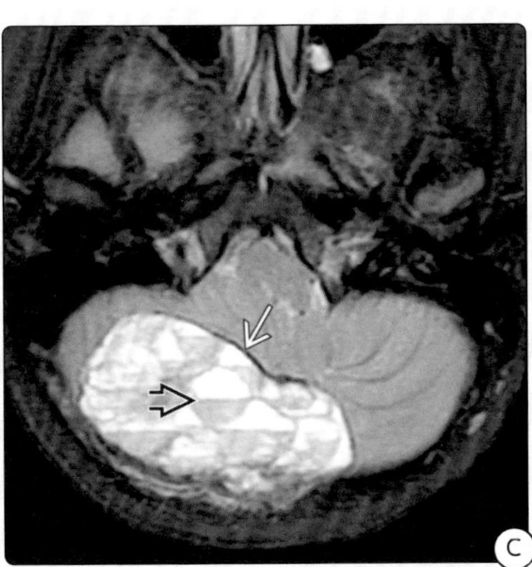


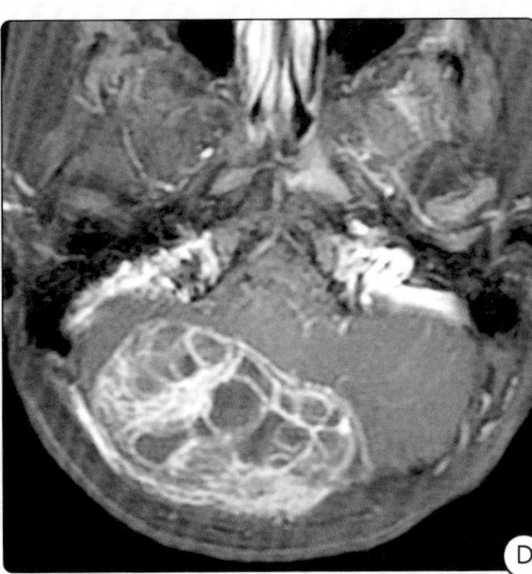


***(33-13C)** T2 MR shows multiple cysts with blood-fluid levels ➡. The thin black line draped over the mass ➡ is the displaced dura. **(33-13D)** T1 C+ FS MR shows the characteristic enhancement of the cyst walls and septations within the tumor.*

# Intracranial Pseudotumors

## Ecchordosis Physaliphora

Ecchordosis physaliphora (EP) is a small (usually < 1 cm), gelatinous soft tissue mass that represents an ectopic notochordal remnant **(33-15)**. Ectopic notochordal rests can occur anywhere along the midline craniospinal axis from the dorsum sellae **(33-14)** to the sacrococcygeal region. EPs are generally asymptomatic and incidental findings at imaging or autopsy. A few reported cases have presented with CSF rhinorrhea of variable duration.

Histopathologically, EPs consist of physaliphorous cells imbedded in a myxoid matrix. The cells are characterized by large mucin-containing intracytoplasmic vacuoles. Necrosis and mitoses are absent.

Imaging features of EPs are quite characteristic. CT demonstrates a well-delineated hypodense, nonenhancing midline intraclival mass with scalloped sclerotic margins **(33-17)**.

The key imaging feature of EP that distinguishes it from other similar-appearing lesions is the presence of a small pedicle or stalk that connects the clival lesion to an intradural component in the prepontine cistern. Best demonstrated on MR, EPs are hypointense to brain on T1WI **(33-16A)** and hyperintense relative to CSF on T2WI **(33-16B)**. EPs do not suppress on FLAIR nor enhance following contrast administration **(33-18)**. Follow-up studies show no change in lesion size.

The major differential diagnosis of EP in the basisphenoid bone is **clival chordoma.** Chordomas are permeative destructive lesions. Other prepontine cistern lesions that can mimic EP include arachnoid, neurenteric, epidermoid, and dermoid cysts. **Arachnoid cysts** are much more common in

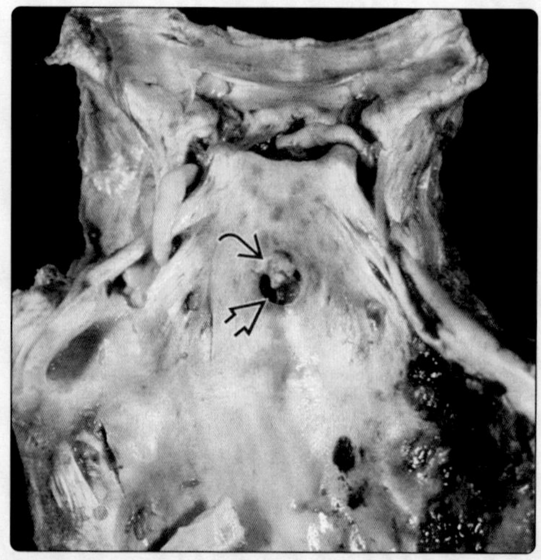

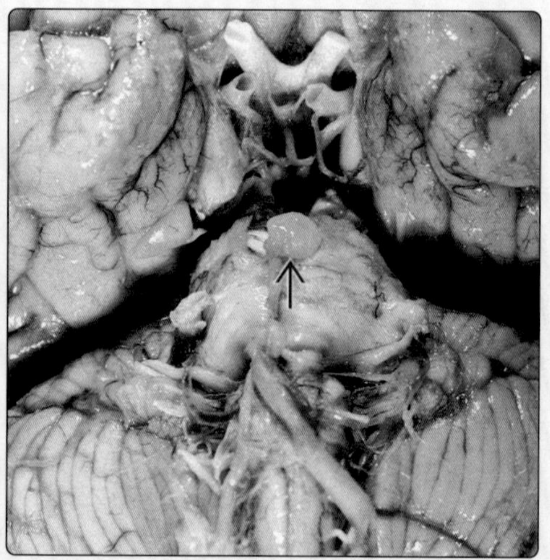

***(33-14)** Focal defect of bone and dura in the midclivus ⇨ is associated with a small ecchordosis physaliphora ⇨. (Courtesy R. Hewlett, MD.) **(33-15)** Gelatinous-appearing nodule ⇨ is in front of the pons. Incidental finding is physaliphorous ecchordosis. (Courtesy R. Hewlett, MD.)*

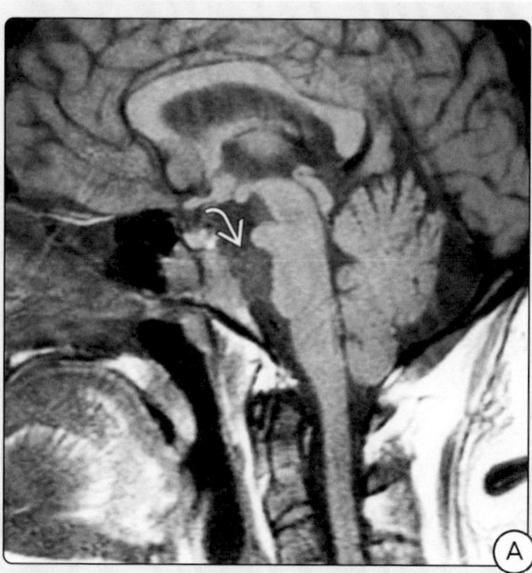


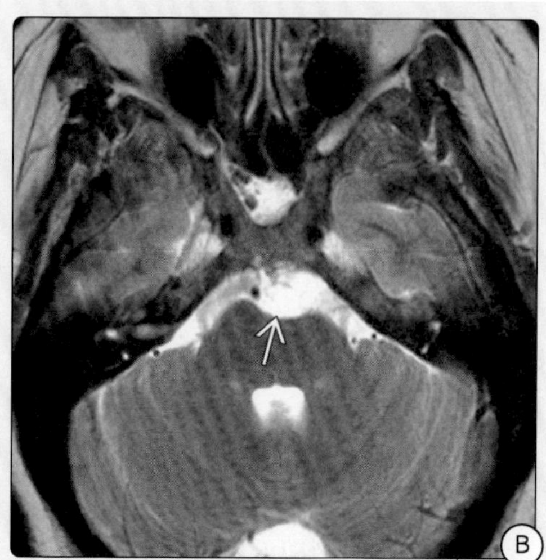


***(33-16A)** Sagittal T1 MR in a 26-yo woman with headaches shows an extraaxial mass ⇨ anterior to and indenting the pons. The mass is slightly hyperintense relative to CSF. **(33-16B)** T2 MR shows lobulated, well-delineated, hyperintense midline mass ⇨ indenting the pons. This is physaliphorous ecchordosis.*

the cerebellopontine angle cisterns and behave exactly like CSF on all sequences.

**Neurenteric cysts** are often slightly off-midline and somewhat lower, adjacent to the pontomedullary junction. **Epidermoid cysts** (ECs) are irregular, somewhat frond-like lesions that restrict on DWI. ECs are more common in the cerebellopontine angle cisterns. **Dermoid cysts** usually follow fat signal, not CSF.

## Intracranial Foreign Body Granuloma

Retained surgical elements, such as cotton balls and Gelfoam, may induce an excessive inflammatory reaction that may be difficult to distinguish from recurrent or residual tumor on neuroimaging studies.

### Terminology

Intracranial **foreign body granuloma** (FBG) is a rare inflammatory reaction to retained surgical materials that can appear months to years following the initial procedure.

FBG (a.k.a. textiloma) refers to a mass created by a retained surgical element (inadvertently or deliberately left behind) and its associated foreign body inflammatory reaction. The terms gossypiboma, gauzoma, and muslinoma refer specifically to retained nonresorbable cotton or woven materials.

### Etiology

Hemostatic agents can be resorbable or nonresorbable. All classes of resorbable and nonresorbable agents may produce textilomas as an allergic response.

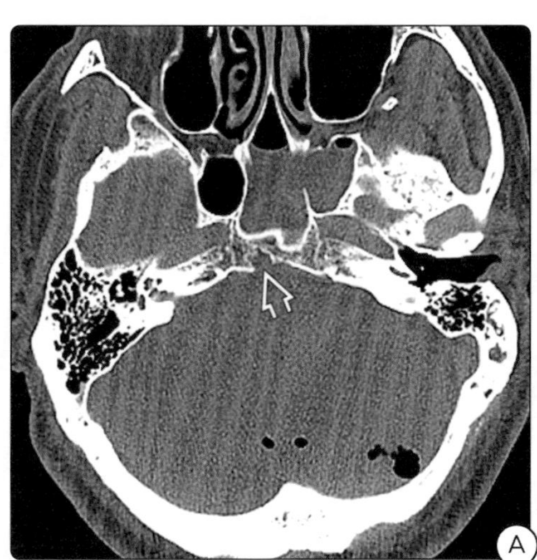

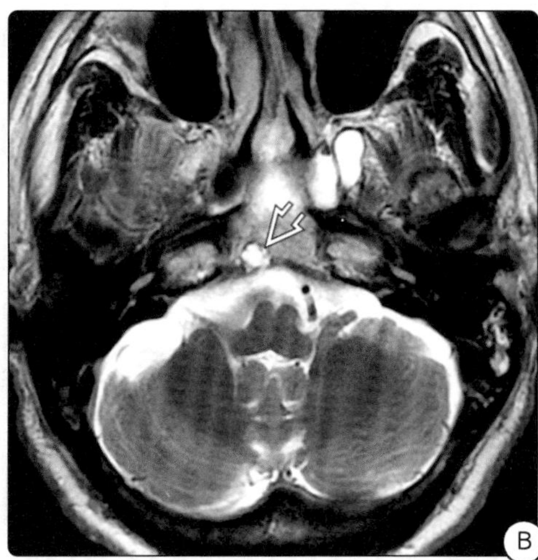

***(33-17A)** Axial bone CT in a patient with trauma shows a focal corticated defect ➡ in the clivus. **(33-17B)** Follow-up T2 MR obtained several days later shows that the well-corticated clival lesion ➡ is extremely hyperintense. This is physaliphora ecchordosis, an incidental finding.*

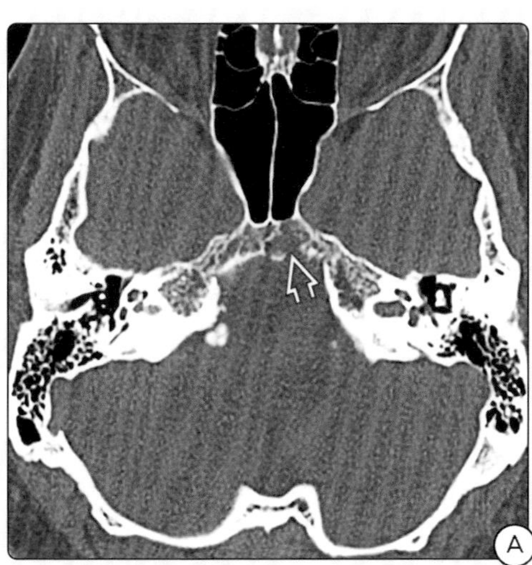

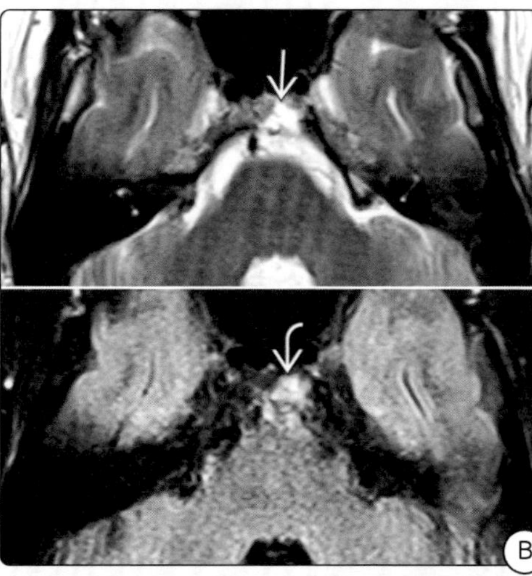

***(33-18A)** Bone CT shows a scalloped, lytic, corticated lesion ➡ in the clivus. **(33-18B)** T2 MR (top) shows that the clival lesion ➡ is well-delineated and very hyperintense. The lesion does not suppress on FLAIR ➡ (bottom). This is physaliphora ecchordosis.*

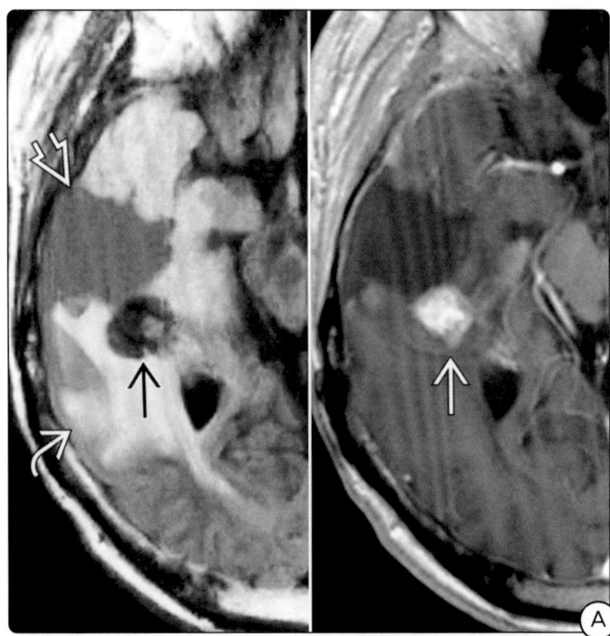

*(33-19A) (L) Axial FLAIR MR after right middle fossa surgery for meningioma shows a hypointense mass ⇒ with edema ➡ next to tumor resection cavity ⇨. (R) The lesion demonstrates enhancement ➡ on T1 C+ MR.*

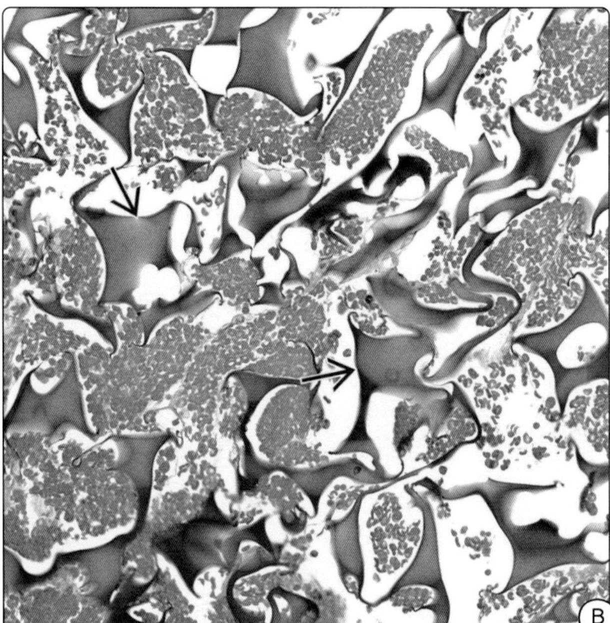

*(33-19B) Histology from the resected specimen shows amorphous spicules ⇒ surrounded by blood. This is a Gelfoam foreign body granuloma a.k.a. textiloma. (Courtesy B. K. Kleinschmidt-DeMasters, MD.)*

Resorbable agents include gelatin sponge, oxidized cellulose, and microfibrillar collagen. Nonresorbable agents include various forms of cotton pledgets, cloth (i.e., muslin), and synthetic rayon. Although bioabsorbable hemostats are often left in place, nonresorbable agents are typically removed prior to surgical closure. Any of these materials may induce an inflammatory reaction, creating a textiloma.

Rare FBGs have been reported following endovascular coil embolization, mechanical thrombectomy, or use of hydrophilic polymers.

## Pathology

Most FBGs occur within surgical resection sites or around muslin-reinforced aneurysms. Histologic examination typically shows a core of degenerating inert hemostatic agent surrounded by inflammatory reaction. Foreign body giant cells and histiocytes are often present. Each agent exhibits distinctive histologic features, often permitting specific identification **(33-19B)**.

## Clinical Issues

Intracranial FBGs are rare with around 100 cases reported in the literature. Most reported cases following brain tumor resection were diagnosed within the first 3 postsurgical months and were often identified incidentally during routine follow-up imaging.

## Imaging

Intracranial FBGs are located adjacent to the resection cavity and are almost always iso- or hypointense on T1WI. Approximately 45% are iso- and 40% are hypointense on T2/FLAIR **(33-19A)**. Some "blooming" on T2* may be present. All reported cases enhance on postcontrast scans **(33-20)**. Ring and heterogeneous solid enhancement patterns occur almost equally. Central diffusion restriction is common.

FBGs occurring after cerebral embolization procedures may show multiple foci of FLAIR hyperintensity and contrast-enhanced nodular lesions in the affected vascular distribution.

## Differential Diagnosis

The major differential diagnosis is **recurrent neoplasm** or **radiation necrosis**. Residual or recurrent tumor can coexist with textiloma. If present, T2 hypointensity helps distinguish textiloma from neoplasm or **abscess**. Definitive diagnosis typically requires biopsy and histologic examination with both routine stains and polarized light.

# Calcifying Pseudoneoplasm of Neuraxis

## Terminology

Calcifying pseudoneoplasm of the neuraxis (CAPNON) is a rare nonneoplastic lesion of the CNS. Calcifying pseudoneoplasms are also known as fibroosseous lesions, cerebral calculi, brain stones, brain rocks, and crudoma.

## Etiology

The precise origin of CAPNONs is unknown. They have been attributed to a reactive proliferative process induced by infection, inflammation, degeneration, or injury, although many are discovered incidentally on imaging studies without an identifiable etiology.

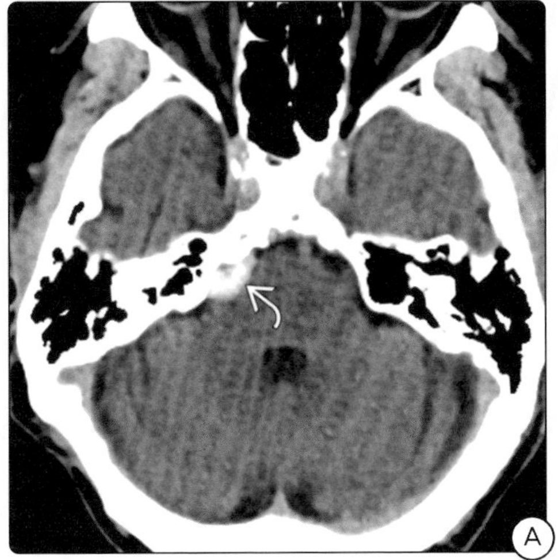


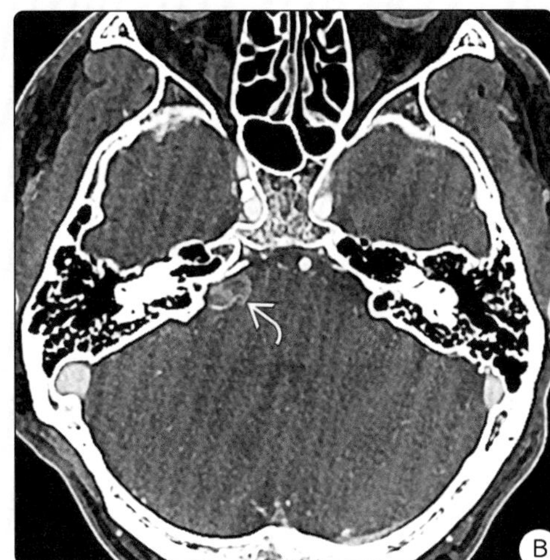


***(33-20A)** NECT in a 72-yo man in the ER initially obtained to "rule out stroke" shows a hyperdense, extraaxial mass in the right cerebellopontine angle (CPA) cistern.* ***(33-20B)** Image from emergent CTA obtained as part of the emergent stroke protocol shows the CPA mass is mixed iso- and hyperdense.*

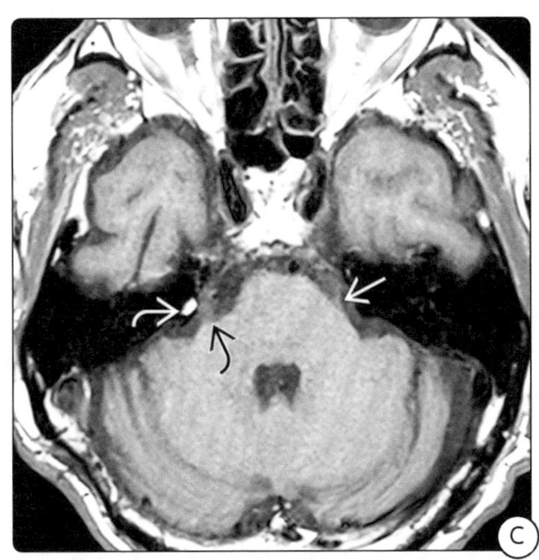


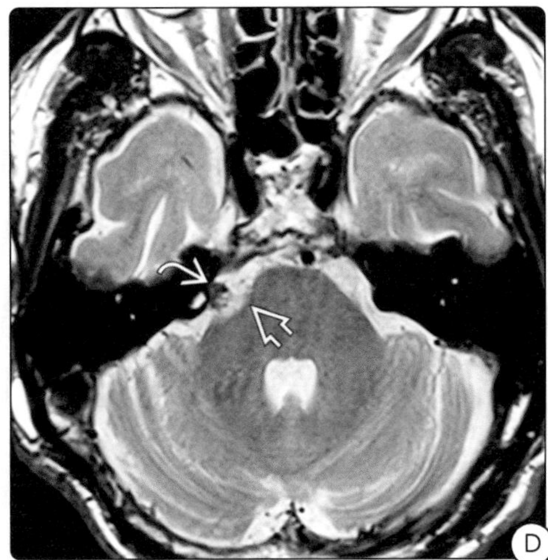


***(33-20C)** T1 MR shows a normal-appearing left trigeminal nerve. The right trigeminal nerve appears thickened and slightly irregular. There is a small hyperintense focus adjacent to the nerve, and the pons appears somewhat deformed.* ***(33-20D)** T2 MR shows that the mass is hypointense. Note focal deformity of the adjacent pons.*

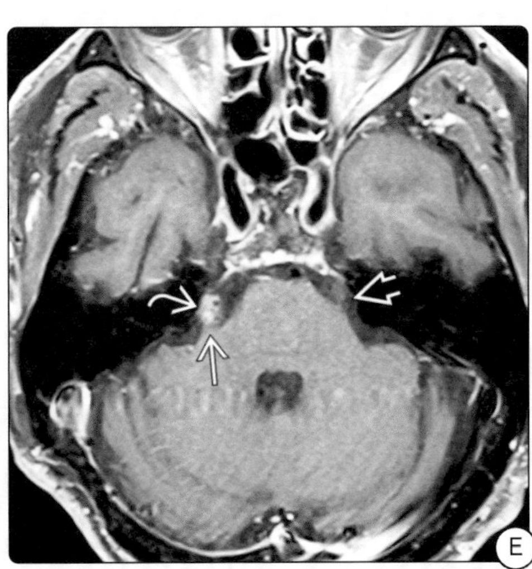


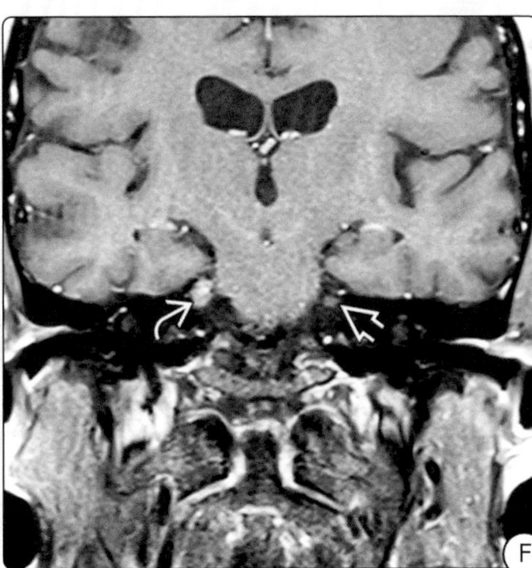


***(33-20E)** T1 C+ FS MR shows that the mass enhances and is adjacent to the root entry zone of the right trigeminal nerve. The left CNV appears normal.* ***(33-20F)** Coronal T1 C+ FS MR shows that the enhancing mass appears to encase the right trigeminal nerve. The left CNV appears normal. The patient had prior trigeminal neuralgia surgery. This is a textiloma.*

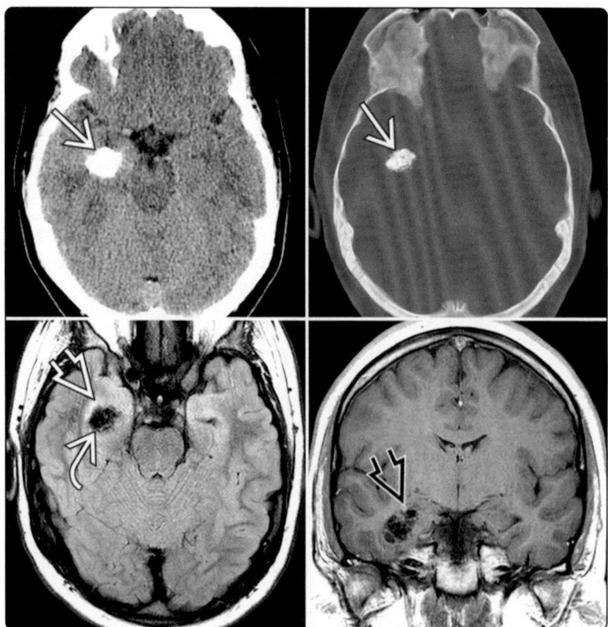

***(33-21) NECT (upper L) and bone CT (upper R) show densely calcified mass ➡. FLAIR MR (lower L) shows that hypointense mass ➡ is surrounded by edema ➡ and does not enhance ➡ (lower R). This is CAPNON. (Courtesy S. Blaser, MD.)***

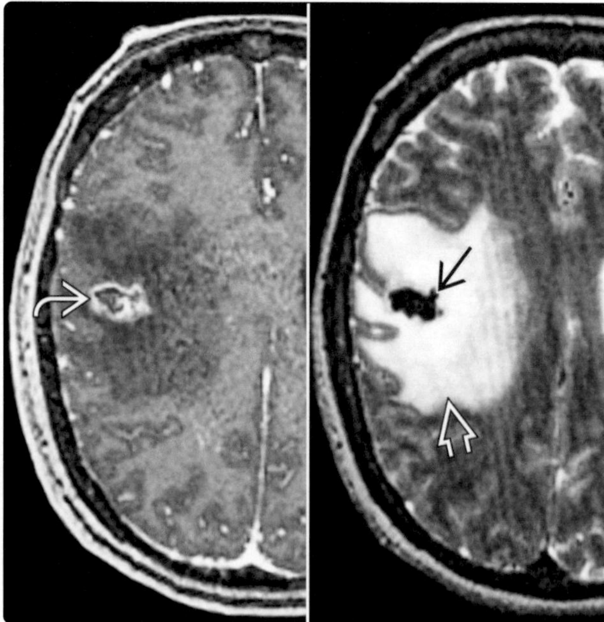

***(33-22) Sometimes, intraaxial CAPNONs are extremely hypointense ➡ on T2 MR, incite intense edema ➡, and exhibit rim enhancement ➡. (Courtesy B. K. Kleinschmidt-DeMasters, MD.)***

## Pathology

CAPNONs are discrete nonneoplastic, noninflammatory lesions. Most are solitary; multiple lesions have been described but are uncommon. CAPNONs can occur anywhere in the CNS, including the spine. Most are extraaxial, but intraparenchymal and even intraventricular CAPNONs do occur.

Grossly, CAPNONs are well-demarcated, white, firm/gritty, intra- or extraaxial masses. They contain various combinations of chondromyxoid and fibrovascular stroma, metaplastic calcification, and—in some cases—even ossification with the appearance of mature bone.

CAPNONs are often surrounded peripherally by palisading spindle/epithelioid cells ("cortical layer") resembling arachnoid cells. Positive immunoreactivity to vimentin and epithelial membrane antigen (EMA) are typical. GFAP and S100 protein are typically negative, helping distinguish CAPNON from astrocytic neoplasms and meningioma.

Rarely, CAPNONs exhibit characteristics of foreign body reactions with giant cells, tissue ossification, and the formation of lamellar bone or scattered psammoma bodies. The surrounding brain may exhibit inflammatory changes with gliosis and edema leading to mass effect.

## Clinical Issues

Although age at diagnosis ranges from 2 to 90 years, CAPNONs affect mostly middle-aged adults and are rare in the pediatric population. There is a slight male predominance.

Presentation is site dependent. Some intracranial CAPNONs are asymptomatic and discovered incidentally on imaging studies, although seizures and headache have been reported.

A few cases have been reported in association with meningioangiomatosis and neurofibromatosis type 2.

## Imaging

CAPNONs are heavily calcified, well-delineated, leptomeningeal (extraaxial) **(33-23)** or parenchymal (intraaxial) masses resembling fibroosseous lesions. NECT scans demonstrate a heavily calcified leptomeningeal, deep intrasulcal, or brain parenchymal "rock" **(33-21)**. The calcifications can be solid or partial, peripheral or central.

On MR, typical CAPNONs demonstrate little mass effect, are iso- to hypointense on T1WI, and are uniformly hypointense on T2WI and FLAIR. Mild "blooming" is seen on T2* GRE and SWI **(33-23)**.

Perilesional edema varies from none to extensive in some cases of intraaxial CAPNONs **(33-22)**. Enhancement varies from none to moderate. Solid, linear, serpiginous, and peripheral rim-like enhancement patterns have all been reported.

## Differential Diagnosis

The differential diagnosis of CAPNON includes an ossified vascular lesion—most often a **cavernous malformation.** Although heavily calcified cavernous malformations can often be distinguished by their "popcorn" mixed hyperintensity on T2WI, blood-fluid levels, and hemosiderin rim, biopsy is usually necessary for definitive diagnosis. Residua of infection, such as calcified **tuberculous granuloma** or **neurocysticercosis**, can also resemble CAPNONs.

CAPNON can mimic densely calcified neoplasms, such as **oligodendroglioma, meningioma**, and **polymorphous low-**

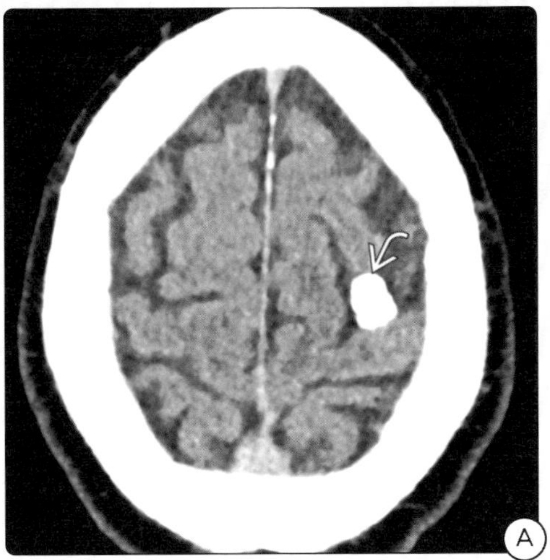

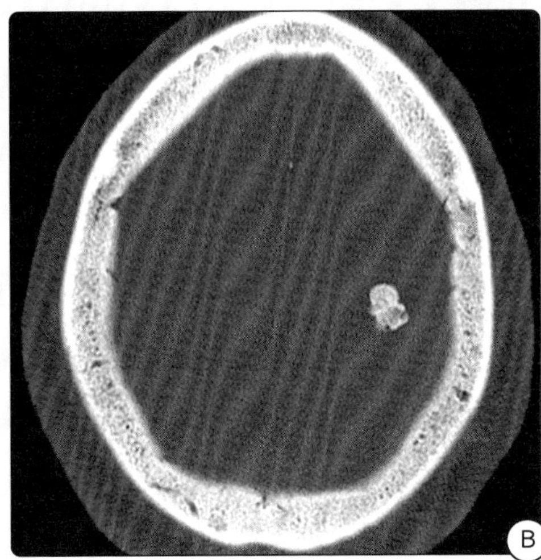

***(33-23A)** NECT in a 37-yo man obtained for minor head trauma shows a hyperdense extraaxial lesion ➡ adjacent to the vertex of the left cerebral hemisphere. **(33-23B)** Bone CT shows that the lesion is densely calcified and resembles bone.*

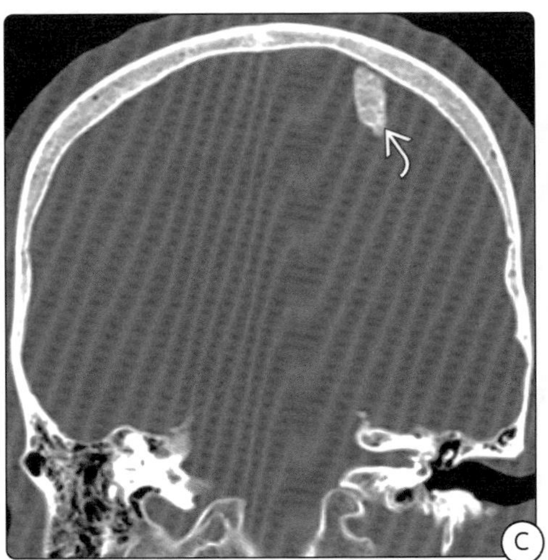

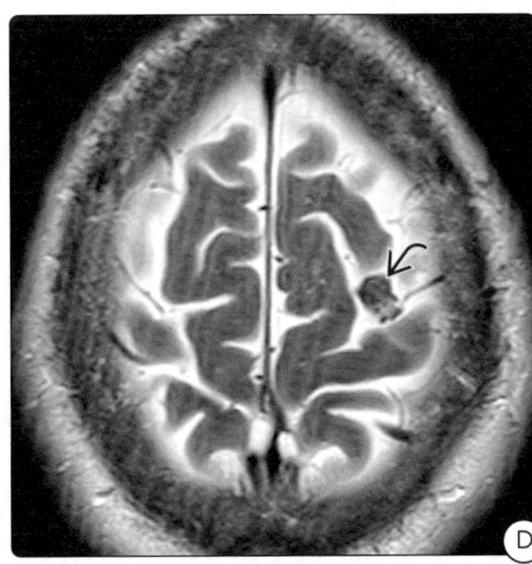

***(33-23C)** Reformatted bone CT shows that the lesion ➡ resembles calvarium but is clearly separated from it. **(33-23D)** T2 MR shows that the lesion ➡ is very hypointense relative to both brain and CSF.*

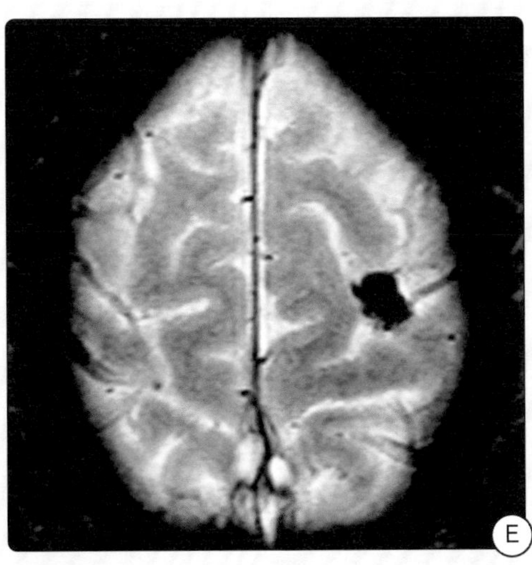

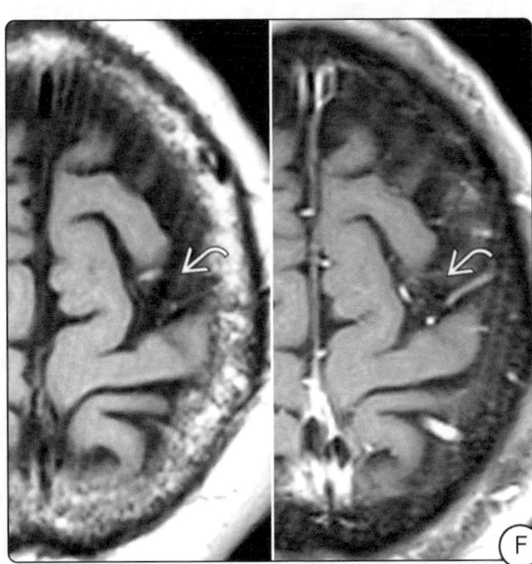

***(33-23E)** The lesion is very hypointense on T2* GRE MR. **(33-23F)** Precontrast T1 (L) and T1 C+ FS (R) MR sequences show that the lesion ➡ is hypointense and does not enhance. This is CAPNON.*

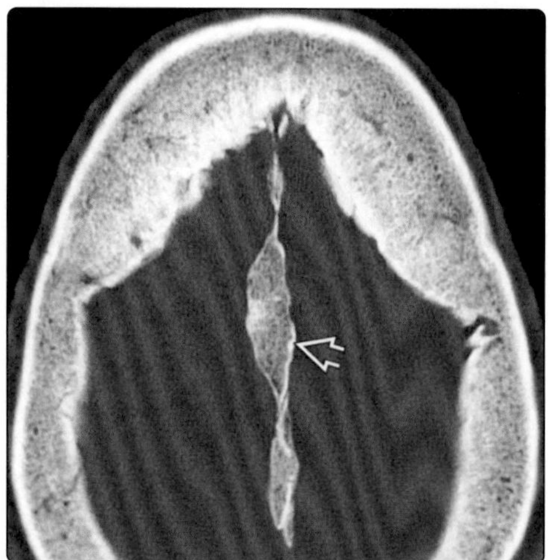

***(33-24)** Bone CT shows falx osseous metaplasia. Note bony cortex ➡ surrounds marrow identical to that of calvarium. (Courtesy M. Jhaveri, MD.)*

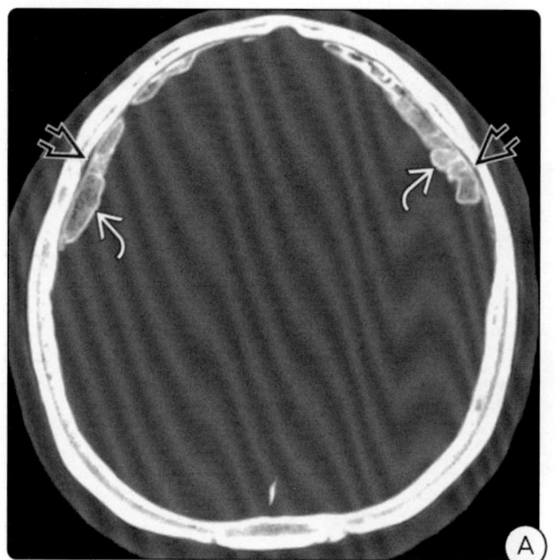


***(33-25A)** Bone CT in a 39-yo woman shows bilateral nodules of osseous metaplasia ➡. Note separation from the inner table of skull ➡.*

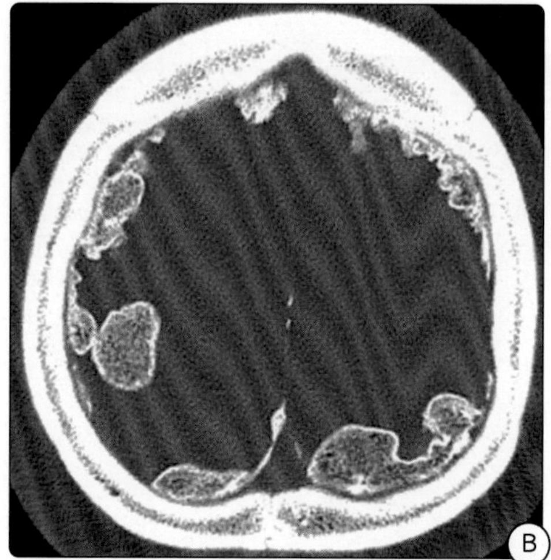


***(33-25B)** More cephalad bone CT with edge enhancement shows multiple nodules of metaplastic bone.*

**grade neuroepithelial tumor of the young (PLNTY)**. The rare intraventricular CAPNON can resemble meningioma or a choroid plexus papilloma with osseous metaplasia.

PLNTYs often have dense central tumoral calcifications and closely mimic CAPNONs. While CAPNONs generally affect middle-aged and older patients, they can occasionally be seen in children and young adults where they may mimic PLNTY.

## Metaplastic Dural Ossification

### Terminology

Physiologic **calcifications** ("plaques") of the intracranial dura are common, age related, and generally of no clinical significance. In contrast, **osseous** metaplasia of the CNS dura involves new bone formation, is relatively rare, and should not be mistaken for neoplastic disease.

### Etiology

The precise etiology of dural osseous metaplasia is unknown. As dura is derived from multipotential mesenchymal cells, activation from trauma, hemorrhage, inflammation, or age-related degeneration might lead to the aberrant formation of bone tissue. Systemic disorders, such as hyperparathyroidism, vitamin D intoxication, and chronic renal failure, have been reported in some cases.

### Pathology

**Location.** Osseous metaplasia of the dura is most common in the spine, where chronic arachnoid inflammation from surgery or trauma can lead to intrathecal ossification ("arachnoiditis ossificans").

In contrast to the spine, dural ossification with new bone formation involving the cranial meninges is rare. By far, the most common site is the falx cerebri; the second most common site is the convexity dura followed by the tentorium cerebelli.

Two types of falx ossification have been identified. In some cases, ossification begins in and is in close proximity to the interior surface of the calvarium with direct continuity to the falx lesion. In others, the ossification is located intracranially without any continuity with the calvarium.

**Size and Number.** Dural ossifications can be solitary or multifocal. Multifocal lesions with numerous confluent or scattered foci present within the dura are more common. Lesions vary in size from a few millimeters to rare cases > 10 cm in length and width up to 1-2 cm **(33-24)**.

**Gross Pathology.** Sheets or nodules of hard white material with a shell of dense mature cortical bone surrounding normal-appearing marrow are typical. Falx ossifications often have a linear medial border with a slight convex or irregular lateral border. In other locations, the ossification may be nodular, irregular, wavy, or even round in appearance.

**Microscopic Features.** Osseous tissue complete with bone marrow elements is present. The osseous tissue is bounded by rows of spindle cells continuous with adjacent connective tissue cells of the falx.

### Clinical Issues

Fatty marrow development in the falx occurs in 0.5-1.0% of the population and is usually an incidental finding of no clinical significance. Patients are generally middle aged to older (45-85 years).

## Imaging

Most cases of intracranial dural ossification are discovered during routine clinical imaging and are incidental findings of no clinical significance.

**CT Findings.** Membranous bone formed in the intracranial dura behaves like and resembles bone elsewhere. An outer shell of dense cortical bone surrounds an inner core of marrow. These range in size from small solitary or multifocal lesions **(33-25A)** to large, bizarre-appearing bony structures that can extend along much or all of the affected dura **(33-25)**. A thin, hypodense line often separates the metaplastic ossification from the inner table of the skull **(33-25A)**.

**MR Findings.** The central marrow-containing portion of the ossified mass is hyperintense on T1WI **(33-26B)**. The bony cortex is hypointense on T2WI, and the marrow is slightly hyperintense relative to brain. The lesions "bloom" on T2* sequences **(33-26C)**. Enhancement is usually minimal or absent on T1 C+ FS, although hemopoietically active marrow nodules may enhance. Slight thickening with continuous linear enhancement of the adjacent dura is common **(33-26C)**.

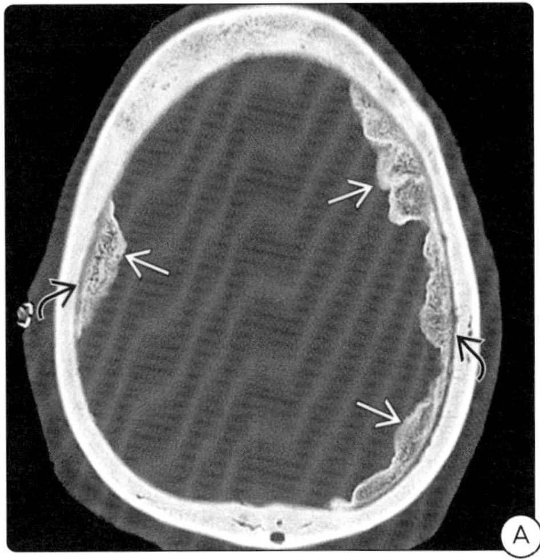

***(33-26A)** Bone CT shows bony masses along inner calvarium ➡. Note thin lucent line ➡ (dura) separates lesions from inner table of the skull.*

## Differential Diagnosis

**Physiologic dural calcifications** are hyperdense, flat plaques that exhibit a laminar pattern of calcification on NECT. No fat or internal marrow cavity is present.

**Hyperostosis frontalis interna** is a benign nodular, continuous overgrowth of the frontal bone that is seen primarily in older postmenopausal females. In contrast to metaplastic dural ossification, the bony overgrowth is continuous with the inner table of the skull.

Dural **osteoma** is a focal lesion with dense, solid calcification. Macroscopic calcification in **meningioma** is common; osseous metaplasia is rare. A densely calcified meningioma (brain "stone") usually exhibits some enhancement on T1 C+ FS.

Calcifying pseudoneoplasm of the neuraxis **(CAPNON)** is rare and can be intra- or extraaxial. Extraaxial CAPNONs tend to be rounded, focal lesions with dense calcification, not osseous metaplasia, and located within a sulcus rather than directly adjacent to the dura.

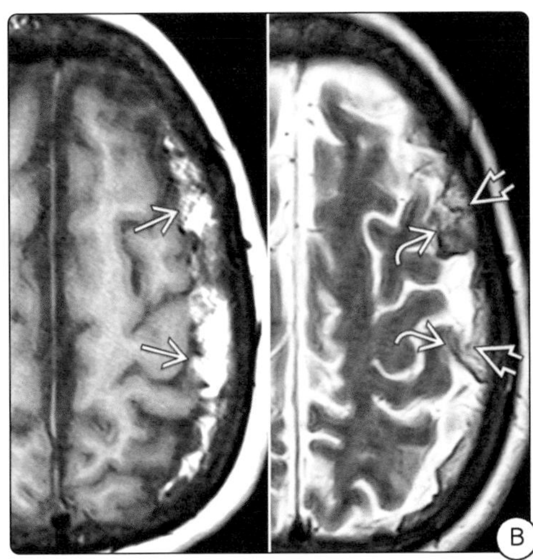

***(33-26B)** (L) T1 hyperintensity in lesions ➡ suggests fatty marrow. (R) Rims are hypointense ➡, centers hyperintense ➡ on T2.*

### INTRACRANIAL PSEUDOTUMORS

**Textiloma**
- Foreign body reaction (Gelfoam, gauze, etc.)
- Iso-/hypointense on T2WI
- Ring, heterogeneous enhancement on T1 C+

**Calcifying Pseudoneoplasm of Neuraxis (CAPNON)**
- Chondrocalcific or ossified mass on NECT
    - Extraaxial (usually in sulcus) > intraaxial
- Very hypointense on T2/FLAIR
- Enhancement varies (none to rim-like)

**Metaplastic Dural Ossification**
- Dense cortical bone surrounds fatty marrow core
- Can be solitary or multifocal, small or extensive
- Anterior/middle falx > > convexity, tentorium

*Selected References: The complete reference list is available on the eBooks+ version included with purchase.*

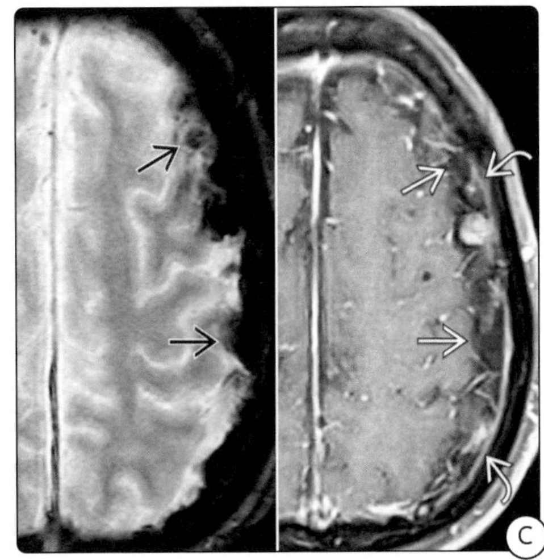

***(33-26C)** (L) Lesions bloom on T2* ➡ and mostly suppress on T1 C+ FS ➡ (R). Note diffuse dural thickening ➡. Ossifying metaplasia of the dura.*

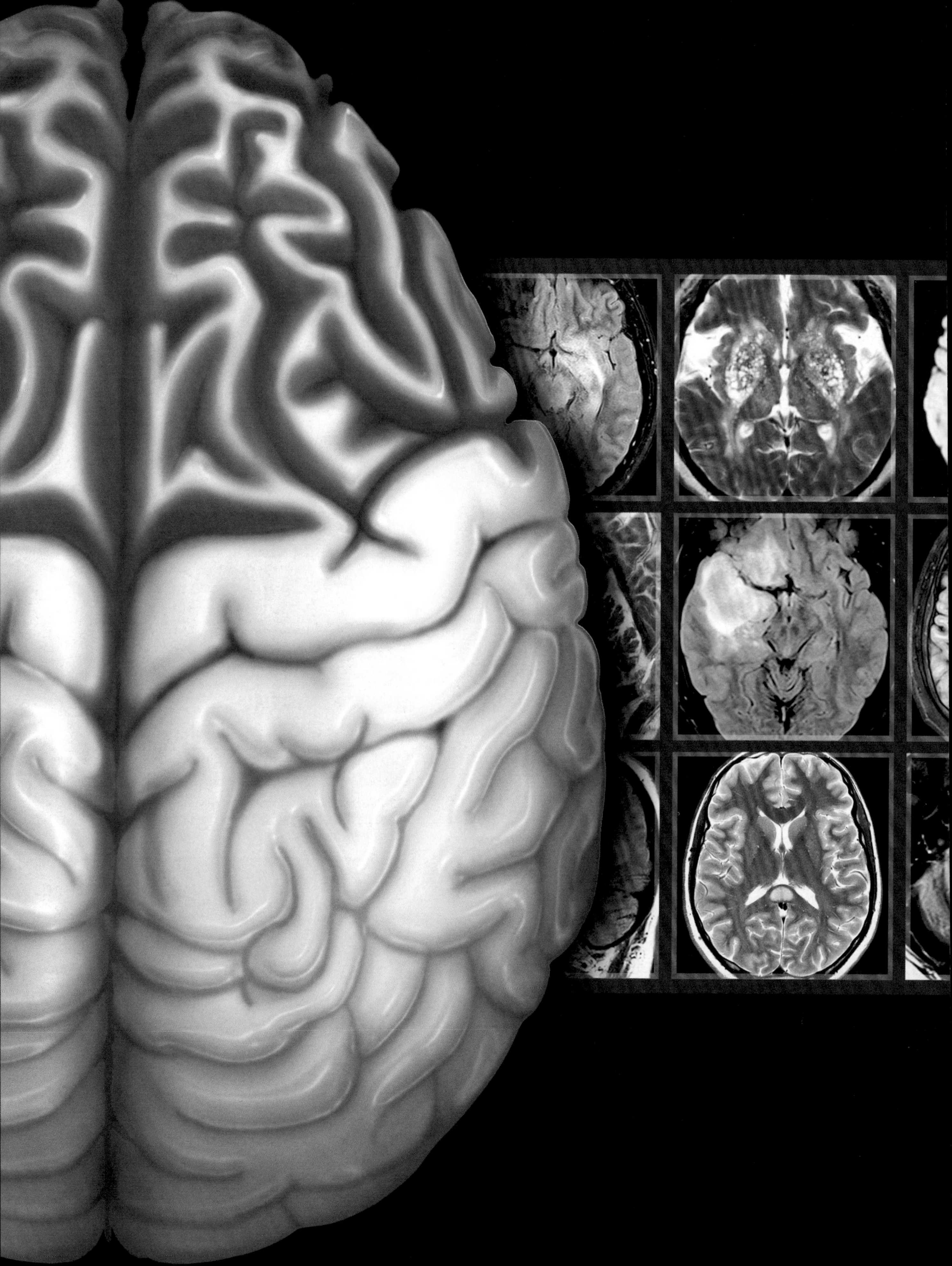

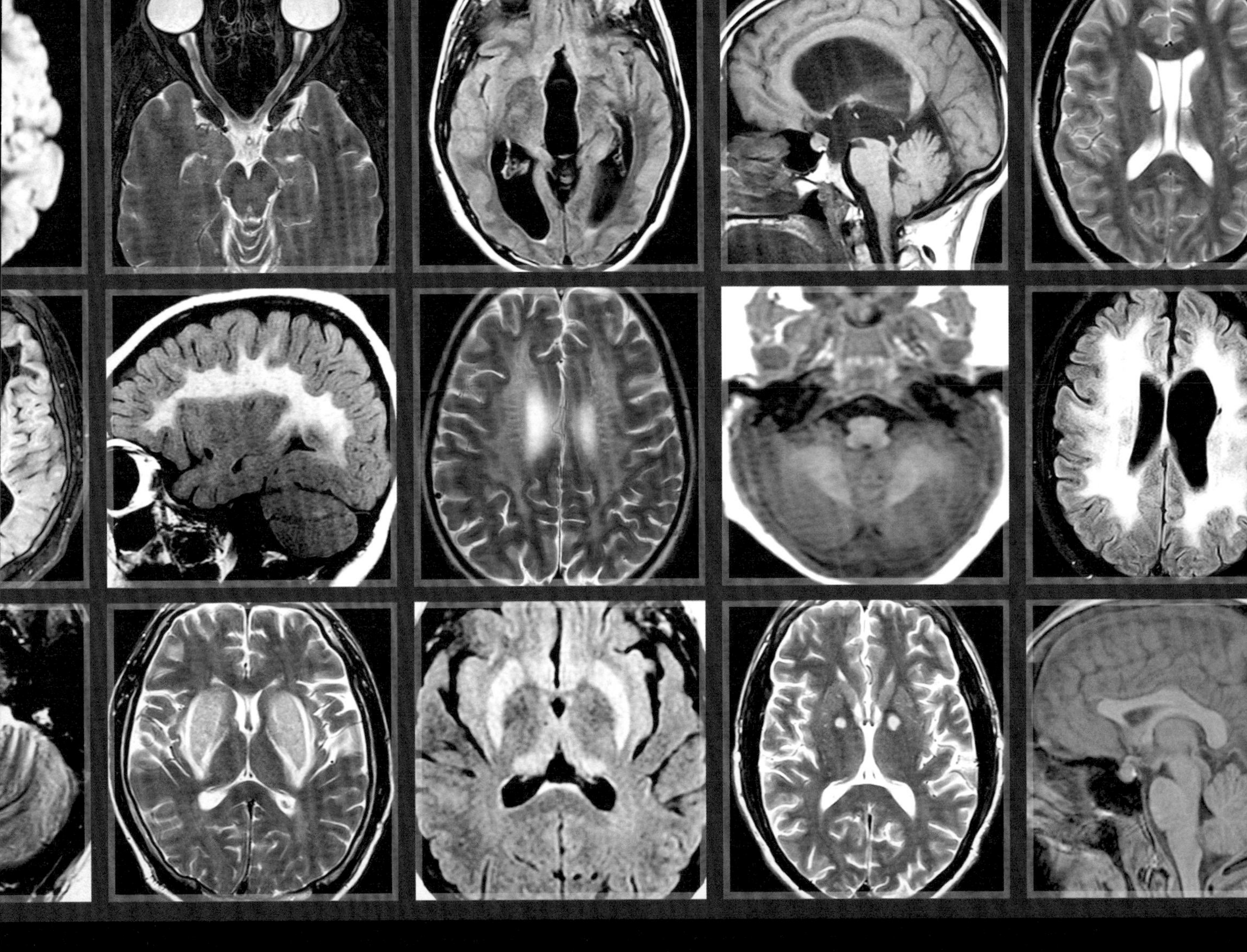

SECTION 5

# Toxic, Metabolic, Degenerative, and CSF Disorders

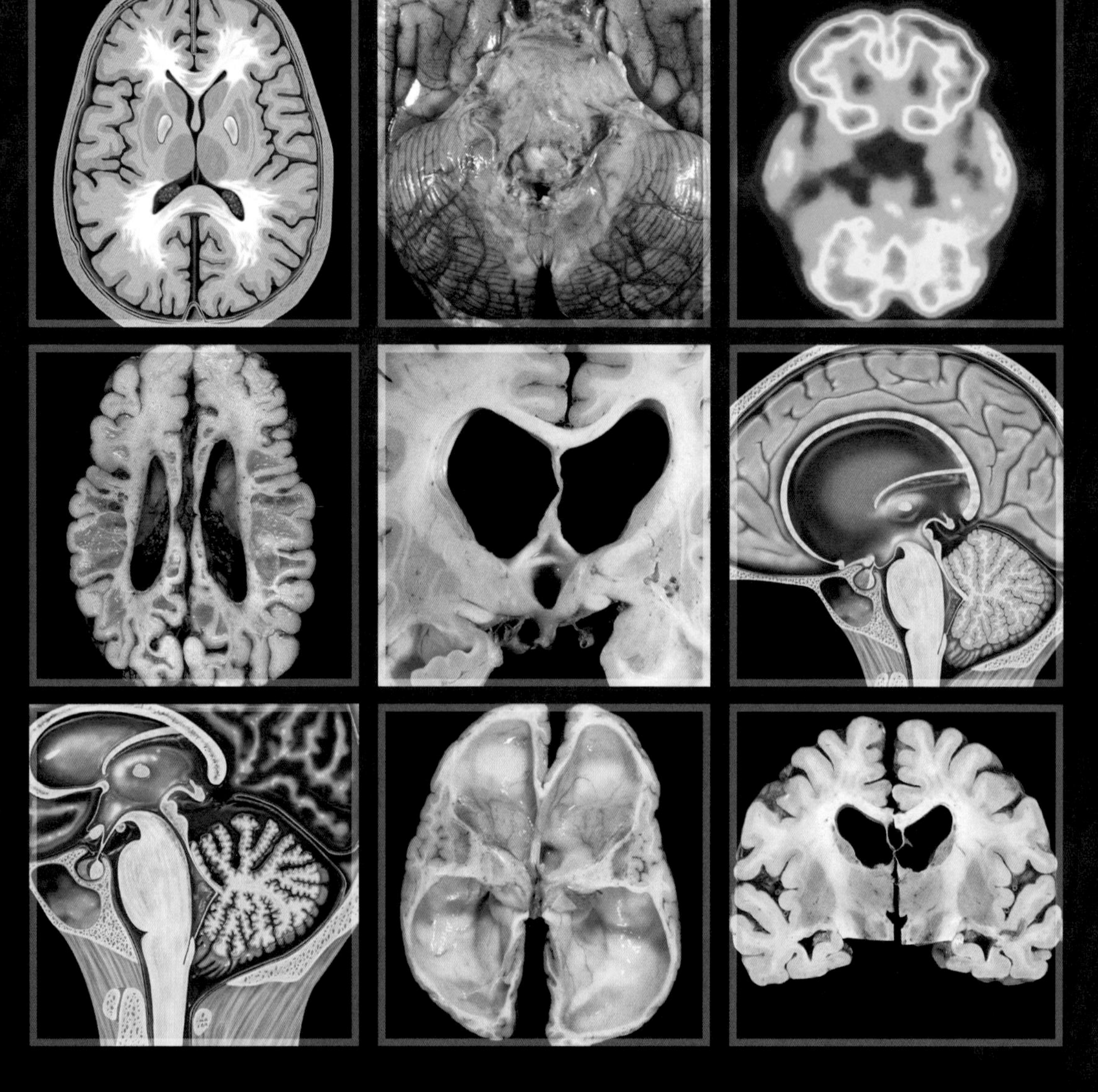

SECTION 5

# Toxic, Metabolic, Degenerative and CSF Disorders

# Approach to Toxic, Metabolic, Degenerative, and CSF Disorders

*Metabolic disorders are relatively uncommon but important diseases in which imaging can play a key role in early diagnosis and appropriate patient management. Drug and alcohol abuse are increasing around the world, and the list of environmental toxins that can affect the CNS continues to increase. Recognizing toxic and metabolic-induced encephalopathies has become a clinical and imaging imperative. The two etiologies are often linked because many toxins induce metabolic derangements and some systemic metabolic diseases have a direct toxic effect on the brain.*



With rapidly increasing numbers of aging people, the prevalence of dementia and brain degeneration is also becoming a global concern. Brain scans in older patients with mental status changes are now some of the most frequently requested imaging examinations, so normal and pathologic age-related CNS changes are discussed in this section.

## Anatomy and Physiology of the Basal Ganglia and Thalami

### Physiologic Considerations

By weight and volume, the brain is a small structure. However, relative to its size, the brain is one of the most metabolically active of all organs. It normally receives ~ 15% of total cardiac output, consumes ~ 20% of blood oxygen, and metabolizes up to 20% of blood glucose.

Because of its high intrinsic metabolic demands, the brain is exquisitely sensitive to processes that decrease delivery or utilization of blood, oxygen, and glucose. A variety of toxic substances do exactly that.

Two areas of the brain are especially susceptible to toxic and metabolic damage: The deep gray nuclei and the cerebral white matter (WM). The basal ganglia (BG) are highly vascular, rich in mitochondria, and loaded with neurotransmitters. The BG—especially the putamen and globus pallidus (GP)—are particularly susceptible to hypoxia or anoxia and are also commonly affected by toxins and metabolic derangements. The cerebral WM is particularly vulnerable to lipophilic toxic substances.

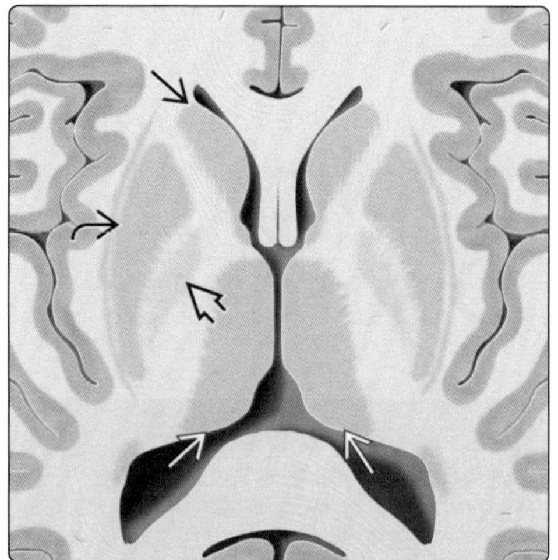

(34-1) Graphic shows basal ganglia, CNuc ➔, putamen ➔, and globus pallidus (GP) ➔. Thalami ➔ form borders of the 3rd ventricle.

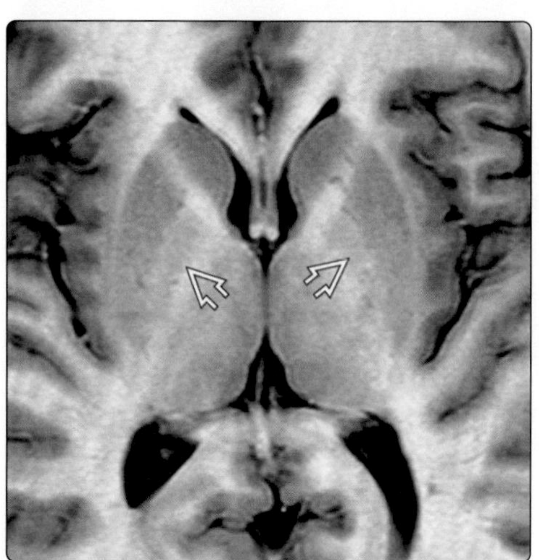

(34-2) Axial T1WI shows basal ganglia, thalami as isointense with gray matter. GPs ➔ are slightly hyperintense to caudate and putamen.

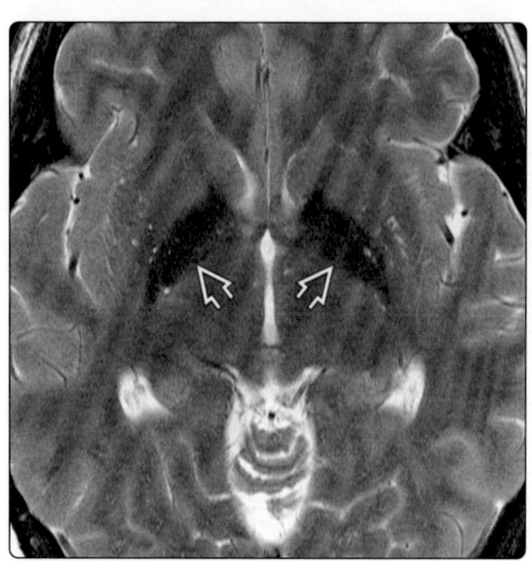

(34-3) On T2WI, the GPs ➔ are more hypointense than putamen, caudate. Putamen reaches same hypointensity in 7th or 8th decade.

## Normal Gross Anatomy

The **BG** are symmetric paired subcortical (deep gray matter) nuclei that form the core of the extrapyramidal system and control motor activity. The BG consist of (1) the caudate nucleus (CNuc), (2) the putamen, and (3) the GP **(34-1)**.

The thalami are the largest and most prominent of the deep gray matter nuclei but are generally not included in the term "basal ganglia."

## Normal Imaging Anatomy

NECT

The BG and thalami are symmetrically hyperdense compared to normal WM. Physiologic calcifications in the GPs are common in adults **(34-9)**.

### T1WI

The CNuc, putamina, and thalami are isointense with cortex on T1 scans **(34-2)**. As the site of both physiologic calcification and age-related iron deposition, the GP segments vary in signal intensity. Calcification may cause T1 shortening and mild hyperintensity in the medial segment.

### T2WI

The CNuc, putamina, and thalami are isointense with cortical gray matter on T2 scans **(34-3)**. Increasing iron deposition occurs with aging, and the putamen becomes progressively more hypointense. A "dark" putamen is normal by the seventh or eighth decade of life.

### T2*

The GP is hypointense relative to cortex on GRE or SWI imaging. By the seventh or eighth decade of life, iron deposition in the putamen "blooms," and the lateral putamen appears hypointense relative to the thalami but not as intensely hypointense as the GP.

# Toxic and Metabolic Disorders

Many toxic, metabolic, systemic, and degenerative diseases affect the BG and thalami in a strikingly symmetric fashion **(34-15)**. Lesions are most often secondary to diffuse systemic or metabolic derangements **(34-11)**. Patchy, discrete, focal, and asymmetric lesions are more commonly infectious, postinfectious, traumatic, or neoplastic in origin **(34-12)**.

## Differential Diagnoses of Bilateral Basal Ganglia Lesions

The most common bilateral BG lesions are normal variants (e.g., physiologic calcification and prominent perivascular spaces). Vascular disease, hypoxic-ischemic insults, and common metabolic disorders, such as chronic liver failure, are the most frequent causes **(34-11)**. Infection, toxins, drug abuse, or metabolic disorders, such as osmotic demyelination and Wernicke encephalopathy, are less common causes of bilateral BG lesions **(34-12)**.

### COMMON BILATERAL BASAL GANGLIA LESIONS

**Normal Variants**
- Physiologic mineralization
  - Medial globus pallidus (GP) > > caudate, putamen
- Prominent perivascular spaces
  - Follow CSF, suppress on FLAIR

**Vascular Disease**
- Lacunar infarcts
  - Multiple bilateral, scattered, asymmetric
- Diffuse axonal/vascular injury
  - Hemorrhage, other lesions

**Hypoxic-Ischemic Injury**
- Hypoxic-ischemic encephalopathy (HIE)
  - Basal ganglia (BG) ± cortex/watershed, hippocampi, thalami

**Metabolic Disorders**
- Chronic liver disease
  - GP, substantia nigra hyperintensity

### LESS COMMON BILATERAL BASAL GANGLIA LESIONS

**Infection/Post Infection**
- Viral
  - Especially flaviviral encephalitides (West Nile virus, Japanese encephalitis, etc.)
- Post virus, post vaccination
  - Acute disseminated encephalomyelitis (ADEM): Patchy > confluent; white matter (WM), thalami, cord often involved
  - Acute striatal necrosis

**Toxic Poisoning and Drug Abuse**
- Carbon monoxide
  - GP (WM may show delayed involvement)
- Heroin
  - BG, WM ("chasing the dragon")
- Methanol
  - Putamen, WM
- Cyanide
  - Putamen (often hemorrhagic)
- Nitroimidazole
  - Dentate nuclei, inferior colliculi, splenium, BG

**Metabolic Disorders**
- Osmotic ("extrapontine") demyelination
  - BG, ± pons, WM
- Wernicke encephalopathy
  - Medial thalami, midbrain (periaqueductal), mammillary bodies

**Vascular Disease**
- Internal cerebral vein/vein of Galen/straight sinus thrombosis
  - BG, deep WM
- Artery of Percheron infarct
  - Bilateral thalami, midbrain (V sign)

**Neoplasm**
- Primary CNS lymphoma
  - Periventricular (WM, BG)
- Astrocytoma
  - Bithalamic "glioma"

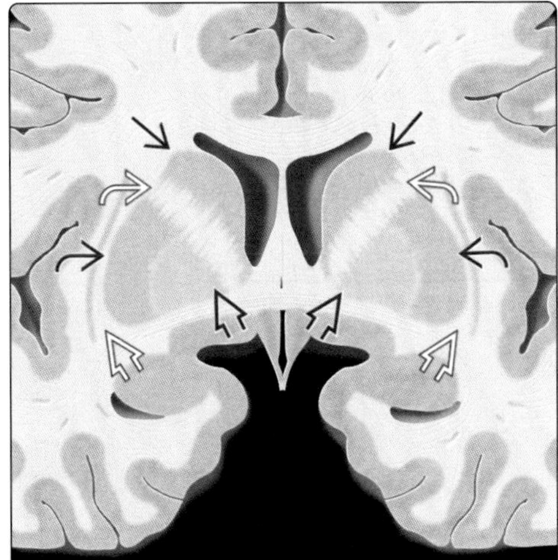

***(34-4)** Coronal graphic through frontal horns shows CNucs ➔, putamen ➔, GPs ➔, external capsule ➔, and internal capsule ➔.*

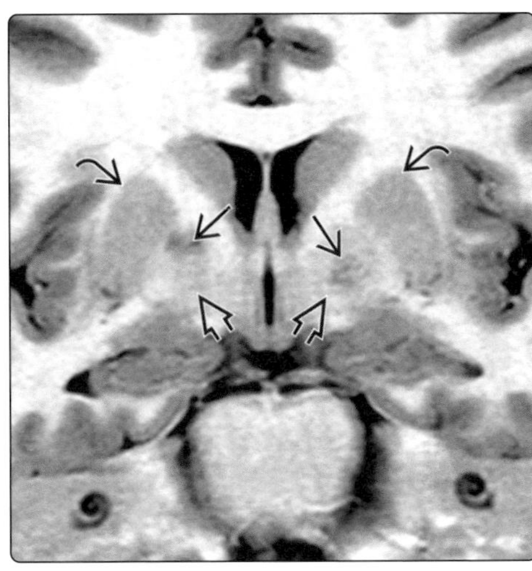

***(34-5)** GPs ➔ are slightly hyperintense to putamina ➔. Punctate hypointensities ➔ are caused by physiologic calcifications.*

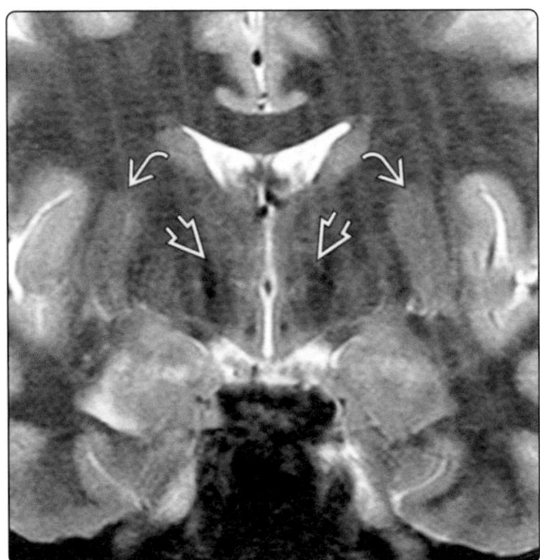

***(34-6)** Coronal T2WI shows medial GPs ➔ are the most hypointense of the basal ganglia. Putamina ➔ are isointense with cortex.*

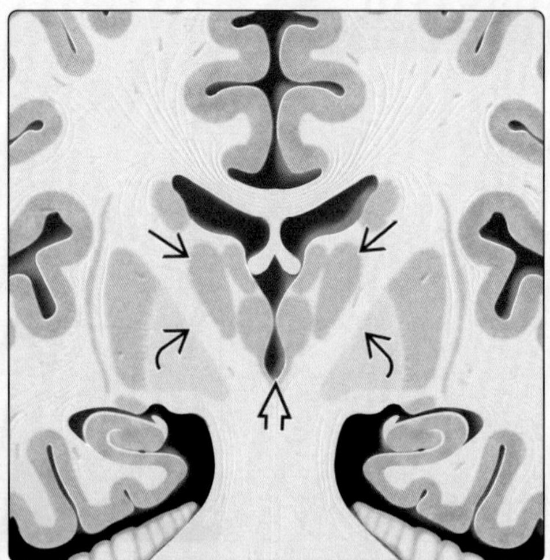

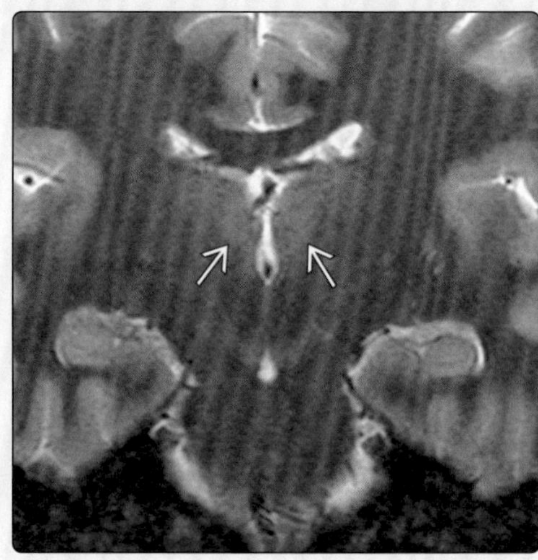

*(34-7) Coronal graphic depicts the major thalamic subnuclei ⇒ and their relationship to the 3rd ventricle ⇒ and internal capsules ↗. (34-8) Coronal T2WI through the posterior 3rd ventricle shows that thalami ➡ are mostly isointense with the cortex.*

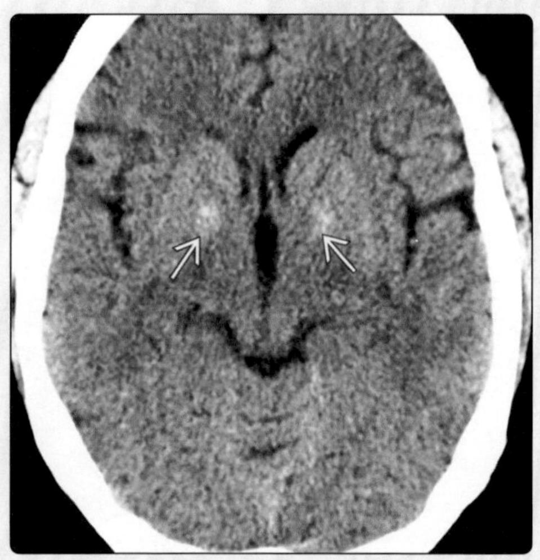

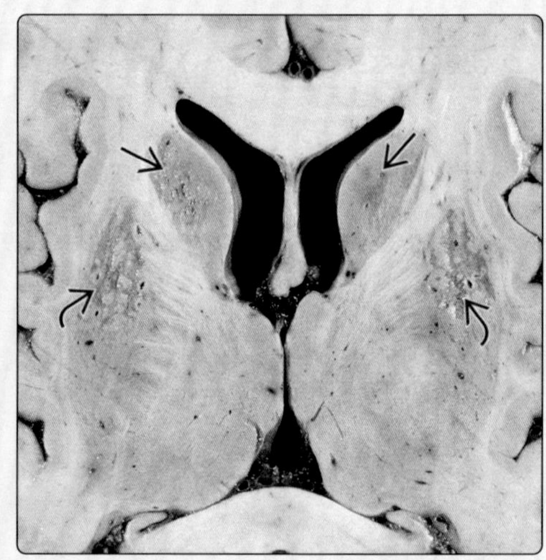

*(34-9) NECT in a 34-year-old woman with headaches shows normal bilateral symmetric physiologic calcifications in the medial GP ➡. (34-10) Autopsy of hypoxia with acute striatal necrosis shows bilateral symmetric CNucs ⇒ and putaminal ↗ lesions. The GP and thalami are spared. (Courtesy R. Hewlett, MD.)*

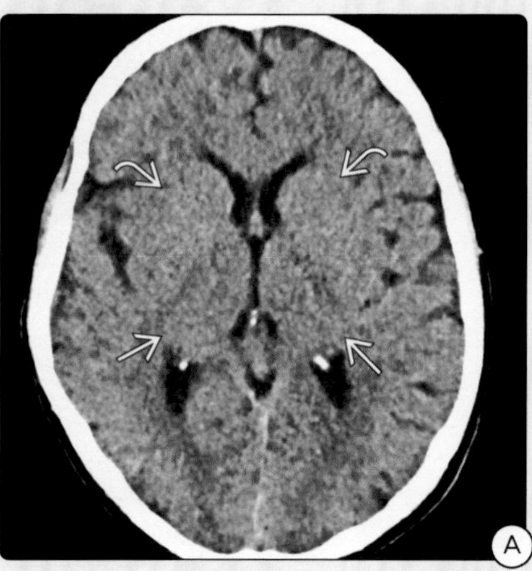

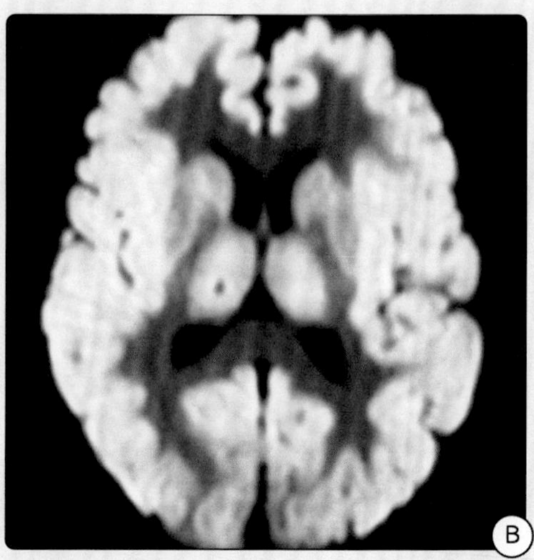

*(34-11A) NECT in a 23-year-old man with confusion, obtundation after a choking episode shows "disappearing" basal ganglia ➡, thalami ➡ with loss of normal gray matter hyperdensity (compare to Fig. 34-9). (34-11B) DWI MR 2 days later shows symmetric restricted diffusion in the basal ganglia, thalami, and cortex of both hemispheres. Only the white matter (WM) is spared.*

RARE BUT IMPORTANT BILATERAL BASAL GANGLIA LESIONS

**Metabolic Disorders**
- Acute diabetic uremia
  - GP, putamen, caudate
- Acute hyperammonemia
  - Acute liver failure
  - Ornithine transcarbamylase deficiency, etc.
- Acute hyperglycemia
  - GP, caudate
- Severe hypoglycemia
  - Occipital cortex, hippocampi, ± WM

**Infection and Inflammation**
- Toxoplasmosis
  - Often HIV-positive, other ring-enhancing lesions
- Behçet disease
  - Midbrain often involved
  - Orogenital aphthous ulcers
- Chronic longstanding multiple sclerosis (MS)
  - BG become very hypointense
  - Putamina, thalami > GP, caudate nucleus (CNuc)
  - Extensive WM disease, volume loss
- Creutzfeldt-Jakob disease (CJD)
  - Anterior BG (caudate, putamen)
  - Posteromedial thalami (T2-/FLAIR-hyperintense hockey stick sign)
  - Variable cortical (occipital = Heidenhain variant)

**Inherited Disorders**
- Neurofibromatosis type 1 (NF1)
  - GP T1 hyperintensity, T2-hyperintense foci
- Mitochondrial encephalopathies
  - Mitochondrial encephalopathy with lactic acidosis and stroke-like episodes (MELAS), myoclonic epilepsy with ragged red fibers (MERRF)
  - Leigh disease (putamen, periaqueductal region, cerebral peduncles)
- Wilson disease
  - Putamina, CNuc, ventrolateral thalami
- Pantothenate kinase-associated neurodegeneration (PKAN)
  - GP ("eye of the tiger")
- Huntington disease
  - Atrophic CNuc, putamina
- Fahr disease
  - Dense symmetric BG, thalami, dentate nuclei, subcortical WM calcification
- Iron storage disorders
  - Symmetric BG "blooming" hypointensity

## Putamen Lesions

Toxic, metabolic, and hypoxic-ischemic events and degenerative disorders account for the vast majority of symmetric putamen lesions. In general, the putamina are less commonly affected than either the GPs or thalami. The most common lesion to affect the putamen is hypertensive hemorrhage. Acute hypertensive bleeds are usually unilateral, although T2* scans often disclose evidence of prior hemorrhages.

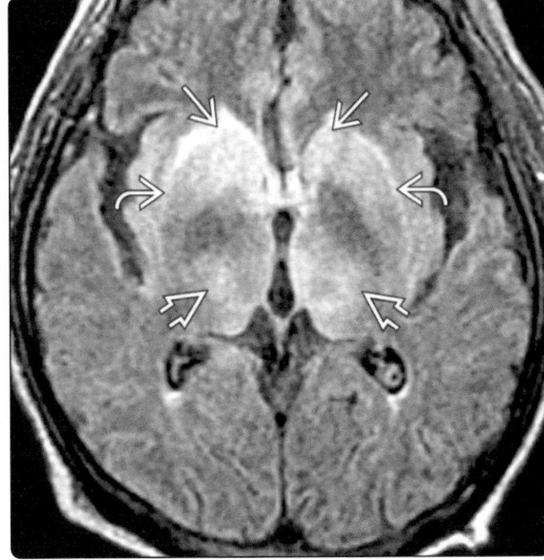

*(34-12) FLAIR MR shows bilateral CNuc ➡, putamina ➡, thalamic hyperintensity ➡; West Nile encephalitis. (Courtesy M. Colombo, MD.)*

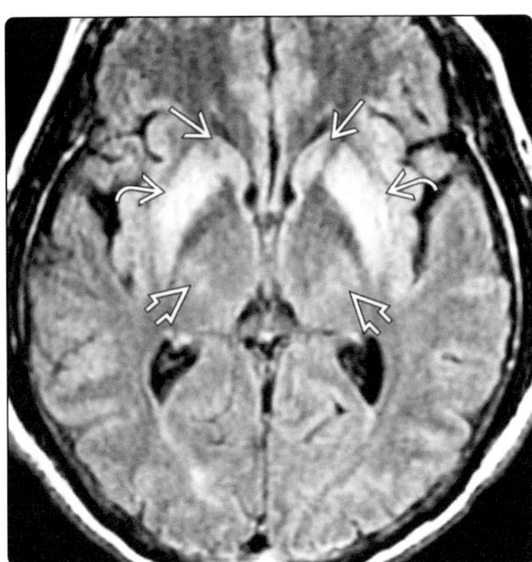

*(34-13) Axial FLAIR shows CNuc ➡, putamina ➡, thalamic ➡ symmetric hyperintensity. This is extrapontine osmotic myelinolysis.*

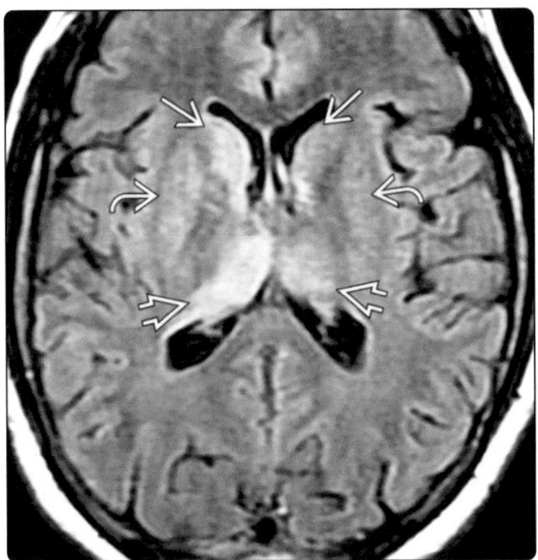

*(34-14) Axial FLAIR MR shows bilateral but asymmetric CNuc ➡, putamen ➡, thalamic ➡ hyperintensity. This is deep vein occlusion.*

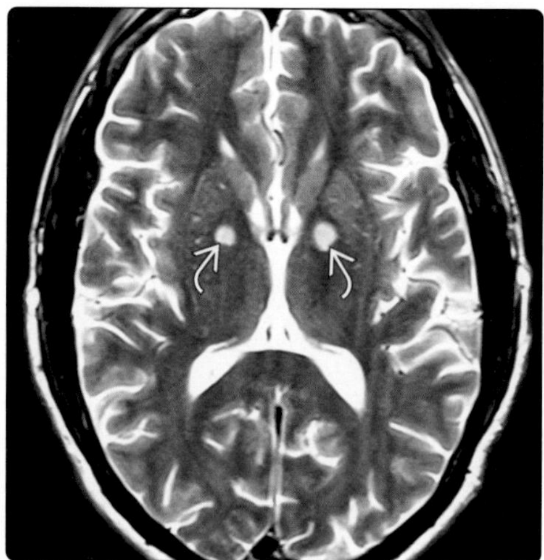

*(34-15) T2 MR in a 42-year-old man with drug overdose and cardiopulmonary arrest shows bilateral GP hyperintensities ➡.*

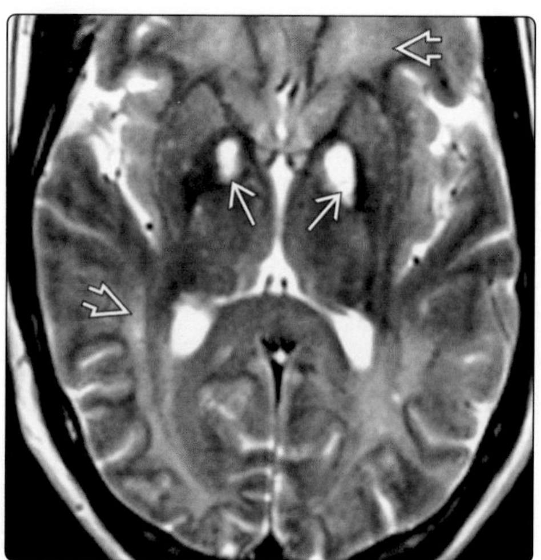

*(34-16) T2 MR shows bilateral medial GP hyperintensities ➡, confluent WM hyperintensity ➡; this is carbon monoxide poisoning.*

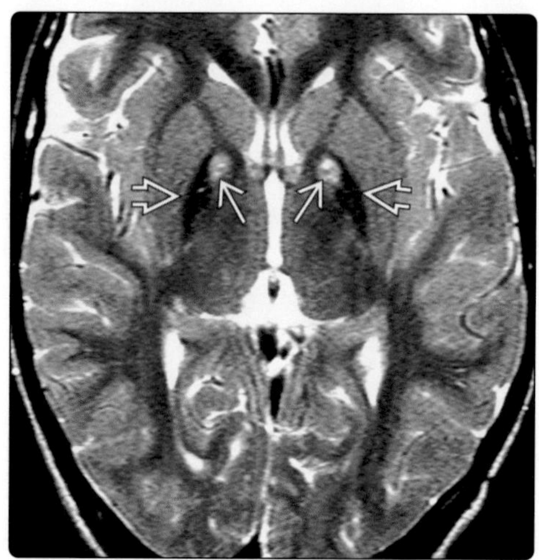

*(34-17) T2 MR shows classic "eye of the tiger" with medial GP hyperintensities ➡ surrounded by well-defined hypointensity ➡. This is PKAN.*

### COMMON PUTAMEN LESIONS

**Metabolic Disorders**

- Hypertensive hemorrhage
  - Lateral putamen/external capsule

**Hypoxic-Ischemic Encephalopathy**

- HIE in term infants
- Hypotensive infarction

Bilateral symmetric putamen lesions usually occur with more generalized BG involvement. However, there are some lesions that predominantly or almost exclusively involve the putamina **(34-22)**.

### LESS COMMON PUTAMEN LESIONS

**Toxic Disorders**

- Methanol toxicity*
  - Often hemorrhagic
  - ± subcortical WM
- Osmotic demyelination
  - Extrapontine myelinolysis

**Inherited Disorders**

- Leigh disease
- Neuroferritinopathy
  - Putamina, GP, dentate

**Predominantly or almost exclusively involves putamina*

### RARE BUT IMPORTANT PUTAMEN LESIONS

**Degenerative Diseases**

- Huntington disease
  - CNuc, putamina
- Parkinson disease
  - Putamen hypointensity
- Multiple system atrophy
  - Parkinsonian type* (hyperintense putaminal rim)

**Miscellaneous**

- CJD*
  - Anterior putamina, CNuc
  - Posteromedial thalami
  - Variable cortex (± predominant or exclusive involvement)

**Predominantly or almost exclusively involves putamina*

## Globus Pallidus Lesions

The globus pallidus (GP) is the part of the BG that is most sensitive to hypoxia. The GPs are rich in mitochondria, vascular supply, and neurotransmitters. Their high metabolic activity makes them especially vulnerable to numerous metabolic abnormalities and systemic/generalized disease processes.

The vast majority of symmetric GP lesions are secondary to hypoxic, toxic, or metabolic processes that diminish blood flow, oxygen supply, &/or energy availability. Most cause bilateral symmetric abnormalities on imaging studies **(34-15) (34-16) (34-17)**.

## COMMON GLOBUS PALLIDUS LESIONS

**Normal Variant**
- Physiologic calcification
  - Medial GP

**Hypoxic-Ischemic Encephalopathy**
- Anoxia, hypoxia (near drowning, cerebral hypoperfusion)
- Neonatal HIE (profound acute)

**Toxic/Metabolic Disorders**
- Chronic liver disease
  - T1 hyperintensity, T2* hypointensity
- Carbon monoxide
  - T2-hyperintense medial GP

## LESS COMMON GLOBUS PALLIDUS LESIONS

**Toxic/Metabolic Disorders**
- Opioid use disorder
  - Often combined with HIE
- Hyperalimentation
  - Manganese deposition, short T1
- Chronic hypothyroidism
  - Punctate calcification
  - T1 hyperintensity, T2 hypointensity

**Inherited Disorders**
- NF1
- Leigh disease

## RARE BUT IMPORTANT GLOBUS PALLIDUS LESIONS

**Toxic/Metabolic Disorders**
- Kernicterus
  - T1 shortening
- Cyanide poisoning
  - Hemorrhagic GP, laminar cortical necrosis

**Inherited Disorders**
- Fahr disease
  - Dense symmetric confluent calcification
- Wilson disease
  - T2 hyperintensity in GP, putamen
  - Face of giant panda sign in midbrain
- PKAN
  - "Eye of the tiger" (central T2 hyperintensity, peripheral hypointensity)
  - Not always present!
- Neurodegeneration with brain iron accumulation (NBIA)
  - GP, substantia nigra hypointensity ± putamen
- Maple syrup urine disease (MSUD)
  - Edema (GP, brainstem, thalami, cerebellar WM)
- Methylmalonic acidemia (MMA)
  - Symmetric GP T2 hyperintensity ± WM

**Degenerative Diseases**
- Hepatocerebral degeneration
  - 1% of patients with cirrhosis, portosystemic shunts
  - T1 shortening
- Progressive supranuclear palsy
  - Also affects subthalamic nucleus, substantia nigra

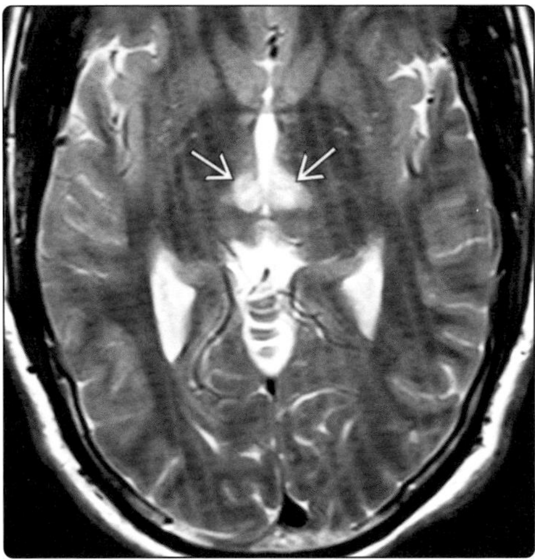

***(34-18)** Axial T2 MR shows bilateral medial thalamic infarcts ➡ caused by artery of Percheron occlusion.*

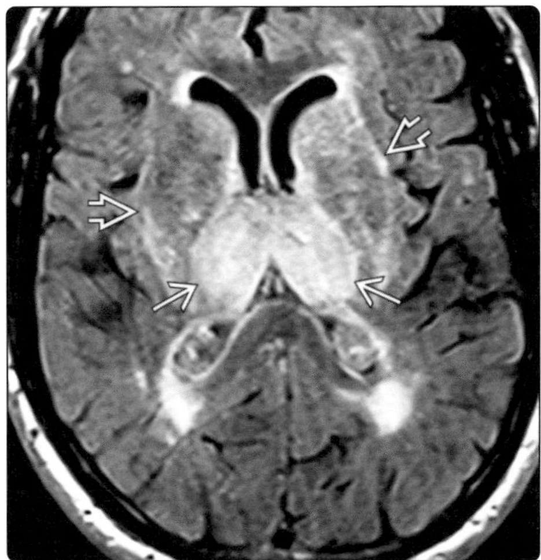

***(34-19)** Axial FLAIR shows bithalamic lesions ➡ with less extensive involvement of putamina ➡ and GP. This is internal cerebral vein occlusion.*

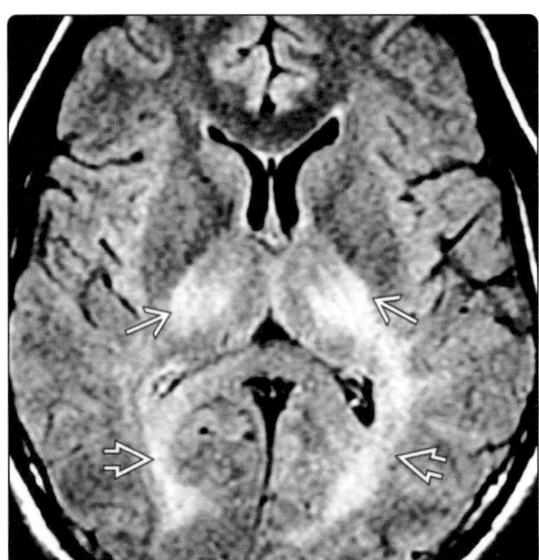

***(34-20)** FLAIR MR in a patient with Epstein-Barr virus encephalitis shows bithalamic ➡ and occipital WM involvement ➡.*

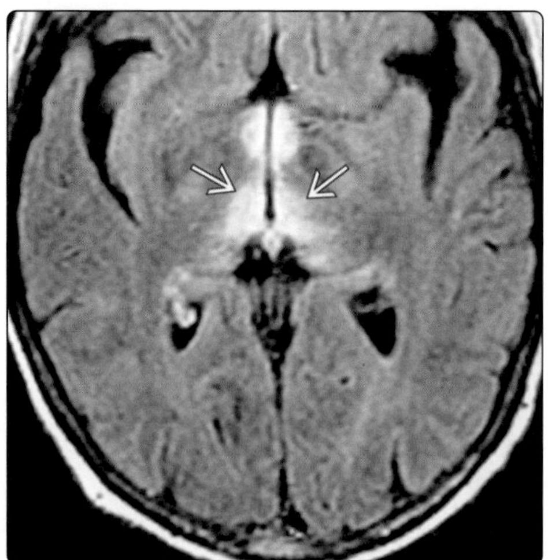

(34-21) FLAIR MR in a patient with Wernicke encephalopathy shows symmetric lesions in both medial thalami ➡.

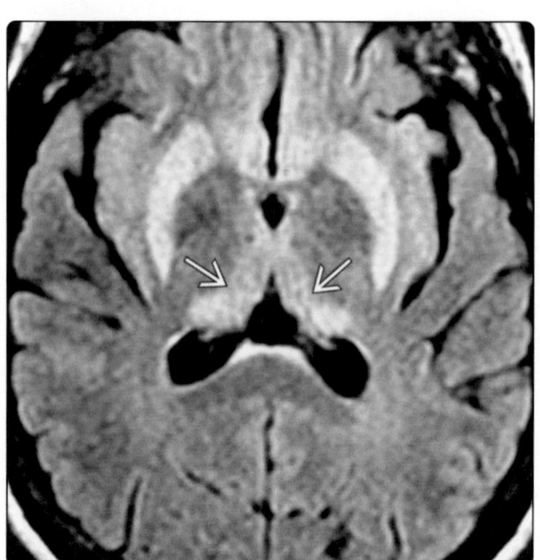

(34-22) FLAIR MR in a patient with CJD shows classic hockey stick sign ➡ as well as anterior caudate and putamen hyperintensity.

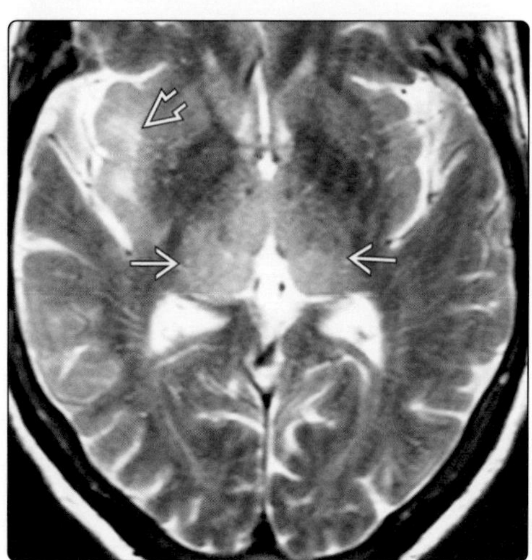

(34-23) T2 MR shows bithalamic ➡ and right insular ➡ hyperintensity in a patient with gliomatosis cerebri, WHO grade 2 astrocytoma.

## Globus Pallidus Lesions by Appearance

Some GP lesions can be distinguished by their typical attenuation on CT or signal intensity on MR.

**GLOBUS PALLIDUS LESIONS BY CHARACTERISTIC APPEARANCE**

**NECT Hypodensity**
- HIE
- Carbon monoxide poisoning

**NECT Hyperdensity**
- Physiologic calcification
- Hypothyroidism
- Fahr disease

**T1 Hyperintensity**
- Chronic hepatic encephalopathy
- Hyperalimentation (manganese deposition)
- NF1
- Hypothyroidism
- Kernicterus (acute)
- Wilson disease

**T2 Hyperintensity**
- HIE
- Drug abuse
- Carbon monoxide poisoning
- NF1
- Leigh disease
- Kernicterus (chronic)
- Wilson disease
- PKAN, MSUD, MMA

# Thalamic Lesions

Because lacunar infarcts and hypertensive bleeds are so common, *unilateral* thalamic lesions are much more common than bilateral symmetric abnormalities.

**UNILATERAL THALAMIC LESIONS**

**Common**
- Lacunar infarction
- Hypertensive intracranial hemorrhage

**Less Common**
- NF1
- Diffuse astrocytoma (low-grade fibrillary)
- Glioblastoma multiforme
- Anaplastic astrocytoma
- ADEM

**Rare but Important**
- MS
- Unilateral internal cerebral vein thrombosis
- Germinoma

In contrast, *bilateral* symmetric thalamic lesions are relatively uncommon and have a somewhat limited differential diagnosis. As with the symmetric BG lesions, bilateral thalamic lesions tend to be toxic, metabolic, vascular, infectious, or hypoxic-ischemic **(34-18) (34-19) (34-20) (34-21) (34-22)** rather than neoplastic **(34-23)**.

### COMMON BITHALAMIC LESIONS

**Vascular Lesions**
- Deep venous occlusion
  - Thalami > GP, putamina
  - CNuc ± deep WM
- Arterial ischemia
  - Artery of Percheron infarct
  - "Top of the basilar" thrombosis
- Vasculitis

**Hypoxic-Ischemic Encephalopathy**
- Profound hypoperfusion
  - BG, hippocampi, cortex
- Usually occurs in full-term neonates

### LESS COMMON BITHALAMIC LESIONS

**Infection/Postinfection/Inflammatory Disorders**
- ADEM
  - Usually with WM lesions
- Viral encephalitis
  - *Many* agents affect thalami
  - Epstein-Barr virus, West Nile virus, Japanese encephalitis, etc.
- CJD
  - Hockey stick sign
  - Pulvinar, medial thalami

**Toxic/Metabolic Disorders**
- Osmotic myelinolysis
  - Extrapontine involvement variable
  - Thalami
  - External capsules, putamina, CNuc
- Wernicke encephalopathy
  - Medial thalami (around 3rd ventricle)
  - Pulvinar
  - Midbrain (periaqueductal)
  - Mammillary bodies
  - Cortex variable
- Solvent inhalation
  - Toluene
  - Glue
  - Ethylene glycol
- Acute hypertensive encephalopathy [posterior reversible encephalopathy syndrome (PRES)]
  - Occipital lobes, watershed zones
  - "Atypical" PRES may involve BG, thalami
- Status epilepticus
  - Pulvinar
  - Corpus callosum splenium (usually transient excitotoxic)
  - Often hippocampi ± cortex

**Neoplasms**
- Bithalamic low-grade astrocytoma
- Germinoma
- Lymphoma

### RARE BUT IMPORTANT BITHALAMIC LESIONS

**Infection/Postinfection/Inflammatory Disorders**
- MS (severe, chronic)
  - Hypointense BG on T2*
- Acute necrotizing encephalopathy of childhood
- Flavivirus encephalitis
- Neuro-Behçet

**Inherited Disorders**
- Mitochondrial disorders
- Lysosomal disorders (GM1/2, Krabbe)
- Krabbe disease
  - Hyperdense on CT, hypointense on T2
- Wilson disease
  - Putamina, CNuc > thalami
- Primary familial brain calcification (Fahr disease)
  - GP > thalami
- Fabry disease
  - T1-hyperintense posterior thalamus ("pulvinar")
  - M > > F
  - Strokes (territorial, lacunar)
  - Renal, cardiac disease

**Neoplasm**
- Glioblastoma
- Diffuse midline glioma, H3 K27-altered
- Rosette-forming glioneuronal tumor
  - Look for multiple "satellite" lesions

**Paraneoplastic Syndromes**
- Paraneoplastic can mimic prion disease (variant of CJD)
- Limbic involvement not always present

# Degenerative and CSF Disorders

With worldwide populations aging, identifying risk and maintaining cognitive health for successful aging is increasingly important. Imaging studies are frequently obtained in older patients with altered mental status and cognitive decline. Degenerative disorders of the brain must be distinguished from normal age-related changes in brain structure, function, connectivity, and volume that occur throughout the lifespan.

## Age-Related Changes

In the past few decades, our understanding of the molecular and cellular mechanisms underlying the changes associated with normal adaptive brain aging and age-related pathologic disorders has expanded significantly.

Normal age-related changes in the brain occur throughout the lifespan. Understanding the different stages of brain formation and the normal progression of myelination in the developing infant is essential to diagnosing inherited metabolic disorders.

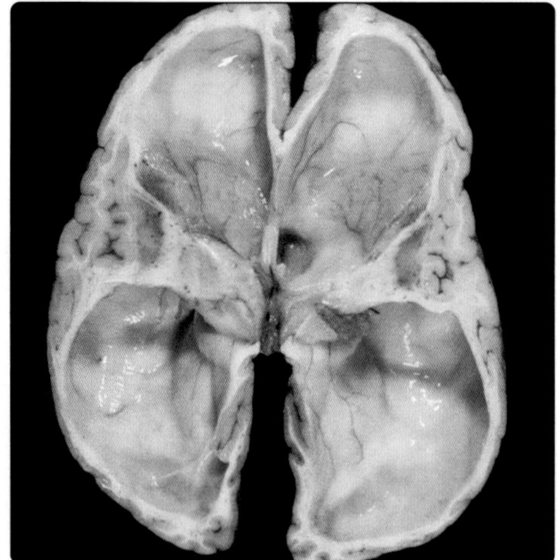

*(34-24) Autopsy of severe compensated obstructive hydrocephalus shows symmetrically enlarged lateral ventricles.*

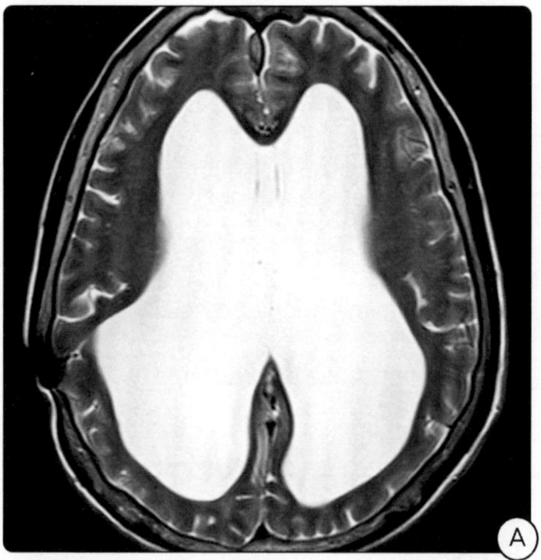

*(34-25A) T2 MR in longstanding compensated shunted hydrocephalus shows symmetric enlargement of both lateral ventricles.*

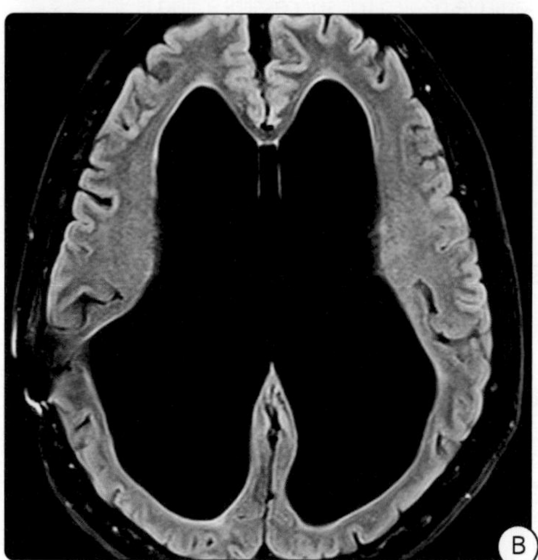

*(34-25B) FLAIR MR in the same patient shows no evidence for periventricular fluid accumulation in the case of longstanding shunted hydrocephalus.*

At the opposite end of the age spectrum, volume is normally lost in some parts of the brain while other areas remain relatively intact. Abnormal mineral deposition in the BG can be a clue to degenerative and metabolic disorders. Understanding what is normal heavy metal deposition in different decades is a prerequisite to diagnosing these abnormalities on imaging studies.

## Dementia and Brain Degeneration

Once an understanding of the normal aging brain is established, we discuss the pathology and imaging manifestations of dementia. Although identifying a lobar-predominant pattern of volume loss on CT and standard MR can be accomplished in some cases, these are usually late-stage manifestations. The use of commercially available automated volumetric analyses has become standard in many neurology practices. Identifying early preclinical manifestations of dementing disorders is increasingly important as pharmacologic intervention becomes more common.

## Hydrocephalus and CSF Disorders

In this section, we first review normal anatomy of the ventricles and CSF spaces as well as imaging variants that can be mistaken for disease. A brief discussion of the production, circulation and absorption of CSF and the role of aquaporin-4 (AQP4) in regulating water homeostasis in the brain's "glymphatic" system follows. The concept that "hydrocephalus" (literally "water brain") is an imaging observation—not a diagnosis—is presented together with imaging-based strategies to determine its etiology **(34-24)** **(34-25)** (see next shaded box).

### ABNORMALLY LARGE VENTRICLES: ETIOLOGIES

**Common**
- Aging brain (secondary to parenchymal volume loss)
- Generalized encephalomalacia
  - Posttraumatic, infectious, etc.
- Extraventricular obstructive hydrocephalus
  - Meningitis, subarachnoid hemorrhage, etc.
- Dementias
  - Alzheimer, frontotemporal dementia, etc.

**Less Common**
- Intraventricular obstructive hydrocephalus
  - Colloid cyst, intraventricular neoplasm
  - Aqueductal stenosis
- Normal pressure hydrocephalus
- Shunt failure
- Disturbed CSF:ISF homeostasis
- Aquaporin-4 (AQP4) abnormalities

**Rare but Important**
- Overproduction of CSF (choroid plexus papilloma)
- Megalencephaly syndromes

*Selected References: The complete reference list is available on the eBooks+ version included with purchase.*

# Toxic Encephalopathy

*The list of toxins and poisons that affect the CNS is long and continues to grow. Some agents are deliberately injected, inhaled, or ingested, whereas others are accidentally encountered or administered in a controlled medical setting. Some toxins accumulate slowly, so their clinical manifestations are subtle and onset insidious. Others cause profound, virtually immediate CNS toxicity with rapid onset of coma and death. Still, others—such as ethanol—have both acute and chronic effects.*



Use of "street" drugs, opioids, synthetic "designer" drugs and the emergence of fentanyl are fueling a worldwide epidemic. Overdoses (ODs) are increasingly common. An accurate history is often difficult to obtain in patients with suspected OD, and clinical symptoms are frequently nonspecific. Presentation may also be confounded by "polydrug" abuse and secondary effects, such as hypoxia, that mask the underlying pathology.

The vast majority of toxins with CNS manifestations cause bilateral, relatively symmetric lesions. Symmetric abnormalities in the deep gray nuclei (basal ganglia, thalamus) with varying white matter (WM) involvement are suggestive of toxic-metabolic etiologies.

In this chapter, we first focus on the most common types of toxic encephalopathies, beginning with the acute and long-term effects of alcohol and similar substances on the brain together with a discussion of Wernicke encephalopathy (WE). We follow with a consideration of drug abuse. Inhaled gases and toxins (such as carbon monoxide and cyanide) and heavy metal poisoning are then considered. We conclude with a brief discussion of treatment-related disorders.

## Alcohol and Related Disorders

Alcohol [ethanol (EtOH)] is one of the most commonly abused substances in the world, estimated to affect 4% of the global population. The most recent Diagnostic and Statistical Manual of Mental Disorders (DSM5) estimates that in the USA, 36% of the male and 23% of the female population met the DSM criteria for alcohol use disorder (AUD) at least once during their lifetime.

AUD can affect more than 60 bodily systems, causing different effects on different organs. Although the gastrointestinal system is exposed to higher concentrations of alcohol than any other tissue, ethanol easily crosses the blood-brain barrier and is a potent neurotoxin. Both its short- and long-term effects on the CNS are profound.

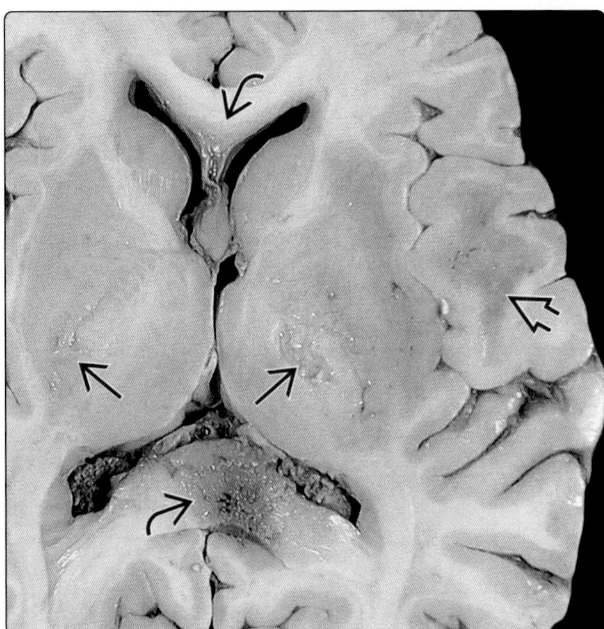

*(35-1) Alcohol [ethanol (EtOH)] poisoning shows brain swelling with white matter (WM) necrosis ➡, especially marked in the corpus callosum ➡. Basal ganglia (BG)/thalami are swollen, pale, infarcted ➡. (Courtesy R. Hewlett, MD.)*

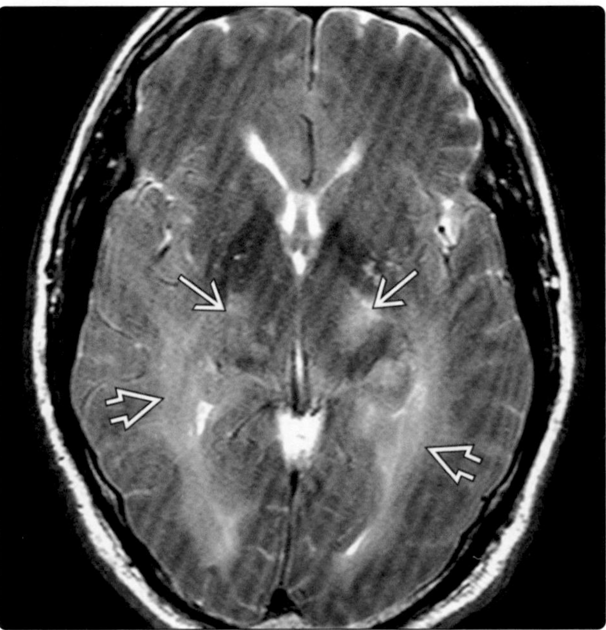

*(35-2) T2 MR in a comatose patient who drank 1 gallon of vodka or whisky daily for a full week shows diffuse brain swelling, hyperintense WM ➡, bithalamic lesions ➡. This is acute alcohol poisoning.*

We begin our discussion of alcohol and the brain by briefly considering the acute effects of alcohol poisoning. We then consider chronic alcoholic encephalopathy before turning to other complications of alcohol abuse, including alcohol-induced demyelination syndromes and Wernicke encephalopathy (WE).

We close this section with two less common forms of related abuse, i.e., methanol intoxication and ethylene glycol (antifreeze) ingestion.

## Acute Alcohol Poisoning

### Etiology

Acute EtOH exposure has deleterious effects on neuronal activity across the striatum, hippocampus, cerebellum, amygdala, substantia nigra, and ventral tegmental area. EtOH also drives changes in both GABAergic and glutamatergic signaling, leading to changes in long-term potentiation and depression across the entire CNS. Significant changes in neuronal networks and depression of glymphatic function, impaired normal immune cell function, increased inflammation, and aberrant microglia activation are also associated with acute EtOH exposure.

EtOH effects can be modulated by many factors, including age when drinking. The acute effects of binge drinking—and its complication, acute alcohol poisoning—are striking. EtOH inhibits Na+/K+ activity. Cellular swelling, life-threatening cytotoxic cerebral edema, and nonconvulsive status epilepticus may ensue **(35-1)**. A blood alcohol concentration of 0.40% typically results in unconsciousness, and a level exceeding 0.50% is usually lethal.

Acute alcohol poisoning is a complication of binge drinking and is most common in adolescents and young adults. The adolescent brain is also still undergoing structural maturation and has a unique sensitivity to alcohol. Binge drinking-induced neurotoxicity damages the cortical and subcortical brain microstructure, especially in areas of the prefrontal and parietal regions that mediate reward-related motivation.

Co-use of ethanol with CNS depressant recreational drugs increases the adverse effects of both. Lower Glasgow Coma Scale (GCS) score, agitation/aggression, hypotension, and increased admission to intensive care units are significantly correlated with co-use of ethanol and recreational drug use.

### Imaging

Imaging findings in patients with acute alcohol poisoning include diffuse brain swelling and confluent hyperintensity in supratentorial subcortical and deep WM on T2/FLAIR **(35-2)**. Seizure-induced changes in cortex with gyral hyperintensity and diffusion restriction may also be associated.

## Chronic Alcoholic Encephalopathy

The long-term adverse effects of ethanol on the brain are much more common than those of acute alcohol poisoning. These effects are even more pronounced in immature brains. Even moderate repeated alcohol consumption can adversely affect the developing functional architecture of adolescent brains.

AUD in adults causes increased apoptosis, dysregulated synaptic connectivity, and widespread volume loss throughout the brain, especially in the middle frontal, cingulate, superior temporal and cerebellar cortices.

Chronic alcohol-related brain damage can be divided into primary and secondary effects. We begin our discussion with the effects of EtOH itself on the brain and then consider secondary remote effects, which are mostly related to the sequelae of liver disease, malnutrition, malabsorption, and electrolyte disturbances.

## Etiology

As ethanol readily crosses the blood-brain barrier, both direct and indirect neurotoxicity may ensue. Upregulation and expression of inflammatory factors contribute to CNS hyperexcitability and aberrant excitotoxicity. Longer-term neurotoxic effects include neuronal loss and reduction of WM volume.

## Pathology

Chronic excessive EtOH consumption causes brain atrophy, evidenced by enlarged ventricles and sulci **(35-6)**. Alcohol-induced cerebellar degeneration is also common. The folia of the rostral vermis and anterosuperior aspects of the cerebellar hemispheres are atrophic, seen as widened interfolial sulci.

## Imaging

**CT Findings.** NECT scans show generalized ventricular and sulcal enlargement **(35-3A)**. The great horizontal fissure of the cerebellum and the superior vermian folia are unusually prominent relative to the patient's age **(35-3)** **(35-4)**.

**MR Findings.** Overall brain volume loss, especially in the prefrontal cortex, is common as is more focal atrophy of the superior vermis **(35-5)**. Volumetric studies show selective frontal, parietal, and temporal gyri are affected along with the insula, cingulate cortex, hippocampus, thalamus, and pallidum. Focal and confluent cerebral WM hyperintensities on T2/FLAIR sequences are frequently present.

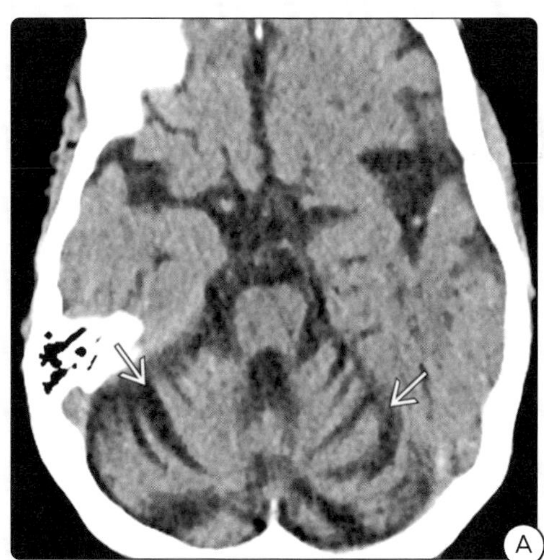


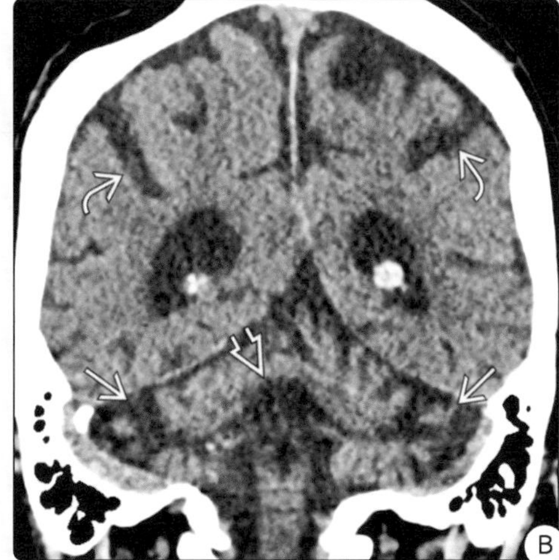


***(35-3A)** NECT in a 56-year-old woman with chronic alcoholism and multiple falls shows severe cerebellar atrophy with grossly enlarged sulci ➡. **(35-3B)** Coronal NECT in the same case shows the striking cerebellar volume loss ➡. Note enlarged 4th ventricle ➡. The cerebral hemispheres also appear moderately atrophic with prominent superficial sulci ➡.*

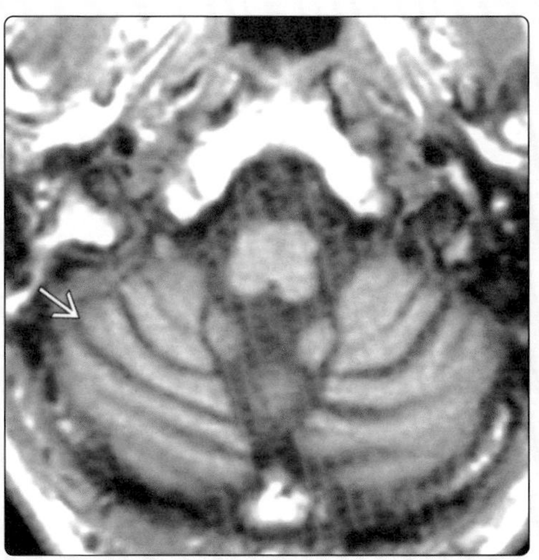

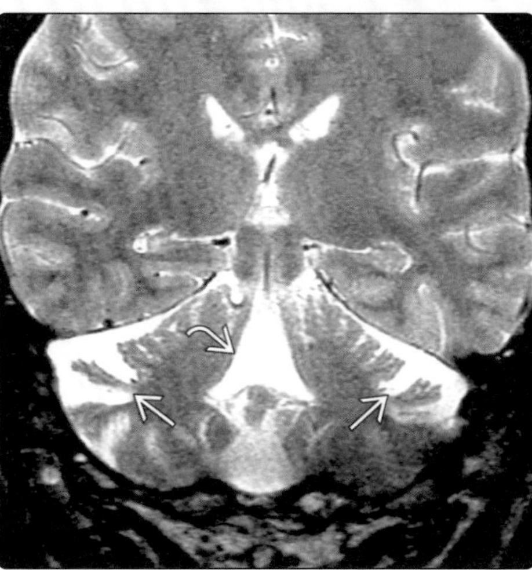

***(35-4)** Axial T1 MR in chronic alcohol use disorder (AUD) shows atrophic cerebellar hemispheres with shrunken folia, enlarged horizontal fissures ➡. **(35-5)** Coronal T2 MR in a 41-year-old man with chronic AUD shows marked atrophy of the superior cerebellum with enlarged 4th ventricle ➡ and striking widening of the horizontal fissures ➡. Note relative sparing of the supratentorial brain.*

DTI may demonstrate low fractional anisotropy (FA) and increased mean diffusivity, reflecting compromised fiber tract integrity. The frontal and superior tracts are most affected with relative sparing of posterior and inferior tracts.

MRS may show reduced NAA:tCr and Cho:tCr ratios in the frontal and medial temporal lobes, cerebellum, and thalami. Metabolic changes associated with AUD may normalize with discontinuation of alcohol consumption.

Chronic liver failure secondary to cirrhosis may cause basal ganglia hyperintensity on T1WI, probably secondary to manganese accumulation. Increased iron deposition in the basal ganglia and dentate nuclei may also occur.

## ACUTE/CHRONIC ALCOHOLIC ENCEPHALOPATHY

**Acute Alcohol Poisoning**
- Rare
  - Usually caused by binge drinking
- Imaging
  - Diffuse cerebral edema
  - Acute demyelination

**Chronic Alcoholic Encephalopathy**
- Primary toxic effect on neurons
- Secondary effects related to liver, GI disease
  - Hepatic encephalopathy
  - Malnutrition, malabsorption, electrolyte imbalance
- Imaging
  - Atrophy (superior vermis, cerebellum, generalized)
  - WM myelinolysis

*(35-6) Graphic shows pathologic spectrum of chronic AUD with cortical ➾, superior vermian atrophy ➾, corpus callosum necrosis [Marchiafava-Bignami disease (MBD)] ➾. Mammillary body ➾ and periaqueductal gray necrosis ➾ are characteristic of Wernicke encephalopathy (WE). (35-7) Autopsy of MBD shows necrosis in the middle layers of the corpus callosum ➾.*

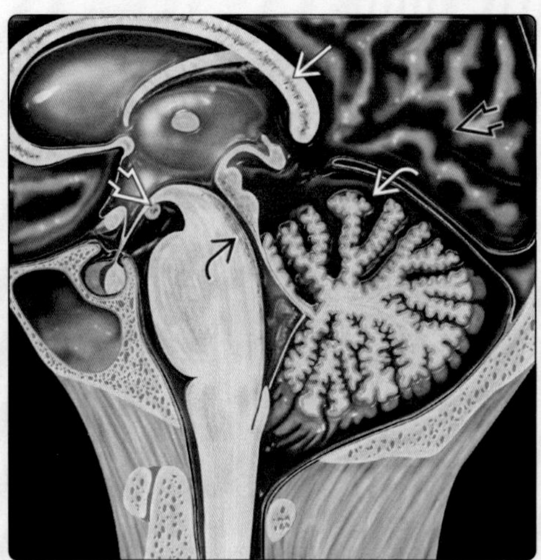

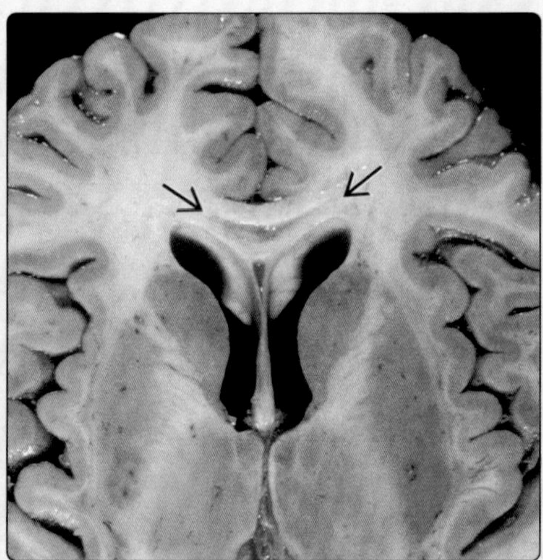

*(35-8A) CECT in a 43-year-old man with chronic alcoholism and MBD shows generalized cerebral atrophy ➾ and striking hypodensity in the corpus callosum genu ➾ and adjacent WM ➾. (35-8B) Sagittal T1 MR in the same case of MBD shows hypointensity in the entire middle corpus callosum ➾. Mammillary bodies ➾ and superior vermis ➾ are also atrophic. (Courtesy A. Datir, MD.)*

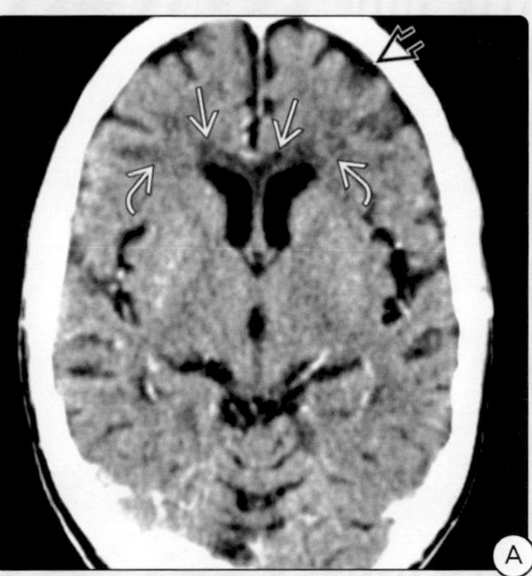


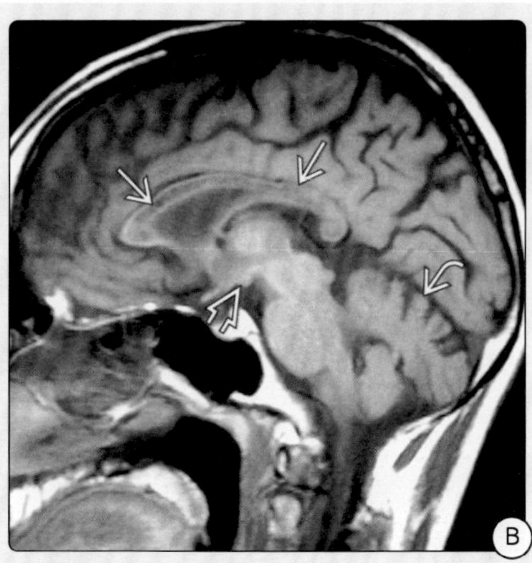

## Marchiafava-Bignami Disease

Marchiafava-Bignami disease (MBD) is a rare disorder characterized by osmotic demyelination (and later necrosis) of the corpus callosum **(35-7)**. MBD is seen most frequently in patients with a history of severe alcohol abuse but can also occur in nonalcoholic patients with malnourishment, poorly controlled diabetes mellitus, or osmotic stresses.

### Terminology

MBD is also (incorrectly) known as "red wine drinkers' encephalopathy."

### Etiology

Alcohol-induced neurotoxicity is the most common associated condition. Vitamin B complex deficiency (i.e., all eight B vitamins, in contrast to the more specific B1 deficiency of WE) has been reported in nonalcoholic patients.

### Pathology

Myelinolysis with selective involvement of the middle layers of the corpus callosum along its entire length is strongly suggestive of MBD **(35-9)**. Cases with extracallosal extension into the hemispheric WM, basal ganglia, internal capsule, and middle cerebellar peduncles have been reported.

### Clinical Issues

MBD is rare. Most reported cases are found in middle-aged men (40-60 years old). A history of malnutrition and alcohol dependence with neuropsychiatric symptoms is common.

The clinical diagnosis of MBD is difficult and often confused with WE, so diagnosis is mainly based on imaging manifestations.

Three clinical subtypes of MBD based on acuteness of onset and disease progression have been described. Acute-onset

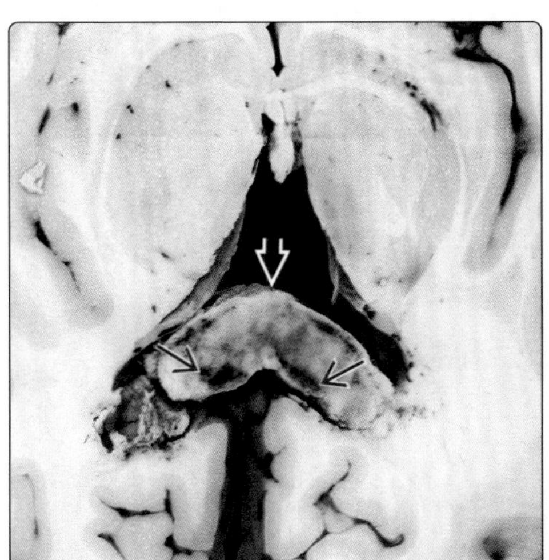

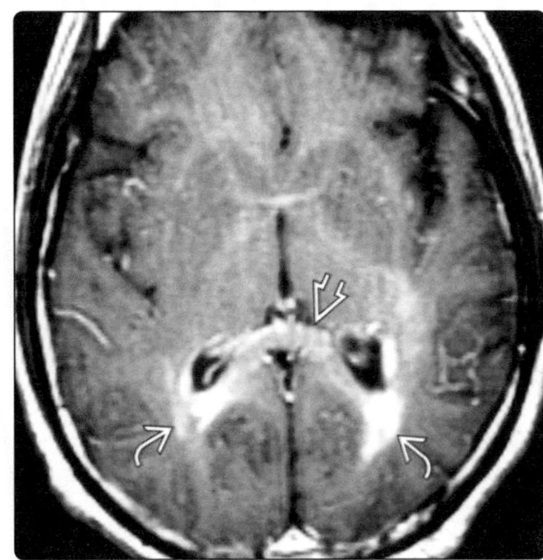

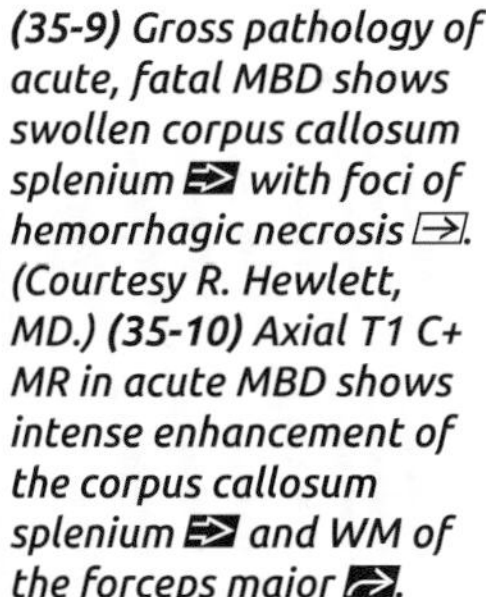

***(35-9)** Gross pathology of acute, fatal MBD shows swollen corpus callosum splenium ➡ with foci of hemorrhagic necrosis ⇨. (Courtesy R. Hewlett, MD.) **(35-10)** Axial T1 C+ MR in acute MBD shows intense enhancement of the corpus callosum splenium ➡ and WM of the forceps major ↪.*

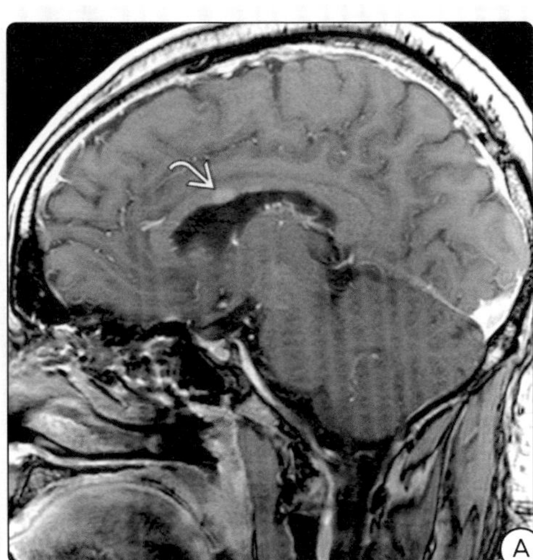

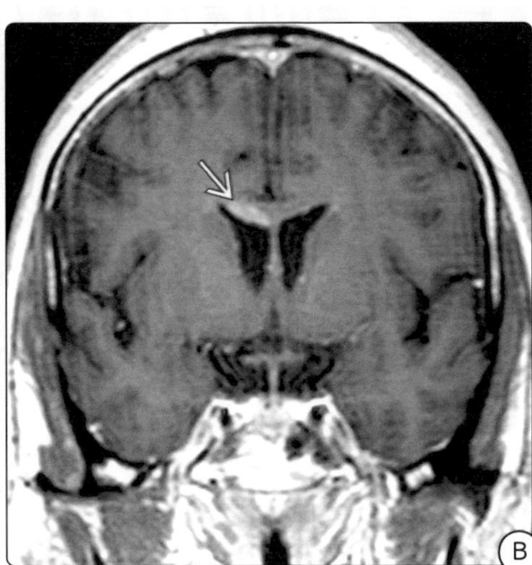

***(35-11A)** Sagittal T1 C+ MR in an encephalopathic middle-aged man who "drinks like a fish" shows enhancement in the corpus callosum splenium ↪. **(35-11B)** Coronal T1 C+ MR in the same case shows enhancement in the corpus callosum ➡.*

MBD presents with sudden loss of consciousness, seizures, and rapid progression to coma. Subacute forms have varying prodromes ranging from depression to ataxia or spasticity. Chronic MBD presents as a progressive dementia with behavior abnormalities, hallucinations, and delusions.

## Imaging

**General Features.** Imaging findings vary with disease stage. The early stages of MBD are characterized by diffuse edema and swelling of the corpus callosum. The subacute and chronic stages are characterized by diffuse volume loss and selective necrosis of the middle layers of the corpus callosum spreading from the genu through the body to the splenium.

**CT Findings.** CT may be normal in acute MBD. Chronic MBD shows linear hypodensity in the corpus callosum that, in the setting of chronic AUD, is highly suggestive of the diagnosis **(35-8A)**.

**MR Findings.** Imaging findings vary with disease stage. The early stages of MBD are characterized by diffuse callosal swelling with T1 hypo- and T2 hyperintensity. **Acute** MBD is best seen on sagittal FLAIR. Hyperintensity in the genu and frontoparietal cortex appear first and are followed by extension into the splenium. Involvement of the adjacent hemispheric WM and basal ganglia occurs but is less common.

Acute lesions of the corpus callosum and adjacent deep WM may exhibit petechial hemorrhages, restrict on DWI, and enhance on T1 C+ **(35-10)**. Both solid and ring-enhancing patterns have been reported **(35-11)**.

**Chronic** MBD with frank callosal necrosis is seen as thinning of the corpus callosum on sagittal T1WI with linear hypointensities in the middle layers **(35-8B)**. T2* GRE or SWI sequences may demonstrate multiple microbleeds in the cortical-subcortical WM and corpus callosum. DTI shows a substantial decrease in fibers crossing through the corpus callosum. Other changes associated with chronic alcohol

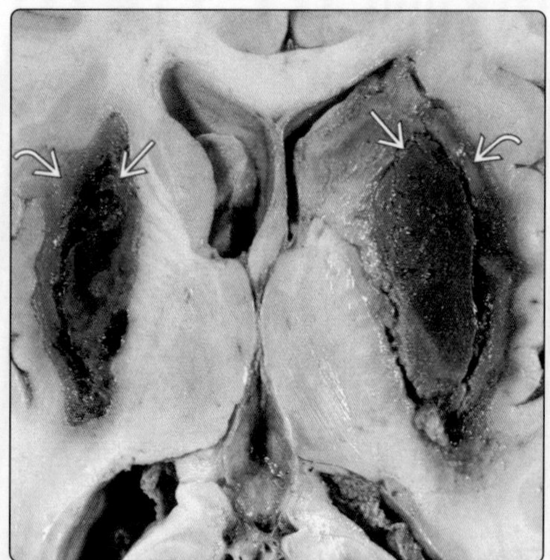

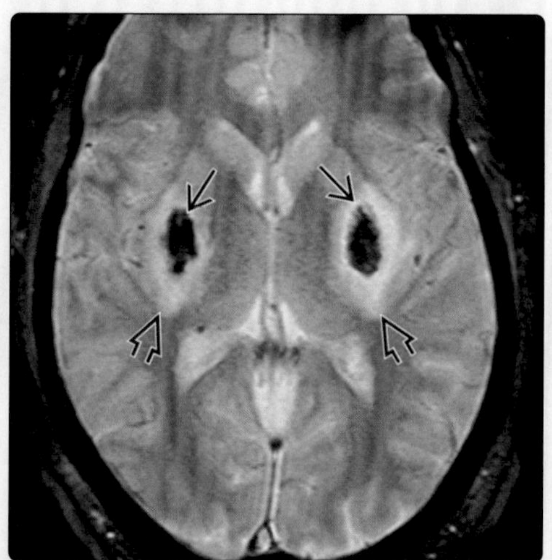

*(35-12) Gross pathology of acute methanol poisoning shows hemorrhagic necrosis in both putamina ➡ and the subinsular WM ⮫. (Courtesy R. Hewlett, MD.) (35-13) T2* GRE MR in a patient with acute methanol poisoning shows bilateral, symmetric putaminal hemorrhages ➡ surrounded by striatal edema ⮫.*

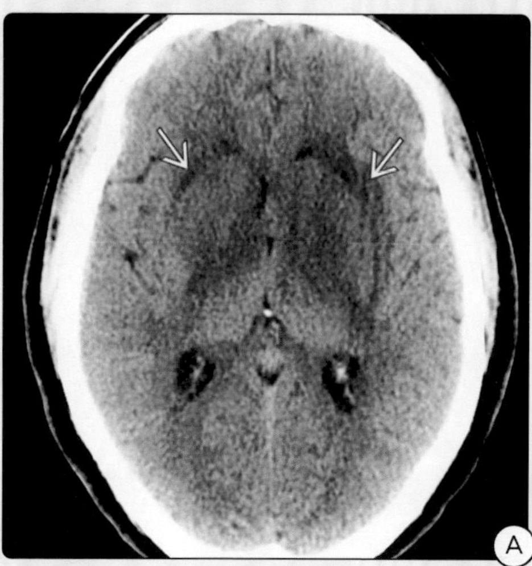

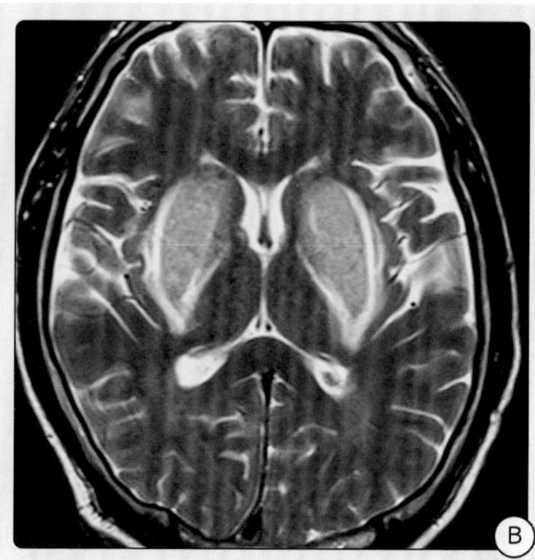

*(35-14A) NECT in a 52-year-old man with acute methanol poisoning shows diffuse, symmetric hypodensity in the BG centered on the putamina ➡. Edema extends into both external and internal capsules but spares the thalami. (35-14B) T2 MR in the same case shows symmetric hyperintense BG from acute methanol poisoning.*

abuse, such as cortical, cerebellar, and mammillary body atrophy, are common.

## Differential Diagnosis

The main differential diagnosis of **acute** MBD is **WE**. WE and acute MBD may coexist. Involvement of the medial thalami and periaqueductal gray matter as well as the mammillary bodies is more common in WE. In the setting of AUD, volume loss with necrosis of the middle layers of the corpus callosum is highly suggestive of **chronic** MBD.

Other diseases that may affect the corpus callosum include **multiple sclerosis** and other demyelinating disorders, **traumatic axonal injury**, and **lacunar infarction** (rare because of rich blood supply). All have patchy, discontinuous lesions and rarely involve the entire length of the corpus callosum.

### MARCHIAFAVA-BIGNAMI DISEASE

**Acute MBD**
- Corpus callosum swelling
- Variable extracallosal extension
  - ± adjacent hemispheric WM, basal ganglia
- ± DWI restriction, focal hemorrhages
- Enhancement common
- May coexist with WE

**Chronic MBD**
- Corpus callosum thinned
- Middle layers encephalomalacic
- Look for associated findings of chronic AUD
  - Generalized hemispheric volume loss
  - Superior vermian atrophy
  - Enlarged cerebellar fissures
- May coexist with chronic hepatic encephalopathy

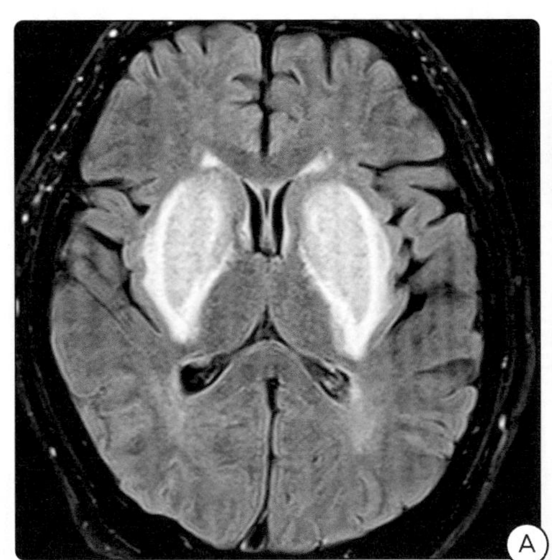


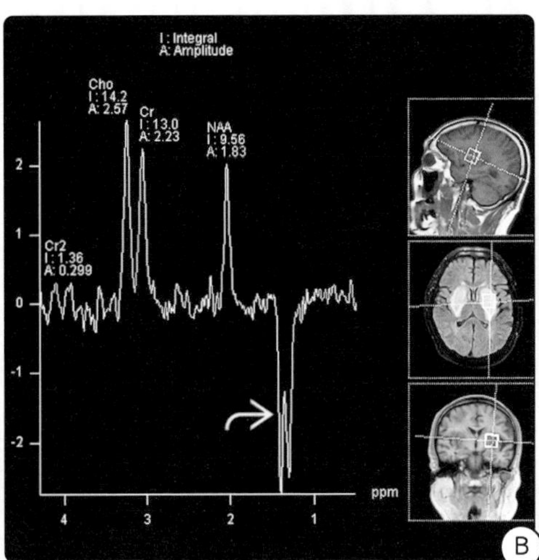


***(35-15A)** Axial FLAIR MR in a 47-year-old man with methanol poisoning shows bilateral, symmetric lesions in the putamina.* ***(35-15B)** MRS in the same case shows reduced NAA and a huge lactate doublet →.*

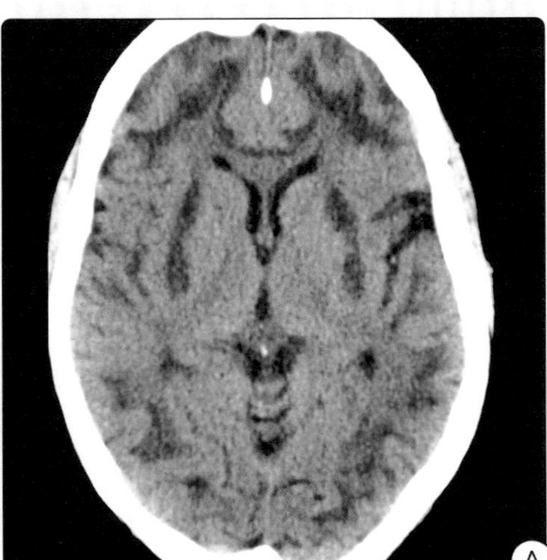


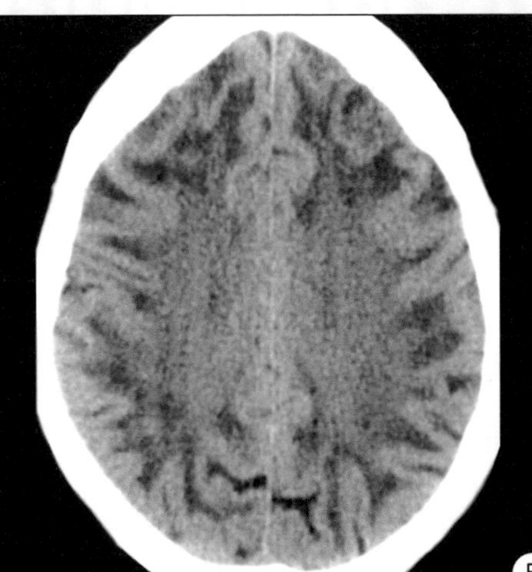


***(35-16A)** Axial NECT in a patient who survived acute methanol poisoning shows shrunken, hypodense putamina and bilateral symmetric hypodensities in the subcortical WM.* ***(35-16B)** More cephalad NECT in the same case shows that the severe, symmetric hypodensities in the subcortical WM spares the cortex.*

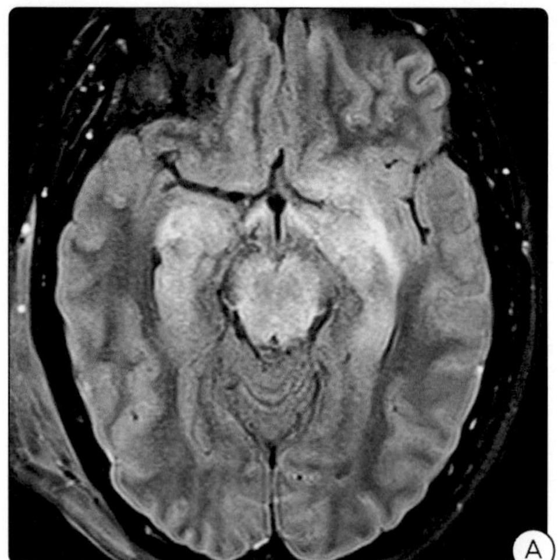
*(35-17A) A 23-yo man ingested antifreeze and presented to the ED in status epilepticus. FLAIR MR shows hippocampi, midbrain hyperintensity.*

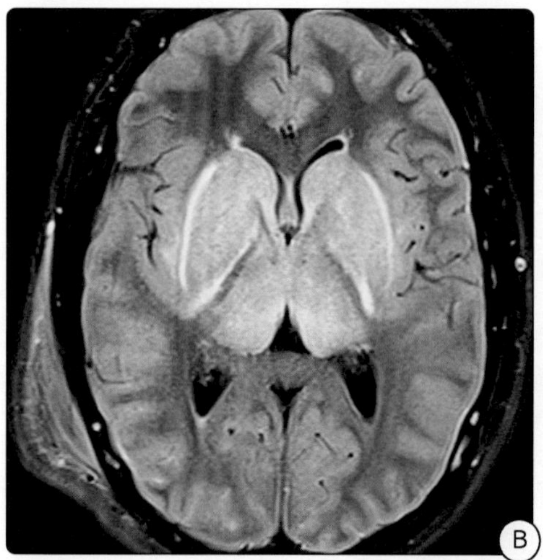
*(35-17B) More cephalad FLAIR MR shows symmetric hyperintensity in the BG and thalami.*

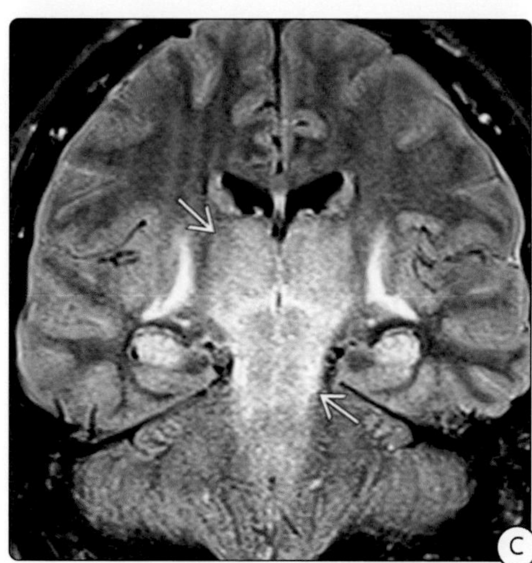
*(35-17C) Coronal FLAIR MR shows "olympic torch" ➡ of hyperintensity in the BG, midbrain, and pons.*

## Methanol Intoxication

Methanol (MtOH) is a strong CNS depressant. Patients are often comatose, and an accurate history may be impossible to obtain. Moreover, few hospitals include methanol in their standard toxicology screens. Therefore, delayed diagnosis is common, and morbidity and mortality remain high.

### Etiology

MtOH intoxication typically occurs as accidental ingestion of adultered illicit spirits ("moonshine") containing methanol. Rumored efficacy of ingesting alcohol, disinfectants, or sanitizers in an attempt to prevent or cure infection during the COVID-19 epidemic resulted in a worldwide spate of cases with methanol poisoning.

Methanol is metabolized to formic and lactic acid, causing high anion gap severe metabolic acidosis and end-organ damage with arterial pHs ranging from 6.8 to 7.1. Formic acid inhibits cytochrome oxidase and disrupts oxidative phosphorylation.

### Pathology

Hemorrhagic and nonhemorrhagic bilateral basal ganglia necrosis is the most characteristic feature of MtOH poisoning. Selective putamina involvement with relative sparing of the globi pallidi is common **(35-12)**. Diffuse necrosis of the subinsular and subcortical WM as well as the cerebellum and optic nerves may occur in severe cases. Hemorrhagic transformation is variable and can occur immediately or as a delayed phenomenon.

### Clinical Issues

The triad of visual impairment, gastrointestinal symptoms, and metabolic acidosis occur in 6-24 hours following methanol ingestion. Increased anion and osmolar gaps are important laboratory clues to the presence of MtOH toxicity. Approximately 25% of cases are comatose at presentation and may not be able to provide a suggestive history of MtOH intoxication.

### Imaging

**CT Findings.** The initial NECT scan is often normal in many patients with MtOH poisoning. Most patients who survive for more than 24 hours demonstrate bilateral symmetric hypodense lesions in the putamina, globi pallidi, and sometimes the subcortical and deep cerebral WM **(35-14A)**. Hemorrhagic putaminal necrosis is seen in 15-45% of cases. If the patient survives, cystic cavities may form within the putamina, representing the chronic sequelae of MtOH poisoning **(35-16)**.

**MR Findings.** Bilateral putaminal and basal ganglia necrosis with variable WM involvement is present. T2/FLAIR hyperintensity is seen **(35-14B)**. Up to 25% of patients exhibit "blooming" hemorrhagic foci on T2* GRE or susceptibility imaging **(35-13)**.

DWI shows restricted diffusion in the acute stage of MtOH poisoning. MRS shows reduced NAA and markedly elevated lactate **(35-15)**.

### Differential Diagnosis

Bilateral symmetric putaminal lesions are not specific for MtOH and can be seen in **Wilson disease** and the **mitochondrial encephalopathies**. **Hypoxic-ischemic encephalopathy** involves the caudate and other deep gray nuclei in addition to the putamina. Acute **cyanide poisoning** is rare but can

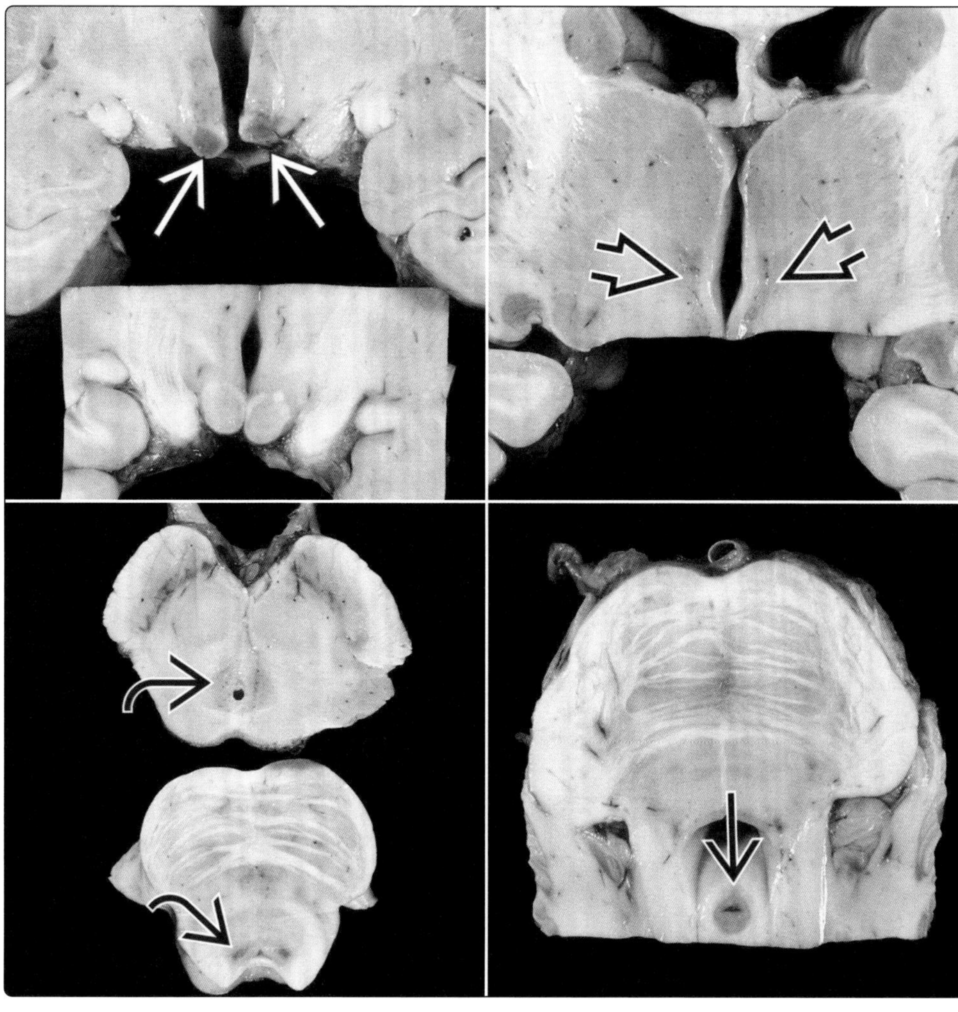

*(35-18) Autopsy specimens are from a patient with Wernicke encephalopathy. (Upper left) Coronal section through the mammillary bodies shows hemorrhagic mammillary body necrosis ➡. Inset below the pathologic section shows normal mammillary bodies for comparison. (Upper right) Coronal section through the 3rd ventricle shows bithalamic necrosis around walls of the 3rd ventricle ⇨. (Lower left and right) Sections through the midbrain and upper pons show necrosis in the periaqueductal gray matter ↗ and the bottom of the tectum ➡. (Courtesy R. Hewlett, MD.)*

resemble MtOH encephalopathy. **Carbon monoxide poisoning** generally affects the globi pallidi rather than the putamina.

## Ethylene Glycol Poisoning

Ethylene glycol is the third most common chemical responsible for deaths by nonpharmaceutical poisoning (following ethanol and carbon monoxide).

Ethylene glycol is a poisonous form of alcohol that is a common ingredient in many household products, such as antifreeze, deicing solutions, and windshield wiper fluids. It can be accidentally ingested by children and animals. Intake of even a small volume can be lethal.

Imaging findings of acute ethylene glycol toxicity include symmetric edema in the basal ganglia, thalami, midbrain, and upper pons. Symmetric hyperintensity in these areas on coronal T2/FLAIR scans has been likened to an Olympic torch **(35-17)**.

## Wernicke Encephalopathy

### Terminology

Wernicke encephalopathy (WE) is also known as Wernicke-Korsakoff syndrome. WE is a neuropsychiatric syndrome caused by thiamine deficiency.

### Etiology

*Both alcohol-related and nonalcoholic WE can occur!* WE is caused by thiamine (vitamin B1) deficiency. Approximately 50% of WE cases are AUD-related nutritional deficiencies with inadequate thiamine intake, decreased gastrointestinal absorption, &/or poor intracellular thiamine utilization.

Nonalcoholic WE may occur with hyperemesis (pregnancy- or chemotherapy-related vomiting), eating disorders, bariatric surgery, and prolonged hyperalimentation. A WE-like encephalopathy has also been reported with some drugs, including antineoplastic agents.

### Pathology

The mammillary bodies, hypothalamus, medial thalamic nuclei (adjacent to the third ventricle), tectal plate, and

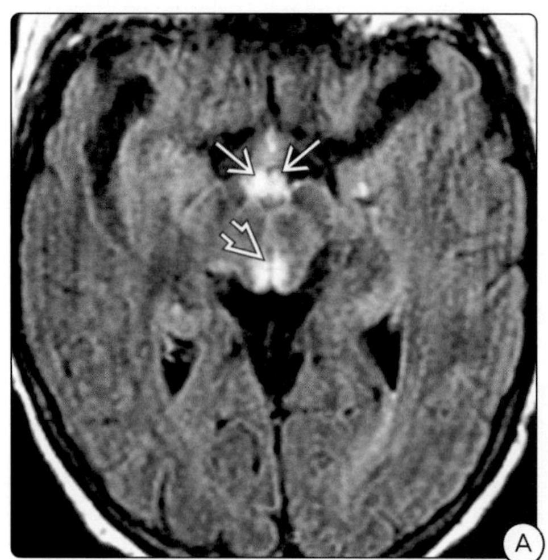

*(35-19A) FLAIR MR in acute WE shows periaqueductal gray matter ➡ and mammillary body hyperintensity ➡.*

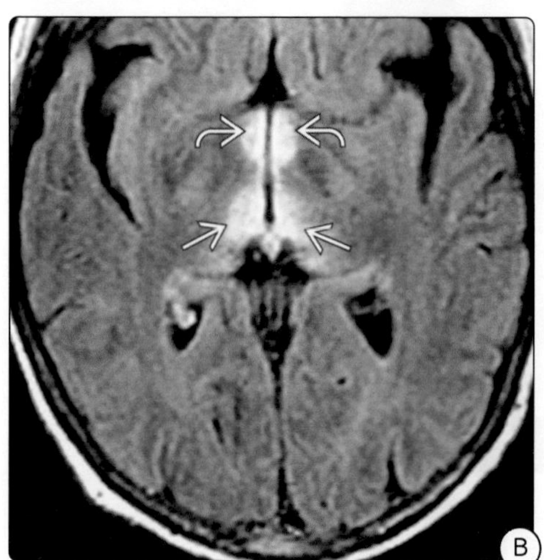

*(35-19B) Hyperintensity in the medial thalami around the walls of the 3rd ventricle ➡ is shown. The hypothalamus ➡ is also involved.*

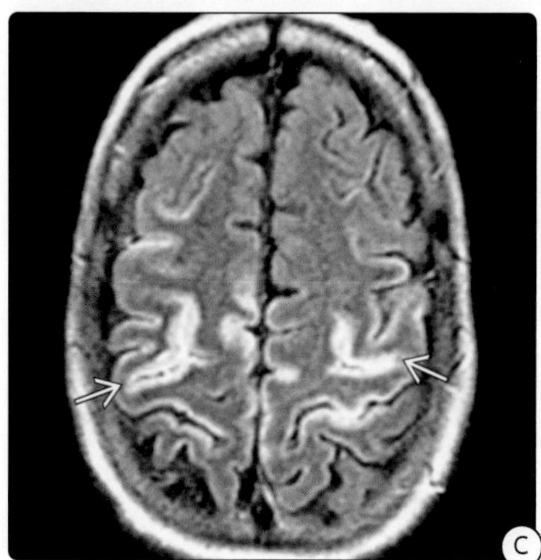

*(35-19C) FLAIR MR through the cerebral convexities shows bilateral, relatively symmetric cortical hyperintensities ➡.*

periaqueductal gray matter are most commonly affected **(35-18)**. Less commonly involved areas include the cerebellum (especially the dentate nuclei), red nuclei, corpus callosum splenium, and cerebral cortex.

Demyelination and petechial hemorrhages are common in the acute stage of WE. Callosal necrosis, WM rarefaction with brain volume loss, and mammillary body atrophy can be seen in chronic WE.

## Clinical Issues

Alcohol abuse is the most common cause of WE. However, *almost 1/2 of all WE cases occur in nonalcoholics.* Although nonalcoholic WE is generally more common in adults, it *can and does occur in children.*

The underlying pathophysiology of **nonalcoholic** WE is identical to that of alcoholic WE, but the etiology is different. Malnutrition secondary to hyperemesis gravidarum (pregnancy-related vomiting), eating disorders, parenteral therapy, or bariatric surgery with drastically reduced thiamine intake is typical. Hyperemesis (e.g., pregnancy, chemotherapy) and prolonged hyperalimentation are other common causes of nonalcoholic WE.

WE can be challenging to diagnose clinically or biochemically. *Only 30% of patients demonstrate the classic WE clinical triad* of (1) oculomotor dysfunction (e.g., nystagmus, conjugate gaze palsies, ophthalmoplegia), (2) cerebellar dysfunction (ataxia), and (3) altered sensorium. Nearly 20% of confirmed WE cases do not display any of these symptoms. In some cases, seizure may be the main manifestation, especially in nonalcoholic WE.

Mortality of untreated WE is high. Untreated, undiagnosed WE can lead to permanent neurologic damage, psychiatric sequelae, and death. Rapid high-dose intravenous thiamine administration is imperative to prevent the most severe sequelae of WE.

## Imaging

MR is the procedure of choice in evaluating patients with possible WE, although up to 1/3 of reported cases have normal initial studies on admission.

T1WI may show hypointensity around the third ventricle and cerebral aqueduct. In severe cases, petechial hemorrhages are present and may cause T1 hyperintensities in the medial thalami and mammillary bodies. T2* SWI sequences may be helpful in detecting microhemorrhages in the affected areas.

During the acute phase, T2/FLAIR hyperintensity can be seen in the affected areas **(35-19)**. Bilateral symmetric lesions in the putamina and medial thalami around the third ventricle are present in up to 85% of confirmed cases **(35-20)**. The tectal plate and periaqueductal gray matter are involved in nearly 2/3 of cases. T2/FLAIR hyperintensity in the mammillary bodies is seen in 50-60% of cases **(35-19A)**.

Less commonly, the dorsal medulla is affected **(35-20A)**. Bilateral but asymmetric cortical hyperintensities ("ribboning") can be present **(35-19C)** **(35-20C)**.

DWI shows corresponding restricted diffusion in the affected areas. Some cases show an isolated transient focus of diffusion restriction ("cytotoxic lesion") in the corpus callosum splenium.

In ~ 1/2 of all alcoholic WE cases, postcontrast scans demonstrate enhancement of the periventricular and periaqueductal lesions. Strong uniform enhancement of the mammillary bodies is seen in up to 80% of acute cases and is considered pathognomonic of WE. With chronic WE, mammillary body atrophy ensues.

## Differential Diagnosis

The medial thalami and midbrain can be symmetrically involved in **artery of Percheron (AOP) infarct** and **deep cerebral vein thrombosis (CVT)**. **Viral infections**, such as influenza A and West Nile virus meningoencephalitis, cause symmetric medial thalamic and midbrain lesions that may mimic WE. Mammillary bodies are usually not involved.

A rare but reported imaging differential diagnosis is demyelination in **neuromyelitis optica spectrum disorder (NMOSD)**. Therefore, measurement of aquaporin-4 antibodies should be considered if no obvious cause for thiamine deficiency is present.

**Biotin-thiamine-responsive basal ganglia disease** (BTBGD) is a rare, autosomal recessive, pan-ethnic treatable metabolic disorder of childhood (age 3-10 years) associated with biallelic pathogenic variations in *SLC19A3*. Bilateral symmetric lesions in the caudate nuclei, putamen, and medial thalami with variable extension into the brainstem, cortex, and cerebellum are typical. Sparing of the mammillary bodies and more extensive cortical involvement is helpful in distinguishing BTBGD from nonalcoholic WE. Treatment with high-dose biotin and thiamine is given orally as early in the disease course as possible and is continued lifelong.

### WERNICKE ENCEPHALOPATHY

**Etiology**
- Thiamine (vitamin B1) deficiency
- Alcohol related (50%), nonalcoholic (50%)

**Pathology**
- Acute: Petechial hemorrhages (especially mammillary bodies), demyelination
- Chronic: Callosal necrosis, mammillary atrophy

**Clinical Issues**
- Classic triad: Ocular dysfunction, ataxia, altered mental status
- Can occur in children
- Intravenous thiamine imperative

**Imaging**
- MR > > CT (usually unhelpful)
- T2/FLAIR hyperintensity, DWI restriction
    - Common: Medial thalami (85%), periaqueductal gray matter (65%), mammillary bodies (60%), tectum (30%)
    - Less common: Dorsal medulla (8%), cerebellum/cranial nerve nuclei (1%), corpus callosum splenium
- SWI may show microhemorrhages
- Enhancement varies
    - More common in alcoholic WE
    - Mammillary body enhancement pathognomonic

**Differential Diagnosis**
- AOP infarct, deep CVT
- Viral infection (e.g., influenza A, West Nile virus)
- Neuromyelitis optica
- BTBGD
    - Children 3-10 years old

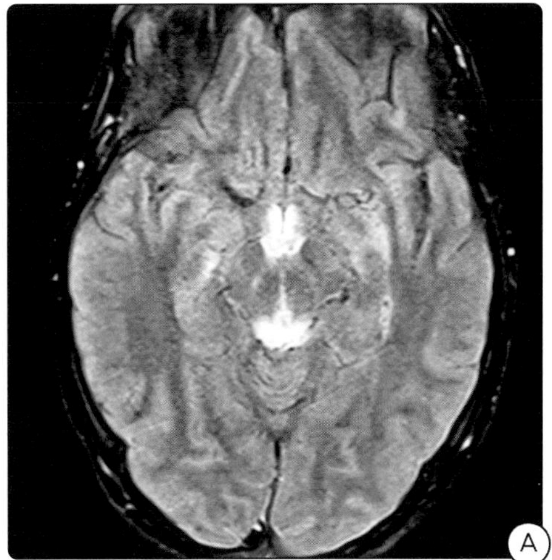


***(35-20A)** Nonalcoholic WE after 3 weeks of vomiting shows FLAIR hyperintensity in the hypothalamus and dorsal midbrain.*

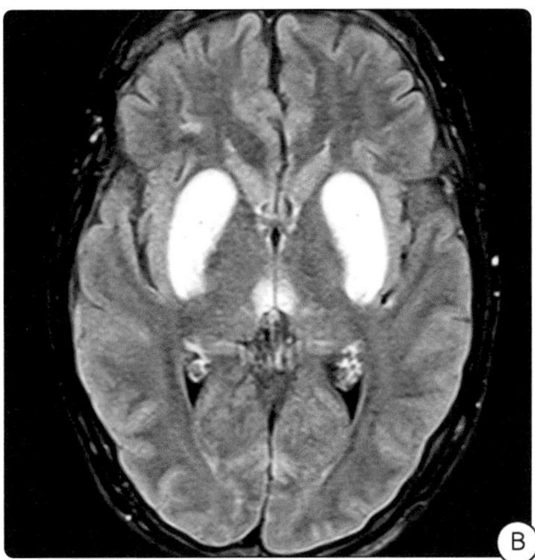


***(35-20B)** More cephalad FLAIR MR shows symmetric hyperintensity in the BG and medial thalami.*

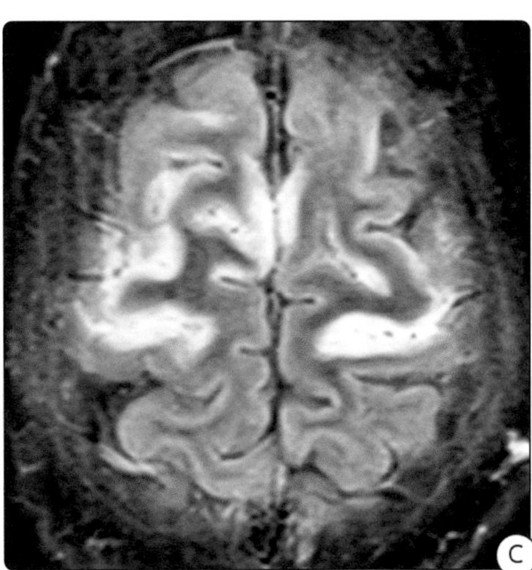


***(35-20C)** More cephalad FLAIR MR shows cortical hyperintensity. All hyperintensities exhibited restricted diffusion (not shown).*

# Medication-Related Toxic Encephalopathies

A number of common medications may exert toxicity in the CNS. While a detailed discussion of drug side effects on the CNS is beyond the scope of this text, we focus on identifying some common recognizable medication-related MR patterns that present acutely (metronidazole, acetaminophen, and antiepileptics).

## Metronidazole-Induced Encephalopathy

Metronidazole is an antibiotic commonly used in the treatment of some parasitic and microbial infections (e.g., amebiasis and *Clostridium difficile*). The drug is usually well tolerated, but patients occasionally develop serious neurologic impairment, including peripheral neuropathy, cerebellar dysfunction, vestibular &/or cochlear toxicity, ataxia, dysarthria, nystagmus, seizures, and sometimes severely altered mental status.

MR shows symmetrical T2/FLAIR hyperintensity in the dentate nuclei of the cerebellum and dorsal midbrain in > 90% of cases **(35-21)**. Involvement of the dorsal medulla, cerebellar peduncles, olivary nuclei, corpus callosum splenium, internal capsules, thalami, globi pallidi, and cerebral WM have also been reported in some cases. Imaging findings usually resolve after metronidazole discontinuation.

## Acute Acetaminophen Intoxication

Acetaminophen (APAP), a.k.a. paracetamol in Europe, is one of the most common nonprescription medications for pain and fever reduction. In the USA, more than 25 billion doses are sold yearly as 325-mg and 500-mg immediate-release tablets,

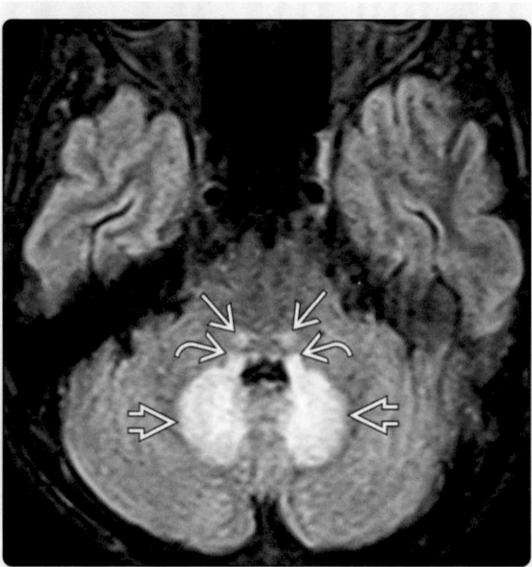

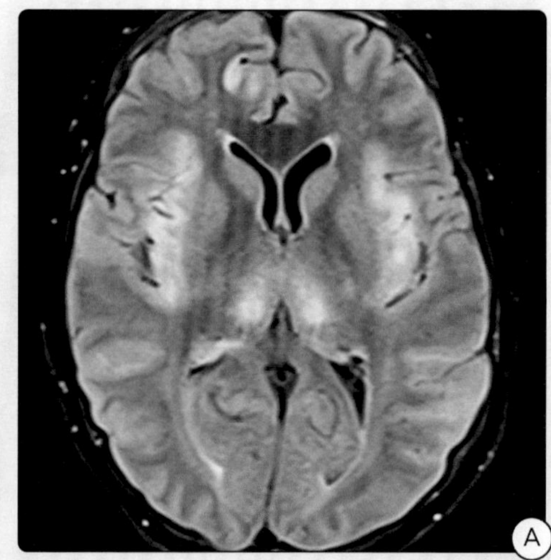

***(35-21)** A 34-yo man treated with metronidazole for refractory Clostridium difficile colitis developed acute onset of ataxia and visual difficulties. FLAIR shows symmetric hyperintensity in the dentate nuclei ➡, vestibular ➡ and superior olivary ➡ nuclei. **(35-22A)** A 46-yo woman became acutely confused and then comatose following acetaminophen OD. FLAIR shows symmetric hyperintensity in the medial thalami, insular cortices.*

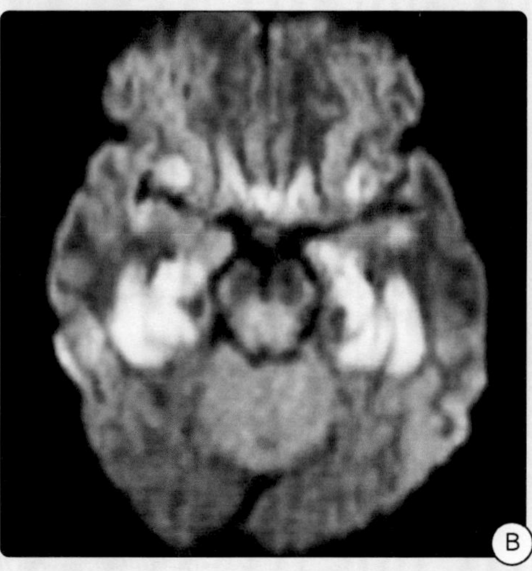

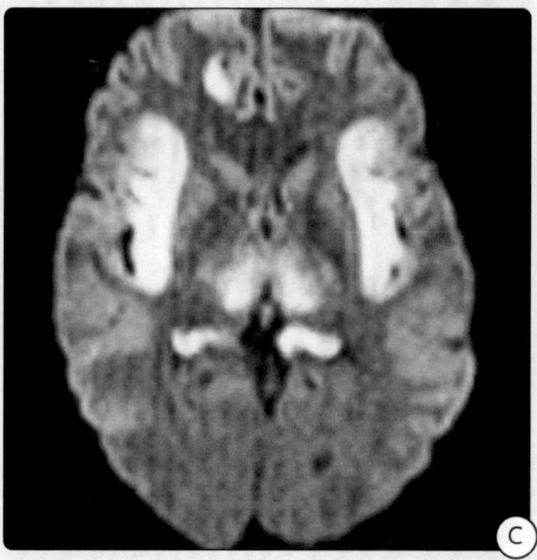

***(35-22B)** DWI MR in the same case shows symmetric restricted diffusion in the hippocampi. **(35-22C)** More cephalad DWI MR shows symmetric restricted diffusion in the medial thalami, insular cortex, and hippocampi. Acetaminophen OD caused acute hepatic encephalopathy.*

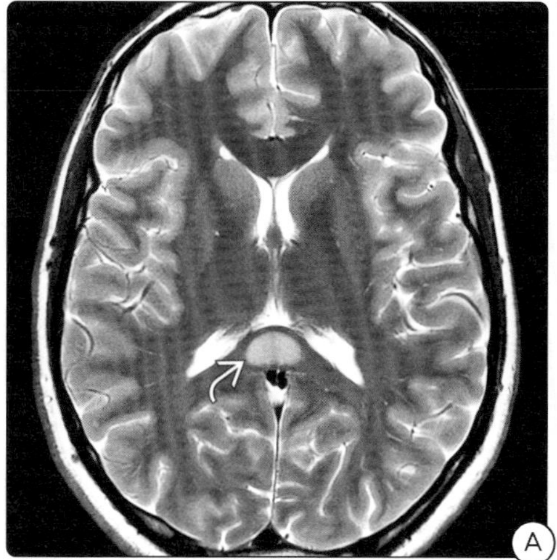

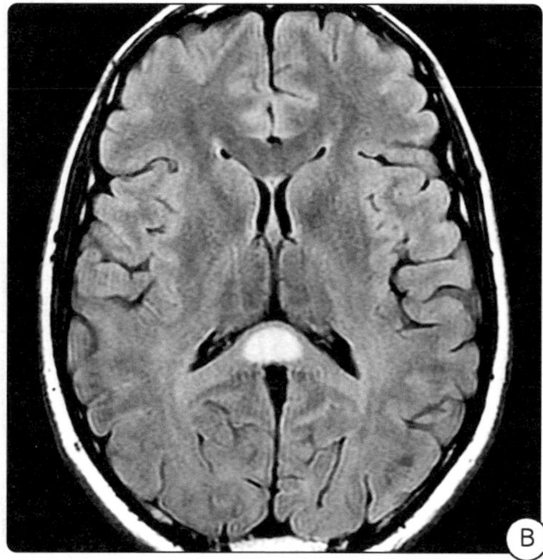

***(35-23A)** T2 MR in a 31-yo man with migraine headaches and acute respiratory illness shows an ovoid hyperintensity ➡ in the middle of the corpus callosum splenium. **(35-23B)** FLAIR MR shows there are no other lesions in the hemispheric WM.*

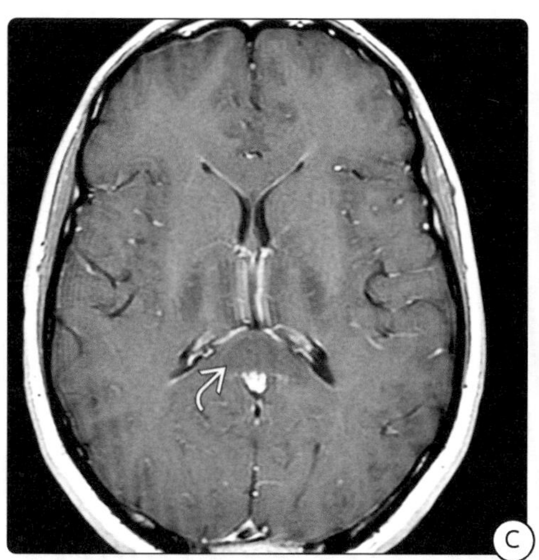

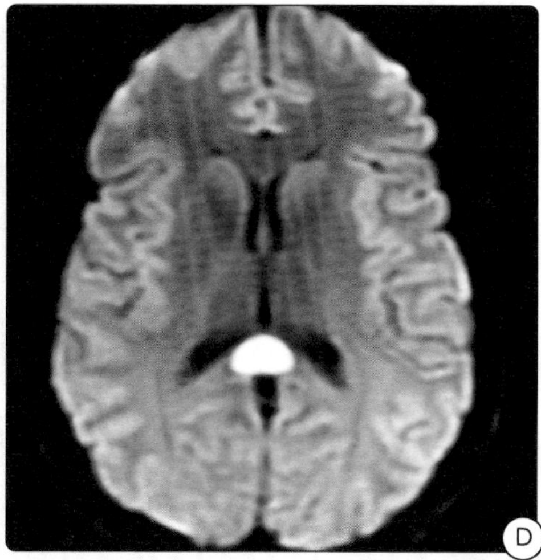

***(35-23C)** T1 C+ FS MR shows the faintly hypointense lesion ➡ does not enhance. **(35-23D)** The lesion restricts strongly on DWI MR. The lesion resolved completely on follow-up imaging.*

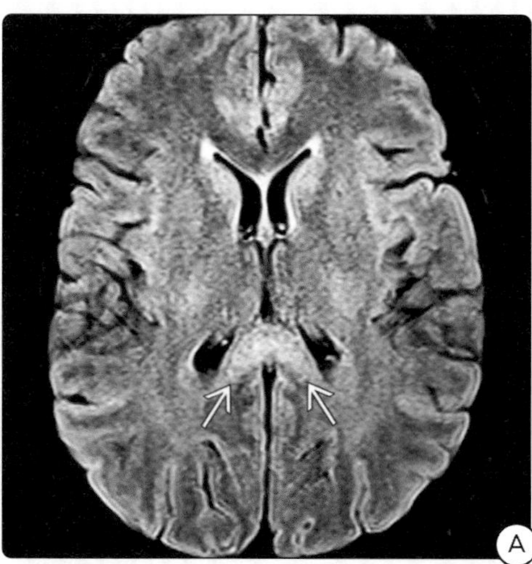

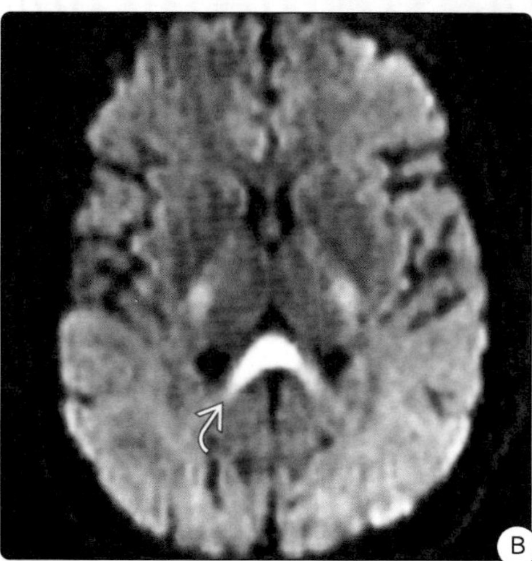

***(35-24A)** FLAIR MR in a 33-yo woman with seizures shows a "boomerang" hyperintense corpus callosum splenium ➡. **(35-24B)** DTI trace DWI clearly shows the distinct boomerang-shaped area of restricted diffusion ➡. The lesion resolved completely on follow-up imaging.*

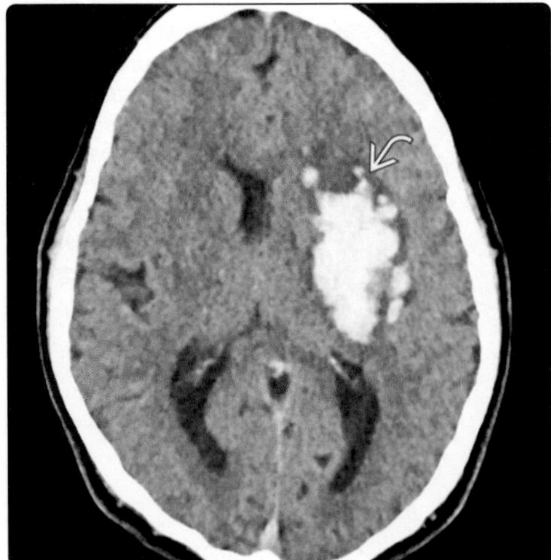

*(35-25) NECT in 61-yo man with right hemiparesis following meth and cocaine abuse shows left basal ganglionic hemorrhage ➡.*

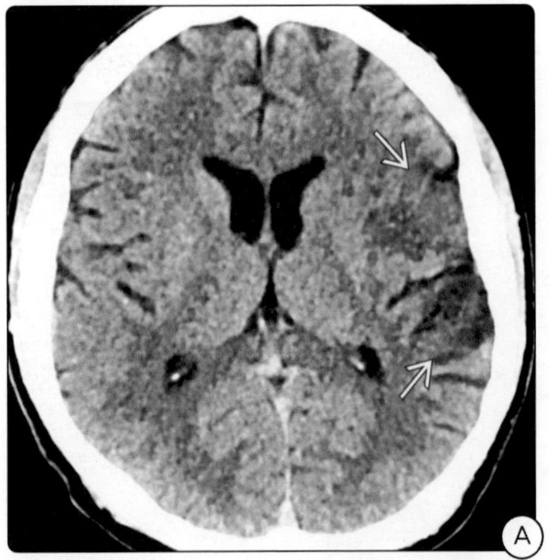


*(35-26A) NECT shows patchy ischemic infarction in the left MCA distribution ➡ of a 42-yo methamphetamine abuser.*

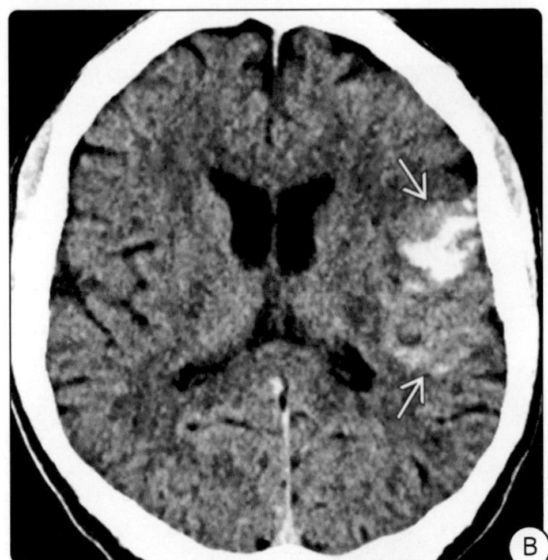


*(35-26B) Repeat NECT obtained 6 hours later following clinical worsening shows early hemorrhagic transformation ➡ in the infarct.*

and high-dose (650-mg) extended release tablets are often used for the treatment of arthritis.

If used in proper therapeutic doses, APAP has an excellent safety profile. Because APAP is metabolized in the liver, acute hepatotoxicity can occur after accidental or intentional overdose (OD). APAP poisoning is the most common cause of acute liver failure in the USA. Nearly 1/2 of all ODs are unintentional. APAP OD can occur at *any* age, including infants and children.

APAP OD breaches the blood-bile barrier, causing massive oxidative stress and hepatocyte death. Only one drug, N-acetylcysteine, is approved for the treatment of APAP OD and must be given within 8 hours after ingestion.

Imaging findings are those of acute liver failure with hyperammonemia (acute hyperammonemic encephalopathy). Symmetrical, extensive cortical T2/FLAIR hyperintensity involving the insular, cingulate, and frontoparietal cortices (cortical ribbon sign) with sparing of the occipital and perirolandic areas is typical. Both thalami are often affected. Affected areas show restricted diffusion **(35-22)**.

## Reversible Splenial Lesions

### Terminology

Reversible splenial lesions (RSLs) are also known as cytotoxic lesions of the corpus callosum (CLCCs). These are acquired, usually transient or reversible lesions that are associated with a number of different entities and often characterized by a nonspecific encephalopathy.

### Etiology

While RSLs/CLCCs have been associated with a number of conditions, most are related to seizures, withdrawal of antiepileptic or psychotropic medications, metabolic derangements, and infections, such as viral encephalitis.

### Clinical Issues

RSLs/CLCCs themselves are usually asymptomatic and discovered incidentally on imaging studies. Most resolve spontaneously and disappear.

### Imaging

RSLs are most often round, ovoid, or boomerang-shaped lesions **(35-24)** centered on the middle of the corpus callosum splenium **(35-23)**. Rarely, CLCCs extend anteriorly from the splenium into the corpus callosum body. Mass effect is absent or minimal.

RSLs/CLCCs are iso- to mildly hypointense on T1WI, homogeneously hyperintense on T2/FLAIR, and do not enhance following contrast administration **(35-23)**. Most demonstrate restricted diffusion **(35-23D)**. Lesions typically resolve completely within a few days or weeks, and follow-up imaging studies are normal.

### Differential Diagnosis

The differential diagnosis is limited. **Glioblastoma** and **primary CNS lymphoma** may involve the corpus callosum splenium but cause mass effect and typically enhance strongly on T1 C+.

# Amphetamines and Derivatives

CNS stimulants include cocaine, amphetamine, methamphetamine (MA), methylenedioxymethamphetamine (MDMA), and methylphenidate. Although not a classic CNS stimulant, nicotine is a prototypic drug that is avidly self-administered and has some stimulating properties. All of these drugs have a high human abuse liability.

Most addictive drugs are excitotoxic and cause two major types of pathologies: Vascular events (e.g., ischemia, hemorrhage) and leukoencephalopathy.

## Methamphetamine

Methamphetamine (MA or "meth") is a highly addictive psychostimulant drug. "Crystal" MA abuse has been steadily increasing over the past decade. Even a single acute exposure to MA can result in profound changes in cerebral blood flow. Both hemorrhagic **(35-25)** and ischemic strokes **(35-26)** occur.

MR in chronic adult MA users demonstrates lower gray matter volumes on T1WI, especially in the frontal lobes, and more WM hyperintensities on T2/FLAIR scans than are appropriate for the patient's age. MRS shows increased choline and myoinositol levels in the frontal lobes. DTI shows lower FA in the frontal lobes and higher ADC values in the basal ganglia.

## MDMA ("Ecstasy")

3-,4-Methylenedioxymethamphetamine is also known as **MDMA** or **ecstasy**. MDMA can cause arterial constriction, vasculitis, or prolonged vasospasm with acute ischemic infarcts. MDMA-induced ischemia is most pronounced in serotonin-rich brain areas, such as the globus pallidus and occipital cortex, which are especially vulnerable.

## Benzodiazepines

Benzodiazepines, sometimes called **"benzo,"** are psychoactive drugs used to treat anxiety, insomnia, seizures, muscle spasms, and alcohol withdrawal. Benzodiazepines, such as temazepam and midazolam, act selectively on GABA-A receptors in the brain, inhibiting or reducing the activity of neurons.

Benzodiazepine OD has been associated with hypoxic-ischemic encephalopathy **(35-27)** **(35-28)**, hemorrhagic ischemic strokes, and delayed toxic leukoencephalopathy.

## Cocaine

Cocaine can be sniffed/snorted, smoked, or injected. In its most common form (cocaine hydrochloride), it is ingested via the nasal mucosa. "Crack," the alkaloidal freebase form of cocaine hydrochloride, can also be smoked.

Regardless of the route of administration, the adverse impact of cocaine on the brain is largely related to its vascular effects. Systemic hypertension can be extreme, causing spontaneous hemorrhagic strokes.

### Etiology

Nearly 1/3 of strokes in patients younger than 45 years old are drug related with 80-90% occurring in the fourth and fifth decades. Stroke risk is highest within the first six hours after drug use.

Rupture of a preexisting aneurysm or underlying vascular malformation accounts for nearly 1/2 of all cocaine-related hemorrhagic strokes. Cocaine

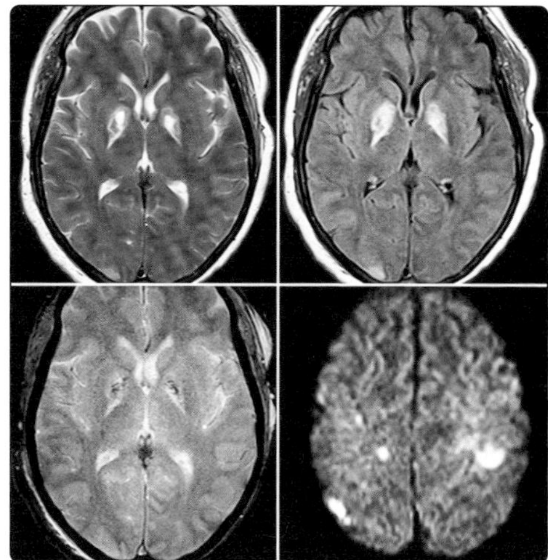

***(35-27)** MR in opiate, benzodiazepine OD shows globi pallidi (GP), cortical infarcts. Patient also had hemorrhagic cerebellar infarcts (not shown).*

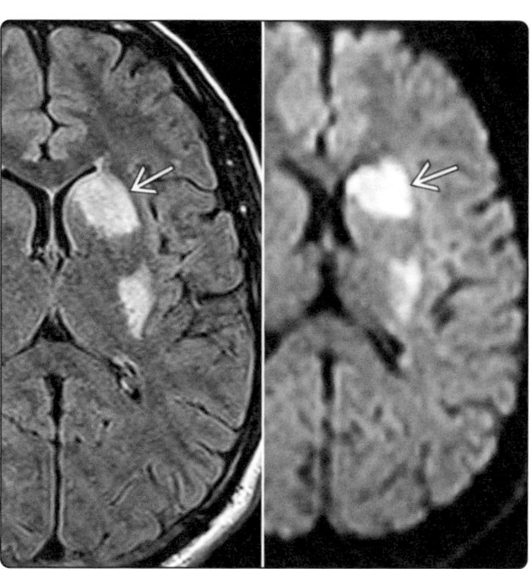

***(35-28)** FLAIR (left) and DWI (right) show acute cocaine-induced BG infarcts ➡.*

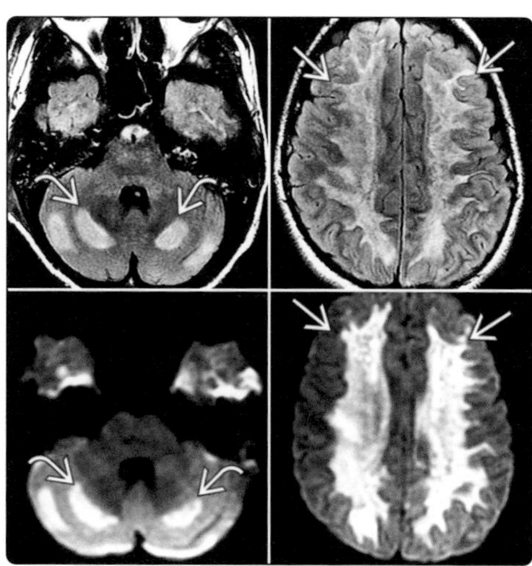

***(35-29)** FLAIR (top), DWI (bottom) in oxycodone OD shows symmetric cerebellar infarcts ➡ and toxic hemispheric leukoencephalopathy ➡.*

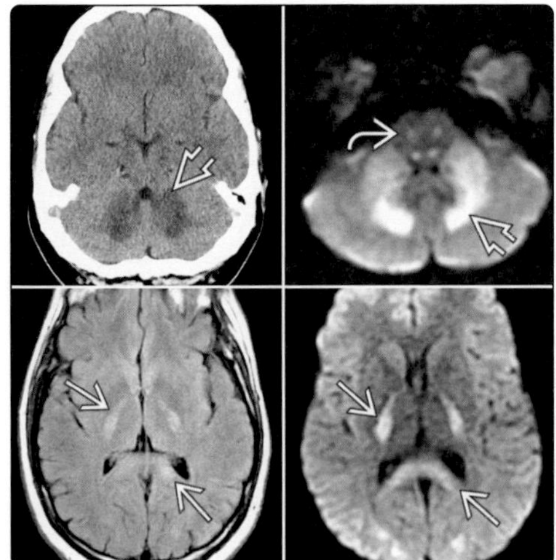

*(35-30) Inhaled heroin results in abnormalities in pons ➡, cerebellum ➡, corpus callosum, and internal capsules ➡. (Courtesy K. Nelson, MD.)*

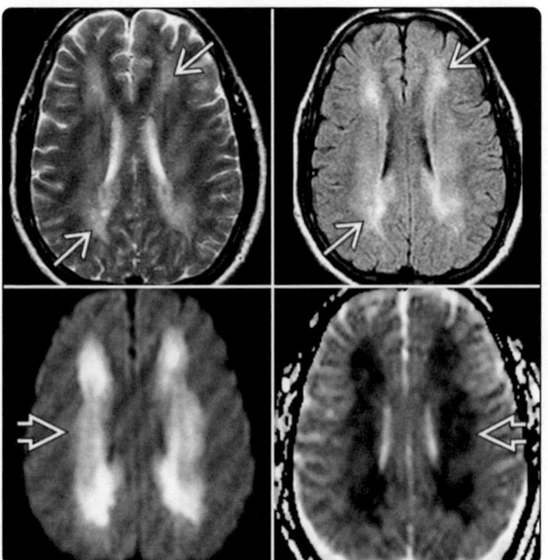

*(35-31) Heroin "chasing the dragon" shows hyperintensity ➡ and restricted diffusion ➡ in periventricular WM. (Courtesy M. Michel, MD.)*

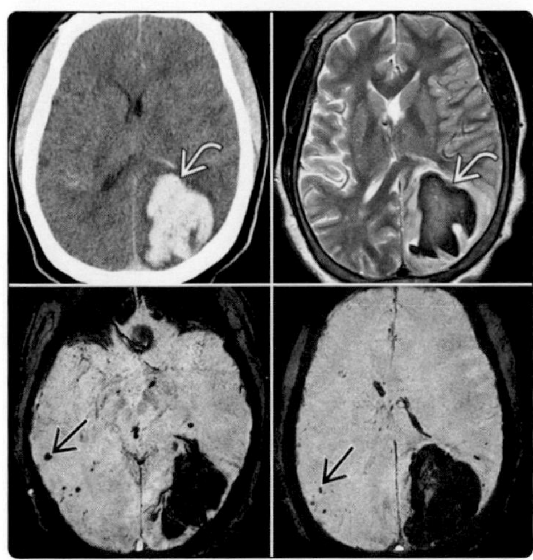

*(35-32) Polydrug abuse shows sICH ➡. SWI also shows microbleeds ➡, "unmasking" of multiple cavernous malformations.*

also facilitates platelet aggregation and may lead to thrombotic vascular occlusion.

Acute cerebral vasoconstriction &/or cocaine-induced vasculopathy may lead to ischemic strokes. Snorted cocaine causes severe vasoconstriction in the vascular plexus of the nasal septal mucosa (Kiesselbach plexus). Chronic abuse may lead to septal necrosis and perforation.

## Imaging

Strokes—both ischemic and hemorrhagic—are the major manifestations of cocaine-induced brain damage **(35-28)**. The hemorrhages can be parenchymal (secondary to hypertension or vascular malformation) or subarachnoid (aneurysm rupture) **(35-32)**. Hypertensive bleeds are usually centered in the external capsule/putamen or in the thalamus.

Ischemic strokes can be caused by vasospasm, cocaine-induced vasoconstriction, vasculitis, or thrombosis. Bilateral globus pallidus infarction has also been reported as a stroke subtype in cocaine abuse.

Acute cocaine-induced strokes are positive on DWI. MRA, CTA, or DSA may show focal areas of arterial narrowing and irregularity.

Acute hypertensive encephalopathy with posterior reversible encephalopathy (PRES-like syndrome) can also occur. Vasogenic edema in the occipital lobes is the most common finding.

## Differential Diagnosis

Unexplained parenchymal hemorrhage in young and middle-aged adults should prompt evaluation for possible drug abuse. **Embolic infarcts** as well as **vasculitis** may appear identical to cocaine vasculopathy.

### COCAINE AND AMPHETAMINE EFFECTS ON THE BRAIN

**Amphetamines**

- MA ("meth")
  - Hemorrhagic, ischemic strokes
- MDMA ("ecstasy")
  - Vasospasm, infarcts
  - Location: Occipital cortex, globus pallidus
- Benzodiazepines
  - Delayed toxic leukoencephalopathy

**Cocaine**

- Intracranial hemorrhage
  - Hypertensive intracranial hemorrhage (50%)
  - "Unmasked" aneurysm or arteriovenous malformation (50%)
- Ischemic stroke
  - Vasospasm, vasculitis
- Acute hypertensive encephalopathy
  - PRES
  - Vasogenic edema (typically bioccipital)

# Opioids and Derivatives

The 10 drugs most frequently involved in OD deaths include several opioids and synthetic opioids: **Heroin, oxycodone, methadone, morphine, hydrocodone**, and **fentanyl**. Deaths typically result from respiratory depression.

## Heroin

Heroin is usually injected intravenously. The most common acute complication of *injected* heroin is stroke. Globus pallidus ischemia, very similar to that seen in carbon monoxide poisoning, is common.

The most dramatic acute effects occur with *inhaled* heroin. The freebase form is heated over aluminum foil and the vapors inhaled (**"chasing the dragon"**). Heroin vapor inhalation causes a striking toxic leukoencephalopathy.

Acute CNS toxicity from inhaled heroin ("chasing the dragon") is characterized by symmetric hypodensities in the cerebellar WM, sometimes described as a butterfly wing pattern **(35-30)**. The cerebral WM, posterior limb of the internal capsule, and globi pallidi are also commonly affected. The anterior limb of the internal capsule is typically spared.

T2 and FLAIR scans in patients with early heroin-related leukoencephalopathy show symmetric hyperintensity in the cerebellar WM with relative sparing of the dentate nuclei **(35-30)**. There is often selective symmetric involvement of the posterior limb of the internal capsule, the corticospinal tract, the medial lemniscus, and the tractus solitarius **(35-30)**.

Confluent hyperintensity in the cerebral WM, including the corpus callosum, is common in severe cases of heroin vapor encephalopathy **(35-31)**. DWI shows acute diffusion restriction in the affected areas; MRS shows a lactate peak in the cerebral WM.

## Methadone

So-called substitute drugs, such as the synthetic opioid methadone, are used in the medication-assisted therapy for drug abuse/dependence as well as in the management of intractable pain. With increasing use and availability, methadone OD is likewise growing.

A postopioid delayed toxic leukoencephalopathy similar to that caused by inhaled heroin has been reported with methadone. Diffuse, symmetric, confluent hyperintensity in the cerebral WM on T2/FLAIR is seen **(35-33)**. Sparing of the subcortical U-fibers is typical. In contrast to heroin toxicity, cerebellar and brainstem changes are subtle or absent in adults. MRS shows elevated choline, decreased NAA, and increased lactate.

## Oxycodone

Imaging in the few reported cases of oxycodone and OxyContin OD shows restricted diffusion in the cerebellar hemispheres and globi pallidi **(35-29) (35-35)**.

## Fentanyl

The rise of fentanyl-based counterfeit opioids is a key driver of the deadliest-to-date wave of the opioid crisis. Toxic spongiform leukoencephalopathy similar to heroin OD has been reported to have changes associated with delayed hypoxic-ischemic encephalopathy.

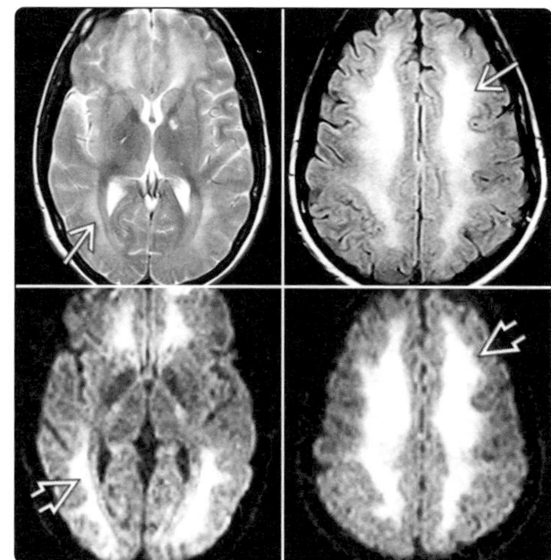

***(35-33)** Methadone OD shows symmetric confluent hyperintensity (leukoencephalopathy) on FLAIR ➡ and restricted diffusion on DWI ➡.*

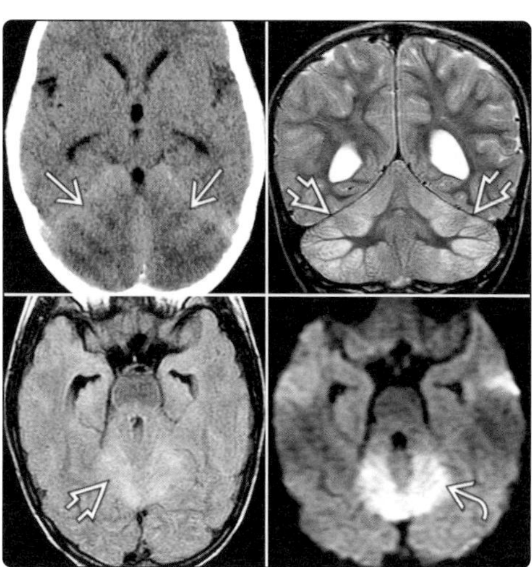

***(35-34)** Methadone poisoning in a child shows cerebellar hypodensity on NECT ➡, T2/FLAIR hyperintensity ➡, and restricted diffusion ➡.*

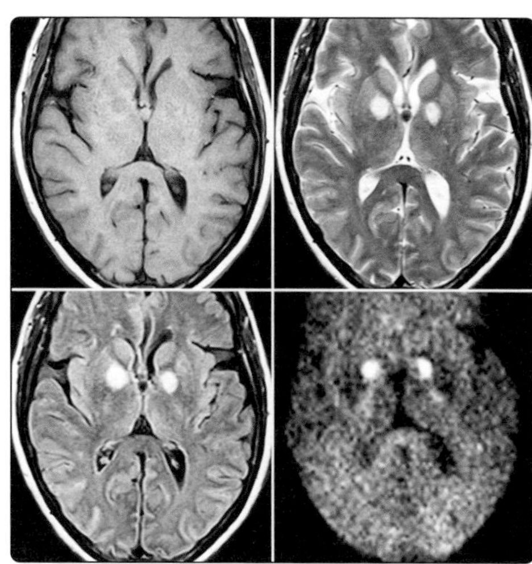

***(35-35)** Opioid, benzodiazepine OD shows symmetric GP lesions mimicking carbon monoxide (CO) poisoning.*

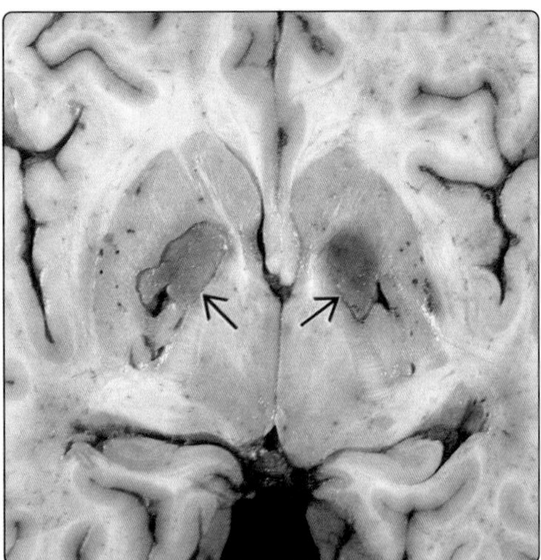

*(35-36) Autopsy of CO poisoning shows symmetric coagulative (nonhemorrhagic) necrosis of both medial GP ⇒. (Courtesy R. Hewlett, MD.)*

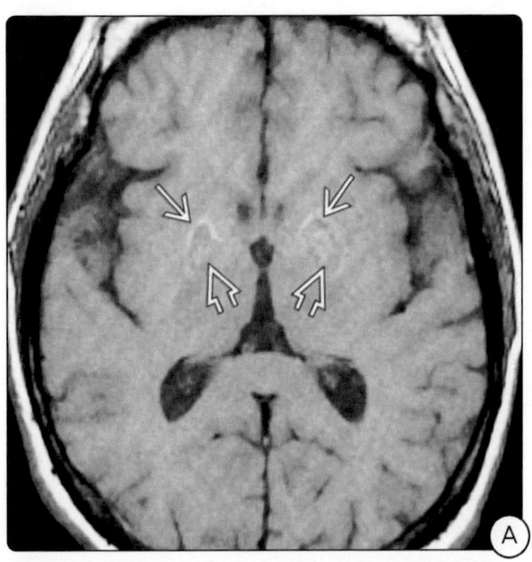

*(35-37A) CO poisoning shows symmetric lesions in both medial GP ⇒ with faint hyperintense rim ⇒.*

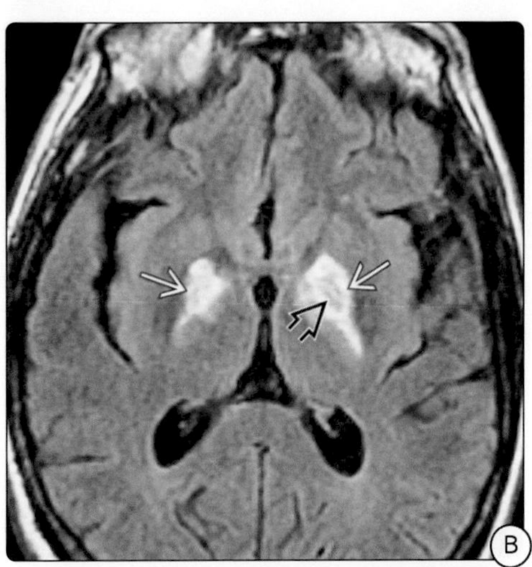

*(35-37B) FLAIR MR shows hyperintense lesion ⇒ with isointense core ⇒. The isointense parts of the lesions enhanced on T1 C+ (not shown).*

OPIOID DRUGS

**Heroin**
- Injected
  - Most common: Ischemic strokes
  - Globi pallidi, WM (resembles carbon monoxide poisoning)
- Inhaled
  - "Chasing the dragon"
  - Most common: Leukoencephalopathy
  - Cerebellum, cerebral WM

**Methadone**
- Adults
  - Toxic leukoencephalopathy
- Children
  - Usually accidental ingestion
  - Cerebellar edema

**Oxycodone**
- Cerebellar, globus pallidus ischemia
- Less common: Toxic leukoencephalopathy

**Fentanyl**
- Leukoencephalopathy (like "chasing the dragon")
- Hypoxic-ischemic changes in basal ganglia, WM

# Inhaled Gases and Toxins

Carbon monoxide (CO) and nitrous oxide ($N_2O$) are purely inhaled toxins. Some toxins, such as cyanide, can be inhaled, ingested, or absorbed transdermally. Inhaled vapors from volatile, intrinsically liquid agents include amyl nitrite ("poppers") and industrial solvents (e.g., toluene).

## Carbon Monoxide Poisoning

CO is a colorless, odorless, tasteless gas that is produced by the incomplete combustion of various fuels. CO poisoning is caused by deliberate (suicide) or accidental (inadequate ventilation) inhalation.

### Etiology

CO combines reversibly with hemoglobin (Hgb) with over 250x higher affinity than that of oxygen and Hgb. If carboxyhemoglobin (CO-Hgb) levels exceed 20%, brain and cardiac damage are common.

### Pathology

Because the globi pallidi are exquisitely sensitive to hypoxia, the hallmark of acute CO poisoning is symmetric globus pallidi necrosis **(35-36)**. The cerebral WM is the second most commonly affected and often shows delayed demyelination and necrosis that may appear several weeks after the initial insult **(35-38)**.

In addition to bilateral globi pallidi and cerebral WM, various sites, such as the cerebral cortex, cerebellum, hippocampus, amygdala, corpus callosum splenium, and insula, are often involved.

### Clinical Issues

Acute CO poisoning initially causes nausea, vomiting, headache, and impaired consciousness. Outcome depends on both duration and intensity of exposure. Seizures, coma, and death may ensue.

Up to 30% of patients who survive acute CO intoxication develop delayed encephalopathy. Parkinson-like symptoms, memory deficits, and cognitive disturbances are common.

## Imaging

**CT Findings.** Early NECT scans may be normal. Symmetric hypodensity in both globi pallidi develops within a few hours. Gross hemorrhage is rare. Variable diffuse hypodensity in the hemispheric WM can be seen in severe cases.

**MR Findings.** Multiplanar MR (e.g., FLAIR, T2WI, and DWI) is the most sensitive technique for early detection of changes caused by CO poisoning. T1WI shows subtle hypointensity in the globi pallidi. A faint rim of hyperintensity caused by hemorrhage or coagulative necrosis may be present **(35-37A)**.

T2/FLAIR shows bilateral hyperintensities in the medial globi pallidi **(35-37B)** with the putamina and caudate nuclei less commonly affected. A thin hypointense rim around the lesion may be present.

In addition to the hyperintense areas seen on T2WI, FLAIR imaging may disclose subtle involvement of the caudate nuclei, thalami, hippocampi, corpus callosum, fornices, and cerebral cortex.

DWI/ADC maps show restricted diffusion in the affected areas. Bilateral globi pallidi hyperintensities as well as foci of restricted diffusion in the subcortical WM are typical. ADC in the cerebral WM increases significantly, reflecting extensive microstructural tissue damage. DTI shows FA decline in associated cortical areas.

T2* GRE or SWI may show hypointensity in the globi pallidi, suggestive of petechial hemorrhage.

Within a week after exposure, MRS shows elevated Cho:Cr and lowered NAA:Cr ratios, indicating increased membrane metabolism and decreased neuroaxonal viability.

Up to 1/3 of CO patients develop a **delayed leukoencephalopathy** with progressive WM demyelination, the "interval" (subacute) form of CO poisoning. Extensive bilateral symmetric confluent areas of hyperintensity on T2/FLAIR are characteristic findings **(35-39)**.

## Differential Diagnosis

The major differential diagnoses of CO poisoning are **hypoxic-ischemic encephalopathy** (HIE) and **drug abuse**. As they share some common pathophysiology, imaging findings often overlap. HIE generally affects the entire basal ganglia and hippocampi and less often affects the WM or only the globi pallidi.

# Nitrous Oxide

$N_2O$ OD irreversibly oxidizes the cobalt ion of vitamin B12. Repeated recreational abuse causes progressive myelopathy with **subacute combined degeneration of the spinal cord**. The dorsal columns and corticospinal tracts are preferentially affected **(35-40)**. Brain lesions are rare, but reversible splenial lesions have been reported.

# Toluene Abuse

Toluene is a colorless lipophilic liquid found in glues, paint thinners, inks, and other industrial products. The common methods of abuse are "sniffing" (direct inhalation from a container), "huffing" (inhalation from a soaked rag

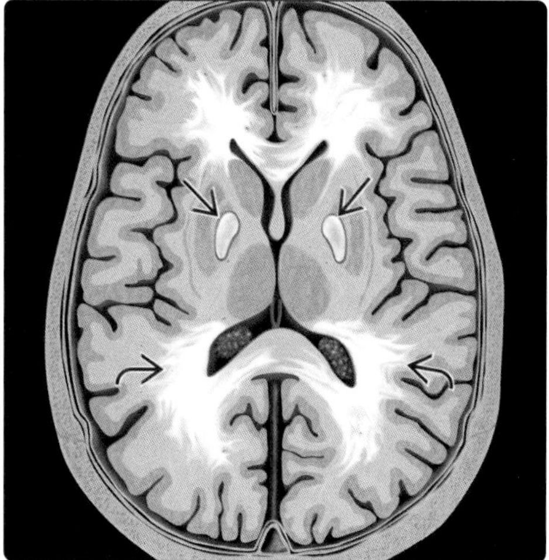

***(35-38)** Graphic of CO poisoning pathologically shows necrosis of the GP ➡ with variable areas of necrosis and demyelination in the WM ⮫.*

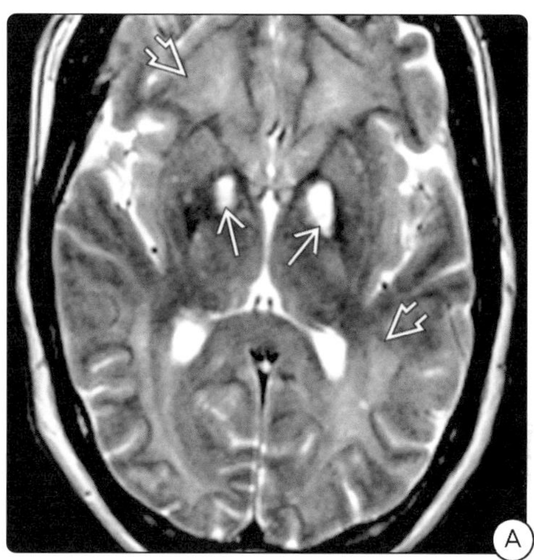

***(35-39A)** T2 MR 2 weeks after CO poisoning shows hyperintensities in GP ➡ and the cerebral WM ⮫, sparing the subcortical U-fibers.*

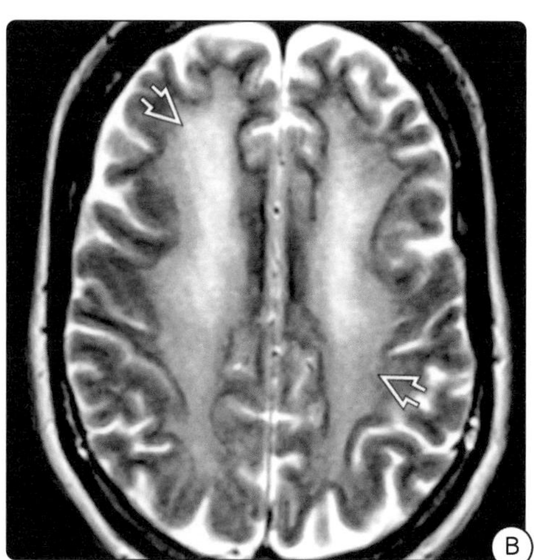

***(35-39B)** Cephalad T2 MR shows involvement of the corona radiata ⮫, sparing of subcortical WM. "Interval" (subacute) form of CO poisoning.*

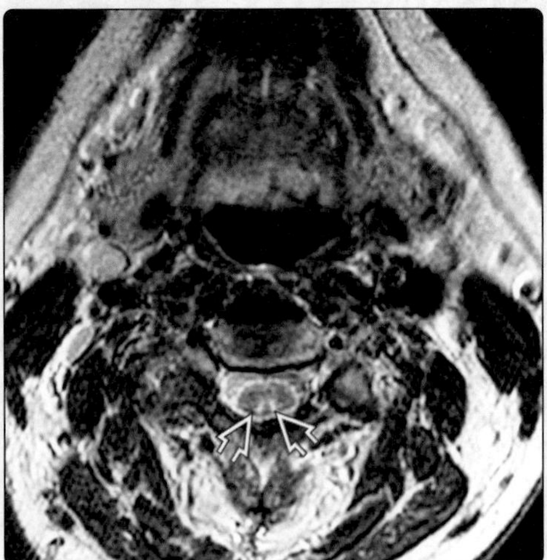

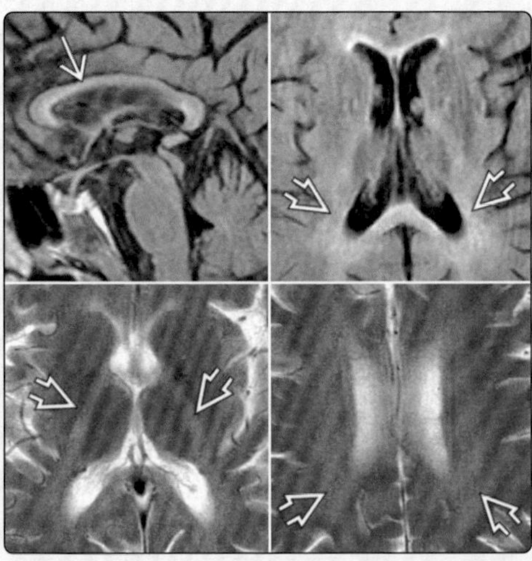

***(35-40)*** *Nitrous oxide abuse shows subacute combined degeneration of the posterior columns* ➡. *(Courtesy C. Glastonbury, MBBS.)* ***(35-41)*** *Thinned corpus callosum* ➡, *T2/FLAIR confluent WM hyperintensity* ➡ *are from toluene toxicity (glue sniffing). (Courtesy S. Lincoff, MD.)*

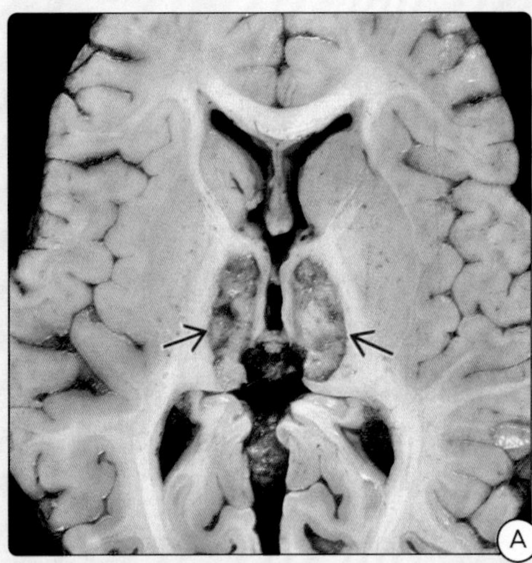

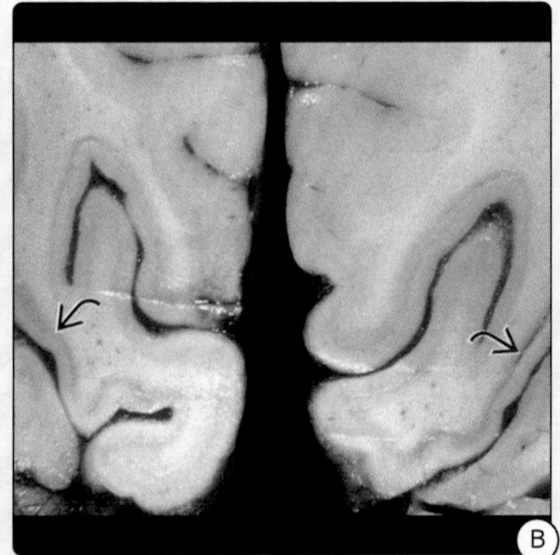

***(35-42A)*** *Autopsy specimen from a patient with smoke inhalation, possibly from burning trash with vaporized cyanide, shows bilateral thalamic necrosis* ➡. ***(35-42B)*** *The occipital lobes in the same case show cortical laminar necrosis* ➡. *(Courtesy R. Hewlett, MD.)*

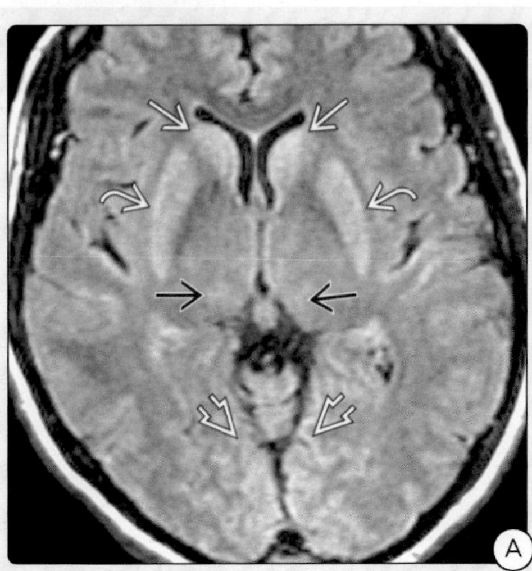

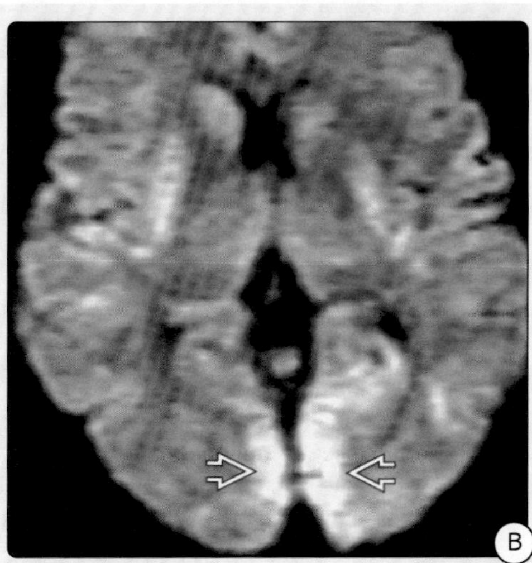

***(35-43A)*** *Axial FLAIR MR in cyanide poisoning from burning trash shows symmetric hyperintensities in the putamina* ➡, *caudate nuclei* ➡, *and occipital cortex* ➡ *with less prominent hyperintensity in the medial thalami* ➡. ***(35-43B)*** *DWI MR shows mild symmetric restricted diffusion in the BG and thalami and striking symmetric restricted diffusion in the occipital cortices* ➡.

held over the nose and mouth), and "bagging" (inhalation from a plastic bag). Solvent abuse is particularly prevalent among adolescents and young adults.

Imaging abnormalities are typically seen only after several years of chronic inhalant abuse. Diffuse WM lesions are seen in nearly 1/2 of all patients, initially seen as T2/FLAIR hyperintensity in the deep periventricular WM with subsequent spread into the centrum semiovale and subcortical areas. The internal capsule, cerebellum, and pons are often affected **(35-41)**.

## Cyanide Poisoning

Cyanide (CN) exists in gas, solid, and liquid form. CN poisoning can occur by inhalation, ingestion, or transdermal absorption **(35-42)**. Combustion of many common materials releases a combination of carbon dioxide, carbon monoxide, and hydrogen CN. Cyanogenic compounds are also found in some foods, including almonds, stone fruit pits, lima beans, and cassava root.

Patients who survive the initial insult show symmetric hyperintensity in the basal ganglia and linear cortical hyperintensity on T2WI and FLAIR **(35-43)**. Sodium nitrite ($NaNO_2$) is a universal antidote, although its use has serious safety drawbacks.

The most important differential diagnosis of CN poisoning is **HIE**. It may complicate CN poisoning. CN poisoning usually spares the hippocampi, but other features often overlap because the basal ganglia are affected in both disorders.

### INHALED GASES AND TOXINS

**Carbon Monoxide Poisoning**
- Acute: Symmetric globi pallidi necrosis
- Subacute ("interval"): Confluent leukoencephalopathy

**Nitrous Oxide Abuse**
- Brain lesions rare
- Subacute combined degeneration of spinal cord
  - Hyperintensity in dorsal columns

**Toluene (Solvent) Abuse**
- Chronic, repeated use
  - Atrophy, WM lesions
  - Thalami, substantia nigra, red nuclei, dentate lesions

**Cyanide Poisoning**
- Suicide, smoke inhalation
- Basal ganglia hemorrhage, necrosis
- Laminar cortical necrosis

# Metal Poisoning and Toxicity

A variety of metals can cause serious neurologic dysfunction when deposited in excess amounts in the CNS. **Manganese** accumulation is most common in the setting of chronic liver failure (see Chapter 37). Other environmental toxins, such as **lead** and **mercury**, are rare causes of neurotoxicity.

Gadolinium-based contrast agents (GBCAs) have been used routinely in clinical neuroimaging for nearly 30 years. **Gadolinium** brain deposition is now an increasingly common cause of heavy metal toxicity.

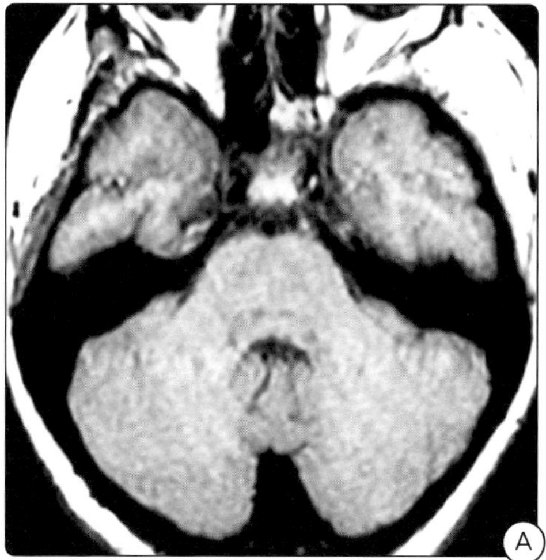


***(35-44A)** Baseline axial T1 MR through the 4th ventricle in a patient with multiple meningiomatosis shows no abnormalities.*

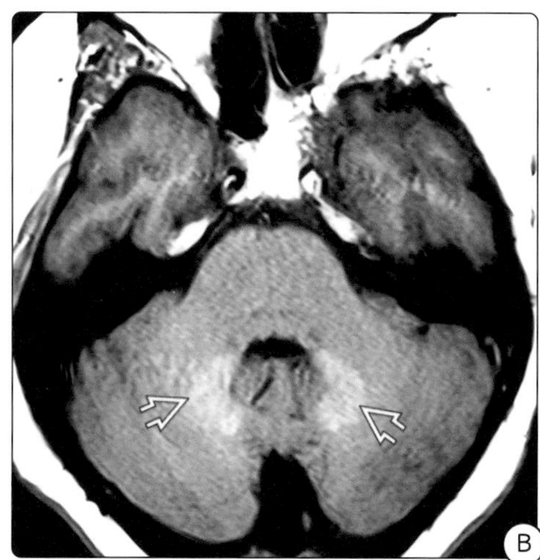


***(35-44B)** After 30+ contrast-enhanced MRs over 15 years, T1 MR shows symmetric hyperintensity in both dentate nuclei ➡.*

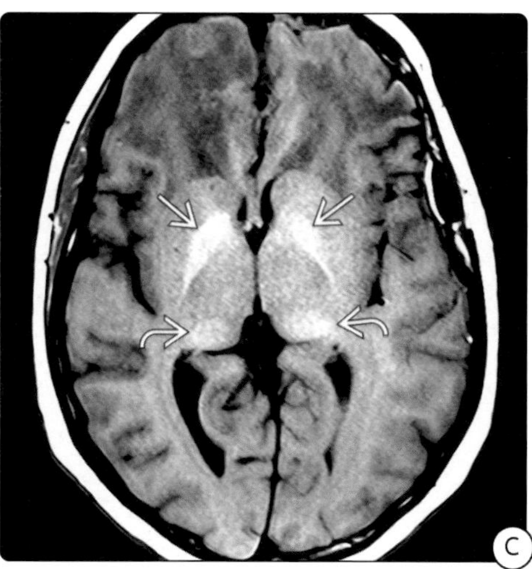


***(35-44C)** Symmetric hyperintensity is present in GP ➡ and thalami ➡. Gadolinium deposition is from repeated use of GBCAs.*

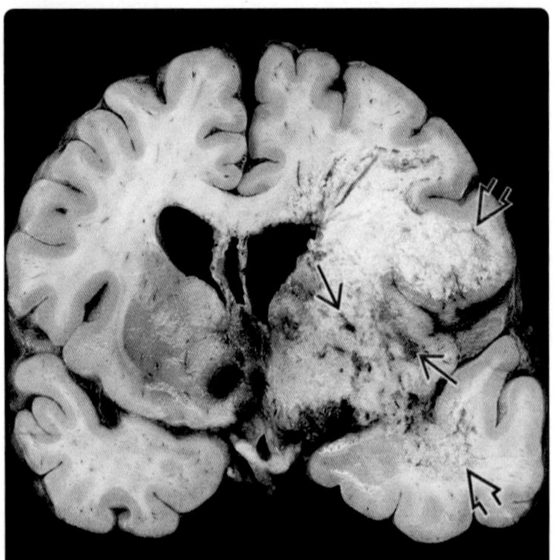

**(35-45)** *Autopsy shows XRT-induced necrotizing leukoencephalopathy ⇒, hemorrhagic vascular malformations →. (Courtesy R. Hewlett, MD.)*

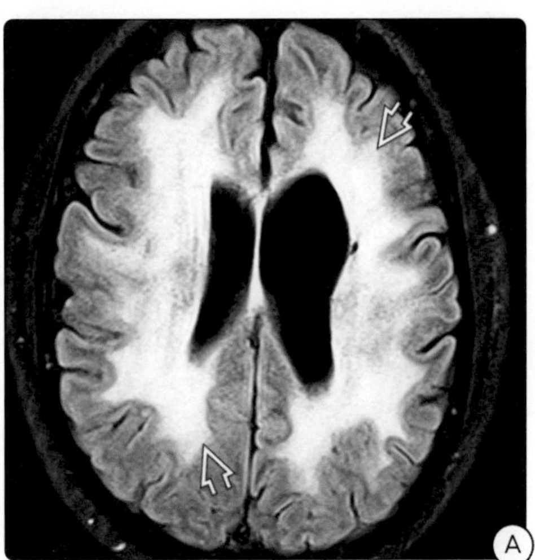

**(35-46A)** *FLAIR MR in a patient with cognitive decline 3 years after whole-brain XRT for leukemia shows confluent WM hyperintensity ⇒.*

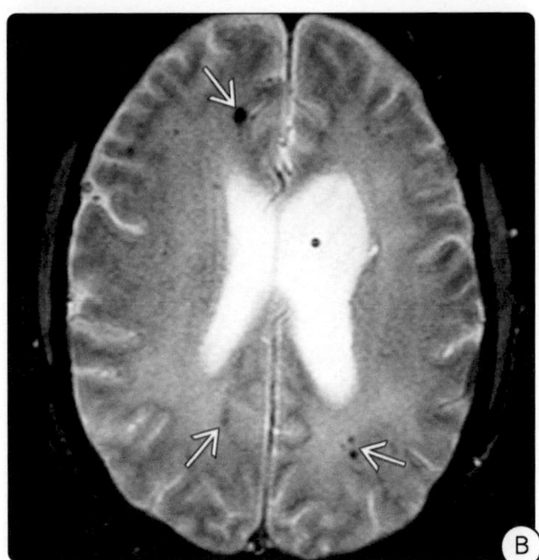

**(35-46B)** *T2* MR shows multiple foci of gradient "blooming" →, necrotizing leukoencephalopathy with XRT-induced vascular malformations.*

## Gadolinium Deposition

### Gadolinium Physiology

Gadolinium is a rare earth heavy metal in the lanthanide series. Its seven unpaired electrons induce a strong paramagnetic effect, reflected in its widespread use for contrast-enhanced MR sequences. Free gadolinium is extremely toxic so various chelating ligands are used to avoid the adverse effects of free gadolinium. Gadolinium in the blood must remain in chelated form until it is excreted by the kidneys. GBCAs are drained from the CSF through olfactory nerves via the "glymphatic" system.

### Gadolinium-Based Contrast Agents

GBCAs are divided into two categories: Linear and macrocyclic. In macrocyclic molecules, free gadolinium is isolated within the cage-like structure of the ligand agent. Ionic agents are chemically more stable than nonionic agents because the donor chelates are stronger in ionic agents. Laboratory evidence has shown that retained gadolinium from linear GBCAs is 10x higher than with macrocyclic GBCAs.

Life-threatening adverse reactions to GBCA are very rare. Potentially lethal nephrogenic systemic fibrosis (NSF) due to GBCA use in patients with renal failure were first described in 2006.

### GBCA Brain Deposition

Dechelation of free gadolinium from an intact GBCA is the initial step in the mechanism of gadolinium deposition in the brain. GBCA brain deposition was first reported in 2014, and investigators have confirmed the association of repeated administration of GBCAs and high T1 signal intensity in the dentate nucleus and globi pallidi **(35-44)**. These iron-rich areas are the same sites specifically affected by neurodegenerative disorders with iron and manganese accumulation, namely the dentate nucleus, globus pallidus interna, and pulvinar of the thalamus. Signal intensity change seems to be significantly related to the use of linear agents, although low levels of deposition have also been recently reported with macrocyclic contrast agents.

To date, there is no strong evidence for harmful CNS effects of retained GBCAs, although elevated concentrations of Cr, lactate, and lipids without altered levels of NAA and choline have been reported in the dentate nuclei using MRS. Many clinical practices now exclusively utilize macrocyclic GBCAs except in rare cases (e.g., prior allergic reaction).

# Treatment-Related Disorders

A comprehensive treatment of all iatrogenic abnormalities in the brain is far beyond the scope of this text. Here, we discuss the most common disorders with a focus on treatment effects that must be recognized on imaging studies, namely radiation and chemotherapy.

## Radiation Injury

Many investigators divide radiation-induced injury (RII) into three temporal phases: Acute (early) injury, early delayed injury, and late delayed injury. Pathologically, radiation injury varies from mild transient vasogenic edema to frank necrosis **(35-45)**. The damage that results from XRT depends on a number of variables, including total dose, field size, number/frequency/fractionation of doses, and whether chemotherapy is used in conjunction with XRT.

Vascular endothelial cells, oligodendrocytes, astrocytes, microglia, and neurons probably all interact in the brain's response to radiation injury. Oligodendrocytes are especially vulnerable.

## Acute Radiation Injury

Acute RII occurs days to weeks after irradiation and is very rarely encountered with modern XRT regimens. Standard imaging studies are usually normal, although MRS, DTI, and fMRI may detect changes before neurocognitive symptoms or anatomic alterations emerge. Occasionally, transient WM edema can be seen on T2/FLAIR sequences. Enhancement is absent.

## Early Delayed Radiation Injury

In early delayed RII, imaging abnormalities can be detected as early as 1-6 months after XRT is completed. Early delayed RII is characterized pathologically by transient demyelination and clinically by somnolence, attention deficits, and short-term memory loss.

Confluent hypodense areas on NECT and periventricular WM hyperintensity on T2/FLAIR are typical abnormalities. Patchy areas of non-mass-like gray matter enhancement may appear. At this stage, RII changes are generally mild and reversible, often resolving spontaneously.

## Late Delayed Radiation Injury

Late delayed RII is usually not observed until at least 6 months post irradiation. These late delayed injuries are viewed as progressive and largely irreversible, resulting from loss of glial and vascular endothelial cells.

Coagulative necrosis in a mosaic pattern with coalescing foci produces a necrotizing leukoencephalopathy in the deep cerebral WM. The subcortical association or U-fibers and corpus callosum are typically spared **(35-46A)**. Vascular changes include fibrinoid necrosis, hyalinization, and sclerosis with thrombosis. Late delayed radiation necrosis is initially expansile and mass-like with necrosis largely confined to WM.

Initially, late delayed RII shows mass-like areas of necrosis, often with irregular peripheral "feathery" enhancement surrounded by coalescent WM hyperintensity. Later, foci of volume loss, WM spongiosis with confluent hyperintensity, and dystrophic calcifications can be seen **(35-46)**.

## Long-Term Sequelae of Radiation Injury

In addition to **necrotizing leukoencephalopathy**, long-term complications of XRT include vasculopathy, mineralizing microangiopathy, telangiectasis (XRT-induced vascular malformations) **(35-49)**, and radiation-induced neoplasms.

**Radiation-induced vasculopathy** with endothelial hyperplasia results in diffusely narrowed large and medium-sized arteries. Ischemic strokes and moyamoya-like disease may result **(35-47)**.

**Mineralizing microangiopathy** is usually seen in patients treated with combination XRT and chemotherapy and generally does not appear until at least two years following treatment. Calcifications in the basal ganglia and subcortical WM are typical findings **(35-48)**.

**Radiation-induced vascular malformations** (RIVMs) are primarily capillary telangiectasias or cavernous malformations most commonly seen in children who have received whole-brain radiotherapy for acute lymphoblastic leukemia. T2* (GRE, SWI) sequences demonstrate "blooming" microhemorrhages in the majority of patients **(35-46B)**. RIVMs rarely occur

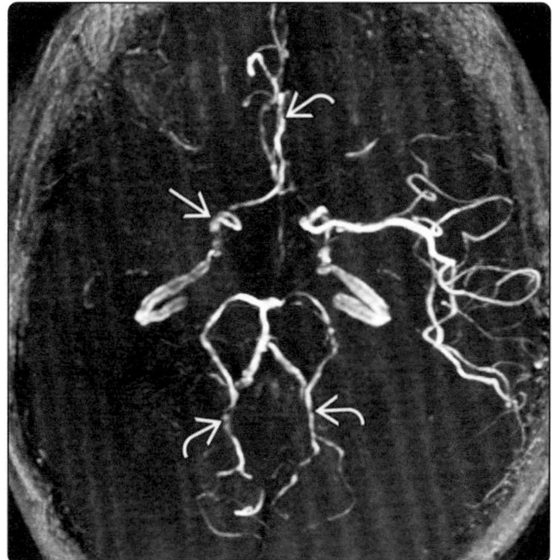

***(35-47)** MRA years after XRT shows postradiation vasculopathy ➡, right MCA occlusion ➡. (Courtesy P. Hildenbrand, MD.)*

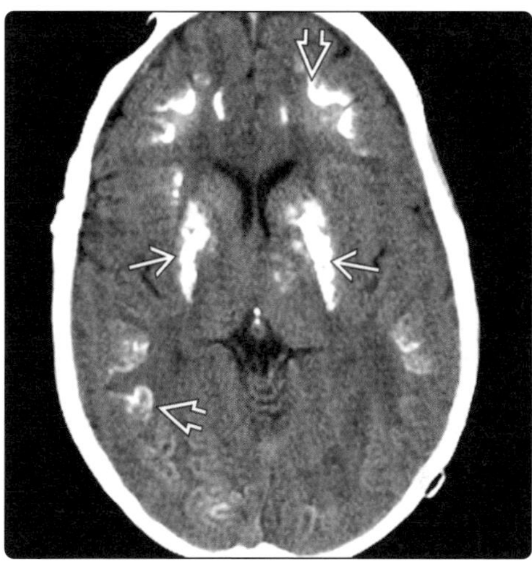

***(35-48)** NECT years after XRT/chemo shows BG ➡, subcortical WM $Ca^{++}$ ➡ of mineralizing microangiopathy. (Courtesy P. Chapman, MD.)*

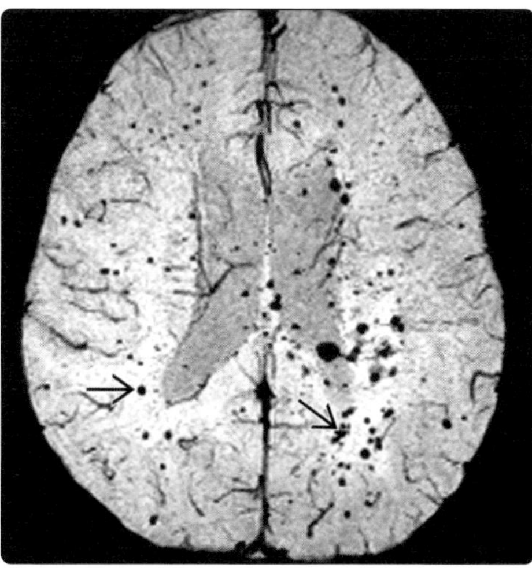

***(35-49)** SWI years after whole-brain radiation shows multiple "blooming" hypointense foci ➡, characteristic of capillary telangiectasias.*

more than three years following XRT. Children under 10 years of age at the time of irradiation are at higher risk.

**Radiation-induced neoplasms** are rare but often devastating. XRT is the single most important risk factor for developing a new primary CNS neoplasm. Approximately 70% are meningiomas, 20% are malignant astrocytomas or medulloblastomas, and 10% are sarcomas. Meningiomas occur an average of 17-20 years after treatment, whereas gliomas occur at a mean of nine years. Sarcomas have a mean latency of seven or eight years following XRT.

### RADIATION-INDUCED BRAIN INJURY

**Pathology**
- Microglial activation; proinflammatory cytokines

**3 Phases of Radiation-Induced Injury**
- Acute radiation injury
  - Rare
  - T2/FLAIR may show WM edema
  - TSPO-PET may show neuroinflammation
- Early delayed injury (at least 6 months)
  - Necrotizing leukoencephalopathy
  - Confluent hyperintensity
- Long-term sequelae
  - Necrotizing leukoencephalopathy
  - Vasculopathy, mineralizing microangiopathy
  - Vascular malformations (T2* "black dots")
  - Radiation-induced neoplasms

## Chemotherapy Effects

Currently, the most common chemotherapy agents implicated in CNS toxicity are methotrexate, cytarabine, vincristine, asparaginase, and corticosteroids. Unlike radiation injury, chemotherapy-associated acute toxic CNS injury is common. The two most frequent abnormalities are posterior reversible encephalopathy syndrome and treatment-induced leukoencephalopathy.

**Posterior reversible encephalopathy syndrome** (PRES) is addressed in detail in Chapter 37. In chemotherapy-related PRES, imaging findings are often atypical. The occipital lobes are frequently spared, whereas the cerebellum, brainstem, and basal ganglia are frequently involved. Hemorrhage, contrast enhancement, and diffusion restriction—all relatively rare in "typical" PRES—are common.

**Treatment-induced leukoencephalopathy** is especially common in patients treated with methotrexate. Acute neurotoxicity occurs in 5-18% of children treated for acute lymphoblastic leukemia. Bilateral, relatively symmetric, confluent areas of T2/FLAIR hyperintensity in the periventricular WM are typical. Imaging abnormalities typically resolve after treatment.

**Transient lesions of the corpus callosum splenium** with acute neurologic symptoms have also been reported with antineoplastic agents, both without and with accompanying lesions in the hemispheric WM. The lesions reversed after discontinuation of treatment.

### CHEMOTHERAPY EFFECTS ON THE BRAIN

**Clinical Issues**
- Acute effects common; often reversible

**Imaging**
- PRES common
  - Atypical > typical imaging findings
  - Occipital lobes often spared
  - Hemorrhage, enhancement, restricted diffusion common
- Acute leukoencephalopathy
  - Reflects acute neurotoxicity
  - Transient T2/FLAIR periventricular hyperintensity

*Selected References: The complete reference list is available on the eBooks+ version included with purchase.*

# Inherited Metabolic Disorders

***Inherited metabolic disorders**—a.k.a. **inborn errors of metabolism**—represent conditions in which a genetic defect leads to a deficiency of a protein (e.g., enzyme or nonenzyme protein) that subsequently affects mechanisms of synthesis, degradation, transport, &/or storage of molecules in the body. Inherited metabolic disorders can present at virtually any age from infancy well into the fifth and sixth decades, although infantile and childhood presentation are most common.*



Inherited metabolic disorders (IMDs) are relatively uncommon diseases. The informed radiologist can merge their understanding of the pathogenetic and pathomorphologic underpinnings of the various IMDs with imaging observations. Specifically, we observe *what part of the brain is involved* [e.g., gray matter (GM) vs. white matter (WM)], *what kind of involvement is present* (e.g., cortex, basal ganglia, WM—subcortical, deep, or periventricular), and *what locations are most affected* (e.g., frontal lobes). Additional information, such as the presence of cysts, calcifications, diffusion restriction, and pathologic enhancement, aids in crystallizing the imaging differential diagnosis.

Because WM abnormalities form a constant part of many, if not most, **inborn metabolic diseases**, familiarization with the normal progression of WM myelination is a prerequisite for detecting and understanding IMDs. We therefore begin this chapter with a brief review of how normal myelination progresses from birth through two years of life.

Once we have reviewed the patterns of normal myelination as assessed with MR, we continue with an overview and introduction of the IMDs. A discussion of classification systems and a practical approach to analyzing imaging is delineated. A detailed discussion of the leukodystrophies and nonleukodystrophic WM disorders is beyond the scope of this text, but selected IMDs representative of their groupings will be presented.

# Normal Myelination and White Matter Development

## General Considerations

### Myelination

Myelination is an orderly, highly regulated, multistep process that begins during the fifth fetal month and is largely complete by 18-24 postnatal

## Selected Myelination Milestones

| Age | T1 Hyperintensity | T2 Hypointensity |
|---|---|---|
| **Birth** | | |
| | Dorsal brainstem | Dorsal brainstem |
| | Posterior limb IC | Partial posterior limb IC |
| | Perirolandic gyri | Perirolandic gyri |
| | Corticospinal tracts | Corticospinal tracts |
| **3-4 Months** | | |
| | Ventral brainstem | Posterior limb IC |
| | Anterior limb IC | |
| | CC splenium | |
| | Central, posterior corona radiata | |
| **6 Months** | | |
| | Cerebellar WM | Ventral brainstem |
| | CC genu | Anterior limb IC |
| | Parietal, occipital WM | CC splenium, genu by 8-9 months |
| | Frontal WM by 9 months | |
| **12 Months** | | |
| | Posterior fossa (≈ adult) | Most of corona radiata |
| | Most of corona radiata | Posterior subcortical WM |
| | Posterior subcortical WM | Occipital WM |
| **18 Months** | | |
| | All WM except temporal, frontal U-fibers | All WM except temporal, frontal U-fibers, occipital radiations |
| **24 Months** | | |
| | Anterior temporal, frontal U-fibers | Anterior temporal, orbital frontal U-fibers |

***(Table 36-1)*** *CC = corpus callosum; IC = internal capsule; WM = white matter. WM maturation is seen earlier on T1WI.*

months. Some structures (e.g., cranial nerves) myelinate relatively early in fetal development, whereas others (e.g., optic radiations and fibers to/from association areas) often do not completely myelinate until the third or even the fourth decade of life.

Brain myelination follows a typical topographic pattern, progressing from **inferior to superior, central to peripheral**, and **posterior to anterior**. For example, the brainstem myelinates before the peripheral cerebellar hemispheres, the posterior limbs of the internal capsules myelinate before the anterior limbs, and the deep periventricular WM myelinates before the subcortical U-fibers. The dorsal brainstem myelinates before the anterior brainstem, and—with the exception of the parietooccipital association tracts—occipital WM myelinates earlier than WM in the anterior temporal and frontal lobes.

## CT

At birth, the WM is largely unmyelinated, so it appears symmetrically hypoattenuating compared with regional GM due to the comparatively high water content of unmyelinated WM.

## MR

The MR appearance of WM maturation varies with two important factors, i.e., **patient age** and the **imaging sequence** employed. Unmyelinated WM is hypointense relative to GM on T1WI and hyperintense to GM on T2WI.

As WM matures, it becomes more hyperintense on T1WI. Progressive T2 shortening (hypointensity) occurs in the first two years of life as myelin matures and proton density decreases.

During the first 6-8 months, T1 hyperintensity occurs earlier and is more conspicuous than T2 hypointensity, so T1WIs are best to evaluate both WM maturation and brain morphology **(36-1)** **(36-2)**. Heavily weighted T2 sequences are sensitive to follow WM maturation between 6-18 months. Fully myelinated WM has high T1 signal and low T2 signal.

Selected major milestones of normal myelination on T1- and T2-weighted images are summarized in the accompanying table **(Table 36-1)**.

# Classification of Inherited Metabolic Disorders

## Overview

An exhaustive discussion of IMDs is far beyond the scope of this book. The interested reader is referred to the superb definitive texts by A. James Barkovich. In this chapter, we consider the major inherited neurometabolic diseases, summarizing the pathoetiology, genetics, demographics, clinical presentation, and key imaging findings of each.

There are several strategies that can be used to conceptually frame IMDs. One way is to divide IMDs according to which cellular organelle (e.g., mitochondria, lysosomes) is predominantly affected. Another characterizes them by defects in a specific metabolic pathway (e.g., disorders of carbohydrate metabolism). However, these methods lack the pragmatic approach needed by the radiologist to be a contributing member of the clinical care team. We therefore emphasize—and advocate the use of—an approach to imaging analysis pioneered by A. James Barkovich that is primarily based on anatomic location and specific imaging features with an emphasis on MR—the **imaging-based approach**.

## Organelle-Based Approach

Three cellular organelles are primarily affected in IMDs, i.e., the lysosomes, peroxisomes, and mitochondria. Classifying IMDs according to the affected organelle has the benefit of conceptual simplicity, but many IMDs do not arise from disordered organelle formation or function, making this classification scheme less than comprehensive. The organelle-based approach to IMDs is summarized in the accompanying box.

**ORGANELLE-BASED CLASSIFICATION OF INHERITED METABOLIC DISORDERS**

**Lysosomal Disorders**
- Mucopolysaccharidoses
- Gangliosidoses
- Metachromatic leukodystrophy
- Krabbe disease
- Fabry disease

**Peroxisomal Disorders**
- Abnormal peroxisomal formation
  - Zellweger syndrome
  - Neonatal adrenoleukodystrophy
  - Infantile Refsum disease
- Abnormal peroxisomal function
  - X-linked adrenoleukodystrophy
  - Classic Refsum disease

**Mitochondrial Disorders**
- Leigh syndrome
- **M**itochondrial **e**ncephalomyopathy with **l**actic **a**cidosis and **s**troke-like episodes (MELAS)
- **M**yoclonic **e**pilepsy with **r**agged **r**ed **f**ibers (MERRF)
- Kearns-Sayre
- Glutaric aciduria types 1 and 2

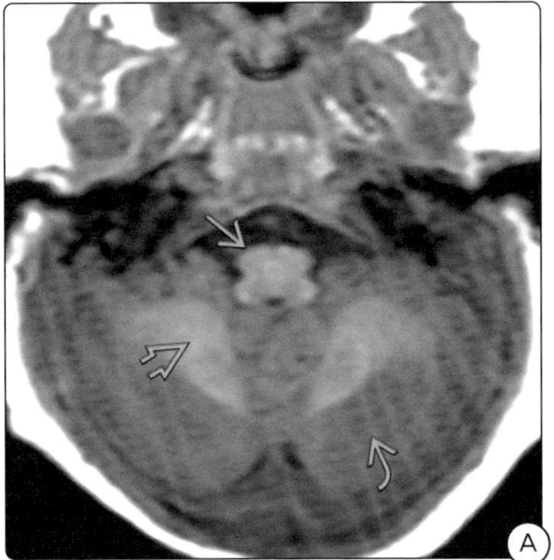


***(36-1A)** T1WI at 4 months shows hyperintense medulla ➙, deep cerebellar WM ➙, while peripheral unmyelinated WM is hypointense ➙.*

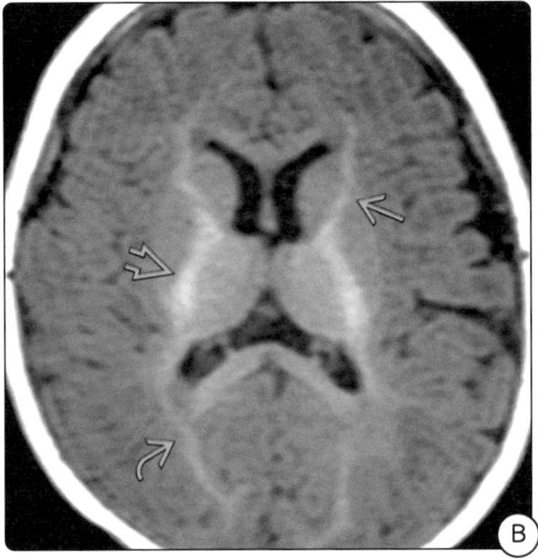


***(36-1B)** T1 MR shows normal T1 shortening in PLIC ➙, subtle in ALIC ➙. The optic radiation WM is beginning to myelinate ➙.*

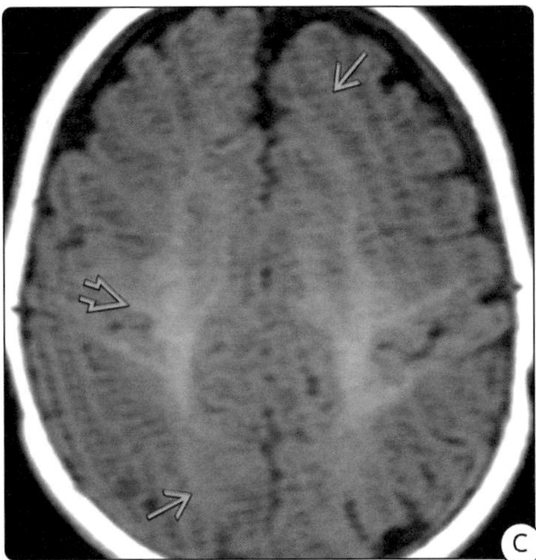


***(36-1C)** T1 MR shows myelin in the perirolandic region ➙, but more anterior and posterior corona radiata remains unmyelinated ➙.*

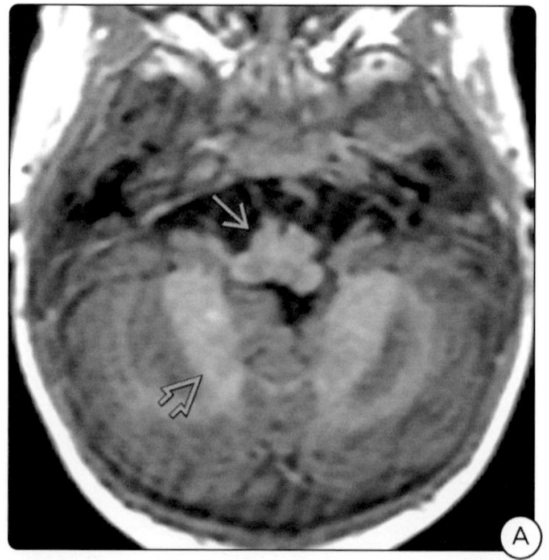

(36-2A) T1 MR at 8 months shows near-complete myelination of the brainstem ➡ and cerebellar hemispheres ➡.

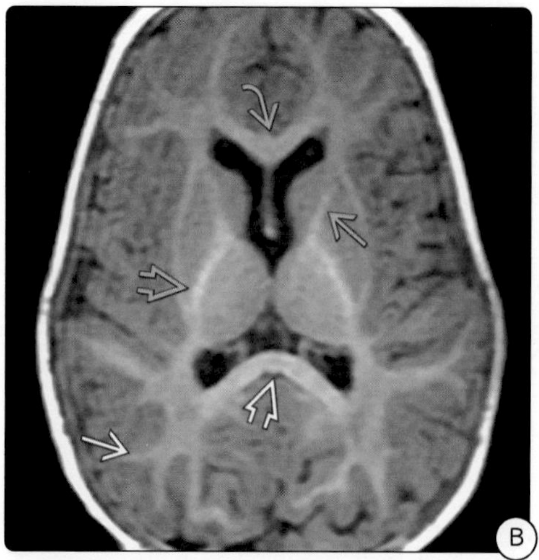

(36-2B) T1 MR shows myelinated WM in PLIC ➡, ALIC ➡, callosal splenium ➡, genu ➡. Subcortical WM is partially myelinated ➡.

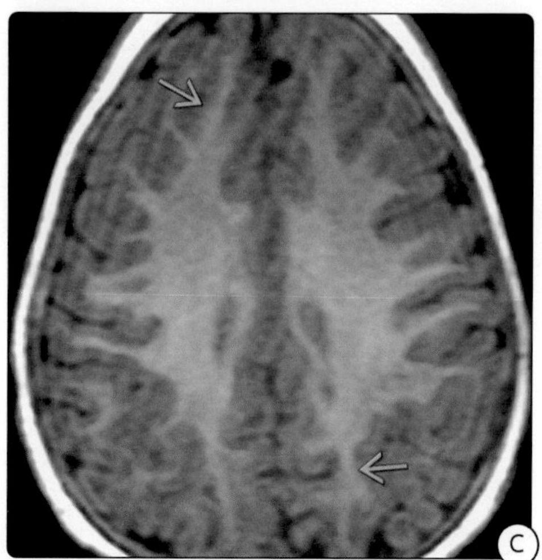

(36-2C) T1 MR shows hyperintensity extends to subcortical WM, especially parietal, occipital lobes ➡; striking change compared to 4 months.

## Imaging-Based Approach

Barkovich et al have elaborated a practical imaging-based approach to the diagnosis of IMDs derived from the seminal work of van der Knaap and Valk. This approach is based on determining whether the disease involves primarily or exclusively (1) WM, (2) mostly GM, or (3) both. Furthermore, a heightened awareness of the region of the brain most heavily involved (e.g., periventricular WM vs. subcortical WM or frontal lobe vs. parietal occipital lobes) and the presence of miscellaneous findings (e.g., cysts &/or calcifications) leads to greater specificity.

In this text, we follow the **imaging-based approach**, the clinically practical classification based on three categories of predominant imaging features (e.g., WM, GM, or both being involved). We then discuss the major diagnostic entities in each imaging-based group.

# Inherited Metabolic Disorders Predominantly Affecting White Matter

Historically, nearly all abnormalities of the WM have been described as "leukodystrophies." *Leukodystrophies* have been divided into three categories: (1) *Dys*myelinating disorders (i.e., normal myelination does not occur), (2) *de*myelinating disease (i.e., myelin forms normally, is deposited around axons, but later breaks down or is destroyed), and (3) *hypo*myelinating diseases (i.e., here, the WM may partially myelinate but never myelinates completely). Hypomyelinating leukoencephalopathies represent an important yet uncommon group of genetic disorders that cause delayed myelin maturation or undermyelination.

From an imaging perspective, it can be difficult to determine whether a disorder is *dys*myelinating, *de*myelinating, or *hypo*myelinating. In structuring a differential diagnosis, it is important to determine whether the disorder primarily affects *deep* (periventricular) WM or the *subcortical* short association WM fibers (U-fibers). In a few diseases, both the deep and peripheral WM are affected.

Examples of leukodystrophies that exhibit early *deep* WM predominance include metachromatic leukodystrophy (MLD) and X-linked adrenoleukodystrophy (X-ALD). Leukodystrophies that involve the *subcortical* U-fibers early in the disease course include megaloencephalic leukoencephalopathy with cysts and infantile Alexander disease (AxD). The latter two diagnoses also present with a large head.

Diseases in which virtually *all* the WM (both periventricular *and* subcortical) remains unmyelinated are rare. The imaging appearance in these disorders resembles that of a normal newborn brain with immature, almost completely unmyelinated, WM. Here, the entire WM—including the subcortical U-fibers—appears uniformly hyperintense on T2WI.

## Hypomyelinating Disorders

The list of hypomyelinating disorders is long and beyond the scope of this book, but it is worth being aware of the imaging findings that may accompany such disorders. The prototypical hypomyelinating disorder is **Pelizaeus-Merzbacher disease (PMD)**, which may result in complete lack of myelination or hypomyelination, depending on severity.

### Pelizaeus-Merzbacher Disease

#### Etiology

Caused by a mutation in *PLP1*, which codes for proteolipid protein 1 and DM20, two primary components of myelin.

#### Clinical Issues

The classic form is X-linked. A more severe "connatal" form presents earlier and generally has a more severe clinical course. Patients usually present in the first year of life. Symptoms include nystagmus, delayed cognitive and motor development, and ataxia.

#### Imaging

CT typically shows decreased attenuation throughout the WM.

MR shows absent or significantly reduced myelination for age with lack of bright T1 signal and dark T2 signal that would be expected with normal myelination **(36-3)**. In milder forms, there may be some degree of myelination in the internal capsules and optic radiations. Cerebellar atrophy may be present.

#### Differential Diagnosis

Primary differential diagnosis includes other hypomyelinating disorders, such as **18q syndrome, fucosidosis**, and **Tay syndrome**, among others. In very young patients, it is important to know the gestational age so as not to mistake the normal brain appearance of **prematurity** for lack of myelination.

## Periventricular White Matter Predominance

The prototypical disorder that typically begins with symmetric deep WM involvement and spares the subcortical U-fibers until late in the disease course is MLD. Others with a similar pattern of periventricular predominance include Krabbe disease (globoid cell leukodystrophy), X-ALD, and vanishing WM disease (VWMD).

**MAJOR INHERITED METABOLIC DISORDERS WITH PERIVENTRICULAR WHITE MATTER PREDOMINANCE**

**Common**
- Metachromatic leukodystrophy
- Classic X-linked adrenoleukodystrophy

**Less Common**
- Globoid cell leukodystrophy (Krabbe disease)
- Vanishing WM disease

**Rare but Important**
- Phenylketonuria
- Maple syrup urine disease
- Merosin-deficient congenital muscular dystrophy

### Metachromatic Leukodystrophy

**Etiology.** MLD is a devastating lysosomal storage disease caused by a reduction in or complete absence of arylsulfatase A (ARSA). Reduced or absent ARSA leads to increased lysosomal storage of sulfatide and, eventually, lethal demyelination.

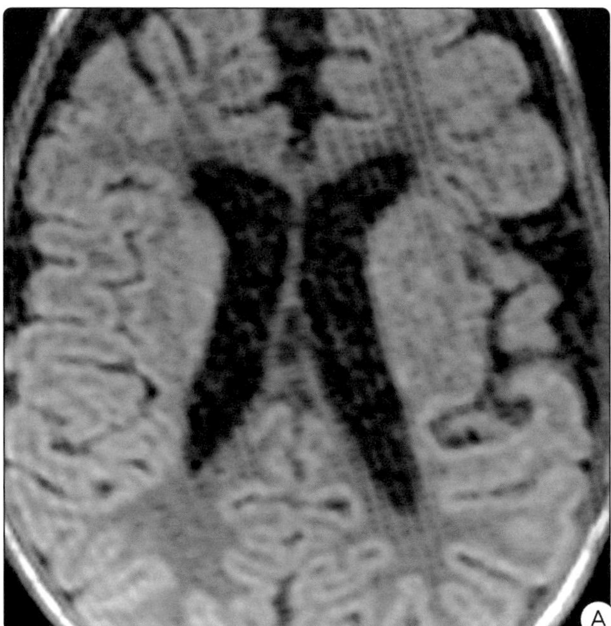

***(36-3A)** Axial T1 in a 3-yo with PMD shows complete absence of myelinated WM. There is an inversion of the normal GM-WM signal intensities for a patient of this age.*

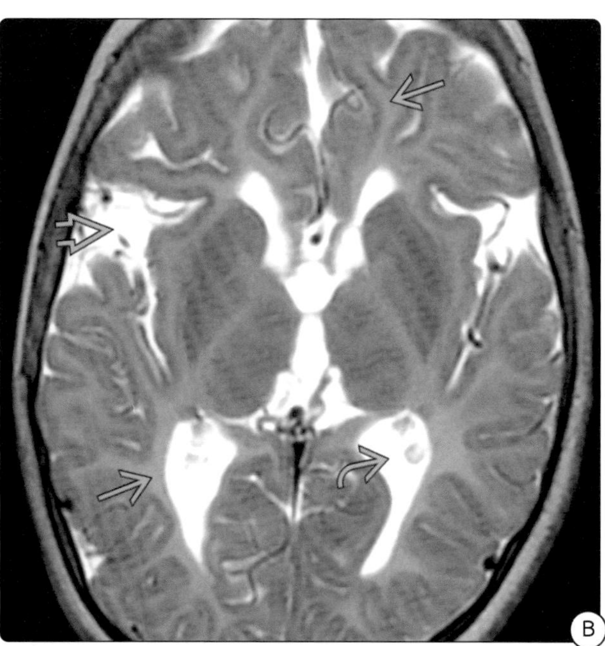

***(36-3B)** Axial T2 in the same patient shows diffusely bright WM ➡ due to absence of myelin. Also note some overall WM volume loss with resultant ventricular ➡ and subarachnoid space ➡ enlargement.*

**Pathology.** Sulfatide deposition occurs within glial cells, plasma membranes, inner layer of myelin sheath, neurons, Schwann cells, and macrophages. The periventricular WM shows a grayish discoloration (e.g., tigroid or leopard pattern) with relatively normal-appearing subcortical U-fibers.

**Clinical Issues.** MLD is one of the most common of all inherited WM disorders. Three distinct clinical forms are currently recognized: Late infantile (onset earlier than three years), juvenile (onset earlier than 16 years), and adult MLD. The *late infantile form* is the most common and typically presents in the second year of life with visuomotor impairment, gait disorder, and abdominal pain. Progressive decline and death within four years are expected. The *juvenile form* presents between 5-10 years, often with deteriorating school performance. Survival beyond 20 years is rare. The *adult form* may present with early-onset dementia, MS-like symptoms, and progressive cerebellar signs.

### Imaging

***CT Findings.*** Early NECT shows symmetric diminished attenuation involving the central hemispheric WM **(36-4)**.

***MR Findings.*** The typical MR features of early MLD are confluent, symmetric, butterfly-shaped T2/FLAIR hyperintensities involving the periventricular WM **(36-8)**. The subcortical U-fibers and cerebellum are typically spared until late in the disease.

With disease progression, centrifugal spread of demyelination involves the corpus callosum (i.e., splenium), parietooccipital WM, and the frontal and then the temporal WM. Islands of normal myelin around medullary veins in the WM may produce a striking tiger, tigroid, or leopard pattern with linear hypointensities in a sea of confluent hyperintensity **(36-5)** **(36-6)**. WM signal abnormalities show no enhancement. Another important finding of MLD is cranial nerve enhancement, which is often striking **(36-7)**.

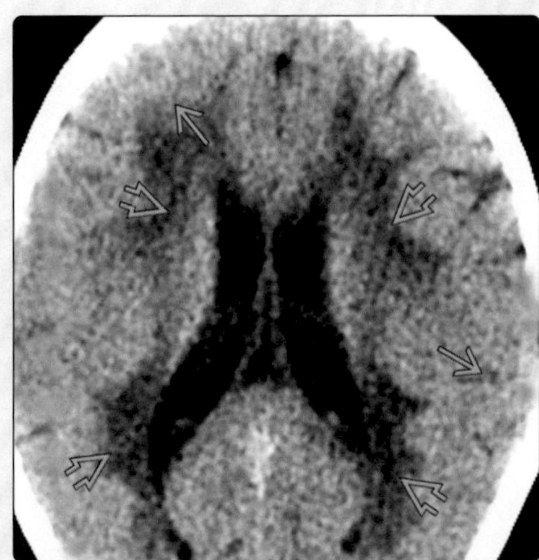

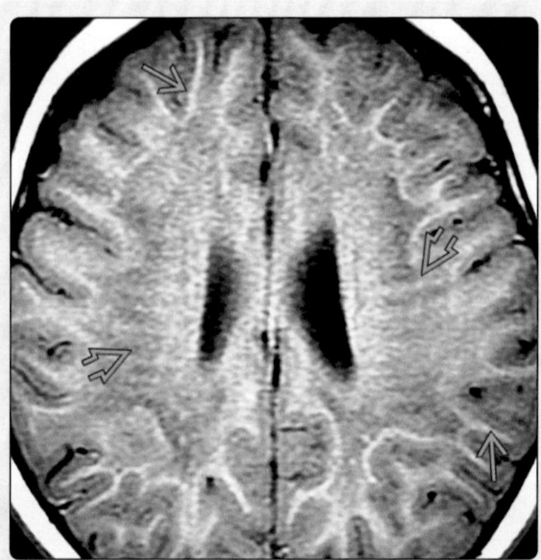

***(36-4)** Axial NECT in a 6-yo boy with MLD shows periventricular WM hypoattenuation ⇒. The subcortical U-fibers ⇒ are spared. **(36-5)** Axial T1 MR shows MLD in a 2-yo boy with sparing of U-fibers ⇒. The tigroid pattern ⇒ arises from preserved areas of myelin surrounding venules, which appear as stripes in the background of WM myelin destruction.*

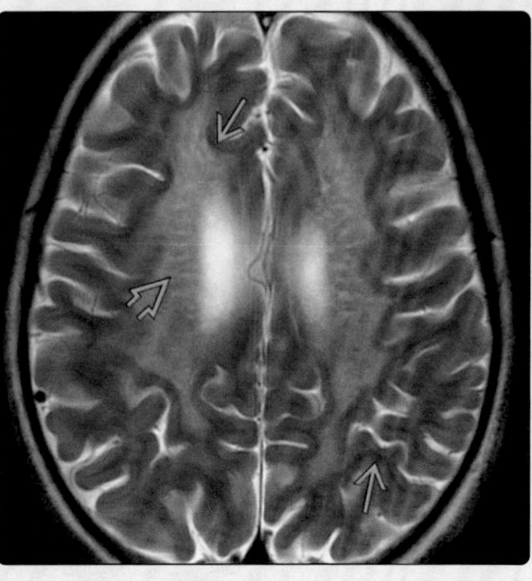

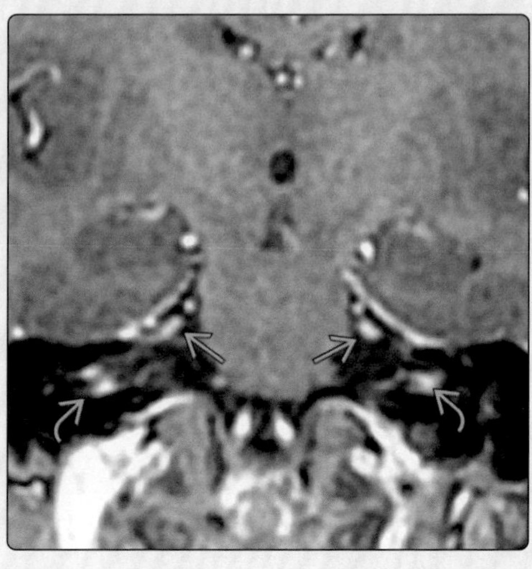

***(36-6)** Axial T2 MR in a 10-yo with MLD shows the typical striped pattern ⇒ of WM involvement with sparing of the subcortical U-fibers ⇒. Early in the disease process, the U-fibers are spared but become involved later. **(36-7)** Coronal T1 C+ MR in a 2-yo with MLD shows avid enhancement of the CNV ⇒ and CNVII and VIII ⇒ within the internal auditory canals. Enhancing cranial nerves are an important finding to suggest a diagnosis of MLD.*

**METACHROMATIC LEUKODYSTROPHY**

**Etiology and Pathology**
- Lysosomal storage disorder
- Decreased ARSA → sphingolipid accumulation
- Periventricular demyelination

**Clinical Issues**
- Most common inherited leukodystrophy
- 3 forms
  - Late infantile (most common)
  - Juvenile
  - Adult (late onset)

**Imaging**
- Centrifugal spread of demyelination
  - Starts in corpus callosum splenium, deep parietooccipital white matter
  - Frontal, temporal white matter affected later
  - Spares subcortical U-fibers, cerebellum
- Classic = butterfly pattern
  - Symmetric hyperintensities around frontal horns, atria
- Tiger pattern
  - "Stripes" of perivenular myelin sparing in white matter

**Differential Diagnosis**
- Other disorders that predominantly affect periventricular white matter
  - Globoid cell leukodystrophy (Krabbe disease)
  - Pelizaeus-Merzbacher disease
  - Vanishing white matter disease
- Destructive disorders
  - Periventricular leukomalacia

***Miscellaneous Imaging.*** Reduction of diffusivity in zones of active demyelination is seen. Regions of "burned-out," aging or chronic demyelination demonstrate increased diffusivity. MRS is nonspecific; choline and myoinositol may be elevated in early and active disease.

**Differential Diagnosis.** The major differential diagnosis of MLD includes other IMDs that primarily affect the periventricular WM. Globoid cell leukoencephalopathy **(Krabbe disease)** shows bithalamic hyperattenuation on NECT, involves the cerebellum early, and often demonstrates enlarged optic nerves and optic chiasm.

**PMD** usually presents in neonates and shows almost a total lack of myelination that does not show interval improvement on serial MRs. The cerebellum may be markedly atrophic.

**Periventricular WM injury (PVL)** is associated with a history of low-birth-weight/preterm deliveries and clinical static spastic di- or quadriparesis and shows nonprogressive periventricular volume loss and T2/FLAIR hyperintensity.

**VWMD** begins in the periventricular WM but eventually involves all of the hemispheric WM. VWMD often cavitates and does not enhance.

## X-Linked Adrenoleukodystrophy

**Etiology.** X-ALD is an inherited disorder of peroxisomal metabolism. Absent or deficient acyl-CoA synthetase leads to impaired oxidation of very-long-chain fatty acids (VLCFAs). VLCFAs accumulate in the WM, causing severe inflammatory demyelination ("brittle" myelin). Axonal degeneration in the posterior fossa and spinal cord are also typical of the disease. The definitive diagnosis of X-ALD is established by tissue assays for increased amounts of VLCFAs.

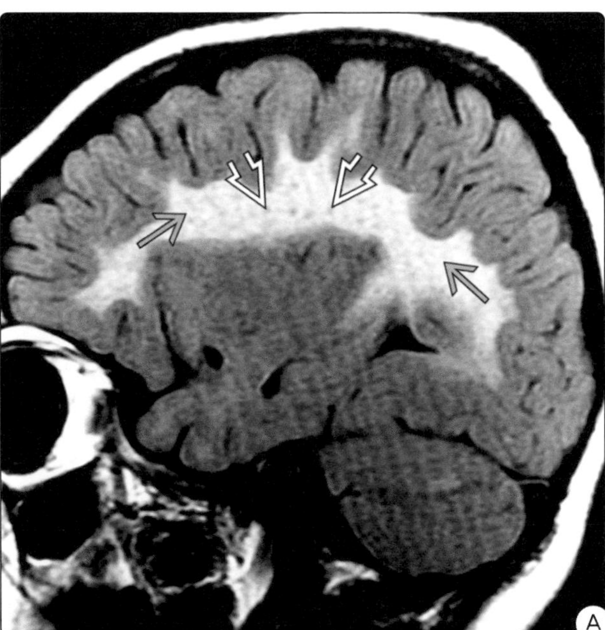


***(36-8A)** Sagittal FLAIR MR shows hypointense dots (leopard pattern) of preserved myelin ➡ along venules surrounded by demyelinated WM ⇨.*

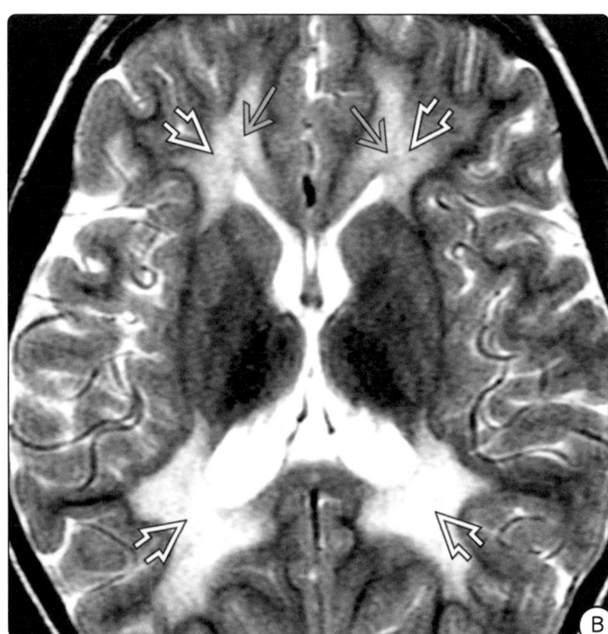


***(36-8B)** Axial T2 MR in a child with MLD shows WM demyelination (hyperintensity) ➡. Note "granular" hypointense frontal perivenular myelin sparing ⇨. Early in the disease process, the internal and external capsules may be spared.*

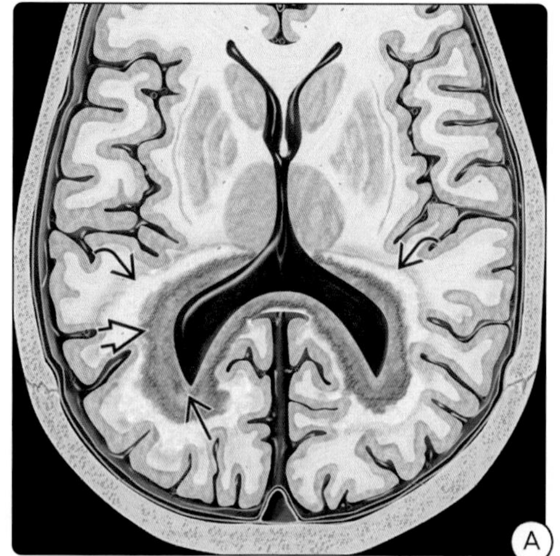


***(36-9A)** X-ALD with burned-out deep zone ➔, intermediate zone of active demyelination ➔, advancing demyelinating edge ➔ are shown.*

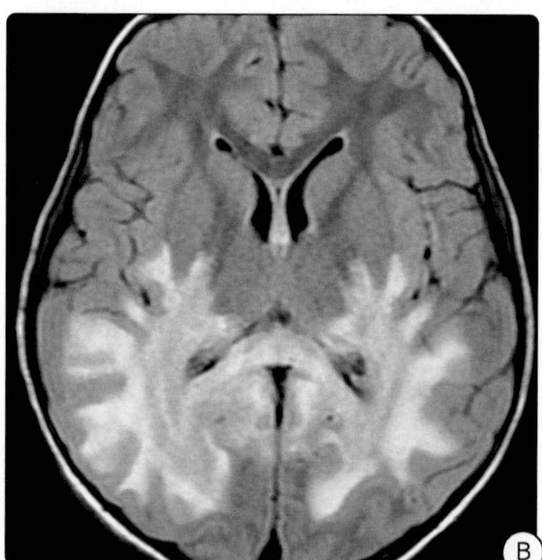


***(36-9B)** Axial FLAIR in a 9-yo boy shows symmetric posterior WM ↑ signal to include the corpus callosum and internal capsules.*

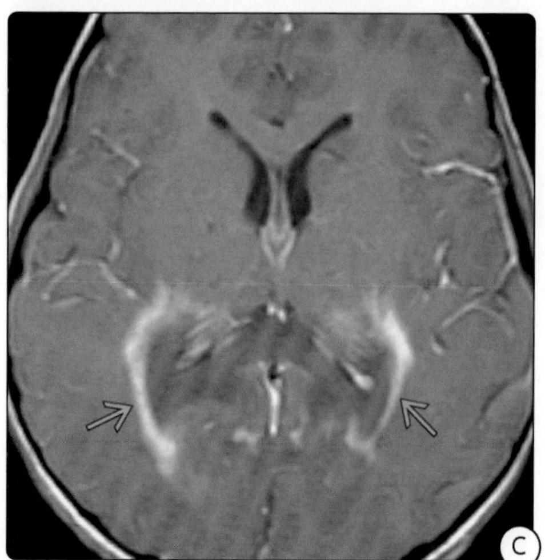


***(36-9C)** Axial T1 C+ MR in the same patient shows enhancement within the active demyelination zone ➔.*

**Pathology.** Three distinct zones of myelin loss are seen in adrenoleukodystrophy (ALD) **(36-9A)**. The *innermost zone* consists of a necrotic core of demyelination with astrogliosis, ± calcification. An *intermediate zone* of active demyelination and perivascular inflammation lies just outside the necrotic, "burned-out" core of the lesion. The most *peripheral zone* represents the advanced edge of ongoing demyelination without inflammatory changes.

### ADRENOLEUKODYSTROPHY: ETIOLOGY, PATHOLOGY, AND CLINICAL ISSUES

**Etiology**
- Peroxisomal disorder
- Impaired oxidation of very-long-chain fatty acids

**Pathology**
- Severe inflammatory demyelination
- 3 zones
  - Necrotic, "burned-out" core
  - Intermediate zone of active demyelination + inflammation
  - Peripheral demyelination without inflammation

**Clinical Issues**
- Classic X-linked adrenoleukodystrophy
  - Most common form (45%)
  - Preteen boys
  - Deteriorating cognition, school performance
- Adrenomyeloneuropathy
  - 2nd most common form (35%)
  - Most common in male patients
- Addison disease without CNS involvement (20%)

**Clinical Issues.** X-ALD is the most common single protein or enzyme deficiency disease to present in childhood. Several clinical forms of ALD and related disorders have been described. **Classic X-ALD** is the most common form (45%) and is seen almost exclusively in boys 5-12 years of age. Behavioral difficulties and deteriorating school performance are common. Approximately 10% of affected patients present acutely with seizures, adrenal crisis, acute encephalopathy, or coma.

**Adrenomyeloneuropathy** (AMN) is the second most common type (35%). It is another X-linked disorder that occurs primarily in male patients. It presents between 14-60 years, thus presenting later than classic X-ALD. AMN is characterized by axonal degeneration in the spinal cord more than the brain and peripheral nerves.

**Imaging.** Although CT scans are sometimes obtained as an initial screening study in children with encephalopathy of unknown origin, MR ± IV contrast is the procedure of choice.

***CT Findings.*** NECT scans demonstrate hypoattenuation involving the corpus callosum splenium and WM around the atria and occipital horns. Calcification in the affected WM may be seen. CECT typically shows enhancement around the central hypoattenuating WM.

***MR Findings.*** A *posterior-predominant* pattern is seen in 80% of patients with X-ALD **(36-9)**. The earliest finding is T2/FLAIR hyperintensity in the middle of the corpus callosum splenium. As the disease progresses, hyperintensity spreads from posterior to anterior and from the center to the periphery. The peritrigonal WM, corticospinal tracts, fornix, commissural fibers, + the visual and auditory pathways can all eventually become involved.

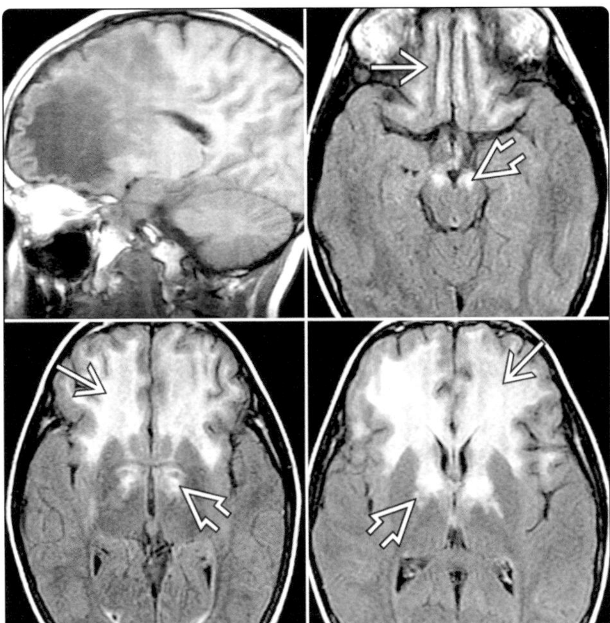

*(36-10) MR multiplanar images of an atypical variant of ALD show symmetric confluent frontal lesions ➡ with sparing of parietooccipital WM. Note the involvement of internal capsules and cerebral peduncles ➪.*

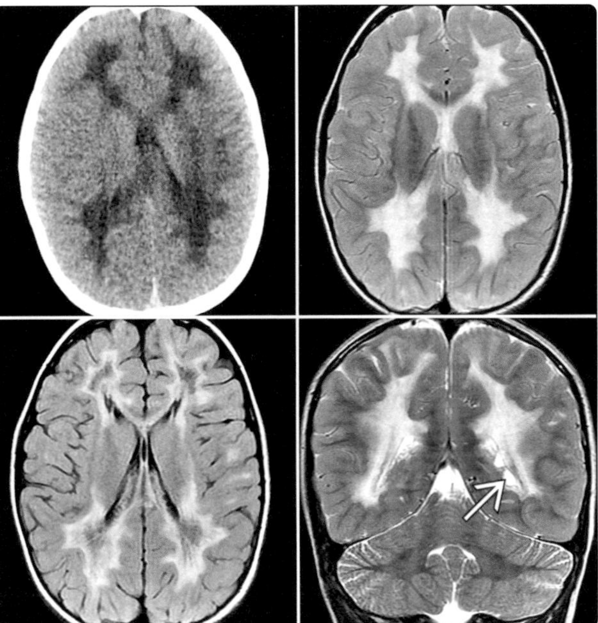

*(36-11) Images show vanishing WM disease in a 5-yo boy originally diagnosed with MLD. Note the symmetric periventricular disease, spared U-fibers, and early cyst formation ➡. (Courtesy S. Harder, MD.)*

The leading edge of demyelination appears hyperintense on T1WI but does not enhance. The intermediate zone of active inflammatory demyelination typically enhances on T1 C+ **(36-9C)**.

X-ALD may present at an atypical age, demonstrate atypical sites of involvement, and lack enhancement. Approximately 10-15% of all patients with classic X-ALD have an *anterior-predominant* demyelination; T2/FLAIR hyperintensity initially appears in the corpus callosum genu (not the splenium) and spreads into the frontal lobe WM **(36-10)**.

In patients with AMN, the cerebral hemispheres are relatively spared with predominant involvement of the cerebellum, corticospinal tracts, and spinal cord. Enhancement is typically absent.

DWI/DTI shows reduced diffusivity in active zones of demyelination and increased diffusivity in regions of "burned-out" demyelination. DTI shows reduced connectivity (i.e., loss of fractional anisotropy) in WM that MR demonstrates as abnormal and in "normal" WM.

MRS shows, at TE of 35 ms, peaks at 0.8-1.4 (i.e., cytosolic amino acids and VLCFA macromolecules). Reduced *N*-acetyl-L-aspartate (NAA) may be detected prior to observed MR abnormality and predicts progression. Increased myoinositol, choline, and lactate doublet are typical findings.

**Differential Diagnosis.** When X-ALD presents in patients of classic age and sex (i.e., 5- to 12-year-old boys) and with typical posterior predominance on imaging studies, the differential diagnosis is very limited.

### ADRENOLEUKODYSTROPHY: IMAGING AND DIFFERENTIAL DIAGNOSIS

**Imaging**

- X-linked adrenoleukodystrophy posterior predominance in 80%
    - Earliest finding: Corpus callosum splenium hyperintensity
    - Spreads posterior to anterior, center to periphery
    - Intermediate zone often enhances, restricts
- Variant patterns
    - X-linked adrenoleukodystrophy with anterior predominance (10-15%)
    - Adrenomyeloneuropathy involves corticospinal tracts, cerebellum, cord more than hemispheric white matter

**Differential Diagnosis**

- X-linked adrenoleukodystrophy pathognomonic if sex, age, imaging findings classic

## Vanishing White Matter Disease

Vanishing WM disease (VWMD) has become recognized as one of the most prevalent inherited leukoencephalopathies. VWMD is characterized by diffusely abnormal cerebral WM that literally "vanishes" over time. VWMD is an autosomal recessive disorder caused by point mutation of genes responsible for encoding any of the five subunits of the eukaryotic translation inhibiting factor 2B (EIF2B).

**Pathology.** VWMD is a slowly progressive, eventually cavitating WM disease that predominately involves the deep frontoparietal with lesser involvement of the temporal lobes.

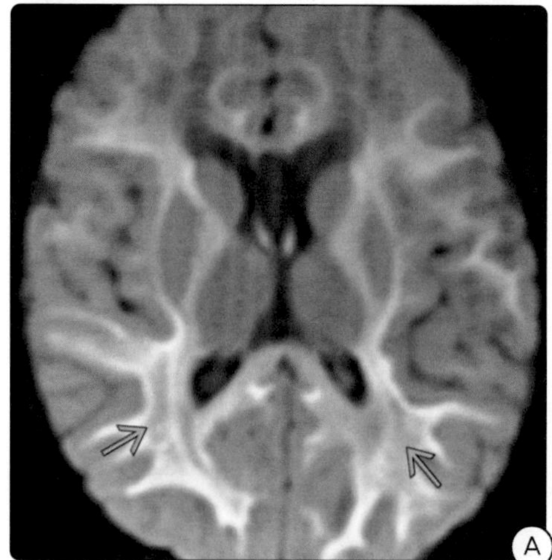

*(36-12A) Axial DWI in an 8-month-old with vanishing WM disease shows symmetric cytotoxic edema ➡ throughout the WM.*

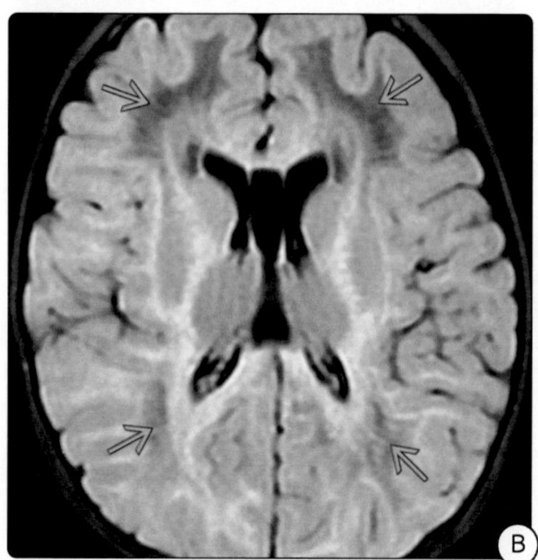

*(36-12B) Axial FLAIR shows suppression of signal (↓ signal) in the most severely affected areas ➡, as if the WM is "vanishing" and replaced by fluid.*

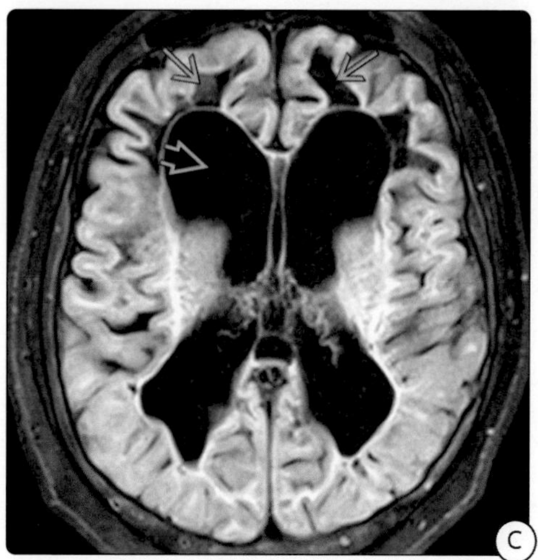

*(36-12C) Axial FLAIR in a 19-yo with chronic vanishing WM disease shows near-complete loss of WM ➡ with ex vacuo ventriculomegaly ➡.*

The basal ganglia, corpus callosum, anterior commissure, internal capsules, and cortex are characteristically spared. The eventual appearance is areas of cystic degeneration with frank WM cavitation.

**Clinical Issues. Classic VWMD** presents in children 2-5 years of age. Development is initially normal, but progressive motor and cognitive impairment with cerebellar and pyramidal signs follow. Progression is typically slow. Death by adolescence is typical.

Approximately 15% of VWMD cases occur in adolescents and adults. Mean age of late-onset VWMD is 30 years.

**Imaging.** WM hypoattenuation without calcifications is typical in the early stages of VWMD **(36-12B)**. Eventually, profound WM volume loss is seen **(36-12C)**.

Extensive confluent WM T1 hypointensity with T2/FLAIR hyperintensity is typical. The disease is initially periventricular but later spreads to involve the subcortical arcuate fibers. Over time, the affected WM undergoes rarefaction. Cavitary foci of CSF-like signal intensity eventually develop **(36-12C)**. Diffuse volume loss with enlarged ventricles and sulci is seen on serial studies. DWI typically shows diffusion restriction in active areas of WM destruction and facilitated diffusion in the CSF-like cavitary areas **(36-12A)**. VWMD does not enhance.

**Differential Diagnosis.** VWMD is not the only leukoencephalopathy that causes "melting away" or "vanishing" of the cerebral WM. AxD and mitochondrial encephalopathies can be associated with WM rarefaction and cystic degeneration. **AxD** presents with macrocephaly and is not associated with the episodic neurologic deterioration characteristic of VWMD; it demonstrates a frontoparietal gradient of disease. Frontal WM cysts can occur in end-stage disease. Approximately 10% of **mitochondrial encephalopathies** predominantly affect the WM and may form cavitations.

## Phenylketonuria

Phenylketonuria (PKU) is the most common inborn error of amino acid metabolism. Phenylalanine (Phe) accumulates and is toxic to the developing brain. Newborns are usually asymptomatic and most cases are diagnosed with newborn metabolic disease-screening programs. With adherence to dietary protein restriction, mitigation of the ravages of this disease occurs. Early treatment is key to minimizing cognitive impairment.

Initial imaging in PKU can appear normal! When abnormality is detected, T2/FLAIR imaging shows hyperintensity in the periventricular WM, particularly frontal and peritrigonal regions **(36-13)**. The subcortical arcuate fibers are spared. There is no enhancement following contrast administration. *Centrifugal* progression eventually leads to end-stage disease. MRS shows a Phe peak resonating at 7.37 ppm (which is missed on routine clinical MRS that only displays to 4 ppm).

The differential diagnoses include **PVL** (at-risk population of low-birth-weight, premature neonates who eventually manifest signs and symptoms of cerebral palsy, **MLD** (demonstrating more confluent zones of deep WM T2/FLAIR hyperintensity), and **Krabbe disease** (optic and cranial nerve enlargement, thalamic hyperattenuation on NECT, MR showing T2/FLAIR hyperintensity in corticospinal tracts, deep cerebral WM, and early cerebellar involvement).

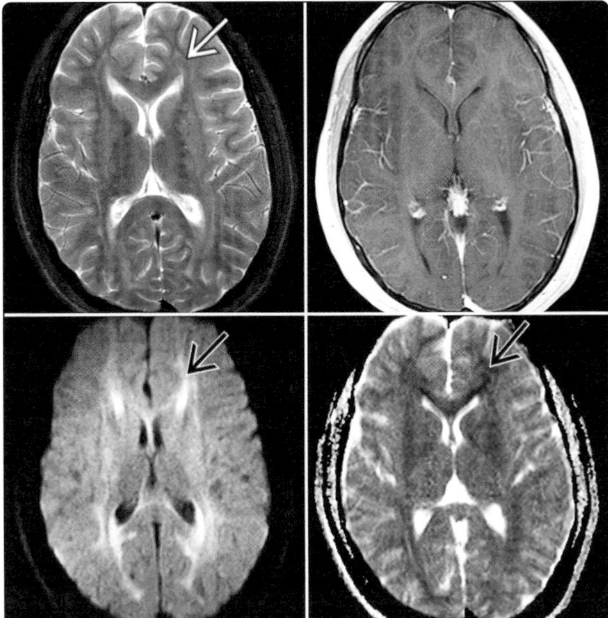

***(36-13)** Axial MR scans in a 13-yo girl with PKU, mild cognitive impairment show subtle periventricular hyperintensity ➡, no enhancement, and restriction on DWI ➡.*

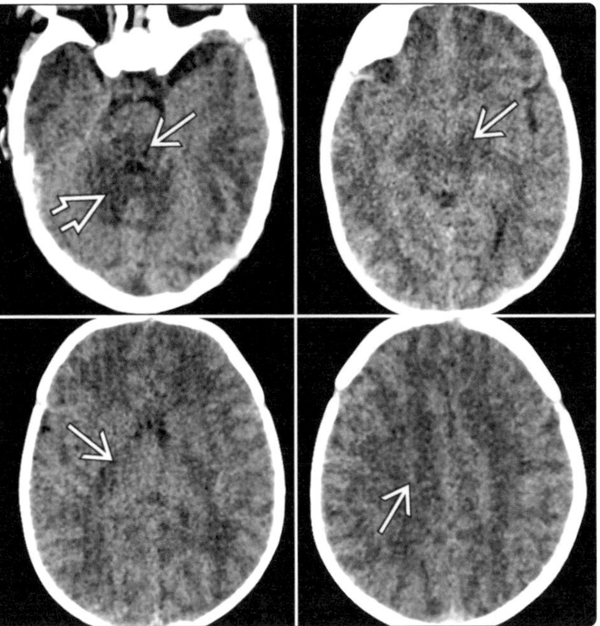

***(36-14)** Axial NECTs in a 13-day-old boy with MSUD show edema (low attenuation) ➡ in the dorsal midbrain and central cerebellar WM ➡, cerebral peduncles (upper R), internal capsules (lower L), and centrum semiovale.*

## Maple Syrup Urine Disease

Maple syrup urine disease (MSUD) is an autosomal recessive disorder of branched-chain amino acid (leucine, isoleucine, valine) metabolism. Elevated levels of leucine and other leukotoxic metabolites induce cytotoxic or intramyelinic edema and spongiform degeneration.

Infants with classic MSUD are initially normal. Within days after birth, poor feeding, lethargy, vomiting, seizures, and encephalopathy may occur. In severe cases, the urine smells of maple syrup or burned sugar.

NECT scans show profound hypoattenuation within the myelinated WM as well as within the dorsal brainstem, cerebellum, cerebral peduncles, and posterior limb of the internal capsule **(36-14)**. MR shows striking T2/FLAIR hyperintensity involving the cerebellar WM, dorsal brainstem, cerebral peduncles, thalami, globi pallidi (GP), posterior limbs of internal capsule, internal medullary lamina, and pyramidal and tegmental tracts.

MRS shows a peak at 0.9 ppm caused by accumulation of branched-chain α-keto amino acids. This peak is present at short (35 ms), intermediate (144 ms), and long (288 ms) PRESS MRS acquisitions, distinguishing them from the broad cytosolic amino acid peaks that only resonate at a short TE (35 ms).

The differential diagnosis includes **AxD** (T2 hyperintensity of the frontal WM and enhancement), **hypoxic-ischemic injury** (HIE) (with history of periparturitional distress, no significant symptom-free period), and **mitochondrial cytopathy** (episodic stroke-like clinical events of varied severity depending on the genotype of the disorder).

# Subcortical White Matter Predominance

IMDs that initially or predominantly affect the subcortical WM are much less common than those that begin with deep periventricular involvement. The most striking IMD with preferential involvement of the subcortical WM is megaloencephalic leukoencephaly with subcortical cysts (MLC).

## Megaloencephalic Leukodystrophy With Subcortical Cysts

MLC, a.k.a. vacuolating megaloencephalic leukoencephalopathy, is a rare autosomal recessive disorder with characteristic MR features.

**Pathology, Clinical Features.** Gross pathology shows a swollen cerebral hemispheric WM, relative occipital sparing, variable involvement of the subcortical arcuate fibers, frequent involvement of the external capsules, and sparing of the internal capsules. Multiple variably sized subcortical cysts, initially involving the temporal lobes, are typical **(36-15) (36-16)**.

MLC is distinguished clinically from other leukoencephalopathies by its remarkably slow course of neurologic deterioration. Infantile-onset macrocephaly is characteristic, but neurologic deterioration is often delayed. Age at symptom onset varies widely, ranging from birth to 25 years. Slow cognitive decline is observed as the disease progresses.

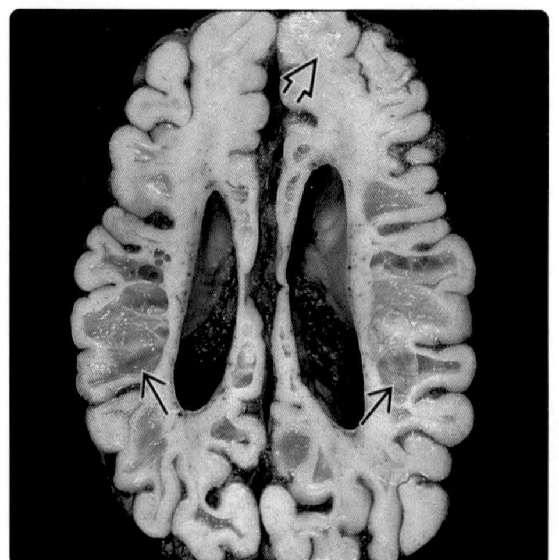

(36-15) MLC autopsy shows multiple subcortical cysts ➡ and WM rarefaction ➡ in frontal subcortical WM. (Courtesy R. Hewlett, MD.)

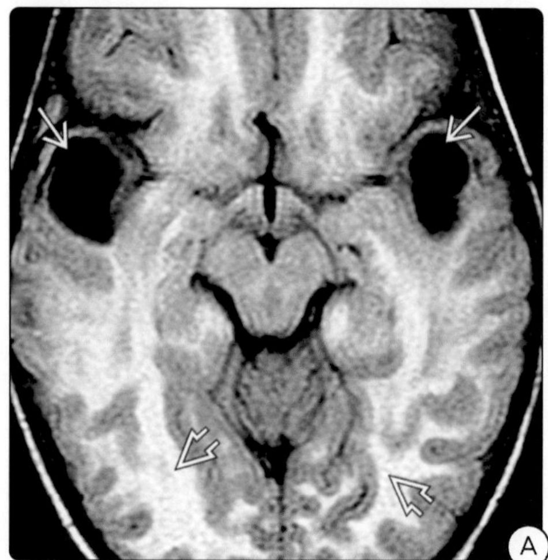

(36-16A) Axial FLAIR in a 22-month-old child with MLC shows swollen, hyperintense, "watery" WM ➡ and CSF-like temporal subcortical cysts ➡.

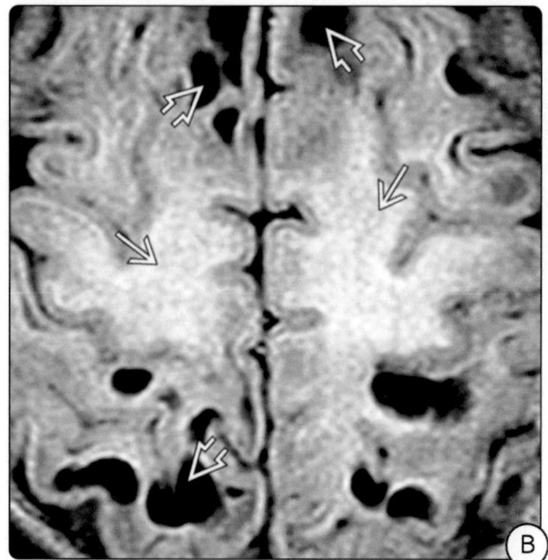

(36-16B) Axial FLAIR MR in a 2-yo child with MLC shows swollen, hyperintense subcortical WM ➡. Note fluid-filled subcortical hypointense cysts ➡.

**Imaging.** Cranial US in symptomatic infants shows unexplained hyperechogenicity of affected WM. NECT will demonstrate hypoattenuation of the cerebral hemispheric WM.

The diagnosis of MLC is typically established by MR. Macrocephaly with diffuse confluent WM T2/FLAIR hyperintensity in the subcortical WM is typical. The affected subcortical WM appears "watery" and swollen. The overlying gyri seemingly stretch over the swollen WM. The optic radiations, occipital subcortical WM, corpus callosum, as well as the basal ganglia and internal capsule, are usually spared.

Characteristic CSF-like subcortical cysts develop in the anterior temporal lobes followed in frequency by frontoparietal cysts. Unlike the "watery" WM, which exhibits T2/FLAIR hyperintensity, the cysts approximate the signal intensity of CSF on FLAIR. The number and size of the cysts may increase over time. The abnormal WM and cysts do not enhance on T1 C+.

**Differential Diagnosis.** MLC must be distinguished from other IMDs with macrocrania. The two major considerations are **Canavan disease** (CD) and **AxD**, both of which are characterized by much greater clinical disability.

**CD** almost always involves the basal ganglia, lacks the development of subcortical cysts, and demonstrates a large NAA peak on MRS. CD also shows very early involvement of the subcortical U-fibers, which may appear uninvolved in the early presentation of MLC.

**AxD** demonstrates a *frontal* WM gradient, involves the basal ganglia, and often enhances following contrast administration.

# Inherited Metabolic Disorders Predominantly Affecting Gray Matter

Inherited metabolic disorders (IMDs) that involve the gray matter (GM) without affecting the white matter (WM) can be subdivided into those that involve the cortex and those that mostly affect the deep gray nuclei. Inherited GM disorders that involve the deep gray nuclei are significantly more common than those that primarily affect the cortex.

## Inherited Metabolic Disorders Primarily Affecting Deep Gray Nuclei

A number of inherited disorders affect mostly the basal ganglia and thalami. Three inborn errors of metabolism with specific predilection for the deep gray nuclei include (1) *pantothenate kinase-associated neurodegeneration* (PKAN), (2) *creatine deficiency syndromes*, and (3) a cytosine-adenine-guanine (CAG) repeat disorder called *Huntington disease* (HD).

We begin this section with an overview of brain iron accumulation disorders before turning our attention specifically to **PKAN** and **HD**. We close the section with a discussion of the most important inherited disorder with abnormal copper metabolism, **Wilson disease** (WD).

### Brain Iron Accumulation Disorders

Some iron accumulation within the basal ganglia and dentate nuclei occurs as part of normal aging (see Chapter 38). Neurodegeneration with brain iron accumulation (NBIA) represents a clinically and genetically heterogeneous group of conditions characterized by progressive neurodegeneration and abnormally elevated brain iron. We focus our discussion on PKAN, the most common type of NBIA, and HD.

MR is especially useful in diagnosing NBIAs. All feature iron deposition in the GP but differ in other associated findings. The distribution of T2 or T2* hypointensity can help distinguish between the different NBIA subtypes (see accompanying box).

### NBIA: T2* HYPOINTENSITY

**Pantothenate Kinase-Associated Neurodegeneration**
- Globus pallidus, substantia nigra, dentate nuclei
- Eye of the tiger sign variable
- *Spares* cortex

**Infantile Neuroaxonal Dystrophy**
- Cerebellar atrophy (95%)
- T2* hypointensity in globus pallidus, substantia nigra (50%)
- *Spares* cortex

**Neuroferritinopathy**
- T2* hypointensity in globus pallidus, substantia nigra
- Then dentate/caudate nuclei, thalami
- *Affects* cortex

**Aceruloplasminemia**
- Globus pallidus, caudate nuclei, putamen, thalamus
- Red nucleus, substantia nigra, dentate nuclei
- *Affects* cerebral, cerebellar cortices

### Pantothenate Kinase-Associated Neurodegeneration

***Terminology and Etiology.*** PKAN, formerly known as Hallervorden-Spatz disease, is a rare familial autosomal recessive disorder characterized by excessive iron deposition in the GP and substantia nigra (SN).

***Pathology.*** Grossly, PKAN is characterized by shrinkage and rust-brown discoloration of the medial GP, the reticular zone of the SN, and, sometimes, the dentate nuclei. The red nuclei are generally spared. Microscopically, increased iron content is found in the GP interna and pars reticulata SN. Iron deposition is found within astrocytes, microglial cells, neurons, and around vessels. The "eye of the tiger" corresponds to regions of reactive astrocytes, dystrophic axons, and vacuoles in the anteromedial GP.

***Clinical Issues.*** PKAN, or NBIA type 1, can develop at any age. Most cases are diagnosed late in the first decade or during early adolescence. The disorder classically begins with slowly progressive gait disturbances and delayed psychomotor development. Progressive mental deterioration finally leads to dementia.

***Imaging.*** Imaging findings reflect the anatomic distribution of the excessive iron accumulation. T2WI demonstrates marked hypointensity in the GP and SN. A small focus of central hyperintensity in the medial aspect of the very hypointense GP (the classic eye of the tiger sign) is caused by tissue gliosis and vacuolization **(36-17)**. Note that *not all cases of PKAN demonstrate the "eye of the tiger"* **(36-18)**.

PKAN does not enhance on T1 C+ nor does it demonstrate restricted diffusion.

***Differential Diagnosis.*** Abnormal iron deposition in the basal ganglia occurs with PKAN as well as other NBIAs. **Aceruloplasminemia** and **neuroferritinopathy** are both adult-onset disorders. Both involve the cortex, which is spared in PKAN.

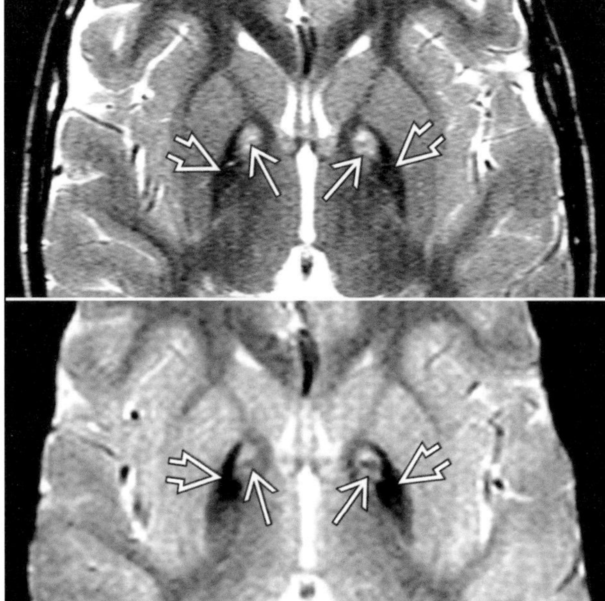

***(36-17) T2 MR (top), GRE (bottom) in a patient with PKAN show classic eye of the tiger sign with bilateral hyperintense central foci ➡ in the medial GP surrounded by striking hypointensity ➡.***

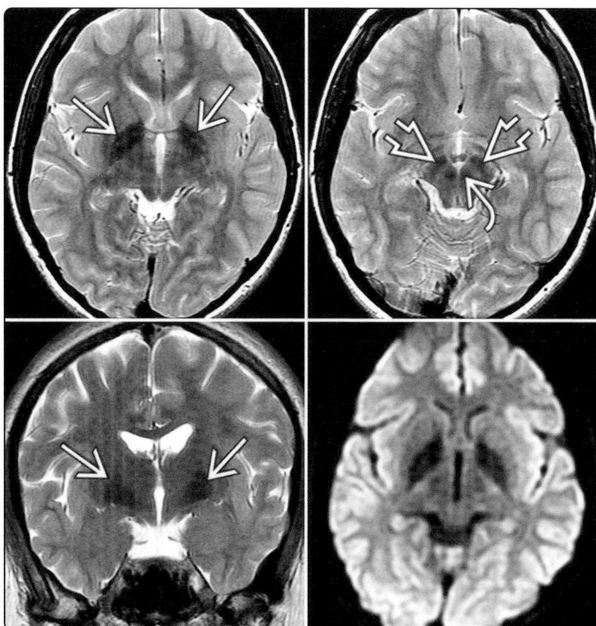

***(36-18) Multiplanar MR shows a 19-yo woman with documented PKAN. Note the profound hypointensity in the GP ➡, SN ➡, red nuclei ➡, and the lack of an eye of the tiger sign. DWI is normal (bottom R).***

Disorders with increased T2 signal within the GP can be grouped within *metabolic* derangements and *toxic/ischemic* insults. These entities lack pallidal GRE and SWI "blooming."

**IMDs** to consider in the differential diagnosis of basal ganglia T2 hyperintensity include **neuroferritinopathy** (variable GP T2 hyperintensity), **WD, Leigh syndrome, infantile bilateral striatal necrosis**, and **mitochondrial encephalopathies**, which show striatal hyperintensity (not hypointensity or "blooming"). These disorders predominantly involve the caudate and putamen, not the medial GP.

**Toxic/ischemic insults** include **HIE** (positive health history, T2 hyperintensity involving striatum, GP, thalami, corticospinal tracts, ± cortical involvement), **CO poisoning** (increased T2 signal involving GP, other deep nuclei, cortex, and WM), **cyanide toxicity** (T2 increased within basal ganglia ± hemorrhagic necrosis), and **kernicterus** (neonate) (increased T1/T2 GP).

## Huntington Disease

**Terminology and Etiology.** HD is an autosomal dominant chronic hereditary neurodegenerative disorder with complete penetrance. The huntingtin gene includes a repeating CAG trinucleotide segment of variable length. The presence of > 38 repeats confirms the diagnosis of HD.

**Pathology.** The most characteristic gross abnormality is volume loss with rarefaction of the caudate nucleus, putamen, and GP **(36-19)** **(36-20)**. The cerebellum is also atrophic in juvenile-onset HD.

**Clinical Issues.** Mean age at symptom onset is 35-45 years. Only 5-10% of patients present before the age of 20 years (juvenile-onset HD). CAG repeat length and age influence both the expression and the progression of HD.

Adult-onset HD is characterized by progressive loss of normal motor function, development of stereotypic choreiform movements, and declining cognition. Once symptoms appear, HD typically results in death within 10-20 years.

### HUNTINGTON DISEASE

**Etiology**
- Autosomal dominant, complete penetrance
- CAG trinucleotide repeat disorder

**Pathology**
- Caudate nuclei, putamina, globus pallidus
  - Huntingtin protein nuclear inclusions
  - Neuronal loss, gliosis, iron accumulation

**Clinical**
- Adult-onset Huntington disease (35-45 years): 90%
- Juvenile-onset Huntington disease (< 20 years): 10%

**Imaging**
- Caudate nuclei, putamina T2/FLAIR hyperintense
- Frontal horns outwardly convex

**Imaging.** NECT scans show caudate atrophy with enlarged, outwardly convex frontal horns and variable generalized diffuse atrophy **(36-21)** ± cerebellar atrophy.

MR shows volume loss in the frontal lobes and caudate heads. Caudate and putaminal T2/FLAIR signal is also common **(36-22)**. MR volumetric studies may demonstrate decreased basal ganglia volumes years before the onset of motor disturbances.

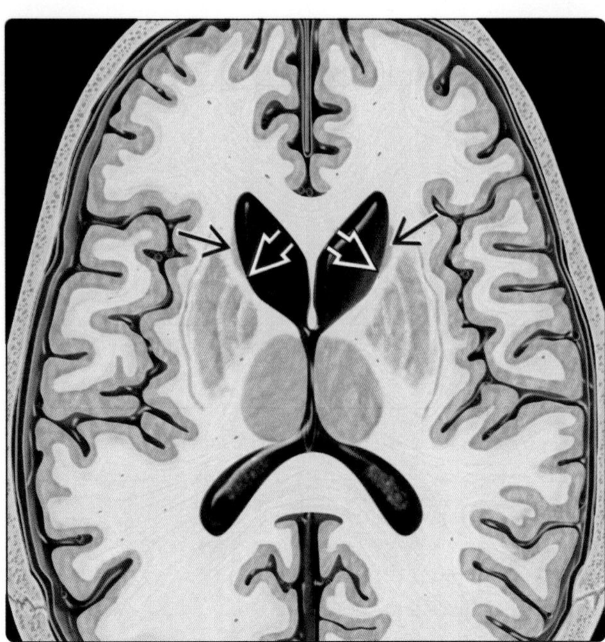

***(36-19)** Axial graphic shows shrunken, atrophic caudate nuclei ⇨ with the outwardly convex frontal horns ➡ that are typical of HD.*

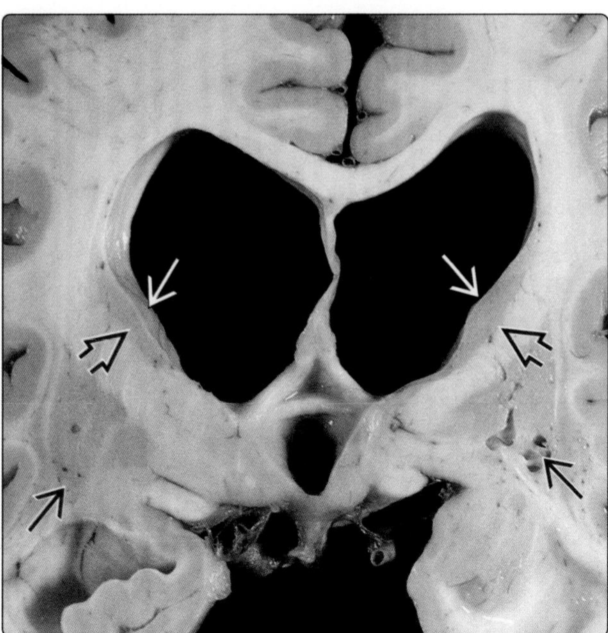

***(36-20)** Coronal autopsy of HD shows outwardly convex frontal horns ➡, severely shrunken caudate nuclei ⇨, and atrophic putamina ⇨. (Courtesy R. Hewlett, MD.)*

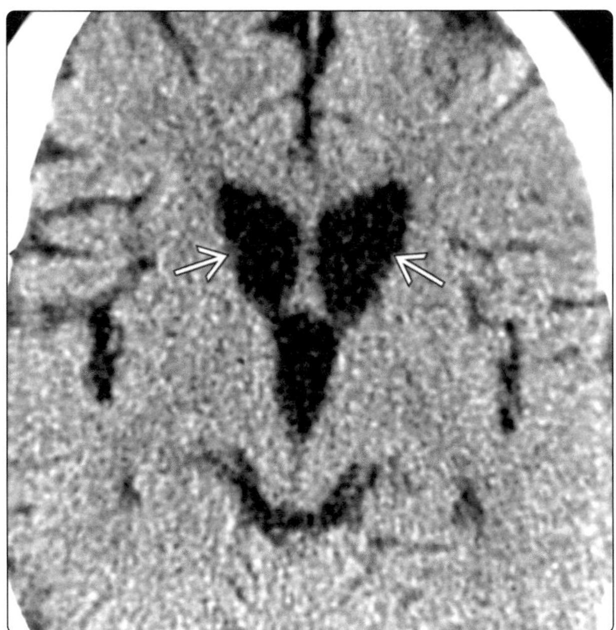

*(36-21) Axial NECT of a patient with HD shows moderate generalized, severe caudate atrophy seen as outwardly convex frontal horns ➔. (Courtesy M. Huckman, MD.)*

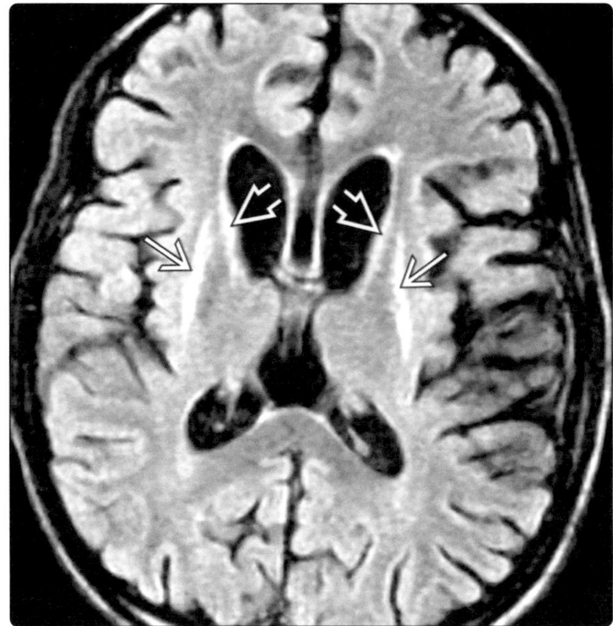

*(36-22) Axial FLAIR MR in a patient with HD shows almost nonexistent caudate heads ➔, basal ganglia atrophy, and thinned atrophic hyperintense putamina ➔.*

**Differential Diagnosis.** *Adult* HD mimics include **multiple system atrophy** (MSA), **corticobasal degeneration**, and **frontotemporal lobar dementia**. These disorders are often accompanied by basal ganglia atrophy. Unlike HD, the caudate nuclei are not disproportionately affected.

## Disorders of Copper Metabolism

Copper homeostasis is a delicate balance that requires both adequate dietary intake and proper excretion. Excess copper is neurotoxic. The most common disorder of copper metabolism—WD—has striking CNS manifestations. The major manifestations of WD are found in the basal ganglia, midbrain, and dentate nucleus of the cerebellum.

### Wilson Disease

***Etiology.*** WD is an uncommon autosomal recessive disorder of copper trafficking. The mutation causes defective incorporation of copper into ceruloplasmin and impaired biliary copper excretion. There is excessive accumulation of copper in hepatocytes, which later spills into the circulation. Copper deposition results in oxidative damage primarily to the liver, brain, kidney, skeletal system, and eye **(36-23)**.

***Pathology.*** Selective vulnerability of the corpus striatum to mitochondrial dysfunction accounts for the predominant basal ganglia volume loss seen in WD **(36-24)**. Gross pathologic features are nonspecific with ventricular enlargement and widened sulci seen at autopsy in severe cases.

***Clinical Issues.*** WD most commonly affects children and young adults. Symptoms of early-onset WD (8-16 years of age) are usually related to liver failure. Later onset WD symptoms are primarily neurologic and are generally recognized in the second or third decade. Dysarthria, dystonia, tremors, ataxia, Parkinson-like symptoms, and behavioral disturbances are common. Copper deposition in the cornea causes the characteristic greenish yellow Kayser-Fleischer rings seen on slit-lamp examination **(36-23)**.

#### WILSON DISEASE

**Etiology**
- Abnormal copper metabolism
- Autosomal recessive
- *ATP7B* gene mutations

**Pathology**
- Copper accumulates in hepatocytes, brain, eye
- Mitochondrial dysfunction damages basal ganglia

**Clinical Issues**
- Childhood Wilson disease: Liver disease
- Young adults: Parkinson-like
- Kayser-Fleischer rings

**Imaging**
- T2/FLAIR hyperintensity
  - Putamina, caudate, thalami, midbrain
- T2* "blooming"

**Differential Diagnosis**
- Leigh syndrome
- Pantothenate kinase-associated neurodegeneration

***Imaging.*** NECT scans may be normal, especially early in the disease course. Signal intensity on T1WI is variable. Some cases demonstrate T1 shortening similar to that seen in chronic

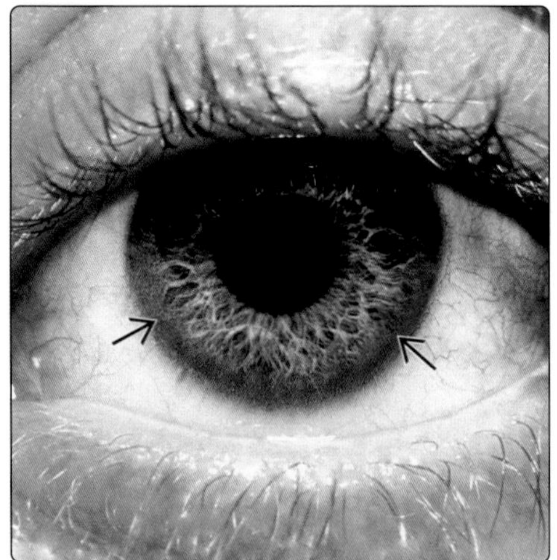

(36-23) WD is shown with classic peripheral greenish yellow Kayser-Fleischer ring ➡. (Courtesy AFIP Archives.)

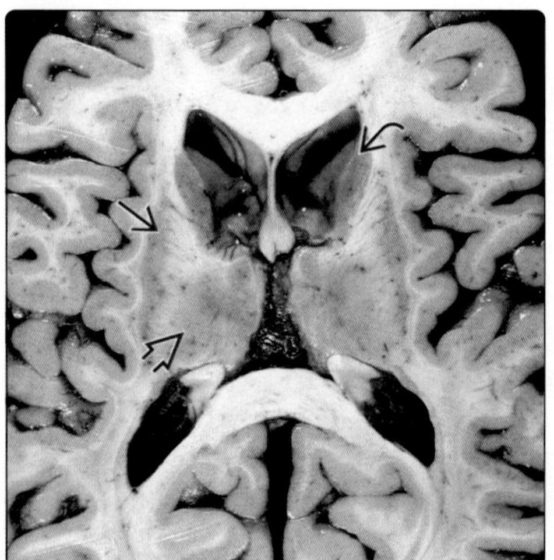

(36-24) Autopsy in WD shows atrophic putamina ➡, caudate ➡, and basal ganglia ➡, characteristic of WD. (Courtesy R. Hewlett, MD.)

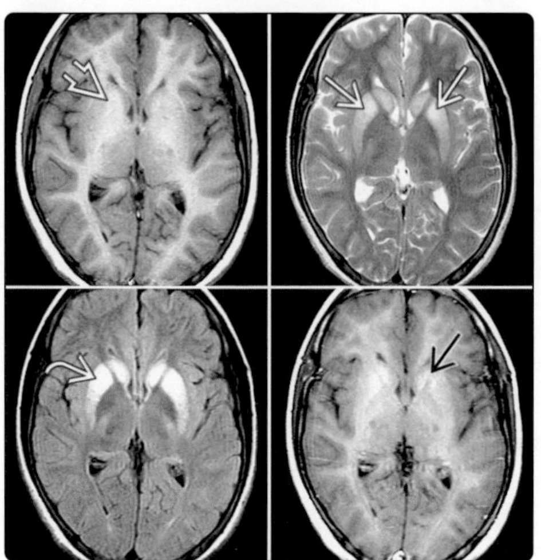

(36-25) Acute WD shows hyperintensity on T1 ➡ and T2 ➡, DWI restriction ➡, and no enhancement ➡. (Courtesy M. Ayadi, MD.)

hepatic encephalopathy (see Chapter 37). Basal ganglia T2 signal reflects paramagnetic effects of copper.

The most common imaging finding of WD on MR is bilaterally symmetric T2/FLAIR hyperintensity (sometimes heterogeneous) in the putamina (70%), caudate nuclei (60%), ventrolateral thalami (55-60%), and midbrain (50%) **(36-25)**. Hyperintensity can sometimes be seen in the pons (20%), medulla (10-15%), and cerebellum (10%). The cerebral (25%) and cerebellar WM (10%) can show focal or diffuse confluent hyperintensities.

In 10-12% of cases, diffuse tegmental (midbrain) hyperintensity with sparing of the red nuclei gives an appearance that has been termed the **"face of a giant panda."**

T2* (GRE, SWI) sequences show "blooming" in the putamina, caudate nuclei, ventrolateral thalami, and often the dentate nuclei. Contrast enhancement is typically absent. Restricted diffusion in the corpus striatum can be seen in the early stages of WD.

PET shows markedly reduced glucose metabolism and diminished dopa-decarboxylase activity indicative of striatonigral dopaminergic pathway dysfunction.

***Differential Diagnosis.*** The differential diagnoses of WD include other IMDs that affect the basal ganglia, such as Leigh syndrome, NBIAs, the organic acidurias, and Japanese encephalitis (JE). **Leigh syndrome** (subacute necrotizing encephalomyelopathy) shows bilateral, symmetric, spongiform, and hyperintense lesions, particularly in the *putamen* and brainstem. The WM is often affected in Leigh syndrome, whereas the caudate and thalamus are less commonly involved. MRS demonstrates elevated lactate levels in the basal ganglia.

**PKAN** can also resemble WD. WD predominantly affects the putamina and caudate nuclei rather than the medial GP and lacks the eye of the tiger sign often seen in PKAN.

# Disorders Affecting Both Gray Matter and White Matter

In the last section of this chapter, we discuss IMDs that affect *both* GM and WM.

## Mucopolysaccharidoses

### Terminology and Etiology

The mucopolysaccharidoses (MPSs) are lysosomal storage disorders characterized by incomplete degradation and progressive accumulation of toxic glycosaminoglycan (GAG) in various organs. In the brain, this accumulation includes GAG deposits in the perivascular spaces (PVSs), leptomeninges, and craniocervical junction ligamentous structures.

The MPSs have a classification of 1-9. Each has a specific enzyme deficiency and gene defect that leads to the inability to break down GAG. For example, MPS 1H (Hurler) has an α-L-iduronidase (4p16.3) deficiency, while MPS 2 (Hunter disease) is characterized by iduronate 2-sulfatase deficiency (Xq28).

### Pathology

The two distinctive gross features of the MPSs are thickened meninges and dilated PVSs packed with undegraded GAG **(36-27)**. The enlarged PVSs give a cribriform appearance to the brain on both pathology and imaging **(36-26)**.

## Clinical Issues

Each MPS subtype has different clinical phenotypes. Age at presentation varies, as do sex predilection and prognosis based on the inherited MPS type.

Hurler (MPS 1H) and Hunter (MPS 2) diseases are two of the most common "prototypical" MPSs. Hurler patients appear normal at birth but soon develop CNS symptoms, including delayed development and intellectual disability. Untreated Hurler disease typically results in death by age 10.

MPS 2 (Hunter disease) is an X-linked disorder and is seen only in male patients. Hunter disease is characterized by progressive multisystem involvement in the CNS, joints, bones, heart, skin, liver, eyes, and other organs. Patients often survive into their midteens but usually expire from cardiac disease.

## Imaging

The prototypical imaging findings in MPSs are illustrated by Hurler (MPS 1H) and Hunter (MPS 2) diseases.

**Macrocephaly.** NECT and MR scans show an enlarged head, often with metopic "beaking" and scaphocephalic configuration. Sagittal MR scans also demonstrate a large head with craniofacial disproportion. Pannus of ligaments at craniocervical junction can be seen.

**Enlarged Perivascular Spaces and White Matter Abnormalities.** A striking sieve-like cribriform appearance in the posterior cerebral WM and corpus callosum is characteristic and caused by numerous dilated PVSs **(36-28)** **(36-29)**. Although sometimes called "Hurler holes," these

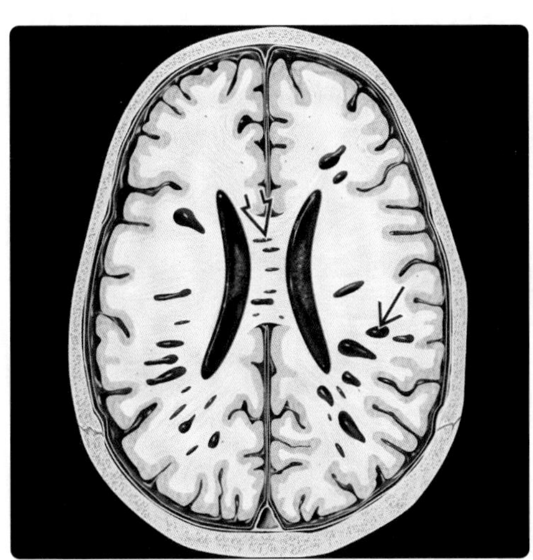

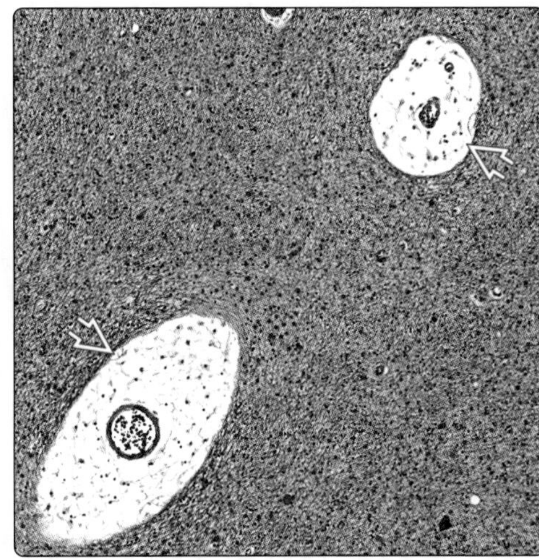

***(36-26)** MPS with dilated PVSs ⇨ is radially oriented in the WM. Posterior predominance and involvement of the corpus callosum ⇨ are frequently seen. Sometimes giant PVSs are seen in the inferior basal ganglia. **(36-27)** MPS 1HS (Hurler-Scheie) myelin stain shows large PVSs ➡ packed with undegraded mucopolysaccharides. (Courtesy P. Shannon, MD.)*

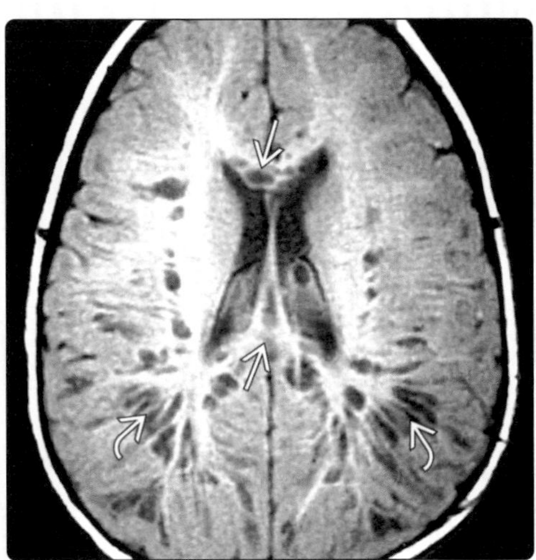

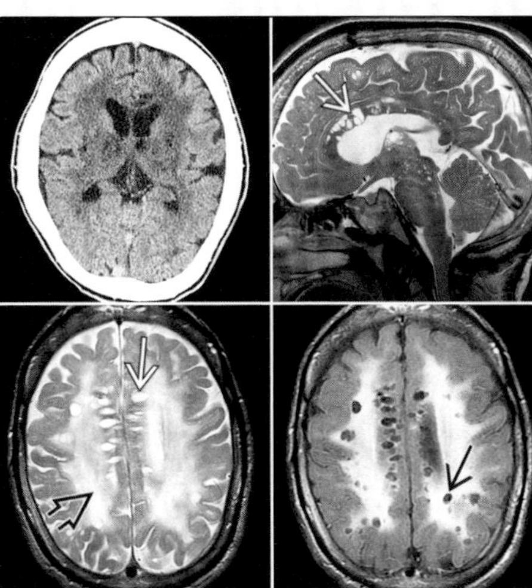

***(36-28)** T1 MR in a toddler with MPS 1H (Hurler disease) shows markedly enlarged WM ➡ PVSs, including the corpus callosum ➡. **(36-29)** MPS 2 (Hunter) shows enlarged PVSs in corpus callosum ➡, confluent WM disease ⇨. PVSs suppress on FLAIR ⇨; WM disease is hyperintense on T2/FLAIR and T1 hypointense.*

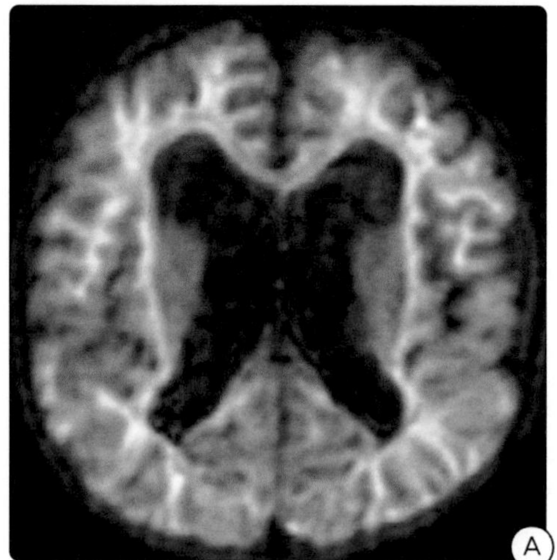


***(36-30A)** Axial DWI in a 3-yo boy with Canavan disease shows diffusion restriction throughout the WM.*

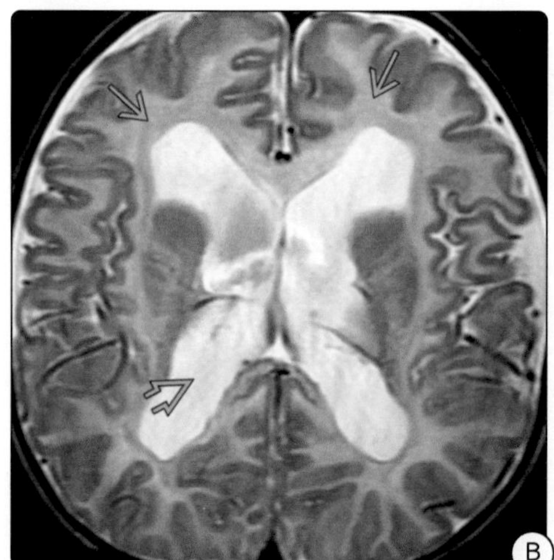


***(36-30B)** Axial T2 MR in the same patient shows increased signal throughout the WM ➡ and ventriculomegaly ➡ from WM volume loss.*

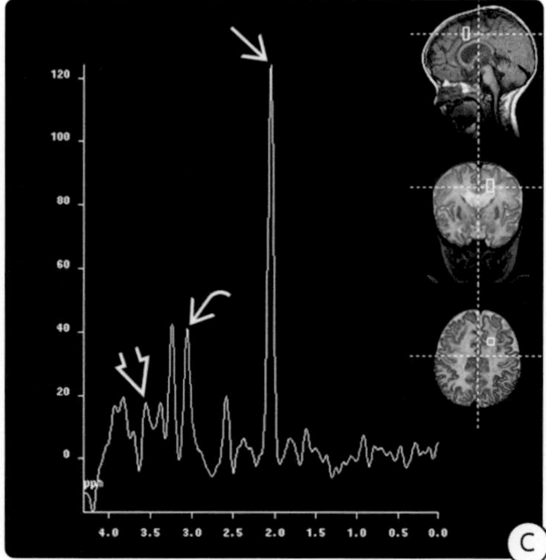


***(36-30C)** MRS with TE = 135 ms shows elevated NAA peak at 2.0 ppm ➡. Cr ➡ is significantly reduced. A small myoinositol peak ➡ is present.*

enlarged PVSs are typical of both Hurler and Hunter diseases. They are much less common in the other MPSs.

T2 scans show CSF-like hyperintensity in the enlarged PVSs. The PVSs themselves suppress completely on FLAIR. The enlarged PVSs do not "bloom" on T2* and do not enhance following contrast administration.

**Pachymeningopathy.** The meninges, especially around the craniovertebral junction, are often thickened and appear very hypointense on T2-weighted images. In severe cases, the thickened meninges can compress the medulla or upper cervical cord. Odontoid dysplasia and a short C1 posterior arch—common in the MPSs—can exacerbate the craniovertebral junction stenosis, causing progressive myelopathy.

### Differential Diagnosis

The differential diagnosis of MPS is limited. **Prominent PVSs** can be normal findings in patients of any age but are more common in middle-aged and older patients. No macrocephaly is present with this normal variant.

## Canavan Disease

Canavan disease (CD) is a fatal autosomal recessive neurodegenerative disorder and the only identified genetic disorder caused by a defect in a metabolite—*N*-acetyl-L-aspartate (NAA)—that is produced exclusively in the brain. Mutations in the *ASPA* gene, located on the long arm of chromosome 17, cause abnormal NAA accumulation in the brain and result in CD.

### Pathology

The brain in CD appears grossly swollen. Microscopic analysis shows spongiform WM degeneration with swollen astrocytes in the GP and thalami.

### Clinical Issues

Three clinical variants of CD are recognized. The *congenital form* presents within the first few days of life and leads to profound hypotonia with poor head control. Death rapidly ensues. The most common form by far is *infantile CD*. Infantile CD presents between 3-6 months and is characterized by hypotonia, macrocephaly, and seizures. Death between 1-2 years is typical. *Juvenile-onset CD* begins between 4-5 years of age and is the most slowly progressive form.

### Imaging

NECT shows a large head with diffuse WM hypoattenuation in the cerebral hemispheres and cerebellum. The GP also appear hypoattenuating.

MR eventually shows virtually complete absence of myelination with confluent T2/FLAIR hyperintensity throughout the WM and GP **(36-30B)**. The gyri may appear swollen, and the subcortical U-fibers are involved early in the disease course. As the disease progresses, widespread volume loss with ventricular and sulcal enlargement ensues.

DWI reveals bright DWI signal with normal to reduced ADC values in the involved areas. This diffusion restriction may persist indefinitely and is thought to be due to the gelatinous state of brain tissue due to diffuse vacuolization **(36-30A)**. CD does not enhance.

**MRS is the key to the definitive imaging diagnosis of CD**. Markedly elevated NAA is seen in virtually all cases **(36-30C)**. Cr is reduced. An elevated myoinositol peak is sometimes present. The choline:creatine (Ch:Cr) ratio is reduced.

## Differential Diagnosis

The major differential diagnosis of CD is **AxD**. Both CD and AxD cause macrocephaly, but an elevated NAA peak on MRS and enhancement on T1 C+ distinguish the two disorders.

**MLC** involves the subcortical arcuate fibers, as does CD; however, the basal ganglia are not affected. **PMD** demonstrates virtually complete lack of myelination but does not cause macrocephaly and does not affect the basal ganglia.

# Alexander Disease

## Etiology

More than 95% of AxD patients have de novo heterozygous dominant mutations in the *GFAP* gene (17q21). *GFAP* encodes for glial fibrillary acidic protein, a protein that is expressed only in astrocytes. *GFAP* mutations cause accumulation of mutant GFAP aggregates, which begins during fetal development.

## Pathology

The brains of infants with AxD have markedly increased astrocytic density and are grossly enlarged. Dramatic myelin loss makes the WM—especially in the frontal lobes—appear very pale. In severe cases, the WM appears partially or almost entirely cystic. In contrast to CD, the subcortical arcuate fibers are relatively spared.

The hallmark histopathologic feature of AxD is the presence of enormous numbers of Rosenthal fibers (RFs) in astrocytes. The striking lack of nearly all myelin in AxD is considered a secondary phenomenon that arises from severely disrupted astrocyte-derived myelination signaling.

## Clinical Issues

*Three clinical forms are recognized*: Infantile, juvenile, and adult. In the infantile form, which is the most common, patients younger than two years old present with megalencephaly, progressive psychomotor delay, and seizures. Spasticity and eventually quadriplegia often develop. All forms eventually lead to death. Care is supportive.

## Imaging

NECT scans of infants with AxD show a large head with symmetric WM hypoattenuation in the frontal lobes that extends posteriorly into the caudate nuclei and internal/external capsules. Intense bifrontal periventricular enhancement can be seen on CECT scans early in the disease course.

MR shows macrocephaly, T1 hypointensity, and T2/FLAIR hyperintensity involving the frontal WM, caudate nuclei, and anterior putamina. Although infantile AxD involves the subcortical U-fibers early in the disease course, the periventricular WM is more severely affected in the juvenile and adult forms **(36-31)**. A classic finding is a T1-hyperintense, T2-hypointense rim around the frontal horns. FLAIR scans may demonstrate cystic encephalomalacia in the frontal WM in more severe, protracted cases.

*A unique finding in AxD* is enlargement of the caudate heads and fornices, which appear swollen and hyperintense. The thalami, GP, brainstem, and cerebellum are less commonly affected.

**AxD is one of the few IMDs that demonstrates enhancement on T1 C+**. Rims of intense enhancement can be

***(36-31)** Axial T2 MR in a 10-month-old with AxD shows frontal-predominant signal abnormality involving periventricular and deep WM ⇒. Also note the subtle signal abnormality within the caudate nuclei ↪ and putamina ⇨.*

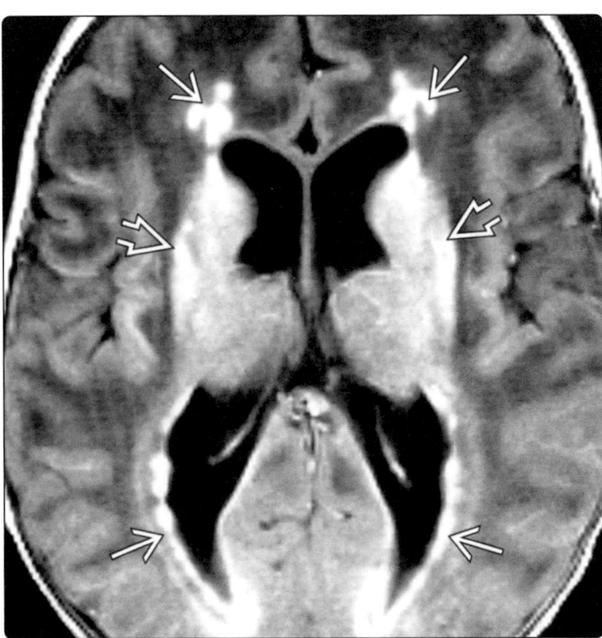

***(36-32)** Axial T1 C+ MR in 6-month-old boy with AxD shows enhancement in the periventricular WM ➡ and basal ganglia ➡. AxD is one of the few metabolic diseases that shows enhancement of affected regions.*

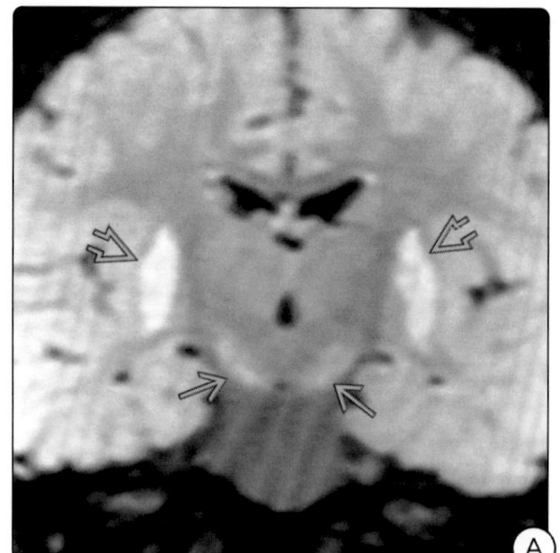

*(36-33A) Coronal FLAIR in a 1-yo with Leigh syndrome shows increased signal in the bilateral putamina ➾ and cerebral peduncles ➾.*

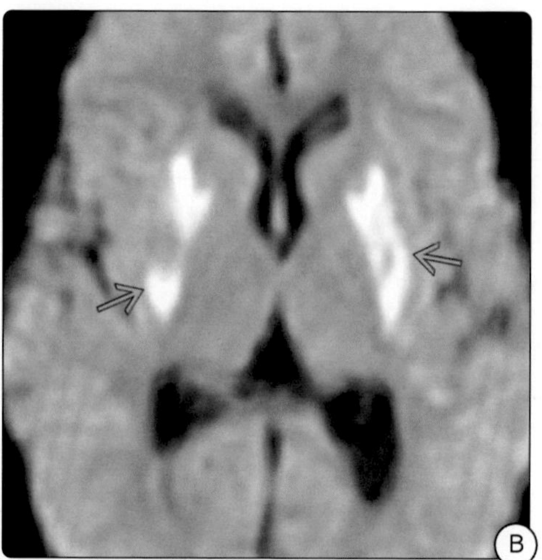

*(36-33B) Axial DWI in the same patient shows diffusion restriction ➾ in the areas of signal abnormality, reflecting cytotoxic edema.*

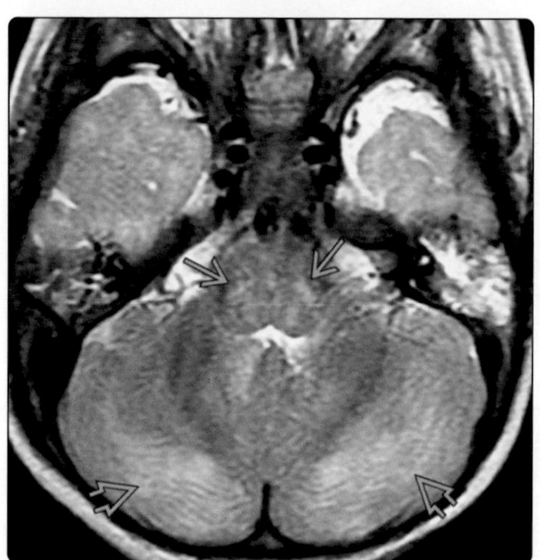

*(36-34) T2 MR in another Leigh syndrome example shows symmetric ↑ signal in the cerebellar WM ➾ and medulla ➾.*

seen around the surfaces of the swollen caudate nuclei and affected frontal lobe WM **(36-32)**. In the juvenile and adult forms, brainstem and cerebellar involvement can be striking and may even mimic a neoplasm.

## Differential Diagnosis

The major differential diagnoses of AxD are other inherited leukodystrophies with macrocephaly. These primarily include **CD** and the **MPSs**. Although both AxD and CD show almost complete lack of myelination with T2/FLAIR WM hyperintensity, the predilection of AxD for the frontal lobes, caudate heads, and enhancement help distinguish it from CD.

The MPSs, especially Hurler and Hunter diseases, display a striking cribriform appearance of the WM and corpus callosum caused by enlarged PVSs. Deep gray involvement is absent, and the lesions do not enhance. Dural thickening is also absent in AxD.

### DIFFERENTIAL DIAGNOSIS: CHILD WITH A LARGE HEAD

**Common**

- Normal variant
- Benign familial macrocrania
- Benign macrocrania of infancy

**Less Common**

- Nonaccidental trauma with subdural hematomas

**Rare but Important**

- Inherited metabolic disorder
  - Canavan disease
  - Alexander disease
  - Mucopolysaccharidoses
  - Megalencephaly with leukoencephalopathy and cysts
  - Glutaric aciduria type 1

# Mitochondrial Diseases (Respiratory Chain Disorders)

The mitochondria are cellular organelles that are the "power plants" responsible for energy production. Mitochondrial disorders are caused by mitochondrial DNA (mtDNA) mutations and are among the most common of all IMDs. Although virtually every organ or tissue of the body can be affected, the nervous system and skeletal muscle are especially vulnerable because of their high energy demands.

Four major encephalomyopathic syndromes have been described: *Leigh syndrome, Kearns-Sayre syndrome, mitochondrial encephalomyopathy with lactic acidosis and stroke-like episodes* (MELAS), and *myoclonic epilepsy with ragged red fibers* (MERRF). Two other less common disorders, glutaric aciduria types 1 and 2, are also caused by mtDNA-mediated enzyme abnormalities.

Mitochondrial disorders have significant clinical and imaging overlap and are challenging to distinguish from each other. We focus on Leigh syndrome, MELAS, and type 1 glutaric aciduria.

## Leigh Syndrome

**Terminology and Pathology. Leigh syndrome**, a.k.a. subacute necrotizing encephalopathy, demonstrates brownish gray gelatinous or cavitary foci within the basal ganglia, brainstem, dentate nuclei, thalami, and spinal cord with variable WM spongiform degeneration and demyelination.

**Clinical Issues.** Clinical manifestations of Leigh syndrome are variable. Most patients with Leigh syndrome present in infancy or childhood with failure to thrive, central hypotonia, developmental regression, ataxia, bulbar dysfunction, and ophthalmoplegia. Serum &/or CSF lactate levels are increased.

**Imaging.** MR in Leigh syndrome shows bilaterally symmetric areas of T2/FLAIR hyperintensity (often *speckled)* in the basal ganglia **(36-33A)**. The putamina (especially the posterior segments) are consistently affected, as are the caudate heads. The dorsomedial thalami can also be involved, whereas the GP are less commonly affected. Acute lesions show swelling of the basal ganglia.

Mid- and lower brainstem (pons/medulla) lesions are typical in Leigh syndrome and, in a few cases, can be the *only* finding. Symmetric lesions in the cerebral peduncles are common, and the periaqueductal GM is frequently affected. Brainstem lesions are especially common in cytochrome-C oxidase deficiency. The cerebellum is often involved **(36-34)**.

Acute lesions restrict on DWI but do not enhance **(36-33B)**. MRS of the brain and CSF typically shows a lactate doublet at 1.3 ppm. Lactate resonates above baseline at short (35 ms) and long (288 ms) TEs and inverts at an intermediate TE (144 ms).

**Differential Diagnosis.** As their imaging findings often overlap, the differential diagnosis of Leigh syndrome includes the other mitochondrial encephalomyopathies. Another important differential consideration is that of vigabatrin toxicity, which shows reversible diffusion restriction in the deep gray nuclei and brainstem similar to Leigh syndrome.

## MELAS

**Terminology and Etiology. M**itochondrial **e**ncephalomyopathy with **l**actic **a**cidosis and **s**troke-like episodes (MELAS) is caused by several different point mtRNA mutations.

**Clinical Issues.** MELAS is an uncommon but important cause of childhood stroke. The diagnosis of MELAS should always be considered when encountering a child or young adult with atypical stroke and encephalitis presenting with seizures.

The clinical triad of lactic acidosis, seizures, and stroke-like episodes is the classic presentation. Other common symptoms include progressive sensorineural hearing loss, migraines, episodic vomiting, alternating hemiplegia, and progressive brain injury. Cardiac abnormalities, renal dysfunction, GI motility disorders, and generalized muscle weakness are also common.

Mean age at symptom onset is 15 years, although some patients may not become symptomatic until 40-50 years of age.

**Imaging.** Imaging findings vary with disease acuity **(36-35)**. *Acute* MELAS often shows swollen T2-/FLAIR-hyperintense gyri. The underlying WM is normal, and the cortical abnormalities cross arterial territories, distinguishing MELAS from acute cerebral infarction **(36-35B)**. The parietal and occipital lobes are most commonly affected.

The appearance of *strokes of differing ages* is often a clue to the diagnosis of MELAS **(36-35)**. Gyral enhancement on T1 C+ is typical. MRA in MELAS shows no evidence of major vessel occlusion. DWI shows diffusion restriction in active areas of metabolic injury, while chronic areas of injury and encephalomalacia show facilitated diffusion. Perfusion imaging shows increased perfusion in acute metabolic injury and decreased perfusion in areas of chronic injury **(36-35C)**.

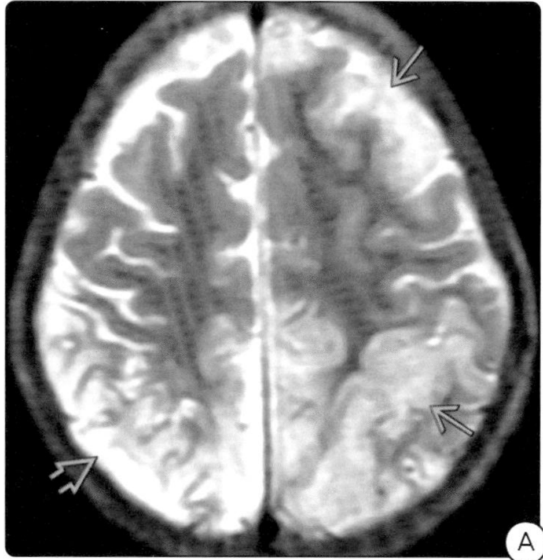


***(36-35A)** Axial T2 in a 7-yo with MELAS shows acute metabolic injury → in the left frontal and parietal lobes with older right parietal injury ⇨.*

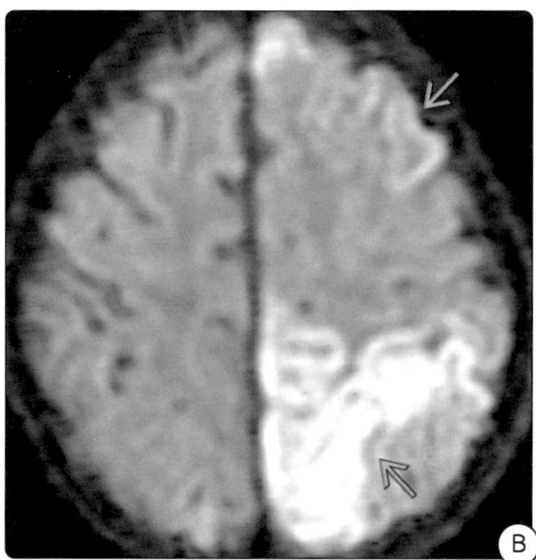


***(36-35B)** Axial DWI shows diffusion restriction in the areas of acute injury →. Note how the injury is not confined to arterial territories.*

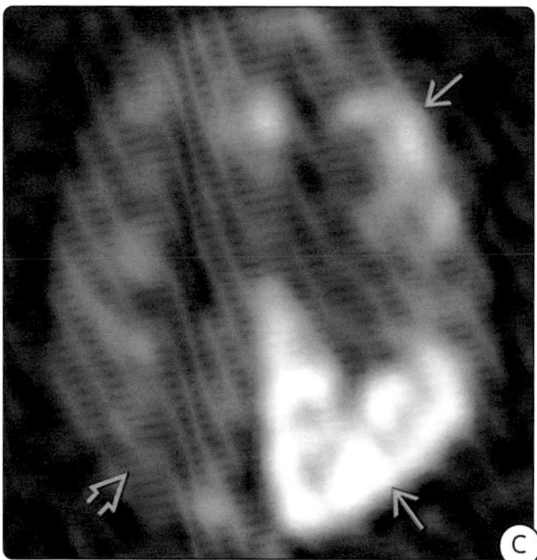


***(36-35C)** Axial ASL perfusion image shows ↑ perfusion (CBF) in the areas of acute metabolic injury → and ↓ CBF in areas of chronic injury ⇨.*

*Chronic* MELAS shows multifocal lacunar-type infarcts, symmetric basal ganglia calcifications, WM volume loss, and progressive atrophy of the parietooccipital cortex.

MRS is extremely helpful in the diagnosis of most mitochondrial encephalopathies. Nearly 2/3 of cases with MELAS show a prominent lactate "doublet" at 1.3 ppm in otherwise normal-appearing brain. **Caution**: 1/3 of cases show no evidence for elevated lactate levels in the brain parenchyma.

**Differential Diagnosis.** The differential diagnosis of acute MELAS includes territorial **arterial infarction**. MELAS spares the subcortical and deep WM and *crosses vascular distributions* (often the middle and posterior cerebral territories). **Prolonged seizures** can cause gyral swelling, hyperintensity, and enhancement that appears identical to MELAS. MRS shows no evidence of elevated lactate levels in normal-appearing brain.

**MERRF** shows a propensity to involve the basal ganglia, caudate nuclei, and vascular watershed zones.

## Glutaric Aciduria Type 1

**Etiology and Pathology.** Glutaric aciduria type 1 is an autosomal recessive IMD caused by deficiency of the mitochondrial enzyme, *GCDH*. The accumulation of excess glutaric acid is neurotoxic. Cells in the basal ganglia and WM are especially vulnerable. Spongiform changes with neuronal loss, myelin splitting and vacuolation, and intramyelinic fluid accumulation are typical pathologic features of glutaric aciduria type 1.

**Clinical Issues.** The majority of infants with glutaric aciduria type 1 exhibit macrocephaly at birth. More than 85% of glutaric aciduria type 1 patients present during the first year of life, usually with acute encephalopathy, seizures, dystonia, choreoathetosis, vomiting, &/or opisthotonus. These episodic crises are often triggered by febrile illness or immunization.

*(36-36) Graphic depicts typical findings of GA1. Note the symmetrically enlarged ➔ basal ganglia and the bilateral "open" sylvian or lateral cerebral fissures ➔. The thalami ➔ appear normal. (36-37) Axial T2 MR in a 7-month-old with GA1 shows enlarged, hyperintense caudate nuclei, putamina, and GP ➔ with thalamic sparing. Sylvian fissures ➔ are enlarged. The hemispheric WM myelination ➔ is grossly delayed.*

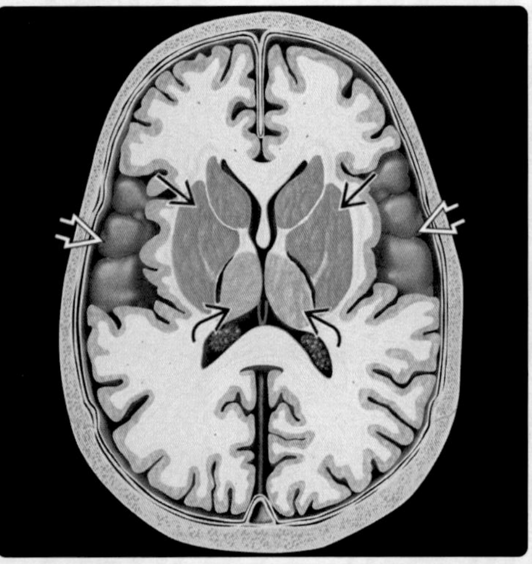

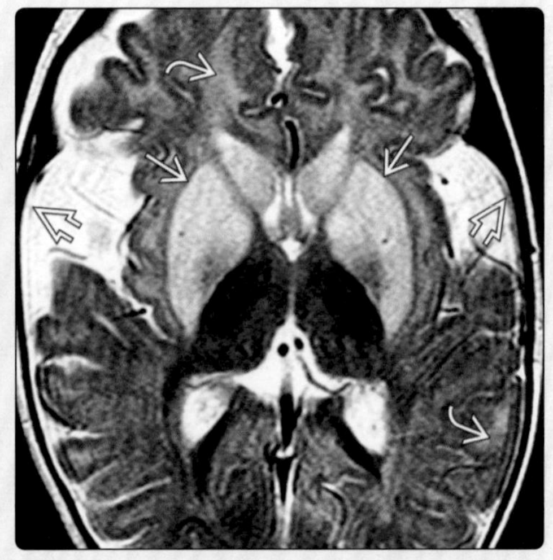

*(36-38A) NECT of GA1 in a 7-month-old infant with a large head and delayed development shows "open" sylvian (lateral cerebral) fissures ➔ and large bifrontal hypoattenuating chronic subdural hematomas (cSDH) ➔. (36-38B) Axial T2 MR in the same patient shows the "open" sylvian fissures ➔, membrane-bound ➔ subdural fluid collections ➔, and significantly delayed myelination for a child 7 months of age. GP shows T2 hyperintensity ➔.*

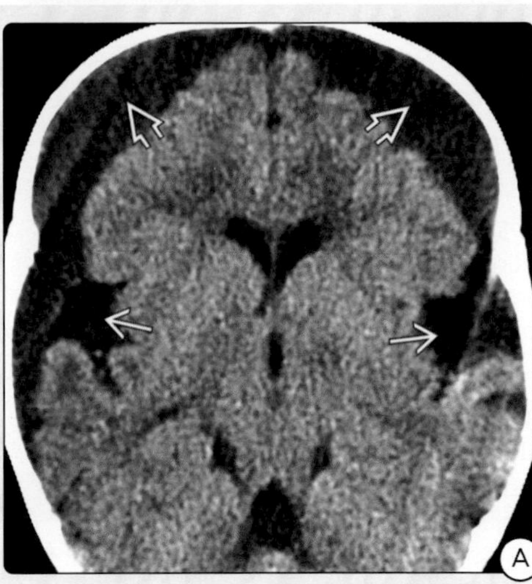


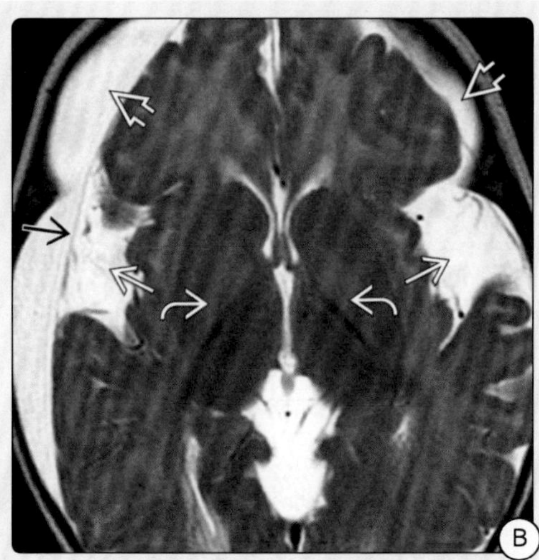

Patients may also develop an acute Reye-like encephalopathy with ketoacidosis and vomiting.

**Imaging.** The three "signature" imaging findings of classic glutaric aciduria type 1 are (1) macrocrania, (2) bilateral widened ("open") lateral cerebral (sylvian) fissures, and (3) bilaterally symmetric basal ganglia lesions **(36-36)**. Severe glutaric aciduria type 1 may also cause diffuse hemispheric WM abnormalities (i.e., central and periventricular).

Glutaric aciduria type 1 infants in metabolic crisis often present with acute striatal necrosis. Bilateral diffusely swollen basal ganglia that are T2/FLAIR hyperintense **(36-37)** and that restrict on DWI are typical.

Chronic glutaric aciduria type 1 causes enlarged CSF spaces and cerebral atrophy. Volume loss leads to tearing of cortical dural bridging veins, resulting in recurrent subdural hematomas **(36-38)**.

Glutaric aciduria type 1 does not enhance on T1 C+ scans. DWI in the acute phase or during crises shows restricted diffusion within the GP. MRS is nonspecific.

**Differential Diagnosis.** The major differential diagnosis of glutaric aciduria type 1 is **subdural hemorrhage** in **abusive head trauma**. However, glutaric aciduria type 1 is not associated with fractures, exhibits basal ganglia lesions, and the associated subdural hematomas do not occur in the absence of enlarged CSF spaces.

## Urea Cycle/Ammonia Disorders

Urea cycle disorders result in elevated serum ammonia, which readily crosses the blood-brain barrier and causes diffuse cerebral edema. The two most common disorders are ornithine transcarbamylase deficiency **(OTCD)** and **citrullinemia**.

Both OTCD and citrullinemia are characterized by diffuse brain swelling. MR shows basal ganglia and cortical swelling with T2/FLAIR hyperintensity. The periinsular cortex is usually affected first (cortical T2/FLAIR hyperintensity and restricted diffusion) **(36-39)**. Involvement progresses into the frontal, parietal, temporal, and (finally) the occipital lobes. The GP, putamina, and thalami are affected with prolonged hyperammonemia and may show restricted diffusion.

The major imaging differential diagnosis of acute hyperammonemia is **HIE**. Infants with HIE typically have more thalamic and perirolandic cortical abnormalities.

## Fabry Disease

Fabry disease is a rare but important cause of strokes in young children and adult men with cryptogenic stroke.

### Etiology and Pathology

Fabry disease is an X-linked lysosomal storage disorder of glycosphingolipid metabolism. Mutation in α-galactosidase leads to glycosphingolipid deposition in the vascular endothelium and smooth muscle cells. Impaired endothelial function results in progressive multisystem vasculopathy. The renal, cardiac, and cerebral vessels are severely affected. Cardiac emboli, large vessel arteriopathy, and microvascular disease all occur.

### Clinical Issues

Late-onset Fabry disease is difficult to diagnose. Although mean onset of first stroke is 39 years in men and 45 years in women, nearly 22% of patients are younger than 30 years at initial presentation. Over 85% of strokes in Fabry disease are ischemic strokes. Hemorrhagic strokes are less common and usually occur secondary to renovascular hypertension.

### Imaging

NECT scans show bilateral, often symmetric, calcifications in the basal ganglia and thalami **(36-40A)**. Multifocal deep WM hypodensities consistent with lacunar infarcts can be identified in some cases. Patients with longstanding Fabry disease show volume loss with enlarged ventricles and sulci.

MR may show T1 shortening in the basal ganglia and posterior thalami (pulvinar sign) **(36-40B)**, a rare but typical finding of Fabry disease. 45-50% of adult patients with Fabry disease have patchy multifocal T2/FLAIR hyperintensities in the basal ganglia, thalami, and cerebral WM **(36-41)**. 10% demonstrate "blooming" hypointensities on T2* (GRE, SWI) due to microbleeds.

### Differential Diagnosis

Other disorders marked by basal ganglia calcifications include **Fahr disease**, which causes bilateral, dense, thick calcifications in the basal ganglia and thalami. The cerebellum and GM-WM interfaces are usually not involved in Fabry disease. Hyperparathyroidism, hypoparathyroidism, and hypothyroidism may have similar calcifications but lack the multifocal infarcts typical of Fabry disease. A pulvinar sign can be seen in variant Creutzfeldt-Jakob disease.

*Selected References: The complete reference list is available on the eBooks+ version included with purchase.*

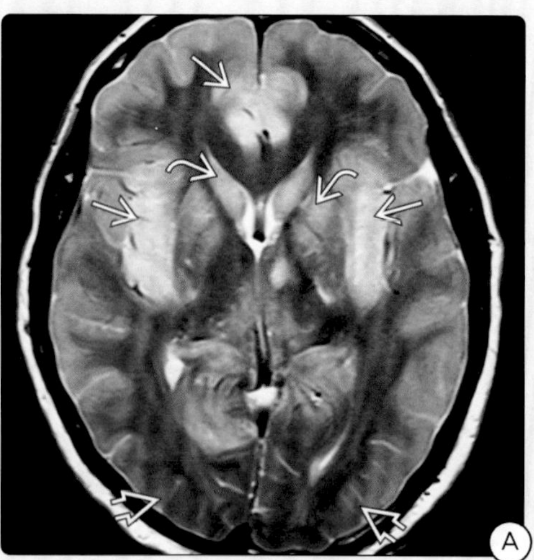

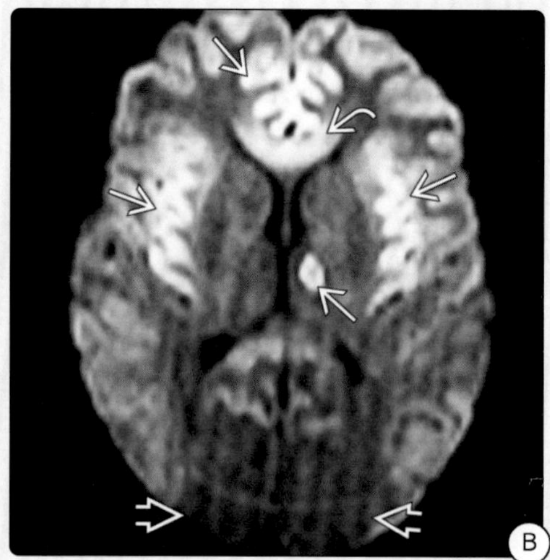

*(36-39A) Axial T2 in a patient with ornithine OTCD shows basal ganglia ➪, cortical hyperintensity, most striking in periinsular and frontal cortices ➡. Note that occipital lobes ➪ are relatively spared. (36-39B) Axial DWI in the same patient shows diffusion hyperintensity in periinsular and frontal cortices ➡ and left thalamus with less striking involvement of corpus callosum ➪. Occipital lobes ➪ show no evidence of restricted diffusion.*

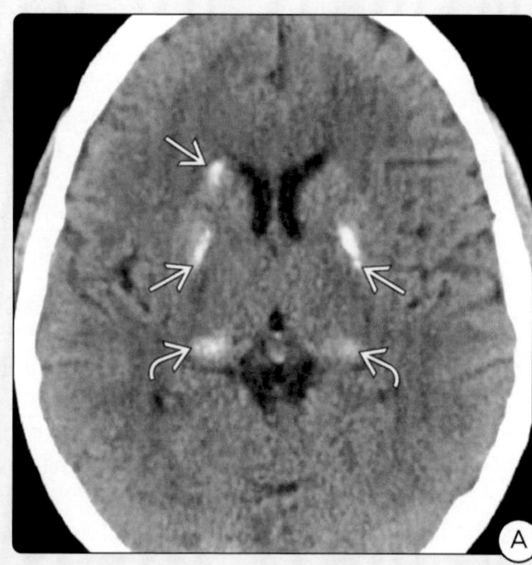

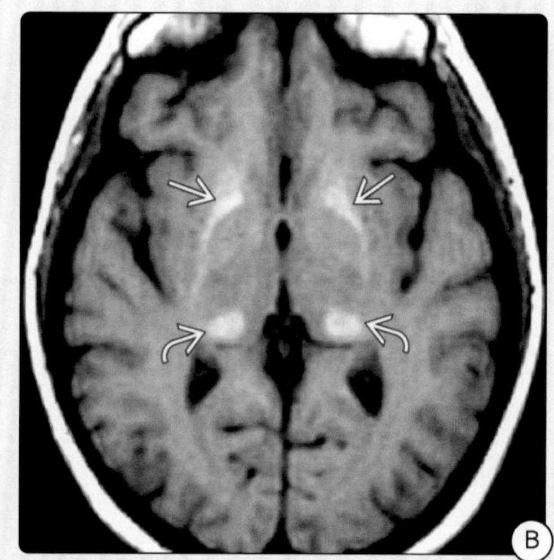

*(36-40A) NECT in a patient with Fabry disease shows symmetric calcifications in the basal ganglia ➡, posterior thalami (pulvinars) ➪. (36-40B) T1 MR in the same case shows symmetric T1 shortening in the basal ganglia ➡. The T1 shortening in the pulvinars of both thalami ➪ is particularly striking.*

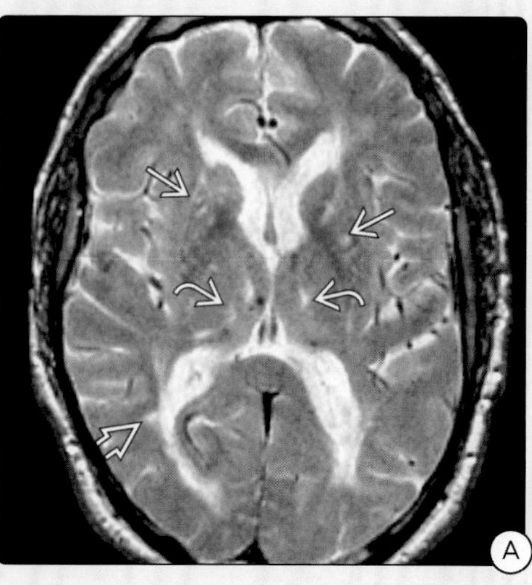

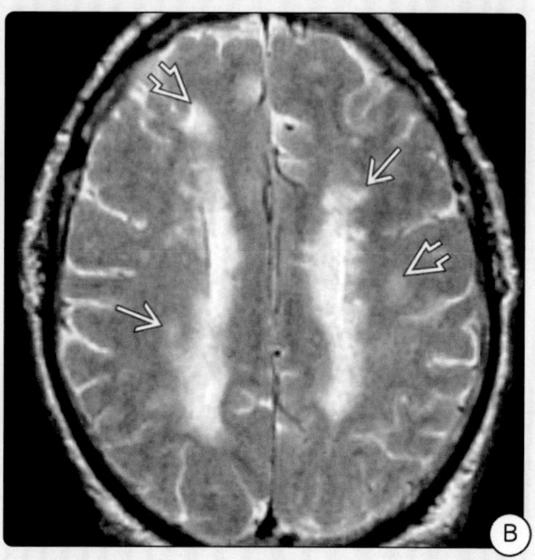

*(36-41A) T2 MR in a 50-yo man with multiple cryptogenic lacunar infarcts shows hyperintense foci in the basal ganglia ➡, thalami ➪, and deep periventricular WM ➪. (36-41B) More cephalad T2 MR in the same case shows multiple subcortical ➪, deep periventricular ➡ lacunar infarcts. This is Fabry disease.*

# Acquired Metabolic and Systemic Disorders

*In this chapter, we focus on acquired metabolic and systemic disorders that involve the CNS. We begin with the most common—hypertension—before turning our attention to abnormalities of glucose metabolism and thyroid/parathyroid function.*

We then discuss seizure disorders, as sustained ictal activity with hypermetabolism can have profound effects on the brain. We finish the section by exploring cytotoxic corpus callosum injury and transient global amnesia.

We close with miscellaneous but important acquired metabolic diseases, such as hepatic encephalopathy (HE) (both acute and chronic) and the osmotic demyelination syndromes.



## Hypertensive Encephalopathies

If not recognized and treated, the effects of both acutely elevated blood pressure and chronic hypertension (HTN) on the brain can be devastating. We begin this section with a discussion of acute hypertensive encephalopathy, then delve into the CNS damage caused by chronic HTN.

### Acute Hypertensive Encephalopathy

#### Terminology

The most common manifestation of acute hypertensive encephalopathy is **p**osterior **r**eversible **e**ncephalopathy **s**yndrome **(PRES)** **(37-1)**. Despite the syndrome's name, lesions are rarely limited to the "posterior" (parietooccipital) aspects of the brain, and atypical is more common than "classic" PRES **(37-3)**.

#### Etiology

**General Concepts.** The pathogenesis of PRES is not yet completely understood. The most common explanation is that severe HTN leads to failed cerebral autoregulation and breakthrough hyperperfusion with *vasodilatation*. However, between 15-20% of patients with PRES are normotensive or even hypotensive, whereas < 1/2 have a mean arterial pressure > 140-150 mm Hg.

Alternative theories for the development of PRES invoke vasculopathy with vascular endothelial injury and dysfunction.

**Associated Conditions.** PRES is associated with a multitude of diverse clinical entities, the most common of which are **eclampsia, HTN**, and **immunosuppressive treatment**.

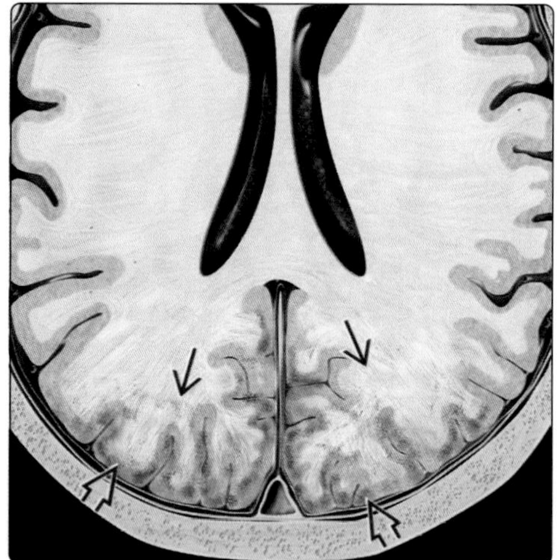

***(37-1)** Axial graphic show PRES with cortical & subcortical vasogenic edema ➔ in the posterior circulation with some petechial hemorrhage ➔.*

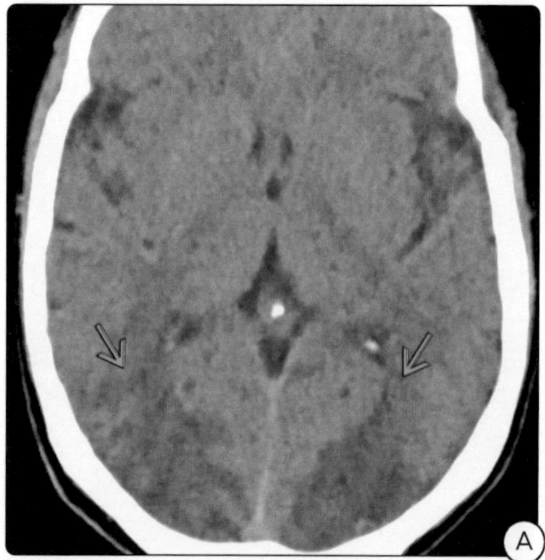


***(37-2A)** NECT in severe hypertension (HTN) shows bioccipital hypodensities in the subcortical white matter (WM) ➔. Initial CT may be normal.*

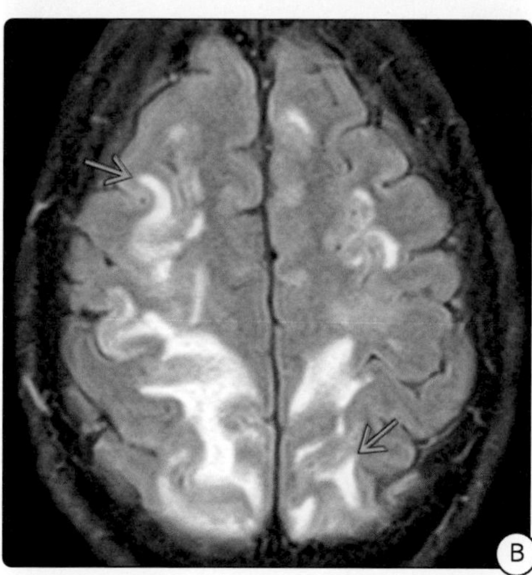


***(37-2B)** Axial FLAIR MR in the same case shows symmetric hyperintensity in the frontal & parietal subcortical WM ➔ related to PRES.*

Other conditions associated with PRES include renal failure with hemolytic-uremic syndrome (HUS), thrombotic thrombocytopenic purpura (TTP), autoimmune disorders (e.g., lupus nephropathy and acute glomerulonephritis), shock/sepsis syndrome, postcarotid endarterectomy with reperfusion syndrome, endocrine disorders, stimulant drugs, such as ephedrine and pseudoephedrine, and ingestion of some food products (e.g., licorice).

## Pathology

Autopsied brains from patients with complicated PRES show diffuse cerebral edema. Intracranial hemorrhage complicates 15-25% of PRES cases. The most common finding is multiple bilateral petechial microhemorrhages in the occipital lobes **(37-1)**.

Microvascular pathology includes fibrinoid arteriolar necrosis with petechial hemorrhages, proteinaceous exudates, and macrophage infiltration along the perivascular spaces.

Pathologic evidence of partial irreversible damage has been documented in PRES despite radiographic resolution of abnormalities. Scattered microinfarcts, white matter (WM) rarefaction with subpial gliosis, and hemosiderin deposition—especially in the posterior cerebrum—have been reported.

**POSTERIOR REVERSIBLE ENCEPHALOPATHY SYNDROME: TERMINOLOGY, ETIOLOGY, AND CLINICAL ISSUES**

**Terminology**

- **P**osterior **r**eversible **e**ncephalopathy **s**yndrome (PRES)
- *Lesions often not* just *posterior, not always reversible!*

**Etiology**

- HTN-induced dysautoregulation vs. vasospasm, ↓ perfusion
- ↑ ↑ BP → failed autoregulation → hyperperfusion
  - Vasogenic (not cytotoxic) edema
  - Endothelial dysfunction ± excessive circulating cytokines → "leaky" blood-brain barrier
  - Fluid, macromolecules ± blood extravasate
- Causes (HTN typical but not invariable)
  - Preeclampsia/eclampsia
  - Chemotherapy, immunosuppressive drugs
  - Thrombotic microangiopathies (e.g., HUS/TTP)
  - Renal failure
  - Shock/sepsis
  - Tumor lysis syndrome
  - Food-/drug-induced mineralocorticoid excess

**Clinical Issues**

- All ages (peak = 20-40 years)
- F >> M
- BP usually ↑ ↑ **but**
  - < 50% have **mean** arterial pressure > 140-50 mm Hg
  - 15-20% normotensive or hypotensive
- Usually resolves completely with BP normalization

## Clinical Issues

**Epidemiology and Demographics.** Although the peak age of onset is 20-40 years, PRES can affect patients of all ages from infants to older adults. There is a moderate female predominance, largely because of the strong association of PRES and preeclampsia.

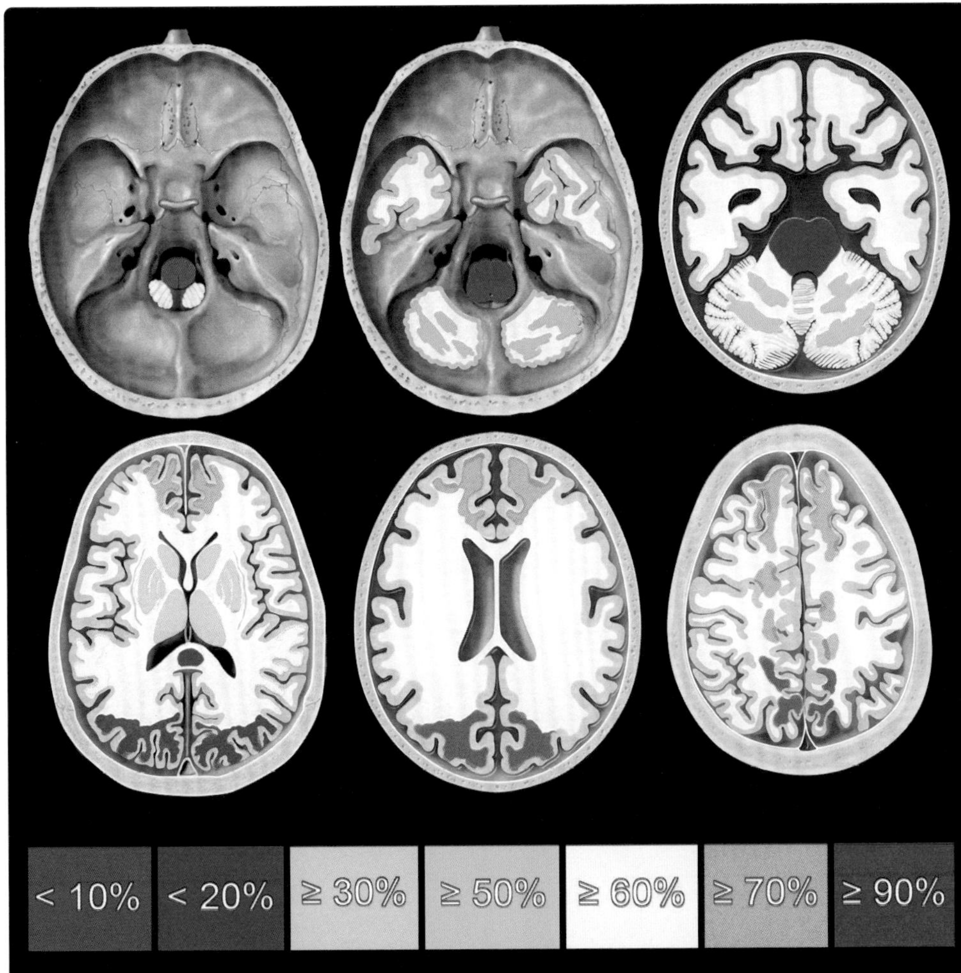


*(37-3) Graphic shows location, relative frequency of PRES lesions. Although > 90% have lesions in the parietooccipital subcortical WM (classic PRES, shown in red), note that multifocality is the rule, not the exception. Most cases of PRES also have lesions in areas other than the classic parietooccipital location. Both classic PRES (red) & the superior frontal sulcus pattern (orange) are frequently combined with additional lesions distributed along the hemispheric cortical (superficial) watershed zones (depicted in the lower right image). The cerebellum is affected in nearly 1/2 of PRES cases, whereas ~ 1/3 have basal ganglia & thalamic lesions (light blue). The pons, medulla, cervical spinal cord, & corpus callosum splenium are less common sites involved by PRES, although, in some cases, only the posterior fossa is affected. Remember: Atypical PRES is actually more common than the classic isolated parietooccipital involvement! (Adapted from Ollivier et al.)*

**Preeclampsia** is the most common overall cause of PRES. HTN (blood pressure > 140/90 mm Hg) and proteinuria are typical. Progression from preeclampsia to **eclampsia** (mean systolic ≥ 160 mm Hg) occurs in 0.5% of patients with mild and 2-3% of patients with severe preeclampsia.

**Presentation.** Although 92% of patients with PRES have acutely elevated blood pressure, *PRES can also occur in the absence of HTN.* The most common clinical symptoms and signs in patients with PRES are encephalopathy (50-80%), seizure (60-75%), headache (50%), visual disturbances (33%), and focal neurologic deficit (10-15%).

**Natural History and Treatment Options.** Reversibility is a typical feature of PRES and is associated with good prognosis. If the inciting substances or precipitating conditions are eliminated and any existing HTN is promptly treated, PRES often resolves with minimal or no residual abnormalities.

Extensive vasogenic edema, hemorrhage, and restricted diffusion on initial imaging are associated with worse clinical outcomes. Severe PRES can be life threatening. In rare cases, lesions are irreversible and permanent damage occurs, typically hemorrhagic cortical/subcortical or basal ganglionic infarcts.

## Imaging

**General Features.** Three distinct imaging patterns of PRES have been described. The most common is a dominant **parietal-occipital pattern** (classic or typical PRES). Two less common (atypical) patterns are a **superior frontal sulcus pattern** (involvement of the mid and posterior aspects of the superior frontal sulcus) and a **holohemispheric watershed pattern** (involvement of the frontal, parietal, and occipital lobes along the internal watershed zones). Combinations of these three patterns as well as involvement of other anatomic areas are also common **(37-3)**.

The parietooccipital lobes are involved in > 90% of PRES cases **(37-1) (37-2) (37-4B)**. The frontal lobes are involved in 75-77% of cases with the temporal lobes (65%) and cerebellum (50-55%) also commonly affected. Other atypical distributions include the basal ganglia and thalami, deep WM, corpus callosum splenium, brainstem, and cervical spinal cord.

**CT Findings.** NECT scans are commonly obtained as an initial screening study **(37-4A) (37-2A)**. It is therefore extremely important to identify even subtle abnormalities that may be suggestive of PRES. **If the screening NECT is normal and PRES is suspected on clinical grounds, an MR scan with DWI**

**and T2* in addition to the routine sequences (T1 and T2/FLAIR) should be obtained.**

Screening NECTs are normal in ~ 1/4 of all PRES cases **(37-4)**. Subtle, patchy cortical/subcortical hypodensities—usually in the parietooccipital lobes, watershed zones, &/or cerebellum—may be the only visible abnormalities on NECT **(37-2A)**. PRES-associated intracranial hemorrhage is uncommon.

**MR Findings.** PRES has both classic and atypical (i.e., variant) MR features. Keep in mind that (1) atypical PRES is actually more common than classic (i.e., purely parietooccipital) PRES; (2) PRES is rarely *just* posterior; and (3) PRES is *not always reversible.*

*Classic* PRES demonstrates bilateral parietooccipital cortical/subcortical hypointensities that are hypointense on T1WI and hyperintense on T2/FLAIR **(37-2B)** **(37-4B)**. T2* (GRE or SWI) sequences may demonstrate hemorrhagic foci. Transient patchy cortical-subcortical enhancement on T1 C+ may occur.

Imaging findings in *atypical* PRES include involvement of the frontal lobes, watershed zones, basal ganglia &/or thalami, brainstem, cerebellum, and even the spinal cord **(37-6)** **(37-7)**. Findings of both classic and atypical PRES very commonly occur together.

In unusual cases, brainstem &/or cerebellar lesions may be the *only* abnormality present. The spinal cord has been reported as a rare site of isolated PRES involvement.

Frank infarction is quite rare in PRES. Because most cases of PRES are caused by vasogenic—not cytotoxic—edema, DWI is usually negative **(37-5)**. However, PRES with restricted diffusion occurs in 15-30% of cases and is usually seen as small foci of restricted diffusion within larger regions of nonrestricting vasogenic edema.

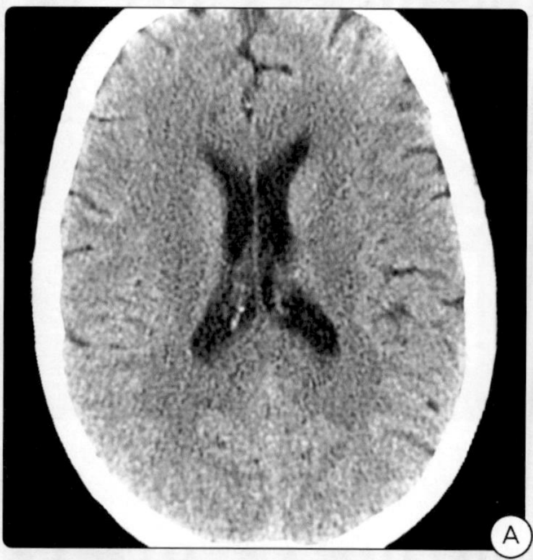


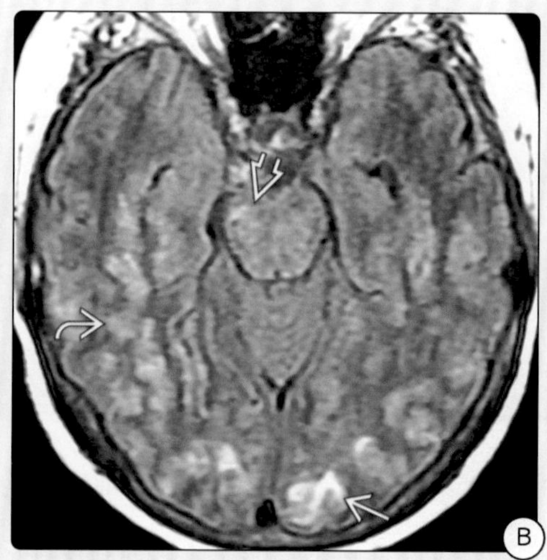


***(37-4A)** A 63-yo woman with end-stage renal disease had a seizure, then fell. Blood pressure on admission was 220/140. NECT performed to evaluate for intracranial hemorrhage shows no focal abnormality. **(37-4B)** MR was ordered for suspected PRES. FLAIR MR obtained 1 hour after the NECT shows multifocal patchy hyperintensities in the midbrain ➡, posteroinferior temporal lobe WM ➡, & occipital cortex ➡.*

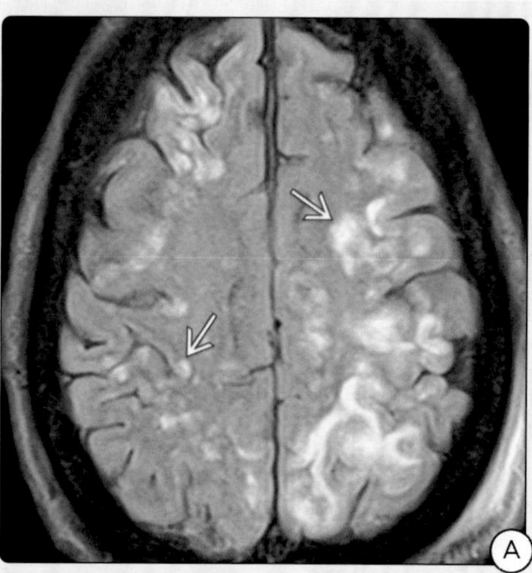


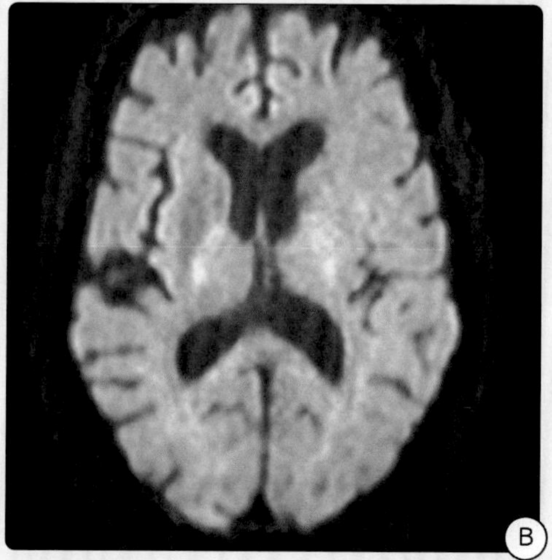


***(37-5A)** FLAIR MR in a 73-yo found down & hypertensive shows asymmetric hyperintensity in the subcortical WM & cortex of the frontal & parietal lobes ➡ related to PRES. **(37-5B)** DTI MR (same patient) shows no diffusion restriction. DWI/DTI images are usually, though not always, normal in PRES, as the edema is predominantly vasogenic, not cytotoxic. Complicated PRES may show DTI abnormality.*

Following blood pressure normalization, imaging findings in most cases of PRES resolve completely. Irreversible lesions are relatively uncommon, occurring in ~ 15% of cases.

## Differential Diagnosis

The major differential diagnoses of PRES include acute cerebral ischemia-infarction, vasculitis, hypoglycemia, status epilepticus (SE), sinovenous thrombosis, reversible cerebral vasoconstriction syndrome (RCVS), and the thrombotic microangiopathies.

PRES rarely involves *just* the posterior circulation, so **acute cerebral ischemia-infarction** is often easily distinguished. **Vasculitis** can resemble PRES-induced vasculopathy on CTA or DSA.

The distribution of lesions in vasculitis is much more random and less symmetric, usually does not demonstrate the parietooccipital predominance seen in PRES, and more often enhances following contrast administration. Vasculitis may have associated hemorrhage. In contrast to vasculitis, high-resolution vessel wall imaging is usually negative in PRES.

**Hypoglycemia** typically affects the parietooccipital cortex and subcortical WM, so the clinical laboratory findings (i.e., low serum glucose, lack of systemic HTN) are important differentiating features. **SE** can cause transient gyral edema but is rarely bilateral and can affect any part of the cortex.

Less common entities that can mimic PRES include **RCVS**. RCVS shares some features (e.g., convexal subarachnoid hemorrhage) with PRES but is typically limited to a solitary sulcus or just a few adjacent sulci. On DSA, RCVS involves large and medium-sized arteries with diffuse, multifocal, segmental narrowing. Small infarcts are often seen on DWI/DTI.

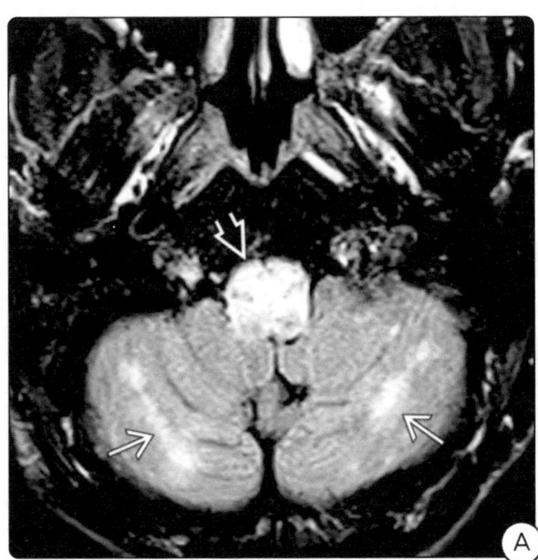


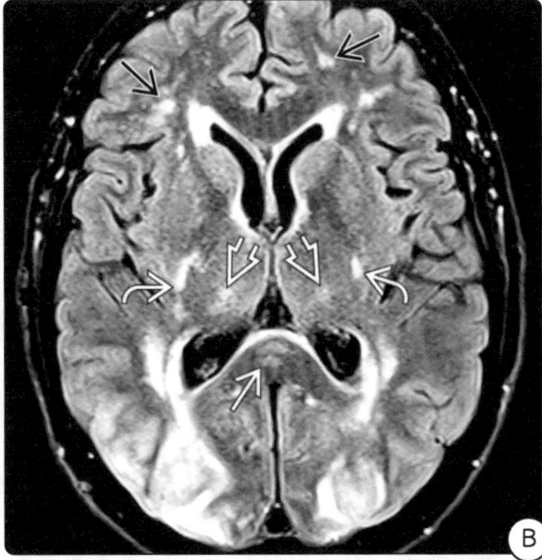


***(37-6A)** Axial FLAIR MR in a 50-yo man with severe HTN (blood pressure = 200/120) shows confluent hyperintensity involving the entire medulla ➡. Note patchy hyperintensities in the WM of both cerebellar hemispheres ➡. **(37-6B)** Additional lesions are present in the thalami ➡, internal capsules ↪, corpus callosum splenium ➡, & frontal WM ⇨.*

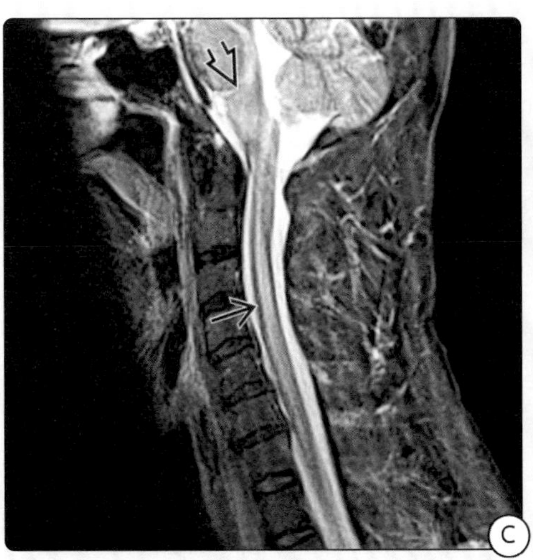


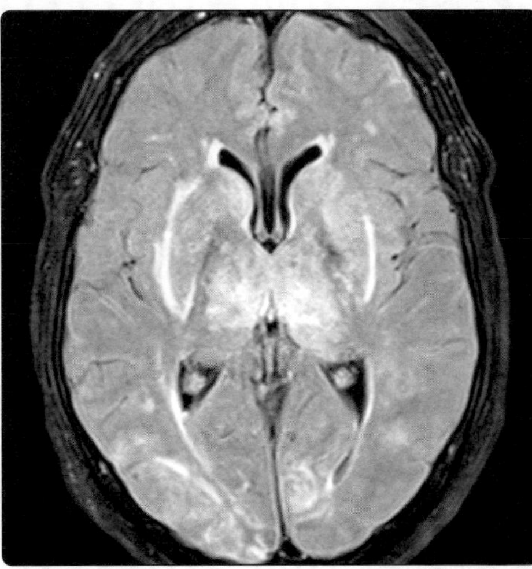

***(37-6C)** Sagittal STIR of the cervical spine shows confluent hyperintensity extending from the medulla ⇨ inferiorly throughout the entire cervical spinal cord ⇨. This is atypical PRES. Remember: "Atypical" PRES is more common than "classic" PRES! **(37-7)** Axial FLAIR MR in a patient with seizures & HTN shows hyperintensity in the deep gray nuclei & occipital lobes related to PRES.*

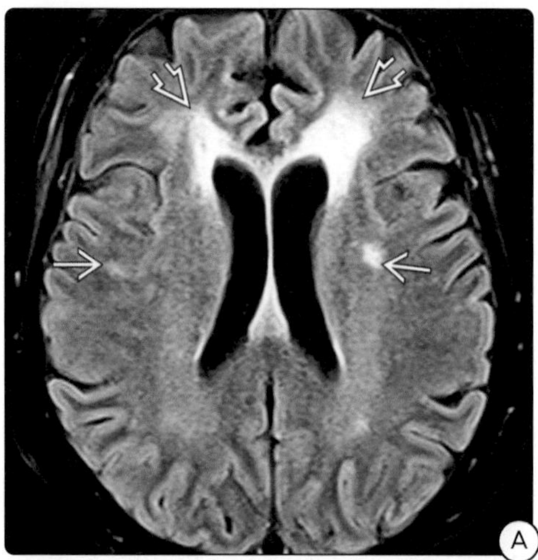

*(37-8A) FLAIR in 54-yo woman with chronic renal failure, TTP, confusion shows bifrontal confluent ➡, scattered WM ➡ hyperintensities.*

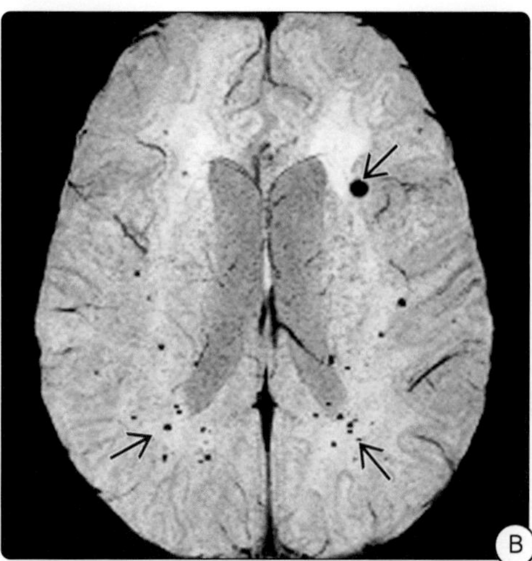

*(37-8B) SWI shows multiple "blooming" foci ➡, microhemorrhage throughout the WM with cortex sparing. Malignant HTN.*

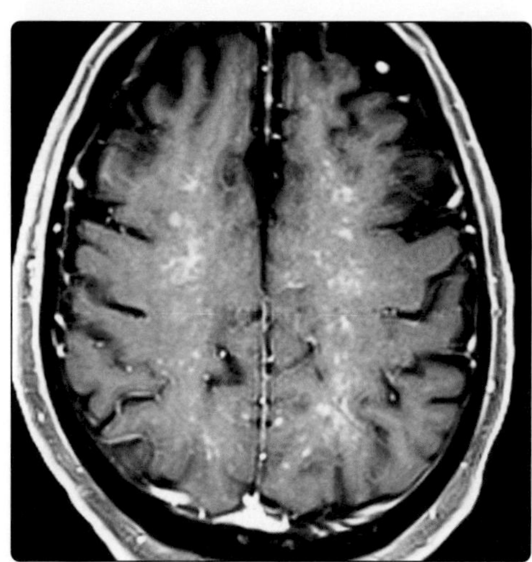

*(37-9) T1 C+ FS shows extensive patchy enhancement in the WM of both hemispheres in malignant HTN.*

**POSTERIOR REVERSIBLE ENCEPHALOPATHY SYNDROME: IMAGING AND DIFFERENTIAL DIAGNOSIS**

**3 Anatomic Patterns**

- Classic PRES
  - **Parietooccipital pattern** (> 90%)
- Variant PRES
  - **Superior frontal sulcus pattern** (70%)
  - **Holohemispheric watershed pattern** (50%)
  - Other: Cerebellum (50%), basal ganglia (30%), brainstem (20%), spinal cord (< 10%)
- Combinations *very* common (> 90%)

**CT**

- Can be normal or only subtly abnormal
  - If PRES suspected and CT normal, get MR!
- Posterior cortical/subcortical hypodensities
- Gross hemorrhage rare (parenchymal > convexal subarachnoid hemorrhage)

**MR**

- T2/FLAIR hyperintensity (parietooccipital most common)
- T2* (GRE/SWI) shows hemorrhage in 15-25%
- DWI usually but not invariably negative
- Enhancement none/mild (unless severe PRES)

**Differential Diagnosis**

- Posterior circulation ischemia-infarction
  - Top of basilar syndrome
- Vasculitis
- SE
- Hypoglycemia
- Thrombotic microangiopathy
  - Primary (ADAMTS13-mediated thrombotic microangiopathy/TTP, Shiga toxin-mediated HUS)
  - Secondary (malignant HTN, HELLP syndrome, autoimmune disorders, DIC)
- Sinovenous thrombosis
  - Internal cerebral veins, vein of Galen/straight sinus
- RCVS

## Malignant Hypertension

### Terminology and Etiology

**Malignant HTN** (mHTN), a.k.a. acute hypertensive crisis, is characterized clinically by extreme blood pressure elevation and papilledema. Diastolic levels often exceed 130-140 mm Hg. **The abruptness of blood pressure elevation seems to be more important than the absolute level of either systolic or mean arterial blood pressure**.

### Pathology

Macroscopically, the brain appears swollen and edematous. Gross parenchymal hematomas and perivascular petechial microhemorrhages may be present. Acute microinfarcts, especially in the basal ganglia and pons, are common.

### Imaging

Imaging findings in mHTN range from classic PRES to "atypical" features. "Atypical" features are more common in mHTN. Brainstem-dominant hypertensive encephalopathy and basal ganglia &/or watershed lesions are common cerebral manifestations of mHTN.

Lobar &/or multifocal parenchymal microhemorrhages in the cortex, basal ganglia, pons, and cerebellum are common in mHTN and are best seen as "blooming" foci on T2* sequences (GRE, SWI) **(37-8)**. Convexal subarachnoid hemorrhage has been reported in a few cases of mHTN. Contrast images may show striking multifocal patchy enhancement related to widespread blood-brain barrier disruption **(37-9)**.

**ACUTE HYPERTENSIVE ENCEPHALOPATHY**

**Terminology**
- a.k.a. mHTN, hypertensive crisis

**Etiology**
- Abrupt rise in BP > absolute value of BP
- Many causes (uncontrolled HTN, drug abuse, etc.)

**Imaging**
- Brainstem, basal ganglia > > cortex, watershed
- Microbleeds on T2* (GRE, SWI) common

**Differential Diagnosis**
- Major differential diagnosis is PRES (can, often does, overlap)

## Chronic Hypertensive Encephalopathy

Although the clinical and imaging manifestations of PRES and mHTN can be dramatic and life threatening, the effects of longstanding untreated or poorly treated HTN on end-organ function can be equally devastating and are far more common.

### Pathology

The most consistent histopathologic feature of chronic hypertensive encephalopathy is a microvasculopathy characterized by arteriolosclerosis and lipohyalinosis (see Chapter 10). The microvasculopathy is accompanied by myelin pallor, gliosis, and spongiform WM volume loss. Multiple lacunar infarcts are common.

### Clinical Issues

Chronic hypertensive encephalopathy is most common in middle-aged and older adult patients. In addition to age and chronically elevated blood pressure, smoking is an independent risk factor as is metabolic syndrome (impaired glucose metabolism, elevated blood pressure, central obesity, and dyslipidemia).

### Imaging

The two cardinal imaging features of chronic hypertensive encephalopathy are (1) diffuse patchy &/or confluent WM lesions and (2) multifocal microbleeds. The WM lesions are concentrated in the corona radiata and deep periventricular WM—especially around the atria of the lateral ventricles. The damaged WM appears hypodense on NECT scans and hyperintense on T2/FLAIR imaging.

Multiple petechial bleeds ("microhemorrhages") are the second most common manifestation of chronic hypertensive encephalopathy. These are not usually identifiable on NECT and may be invisible on standard MR sequences (FSE T2WI and FLAIR). T2* (GRE, SWI) scans show multiple "blooming" hypointensities ("black dots") that tend to be concentrated in the basal ganglia and cerebellum **(37-10)**.

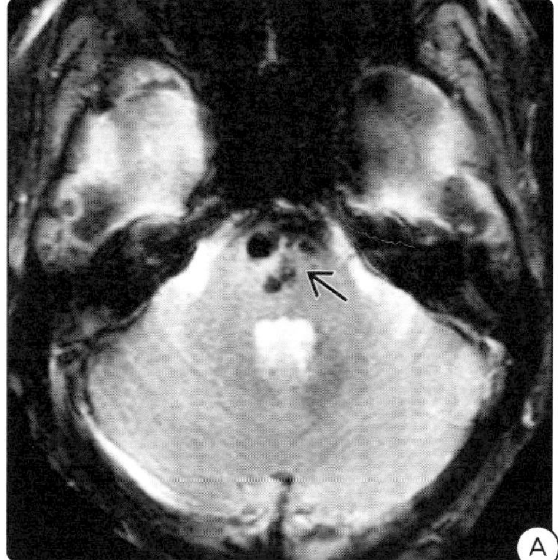


***(37-10A)*** *T2* GRE in a 37-yo woman with longstanding, poorly treated HTN shows multiple "blooming" foci in the pons ⇨.*

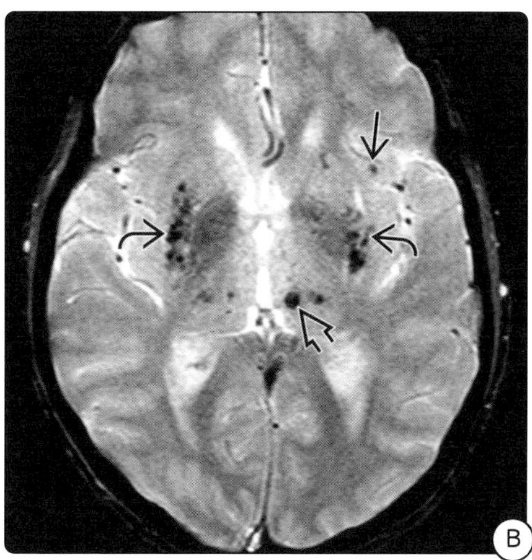


***(37-10B)*** *Numerous hypointensities in the basal ganglia ⇨ & thalami ⇨ & a single lesion in the left insular cortex ⇨ are present.*

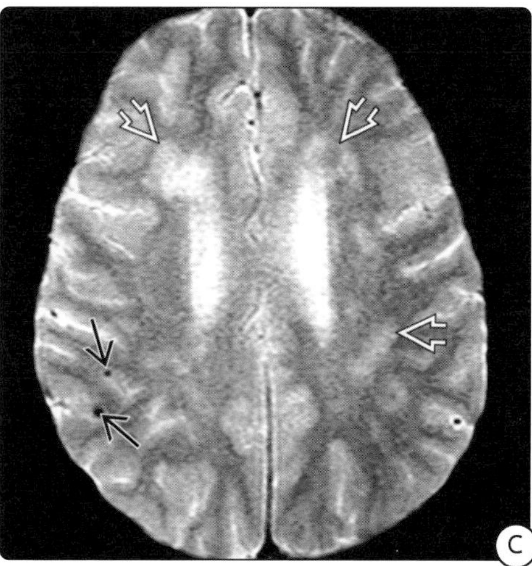


***(37-10C)*** *Scattered foci of gradient susceptibility in the cortex ⇨, extensive periventricular WM hyperintensities ⇨ are present. Chronic HTN.*

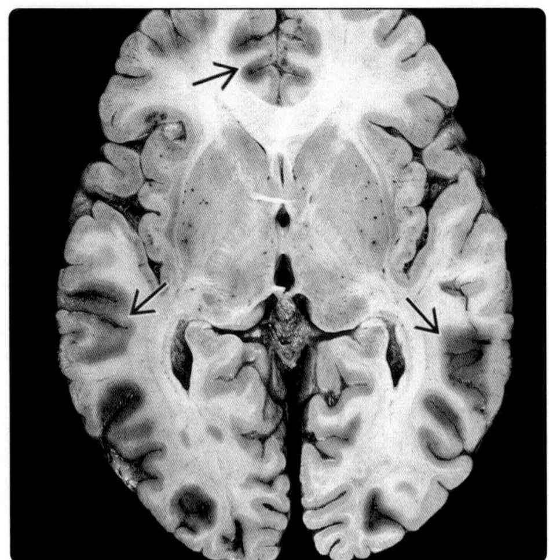

*(37-11) Autopsy of severe hypoglycemia shows bilateral symmetric parietooccipital, frontal cortical necrosis ➡. (Courtesy R. Hewlett, MD.)*

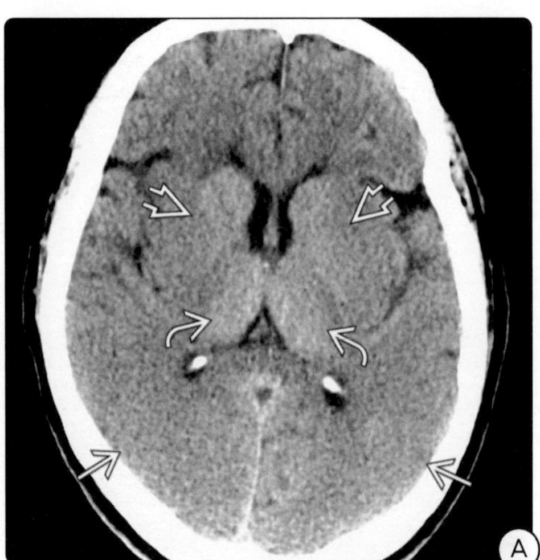

*(37-12A) NECT shows typical changes of hypoglycemia with parietooccipital gyral swelling ➡, putamen hypodensity ➡, spared thalami ➡.*

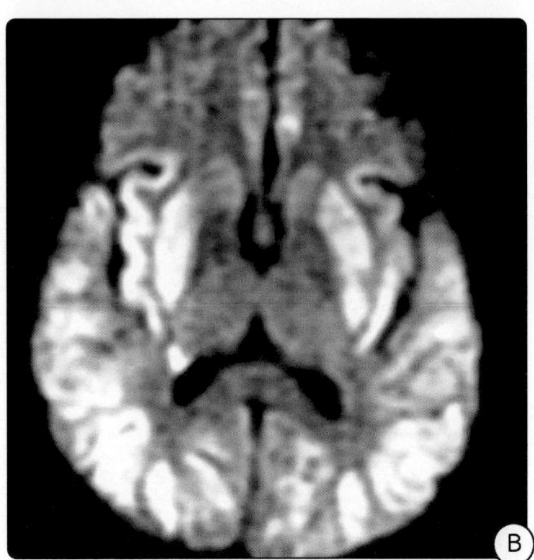

*(37-12B) DWI in the same case of typical acute HE shows restricted diffusion in parietooccipital cortex, putamina with thalamic & WM sparing.*

## Differential Diagnosis

The major differential diagnosis of chronic hypertensive encephalopathy is **cerebral amyloid angiopathy** (CAA). The WM lesions in both diseases often appear similar, and both disorders can cause hemorrhagic microangiopathy. The microbleeds of CAA are more often peripheral (e.g., cortex, siderosis of the leptomeninges) and rarely affect the brainstem or cerebellum. Hypertensive microhemorrhages are most common in the basal ganglia, pons, and cerebellum.

**Cerebral autosomal dominant arteriopathy without subcortical infarcts and leukoencephalopathy** (CADASIL) can also mimic chronic hypertensive encephalopathy. CADASIL typically presents in younger patients and causes multiple subcortical lacunar infarcts. Lesions in the anterior temporal lobes and external capsules are classic imaging findings of CADASIL.

**CHRONIC HYPERTENSIVE ENCEPHALOPATHY**

**Pathology**
- Microvasculopathy
  - Arteriolosclerosis, lipohyalinosis
  - Myelin pallor, lacunar infarcts
  - Microbleeds (cerebellum, basal ganglia/thalami > cortex)

**Clinical Issues**
- Metabolic syndrome, headaches
- Can have "acute-on-chronic" HTN with encephalopathy

**Imaging**
- Diffuse patchy &/or confluent WM lesions
- Microbleeds on T2* (basal ganglia, cerebellum)

**Differential Diagnosis**
- Amyloid angiopathy (cortex > basal ganglia, cerebellum)
- CADASIL (younger patients, anterior temporal/external capsule WM lesions)

# Glucose Disorders

The brain is a glucose glutton, consuming > 1/2 of the body's total glucose. Because the brain does not store excess energy as glycogen, CNS function is highly dependent on a steady, continuous supply of blood glucose (see next box).

Blood glucose levels are tightly regulated and are normally maintained within a narrow physiologic range. Disorders of glucose metabolism—both *hypo*glycemia and *hyper*glycemia—can injure the CNS.

The neurologic manifestations of deranged glucose metabolism range from mild, reversible focal deficits to SE, coma, and death. Because the clinical and imaging manifestations differ in neonates from those of older children and adults, hypoglycemia in these two age groups is discussed separately.

## Pediatric/Adult Hypoglycemic Encephalopathy

### Terminology

**Hypoglycemia** literally means low blood sugar and is caused by an imbalance between glucose supply and glucose utilization. Acute hypoglycemic brain injury is called hypoglycemic encephalopathy.

## Etiology

Childhood hypoglycemic encephalopathy is most commonly associated with type 1 diabetes mellitus. In its most common adult setting—advanced type 2 diabetes—hypoglycemia typically results from the interplay between absolute or relative insulin excess and compromised glucose counterregulation; insulin in and of itself is not neurotoxic. Most cases of adult hypoglycemia occur as a side effect of diabetes treatment with insulin and sulfonylureas.

## Pathology

Cortical necrosis is the most common gross finding in hypoglycemic encephalopathy. Although the entire cortical ribbon can be affected, the parietooccipital regions are usually the most severely involved **(37-11)**. Other especially vulnerable areas include the basal ganglia, hippocampi, and amygdalae. The thalami, WM, brainstem, and cerebellum are typically spared.

## Clinical Issues

The typical hypoglycemic patient is an older diabetic patient on insulin replacement therapy with altered dietary glucose intake. Deliberate or accidental insulin overdose is more common in children and young or middle-aged adults.

## Imaging

**CT Findings.** NECT scans typically show symmetrically hypodense parietal and occipital lobes. The putamina frequently appear hypodense, whereas the thalami are spared **(37-12A)**. In severe cases, diffuse cerebral edema with near-total sulcal effacement and blurred gray matter (GM)-WM interfaces can be seen.

**MR Findings.** T2/FLAIR hyperintensity in the parietooccipital cortex and basal ganglia is typical of acute hypoglycemic encephalopathy. The thalami, subcortical/deep WM, and cerebellum are generally spared. T2* scans generally show minimal or no "blooming" to suggest hemorrhage. Enhancement on T1 C+ is variable and, when present, usually mild.

DWI scans show restricted diffusion in the affected areas, predominately the posterior parietal and occipital cortex **(37-12B)**. Cytotoxic corpus callosum splenium lesions with restricted diffusion have also been reported in association with hypoglycemia.

## Differential Diagnosis

The most important differential diagnosis of hypoglycemic encephalopathy is **hypoxic-ischemic encephalopathy** (HIE). HIE typically occurs following cardiac arrest or global hypoperfusion. In contrast to hypoglycemic encephalopathy, the thalami and cerebellum are often affected in HIE. **Acute cerebral ischemia-infarction** is wedge-shaped, involving both the cortex and underlying WM. **Acute hypertensive encephalopathy** typically affects the parietooccipital cortex but spares most of the underlying WM and rarely restricts on DWI.

# Neonatal/Infantile Hypoglycemia

Unlike older children and adults, neonates have lower absolute glucose demands and can utilize other substrates, such as lactate, to produce energy. Nevertheless, prolonged &/or severe hypoglycemia can result in devastating brain injury in newborn infants.

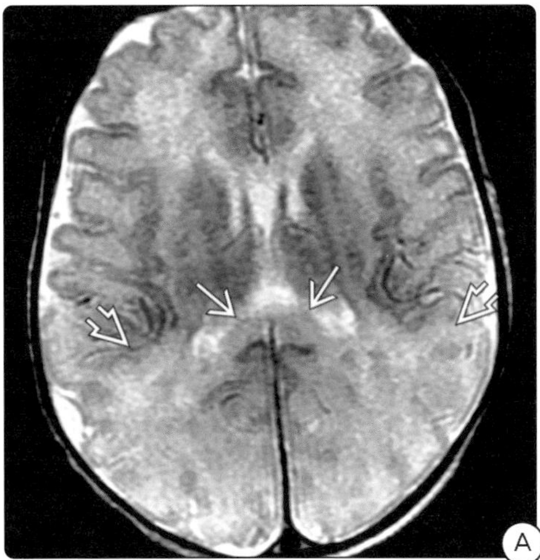


***(37-13A)*** *T2 MR in 5-day-old hypoglycemic infant shows edematous, hyperintense parietooccipital lobes ➡, corpus callosum splenium ➡.*

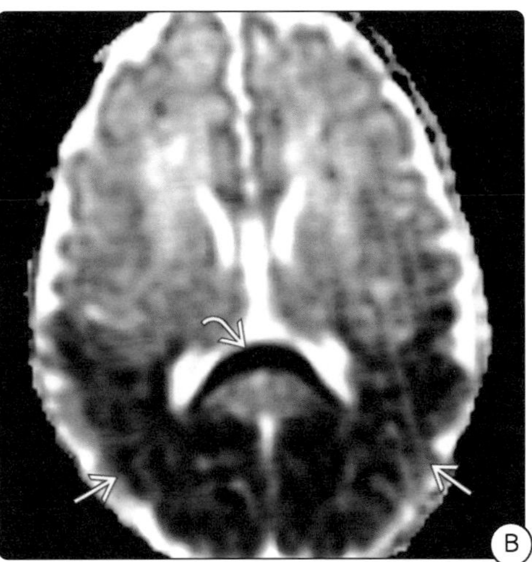


***(37-13B)*** *ADC shows profound restricted diffusion in the parietal & occipital lobes ➡ & corpus callosum splenium ➡.*

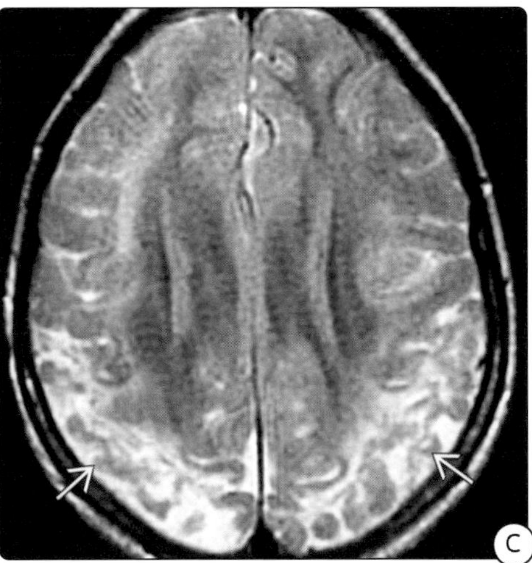


***(37-13C)*** *T2 MR at 1 year shows shrunken, hyperintense parietooccipital lobes with cortical loss & encephalomalacic-appearing WM ➡.*

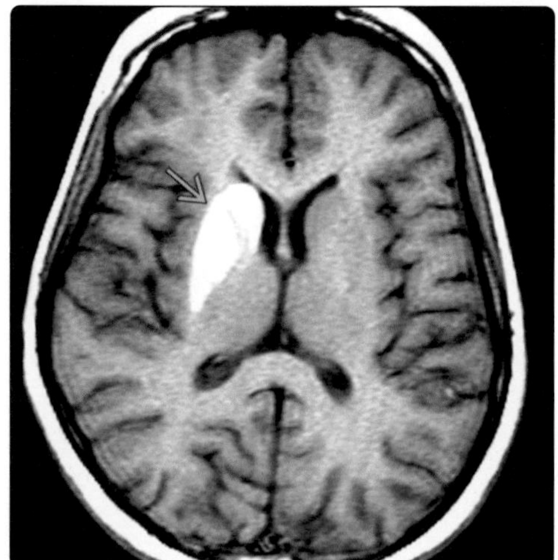

***(37-14) Axial T1 MR shows unilateral hyperintense basal ganglia ➙ in severe hyperglycemia (HIHH). (Courtesy K. K. Oguz, MD.)***

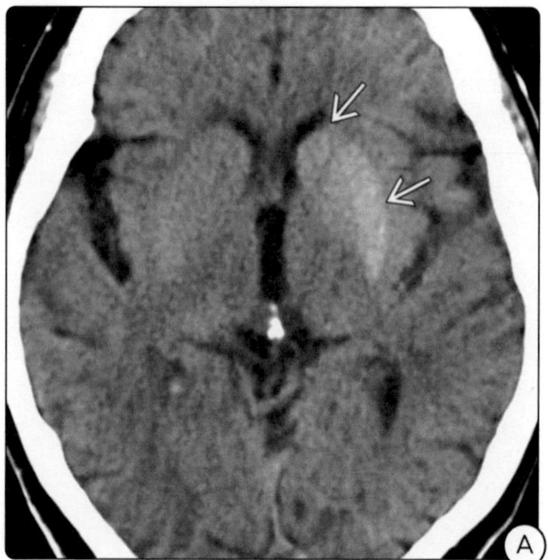

***(37-15A) Axial CT in an adult with involuntary unilateral movements shows hyperdensity ➙ in the caudate & putamen.***

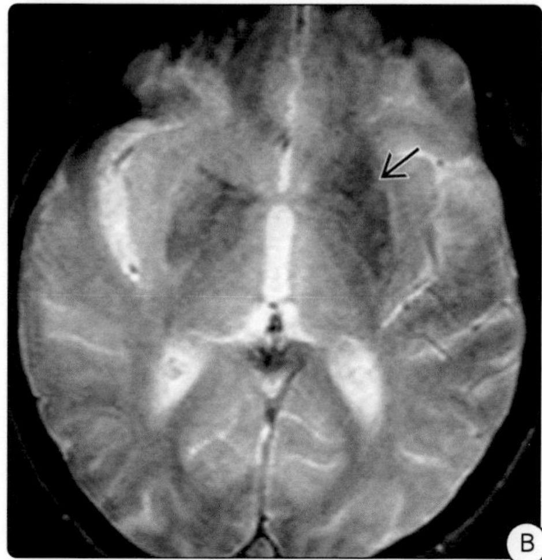

***(37-15B) Axial T2* GRE in the same patient shows mild hypointensity ➙ in the left basal ganglia related to HIHH. Patient with uncontrolled DM2.***

Neonatal/infantile hypoglycemic encephalopathy typically presents in the first three days of life, usually within the first 24 hours, and is most often caused by maternal diabetes with poor glycemic control. Uncontrolled maternal diabetes leads to chronic fetal hyperglycemia in utero. This results in *transient* neonatal hyperinsulinemia and hypoglycemia of varying severity. Congenital hyperinsulinism (HI) is the most common, most severe cause of *persistent* hypoglycemia in neonates and children.

MR scans in the acute stages of neonatal hypoglycemic encephalopathy show T2/FLAIR hyperintensity and restricted diffusion in the parietooccipital cortex, subcortical WM, and corpus callosum splenium **(37-13)**.

## HYPOGLYCEMIA

**General Concepts**

- Imbalance between glucose supply, utilization → hypoglycemia
- Can be mild, transient, asymptomatic
- Extent of brain injury depends on
  - Degree, duration of hypoglycemia
  - CBF, glucose utilization
  - Availability/utilization of alternative energy sources (e.g., lactate)
  - Exacerbating factors (e.g., hypoxia)
  - Recognition, prompt/appropriate treatment

**Pediatric/Adult Hypoglycemia**

- Etiology
  - Usually associated with diabetes
  - Absolute/relative insulin excess or glucose insufficiency
  - Energy production/$O_2$ utilization ↓, excitotoxic neurotransmitters ↑
- Pathology
  - Cortical necrosis
- Imaging
  - Hypodense/hyperintense parietooccipital cortex, basal ganglia
  - WM, thalami, cerebellum generally spared
  - Restricted diffusion common
  - May cause reversible corpus callosum splenium lesion

**Neonatal/Infantile Hypoglycemia**

- Etiology
  - Most common cause of transient hypoglycemia = maternal diabetes
  - Fetal hyperglycemia → neonatal hyperinsulinemia → hypoglycemia
  - Most common cause of severe, persistent hypoglycemia = congenital hyperinsulinemia (KATP mutation in 60%)
- Clinical issues
  - Usually presents in first 3 postnatal days
  - Glucose levels variable
- Imaging
  - Often similar to adult (posterior predominance)
  - Different: Subcortical WM, thalami often involved
- Differential diagnosis
  - Term HIE
  - Mitochondrial encephalopathy (mitochondrial encephalopathy with lactic acidosis and stroke-like episodes)

As with older children and adults, the major differential diagnosis of neonatal hypoglycemic encephalopathy is **term hypoxic-ischemic injury** (HII). Hypoglycemic encephalopathy and HII often coexist, potentiating the extent of brain injury. Imaging findings in the two disorders may be indistinguishable.

Inherited mitochondrial disorders, such as **mitochondrial encephalopathy with lactic acidosis and stroke-like episodes** (MELAS), may present with cortical swelling that spares the underlying WM. MELAS is rarely bilaterally symmetric and demonstrates much more markedly elevated lactate on MRS.

## Hyperglycemia-Associated Disorders

Hyperglycemia-induced brain injury can be chronic or acute. With the worldwide rise in obesity and the soaring prevalence of diabetes mellitus type 2 (DM2), the effects of *chronic* hyperglycemia on the brain are increasingly recognized. Patients with DM2 have accelerated arteriolosclerosis and lipohyalinosis with silent infarcts, brain volume loss, and decreased cognitive functioning.

MR in chronic hyperglycemia shows increased numbers of T2/FLAIR subcortical and periventricular hyperintensities, especially in the frontal WM, pons, and cerebellum. DTI demonstrates loss of microstructural integrity with decreased fractional anisotropy. Elevated myoinositol on MRS reflects gliosis, an indicator of brain injury.

*Acute* hyperglycemic brain injury can manifest as diabetic ketoacidosis (DKA). Imaging is nonspecific with vasogenic cerebral edema the most common abnormality. Hyperglycemic hyperosmolar state with overrapid correction may also develop osmotic demyelination with typical findings of central pontine myelinolysis.

Hyperglycemia-induced hemichorea-hemiballismus (HIHH), a.k.a. delayed-onset diabetic striatopathy, is characterized by involuntary unilateral movements. It is a complication of nonketotic hyperglycemia. MR classically shows T1 shortening in the unilateral basal ganglia with sparing of thalamus **(37-14)**. T2 may show hyperintensity and T2* may show hypointensity in the affected striatum **(37-15B)**. CT may show unilateral basal ganglia hyperdensity **(37-15)**.

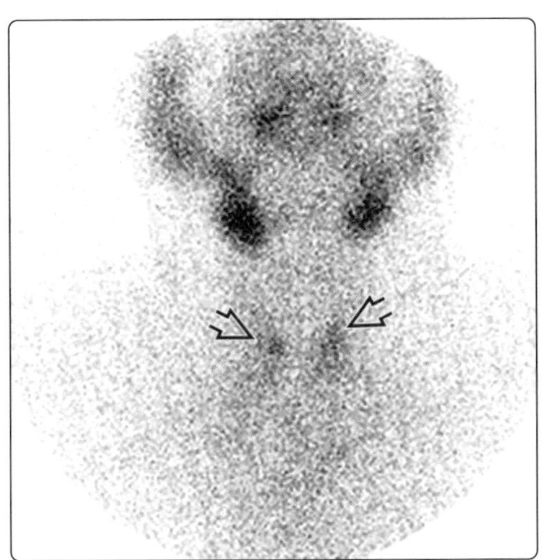

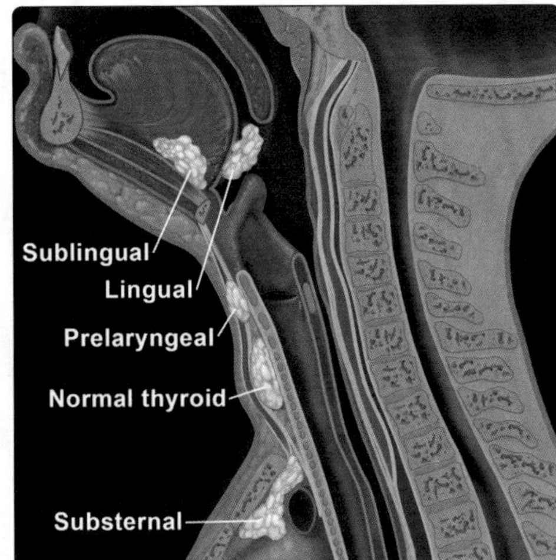


***(37-16)** Nuclear medicine Tc-99 in hypothyroidism related to inborn error of thyroid hormone metabolism shows low uptake ⇒ in a bilobed thyroid gland. Evaluation of congenital hypothyroidism often requires nuclear medicine study & ultrasound. (Courtesy J. P. O'Malley, MD.) **(37-17)** Graphic depicts typical locations of ectopic thyroid, primarily along the thyroglossal duct, though ectopic tissue may rarely occur elsewhere (i.e., substernal).*

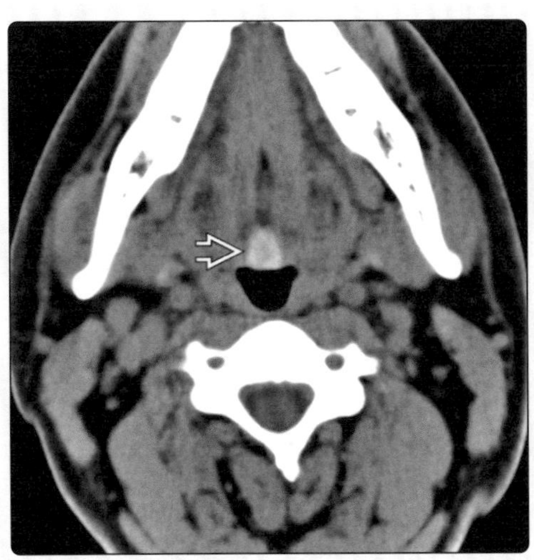

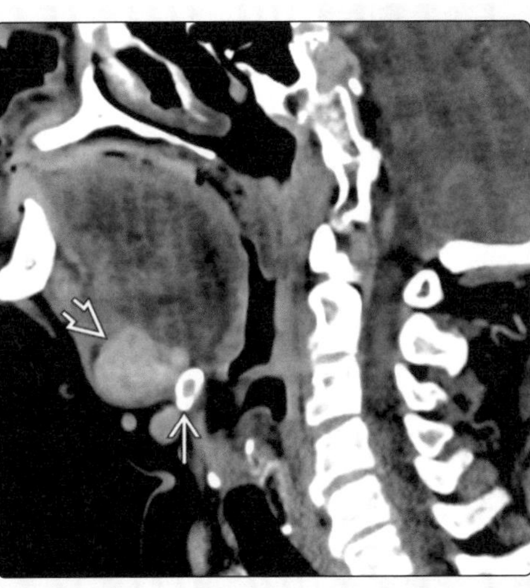

***(37-18)** Axial NECT in a 26-yo trauma patient shows a typical lingual thyroid as a midline hyperdense mass ➡ in the oral cavity, the most common location of ectopic thyroid. **(37-19)** Sagittal CECT shows a round enhancing mass ➡ related to ectopic thyroid anterior to the hyoid bone ➡. Ectopic thyroid may be seen from the tongue base to the superior mediastinum. In 75% of patients, lingual thyroid is only functioning thyroid tissue.*

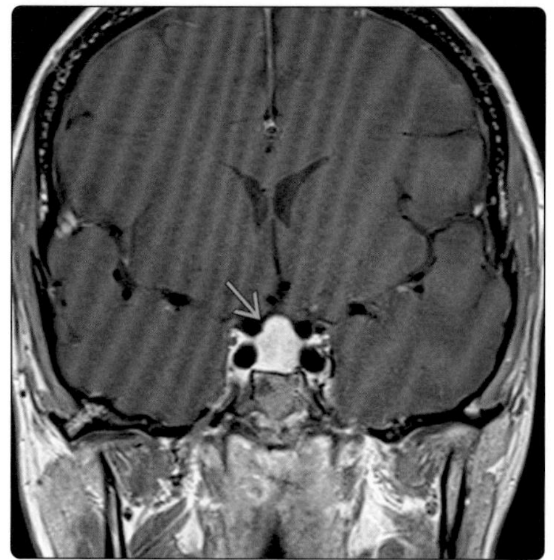
(37-20) Axial T1 C+ MR shows enlargement of the pituitary gland ⊟ in a 16-yo girl with hypothyroidism related to pituitary hyperplasia.

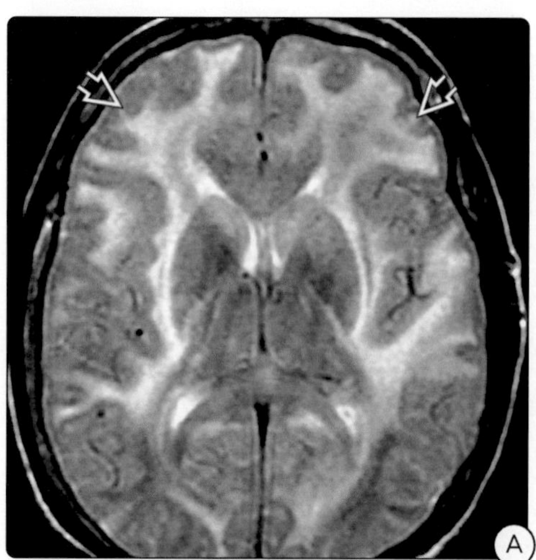

(37-21A) T2 MR of acute Hashimoto encephalopathy shows confluent, symmetric hyperintensity in the subcortical, deep WM ⊟.

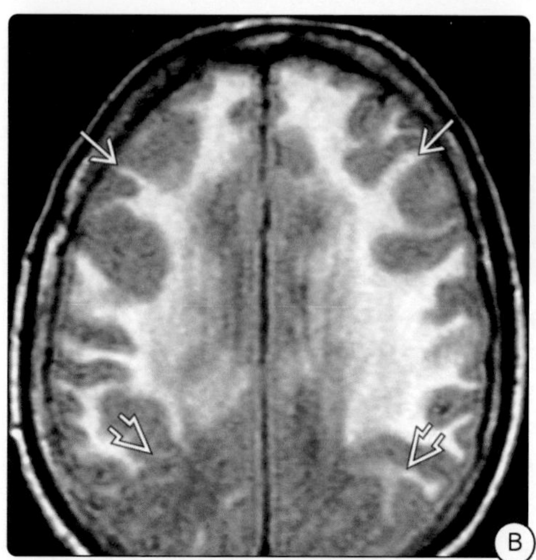

(37-21B) FLAIR MR through corona radiata shows frontal subcortical/deep WM edema ⊟ with marked sparing of the occipital lobes ⊟.

# Thyroid Disorders

Thyroid disorders are relatively common metabolic disturbances that are usually mild and rarely affect brain function. However, several imaging findings—some of them striking—have been associated with thyroid disease. Some can be mistaken for more serious disease (e.g., hypothyroid-induced pituitary hyperplasia mimicking pituitary adenoma), and a few (e.g., Hashimoto encephalopathy) can be life threatening. Hypothyroidism may be congenital or acquired.

## Congenital Hypothyroidism

Hypothyroidism is one of the most frequent congenital endocrine disorders. It occurs in 1:2,000-4,000 newborns and is one of the most common preventable causes of intellectual disability. In resource-rich countries, infant screening programs allow early identification of congenital hypothyroidism. If treated within a few weeks of birth, neurodevelopmental outcome is generally normal.

Newborns with congenital hypothyroidism normally have some initial thyroid function related to the maternal T4, which crosses the placenta to the fetus. Congenital hypothyroidism may be caused by thyroid dysgenesis, dyshormonogenesis, or central hypothyroidism **(37-16)**. **Maternal factors** may cause transient hypothyroidism in preterm infants in areas with endemic iodine deficiency or in families with a goiter history.

**Thyroid dysgenesis** is the most common cause of congenital hypothyroidism, representing 70-75% of cases. There is failure of normal thyroid gland development, which includes both abnormal gland formation and aberrant descent.

**Ectopic thyroid tissue** represents 25-50% of cases with thyroid dysgenesis. Ectopia may occur anywhere along the embryonic thyroglossal duct, the path the developing thyroid follows as it descends from the tongue to the infrahyoid neck. Rarely, ectopic thyroid tissue may occur in the substernal region or superior mediastinum **(37-17)**. Hormone production in ectopic thyroids is often low but not absent.

**Thyroid agenesis** or **hypoplasia** accounts for 20-50% and causes severe hypothyroidism. **Dyshormonogenesis**, a.k.a. inborn errors of thyroid hormone biosynthesis, accounts for 5-15% of congenital hypothyroidism. **Central hypothyroidism**, a.k.a. secondary hypothyroidism related to pituitary or hypothalamic disfunction, causes 10-15% of cases.

**Imaging studies** of the face and neck demonstrate an ectopic thyroid in up to 50% of congenital hypothyroid cases. Nearly 90% occur at the tongue base as a midline hyperdense mass on NECT **(37-18)** and a T2-hyperintense mass on MR. Avid enhancement is typical following contrast **(37-19)**. Nuclear medicine studies (Tc-99m pertechnetate or I-123 thyroid scan) are best for diagnosis of agenesis or hypoplasia. In agenesis, there is no focal radiotracer uptake between the base of tongue and upper chest. In hypoplasia/partial agenesis, there is decreased or normal uptake in a small, abnormally shaped gland in a normal location.

## Acquired Hypothyroid Disorders

Acquired hypothyroidism is much more common than the congenital variety. Acquired hypothyroidism has two important imaging manifestations: **Pituitary hyperplasia** and **Hashimoto thyroiditis/encephalopathy**.

## Pituitary Hyperplasia

Physiologically enlarged pituitary glands are common in young menstruating female patients and pregnant/lactating female patients. *Non*physiologic increase in pituitary volume—pathologic pituitary enlargement—is much less common and typically occurs in response to end-organ failure **(37-20)**.

Both physiologic and nonphysiologic pituitary hyperplasia are discussed in detail in Chapter 30. Most cases of hypothyroid-induced pituitary hyperplasia reverse with thyroid hormone replacement therapy (see Fig. 30-5). Caution: Any prepubescent male patient thought to harbor a "pituitary macroadenoma" on imaging studies should undergo comprehensive endocrine evaluation, as macroadenomas are exceptionally rare in this age group!

## Hashimoto Encephalopathy

Hashimoto encephalopathy is a rare but treatable condition typically associated with Hashimoto thyroiditis. Hashimoto encephalitis is also called "steroid-responsive encephalopathy with autoimmune thyroiditis." It is a well-recognized neurologic complication of autoimmune thyroid disease and is the most common cause of acquired hypothyroidism.

Hashimoto encephalopathy occurs in both children and adults. Psychiatric symptoms ("myxedema madness") are common. Approximately 50% of patients demonstrate imaging abnormalities. The most typical MR findings are diffuse confluent or focal T2/FLAIR hyperintensities in the subcortical and deep periventricular WM with sparing of the occipital lobes **(37-21)**.

## Hyperthyroidism

The most common manifestation of hyperthyroidism in the head and neck is thyroid ophthalmopathy (Graves disease). Brain involvement in hyperthyroidism occurs but is very rare. A few cases of **acute idiopathic intracranial HTN** ("pseudotumor cerebri") associated with hyperthyroidism have been reported.

Because of its effect on factor VIII activity, hyperthyroidism has also been reported as an independent risk factor for **dural venous sinus thrombosis**. Graves disease has been reported as a rare cause of **transient corpus callosum splenium hyperintensity** and an **MS-like multiphasic demyelinating autoimmune syndrome**.

# Parathyroid and Related Disorders

Metabolic abnormalities related to parathyroid hormone (PTH) dysfunction include primary and secondary hyperparathyroidism (HPTH) as well as hypoparathyroidism (HP), pseudohypoparathyroidism (PHP), and pseudo-pseudohypoparathyroidism (PPHP).

## Hyperparathyroidism

The parathyroid glands control calcium metabolism by producing PTH. HPTH is the classic disease of bone resorption, so imaging abnormalities may be seen in both the skull and brain. The most common cause of primary HPTH is a parathyroid adenoma, representing 75-85% of cases.

HPTH can be an acquired (common) or inherited disorder (rare). HPTH can also be primary, secondary, or even tertiary. Because of the increasing number of patients on dialysis, the most common type is now secondary

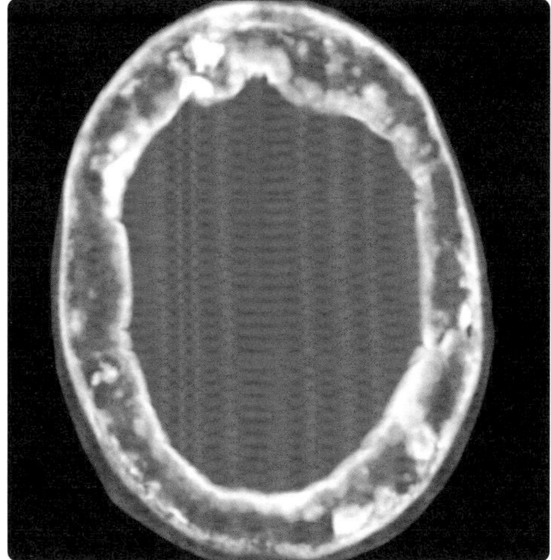

*(37-22) NECT of the skull in a patient with HPTH shows the characteristic alternating salt & pepper foci of resorption & sclerosis.*

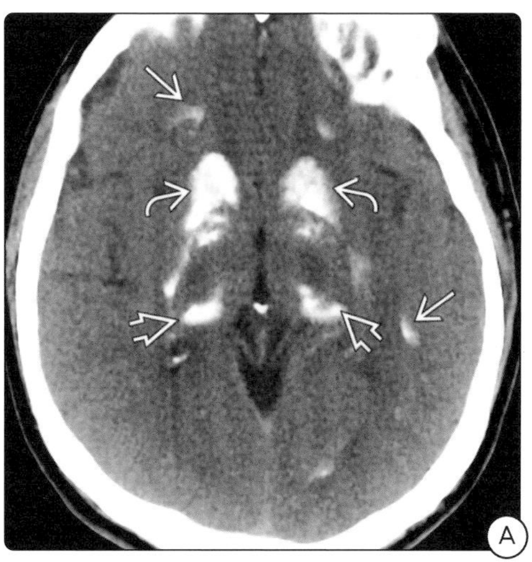


*(37-23A) NECT in a 54-yo man with HPTH shows extensive symmetric calcifications in basal ganglia ➡, thalami ➡, cortex ➡.*

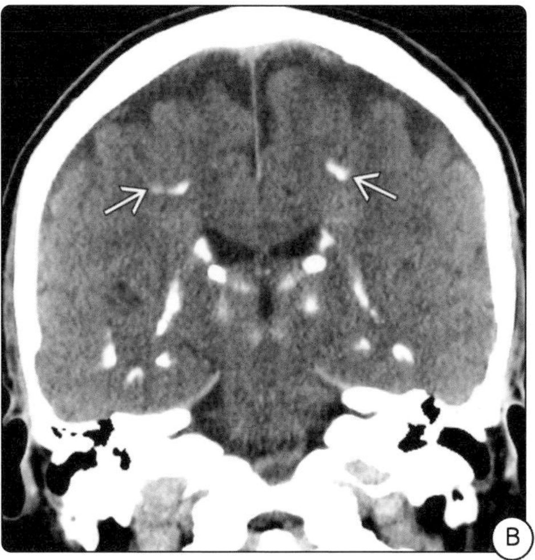


*(37-23B) Coronal NECT in the same case shows how symmetric the basal calcification is. Note GM-WM interface calcifications ➡.*

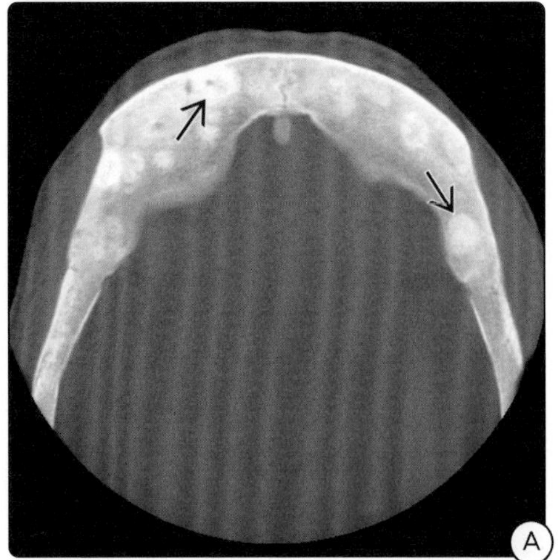

***(37-24A)*** *Axial bone CT in a patient with 2° HPTH shows leontiasis ossea with marked calvarial thickening, focal sclerotic "brown tumors" ⇨.*

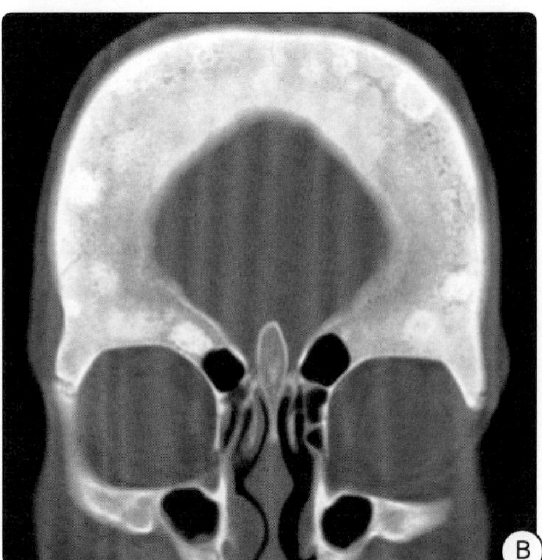

***(37-24B)*** *Coronal bone CT in the same patient demonstrates the striking calvarial thickening and more focal "brown tumors."*

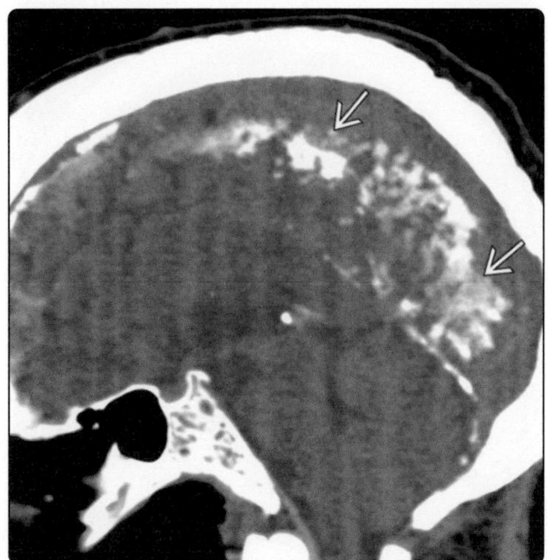

***(37-25)*** *NECT in a 40-yo with end-stage renal disease shows markedly thickened, plaque-like deposits along the falx ➡. Note thick calvarium.*

HPTH. Sporadic primary HPTH is more common than hereditary. The most important syndromes associated with primary HPTH are **multiple endocrine neoplasia (MEN)** type 1, MEN type 2A, and familial isolated HPTH. Major features of **MEN1** include parathyroid tumors (95%), pancreatic neuroendocrine tumor (40%), and pituitary neoplasms (30%). **MEN2a** is characterized by medullary thyroid carcinoma (99%), pheochromocytoma (50%), and parathyroid tumors (20-30%).

## Primary Hyperparathyroidism

Primary HPTH is most common in middle-aged to older adults and relatively rare in children. There is a striking female predominance. Primary HPTH is characterized by hypercalcemia and hypophosphatemia (serum calcium is elevated; serum phosphorus is normal or decreased). HPTH is usually asymptomatic. General signs of symptomatic HPTH have been characterized as "stones, bones, abdominal groans, and psychic moans."

Bone CT demonstrates diffuse patchy **salt and pepper lesions** in the skull **(37-22)**. Foci of bone resorption are interspersed with variable patchy sclerosis. The most common findings in the brain are **basal ganglia calcifications** on NECT. Bilateral symmetric deposits in the globi pallidi, putamen, and caudate nuclei are typical. The thalami, subcortical WM, and dentate nuclei may also be affected **(37-23)**.

MR shows symmetric T1 shortening and T2 hypointensity in the basal ganglia. Mild to moderate "blooming" on T2* (GRE, SWI) sequences is typical. **"Brown tumors"**—solitary or multiple nonneoplastic lesions in the skull—are common **(37-24)**.

## Secondary Hyperparathyroidism

The most common cause of secondary HPTH is chronic renal disease (CRD). The majority of dialysis patients eventually develop secondary HPTH. Other etiologies of secondary HPTH include dietary calcium deficiency, vitamin D disorders, disrupted phosphate metabolism, and hypomagnesemia.

Most patients with secondary HPTH are older than 40 years at the time of initial diagnosis. Serum calcium is normal or low, serum phosphorus is increased, and calcium-phosphate product is elevated. Vitamin D is low, almost always secondary to renal disease rather than dietary deficiency.

A common manifestation of CRD is renal osteodystrophy. Massive thickening of the calvarium and skull base narrows neural and vascular channels. Progressive cranial nerve involvement—most commonly compressive optic neuropathy—and carotid stenosis with ischemic symptoms are typical.

Secondary HPTH primarily affects the skull and dura; the brain parenchyma itself is usually normal. NECT scans show markedly thickened skull and facial bones, a condition sometimes referred to as **"uremic leontiasis ossea"** or "big head disease" **(37-24)**.

**"Brown tumors"** can be seen in both primary and secondary HPTH. Fibrous replacement, hemorrhage, and necrosis lead to formation of brownish-appearing cysts. Solitary or multiple "brown tumors" are seen on bone CT as focal, expansile, lytic lesions with nonsclerotic margins. Signal intensity on MR is highly variable, reflecting the age and amount of hemorrhage as well as the presence of fibrous tissue and cyst formation.

The classic intracranial finding in secondary HPTH is unusually extensive, **plaque-like dural thickening (37-25)**. Longstanding CRD can also result in extensive **"pipestem" calcifications** in the internal and external carotid arteries.

## Hypoparathyroid Disorders

Three types of hypoparathyroid disorders are recognized: HP, PHP, and PPHP. All three disorders share common features on brain imaging, although their clinical presentation and laboratory findings vary.

**HP** is characterized by brain calcifications. The basal ganglia and thalami are the most common sites **(37-26)** followed by the cerebrum and cerebellum.

**PHP** is characterized by *elevated* PTH levels and PTH-resistant hypocalcemia and hyperphosphatemia. Bilateral symmetric calcifications in the basal ganglia and thalami **(37-27)**, cerebellar hemispheres, subcortical WM, and, occasionally, the cerebral cortex are typical findings in both PHP and PPHP. **PPHP** typically shows no laboratory abnormalities, so calcium and phosphate levels are normal.

### PARATHYROID DISORDERS

**Hyperparathyroidism**
- Primary HPTH (parathyroid adenomas)
  - Salt and pepper skull, "brown tumors"
  - Basal ganglia calcifications
- Secondary HPTH (chronic renal failure)
  - Thick skull, face ("big head" disease) ± "brown tumors"
  - Plaque-like dural thickening, calcification

**Hypoparathyroid Disorders**
- 3 types (distinguished by clinical, laboratory findings)
  - HP
  - PHP
  - PPHP
- All have calcifications in basal ganglia > cerebrum, cerebellum

## Primary Familial Brain Calcification (Fahr Disease)

Primary familial brain calcification (PFBC), formerly termed Fahr disease, is an inherited disorder that results in striking brain calcifications. Calcium deposition begins in the third decade, but symptoms develop one or two decades later, usually between 30-60 years of age. Schizophrenic-like psychosis in young adults and extrapyramidal symptoms with subcortical dementia in patients over the age of 50 are typical.

NECT discloses extensive bilateral, relatively symmetric basal ganglia calcification. The lateral globus pallidus (GP) is the most severely affected with relative sparing of the medial GP. The putamen, caudate, thalami, dentate nuclei of the cerebellum, and both the cerebral and cerebellar WM (including the internal capsule) are commonly affected **(37-28)**.

MR signal intensity varies according to disease stage and the amount of calcification and heavy metal deposition. Calcification is typically hyperintense on T1WI **(37-29A)** **(37-29C)** but can be quite variable on T2WI. T2/FLAIR scans may appear normal or mildly abnormal. They may also show extensive foci of T2 prolongation in the cerebral WM that can be so striking as to mimic toxic/metabolic demyelination **(37-29D)**.

T2* (GRE, SWI) scans show profound susceptibility changes with "blooming" hypointensity secondary to iron deposition **(37-29B)**. Fahr disease does not enhance on T1 C+ sequences.

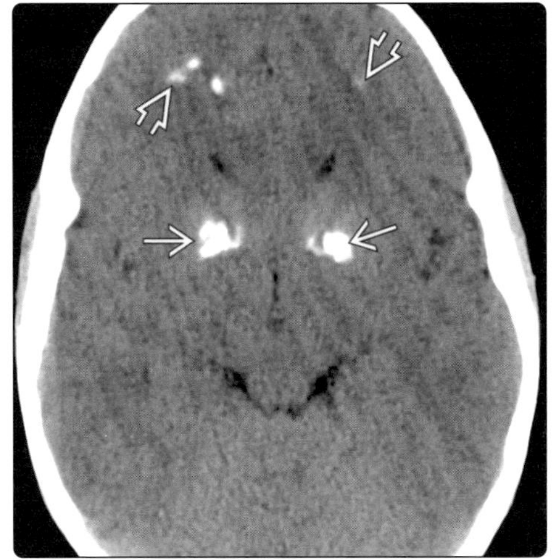

***(37-26)** NECT in 7-yo with hypoparathyroidism shows calcifications in the globi pallidi ➡ with smaller calcific foci at the GM-WM interfaces ⇨.*

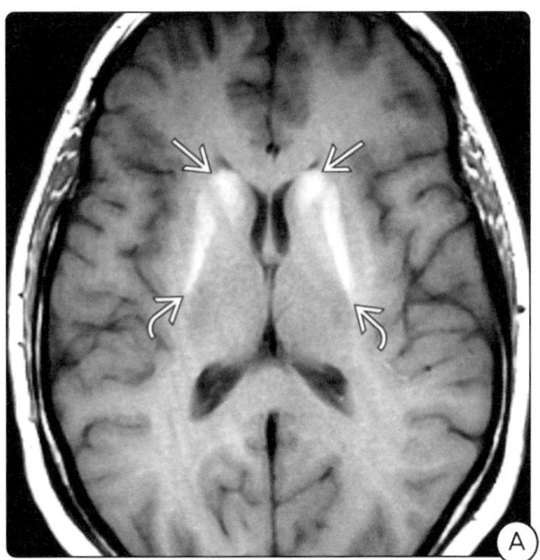


***(37-27A)** Axial T1 MR in 34-yo woman with PPHP on calcitriol shows symmetric T1 shortening in both caudate nuclei ➡ & putamina ⇨.*

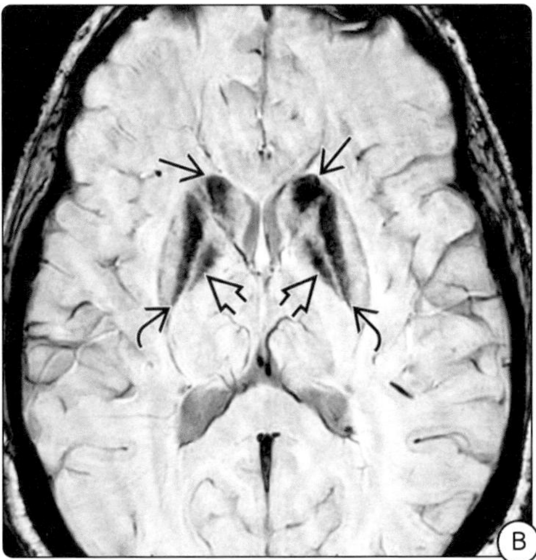


***(37-27B)** T2* SWI shows symmetric hypointensity in both caudate nuclei ➡, putamina ⇨, & the globi pallidi ⇨. (Courtesy P. Hildenbrand, MD.)*

**PRIMARY FAMILIAL BRAIN CALCIFICATION**

**Pathoetiology, Clinical Features**
- a.k.a. Fahr disease
- Caused by 4 gene mutations (*SLC20A2* most common)
- Usually presents between 30-60 years
  - Extrapyramidal symptoms, dementia

**Imaging Findings**
- NECT
  - Extensive bilateral basal ganglia calcifications
  - Putamen, caudate, thalami, dentate nuclei
  - WM of hemispheres, cerebellum
- MR
  - T1 shortening in areas of calcification
  - ± T2/FLAIR WM hyperintensity, cysts
  - Extensive "blooming" on T2* (GRE/SWI)
  - Differential diagnoses = physiologic calcification, PHP/PPHP

The major differential diagnosis of PFBC is normal **physiologic calcification of the basal ganglia**. Age-related ("senescent") calcification in the basal ganglia is common, typically localized in the *medial* GP. PFBC has much heavier, far more extensive calcification.

# Seizures and Related Disorders

Seizures can be precipitated by many infective, metabolic, toxic, developmental, neoplastic, or degenerative conditions and can affect numerous different areas of the brain. The temporal lobe is the most affected site for seizures, so we will start with a brief discussion of the temporal lobe anatomy. We will then look at the imaging manifestations of two classic disorders, the effects of (1) chronic repeated seizures (mesial

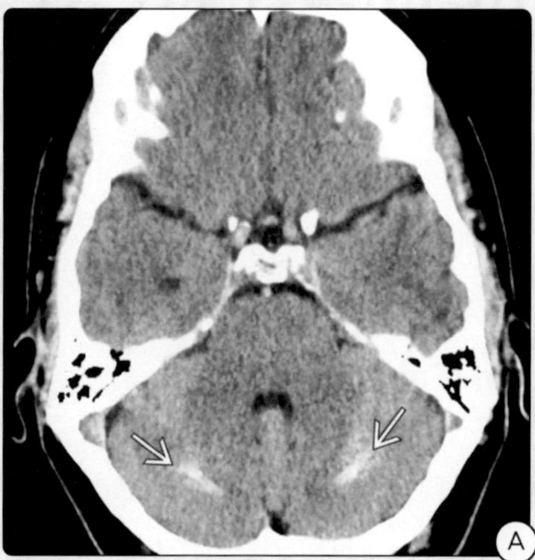

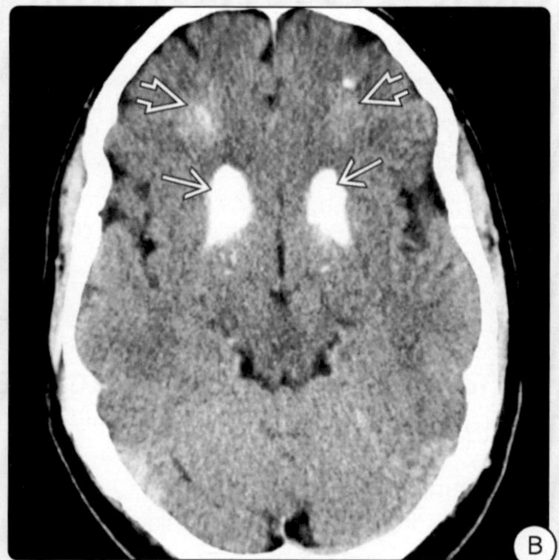

***(37-28A)** Series of axial NECT scans in a 51-yo man with Fahr disease shows bilaterally symmetric calcifications in the cerebellar WM. **(37-28B)** NECT shows very dense calcifications in both caudate nuclei & globi pallidi, as well as more faint calcification in the frontal WM.*

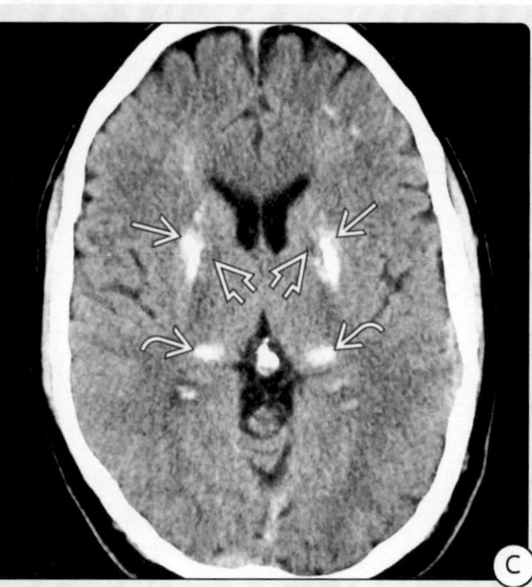

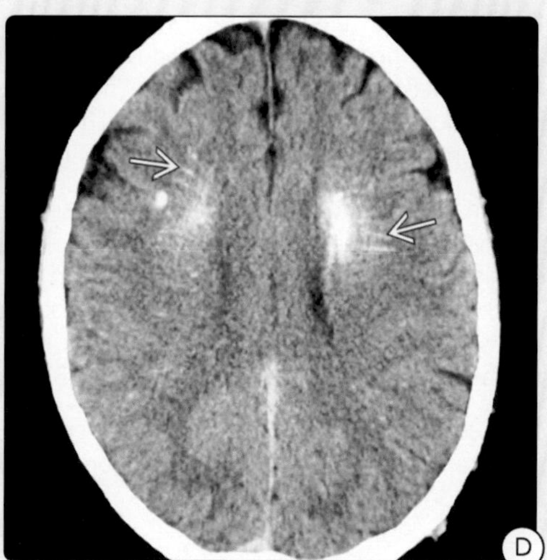

***(37-28C)** More cephalad NECT in the same patient shows calcification in the putamina & lateral globi pallidi with relative sparing of the most medial globus pallidus. Calcification is present in the pulvinars of both thalami. Punctate calcification is seen in the cerebral WM. **(37-28D)** NECT shows linear calcification extending perpendicularly from the caudate nuclei into the cerebral WM.*

temporal sclerosis) and (2) prolonged acute seizure activity (SE).

Next, we discuss cytotoxic lesions of the corpus callosum that can be seen with seizures (as well as a variety of other disorders). The section concludes with a consideration of imaging findings in transient global amnesia, which specifically affects the hippocampus.

## Temporal Lobe Anatomy

The temporal lobe lies inferior to the sylvian fissure. Its lateral surface has three gyri: The **superior** temporal gyrus (contains primary auditory cortex), **middle** temporal gyrus (connects with auditory, somatosensory, visual association pathways), and the **inferior** temporal gyrus (contains the higher visual association area). The temporal lobe also includes the major subdivisions of the **limbic system**. The parahippocampal gyrus is present along the temporal lobe medial surface and merges into the uncus.

The **hippocampus** plays a major role in memory. The hippocampus is part of the limbic system, which includes three nestled, C-shaped arches that surround the diencephalon and basal ganglia. The hippocampus has three anatomic subdivisions: The **head** (pes hippocampus, digitated anterior part), the **body** (cylindrical), and the posterior **tail** that narrows and then curves around the corpus callosum splenium **(37-30)**.

The hippocampus body on coronal sections consists of two interlocking, U-shaped GM structures, the hippocampus proper (Ammon horn) forms more superolateral, upside-down U, and the dentate gyrus forms the inferomedial U. The WM of the alveus and fimbria is external to the GM of the Ammon horn **(37-31)**.

The Ammon horn is subdivided into four zones based on width, cell size, and cell density. These zones are designated as

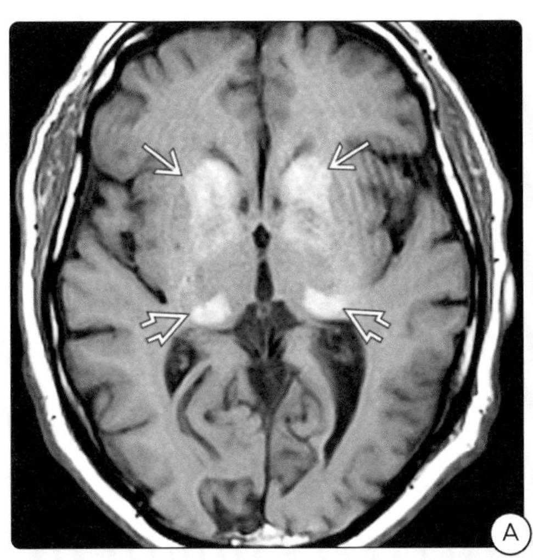


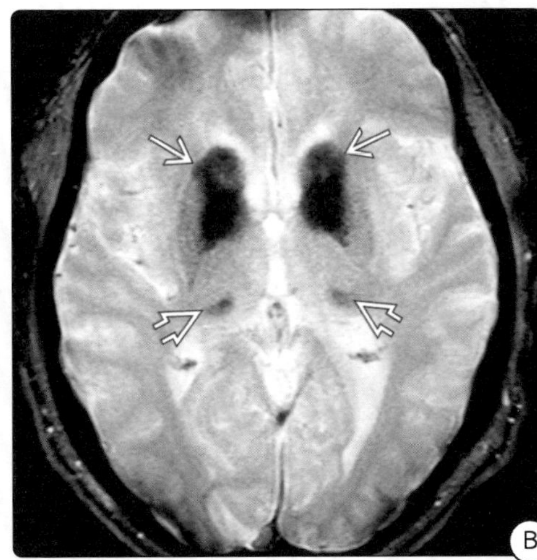


***(37-29A)** Axial T1 MR in a 67-yo man with epilepsy & known Fahr disease shows symmetric T1 shortening in the basal ganglia ➔ & pulvinars ➔ of both thalami. **(37-29B)** T2* GRE in the same case shows dense susceptibility "blooming" in the basal ganglia ➔ & thalami ➔, corresponding to the areas of T1 shortening.*

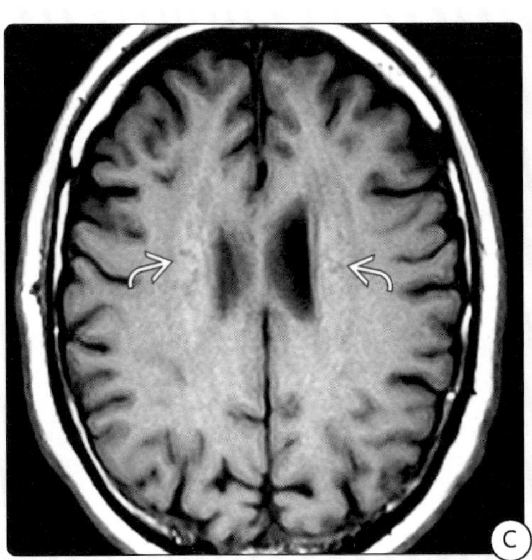


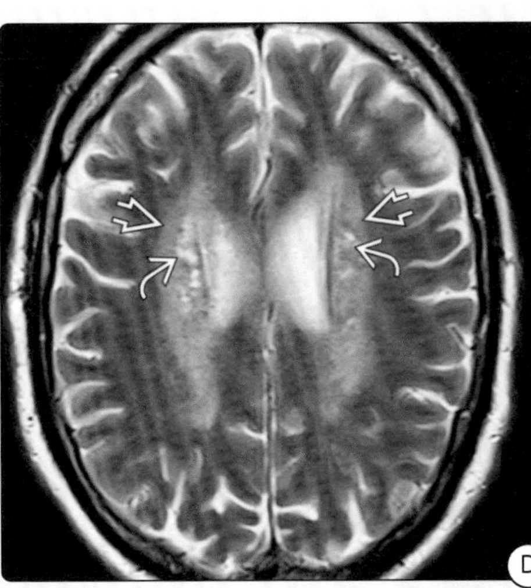


***(37-29C)** More cephalad T1 MR in the same case shows mixed foci of T1 shortening & hypointensity in the caudate nuclei & deep periventricular WM ➔. **(37-29D)** T2 MR in the same case shows extensive confluent areas of T2 hyperintensity in the deep WM ➔ intermixed with areas of cystic degeneration ➔ & hypointense foci. This pattern of WM cysts with leukodystrophy is characteristic for PDGFB mutation.*

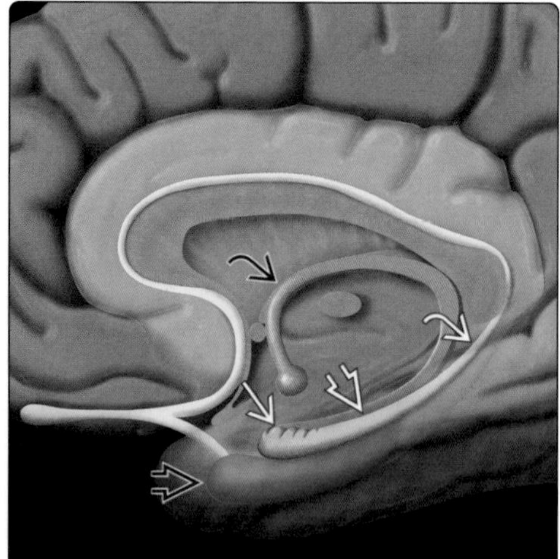

(37-30) Graphic shows 3 nested arches of limbic system. Hippocampus (yellow) has an anterior head ➡, body ➡, & tail ➡. Fornix ➡. Uncus ➡.

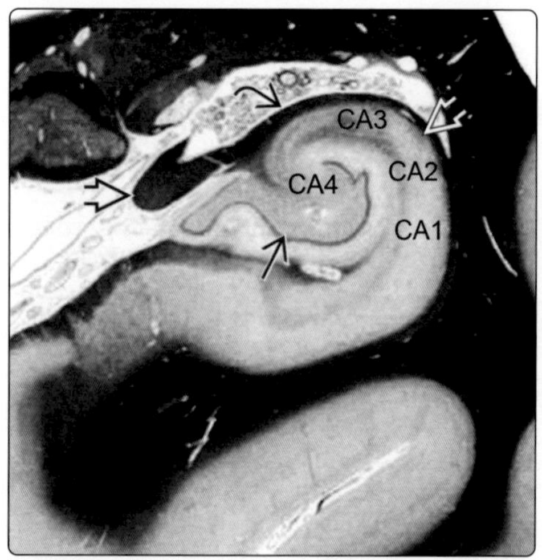


(37-31) Coronal histology shows CA1-4 zones of Ammon horn ➡ & dentate gyrus ➡ of the hippocampus. Alveus ➡ & fimbria ➡ WM.

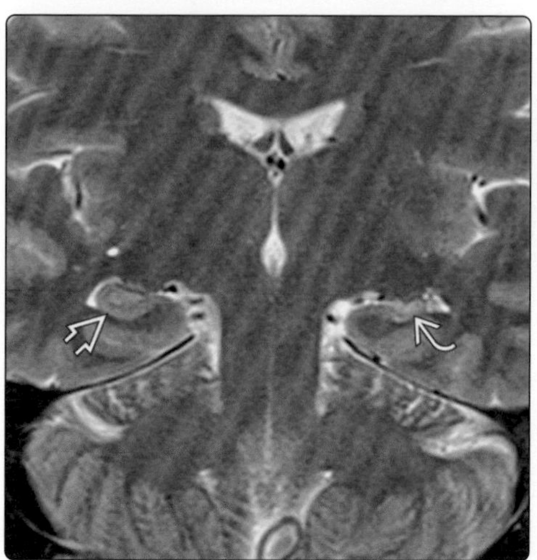

(37-32) Coronal T2 MR shows a normal right hippocampus ➡ with preserved internal architecture & a small left hippocampus, MTS ➡.

CA1, CA2, CA3, and CA4. CA1 is the most lateral zone and is most vulnerable to anoxia and is affected with mesial temporal sclerosis.

## Mesial Temporal (Hippocampal) Sclerosis

Mesial temporal sclerosis (MTS), a.k.a. hippocampal sclerosis (HS) **(37-32)** **(37-33)**, is the most common type of localization-related epilepsy and accounts for the majority of patients undergoing temporal lobectomy for seizure disorder.

### Etiology and Pathology

A variety of events, such as trauma or infection, may precipitate intractable complex partial seizures. The end result is MTS. MTS is characterized grossly by atrophy of the hippocampus and adjacent structures. The hippocampal body—particularly the CA1 and CA4 areas—is the most susceptible to hypoxic-ischemic damage, but all regions of the hippocampus can be affected. Approximately 15-20% of cases are bilateral but usually asymmetric.

### Clinical Issues

Nearly 10% of all individuals experience a seizure in their lifetime. 2/3 of these are nonrecurrent febrile/nonfebrile seizures. Peak prevalence is bimodal (< 1 year and > 55 years of age). 1/3 of patients develop repeated seizures ("epilepsy").

### Imaging

**MR Findings.** Imaging markers of MTS are found in 60-70% of patients with temporal lobe epilepsy (TLE). True coronal IR or 3D SPGR sequences show a shrunken hippocampus with atrophy of the ipsilateral fornix and widening of the adjacent temporal horn &/or choroid fissure. Abnormal T2/FLAIR hyperintensity with obscuration of the internal hippocampal architecture is typical **(37-34)**. MTS typically does not enhance following contrast administration.

**Nuclear Medicine Findings.** FDG PET is one of the most sensitive imaging procedures for diagnosing MTS. Temporal lobe hypometabolism is the typical finding. SPECT shows hyperperfusion in the epileptogenic zone during seizure activity; hypoperfusion in the interictal period is common.

### Differential Diagnosis

The major differential diagnosis of MTS is SE. **SE** can be subclinical and may cause transient gyral edema with T2/FLAIR hyperintensity &/or enhancement in the affected cortex as well as the hippocampus.

A **glioma** (astrocytoma, IDH-mutant, or oligodendroglioma, IDH-mutant, 1p/19q codeleted, WHO grade 2) in the temporal lobe can cause drug-resistant TLE **(37-35)**. Gliomas are usually T2/FLAIR hyperintense and cause mass effect, not volume loss. Cortically based neoplasms associated with TLE include **dysembryoplastic neuroepithelial tumor (DNET)**. DNET is typically a well-demarcated, "bubbly" mass that is often associated with adjacent cortical dysplasia. **Cortical dysplasia** is isointense with GM but frequently causes T2 hyperintensity in the underlying temporal lobe WM.

Cystic-appearing lesions in the temporal lobe that are hyperintense on T2WI include **prominent perivascular spaces, hippocampal sulcus remnants**, and **choroid fissure cysts**. These "leave me alone" lesions all behave like CSF and suppress on FLAIR.

## Status Epilepticus

### Etiology and Pathophysiology

Status epilepticus (SE) is a prolonged (> 30 minutes), continuously active seizure with EEG-demonstrated seizure activity. SE can be focal or generalized, clinical or subclinical (silent). Generalized convulsive SE is potentially life threatening if not controlled.

Prolonged ictal activity induces hypermetabolism with increased glucose utilization. Perfusion increases but is still insufficient to match glucose demand. The result is compromised cellular energy production, cytotoxic cell swelling, and vasogenic edema. With prolonged severe seizure activity, the blood-brain barrier may become permeable, permitting leakage of fluid and macromolecules into the extracellular spaces.

### Imaging

**CT Findings.** Initial NECT scans may be normal or show gyral swelling with sulcal effacement, parenchymal hypodensity, and lack of GM-WM differentiation.

**MR Findings.** Periictal MR shows T2/FLAIR hyperintensity with gyral swelling **(37-38A)**. Subcortical and deep WM is relatively spared. Ipsilateral thalamic hyperintensity is common in SE.

Gyriform enhancement on T1 C+ varies from none to striking **(37-37B)**. DWI may show restricted diffusion with uni- or bilateral hippocampal, thalamic, and cortical lesions **(37-36)** **(37-37A)**. Perfusion imaging shows marked hyperemia in region of epileptic focus with elevated rCBF and rCBV maps **(37-38B)**.

Follow-up scans in severe cases may show permanent abnormalities, including focal brain atrophy, cortical laminar necrosis, and mesial temporal sclerosis.

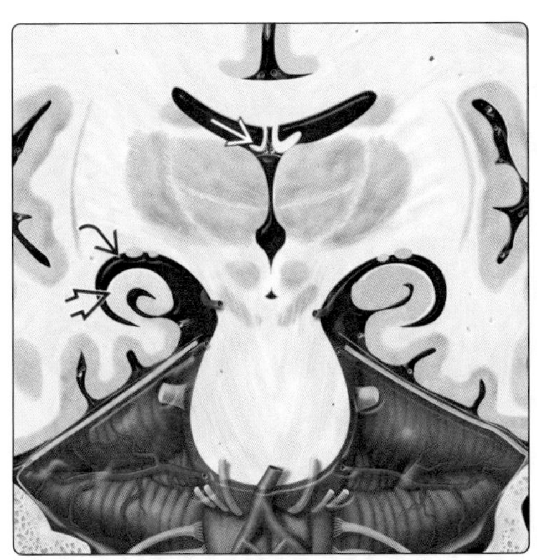

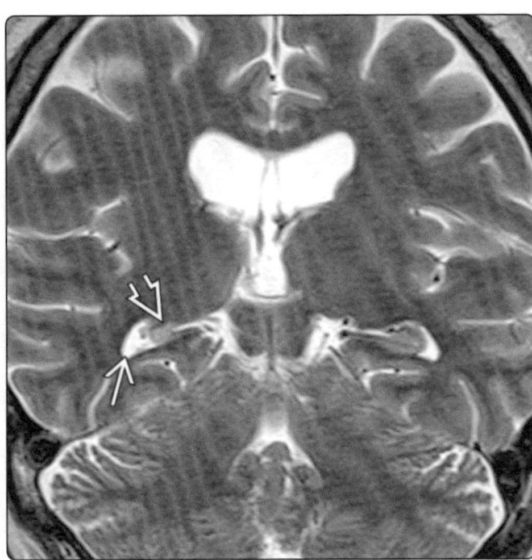

***(37-33)** Coronal graphic shows typical MTS. The hippocampus ⊟ is atrophied, sclerotic with loss of normal internal architecture. Temporal horn ⊟ is enlarged, ipsilateral fornix ➡ & mammillary body are small. **(37-34)** Coronal T2 MR in a 48-yo with complex partial seizures shows classic MTS as a small, hyperintense hippocampus ➡ with loss of internal architecture. Note the enlarged temporal horn ➡.*

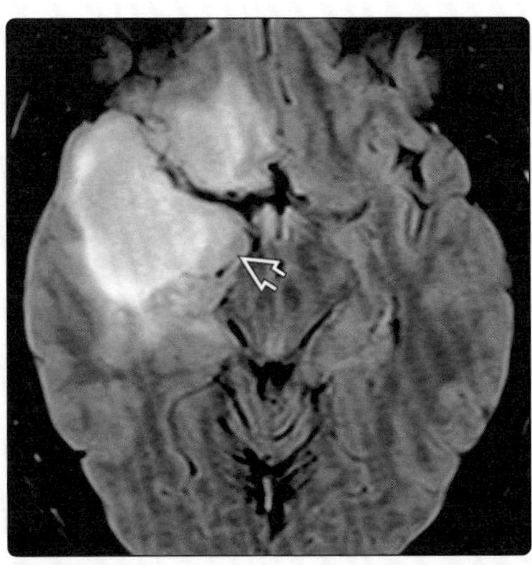

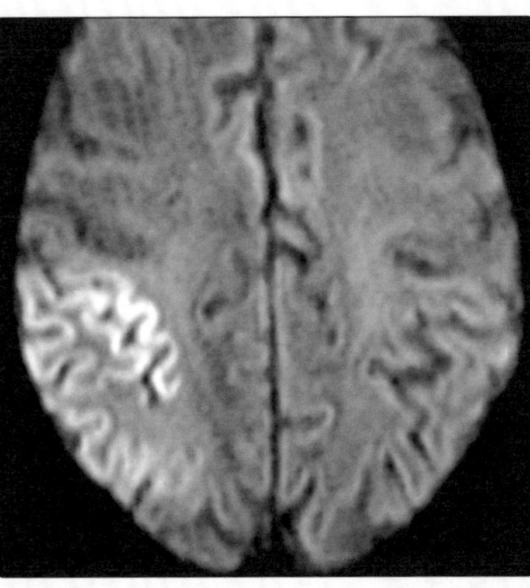

***(37-35)** Axial FLAIR MR in a patient with new-onset drug-refractory seizures shows mass-like hyperintensity in the medial temporal lobe ➡ & frontal lobe. Astrocytoma, IDH-mutant, was found at resection. **(37-36)** Axial DTI trace MR in a status epilepticus patient shows hyperintensity (diffusion restriction) related to hypermetabolism. T2 hyperintensity & gyriform enhancement were present (not shown).*

## Differential Diagnosis

The major differential diagnosis of periictal brain swelling is **acute cerebral ischemia-infarction**. Acute cerebral ischemia occurs in a typical vascular territorial distribution, is wedge-shaped (involving both GM and WM), and is positive on DWI *before* T2/FLAIR hyperintensity develops. In ongoing SE, DWI and T2 signal changes typically occur simultaneously.

**Cerebritis** may cause a T2-/FLAIR-hyperintense mass that restricts on DWI. Cerebritis typically involves the subcortical WM as well as the cortex. **Herpes encephalitis** is confined to the limbic system and temporal lobes, has acute onset, and may have blood products and enhancement. Acute onset of **MELAS** may affect the cortex in a nonvascular distribution.

# Cytotoxic Lesions of Corpus Callosum

## Terminology and Etiology

Cytotoxic lesions of the corpus callosum (CLCCs) are acquired lesions that have been associated with a number of different entities. Because they are (1) often reversible and (2) most common in the corpus callosum splenium, they have also been called transient or reversible splenial lesions.

Most investigators believe CLCCs are a cytokinopathy with secondary excitotoxic glutaminergic-associated intracellular edema. The corpus callosum—especially the splenium—has a high density of excitatory amino acid, toxin, and drug receptors and is hence more vulnerable to the development of cytotoxic edema.

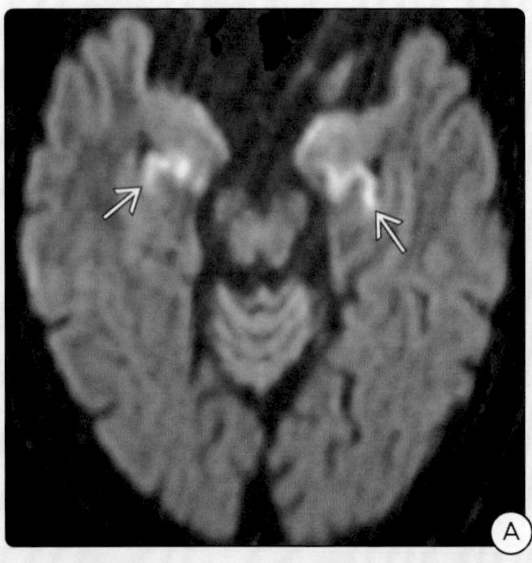

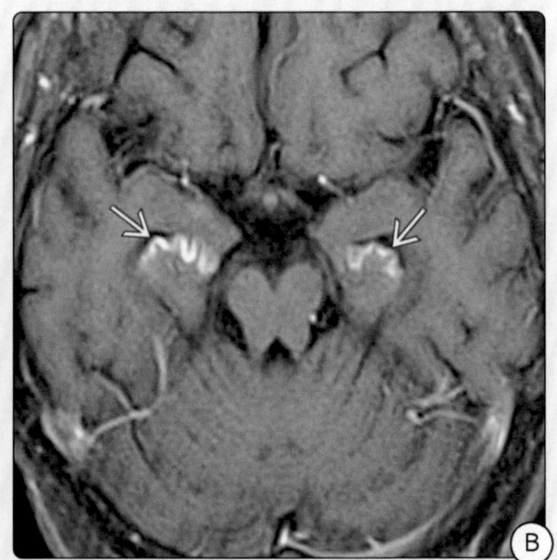


***(37-37A)** Axial DTI trace MR in a young patient with status epilepticus shows hyperintensity (diffusion restriction) in the bilateral hippocampi ➡. **(37-37B)** Axial T1 C+ FS in the same patient shows gyriform enhancement ➡. Findings are related to hypermetabolism with increased glucose utilization & blood-brain barrier breakdown. Differential considerations include cerebritis, infarct, viral encephalitis, or, in some cases, neoplasm.*

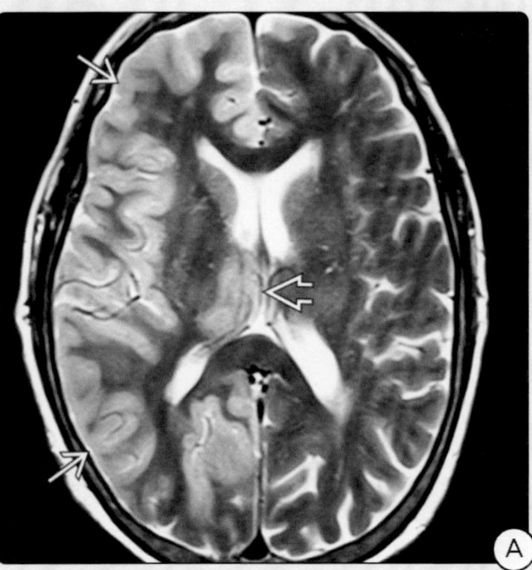

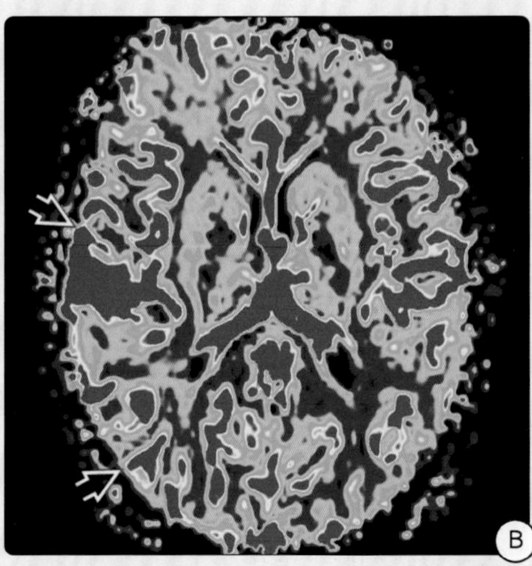


***(37-38A)** T2 MR in a 52-yo woman in status epilepticus for 24 hours shows diffuse gyral ➡ & right thalamic ➡ edema & hyperintensity. Status epilepticus MR findings are typically transient & involve cortex & subcortical WM. **(37-38B)** The rCBV map shows increased blood volume in the right hemisphere ➡ compared with the left. Increased perfusion with marked hyperemia, increased rCBF & rCBV may be seen in the ictal state.*

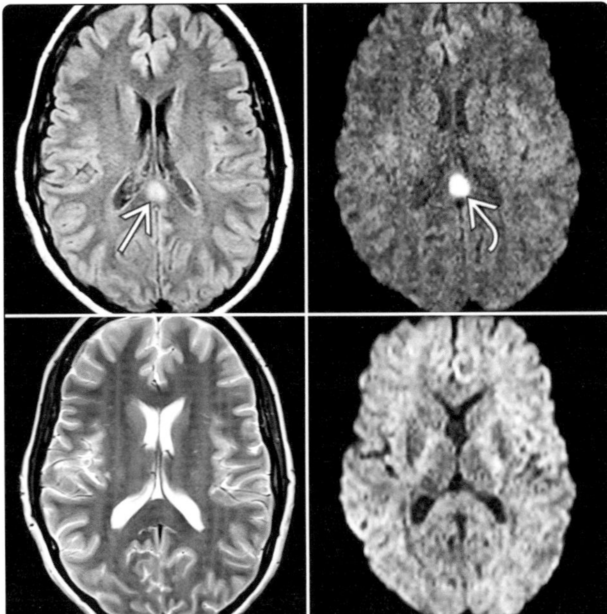

*(37-39) A patient taken off antiseizure medications 3 weeks prior to imaging shows round, FLAIR-hyperintense lesion in corpus callosum splenium (top L) that restricts on DWI (top R). Repeat scan 2 weeks later shows lesions have resolved. CLCC.*

*(37-40) Series of FLAIR MR scans in viral encephalitis shows lesions in pons, peduncles, & cerebellar hemisphere. Corpus callosum splenium lesion restricts on DWI. This is virus-associated CLCC.*

## Associated Conditions

The most common causes of CLCCs are **drug associated**. CLCCs were initially reported as a reversible phenomenon associated with the use and subsequent withdrawal of antiepileptic drugs (e.g., carbamazepine). Other drugs, such as metronidazole, have been associated with CLCCs.

The second most common cause of CLCC is **infection**, usually a viral encephalitis that may also cause a mild febrile encephalopathy. Influenza virus, measles, human herpesvirus-6, West Nile virus, Epstein-Barr virus, varicella-zoster virus, mumps, and adenoviruses have all been reported with CLCCs.

**Metabolic derangements**, such as hypoglycemia and hypernatremia, acute alcohol poisoning, malnutrition, and vitamin B12 deficiency, are the third most common group of CLCC-associated disorders.

Miscellaneous reported associations include migraine headache, trauma, high-altitude cerebral edema, systemic lupus erythematosus, internal cerebral vein occlusion, Charcot-Marie-Tooth disease, and neoplasms.

## Imaging

Typical CLCCs are round to ovoid, homogeneous, nonhemorrhagic lesions centered in the corpus callosum splenium. They are mildly hypointense on T1WI, hyperintense on T2/FLAIR, do not enhance, and demonstrate restricted diffusion **(37-39)** **(37-40)**. A variant type of CLCC that involves the entire corpus callosum splenium and extends into the forceps major has been termed the boomerang sign. Rarely, CLCCs extend anteriorly from the splenium into the corpus callosum body.

Most CLCCs resolve spontaneously and disappear completely within a few days or weeks. Follow-up imaging studies are typically normal.

### CYTOTOXIC LESIONS OF CORPUS CALLOSUM

**Pathoetiology**
- Cytokinopathy with glutamate-induced intracellular edema
- Associated with
  - Seizures
  - Drugs (antiepileptic, metronidazole, etc.)
  - Infections (often, but not invariably, viral)
  - Metabolic disorders (alcohol, Wernicke, osmotic)
  - Neoplasms, chemotherapy
  - Trauma

**Clinical Features**
- Usually asymptomatic, incidental
- Typically (but not invariably) resolve spontaneously

**Imaging Findings**
- Round, ovoid, or boomerang-shaped lesion
- Splenium > > > body, central > > eccentric
- T2/FLAIR hyperintense
- Restricts on DWI
- Does not enhance

# Transient Global Amnesia

## Terminology and Clinical Features

Transient global amnesia (TGA) is a unique neurologic disorder characterized by (1) sudden memory loss without other signs

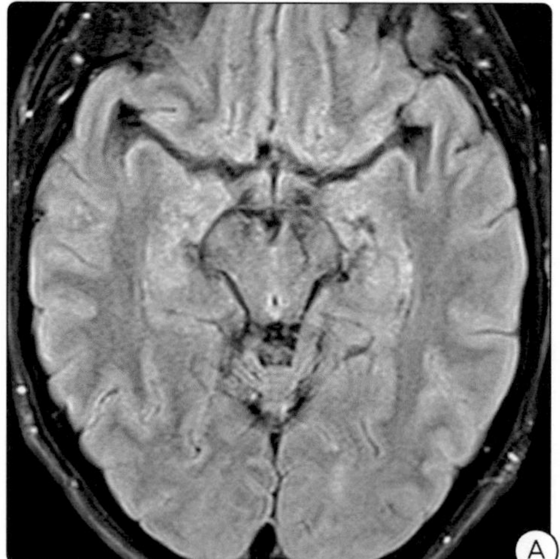


***(37-41A)** Axial FLAIR MR in a 52-yo woman with sudden onset of confusion & amnesia is normal.*

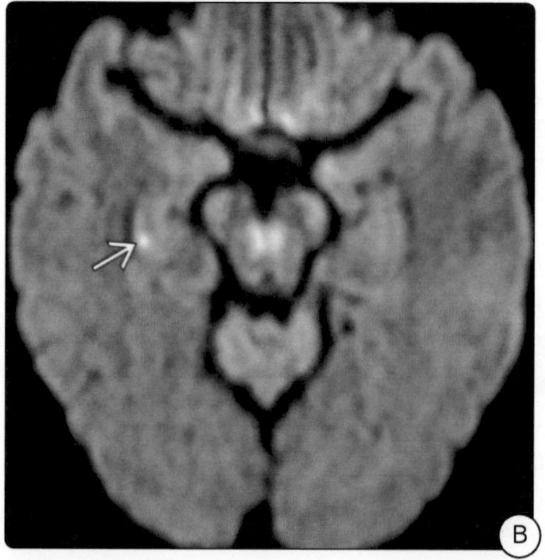


***(37-41B)** DWI MR in same patient shows a small focus of hyperintensity in the right hippocampus ➡ related to TGA.*

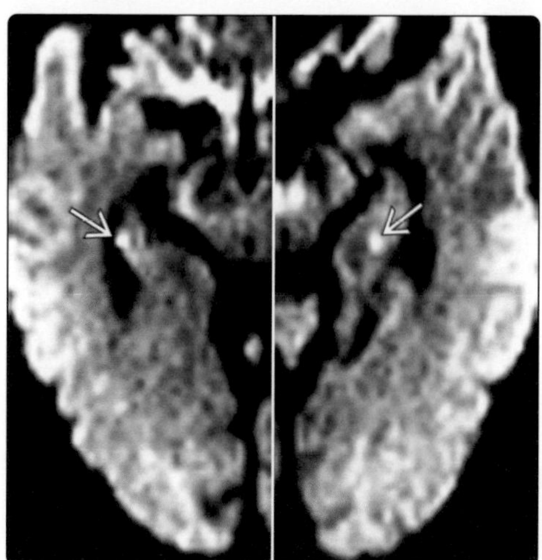

***(37-42)** DWI MR in 65-yo man with sudden anterograde memory loss shows foci of restricted diffusion in both hippocampi ➡. This is TGA.*

of cognitive or neurologic impairment and (2) complete clinical recovery within 24 hours. The underlying etiology of TGA is unknown.

Most TGA patients are between 50-70 years old; TGA is rare under the age of 40. Isolated anterograde amnesia with preserved alertness, attention, and personal identity are consistent features. EEGs are normal in 80-90% of cases with the remainder showing minor nonepileptiform activity. Symptoms resolve in 24 hours or less. Recurrences are relatively rare.

### Imaging

CT scans are invariably normal, and standard MR sequences (T2/FLAIR) typically show no abnormalities. DWI shows punctate or dot-like foci of restricted diffusion in the CA1 area of the hippocampus along the lateral aspect of the hippocampus just medial to the temporal horn. Lesions can be single (55%) **(37-41B)** or multiple (45%), unilateral (50-55%) or bilateral (45-50%) **(37-42)**. The body of the hippocampus is most commonly involved followed by the head.

DWI abnormalities in TGA increase significantly with time following symptom onset. Between 0-6 hours, 34% show foci of restricted diffusion. This increases to 62% in patients imaged between 6-12 hours and to 67% of patients between 12-24 hours. By day three, 75% of patients demonstrate abnormalities. Follow-up scans typically show complete resolution by day 10.

### Differential Diagnosis

The two major differential diagnoses of TGA are stroke and seizure. Their exclusive location in the hippocampus mitigates against typical embolic infarcts. However, acute **isolated punctate hippocampal infarction** can be indistinguishable from TGA based on imaging studies alone.

Seizures can cause transient diffusion restriction but typically involve moderate to large areas of the cortex. The dot-like lesions in TGA are distinctly different from the cortical gyriform ribbons of restricted diffusion seen in **SE** and the posterior-predominant lesions seen in **hypoglycemic seizures**.

# Miscellaneous Disorders

## Hepatic Encephalopathy

Hepatic encephalopathy (HE) is an important cause of morbidity and mortality in patients with severe liver disease. HE is classified into three main groups: Minimal HE (a.k.a. latent or subclinical HE), chronic HE, and acute HE.

Although the precise mechanisms responsible for HE remain elusive, elevated blood and brain ammonia levels have been strongly implicated in the pathogenesis of HE.

Ammonia is metabolized primarily in the liver via the urea cycle. When the metabolic capacity of the liver is severely diminished, ammonia detoxification is compromised. Nitrogenous wastes accumulate and easily cross the blood-brain barrier. Ammonia and its principal metabolite, glutamine, interfere with brain mitochondrial metabolism and energy production. Increased osmolarity in the astrocytes causes swelling and loss of autoregulation and results in cerebral edema.

We first discuss chronic HE, then focus on the acute manifestations of liver failure and its most fulminant manifestation, hyperammonemic encephalopathy.

## Chronic Hepatic Encephalopathy

**Chronic HE** is a potentially reversible clinical syndrome that occurs in the setting of chronic severe liver dysfunction. Both children and adults are affected. Most patients have a longstanding history of cirrhosis, often accompanied by portal HTN and portosystemic shunting.

NECT scans are typically normal or show mild volume loss. In the vast majority of cases, MR scans show bilateral symmetric hyperintensity in the GP and substantia nigra on T1WI, probably secondary to manganese deposition **(37-43A)**. T1 hyperintensity has also been reported in the pituitary gland and hypothalamus but is less common. The T1 hyperintensity in the striatopallidal system may decrease or even disappear completely after liver transplantation.

## Acute-on-Chronic Liver Failure

**Acute-on-chronic liver failure** (ACLF) is acute deterioration in liver function in an individual with preexisting chronic liver disease, commonly cirrhosis. Hepatic and extrahepatic organ failure—often renal dysfunction—is common in ACLF and is associated with substantial short-term mortality. Precipitating factors include bacterial and viral infections, alcoholic hepatitis, and surgery. In > 40% of cases, no precipitating event is identified.

Changes in consciousness as a result of acute HE are common and range from mild confusion to coma. Imaging reflects a combination of chronic liver disease and superimposed changes of acute liver dysfunction, such as hyperammonemia with cortical edema or Wernicke encephalopathy **(37-43)**.

## Acute Hepatic Encephalopathy and Hyperammonemia

**Terminology. Acute HE** is caused by hyperammonemia, which can be both hepatic *and* nonhepatic. Hyperammonemia, systemic inflammation (including sepsis, bacterial translocation, and insulin resistance), and oxidative stress are key factors mediating clinical deterioration.

**Etiology.** Although acute hepatic decompensation is the most common cause of hyperammonemia in adults, drug toxicity is also an important consideration. Valproate, asparaginase, acetaminophen, and chemotherapy have all been implicated in the development of hyperammonemic encephalopathy. Other important nonhepatic causes of hyperammonemia include hematologic disease, parenteral nutrition, bone marrow transplantation, urinary tract infection, and fulminant viral hepatitis.

Inherited urea cycle abnormalities or organic acidemias, such as citrullinemia and ornithine transcarbamylase deficiency, are other potential causes of acute hyperammonemic encephalopathy (see Chapter 36).

**Imaging.** Bilaterally symmetric T2/FLAIR hyperintensity in the insular cortex, cingulate gyri, and basal ganglia is typical, as is relative sparing of the perirolandic and occipital regions. The hemispheric WM is typically spared. Acute HE restricts strongly on DWI.

**Differential Diagnosis.** The major differential diagnoses of acute HE/hyperammonemia are HIE, hypoglycemia, SE, and Wernicke encephalopathy. **HIE** may be difficult to distinguish from acute HE on imaging alone. Symmetric involvement of the insular cortex and cingulate gyri should suggest acute HE.

**Hypoglycemia** is a common comorbidity in patients with chronic HE. Acute hypoglycemia typically affects the parietooccipital GM, whereas early acute HE may spare the posterior cortex. Serum glucose is low, and ammonia is normal. **SE** is usually unilateral, and, although the thalamus is often involved, the basal ganglia are generally spared. **Wernicke encephalopathy** affects

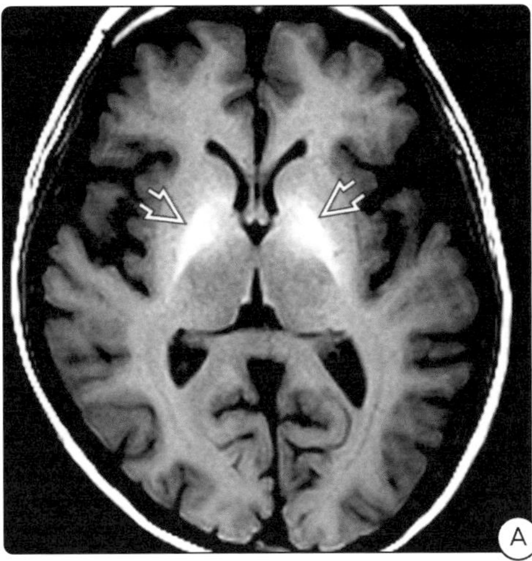


***(37-43A)** T1 MR in chronic liver failure with acute onset of encephalopathy shows striking, symmetric T1 shortening in the globi pallidi ➾.*

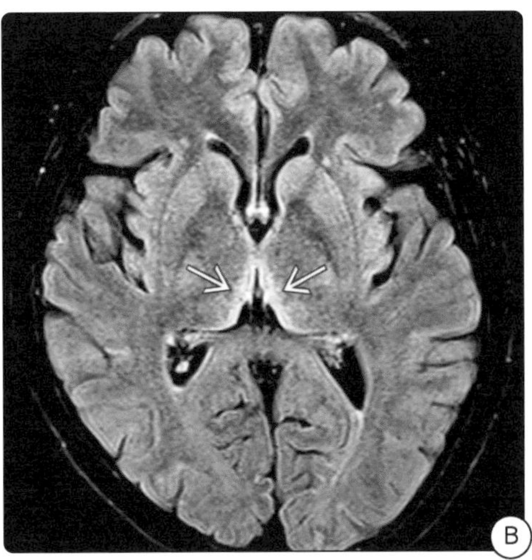


***(37-43B)** Axial FLAIR MR in the same case shows symmetric hyperintensity ➾ in the medial thalami around the 3rd ventricle.*

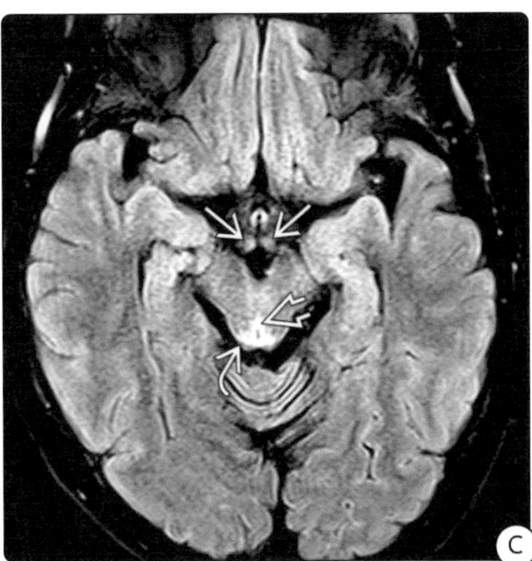


***(37-43C)** Hyperintensity in periaqueductal gray ➾, tectum ➾, both mammillary bodies ➾. Acute WE superimposed on chronic liver failure.*

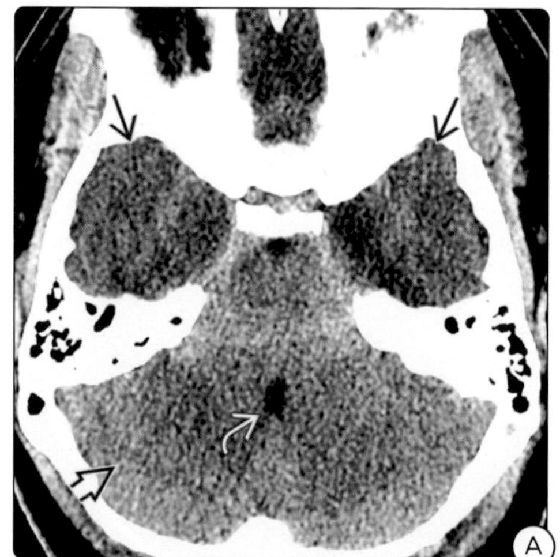


***(37-44A) NECT of heatstroke 6 days after admission shows swollen temporal lobes, cerebellum, compressed 4th ventricle.***

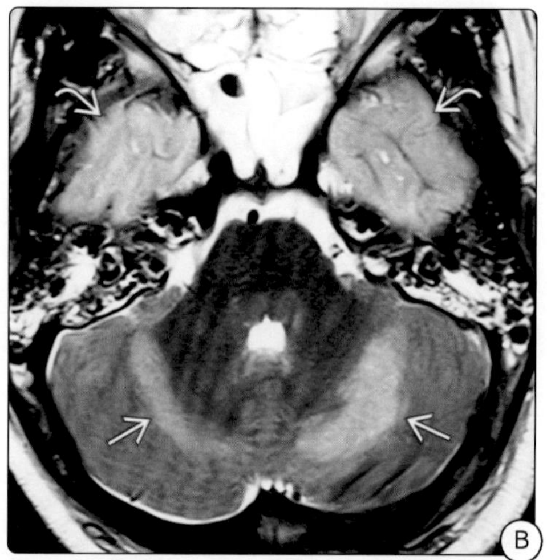


***(37-44B) T2 MR shows diffuse swelling & hyperintensity of both temporal lobes. The cerebellar WM is also hyperintense.***

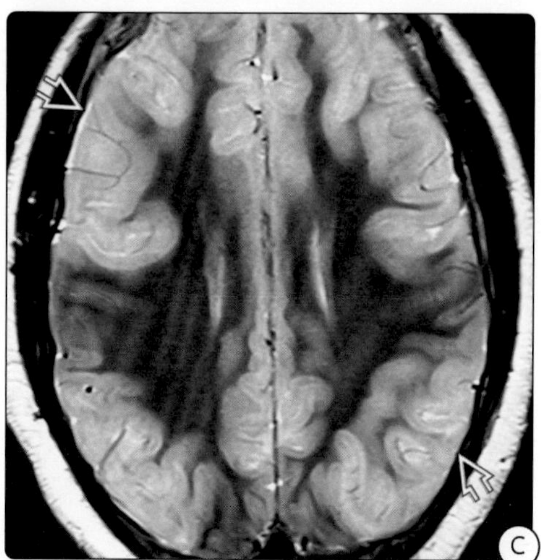


***(37-44C) More cephalad T2 MR shows diffuse cortical hyperintensity. This is heat stroke. (Courtesy P. Hudgins, MD.)***

the medial thalami, mammillary bodies, tectal plate, and periaqueductal GM. The cerebral cortex and basal ganglia are less commonly involved.

## Hyperthermic Encephalopathy

Acute heat-related illness is a spectrum of disorders that ranges from minor heat cramps and heat exhaustion to life-threatening heat stroke. It can cause delirium, seizures, and coma.

Heat stroke is defined clinically as a core body temperature > 40 °C. Risk factors include high ambient temperature and humidity, dehydration, alcohol abuse, and some medications (antihypertensive or psychiatric). Both ends of the age spectrum—infants and the very old—are especially susceptible. Morbidity and mortality in patients suffering from heat stroke range between 10-50%.

Purkinje cells in the cerebellum are especially susceptible to thermic injury. MR may demonstrate T2/FLAIR hyperintensity in the cerebellum, basal ganglia/thalami, hippocampus, and cerebral cortex **(37-44)**. Restricted diffusion in the affected areas is common.

## Uremic Encephalopathy

Uremic encephalopathy is a toxic-metabolic encephalopathy in patients with **severe renal failure**. Most commonly, patients with renal failure present with cortical and subcortical hyperintensities in a posterior distribution, as seen with PRES. Other less common presentations include the lentiform fork sign, which is a hyperintense rim delineating the lateral and medial boundaries of the putamina resembling a fork **(37-45)**. Centrum semiovale involvement with T2/FLAIR hyperintensity and variable diffusion restriction is a rare manifestation of acute uremic encephalopathy.

Patients often have a history of diabetes and renal failure. Symptoms are typically associated with accumulation of uremic toxins (creatinine and guanidine) and a metabolic acidosis. Dialysis and correction of metabolic acidosis is often required for treatment. There is typically complete reversal of imaging findings with normalization of the serum creatinine.

Differential considerations include other **toxic-metabolic encephalopathies**, including carbon monoxide, cyanide, cocaine, opiates, and Wilson disease. The lentiform fork sign has also been described in patients with methanol intoxication. The other main differential consideration is **hypoglycemia** with parietooccipital edema and diffusion restriction. Imaging may be identical, so history is often key to diagnosis. Lastly, **HII** may mimic uremic encephalopathy or may occur in addition to findings related to uremic encephalopathy. HII typically presents with bilateral diffusion restriction and T2/FLAIR hyperintensities.

## Osmotic Encephalopathy

The most common hypoosmolar state is hyponatremia, and the most common osmotic encephalopathy is **osmotic demyelination syndrome** (ODS).

### Terminology and Etiology

ODS was formerly called **central pontine myelinolysis** (when it affected only the pons) or, if it involved both the pons and **extrapontine myelinolysis**, osmotic myelinolysis. ODS is now the preferred term.

ODS occurs with osmotic stress, classically occurring when wide fluxes in serum sodium levels are induced by too-rapid correction of hyponatremia.

ODS occurs with other disorders, such as organ transplantation (particularly liver), hemodialysis, and correction of hypoglycemia.

## Pathology

ODS is traditionally considered primarily a pontine lesion **(37-46)**. However, multifocal involvement is common and typical. Only 50% of ODS cases have isolated pontine lesions. In 30% of cases, myelinolytic foci occur both outside and inside the pons. The basal ganglia and hemispheric WM are common sites. WM demyelination is exclusively extrapontine in 20-25% of cases.

Other parts of the CNS that can be involved in ODS include the cerebellum (especially the middle cerebellar peduncles), basal ganglia, thalami, lateral geniculate body, and hemispheric WM. Some ODS cases involve the cortex.

Grossly, the central pons is abnormally soft and exhibits a rhomboid or trident-shaped area of grayish-tan discoloration. The peripheral pons is spared. Laminar cortical necrosis can occur in ODS, either primarily or in association with hypoxia or anoxia. In such cases, the affected cortex appears soft and pale.

## Clinical Issues

ODS is rare. It can occur at any age but is most common in middle-aged patients (peak = 30-60 years). Pediatric patients with ODS typically have diabetes or anorexia. The most common presenting symptoms of ODS are altered mental status and seizures. ODS outcome varies significantly, ranging from complete recovery to coma, "locked-in" syndrome, and death.

*ODS may also occur (1) in normonatremic patients and (2) independent of changes in serum sodium!*

## Imaging

Imaging findings in ODS typically lag one or two weeks behind clinical symptoms.

**CT Findings.** NECT scans can be normal or show hypodensity in the affected areas, particularly the central pons **(37-48A)**.

**MR Findings.** Standard MR sequences may be normal in the first several days. Eventually, ODS becomes hypointense on T1WI **(37-48B)** and hyperintense on T2/FLAIR **(37-48C)**. The lesions are typically well demarcated and symmetric. Pontine ODS is often round or sometimes trident-shaped **(37-47)**. The peripheral pons, corticospinal tracts, and transverse pontine fibers are spared **(37-46)**. Involvement of the basal ganglia and hemispheric WM or cortex is seen in at least 1/2 of all cases ("extrapontine myelinolysis") **(37-50)**.

DWI is the most sensitive sequence for acute ODS and can demonstrate restricted diffusion when other sequences are normal **(37-49D) (37-50)**. DTI shows disruption of central pontine WM with sparing of peripheral, transverse tracts.

In ~ 20% of acute ODS cases, enhancement in midline and rim of affected region may form a distinct trident-shaped lesion. Late acute or subacute ODS lesions may demonstrate moderate confluent enhancement on T1 C+ **(37-49)**. Enhancement typically resolves within a few weeks after onset.

## Differential Diagnosis

The major differential diagnosis of "central" ODS is pontine ischemia-infarction. **Basilar perforating artery infarcts** involve the surface of the pons and are usually asymmetric. Infarcts are typically diffusion restricting

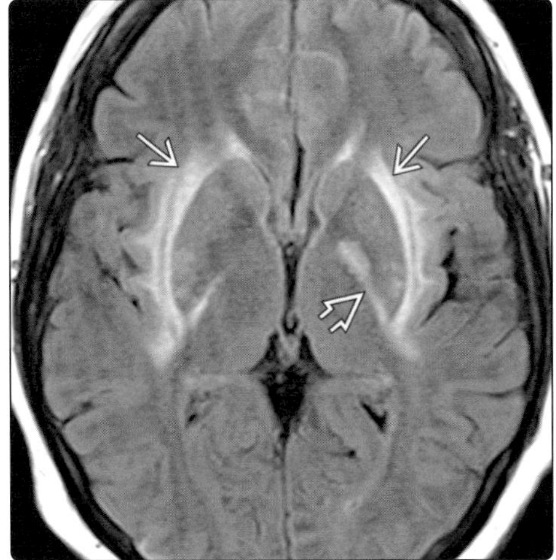

***(37-45)** Axial FLAIR MR in a renal failure patient shows the lentiform fork sign with hyperintensity along the lateral ➡ & medial ➡ putamina.*

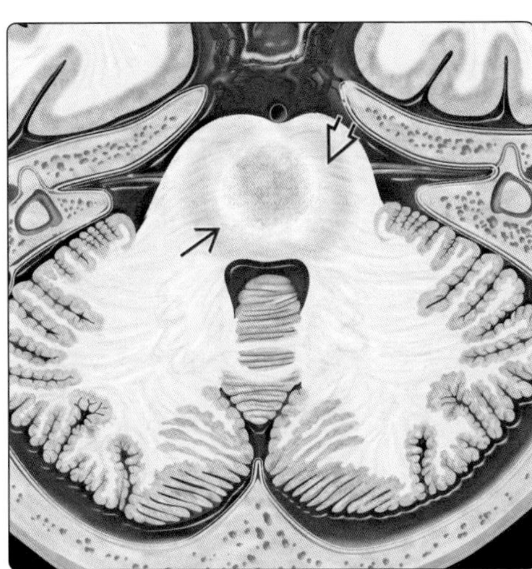

***(37-46)** Graphic shows acute osmotic central pontine demyelination ➡. Note sparing of peripheral WM, traversing corticospinal tracts ➡.*

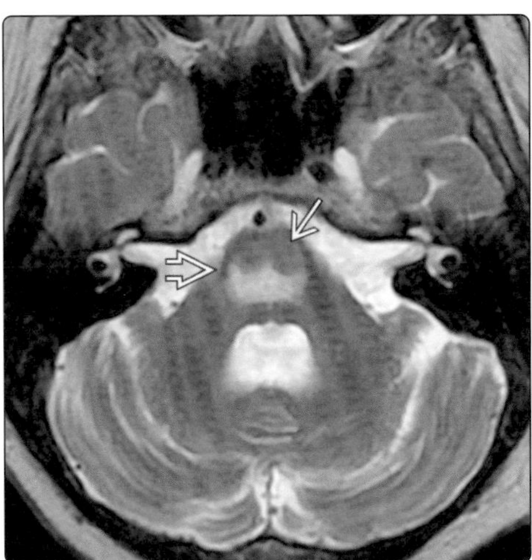

***(37-47)** T2 MR shows CPM ➡ as a trident with sparing of the peripheral pons, corticospinal tracts ➡, & transverse pontine fibers.*

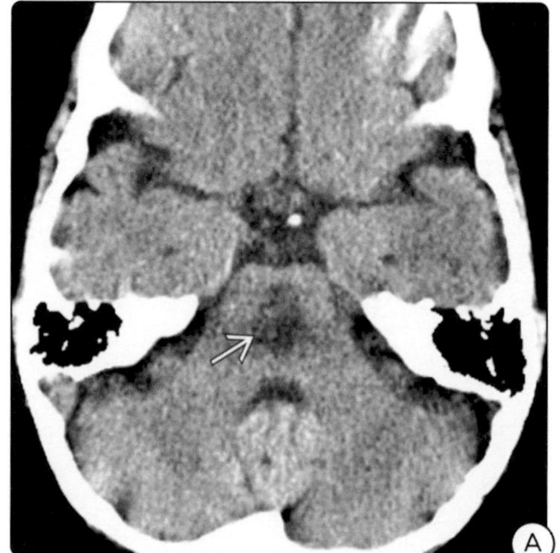

*(37-48A) NECT in a 37-yo woman with osmotic demyelination syndrome shows a triangular central pontine hypodensity ➡.*

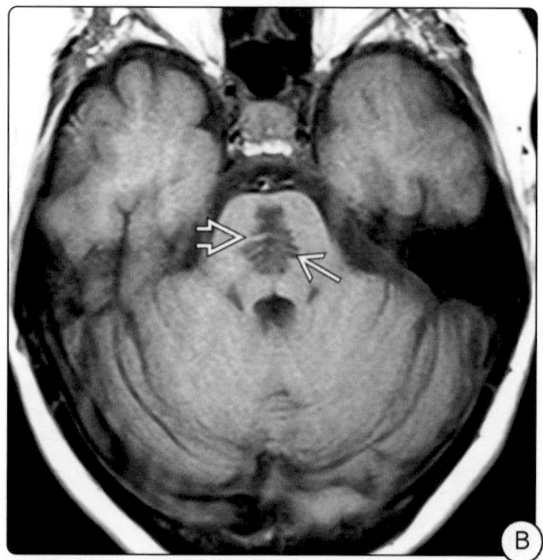

*(37-48B) T1 MR shows that the lesion is hypointense ➡. Transverse pontine fibers are spared, seen here as lines of preserved brain ➡.*

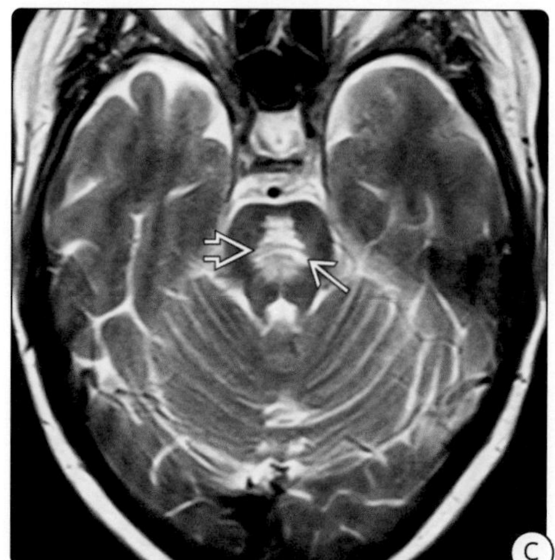

*(37-48C) T2 MR through the upper pons shows the lesion ➡ with "stripes" of preserved myelinated transverse pontine tracts ➡.*

and T2/FLAIR hyperintense. **Demyelinating disease** can involve the pons but is rarely symmetric. Acute demyelinating disease often shows diffusion restriction, T2/FLAIR hyperintensity and enhancement.

The major differential diagnosis of extrapontine ODS with basal ganglia &/or cortical involvement is metabolic disease. **Hypertensive encephalopathy** (PRES) can involve the pons but does not spare the peripheral WM tracts. PRES typically does not show diffusion restriction. The basal ganglia are affected in **Wilson disease** and **mitochondrial disorders**, but the pons is less commonly involved.

## OSMOTIC DEMYELINATION SYNDROMES

**Terminology, Etiology**

- ODS (formerly pontine, extrapontine myelinolysis)
- Serum hypotonicity → cells lose osmoles, shrink
- Oligodendrocytes especially vulnerable to osmotic stress
- Note: Can occur without serum sodium disturbances!

**Location**

- 50% pons (spares periphery, transverse pontine tracts)
- 30% pons + extrapontine (basal ganglia, thalami, WM)
- 20-25% exclusively extrapontine
- ± cortical laminar necrosis

**Imaging**

- Hypointense on T1, hyperintense on T2
    - Trident sign on T2WI, T1 C+ in acute ODS
- May restrict on DWI

*Selected References: The complete reference list is available on the eBooks+ version included with purchase.*

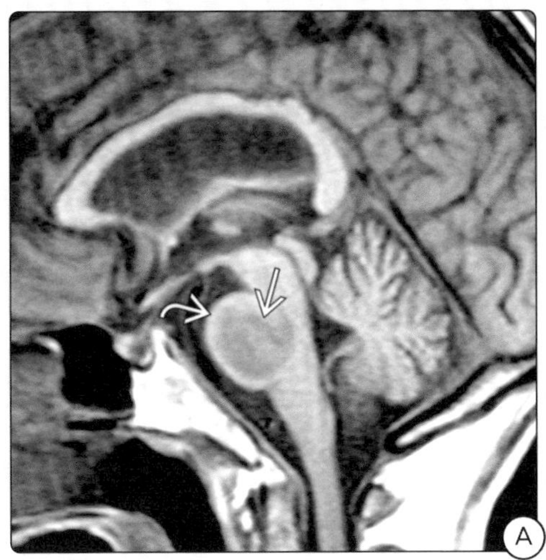

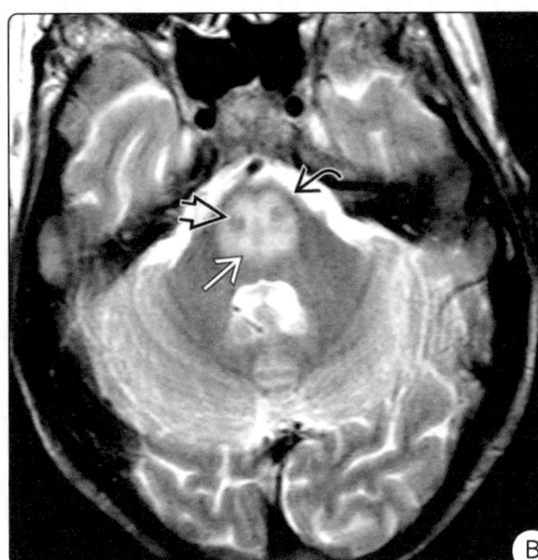

***(37-49A)** Sagittal T1 MR shows a 44-yo alcoholic man with vomiting, seizures, & acutely altered mental status. The central pons is slightly swollen & hypointense, whereas the peripheral pons is spared. **(37-49B)** T2 MR in the same patient shows symmetric central hyperintensity with sparing of the peripheral pons & corticospinal tracts.*

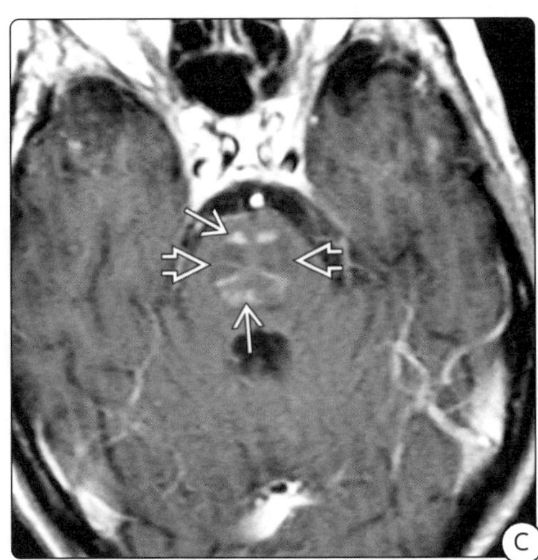

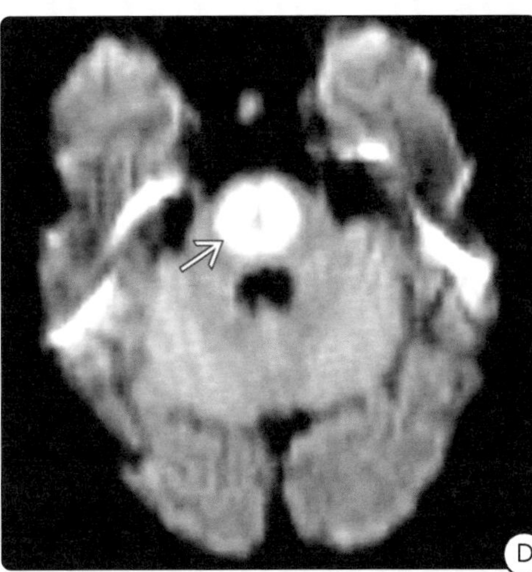

***(37-49C)** Axial T1 C+ MR in the same patient shows patchy but symmetric enhancement in the affected WM with sparing of the corticospinal tracts. **(37-49D)** DWI MR in the same patient shows acutely restricted diffusion. Osmotic demyelination syndrome with acute demyelination can both enhance & restrict.*

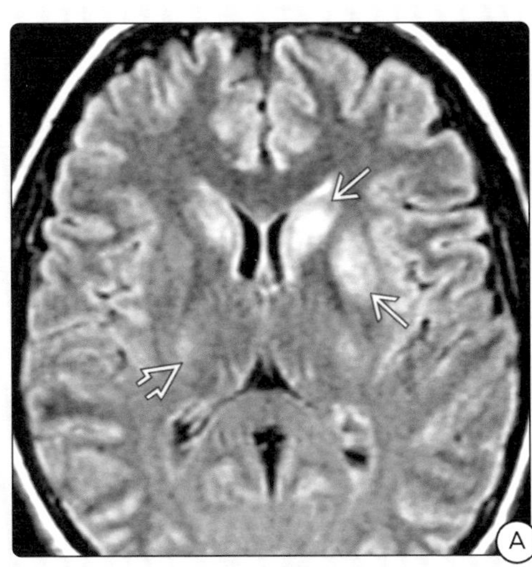

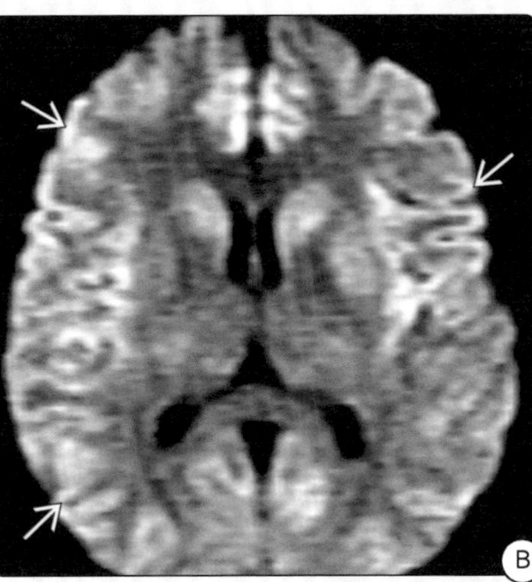

***(37-50A)** A variant case of osmotic demyelination syndrome is illustrated by this axial FLAIR MR in a 56-yo man with confusion after rapid correction of hyponatremia. Note hyperintensity in the basal ganglia & both thalami. **(37-50B)** DWI MR shows that the cortex is also diffusely but somewhat asymmetrically affected. Cortical laminar necrosis can sometimes be seen in osmotic demyelination syndrome.*

# Dementias and Brain Degenerations

*One in three adults over 85 years old suffers from Alzheimer disease or other forms of dementia. New treatments to slow progression of this devastating disease are being developed; most rely on early identification of at-risk individuals before clinical symptoms emerge.*



Innovative technologies, such as tau imaging and MR connectivity analyses, represent new, exciting frontiers in the early identification of dementing disorders. While some illustrative case examples are included here, the overall purpose of this chapter is to discuss normal and abnormal brain aging changes on imaging modalities that are generally available to practicing neuroradiologists.

After our discussion of the normal aging brain, we turn our attention to dementias and brain degenerative disorders. **Dementia** is a loss of brain function that affects memory, thinking, language, judgment, and behavior. Dementia has many causes but most often occurs secondary to degenerative processes in the brain.

**Neurodegeneration** occurs when neurons in specific parts of the brain, spinal cord, or peripheral nerves die. Although dementia always involves brain degeneration, not all neurodegenerative disorders are dementing illnesses. Some neurodegenerative disorders [e.g., Parkinson disease (PD)] can have associated dementia, but most do not.

## The Normal Aging Brain

### Introduction to the Normal Aging Brain

Age-related changes take place in virtually all parts of the brain and occur at all ages. Understanding the biology and imaging of normal aging is a prerequisite to understanding the pathobiology of degenerative brain diseases.

#### Terminology

The term **normal aging brain**, as used in this chapter, refers to the spectrum of normal age-related neuroimaging findings as delineated by longitudinal population-based studies, such as the Rotterdam Scan Study (RSS).

#### Genetics

Genetic factors definitely affect brain aging and contribute to age-related cognitive decline. Apolipoprotein E (specifically *APOE*-ε4) and other risk-associated single-nucleotide polymorphisms are genetic variants that are

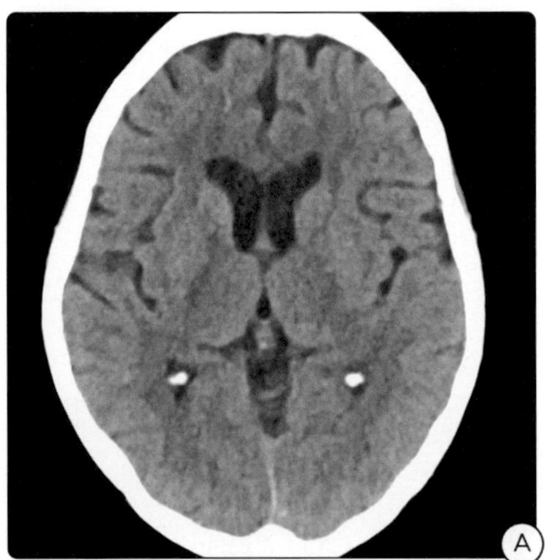

*(38-1A) NECT in an 80-year-old cognitively intact woman shows mildly enlarged ventricles and sulci with normal-appearing WM.*

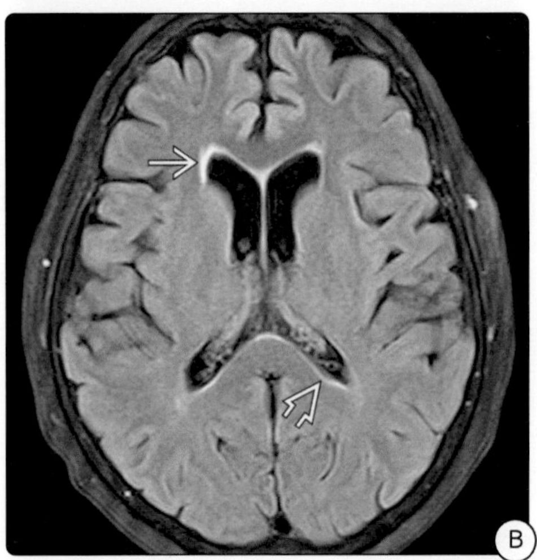

*(38-1B) FLAIR MR in the same patient shows frontal periventricular "caps" ➡ and a thin hyperintense rim around the lateral ventricles ➡.*

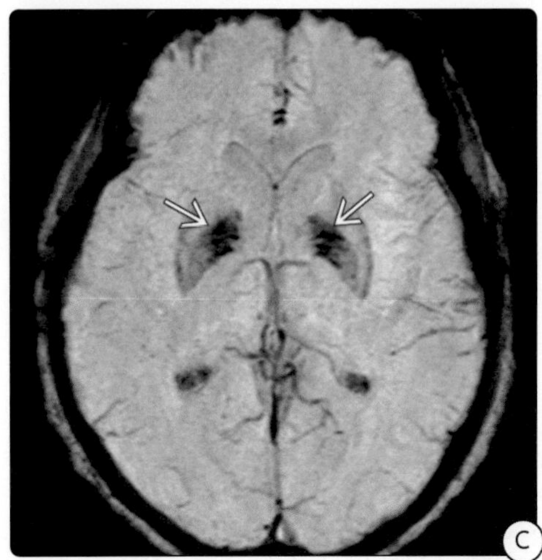

*(38-1C) SWI shows hypointensity in globi pallidi ➡ but not in putamina, thalami. No microbleeds are present. Normal "successfully" aging brain.*

robustly associated with brain pathology on MR. Epigenetic dysregulation has also been identified as a pivotal player in aging as well as age-related cognitive decline and degenerative disorders.

## Pathology

**Gross Pathology.** Overall brain volume decreases with advancing age and is indicated by a relative increase in the size of the CSF spaces. Widened sulci with proportionate enlargement of the ventricles are common. Although minor thinning of the cortical mantle occurs with aging, the predominant neuroanatomic changes occur in the subcortical white matter (WM).

**Microscopic Features.** The subcortical WM demonstrates decreased numbers of myelinated fibers, increased extracellular space, and gliosis. Perivascular (Virchow-Robin) spaces in the subcortical and basal ganglia enlarge.

Three histologic markers are associated with dementias: **Senile plaques (SPs), neurofibrillary tangles (NFTs)**, and **Lewy bodies**. **SPs** are extracellular amyloid deposits that accumulate in cerebral gray matter. Nearly 1/2 of cognitively intact older individuals demonstrate moderate or frequent SP density.

**NFTs** are caused by tau aggregations within neurons. **Lewy bodies** are intraneuronal clumps of α-synuclein and ubiquitin proteins. They are found in 5-10% of cognitively intact individuals.

## Clinical Issues

Although the incidence of dementias increases dramatically with aging, nearly 2/3 of patients over 85 years of age remain neurologically intact and cognitively normal.

# Imaging the Normal Aging Brain

Imaging plays an increasingly central role in evaluating older patients for "altered mental status" and early signs of dementia.

## CT Findings

Screening NECT scans are often obtained in older patients for nonspecific indications, such as "altered mental status." The normal aging brain demonstrates mildly enlarged ventricles and widened sulci on NECT scans **(38-1A)**. A few scattered patchy WM hypodensities are common, but confluent subcortical hypointensities, especially around the atria of the lateral ventricles, are a marker of arteriolosclerosis ("microvascular disease").

## MR Findings

**T1WI.** T1-weighted images show mild but symmetric ventricular enlargement and proportionate prominence of the subarachnoid spaces.

**T2/FLAIR.** WM hyperintensities (WMHs) and lacunar infarcts on T2/FLAIR scans are highly prevalent in older adults. They are associated with cardiovascular risk factors, such as diabetes and hyperlipidemia. "Successfully" aging brains may demonstrate a few scattered nonconfluent WMHs (a reasonable number is one WMH per decade, but the prevalence rises more steeply after age 50).

Perivascular spaces increase in prevalence and size with aging and are seen on T2WI as well-delineated round, ovoid, or linear CSF-like collections in the basal ganglia, subcortical WM, midbrain, etc. (see Chapter 32). Perivascular spaces suppress completely on FLAIR. Between 25-30% may display a thin, smooth, hyperintense rim. Lacunar infarcts typically demonstrate an irregular hyperintense rim around the lesions.

FLAIR scans in normal older patients demonstrate a smooth, thin, periventricular hyperintense rim around the lateral ventricles that probably represents increased extracellular interstitial fluid in the subependymal WM **(38-1B)**. A "cap" of hyperintensity around the frontal horns is common and normal.

**T2* (GRE, SWI). Ferric iron deposition** in the basal ganglia increases with age and is best demonstrated on T2* sequences. Hypointensity on T2* scans is normal in the medial globus pallidus **(38-1C)**. Putaminal hypointensity is typically less prominent until the eighth decade. The caudate nucleus shows a scarce iron load at any age. The thalamus does not normally exhibit any hypointensity on T2* sequences.

**Microbleeds** on T2* scans are common in the aging brain. GRE and SWI sequences demonstrate cerebral microbleeds in 20% of patients over age 60 and 1/3 of patients aged 80 and older. Although common and therefore *statistically* "normal," microbleeds are not characteristic of *successful* brain aging. Basal ganglia and cerebellar microbleeds are usually indicative of chronic hypertensive encephalopathy. Lobar and cortical microbleeds are typical of amyloid angiopathy and are associated with worse cognitive performance.

## Differential Diagnosis

The correlation between cognitive performance and brain imaging is complex and difficult to determine. Therefore, the major differential diagnosis of a normal aging brain is **mild cognitive impairment (MCI)** and early "preclinical" **Alzheimer disease (AD)**. WMHs are markers of microvascular disease, so there is considerable overlap between normal brains and those with **subcortical arteriosclerotic encephalopathy**.

# Dementias

The three most common dementias are **AD, dementia with Lewy bodies**, and **vascular dementia (VaD)**. Together, they account for the vast majority of all dementia cases. Less frequent causes include **frontotemporal lobar degeneration (FTLD)** (formerly known as Pick disease) and **corticobasal degeneration (CBD)**. It can be difficult to distinguish between the various dementia syndromes because clinical features frequently overlap and so-called mixed dementias are common.

## Alzheimer Disease

AD remains the only leading cause of death for which no disease-modifying treatment currently exists and age is by far the greatest risk factor. At least 1/3 of older individuals in the USA will die with dementia, largely due to AD.

### Terminology

AD is a progressive neurodegenerative condition that leads to cognitive decline, impaired ability to perform the activities of daily living, and a range of behavioral and psychologic conditions.

There is increasing evidence that AD represents a continuum of severity. The pathogenic process is prolonged and may extend over several decades. A prodromal **preclinical/asymptomatic disease** (i.e., pathology is present, but cognition remains intact) may exist for years before evidence of **MCI** develops.

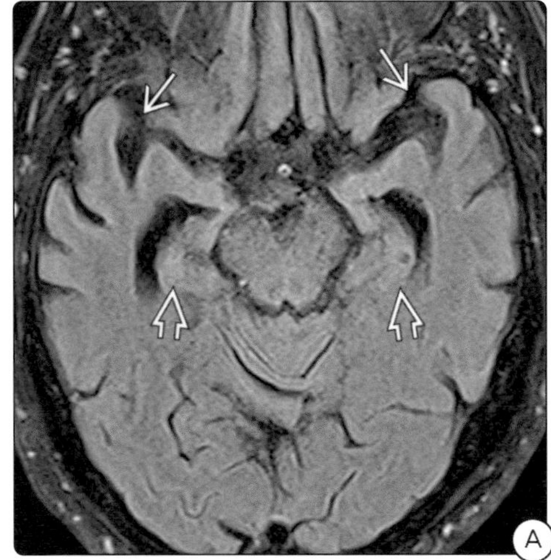


***(38-2A)** FLAIR in 74-year-old with AD shows shrunken hippocampi ➡ and medial temporal lobes with prominent sylvian fissures ➡.*

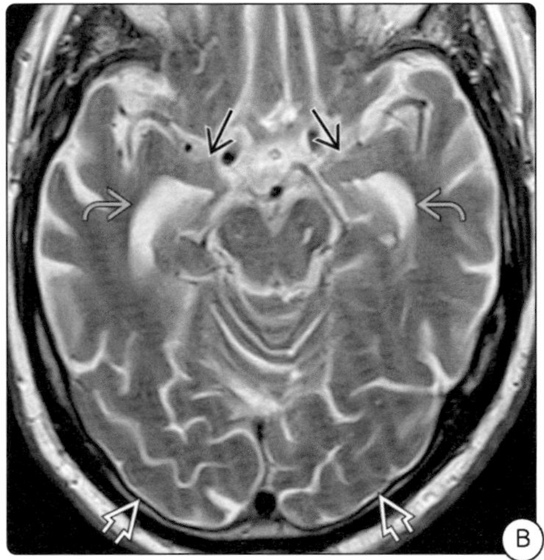


***(38-2B)** T2 MR shows enlarged temporal horns ➡, volume loss in the temporal lobes ➡, and normal-appearing occipital lobes ➡.*

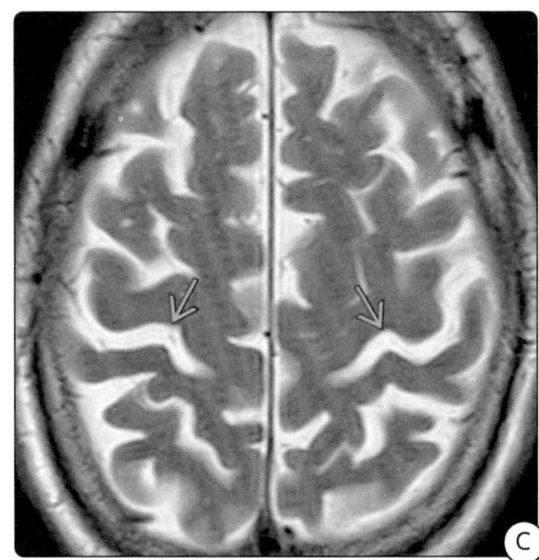


***(38-2C)** T2 MR in same patient at the upper cerebral hemispheres shows symmetric parietal lobe atrophy with enlarged central sulci ➡.*

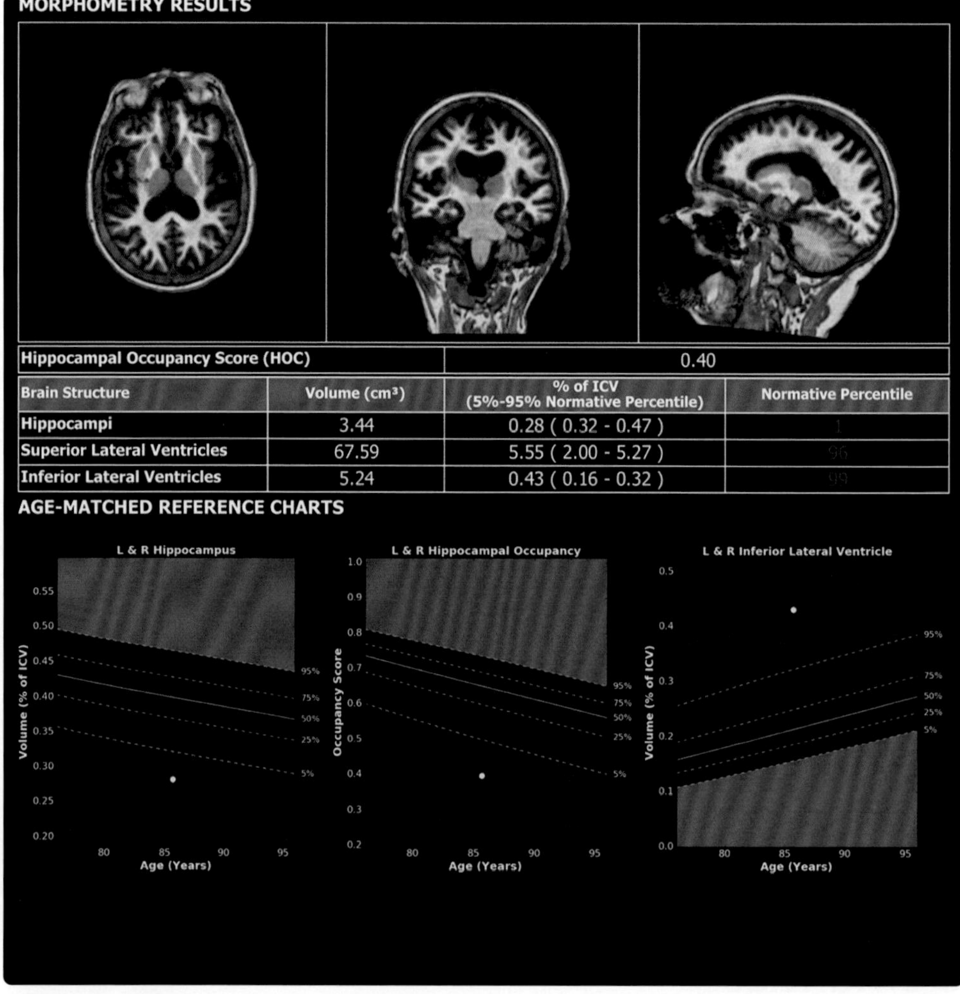

MORPHOMETRY RESULTS
Hippocampal Occupancy Score (HOC) 0.40
Brain Structure | Volume (cm³) | % of ICV (5%-95% Normative Percentile) | Normative Percentile
Hippocampi | 3.44 | 0.28 ( 0.32 - 0.47 ) | 1
Superior Lateral Ventricles | 67.59 | 5.55 ( 2.00 - 5.27 ) | 96
Inferior Lateral Ventricles | 5.24 | 0.43 ( 0.16 - 0.32 ) | 99
AGE-MATCHED REFERENCE CHARTS
L & R Hippocampus
L & R Hippocampal Occupancy
L & R Inferior Lateral Ventricle
Volume (% of ICV)
Occupancy Score
Age (Years)


***(38-3)** NeuroQuant morphometry obtained using thin-section MP-RAGE and age-matched controls shows a hippocampal occupancy score (HOC) of 0.40. The hippocampal volumes are at the 1st percentile, and the inferior lateral ventricle volumes are at the 99th percentile for age. The mesial temporal lobes are > 2 standard deviations below normal. This volumetric data can be helpful in evaluating hippocampal volumes in patients with suspected AD.*

## Etiology

**General Concepts.** AD is characterized by an "amyloid cascade." Reduced clearance of amyloid-β (Aβ) results in its aggregation in neurons. The **Aβ**42 residue is both insoluble and highly neurotoxic. Aβ42 clumps form **SPs** in the cortical gray matter. Aβ42 deposits also thicken the walls of cortical and leptomeningeal arterioles, causing **amyloid angiopathy**.

Another key feature of AD is **tauopathy**. Abnormal phosphorylation of a microtubule-associated protein known as "tau" eventually leads to the development of **NFTs** and **neuronal death**.

**Genetics.** Approximately 10% of AD cases have a strong family history of the disorder. The ε4 allele is the ancestral form of apolipoprotein E (*APOE*) and is associated with both higher absorption of cholesterol at the intestinal level and higher plasma cholesterol levels in carriers. Both the ε4 and *MTHFR* polymorphisms are known risk factors for late-onset AD (the most common type) and cerebrovascular disease (including VaD; see later discussion).

## Pathology

**Gross Pathology.** Brains affected by AD show generalized (whole-brain) atrophy with shrunken gyri, widened sulci, and ventricular expansion (especially the temporal horns). Changes are most marked in the medial temporal and parietal lobes **(38-6)**. The frontal lobes are commonly involved, whereas the occipital lobes and motor cortex are relatively spared.

**Microscopic Features.** The three characteristic histologic hallmarks of AD are SPs, NFTs, and exaggerated neuronal loss. All are characteristic of—but none is specific for—AD.

AD also often coexists with other pathologies, such as vascular disease or Lewy bodies. Variable amounts of amyloid deposition in arterioles of the cortex and leptomeninges (amyloid angiopathy) are present in > 90% of AD cases.

**Staging, Grading, and Classification.** One of the most widely used systems—the Braak and Braak system—is based on the topographic distribution of NFTs and neuropil threads with grades 1-6.

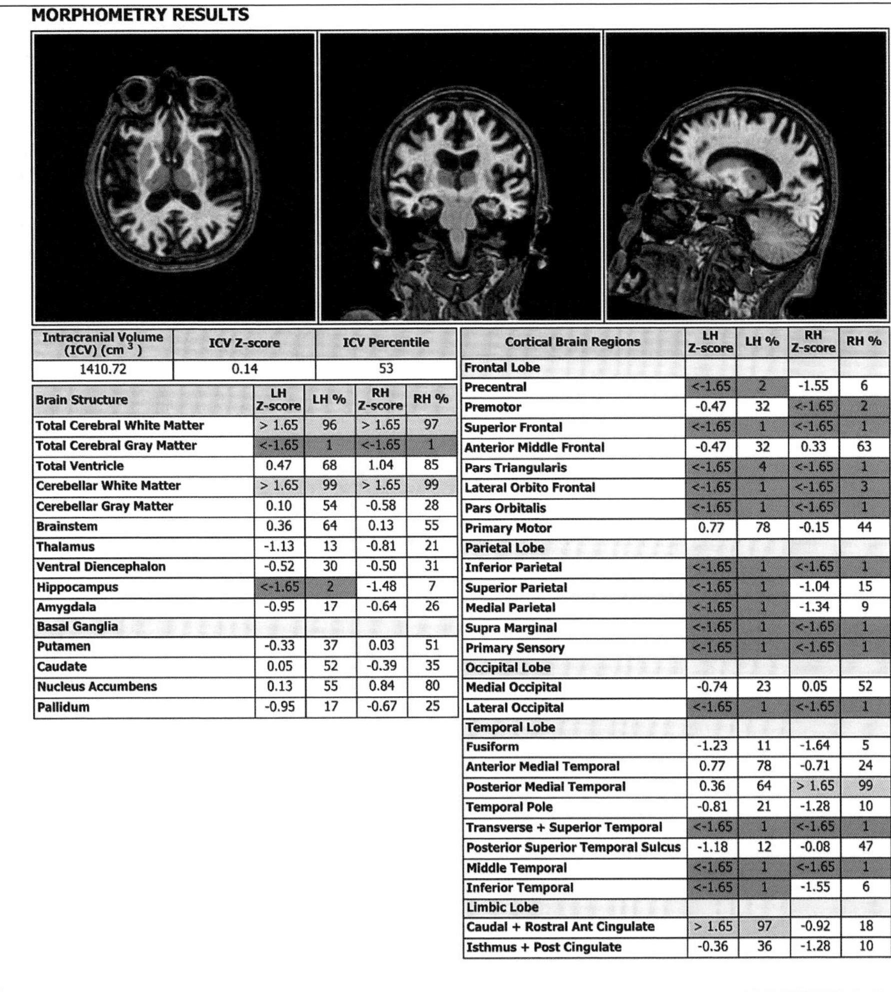

MORPHOMETRY RESULTS

| Intracranial Volume (ICV) (cm 3 ) | ICV Z-score | ICV Percentile |
|---|---|---|
| 1410.72 | 0.14 | 53 |

| Brain Structure | LH Z-score | LH % | RH Z-score | RH % |
|---|---|---|---|---|
| Total Cerebral White Matter | > 1.65 | 96 | > 1.65 | 97 |
| Total Cerebral Gray Matter | <-1.65 | 1 | <-1.65 | 1 |
| Total Ventricle | 0.47 | 68 | 1.04 | 85 |
| Cerebellar White Matter | > 1.65 | 99 | > 1.65 | 99 |
| Cerebellar Gray Matter | 0.10 | 54 | -0.58 | 28 |
| Brainstem | 0.36 | 64 | 0.13 | 55 |
| Thalamus | -1.13 | 13 | -0.81 | 21 |
| Ventral Diencephalon | -0.52 | 30 | -0.50 | 31 |
| Hippocampus | <-1.65 | 2 | -1.48 | 7 |
| Amygdala | -0.95 | 17 | -0.64 | 26 |
| Basal Ganglia | | | | |
| Putamen | -0.33 | 37 | 0.03 | 51 |
| Caudate | 0.05 | 52 | -0.39 | 35 |
| Nucleus Accumbens | 0.13 | 55 | 0.84 | 80 |
| Pallidum | -0.95 | 17 | -0.67 | 25 |

| Cortical Brain Regions | LH Z-score | LH % | RH Z-score | RH % |
|---|---|---|---|---|
| Frontal Lobe | | | | |
| Precentral | <-1.65 | 2 | -1.55 | 6 |
| Premotor | -0.47 | 32 | <-1.65 | 2 |
| Superior Frontal | <-1.65 | 1 | <-1.65 | 1 |
| Anterior Middle Frontal | -0.47 | 32 | 0.33 | 63 |
| Pars Triangularis | <-1.65 | 4 | <-1.65 | 1 |
| Lateral Orbito Frontal | <-1.65 | 1 | <-1.65 | 3 |
| Pars Orbitalis | <-1.65 | 1 | <-1.65 | 1 |
| Primary Motor | 0.77 | 78 | -0.15 | 44 |
| Parietal Lobe | | | | |
| Inferior Parietal | <-1.65 | 1 | <-1.65 | 1 |
| Superior Parietal | <-1.65 | 1 | -1.04 | 15 |
| Medial Parietal | <-1.65 | 1 | -1.34 | 9 |
| Supra Marginal | <-1.65 | 1 | <-1.65 | 1 |
| Primary Sensory | <-1.65 | 1 | <-1.65 | 1 |
| Occipital Lobe | | | | |
| Medial Occipital | -0.74 | 23 | 0.05 | 52 |
| Lateral Occipital | <-1.65 | 1 | <-1.65 | 1 |
| Temporal Lobe | | | | |
| Fusiform | -1.23 | 11 | -1.64 | 5 |
| Anterior Medial Temporal | 0.77 | 78 | -0.71 | 24 |
| Posterior Medial Temporal | 0.36 | 64 | > 1.65 | 99 |
| Temporal Pole | -0.81 | 21 | -1.28 | 10 |
| Transverse + Superior Temporal | <-1.65 | 1 | <-1.65 | 1 |
| Posterior Superior Temporal Sulcus | -1.18 | 12 | -0.08 | 47 |
| Middle Temporal | <-1.65 | 1 | <-1.65 | 1 |
| Inferior Temporal | <-1.65 | 1 | -1.55 | 6 |
| Limbic Lobe | | | | |
| Caudal + Rostral Ant Cingulate | > 1.65 | 97 | -0.92 | 18 |
| Isthmus + Post Cingulate | -0.36 | 36 | -1.28 | 10 |

***(38-4)*** *NeuroQuant morphometry results in a patient with clinical probable AD shows marked cerebral atrophy. Detailed analyses of total cerebral GM, hippocampi, and several cortical brain regions (frontal, parietal, temporal) are grossly abnormal, highlighted in red. The average hippocampal volume reduction in AD is 20-25%. Volume loss of hippocampal regions with NeuroQuant and Neuroreader is extremely valuable in the prediction of AD from MCI at 3-year follow-up compared with other regions.*

## Clinical Issues

**Epidemiology and Demographics.** AD accounts for ~ 50-60% of all dementias. Age is the biggest risk factor for developing AD. The prevalence of AD is 1-2% at age 65 and increases by 15-25% each decade. In the "oldest-old" patients (> 90 years), mixed pathologies—typically AD + VaD—predominate.

**Diagnosis.** AD represents a disease spectrum that ranges from cognitively normal individuals with elevated Aβ through those who exhibit the very first, minimal signs of cognitive impairment (MCI) to frank AD.

Historically, the *definitive* diagnosis of AD was made only by biopsy or autopsy. The *clinical* diagnosis of AD defines three levels of certainty: Possible, probable, and definite AD. The diagnosis of definite AD currently requires the clinical diagnosis of probable AD *plus* neuropathologic confirmation.

The Alzheimer Disease Neuroimaging Initiative (ADNI) standardized datasets are currently the most commonly used references for the computer-aided diagnosis of dementia.

**Natural History.** AD is a chronic disease. Progression is gradual, and patients live an average of 8-10 years after diagnosis. Between 5-10% of patients with MCI progress to probable AD each year.

## Imaging

**General Features.** One of the most important goals of routine CT and MR is to identify specific abnormalities that could support the clinical diagnosis of AD. The other major role is to exclude alternative etiologies that can mimic AD clinically, i.e., "causes of reversible dementia."

The introduction of radiotracers for the noninvasive in vivo quantification of Aβ burden in the brain has revolutionized the approach to the imaging evaluation of AD.

**CT Findings.** NECT is used to exclude potentially reversible or treatable causes of dementia, such as subdural hematoma, but are otherwise uninformative, especially in the early stages of AD. Medial temporal lobe atrophy is generally the earliest identifiable finding on CT.

**MR Findings.** The current role of conventional MR in the evaluation of patients with dementing disorders is to (1) exclude other causes of dementia, (2) identify region-specific patterns of brain volume loss (e.g., "lobar-predominant" atrophy), and (3) identify imaging markers of comorbid vascular disease, such as amyloid angiopathy.

The most common morphologic changes on standard MR are thinned gyri, widened sulci, and enlarged lateral ventricles.

The medial temporal lobe—particularly the hippocampus and entorhinal cortex—are often disproportionately affected **(38-2)**, as are the posterior cingulate gyri.

T1-weighted MP-RAGE data can be used to quantify regional brain atrophy using open-source (i.e., FreeSurfer), proprietary, or commercial (i.e., NeuroQuant) automated volumetric analyses **(38-3)**. 7T MR can identify abnormalities in the hippocampal subfields. The most consistent finding is reduction in CA1 volume (specifically CA1-SRLM) **(38-4)**. Volume loss of hippocampal regions with NeuroQuant and Neuroreader is valuable in the prediction of AD from MCI at three-year follow-up compared with other regions.

T2* (GRE, SWI) sequences are much more sensitive than standard FSE in detecting cortical microhemorrhages that may suggest comorbid amyloid angiopathy.

**Functional Neuroimaging.** fMRI shows decrease in intensity &/or extent of activation in the frontal and temporal regions in cognitive tasks. pMR may demonstrate subtly reduced rCBV in the temporal and parietal lobes in MCI patients.

**Nuclear Medicine. F-18 FDG PET** demonstrates areas of regional hypometabolism **(38-5)** and helps distinguish AD from other lobar-predominant dementias (e.g., FTLD). Early-stage AD shows decreased metabolism in the parietotemporal association cortices, posterior cingulate, and precuneus regions. With moderate to severe AD, there is additional frontal lobe involvement.

**Amyloid (Aβ) PET** using amyloid-binding radiotracers has emerged as one of the best techniques for early AD diagnosis. Aβ deposition occurs well before symptom onset and likely represents preclinical AD in asymptomatic individuals and prodromal AD in patients with MCI. F-18 florbetapir, flutemetamol, and florbetaben tracers are FDA approved for clinical use. A positive Aβ PET scan shows loss of gray matter-WM distinction due to tracer uptake in the cortex, typically temporal, parietal, and frontal lobes **(38-7)**.

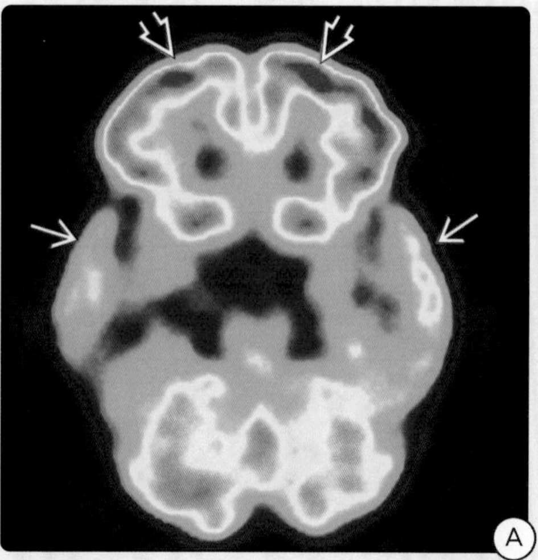


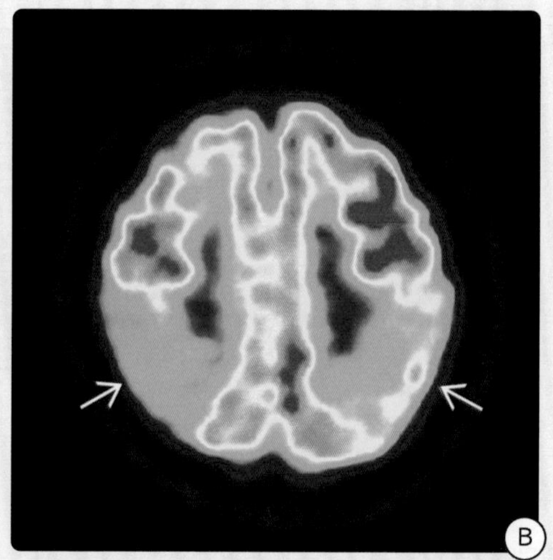


***(38-5A)** F-18 FDG PET in AD shows markedly reduced metabolism in both temporal lobes (yellow, green) ➡ with comparatively normal frontal lobes ➡. **(38-5B)** There is hypometabolism ➡ (yellow, green cortex) in the parietal lobes on F-18 FDG PET. Early-stage AD shows ↓ metabolism in parietotemporal association cortices, posterior cingulate, and precuneus regions. Moderate to severe AD shows additional frontal lobe involvement.*

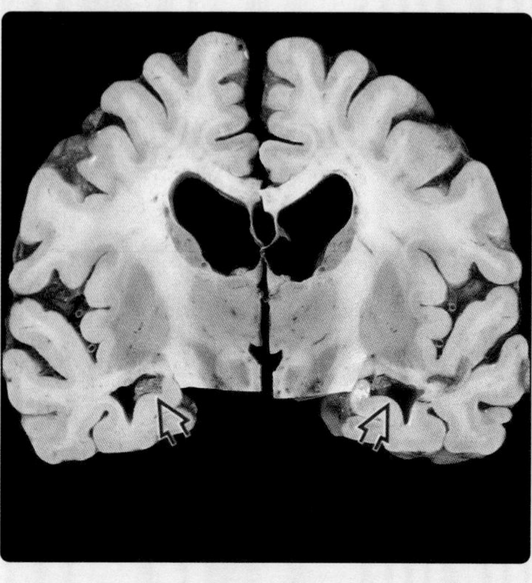

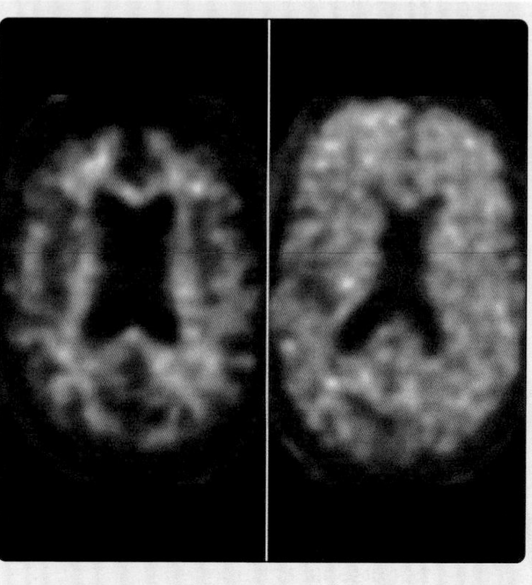

***(38-6)** Autopsy in proven early AD shows enlarged lateral ventricles. Hippocampi ➡ appear mildly atrophic. (Courtesy R. Hewlett, MD.) **(38-7)** F-18 AV-45 (florbetapir) PET (amyloid PET) in a healthy control (left) shows normal nonspecific WM uptake and preserved GM-WM differentiation. In a patient with AD (right), there is marked cerebral GM uptake (Aβ deposition) with loss of GM-WM differentiation. (Courtesy A. Ali, MD.)*

## Differential Diagnosis

The most difficult distinction is differentiating **normal age-related degenerative processes** and early "preclinical" AD.

"Mixed dementias" are common, especially in patients over the age of 90 years old. **VaD** is the most common dementia associated with AD. Lacunar and cortical infarcts are typical findings in VaD. **Cerebral amyloid angiopathy** often coexists with AD. Cerebral amyloid angiopathy is characterized by WM lesions and multiple T2*/GRE/SWI hypointensities related to hemosiderin. **Lewy bodies** are sometimes found in AD patients ("Lewy body variant of AD").

**FTLD** shows frontal &/or anterior temporal atrophy and hypometabolism; the parietal lobes are generally spared. **Dementia with Lewy bodies** typically demonstrates generalized, nonfocal hypometabolism. Patients with **CBD** have prominent extrapyramidal symptoms.

**Causes of reversible dementia** that can be identified on imaging studies include mass lesions, such as chronic subdural hematoma or neoplasm, vitamin deficiencies (thiamine, B12), endocrinopathy (e.g., hypothyroidism), and normal pressure hydrocephalus.

### ALZHEIMER DISEASE

**Pathoetiology**
- Neurotoxic "amyloid cascade"
  - Aβ42 accumulation → senile plaques, amyloid angiopathy
- Tauopathy → neurofibrillary tangles, neuronal death

**Clinical Issues**
- Most common dementia (50-60% of all cases)
- Prevalence increases 15-25% per decade after 65 years
- Pathology begins *at least* 1 decade before clinical symptoms emerge
  - "Clinically normal" on preclinical Alzheimer cognitive composite
  - Aβ in clinically normal patients predicts significant longitudinal decline

**Imaging**
- Frontoparietal dominant lobar atrophy
  - Hippocampus, entorhinal cortex
  - FDG PET shows hypometabolism
  - Amyloid-binding markers show loss of gray matter-white matter distinction
- Amyloid angiopathy
  - Present in > 95% of cases
  - T2* cortical "blooming black dots"
  - ± cortical siderosis

**Differential Diagnosis**
- Exclude reversible dementias!
  - Subdural hematoma
  - Normal pressure hydrocephalus
- Differential diagnoses
  - Normal aging
  - Vascular dementia (VaD)
  - Frontotemporal lobar degeneration (FTLD)
  - Alzheimer disease (AD) often mixed with other dementias (especially vascular)

## New Alzheimer Disease Therapies and Imaging

Recently, **monoclonal antibodies** against Aβ have become available in both clinical trials and early clinical practice for the AD treatment. These new

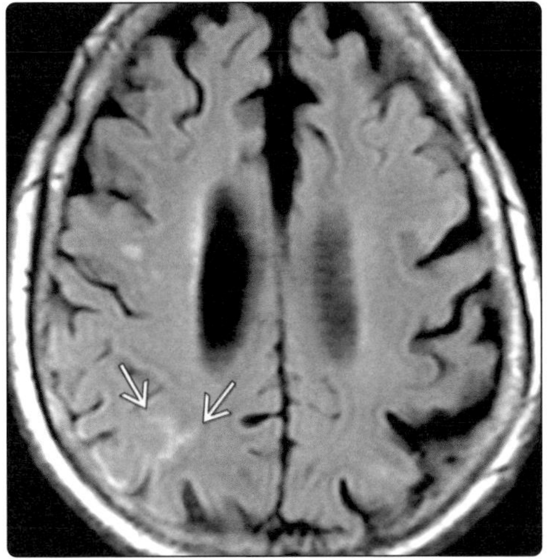

*(38-8) Axial FLAIR MR in an 83-year-old on AD treatment with monoclonal antibody shows focal leptomeningeal proteinaceous fluid ➡, ARIA-E.*

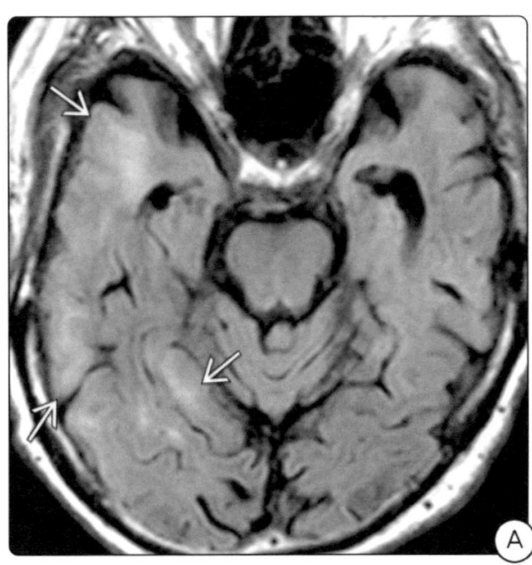


*(38-9A) Axial FLAIR MR shows parenchymal hyperintensity ➡ in the temporal and occipital lobes and mild local mass effect, ARIA-E.*

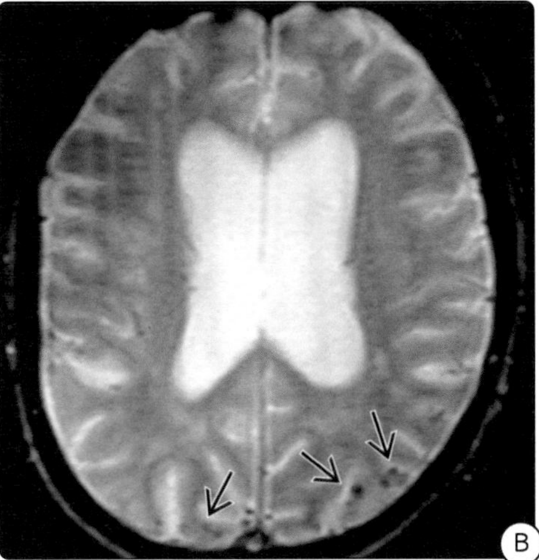


*(38-9B) Axial GRE in the same patient being treated for AD shows multiple new hypointense foci ➡ related to ARIA-H.*

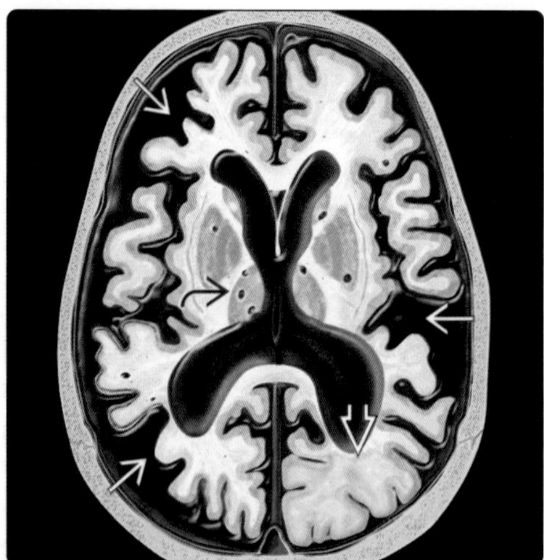

(38-10) Graphic of VaD shows multiple chronic infarcts ➡, acute occipital lobe infarct ➡, and small basal ganglia, thalamic lacunar infarcts ➡.

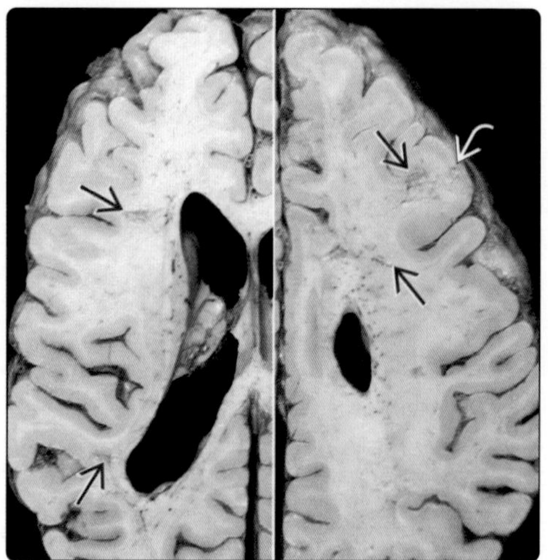

(38-11) VaD shows multiple WM ➡, cortical ➡ lacunae at the level of the lateral ventricle (L), corona radiata (R). (Courtesy R. Hewlett, MD.)

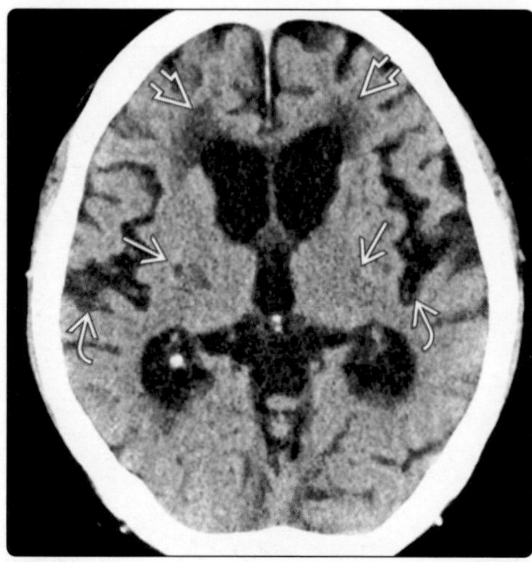

(38-12) NECT in 72-year-old man with VaD shows enlarged ventricles, sulci ➡, WM rarefaction ➡, and old lacunar infarcts ➡.

therapies require brain MR imaging to detect contraindications to treatment and to monitor for adverse events associated with treatment. The new agents include monoclonal antibodies: Bapineuzumab, aducanumab, donanemab, lecanemab, and gantenerumab. These therapies have been shown to reduce amyloid plaque.

The main imaging findings of these new treatment complications are called **amyloid-related imaging abnormalities (ARIA)** and are reported for several agents that target cerebral Aβ burden. ARIA includes **ARIA-E** for edema or effusion and **ARIA-H** for microhemorrhages and hemosiderosis.

FLAIR MR of AIRA-E shows parenchymal &/or sulcal hyperintensities **(38-8)** **(38-9A)**. ARIA-H shows areas of hypointense signal on GRE/T2* or SWI indicative of hemosiderin deposition or superficial siderosis **(38-9B)**. These MR findings typically resolve spontaneously or after the therapy is decreased or discontinued.

The main imaging differential for ARIA is **cerebral amyloid angiopathy-related inflammation (CAA-RI)**. CAA-RI is an inflammatory condition that occurs in patients with cerebral amyloid angiopathy and responds to steroid treatment or immunosuppression. ARIA only occurs secondary to monoclonal antibody therapy. CAA-RI and ARIA have similar imaging findings of sulcal effusion and parenchymal edema as well as microhemorrhages and siderosis. Clinical history is key.

Risk factors for developing ARIA are drug exposure, *APOE*-ε4 allele carriership, and pretreatment microhemorrhages. It is noted that the risk for developing ARIA is reduced if patients are started at a low drug dose and progressively titrated over time to the higher optimal treatment dose.

## Vascular Dementia

Cerebrovascular disease is a common cause of cognitive decline. The burden of "silent" microvascular disease and its long-term deleterious effect on cognition are becoming increasingly well recognized, as is its link with AD as a significant comorbidity.

### Terminology

VaD is sometimes also called multiinfarct dementia, vascular cognitive disorder, vascular cognitive impairment, subcortical ischemic VaD, and poststroke dementia.

### Etiology

**Inherited Vascular Dementias.** Monogenic disorders are estimated to cause ~ 5% of all strokes and 10% of VaDs. The most common inherited disorders that can cause VaD are CADASIL and Fabry disease.

**Sporadic Vascular Dementias.** Most cases of VaD are sporadic and caused by the cumulative burden of cerebrovascular lesions. Risk factors for VaD include hypertension, dyslipidemia, and smoking. Mutations in the *MTHFR* gene correlate with elevated levels of plasma homocysteine and are associated with both AD and vasculogenic cognitive impairment.

### Pathology

**Gross Pathology.** The most common, readily identifiable gross finding in VaD is multiple infarcts with focal atrophy **(38-10)**. Multiple subcortical lacunar infarcts **(38-11)** &/or widespread WM ischemia are more common than cortical branch occlusions or large territorial infarcts **(38-40)**.

**Microscopic Features. Arteriolosclerosis** and **amyloid angiopathy** are the major underlying pathologies in VaD. So-called **microinfarcts**—minute foci of neuronal loss, gliosis, pallor, or frank cystic degeneration—are seen at autopsy in nearly 2/3 of patients with VaD and > 1/2 of all cases with other dementing disorders (e.g., AD, dementia with Lewy bodies). Lesions are found in all brain regions and are especially common in the cortex, subcortical WM, and basal ganglia.

## Clinical Issues

**Epidemiology and Demographics.** VaD is the second most common cause of dementia (after AD) and accounts for ~ 10% of all dementia cases in resource-rich countries. VaD is a common component of "mixed" dementias and is especially prevalent in patients with AD.

The incidence of VaD increases with age. Risk factors include hypertension, diabetes, dyslipidemia, and smoking. There is a moderate male predominance.

**Natural History.** Progressive, episodic, stepwise neurologic deterioration interspersed with intervals of relative clinical stabilization is the typical pattern of VaD.

## Imaging

**General Features.** The general imaging features of VaD are those of multifocal infarcts and WM ischemia.

**CT Findings.** NECT scans often show generalized volume loss with multiple cortical, subcortical, and basal ganglia infarcts. Patchy or confluent hypodensities in the subcortical and deep periventricular WM, especially around the atria of the lateral ventricles, are typical **(38-12)**.

**MR Findings.** T1WI often shows greater than expected generalized volume loss. Multiple hypointensities in the basal ganglia and deep WM are typical. Focal cortical and large territorial infarcts with encephalomalacia can be identified in many cases.

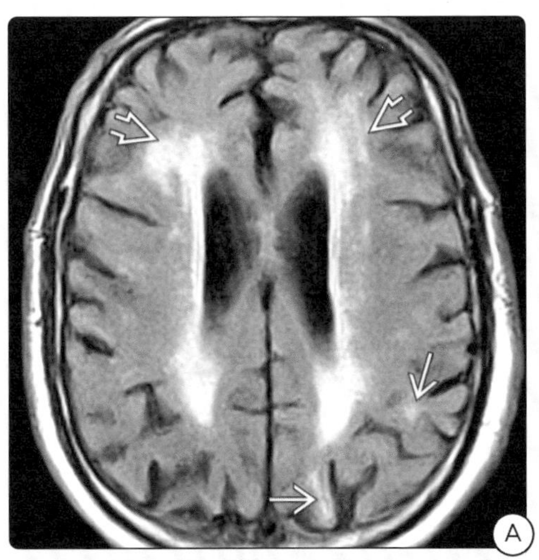

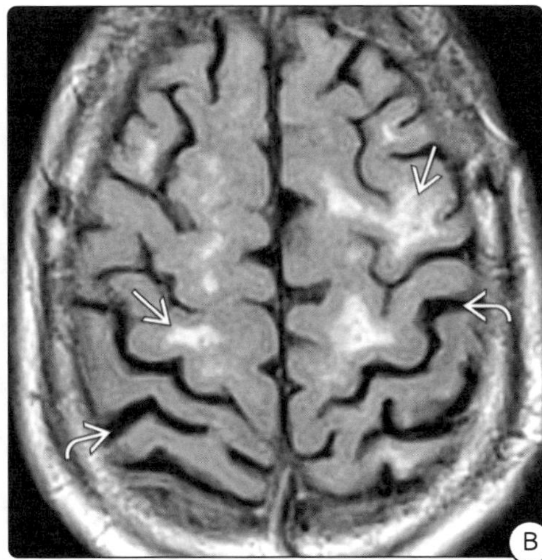

***(38-13A)** FLAIR MR in a 76-year-old normotensive man with dementia shows multifocal confluent hyperintensities in the subcortical → and deep periventricular WM →. **(38-13B)** More cephalad FLAIR MR in the same patient shows significant lesion burden in the subcortical WM →. Note the enlarged parietal sulci →.*

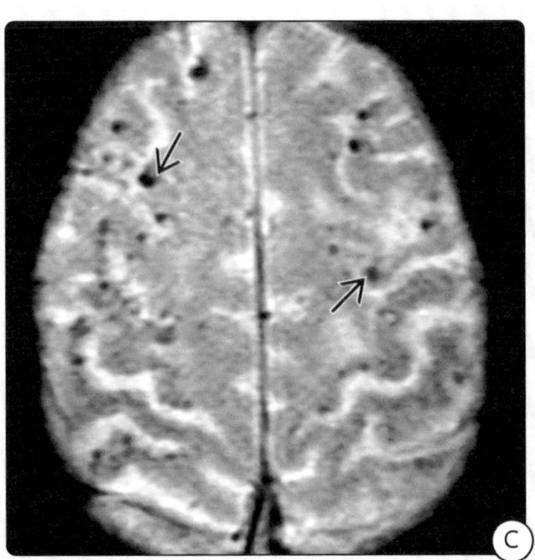

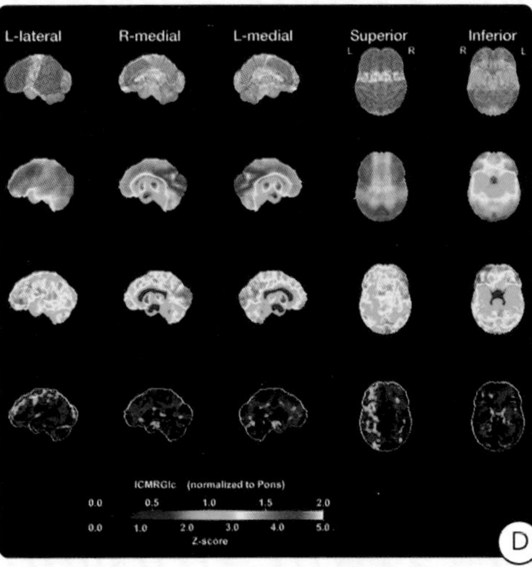


***(38-13C)** T2* GRE MR in the same patient shows multifocal cortical "blooming" hypointensities → related to hemosiderin deposition, characteristic of cerebral amyloid angiopathy. **(38-13D)** PET scan in the same patient shows multifocal areas of ↓ glucose metabolism (3rd row) compared with age-matched normal controls (2nd row). Z-score map (bottom row) shows the diffuse nature of the lesions seen in VaD. (Courtesy N. Foster, MD.)*

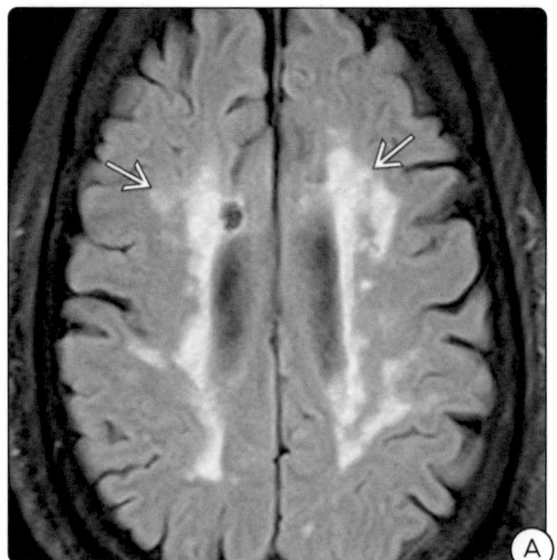

***(38-14A)** Axial FLAIR MR in a 64-year-old man with a history of multiple strokes shows volume loss and confluent subcortical WMHs ➡.*

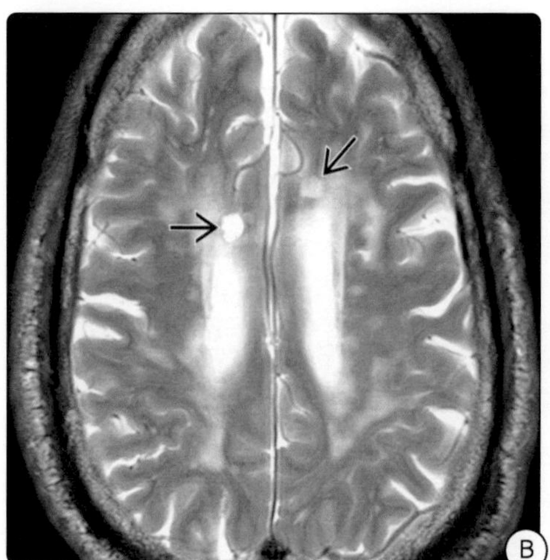

***(38-14B)** Axial T2 in the same patient shows the chronic WM disease and chronic lacunar infarcts ➡.*

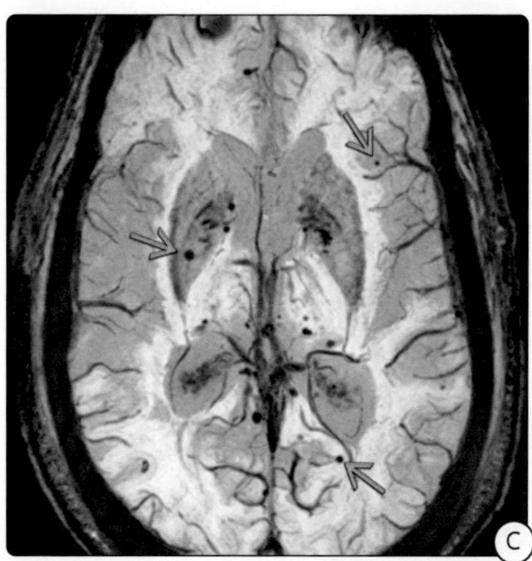

***(38-14C)** Axial SWI in the same patient shows multiple foci of "blooming" related to hemosiderin deposition ➡. VaD.*

T2/FLAIR scans show multifocal diffuse and confluent hyperintensities in the basal ganglia and cerebral WM. The cortex and subcortical WM are commonly affected **(38-13)** **(38-14)**. T2* sequences may demonstrate multiple "blooming" hypointensities in the cortex and along the pial surface of the hemispheres **(38-13C)** **(38-14C)**.

**Nuclear Medicine.** FDG PET shows multiple diffusely distributed areas of hypometabolism, generally without specific lobar predominance **(38-13D)**.

## Differential Diagnosis

The major differential diagnosis of VaD is **AD**. The two disorders overlap and often coexist. AD typically shows striking and selective volume loss in the temporal lobes, especially the hippocampi. The basal ganglia are typically spared in AD, whereas they are often affected in VaD.

**CADASIL** is the most common *inherited* cause of VaD. Onset is typically earlier than in *sporadic* VaD. Anterior temporal and external capsule lesions are highly suggestive of CADASIL.

**FTLD** is characterized by early onset of behavior changes, whereas visuospatial skills remain relatively unaffected. Frontotemporal atrophy with knife-like gyri is classic. **Dementia with Lewy bodies** may be difficult to distinguish from VaD without biopsy. FDG PET shows hypometabolism of the entire brain, especially the visual cortex. **Cerebral amyloid angiopathy** commonly coexists with both AD and VaD and may be indistinguishable without biopsy. It is characterized by multiple microhemorrhages on T2*/GRE/SWI.

### VASCULAR DEMENTIA: IMAGING AND DIFFERENTIAL DIAGNOSIS

**Imaging**
- General features
  - Multifocal infarcts (lacunae, cortical > large territorial)
  - White matter ischemia (patchy &/or confluent T2/FLAIR hyperintensities)
  - T2* "blooming black dots" (amyloid or hypertension)

**Differential Diagnosis**
- AD
- CADASIL (most common *inherited* vascular dementia)
- FTLD
- Lewy body disease
- Cerebral amyloid angiopathy

# Frontotemporal Lobar Degeneration

## Terminology

FTLD is a clinically, pathologically, and genetically heterogeneous group of disorders—sometimes called frontotemporal dementias (FTDs)—that principally affect the frontal and temporal lobes. The FTLD spectrum also includes PD with dementia and amyotrophic lateral sclerosis (ALS).

## Etiology

**Genetics.** Mutations in three major genes, *MAPT*, *GRN*, and *C9orf72*, account for most cases of FTLD. Tau protein is the product of *MAPT*, and abnormal tau accumulation in neurons &/or glia is known as Pick bodies.

## Pathology

**Gross Pathology.** FTLDs are characterized by severe frontotemporal atrophy with neuronal loss, gliosis, and spongiosis of the superficial cortical layers **(38-15)**. The affected gyri are thinned and narrowed, causing the typical appearance of knife-like gyri **(38-16)**. The posterior brain regions, especially the occipital poles, are relatively spared until very late in the disease process **(38-16)**.

**Microscopic Features.** The three principal FTLD histologies are characterized by neuronal accumulations of aggregated proteins. They are (1) tau, (2) TDP-43, and (3) FUS proteins. Intraneuronal tau occurs as either Pick bodies or NFT-like structures.

## Clinical Issues

**Epidemiology and Demographics.** FTLD is the second most common cause of "presenile dementia," accounting for 20% of all cases in patients under the age of 65 years. FTLD is the third most common overall cause of dementia (after AD and VaD), constituting 10-25% of all dementia cases. Average age at disease onset is typically around 60 years, younger than seen in AD and other neurodegenerative disorders.

**Presentation.** Three different classic *clinical* subtypes of FTLD are recognized. The most common is **behavioral variant FTD (bvFTD)**, which accounts for > 1/2 of all cases. bvFTD shows progressive behavior and cognition deterioration.

**Primary progressive aphasia** (PPA) syndromes are divided into three separate syndromes. The second, less common syndrome after bvFTD is **semantic variant PPA (sv-PPA)**, previously known as semantic dementia. sv-PPA dementia presents with impaired single-word comprehension and object naming with preserved fluency, repetition, and grammar. It is associated with left frontotemporal dysfunction. The third clinical syndrome is termed **progressive nonfluent/agrammatic variant (nfv-PPA)**, formerly known as progressive nonfluent aphasia. Patients with nfv-PPA present with impaired complex sentence comprehension but preserved single-word comprehension. It is associated with frontotemporal dysfunction. Lastly, there is a controversial **logopenic variant (lv-PPA)** dementia that presents with impaired word finding and repetition with errors in speech and naming. This variant is more often classified as an atypical variant of AD.

Recently, there has been a shift to include a category of FTD with motor symptoms. Within this category, the following degenerations are included: CBD, progressive supranuclear palsy (PSP), FTD with motor neuron disease, and ALS. However, these entities are discussed later in the chapter.

## Imaging

**General Features.** Neuroimaging features of the FTDs should be assessed according to whether they produce focal temporal or extratemporal (e.g., frontal) atrophy, whether the pattern is relatively symmetric or strongly asymmetric, and which side (left vs. right) is most severely affected. FTLD is characterized by frontal and temporal lobe atrophy that occurs with relative preservation of posterior areas, which is the imaging hallmark of the disease group. Occasionally, focal atrophy manifests with a knife edge appearance due to the marked brain volume loss **(38-17)**.

**CT Findings.** Abnormalities on CT represent late-stage FTLD. Severe symmetric atrophy of the frontal lobes with lesser volume loss in the temporal lobes is the most common finding.

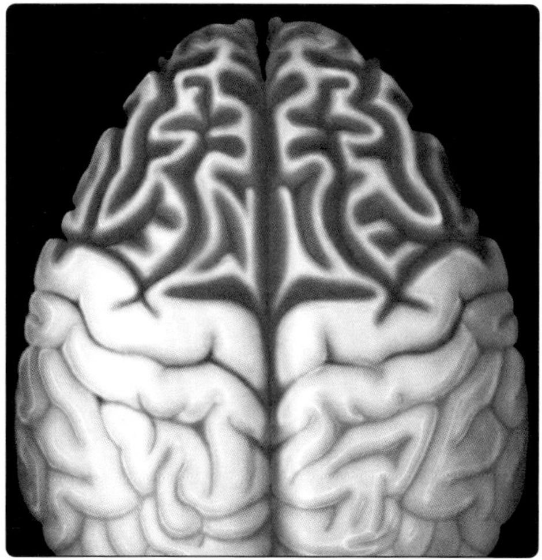

***(38-15)** Graphic shows frontal atrophy in late-stage FTLD with knife-like gyri. Parietooccipital lobes are spared.*

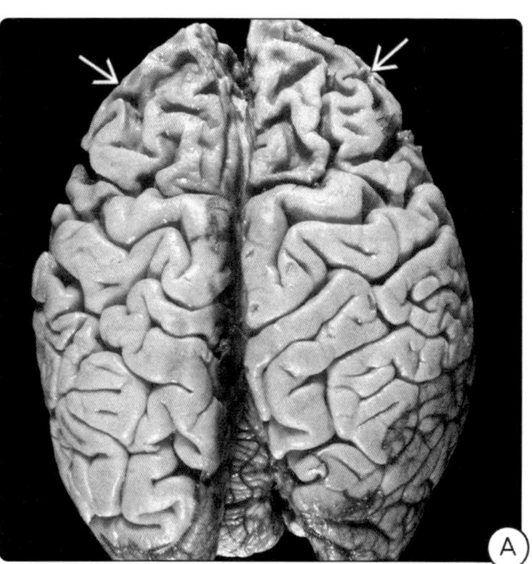


***(38-16A)** Autopsy of FTLD shows striking atrophy of the frontal gyri ➡ and normal-appearing parietal and occipital lobes.*

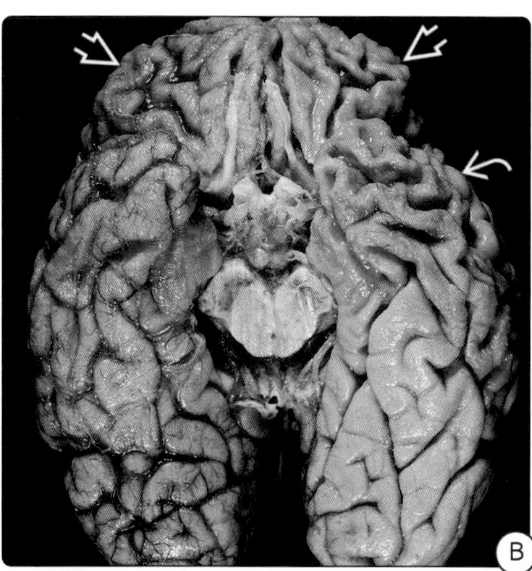


***(38-16B)** Submentovertex view in the same case shows striking frontal ➡ and temporal lobe atrophy ➡. (Courtesy R. Hewlett, MD.)*

**MR Findings.** Whereas standard T1 scans may show generalized frontotemporal volume loss, voxel-based morphometry can discriminate between various *pathologic* subtypes. For example, FTLD-tau is associated with strongly asymmetric atrophy involving the temporal &/or extratemporal (i.e., frontal) regions. FTLD is characterized by frontal and temporal lobe atrophy that occurs with relative preservation of posterior areas, which is the imaging hallmark of the disease group.

*Clinical* FTLD subtypes also correlate with frontal vs. temporal and left vs. right atrophy predominance. The **bvFTD** is characterized by atrophy of the frontal and temporal lobes with involvement of the anterior insula, anterior cingulate, orbitofrontal cortex, and amygdala **(38-17)**. Early changes often affect the right hemisphere. The **sv-PPA** typically shows left anterior temporal lobe atrophy, though may show the entire temporal lobe involved **(38-19)**. sv-PPA may also involve the frontal lobes. Involvement of the bilateral temporal lobes may be seen as the disease progresses **(38-18)**. **nfv-PPA** demonstrates bilateral frontal and temporal volume loss, but the left hemisphere is most affected in nfv-PPA. With lv-PPA, there is predominant atrophy of the left posterior temporal cortex and parietal lobe.

Newer MR imaging techniques with DTI show DTI tract differences between bvFTD and the PPAs. The bvFTD shows abnormalities in the uncinate fasciculus, genu, and cingulum. The PPA have abnormalities in the longitudinal fasciculus.

**Nuclear Medicine Findings.** F-18 FDG PET scans show hypoperfusion and glucose hypometabolism in the frontal and temporal lobes **(38-20)**. Initially, the hypometabolism is within the frontal lobes with progression to include regions of temporal and parietal lobes. The anterior cingulate cortex, frontal insula, caudate nuclei, thalamus may also have hypometabolism bilaterally. There is relative sparing of the motor cortex. Hemispheric metabolic asymmetry may be present in a similar pattern to the MR findings of each type of

*(38-17A) Axial FLAIR MR in a 67-year-old man with severe dementia shows prominent frontal ➡ and temporal lobe ↪ atrophy with knife-like gyri. (38-17B) Axial T2 MR in the same patient shows frontal ➡ and temporal lobe ↪ atrophy with enlarged frontal horns. FDG PET showed ↓ metabolism in the same regions. bvFTD was ultimately diagnosed. Right hemisphere involvement may be seen early in the disease.*

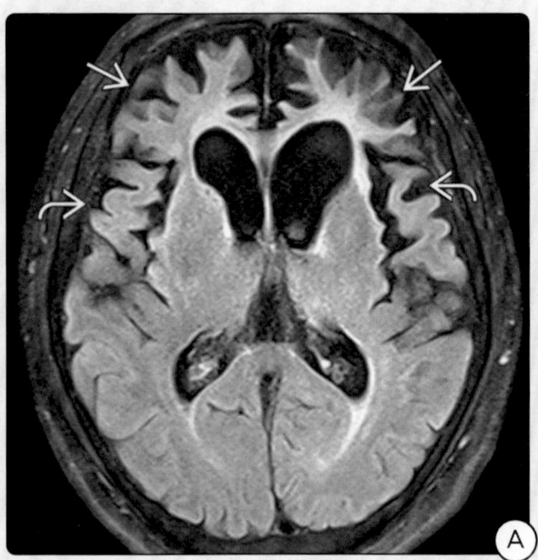

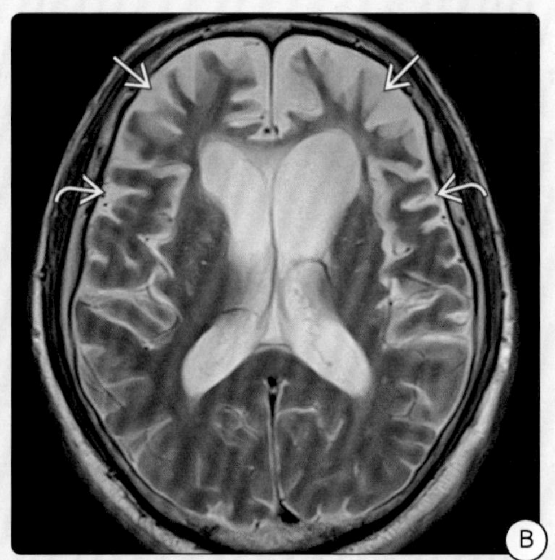

*(38-17C) Axial FLAIR MR in the same patient shows the severe atrophy in the inferior frontal lobes ➡ and anterior temporal lobes with prominent sylvian fissures ↪. (38-18) T2 MR shows symmetric temporal lobe atrophy, knife-like gyri ➡, and large temporal horns ↪ with normal occipital lobes ➡. sv-PPA FTLD. Left hemisphere involvement is typical of sv-PPA.*

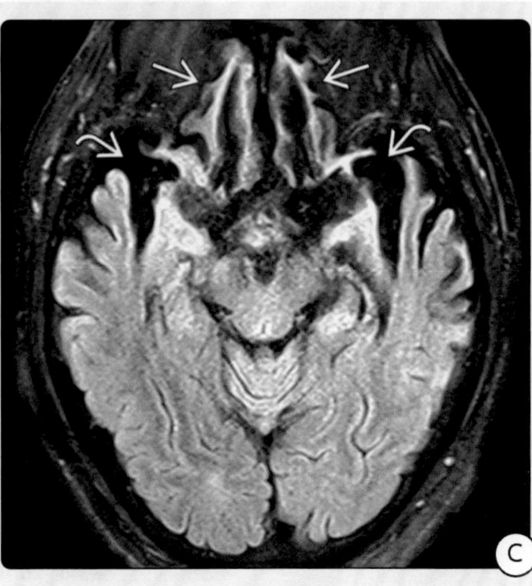

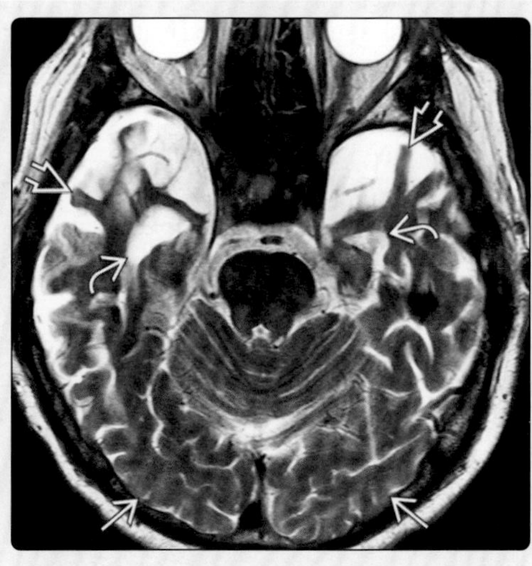

FTD. This hypometabolism typically occurs before atrophy is visualized on CT or MR.

**Differential Diagnosis.** The major differential diagnoses of FTLD are AD and VaD. **AD** shows atrophy of the parietal and temporal lobes and hippocampi more than frontal lobe. Early F-18 FDG hypometabolism in the parietotemporal and posterior cingulate cortices and positivity on amyloid PET helps make the AD diagnosis. **VaD** is characterized by global atrophy with diffuse WM lesions related to infarcts and chronic microvascular ischemia. Deep gray nuclei lacunar infarcts are also typical.

**FRONTOTEMPORAL LOBAR DEGENERATION**

**Pathology**
- 3 major types
  - FTLD-tau (45%)
  - FTLD-TDP (50%)
  - FTLD-FUS (5%)

**Clinical Issues**
- 2nd most common cause of "presenile" dementia
- Accounts for 20% of all cases < 65 years of age
- 3 major subtypes
  - **Behavioral variant frontotemporal dementia**
  - **Semantic variant primary progressive aphasia**, previously semantic dementia
  - **Nonfluent/agrammatic variant primary progressive aphasia**, previously progressive nonfluent aphasia

**Imaging**
- Classify atrophy (volumetric MR best)
  - Temporal vs. extratemporal (frontal) predominance
  - Symmetric or asymmetric
- F-18 FDG PET
  - Frontotemporal hypometabolism
  - Hypometabolism often occurs before atrophy on CT/MR

**Differential Diagnosis**
- AD (parietal, temporal > frontotemporal)
- VaD
  - Multifocal infarcts
  - White matter ischemic changes

## Miscellaneous Dementias

### Creutzfeldt-Jakob Disease

Transmissible spongiform encephalopathies (TSEs), a.k.a. **prion diseases**, are a group of neurodegenerative disorders that includes **Creutzfeldt-Jakob disease** (CJD). Animal TSEs include bovine spongiform encephalopathy ("mad cow" disease).

CJD is the most common human TSE and has a worldwide distribution. CJD is unique, as it is both an infectious and neurogenetic dementing disorder. CJD is the archetypal human TSE.

**Etiology.** CJD is a rapidly progressive neurodegenerative disorder caused by an abnormal, misfolded prion protein, PrP(Sc). The abnormal form propagates itself by recruiting its normal isoform and imposing its conformation on the homologous host cell protein. *The conformational conversion of PrP(C) to PrP(Sc) is the fundamental event underlying all prion diseases.*

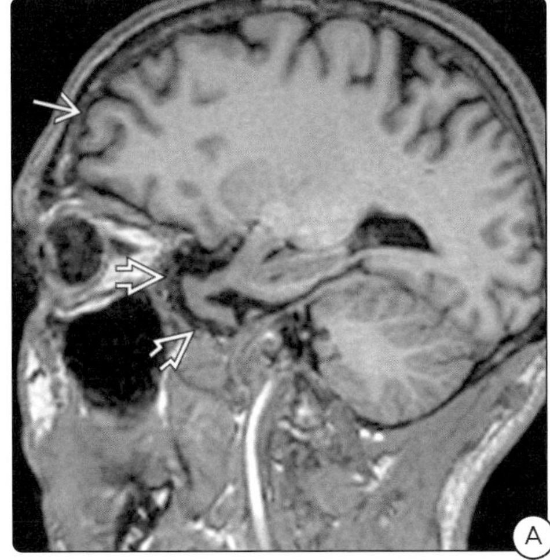


***(38-19A)** Sagittal T1 MR in a 55-year-old with dementia shows temporal lobe volume loss ➡ with well-preserved frontal gyri ➡.*

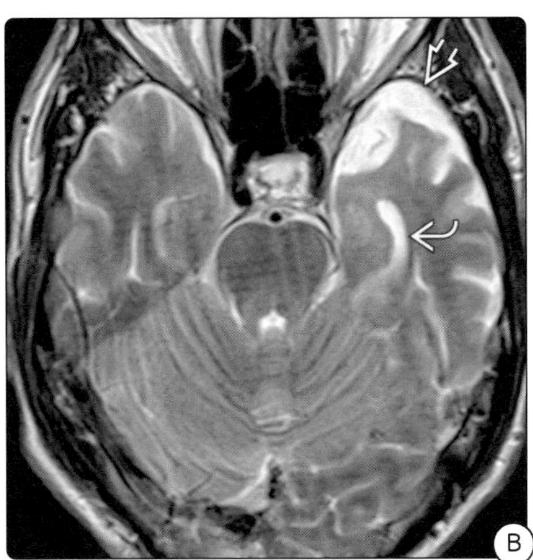


***(38-19B)** Axial T2 MR in same patient shows left temporal lobe atrophy ➡, large temporal horn ➡. sv-PPA subtype FTLD.*

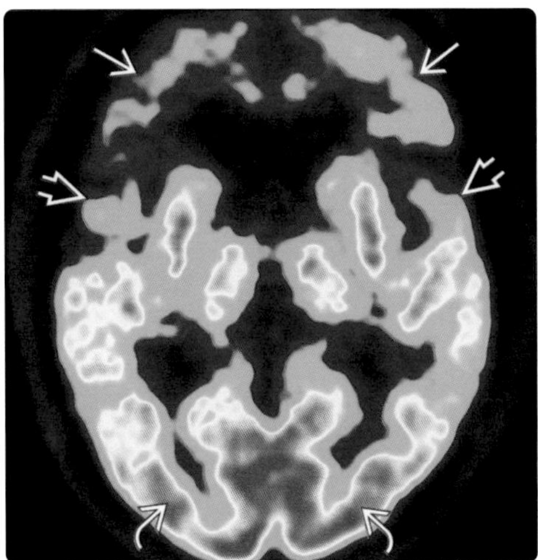

***(38-20)** FDG PET in FTLD shows severe frontal ➡, moderate temporal lobe ➡ hypometabolism. Both occipital lobes appear normal ➡.*

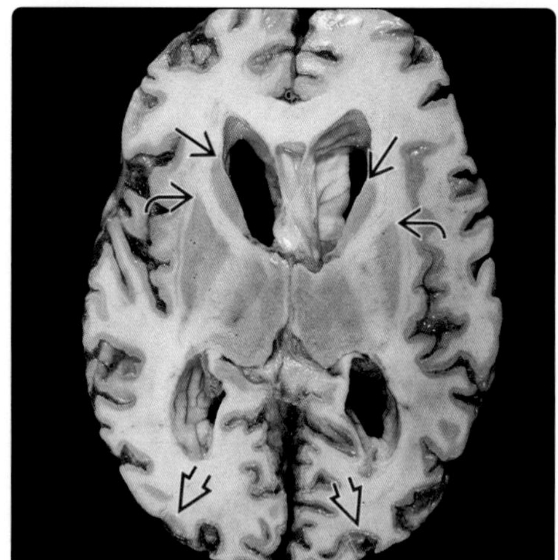

*(38-21) sCJD shows caudate ⇒, anterior basal ganglia atrophy ⇒, cortical thinning, especially in occipital lobes ⇒. (Courtesy R. Hewlett, MD.)*

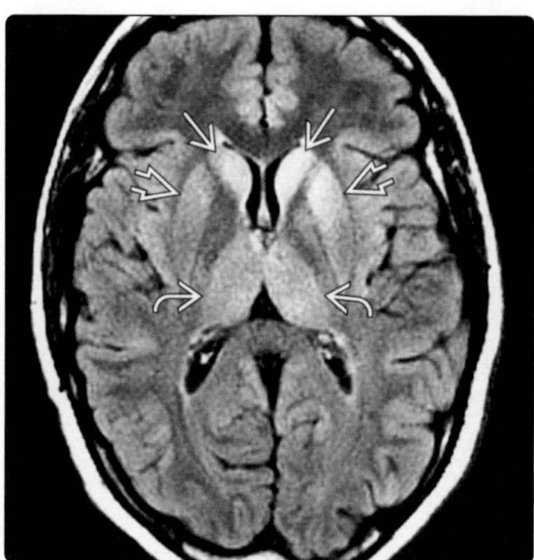

*(38-22) Axial FLAIR MR shows classic findings of sCJD with hyperintense caudate nuclei ⇒, anterior putamina ⇒, and thalami ⇒.*

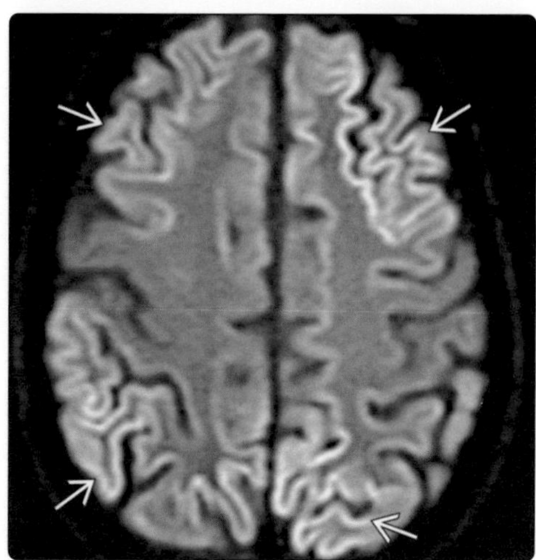

*(38-23) Axial FLAIR MR in a patient with rapidly progressive dementia shows hyperintensity in the bilaterally cortex ⇒. This is sCJD.*

Four types of CJD are recognized: **Sporadic** (sCJD), **familial** or **genetic** (gCJD), **iatrogenic** (iCJD), and **variant** (vCJD). sCJD is the most common type. gCJD is caused by diverse mutations in the *PRNP* gene. iCJD is caused by prion-contaminated materials (e.g., surgical instruments, dura mater grafts). vCJD typically results from the transmission of bovine spongiform encephalopathy from cattle to humans.

**Pathology.** Gross pathology shows ventricular enlargement, caudate atrophy, and variable cortex volume loss **(38-21)** with relative sparing of the WM. The classic triad of histopathologic findings is marked neuronal loss, spongiform change, and striking astrogliosis. PrP(Sc) immunoreactivity is the gold standard for the neuropathologic diagnosis of human prion diseases.

### HUMAN PRION DISEASES

**Sporadic (Idiopathic) Prion Diseases (85%)**
- Sporadic Creutzfeldt-Jakob disease (sCJD)
- Sporadic fatal insomnia, variably protease-sensitive prionopathy

**Acquired (Infectious) Prion Diseases (2-5%)**
- Iatrogenic Creutzfeldt-Jakob disease (iCJD) (due to medical interventions)
- Kuru
- Variant Creutzfeldt-Jakob disease (vCJD)

**Familial (Inherited/Genetic) Prion Diseases (5-15%)**
- iCJD
- Gerstmann-Sträussler-Scheinker syndrome
- Fatal familial insomnia

**Epidemiology and Demographics.** CJD now accounts for > 90% of all human prion diseases. Approximately 85% of CJD cases are sporadic (sCJD). Peak age of onset is 55-75 years. gCJD causes most of the remaining cases (5-15%). vCJD and iCJD are now rare.

**Clinical Issues.** CJD is a progressive, fatal illness. Over 90% of patients progress from normal function to death in under a year. Median survival is ~ 4 months, although vCJD progresses more slowly.

Several clinicopathologic subtypes of sCJD have been identified. In the most common subtype, rapidly worsening dementia is followed by myoclonic jerks and akinetic mutism. In 2/3 of sCJD cases, EEG shows a characteristic pattern of periodic bi- or triphasic complexes. The **Heidenhain variant** occurs as pure visual impairment leading to cortical blindness.

**Imaging.** CJD primarily involves the gray matter structures of the brain. MR with DWI is the imaging procedure of choice. T1 scans are often normal but may show faint hyperintensities in the posterior thalami **(38-25)**. FLAIR hyperintensity or restricted diffusion in the caudate nucleus and putamen or in at least two cortical regions (temporal-parietal-occipital "cortical ribboning") are considered highly sensitive and specific (96% and 93%, respectively) for the diagnosis of sCJD **(38-22)** **(38-23)**. Occipital lobe involvement predominates in the Heidenhain variant.

T2/FLAIR hyperintensity in the posterior thalamus (pulvinar sign) or posteromedial thalamus (hockey stick sign) is seen in 90% of vCJD cases but can also occur in sCJD **(38-24)**. CJD does not enhance on T1 C+.

**Differential Diagnosis.** CJD must be distinguished from other causes of rapidly progressive dementia, such as **viral encephalitis, paraneoplastic limbic encephalitis**, and **autoimmune-mediated inflammatory disorders**, such as LGI1, NMDAR, or GABA encephalopathies. These CJD "mimics" can usually be excluded with appropriate serologic examination.

Other dementias, such as **AD** and **FTLD**, are more insidiously progressive. The basal ganglia involvement in CJD is a helpful differentiating feature. Unlike most dementing diseases, CJD also shows striking diffusion restriction.

**CREUTZFELDT-JAKOB DISEASE**

**Pathology and Etiology**

- Most common human transmissible spongiform encephalopathy
- Creutzfeldt-Jakob disease (CJD) is prion disease
  - Proteinaceous particles without DNA, RNA ("prions")
  - Misfolded isoform PrP(Sc) of normal host PrP(C)
  - Propagated by conformational conversion of PrP(C) to PrP(Sc)
- 4 CJD types recognized
  - sCJD (85%)
  - Genetic/familial CJD (gCJD) (5-15%)
  - iCJD (2-5%)
  - vCJD ("mad cow" disease) (< 1%)

**Clinical Issues**

- Peak age = 55-75 years
- Rapidly progressive dementia, death in sCJD within 4 months

**Imaging**

- T2/FLAIR hyperintensity
  - Basal ganglia, thalami, cortex
  - Pulvinar sign: Posterior thalami
  - Hockey stick sign: Posteromedial thalami
  - Occipital cortex in Heidenhain variant
- Restricted diffusion

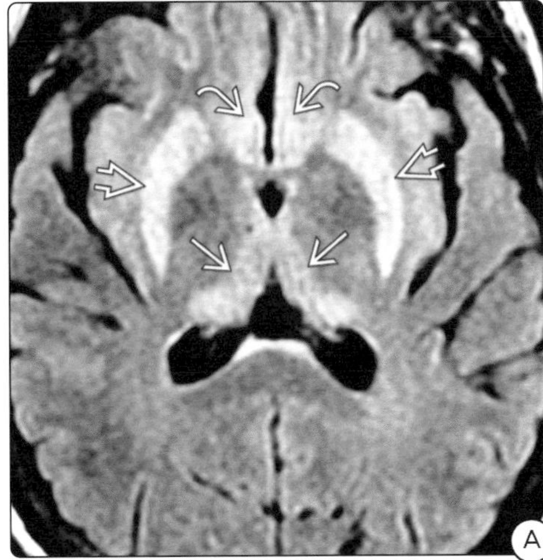

***(38-24A)** FLAIR in sCJD shows the classic hockey stick sign in thalami ➡. Anterior caudate nuclei ➡ and both putamina ➡ are also involved.*

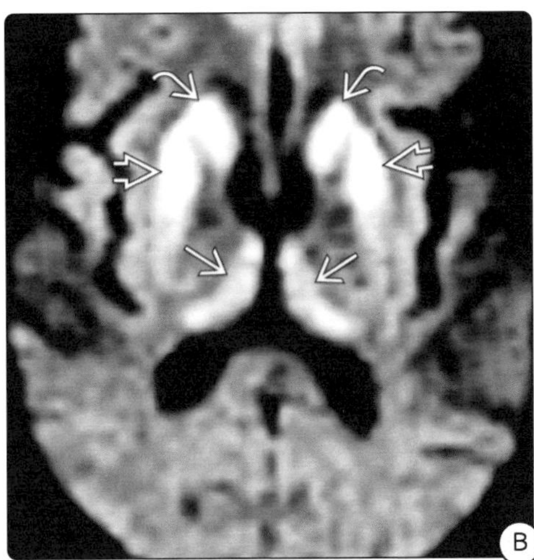

***(38-24B)** DWI MR shows corresponding strong diffusion restriction in the posteromedial thalami ➡, caudate nuclei ➡, and putamina ➡.*

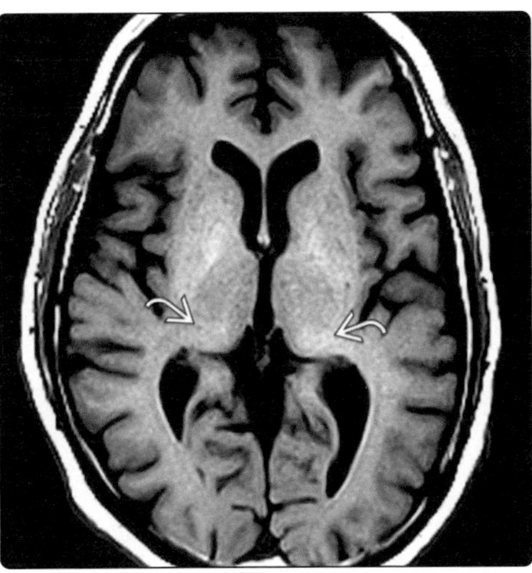

***(38-25)** Axial T1 MR in a 64-year-old man with biopsy-proven sCJD shows faint hyperintensities ➡ in the pulvinars of both thalami.*

# Degenerative Disorders

In this section, we consider a range of brain degenerations. Although some [such as Parkinson disease (PD)] can be associated with dementia, most are not. Because PD occurs more often as a movement disorder than a dementing illness, it is discussed with other degenerative diseases.

The use of deep brain stimulators (DBSs) in treating patients with disabling akinetic-rigid PD is increasingly common, so a brief review of the dopaminergic striatonigral system and its relevant anatomy will be helpful before we discuss PD.

## Parkinson Disease

### Terminology

**PD** is a neurodegenerative disorder. The constellation of resting tremor, bradykinesia, and rigidity is often termed **parkinsonism**. When PD is accompanied by dementia, it is referred to as **PD dementia** (PDD). PDD is a synucleinopathy, like Lewy body dementia.

### Etiology

Aging is the most significant known risk factor for PD. Degeneration of dopaminergic neurons in the SNPc reduces dopaminergic input to the striatum. By the time clinical symptoms develop, over 60% of dopaminergic neurons are lost and 80% of striatal dopamine is already depleted.

Between 10-20% of cases of PD are familial, but most are sporadic. The vast majority of cases are genetically complex but only 5-10% of patients have a monogenic form of PD.

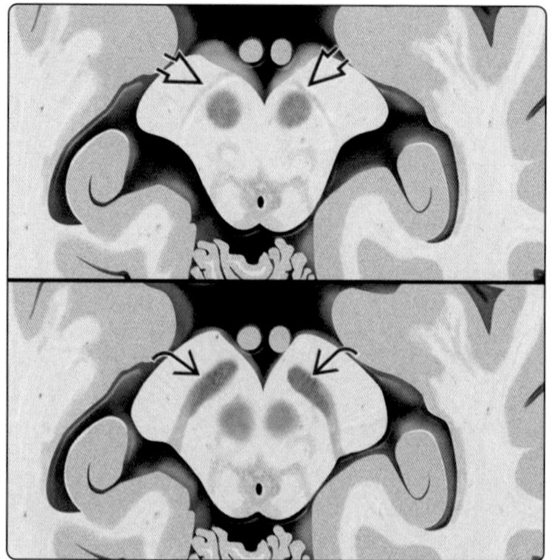

(38-26) PD midbrain atrophy, SN narrowed, depigmented ➡; pars compacta between red nuclei, SN ↓ (top). Normal STN ➡ on bottom.

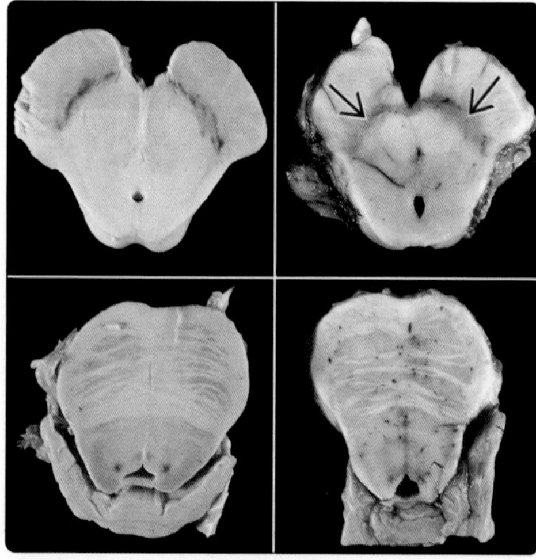

(38-27) Normal midbrain (L), PD (R). Midbrain volume loss in PD, abnormal pallor of the SN ➡. (Courtesy R. Hewlett, MD.)

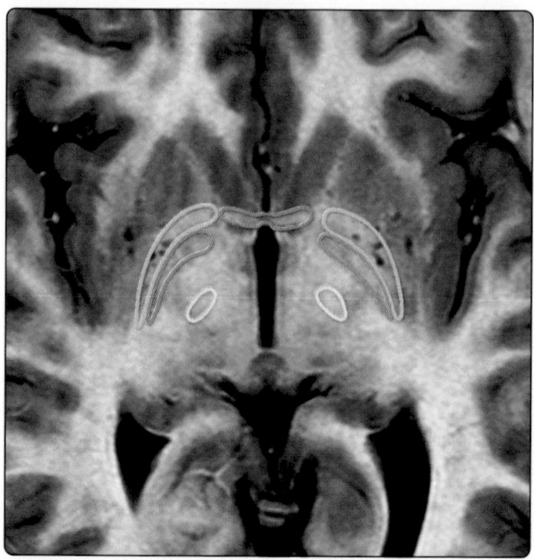

(38-28) Normal 3T T1 MR shows approximate locations of globus pallidus externa (green), interna (red), and STNs (orange).

## Pathology

**Gross Pathology.** The midbrain may appear mildly atrophic with a splayed or butterfly configuration of the cerebral peduncles **(38-27)**. Depigmentation of the substantia nigra is a common pathologic feature of PD **(38-27)**.

**Microscopic Features.** The two histopathologic hallmarks of PD are (1) severe depletion of dopaminergic neurons in the pars compacta of the substantia nigra and (2) the presence of Lewy bodies in the surviving neurons.

## Clinical Issues

**Epidemiology and Demographics.** PD is both the most common movement disorder and the most common of the Lewy body diseases. Peak age at onset is 60 years. PD typically follows a slowly progressive course with an overall mean duration of 13 years.

**Presentation.** PD diagnosis depends on a constellation of symptoms. The three cardinal clinical features of PD are (1) resting tremor, (2) rigidity, and (3) bradykinesia (slowness in executing movements). Other classic symptoms are "pill-rolling" tremor, "cogwheel" or "lead pipe" rigidity. Dementia eventually develops in 40% of PD patients.

**Treatment Options.** A number of medications are available to control PD symptoms. Levodopa was introduced > 40 years ago and remains the most efficacious treatment.

DBS has become the preferred technique for treating a gamut of advanced PD-related symptoms. As the subthalamic nucleus (STN) is often difficult to identify on standard MR, many neurosurgeons identify the red nucleus and position the DBSs slightly anterolateral to it.

High-frequency ultrasound (HIFU) is a new ablative therapy for PD and essential tremor.

## Imaging

**CT Findings.** CT is used primarily following DBS placement to evaluate electrode position and to check for surgical complications. The STN is the usual target, and electrode tips are located ~ 9 mm from the midline, just inside the upper margin of the cerebral peduncles **(38-28)**. Complications are rare and include hemorrhage and ischemia. Transient inflammation may develop, appearing within a few weeks as hypodensity around the electrodes. Changes gradually resolve.

**MR Findings.** Mild midbrain volume loss with a butterfly configuration can be seen at 1.5T in some *late*-stage cases of PD. Findings that may support the diagnosis of PD include thinning of the pars compacta (with "touching" red nuclei and "smudging" of the substantia nigra) **(38-29)** and loss of normal substantia nigra hyperintensity on T1WI.

**Nuclear Medicine.** The most sensitive imaging techniques for an *early* diagnosis of parkinsonian syndromes are SPECT and PET. DaT-SPECT is used to assess integrity of presynaptic dopaminergic nerve cells in patients with movement disorders **(38-30)**. Decreased uptake of I-123 FP-CIT is considered highly suggestive of PD **(38-31)** but is also seen in other parkinsonian degenerations.

## Differential Diagnosis

DaT-SPECT imaging enables differentiation of neurodegenerative causes of parkinsonism from other movement or tremor disorders in which the study is typically normal. When dementia is present, the major differential diagnosis of PDD is **dementia with Lewy bodies**.

### PARKINSON DISEASE

**Etiology and Pathology**
- Degeneration of dopaminergic neurons in SNPc
  - Reduced dopaminergic input to striatum
  - 60% of SNPc neurons lost
  - 80% striatal dopamine depleted before clinical Parkinson disease (PD) develops
- Substantia nigra becomes depigmented
- Pars compacta thins
- Synucleinopathy with Lewy bodies develops
  - PD is most common Lewy body disease

**Clinical Issues**
- Peak age = 60 years
- 3 cardinal features
  - Resting tremor
  - Rigidity
  - Bradykinesia

**Treatment Options**
- Medical
  - Levodopa (L-dopa), other drugs
- Surgical
  - Deep brain stimulation (DBS)
  - Electrodes implanted into subthalamic nuclei
  - Should be ≈ 9 mm from midline
  - Just inside upper margin of cerebral peduncles
  - Complications = ischemia, hemorrhage, transient inflammation around electrodes

**Imaging**
- Difficult to diagnose on standard MR
  - ± midbrain atrophy
  - ± thinned, irregular substantia nigra
  - ± "touching" substantia nigra, red nuclei
- Dopamine transporter (DaT) imaging
  - PET or SPECT can show decreased uptake

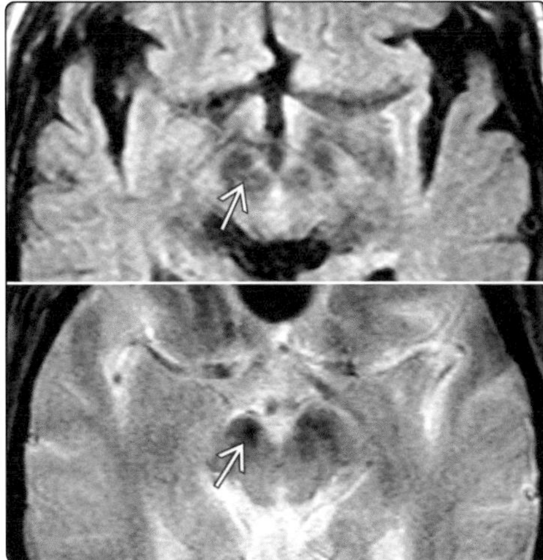

***(38-29)** FLAIR (top), T2* GRE (bottom) in PD shows mild midbrain atrophy with narrowed SNPc ➡ between SN, red nucleus.*

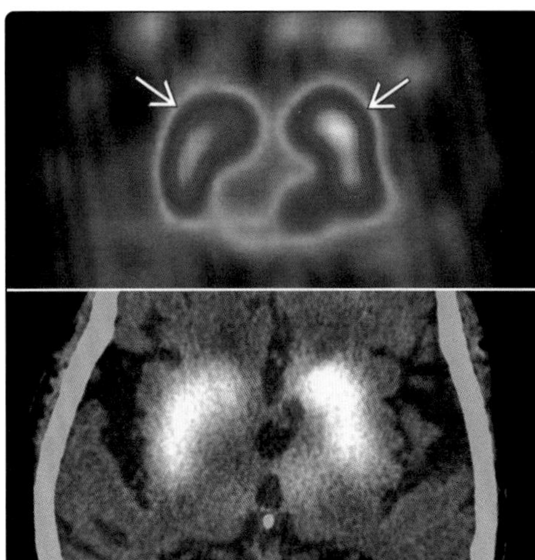

***(38-30)** Normal DaT scan (top) with double comma-shaped configuration ➡. (Bottom) Fused PET/CT is negative for PD.*

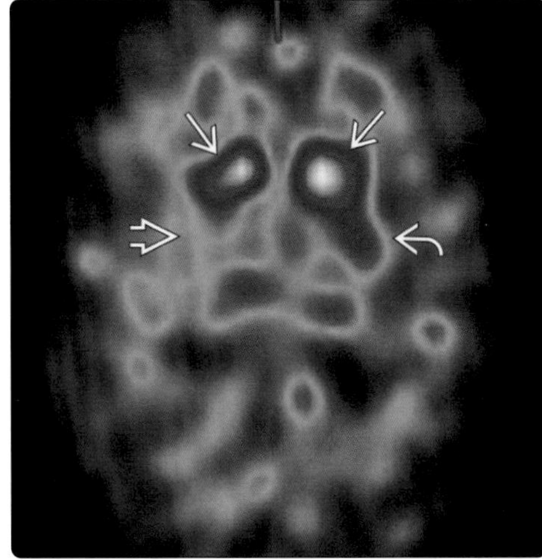

***(38-31)** DaT scan in PD shows normal caudate heads ➡, absent uptake in right putamen ➡, markedly reduced uptake in the left putamen ➡.*

## Multiple System Atrophy

### Terminology

**Multiple system atrophy** (MSA) is an adult-onset sporadic neurodegenerative disorder that is one of the more common **Parkinson-plus** syndromes. There are three MSA subtypes. When extrapyramidal (i.e., parkinsonian) symptoms predominate, the disease is designated **MSA-P**. If cerebellar symptoms, such as ataxia, predominate, the disorder is designated **MSA-C**. MSA with signs of autonomic failure **(MSA-A)** is the rarest subtype.

### Pathology

Gross pathology shows two distinct atrophy patterns. MSA-P shows depigmentation and pallor of the substantia nigra. The putamen may be atrophic and show a grayish discoloration secondary to lipofuscin pigment accumulation. In MSA-C, marked volume loss in the cerebellum, pons, middle cerebellar peduncles (MCPs), and medulla gives the pons a beaked appearance. MSA-A may demonstrate a combination of these patterns. Like PD and dementia with Lewy bodies, MSA is a synucleinopathy.

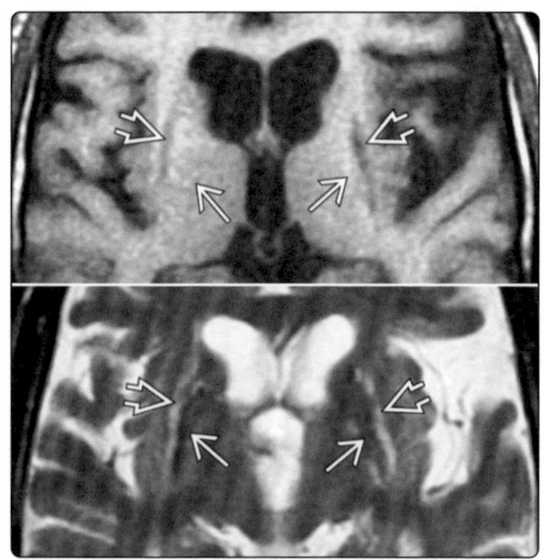

*(38-32) MSA-P shows large ventricles/sulci and thinned, atrophic putamina ➡ with an irregular lateral rim of hypo- and hyperintensity ⇨.*

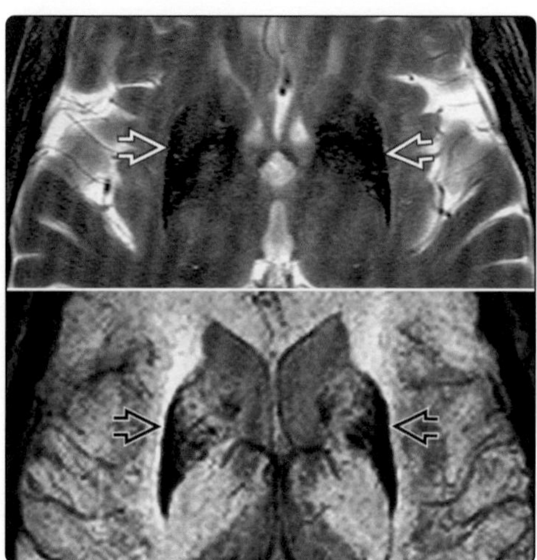

*(38-33) MSA-P shows putaminal hypointensity on T2 MR ⇨, SWI with shrunken, hypointense putamina and irregular lateral margins ⇨.*

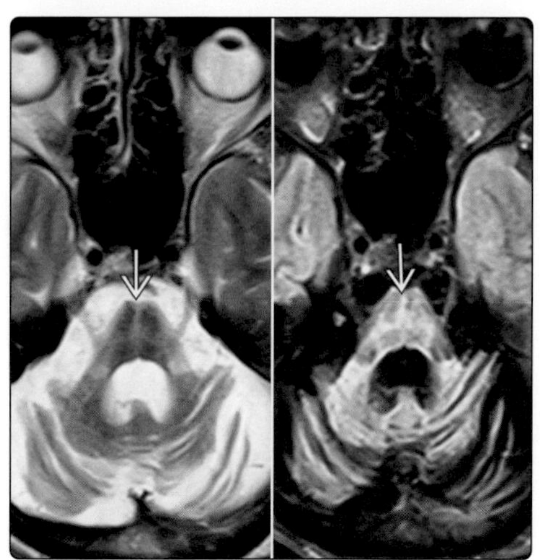

*(38-34) (L) T2 and (R) FLAIR MR in MSA-C show severe pontine, cerebellar atrophy with a distinct hyperintense hot cross bun sign ➡.*

## Clinical Issues

Mean age of onset is 58 years; mean disease duration is 5.8 years.

Parkinson-like features are present in 85-90% of all MSA patients, regardless of subtype. Nearly 2/3 of MSA cases are classified as parkinsonian type (MSA-P) and 32% as MSA-C. Less than 5% of MSA patients have MSA-A.

## Imaging

**CT Findings.** NECT scans in MSA-C show cerebellar atrophy with the hemispheres more severely affected than the vermis. A small flattened pons and an enlarged fourth ventricle are common associated findings. Cortical atrophy—especially involving the frontal and parietal lobes—may be present. Findings in MSA-P are less obvious; NECT may demonstrate shrunken putamina with flattened lateral margins.

### MR Findings

***MSA-P.*** In patients with MSA-P, the putamina appear small and hypointense on T2WI and often have a somewhat irregular high signal intensity rim along their lateral borders on 1.5T scans (**hyperintense putaminal rim** sign) **(38-32)**. This finding is nonspecific, as it can be seen in some cases of CBD as well as in > 1/3 of normal patients.

T2* (GRE, SWI) scans show significantly higher iron deposition in the putamen compared with both age-matched controls and patients with PD **(38-33)**. DTI shows decreased fractional anisotropy (FA) in the pons and MCP.

***MSA-C.*** T1 scans in MSA-C show a shrunken pons and medulla, symmetric cerebellar atrophy, small concave-appearing MCPs, and an enlarged fourth ventricle.

T2/FLAIR scans demonstrate a cruciform hyperintensity in the pons termed the **hot cross bun** sign **(38-34)**. The hot cross bun sign results from selective loss of myelinated transverse pontocerebellar fibers and neurons in the pontine raphe.

**Nuclear Medicine.** DaT scans are usually normal in MSA.

## Differential Diagnosis

The major differential diagnosis of MSA is **PD**. Clinical findings often overlap. Imaging shows that the width of the MCPs is diminished in MSA-C but not PD. Putaminal iron deposition appears earlier and is more prominent in MSA-P compared with PD. DTI also shows decreased FA in the middle cerebral peduncles in MSA-P.

# Progressive Supranuclear Palsy

## Terminology

Progressive supranuclear palsy (PSP) is a neurodegenerative disease characterized by supranuclear gaze palsy, postural instability, and mild dementia.

## Etiology and Pathology

PSP is a **tauopathy**. PSP shares many clinical, pathologic, and genetic features with other tau-related diseases, such as tau-positive FTLD.

The major gross pathologic findings are substantia nigra depigmentation and midbrain atrophy. Variable atrophy of the pallidum, thalamus, and STN together with mild symmetric frontal volume loss may also be present **(38-35) (38-36)**.

## Clinical Issues

PSP is the second most common form of parkinsonism (after idiopathic PD) and is the most common of the so-called Parkinson-plus syndromes.

PSP symptom onset is insidious, typically beginning in the sixth or seventh decade. Peak onset is 63 years, and no cases have been reported in patients under the age of 40 years.

## Imaging

**CT Findings.** NECT scans show variable midbrain volume loss with prominent interpeduncular and ambient cisterns. Mild to moderate ventricular enlargement is common.

**MR Findings.** Sagittal T1- and T2-weighted images show midbrain atrophy with a concave upper surface (the **penguin** or **hummingbird sign**) **(38-37)**. Axial scans show a widened interpeduncular angle and abnormal concavity of the midbrain tegmentum.

The quadrigeminal plate is often thinned, especially the superior colliculi. Cerebellar atrophy is common, and the *superior* cerebellar peduncles also frequently appear atrophic.

## Differential Diagnosis

The major differential diagnosis includes **other tauopathies**, such as some FTLD subtypes. All share common molecular mechanisms and are therefore probably part of the same disease spectrum. **AD, PD**, and **MSA-P** usually do not exhibit severe atrophy of the superior colliculi that is seen with PSP.

# Corticobasal Degeneration

## Terminology

Corticobasal degeneration (CBD) is an uncommon sporadic neurodegenerative and dementing disorder with evolving characterization. Patients typically present with cognitive dysfunction and progressive "asymmetrical" parkinsonism.

## Pathology and Clinical Issues

CBD is characterized pathologically by cortical and striatal tau protein accumulation (tauopathy). Patients are affected between 50-70 years of age. They typically present with unilateral or asymmetrical parkinsonism, often involving the arm, dystonia, or tremors. An "alien limb" phenomenon has been reported in ~ 50% of cases.

## Imaging

Classic imaging shows severe focal asymmetric cortical atrophy with involvement of the perirolandic regions, posterior frontal and parietal cortex **(38-38)**. There is relative sparing of the temporal and occipital regions. There is often T2/FLAIR hyperintensity in the frontal &/or parietal subcortical WM. Abnormal T2 hypointensity in the putamen and globus pallidus may be present. MR voxel-based morphometry shows atrophy predominantly in the frontal lobes, basal ganglia, and midbrain.

F-18 FDG PET shows decreased uptake in the cortical and subcortical regions of the frontal, temporal, sensorimotor, and parietal association cortices, caudate, lentiform nucleus, and thalamus.

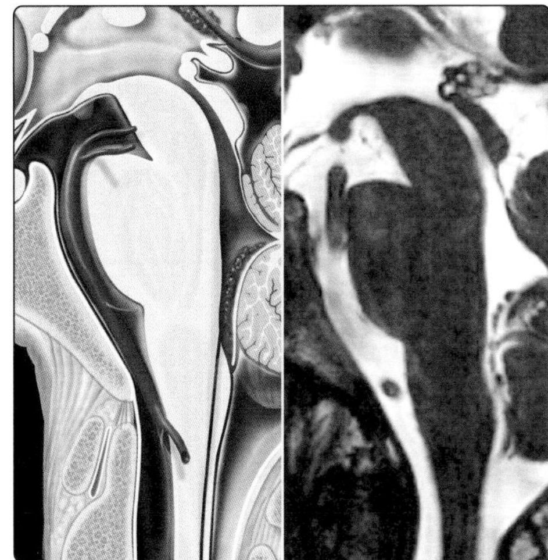

***(38-35) Sagittal graphic (L) and high-resolution T2 MR (R) together show normal midbrain and pons.***

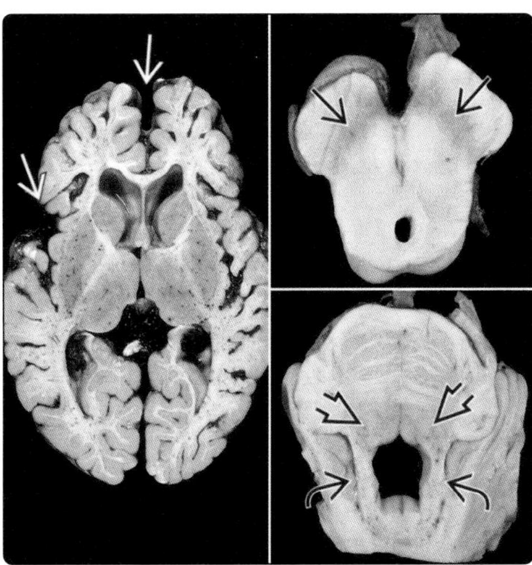

***(38-36) PSP with frontotemporal atrophy ➡, depigmented SN ⇨, locus ceruleus ⇨, small superior peduncles ⇨. (Courtesy R. Hewlett, MD.)***

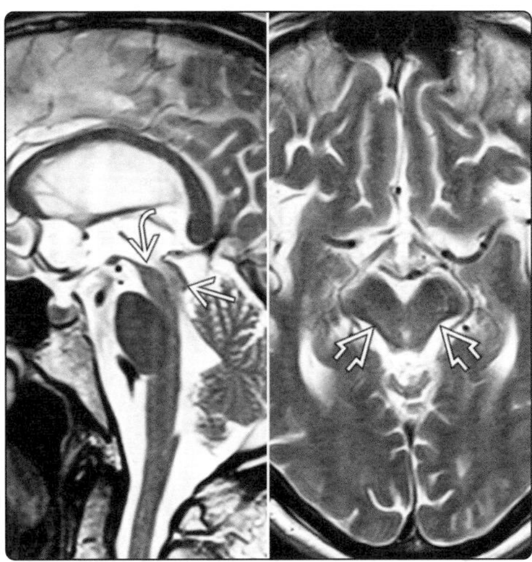

***(38-37) PSP shows small midbrain with upper concavity and penguin or hummingbird sign ➡, tectal atrophy ➡, and concave midbrain ➡.***

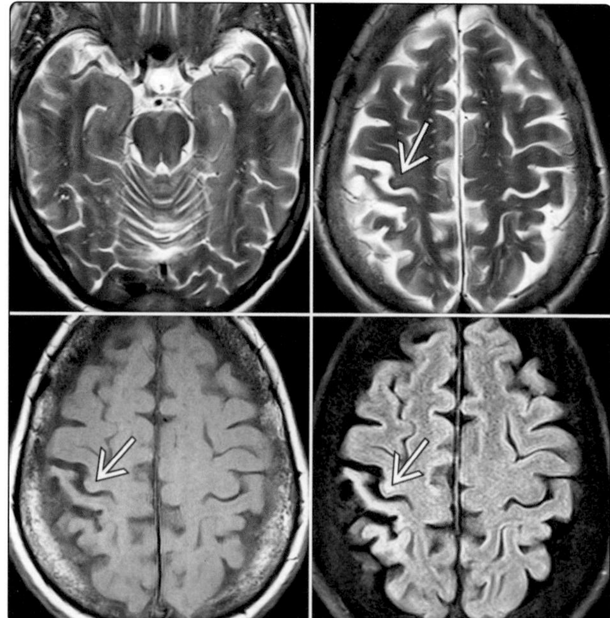

*(38-38) CBD in a 66-year-old woman with a spastic left arm shows asymmetric atrophy, thin cortex, and hyperintense WM signal in the right perirolandic region ➡. Frontoparietal atrophy is typical in CBD, contralateral to the symptomatic side.*

*(38-39) Axial T2 MR in a patient with ALS shows hyperintense signal along the corticospinal tracts ➡. ALS is a motor neuron disease that affects the upper and lower motor neurons.*

### Differential Diagnosis

The clinical differential diagnosis of corticobasal degeneration includes **PD, PSP**, and **MSA**. PD shows "blurring" and thinning of the pars compacta between two hypointense structures (pars reticulata of substantia nigra and red nucleus). As a result, the red nuclei and substantia nigra are almost touching. PSP is characterized by prominent atrophy of the midbrain ± pons (penguin silhouette sign). Other imaging differential considerations are **FTLD**, which shows frontal and anterior temporal lobe atrophy. **AD** shows parietotemporal lobe atrophy with involvement of the entorhinal cortex and hippocampus.

## Amyotrophic Lateral Sclerosis

### Etiology and Pathology

Amyotrophic lateral sclerosis (ALS), a.k.a. Lou Gehrig disease, is caused by selective degeneration of the somatic motor neurons of the brainstem, spinal cord, and large pyramidal neurons of the motor cortex. There is eventual loss of the corticospinal tract (CST) fibers.

ALS is characterized by progressive degeneration of the motor neurons in both the brain and spinal cord.

### Clinical Issues

ALS is the most common motor neuron disease, representing ~ 90% of all cases. ALS is predominantly sporadic with 5-10% of cases familial. Patients often present with upper motor neuron signs, including hypertonicity, spasticity, and hyperreflexia. Lower motor neuron signs include asymmetric muscle weakness, atrophy, fasciculations, and hyporeflexia. Median survival from diagnosis to death is 3-4 years.

### Imaging

Imaging in ALS is often normal. T2/FLAIR may show hyperintensity in the CSTs **(38-39)**. The hyperintensity can occur anywhere from the subcortical WM of the precentral gyrus to the posterior limb of the internal capsules, cerebral peduncles, and pons. Hypointense gray matter has also been described in the precentral gyrus (motor cortex).

### Differential Diagnosis

The main differential diagnosis of ALS is the **normal hyperintense signal** in compact, fully myelinated WM tracts. The CST is typically slightly hyperintense on T2 MR, especially at 3T. Other considerations include **primary lateral sclerosis**, which is an upper motor neuron disease where there are T2-hyperintense changes in the motor pathways. **Wallerian degeneration (WaD)** shows unilateral hyperintense signal along the CSTs in patients with various cortical and subcortical lesions.

## Wallerian Degeneration

### Terminology

WaD is an intrinsic anterograde degeneration of distal axons and their myelin sheaths caused by detachment from—or injury to—their proximal axons or cell bodies.

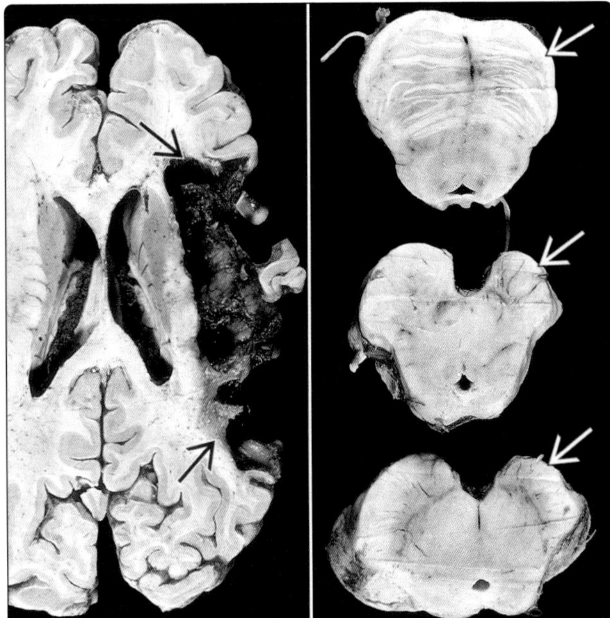

*(38-40) Autopsy specimen from a patient with chronic WaD following large left MCA infarct* ⇨ *shows volume loss in the left cerebral peduncle and upper pons* ➡. *(Courtesy R. Hewlett, MD.)*

*(38-41) NECT (upper left) and a series of T2 scans demonstrate changes of chronic WaD following major territorial infarction. Note atrophy of the left cerebral peduncle, upper pons, and midbrain* ➡.

## Etiology

In the brain, WaD most often occurs after trauma, infarction, demyelinating disease, or surgical resection. Descending WM tracts ipsilateral to the injured neurons degenerate—but not immediately. Axons may stay morphologically stable for the first 24-72 hours. The distal part of the axon then undergoes progressive fragmentation that proceeds directionally along the axon stump.

## Pathology

Virtually any WM tract or nerve in the brain, spinal cord, or peripheral nervous system can exhibit changes of WaD. The descending CST is the most common site of visible brain involvement. In chronic WaD, midbrain and pons volume loss ipsilateral to a destructive lesion (e.g., a large territorial infarct) is grossly visible **(38-40)**.

## Imaging

**CT Findings.** Chronic changes of WaD include foci of frank encephalomalacia with volume loss of the ipsilateral peduncle, rostral pons, and medullary pyramid **(38-41)**.

**MR Findings.** The development of visible WaD following stroke, trauma, or surgery is unpredictable. Fewer than 1/2 of all patients with motor deficits following acute cerebral infarction demonstrate T2/FLAIR hyperintensities or diffusion restriction in the CST that might herald WaD. Transient restricted diffusion in the CST may develop in acute ischemic stroke within 48-72 hours.

When it does develop, T2/FLAIR hyperintensity along the CST ipsilateral to the damaged cortex may occur as early as three days after major stroke onset ("pre-WaD") but more typically becomes visible between 3-4 weeks later **(38-41)**. The hyperintensity may be transient or permanent.

Other WM tracts can undergo WaD with an insult to their neuronal cell bodies. These include the corticopontocerebellar tract, dentate-rubro-olivary pathway (Guillain-Mollaret triangle), posterior column of the spinal cord, limbic circuit, and optic pathway.

## Differential Diagnosis

The major differential diagnosis of WaD is primary neurodegenerative disease. The T2/FLAIR hyperintensity sometimes seen in **ALS** is bilateral and extends from the subcortical WM adjacent to the motor cortex into the brainstem. High-grade infiltrating primary brain tumors (typically **anaplastic astrocytoma** or **glioblastoma multiforme**) infiltrate along compact WM tracts but cause expansion, not atrophy.

# Hypertrophic Olivary Degeneration

## Anatomy of the Medulla and Guillain-Mollaret Triangle

The **Guillain-Mollaret triangle** consists of the **ipsilateral inferior olivary nucleus** (ION), **contralateral dentate nucleus** (DN), and **ipsilateral red nucleus** together with their three connecting neural pathways, i.e., the **olivocerebellar tract, dentatorubral tract**, and **central tegmental tract**.

Olivocerebellar fibers from the ipsilateral ION cross the midline through the inferior cerebellar peduncle, connecting it with the contralateral DN and cerebellar cortex.

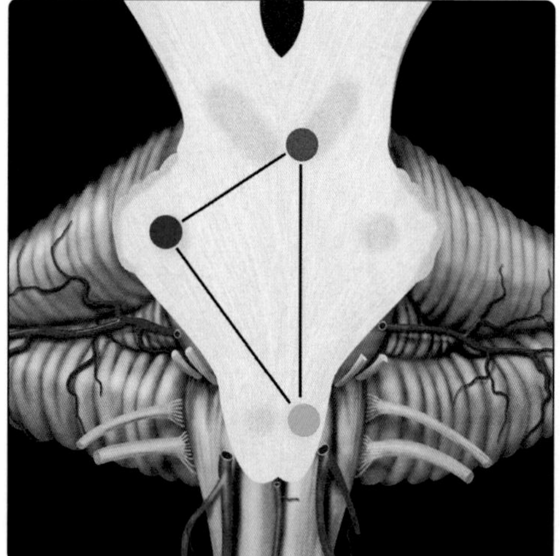

*(38-42) Guillain-Mollaret triangle = ipsilateral olivary nucleus (green), contralateral dentate nucleus (blue), ipsilateral red nucleus (red).*

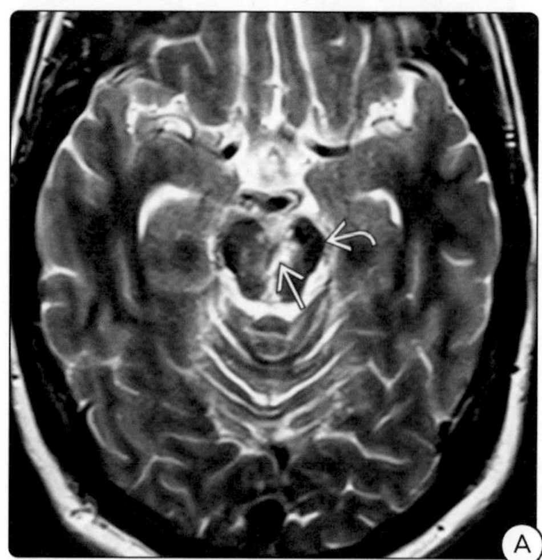

*(38-43A) T2 MR in 24-year-old man shows palatal myoclonus from remote midbrain infarct ➡. Note volume loss in the left side of midbrain ➡.*

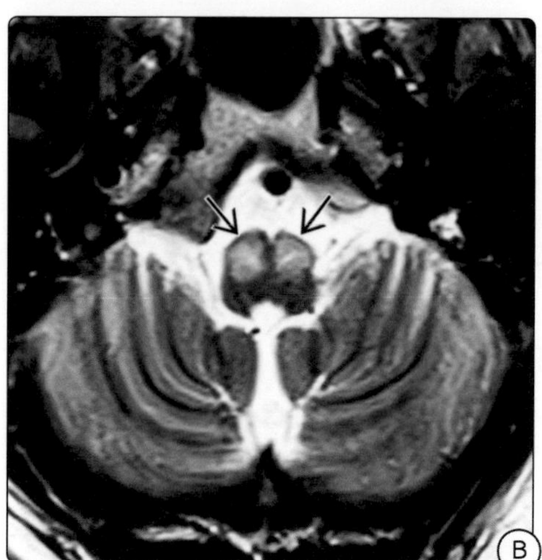

*(38-43B) T2 MR shows expansion, hyperintensity of both olives ➡. This is acute hypertrophic olivary degeneration.*

Dentatorubral fibers then enter the superior cerebellar peduncle (brachium conjunctivum) and decussate in the midbrain to connect to the opposite red nucleus. The ipsilateral central tegmental tract then descends from the red nucleus to the ipsilateral ION, completing the Guillain-Mollaret triangle **(38-42)**.

## Terminology

Hypertrophic olivary degeneration (HOD) is a transsynaptic degeneration caused by injury to the dentato-rubro-olivary pathway. Interruption of the dentato-rubro-olivary pathway at any point can cause HOD, which can be uni- (75%) or bilateral (25%).

## Etiology

Unlike other degenerations, in HOD, the degenerating structure (the olive) becomes hypertrophic rather than atrophic. Cerebellar symptoms and olivary hypertrophy typically develop many months after the inciting event.

The primary causative lesion in developing HOD is often **hemorrhage**, either from hypertension, surgery, vascular malformation, or trauma. **Pontomesencephalic stroke** also occasionally causes HOD. **Postoperative pediatric cerebellar mutism** (POPCMS) is a well-recognized complication that affects children undergoing posterior fossa brain tumor resection. Interruption of the dentato-thalamo-cortical pathway is recognized as its anatomic substrate. The proximal structures of the dentato-thalamo-cortical pathway also form a segment of the Guillain-Mollaret triangle, so bilateral HOD is common in patients with POPCMS.

## Pathology

**Location.** Three distinct patterns develop, all related to the location of the inciting lesion. In **ipsilateral HOD**, the primary lesion is limited to the central tegmental tract of the brainstem. In **contralateral HOD**, the primary lesion is located within the cerebellum (either the DN or the superior cerebellar peduncle). In **bilateral HOD**, the lesion involves both the central tegmental tract and the superior cerebellar peduncle.

**Gross Pathology.** Olivary hypertrophy is seen grossly as asymmetric enlargement of the anterior medulla. In chronic HOD, the ipsilateral ION and contralateral cerebellar cortex may be shrunken and atrophic.

**Microscopic Features.** Interruption of the Guillain-Mollaret triangle functionally deafferents the olive. The result is vacuolar cytoplasmic degeneration, neuronal enlargement, and proliferation of gemistocytic astrocytes. The enlarged neurons and proliferating astrocytes cause the initial hypertrophy. Over time, the affected olive atrophies.

## Clinical Issues

HOD is rare. It has been reported in patients of all ages, from young children to older adults. The classic clinical presentation of HOD is palatal myoclonus, typically developing 4-12 months following the brain insult.

## Imaging

The development of HOD is a delayed process. Although changes can sometimes be detected within three or four weeks after the initial insult, maximum hypertrophy occurs between 5-15 months. The hypertrophy typically resolves in 1-3 years, and the ION eventually becomes atrophic.

T1 scans are usually normal or show mild enlargement of the ION. T2/FLAIR hyperintensity without enlargement of the ION occurs in 4-6 months but may be detectable as early as three weeks after the initial insult.

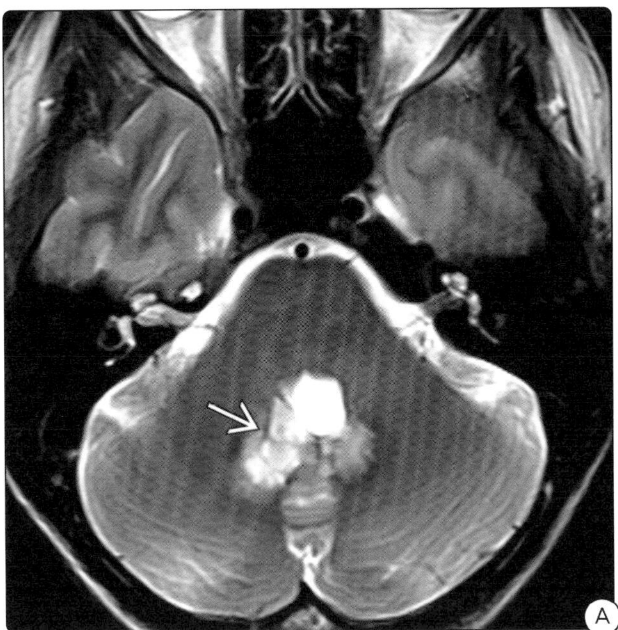

***(38-44A)** Axial T2 MR in a patient who developed palatal myoclonus 6 months after medulloblastoma resection shows surgical changes in the right dentate nucleus ➡.*

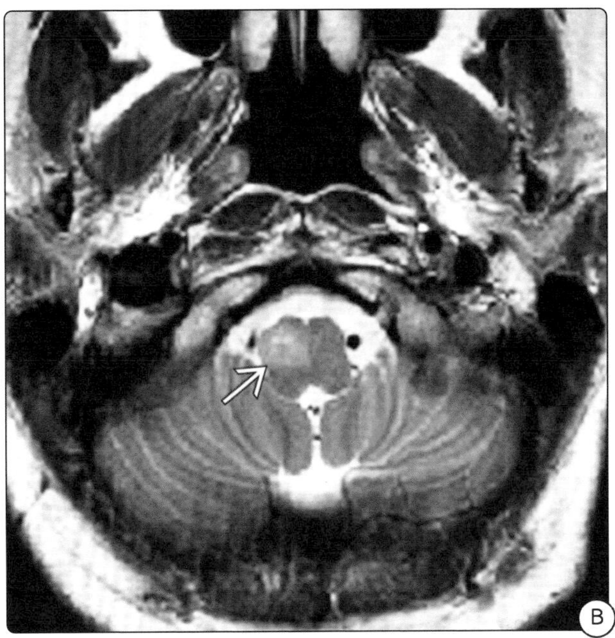

***(38-44B)** Axial T2 MR through the medulla in the same patient shows unilateral hypertrophic olivary degeneration ➡. When unilateral, hypertrophic olivary degeneration may mimic a neoplasm.*

Between six months and several years later, the ION appears both hyperintense and hypertrophied **(38-43B) (38-44)**. HOD does not enhance on T1 C+. The hypertrophy typically resolves and atrophy ensues, but the hyperintensity may persist indefinitely.

### HYPERTROPHIC OLIVARY DEGENERATION

**Etiology**

- Interruption of Guillain-Mollaret triangle

**Pathology**

- Inferior olives hypertrophy
  - Can be uni- or bilateral
  - Ipsi- or contralateral to primary lesion

**Imaging**

- Maximum hypertrophy at 5-15 months
  - Usually resolves in 1-3 years
  - Then inferior olivary nucleus (ION) atrophies
- ION T2/FLAIR hyperintensity
- Does not enhance

**Differential Diagnosis**

- Multiple sclerosis, neoplasm
- Perforating artery infarct
- Metronidazole neurotoxicity

## Differential Diagnosis

Other lesions with T2/FLAIR hyperintensity in the medulla include **demyelinating disease, neoplasm**, and **perforating artery infarction.** Most medullary infarctions occur in the posterior inferior cerebellar artery (PICA) territory and involve the posterolateral medulla, often related to a vertebral artery dissection. Alternatively, medullary infarcts are related to perforating branches of the anterior spinal or vertebral arteries and have a paramedial location. **Metronidazole neurotoxicity** exhibits bilateral, symmetric T2-/FLAIR-hyperintense lesions in the corpus callosum splenium and red nucleus as well as the caudate, lentiform, olivary, and dentate nuclei.

*Selected References: The complete reference list is available on the eBooks+ version included with purchase.*

# Hydrocephalus and CSF Disorders

*The brain CSF spaces include the ventricular system—a series of interconnected, CSF-filled cavities—and the subarachnoid space. This chapter begins with a brief discussion of the normal ventricles and CSF spaces.*

We describe normal variants, which should not be mistaken for disease, then turn our attention to hydrocephalus and the manifestations of elevated CSF pressure, including idiopathic intracranial hypertension (IIH) ("pseudotumor cerebri"). We close the chapter with a discussion of CSF leaks and intracranial hypotension.



## Normal Anatomy of Ventricles and Cisterns

### Ventricular System

The ventricular system is composed of four interconnected, ependyma-lined cavities that lie deep within the brain **(39-1)** **(39-3)**. Each lateral ventricle is C-shaped with a body, atrium, and three projections or "horns": The frontal horns, temporal horns, and occipital horns. The paired lateral ventricles communicate with the third ventricle via the Y-shaped interventricular foramen known as the foramen of Monro. The third ventricle is a single, midline cavity that lies between the thalami. The anterior commissure lies along the anterior border of the third ventricle. The floor of the third ventricle is formed by the optic chiasm, hypothalamus, mammillary bodies, and roof of the midbrain tegmentum. The third ventricle communicates with the fourth ventricle via the cerebral aqueduct (of Sylvius). In turn, the fourth ventricle communicates with the subarachnoid space (SAS).

### Choroid Plexus, CSF, and Brain Interstitial Fluid

The CSF space is a dynamic pressure system with a hydrostatic balance between CSF production and absorption. The choroid plexus (CP) has two major functions: CSF production and maintenance of the blood-CSF barrier. In adult humans, the CP epithelium forms CSF at a rate of ~ 0.4 mL per minute or ~ 500-600 mL every 24 hours. CSF is turned over about four times a day, allowing for the removal of waste products.

Brain interstitial fluid (ISF) in the extracellular spaces is also a significant extrachoroidal source of CSF.

The CP maintains the blood-CSF barrier via tight junctions between epithelial cells. The exchange of substances between the brain ISF and the CSF across

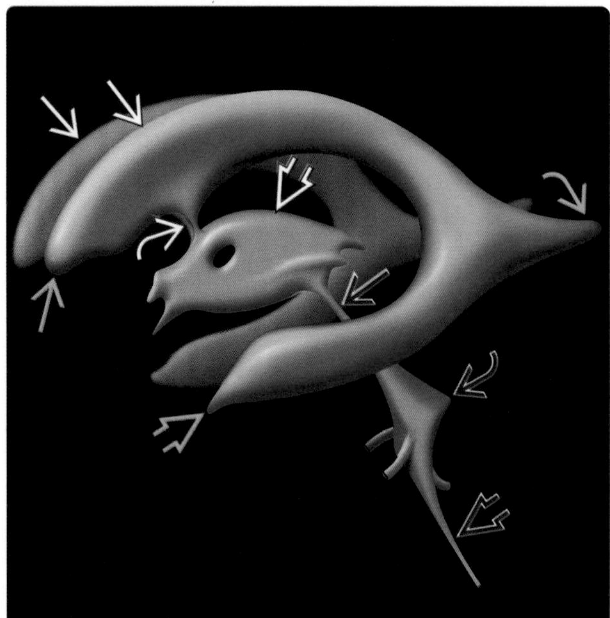

*(39-1) Graphic shows paired lateral ventricles ➡ with frontal ➡, temporal ➡, & occipital ➡ horns, foramen of Monro ➡, 3rd ventricle ➡, cerebral aqueduct ➡, & 4th ventricle ➡ with foramina of Magendie & Luschka & inferiorly directed obex ➡.*

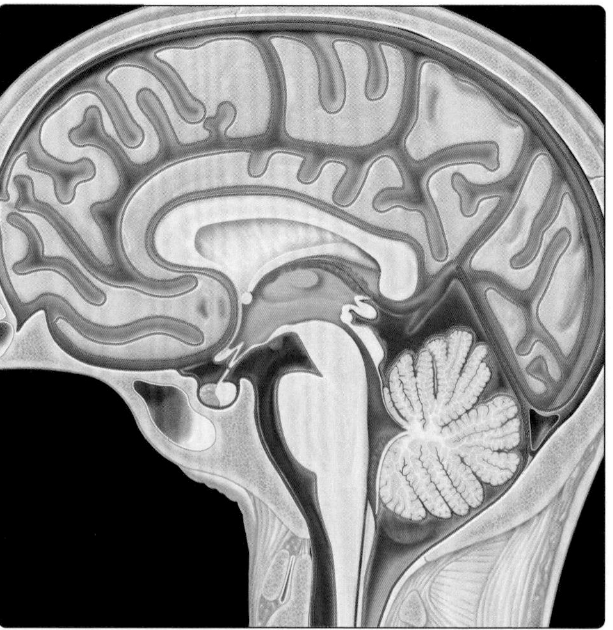

*(39-2) Sagittal graphic depicts subarachnoid spaces (SASs) with CSF (blue) between the arachnoid (purple) & pia (orange). The pia is closely adherent to the brain, while the arachnoid loosely adheres to the dura.*

the blood-CSF barrier is highly regulated. Specialized subpopulations of CP epithelial cells are responsible for the transfer of plasma proteins from blood to the CSF.

## CSF Circulation and Homeostasis

**Traditional Model of CSF Homeostasis.** The longstanding, classic model of CSF homeostasis was based on the *circulation theory*, in which the majority of CSF is produced by the CP, then circulates from the ventricles into the SASs **(39-2)** **(39-4)**. In this model, CSF flow in the ventricular cavities is unidirectional and rostrocaudal. CSF exits the fourth ventricle into the SASs through the medial foramen (of Magendie) and the two lateral foramina (of Luschka), which form the only natural communications between the ventricles and the SAS **(39-4)**.

**Updated Model of CSF and ISF Homeostasis.** New evidence suggests that the traditional model of CSF production, circulation, and function is too simplistic and much more complex than previously thought. It is now recognized that CSF plays an essential role in the maintenance of brain ISF homeostasis and that the two are intimately interrelated in maintaining normal brain function. The main sources of ISF are the blood and CSF.

In the updated CSF-ISF model, the brain perivascular spaces (PVSs) (Virchow-Robin) and paravascular spaces play a critical role in CSF homeostasis. The PVSs form a key component of the brain's "protolymphatic" or "*glymphatic*" system. The PVSs are lined with leptomeningeal (pial) cells that coat the PVSs as well as arteries and veins in the SAS, thus separating CSF in the SAS from the brain parenchyma and PVSs.

ISF diffuses through the brain's extracellular spaces and then drains via bulk flow along the basement membranes of cerebral capillaries. ISF circulation likely occurs through the water-selective aquaporin (AQP) channels of the glymphatic system, key factors in regulating extracellular space water homeostasis. AQP4 is highly expressed in astrocytic end-feet and also appears to be crucial for fluid exchange between the CSF and ISF.

Finally, in this model of CSF and ISF homeostasis, drainage of extracellular fluids in the CNS and integrity of the brain glymphatic system is important for not only volume regulation, but also clearance of waste products, such as amyloid-β (Aβ), from the brain parenchyma.

## Subarachnoid Spaces/Cisterns

The **subarachnoid spaces** (SASs) lie between the pia and arachnoid **(39-2)**. The **sulci** are small, thin SASs that are interposed between the gyral folds. Focal expansions of the SASs form the brain CSF cisterns. Numerous pial-covered septa cross the SASs from the brain to the arachnoid, which is loosely attached to the inner layer of the dura. All SASs normally communicate freely with each other and the ventricular system.

# Normal Variants

## Age-Related Changes

Increase in lateral ventricular volume is a constant, linear function of age throughout life.

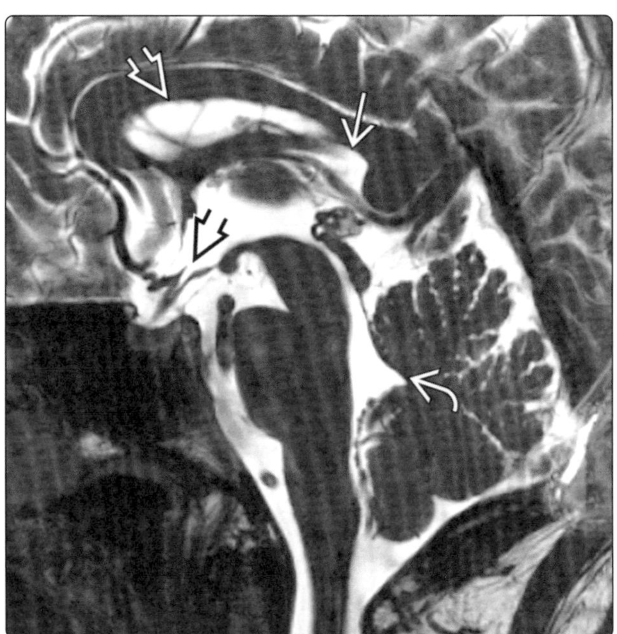

*(39-3) Sagittal T2 MR shows the lateral ventricle, velum interpositum, anterior 3rd ventricle optic & infundibular recesses, & the fastigium of the 4th ventricle. Midline sagittal sequences are helpful in evaluating hydrocephalus.*

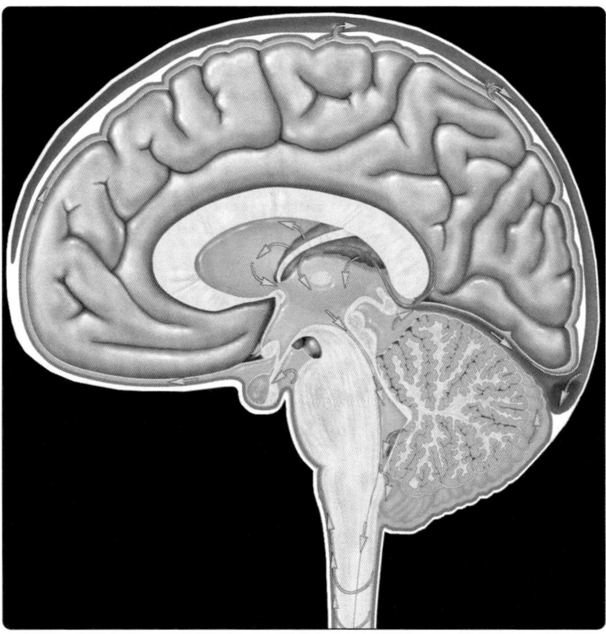

*(39-4) Classic model of CSF circulation: CSF produced by choroid plexus, flows in a unidirectional manner through the ventricles & subarachnoid cisterns & is absorbed by arachnoid granulations. New model suggests CSF-ISF homeostasis.*

## Asymmetric Lateral Ventricles

Asymmetric lateral ventricles can be identified on imaging studies in ~ 5-10% of normal patients. The asymmetry is typically mild to moderate. Bowing, deviation, or displacement of the septi pellucidi across the midline is common; by itself, it neither indicates pathology nor implicates an etiology for nonspecific headache.

## Cavum Septi Pellucidi and Vergae

A **cavum septi pellucidi** (CSP) is a fluid-filled cavity that lies between the frontal horns of the lateral ventricles **(39-5)**. A **cavum vergae** (CV) is an elongated, finger-like posterior extension from the CSP that lies between the fornices **(39-6)**.

A CSP may occur in isolation, but a CV occurs only in combination with a CSP. When the two occur together, the correct Latin terminology is "cavum septi pellucidi et vergae." In common usage, the combination is often referred to simply as a CSP.

The appearance of CSPs and CVs on CT and MR varies from an almost inapparent, slit-like cavity to a prominent collection measuring several millimeters in diameter. A CSP is isodense with CSF on NECT and follows CSF signal intensity exactly on MR. It suppresses completely on FLAIR.

## Cavum Velum Interpositum

The velum interpositum (VI) is a thin, translucent membrane formed by two infolded layers of pia-arachnoid. The VI extends laterally over the thalami to become continuous with the CP of the lateral ventricles. Together with the fornices, the VI forms the roof of the third ventricle.

The VI is often CSF filled and open posteriorly, communicating directly with the quadrigeminal cistern. In such cases, it is called a cavum velum interpositum (CVI) **(39-7)**. A CVI is considered a normal anatomic variant.

On imaging studies, a CVI appears as a triangular CSF space that curves over the thalami between the lateral ventricles. Its apex points toward the foramen of Monro **(39-8)**. A CVI is isodense with CSF on NECT and isointense on all MR sequences. It suppresses completely on FLAIR, does not enhance, and does not restrict on DWI.

## Enlarged Subarachnoid Spaces

Enlarged SASs occur in three conditions: Extraventricular obstructive ("communicating") hydrocephalus (EVOH), brain atrophy, and benign enlargement of the SASs (BESS) **(39-9)**. Obstructive hydrocephalus (both the intra- and extraventricular types) is discussed in the hydrocephalus section below. Brain volume loss is a manifestation of both normal aging and brain degeneration. In this section, we discuss benign physiologic enlargement of the SAS.

### Terminology

Idiopathic enlargement of the SASs with normal to slightly increased ventricular size is common in infants. Large CSF spaces in developmentally and neurologically normal children with or without macrocephaly is termed **BESS**.

### Etiology and Pathology

The etiology of BESS in infants is unknown but probably related to immature CSF drainage pathways. Approximately

80% of infants with BESS have a family history of macrocephaly.

Grossly, the SASs appear deep and unusually prominent but otherwise normal. There are no subdural membranes present that would suggest chronic subdural hematomas or effusions.

## Clinical Issues

BESS typically presents between 3-8 months. There is a 4:1 M:F predominance. There are no findings indicative of elevated ICP or nonaccidental trauma.

BESS is reported on 2-65% of imaging studies for macrocrania in children under one year of age. BESS is a self-limited phenomenon that typically resolves by 12-24 months without intervention. The associated macrocephaly may resolve by two years, but it often levels off, remaining at the 98th percentile.

## Imaging

Bifrontal and anterior interhemispheric SASs are > 5 mm in diameter **(39-10)**. The suprasellar/chiasmatic cistern and sylvian fissures are also prominent. The lateral and third ventricles can be mildly enlarged. CECT scans demonstrate bridging veins traversing the SAS **(39-10)**. There is **no** evidence of thickened enhancing membranes to suggest subdural hematoma or hygroma.

Fluid in the enlarged frontal SASs exactly parallels CSF on all MR sequences because it *is* CSF **(39-11)**. The fluid suppresses completely on FLAIR. Bridging veins can be seen crossing the prominent SASs on T1 C+.

## Differential Diagnosis

The major differential diagnoses of BESS are atrophy, EVOH, and nonaccidental trauma. Occasionally, infants with BESS have minor superimposed hemorrhagic subdural collections

***(39-5)** Coronal graphic with axial inset shows a classic cavum septi pellucidi (CSP) with cavum vergae (CV) ➲. The CSP appears triangular on the coronal image but finger-like on the axial view. **(39-6)** Axial T2 MR shows a CSP ➡ with CV ➲. The leaves of the septum pellucidum ➡ & bodies of the fornices ➡ are splayed apart by a contiguous CSF-containing cavity that lies between them. The CSP & CV are continuous in this normal variant.*

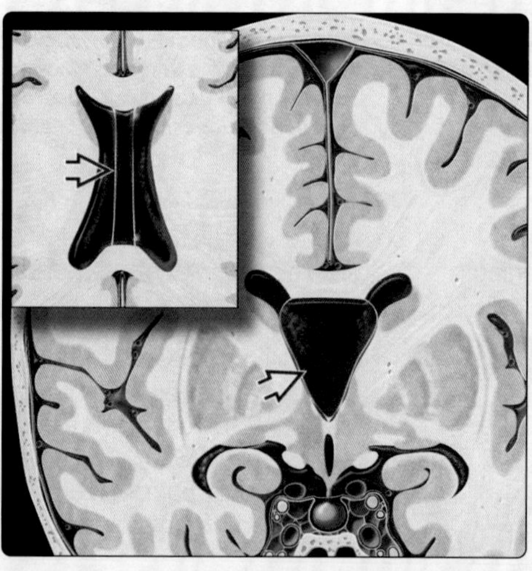

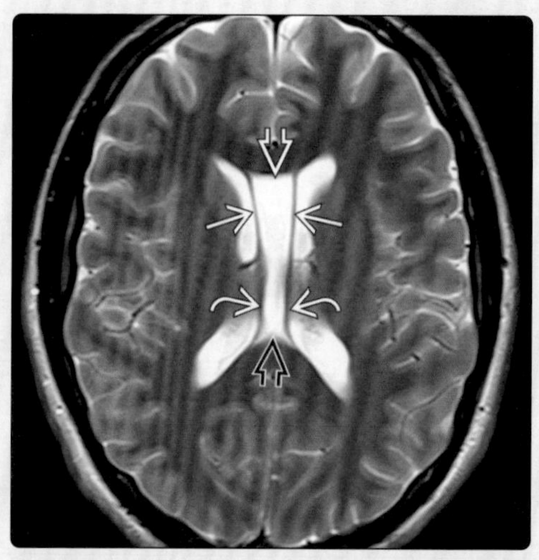

***(39-7)** Sagittal graphic with axial inset shows a cavum vellum interpositum (CVI). Note the elevation & splaying of the fornices ➡. Also noted is the inferior displacement of the internal cerebral veins & 3rd ventricle ➡. **(39-8)** On axial T2 MR, a CVI is triangular & separates the fornices ➲. On the sagittal image, CVI ➡ flattens the internal cerebral veins inferiorly ➡ but elevates & displaces the fornix superiorly ➡.*

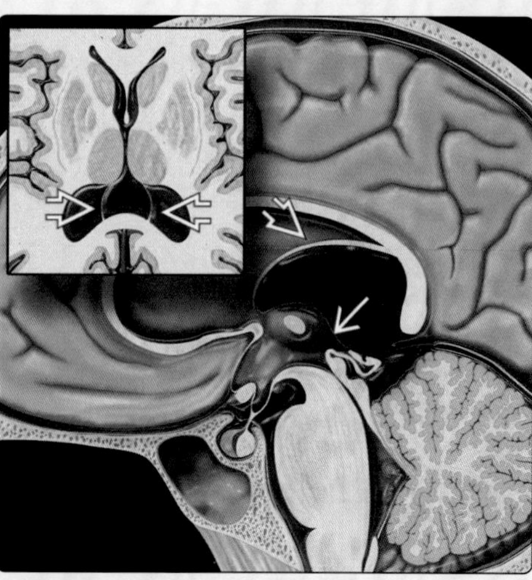

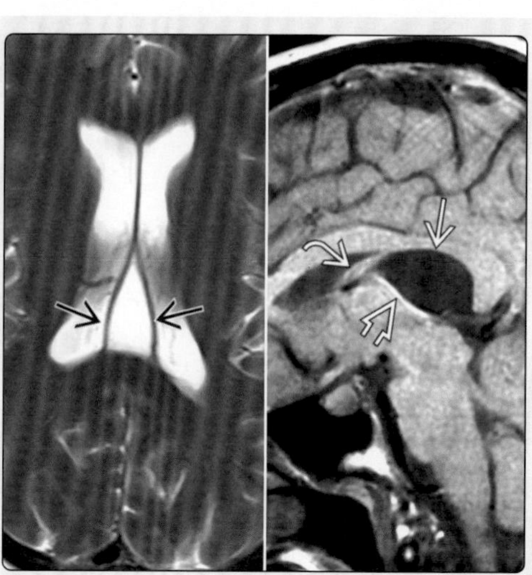

similar to those sometimes observed with arachnoid cysts. In such infants, **abusive head trauma** must be a consideration until careful screening discloses no substantiating evidence of inflicted injury.

# Hydrocephalus

The term "hydrocephalus" literally means "water head." The term "ventriculomegaly" means enlargement of the ventricular system. Remember: The terms **"hydrocephalus" and "ventriculomegaly" are descriptive findings, not a diagnosis**! The role of imaging is to **find the etiology of the ventricular enlargement**.

Hydrocephalus has traditionally been regarded as an abnormality in the formation, flow, or resorption of CSF. If normal CSF flow is impeded by a blockage within the ventricular system, CSF production continues and the ventricles enlarge. In the classic model, hydrocephalus can also result from an imbalance between CSF production and absorption. When CSF absorption through the arachnoid granulations is compromised, the ventricles enlarge and hydrocephalus results. Absorption can be blocked at any level within the subarachnoid cisterns, e.g., within the cisterna magna, at the basilar cisterns, or along the cerebral convexities.

In the newest attempt to understand the development of hydrocephalus, aquaporin (AQP)-mediated brain water homeostasis &/or clearance of both CSF and ISF into the PVSs and blood are compromised. The molecular mechanisms that drive AQP4 modifications in hydrocephalus that fail to facilitate removal of excess water are still relatively unknown.

## Terminology

We follow the common approach of subclassifying hydrocephalus by the *presumed* site of CSF obstruction, i.e., inside [**intraventricular obstructive hydrocephalus** (IVOH)] or outside the ventricles [**extraventricular obstructive hydrocephalus** (EVOH)]. The outdated term "ex vacuo hydrocephalus," referring to ventricular and cisternal enlargement caused by parenchymal volume loss, is no longer used.

## Etiology

When abnormally large cerebral ventricles are identified on imaging studies, the diagnostic imperative is to find the cause of the hydrocephalus.

In the pediatric age group, a majority of cases are caused by congenital defects of the CSF pathway or as a complication of hemorrhage, infection, or neoplasms. Adult-onset hydrocephalus is usually secondary to different pathologies that encompass a heterogeneous group of disorders, such as intracranial hemorrhage (most commonly aneurysmal subarachnoid hemorrhage; ~ 45%) and neoplasms (~ 30%). Normal pressure hydrocephalus (NPH) accounts for ~ 11% of cases.

# Intraventricular Obstructive Hydrocephalus

## Terminology

IVOH is used to designate physical obstruction at, or proximal to, the fourth ventricular outlet foramina. The term "noncommunicating hydrocephalus" is no longer used.

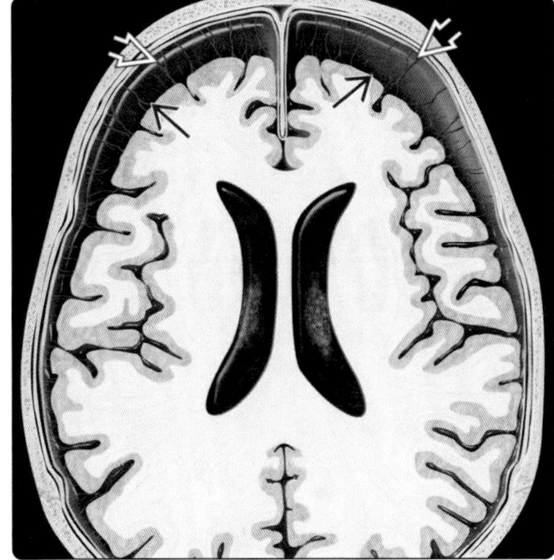

***(39-9)** Graphic depicts benign enlarged frontal SASs ⇒. Posterior SASs are normal. Note cortical veins crossing the prominent SASs ⇒.*

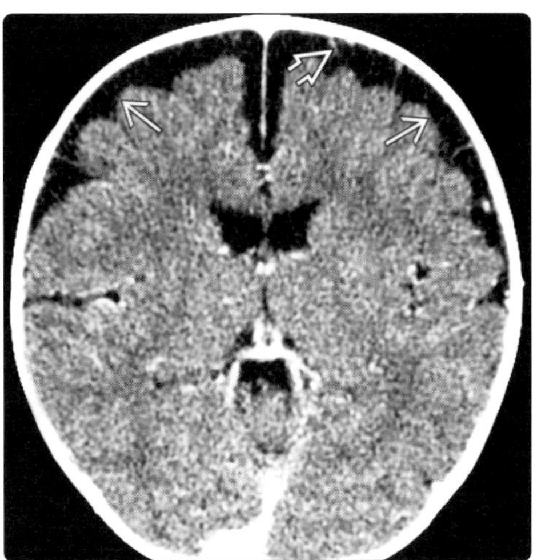

***(39-10)** CECT in a 7-month-old infant shows prominent bifrontal, interhemispheric SASs ⇒ & bridging veins ⇒.*

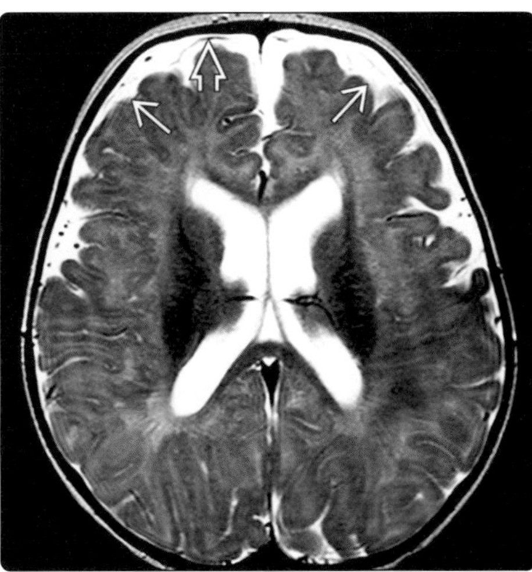

***(39-11)** Axial T2 shows prominent frontal & interhemispheric SASs ⇒ & bridging veins ⇒. Benign enlarged SASs.*

## Etiology

**General Concepts.** IVOH can be **congenital** or **acquired**, **acute** (aIVOH) or **chronic** (cIVOH). Congenital IVOH occurs with disorders like aqueductal stenosis.

When the ventricles become obstructed, CSF outflow is impeded. As CSF production continues, the ventricles expand. As the ventricles expand, increased pressure is exerted on the adjacent brain parenchyma. Increased intraparenchymal pressure compromises cerebral blood flow, reducing brain perfusion. The increased pressure also compresses the subependymal veins, which reduces absorption of brain ISF via the deep medullary veins and PVSs. The result is **periventricular interstitial edema**. Whether the edema results from CSF extruding across the ventricular ependyma **("transependymal CSF flow")** or accumulation of brain extracellular fluid is unknown.

In chronic "compensated" IVOH, the ventricles expand slowly enough that CSF homeostasis is relatively maintained. Periventricular interstitial edema is minimal or absent.

Causes of obstructive hydrocephalus include developmental/genetic lesions, intracranial hemorrhage, infection, trauma, neoplasms, and cysts. The most common cause of acquired IVOH is intraventricular inflammatory or posthemorrhagic membranous obstruction. The next most common cause of acquired IVOH is intraventricular masses. Colloid cyst is the most common mass found at the foramen of Monro **(39-12)**. These benign masses may result in aIVOH. Other masses in this location include subependymal giant cell astrocytomas in tuberous sclerosis patients. Other common neoplasms to cause obstruction at the cerebral aqueduct include tectal plate gliomas and pineal region neoplasms, such as pineal parenchymal tumors or germ cell tumors **(39-13)**. Masses that may cause obstruction at the fourth ventricle level include medulloblastoma and ependymoma in children

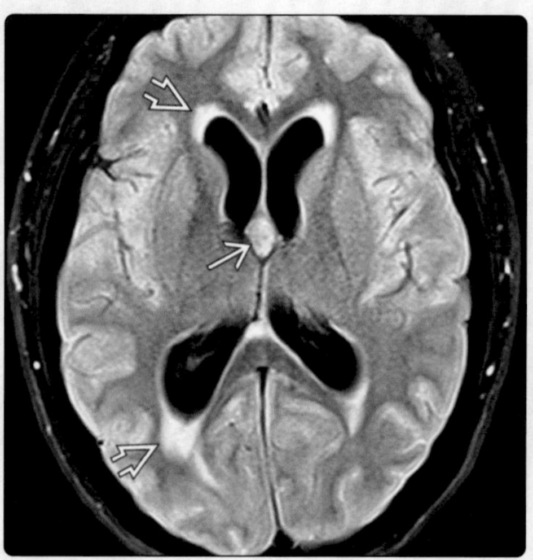

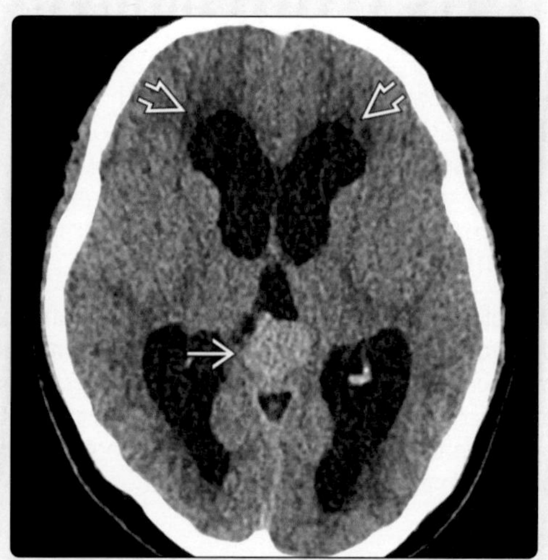

***(39-12)** Axial FLAIR MR shows a colloid cyst ➡ at the foramen of Monro with associated acute hydrocephalus. Note the classic periventricular halo ⇨ along the lateral ventricle margins related to periventricular interstitial edema. **(39-13)** Axial CT shows a hyperdense germinoma ➡ at the posterior 3rd ventricle, resulting in acute hydrocephalus. Note the classic ballooned ventricles & periventricular halo ⇨. This is IVOH.*

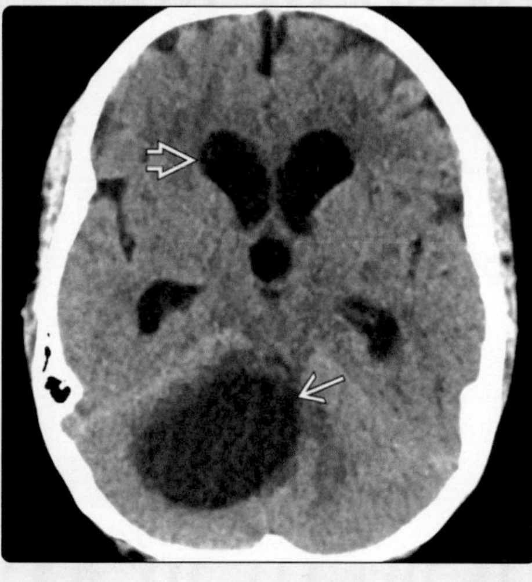

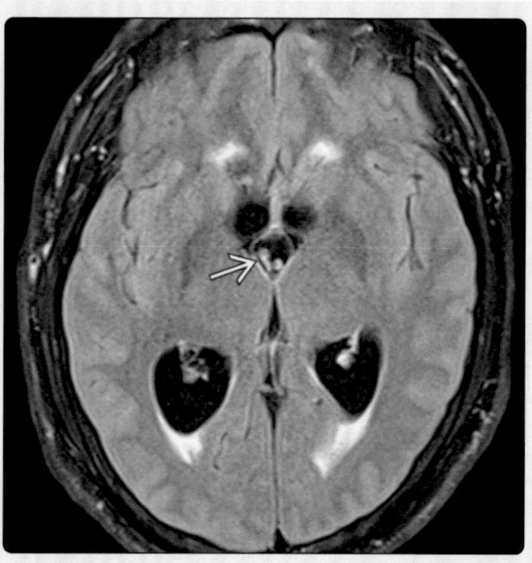

***(39-14)** Axial CT shows a cystic posterior fossa mass ➡ related to hemangioblastoma with classic ballooned ventricles ⇨. This is IVOH. **(39-15)** Axial FLAIR MR shows a cystic mass ➡ at the foramen of Monro with IVOH. Note the small nodules in the cyst related to a scolex in this patient with neurocysticercosis (NCC). Inflammatory cysts may occur anywhere in the ventricular system & at any age.*

and metastases and hemangioblastomas in adults **(39-14)**. Inflammatory cysts, including neurocysticercosis, may occur throughout the ventricular system at any age **(39-15)**.

## Pathology

Grossly, the ventricles proximal to the obstruction appear ballooned **(39-16)**. The ependyma is thinned and may be focally disrupted or even absent. The corpus callosum (CC) is thinned and compressed superiorly against the falx cerebri. The ependymal lining is discontinuous or inapparent, the periventricular extracellular space is increased, and the surrounding white matter (WM) is rarefied and stains pale.

## Clinical Issues

The presentation of IVOH varies with acuity and severity. Headache is the most common overall symptom, and papilledema is the most common sign. Nausea, vomiting, and CNVI palsy are also common with aIVOH.

Most cases are typically progressive unless treated. Untreated severe aIVOH can result in brain herniation with coma and even death. Some patients with slowly developing compensated IVOH may not present until late in adult life (e.g., the recently recognized syndrome of late-onset aqueductal stenosis).

CSF diversion (shunt, ventriculostomy, endoscopic fenestration of the third ventricle floor) is common, often performed as a first step before definitive treatment of the obstruction (e.g., removal of a colloid cyst or resection of an intraventricular neoplasm).

## Imaging

**CT Findings.** Imaging findings vary with acuity and severity. NECT scans in aIVOH demonstrate enlarged lateral and third ventricles, whereas the size of the fourth ventricle varies. The temporal horns are prominent, the frontal horns are "rounded," and the margins of the ventricles appear indistinct or "blurred." Periventricular fluid—whether from compromised drainage of ISF or transependymal CSF migration—causes a "halo" of low density in the adjacent WM. The sulci and basal cisterns appear compressed or indistinct.

**MR Findings.** Axial T1WI shows that both lateral ventricles are symmetrically enlarged. On sagittal views, the CC appears thinned and stretched superiorly **(39-18A)**, whereas the fornices and internal cerebral veins are displaced inferiorly.

In aIVOH, T2 scans may demonstrate "fingers" of CSF-like hyperintensity extending outward from the lateral ventricles into the surrounding WM **(39-17)**. Fluid in the periventricular "halo" does not suppress on FLAIR **(39-17B)**. In longstanding chronic "compensated" hydrocephalus, the ventricles appear enlarged and the WM attenuated but without a thick periventricular "halo" **(39-18)**.

**Complications of Hydrocephalus.** In severe cases of IVOH, the CC becomes compressed against the free inferior margin of the falx **(39-19)** **(39-20)**. This can cause pressure necrosis and loss of callosal axons, the so-called **CC impingement syndrome** (CCIS) **(39-26B)**. In acute CCIS, the CC may initially appear swollen and hyperintense on T2WI and FLAIR. Subacute and chronic changes are seen as encephalomalacic foci in a shrunken, atrophic-appearing CC. In 15% of treated IVOH cases, the CC shows T2/FLAIR hyperintensity after decompression. In rare cases, the hyperintensity extends beyond the CC itself into the periventricular WM **(39-21)**.

Massive ventricular enlargement may weaken the medial wall of the lateral ventricle enough that a pulsion-type diverticulum of CSF extrudes through the inferomedial wall of the atrium. Such **medial atrial diverticula** may

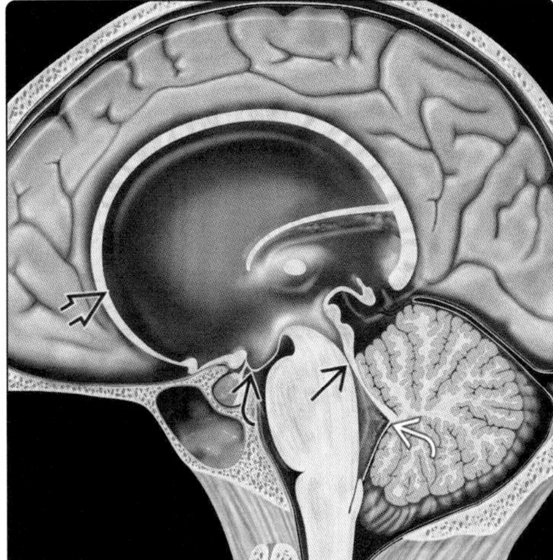

***(39-16)** Note aqueductal stenosis ➡, IVOH with enlarged lateral ➡ & 3rd ➡ ventricles, stretched CC, & normal 4th ventricle ➡.*

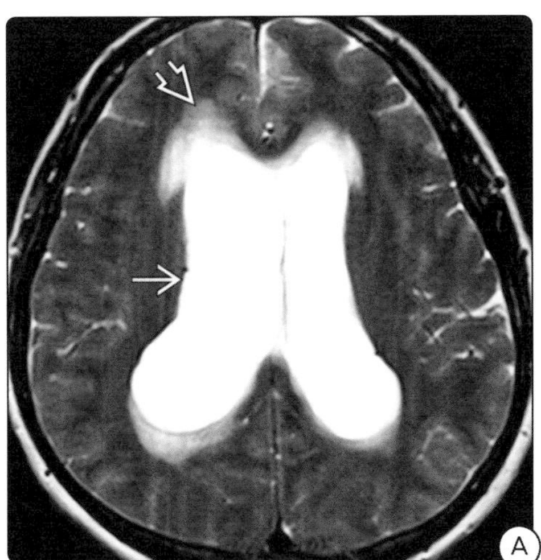


***(39-17A)** Axial T2 MR in patient with severe headaches shows large lateral ventricles ➡ with extensive periventricular fluid accumulation ➡.*

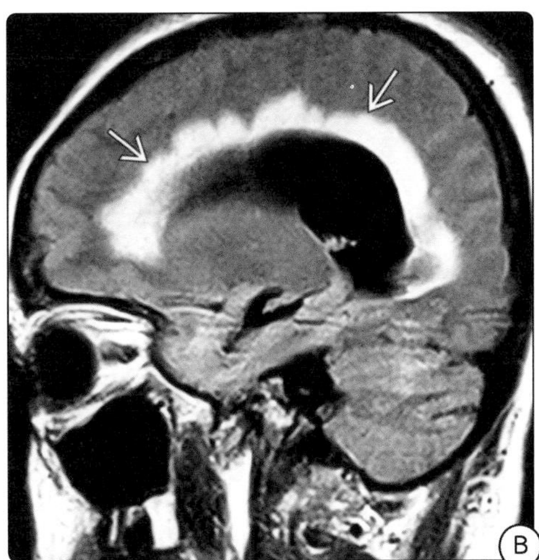


***(39-17B)** Sagittal FLAIR MR shows hyperintense "fingers" ➡ extending along the entire margin of the lateral ventricle. This is acute IVOH.*

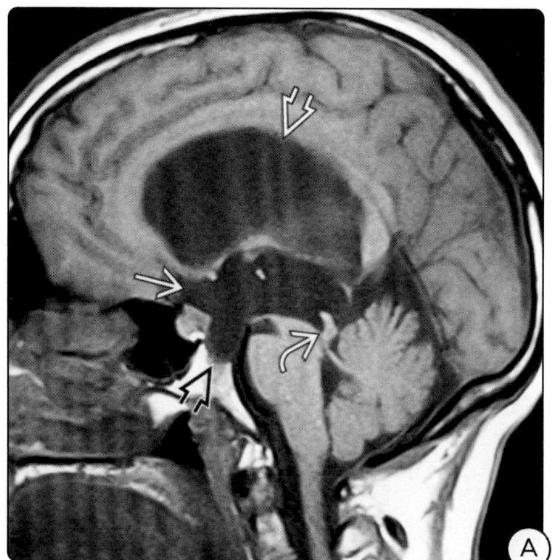

***(39-18A)** T1 MR in a 22-yo with longstanding aqueductal stenosis ➡ shows enlarged lateral ➡ & 3rd ➡ ventricles with remodeled clivus ⇨.*

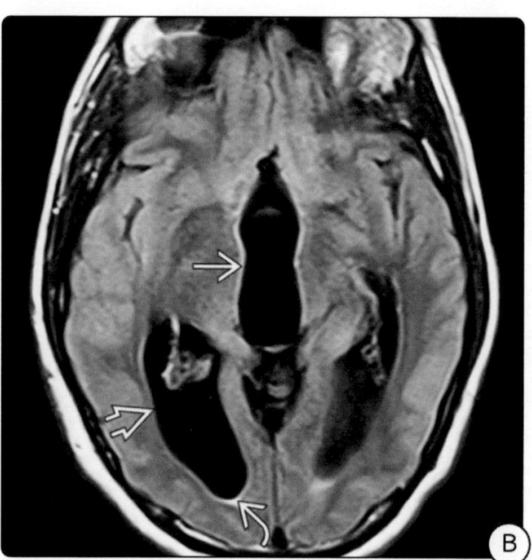

***(39-18B)** Axial FLAIR MR in the same patient shows enlarged 3rd ➡ & lateral ➡ ventricles with minimal hyperintense rim ➡.*

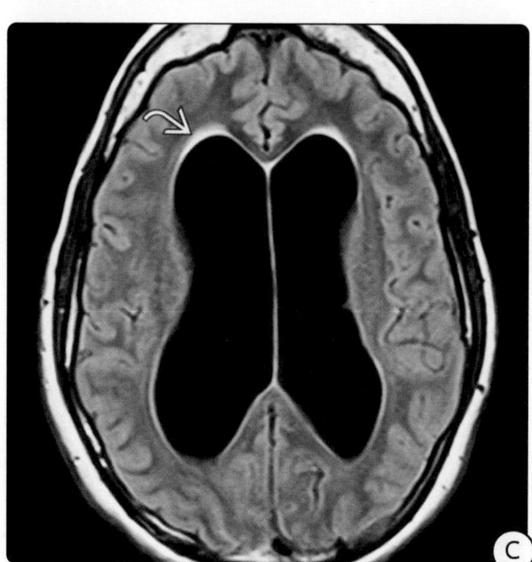

***(39-18C)** More cephalad FLAIR MR shows marked, symmetrically enlarged ventricles & thin fluid rim ➡. This is chronic compensated IVOH.*

cause significant mass effect on the posterior third ventricle, tectal plate, and aqueduct. Large atrial diverticula can herniate inferiorly through the tentorial incisura into the posterior fossa, compressing the vermis and fourth ventricle.

## Differential Diagnosis

The major differential diagnosis of IVOH is **EVOH**. **Parenchymal volume loss** causes secondary dilatation of the ventricles (ventriculomegaly) with proportional enlargement of the surface sulci and cisterns.

A helpful feature to distinguish obstructive hydrocephalus from atrophy is the appearance of the temporal horns. In obstructive hydrocephalus, they appear rounded and moderately to strikingly enlarged. Even with relatively severe volume loss, the temporal horns retain their normal kidney bean shape and are only minimally to moderately enlarged.

**NPH** is typically a disorder of older adults and is typified clinically by progressive dementia, gait disturbance, and incontinence. The ventricles often appear disproportionately enlarged relative to the sulci and cisterns.

### INTRAVENTRICULAR OBSTRUCTIVE HYDROCEPHALUS

**Terminology, Etiology**
- Proximal to 4th ventricle outlet foramina
- Can be congenital or acquired, acute or chronic
    - Post inflammation/post hemorrhage
    - Obstructing intraventricular mass

**Acute Obstructive Hydrocephalus**
- Ventricles proximal to obstruction are ballooned
- "Blurred" margins of ventricles
- Periventricular fluid accumulation (CSF, ISF, or both)
    - "Halo" ± "fingers" of fluid around ventricles
    - T2 hyperintense; does not suppress on FLAIR

**Chronic Compensated Obstructive Hydrocephalus**
- Large ventricles, no periventricular "halo"
- ± callosal impingement, atrial diverticula

# Extraventricular Obstructive Hydrocephalus

## Terminology

In EVOH, the obstruction is located *outside* the ventricular system.

## Etiology

The obstruction causing EVOH can be located at any level from the fourth ventricular outlet foramina to the arachnoid granulations. Subarachnoid hemorrhage—whether aneurysmal or traumatic—is the most frequent cause. Other common etiologies include purulent meningitis, granulomatous meningitis, and disseminated CSF metastases.

As with IVOH, the presentation of EVOH varies with acuity and severity. Headache is the most common symptom followed by signs of increased ICP, including nausea, vomiting, papilledema, and diplopia.

## EXTRAVENTRICULAR OBSTRUCTIVE HYDROCEPHALUS

**Terminology**
- Formerly called "communicating" hydrocephalus
- Obstruction outside ventricular system
  - Any site from 4th ventricle foramina to arachnoid granulations

**Etiology**
- Most common
  - Subarachnoid hemorrhage (aneurysm > trauma)
- Less common
  - Meningitis (bacterial, granulomatous)
  - Metastases

**Imaging**
- > 50% show no discernible etiology
- Use CISS to look for obstructing membranes

## Imaging

The classic appearance of EVOH on NECT scans is that of symmetric, proportionally enlarged lateral, third, and fourth ventricles. CECT scans may demonstrate enhancement in cases of EVOH secondary to infection or neoplasm.

The same imaging sequences used in IVOH apply to the evaluation of EVOH **(39-22)**. If the hydrocephalus is caused by acute subarachnoid hemorrhage or meningitis, the CSF appears "dirty" on T1WI and hyperintense on FLAIR. T1 C+ scans may demonstrate sulcal-cisternal enhancement **(39-23)**.

In contrast to IVOH, > 1/2 of EVOH cases have no discernible cause for the obstruction on standard MR sequences. In such cases, it is especially important to identify subtle, thin membranes that may be causing the extraventricular obstruction.

# Overproduction Hydrocephalus

Overproduction hydrocephalus is uncommon and results from excessive CSF formation. **CP papillomas** (CPPs) are the most common cause of overproduction hydrocephalus (see Fig. 22-8). CP carcinomas may also result in overproduction hydrocephalus. **Diffuse villous hyperplasia of the CP** (DVHCP) is a rare cause of overproduction hydrocephalus. Imaging studies in DVHCP show severe hydrocephalus with massive enlargement of the entire CP.

# Normal Pressure Hydrocephalus

There are no currently accepted evidence-based guidelines for either the diagnosis or treatment of normal pressure hydrocephalus (NPH). In this section, we briefly review the syndrome and summarize the spectrum of imaging findings that—in conjunction with clinical history and neurologic examination—may suggest the diagnosis.

## Terminology

NPH is characterized by ventriculomegaly with normal CSF pressure but altered CSF hydrodynamics. **Primary** or **idiopathic NPH** (iNPH) is distinguished from **secondary NPH** (sNPH), in which there is a known antecedent, such as subarachnoid hemorrhage, traumatic brain injury, or meningitis.

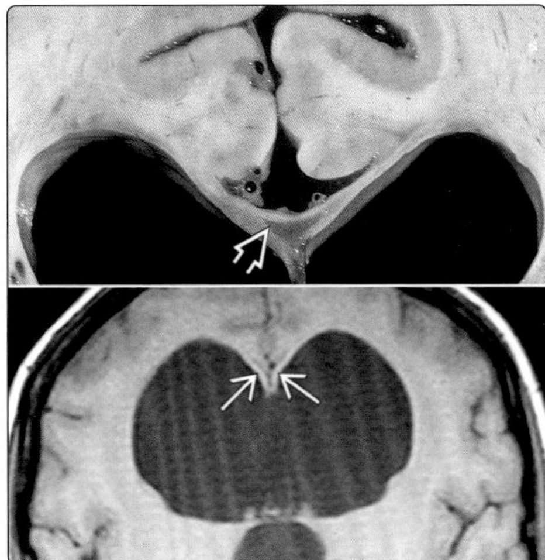

***(39-19)** (Top) IVOH, thinned encephalomalacic CC ➡ is caused by falx impingement. (Bottom) T1 MR shows CC impingement ➡.*

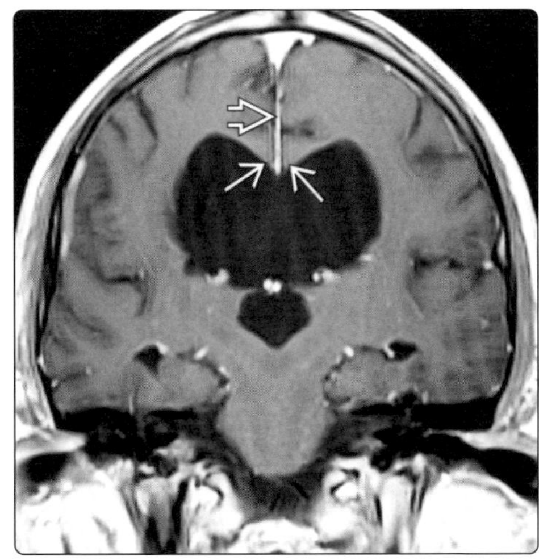

***(39-20)** Coronal T1 C+ MR of longstanding IVOH shows the lateral ventricles ➡ & CC are forced upward against the falx cerebri ➡.*

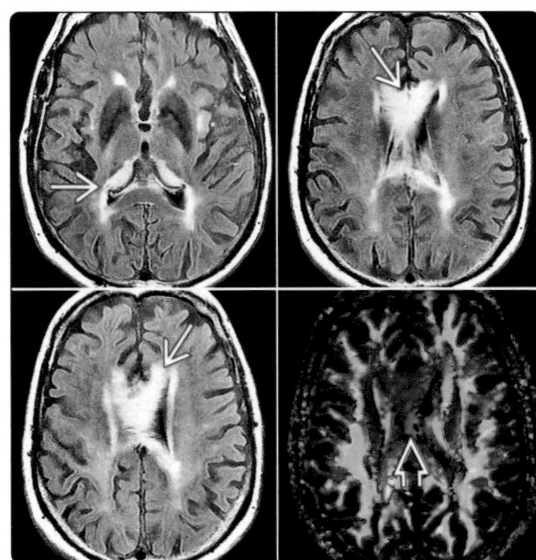

***(39-21)** CCIS with decompression, postshunt FLAIR shows hyperintensity in CC, periventricular WM ➡, disrupted fibers on DTI ➡.*

## Etiology

The pathogenesis of NPH is poorly understood and remains controversial. Recent studies of NPH suggest altered CSF dynamics (production, kinetics, reabsorption), and ISF stasis disrupts the balance between hydrostatic and osmotic pressures, reversing ISF flow and causing ventricular enlargement. Newer studies suggest involvement of the glymphatic system in NPH.

## Pathology

The ventricles appear grossly enlarged. The periventricular WM often appears abnormal with or without frank lacunar infarction. Neurofibrillary tangles and other microscopic changes, typically found in Alzheimer disease, are seen in 20% of cases.

## Clinical Issues

NPH accounts for ~ 5-6% of all dementias. The nature and severity of symptoms and the disease course vary. Impaired gait and balance are the typical initial symptoms. The classic triad of dementia, gait disturbance, and urinary incontinence is present in a minority of patients and typically represents advanced disease.

Some patients initially respond dramatically to ventricular shunting ("shunt-responsive" NPH). The favorable response to shunting varies from ~ 35-40% in patients with clinically "possible" NPH to 65% in patients diagnosed with "probable" NPH. The responsiveness is often improvement in gait and incontinence. The predictors of positive response to shunting remain elusive.

*(39-22A) Sagittal T1 MR in a patient with headaches & a remote history of meningitis shows enlarged 4th, 3rd, & lateral ventricles & the cerebral aqueduct related to postinflammatory hydrocephalus. Subarachnoid hemorrhage is the most common cause of EVOH. (39-22B) T2 MR shows marked enlargement of 4th ventricle & lateral recesses with CSF migration into the adjacent cerebellum.*

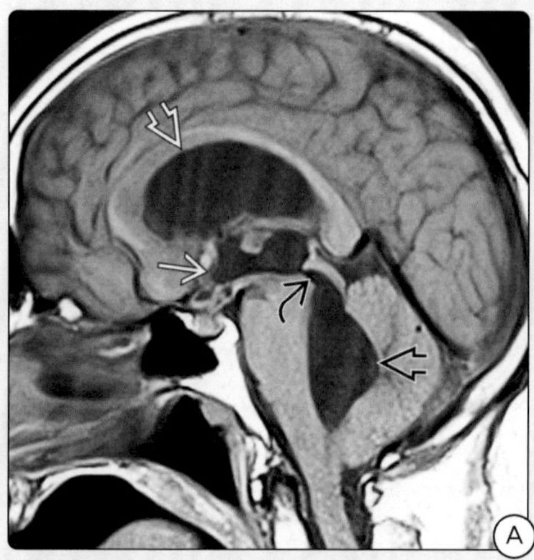


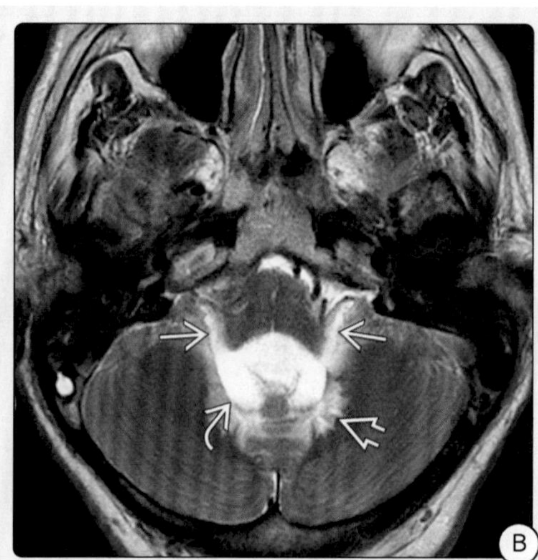


*(39-22C) Contrast injected via ventriculostomy in the same patient fills the 4th ventricle & lateral recesses but is obstructed at the outlet foramina. This is EVOH. (39-23) Gross autopsy specimen shows extensive tuberculous meningitis with thick exudate filling the basal cisterns. The basal location of the exudate results in occlusion of the foramina of Magendie & Luschka. (Courtesy R. Hewlett, MD.)*

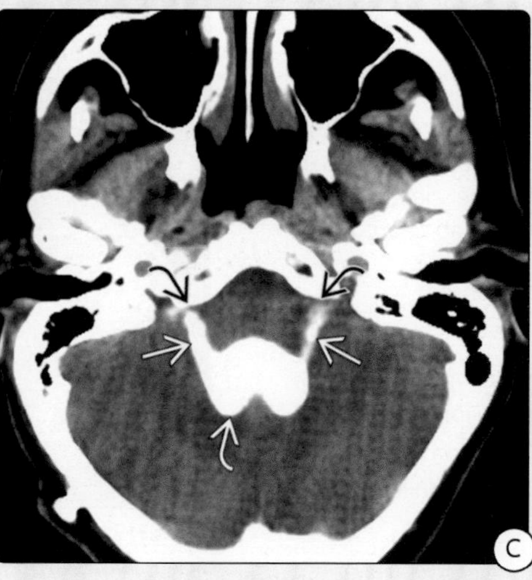


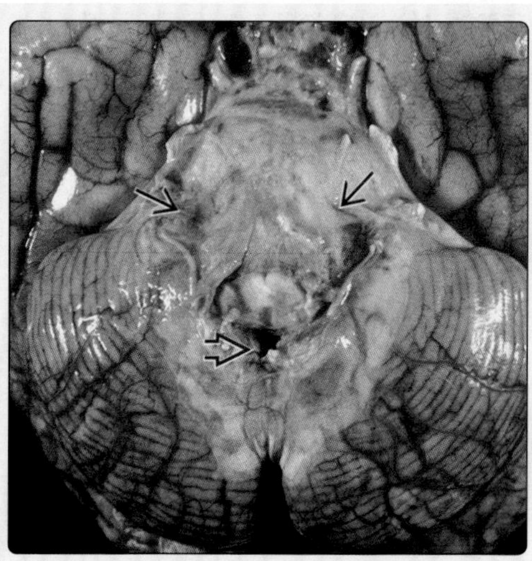

## Imaging

**General Features.** Imaging studies in suspected NPH are necessary but insufficient to establish the definitive diagnosis of NPH. The goal of identifying patients who are likely to improve following ventriculoperitoneal shunting likewise remains elusive.

The most common general imaging feature of NPH is ventriculomegaly that appears out of proportion to sulcal enlargement ("ventriculosulcal disproportion") **(39-24)**.

Additional helpful imaging findings include a prominent cerebral aqueduct flow void **(39-24A)** **(39-25)** and enlarged lateral and third ventricles with the fourth ventricle relatively normal. Disproportionately enlarged subarachnoid space hydrocephalus (DESH), particularly involving the sylvian fissures and basal cisterns, as well as a high tight convexity with effacement of sulci at the brain vertex have also been described as imaging features suggestive of NPH.

**CT Findings.** NECT scans show enlarged lateral ventricles with rounded frontal horns **(39-28)**. The third ventricle is moderately enlarged, whereas the fourth ventricle appears relatively normal. Compared with the degree of ventriculomegaly, generalized sulcal enlargement is mild. Periventricular hypodensity is common and often represents a combination of increased ISF and WM rarefaction secondary to microvascular disease.

**MR Findings.** T1 scans show large lateral ventricles. The convexity and medial SASs may appear decreased or "tight," whereas the basal cisterns and sylvian fissures are often enlarged. The CC is usually thinned. Most patients have a mild to moderate periventricular "halo" on T2/FLAIR **(39-26A)**.

A prominent, exaggerated "hyperdynamic" aqueductal "flow void" may be present **(39-24A)** **(39-25)**. Recent studies show some NPH patients have hyperdynamic CSF flow with increased velocity and volume in *both* systole and diastole. Net flow direction is caudocranial, the reverse of normal.

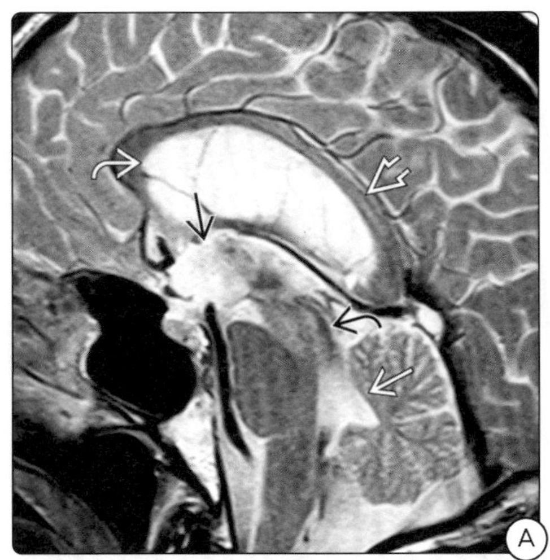


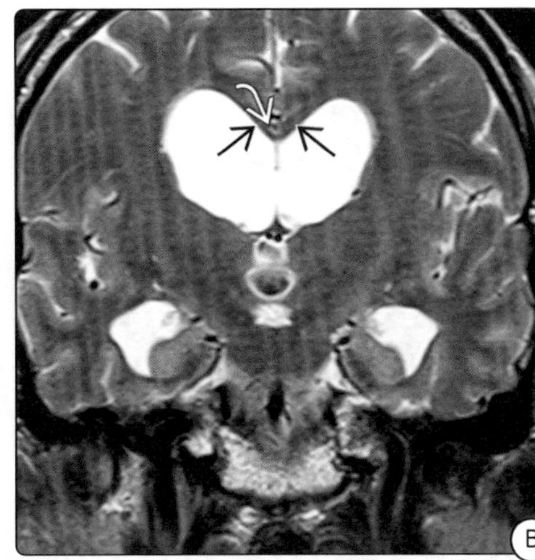


***(39-24A)** Sagittal T2 MR shows large lateral ⇨, 3rd →, & 4th ➡ ventricles with an exaggerated aqueductal "flow void" ↷. Thinning of the hyperintense CC ➡ is also present in this patient with gait abnormality & incontinence. CSF diversion may improve symptoms. **(39-24B)** Coronal T2 MR shows enlarged lateral ventricles → that push the thin, encephalomalacic CC against the falx ↷. (See Fig. 34-19).*

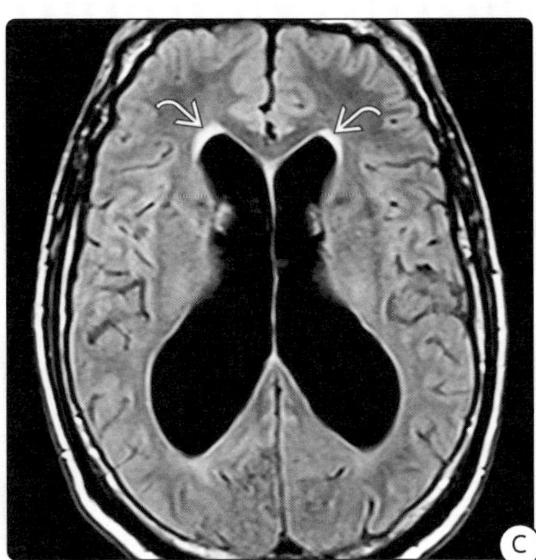


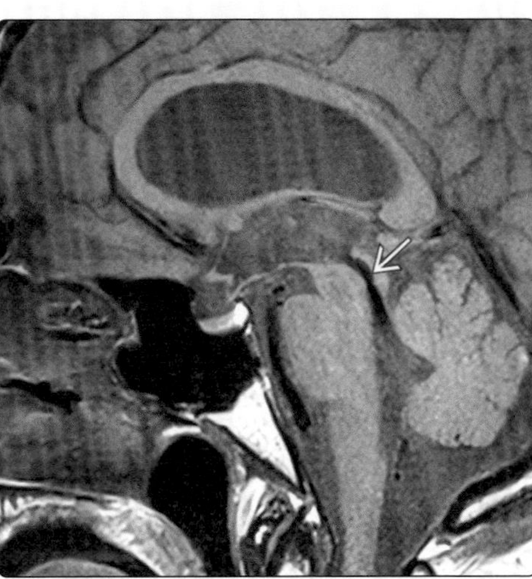

***(39-24C)** FLAIR shows a thin rim of periventricular fluid accumulation ↷. Aqueductal stroke volume was 72 µL. This patient had shunt-responsive NPH. **(39-25)** Sagittal T1 MR in a patient with symptoms of NPH shows a prominent "aqueductal flow void" ➡. This feature is often most prominent on T2 sequences & supports the clinical diagnosis of NPH. The patient underwent a large-volume LP & CSF shunt with improved symptoms.*

Two useful measurements to help evaluate for the presence of NPH on CT or MR include the Evans index, which is a ratio of the widest diameter of the frontal horns:the widest diameter of the transverse internal skull measured on the same axial slice with a value of ≥ 0.3 considered abnormal **(39-27)**. The callosal angle is the angle between the lateral ventricles on coronal imaging at the level of the posterior commissure with a value of < 90° considered abnormal **(39-28)**. Together, the Evans index and the callosal angle have shown a high accuracy rate for identifying those patients with NPH.

**Nuclear Medicine.** Prominent ventricular activity at 24 hours on In-111 DTPA cisternography is considered a relatively good indicator of NPH. F-18 FDG PET shows decreased regional cerebral metabolism.

**Spine Intervention.** Prior to CSF diversion surgery, patients will often undergo a large-volume lumbar puncture (LP) to assess the patient's response to CSF removal. Typically, during the LP, ~ 30-50 mL of CSF are removed. The patient's gait and cognitive function are evaluated before the LP and again at 3-4 hours after the LP. This "tap procedure" has a high positive predictive value (73-100%) for those patients who might benefit from CSF shunt placement.

## Differential Diagnosis

A major difficulty in diagnosing NPH is distinguishing it from other neurodegenerative disorders, such as **Alzheimer disease, vascular dementia**, and **age-related atrophy**. Recent studies suggest CSF biomarkers, such as AQP4, T-tau, and Aβ40, may be helpful in separating NPH from cognitive and movement disorder mimics.

# Arrested Hydrocephalus

Arrested hydrocephalus (AH) has also been called compensated hydrocephalus, ventriculomegaly of adulthood, and late-onset idiopathic aqueductal stenosis. Patients rarely present with symptoms or stigmata of elevated ICP, and the

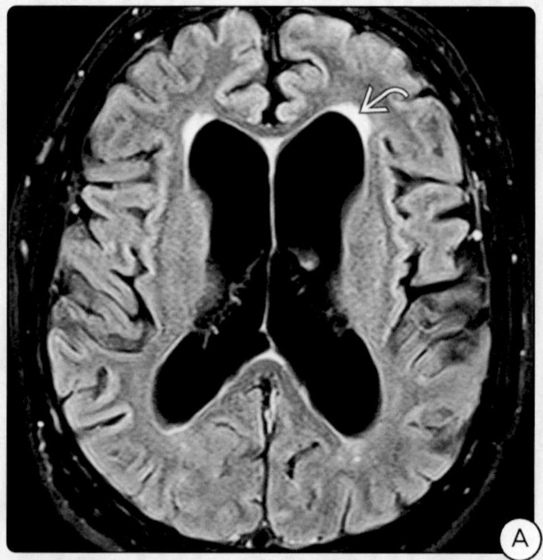


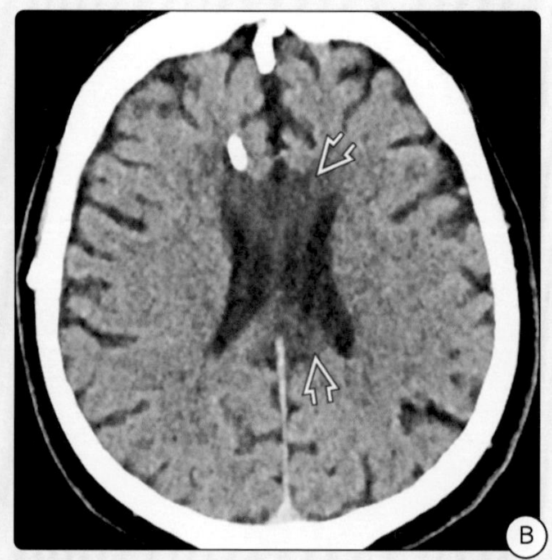


***(39-26A)** FLAIR MR in 72-yo man with NPH shows enlarged lateral ventricles out of proportion to the volume loss. Prominent hyperintense rim ➪ surrounds the ventricles. **(39-26B)** Follow-up NECT after shunting shows a hypodense CC ➪. This is NPH with callosal impingement syndrome. After CSF shunting, the ventricles may be stable or decreased in size. Gait abnormalities are most likely to respond to CSF shunting.*

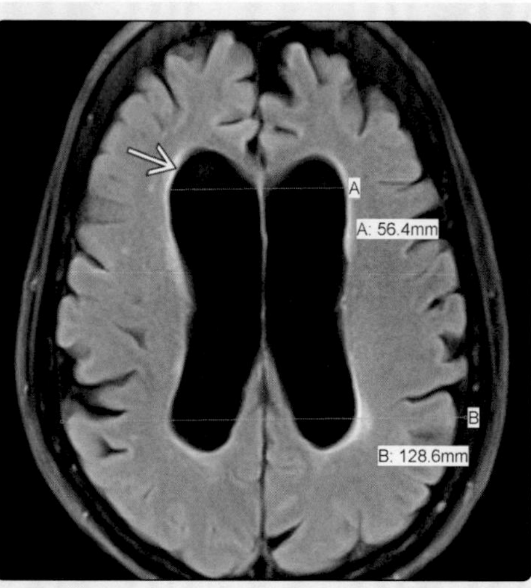


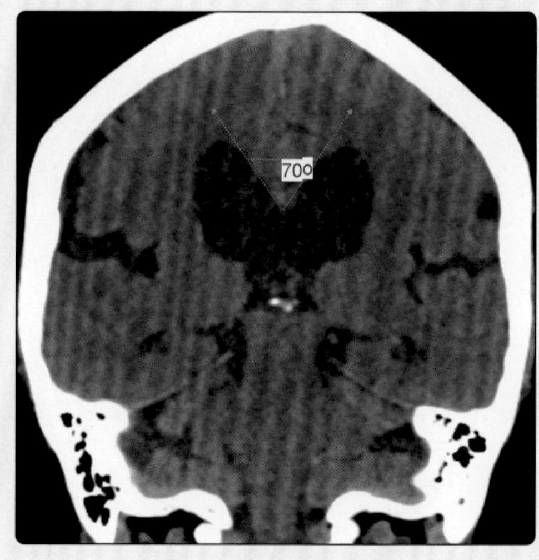


***(39-27)** Axial FLAIR MR in a NPH patient shows enlarged lateral ventricles ➪. The Evans index, a ratio of widest diameter of the frontal horns:widest diameter of the transverse inner table of the skull, is 56.4/128.6 = 0.4. A value of ≥ 0.3 is considered abnormal. **(39-28)** Coronal CT in the same patient shows an abnormal callosal angle of 70°. An angle < 90° is considered abnormal. Together, Evans index & callosal angle support a diagnosis of NPH.*

diagnosis of hydrocephalus is often incidental and unexpected. Moderate to severe triventricular enlargement without evidence for periventricular fluid accumulation is present on imaging studies and may remain stable for years.

## Idiopathic Intracranial Hypertension

### Terminology

Idiopathic intracranial hypertension (IIH) is preferred to the term **pseudotumor cerebri**. IIH is characterized by unexplained elevation of ICP not related to an intracranial mass lesion, a meningeal process, or cerebral venous thrombosis. Patients with a known cause of elevated ICP (e.g., dural venous sinus stenosis) are nonetheless often still classified as having IIH.

### Etiology and Pathology

The precise etiology of IIH is unknown. An obese phenotype with elevated body mass index is common. Disturbed CSF-ISF drainage through the "glymphatic pathway" has been invoked by some investigators.

It is unclear whether the dural venous sinus stenosis found in the vast majority of IIH patients is a cause (from venous outflow obstruction) or an effect (from extrinsic compression) of elevated ICP, or both. The venous sinus stenosis is typically at the junction of the transverse and sigmoid sinuses and may be seen on CTV, MRV, or conventional angiography **(39-32)** **(39-33)**.

### Clinical Issues

Classically, IIH presents in overweight women who are 20-45 years of age, although recent studies have confirmed a rising incidence in obese children, especially girls.

Headache is the most constant symptom (90-95%) followed by tinnitus and visual disturbances. Papilledema is the most common sign on neurologic examination **(39-29)**. Cranial nerve deficits, usually limited to CNVI, are common. Patients may also present with transient vision loss, diplopia, or vertigo.

The definitive diagnosis of IIH is established by LP, which demonstrates elevated ICP (> 20 cm $H_2O$ in adults or 28 cm $H_2O$ in children) with normal CSF composition.

Visual loss is the major morbidity in IIH. In fulminant IIH, visual loss can progress rapidly and become irreversible **(39-29)**. Serial CSF removal (10-20 mL at initial LP) often temporarily ameliorates IIH-associated headache. Venous sinus stenting in patients who have transverse sinus stenosis has been successful in improving symptoms and reducing papilledema in some cases, though this remains controversial **(39-32)**. Other treatments include weight loss, carbonic anhydrase inhibitors, and therapeutic LP. Surgical treatment, including lumboperitoneal shunt and optic nerve sheath fenestration, is reserved for patients who continue to experience vision loss despite conservative management and those initially presenting with rapid vision loss.

### Imaging

Neuroimaging is used to (1) exclude identifiable causes of increased ICP (e.g., neoplasm, venous thrombosis, or obstructive hydrocephalus) and (2) detect findings associated with IIH.

The most significant imaging findings of IIH include **flattening of the posterior globes, distention of the perioptic SAS with or without a tortuous optic nerve, intraocular optic nerve protrusion, partial empty**

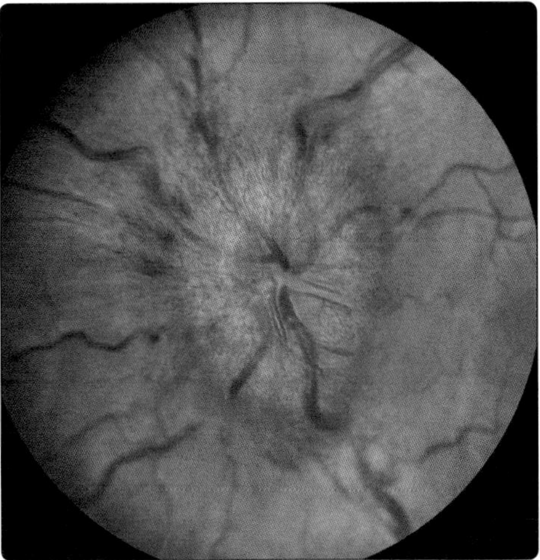

***(39-29)** Funduscopic image shows findings of severe papilledema with elevated, blurred optic disc. (From K. Digre, MD, Imaging in Neurology.)*

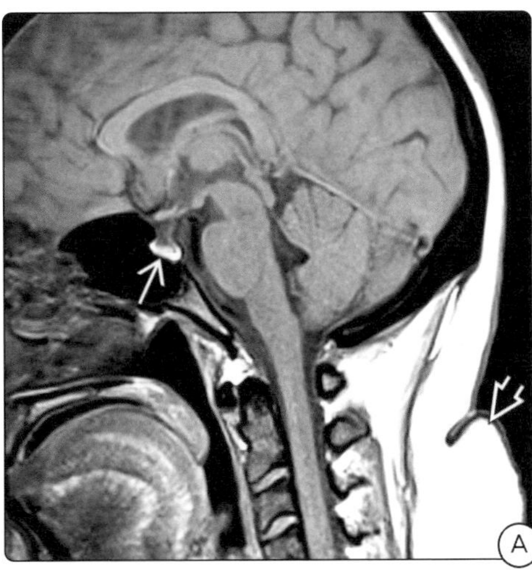


***(39-30A)** Sagittal T1 MR in a 33-yo obese woman shows excessive subcutaneous fat ➪ & a partial empty sella ➡.*

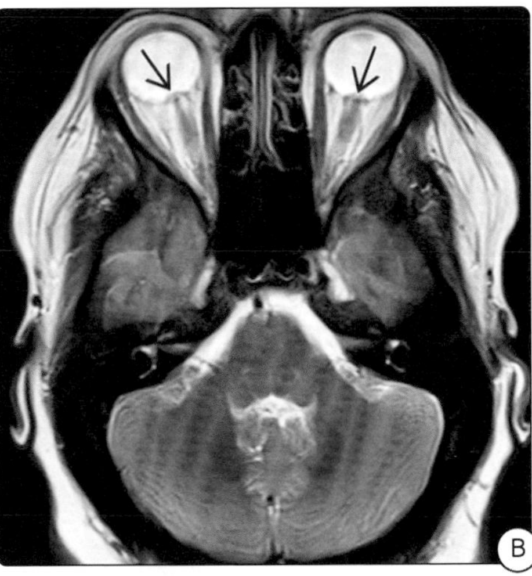


***(39-30B)** T2 MR shows flattening of the globes, intraocular protrusion of optic nerve heads ➡. At LP, opening pressure 44 cm $H_2O$. This was IIH.*

**sella, and transverse venous sinus stenosis** on CTV/MRV or DSA **(39-30) (39-32) (39-34) (39-33) (39-31)**. The presence of one or a combination of these signs—especially transverse sinus stenosis—significantly increases the odds of IIH, but their absence does not rule out IIH.

The prevalence of other reported findings, such as slit-like or "pinched" ventricles (10%), "tight" SASs (small sulci and cisterns), and inferiorly displaced tonsils, may be present. Cerebellar tonsillar ectopia **(39-31)** may be present and sometimes even peg-like in configuration, mimicking a Chiari 1 malformation or intracranial **hypo**tension. It is key to make the correct diagnosis and not confuse these other entities with IIH, as the treatments are vastly different.

Meningoceles or cephaloceles protruding through osseous-dural defects in the skull base are common, especially in extremely obese patients. CSF leaks are common, and CT or gadolinium MR cisternography may identify which of several bony defects is leaking.

## Differential Diagnosis

The most important differential diagnosis in patients with suspected IIH is **secondary intracranial hypertension** (i.e., increased ICP with an identifiable cause). Ventriculomegaly is more common in secondary intracranial hypertension, whereas the ventricles are usually normal to small in IIH.

**Dural sinus thrombosis** is a major consideration. T2* (GRE, SWI) shows "blooming" thrombus in the affected sinuses. Dural venous sinus thrombosis most commonly involves the transverse sinuses. Noncontrast CT usually shows a hyperdense sinus, > 70 HU. A filling defect is typically seen on CTV or MRV. Only ~ 50% of venous thrombosis patients will have an associated venous infarct.

Other differential considerations include secondary intracranial hypertension from vascular etiologies, including bilateral jugular vein thrombosis, superior vena cava syndrome, or arteriovenous fistula. Medications, including

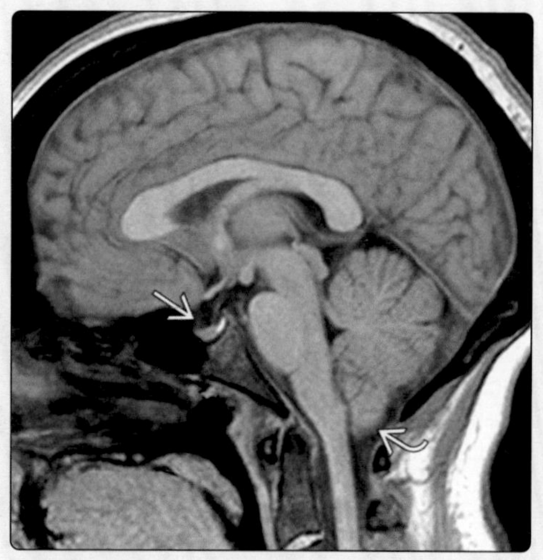

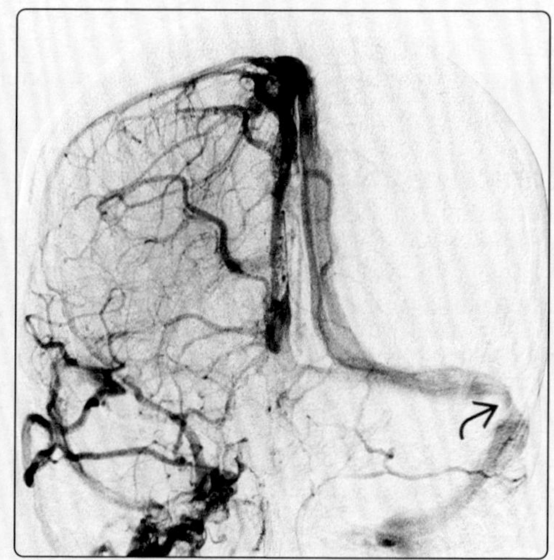

***(39-31)** Sagittal T1 MR in severe headache patient shows a partial empty sella ➡ & low-lying tonsils ➡. It is key to make the correct diagnosis, IIH. Low-lying tonsils may be seen in IIH, intracranial hypotension, & Chiari malformations. **(39-32)** AP DSA shows a transverse sinus stenosis ➡ with 10 mm Hg gradient. Stenting resolved the patient's severe headaches. Venous stenting may benefit some patients, though it remains controversial.*

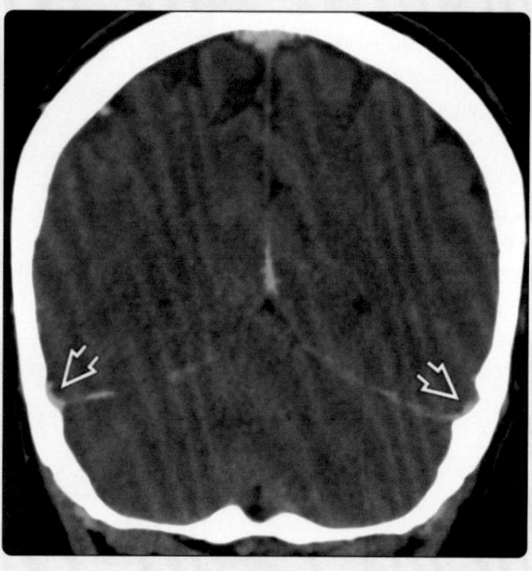

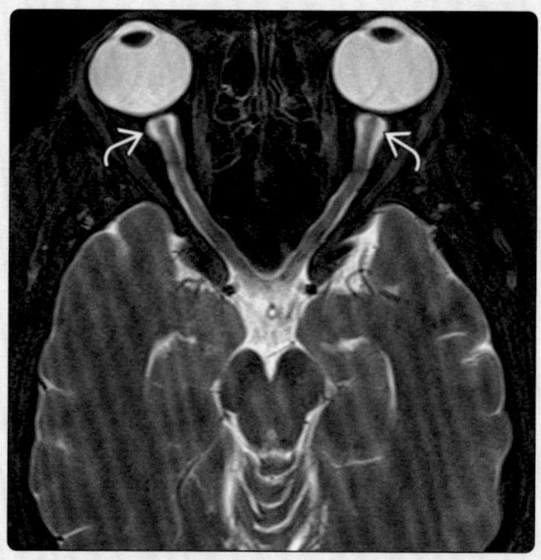

***(39-33)** Coronal CTV in a 39-yo woman with severe headaches shows marked stenosis of the transverse-sigmoid sinus junctions ➡. Her opening pressure at LP was 36 cm $H_2O$ (IIH). Sinus stenosis may be visualized on CTV, MRV, or DSA. **(39-34)** Axial STIR MR shows optic nerve sheath enlargement ➡ & mild tortuosity of the optic nerves in this IIH patient with opening pressure of 31 cm $H_2O$. Treatment is to preserve vision & improve headaches.*

tetracycline, minocycline, vitamin A, lithium, retinoids, and anabolic steroids, have been associated with intracranial hypertension. Elevated ICP may also result from endocrine disorders, including Addison disease and hypoparathyroidism.

**IDIOPATHIC INTRACRANIAL HYPERTENSION**

**Terminology and Etiology**
- a.k.a. benign intracranial hypertension
- Often no cause identified (idiopathic)

**Clinical Issues**
- F > M; obesity = definite risk
- Peak: 20-45 years
- Headache, tinnitus, vision loss, LP > 20 cm $H_2O$

**Imaging**
- Dilated optic nerve sheaths
- Intraoptic disc protrusion
- Flat posterior globe
- Partial empty sella
- "Tight" brain, ± tonsillar herniation
- ± dural sinus stenosis, thrombosis

## CSF Shunts and Complications

Imaging is a key component in evaluating patients with CSF diversions. Shunt failure can result in either enlarging or collapsing ventricles. The most common imaging manifestation of shunt failure is enlarging ventricles. CT is generally the preferred technique to assess patients with intracranial shunt catheters. Alternative modalities include transfontanelle ultrasound and new rapid MR techniques, such as fast steady-state gradient-recalled-echo (SS-GRE) sequences.

Some shunted hydrocephalus patients exhibit clinical signs of shunt failure without evidence of ventricular enlargement, a condition called **slit ventricle syndrome** (SVS). Comparison to prior imaging studies is essential. NECT scans show that one or both lateral ventricles are small or slit-like.

# CSF Leaks and Sequelae

## CSF Leaks

CSF leaks can occur in patients of all ages. Trauma, prior skull base operation, and sinonasal surgery are common antecedents. Spontaneous CSF leaks usually develop in middle-aged obese women with IIH and are most commonly associated with arachnoid granulations in the lateral sphenoid sinus. In a patient with suspected skull base leak and CSF rhinorrhea, a positive β-2-transferrin test on nasal secretions is extremely valuable.

Bone CT with multiplanar reformations is the procedure of choice and may obviate the need for invasive CT cisternography. A bone defect, with or without an air-fluid level in the adjacent sinus, is the typical finding **(39-35)**. Defects < 3 or 4 mm may be difficult to detect, especially in areas where the bone is normally very thin. If a patient has multiple potential leak sites, a CT cisternogram may be necessary **(39-36B)**.

MR is generally used only if CT is negative or the presence of brain parenchyma within a cephalocele is suspected. T2 scans often disclose an osseous defect with fluid &/or parenchyma in the adjacent sinus cavity **(39-36)**.

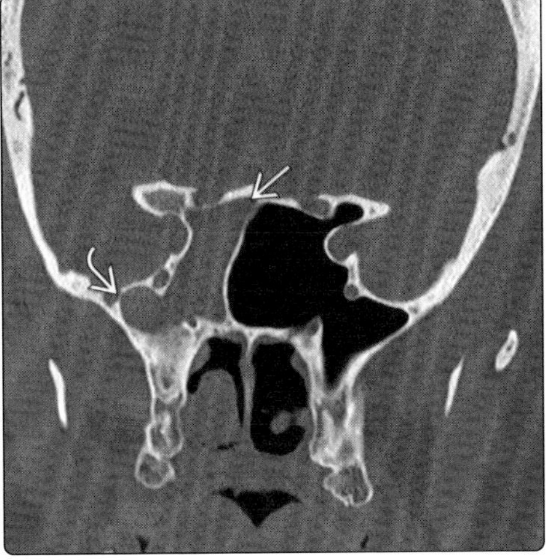

***(39-35)** Coronal CT shows an opacified sphenoid sinus ➡ with a lateral sphenoid defect ➡, in a man with a positive β-2-transferrin test, CSF leak.*

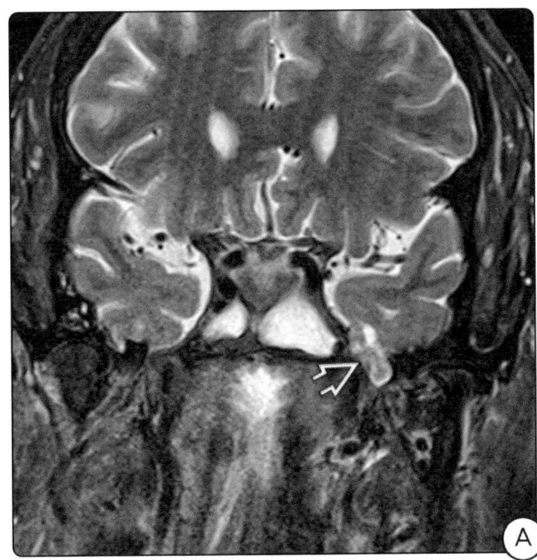


***(39-36A)** Coronal T2 MR in a patient with IIH shows a cephalocele ➡ in the middle cranial fossa floor involving the sphenoid bone.*

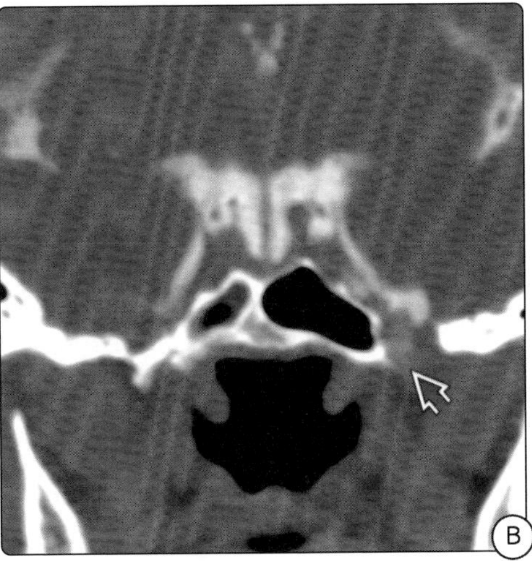


***(39-36B)** CT cisternogram confirms the sphenoid defect ➡ as the patient's CSF leak site. IIH patients may have multiple potential leak sites.*

## Intracranial Hypotension

### Terminology

Intracranial hypotension is also known as **CSF hypovolemia syndrome**.

### Etiology and Pathology

Intracranial hypotension can be spontaneous (SIH) or acquired. Common antecedent causes include LP, spinal surgery, and trauma.

Spinal meningeal diverticula can rupture suddenly and may be responsible for many cases of "spontaneous" intracranial hypotension. In contrast to IIH, skull base CSF leaks rarely cause SIH.

CSF hypovolemia and hypotension (LP opening pressure < 6 cm $H_2O$) result in venous and dural interstitial engorgement with brain descent ("sagging") **(39-37)**. Patients with Marfan and Ehlers-Danlos syndromes have abnormal connective tissue and an increased risk of CSF rupture through the congenitally weakened dura.

### Clinical Issues

Symptoms range widely, from mild headache to coma. The classic presentation is severe orthostatic headache that is relieved by lying down. Most cases of SIH resolve spontaneously. Severe cases may present with progressive encephalopathy, and, in rare cases, severe unrelieved brain descent can result in coma or even death.

Treatment is aimed at restoring CSF volume. Fluid replacement and bed rest can be sufficient in many cases. In others, epidural blood patch or surgical repair may be required.

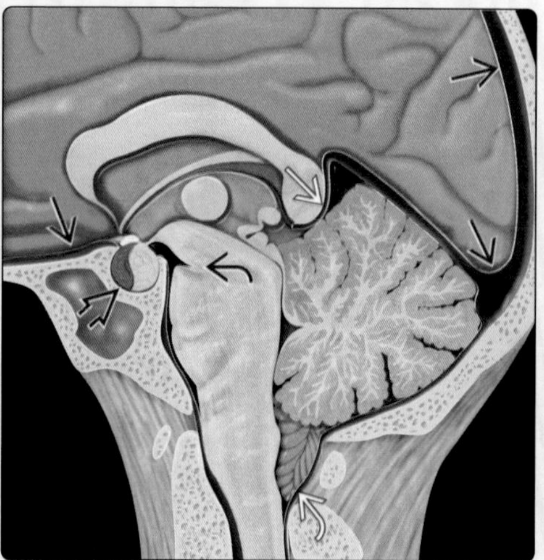

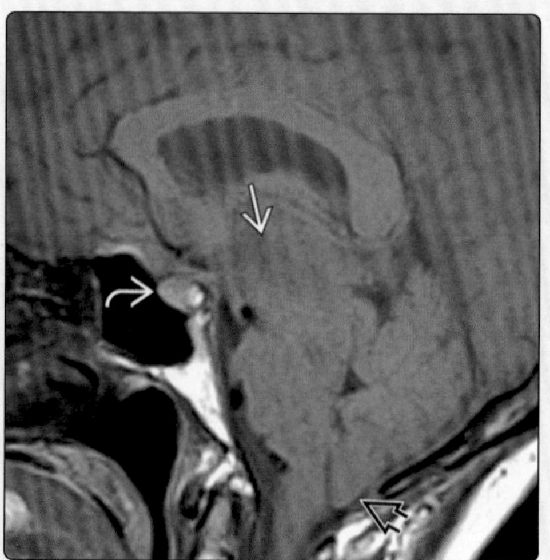

***(39-37)** Intracranial hypotension is shown with distended dural sinuses ➔, enlarged pituitary ➔, & low tonsils ➔. Central brain descent causes midbrain "slumping," inferiorly displaced pons, decreased pons-midbrain angle ➔, splenium depressing ICV/V of G junction ➔. **(39-38)** Sagittal T1 MR in patient with intracranial hypotension shows brainstem "sagging" ➔, "fat" pituitary ➔, & low-lying tonsils ➔.*

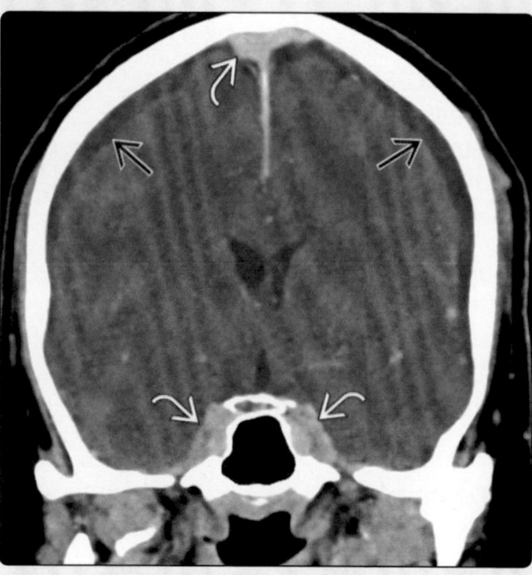

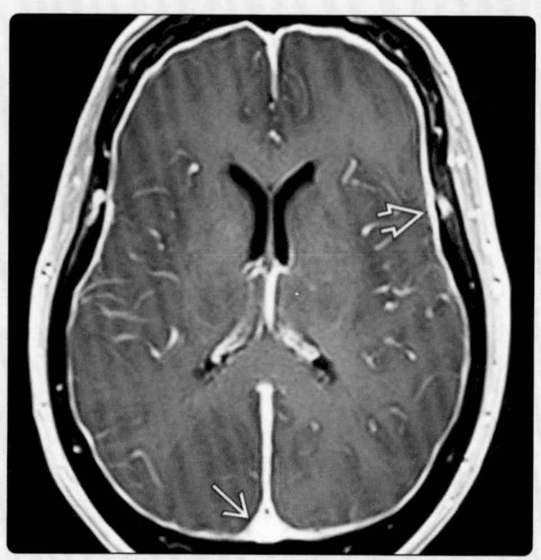

***(39-39)** Coronal CECT in a patient who presents with severe headache shows small bilateral subdural hygromas ➔ & marked venous engorgement ➔, typical for SIH. **(39-40)** Axial T1 C+ MR shows venous engorgement ➔, diffuse dura-arachnoid thickening, & enhancement ➔. This patient's intracranial hypotension is secondary to a spinal CSF leak (not shown).*

Epidural blood patch is often performed on the basis of clinical and brain imaging findings alone. If low- and high-volume patches are unsuccessful, further studies may be necessary to localize precisely the level of the CSF leak.

The Bern scoring system based on MR findings may help to identify CSF leaks that will be found on invasive imaging (CT myelography). The Bern score ranges from 0-9 with 9 having the most MR imaging features suggestive of intracranial hypotension. Those patients with a Bern score of 5-9 have a high likelihood of having a CSF leak identified on dynamic CT myelography **(39-41)**.

## Imaging

Imaging is key to the diagnosis, sometimes providing the first insight into the cause of often puzzling symptoms.

Although CT is often obtained as an initial screening study in patients with severe or intractable headache, MR of the brain and spine is the procedure of choice to evaluate possible SIH.

Between 90-95% of SIH patients have one or more key findings on standard MR scans. A spectrum of findings occurs with SIH; only rarely are *all* imaging signs present in the same patient!

**CT Findings.** CT scans in SIH are often normal. The most obvious findings are subdural fluid collections **(39-39)** **(39-41A)**. Subtle CT clues to the presence of SIH include effacement of the basal cisterns (especially the suprasellar SAS), medial herniation of the temporal lobes into the tentorial incisura, small ventricles with medial deviation of the atria of the lateral ventricles, and a "fat" pons.

### MR Findings

***T1WI.*** Sagittal T1 scans show brain descent in ~ 1/2 of all cases **(39-38)**. Midbrain "sagging" with the midbrain displaced below the level of the dorsum sellae **(39-38)**, decreased angle between the peduncles and pons < 50°, shortened pontomammillary distance < 5.5 mm, and flattening of the pons against the clivus are typical findings **(39-42)**. Caudal displacement of the tonsils is common but not invariably present.

The optic chiasm and hypothalamus are often draped over the sella, effacing the suprasellar cistern. The pituitary gland appears enlarged in at least 50% of all cases **(39-38)** **(39-43)**.

Axial scans show that the basal cisterns are effaced. The pons often appears elongated and "fat." Midbrain anatomy is distorted with decreased width and increased anteroposterior diameter. The temporal lobes are displaced medially over the tentorium into the incisura. The lateral ventricles are usually small and distorted, as they are pulled medially and inferiorly by the brain "sagging."

In cases with severe brain descent, coronal scans may show that the angle between the roof of the lateral ventricles progressively decreases (< 120°) as brain "sagging" increases. The dural sinuses often appear distended with outwardly convex margins and exaggerated "flow voids" **(39-40)** **(39-42)**. 15-50% of cases have subdural fluid collections **(39-39)** (hygromas > hematomas).

***T2/FLAIR.*** The slit-like third ventricle is displaced downward and, on axial scans, appears almost superimposed on the midbrain and hypothalamus.

***T1 C+.*** One of the most consistent findings in SIH, seen in 80-85% of cases, is diffuse dural thickening with intense enhancement. Linear dural thickening

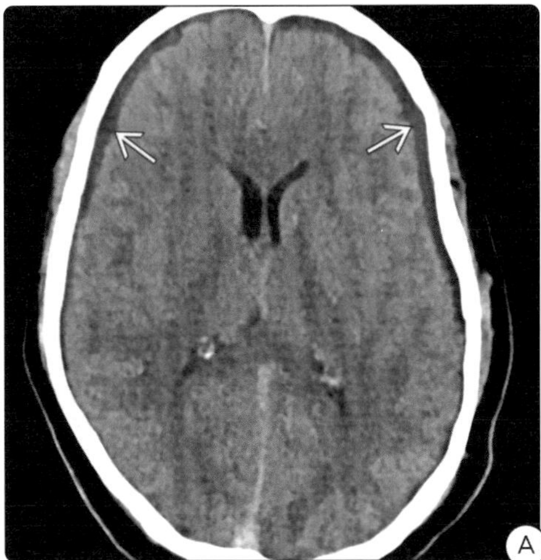


***(39-41A)** CT shows small subdural hygromas ➡ in patient with severe headaches. Additional imaging showed brainstem "slumping."*

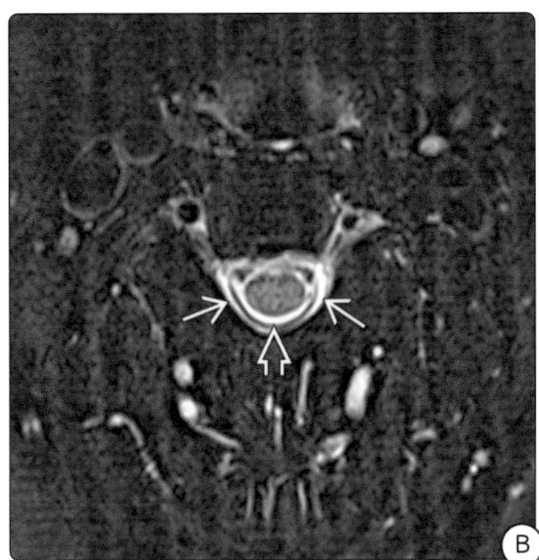


***(39-41B)** Axial T2 FS MR shows an epidural fluid collection ➡ related to CSF leak. The dura ➡ is between the epidural collection & the thecal sac.*

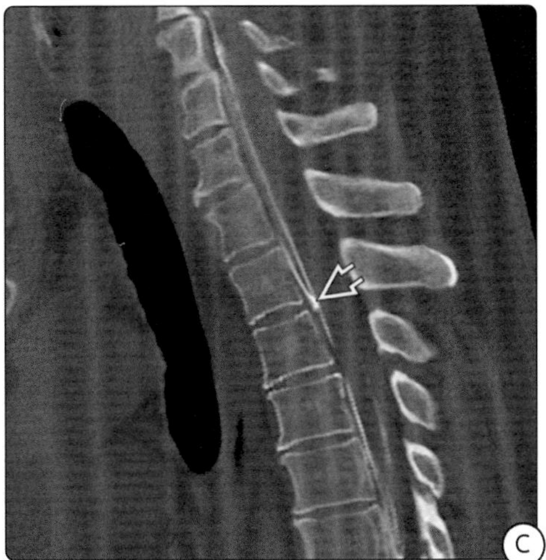


***(39-41C)** Dynamic CT myelography shows a CSF leak at the T2/T3 level ➡ related to a ventral epidural tear from a disc osteophyte complex.*

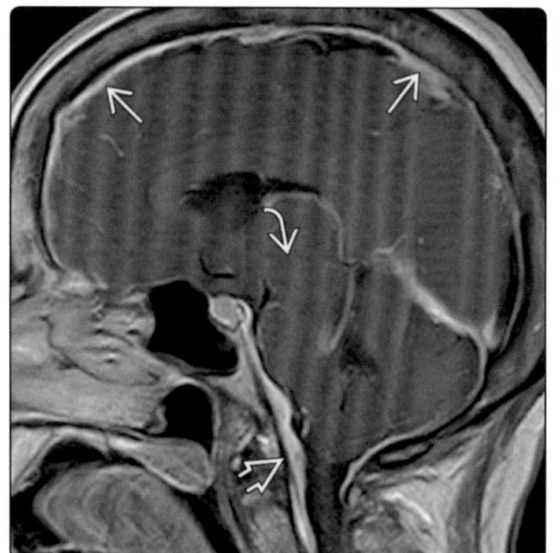

***(39-42)** Sagittal T1 C+ MR shows diffuse dural enhancement ➡ that extends into upper cervical spine ➡ & midbrain "slumping" ➡. This is SIH.*

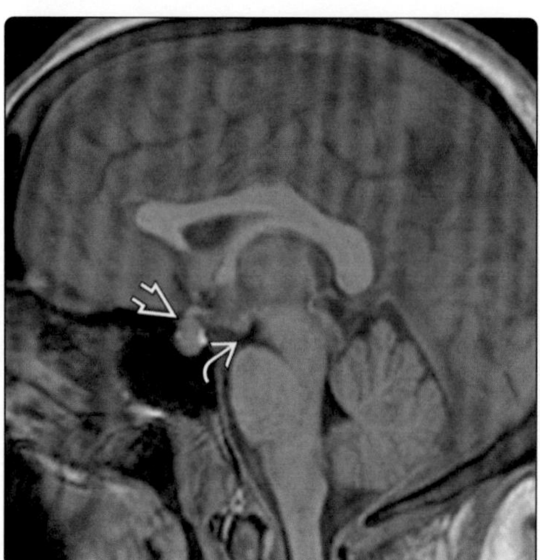

***(39-43)** Sagittal T1 MR shows a decreased mammilopontine distance (< 5.5 mm) ➡ & a large pituitary gland ➡. This is SIH.*

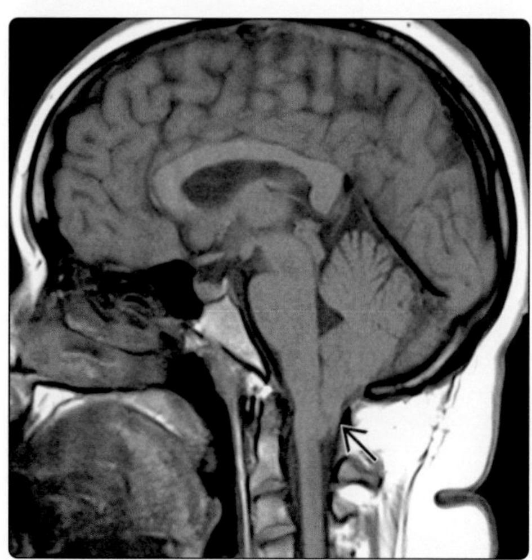

***(39-44)** Sagittal T1 shows Chiari 1 with pointed cerebellar tonsils extending ≥ 5 mm below foramen magnum ➡. Note normal brainstem.*

may extend into the internal auditory canals, down the clivus, and through the foramen magnum into the upper cervical canal **(39-42)**.

***T2* (GRE, SWI).*** Tearing of bridging veins caused by brain "sagging" can result in subarachnoid hemorrhage and superficial siderosis.

## Differential Diagnosis

The major differential diagnosis of intracranial hypotension is **Chiari 1 malformation**. In Chiari 1, the only intracranial abnormality is displaced tonsils **(39-44)**. Other findings of SIH are absent. **Mistaking SIH for Chiari 1 on imaging studies can lead to decompressive surgery, worsening CSF hypovolemia, and clinical deterioration!**

### INTRACRANIAL HYPOTENSION

**Etiology and Pathology**
- CSF hypovolemia leads to brain "sags," dural/venous sinuses increase
- Can be spontaneous (idiopathic) or acquired

**Clinical Issues**
- Most common symptom = headache
  - ± orthostatic
- Severe intracranial hypotension can cause coma, even death

**MR Findings**
- Common
  - Midbrain "sags" down
  - Angle between midbrain, pons decreases (< 50°)
  - Pontomammillary distance: < 5.5 mm
  - Optic chiasm/hypothalamus draped over prominent pituitary
  - Diffusely thickened enhancing dura (reduced with time)
  - "Fat" pituitary
- Less common
  - Pons, midbrain may appear "fat"
  - ± tonsils displaced downward
  - Effaced cisterns/sulci
  - Small lateral ventricles ± atria "tugged" inferomedially
  - ± subdural collections (hygromas > frank hematomas)
  - Enlarged dural sinuses with outwardly bulging (convex) margins
- Rare but important
  - Ventricular angle on coronal imaging decreases
  - Torn bridging cortical veins
  - Subarachnoid hemorrhage, superficial siderosis

*Selected References: The complete reference list is available on the eBooks+ version included with purchase.*

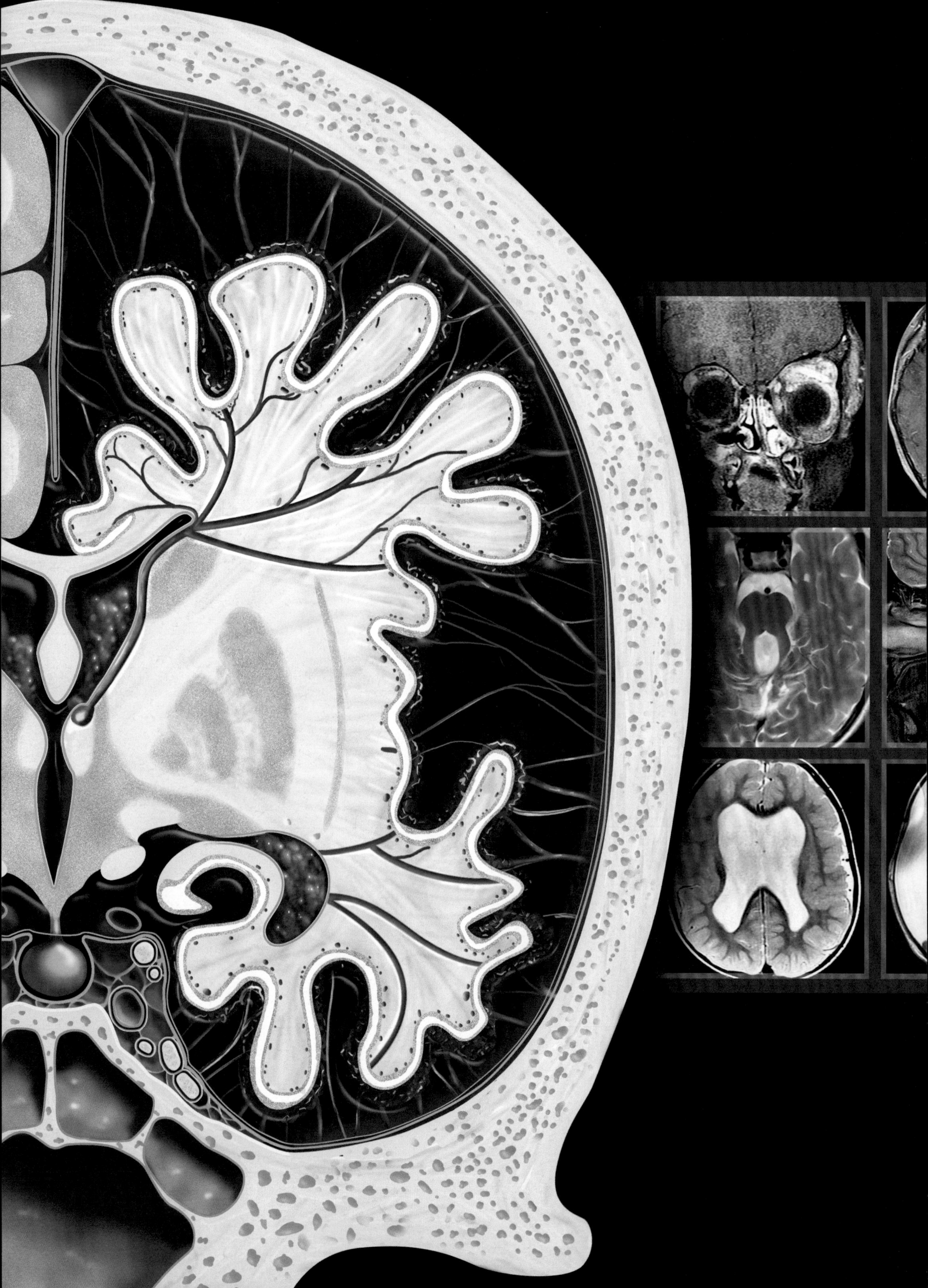

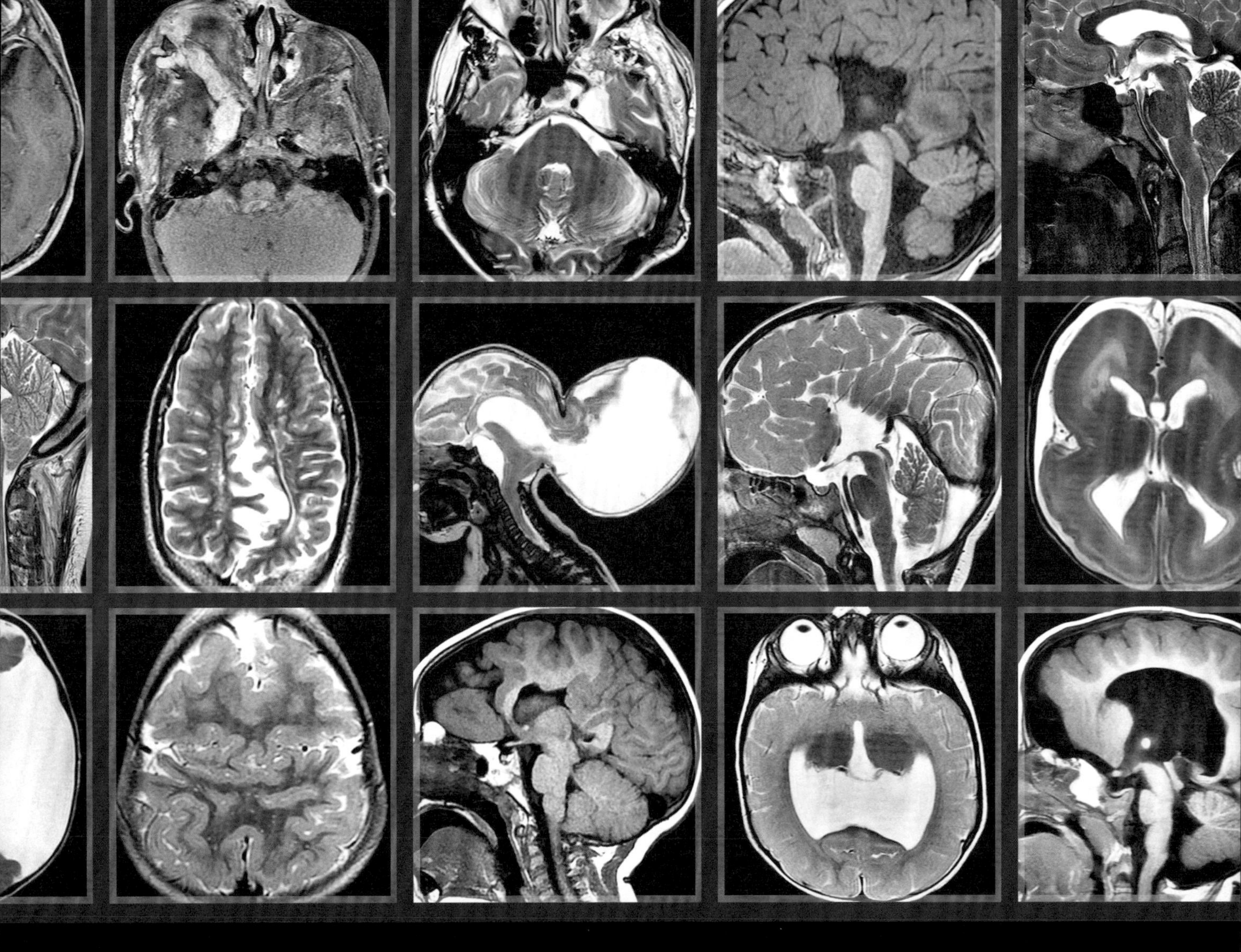

SECTION 6

# Congenital Malformations and Genetic Tumor Syndromes

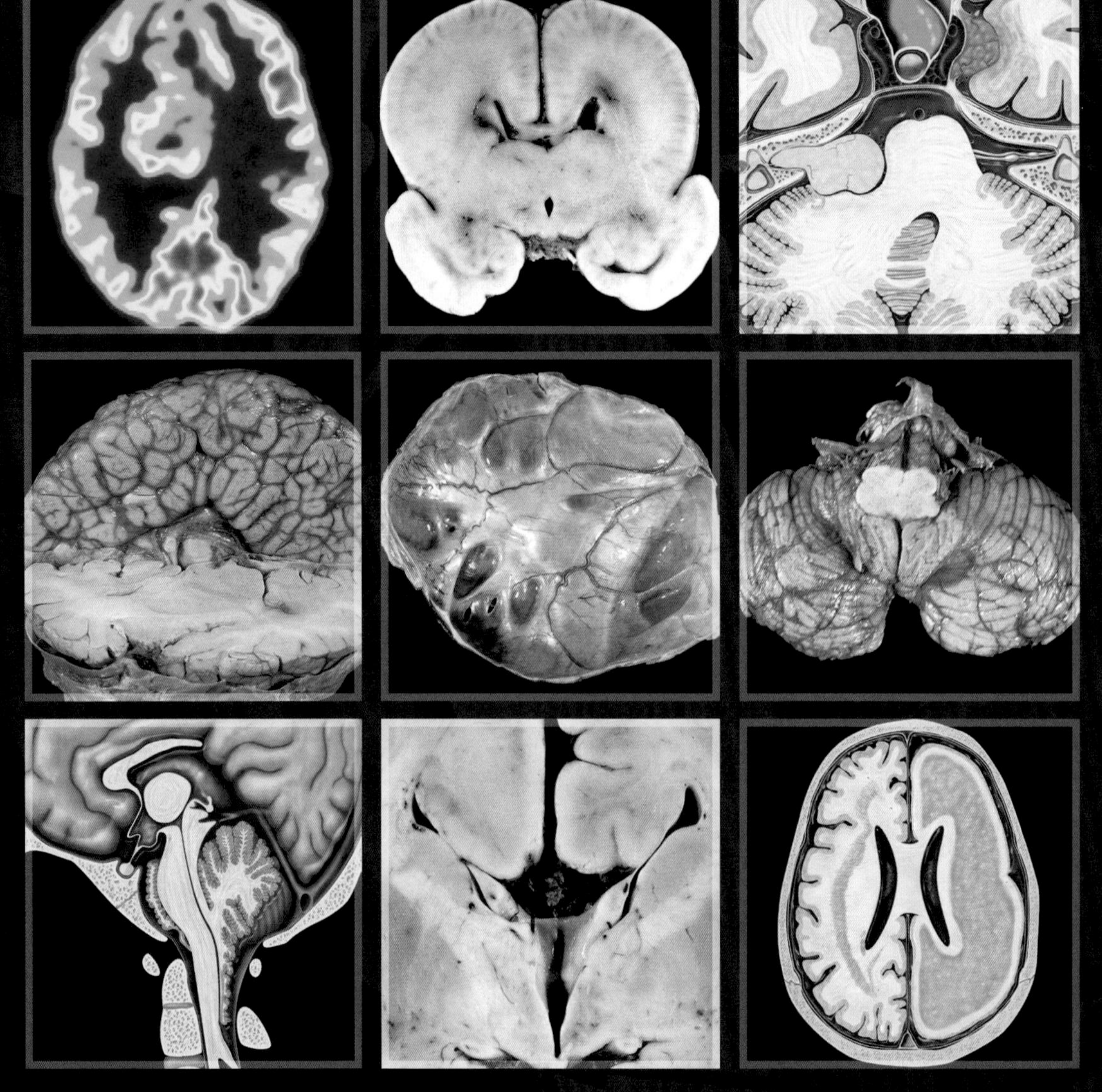

SECTION 6

# Congenital Malformations and Genetic Tumor Syndromes

# Approach to Congenital Malformations

*A basic knowledge of normal brain development and maturation provides the essential foundation for understanding congenital malformations, the subject of the final part of this book.*



Here, we briefly consider normal development of the cerebral hemispheres and cerebellum. We first focus on the basics of neurulation and neural tube closure, then turn our attention to how the neural tube flexes, bends, and evolves into the forebrain, midbrain, and hindbrain. Developmental errors and the resulting malformations that may occur at each stage are briefly summarized.

Cerebral hemisphere growth and elaboration into lobes, development of sulci and gyri, patterns of gray matter migration, and layering of the neocortex are all succinctly delineated.

## Cerebral Hemisphere Formation

The major embryologic events in brain development begin with neurulation, neuronal proliferation, and neuronal migration. The processes of operculization, gyral and sulcal development, and the earliest steps in myelination all take place later, between gestational week 11 and birth.

### Neurulation

#### Neural Tube and Brain Vesicles

The **neural plate** develops at the cranial end of the embryo as a thickening of ectoderm on either side of the midline. The neural plate then indents and thickens laterally, forming the **neural folds**. The neural folds bend upward, meet in the midline, and then fuse to form the **neural tube**. The primitive **notochord** lies ventral to the neural tube. **Neural crest** cells are extruded and migrate laterally. The neural tube forms the brain and spinal cord, whereas the neural crest gives rise to peripheral nerves, roots, and ganglia of the autonomic nervous system **(40-1)**.

The neural tube closes, beginning in the middle and proceeding bidirectionally in a zipper-like fashion along the length of the embryo **(40-2)**.

As the neural tube closes, the neuroectoderm (which will form the CNS) separates from the cutaneous ectoderm in a process known as disjunction. Upon completion of disjunction, the cutaneous ectoderm fuses in the midline, dorsal to the closed neural tube. The brain grows rapidly and begins to bend, forming several flexures. The embryonic brain eventually has five definitive vesicles **(40-3)**.

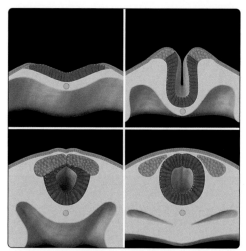

(40-1) *Neural plate (red) forms, folds, & fuses in midline. Neural, cutaneous ectoderm separate. Notochord (green), neural crest (blue) are shown.*

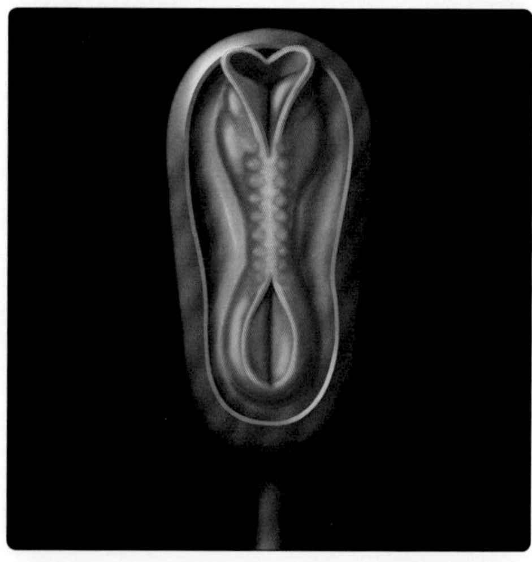

(40-2) *The neural tube closes in a bidirectional, zipper-like manner, starting in the middle & proceeding toward both ends.*

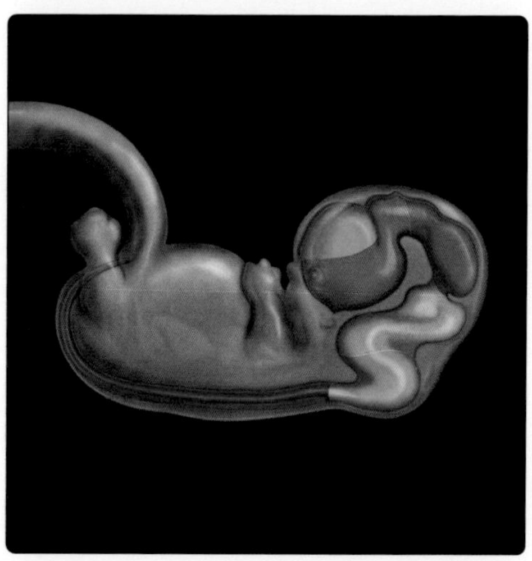

(40-3) *Brain flexures with telencephalon (green), diencephalon (red), mesencephalon (purple), metencephalon (yellow) are shown.*

### Neurulation Errors

Errors in neurulation result in a spectrum of congenital anomalies. The most severe is **anencephaly** (essentially complete absence of the cerebral hemispheres). Various types of **cephaloceles** also result from abnormalities of neurulation.

Incomplete closure of the posterior neuropore results in **spina bifida**. If the neuroectoderm fails to separate completely from the cutaneous ectoderm, **myelomeningocele** results.

## Neuronal Proliferation

### Embryonic Stem Cells

*Pluri*potent embryonic stem cells are derived from the inner cell mass of the 4- to 5-day blastocyst. These cells are able to proliferate and differentiate into all three germ layers (ectoderm, mesoderm, endoderm). MicroRNAs seem to play an important role as genetic regulators of stem cell development, differentiation, growth, and neurogenesis.

### Histogenesis of Neurons and Glia

As the cerebral vesicles develop and expand, layers of stem cells arise around the primitive ventricular ependyma, forming the germinal matrix. These neural stem cells (NSCs) are *multi*potent cells that generate the main CNS phenotypes, i.e., neurons, astrocytes, and oligodendrocytes. NSCs are found primarily in the germinal zones.

*Pluri*potent NSCs in the germinal matrix give rise to "primitive" or "young" **neurons** that migrate outward to form the cortical mantle zone (precursor of the definitive cortex). Axons from the migrating neurons form an intermediate zone between the germinal matrix and cortical mantle that will eventually become the cerebral white matter.

Some NSCs become specialized **radial glial cells** (RGCs) that will eventually span the entire hemisphere from the ventricular ependyma to the pia. RGCs can give rise to both neurons and glia. Elongated cell bodies of the RGCs serve as a "rope ladder" that guides migrating neurons from the germinal matrix to the cortex.

### Errors in Histogenesis

Errors in histogenesis and differentiation result in a number of embryonal neoplasms, including medulloblastoma and primitive neuroectodermal tumors. Problems with NSC proliferation and differentiation also contribute to malformations of cortical development (MCDs).

## Neuronal Migration

Understanding how neurons are formed, migrate, organize, and then connect is essential to recognizing and understanding MCDs.

### Genesis of Cortical Neurons

Once the "young" neurons have been generated in the germinal matrix, they must leave their "home" to reach their final destination (the cortex). The definitive cerebral cortex develops through a highly ordered process of neuronal proliferation, migration, and differentiation.

### Neuronal Migration

**Migration** of newly proliferated neurons occurs along scaffolding provided by the RGCs. Neurons travel from the germinal zone to the cortical mantle in a generally "inside-out" sequence. Cells initially form the deepest layer of the cortex with each successive migration ascending farther outward and progressively forming more superficial layers. Each migrating group passes through layers already laid down by the earlier arriving cells.

Peak neuronal migration occurs between 11-15 fetal weeks, although migration continues up to 35 weeks. From 16-20 weeks, there is a three-layer pattern of the fetal brain on T2WI with germinal matrix, fetal white matter, and cortex from deep to superficial. From 20-30 weeks, there is a five-layer pattern of the fetal brain on T2WI with germinal matrix, subventricular-periventricular fiber-rich zone, subventricular cellular/intermediate zone, subplate, and cortical plate from deep to superficial.

### Errors in Neuronal Migration and Cortical Organization

The primary result of errors at these stages are **MCDs**. Problems with NSC proliferation or differentiation, migration, and cortical organization can all result in developmental anomalies of the neocortex. Examples include **microcephaly, megalencephaly, gray matter heterotopias, cortical dysplasias, and lissencephaly**.

## Operculization, Sulcation, and Gyration

### Lobulation and Operculization

The hemispheres are initially almost featureless; the cortex is thin and smooth. As the hemispheres elongate and rotate, they assume a "C" shape with the caudal ends turning ventrally to form the temporal lobes.

### Sulcation and Gyration

Sulcation and gyration occur relatively late in embryonic development. Shallow triangular surface indentations along the sides of the hemisphere—the beginnings of the lateral cerebral (sylvian) fissures—first become evident at ~ 16 weeks **(40-4)**.

After the sylvian fissures form **(40-6)**, multiple secondary and tertiary gyri begin to develop at 22- to 23-weeks gestation **(40-5)**. The central sulcus is usually visible by 26 weeks. All major sulci are formed by ~ 34 weeks.

### Anomalies in Sulcation and Gyration

Developmental errors in operculization, sulcation, and gyration are relatively common among congenital MCDs. Examples include **microcephaly with simplified gyral pattern** and **polymicrogyria**, which are representative anomalies that result from abnormal sulcation and gyration.

## Myelination

Myelination occurs in an orderly, predictable manner and can be detected as early as 18 fetal weeks.

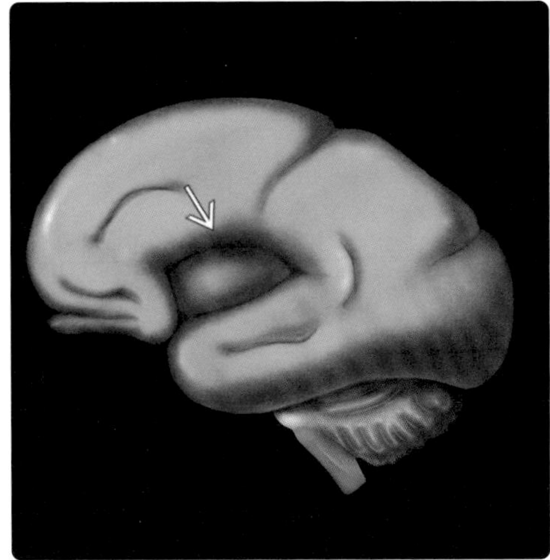

***(40-4)** 22-week fetal brain is mostly agyric with shallow lateral cerebral (sylvian) fissures ➡.*

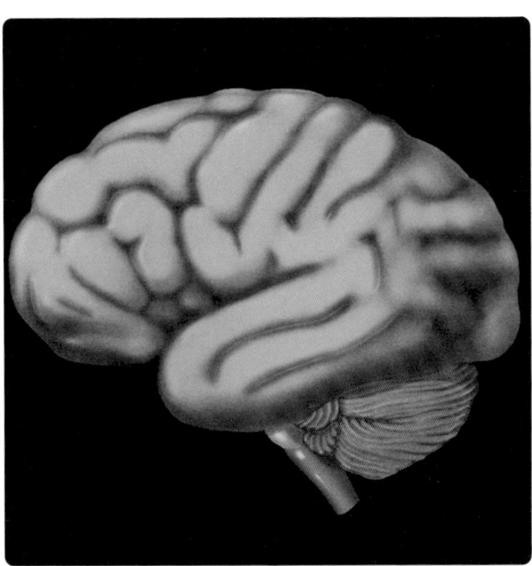

***(40-5)** Multiple secondary & tertiary gyri then develop, & the number & complexity of the cerebellar folia increase.*

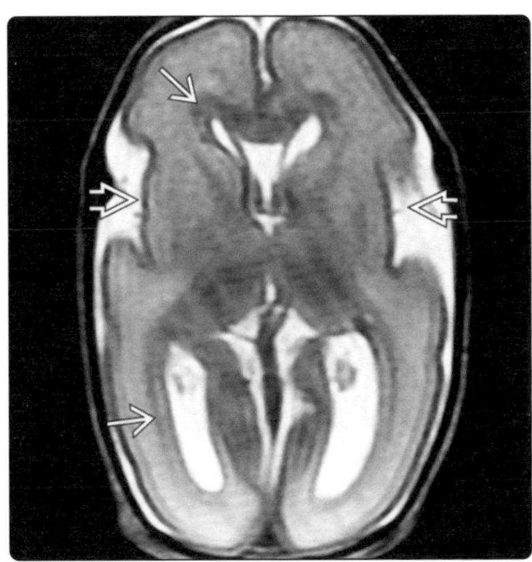

***(40-6)** T2 MR in 26-week-old preemie shows sylvian fissures ➡ are just beginning to form. Germinal matrix ➡ surrounds lateral ventricles.*

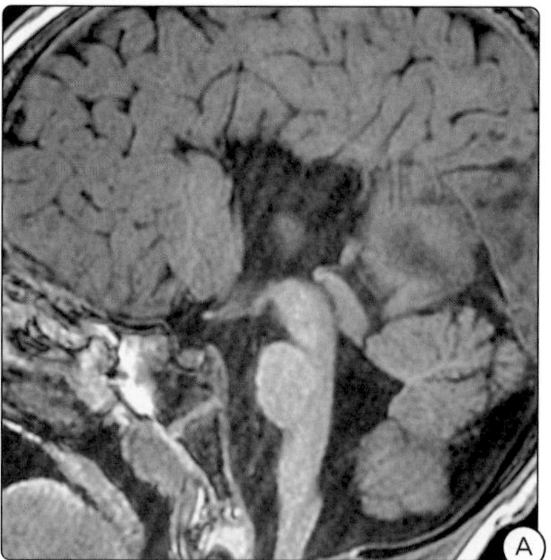

*(40-7A) Sagittal T1WI in a child with callosal agenesis is shown. Note the absence of the cingulate gyrus & extension of sulci centrally.*

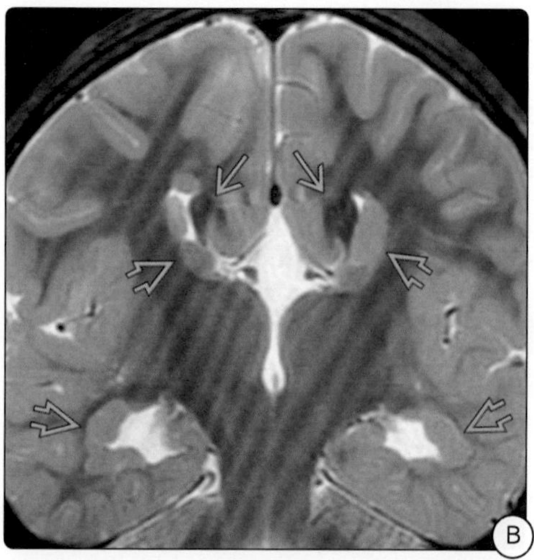

*(40-7B) Coronal T2 MR in the same child shows Probst bundles ⇨ & associated periventricular nodular gray matter heterotopia ⇨.*

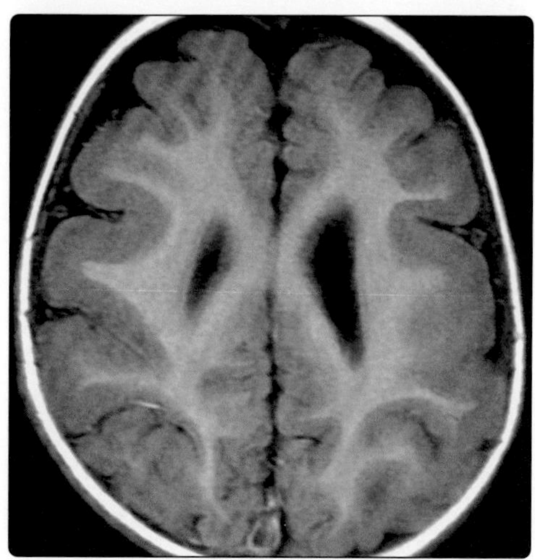

*(40-8) Axial T1 MR in a child with pachygyria & gyral simplification shows smooth cortical thickening & undersulcation of affected cortex.*

# Imaging Approach to Brain Malformations

## Technical Considerations

### CT

Clinicians sometimes order NECT scans as an initial screening examination in a patient with seizures or suspected brain malformation. Although parenchymal calcifications, ventricular size/configuration, and major abnormalities can be identified, subtle abnormalities, such as cortical dysplasia, are difficult to detect and easy to overlook.

Bone CT is helpful in depicting midline facial defects, synostoses, and anomalies of endochondral bone.

### MR

MR is the examination of choice. The two most important factors are gray matter-white matter differentiation and high spatial resolution. Many pediatric neuroradiologists recommend volumetric T1 sequences (e.g., MP-RAGE), and sagittal and coronal heavily T2-weighted sequences with very long TR/TEs. 3D imaging acquisitions allow isotropic orthogonal reformations. FLAIR can be very helpful in identifying focal cortical dysplasia (FCD), but only once the brain is fully myelinated (≥ 2 years).

A T2* sequence (GRE, SWI) can be a helpful addition if abnormal mineralization or vascular anomaly is suspected. DTI tractography is valuable when commissural anomalies are identified on initial sequences.

Contrast-enhanced T1WI generally provides little additional useful information in most congenital malformations, except in the case of associated vascular anomalies. DWI and MRS are useful in evaluating mass lesions and inborn errors of metabolism.

## Image Analysis

The following approach to analyzing imaging studies is modified and adapted from A. James Barkovich's guidelines on imaging evaluation of the pediatric brain.

### Sagittal Images

Begin with the midline section and examine the craniofacial proportion. At birth, the ratio of calvarium:face should be 5:1 or 6:1. At two years, it should be 2.5:1. In adults and children over the age of 10 years, it should be ~ 1.5:1. Assess myelination of midline structures, such as the corpus callosum and brainstem.

The most common of all brain malformations are anomalies of the cerebral commissures (especially the corpus callosum), which can be readily identified on sagittal T1 scans **(40-7A)**. Commissural anomalies are also the most common malformation associated with other anomalies and syndromes, so, if you see one, keep looking! Look for abnormalities of the pituitary gland and hypothalamus. Evaluate the size and shape of the third ventricle, especially its anterior recesses.

Look for other lesions, such as lipomas and cysts. These are often midline or paramidline and can be readily identified. The midline sagittal scan also permits a very nice evaluation of the posterior fossa structures. Does the fourth ventricle appear normal? Can you find its dorsally pointing fastigium?

Evaluate the position of the tonsils and the craniovertebral junction for anomalies.

If the lateral and third ventricles are large and the fourth ventricle appears normal, look for a funnel-shaped aqueduct indicating aqueductal stenosis. If you see aqueductal stenosis in such instances, look for rhombencephalosynapsis, which is seen in ~ 50% of aqueductal stenosis cases.

Sagittal images are also especially useful in evaluating the cerebral cortex. Is the cortex too thick? Too thin? Irregular? "Lumpy-bumpy"? MCDs, such as pachygyria and polymicrogyria associated with brain clefting ("schizencephaly"), are often most easily identified on sagittal images. Finally, note the position and size of the vein of Galen, straight sinus, and torcular Herophili.

## Coronal Images

MCDs are often bilateral. Polymicrogyria may occur anywhere but has a strong predilection for the perisylvian region. Coronal scans make side-to-side comparison relatively easy. Follow the interhemispheric fissure (IHF) all the way from front to back. If the hemispheres are in contiguity across the midline, holoprosencephaly is present. If the IHF appears irregular and the gyri "interdigitate" across the midline, the patient has a deficient falx, which is most commonly encountered in a Chiari 2 malformation.

Evaluate the size, shape, and position of the ventricles. In callosal dysgenesis/agenesis, the third ventricle appears "high riding" and the frontal horns of the lateral ventricles often look like a "Viking helmet" **(40-7B)**.

If the frontal horns appear squared-off or box-like, look carefully for an absent cavum septi pellucidi, a finding seen in septo-optic dysplasia and sometimes associated with polymicrogyria or schizencephaly.

Carefully evaluate the temporal horns and hippocampi to make sure that they are normally folded and oriented horizontally (not vertically, as occurs in many MCDs).

## Axial Images

The combination of a true T1WI together with a long TR/TE T2WI is necessary in evaluating all cases of delayed development to assess myelin maturation. The thickness and configuration of the cortical mantle are well seen **(40-8)**. The size, shape, and configuration of the ventricles are easily evaluated on these sequences.

Isolated FCD and cortical dysplasias associated with tuberous sclerosis complex are often best seen on T1WI in the first few months of life as hyperintense areas in the background of unmyelinated white matter. From approximately a few months of life into the second year of life, such abnormalities can be difficult to identify. Once myelination is complete, FCD is typically best seen on T2 FLAIR imaging **(40-9)**.

Do not forget the posterior fossa! The fourth ventricle in the axial plane is normally shaped like a kidney bean on its side. If the vermis is absent and the cerebellar hemispheres appear continuous from side-to-side, rhombencephalosynapsis is present **(40-10)**. If the fourth ventricle and superior cerebellar peduncles resemble a molar tooth, then a molar tooth malformation is present, suggesting Joubert syndrome and related disorders **(40-11)**.

*Selected References: The complete reference list is available on the eBooks+ version included with purchase.*

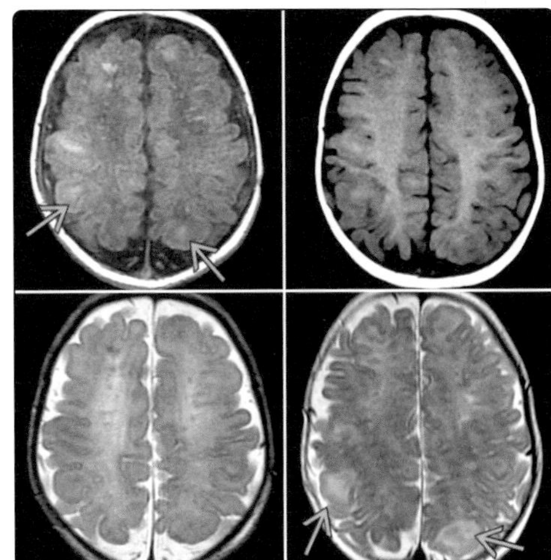

***(40-9)** Axial T1 (top) & T2 (bottom) at birth (left) & 8 months (right). Tubers ⇨ are best seen on T1 at birth, & T2 once myelination occurs.*

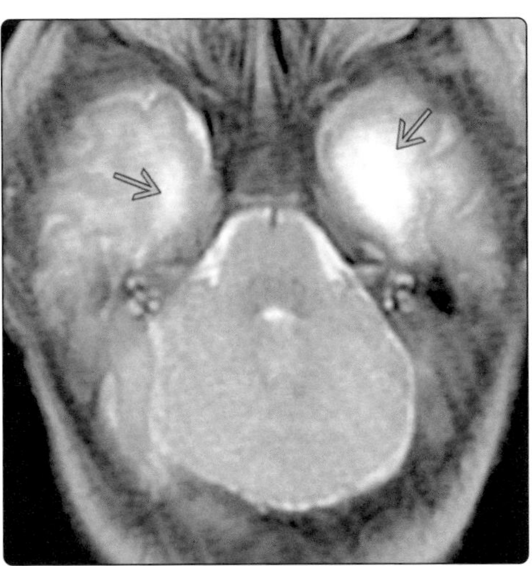

***(40-10)** Axial T2 MR in a neonate with aqueductal stenosis (hydrocephalus ⇨) shows continuity of the cerebellar hemispheres.*

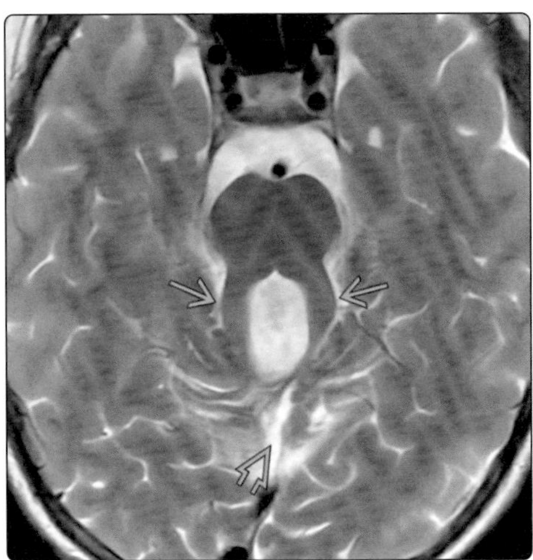

***(40-11)** Axial T2 MR shows thick, elongated superior cerebellar peduncles ⇨ & vermian clefting ⇨ in this case of Joubert syndrome.*

# Posterior Fossa Malformations

*Neural structures in the midbrain and posterior fossa are derived from three sources: (1) The embryonic mesencephalon gives rise to midbrain structures. (2) The embryonic hindbrain (rhombencephalon) gives rise to the posterior fossa structures. (3) Mesodermal elements give rise to the meninges and bone that surround and protect these neural structures. Developmental errors can give rise to a spectrum of midbrain and hindbrain malformations.*



## Chiari Malformations

### Introduction to Chiari Malformations

Chiari 1 and 2 are pathogenetically distinct disorders. **Chiari 1** is inferior dislocation of the cerebellar tonsils **(41-1)** in a typically otherwise normal patient. **Chiari 2** is herniation of the medulla and vermis and is caused by an associated myelodysplasia (spinal cord anomalies) **(41-8)**, usually an open neural tube defect. **Chiari 3** is characterized by herniation of posterior fossa contents through a low occipitocervical bony defect.

### Chiari 1

#### Terminology

Chiari 1 malformation (CM1) is defined as caudal cerebellar tonsillar ectopia. The precise distance of the tonsils below the foramen magnum (FM) required to diagnose CM1 is not agreed upon. Some investigators consider tonsillar ectopia measuring ≥ 5 mm as sufficient to establish the diagnosis of CM1. However, most insist additional abnormalities, such as tonsillar deformity ("pointing"), obliterated CSF spaces at the FM, or altered CSF flow dynamics, should also be present.

#### Etiology

**Abnormal Posterior Fossa.** The primary problem in CM1 is a size mismatch between the bony posterior fossa and the cerebellum. Many patients with CM1 demonstrate abnormal geometry of the bony posterior fossa ("*normal-sized hindbrain housed in a too-small bony envelope*"). Various combinations of congenitally reduced clival length, shortened basiocciput, and craniovertebral junction (CVJ) fusion anomalies may all result in diminished posterior cranial fossa depth &/or an abnormally small posterior fossa volume.

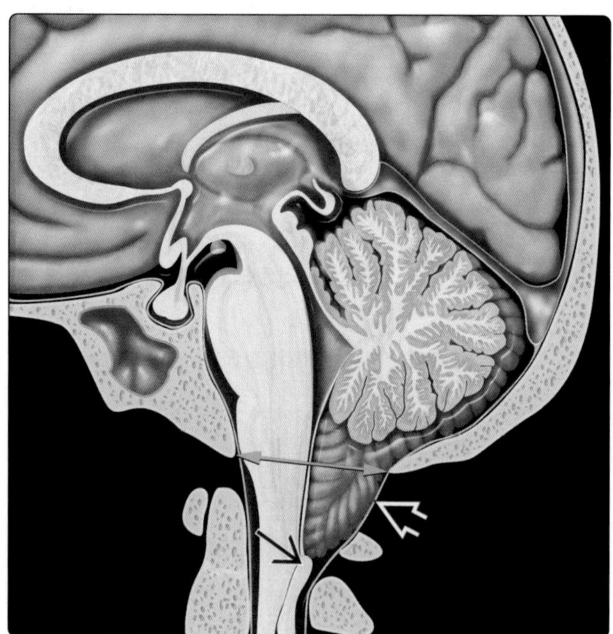

***(41-1)** CM1 shows the basion-opisthion line in green. Note the low-lying, pointed tonsil with vertically oriented folia ➡. The nucleus gracilis ➡ is inferiorly displaced.*

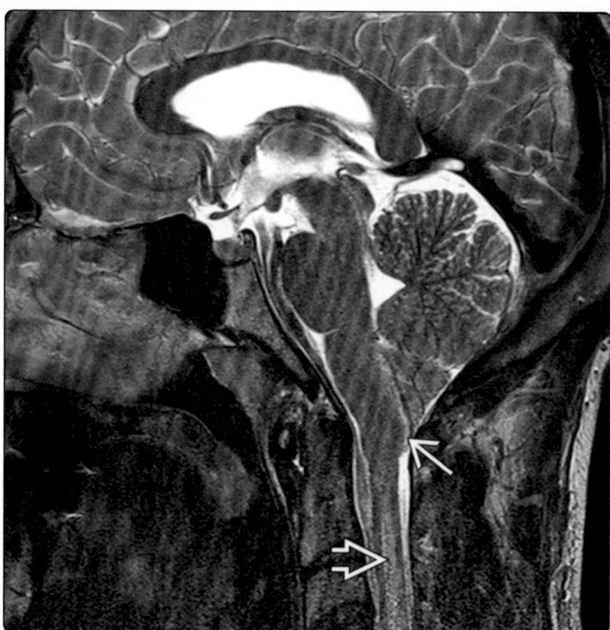

***(41-2)** Sagittal T2 MR in a 23-year-old man with classic CM1 shows a low-lying, pointed tonsil ➡ and normal-sized posterior fossa. Cord T2 hyperintensity ➡ represents the "presyrinx" state.*

**Altered CSF Dynamics.** Descent of the cerebellar tonsils below the FM into the upper cervical spine cases leads to crowding of structures and effacement of CSF spaces. This effacement of CSF spaces leads to reduced CSF flow between the intracranial and spinal compartments, resulting in poor intracranial pressure control during the cardiac cycle. Syringomyelia is present in 40-80% of individuals with symptomatic CM1 who undergo surgical treatment. The exact mechanism for development of syrinx in CM1 is not well understood, but it is likely related to altered CSF flow dynamics at the craniocervical junction and upper cervical spine.

## Pathology

Grossly, the herniated tonsils in CM1 are inferiorly displaced and grooved by impaction against the opisthion **(41-3A)**. In severe cases, they may appear firm and sclerotic. Arachnoid thickening and adhesions around the CVJ are common.

## Clinical Issues

**Epidemiology and Demographics.** CM1 is the most common of the Chiari malformations and can be identified in patients of all ages. When using tonsillar ectopia of > 5 mm as the imaging definition of CM1, the prevalence is quite high, somewhere between 0.24-3.6% of the population.

**Presentation.** While the incidence of an imaging diagnosis of CM1 is quite high, the incidence of symptomatic CM1 is relatively low (~ 0.01% of the population).

Clinical symptoms arise from 1) altered CSF flow through the FM, 2) direct mass effect on the brainstem, or 3) development of a syrinx. The most common symptom in the pediatric age group is an occipitocervical headache (27-70%). However, presentation of symptomatic CM1 differs with age. Children who are two years and younger most commonly present with oropharyngeal dysfunction. Older children more often present with headache and, less frequently, with sleep apnea and ataxia. Children with syrinx may present with scoliosis, motor/sensory deficits, spasticity, hyperreflexia, and poor coordination.

**Natural History.** The vast majority of patients with tonsillar ectopia > 5 mm below the plane of the FM remain asymptomatic. The imaging findings of CM1 may worsen or improve over time, especially in very young children who are undergoing significant head growth.

**Treatment Options.** Asymptomatic CM1 in the absence of an associated syrinx or scoliosis is usually not treated. Surgical treatment of symptomatic CM1 with suboccipital decompression attempts to restore normal CSF fluid dynamics at the FM. Depending on the severity of the tonsillar herniation, a simple bony decompression may be sufficient, whereas a duroplasty and tonsillar reduction may be necessary in more severe cases. When patient symptoms are clearly arising from the CM1, surgery usually results in improved or resolved symptoms. There is usually a decrease or resolution of associated spinal cord syrinx following surgery, although this is not universal.

## Imaging

**General Features.** The basion-opisthion line (BOL) is a line drawn from the tip of the clivus to the posterior rim of the FM **(41-1)**. Measuring the distance from this line to the inferior margin of the cerebellar tonsils on sagittal MR defines tonsillar position.

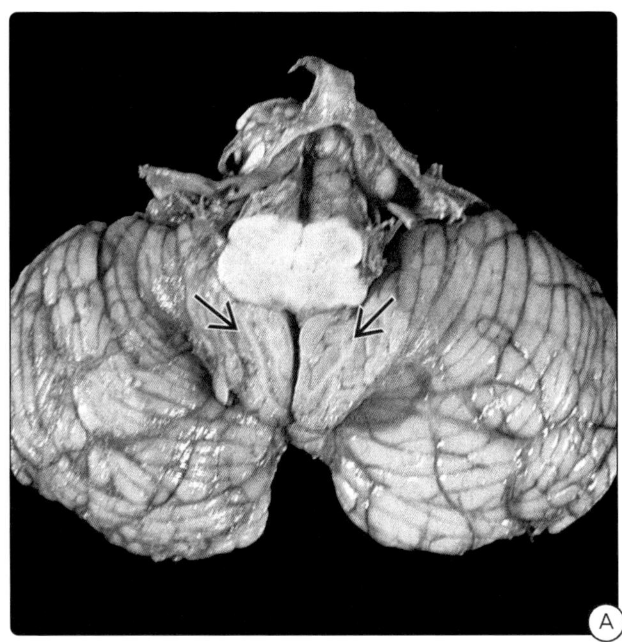


*(41-3A) Semiaxial view of an autopsy case shows CM1. Note inferiorly displaced tonsils with vertically oriented folia ⇒. (Courtesy E. T. Hedley-Whyte, MD.)*

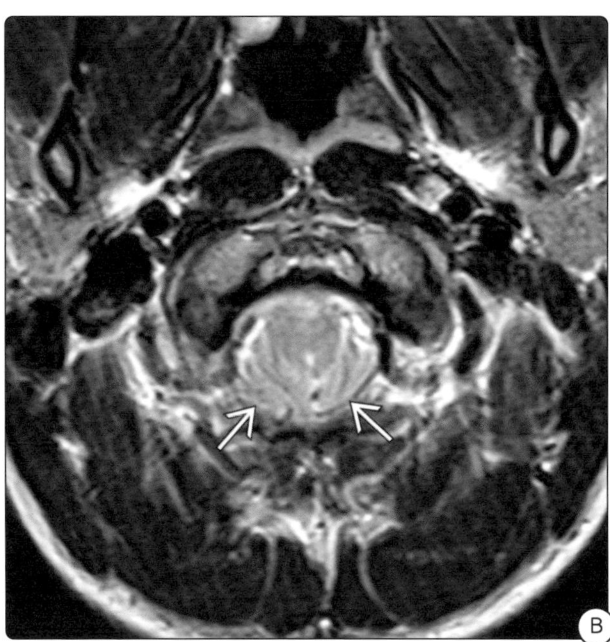


*(41-3B) Axial T2 MR in the same patient shows "crowded" foramen magnum with obliterated retrotonsillar CSF spaces ➡.*

Midline tonsillar descent 5 mm or more below the BOL—often considered diagnostic of CM1—is, by itself, a poor criterion for definitive diagnosis. Tonsils 6 mm below the FM are common during the first decade of life. Almost 15% of normal patients have tonsils that lie 1-4 mm below the FM, and 0.5-1.0% have tonsils that project 5 mm into the upper cervical canal.

Great caution should be exercised in establishing a diagnosis of CM1, especially on the basis of borderline tonsillar ectopia alone. Unless (1) the tonsils appear compressed and pointed (peg-like) instead of gently rounded **(41-2)**, (2) the tonsillar folia are angled obliquely or inferiorly (instead of horizontally), and (3) the retrocerebellar CSF spaces at the FM/C1 level are effaced **(41-3B)**, the diagnosis may not be warranted. Low-lying tonsils that retain their rounded shapes and are surrounded by normal-appearing CSF spaces are usually asymptomatic and of no diagnostic significance.

**CT Findings.** NECT scans may reveal a "crowded" FM and effaced retrotonsillar CSF space. However, beware of streak artifact at the skull base mimicking tonsillar ectopia. Bone CT often demonstrates a combination of undersized, shallow posterior cranial fossa, short clivus, and CVJ assimilation anomalies.

**MR Findings.** Sagittal T1 and T2 scans show "pointed" tonsils with more vertically oriented folia, obliterated FM subarachnoid spaces, and a "crowded" FM **(41-4)** **(41-5)**. The fourth ventricle usually appears normal. In severe cases, the dorsal cervicomedullary junction may be "kinked" or may demonstrate a dorsal "bump," which is typically the result of longstanding pistoning of the tonsils causing remodeling of the dorsal cervicomedullary junction **(41-6)**.

Sagittal phase-contrast CSF flow studies show diminished or absent alternating bright (systolic) and dark (diastolic) signals behind the cervicomedullary junction. Any change in signal intensity of the cerebellar tonsils on phase contrast sequences suggests tonsillar pulsations **(41-7)**, sometimes referred to as "pistoning". Cine MR may directly show this abnormal tonsillar motion/pistoning.

The proximal cervical spinal cord should be carefully examined for the presence of a syrinx. T2/FLAIR parenchymal hyperintensity without frank cyst formation may indicate a "presyrinx" state.

## Differential Diagnosis

*Congenital* tonsillar descent (CM1) must be distinguished from **normal variants** (mild uncomplicated tonsillar ectopia). The most important pathologic differential diagnosis is *acquired* tonsillar herniation caused by increased intracranial pressure **or** intracranial hypotension.

**Increased intracranial pressure** due to supratentorial mass effect with transmission of the pressure cone through the tentorial incisura can be easily distinguished from CM1. Signs of descending transtentorial herniation are present along with downward midbrain displacement. Tonsillar herniation in such cases is a secondary effect and should *not* be termed "acquired Chiari 1."

**Intracranial hypotension** shows a constellation of other findings besides inferiorly displaced tonsils. "Slumping" midbrain, enlarged pituitary gland, draping of the optic chiasm and hypothalamus over the dorsum sellae, engorged venous sinuses, and dura-arachnoid thickening and enhancement are typical abnormalities. *Mistaking intracranial hypotension for*

*CM1 can have disastrous consequences due to the very different treatments and management strategies for each.*

Approximately 20% of patients with **idiopathic intracranial hypertension** exhibit cerebellar tonsillar ectopia ≥ 5 mm. 50% have a peg-like tonsil configuration, and many have a low-lying obex. Looking for other signs of idiopathic intracranial hypertension (e.g., optic nerve head protrusion into the globe) is essential to avoid misdiagnosis as CM1.

## CHIARI 1 IMAGING

**General Features**

- Caudal tonsillar ectopia [≥ 5 mm below foramen magnum (FM)]
- Pointed, peg-like tonsils with angled folia
- "Crowded" FM with effaced CSF spaces
- Diminished/absent CSF flow at FM
- Syrinx prevalence
  - 40-80% symptomatic patients

**Differential Diagnosis**

- Normal "low-lying" tonsils (rounded, no disturbed CSF flow)
- Acquired herniation (elevated intracranial pressure, intracranial hypotension)

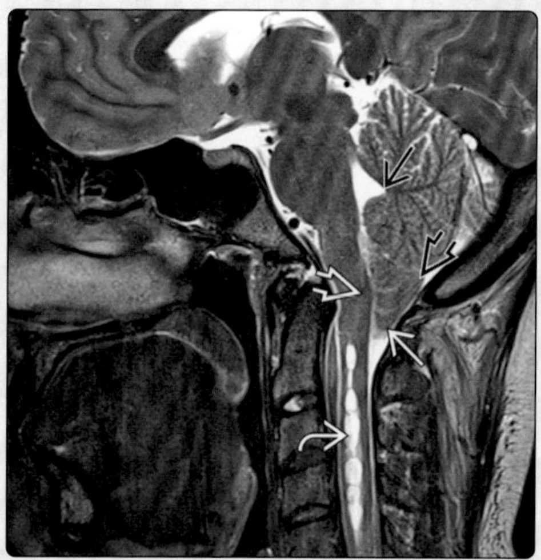

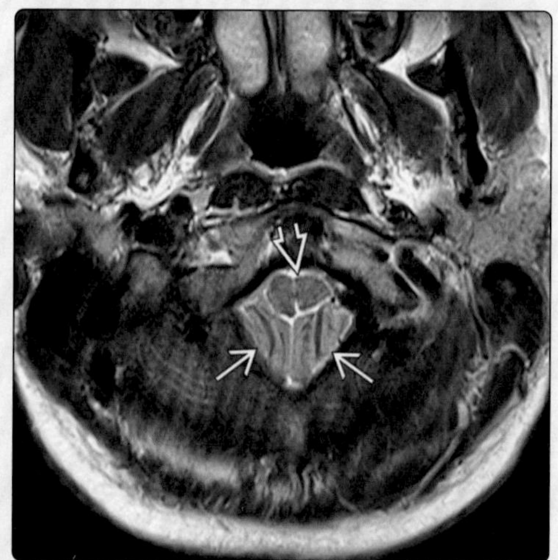

***(41-4)** Sagittal T2 MR of CM1 shows "pointed" tonsil ➔, obliquely oriented tonsillar folia ➔. Multiple septations in a syrinx cavity are clearly seen ➔. The fastigium ➔ is normal, but the inferior 4th ventricle is somewhat elongated, and the nucleus gracilis ➔ is slightly low lying. **(41-5)** T2WI in the same patient shows tonsils ➔ and a compressed and slightly deformed medulla ➔, giving the appearance of the "crowded" foramen magnum typical of CM1.*

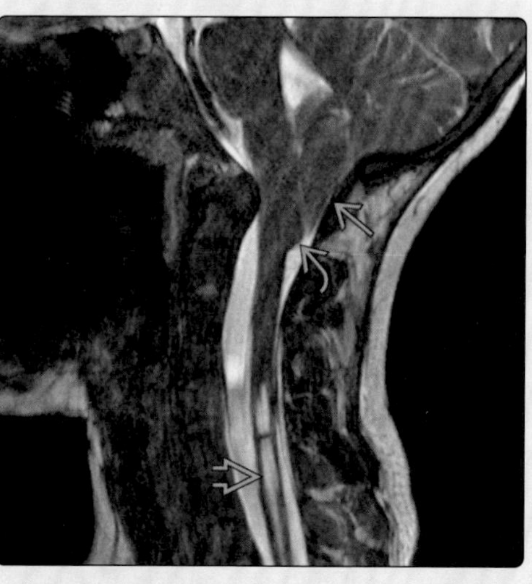

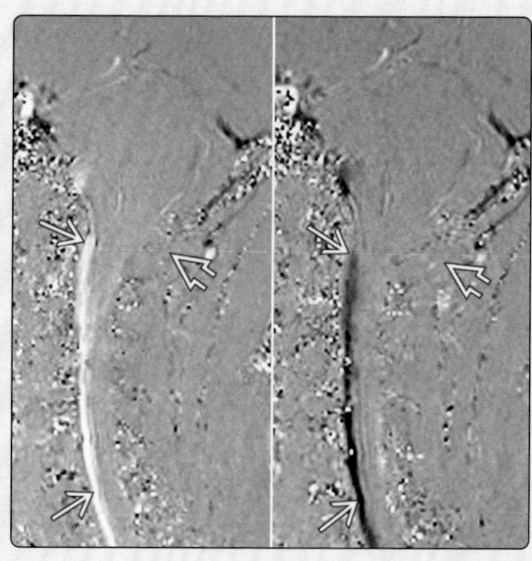

***(41-6)** Sagittal FIESTA in a child with CM1 shows ectopic pointed cerebellar tonsils ➔, severe effacement of CSF spaces, dorsal cervicomedullary bump or kink ➔, and a cervical cord syrinx ➔. **(41-7)** Sagittal phase-contrast CSF flow study in systole (L) and diastole (R) shows normal CSF flow ➔ in front of the cervicomedullary junction and no posterior flow in the foramen magnum ➔. Tonsillar "crowding" and adhesions prevent normal CSF circulation.*

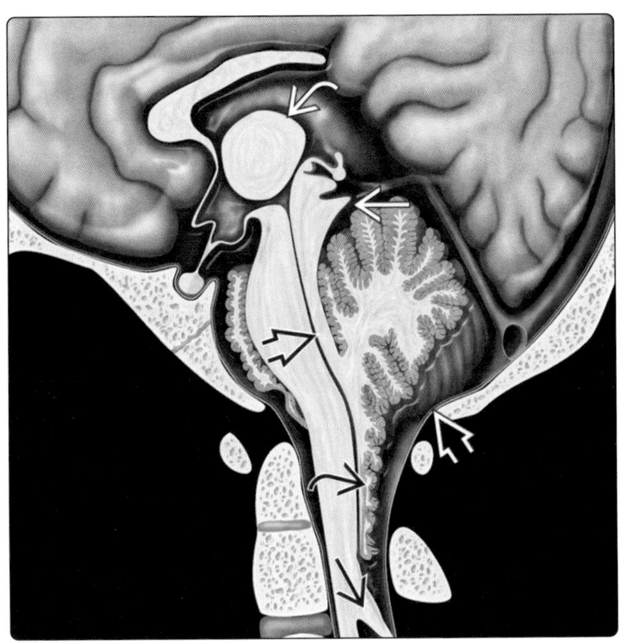

**(41-8)** *Graphic shows CM2 with small posterior fossa ➡, large massa intermedia ➡, "beaked" tectum ➡, callosal dysgenesis, elongated 4th ventricle ➡ with "cascade" of inferiorly displaced nodulus ➡ and choroid plexus, and medullary spur ➡.*

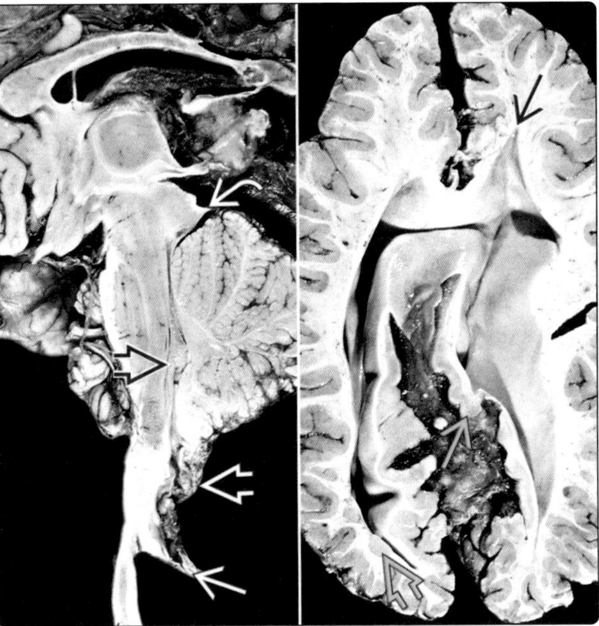

**(41-9)** *(L) CM2 shows medullary spur ➡, nodulus ➡ behind medulla, elongated 4th ventricle ➡, beaked tectum ➡. (R) CM2 has stenogyria ➡, heterotopic GM ➡, pointed lateral ventricles ➡. (Courtesy T. P Naidich, MD and E. T. Hedley-Whyte, MD.)*

# Chiari 2

## Terminology and Definition

Chiari 2 malformation (CM2) is a complex hindbrain malformation that is caused by an associated myelodysplasia (neural tube defect), almost always an open neural tube defect.

## Etiology

**General Concepts.** CM2 is postulated to arise due to fetal brain development in the setting of a CSF leak from the open neural tube defect and resultant intracranial hypotension. The CSF leak leads to collapse of the developing ventricular system and caudal displacement of the posterior fossa structures, resulting in a small posterior fossa and hindbrain structures. The etiology of other associated anomalies, such as callosal dysplasia and falcine deficiency, are not as well understood but are also likely secondary to the neural tube defect.

**Genetics.** Nearly 1/2 of all neural tube closure anomalies have mutations on the methylene-tetra-hydrofolate reductase gene (*MTHFR*). Maternal folate deficiency and teratogens, such as anticonvulsants, have been linked to increased risk of CM2.

## Pathology

Grossly, a broad spectrum of findings can be present in CM2. Myelomeningocele and a small posterior fossa with concave clivus and petrous pyramids are virtually always present **(41-8)**. The cerebellar vermis (typically the nodulus) is displaced inferiorly along the dorsal aspect of the cervical spinal cord. The fourth ventricle, pons, and medulla are elongated and partially dislocated into the cervical spinal canal. The lower medulla may be kinked.

Unlike CM1, supratentorial abnormalities are the rule in CM2, not the exception. Hydrocephalus is present in the majority of cases. Corpus callosum dysgenesis and gray matter anomalies, such as subependymal gray matter heterotopia, are common.

## Clinical Issues

**Epidemiology and Demographics.** The overall prevalence of CM2 is 0.44 in 1,000 live births but has been decreasing with prophylactic maternal folate therapy. A dose of 4 mg per day reduces the risk of CM2 by at least 70%.

**Presentation.** CM2 is identified in utero with ultrasound or fetal screening for elevated α-fetoprotein. At birth, coexistent myelomeningocele and hydrocephalus are dominant clinical features in > 90% of cases. Lower cranial nerve deficits, apneic spells, and bulbar signs may be present. Lower extremity paralysis, sphincter dysfunction, and spasticity often develop later.

**Treatment Options.** Fetal repair of myelomeningocele is increasingly common and may reduce subsequent symptoms. Surgical repair within 72 hours following delivery reduces mortality and morbidity from the open dysraphism.

## Imaging

CM2 affects many regions of the skull, brain, and spine, so a variety of imaging abnormalities may be seen.

**Skull and Dura.** The calvarial vault forms from membranous bone. With failure of neural tube closure and absence of fetal brain distention, normal induction of the calvarial membranous plates does not occur. Disorganized collections of collagen fibers and deficient radial growth of the developing calvarium ensue, resulting in **lacunar skull** (i.e., Lückenschädel) **(41-10)**.

Focal calvarial thinning and a scooped-out appearance are typical imaging findings of lacunar skull. The calvarium appears thinned with numerous circular or oval lucent defects and shallow depressions. The craniofenestra diminish with age and typically resolve by six months, although some scalloping of the inner table often persists into adulthood.

A **small, shallow, bony posterior fossa** with low-lying transverse sinuses is almost always present in CM2. A **large, "gaping" FM** is common. **Concave petrous temporal bones** and a **short concave clivus** are often present **(41-12)**.

Dural abnormalities are common. A widened, open, **heart-shaped tentorial incisura** and **thinned, hypoplastic**, or **fenestrated falx** are frequent findings. The fenestrated falx allows gyri to cross the midline. Interdigitating gyri and the deficient falx result in the appearance of an **irregular interhemispheric fissure** on imaging studies **(41-11C) (41-15)**.

**Midbrain, Hindbrain, and Cerebellum.** Hindbrain and cerebellum anomalies are a constant in CM2. The medulla and inferior cerebellum are displaced downward into the upper cervical canal for a variable distance. A **cervicomedullary "kink"** with a **medullary "spur"** is common in the upper cervical canal but may lie as low as T1-T4 in severe cases **(41-9)**.

On sagittal T1 and T2 scans, the inferiorly displaced vermis, medulla, and choroid plexus form a **"cascade" of tissue** that protrudes downward through the gaping FM to lie behind the spinal cord. The superiorly herniated cerebellum may compress and deform the quadrigeminal plate, giving the appearance of a **beaked tectum (41-13)**.

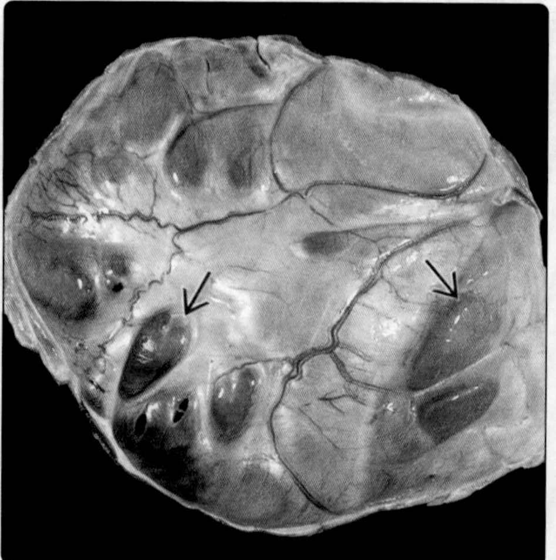

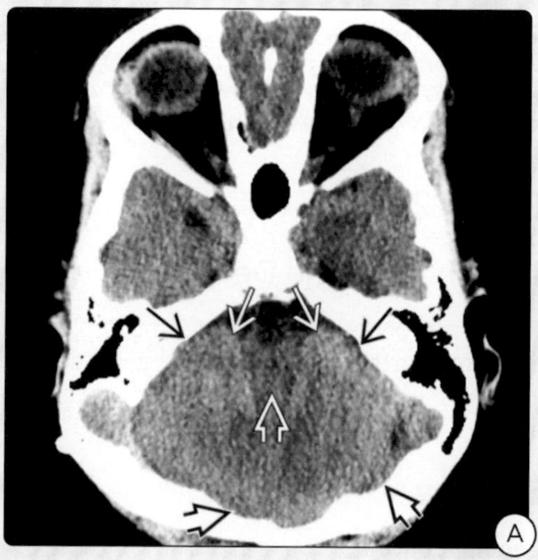


***(41-10)** Autopsy case of lacunar (Lückenschädel) skull in CM2 shows multiple scooped-out foci of thinned, almost translucent bone ➙. (Courtesy R. Hewlett, MD.) **(41-11A)** NECT of CM2 shows small posterior fossa with concave petrous ridges ➙, scalloped inner table ➙, no visible 4th ventricle, and "creeping" cerebellar hemispheres ➙ almost enveloping an elongated, inferiorly stretched medulla ➙.*

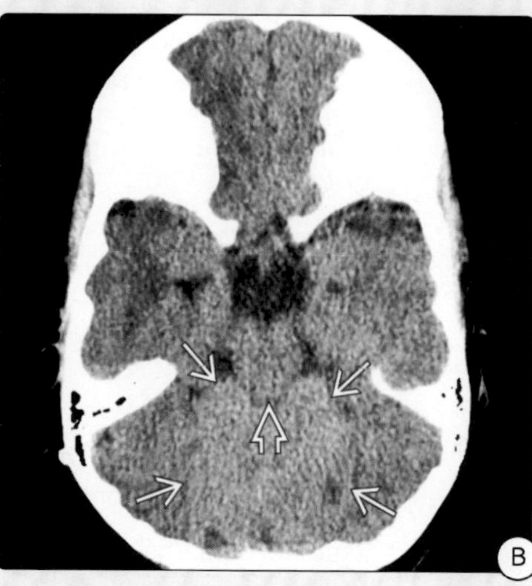


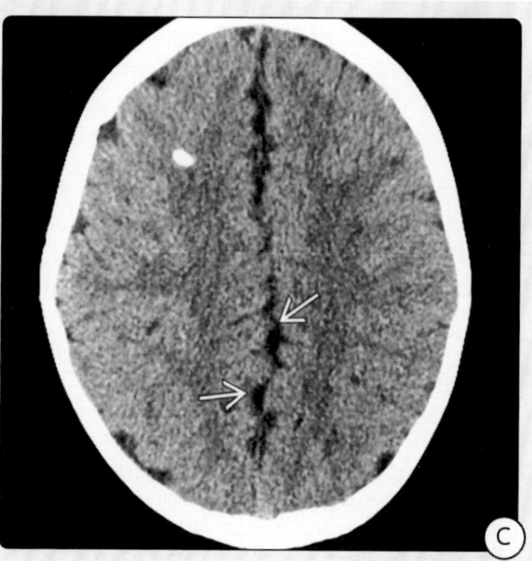


***(41-11B)** NECT in the same patient shows widely gaping, heart-shaped incisura with "towering" cerebellum protruding superiorly ➙ and mild "beaking" of the tectum ➙. **(41-11C)** More cephalad scan in the same patient shows the typical serrated appearance of the interhemispheric fissure ➙ due to the interdigitating gyri typically seen in CM2.*

In addition to the cephalocaudal displacement of posterior fossa contents, the cerebellar hemispheres often curve anteromedially around the brainstem. In severe cases, the pons and medulla appear nearly engulfed by the "creeping" cerebellum on axial imaging studies.

The cerebellar hemispheres are pushed upward through the incisura, giving the appearance of a **towering cerebellum** on coronal T1 and T2 scans.

**Ventricles.** Abnormalities of the ventricles are present in > 90% of CM2 patients. The fourth ventricle is caudally displaced, typically lacks a fastigium (dorsal point), and appears thin and elongated **("soda straw" fourth ventricle) (41-13) (41-14)**. The third ventricle is often large and has a very **prominent massa intermedia (41-13)**.

The lateral ventricles vary in size and configuration. Hydrocephalus is almost always present at birth, but sometimes develops later, and usually requires shunting. The atria and occipital horns are often disproportionately enlarged **("colpocephaly")**, suggesting the presence of callosal and forceps major dysgenesis.

Following shunting, the lateral ventricles frequently retain a **serrated** or **scalloped appearance**. A large CSF space between the occipital lobes often persists.

**Cerebral Hemispheres.** Malformations of cortical development, such as subependymal gray matter heterotopia, are common, especially in cases with hydrocephalus. In those patients with severe hydrocephalus treated with shunting, there is development of numerous and narrow gyri ("stenogyria") **(41-15)**.

**Callosal dysgenesis** is found in nearly 2/3 of all cases, and **abnormalities of the fornices** are also common.

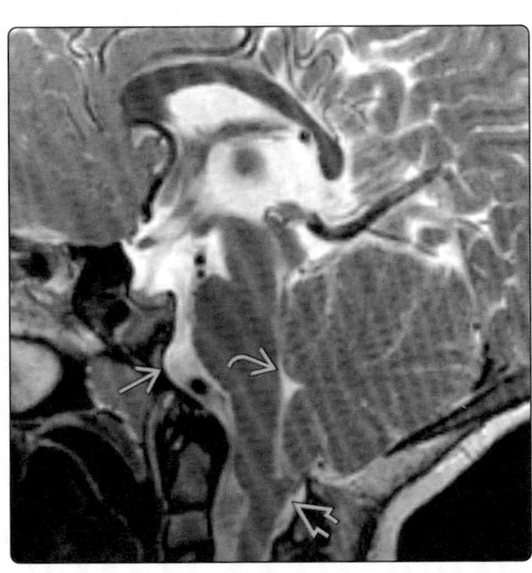

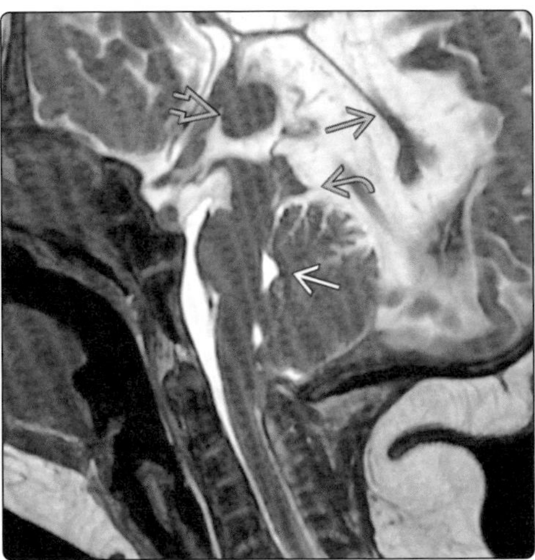

***(41-12)** Sagittal T2 MR shows a mild CM2 with low torcular, scalloped clivus ➙, small 4th ventricle ➙, large foramen magnum, and dorsal cervicomedullary kink ➙. **(41-13)** Sagittal FIESTA in a moderate CM2 shows a small posterior fossa, callosal dysgenesis ➙, large masa intermedia ➙, beaked tectum ➙, and blunted 4th ventricular fastigium ➙.*

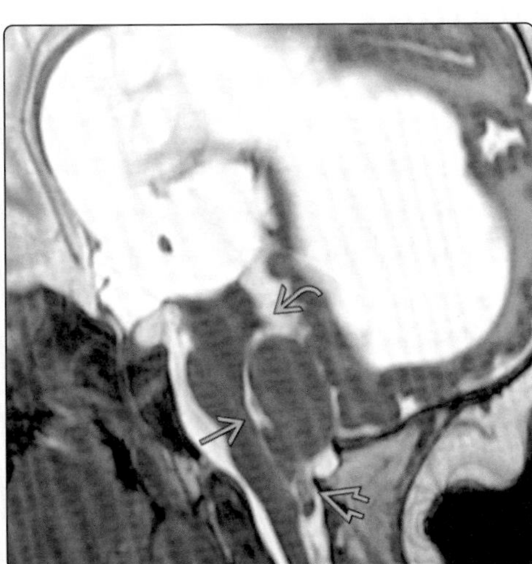

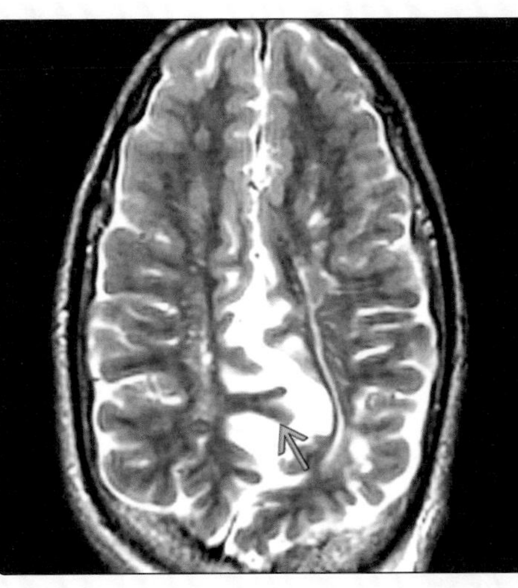

***(41-14)** Sagittal FIESTA in a severe CM2 shows an extremely small posterior fossa and cerebellum with small 4th ventricle ➙, ectopic inferior cerebellum ➙, beaked tectum ➙, and severe hydrocephalus. Hydrocephalus is seen in almost all CM2s, especially without in utero repair. **(41-15)** Axial T2 MR in previously shunted CM2 shows a deficient falx with supernumerary thin gyri ("stenogyria") ➙ interdigitating across the midline.*

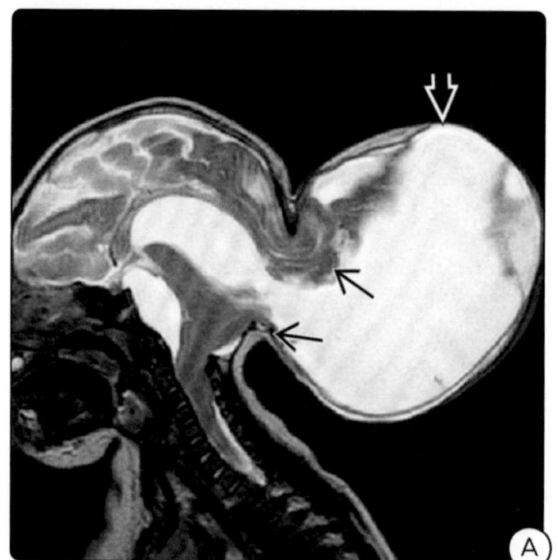

*(41-16A) Sagittal T2 shows CM3 with cephalocele ⇨ that contains herniated dysplastic brain ➡ and CSF in continuity with a lateral ventricle.*

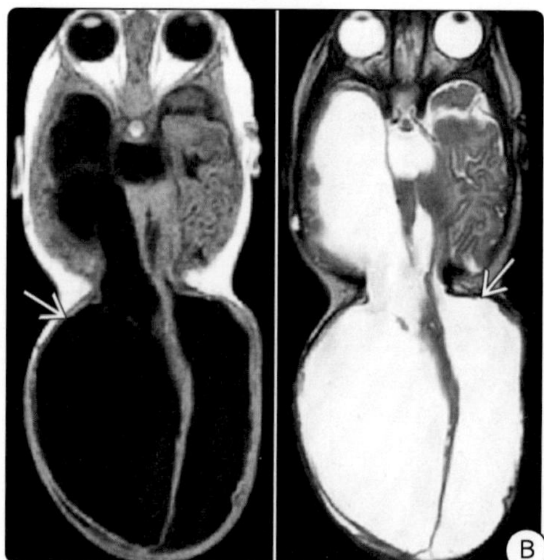

*(41-16B) Axial T1 (L), T2 (R) MRs in the same patient show extension of the lateral ventricles ➡ into the cephalocele.*

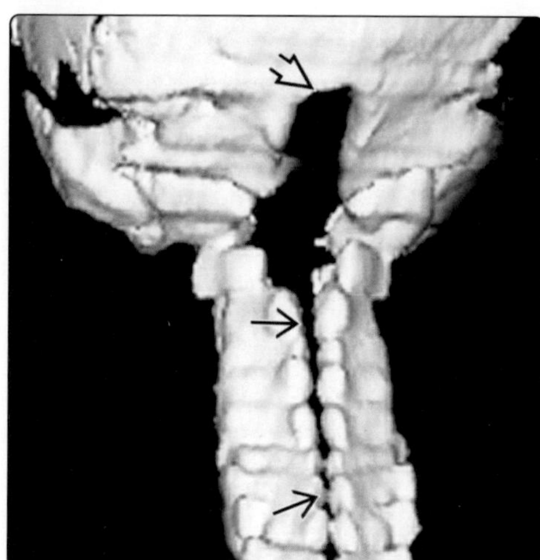

*(41-17) CM3 is shown with extensive cranium bifidum extending from the occipital bone ⇨ through the entire cervical spine ➡.*

**Spine and Spinal Cord.** Open spinal dysraphism with **myelomeningocele** is present in almost all cases of CM2. **Hydrosyringomyelia** is seen in ~ 50%.

## Differential Diagnosis

The major differential diagnosis of CM2 is other Chiari malformations.

In **Chiari 1**, myelomeningocele is absent, and, other than being somewhat small, the posterior fossa and its contents appear relatively normal.

If findings of CM2 + a low occipital or high cervical cephalocele are present, the diagnosis is **Chiari 3**.

### CHIARI 2 MALFORMATION

**Pathoetiology**
- Complex hindbrain malformation with myelomeningocele
  - Posterior neuropore closure disorder
  - Fetal brain forms in setting of CSF leak
  - Results in hindbrain herniation and small posterior fossa

**Clinical Issues**
- Prevalence reduced with maternal folate
- Myelomeningocele, hydrocephalus dominate clinical picture at birth

**Imaging Findings**
- Myelomeningocele (almost always)
- Lacunar skull
- Small posterior fossa
- Abnormal dura (heart-shaped incisura, fenestrated falx)
- Inferiorly displaced medulla and inferior cerebellum
- Cervicomedullary "kink," medullary "spur"
- "Towering" and "creeping" cerebellum
- "Soda straw" 4th ventricle
- Prominent massa intermedia
- Hydrocephalus, shunted ventricles appear scalloped
- Callosal dysgenesis
- Periventricular nodular heterotopia, stenogyria after shunting

# Chiari 3

Chiari 3 malformation (CM3) is the rarest of the Chiari malformations. CM3 consists of a small posterior fossa with a caudally displaced brainstem and variable herniation of meninges/posterior fossa contents through a low occipital or upper cervical bony defect.

The cephalocele contains meninges together with variable amounts of brain tissue, vessels, and CSF spaces. The brain is often featureless, dysplastic-appearing, and disorganized with extensive gliosis and gray matter heterotopias.

NECT scans show bony features similar to those seen in CM2, i.e., a small posterior cranial fossa, short, scalloped clivus, lacunar skull, a defect in the ventral chondral portion of the supraoccipital bone, and low cranium bifidum that may extend inferiorly to involve much of the cervical spine **(41-17)**.

MR best delineates sac contents, which often include dysplastic-appearing cerebellum &/or brainstem, as well as distorted CSF spaces and vessels. A deformed fourth and, sometimes, third ventricle can be partially found within the mass of herniated brain and meninges. Vascular structures, both venous and arterial, are sometimes "pulled" into the defect **(41-16)**.

# Hindbrain Malformations

## Cystic Posterior Fossa Anomalies

### Terminology

Cystic posterior fossa anomalies include a spectrum or "continuum" of cystic abnormalities, including Classic Dandy-Walker malformation (DWM), vermian hypoplasia (VH), Blake pouch cyst (BPC), and mega cisterna magna (MCM). Arachnoid cysts are also considered in the posterior fossa cystic malformation differential diagnosis. Due to overlapping features and inconsistency in definitions, the Dandy-Walker continuum terminology has been a source of confusion for many radiologists. In past iterations, there has been an emphasis on the cystic portion of the malformation and less emphasis on the anatomic changes in the cerebellum, the vermis in particular. A most recent attempt to refine the "Dandy-Walker phenotype" by Whitehead et al has resulted in five distinct diagnoses: **DWM**, **inferior VH (IVH), VH, BPC**, and **VH + BPC**. This newest refinement of neuroimaging criteria is based upon five anatomic features of the posterior fossa: 1) Vermis, 2) tegmentovermian angle (TVA), 3) fastigial recess, 4) tail sign, and 5) taenia/tela choroidea complex/choroid plexus location (TCC/CPL) **(Table 41-1)**. The main goal of the neuroradiologist should be to accurately describe the posterior fossa anatomy **and** identify associated supratentorial abnormalities (e.g., hydrocephalus).

A key component of this system is assessing the vermis and whether it is hypoplastic based upon the major vermian landmarks (i.e., primary fissure).

The traditional definition of the **classic DWM** has focused on cystic enlargement of the posterior fossa with elevation of the torcular Herophili. Whitehead et al have suggested that posterior fossa size and torcular location should no longer be considered diagnostic criteria for this diagnosis. Rather, the

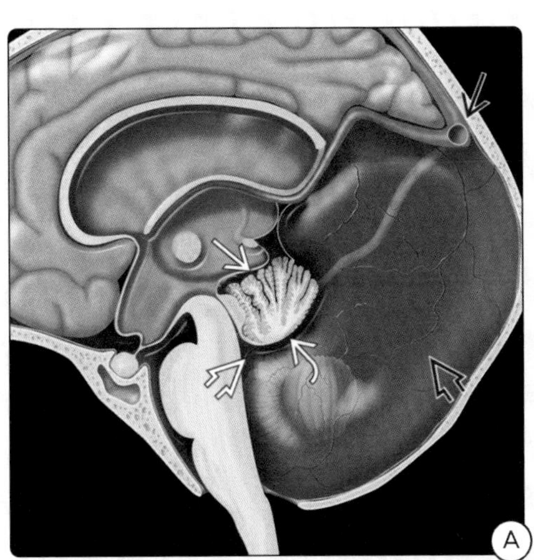


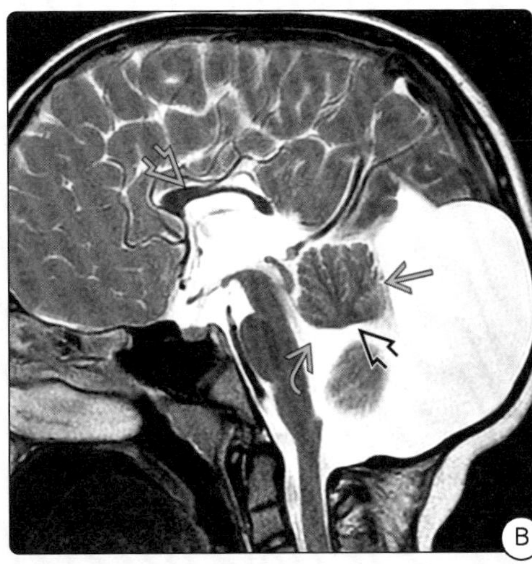


***(41-18A)** Graphic shows typical findings of DWM with IVH, ↑ TVA, and obtuse fastigial angle. The posterior fossa is also enlarged and the torcular Herophili elevated, but these are no longer diagnostic criteria for DWM. **(41-18B)** Sagittal T2 MR shows IVH, ↑ TVA, and obtuse fastigial recess, consistent with DWM. Also note the dysplastic corpus callosum.*

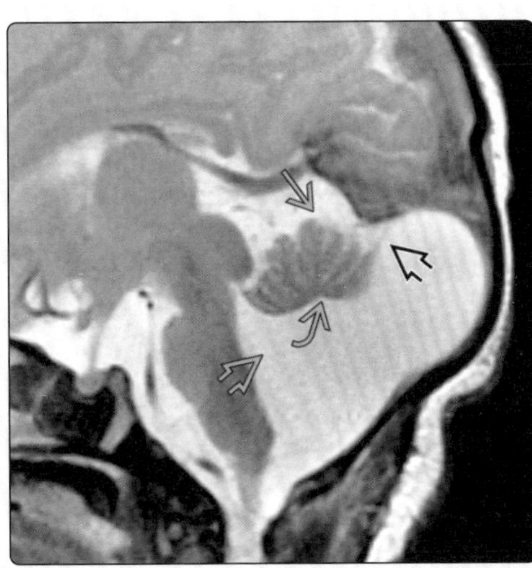

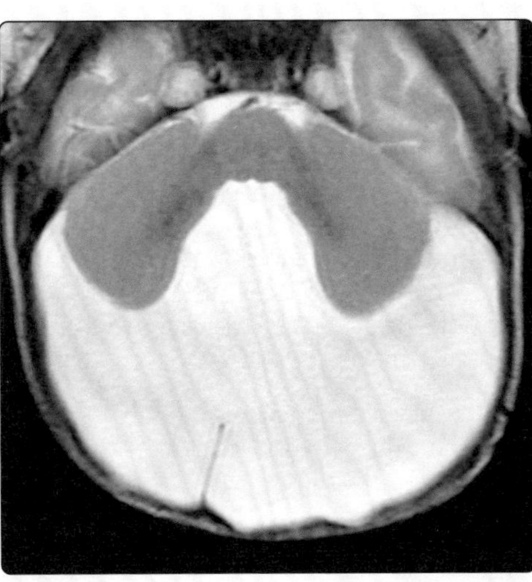

***(41-19)** Sagittal T2 MR in a newborn with DWM shows IVH, obtuse fastigial angle, ↑ TVA, and tail sign. While the posterior fossa is only mildly enlarged, this patient has all the features of DWM. **(41-20)** Axial T2 MR in a 2-month-old with DWM shows marked cystic enlargement of the posterior fossa with splaying of the cerebellar hemispheres in a winged configuration.*

## Refined Dandy-Walker Malformation Neuroimaging Criteria

| Diagnosis | Vermis | TVA | Fastigial Recess | Tail Sign | TTC/CP |
|---|---|---|---|---|---|
| Dandy-Walker malformation | IVH | Increased | Obtuse | Present | Down and out |
| IVH | IVH | Normal | Acute | Absent | Up and in |
| VH | DVH | Normal | Acute | Absent | Up and in |
| BPC | Normal | Increased | Acute | Absent | Up and in |
| VH + BPC | VH | Increased | Acute | Absent | Up and in |

***(Table 41-1)*** *TVA = tegmentovermian angle; TTC/CP = taenia-tela choroidea complex/choroid plexus location; IVH = inferior vermian hypoplasia; VH = vermian hypoplasia; DVH = diffuse vermian hypoplasia; BPC = Blake pouch cyst.*

Whitehead et al: Refining the neuroimaging definition of the Dandy-Walker phenotype. AJNR. 2022.

diagnosis of **DWM** is defined as having IVH + increased TVA + obtuse fastigial recess ± tail sign ± down and out location of the TCC/CPL.

**VH** (old term = "Dandy-Walker variant") is divided into 1) **IVH** and 2) **VH**. The major anatomic landmark of the vermis in the sagittal view is the primary fissure. Approximately 1/3 of the vermis should be above the primary fissure and ~ 2/3 of the vermis should be below the primary fissure. The diagnosis of IVH is made when < 1/2 the vermian tissue is below the primary fissure **(41-21)**. In contrast, VH is defined as a diffusely small vermis with normal proportions of vermian tissue above and below the primary fissure **(41-22)**.

**BPC** is defined as a normal vermis + increased TVA + normal fastigial recess **(41-23)**. A common pitfall is the misdiagnosis of IVH whenever the TVA is increased. If the vermis is normal, but simply rotated up and away, the diagnosis is BPC.

## Etiology

**Etiology and Genetics.** Three main genes have been associated with DWM: *FOXC1* and the linked *ZIC1* and *ZIC4* genes.

DWM is accompanied by > 18 types of chromosomal abnormality and cooccurs with > 40 genetic syndromes. In addition, DWM can arise as a result of maternal diabetes or fetal infection (e.g., cytomegalovirus or Zika virus).

## Pathology

**Gross Pathology.** The most common findings in DWM are (1) an enlarged posterior fossa with (2) upward displacement of the tentorium and accompanying venous sinuses and (3) cystic dilatation of the fourth ventricle. Vermian abnormalities range from complete absence to varying degrees of hypoplasia. The posterior fossa cyst in DWM is typically lined by an outer layer of pia-arachnoid and an inner layer of ependyma.

DWM is frequently associated with other CNS anomalies. Almost 2/3 of patients have gyral abnormalities (e.g., pachy- or polymicrogyria and heterotopic gray matter). Callosal dysgenesis and hydrocephalus are common.

## Clinical Issues

DWM occurs in ~ 1:30,000. The most common presentation is increased intracranial pressure secondary to hydrocephalus.

## Imaging

The spectrum of imaging abnormalities in classic DWM is broad, affecting—to varying degrees—the skull and dura, ventricles and CSF spaces, and brain.

**Skull and Dura, Venous Sinuses.** In contrast to CM2 in which the posterior fossa is abnormally small, the posterior fossa in DWM is usually enlarged, sometimes dramatically so. The straight sinus, sinus confluence, and tentorial apex are usually elevated, sometimes above the lambdoid suture ("lambdoid-torcular inversion"). The transverse sinuses descend at a steep angle from the torcular Herophili toward the sigmoid sinuses **(41-18)**. While posterior fossa size and elevation of the torcular Herophili are not considered diagnostic criteria in the most recent Whitehead et al classification system, they are seen in the vast majority of DWM.

The occipital bone may appear scalloped, focally thinned, and remodeled. Retrocerebellar CSF cysts often demonstrate partially infolded dura-arachnoid (falx cerebelli) on axial T2 scans. The falx cerebelli is often absent in DWM.

**Ventricles and Cisterns.** In DWM and BPC, the fourth ventricle opens dorsally to a variably sized CSF-containing cyst that balloons posteriorly behind and between the cerebellar hemisphere remnants. This causes an increase in the TVA in both DWM and BPC. In DWM, the normal fastigium is absent or significantly attenuated to form an obtuse angle. In all other posterior fossa malformations, the relatively acute angle of the fastigial recess is maintained. Sometimes visible in DWM is a raised and dysplastic fourth ventricle roof, referred to as the tail sign **(41-19)**. In DWM, the choroid plexus is displaces inferiorly and laterally ("down and out").

Generalized obstructive hydrocephalus is present in > 80% of neonates with DWM at birth. If callosal dysgenesis is present, the lateral ventricles are widely separated and may have unusually prominent occipital horns (colpocephaly).

Axial images in DWM often demonstrate marked enlargement of the fourth ventricular vallecula and lateral displacement of the cerebellar hemispheres in a winged appearance **(41-20)**.

**Brainstem, Cerebellum, and Vermis.** The brainstem appears normal in mild forms of DWM but often appears somewhat small in moderate to more severe DWM.

Varying degrees of VH are seen in DWM. In DWM, the vermian remnant is rotated and elevated above the large posterior fossa cyst **(41-18)**.

The cerebellar hemispheres are often hypoplastic in DWM, and, in severe cases, the cerebellar remnants appear "winged" outward and displaced anterolaterally.

A normal vermis should have ~ 2/3 of the vermis inferior/posterior to the primary fissure. The diagnosis of IVH is made when < 1/2 the vermian tissue is below the primary fissure. In contrast, VH is defined as a diffusely small vermis with normal proportions of vermian tissue above and below the primary fissure.

**Associated Abnormalities.** Other CNS abnormalities are present in 70% of DWM. The most common finding is callosal agenesis or dysgenesis. A dorsal interhemispheric cyst may be present. Gray matter abnormalities (e.g., heterotopias, clefts, and pachy- and polymicrogyria) are common associated abnormalities. Hydrocephalus is seen in the majority of DWM cases. Careful attention and description of associated anomalies is important because they often have an equal or greater influence on the patient's prognosis.

## Differential Diagnosis

A **retrocerebellar arachnoid cyst** is an important differential diagnosis and, when small, can be difficult to distinguish from a MCM. It is an arachnoid-lined cyst located behind the vermis and fourth ventricle that does not communicate with the latter. When large, an arachnoid cyst may cause mass effect on adjacent structures. The cerebellum otherwise appears normal. Veins and a falx cerebelli do not traverse the CSF collection.

An **MCM** is the mildest cystic posterior fossa anomaly with an enlarged retrocerebellar CSF collection (> 10 mm). There is no mass effect on the cerebellar hemispheres or vermis. The vermis is well formed and normal. Cerebellar veins and elements of the falx cerebelli can be seen crossing through the MCM, and the adjacent bone can appear scalloped by pulsatile CSF in the MCM **(41-24)**.

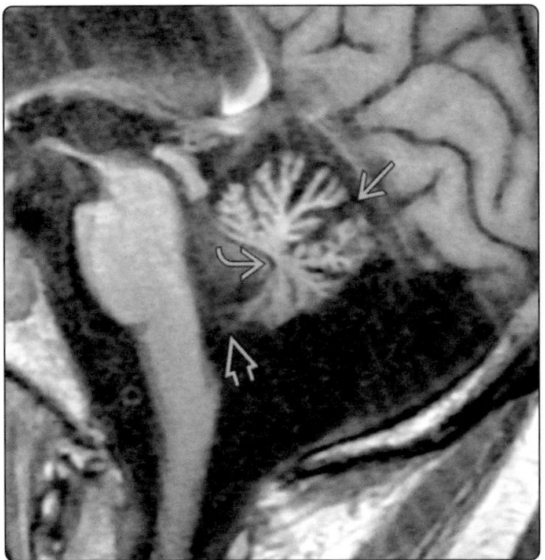

***(41-21)*** *Adult with IVH shows < 1/2 the vermis below the primary fissure ➡. Note the normal fastigium ➡ and TVA ➡.*

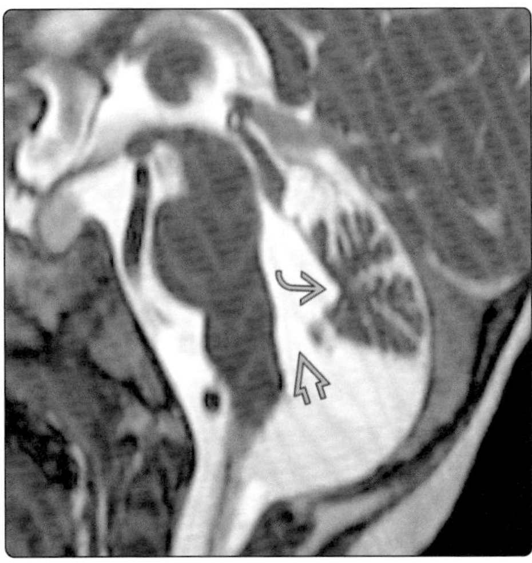

***(41-22)*** *1-year-old with VH shows diffusely small vermis, normal 2:1 inferior:superior vermian ratio, normal fastigium ➡, and TVA ➡.*

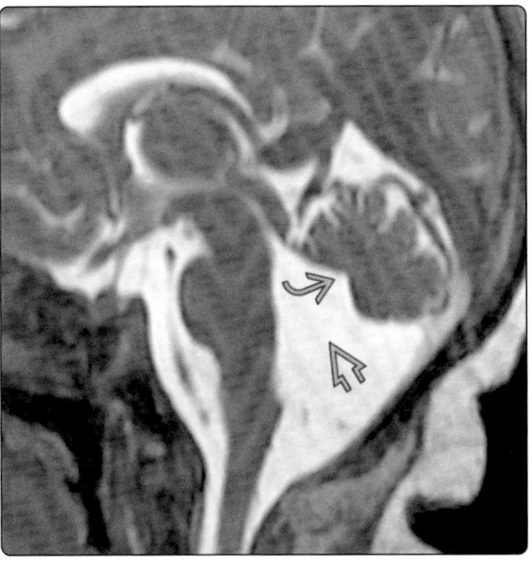

***(41-23)*** *Newborn with BPC shows a normal vermis that is rotated upward with ↑ TVA ➡ and normal fastigial angle ➡.*

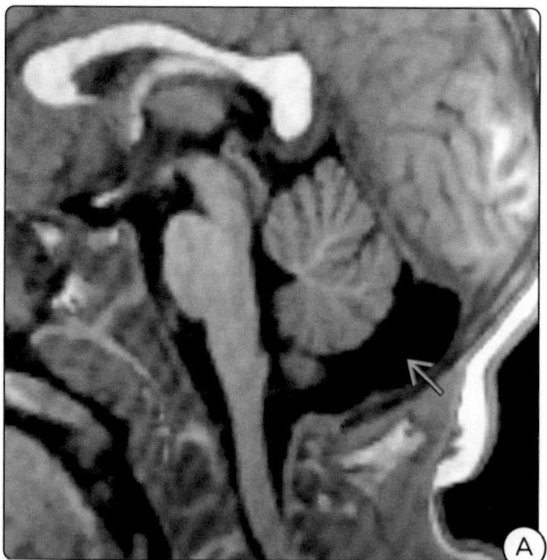

**(41-24A)** *Sagittal T1 MR in a 5-year-old with a mega cisterna magna ➡. Note the lack of mass effect and normal TVA.*

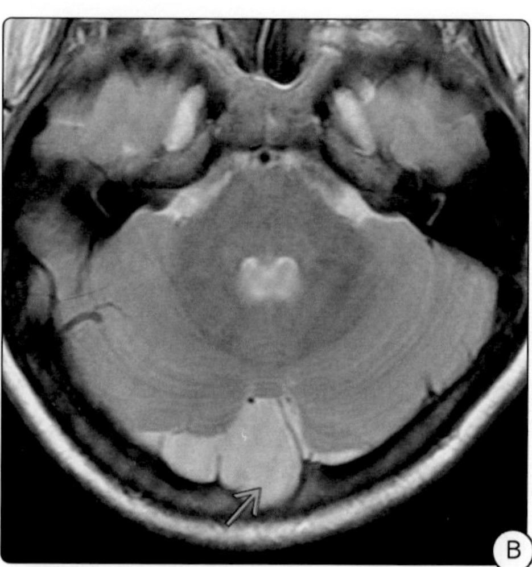

**(41-24B)** *Axial T2 MR in a child with mega cisterna magna (favored) ➡ vs. a small arachnoid cyst.*

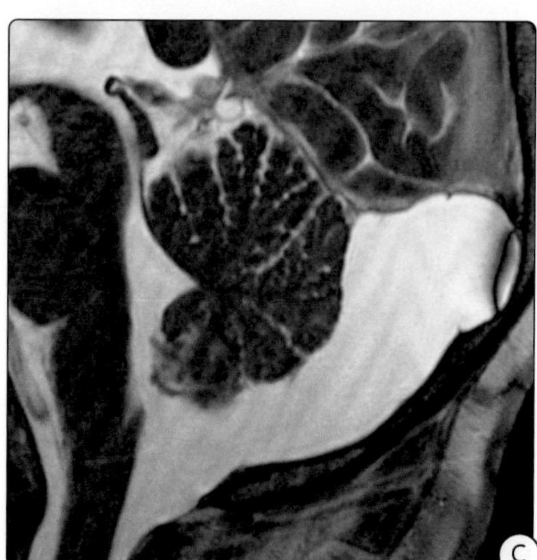

**(41-24C)** *Sagittal FIESTA shows a retrocerebellar cyst without mass effect, mega cisterna magna vs. small arachnoid cyst.*

### DANDY-WALKER CONTINUUM: DIFFERENTIAL DIAGNOSIS

**Dandy-Walker Malformation**
- Inferior vermian hypoplasia of varying degrees
- Increased tegmentovermian angle
- Cyst extending posteriorly from 4th ventricle
- Large posterior fossa
  - Elevated tentorium and torcular
- Cerebellar hemispheres often hypoplastic
  - May appear "winged" outward, displaced anterolaterally

**Inferior Vermian Hypoplasia**
- Reduced vermian tissue below primary fissure
- Normal tegmentovermian angle, fastigial recess

**Vermian Hypoplasia**
- Diffusely hypoplastic vermis
  - Maintains normal 2:1 inferior:superior vermian ratio
- Normal tegmentovermian angle, fastigial recess

**Blake Pouch Cyst**
- Normal vermis with increased tegmentovermian angle
- Normal fastigial recess

**Mega Cisterna Magna**
- Enlarged retrocerebellar CSF (> 10 mm)
- No mass effect on vermis or cerebellum
- Normal vermis
- Fluid crossed by veins, falx cerebelli
- May scallop, remodel occiput

**Arachnoid Cyst**
- When small, it is difficult to distinguish from mega cisterna magna
  - Differentiation not usually clinically significant when small
- More reliable differentiation from mega cisterna magna when large due to mass effect on adjacent structures
- No communication with 4th ventricle and subarachnoid spaces
- No crossing veins or falx cerebelli

# Miscellaneous Malformations

Several less common posterior fossa malformations are largely defined by imaging features. These include rhombencephalosynapsis, Joubert syndrome (JS), and cerebellar hypoplasias/dysplasias.

## Rhombencephalosynapsis

Rhombencephalosynapsis is a midline brain malformation characterized by (1) a "missing" cerebellar vermis and (2) apparent fusion of the cerebellar hemispheres. Dorsal midline continuity of the cerebellar hemispheres is characteristic.

Sagittal MR scans show an upwardly rounded fastigial recess of the fourth ventricle and lack of the normal midline foliar pattern of the vermis. Coronal and axial images show transverse folia and continuity of the cerebellar white matter across the midline **(41-25A)**. Images through the rostral fourth ventricle may demonstrate a diamond or pointed shape.

Aqueductal stenosis and hydrocephalus are seen in ~ 50% of cases **(41-25B)**. Other midline structures may be abnormal, including the cavum septi pellucidi, corpus callosum, optic chiasm/nerves, and olfactory bulbs.

## Joubert Syndrome and Related Disorders

JS and related disorders (JSRD) are a group of syndromes in which the hallmark is the molar tooth sign, a complex mid- and hindbrain malformation that resembles a molar tooth on axial MR scans. Multiple syndromes exhibit "molar tooth" posterior fossa malformations, so genetic analysis may be required to distinguish among different JSRD subtypes.

Midline sagittal MR scans show a small dysmorphic vermis. The fourth ventricle appears deformed with a thin upwardly convex roof and an elongated, rounded fastigium **(41-26)**.

Axial scans demonstrate the classic molar tooth appearance with foreshortened midbrain, narrow isthmus, deep interpeduncular fossa, and thickened elongated superior cerebellar peduncles surrounding an oblong or diamond-shaped fourth ventricle **(41-27)**. The superior vermis is characteristically clefted, usually best seen in the coronal plane. The cisterna magna may appear enlarged.

## Cerebellar Hypoplasia and Unclassified Dysplasias

Unclassified cerebellar dysplasias are not associated with other known malformations or syndromes. In severe cases of cerebellar hypoplasia, the cerebellar hemispheres and vermis are almost completely absent, and the pons is hypoplastic. Remote hemorrhage, infarct, or other insult should always be considered when the cerebellar hemispheres appear hypoplastic or dysplastic, especially when asymmetry is present.

*Selected References: The complete reference list is available on the eBooks+ version included with purchase.*

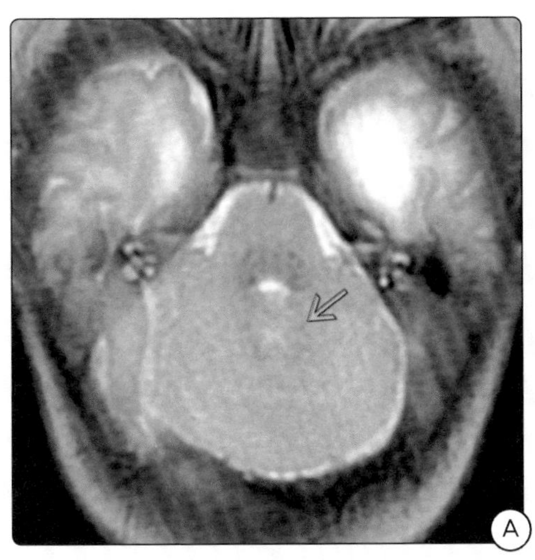


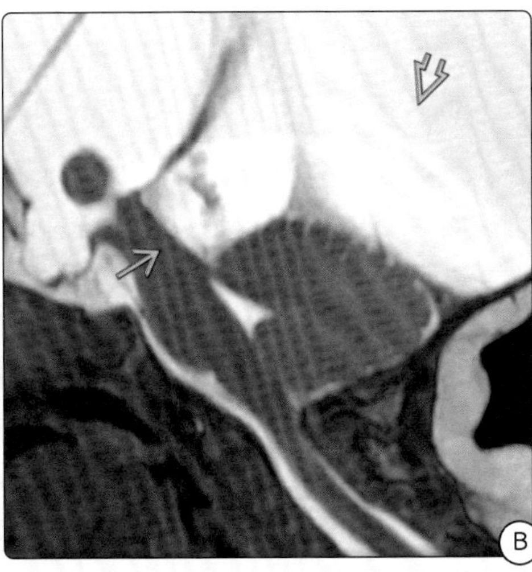


***(41-25A)** Axial T2 MR in a 2-month-old shows fusion of the dentate nuclei ➡ and absent vermis with continuity of the cerebellar hemispheres, consistent with rhombencephalosynapsis. **(41-25B)** Sagittal FIESTA in the same patient with rhombencephalosynapsis shows absence of the normal vermian landmarks (e.g., primary fissure) and associated aqueductal stenosis ➡ with hydrocephalus ⇨.*

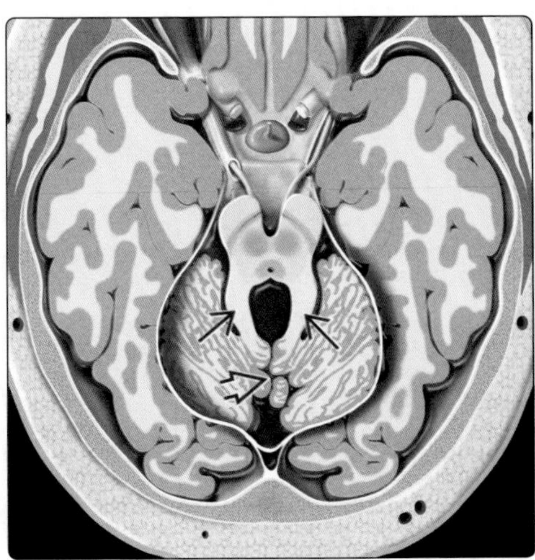

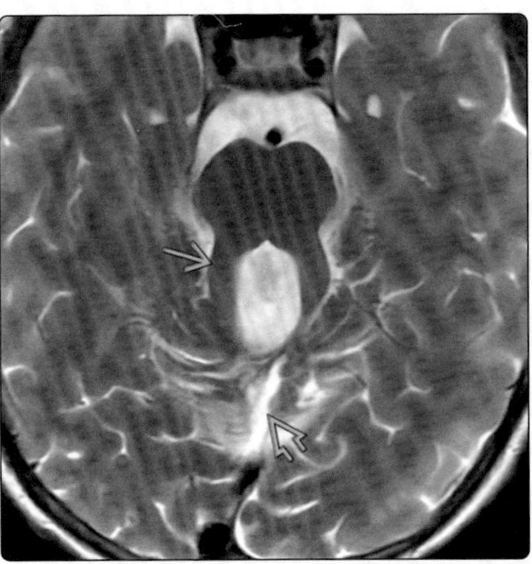

***(41-26)** Axial graphic shows Joubert malformation. Thickened superior cerebellar peduncles ➡ around an elongated 4th ventricle form the classic molar tooth sign. Note cleft cerebellar vermis ⇨. **(41-27)** Axial T2 MR shows thickened and elongated superior cerebellar peduncles ➡ and a superior vermian cleft ⇨ in this child with Joubert syndrome.*

# Commissural and Cortical Maldevelopment

*Corpus callosum dysgenesis and malformations of cortical development are two of the most important congenital brain anomalies. Anomalies of the cerebral commissures are the most common of all congenital brain malformations, and corpus callosum dysgenesis is the single most common malformation that accompanies other developmental brain anomalies.*



Cortical malformations arise when migrating precursor cells fail to reach their target destinations. Malformations of cortical development (MCDs) are intrinsically epileptogenic and may be responsible for 25-40% of all medically refractory childhood epilepsies.

## Commissural Anomalies

### Callosal Dysgenesis Spectrum

#### Terminology

The corpus callosum (CC) can be completely absent (agenesis) **(42-1)** or partially formed (dysgenesis). **Complete CC agenesis** is almost always accompanied by the absence of the hippocampal commissure (HC). The anterior commissure (AC) is usually present and normal. If the CC is dysgenetic, the splenium and rostrum are most frequently affected.

#### Pathology

In *complete* CC agenesis, all five segments are missing. The **cingulate gyrus** is absent on sagittal images and in its place is a radiating **spoke-wheel gyral pattern** extending perpendicularly to the roof of the third ventricle **(42-4)**.

On coronal sections, the **"high-riding" third ventricle** looks as if it opens directly into the interhemispheric fissure. It is actually covered by a thin membranous roof that bulges into the interhemispheric fissure, displacing the fornices laterally. The lateral ventricles have upturned, pointed corners **(42-1)**.

A prominent longitudinal white matter (WM) tract called the **Probst bundle** is situated just medial to the apex of each ventricle **(42-1)**. These bundles consist of the misdirected commissural fibers, which should have crossed the midline but instead course from front to back, indenting the medial walls of the lateral ventricles.

Axial sections show that the lateral ventricles are parallel and nonconverging. The occipital horns are often disproportionately enlarged, a condition termed "colpocephaly."

## Clinical Issues

CC dysgenesis is the most common of all CNS malformations and is present in 3-5% of individuals with neurodevelopmental disorders.

Minor CC dysgenesis/hypogenesis is often discovered incidentally on imaging studies or at autopsy. Major commissural malformations are associated with seizures, developmental delay, and symptoms secondary to disruptions of the hypothalamic-pituitary axis.

### CALLOSAL DYSGENESIS: PATHOETIOLOGY AND CLINICAL ISSUES

**Terminology**

- Complete absence of corpus callosum (CC) = agenesis
  - Hippocampal commissure (HC) absent
  - Anterior commissure (AC) often present
  - All 3 absent = tricommissural agenesis
- Partial absence or hypogenesis of CC segments = dysgenesis
  - Rostrum, splenium most often affected segments
  - Partial posterior agenesis = HC, splenium, ± posterior body

**Clinical Issues**

- Most common CNS malformation
- Found in 3-5% of neurodevelopmental disorders

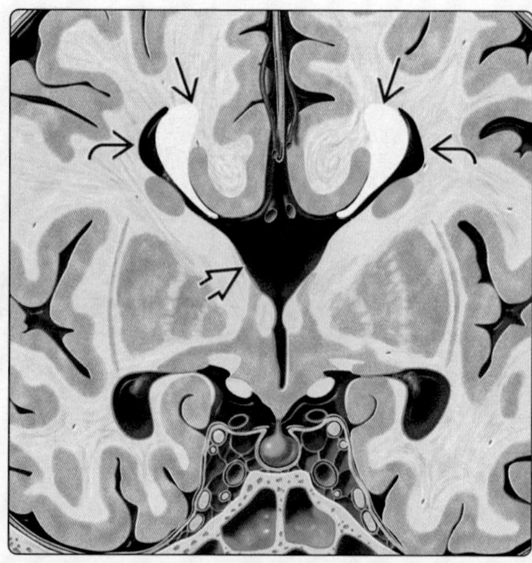

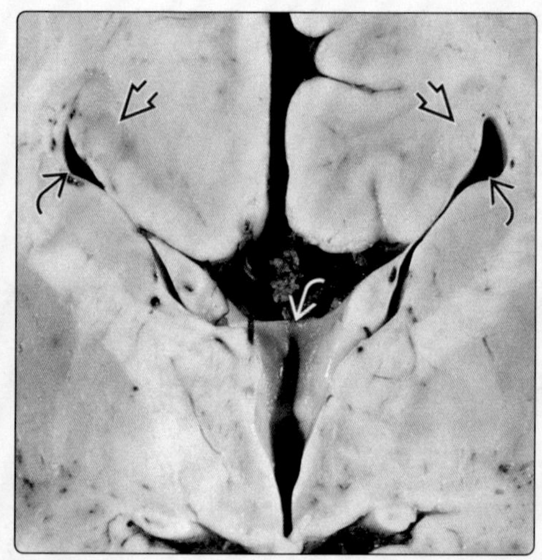

***(42-1)** Agenesis of corpus callosum (ACC) shows "Viking helmet," "high-riding" 3rd ventricle ➡, pointed lateral ventricles ➡, and Probst bundles ➡. **(42-2)** Coronal autopsy in ACC shows Viking helmet configuration. Note thin, "high-riding" 3rd ventricle roof ➡, white matter (WM) tracts ("Probst bundles") ➡ coursing along the medial surfaces of the parallel lateral ventricles ➡.*

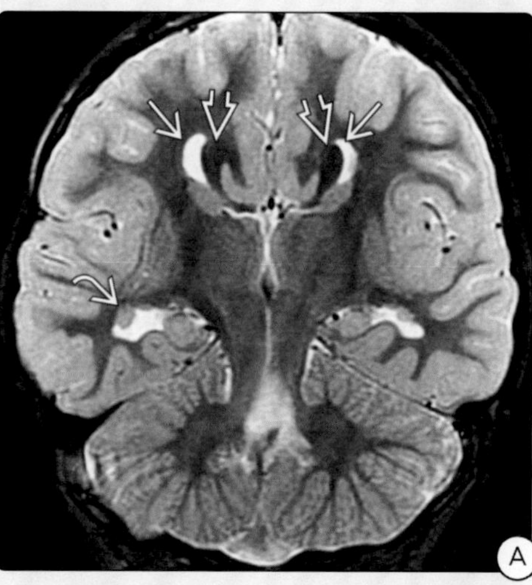

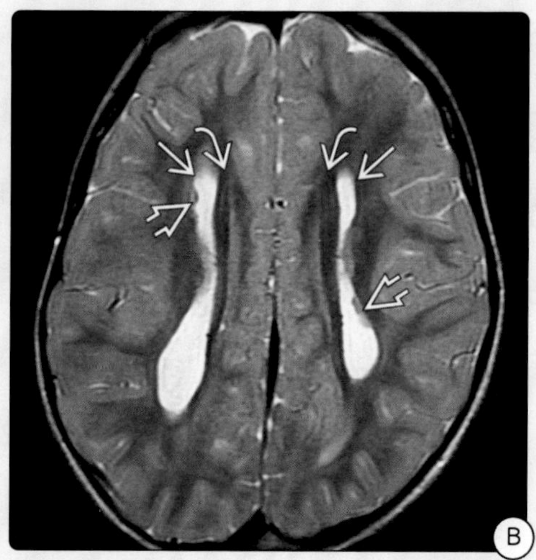

***(42-3A)** Coronal T2 MR shows "Viking helmet" of ACC with curving, upturned lateral ventricles ➡, Probst bundles ➡, and heterotopic gray matter (GM) ➡. **(42-3B)** Axial T2WI in the same case shows parallel, "nonconverging" lateral ventricles ➡ and myelinated, hypointense Probst bundles ➡. Note multiple foci of periventricular nodular heterotopia ➡.*

## Imaging

**MR Findings.** Sagittal T1 and T2 scans best demonstrate complete CC absence or partial dysgenesis.

***Complete Corpus Callosum Agenesis.*** With complete agenesis, the third ventricle appears continuous with the interhemispheric fissure and is surrounded dorsally by fingers of radiating gyri that "point" toward the third ventricle on sagittal images **(42-4)** **(42-5)**. Associated findings include a variable midline interhemispheric cyst and azygous anterior cerebral artery.

Axial scans demonstrate the parallel lateral ventricles especially well. The myelinated tracts of the Probst bundles can appear quite prominent **(42-3B)**.

Coronal scans show a Viking helmet or moose head appearance caused by the curved, upwardly pointed lateral ventricles and "high-riding" third ventricle that expands into the interhemispheric fissure **(42-3A)**. The Probst bundles are seen as densely myelinated tracts lying just lateral to the lateral ventricle bodies. The hippocampi appear abnormally rounded and vertically oriented. Moderately enlarged temporal horns are common. Look for malformations, such as heterotopic gray matter (GM) **(42-3A)**.

DTI allows depiction of the abnormal WM tracts in CC agenesis. The normal red (right-to-left encoded) color of the CC is absent. Instead, prominent front-to-back (green) tracts of the Probst bundles are seen.

***Corpus Callosum Dysgenesis.*** In partial agenesis, the rostrum and splenium are most often affected being either absent or hypoplastic **(42-6)**. The remaining genu and body often have a blocky, thickened appearance. The HC is typically absent, but the AC is generally preserved and often appears quite normal or even larger than usual.

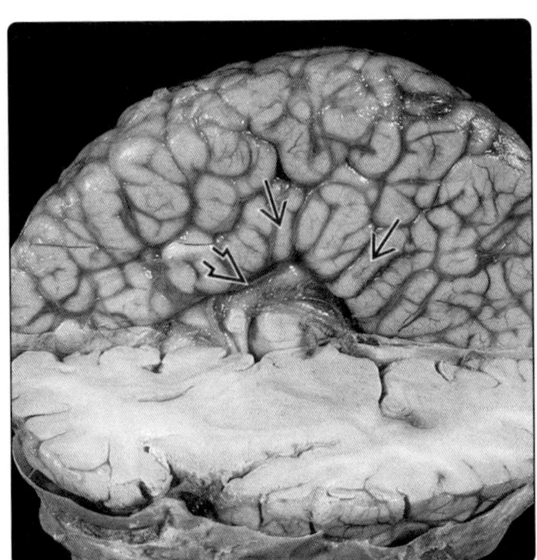

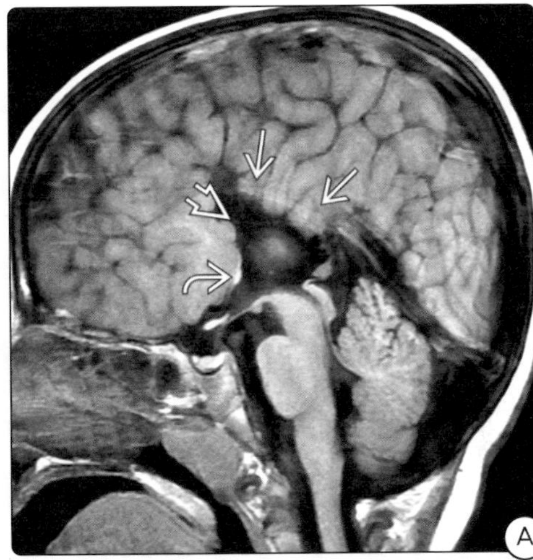


***(42-4)** ACC in Aicardi syndrome shows "radiating" gyri converging on "high-riding" 3rd ventricle. (Courtesy R. Hewlett, MD.) **(42-5A)** Sagittal T1WI shows "spoke-wheel" gyri converging on "high-riding" 3rd ventricle. The anterior commissure is normal. Hippocampal commissure is absent.*

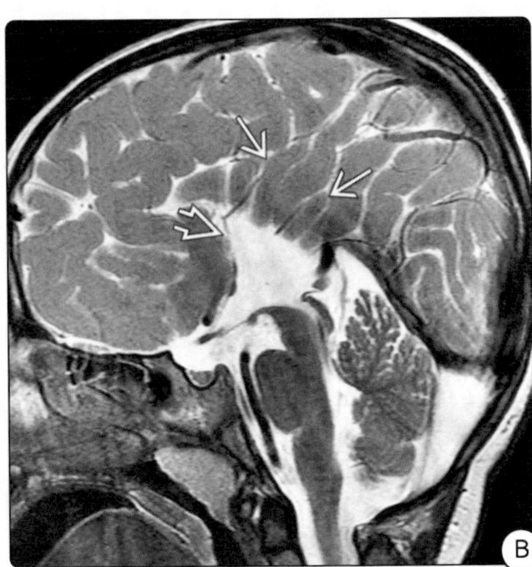


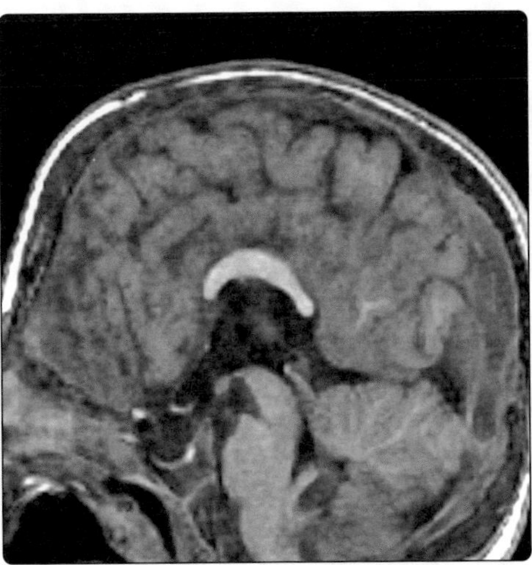

***(42-5B)** Sagittal T2WI in the same case shows the "spoke-wheel" gyri converging on the "high-riding" 3rd ventricle. Complete ACC. **(42-6)** Child with multiple facial anomalies shows a short, dysplastic corpus callosum with absence of the rostrum and splenium.*

## Associated Anomalies and Syndromes

Although CC dysgenesis can occur as an isolated phenomenon, CC anomalies are the single most common malformation associated with *other* CNS anomalies and syndromes. **Chiari 2 malformation, Dandy-Walker spectrum**, syndromic **craniosynostoses, hypothalamic-pituitary** anomalies, and **MCDs** all have an increased prevalence of CC anomalies.

Anomalies of the cerebral commissures have been described in nearly 200 different syndromes and many are linked to mutations in tubulin isotypes. Striking examples include **Aicardi syndrome**, where callosal agenesis is the most common anatomic abnormality.

### CALLOSAL DYSGENESIS: IMAGING

**Sagittal**
- Partial or complete CC agenesis
- 3rd ventricle "open" to interhemispheric fissure
- Cingulate gyrus absent → gyri "radiate" outward from 3rd ventricle

**Axial**
- Lateral ventricles parallel, nonconverging, widely separated
- Probst bundles = white matter (WM) along medial margins of lateral ventricles

**Coronal**
- Viking helmet or moose head appearance
- "High-riding" 3rd ventricle
- Pointed, upcurving lateral ventricles
- Probst bundles

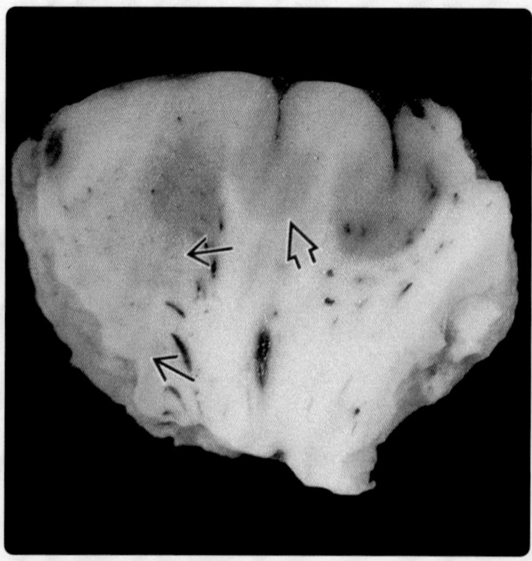

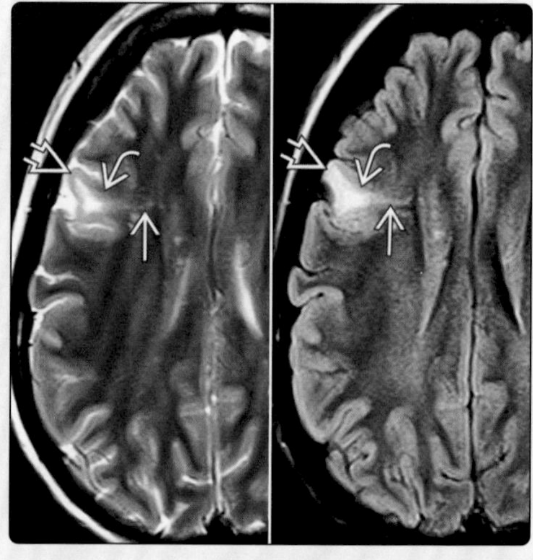

***(42-7)** Classic funnel-shaped area of thickened cortex, blurred GM-WM interface ⇨ in FCD. Contrast with normal sulcus and gyrus ⇨. **(42-8)** (L) T2WI, (R) FLAIR shows pathologically proven FCD IIb. Note funnel-shaped malformation ➡ with indistinct GM-WM interface ➡ and stalk-like transmantle deep extension ➡ (this can also be seen in pediatric-type diffuse low-grade gliomas like angiocentric glioma and PLNTY).*

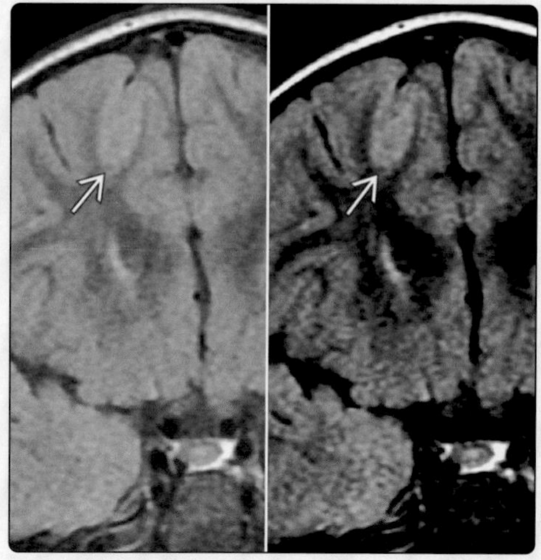

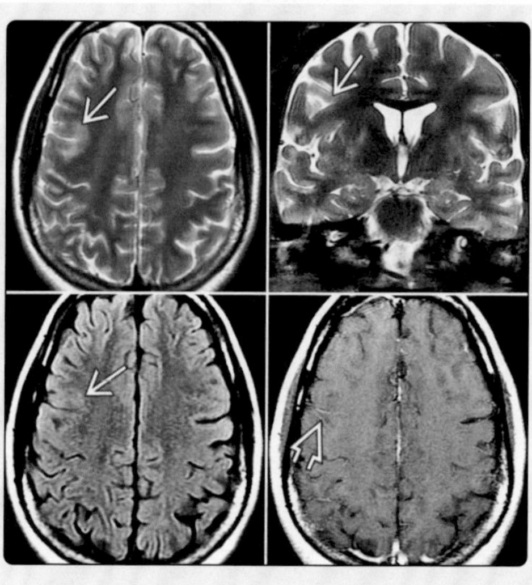

***(42-9)** Coronal FLAIR with varied windowing shows the importance of contrast resolution in making a diagnosis of FCD ➡. This is FCD IIb. **(42-10)** Note FCD ➡. Signal intensity is similar to GM. T1 C+ shows enhancement of "primitive" cortical veins ➡. (Courtesy P. Hildenbrand, MD.)*

# Malformations of Cortical Development

## Focal Cortical Dysplasias

Focal cortical dysplasias (FCDs) are a common cause of medically refractory epilepsy in both children and adults. Surgical resection is an increasingly important treatment option, so recognition and accurate delineation of FCD on imaging studies are key to successful patient management.

### Terminology and International League Against Epilepsy Classification

**FCD type I** is an isolated malformation with abnormal cortical layering that demonstrates either abundant developmental microcolumns (FCD type Ia) or abnormal layering (FCD type Ib) in one or multiple lobes. FCD type Ic is characterized by both vertical and horizontal abnormalities of cortical organization.

**FCD type II** is an isolated lesion characterized by altered cortical layering and dysmorphic neurons either without (type IIa) or with **balloon** (type IIb) **cells**. Type II is the most common type of FCD in surgical epilepsy specimens.

The third type of FCD, **FCD type III**, is a postmigrational disorder associated with principal pathologies, such as ischemia, infection, trauma, etc. In such cases, cytoarchitectural abnormalities occur together with hippocampal sclerosis (FCD type IIIa), epilepsy-associated tumors (FCD type IIIb), vascular malformations (FCD type IIIc), or—in the case of FCD type IIId—other epileptogenic lesions acquired in early life.

### Etiology

The most convincing data implicate mammalian target of rapamycin (mTOR) cascade abnormalities as the cause of FCD. FCD type IIb is considered an "mTORopathy" as is tuberous sclerosis complex (TSC) and the rare hemimegalencephaly syndrome. FCD IIb resembles the cortical tubers seen in TSC.

### Pathology

Mildly thickened, slightly firm cortex with poor demarcation from the underlying WM is characteristic **(42-7)**. The histopathologic hallmarks of FCD are disorganized cytoarchitecture and neurons with abnormal shape, size, and orientation. Prominent balloon cells are typical of type IIb. These balloon cells are histologically identical to giant cells in the tubers from TSC patients.

### Clinical Issues

FCDs are the single most common cause of severe early-onset drug-resistant epilepsy in children and young adults. This is a critical diagnosis to make because successful surgical resection of FCD results in a very high chance of seizure freedom.

### Imaging

MR of FCD type IIb shows a localized area of increased cortical thickness and a funnel-shaped area of blurred GM-WM interface at the bottom of a sulcus extending towards the ventricular margin, the **transmantle MR sign (42-8)**. Signal intensity varies with age. In older patients, FCD most often appears as a wedge-shaped area of T2/FLAIR hyperintensity extending from the bottom of a sulcus into the subcortical and deep WM **(42-9) (42-10)**. In the first few

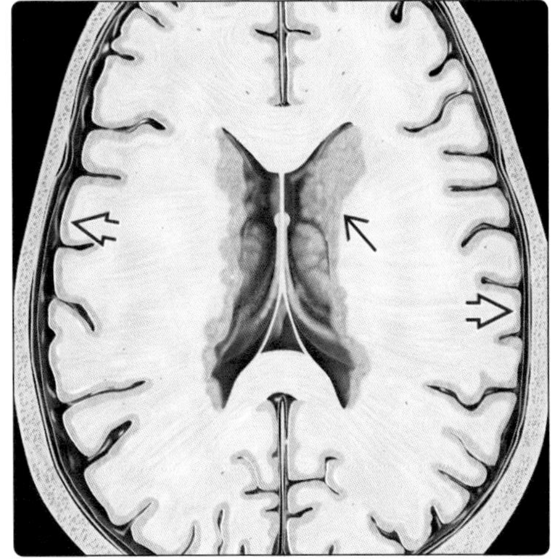

***(42-11)** Extensive subependymal heterotopia ⇨ lines the lateral ventricles. The GM cortical ribbon is thin ⇨; sulci are shallow.*

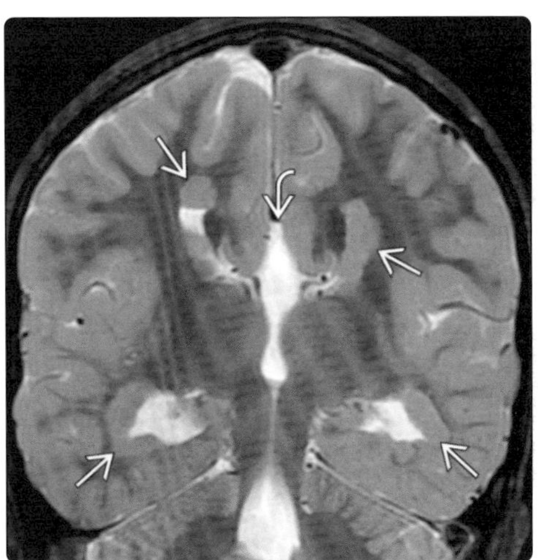

***(42-12)** Coronal T2 MR shows extensive periventricular nodular heterotopia ➡ in this patient with absent corpus callosum ➡.*

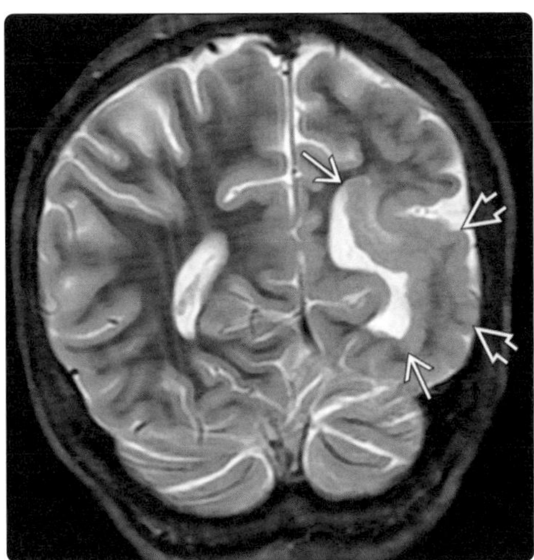

***(42-13)** T2 shows cortical malformation ➡, subependymal GM heterotopia ➡ around distorted lateral ventricle.*

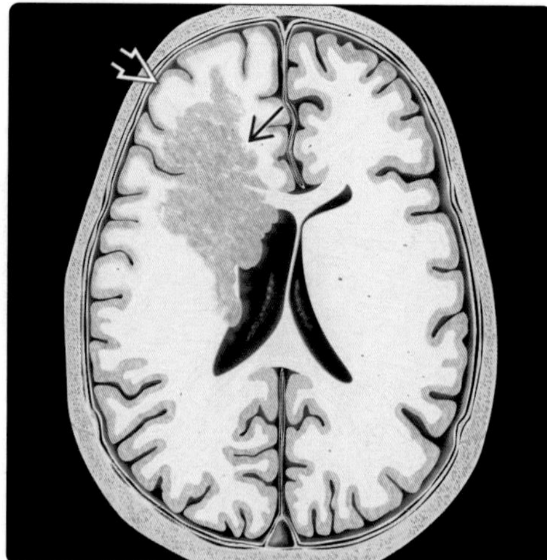

*(42-14) Graphic depicts subcortical heterotopia. The large, focal, mass-like collection of GM ⇒, thin overlying cortex ⇒ are typical.*

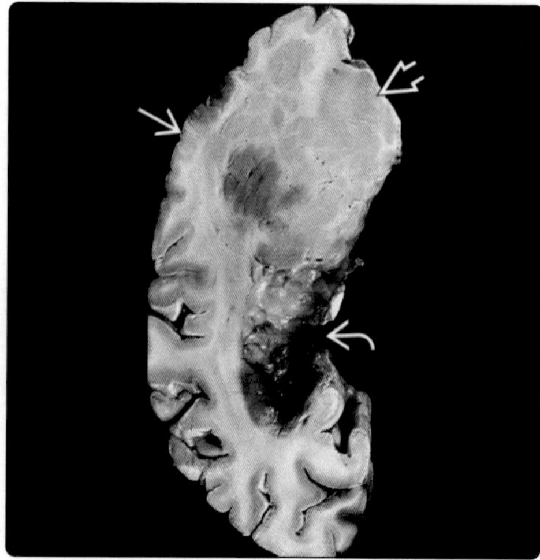

*(42-15) Autopsy dysplastic lateral ventricle ⇒, mass-like GM heterotopias ⇒ under thin, polymicrogyric cortex ⇒. (From AFIP Archives.)*

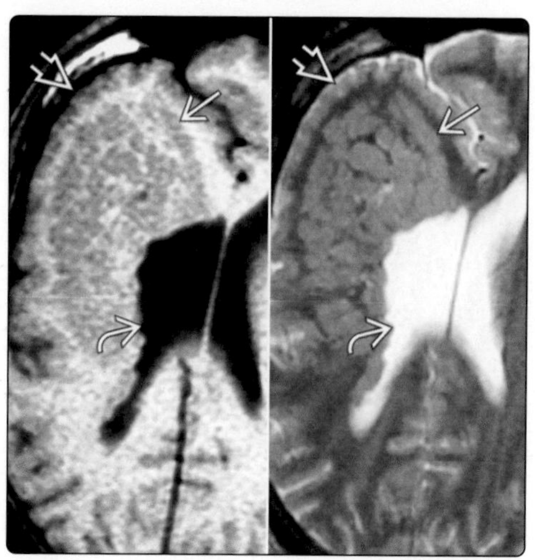

*(42-16) T1 (L), T2 (R) show mass of heterotopic GM ⇒, thin overlying cortex ⇒, deformed underlying ventricle ⇒, mimicking neoplasm.*

months of life prior to myelination, FCD is typically T1 hyperintense and T2 hypointense compared to adjacent unmyelinated WM. Any nonenhancing signal involving both cortex and subcortical WM should prompt consideration of FCD. FCD type IIb does not enhance on T1 C+.

FCD type I is not typically visible on MR.

### Differential Diagnosis

The major differential diagnosis of FCD (especially type IIb) includes epilepsy-associated **neoplasm** (e.g., dysembryoplastic neuroepithelial tumor, ganglioglioma, diffuse astrocytoma) and TSC. Cortical lesions in **TSC** can look very similar to FCD type IIb. TSC usually shows multifocal dysplasias ("tubers") and usually demonstrates other imaging stigmata, such as subependymal nodules.

#### FOCAL CORTICAL DYSPLASIA

**International League Against Epilepsy Classification**

- Most common type is FCD II
  - FCD IIa = without balloon cells
  - FCD IIb = with balloon cells (most common)
- FCD I: Usually not visible on imaging

**Pathology and Clinical Issues**

- Thickened disorganized cortex with indistinct gray matter (GM)-WM junction
- Most common cause of refractory epilepsy in children

**Imaging**

- Focal area of thickened cortex with blurred GM-WM junction
- Cortical and subcortical T2/FLAIR hyperintensity ± transmantle sign

# Abnormalities of Neuronal Migration

The most common abnormalities of neuronal migration are GM heterotopias and lissencephaly (LIS) spectrum disorders.

## Heterotopias

Arrest of normal neuronal migration along the radial glial cells can result in grossly visible masses of "heterotopic" GM. These collections come in many shapes and sizes and can be found virtually anywhere between the ventricles and the pia. They can be solitary or multifocal and exist either as an isolated phenomenon or in association with other malformations.

### Periventricular Nodular Heterotopia

**Periventricular nodular heterotopia** (PVNH) is the most common form of cortical malformation in adults. Here, one or more subependymal nodules of GM line the lateral walls of the ventricles **(42-11)**. PVNH can be unilateral or bilateral, focal or diffuse. Collections of round or ovoid nodules indent the lateral walls of the ventricles, giving them a distinctive lumpy-bumpy appearance **(42-12)**.

PVNH follows GM in density/signal intensity and does not enhance following contrast administration. The overlying cortex may be dysplastic **(42-13)**, but sulcation and gyration of overlying brain are most often grossly normal.

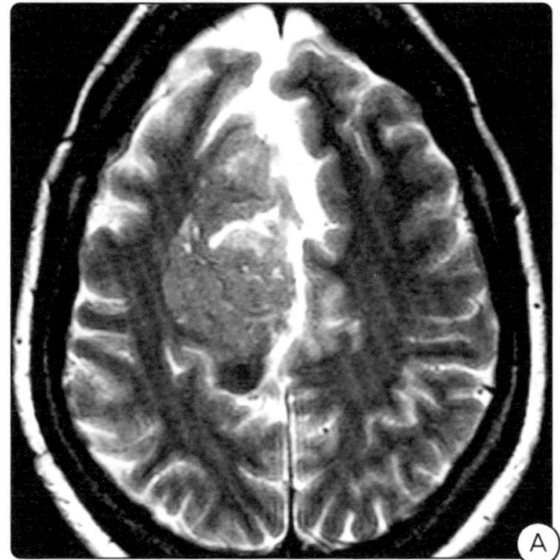

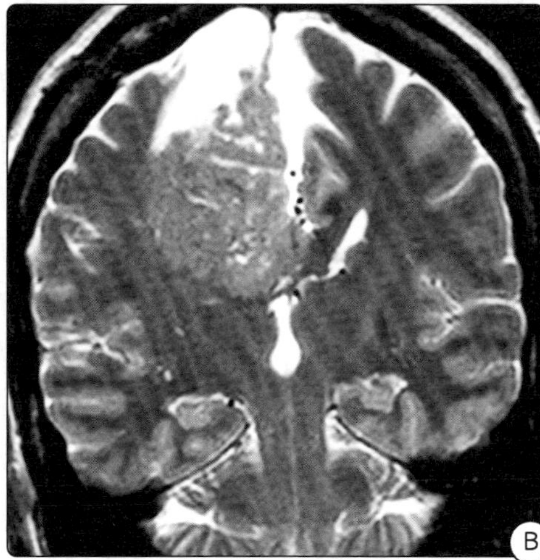

***(42-17A)** Axial T2WI in a 38-yo woman with epilepsy and a history of "brain tumor, not malignant" biopsied 15 years earlier shows a dysplastic-appearing mass in the right medial frontal lobe. Most of the mass is isointense with cortex, and an aberrant CSF-filled sulcus courses through the middle of the mass. **(42-17B)** Coronal T2WI shows the mass-like lesion.*

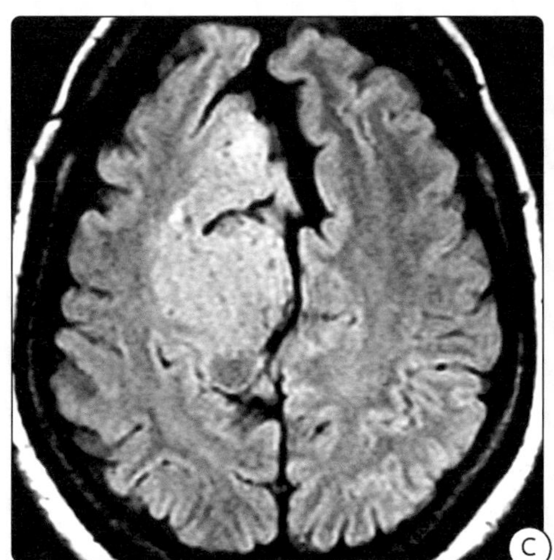

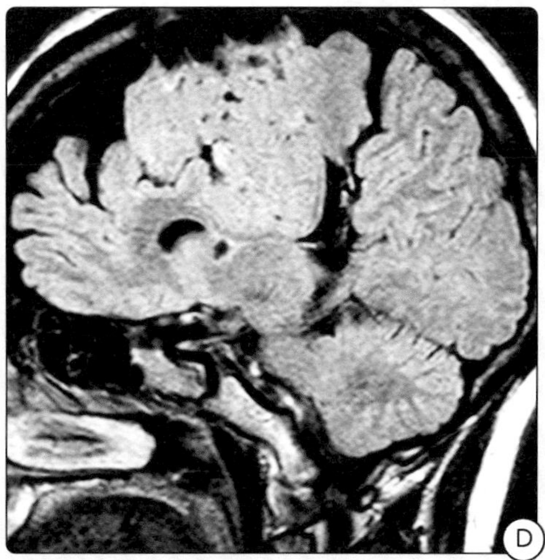

***(42-17C)** The mass is isointense with cortex on FLAIR. CSF in the aberrant sulcus suppresses completely. **(42-17D)** Sagittal FLAIR shows the dysplastic mass.*

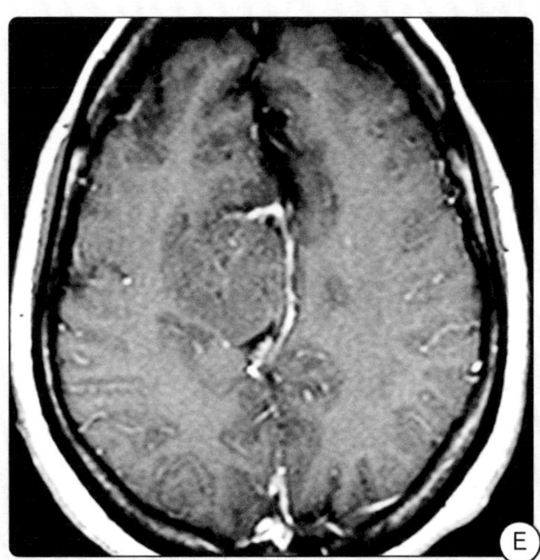

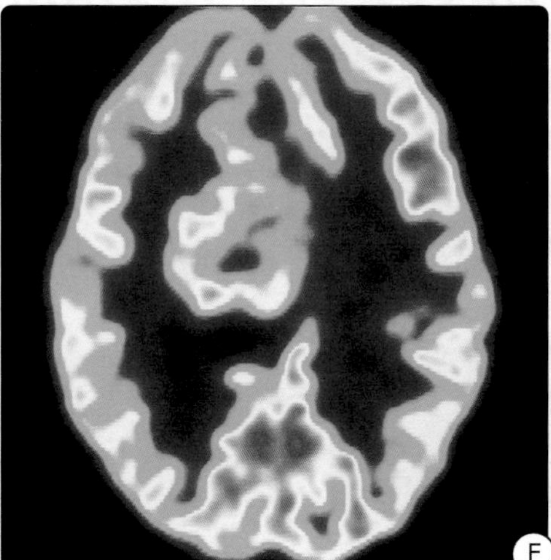

***(42-17E)** T1 C+ shows prominent vessels—possibly an azygous anterior cerebral artery—borders the lesion. The lesion does not enhance. **(42-17F)** FDG PET shows the mass resembles normal cortex. This is mass-like GM heterotopia. Unusual focal mass-like collections of heterotopic GM should not be mistaken for neoplasms.*

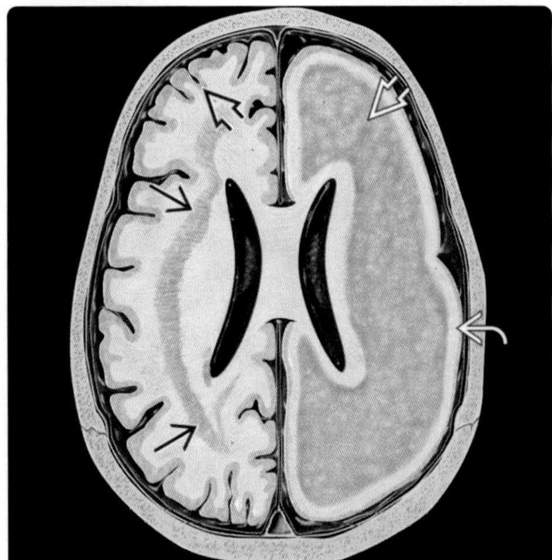

(42-18) cLIS on L shows thick subcortical GM band ➡, thin cortex ➡. R = band heterotopia ("double cortex") ➡ with thin outer cortex ➡.

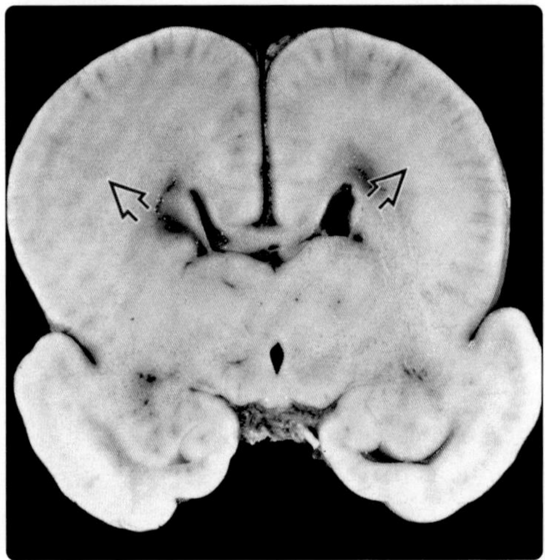

(42-19) Coronal autopsy shows cLIS with "hourglass" smooth brain, thick incompletely layered cortex ➡.

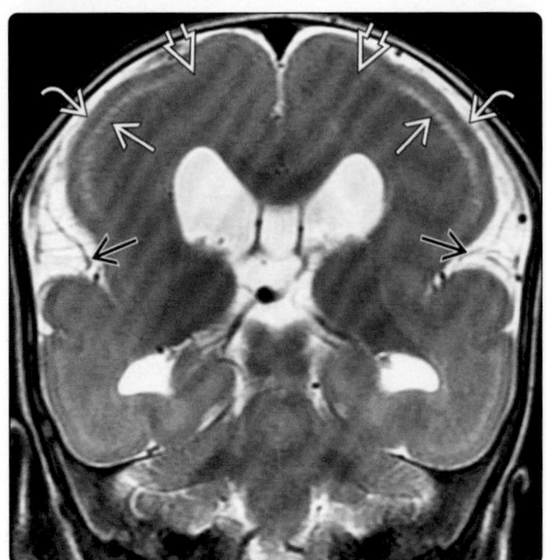

(42-20) T2 of cLIS shows smooth brain with thin cortex ➡, hyperintense "cell-sparse" layer ➡, thick inner band of GM ➡, primitive veins ➡.

The major differential diagnosis of PVNH is the subependymal nodules of **TSC**.

### Subcortical Heterotopias

**Subcortical heterotopias** are malformations in which large, focal, mass-like collections of neurons are found in the cerebral WM anywhere from the ependyma to the cortex **(42-14)**. The involved portion of the affected hemisphere is abnormally small, and the overlying cortex appears thin and sometimes dysplastic **(42-15)**.

In other forms of heterotopia, focal masses of ectopic GM occur in linear or swirling curved columns of neurons that extend through normal-appearing WM from the ependyma to the pia. The overlying cortex is thin, and the underlying ventricle often appears distorted **(42-16)**. The masses follow GM on all sequences, do not demonstrate edema, and do not enhance.

Occasionally, ribbon-like bands of heterotopic GM (**subcortical band heterotopia**) form partway between the lateral ventricles and cortex **(42-18)**. Although these have been described with megalencephaly and polymicrogyria (PMG), most are probably part of the "double cortex" form of LIS.

## Lissencephaly Spectrum

Malformations due to widespread abnormal transmantle migration include **agyria, pachygyria**, and **band heterotopia**. All are part of the **LIS spectrum**.

### Terminology

The term LIS literally means "smooth brain." The spectrum of LISs ranges from severe (agyria) to milder forms, including abnormally broad folds (pachygyria) or a heterotopic layer of GM embedded in the WM below the cortex (subcortical band heterotopia).

In classic LIS (cLIS), the brain surface lacks normal sulcation and gyration. **cLIS** is also called **type 1 LIS** or **four-layer LIS** to differentiate it from cobblestone cortical malformation. Agyria is defined as a thick cortex with absence of surface gyri **("complete" LIS)**.

True agyria with complete loss of all gyri is relatively uncommon. Many cases of LIS spectrum show areas of broad, flat gyri ("pachygyria") and shallow sulci **("incomplete" LIS)**. **Subcortical band heterotopia** is also called **"double cortex" syndrome**.

### Etiology

cLIS is caused by mutation in genes that regulate the outward migration of neuroblasts from the subependymal ventricular zone. Guided by radial glial fibers, postmitotic neuroblasts normally migrate outward to populate the cortical plate.

### Pathology

In cLIS, the external surface of the brain shows a marked lack of gyri and sulci. In the most severe forms, the cerebral hemispheres are smooth with poor opercularization and underdeveloped sylvian fissures. In cLIS, the normal six-layer cortex is replaced by a thick four-layer cortex. Coronal sections demonstrate a markedly thickened cerebral cortex with absent or broad gyri **(42-19)** and reduced volume of the underlying WM **(42-18)**.

## Clinical Issues

Patients with cLIS typically exhibit moderate to severe developmental delay, impaired neuromotor functions, variable intellectual disability, and seizures. Patients with band heterotopia are almost always female.

## Imaging

**General Features.** Imaging in patients with complete cLIS (agyria) shows a smooth, featureless brain surface with shallow sylvian fissures and mildly enlarged ventricles. The cortex is thickened, and the WM is diminished in volume. The normal finger-like interdigitations between the cortical GM and subcortical WM are absent. In some cases, the cerebellum appears hypoplastic.

**CT Findings.** Axial NECT scans in cLIS show an hourglass or figure-eight appearance caused by the flat brain surface and shallow, wide sylvian fissures. A thick band of relatively well-delineated dense cortex surrounds a thinner, smooth band of WM.

CECT scans show prominent primitive-appearing veins running in the shallow sylvian fissures and coursing over the thickened cortices.

### LISSENCEPHALY SPECTRUM

**Classic Lissencephaly**
- Pathology: Thick, 4-layer cortex
  - Thin subpial layer
  - Thin outer cortex
  - "Cell-sparse" zone
  - Broad inner band of disorganized neurons
- Clinical issues
  - Classic lissencephaly (cLIS) + severe facial anomalies = Miller-Dieker
- Imaging
  - Smooth, "hourglass" brain
  - Flat surface, shallow "open" sylvian fissures

**Band Heterotopia ("Double Cortex")**
- Clinical issues
  - Almost always in female patients
- Imaging: Looks like "double cortex"
  - Overlying cortex grossly normal
  - Normal-appearing WM under cortex
  - Ill-defined inner band of GM often following gyri
  - Normal-appearing periventricular WM

**Differential Diagnosis**
- Extremely premature brain
  - cLIS looks like 20- to 24-week fetal brain
- Microcephaly with simplified gyral pattern
  - Brain size ≥ 3 standard deviations below normal
- Cobblestone LISs (type 2 LIS)
  - Associated with congenital muscular dystrophies
  - "Pebbly" (cobblestone) surface, not smooth
- Pachygyria
  - More localized, often multifocal
  - GM-WM interface indistinct
- Congenital cytomegalovirus
  - Often microcephalic
  - Smooth brain, periventricular calcifications

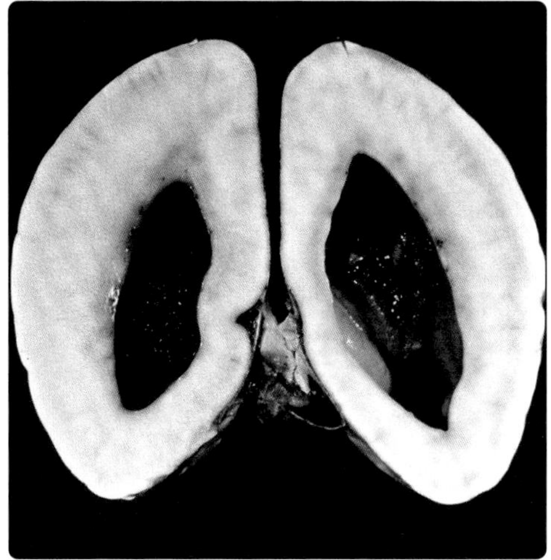

***(42-21)** Coronal gross autopsy of cLIS shows alternating layers of smooth, undifferentiated GM and WM.*

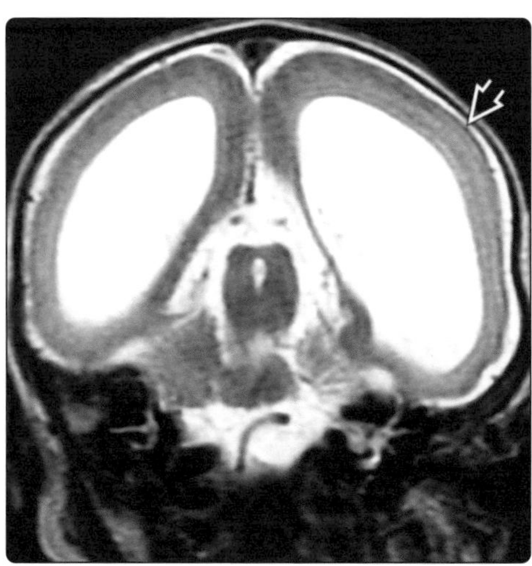

***(42-22)** Coronal T2WI in 1-day-old microcephalic infant shows severe lissencephaly. Layered cortex, WM are barely discernible ➔.*

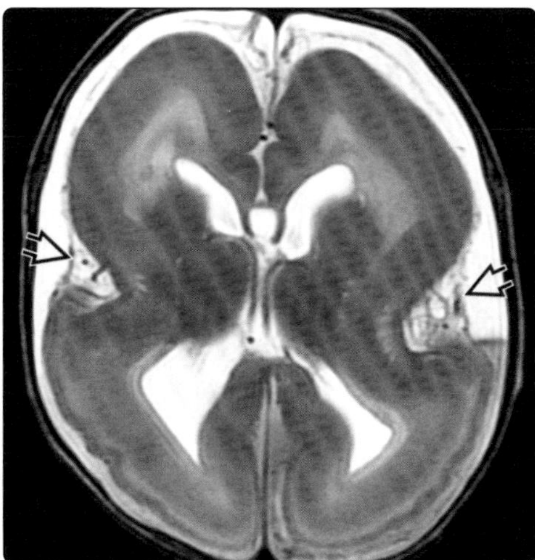

***(42-23)** T2WI shows cLIS with thin cortex, "cell-sparse" layer, thick cortex, and shallow sylvian fissures with primitive veins ➔.*

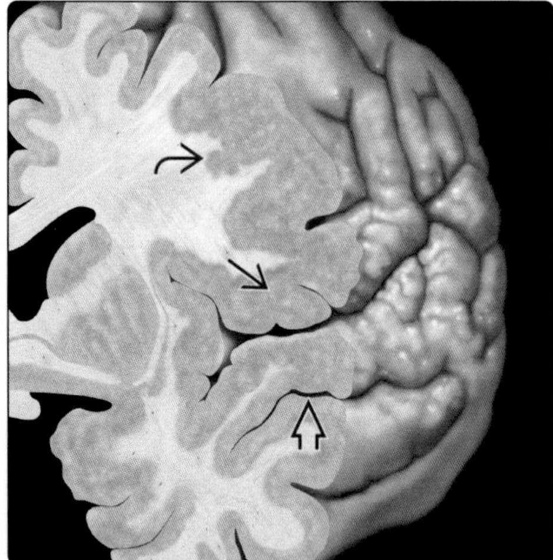

(42-24) Thick, "pebbly" polymicrogyria (PMG) in frontal ➡, temporal ➡ lobes. Note abnormal sulcation, irregular cortical-WM interface ➡.

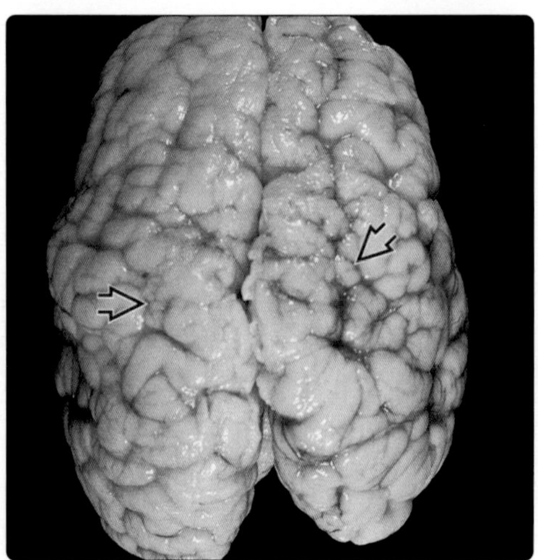

(42-25) PMG with tiny nodules ("gyri piled on top of gyri") ➡ give brain an irregular pebbly appearance. (Courtesy R. Hewlett, MD.)

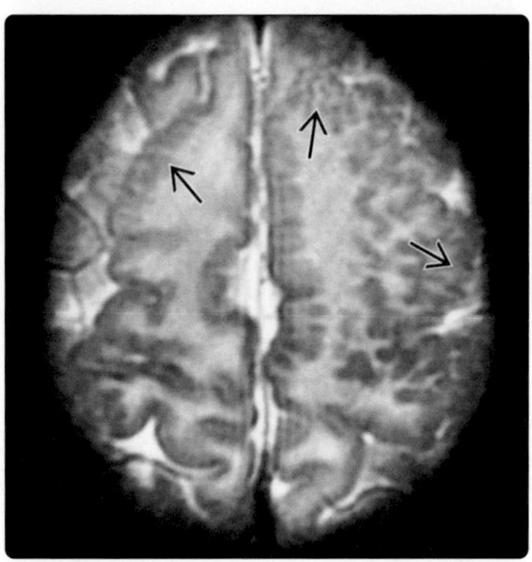

(42-26) T2 MR in a 2-week-old infant shows multiple foci of PMG ➡. Left hemisphere is much more severely affected than the right.

#### MR Findings

***Classic Lissencephaly.*** In **cLIS**, T1 scans show a smooth cortical surface, a thick band of deep GM that is sharply demarcated from the underlying WM, and large ventricles **(42-23)**. T2 sequences are best to distinguish the separate cortical layers. A thin outer cellular layer that is isointense with GM covers a hyperintense "cell-sparse" layer **(42-20)**. The WM layer is smooth and reduced in volume **(42-20)**. A deeper, thick layer of arrested migrating neurons is common and may mimic band heterotopia **(42-23)**. Callosal hypogenesis is common in cLIS.

***Variant Lissencephaly.*** In **variant LIS (vLIS)**, sulcation is reduced, and the cortex appears thick (although not as thick as in cLIS).

***Band Heterotopia or "Double Cortex" Syndrome.*** In **band heterotopia**, a band of smooth GM is separated from a relatively thicker, more gyriform cortex by a layer of normal-appearing WM.

MR scans show a more normal gyral pattern with relatively thicker cortex. The distinguishing feature of band heterotopia is its "double cortex," a homogeneous layer of GM separated from the ventricles and cerebral cortex by layers of normal-appearing WM.

### Differential Diagnosis

**Extremely premature brain** is smooth at 24-26 gestational weeks and normally has a "lissencephalic" appearance. Full sulcation and gyration do not develop completely until term gestation. **Pachygyria** is more localized, often multifocal, and usually asymmetric. In contrast to cLIS, the GM-WM junction along the thickened cortex is indistinct. **Cytomegalovirus**-associated LIS demonstrates periventricular calcifications.

# Malformations Secondary to Abnormal Postmigrational Development

The third major group of cortical malformations is secondary to abnormal postmigrational development and often reflects infectious or ischemic insults. This group was formerly designated "abnormalities of cortical organization." It is currently divided into several subtypes of polymicrogyria (PMG) according to whether clefts (schizencephaly) are present and whether they occur as part of a recognized multiple malformation syndrome, inherited metabolic disease, or genetic disorder.

## Polymicrogyria

The signature feature of PMG is an irregular cortex with numerous small convolutions and shallow or obliterated sulci. The appearance is that of tiny miniature gyri piled on top of other disorganized gyri **(42-24)**.

### Etiology

Both genetic and nongenetic causes of PMG have been identified. Encephaloclastic insults, such as infection (e.g., TORCH, Zika virus infection), intrauterine vascular accident (e.g., middle cerebral artery occlusion), trauma, and metabolic disorders, have been implicated in the development of PMG.

Mutations in > 30 genes are associated with PMG, especially mutations in the tubulin family. The phenotypic spectrum of *TUBA1A* mutations includes bilateral perisylvian PMG with dysmorphic basal ganglia **(42-27)**, cerebellar vermis dysplasia, and pontine hypoplasia.

## Pathology

PMG is characterized by overfolding of the cerebral cortex and abnormal cortical layering. PMG can involve a single gyrus or most of an entire cerebral hemisphere. It can be uni- or bilateral, symmetric or asymmetric, and focal or diffuse. Multiple small, shallow, and abnormally oriented gyri with an undulating surface and complex sulcal branching are typical findings **(42-25)**.

Bilateral perisylvian PMG is the most common location (61% of cases). Generalized (13%), frontal (5%), and parasagittal parietooccipital (3%) sites are less common. Associated periventricular GM heterotopias are found in 11% of cases, and other anomalies, such as schizencephaly, are common.

## Clinical Issues

PMG can present at any age, but many do not present until late in childhood, and some mild cases may remain asymptomatic. PMG is the most common imaging abnormality seen in infants with congenital cytomegalovirus infection. Symptoms depend on the location and extent of PMG, ranging from global developmental delay to focal neurologic deficit(s) and seizures.

## Imaging

Multiplanar MR with high-resolution thin sections is required for complete delineation and detection of subtle lesions. 3D acquisitions with MPRs are ideal. Thickened or overfolded cortex with nodular surfaces and irregular "stippled" GM-WM interfaces are the most characteristic findings **(42-26)**. Detection of PMG is more difficult prior to completion of myelination. Prior to myelination, T2-weighted imaging tends to be the most sensitive sequence for detecting PMG **(42-26)**. Early or asymmetric sulcation in the fetus is a sign of PMG on fetal MR.

## Differential Diagnosis

The major differential diagnosis of PMG is **type 2 LIS** (cobblestone malformation) **(42-27)** **(42-28)**. The absence of congenital muscular dystrophy and Z-shaped brainstem is a helpful clinical distinction.

Sometimes, **pachygyria** can be confused with PMG. In pachygyria, the cortex and GM-WM junction are smooth. In contrast, the cortex in PMG is nodular and excessively folded with an irregular GM-WM junction. In **FCD**, the GM is focally thickened with subtle cortical and subcortical T2/FLAIR hyperintensity, and the GM-WM interface is blurred.

In **schizencephaly**, the dysplastic cortex lining the cleft may appear "pebbled," but the cleft distinguishes it from PMG.

# Schizencephaly

Schizencephaly (literally meaning "split brain") is a GM-lined cleft that extends from the ventricular ependyma to the pial surface of the cortex. The cleft spans the full thickness of the affected hemisphere **(42-29)**. Encephaloclastic in utero insults, including vascular disruptions and infections (e.g., TORCH) occurring before 28 fetal weeks, are the primary etiologies. Schizencephaly can be considered on the severe spectrum of PMG with similar causes and associations (e.g., septo-optic dysplasia).

A schizencephalic brain exhibits a deep cleft that extends from its surface to the ventricle. The cleft is surrounded and lined by disorganized, dysmorphic-appearing GM **(42-30)**. The "lips" of the cleft can be fused or closely apposed ("closed-lip" schizencephaly) **(42-31)** or appear widely separated ("open-lip"

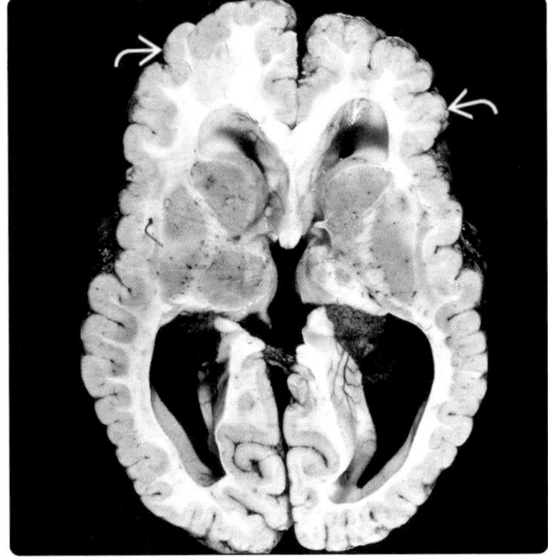

***(42-27)** Tubulinopathy shows PMG ➡, grossly enlarged caudate heads, dysplastic-appearing putamina, small thalami.*

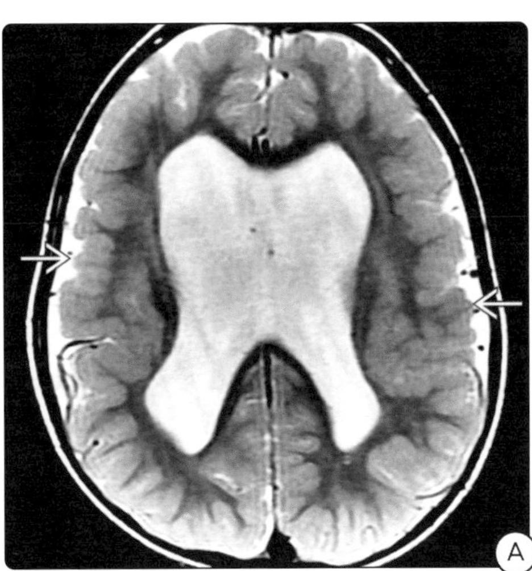


***(42-28A)** T2WI shows tubulinopathy-associated PMG ➡.*

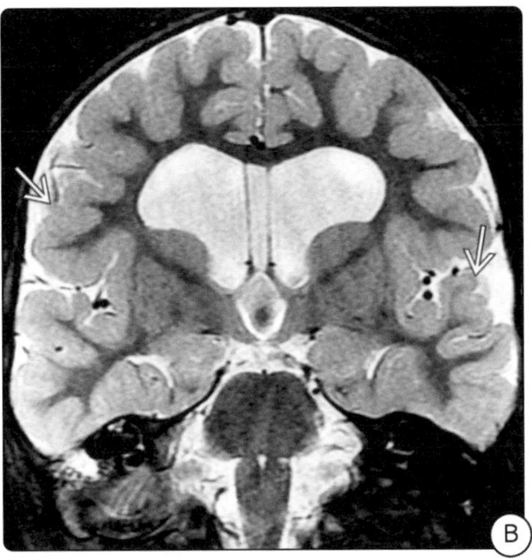


***(42-28B)** Coronal T2WI in the same case shows PMG ➡.*

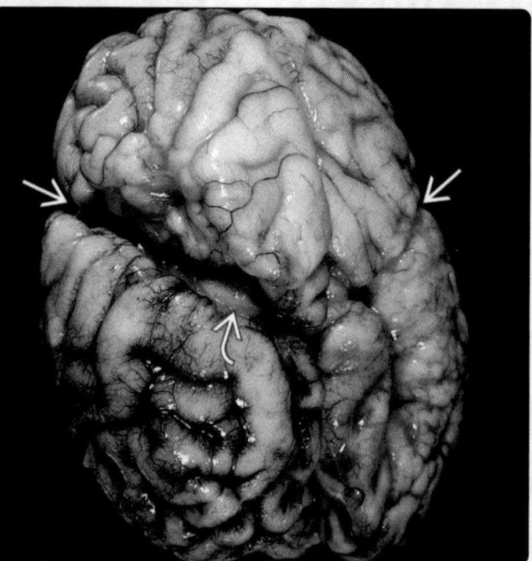

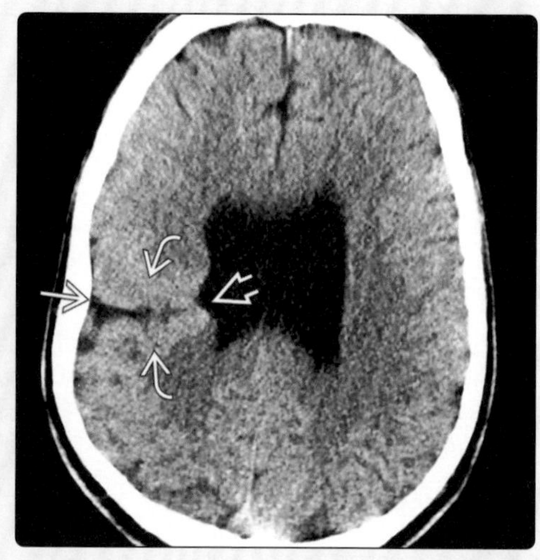

*(42-29) Autopsy shows bilateral schizencephalic clefts ➡. Note that the thick, abnormal cortex curves over the "lips" of the clefts and follows them all the way medially to the ventricular ependyma ↪. (Courtesy R. Hewlett, MD.) (42-30) Unilateral schizencephaly is shown with outpouching of CSF from the lateral ventricle ⇨. Cleft of CSF ➡ is lined with dysplastic GM ↪.*

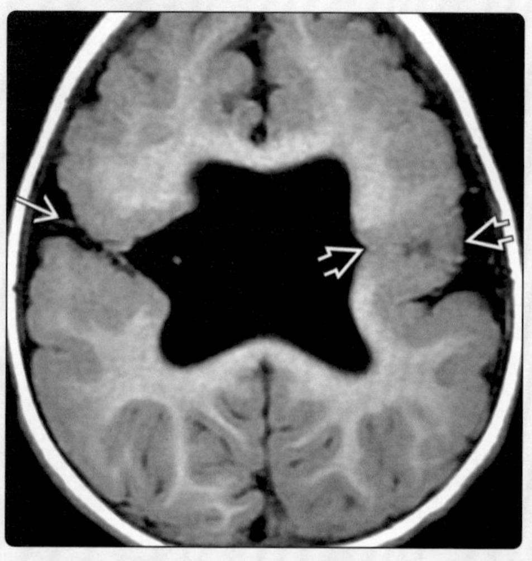

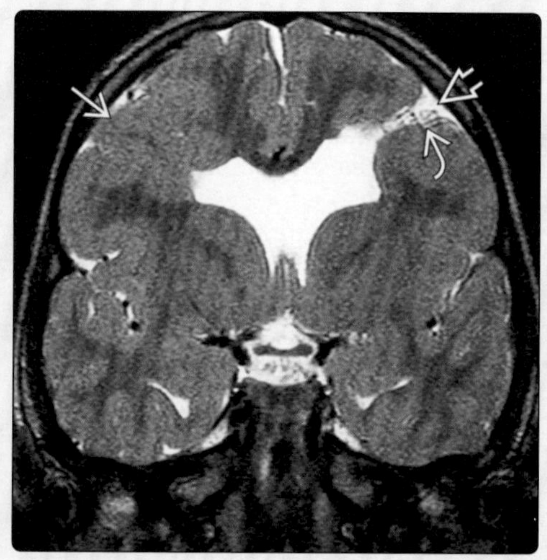

*(42-31) Child with septo-optic dysplasia shows right "open-lip" ➡ and left "closed-lip" ⇨ schizencephaly. (42-32) Coronal T2WI in septo-optic dysplasia, intractable epilepsy shows "open-lip" L ⇨, "closed-lip" R ➡ schizencephalic clefts lined with GM. Note absence of the septum pellucidum, inferiorly pointed frontal horns of the lateral ventricles, and dysplastic veins ↪ in the "open-lip" cleft.*

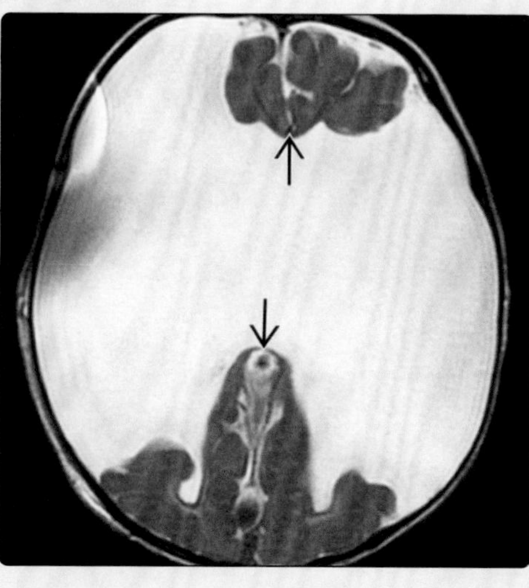

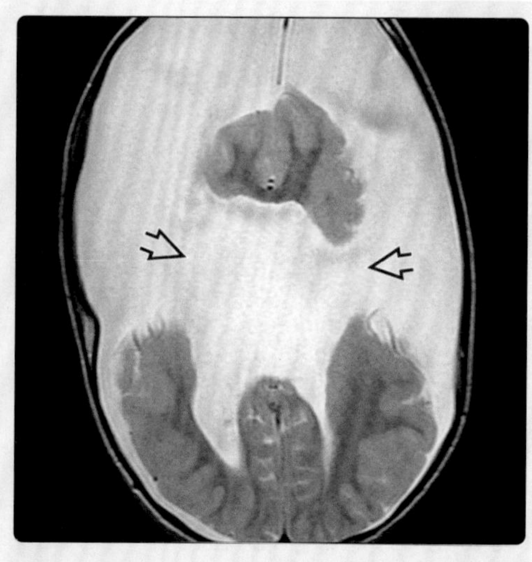

*(42-33) T2WI in extreme "open-lip" schizencephaly shows presence of a falx cerebri →, distinguishing this case from holoprosencephaly. Lack of cortex around the fluid-filled open clefts distinguishes this from holoprosencephaly and maximal hydrocephalus. (42-34) T2WI shows bilateral "open-lip" schizencephaly ⇨ lined with dysplastic GM (do not confuse with large areas of porencephaly, which are lined with gliotic WM).*

schizencephaly) **(42-33)**. Clefts may be associated with a range of other macroscopic abnormalities involving the septi pellucidi, CC, optic chiasm, and hippocampus.

The key imaging features of schizencephaly are (1) a CSF-filled defect extending from the ventricle wall to the pial surface and (2) dysplastic GM lining the cleft.

Imaging studies show a focal V-shaped outpouching or "dimple" of CSF extending outward from the lateral ventricle **(42-30)**. The clefts can be uni- (60%) or bilateral (40%) with prominent ("open") or barely visible ("closed") lips **(42-32)**.

MR is more sensitive than CT in delineating associated abnormalities, such as cortical dysplasia (PMG, pachygyria) and heterotopic GM. The cleft follows CSF signal intensity on all sequences **(42-34)**.

The differential diagnosis includes both developmental and destructive lesions. The major differential diagnosis of schizencephaly is **porencephaly**. In porencephaly, the cleft is lined by gliotic WM, not dysplastic GM. Transmantle **heterotopia** or deeply infolded **PMG** may be difficult to distinguish from schizencephaly with closed, nearly fused "lips." An **arachnoid cyst** displaces the adjacent cortex, which is otherwise normal in appearance.

## POSTMIGRATION DISORDERS

**Polymicrogyria**

- Etiology
  - Acquired [infection (e.g., cytomegalovirus), intrauterine vascular accident]
  - Inherited (tubulin gene mutations)
- Pathology
  - Irregular, "pebbly" cortex
  - Can be uni- or bilateral
  - Symmetric or asymmetric
  - Focal or diffuse
  - Miniature gyri "piled on top of gyri"
- Imaging
  - Bilateral perisylvian most common location
  - Thickened cortex, nodular surfaces
  - Irregular GM-WM interfaces
- Differential diagnosis
  - Type 2 LIS (no congenital muscular dystrophy, Z-shaped brainstem)

**Schizencephaly**

- Etiology
  - Encephaloclastic (TORCH, vascular accident)
- Pathology
  - Full-thickness CSF-containing cleft from ventricle to pia
  - CSF cleft can be closed, open
  - Uni- or bilateral
- Imaging
  - Look for "nipple" outpouching of CSF from ventricle
  - Cleft lined by dysmorphic GM
  - Follows cortex on all sequences
- Differential diagnosis
  - Transmantle heterotopia (no CSF cleft)

*Selected References: The complete reference list is available on the eBooks+ version included with purchase.*

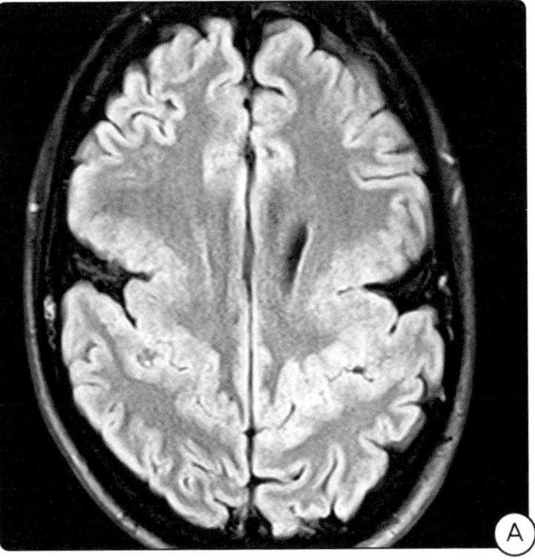


***(42-35A)** FLAIR in 19-yo man with epilepsy shows unusually large open sulcus, more extensive closed sulcus, both lined with heterotopic GM.*

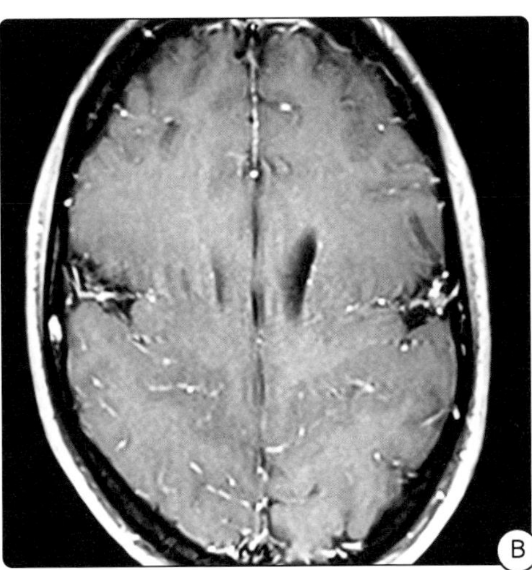


***(42-35B)** T1 C+ FS shows enhancing cortical veins in the clefts. Note the clefts do not extend to the lateral ventricles.*

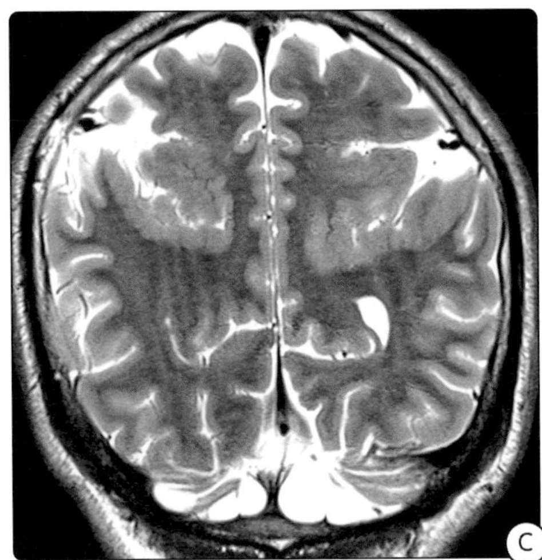


***(42-35C)** Coronal T2WI shows deep sulci with PMG. This is not schizencephaly, which has a cleft from brain surface to lateral ventricle.*

# Holoprosencephalies, Related Disorders, and Mimics

*Holoprosencephalies and variants, such as syntelencephaly, are classified as anomalies of ventral prosencephalon development. Other anomalies of the ventral prosencephalon include septo-optic dysplasia (with or without anomalies of the hypothalamic-pituitary axis) and arrhinencephaly, both of which are discussed in this chapter.*

We conclude the chapter with a brief discussion of hydranencephaly, an in utero acquired destruction of the cerebral hemispheres that can sometimes be confused with alobar holoprosencephaly or severe "open-lip" schizencephaly.



## Holoprosencephaly

Holoprosencephaly (HPE) spans a continuum from alobar to lobar forms. Although each is delineated separately, keep in mind that the HPEs are really a spectrum with no clear boundaries that reliably distinguish one type from another.

### Overview and Etiology

The fetal forebrain starts as a featureless, mostly fluid-filled sac. Outpouchings from the neural tube initially form a single central fluid-filled cavity ("monoventricle"). The fetal forebrain and monoventricle subsequently divide into the two cerebral hemispheres, also forming the definitive ventricles. Failure of this process leads to HPE. "Holoprosencephaly" literally means a single ("holo") ventricle involving the embryonic forebrain (prosencephalon).

HPE is divided into three subtypes based on severity, although HPE is a continuum that ranges from the most severe type [**alobar** HPE (aHPE)] to milder **lobar** forms. In the most severe forms, a central monoventricle is present, and structures, such as the basal ganglia, are fused in the midline.

An intermediate type, **semilobar** HPE (sHPE), is more severe than aHPE but not nearly as well differentiated as the lobar variety. The distinction between these three forms is based primarily on the presence or absence of a midline fissure separating the hemispheres.

### Clinical Issues

HPE is the most common human forebrain malformation. Craniofacial malformations, such as cyclopia or single proboscis, hypotelorism, nasal anomalies, solitary median maxillary central incisor (SMMCI), and facial clefts, occur in ~ 75-80% of cases. The statement "the face predicts the brain" means that the most severe facial defects generally are associated with the most severe intracranial anomalies.

Nearly 3/4 of HPE patients have endocrinopathies. Pituitary insufficiency and congenital anosmia with absent CNI [arrhinencephaly (ARR)] are other common clinical features of HPE.

### General Imaging Features

Imaging findings range from a pancake-like holosphere with central monoventricle (aHPE) to well-differentiated, almost completely separated hemispheres with minimal abnormalities (lobar HPE). The septum pellucidum is absent in all cases of HPE.

## Alobar Holoprosencephaly

### Terminology and Pathology

aHPE is the most severe form of HPE. No midline fissure divides the brain into two separate cerebral hemispheres and no identifiable lobes are seen. The basal ganglia are fused. The falx and sagittal sinus are absent, as are the olfactory bulbs and tracts.

The brain configuration varies from flat ("pancake") to cup- or ball-shaped. The sylvian fissures are unformed, and the brain surface often appears completely agyric or minimally sulcated with shallow sulci and flat, disordered gyri **(43-1)**.

Cut sections demonstrate a single crescent-shaped monoventricle that opens dorsally into a large CSF-filled dorsal cyst.

*(43-1) Autopsy of alobar holoprosencephaly (HPE) shows a large dorsal cyst ➡, fused thalami ➡, and rudimentary hemispheres ➡ with minimal sulcation and gyration. (43-2) NECT scan shows alobar HPE. Small rim of cortex ➡ surrounds "horseshoe" central monoventricle ➡. Thalami are fused ➡. Note the absence of the falx cerebri, interhemispheric fissure, and septum pellucidum.*

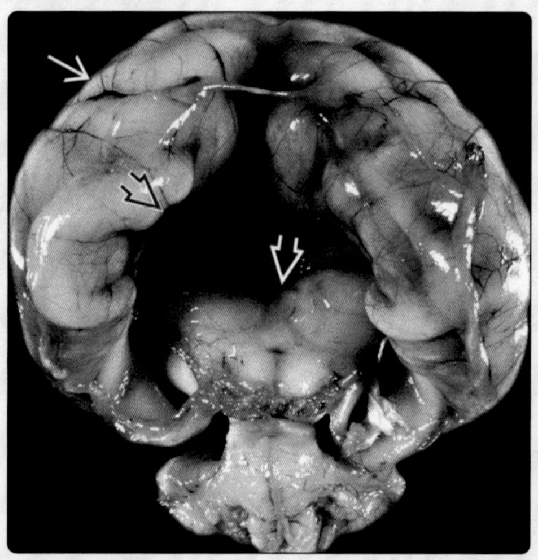

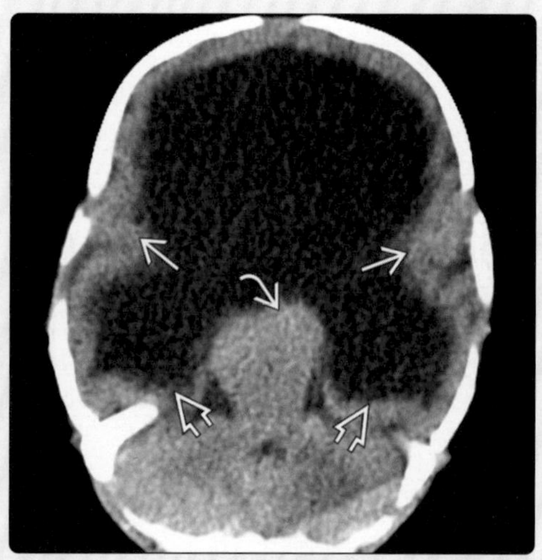

*(43-3) Coronal autopsy of severe sHPE shows H-shaped central ventricle with primitive-appearing temporal horns ➡, fused BG ➡, and rudimentary interhemispheric fissure ➡. (Courtesy R. Hewlett, MD.) (43-4) Axial T2 MR shows severe sHPE with rudimentary posterior interhemispheric fissure ➡, primitive ventricular horns ➡, and anterior midline fusion. Diffuse frontal migration arrest with subcortical heterotopic GM ➡ is also present.*

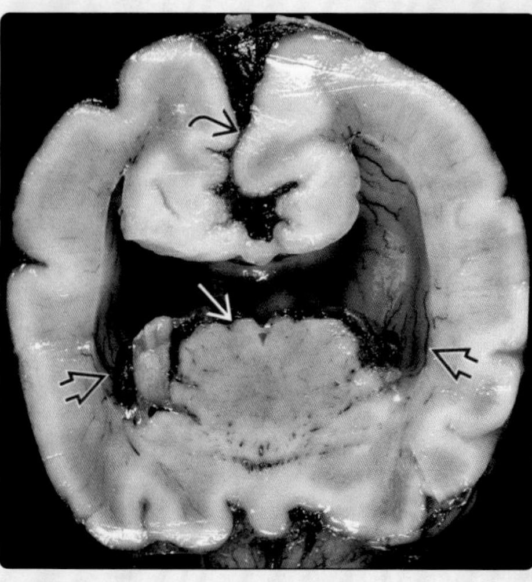

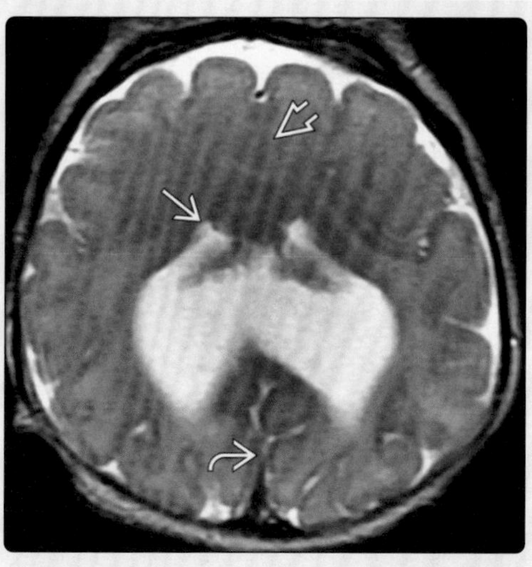

### Clinical Issues

aHPE has a high intrauterine lethality and stillbirth rate. Prognosis in surviving infants is poor. At least 1/2 of all patients with aHPE die in < 5 months, and 80% die before one year of age.

### Imaging

The cardinal feature of aHPE is a CSF-filled, horseshoe-shaped cavity **(43-2)** ("central monoventricle") that is often continuous posteriorly with a large dorsal cyst. Severe facial anomalies, such as cyclopia and proboscis, are more likely in those cases with a more severe spectrum of HPE.

The septum pellucidum and third ventricle are absent, as are the falx cerebri and interhemispheric fissure. The brain is completely fused across the midline without evidence of an anterior interhemispheric fissure. The brain appears thin and almost agyric, although a few shallow sulci may be present.

The basal ganglia are small and fused across the midline. There are no discernible commissures. Associated vascular anomalies, such as azygous anterior cerebral artery, are common.

### Differential Diagnosis

The major differential diagnosis of aHPE is **hydranencephaly**. In hydranencephaly, the face is normal. A falx is present, but most of the cerebral tissue has been destroyed, usually by an intrauterine vascular accident or infection.

## Semilobar Holoprosencephaly

### Terminology and Pathology

sHPE is intermediate in severity between aHPE and lobar HPE. A gradation of findings is present. The most severe sHPE shows a rudimentary interhemispheric fissure and incomplete falx **(43-3)**. The temporal horns of the lateral ventricle may be

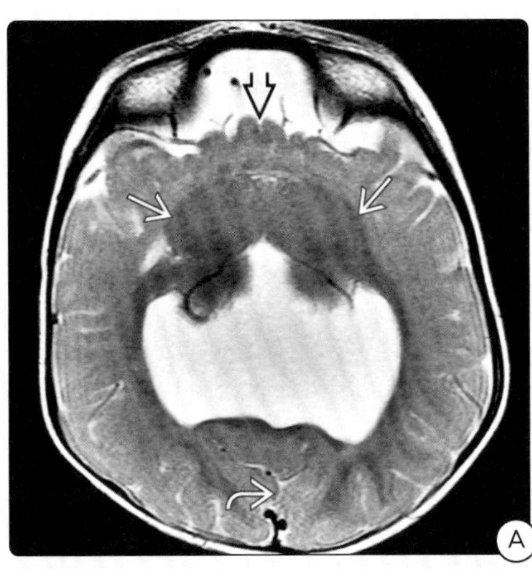


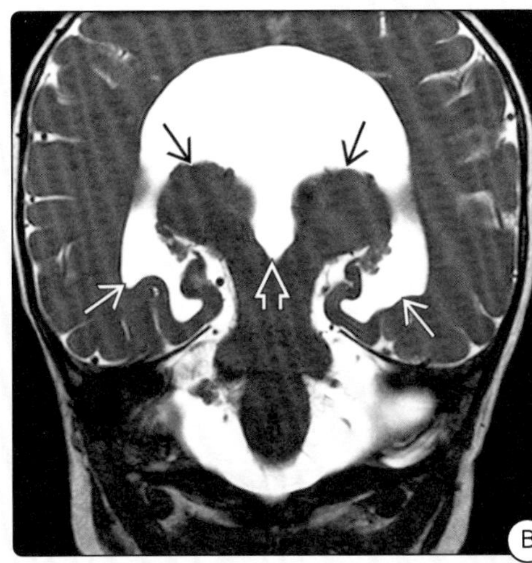


***(43-5A)*** *T2 MR in sHPE shows fused BG ➡, rudimentary posterior interhemispheric fissure ➡, and absence of anterior interhemispheric fissure with the brain fused across the midline ➡.* ***(43-5B)*** *Coronal T2 MR shows the monoventricle with rudimentary temporal horns ➡. A partially formed 3rd ventricle ➡ separates the thalami ➡. The interhemispheric fissure is absent.*

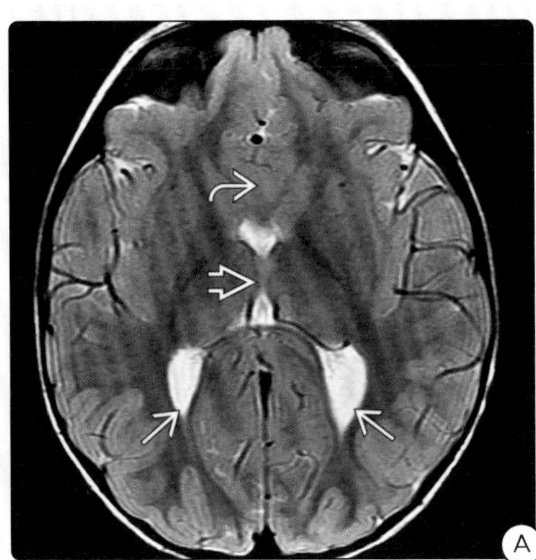


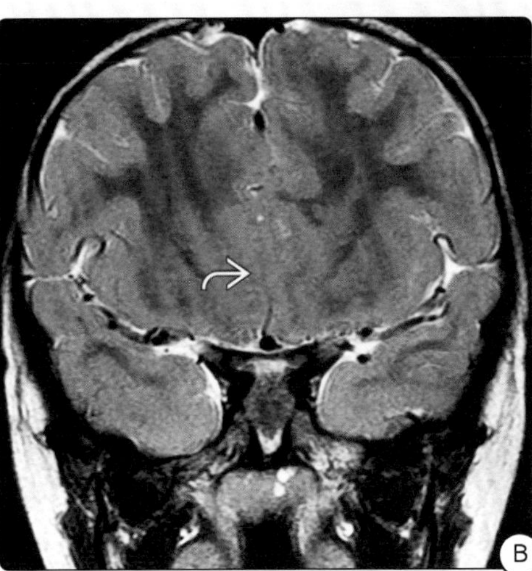


***(43-6A)*** *Axial T2 MR of lobar HPE shows well-developed occipital horns ➡, 3rd ventricle ➡, and minimal anterior midline fusion ➡.* ***(43-6B)*** *Coronal T2 MR shows that the anteroinferior frontal cortex is fused across the midline ➡. While alobar HPE and sHPE are often very obvious, lobar HPE can be so mild and subtle that care must be taken so as not to miss the anterior frontal connection.*

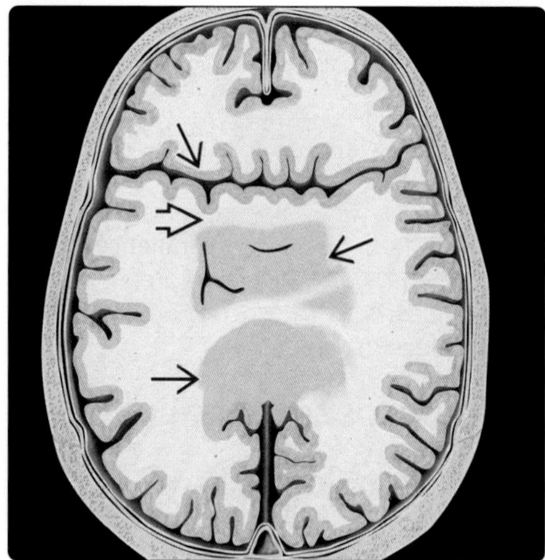

***(43-7)** Syntelencephaly shows absent midsection of interhemispheric fissure, crossing bridges of both GM ➡ and white matter ➡.*

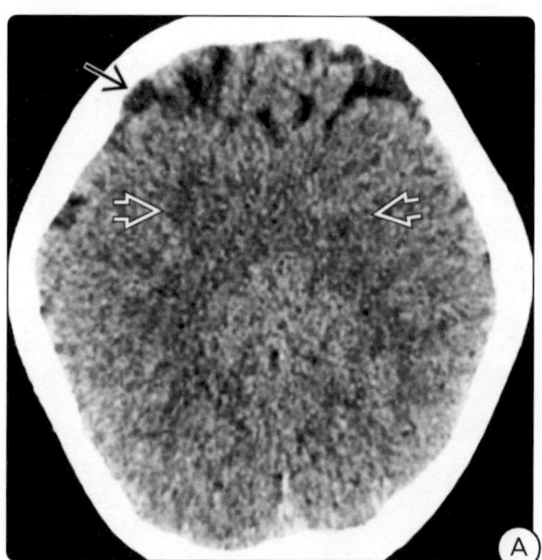

***(43-8A)** NECT shows aberrant fissure ➡, midportions of hemispheres ➡ fused across midline.*

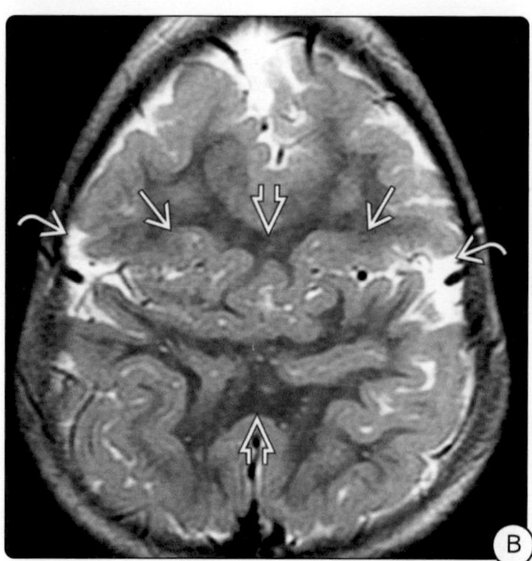

***(43-8B)** T2WI shows absent falx, abnormal sylvian fissures ➡ that meet over convexity with bridging cortex ➡ and white matter ➡.*

partially formed, but the septi pellucidi are absent. A dorsal cyst is often present.

### Imaging

With progressively better-differentiated sHPE, more of the interhemispheric fissure appears formed **(43-4)**. The deep nuclei exhibit various degrees of separation. If a rudimentary third ventricle is present, the thalami may be partially separated. The basal ganglia and hypothalami are still largely fused **(43-5)**. The caudate heads are continuous across the midline.

A corpus callosum splenium is present, but the body and genu are absent. Associated abnormalities include a dorsal cyst (present in 1/3 of cases) and vascular anomalies, such as azygous anterior cerebral artery and rudimentary deep veins.

### Differential Diagnosis

The major differential diagnoses of sHPE are **aHPE and lobar HPE**, depending on the severity of the sHPE.

## Lobar Holoprosencephaly

### Terminology and Pathology

Lobar HPE is the best differentiated of the HPEs. The interhemispheric fissure and falx are clearly developed. The third ventricle and lateral ventricular horns are generally well formed, although the septum pellucidum is absent and the frontal horns almost always appear dysmorphic. The hippocampi are present but often more vertically oriented than normal.

### Clinical Issues

Patients with lobar HPE are less severely affected compared with individuals with sHPE. Mild developmental delay, hypothalamic-pituitary dysfunction, and visual disturbances are the most common symptoms.

### Imaging

In lobar HPE, the cerebral hemispheres—including the thalami and most of the basal ganglia—are mostly separated. At least some of the most rostral and ventral portions of the frontal lobes are continuous across the midline **(43-6)**. The anterior columns of the fornix are fused. The thalami and basal ganglia are separated, although the caudate heads may remain fused.

The frontal horns of the lateral ventricles are present but dysplastic-appearing. The temporal and occipital horns are better defined, and the third ventricle generally appears normal. There is no septum pellucidum.

The corpus callosum is present and can be normal, incomplete, or hypoplastic. The splenium and most of the body can usually be identified, although the genu and rostrum are often absent. In contrast to isolated or syndromic corpus callosum dysgenesis, there are no Probst bundles in any of the HPEs.

The walls of the hypothalamus remain unseparated, and the optic chiasm is often smaller than normal. The olfactory bulbs are present in well-differentiated lobar HPE. The pituitary gland can be flattened, hypoplastic, or ectopic. Associated vascular anomalies include an azygous anterior cerebral artery.

## Differential Diagnosis

The major differential diagnosis of lobar HPE is **septo-optic dysplasia** (SOD). Some authors consider SOD the best differentiated of the HPE spectrum. In contrast to lobar HPE, the frontal horns are well formed in SOD. **ARR** may resemble lobar HPE, but the olfactory bulbs are usually present in lobar HPE.

In the rare **middle interhemispheric variant of HPE (MIH)** (syntelencephaly) **(43-7)**, the corpus callosum genu and splenium are formed; however, the *body* is missing, and the posterior frontal lobes are continuous across the midline.

# Holoprosencephaly Variants

Several holoprosencephaly (HPE) variants have been identified, including syntelencephaly and the septopreoptic HPEs. ARR, which some authors consider a variant of HPE, is considered together with SOD in the related midline disorders section later in the chapter.

## Middle Interhemispheric Variant of Holoprosencephaly

### Terminology

MIH is a mild HPE subtype that is also known as **syntelencephaly**.

### Etiology

HPE is a disorder of ventral induction that results from incomplete midline cleavage of the prosencephalon. In MIH, there is failure of separation of the posterior frontal and parietal lobes **(43-7)**.

Mutations in the *ZIC2* gene have been recognized as a potential cause of MIH.

### Pathology

The MIH variant represents 2-15% of HPE cases. In classic MIH, the callosal genu and splenium are normally formed, but the middle part (the body) is absent.

### Clinical Issues

Patients with MIH often have closely spaced eyes and a depressed or narrowed nasal bridge but otherwise relatively normal facial appearance.

### Imaging

Imaging findings in MIH are diagnostic. Sagittal T1 and T2 scans show that the corpus callosum splenium and genu are present, but the body is absent **(43-9)**.

Axial scans show the anterior and posterior parts of the interhemispheric fissure are present, but the midsection is absent, so the hemispheres are fused across the midline **(43-8B)**. The anterior falx is present or mildly dysplastic but then narrows and disappears in the posterior frontal and anterior parietal regions. In 85% of cases, the sylvian fissures course superiorly and meet in a coronally oriented, cortically lined fissure that is continuous across the midline **(43-8A)**.

On coronal scans, the posterior frontal lobes are continuous across the midline, while the lateral ventricle bodies appear narrow and fused. A single

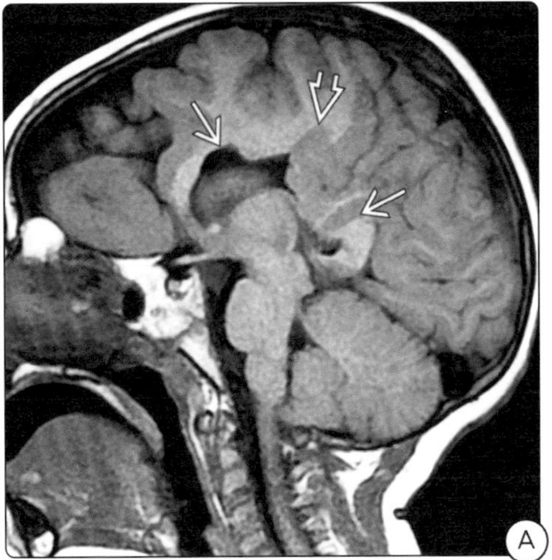


***(43-9A)** T1WI of MIH shows midsection of corpus callosum ➡ is absent. Note dysplastic cortex ➡ deforms lateral ventricle.*

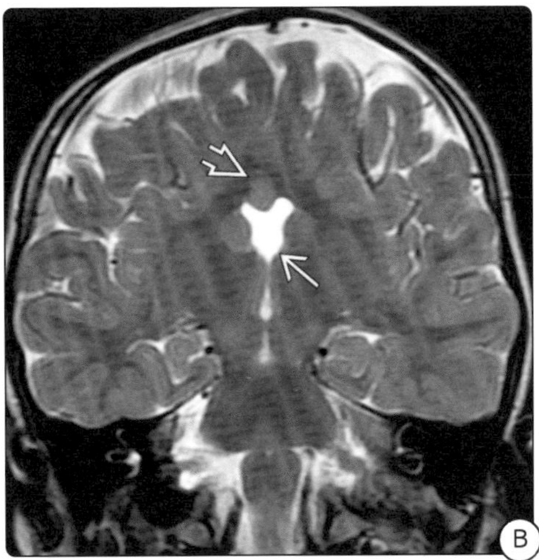


***(43-9B)** Coronal T2WI GM nodule ➡ perched on top of fused, "notched" lateral ventricles ➡. Interhemispheric fissure is absent.*

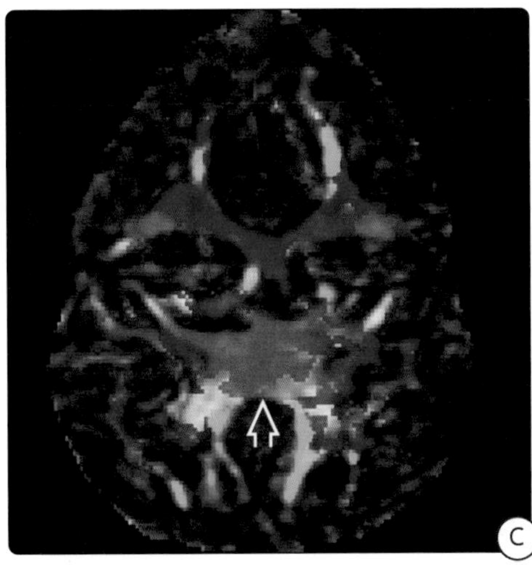


***(43-9C)** Axial DTI shows white matter tracts in the posterosuperior frontal lobes meet and cross in the midline ➡.*

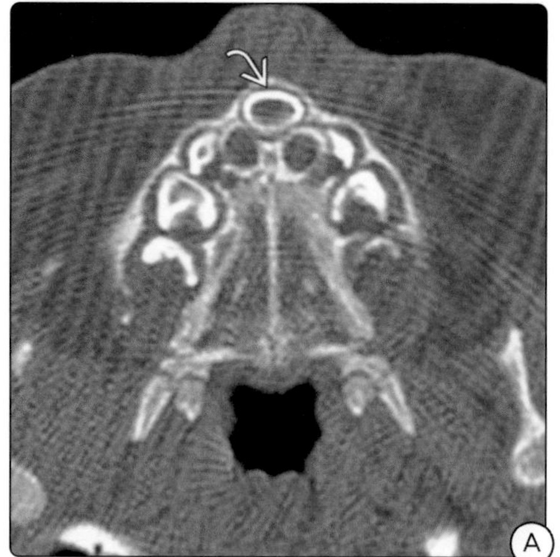

***(43-10A)** Bone CT in a newborn with difficulty breathing shows single midline maxillary incisor* ➯.

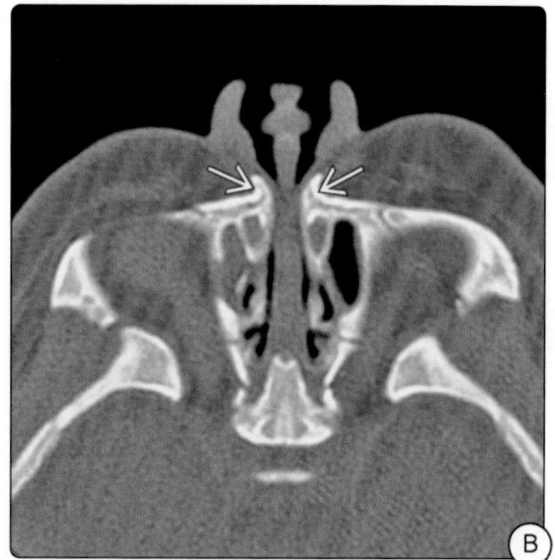

***(43-10B)** More cephalad CT shows pyriform aperture stenosis* ➡.

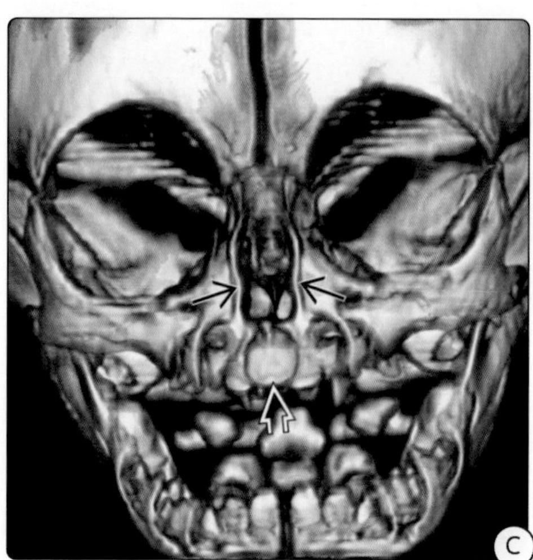

***(43-10C)** AP view of shaded surface display in the same case shows the midline central incisor* ➡, *pyriform aperture stenosis* ⇨.

common ventricle without a septum pellucidum is present. The third ventricle is well formed. A nodule of heterotopic gray matter is often perched along the dorsal aspect of the fused lateral ventricles, forming a characteristic central ventricular "notch" **(43-9B)**. Other foci of heterotopic gray matter are also common.

The hypothalamus and basal ganglia are normally separated in MIH, while the caudate nuclei and thalami are partially fused. An azygous anterior cerebral artery is present in most cases. Other common associated anomalies include cerebellar abnormalities and polymicrogyria.

DTI shows that the callosal body and central cingulum fibers are absent, but all other major white matter tracts have a normal course, thickness, and integrity. The horizontal white matter tracts cross the midline just under the fused cortex **(43-9C)**.

### Differential Diagnosis

In contrast to **classic HPE**, in syntelencephaly, the ventral aspects of the basal forebrain are largely spared, so the basal ganglia and olfactory sulci appear normal.

## Septopreoptic Holoprosencephaly

Several very mild forms of HPE have been described where failure of hemispheric separation is restricted to the septal (subcallosal) &/or preoptic regions or both. Patients with septopreoptic HPE often present with mild midline craniofacial malformations. These include **solitary median maxillary central incisor** (SSMCI) and **congenital nasal pyriform aperture stenosis** (CNPAS) **(43-10)**.

Neonates with SMMCI often present with breathing difficulties secondary to nasal obstruction. Imaging findings range from isolated dental abnormalities with a single maxillary incisor and V-shaped palate to more complex abnormalities that also involve the brain. Anomalies of the fornix, septi pellucidi, and corpus callosum are often present. An azygous anterior cerebral artery is common. Some cases have pituitary stalk hypoplasia.

# Related Midline Disorders

## Septo-Optic Dysplasia

### Terminology and Etiology

Some authors consider SOD simply a very well-differentiated form of lobar HPE.

Several genes connected to the development of the forebrain and related midbrain structures have been implicated in the development of SOD. These include *HESX1*, *SOX2*, *SOX3*, *FGF1*, and *FGF8*.

### Pathology

SOD is characterized by any combination of the following: (1) Optic nerve hypoplasia, (2) pituitary hypofunction, and (3) midline brain abnormalities. Brain abnormalities include dysgenesis of the septum pellucidum &/or corpus callosum or hypoplasia of the pons, vermis, or medulla. Ventral midline fusions are absent. Approximately 1/3 of SOD patients have the full spectrum of manifestations **(43-11A)**.

## Clinical Issues

Individuals with SOD have different manifestations of visual and pituitary-hypothalamic dysfunction. The most common clinical feature of SOD is visual impairment. Nearly 2/3 of SOD patients also develop endocrine abnormalities from hypothalamic-pituitary insufficiency (e.g., hypoglycemic seizures).

## Imaging

Thin-section coronal T1- and T2-weighted images show absent or hypoplastic septum pellucidum. The frontal horns appear "squared-off" or box-like with distinct inferior pointing. The optic chiasm and one or both optic nerves appear small in most cases **(43-11)**. Sagittal images show that the septum pellucidum is absent and the fornices are low-lying, giving the lateral ventricles an empty appearance. The optic nerves and chiasm are hypoplastic.

Isolated absence of the septum pellucidum is relatively rare, so look carefully for other anomalies midline anomalies, such as pituitary malformations (anterior pituitary hypoplasia, ectopic posterior pituitary, and thin/interrupted or absent infundibulum). When associated with malformations of cortical development (e.g., schizencephaly and polymicrogyria), this constellation of findings is referred to as SOD plus **(43-12)**.

### SEPTO-OPTIC DYSPLASIA: IMAGING

**Imaging Findings**
- Absent septum pellucidum
  - "Squared-off" frontal horns, pointed inferiorly on coronal T2WI
- Hypoplastic optic nerves, chiasm
- Look for
  - Malformations of cortical development
  - Thin stalk, small gland, ectopic posterior pituitary

## Differential Diagnosis

The major differential diagnosis of SOD is well-differentiated **lobar HPE**. The cerebral hemispheres and basal ganglia are completely separated in SOD.

# Arrhinencephaly

ARR is a congenital malformation in which the olfactory bulb and tracts are absent **(43-13)** **(43-15)**. ARR can exist in isolation, although most cases occur with other midline facial anomalies, such as cleft palate or lip, and aHPE or sHPE.

When olfactory aplasia/hypoplasia occurs with hypogonadotrophic hypogonadism, it is termed **Kallman syndrome**. Olfactory agenesis occurs in ~ 25% of patients with **CHARGE** syndrome (**c**oloboma, **h**eart malformations, choanal **a**tresia, growth/development **r**estriction, **g**enital anomalies, **e**ar anomalies).

# Holoprosencephaly Mimics

## Hydranencephaly

Although some authors consider hydranencephaly a congenital malformation, it is actually the consequence of severe brain destruction in

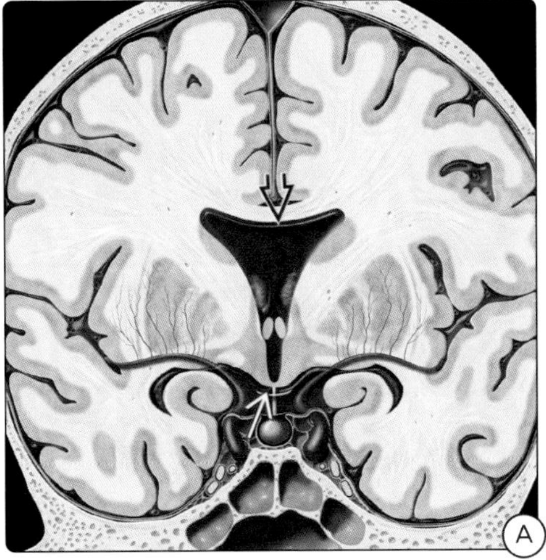

*(43-11A) Coronal graphic shows SOD with absent cavum septi pellucidi with flat-roofed anterior horns ⇨ and small optic chiasm ➡.*

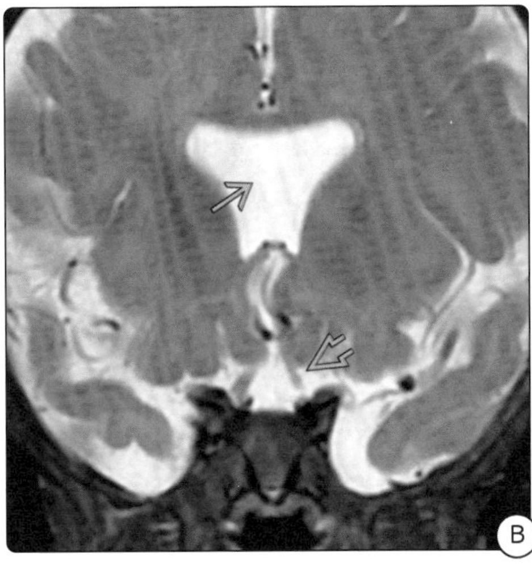

*(43-11B) Coronal T2 MR a 5-month-old with SOD shows absent septum pellucidum ⇨ and small left optic nerve ⇨.*

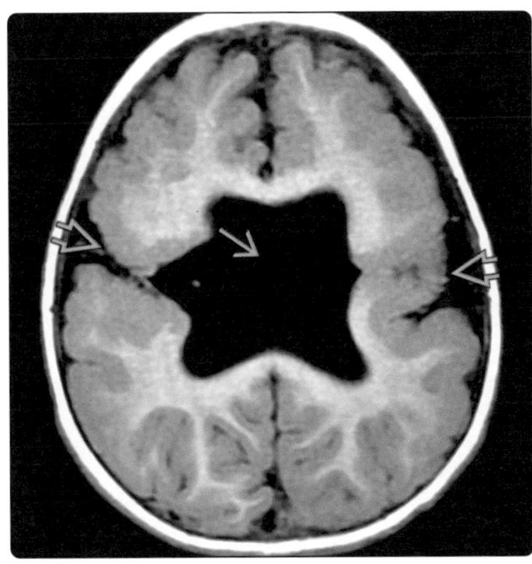

*(43-12) Axial T1 MR in an 11-month-old with SOD plus shows absence of the septum pellucidum ⇨ and bilateral schizencephaly ⇨.*

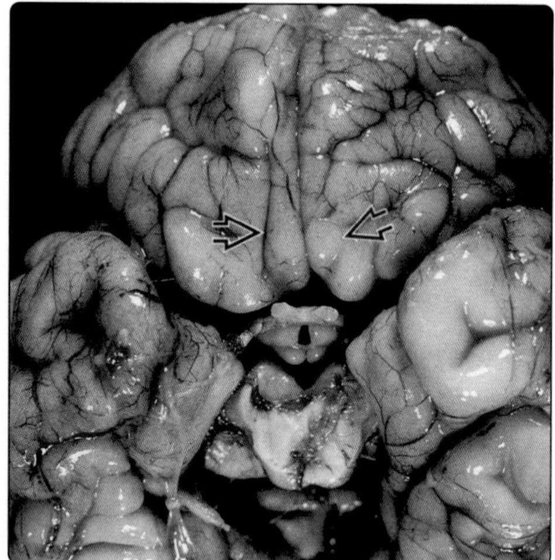

***(43-13)** Autopsied arrhinencephaly shows absent olfactory bulbs, shallow deformed olfactory sulci ⇒. (Courtesy R. Hewlett, MD.)*

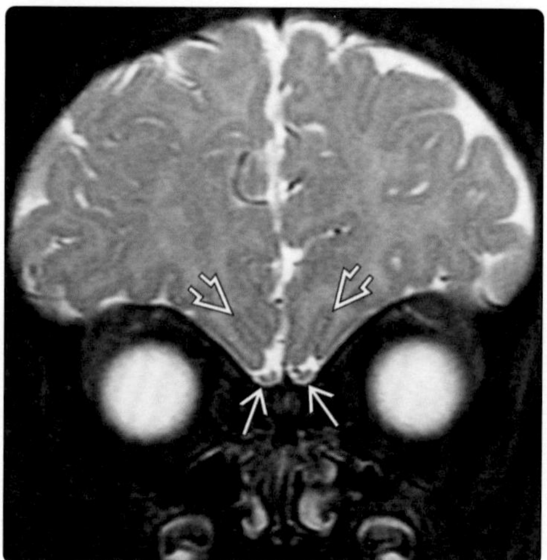

***(43-14)** Coronal T2 FS in a normal newborn shows olfactory bulbs ➡, normal olfactory sulci ⇒.*

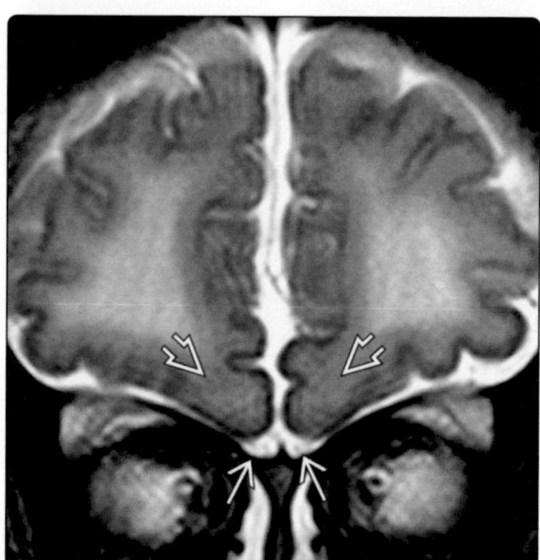

***(43-15)** Coronal T2 FS in newborn with multiple anomalies shows absent olfactory bulbs ➡, no olfactory sulci ⇒. (Courtesy S. Blaser, MD.)*

utero. It is important to distinguish hydranencephaly from other disorders, such as **aHPE** and **maximal hydrocephalus**.

In hydranencephaly, the cerebral hemispheres are completely or almost completely missing. Instead, a membranous sac filled with CSF, glial tissue, and ependyma is present **(43-16)**.

NECT scans show CSF almost completely filling the supratentorial space. The falx cerebri is generally intact within the water-filled cranial vault. The basal ganglia are absent, but the thalami are present. Occipital and temporal cortex within the posterior cerebral artery territory are usually present.

MR demonstrates a largely absent cerebral mantle **(43-17A)**. The falx is easily identified **(43-17B)**. The fluid-filled spaces follow CSF on all sequences.

The most important differential diagnosis of hydranencephaly **(43-17)** is severe, "maximal" **obstructive hydrocephalus** (OH). In severe OH (e.g., secondary to aqueductal stenosis), a thin cortex can be seen compressed against the dura and inner table of the calvarium **(43-18)**.

In **aHPE**, the falx and interhemispheric fissure are absent. The basal ganglia are fused **(43-19)**. Severe **bilateral "open-lip" schizencephaly** has large transmantle CSF clefts that are lined with dysplastic cortex **(43-20)**. The falx and tentorium are normal.

### DIFFERENTIAL DIAGNOSIS OF "WATER-BAG" BRAIN

**"Maximal" Obstructive Hydrocephalus**
- Large head
- Thinned but normal cortex
- Massively enlarged ventricles
- Falx present
- Basal ganglia separated

**Hydranencephaly**
- Large head
- Absent brain; bilateral internal carotid artery territories
- Markedly enlarged ventricles occupy absent brain
- Falx present
- Basal ganglia typically absent; thalami present

**Alobar Holoprosencephaly**
- Small head
- Smooth or minimally sulcated brain
- "Horseshoe" monoventricle
- Absent falx, interhemispheric fissure
- Basal ganglia fused

**"Open-Lip" Schizencephaly**
- Remnant "nubbins" of brain
- No cortex external to huge "open" clefts
- Dysplastic cortex lines sides of open cleft
- Falx, interhemispheric fissure present
- Basal ganglia separated

*Selected References: The complete reference list is available on the eBooks+ version included with purchase.*

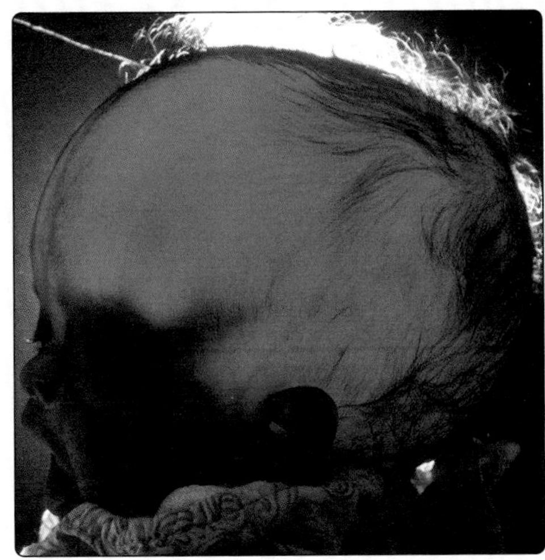

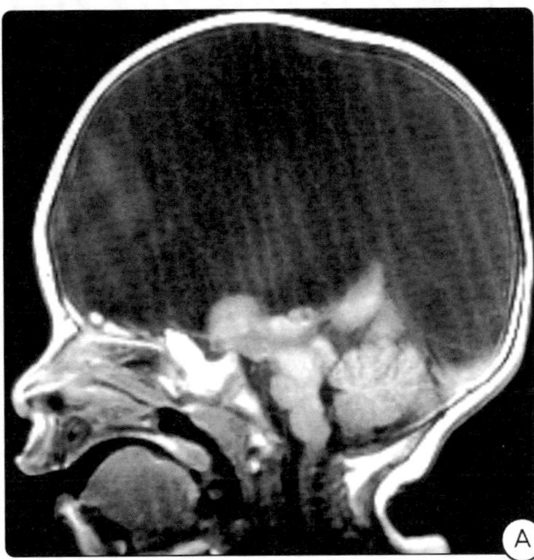

***(43-16)*** *Autopsy of hydranencephaly with transillumination shows most of the enlarged cranium is water filled.* ***(43-17A)*** *T1 MR shows hydranencephaly with macrocephaly; CSF fills the supratentorial spaces. Brainstem and cerebellum are normal.*

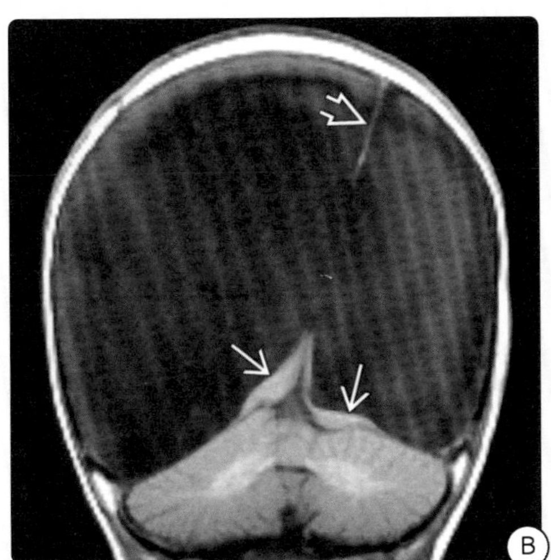

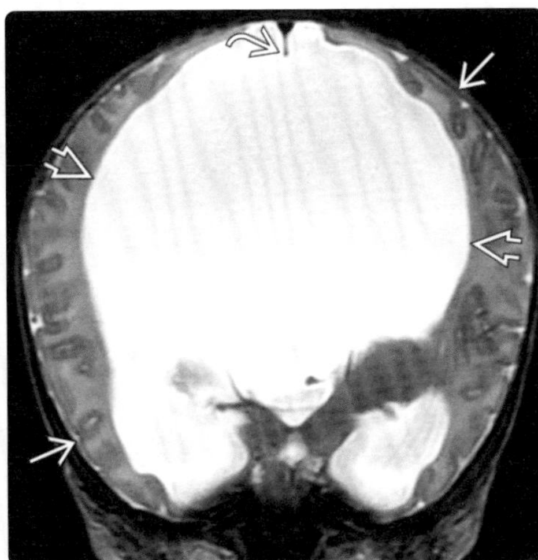

***(43-17B)*** *Coronal T1 MR shows CSF-filled cranial vault and only tiny remnants of brain ➡. A falx is present ➡. (Courtesy A. Illner, MD.)* ***(43-18)*** *In contrast to hydranencephaly, coronal T2 MR in a case of maximal obstructive hydrocephalus shows enlarged lateral ventricles ➡, rim of compressed but normal brain ➡. Falx ➡ is present.*

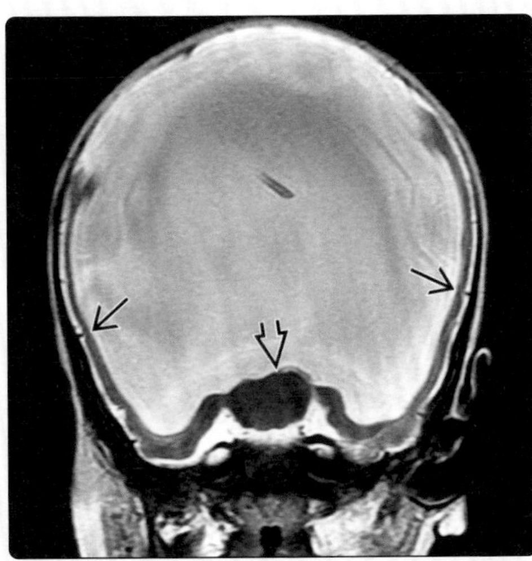

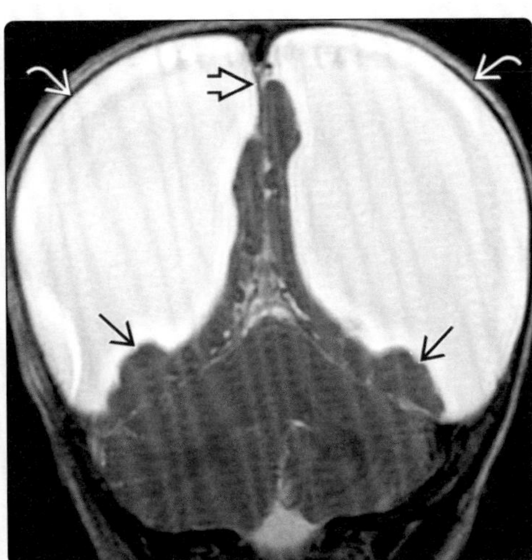

***(43-19)*** *T2 MR shows alobar HPE with horseshoe-shaped monoventricle, fused BG ➡, absent falx, thin, dysplastic-appearing brain ➡.* ***(43-20)*** *Huge "open-lip" schizencephaly with dysplastic brain lining clefts ➡, no cortex external to clefts ➡. Falx ➡ is present.*

# Genetic Tumor Syndromes Involving the CNS

*Historically, few CNS neoplasms were thought to result from a genetic predisposition to tumorigenesis. Within the last decade, new DNA sequencing methods and methylome profiling have led to increasing recognition and definition of high-risk cancer predisposition syndromes. Recent studies identified a cancer predisposition syndrome in 7-15% of pediatric patients with newly diagnosed CNS tumors. In certain tumor types (i.e., choroid plexus carcinoma), the predisposition rate can approach 50%.*



The term **familial cancer predisposition syndrome** is used to describe familial cancers in which a clear mode of inheritance can be established. The CNS and PNS are frequently involved in these disorders. The 2021 WHO now classifies such familial cancers with CNS &/or PNS neoplasms as **genetic tumor syndromes involving the CNS**. While many of the index neoplasms occur sporadically and are described in detail in previous chapters of this book, here we consider the clinical spectrum, pathogenesis, and molecular genetics of syndromic-associated nervous system tumors.

**Cancer predisposition syndromes** are caused by pathogenic variation in genes that primarily function as tumor suppressors and protooncogenes. These variants are found in the germline or constitutional DNA. New insights into the underlying mechanisms of these cancer predisposition syndromes have used CRISPR/Cas9 gene-editing tools to model these disorders.

To date, 19 genetic tumor syndromes involving the CNS—including eight new ones since the 2016 WHO classification of CNS tumors—are formally recognized. In this chapter, we consider the major familial tumor syndromes that involve the nervous system, beginning with the neurofibromatoses. Major attention is also directed to tuberous sclerosis, von Hippel-Lindau disease (VHL), Li-Fraumeni syndrome, and constitutional mismatch repair deficiency (CMMRD) syndromes.

Some uncommon but nevertheless important syndromes, such as Turcot, Gorlin, and Cowden syndromes, rhabdoid tumor predisposition syndrome, *DICER1* syndrome, familial retinoblastoma (RB), and *BAP1* tumor predisposition syndrome, are also briefly considered in this chapter.

## Neurofibromatosis and Schwannomatosis

Neurofibromatoses are the most common CNS tumor predisposition syndromes. Two types of neurofibromatosis are widely recognized:

**Neurofibromatosis type 1 (NF1)** and **neurofibromatosis type 2 (NF2)**. Both are multisystem disorders with neoplastic as well as nonneoplastic manifestations. A third related disorder, **schwannomatosis**, is associated with inactivation of the *NF2* gene in tumors (but not in the germline) and is considered a distinct genetic disease, so it, too, is included in this section.

## Neurofibromatosis Type 1

NF1 is an autosomal dominant inherited genodermatosis and tumor predisposition syndrome with variable expression, a high rate of new mutations (nearly 50%), and virtually 100% penetrance by age 20.

### Etiology

**Genetics.** A pathogenic NF1 variant is detected in > 95% of people with NF1. NF1 is caused by mutation of the *NF1* gene on chromosome 17q11.2. Mutations inactivate the gene that encodes the tumor suppressor protein, **neurofibromin 1**, a negative regulator of the Ras signal transduction pathway that plays a key role in both tumor suppression and regulation of cell growth/proliferation. Neurofibromin also acts as a regulator of neural stem cell proliferation and differentiation; it is required for normal glial and neuronal development **(44-1)**.

Approximately 1/2 of all NF1 cases are familial. Such patients already harbor a heterozygous germline *NF1* mutation and develop neurofibromas upon somatic mutation of the second (wildtype) *NF1* allele. Nearly 1/2 the individuals with NF1 have unaffected parents. These NF1 cases are caused by a pathogenic, de novo mutation in the *NF1* gene.

### Pathology

CNS lesions are found in 15-20% of patients. A variety of nonneoplastic lesions as well as benign and malignant tumors

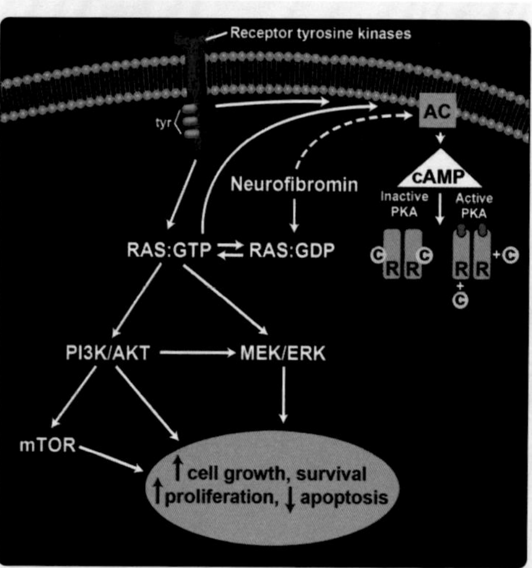


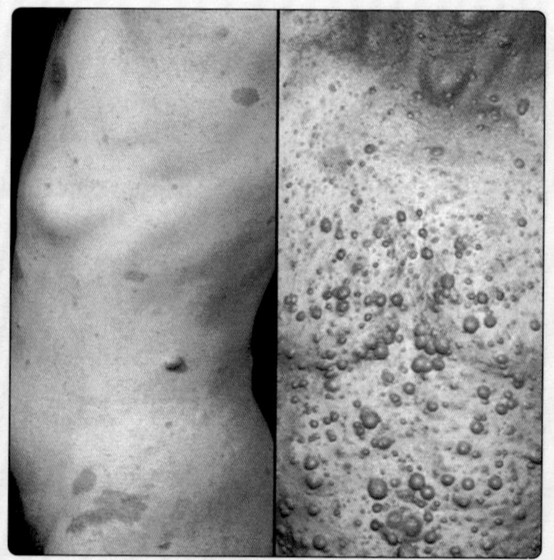

*(44-1) Germline mutations causing neurofibromatosis type 1 (NF1) result in loss of the neurofibromin tumor suppressor, resulting in constitutive RAS/MEK/ERK and PI3K/AKT signaling, as well as altered cAMP levels. (44-2) Photographs show multiple café au lait spots (L) and cutaneous neurofibromas (R) in patients with NF1. (Courtesy A. Ersen, MD.)*

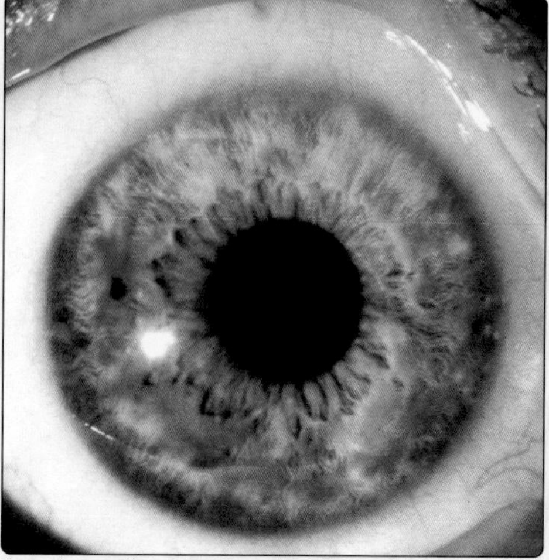

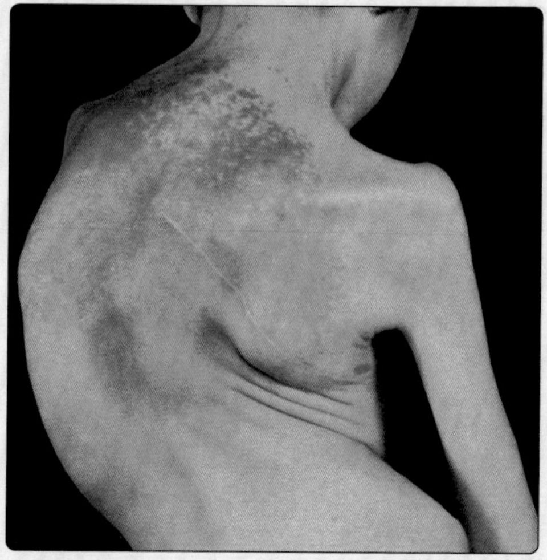

*(44-3) Clinical photograph shows multiple Lisch nodules in a patient with NF1. (Courtesy A. Ersen, MD.) (44-4) Clinical photograph of a patient with NF1 demonstrates extreme kyphoscoliosis and numerous café au lait spots. (From DP: Neuro.)*

are associated with NF1. There is also an increased risk of non-CNS malignancies in NF1 patients.

**Nonneoplastic CNS Lesions.** Multiple waxing and waning cerebral **dysplastic white matter (WM) lesions** on T2/FLAIR are identified in ~ 70% of children with NF1 **(44-9)**. Histopathologically, these benign lesions—also called unidentified bright objects (UBOs) or focal areas of signal intensity (FASIs)—represent zones of myelin vacuolization and dysgenesis, not hamartomas, demyelination, or axonal degeneration **(44-8)**. These lesions do not enhance with contrast and follow a benign course, initially waxing and then completely regressing by 20 years. Similar T2-hyperintense, nonenhancing lesions are seen in the spinal cords of 8% of children with NF1 (all reported cases exhibited similar brain T2 hyperintensities).

**Dural ectasia** may cause dilatation of the optic nerve sheaths, Meckel cave, or internal auditory canals **(44-6)**. Spinal abnormalities, including dural ectasia, meningoceles, and bony deformities, occur in ~ 15% of patients with classic NF1 **(44-5) (44-4)**.

NF1 is associated with CNS **vasculopathy** in 2-6% of cases. A variety of vascular abnormalities, including vessel ectasia, moyamoya, hypoplasia, and vessel narrowing, have been associated **(44-7)**. The most common manifestation is progressive intimal fibrosis with stenoocclusion of the supraclinoid internal carotid arteries, resulting in **moyamoya disease (MMD)**. MMD can cause both ischemic and hemorrhagic strokes.

**CNS Neoplasms.** Patients with NF1 have a high risk for developing a spectrum of neoplasms in the CNS and PNS. CNS tumors occur in ~ 20% of individuals with NF1 and are a pathologically and biologically heterogeneous group of neoplasms.

Optic pathway gliomas (OPGs)—nearly always pilocytic astrocytomas—account for ~ 70% of all CNS tumors in

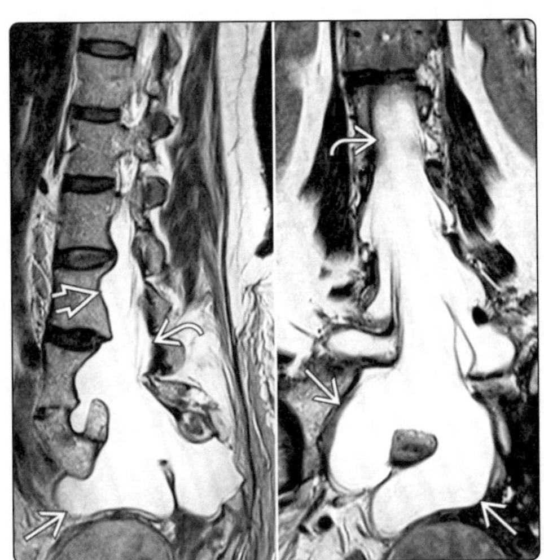

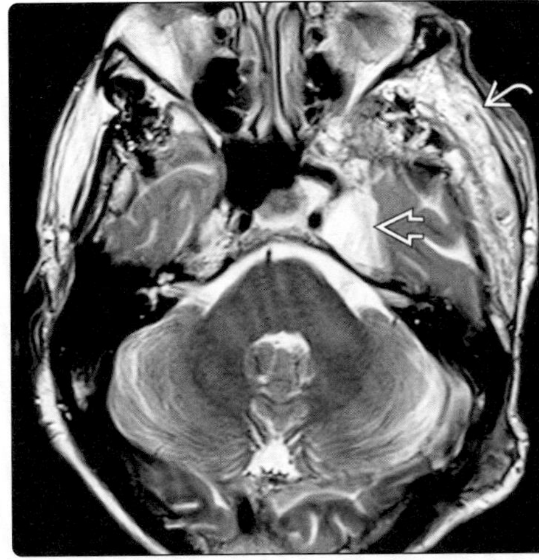

***(44-5)** Sagittal (L) and coronal (R) T2 MRs show NF1 dural ectasia ➡ causing posterior vertebral scalloping ➡ and extensive meningoceles ➡. **(44-6)** T2 MR in NF1 shows scalp plexiform neurofibroma ➡ and patulous left Meckel cave ➡.*

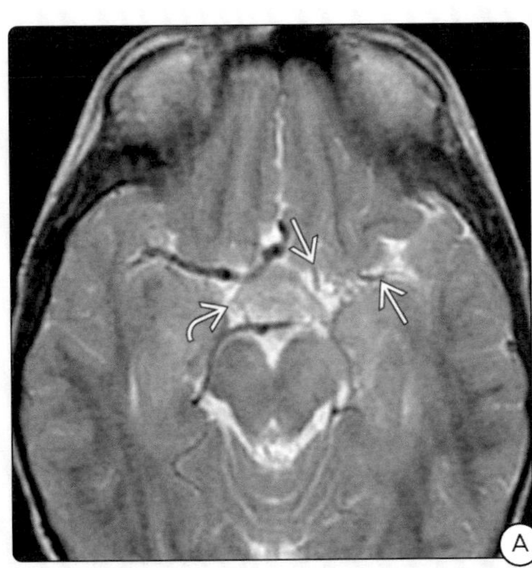



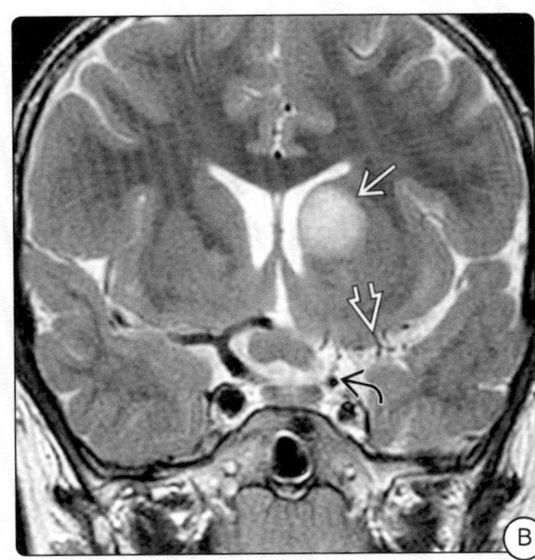



***(44-7A)** Axial T2 MR in a 10-yo boy with NF1 shows glioma of the optic chiasm ➡. The right middle cerebral artery (MCA) appears normal, while the left MCA is attenuated and hypoplastic ➡. **(44-7B)** Coronal T2 MR shows extreme hypoplasia of the left ICA ➡ and MCA ➡, characteristic of NF1-associated vasculopathy. The mass in the left caudate nucleus did not enhance and is an unusual focal area of signal intensity (FASI) ➡.*

children with NF1 **(44-15)**. The second most common brain tumor is brainstem glioma (15-17%).

Benign NF1-related neoplasms include neurofibromas. Malignant tumors include malignant peripheral nerve sheath tumors (MPNSTs) and gliomas.

***Neurofibromas.*** A spectrum of NF1-associated neurofibromas occurs. **Dermal neurofibromas** arise within a peripheral nerve and appear as soft, well-circumscribed, pedunculated or sessile lesions. Most patients develop more tumors as they age, and some have literally thousands of dermal neurofibromas **(44-2)** **(44-22)**. More than 95% of adults with NF1 have at least one lesion.

**Plexiform neurofibromas** (PNFs) are distinct from dermal neurofibromas and are virtually pathognomonic of NF1. PNFs develop in 30-50% of individuals with NF1. PNF and atypical neurofibromatous neoplasm of unknown biologic potential (ANNUBP) are considered precancerous lesions that may develop into MPNSTs.

PNFs are generally large, bulky tumors usually associated with major nerve trunks and plexuses. PNFs are rope-like, diffusely infiltrating, noncircumscribed, transspatial lesions that resemble a bag of worms **(44-10)**. The scalp and orbit are common sites for PNFs. Spinal neurofibromas and PNFs are found in ~ 40% of patients with NF1 **(44-13)**.

***Malignant Peripheral Nerve Sheath Tumors.*** Although most PNFs remain benign, 10-15% become malignant. Individuals with NF1 have an 8-13% cumulative lifetime risk of developing an **MPNST** from a PNF **(44-14)**. MPNST is an aggressive, deadly tumor with a high rate of metastases and poor overall prognosis.

***Gliomas.*** Individuals with NF1 are prone to develop a wide variety of glial neoplasms. Gliomas arising in the setting of NF1 are a heterogeneous group of neoplasms that occur from

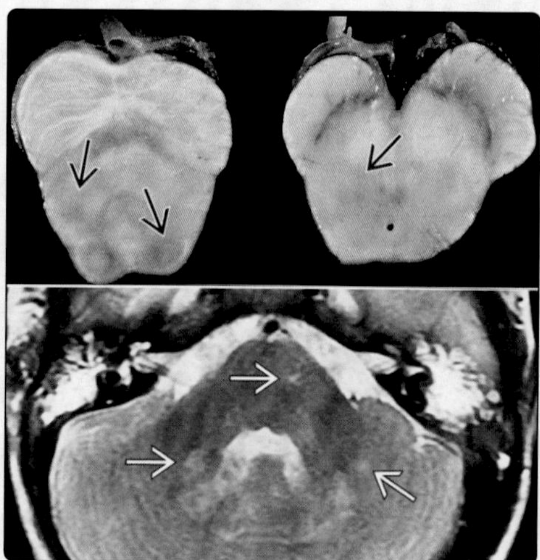

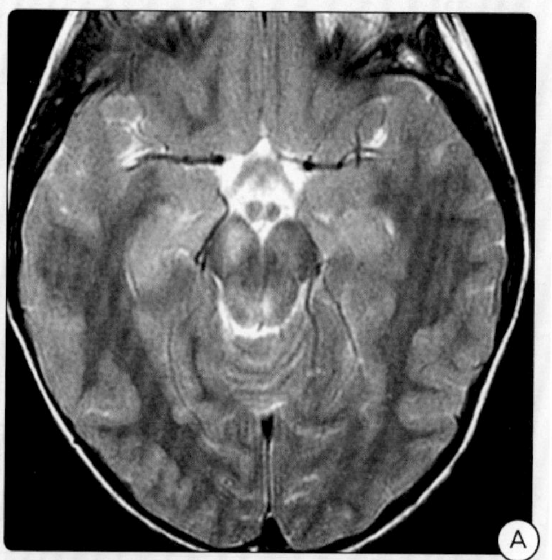


***(44-8)** (Top) Autopsied NF1 shows foci of discolored white matter (WM) ⇒. (Courtesy AFIP Archives.) (Bottom) T2 MR shows hyperintense lesions ➡ in the pons and cerebellum. **(44-9A)** T2 MR in a 7-yo girl with NF1 shows hyperintense foci in the right medial temporal lobe, cerebral peduncle, and dorsal midbrain.*

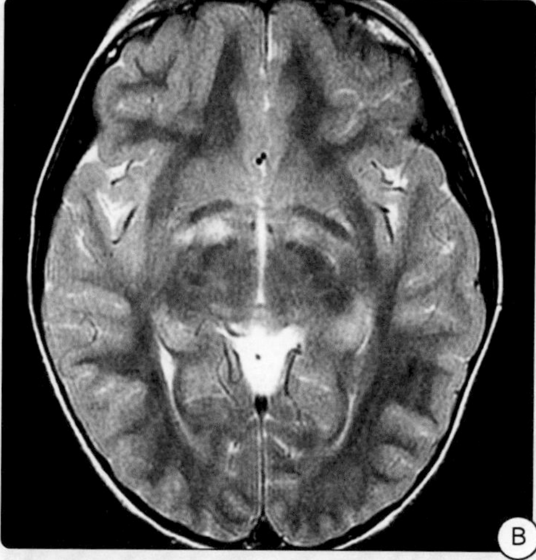


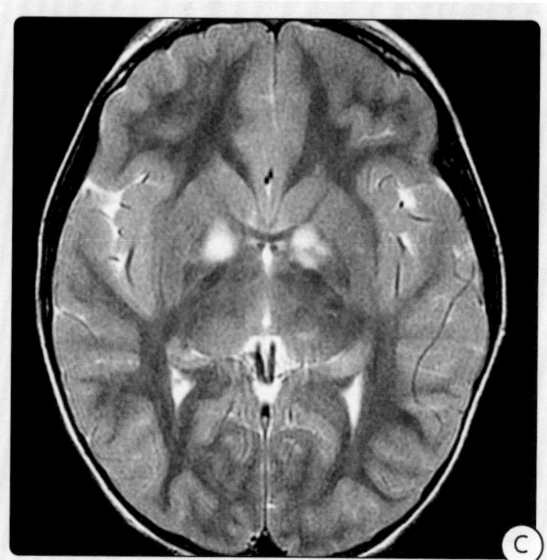


***(44-9B)** More cephalad T2 MR shows FASIs in both internal capsules. **(44-9C)** More cephalad T2 MR shows FASIs in both globi pallidi and left thalamus. No lesions enhanced, and all resolved completely by 15 years of age.*

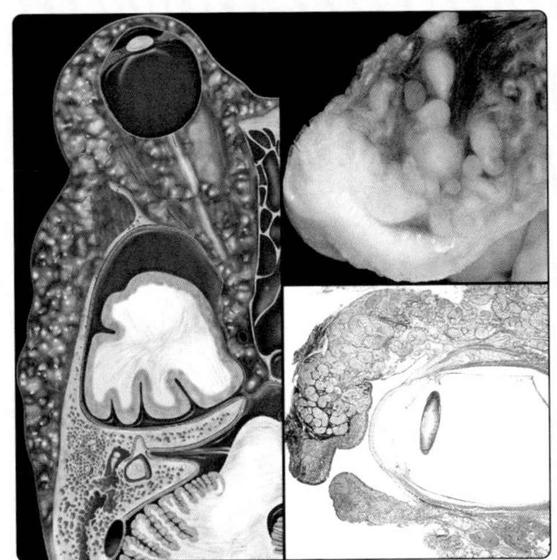

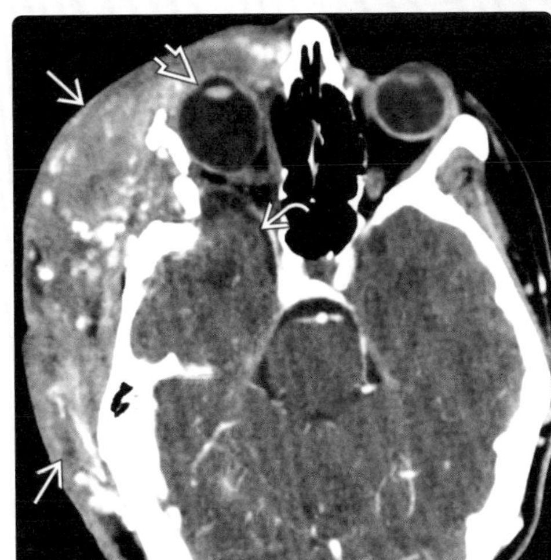

**(44-10)** Graphic (L) and surgical specimens (courtesy AFIP Archives) (R) show typical plexiform neurofibroma of the orbit, eyelid, and scalp. **(44-11)** CECT of NF1 shows sphenoid hypoplasia with temporal lobe protrusion into the orbit ➡, buphthalmos ➡, and plexiform neurofibroma ➡.

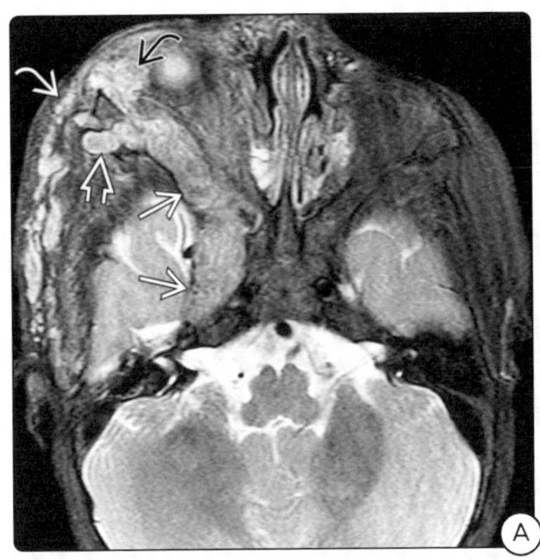

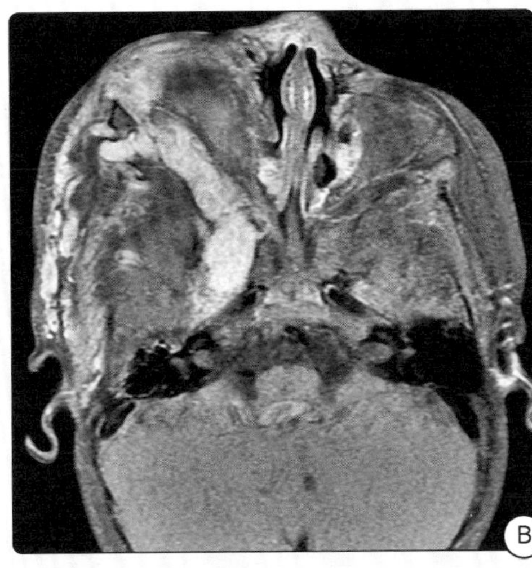

**(44-12A)** T2 MR in NF1 shows plexiform neurofibroma with extensive infiltration into the right orbit ➡, cavernous sinus ➡, pterygopalatine fossa ➡, and scalp ➡. **(44-12B)** T1 C+ FS MR in the same case shows strong but heterogeneous enhancement of the plexiform neurofibroma.

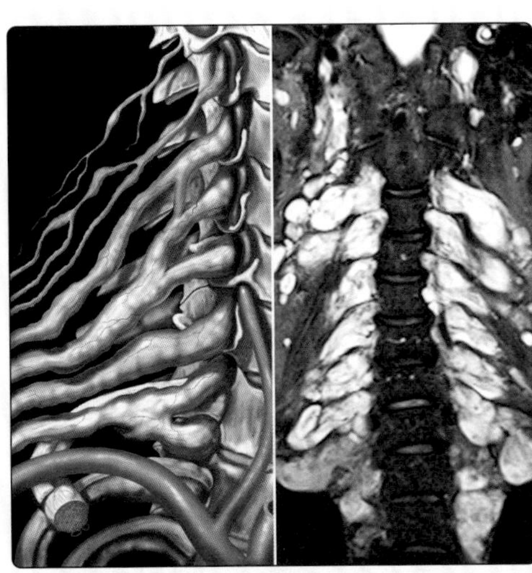

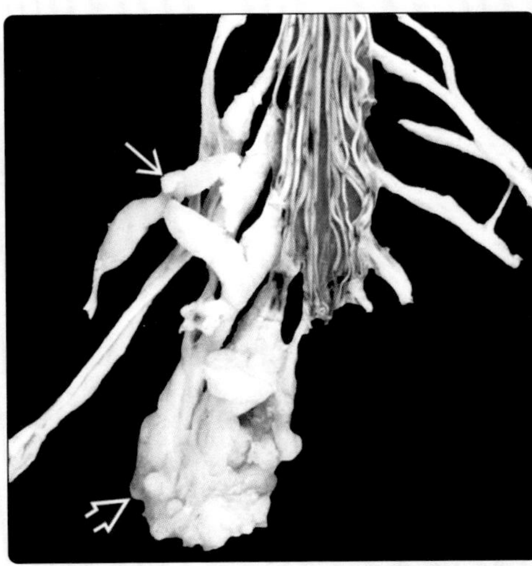

**(44-13)** Plexiform neurofibroma involving cervical nerve roots is depicted in the graphic (L) and on a coronal STIR scan (R). **(44-14)** Gross pathology shows neurofibromas along multiple spinal nerve roots in a patient with NF1 ➡. The large, bulky lesion ➡ is a malignant peripheral nerve sheath tumor. (From DP: Neuro.)

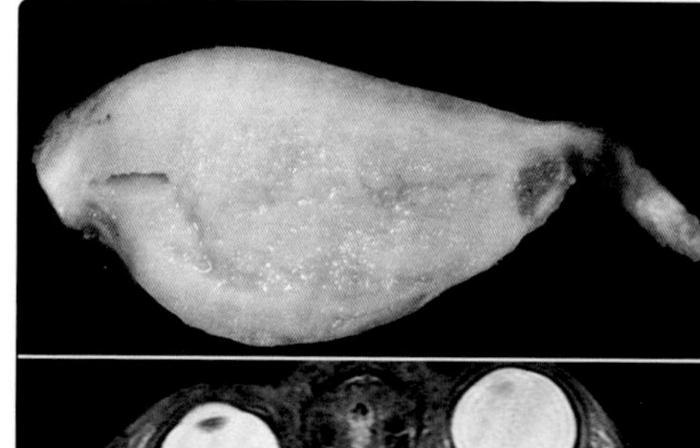
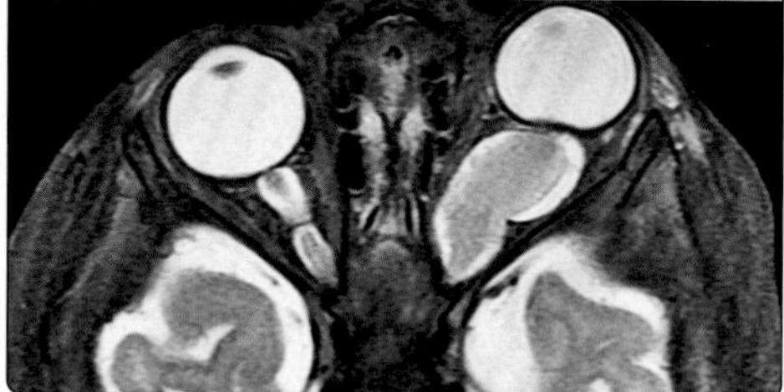

*(44-15) Optic nerve glioma in NF1 (top) and axial T2 MR (bottom) show fusiform enlargement of optic nerve. Nerve sheaths are partly patulous.*

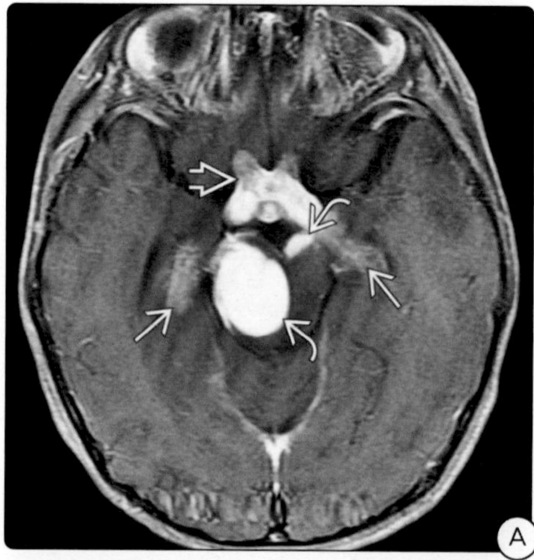


*(44-16A) T1 C+ FS MR in a 7-yo with NF1 shows intense enhancement in an enlarged optic chiasm ➡, medial temporal lobes ➡, and midbrain ➡.*

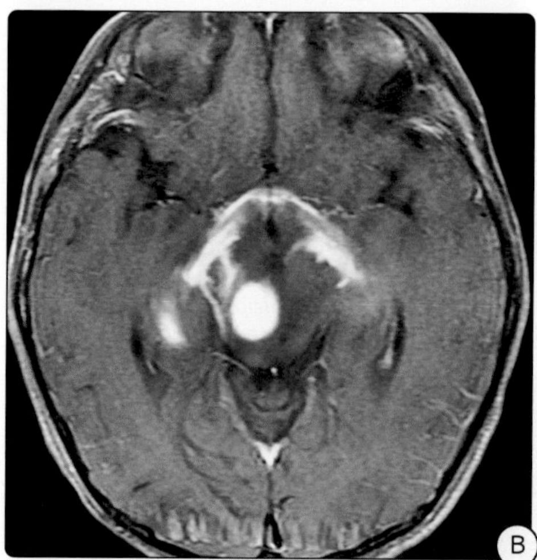


*(44-16B) More cephalad T1 C+ FS MR shows extensive enhancing tumor. Biopsy disclosed pilocytic astrocytoma, CNS WHO grade 1.*

childhood throughout adulthood. NF1-associated gliomas can arise anywhere in the neuraxis, including the optic pathway and spinal cord. These tumors can be histologically low or high grade and vary in biologic behavior from indolent to extremely aggressive.

Two different molecular subgroups of NF1-associated gliomas have been recently identified. Molecular **low-grade NF1-associated gliomas**—usually pilocytic astrocytomas **(44-17)**, less commonly diffuse astrocytomas or gangliogliomas—occur primarily in children, can be found throughout the neuraxis, and generally behave in an indolent manner. The most common site is the optic pathway; the second most common site is the brainstem.

NF1-associated OPGs can be uni- or bilateral and may involve any part of the optic pathway. Some OPGs affect just the optic nerve, whereas others involve the optic chiasm and optic tracts **(44-16)**. 2/3 of children with NF1-associated OPGs will not require an intervention, and some have even been reported to spontaneously regress over time. Less often, other low-grade gliomas in children with NF1 are found in the cerebral hemispheres, thalamus/brainstem, cerebellum, and spinal cord.

Molecular **high-grade NF1-associated gliomas** occur primarily during adulthood (mean age: 28 years), occur outside the optic pathway, and are histologically and genetically more diverse. These tumors are typically *IDH1*-wildtype, independent of histology **(44-18)**. The most common genetic variants are *NF1, EGFR, FGFR3, ATRX, CDKN2A/CDKN2B, TP53, TERT*, and *MSH2/MSH3* mutation.

Over 70% of adult NF1-associated gliomas involve midline structures, including the basal ganglia, thalamus and hypothalamus, corpus callosum, brainstem, cerebellar peduncles/vermis, or spinal cord. Adult NF1-associated gliomas often have an aggressive clinical course even if they are histologically low-grade lesions **(44-19)**.

Most adult NF1-associated neoplasms are **high-grade astrocytomas with piloid features (HGAPs)** or **IDH-wildtype glioblastomas (44-20)**. Whole-genome DNA methylation patterns have identified a specific HGAP subtype that is enriched in patients with NF1, is confined to the posterior fossa, and has decreased progression-free survival **(44-21)**.

Rare NF1-associated tumors also include more difficult-to-classify gliomas with ambiguous features **(44-19)**. Some exhibit morphologic similarities to subependymal giant cell astrocytomas (SEGAs) while others are high-grade astrocytomas, such as giant cell glioblastoma or anaplastic pleomorphic xanthoastrocytoma **(44-24)**.

NF1-associated gliomas of the medulla, tectum, and pons are typically indolent neoplasms.

**Non-CNS Neoplasms.** NF1 is associated with an increased risk of leukemia (especially juvenile myelomonocytic leukemia and myelodysplastic syndromes), gastrointestinal stromal tumors (6%), breast cancers and adrenal or extraadrenal pheochromocytoma (0.1-5.0%). In children with multiple café au lait spots and malignant tumors, such as leukemia, the WHO suggests constitutive mismatch repair deficiency should also be considered.

Patients with NF1 have up to a 5x increased risk of breast cancer before age 50. Recent studies also suggest cutaneous and CNS lymphomas can also be associated with NF1. As these patients often have skin lesions &/or cutaneous/subcutaneous nodules or other tumors like neurofibromas, their prevalence may be underdiagnosed.

## REVISED 2021 DIAGNOSTIC CRITERIA FOR NF1 (Legius et al, 2021)

If child *without* parent diagnosed with NF1, 2 or more of following
- 6 café au lait spots (> 5 mm prepubertal, > 15 mm postpubertal)
- Axillary or inguinal freckling
- ≥ 2 neurofibromas (any type) or 1 plexiform neurofibroma
- Optic pathway glioma
- ≥ 2 Lisch nodules **or** ≥ choroidal anomalies by OTC
- Distinctive osseous lesion, such as
  - Sphenoid wing dysplasia
  - Tibial bowing
  - Long bone pseudarthrosis
- Heterozygous pathogenic *NF1* gene variant in 50% normal tissue (e.g., WBCs)

If child *with* parent who meets above diagnostic criteria
- Only 1 or more of above criteria need be present

## NF1-ASSOCIATED NEOPLASMS

**Common**
- Dermal neurofibromas (95% of adults)
- Plexiform neurofibromas (30-50%)
- Spinal neurofibromas

**Less Common**
- Pilocytic astrocytoma (80% of gliomas)
  - 80% in optic pathway (15-20% of NF1 patients)
  - 15% in brainstem
  - 5% in other locations (cerebellum, cerebral hemispheres)
- Other astrocytomas (20%)
  - Astrocytoma, IDH-mutant (CNS WHO grades 2-4)
  - Glioblastoma, IDH-wildtype (CNS WHO grade 4)
  - High-grade astrocytoma with piloid features
  - Pleomorphic xanthoastrocytoma (PXA)

**Rare but Important**
- Malignant peripheral nerve sheath tumor
  - Develops in 8-13% of plexiform neurofibromas
- Juvenile chronic myeloid leukemia
- Pheochromocytoma

## Clinical Issues

**Presentation.** NF1 is one of the most common CNS single-gene disorders, affecting 1:3,000 live births.

Characteristic features include cutaneous neurofibromas (present in almost all adults with NF1), hyperpigmentary skin abnormalities with café au lait macules (95%) **(44-2)**, inguinal/axillary freckling (65-85%), and iris hamartomas or Lisch nodules **(44-3)**. Funduscopic examination using near-infrared reflectance demonstrates bright, patchy choroidal nodules in 70% of pediatric patients and 80% of adults.

Other less common NF1-associated features include distinctive skeletal abnormalities, such as sphenoid dysplasia (3-11%), long bone deformities (1-4%), pseudarthroses, and progressive kyphoscoliosis **(44-4)**. Cardiovascular anomalies occur in ~ 25% of individuals with NF1. Conotruncal cardiac defects, pulmonary valvular stenosis, and arterial hyperplasia are typical anomalies.

**Clinical Diagnosis.** Criteria for the clinical diagnosis of NF1 were originally established in 1988 by a National Institutes of Health (NIH) consensus

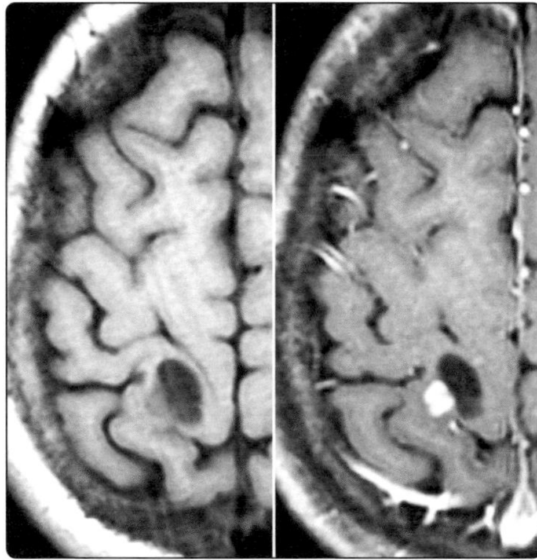

***(44-17)** Pre- (L) and postcontrast (R) T1 MRs in an 18-yo man with NF1 shows hemispheric cyst + nodule. Pilocytic astrocytoma, CNS WHO grade 1.*

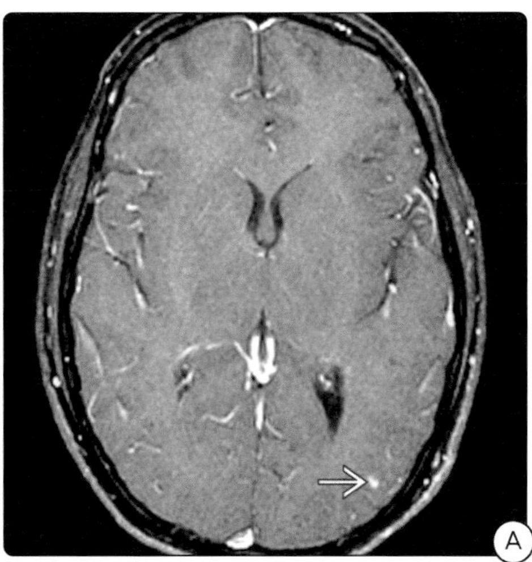


***(44-18A)** Axial T1 C+ MR in a 41-yo woman with NF1 shows a solitary enhancing left parietal lobe nodule ➡.*

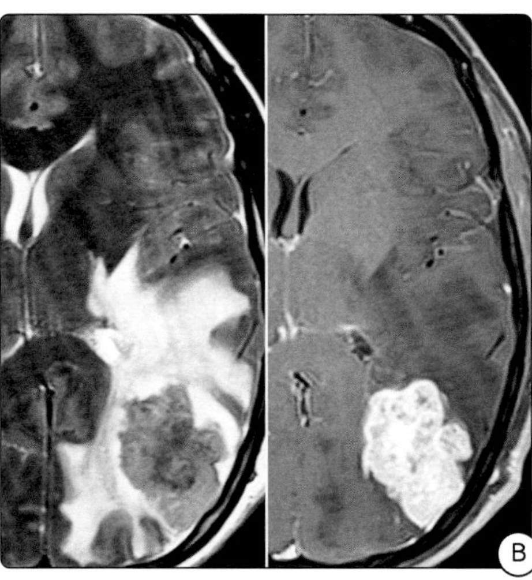


***(44-18B)** The patient was lost to follow-up for 12 years. T2 (L), T1 C+ (R) MRs show glioblastoma, likely arising in a lower grade astrocytoma.*

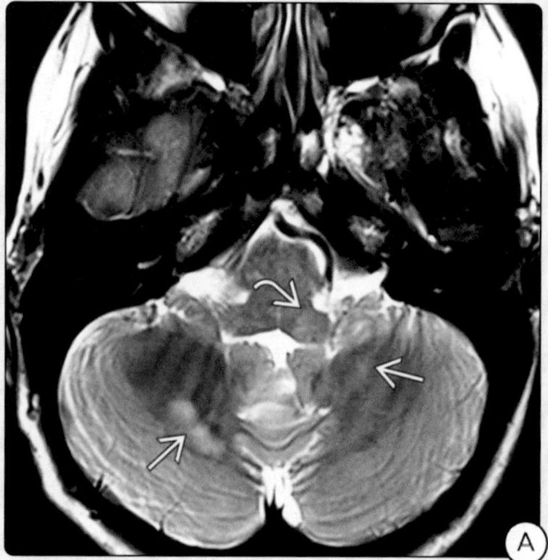

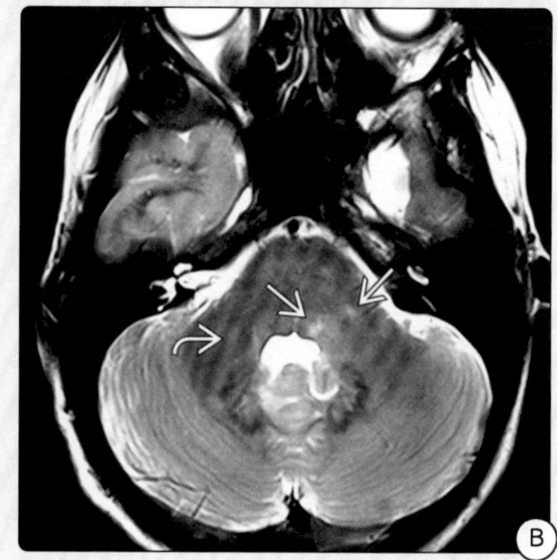

***(44-19A)*** *T2 MR in a 24-yo woman diagnosed with NF1 at age 2 and had a left optic nerve glioma resected shows FASIs in the cerebellar hemispheres ➡ and medulla ➡.* ***(44-19B)*** *More cephalad T2 MR shows additional FASIs in the pons ➡ and brachium pontis ➡.*

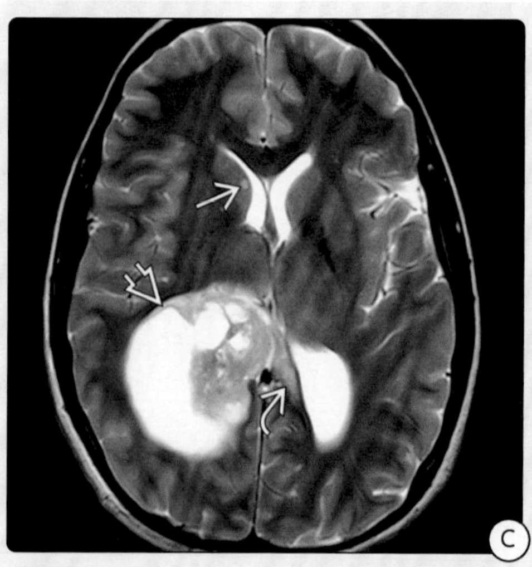

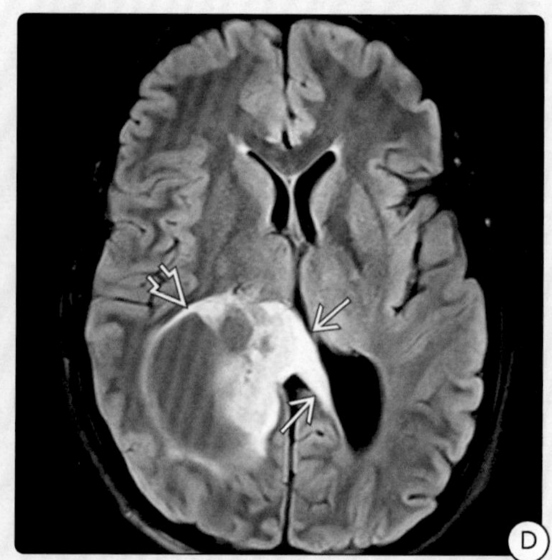

***(44-19C)*** *T2 MR through the lateral ventricles shows a small right caudate FASI ➡ and a large heterogeneously hyperintense mass in the right parietal lobe ➡ that also extends across the corpus callosum ➡.* ***(44-19D)*** *FLAIR MR shows that the mass ➡ suppresses incompletely and thickens and infiltrates the corpus callosum ➡.*

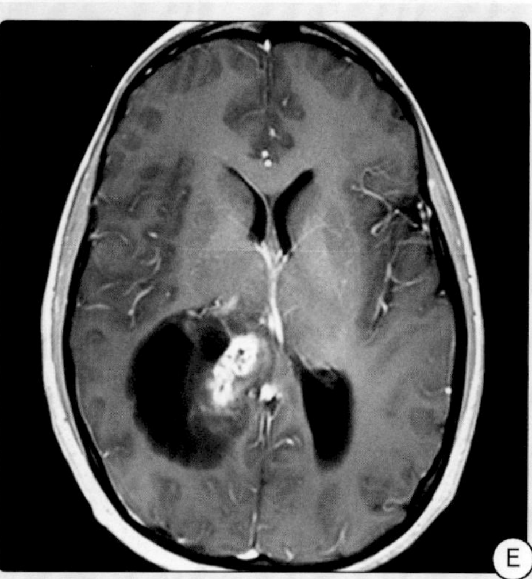

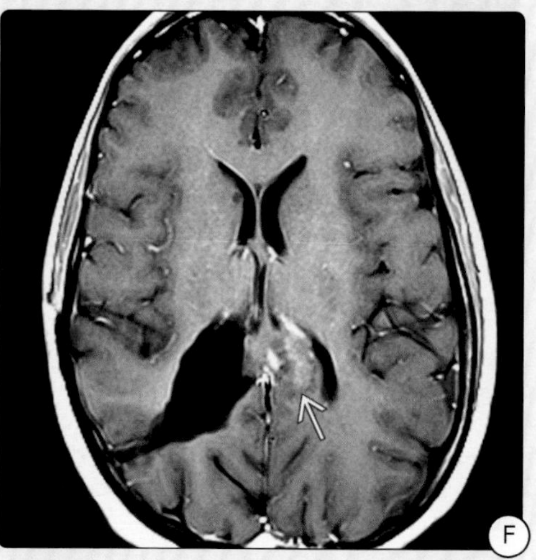

***(44-19E)*** *T1 C+ MR shows that the mass enhances heterogeneously. Resection showed a pilocytic astrocytoma with some atypical features and FGFR and NF1 mutations.* ***(44-19F)*** *Follow-up imaging 1 year later shows new enhancing tumor infiltrating the corpus callosum ➡.*

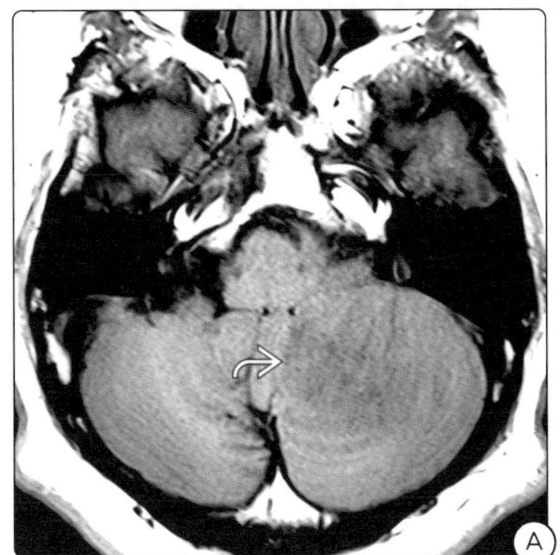
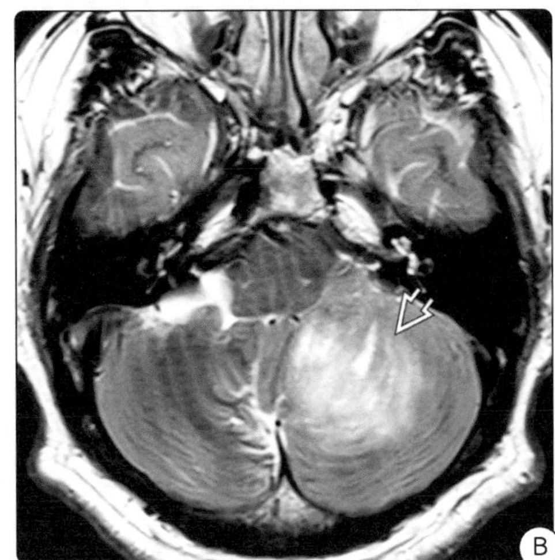

***(44-20A)** Axial T1 MR in a 28-yo man with NF1 shows a hypointense, infiltrating mass in the left cerebellar hemisphere ➲. **(44-20B)** Axial T2 MR shows a hyperintense infiltrating lesion ➲ in the left cerebellar hemisphere infiltrating along the cerebellar folia.*

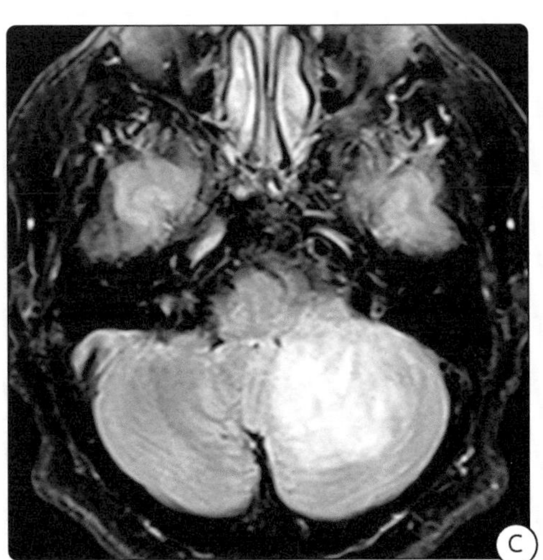
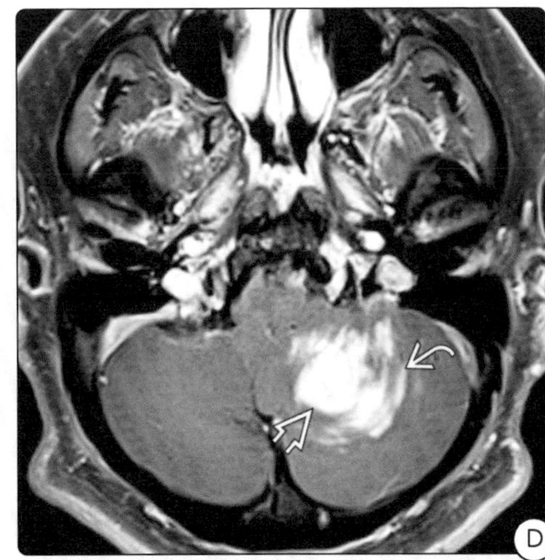

***(44-20C)** The mass is hyperintense and appears more extensive on FLAIR MR. **(44-20D)** T1 C+ FS MR shows the mass ➲ enhances intensely and uniformly, appearing to infiltrate along the cerebellar folia ➲. Biopsy disclosed IDH-wildtype glioblastoma, CNS WHO grade 4. CDKN2A was mutated. The patient died 3 years after diagnosis.*

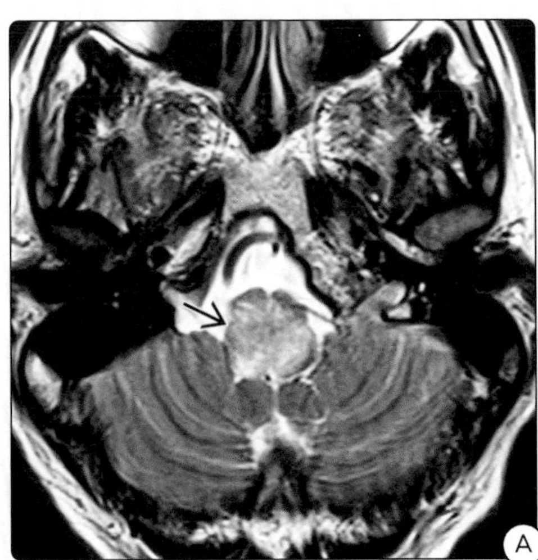
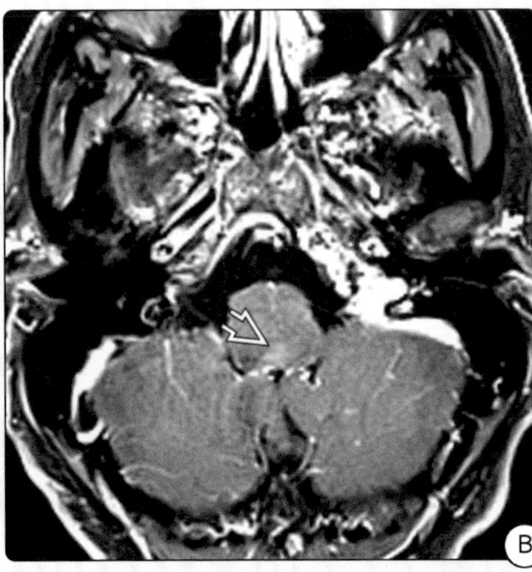

***(44-21A)** Axial T2 MR in a 44-yo man with NF1 shows a hyperintense, expansile mass diffusely infiltrating the medulla ➔. **(44-21B)** T1 C+ FS MR shows some faint enhancement in the dorsal medulla ➲ adjacent to the obex of the 4th ventricle. Biopsy disclosed a high-grade astrocytoma with pilocytic features (HGAP, proved by methylation profiling).*

conference. In the past, two or more of seven listed criteria must be met for a definitive diagnosis of NF1 to be made. However, many of these features are age dependent; nearly 1/2 of patients who are diagnosed with NF1 later in life do not meet these strict diagnostic criteria. Diagnostic consensus criteria for NF1 were revised in 2021 and now include detection of a pathogenic variant in the *NF1* gene, which allows for early diagnosis in young children without a family history of the disease. The revised diagnostic criteria also include choroidal anomalies as a new ophthalmic symptom with high sensitivity and specificity for NF1.

Molecular diagnostic testing can distinguish NF1 from other disorders that share similar phenotypic features. With the exception of PNF, most clinical stigmata of NF1 also occur in other disorders (e.g., multiple café au lait macules in McCune-Albright syndrome). The new 2021 revised consensus criteria for the clinical diagnosis of NF1 are summarized in the next box.

**Natural History.** Prognosis in NF1 is variable and relates to its specific manifestations. Malignant gliomas and MPNSTs represent the two most common causes of cancer-related mortality for NF1 patients.

The foci of myelin vacuolization increase in number and size over the first decade, then regress, and eventually disappear. They are rarely identified in adults.

## Imaging

**Nonneoplastic CNS Lesions. Bone dysplasias** occur in the skull, spine, and long bones (e.g., pseudarthroses). NECT scans may demonstrate a hypoplastic sphenoid wing and enlarged middle cranial fossa, with or without an associated arachnoid cyst **(44-23)**. Protrusion of the anterior temporal lobe may result in ipsilateral proptosis. The globe is frequently enlarged ("buphthalmos") **(44-11)** and a PNF is often present **(44-12)**.

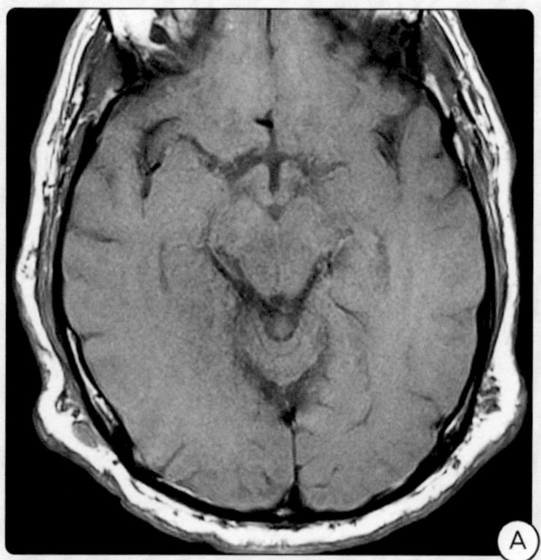


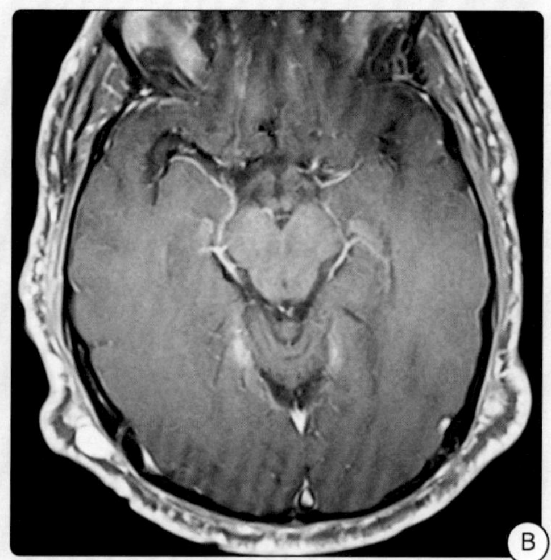


***(44-22A)** T1 MR in a 42-yo man with NF1 shows multiple small cutaneous neurofibromas in the scalp. **(44-22B)** T1 C+ FS MR shows the cutaneous neurofibromas enhance strongly. As they age, patients may develop multiple dermal neurofibromas. More than 95% of adults with NF1 have at least 1 such lesion.*

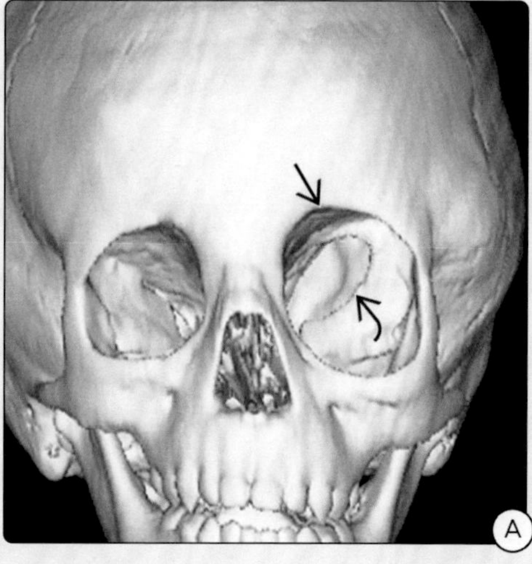


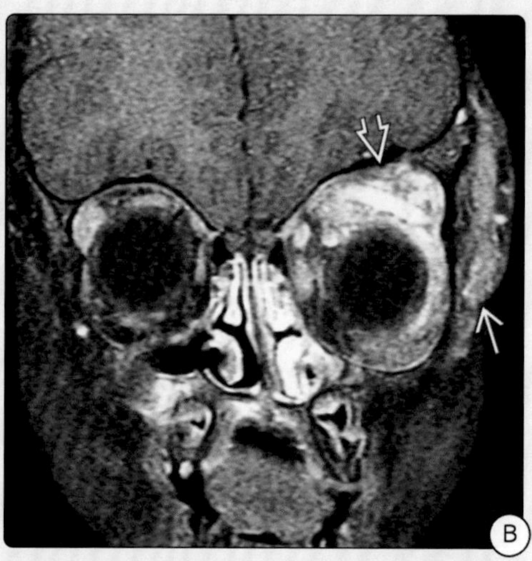


***(44-23A)** 3D bone CT in a patient with NF1 and sphenoid dysplasia shows enlarged left bony orbit → and widened superior orbital fissure ↗. **(44-23B)** Coronal T1 C+ FS MR in the same patient shows enhancing plexiform neurofibroma infiltrating the orbit ⇨ and high deep masticator space ➡.*

**Dural dysplasia** with patulous spinal dura as well as enlarged optic nerve sheaths, internal auditory canals, and Meckel caves can occur **(44-6)**.

**Dysplastic WM lesions** (often termed "FASIs" for **f**oci of **a**bnormal **s**ignal **i**ntensity) are seen as multifocal hyperintensities on T2/FLAIR imaging **(44-8)**. These foci represent zones of myelin vacuolization and are seen in 70% of children with NF1. They generally increase in size and number until ~ 10 years of age but then wane and disappear **(44-9)**.

The most common sites are the globi pallidi (GP), centrum semiovale, cerebellar WM, dentate nuclei, thalamus, and brainstem **(44-8)**. Most are smaller than 2 cm in diameter. Most FASIs are iso- or minimally hypointense on T1WI, although GP lesions are often mildly hyperintense. FASIs do not enhance following contrast administration.

Relentless endothelial hyperplasia can cause progressive stenosis of the intracranial internal carotid arteries, resulting in a **moyamoya** pattern. Careful scrutiny of the intracranial vasculature demonstrates attenuation of the middle cerebral artery "flow voids" **(44-7)**

### CNS Neoplasms

***Neurofibromas.*** Patients with **cutaneous neurofibromas** often demonstrate solitary or multifocal, discrete, round or ovoid scalp lesions that are hypointense to brain on T1WI and hyperintense on T2WI **(44-22)**. A target sign with a hyperintense rim and relatively hypointense center is common. Strong but heterogeneous enhancement following contrast administration is typical.

**PNFs** are most common in the orbit, where they are seen as poorly marginated serpentine masses that infiltrate the orbit, extraocular muscles, and eyelids **(44-10)** **(44-23)**. They often extend inferiorly into the pterygopalatine fossa and buccal spaces as well as superiorly into the adjacent scalp and masticator spaces. PNFs enhance strongly and resemble a bag of worms **(44-12)**.

***Malignant Peripheral Nerve Sheath Tumors.*** **MPNSTs** arising within a PNF can be difficult to detect and to differentiate from the parent tumor. MPNSTs tend to be more heterogeneous in signal intensity, often exhibiting intratumoral cysts, perilesional edema, and peripheral enhancement.

***Gliomas.*** The most common NF1-associated glioma is **pilocytic astrocytoma**. Optic pathway glioma (OPG) is the most frequent type and occurs as a diffuse, fusiform, or bulbous enlargement of one or both optic nerves **(44-15)**. Tumor may extend posteriorly into the optic chiasm, superiorly into the hypothalamus, and involve the optic tracts and lateral geniculate bodies. Extensive lesions can reach the cerebral peduncles and brainstem **(44-16)**.

Most OPGs are isointense with brain on T1WI and iso- to moderately hyperintense on T2WI. Enhancement on T1 C+ FS scans varies from none to striking.

NF1-associated **pediatric-type diffuse low-grade gliomas** can be difficult to distinguish from FASIs. They are usually moderately hypointense on T1WI and hyperintense on T2WI, do not resolve spontaneously, and show slow progression on follow-up imaging.

**High-grade astrocytoma with piloid features** and **glioblastoma** are more aggressive, more heterogeneous tumors that demonstrate relentless progression **(44-18)** **(44-21)**. A progressively enlarging mass that enhances following contrast administration in a child with NF1 should raise suspicion of malignant neoplasm.

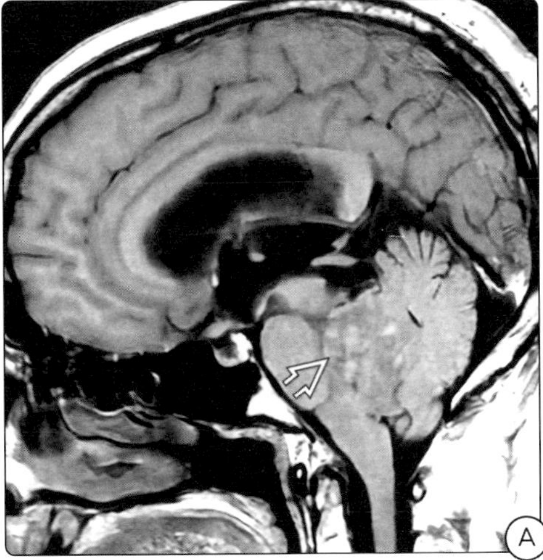


***(44-24A)** Sagittal T1 MR in a 37-yo man with headaches and NF1 shows hydrocephalus with a large, heterogeneous 4th ventricle mass ➲.*

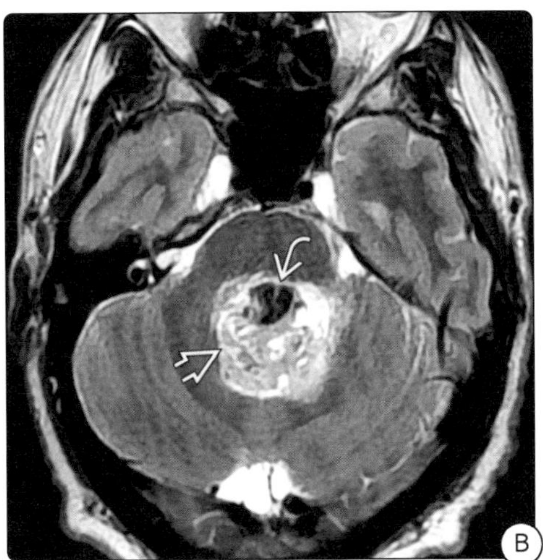


***(44-24B)** T2 MR shows the mass ➲ is very heterogeneous. The hypointensity ➲ was acute hemorrhage on NECT (not shown).*

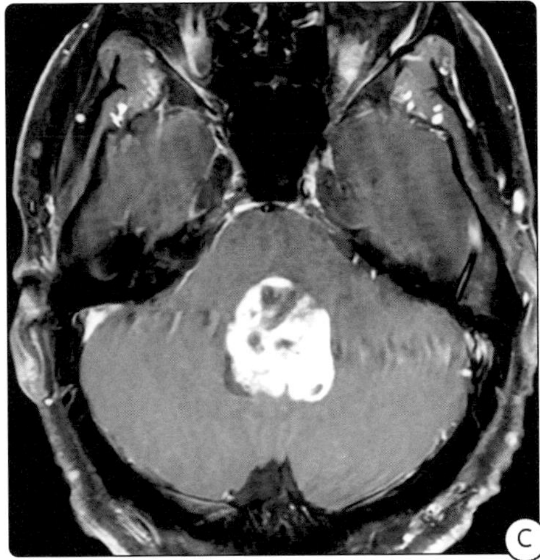


***(44-24C)** The mass enhances intensely on T1 C+ FS MR. Pleomorphic xanthoastrocytoma, CNS WHO grade 2 confirmed by methylation profiling.*

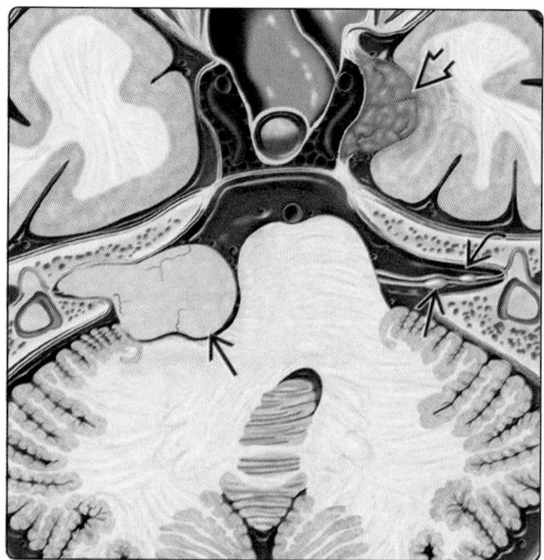

*(44-25) Graphic depicts classic NF2 with bilateral vestibular schwannomas (VSs) ➡, facial schwannoma ➡, and meningioma ➡.*

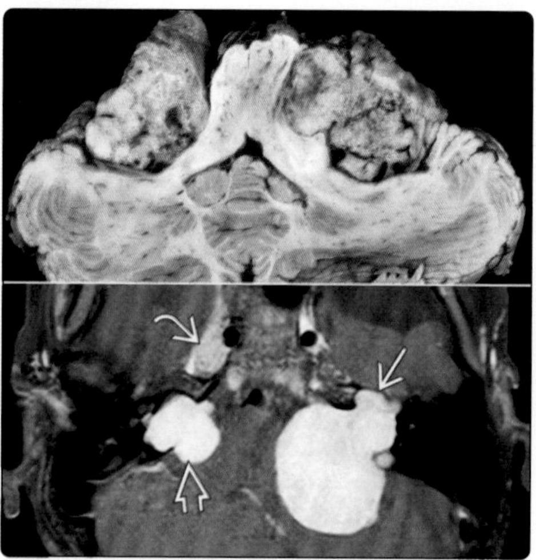

*(44-26) (Top) Bilateral VSs are shown in NF2. (A. Ersen, MD.) (Bottom) T1 C+ shows bilateral VS ➡, facial ➡, and right CNV ➡ schwannomas.*

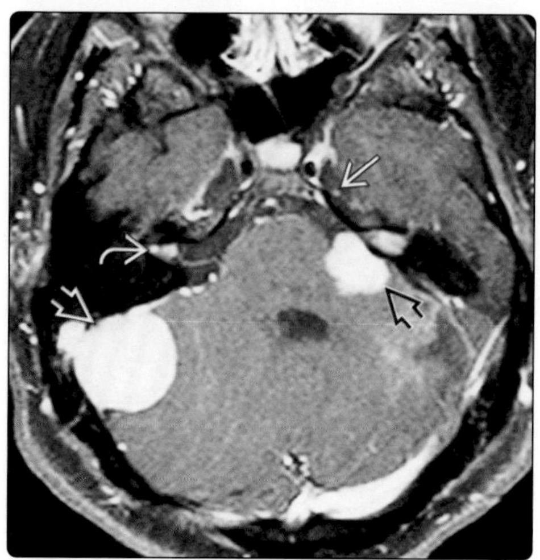

*(44-27) T1 C+ FS MR of NF2 shows large left ➡ and small right ➡ VSs, tiny CNV schwannoma in Meckel cave ➡, and right CPA meningioma ➡.*

### NF1: IMAGING

**Scalp/Skull, Meninges, and Orbit**

- Dermal neurofibromas
  - Solitary/multifocal scalp nodules
  - Increases with age
  - Localized, well circumscribed
- Plexiform neurofibroma
  - Pathognomonic of NF1 (30-50% of cases)
  - Large, bulky, infiltrative transspatial lesions
  - Scalp, face/neck, spine
  - Orbit lesions may extend into cavernous sinus
- Sphenoid wing dysplasia
  - Hypoplasia → enlarged orbital fissure
  - Enlarged middle fossa ± arachnoid cyst
  - Temporal lobe may protrude into orbit
- Dural ectasia
  - Tortuous optic nerve sheath
  - Patulous Meckel caves
  - Enlarged internal auditory canals (IACs)

**Brain**

- Hyperintense T2/FLAIR WM foci (UBOs, FASIs)
  - Wax in 1st decade, then wane
  - Rare in adults > 20 years old
- Gliomas
  - Pilocytic astrocytoma, arising in setting of NF1
  - High-grade astrocytoma with piloid features
  - Glioblastoma, IDH-wildtype
  - Uncommon gliomas (e.g., PXA, SEGA)
  - Ambiguous, difficult-to-classify gliomas

**Arteries**

- Progressive ICA stenosis → moyamoya
- Fusiform ectasias, arteriovenous fistulas
  - Vertebral > carotid

## Differential Diagnosis

In combination with appropriate clinical findings, the presence of FASIs on MR with or without OPG is diagnostic of NF1. Unusually large FASIs can cause mass effect and mimic **neoplasm** (i.e., pilocytic astrocytoma, diffuse astrocytoma). While FASIs and astrocytomas are both part of the NF1 spectrum, FASIs typically do not enhance.

# Neurofibromatosis Type 2

Neurofibromatosis type 2 (NF2) is a distinct syndrome with totally different mutations, clinical features, and imaging findings from NF1. Neurofibromas characterize NF1 and are composed of Schwann cells and fibroblasts. Schwannomas—especially bilateral vestibular schwannomas (VSs)—are the major feature of NF2. Schwannomas contain only Schwann cells.

The associated neoplasms are also different from those in NF1. Astrocytomas are found in NF1, whereas ependymomas and meningiomas are the predominant tumors in NF2.

## Etiology

**General Concepts.** Like NF1, NF2 is an autosomal dominant disorder. About 1/2 of all cases occur in individuals with no family history of NF2 and are caused by newly acquired germline mutations.

**Genetics.** NF2 is caused by mutations of the *NF2* gene on chromosome 22q12.2. The *NF2* gene encodes the protein merlin, which functions as a tumor suppressor gene and is a negative regulator of mTORC1. Inactivating *NF2* mutations cause loss of merlin and result in predominantly benign neoplasms (schwannomas and meningiomas). Biallelic *NF2* inactivation is also detected in 60% of sporadic meningiomas and nearly all schwannomas.

## Pathology

**Location.** The most common NF2-related schwannomas are VSs **(44-25)**. Approximately 50% of patients also have nonvestibular schwannomas (NVSs). The most common locations for NVSs are the trigeminal and oculomotor nerves **(44-27)**. Trochlear and lower cranial nerve schwannomas occur but are rare.

Meningiomas occur in ~ 1/2 of all patients with NF2 and can be found anywhere in the skull and spine. The most frequent sites are along the falx and cerebral convexities.

Intracranial ependymomas are rare in NF2. Most are found in the spinal cord, especially within the cervical cord or at the cervicomedullary junction.

**Size and Number.** NF2-related schwannomas, meningiomas, and ependymomas are often multiple. The presence of bilateral VSs is pathognomonic of NF2 **(44-26)**.

Size varies from tiny to several centimeters. Innumerable tiny schwannomas ("tumorlets") throughout the cauda equina are seen in the majority of patients. Intramedullary ependymomas are often small; multiple tumors are present in nearly 60% of patients.

**Gross Pathology.** NF2 is characterized by multiple schwannomas, meningiomas, and ependymomas. Virtually all patients have bilateral VSs, the hallmark of NF2 **(44-26)**. Most schwannomas are well-delineated, round or ovoid, encapsulated masses that are attached to—but do not infiltrate—their parent nerves.

Multiple meningiomas are the second pathologic hallmark of NF2 **(44-28)**. They are found in ~ 50% of patients and may be the presenting feature (especially in children). Meningiomas appear as unencapsulated but sharply demarcated masses.

**Microscopic Features.** Schwannomas are composed of neoplastic Schwann cells. Areas of alternating high and low cellularity (Antoni A pattern) are admixed with foci that exhibit microcysts and myxoid changes (Antoni B pattern).

**Staging, Grading, and Classification.** NF2-associated schwannomas are CNS WHO grade 1 tumors. Most NF2-associated meningiomas are also WHO grade 1 neoplasms. NF2-associated ependymomas—especially those in the spinal cord—are generally indolent and carry a favorable prognosis.

## Clinical Issues

**Presentation.** NF2 is much less common than NF1. However, individuals with NF2 generally do not become symptomatic until the 2nd-4th decades; < 20% of patients with NF2 present under the age of 15. Multiple tumors may develop throughout the affected individual's lifetime. Progressive sensorineural hearing loss, tinnitus, and difficulties with balance are typical. Other common symptoms include facial pain &/or paralysis, vertigo, and seizures.

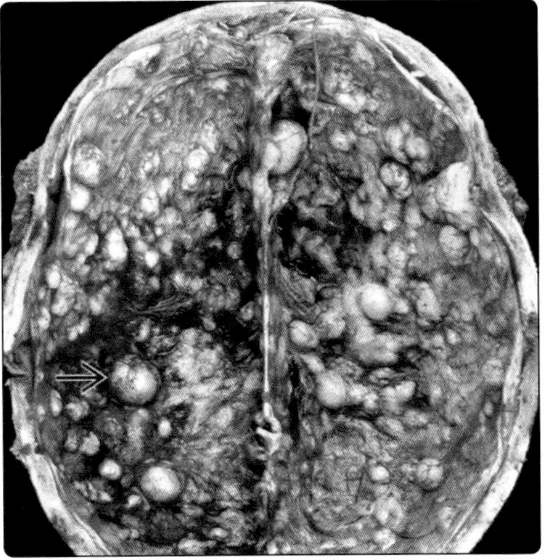

***(44-28)** Autopsy specimen demonstrates innumerable small meningiomas ⇒, a common finding in NF2. (From DP: Neuro.)*

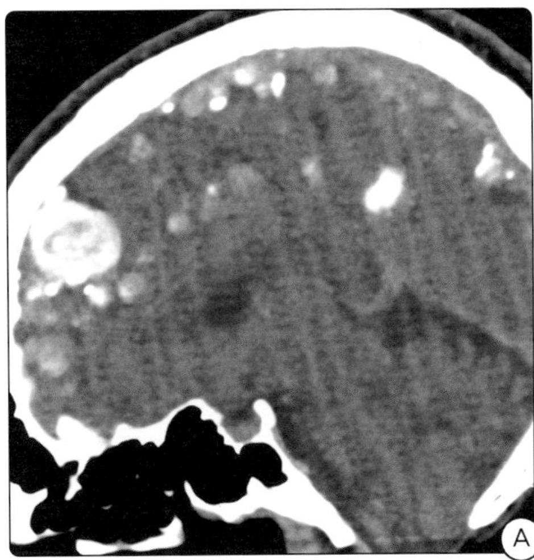

***(44-29A)** NECT shows hyperdense calcified masses that abut the dura and falx, characteristic of NF2-associated meningiomatosis.*

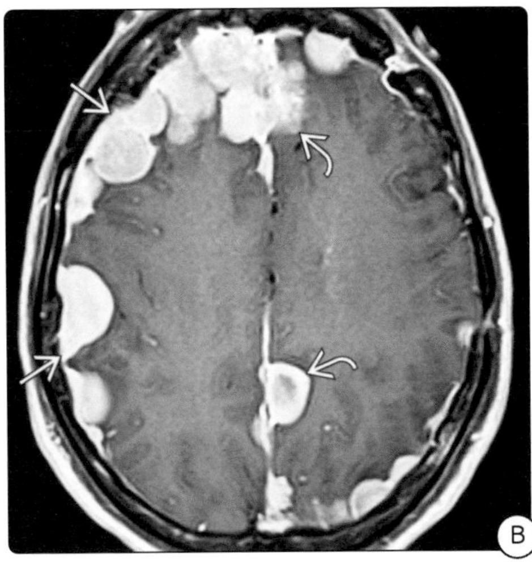

***(44-29B)** T1 C+ FS MR in the same case shows multiple meningiomas along the convexity ➡ and falx ➡.*

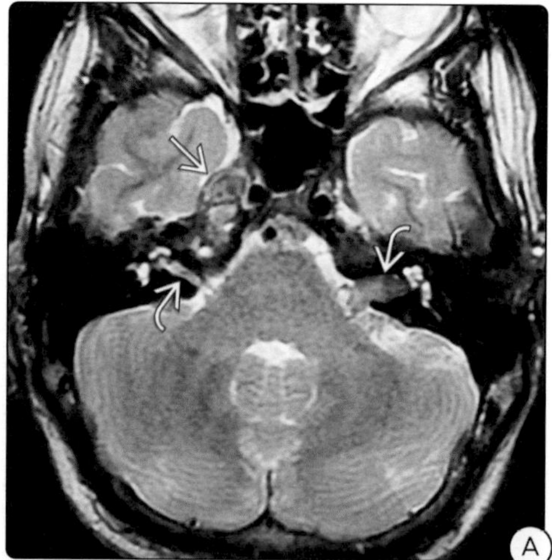
*(44-30A) T2 MR in a 14-yo boy with NF2 reveals lesions in the right cavernous sinus ➡ and both internal auditory canals (IACs) ➡.*

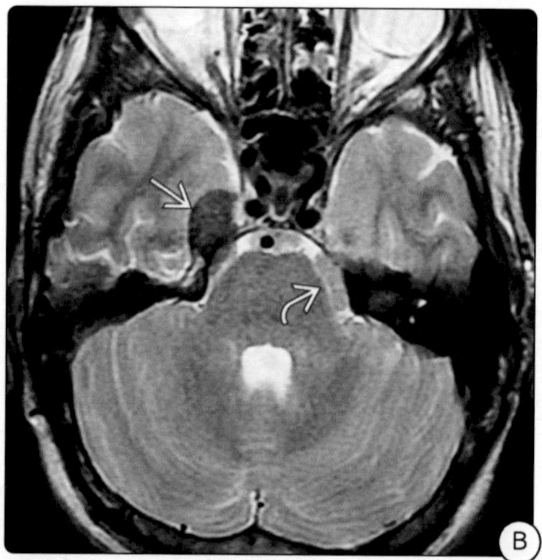
*(44-30B) More cephalad T2 MR in the same case shows a hypodense mass in the right cavernous sinus ➡ and lesions in the left CPA cistern ➡.*

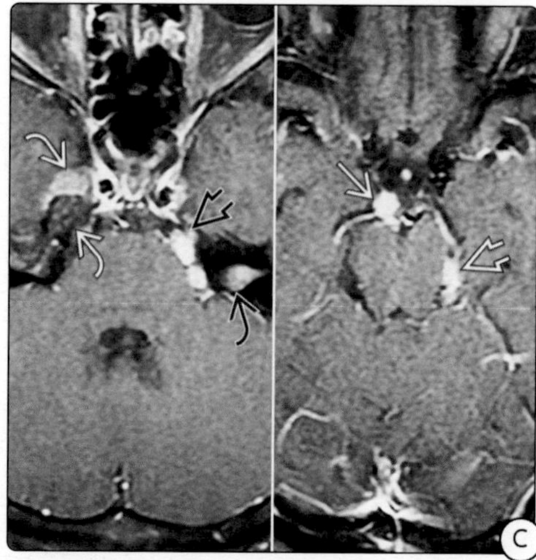
*(44-30C) T1 C+ FS MRs show right cavernous sinus meningioma ➡, CNIII ➡, and left CNIV ➡, V ➡, and VIII ➡ schwannomas.*

Many NF2-related meningiomas are asymptomatic and discovered incidentally on imaging. Spinal cord ependymomas are asymptomatic in 75% of patients.

**Clinical Diagnosis.** The definitive diagnosis of NF2 is established by fulfilling the Manchester diagnostic criteria or by identifying a pathogenic *NF2* mutation. Consensus criteria for the clinical diagnosis of NF2 as recently revised and updated are summarized in the box below.

**REVISED MANCHESTER CRITERIA FOR NF2**

Bilateral VSs (diagnosed < 70 years of age)

1st-degree relative with NF2 **and** unilateral VS diagnosed before 70 years of age

1st-degree relative with NF2 or unilateral VS or 2 of following

- Meningioma
- Cataract
- Schwannoma
- Cerebral calcification
- If unilateral VS and > 2 nonintradermal schwannomas, needs negative *LZTR1* genetic testing

Multiple meningiomas (2 or more) and 2 of

- Unilateral VS
- Cataract
- Ependymoma
- Schwannoma
- Cerebral calcification

Constitutional or mosaic pathogenic *NF2* gene mutation in blood **or** identical mutations in 2 distinct tumors

**Natural History.** NF2-associated intracranial neoplasms often demonstrate a "saltatory" growth pattern characterized by alternating periods of growth and quiescence. As new tumors can develop and radiographic progression and symptom development are unpredictable, continued surveillance is necessary. Current recommended MR surveillance includes imaging at one, five, and 10 years after surgery.

## Imaging

**General Features.** The cardinal imaging feature of NF2 is bilateral VSs.

**CT Findings.** NECT scans typically demonstrate a mass in one or both cerebellopontine angle (CPA) cisterns. Both schwannomas and meningiomas are typically iso- to slightly hyperdense on NECT **(44-29A)** and exhibit strong enhancement following contrast administration.

Nonneoplastic choroid plexus calcifications in atypical locations (e.g., temporal horn) are a rare manifestation of NF2 but can be striking. Bone CT typically shows that one or both internal auditory canals are widened.

**MR Findings.** MR findings of NF2-related schwannomas and meningiomas are similar to those of their sporadic counterparts. If NF2 is suspected on the basis of brain imaging, the entire spine and spinal cord should be screened. High-resolution T2WI and contrast-enhanced sequences disclose asymptomatic tiny schwannomas **(44-30)** **(44-33)** and intramedullary ependymomas **(44-31)** in at least 1/2 of all individuals with NF2 **(44-32)**.

## Differential Diagnosis

The major differential diagnosis of NF2 is *LZTR1*-associated **schwannomatosis**, especially when one VS is present. Schwannomatosis is characterized by multiple **NV**Ss while meningiomas are less common (see box below). **Multiple meningiomatosis** is characterized by multifocal meningiomas without schwannomas.

### NF1 vs. NF2 vs. SCHWANNOMATOSIS

**NF1**

- Common (90% of all neurofibromatosis cases)
- Chromosome 17 mutations
- Almost always diagnosed by age 10
- Cutaneous/eye lesions > 95%
  - Café au lait spots
  - Lisch nodules
  - Cutaneous neurofibromas (often multiple)
  - Plexiform neurofibromas (pathognomonic)
- CNS lesions less common (15-20%)
  - T2/FLAIR hyperintensities (myelin vacuolization; lesions wax, then wane)
  - Sphenoid wing, dural dysplasias
  - Molecularly low-grade gliomas (usually pilocytic astrocytoma)
  - Molecular high-grade gliomas (glioblastoma, high-grade astrocytoma with piloid features)
  - Moyamoya
  - Neurofibromas

**NF2**

- Much less common (10% of all neurofibromatosis cases)
- Chromosome 22 mutations
- Cutaneous, eye lesions less prominent
  - Mild/few café au lait spots
  - Juvenile subcapsular opacities
- CNS lesions in 100%
  - Bilateral vestibular schwannomas (almost all)
  - Nonvestibular schwannomas (50%)
  - Meningiomas (50%)
  - Cord ependymomas (often multiple)
  - Schwannomas ("tumorlets") of spinal nerve roots

**Schwannomatosis**

- Very rare; usually de novo mutation
- Multiple **nonvestibular** schwannomas; meningiomas less common
- *SMARCB1* and *LZTR1* mutations

## Schwannomatosis

Schwannomatosis is related to—but differs from—NF2. Schwannomatosis is characterized by multiple peripheral and spinal schwannomas—less commonly, meningiomas—in the absence of bilateral VSs **(44-34)**. The majority of cases are sporadic; only 15-25% are familial. Peak incidence is between ages 30-60 years (in contrast with NF1—typically diagnosed in the first decade—and NF2, usually diagnosed in the second or third decade).

Familial schwannomatosis is an autosomal dominant disorder characterized by inactivating mutations in the tumor suppressor genes *SMARCB1* and *LZTR1*, which are both located on chromosome 22, centromeric to *NF2*. Tumors typically present in the second and third decades.

Approximately 75% of schwannomas affect the spine, and the peripheral nerves are affected in nearly 90%. Schwannomas of the cranial nerves are uncommon (< 10% of cases), and, when present, they affect mostly the trigeminal nerve. Unilateral VSs may occur; the presence of bilateral vestibular lesions is diagnostic of NF2, not schwannomatosis. Nonneurogenic tumors, such as lipomas and angiolipomas, occur in 5-10% of cases.

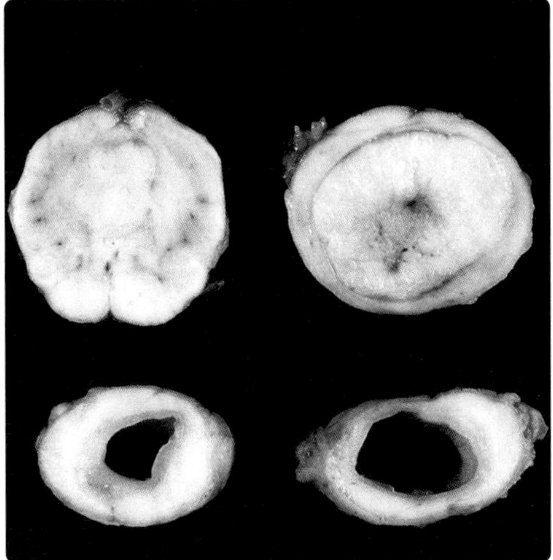

***(44-31)** Axial gross pathology in NF2 shows intramedullary ependymoma with cyst expanding cervical cord. (Courtesy R. Hewlett, MD.)*

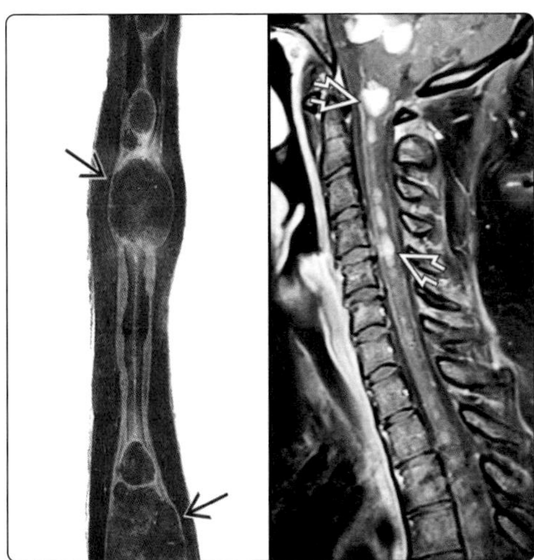

***(44-32)** Autopsy (L) shows intramedullary ependymomas ➙. (Courtesy A. Ersen, MD.) (R) T1 C+ shows multiple cord ependymomas ➡ in NF2.*

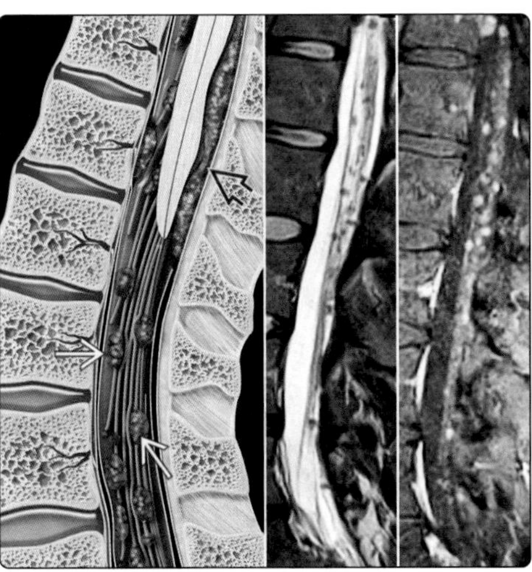

***(44-33)** NF2 graphic (L) depicts spinal "tumorlets" ➡, meningioma ➙. T2 (middle), T1 C+ (R) show cauda equina schwannomas.*

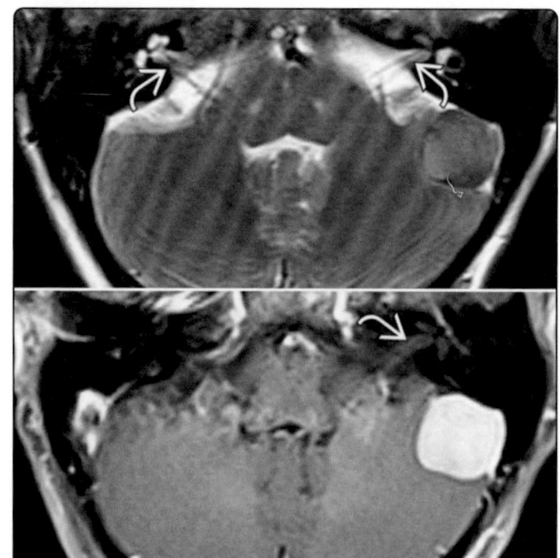

*(44-34) T2 (top), T1 C+ FS (bottom) in SMARCB1 mutation shows normal IACs and an enhancing CPA mass (meningioma).*

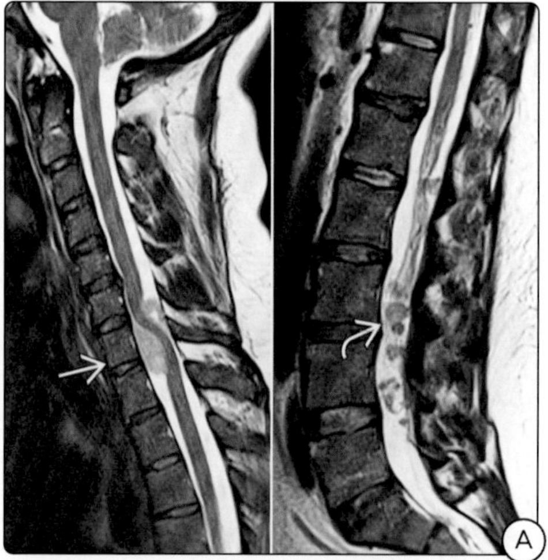


*(44-35A) Sagittal T2 MRs show multiple intradural extramedullary masses in the cervical and lumbar spine.*

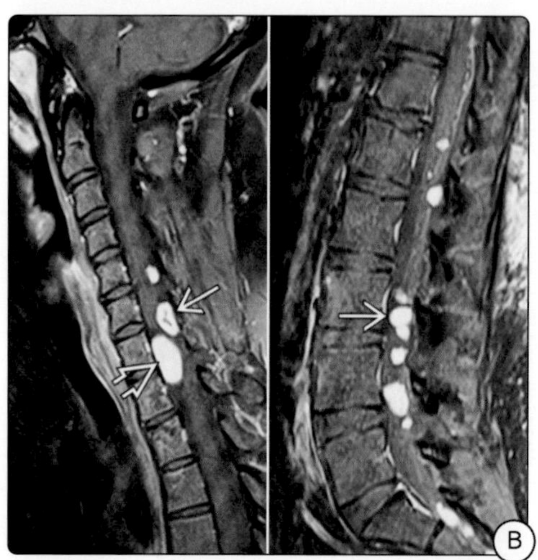


*(44-35B) T1 C+ MR in the same case shows a meningioma and multiple schwannomas. This is schwannomatosis.*

Imaging in schwannomatosis discloses multiple circumscribed, well-defined, round to oval or dumbbell-shaped lesions that are hypo- to isointense on T1WI and hyperintense on T2/FLAIR. Lesions enhance strongly on T1 C+ sequences **(44-35)**. The risk of malignant degeneration is low.

# Other Common Familial Tumor Syndromes

## Tuberous Sclerosis Complex

### Terminology

Tuberous sclerosis complex (TSC) is a neurocutaneous syndrome characterized by the formation of nonmalignant hamartomas and benign neoplastic lesions that affect the CNS and various nonneural tissues.

### Etiology

**Genetics.** Approximately 50% of TSC cases are inherited and follow an autosomal dominant pattern while the other 50% represent de novo mutations. Two separate genes are mutated or deleted in TSC: *TSC1* and *TSC2*. The *TSC1* gene is located on chromosome 9q34 and encodes a protein called **hamartin**. The *TSC2* gene is localized to chromosome 16p13.3 and encodes the **tuberin** protein. Mutations in either gene are identified in 75-85% of patients with TSC.

The TSC protein complex functions as a tumor suppressor. Hamartin/tuberin inhibits the mTORC1 signaling pathway (mammalian target of rapamycin complex 1). Mutations that lead to increased mTORC1 activation promote cellular disorganization, overgrowth, and abnormal differentiation. *TSC2* mutations are associated with a more severe disease phenotype with more and larger tubers, more radial migration lines, and more subependymal nodules (SENs) compared with *TSC1*.

### Pathology

The four major pathologic features of TSC in the brain are **cortical tubers, SENs, WM lesions**, and **SEGA (44-37) (44-36)**.

**Cortical Tubers.** Cortical tubers are glioneuronal hamartomas and are found in > 90% of TS patients. They are firm, whitish, pyramid-shaped, elevated areas of smooth gyral thickening. Cortical tubers grossly resemble potatoes ("tubers").

Cortical tubers consist of giant cells and dysmorphic neurons. Balloon cells similar to those seen in Taylor-type focal cortical dysplasia (FCD type IIb) are also commonly found in tubers. Tubers do **not** undergo malignant transformation.

**Subependymal Nodules.** SENs are located immediately beneath the ependymal lining of the lateral ventricles, along the course of the caudate nucleus.

SENs appear as elevated, rounded, hamartomatous lesions that grossly resemble candle guttering or drippings. They often calcify with increasing age. SENs along the caudothalamic groove adjacent to the foramen of Monro may undergo neoplastic transformation into SEGA.

**White Matter Lesions.** WM lesions are almost universal in patients with TSC. They appear as foci of bizarre dysmorphic neurons and balloon cells in the subcortical WM &/or fine radial lines extending outward from the ependymal ventricular surface toward the cortex. These radial migration lines often terminate in a tuber.

**Subependymal Giant Cell Astrocytoma.** SEGA is seen almost exclusively in the setting of TSC, occurring in 6-9% of patients. Grossly, SEGAs appear as well-circumscribed solid intraventricular masses located near the foramen of Monro **(44-37B)**. SEGAs are CNS WHO grade 1 tumors that often cause obstructive hydrocephalus but do not invade adjacent brain. Although most SEGAs are unilateral, bilateral tumors occur in 10-15% of cases.

## Clinical Issues

**Epidemiology and Demographics.** TSC is the second most common inherited tumor syndrome (after NF1). Almost 80% of cases are diagnosed before the age of 10.

**Presentation.** The classic clinical triad of TSC consists of facial lesions ("adenomata sebaceum"), seizures, and intellectual disability. All cutaneous features are age dependent and may not become apparent until later in childhood. A subset of patients have more subtle symptoms due to variable penetrance of the *TSC1* gene inactivation and may not be diagnosed until adulthood.

Hypomelanotic macules ("ash leaf") spots are seen in > 90% of cases and may be the first visible manifestation of TSC. Other common cutaneous findings, such as facial angiofibromas ("adenoma sebaceum"), and periungual fibromas usually do not appear until after puberty.

**Natural History.** Disease severity and natural course vary widely. Neurologic manifestations—primarily intractable seizures from brain hamartomas and obstructive hydrocephalus secondary to SEGA—are the leading cause of morbidity and mortality.

SEGAs are benign and usually slow-growing neoplasms. Although they can develop at any age, they are most frequent

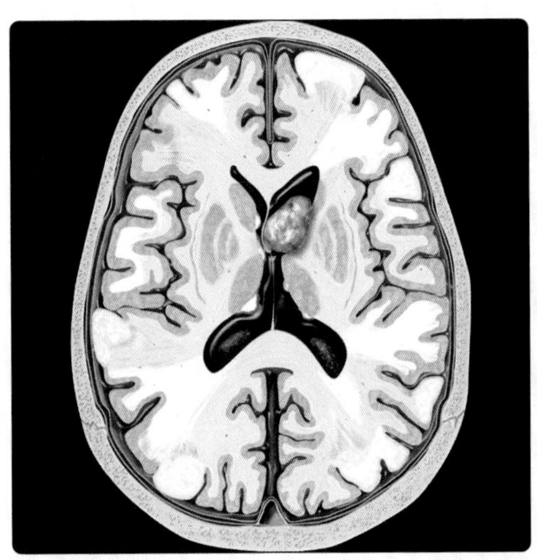

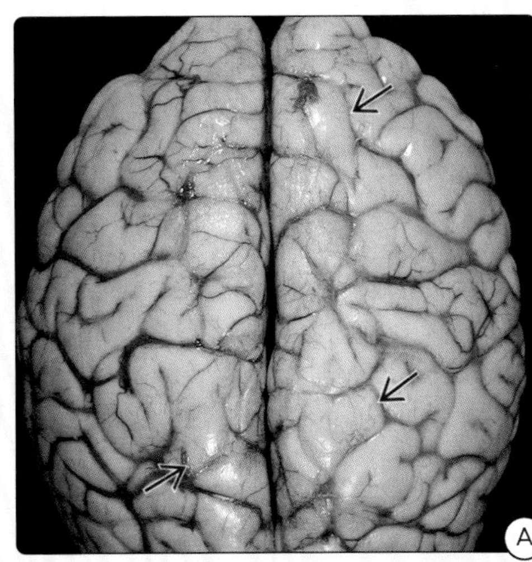

***(44-36)** Graphic shows pathologic findings of tuberous sclerosis complex (TSC). **(44-37A)** Autopsy of TSC shows multiple expanded gyri with the potato-like appearance characteristic of cortical tubers ➙. (Courtesy R. Hewlett, MD.)*

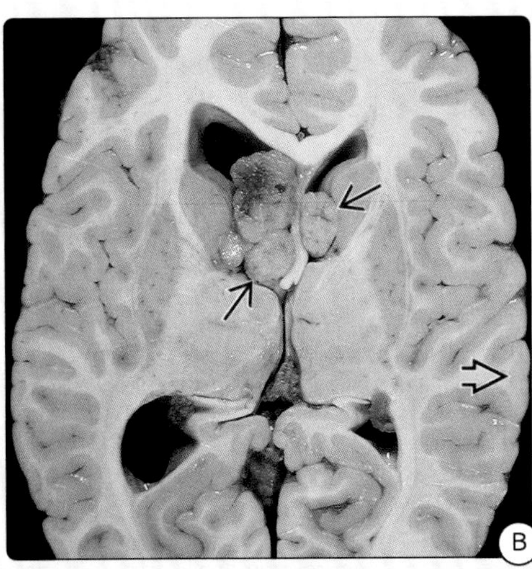

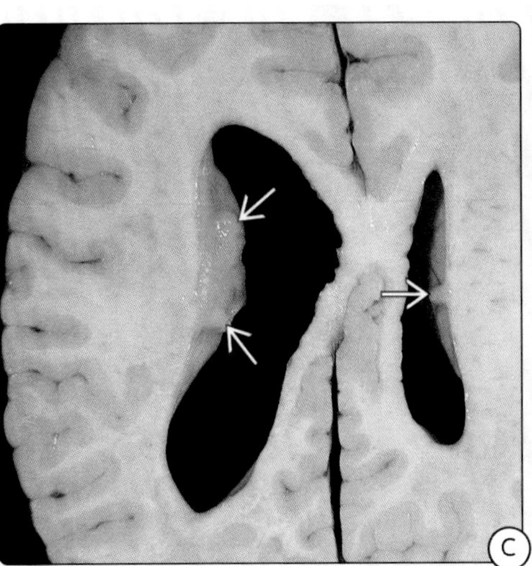

***(44-37B)** Axial cut section from the same case shows bilateral subependymal giant cell astrocytomas (SEGAs) ➙ and cortical tubers ⇨. (Courtesy R. Hewlett, MD.) **(44-37C)** Note "heaped-up" subependymal nodules (SENs) along the striothalamic groove ➡. (Courtesy R. Hewlett, MD.)*

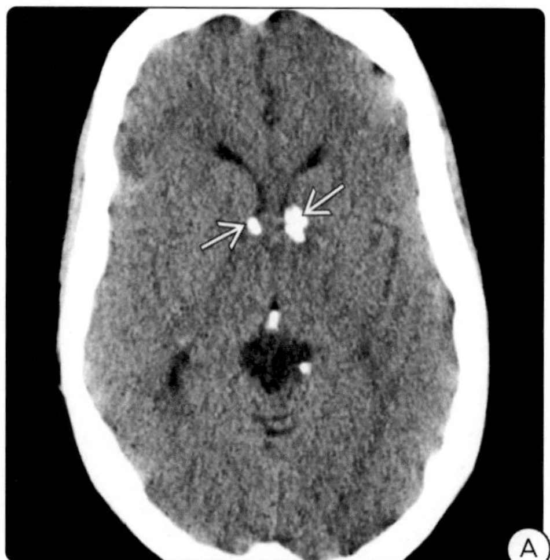

*(44-38A) NECT in a 22-yo woman with TSC demonstrates typical calcifications ➡ seen in SENs.*

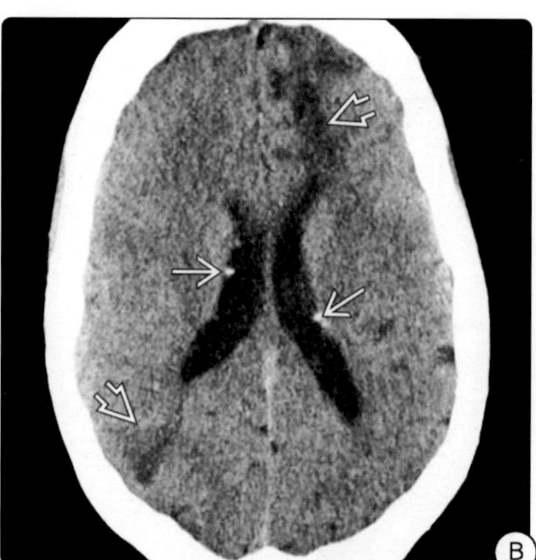

*(44-38B) NECT shows additional calcified SENs ➡ and wedge-shaped hypodensities ➡, characteristic of the WM lesions in TSC.*

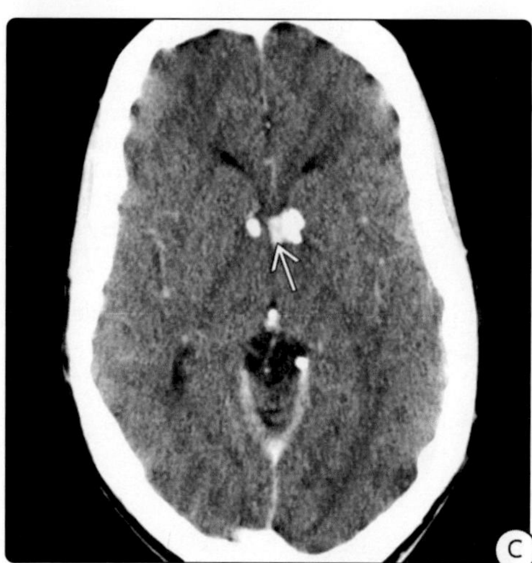

*(44-38C) CECT shows enhancement ➡ adjacent to the foramen of Monro, suspicious for SEGA.*

in patients between 5-19 years of age. Rapamycin inhibitors ("rapalogs"), such as everolimus and sirolimus, have been approved for the treatment of TSC-associated SEGAs in patients with TSC.

**TSC: DIAGNOSTIC CLINICAL FEATURES**

**Diagnosis**
- Definite TSC
  - 2 major **or** 1 major + 2 minor features
- Probable TSC
  - 1 major + 1 minor feature
- Possible TSC
  - 1 major **or** ≥ 2 minor features

**Major Features**
- Identified clinically
  - ≥ 3 hypomelanotic ("ash leaf") macules (97%)
  - Facial angiofibromas (75%) or forehead plaque (15-20%)
  - Shagreen patch (45-50%)
  - Ungual/periungual fibroma (15%)
  - Multiple retinal hamartomas (15%)
- Identified on imaging
  - Subependymal nodules (98%)
  - Cortical tubers (95%)
  - Cardiac rhabdomyoma (50%)
  - Renal angiomyolipoma (50%)
  - Subependymal giant cell astrocytoma (15%)
  - Lymphangioleiomyomatosis (1-3%)

**Minor Features**
- Identified clinically
  - Gingival fibromas (70%)
  - Affected 1st-degree relative (50%)
  - Pitting of dental enamel (30%)
  - Retinal achromic patch (35%)
  - Confetti-like skin macules (2-3%)
- Identified on imaging
  - WM hamartomas, radial migration lines (100%)
  - Hamartomatous rectal polyps (70-80%)
  - Nonrenal hamartomas (40-50%)
  - Bone cysts (40%)
  - Renal cysts (10-20%)

## Imaging

### CT Findings

***Cortical Tubers.*** Neonatal and infantile cortical tubers are initially seen as hypodense cortical/subcortical masses within broadened and expanded gyri. The lucency decreases with age. Calcifications progressively increase with age. By 10 years, 50% of affected children demonstrate one or more globular or gyriform cortical calcifications.

***Subependymal Nodules.*** SENs are a near-universal finding in TSC. Most are found along the caudothalamic groove. The walls of the atria and temporal horns of the lateral ventricles are less common sites.

SENs are rarely calcified in the first year of life. Like cortical tubers, SEN calcifications increase with age. Eventually, 50% demonstrate some degree of globular calcification **(44-38B)**. SENs typically do not enhance on CECT scans. An enhancing or enlarging SEN—especially if located near the foramen of Monro—is suspicious for SEGA **(44-38C)**.

***Subependymal Giant Cell Astrocytoma.*** SEGAs show mixed density on NECT scans and frequently demonstrate focal calcification. Hemorrhage is rare. Moderate enhancement on CECT is typical.

**MR Findings.** In general, MR is much more sensitive than CT in depicting parenchymal abnormalities in TSC. Findings vary with lesion histopathology, patient age, and imaging sequence. Standard T2-weighted sequences, FLAIR, and sometimes T1WI with magnetization transfer contrast are particularly useful in detecting TSC-associated CNS lesions.

***Cortical Tubers.*** In infants, tubers appear as thickened hyperintense cortex compared to the underlying unmyelinated WM on T1WI and become moderately hypointense on T2WI. "Streaky" linear or wedge-shaped T2-/FLAIR-hyperintense bands may extend from the tuber all the way through the WM to the ventricular ependyma **(44-41A)**.

Signal intensity changes after myelin maturation. Tubers gradually become more isointense relative to cortex on T1WI (unless calcification is present and causes T1 shortening). Occasionally, the outer margin of a tuber is mildly hyperintense to gray matter, while the subcortical component appears hypointense relative to WM.

Tubers in older children and adults demonstrate mixed signal intensity on T2/FLAIR. The periphery of the expanded gyrus is isointense with cortex, while the deeper component is strikingly hyperintense **(44-39C)**. Between 3-5% of cortical tubers show mild enhancement on T1 C+ imaging.

Cerebellar tubers are much less common than supratentorial cortical tubers and are rare under the age of eight years. Unique features reported in cerebellar tubers are retraction and "zebra-striped" enhancement.

***Subependymal Nodules.*** SENs are seen as small (generally < 1.3 cm) nodular "bumps" or "candle gutterings" that protrude from the walls of the lateral ventricles **(44-39)**. In the unmyelinated brain, SENs appear hyperintense on T1WI and hypointense on T2WI. With progressive myelination, the SENs gradually become isointense with WM.

Calcified SENs appear variably hypointense on T2WI or FLAIR and are easily identified on T2* sequences (GRE, SWI). They can be distinguished from blood products on the SWI phase map, as calcification is diamagnetic and appears bright, whereas paramagnetic substances (blood products) are hypointense.

Enhancement of SENs following contrast administration is variable **(44-41)**. About 1/2 of all SENs show moderate or even striking enhancement, which—in contrast to enhancement on CECT—does not indicate malignancy.

SENs are stable lesions. However, as SENs near the foramen of Monro may become malignant, close interval follow-up is essential. It is the interval change in size seen on serial examinations—not the degree of enhancement—that is significant. Some investigators suggest an increase of > 20% demonstrated on two consecutive MR scans as defining a SEGA.

***White Matter Lesions.*** WM lesions are seen in 100% of cases. Even though they are considered a "minor" criterion for TSC, their appearance is highly characteristic of the disease. Streaky linear or wedge-shaped lesions extend along radial bands from the ventricles to the undersurfaces of cortical tubers **(44-41)**. In the unmyelinated brain, these linear foci (radial migration lines) appear mildly hyperintense to WM on T1WI. In older children and adults, they are hyperintense on T2/FLAIR sequences **(44-40B)**.

Small, round, cyst-like parenchymal lesions are seen in nearly 50% of TSC cases. They are typically located in the deep periventricular WM **(44-41A)**.

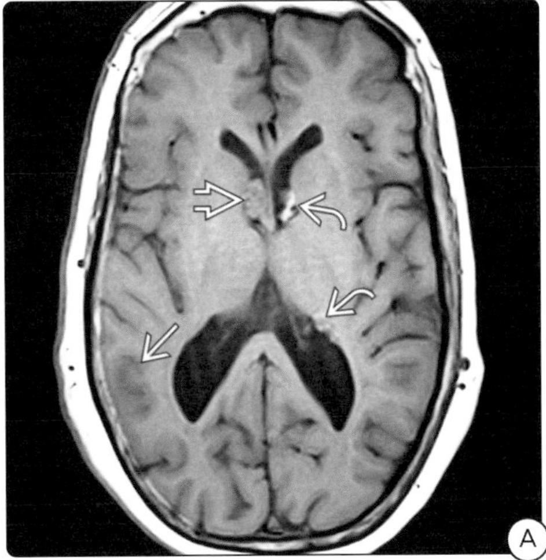


***(44-39A)** T1 MR shows hyperintense calcified SENs ➡ and right SEGA ➡. Note poorly defined GM-WM junctions ➡ of typical cortical tubers.*

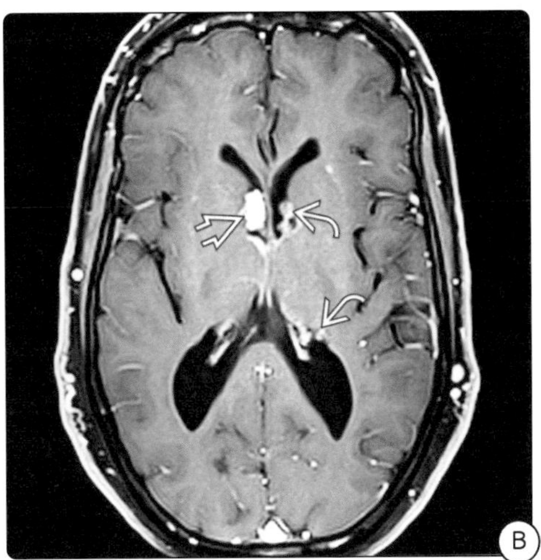


***(44-39B)** T1 C+ FS MR shows that the SEGA ➡ enhances intensely. The SENs ➡ also enhance moderately.*

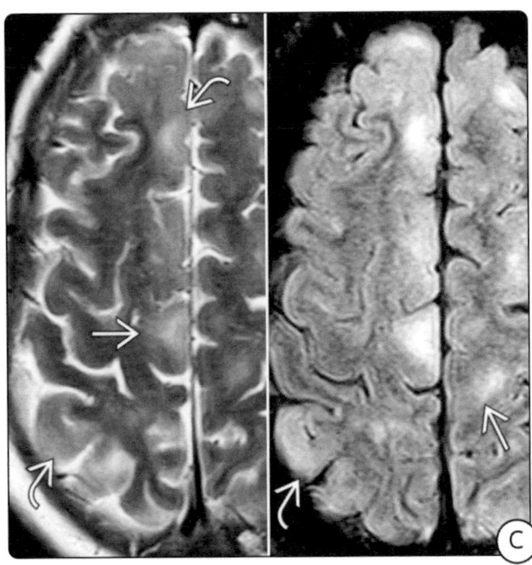


***(44-39C)** T2 (L) and FLAIR (R) MRs show tubers as expanded, hyperintense gyri ➡ with flame-shaped subcortical hyperintensities ➡.*

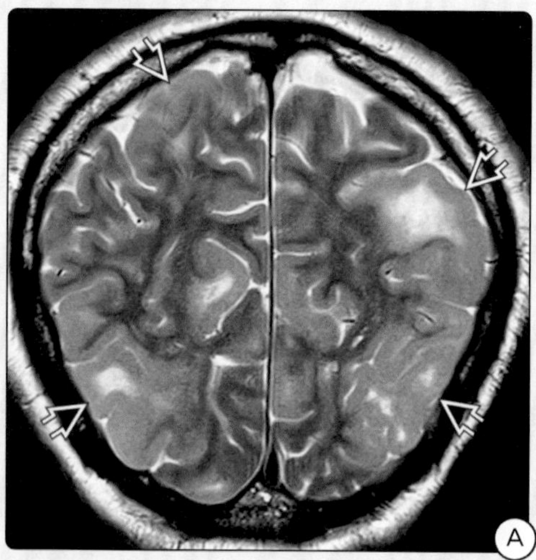

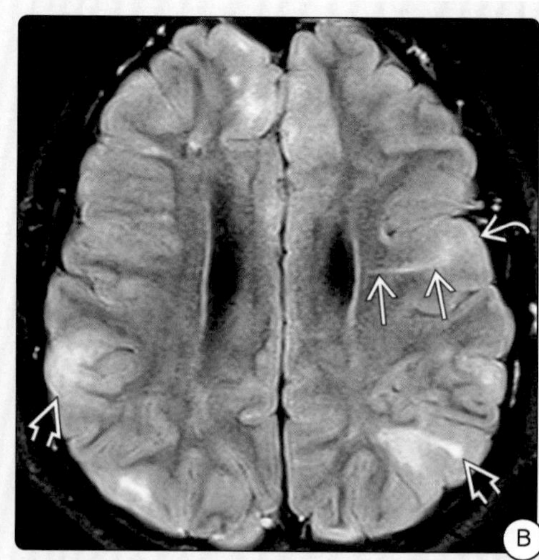

***(44-40A)*** *Coronal T2 MR in a 21-yo man with TSC shows multiple cortical tubers ➩, characterized by thick mildly hyperintense cortex and multiple hyperintense foci in the subcortical WM.* ***(44-40B)*** *FLAIR MR in the same case shows hyperintense cortical tubers ➩. Note hyperintense radial glial band ➡ extending from a cortical tuber ➩ through the WM toward the lateral ventricle.*

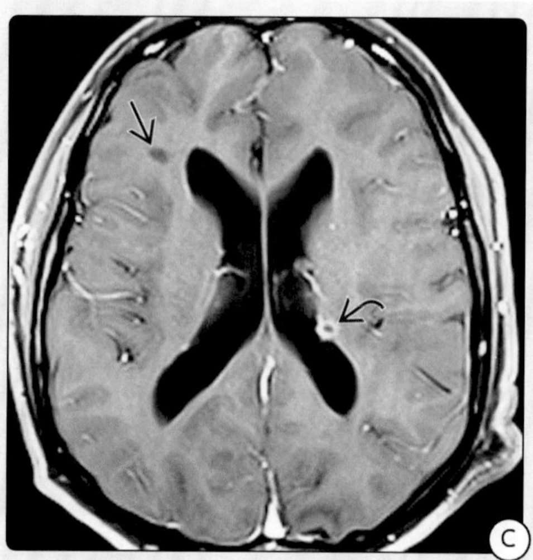

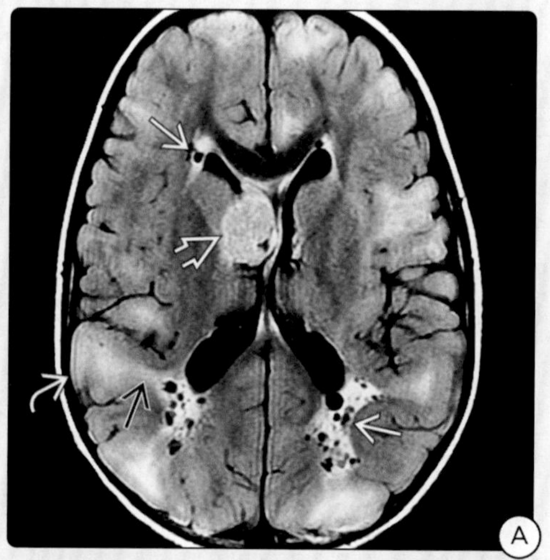

***(44-40C)*** *T1 C+ FS MR in the same case shows an enhancing SEN ➩ and a small nonenhancing cyst ➡ in the WM.* ***(44-41A)*** *FLAIR MR in 5-yo boy shows SEGA ➩, cortical tubers ➩ with WM band ➡, and numerous CSF-like cysts in the deep periventricular WM ➡.*

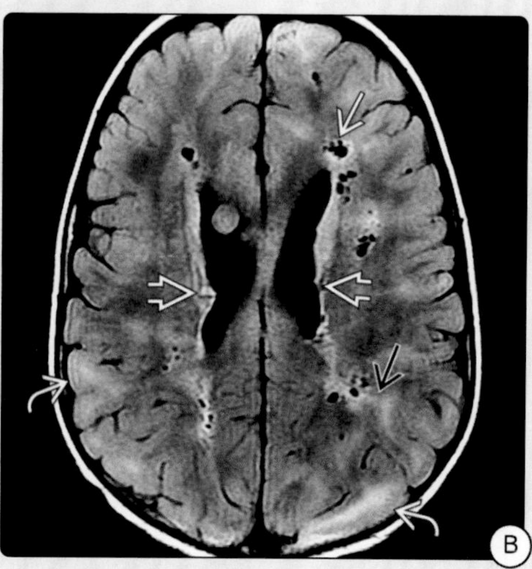

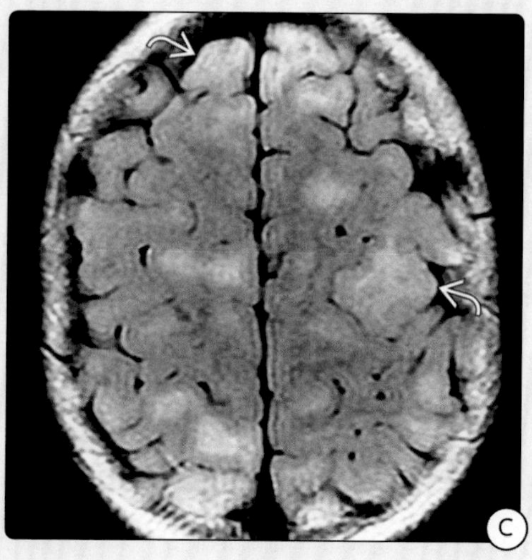

***(44-41B)*** *FLAIR MR shows multiple cortical tubers ➩, WM bands ➡, CSF cysts ➡, and irregular "candle gutterings" ➩ of SENs.* ***(44-41C)*** *More cephalad FLAIR MR in the same case shows multiple hyperintense cortical tubers ➩ with poorly defined GM-WM borders.*

They are often multiple and resemble CSF, i.e., they suppress on FLAIR and do not enhance **(44-42)**.

***Subependymal Giant Cell Astrocytoma.*** Although SEGAs can occur anywhere along the ventricular ependyma, the vast majority are found near the foramen of Monro. SEGAs are of mixed signal intensity on both T1- and T2WI **(44-39)**. Virtually all enhance moderately strongly on T1 C+ scans **(44-39B)**.

SEGAs become symptomatic when they obstruct the foramen of Monro and cause hydrocephalus. Even large SEGAs rarely invade brain.

***Miscellaneous CNS Lesions.*** Cerebellar tubers can be identified in 10-40% of cases and are always associated with supratentorial lesions. Other uncommon abnormalities include hemimegalencephaly, cerebellar malformations, and linear, clump-like, or gyriform parenchymal calcifications. Aneurysms (mostly fusiform aortic and intracranial) are seen in 1% of TSC.

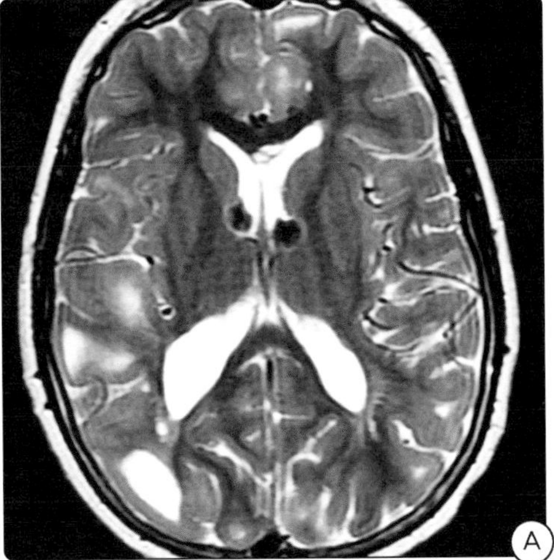


***(44-42A)*** *T2 MR in an 11-yo boy with TSC shows calcified SEGAs and subcortical cysts.*

## Differential Diagnosis

**Focal cortical dysplasia (FCD)** can appear identical to cortical tubers on imaging studies, but lesions are typically solitary, whereas cortical tubers are almost always multiple. Foci of **subependymal heterotopic gray matter** can resemble SENs, but most SENs calcify and often enhance on T1 C+ sequences.

SEGAs can resemble other frontal horn/septum pellucidum lesions, such as **subependymoma**. Subependymomas are tumors of middle-aged and older individuals, and other TSC stigmata, such as cortical tubers and SENs, are absent.

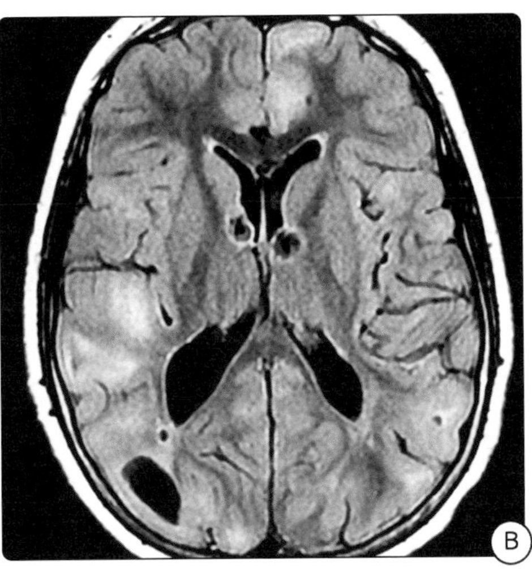


***(44-42B)*** *FLAIR MR shows that fluid in the subcortical cyst suppresses completely.*

### TSC: IMAGING

**Cortical Tubers**
- Broad, expanded gyrus
- CT: Initially hypodense; calcification increases with age
  - 50% of patients eventually develop ≥ 1 calcified tuber(s)
- MR: Periphery isointense, subcortical portion T2/FLAIR hyperintense

**Subependymal Nodules**
- CT: Calcification rare in 1st year; increases with age
  - 50% eventually calcify; do not enhance
- MR: T1 hyper-, T2 hypointense; 50% enhance

**White Matter Lesions**
- T2-/FLAIR-hyperintense radial lines/wedges
- CSF-like cysts in deep periventricular WM

**Subependymal Giant Cell Astrocytoma**
- CT: Mixed-density mass at foramen of Monro, moderate enhancement
- MR: Heterogeneous signal, strong enhancement

**Miscellaneous Lesions**
- Vascular (usually fusiform aneurysms), seen in 1% of cases
- Parenchymal calcifications

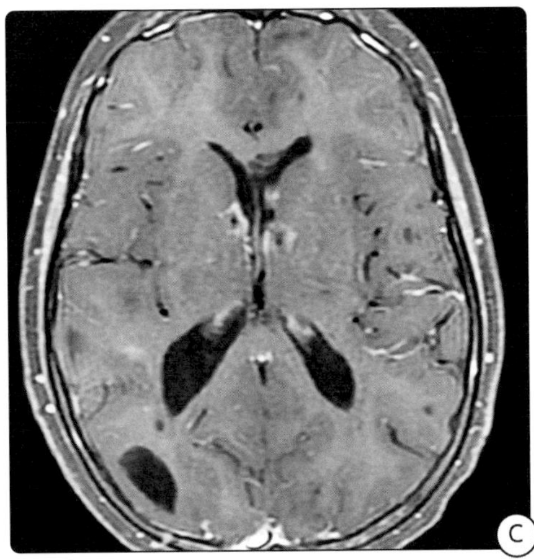


***(44-42C)*** *Axial T1 C+ FS MR shows enhancement around the SENs. The subcortical cyst does not enhance.*

# von Hippel-Lindau Disease

## Terminology

von Hippel-Lindau disease (VHL) is an autosomal dominant hereditary cancer syndrome caused by pathogenic germline variants in the *VHL* tumor suppressor gene. Affected individuals are at risk of developing multiple benign and malignant neoplasms. VHL is characterized by retinal and CNS

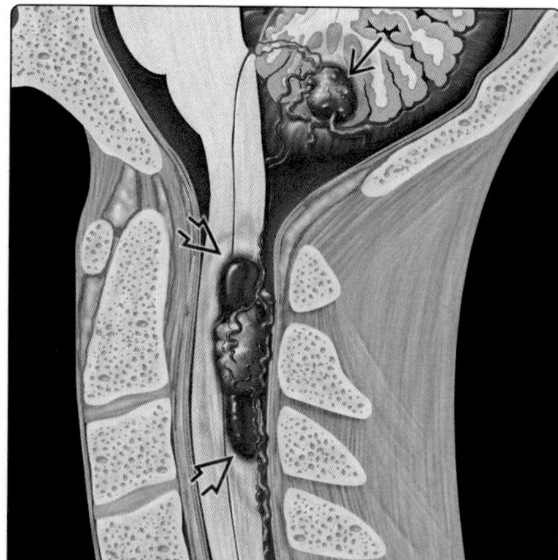

*(44-43) Two HBs in VHL show spinal cord tumor has an associated cyst ⇨, causing myelopathy. Small cerebellar HB ⇨ would be asymptomatic.*

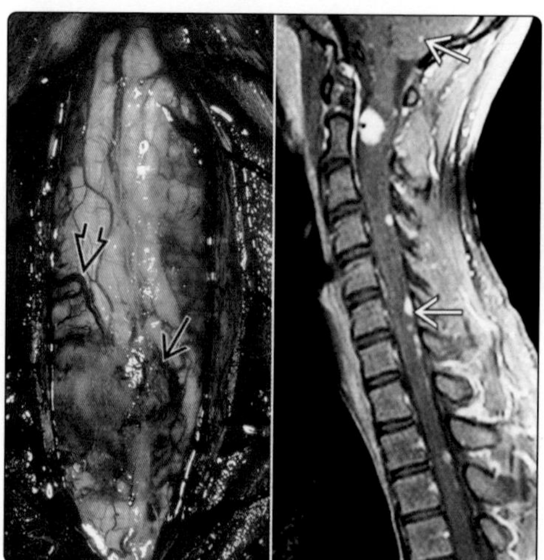

*(44-44) (L) Surgical photo shows typical dorsal subpial location of HB nodule ⇨, prominent vessels ⇨. (R) T1 C+ MR shows multiple HBs ➡.*

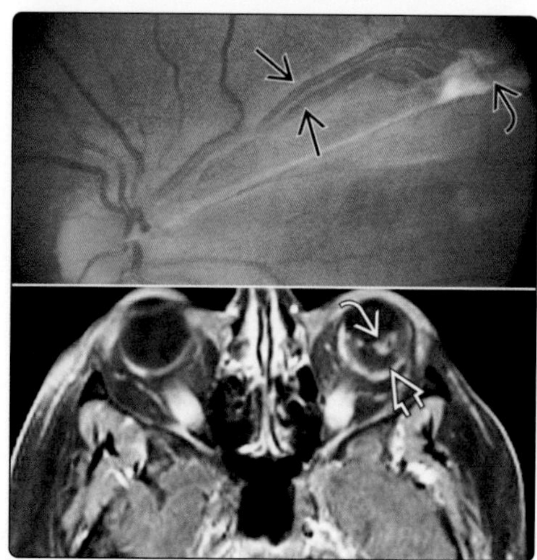

*(44-45) (Top) Retinal angioma ⇨ is supplied by prominent arteries ⇨. (From Imaging in Neuro.) (Bottom) Angioma ➡, retinal detachment ➡.*

hemangioblastomas (HBs) **(44-43)**, endolymphatic sac tumors (ELSTs) **(44-49)**, abdominal neoplasms (adrenal pheochromocytomas, clear cell renal carcinomas), and pancreatic and renal cysts.

## Etiology

**Genetics.** VHL is an autosomal dominant familial tumor syndrome with marked phenotypic variability and age-dependent penetrance. Overall penetrance of patients aged < 60 years is 95%.

Mutations in the *VHL* tumor suppressor gene on chromosome 3p25.3 cause inactivation of the VHL protein (pVHL) and increased expression of factors, such as PDGF and VEGF, which, in turn, leads to angiogenesis and tumorigenesis.

Two VHL phenotypes are recognized, distinguished by the presence or absence of associated pheochromocytoma. Type 1 has a **low risk** of pheochromocytoma and is caused by truncating mutations of the *VHL* gene. Type 2 is caused by missense mutations and has a **high risk** of developing pheochromocytoma. Type 2 VHL is subdivided into type 2A [low risk of renal cell carcinoma (RCC), 2B (high risk of RCC), and 2C (familial pheochromocytoma without either HB or RCC)].

Approximately 20% of tumors in patients with VHL result from de novo germline mutations. Mosaic VHL is rare. In such cases, tests for germline mutations can be negative, but next-generation sequencing (NGS) of tumor tissue is positive for *VHL* somatic mutations.

### VHL: GENETICS

**Type 1 VHL**

- Genotype = truncating mutations
- Phenotype
  - **Low** risk for pheochromocytoma (PCC)
  - Retinal angioma, CNS hemangioblastomas (HBs)
  - Renal cell carcinoma (RCC), pancreatic cysts, neuroendocrine tumors

**Type 2 VHL**

- Genotype = missense mutation
- Phenotypes
  - **All have high risk** of PCC
  - Type 2A (low risk of RCC); retinal angiomas, CNS HBs
  - Type 2B (high risk of RCC); retinal angioma, CNS HBs, pancreatic cysts, neuroendocrine tumor
  - Type 2C (risk for PCC only); no HB or RCC

## Pathology

The great majority of VHL patients harbor significant CNS disease. The two most common VHL-related CNS neoplasms are craniospinal **HBs** (found in 60-80% of all VHL cases) and **ELSTs** (seen in 10-15% of patients).

**Hemangioblastomas.** HBs are well-circumscribed red or yellowish masses that usually abut a pial surface. The vast majority of intracranial HBs are infratentorial; the dorsal 1/2 of the cerebellum is the most common site followed by the medulla.

Approximately 10% are supratentorial; the most common site is the pituitary stalk (30% of all supratentorial HBs and 3% of those in patients with VHL). Most are asymptomatic and do not require treatment. Less common locations are along the optic pathways and in the cerebral hemispheres.

Nearly 1/2 of all VHL-associated HBs occur in the spinal cord. Intraspinal HBs are often multiple and are frequently associated with a syrinx.

Between 1/4-1/3 of HBs are solid; 2/3 are at least partially cystic and contain amber-colored fluid. One or more cysts together with a variably sized mural tumor nodule is the typical appearance. HBs are highly vascular with large arteries and prominent draining veins.

**Retinal Hemangioblastomas ("Angiomas").** Retinal capillary angiomas are the typical ocular lesions of VHL and are seen in 1/2 of all cases **(44-45)**. Retinal angiomas are small but often multifocal, and almost 50% are bilateral.

**Endolymphatic Sac Tumors.** ELSTs are slow-growing, benign but locally aggressive papillary cystadenomatous tumors of the endolymphatic sac **(44-50)**. Sporadic ELSTs are more common than VHL-associated tumors. Approximately 10-15% of VHL patients develop an ELST; of these, 30% are bilateral.

### VHL: PATHOLOGY

**CNS Neoplasms**
- HBs (60-80%)
  - Retinal HBs ("angiomas") (50%)
- ELSTs (10-15%)

**Visceral Lesions**
- Renal lesions (2/3 of all VHL patients)
  - Cysts (50-75%)
  - Clear cell renal carcinomas (25-45%)
- Adrenal PCC (10-20%)
  - Hallmark of type 2 VHL
- Pancreatic cysts (35-70%), nonsecretory islet cell tumors (5-10%)
- Epididymal cysts, cystadenomas (60% of male patients; often bilateral)
- Broad ligament cystadenomas (female patients; rare)

## Clinical Issues

**Presentation and Clinical Diagnosis.** Because all VHL-associated lesions can also occur as sporadic (i.e., nonfamilial) events, a clinical diagnosis of VHL disease in a patient without a positive family history requires the presence of at least two tumors (see next box).

Age at diagnosis varies. Although VHL can present in children and even infants, most patients become symptomatic as young adults. Painless visual loss from retinal angioma-induced hemorrhage is often the first symptom (mean: 25 years).

Tumors are the presenting feature in ~ 40% of cases. HBs, pheochromocytomas, and endolymphatic tumors typically become symptomatic in the 30s, whereas RCCs tend to present somewhat later. Mean age at diagnosis of symptomatic RCCs is 40 years, but asymptomatic tumors are frequently detected earlier on screening abdominal CT.

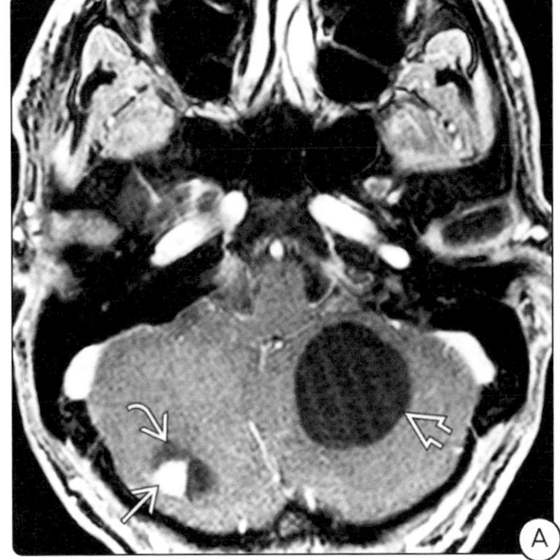


***(44-46A)** T1 C+ FS MR in VHL shows cystic left cerebellar mass and a smaller cyst with enhancing nodule in the right hemisphere.*

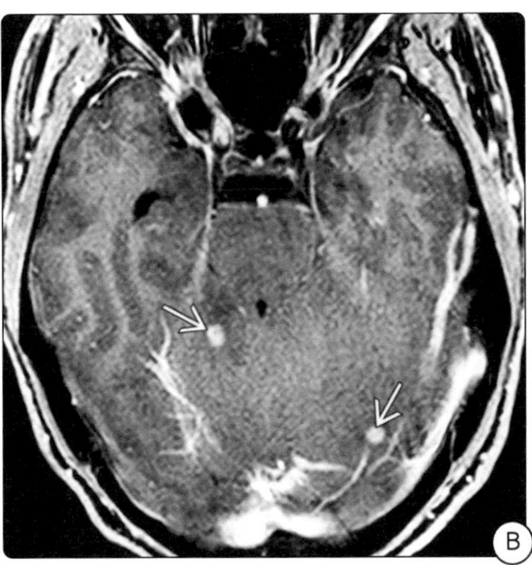


***(44-46B)** More cephalad scan in the same case shows 2 tiny enhancing nodules.*

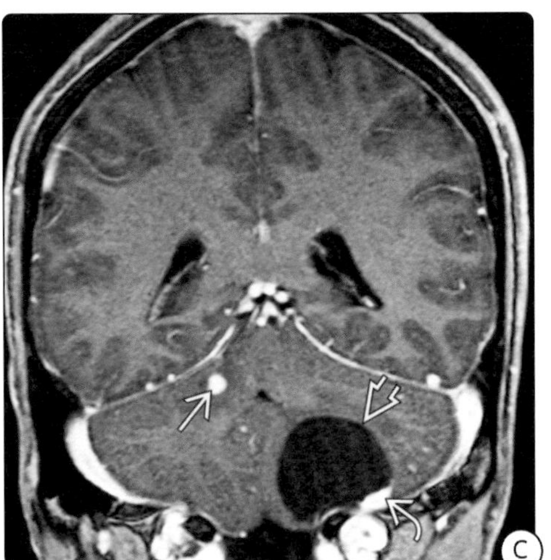


***(44-46C)** Coronal shows enhancing nodule abuts pial surface. Cyst wall does not enhance. Note separate enhancing nodule.*

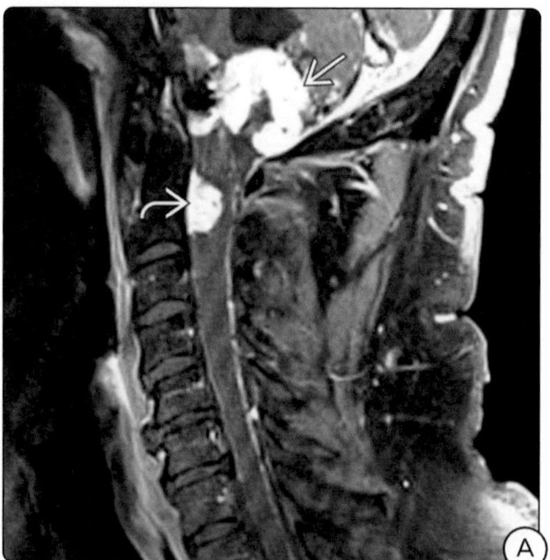

*(44-47A) Sagittal T1 C+ MR in a 38-yo man with VHL shows multiple HBs in the cerebellum ➡ and cervical spinal cord ➡.*

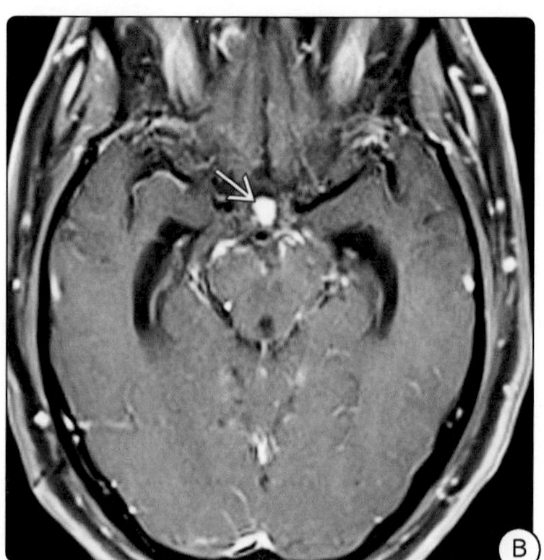

*(44-47B) Axial T1 C+ FS MR in the same case demonstrates an enlarged enhancing pituitary stalk ➡.*

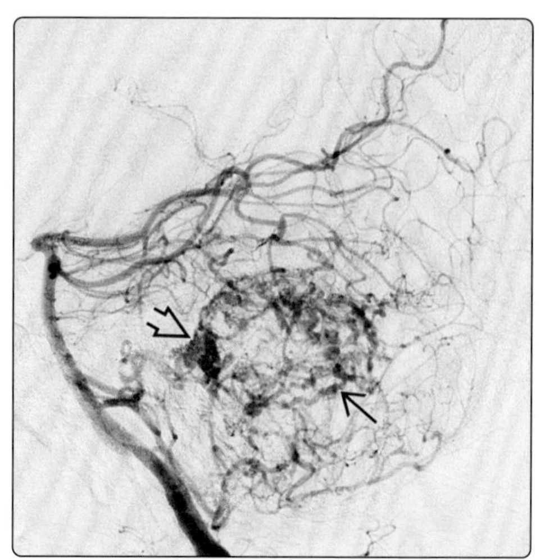

*(44-48) DSA of HGBL shows vascular "stain" ➡ and striking neovascularity with tortuous, irregular-appearing vessels ➡.*

VHL: DIAGNOSTIC CLINICAL FEATURES

**No Family History of VHL**
- ≥ 2 CNS HBs **or**
- 1 CNS HB + visceral tumor

**Positive Family History of VHL**
- 1 CNS HB **or**
- PCC **or**
- Clear cell renal carcinoma

**Natural History.** VHL-associated HBs demonstrate a "saltatory" growth pattern characterized by quiescent periods (averaging slightly over two years) interspersed with periods of growth. Nearly 1/2 of all patients develop de novo lesions after the initial diagnosis of VHL.

The two major causes of death in VHL patients are RCC (50%) and HBs. Overall median life expectancy is 49 years.

**Surveillance Recommendations.** Imaging is crucial in the identification and surveillance of extra-CNS lesions. Identification of RCC is especially important because it is the major malignant neoplasm of VHL and one of the leading causes of mortality.

Patients with a family history of VHL should undergo annual screening (ophthalmoscopy, physical/neurologic examination) beginning in infancy or early childhood. Brain MRs are recommended every 1-3 years starting in adolescence. Abdominal MR or ultrasound screening for RCC and pancreatic tumors is recommended annually, beginning at age 16.

Methods for pheochromocytoma screening vary. Blood pressure should be monitored and 24-hour urine catecholamines obtained annually. More intense surveillance beginning at age eight years should be considered in families at high-risk for pheochromocytoma (i.e., type 2 VHL).

## Imaging

**General Features.** Two or more CNS HBs **(44-46)** or one HB + a visceral lesion or concomitant presence of retinal hemorrhage (highly suggestive of intraocular HB) are the best imaging clues to the diagnosis.

**Hemangioblastomas.** Approximately 2/3 of HBs are cystic; 1/3 are solid or mixed solid/cystic lesions. NECT scans typically demonstrate a hypodense cyst with isodense mural nodule that abuts a pial surface of the cerebellum. The tumor nodule enhances intensely on CECT.

The cyst is slightly to moderately hyperintense to CSF on T1WI and iso- to hyperintense on T2/FLAIR. Signal intensity of the nodule is variable; large lesions may show prominent "flow voids." Hemorrhage is common, and peritumoral edema varies.

Tumor nodules enhance strongly on T1 C+ **(44-47)**. Enhanced scans often demonstrate several tiny nodules in the cerebellum &/or spinal cord **(44-44)**. Supratentorial HBs are uncommon; most occur in the pituitary stalk (the most common supratentorial site) **(44-47B)** or along the optic tracts. Disseminated leptomeningeal hemangioblastomatosis, seen as multiple tumor nodules with diffuse pial enhancement of the spinal cord **(44-47A)** &/or brain, is a rare, late manifestation of VHL.

DSA demonstrates one or more intensely vascular masses with prolonged tumor "blush" and variable arteriovenous shunting **(44-48)**.

Compared to nonsyndromic HBs, VHL-associated CNS HBs are smaller and more often solid, without associated cysts.

**Retinal Hemangioblastomas ("Angiomas").** Retinal angiomas (actually small capillary HBs) are usually visualized as hemorrhagic retinal detachments that are hyperdense compared with normal vitreous on NECT. Tiny enhancing nodules can sometimes be identified on T1 C+ MR **(44-45)**.

**Endolymphatic Sac Tumors.** ELSTs are located along the posterior petrous temporal bone between the internal auditory canal and the sigmoid sinus. The imaging hallmark of ELST is that of a retrolabyrinthine mass associated with osseous erosion. Bone CT shows an infiltrative, poorly circumscribed, lytic lesion with central intratumoral bone spicules **(44-50A)**.

MR demonstrates T1-hyperintense foci in 80% of cases. Signal intensity is mixed hyper- and hypointense on T2WI. Heterogeneous enhancement is seen following contrast administration **(44-50B)**. ELSTs are vascular lesions that may demonstrate prominent "flow voids" on MR and prolonged tumor "blush" on DSA.

**VHL: IMAGING**

**Multiple Hemangioblastomas (Diagnostic of VHL)**
- 2/3 cystic, 1/3 solid
- Nodule abuts pia
- 50% in cord (dorsal > ventral surface)
  - Multiple tiny "tumorlets" along cord common
  - Disseminated leptomeningeal hemangioblastomatosis

**Retinal "Angiomas"**
- Hemorrhagic retinal detachment
  - V-shaped hyperdense posterior globe
- ± enhancing "dots" (tiny HBs)

**Uni- or Bilateral Endolymphatic Sac Tumors**
- Dorsal temporal bone
  - Between IAC, sigmoid sinus
- Infiltrative, lytic, intratumoral bone spicules
- T1 iso-/hyperintense; T2 hyperintense
- Strong enhancement

**Differential Diagnosis**
- Solitary HB
- Vascular metastases

## Differential Diagnosis

The major differential diagnosis of VHL in the brain is **sporadic non-VHL-associated HB**. Between 60-80% of HBs are sporadic tumors **not** associated with VHL. Multiple HBs &/or supratentorial lesions are highly suggestive of VHL.

**Vascular metastases** can mimic multiple HBs but are rarely isolated to the cerebellum &/or spinal cord.

Other neoplasms that commonly have a cyst + nodule configuration include **pilocytic astrocytoma** and **ganglioglioma**. Pilocytic astrocytomas are solitary tumors of childhood, whereas HBs are rarely seen in patients younger than 15 years. In contrast to HB, the tumor nodule in pilocytic astrocytoma typically does not abut a pial surface.

**Ganglioglioma** is typically a tumor of the cerebral hemispheres. While hemispheric HBs can occur, they are rare. When present, they are typically found along the optic pathways.

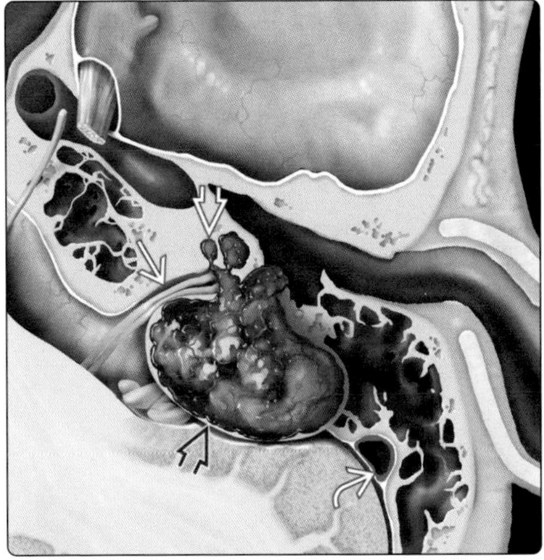

***(44-49)** ELST ➡ is a lytic, vascular, hemorrhagic mass between the IAC ➡ and sigmoid sinus ➡. Note tendency to fistulize inner ear ➡.*

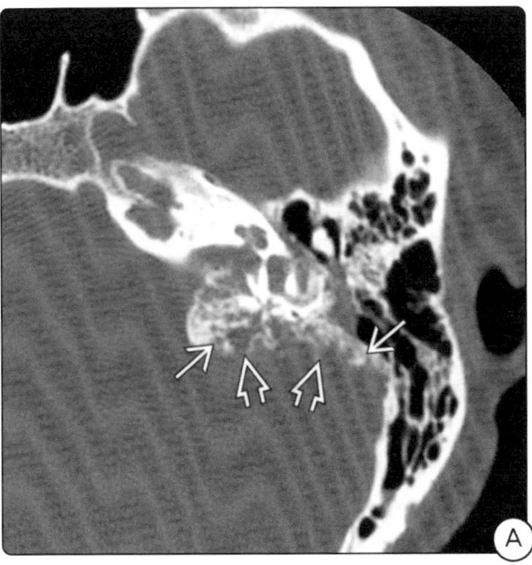


***(44-50A)** Lytic infiltrative lesion ➡ with preserved bond "spicules" ➡; location between the IAC, sigmoid sinus is characteristic for ELST.*

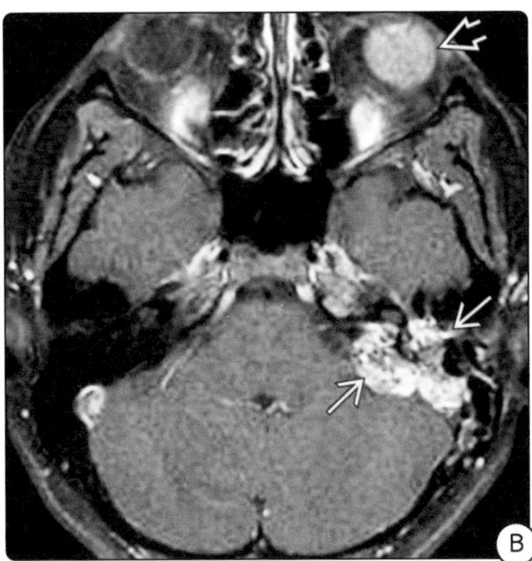


***(44-50B)** T1 C+ FS MR shows lesion ➡ enhances intensely but heterogeneously. Hyperintense retinal hemorrhage ➡ + ELST = VHL.*

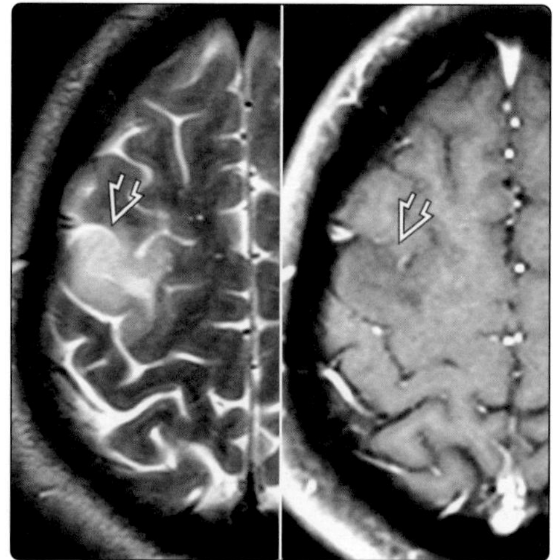

*(44-51) (L) T2, (R) T1 C+ in 23-yo man with LFS, grade 2 IDH-mutant astrocytoma ➡ that slowly progressed to grade 4. He expired after 10 years.*

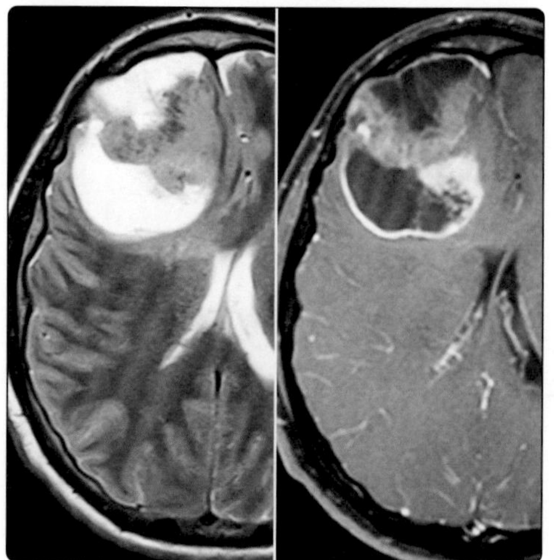

*(44-52) (L) T2, (R) T1 C+ FS in a 22-yo with LFS, diffuse astrocytoma, IDH-mutant, CNS WHO grade 4.*

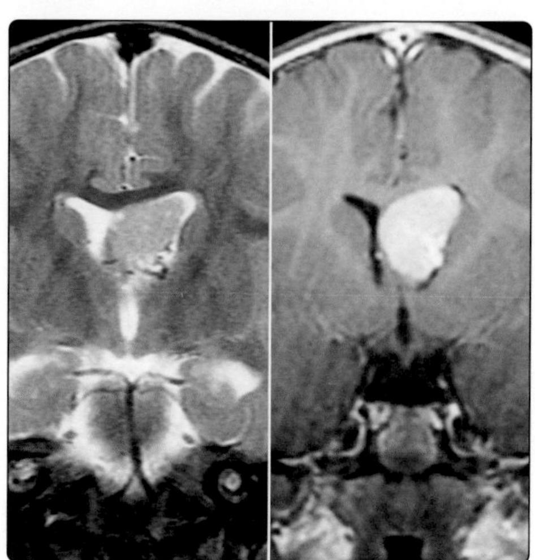

*(44-53) (L) T2, (R) T1 C+ in child with LFS shows intraventricular enhancing mass. This is choroid plexus carcinoma.*

# Less Common Familial Cancer Syndromes

A growing number of cancer predisposition syndromes have been identified in recent years. Up to 10% of pediatric, adolescent, and young adult patients with CNS neoplasms have a genetic predisposition to tumor development. Young patients with CNS malignancies are overall more likely to have an underlying genetic predisposition than patients with other malignancies.

In this section, we briefly consider some of these inherited cancer syndromes. The specific neoplasms associated with these disorders do not differ much, if at all, from their sporadic counterparts. They are histopathologically identical and often feature the same molecular profiles. What sets them apart is the **constellation** of clinical features—often cutaneous lesions—combined with systemic and CNS neoplasms.

We close this chapter with a brief consideration of some of these interesting syndromes.

## Li-Fraumeni Syndrome

### Terminology

Li-Fraumeni syndrome (LFS) is a highly penetrant, early-onset tumor predisposition syndrome characterized by a lifelong risk of developing multiple primary malignant tumors in a variety of organ systems, including the brain.

### Etiology

LFS is an autosomal dominant disorder caused by a pathogenic germline alteration (mutation, rearrangement, or partial/complete deletion) in the *TP53* tumor suppressor gene on chromosome 17.

### Pathology

Tumors classically associated with LFS are soft tissue sarcomas, osteosarcomas, premenopausal breast cancer, CNS neoplasms, and adrenocortical carcinoma.

CNS tumors are the fourth most common tumor type in LFS. The most common LFS-associated CNS neoplasms are choroid plexus carcinoma **(44-53)**, medulloblastoma (usually the SHH-activated, *TP53*-mutant molecular subtype) **(44-51)**, and diffuse astrocytic gliomas, such as glioblastoma **(44-52)**. Other reported CNS neoplasms include ependymomas, meningiomas, and low-grade gliomas.

LFS-associated astrocytomas exhibit distinct age-dependent molecular patterns. Pediatric patients present with IDH-wildtype glioblastomas characterized by frequent *NF1* mutations. Lower grade hemispheric diffuse astrocytic gliomas with *IDH1* and *ATRX* mutations predominate in young adults.

### Clinical Issues

Up to 40% of patients are diagnosed with cancer before age 18. Recent screening guidelines have demonstrated that early tumor detection is associated with improved long-term survival. Some of the strongest supporting evidence for whole-body screening MR in cancer predisposition syndromes has been found in LFS, as a majority of low-grade CNS lesions are found on surveillance protocols in asymptomatic patients.

The classic clinical criteria for LFS are (1) a sarcoma diagnosed before age 45 years **and** (2) at least one first-degree relative with any cancer before age 45 years **and** (3) a first- or second-degree relative with any cancer before age 45 years or a sarcoma at any age.

Some research suggests that low-grade gliomas in LFS patients have a higher risk of transformation into high-grade gliomas than patients with sporadic tumors. Approximately 25% exhibit malignant transformation at five years and 50% at seven years.

### Imaging

Brain imaging in LFS patients with CNS symptoms varies with tumor type. Imaging findings and differential diagnoses in LFS-associated neoplasms are similar to those of their sporadic counterparts.

## Cowden Syndrome

### Terminology

Cowden syndrome (CS) is a.k.a. **multiple hamartoma-neoplasia syndrome** and **PTEN hamartoma tumor syndrome**. The classic brain hamartoma in CS a dysplastic cerebellar gangliocytoma, a.k.a. **Lhermitte-Duclos disease** (LDD).

### Etiology

CS is an autosomal dominant disorder caused by pathogenic germline mutations in the *PTEN* tumor suppressor gene with variable expression and age-related penetrance. Nearly 60-90% of pathogenic variants are inherited.

Other disorders caused by *PTEN* pathogenic variants are Bannayan-Riley-Ruvalcaba syndrome.

### Pathology

Multiple hamartomas involving tissues derived from all three germ cell layers characterize CS. The classic brain hamartoma is adult-onset dysplastic cerebellar gangliocytoma (LDD), considered to be pathognomonic of the disorder.

Affected patients have an elevated lifetime risk of developing endometrial, breast, thyroid, colorectal, or renal carcinomas. The two most common cancers in CS are breast and thyroid carcinomas.

### Clinical Issues

The diagnosis of CS is suggested by clinical criteria and confirmed by genetic testing. Women with CS have a 50% lifetime risk of developing breast cancer, 10% risk of developing follicular thyroid cancer, and 5-10% risk of developing endometrial cancer.

CS patients may have mild macrocrania ≥ 97th percentile **(44-54)**, megalencephaly, hydrocephalus, autism spectrum disorder, intellectual disability, and seizures.

Characteristic mucocutaneous lesions (trichilemmomas, acral keratoses, papillomatous lesions) are present in almost all CS patients by the third decade of life. Other non-CNS features include gastrointestinal polyps as well as various benign breast, thyroid, and uterine lesions.

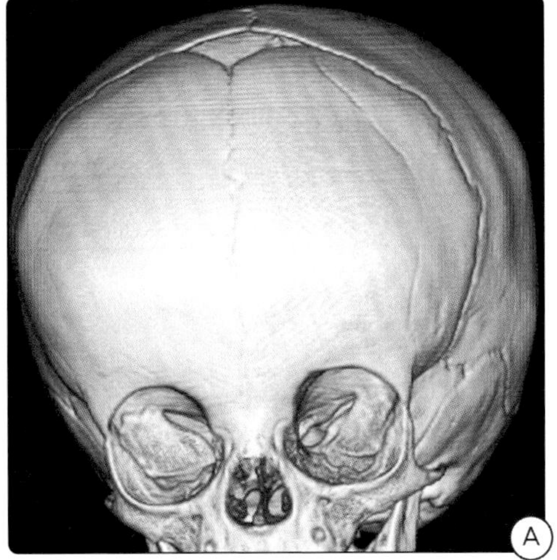


***(44-54A)*** *3D CT in a 16-mo boy with skin lesions characteristic of Cowden syndrome (CS) and PTEN mutation shows gross macrocephaly.*

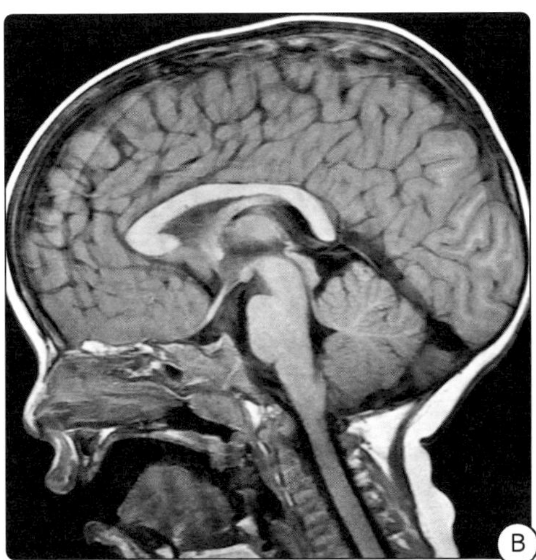


***(44-54B)*** *Sagittal T1 MR in the same case shows severe craniofacial disproportion with prominent frontal bossing.*

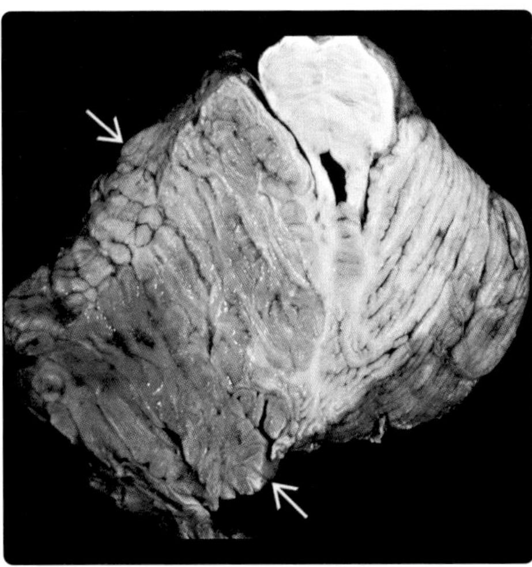

***(44-55)*** *Autopsied cerebellum in a patient who died from breast cancer shows classic LDD ➡. (Courtesy AFIP Archives.)*

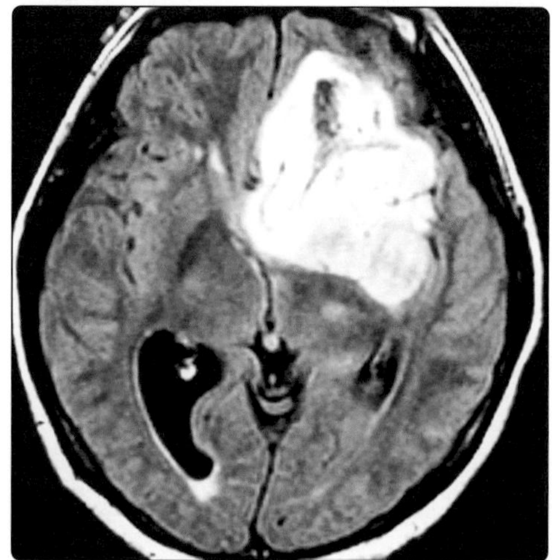

***(44-56)*** *Diffuse astrocytoma, grade 3, is shown in constitutional mismatch repair deficiency syndrome (CMMRD). (Courtesy T. Tihan, MD.)*

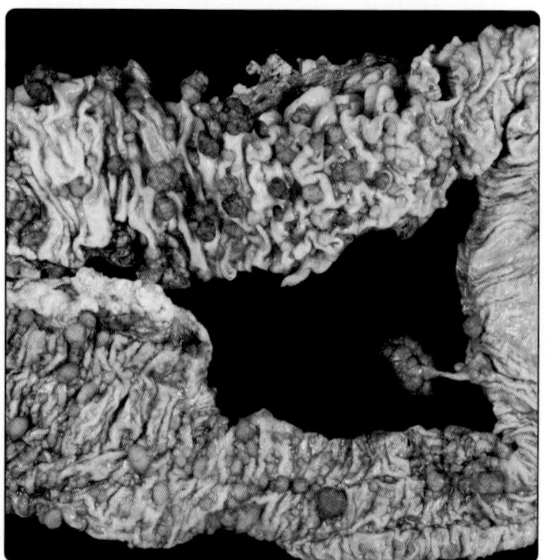

***(44-57)*** *Colon from patient with FAP1 (formerly type 2 Turcot) syndrome shows innumerable small polyps. (Courtesy T. Tihan, MD.)*

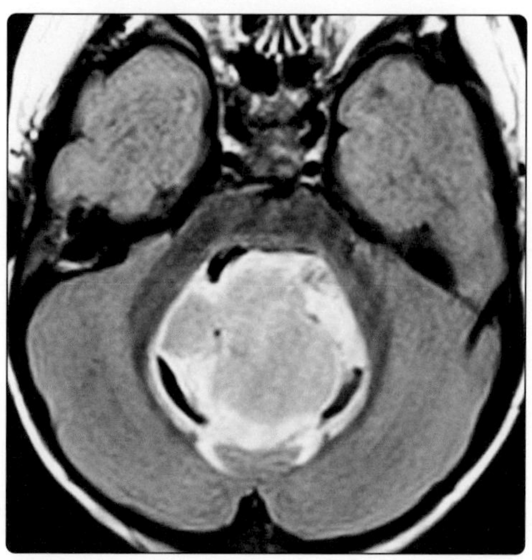

***(44-58)*** *WNT-activated medulloblastoma in FAP1 is seen as a hyperintense mass centered in the 4th ventricle. (Courtesy T. Tihan, MD.)*

### Imaging

Imaging findings of dysplastic cerebellar gangliocytoma in the setting of CS are identical to those of LDD **(44-55)**. An enlarged cerebellar hemisphere with thickened folia in a corduroy or tiger-striped appearance is typical.

### Differential Diagnosis

Patients with LDD should be screened for CS and vice versa. A dysplastic cerebellar gangliocytoma without a characteristic mucocutaneous lesion or other criteria (e.g., breast cancer, thyroid lesions) is simply LDD.

## Constitutional Mismatch Repair Deficiency Syndrome

### Terminology

Constitutional mismatch repair deficiency syndrome (CMMRD) is a rare inherited **autosomal recessive** cancer predisposition syndrome. Individuals with CMMRD develop frequent hematologic, gastrointestinal, and CNS malignancies early in life, including ultrahypermutated malignant gliomas, CNS embryonal tumors, and a variety of other cancers. The term Turcot syndrome is no longer recommended.

### Etiology

CMMRD results from a biallelic germline pathogenic variant of one of four mismatch repair (MMR) genes, *MSH2, MSH6, MLH1*, and *PMS2*. *PMS2* mutations account for 60% of cases.

Monoallelic germline variants in MMR genes cause Lynch syndrome, which predisposes individuals mainly to colorectal cancer, endometrial cancer, and other related malignancies.

### Pathology

The most common CMMRD-associated malignancies are brain tumors, most commonly high-grade gliomas, that usually develop in the first two decades of life **(44-56)**. Medulloblastoma and CNS embryonal tumors have also been associated with CMMRD. All CMMRD-associated brain tumors have a unique ultrahypermutation genotype.

Corpus callosum dysgenesis and developmental venous anomalies have also been reported in children with CMMRD.

### Clinical Issues

CMMRD primarily affects children and adolescents. A family history of cancer is often lacking. The presence of café au lait macules or hyperpigmented skin alterations > 1 cm and gastrointestinal cancers in a child or adolescent should raise suspicion for CMMRD.

Slightly over 1/2 of all CMMRD patients develop brain tumors with a mean age at diagnosis of nine years. In rare cases, a malignant brain tumor is the initial presentation of CMMRD.

### Imaging

Imaging findings are similar to those of their nonsyndromic counterparts.

### Differential Diagnosis

CMMRD should not be confused with **Lynch syndrome** [formerly called hereditary nonpolyposis colorectal cancer (HNPCC) or **Turcot syndrome**

**type 1**]. Lynch syndrome is also an MMR disorder but is an autosomal dominant syndrome with heterozygous germline mutations, most commonly in *MLH1* or *MSH2*. Onset is typical later than CMMRD. Associated neoplasms are typically high grade, mostly glioblastoma.

## Familial Adenomatous Polyposis 1

Familial adenomatous polyposis 1 (FAP1)—formerly called **Turcot syndrome**—is an autosomal dominant multiorgan cancer predisposition syndrome with a pathogenic germline mutation in the *APC* gene. The germline *APC* mutation, together with the progressive accumulation of mutations involving other oncogenes and tumor suppressor genes, will alter genomic stability. Such alterations give rise to chromosomal instability, a distinctive characteristic of *APC*-altered cancers.

Only 20% of patients have a positive family history of the disease. Affected patients develop multiple colorectal adenomatous polyps at different stages of development that, when untreated or undiagnosed, may progress to carcinoma by the time the patient reaches 40 years of age **(44-57)**. Therefore, endoscopic evaluation is paramount in surveillance strategies for diagnosis as well as therapeutic interventions.

FAP patients are also prone to a wide range of systemic extraintestinal manifestations that must be monitored. More than 70% will develop extracolonic neoplasms, such as osteomas, thyroid cancers, and hepatoblastoma.

A subset of patients with FAP1 develop a brain tumor, which is also termed brain tumor polyposis syndrome 2 (BTP2). WNT-activated medulloblastoma without *CTNNB1* mutation is the only tumor clearly associated with this syndrome **(44-58)**.

## Nevoid Basal Cell Carcinoma Syndrome

### Terminology

Nevoid basal cell carcinoma syndrome (NBCCS), a.k.a. Gorlin or Gorlin-Goltz syndrome, is a multisystem disorder caused by germline mutations in the hedgehog signaling pathway. This pathway is involved in embryogenesis and tumorigenesis, and PTCH1 protein loss of function produces an aberrant increase in hedgehog signaling pathway activity.

### Etiology

NBCCS results from inactivating germline mutations in *PTCH1*, its paralog *PTCH2*, or *SUFU*. *PTCH1* and *SUFU* are classic tumor suppressor genes. Inactivation leads to pathologic activation of the sonic hedgehog (SHH) signaling pathway.

### Pathology

The most common manifestations of NBCCS are basal cell carcinomas and jaw odontogenic keratocysts, found in > 90% of affected individuals by age 40 years **(44-59)**. Approximately 20% of patients with germline *SUFU* pathogenic variants develop a medulloblastoma with SHH activation. Almost all are desmoplastic/nodular or extensive nodular histologic types **(44-61)**.

### Clinical Issues

Clinical features of NBCCS manifest at different points of life. Macrocephaly and rib anomalies can be detected at birth. Medulloblastomas typically develop within the first three years of life. Jaw cysts are rare before eight

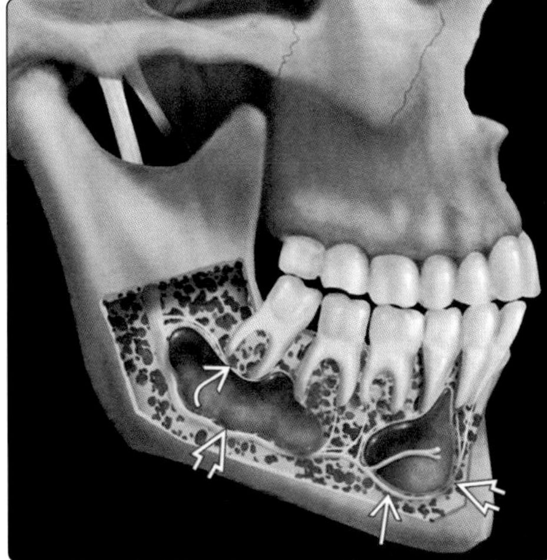

***(44-59)** NBCCS with multiple odontogenic keratocysts ➡ is shown. Lesions splay teeth roots ➡ and displace nerves ➡.*

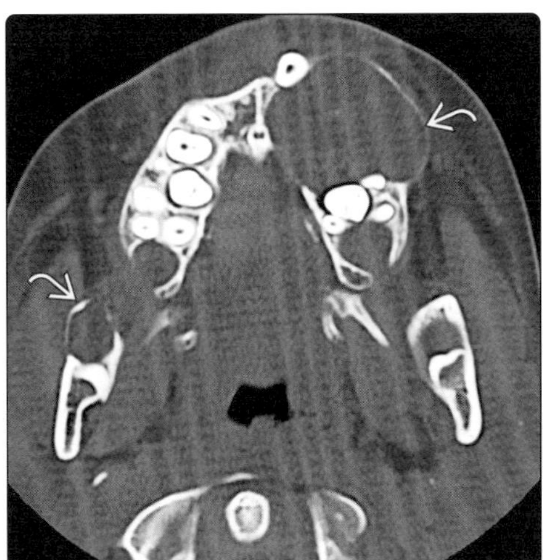

***(44-60)** Bone CT in 9-yo boy with NBCCS shows multiple lytic lesions in the maxilla and mandible ➡. These are typical odontogenic keratocysts.*

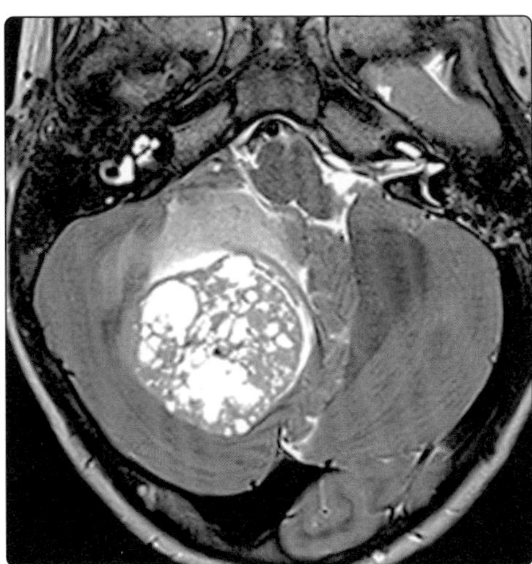

***(44-61)** T2 MR in a 6-yo boy with NBCCS shows cerebellar desmoplastic medulloblastoma, SHH subtype, PTCH1 mutation.*

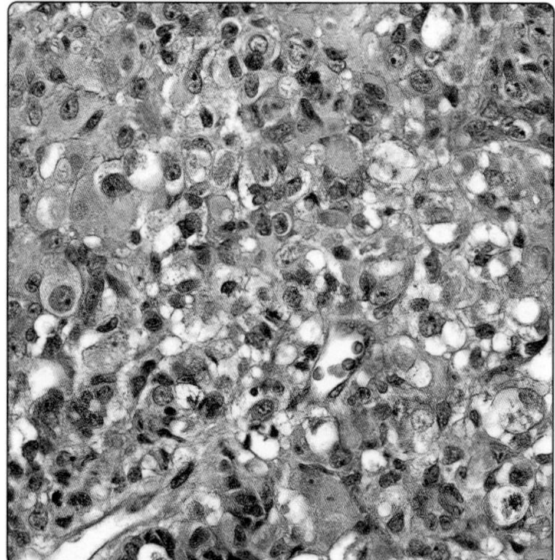

*(44-62) Micrograph of AT/RT with SMARCA4 mutation shows classic rhabdoid tumor morphology. (From DP: Neuro.)*

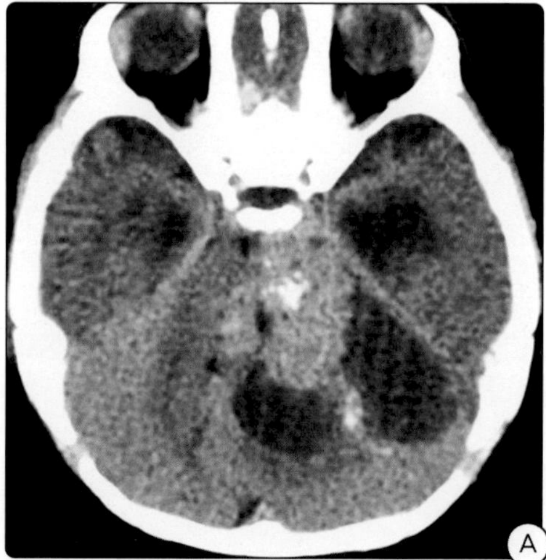

*(44-63A) NECT in a 4-mo infant with vomiting, bulging fontanelles shows a large mixed solid/cystic posterior fossa mass.*

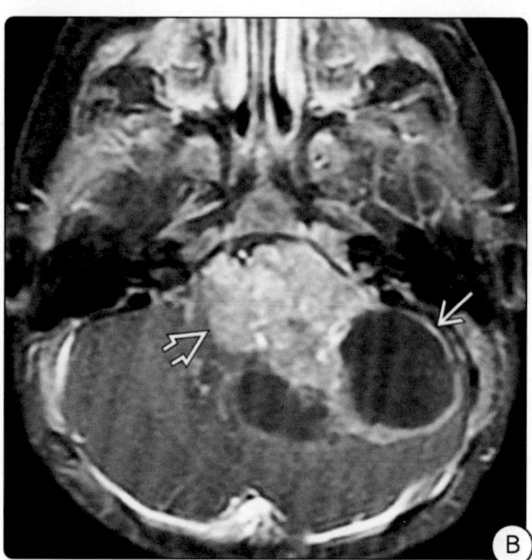

*(44-63B) T1 C+ FS MR shows solid portion of the mass ➲ and cyst walls ➲ enhance strongly. This is AT/RT in rhabdoid predisposition syndrome.*

years of age **(44-60)**. Multiple early-onset (< 30 years) basal cell carcinomas are common.

The prognosis of NBCCS-associated medulloblastomas seems to be better than that of sporadic cases, although patients with a *SUFU* pathogenic variant may have a somewhat worse prognosis.

### Imaging

Lamellar (sheet-like) calcifications of the falx and jaw keratocysts are two of the five major diagnostic criteria for NBCCS. Minor criteria include macrocephaly with an occipitofrontal circumference > 97th percentile and childhood medulloblastoma.

### Differential Diagnosis

The major differential diagnosis of the abnormal calcifications in NBCCS is **physiologic-** or **metabolic-related dural calcifications** (e.g., as occurs with secondary hyperparathyroidism). Physiologic calcification is much less striking. **Metaplastic dural ossification** causes prominent new bone formations with both dense cortex and fatty marrow.

The main differential diagnoses of NBCCS-associated medulloblastomas are **sporadic (i.e., nonsyndromic) medulloblastoma** and **atypical teratoid/rhabdoid tumor**. Their imaging features are identical, so look for other differentiating features, such as atypically prominent dural calcifications and jaw cysts.

## Rhabdoid Tumor Predisposition Syndrome

Rhabdoid tumor predisposition syndrome (RTPS) is characterized by markedly increased risk of developing malignant rhabdoid tumors due to constitutional loss or inactivation of *SMARCB1* (RTPS1) or, less commonly, *SMARCA4* (RTPS2).

The most common CNS tumor in RTPS is **atypical teratoid/rhabdoid tumor**. Malignant rhabdoid tumors of the kidney are the most common extraneural manifestation.

Atypical teratoid/rhabdoid tumor is composed of poorly differentiated neuroectodermal and mesenchymal elements. Approximately 60% are found in the posterior fossa as large bulky masses with mixed cystic and solid components **(44-63)**. Enhancement is variable. Dissemination at the time of initial diagnosis is common.

The macroscopic appearance, histopathology, and cytology of RTPS-associated neoplasms is similar to that of their sporadic counterparts.

Whether tumors, such as choroid plexus carcinoma (which shares the same *SMARCB1*-inactivating mutation), medulloblastoma, and other embryonal neoplasms, are associated with RTPS is controversial **(44-62)**.

## *DICER1* Syndrome

*DICER1* syndrome is an autosomal dominant tumor predisposition syndrome caused by germline pathogenic variants in the *DICER1* gene. *DICER1* is an endoribonuclease that is critical for correct processing of precursor micro-RNA. Failure of dicing pre-miRNA is a critical event in most *DICER1*-associated tumors.

*DICER1* syndrome is a tumor susceptibility syndrome that carries increased risk of both benign and malignant neoplasias in multiple organ systems, including the pleura, ovaries, thyroid, pituitary, pineal gland, and mesenchymal tissues. Over 30 different neoplastic lesions, usually affecting children and adolescents, have been described.

There are no well-established clinical algorithms for the diagnosis of *DICER1* syndrome, although the presence of a pleuropulmonary blastoma should prompt germline testing.

The most common CNS manifestation of *DICER1* syndrome is metastasis of a pleuropulmonary blastoma to the CNS. The primary CNS tumors are pineoblastoma, pituitary blastoma, embryonal tumor with multilayered rosettes (ETMR), and *DICER1*-mutant primary intracranial spindle cell sarcoma **(44-64)**. All these tumors are indistinguishable on imaging studies from their sporadic counterparts.

## Familial (Hereditary) Retinoblastoma

Retinoblastoma (RB) is the most common intraocular malignancy in children. Approximately 40% of RBs are hereditary. Inheritance is autosomal dominant with high penetrance; 60-80% of carriers develop RB(s). Familial RB is caused by pathogenic germline variants in the *RB1* tumor suppressor gene but is also driven by genomic and epigenomic alterations outside the locus.

The large majority (80%) of cases are diagnosed before three years of age. A "white" fundus (leukocoria) is the classic clinical finding **(44-65)**. Mean age at presentation is 12 months vs. 18-24 months for sporadic, noninherited RBs.

About 60% of patients develop bilateral tumors **(44-66)**. So-called trilateral RB occurs when a child with bilateral RB develops a germline mutation-related pineoblastoma. Approximately 5% develop these synchronous or metachronous malignancies in the pineal or suprasellar region. Intracranial RBs are identical to pineoblastomas and have a distinct DNA methylation profile that differs from other pineal tumors.

Patients with treated RBs have survival rates approaching 95-98% in industrialized countries, but mortality is high in resource-limited countries. Untreated RBs are fatal. Extensive retrolaminar optic nerve invasion and massive choroidal invasion are high-risk pathologic findings.

## *BAP1* Tumor Predisposition Syndrome

*BAP1* tumor predisposition syndrome is an autosomal dominant disorder with high penetrance caused by inactivating germline mutations in the *BAP1* tumor suppressor gene. *BAP1*-associated neoplasms include uveal and cutaneous melanoma, malignant mesothelioma, clear cell renal cell carcinoma, and rhabdoid meningioma **(44-67)**.

Median age of tumor onset is younger in people with *BAP1* predisposition syndrome compared to the general population. Lifetime risk of developing cancer is estimated at 80-100%. Uveal melanomas in patients < 30 years and meningiomas are the most common neoplasms affecting the CNS. Many BAP1-mutant meningiomas have overt rhabdoid &/or papillary features and exhibit aggressive behavior with frequent recurrences. BAP1 mutations have recently been cited as genetic factors in the rare malignant transformation of adamantinomatous craniopharyngiomas.

Imaging features are similar to those of comparable sporadic tumors.

*Selected References: The complete reference list is available on the eBooks+ version included with purchase.*

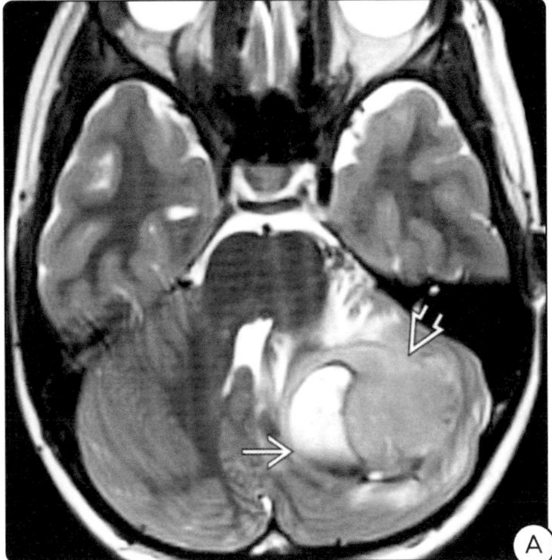


***(44-64A)** T2 MR in a child shows a large, very heterogeneous-appearing cerebellar hemispheric mass ➔ with a blood-fluid level ➔.*

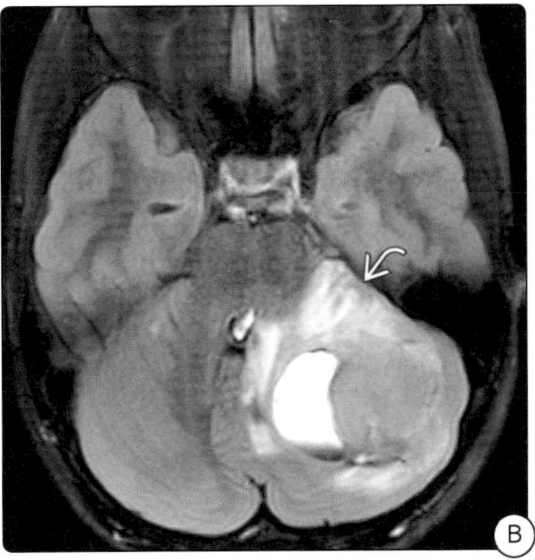


***(44-64B)** FLAIR MR in the same case shows significant peritumoral edema ➔.*

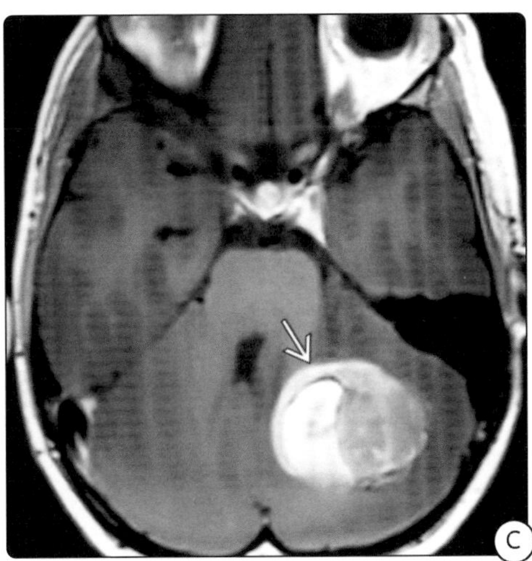


***(44-64C)** T1 C+ MR shows heterogeneous enhancement ➔. Primary intracranial sarcoma, DICER1-mutant. (Courtesy T. Poussaint, MD.)*

*(**44-65**) Gross pathology of retinoblastoma shows white posterior segment mass that is responsible for leukocoria. Retinoblastoma is the main tumor that develops in infants with germline RB1 mutations. (From DP: Neuro.) (**44-66A**) Coronal T1 C+ FS MR in an 18-mo infant with bilateral leukocoria shows enhancing masses in both globes.*

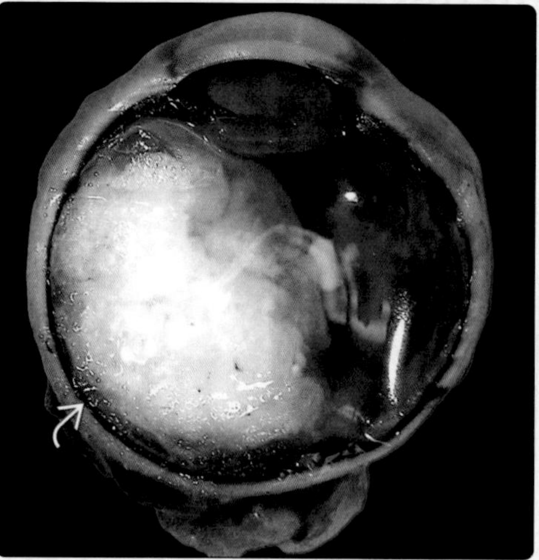

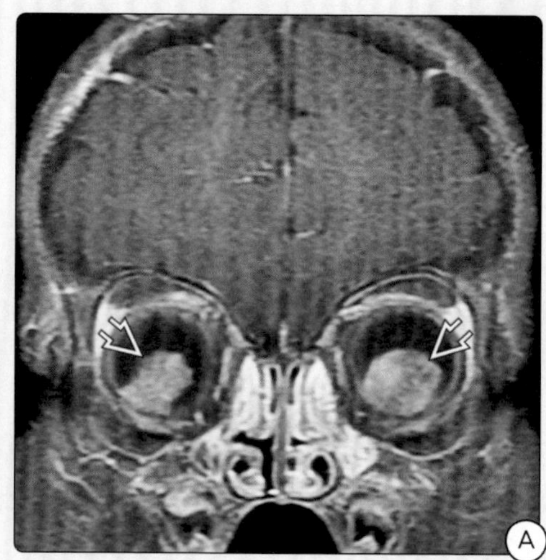


*(**44-66B**) Sagittal T1 C+ FS MR in the same case shows a small enhancing pineal mass. This is trilateral retinoblastoma with germline RB1 mutation (hereditary retinoblastoma syndrome). (**44-67A**) T2 MR shows a hyperintense mass straddling the falx and invading the SSS. Note significant adjacent edema.*

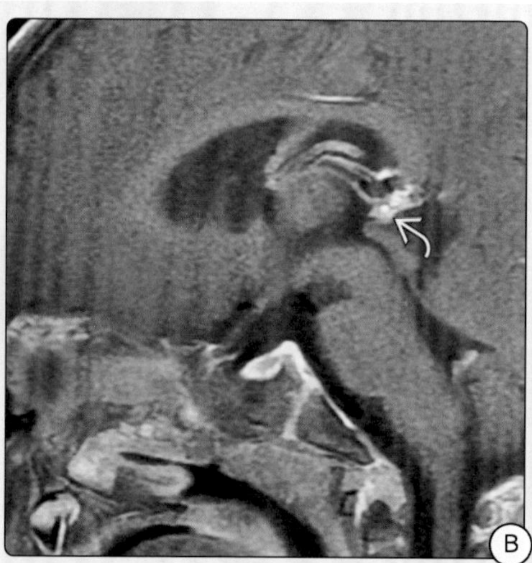


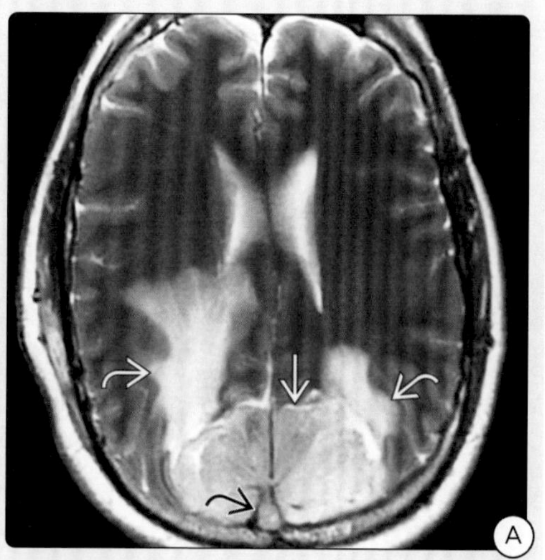


*(**44-67B**) T1 C+ MR shows the mass enhances uniformly and invades and occludes the SSS. (**44-67C**) Coronal T1 C+ MR shows the bilateral mass surrounding the falx. This is BAP1-mutant rhabdoid meningioma, CNS WHO grade 3.*

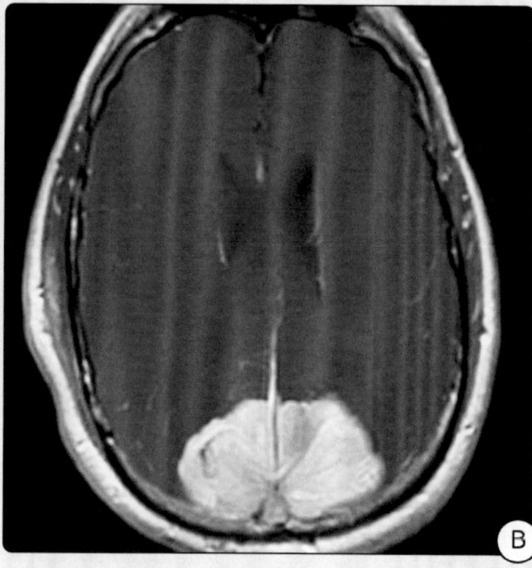


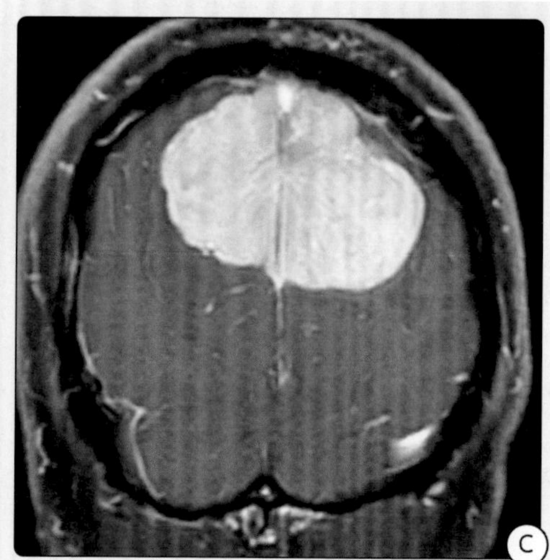

# Vascular Neurocutaneous Syndromes

*A number of syndromes with prominent cutaneous manifestations occur* ***without*** *associated neoplasms and can be inherited or occur spontaneously. Many of these are disorders in which both cutaneous and intracranial vascular lesions are the predominant features.*



Some vascular neurocutaneous syndromes [e.g., Sturge-Weber syndrome (SWS)] are present at birth (i.e., congenital) but have somatic mutations and are **not** inherited. Others, including hereditary hemorrhagic telangiectasia, have specific gene mutations with known inheritance patterns.

In the most recent (2018) classification scheme adopted by the International Society for the Study of Vascular Anomalies (ISSVA), vascular malformations are nonneoplastic structural anomalies that are distinguished from true vascular tumors that result from neoplastic proliferation of vascular endothelial cells). Port-wine stains and associated syndromes (e.g., SWS and others) are classified as low-flow vascular malformations and then grouped under the heading of "clinical syndromes with low-flow vascular malformations associated with other anomalies."

## Capillary Malformation Syndromes

Capillary malformations (CMs) are the most common cutaneous vascular anomalies. Most CMs occur sporadically without any syndromic findings. Genetic disorders that feature CMs include Sturge-Weber syndrome (SWS), diffuse CM with overgrowth (DCMO), Klippel-Trenaunay syndrome (KTS), and CLOVES syndrome (among others).

### Sturge-Weber Syndrome

SWS is one of the very few neurocutaneous syndromes that are sporadic, i.e., not familial and not inherited. It is also one of the most disfiguring syndromes, as a prominent facial CM (commonly referred to as port-wine birthmark [PWB]) is seen in the vast majority of cases.

#### Terminology

SWS is a congenital neurocutaneous syndrome that is also known as **encephalo-trigeminal angiomatosis**. Its hallmarks are variable combinations of (1) a facial capillary-venular malformation (the PWB) in the sensory distribution of the trigeminal nerve, (2) retinal choroidal angioma (either with or without glaucoma), and (3) a cerebral capillary-venous leptomeningeal angioma.

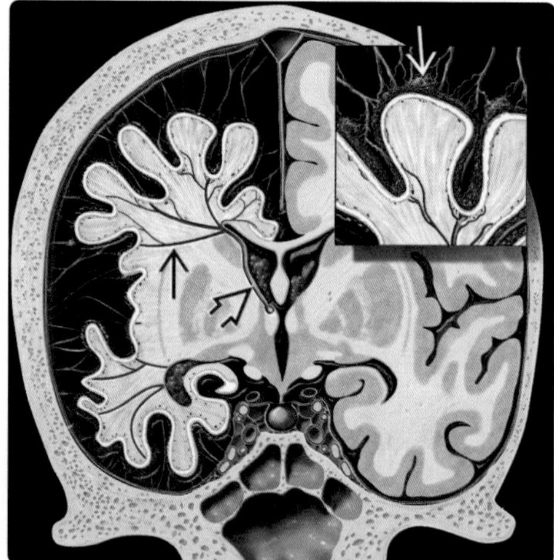

(45-1) SWS shows pial angiomatosis ➡, deep medullary collaterals ⇨, enlarged choroid plexus ⇨, and atrophy of the right cerebral hemisphere.

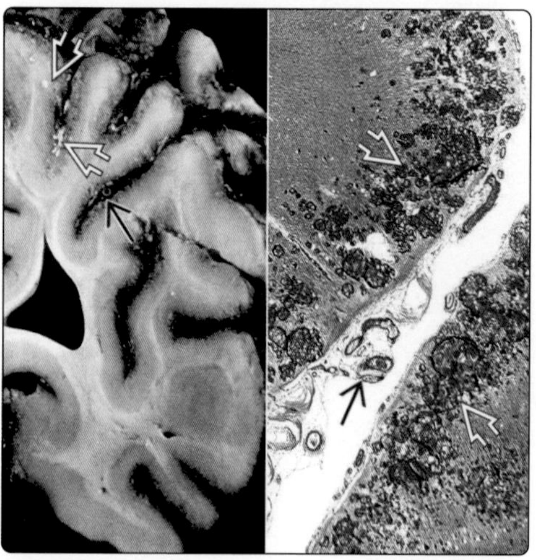

(45-2) Gross image (L), photomicrograph (R) of SWS show cortical atrophy, calcifications ➡, and pial angioma ⇨ within sulci. (AFIP Archives.)

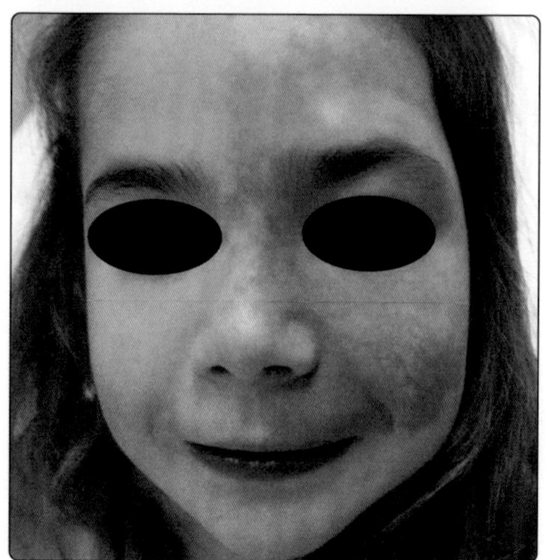

(45-3) Photograph shows the classic CNV1-V2 nevus flammeus characteristic of SWS.

## Etiology

Approximately 80-90% of patients with SWS have a pathogenic, somatic mosaic R183Q *GNAQ* or *GNA11/GNAB2* missense mutation. Germline variants in *RASA1*, *EPHB4*, or *KIT* have been reported in patients with atypical clinical characteristics, so broad germline and somatic genetic testing in these patients may have implications for medical care, prognosis, and trial eligibility.

*GNAQ* mutations cause a spectrum of vascular and melanocytic birthmarks. Depending on when they occur, they can lead to differing dermal phenotypes, either vascular alone (SWS), pigmentary alone (extensive dermal melanocytosis), or both.

## Pathology

A tangle of thin-walled vessels—multiple enlarged capillaries, small veins, and postcapillary venules—forms the characteristic leptomeningeal (pial) angioma. The angioma covers the brain surface, dipping into the enlarged sulci between shrunken apposing gyri **(45-1)** **(45-2)**.

The most common location is the parietooccipital region followed by the frontal and temporal lobes. Part or all of one hemisphere can be affected. SWS is unilateral in 80% of cases and is typically ipsilateral to the facial angioma. Bilateral involvement is seen in 20% of cases. Infratentorial lesions are seen in 11% of cases.

Dystrophic laminar cortical calcifications are typical **(45-2)**. Frank hemorrhage and large territorial infarcts are rare.

## Clinical Issues

**Presentation.** The vast majority of SWS patients exhibit a facial CM—formerly termed a facial "angioma" or "port-wine stain"—that is plainly visible at birth. It can be uni- (63%) or bilateral (31%) and is distributed over the skin innervated by one or more sensory branches of the trigeminal nerve. CNV1 (forehead &/or eyelid) or a combination of CNV1-V2 (plus cheek) are the most common sites **(45-3)**. All three trigeminal divisions are involved in 13% of cases. Approximately 1/3 of patients have ocular or orbital abnormalities, such as a diffuse choroidal hemangioma ("tomato catsup fundus"), congenital glaucoma with an enlarged globe (buphthalmos), and optic disc colobomas.

Occasionally, the facial vascular malformation involves the midline and may even extend to the chest, trunk, and limbs. *Approximately 10% of patients have isolated SWS brain or eye involvement without a facial PWB so lack of a visible port-wine nevus does not rule out SWS!*

Similarly, the presence of a PWB is *not* sufficient in and of itself for the definitive diagnosis of SWS. Patients with PWBs in the CNV1 distribution have only a 10-20% risk of SWS, although the risk increases with size, extent, and bilaterality of the nevus flammeus.

Seizures developing in the first year of life (75-90%), glaucoma (70%), hemiparesis (30-65%), and migraine-like headaches are other common manifestations of SWS.

## Imaging

**General Features.** Neuroimaging is used to identify the intracranial pial angioma and the sequelae of longstanding venous ischemia. *Findings may be minimal or absent in newborn/young infants, so serial imaging is necessary in suspected cases.*

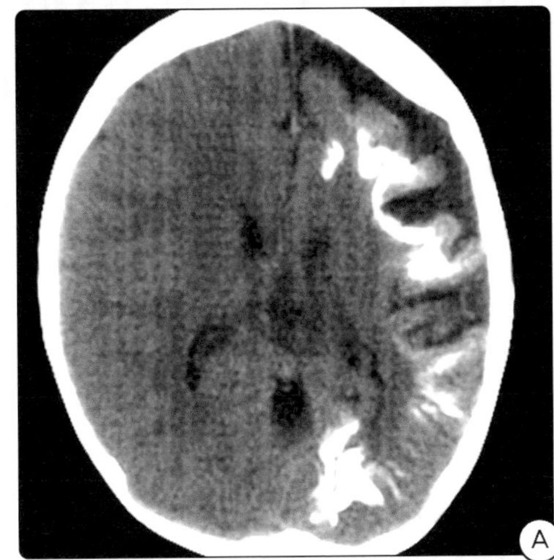

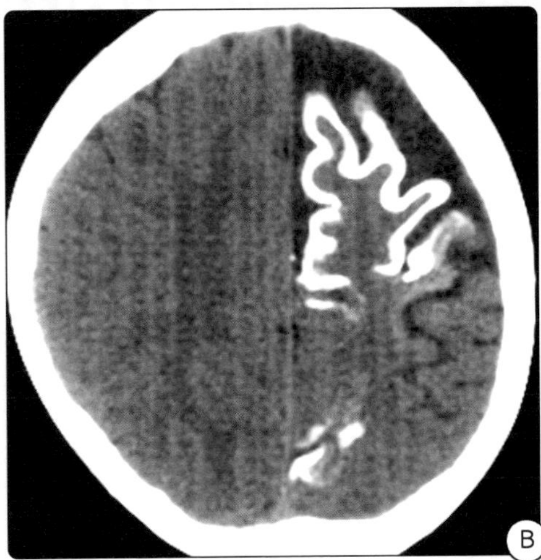

***(45-5A)** NECT in an 8-year-old girl with SWS shows striking cortical atrophy and extensive calcifications in the cortex and subcortical white matter (WM) throughout most of the left cerebral hemisphere. **(45-5B)** More cephalad NECT shows the typical serpentine gyral calcifications together with significant volume loss.*

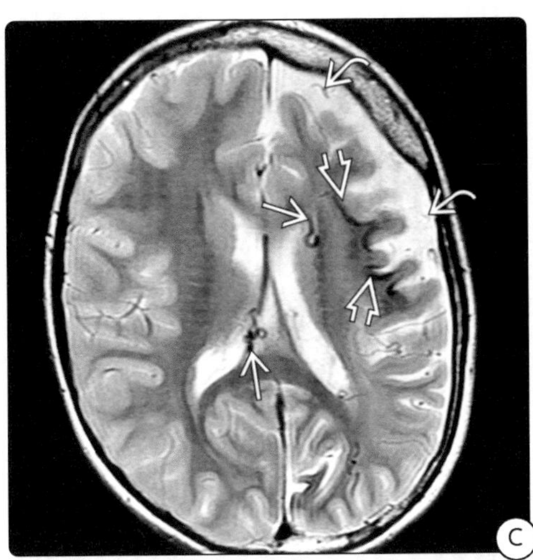

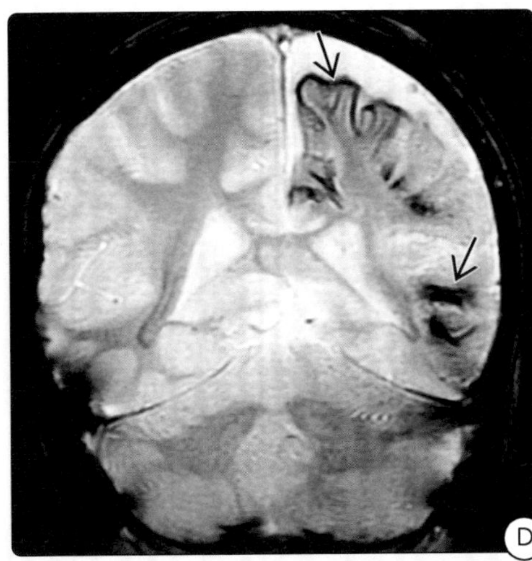

***(45-5C)** T2 MR shows atrophy with thinned cortex, extensive curvilinear hypointensity in the GM-WM interface . Note the prominent "flow voids" in the subependymal veins . The CSF in the enlarged subarachnoid space appears somewhat "dirty" with enlarged traversing trabeculae and veins . **(45-5D)** Coronal T2* GRE MR shows "blooming" of the extensive cortical/subcortical calcifications .*

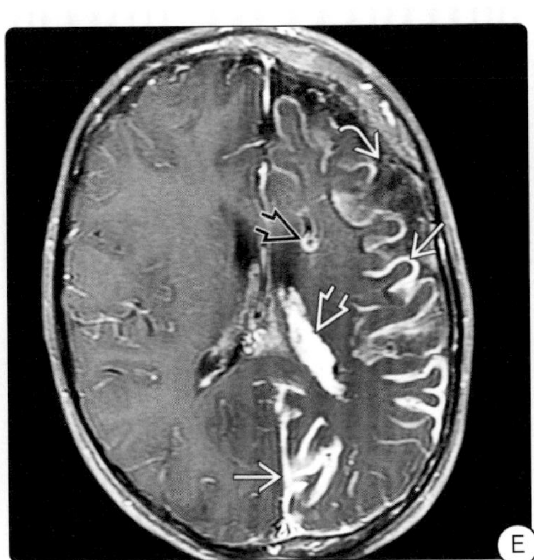

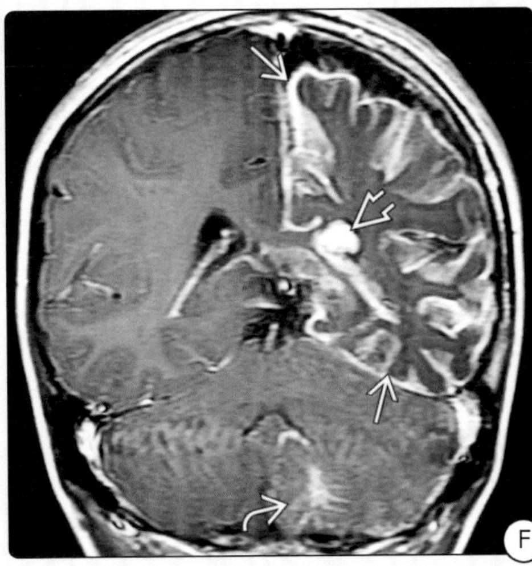

***(45-5E)** T1 C+ FS MR shows serpentine enhancement covering gyri, filling sulci  with grayish "dirty" CSF . Note enlargement, enhancement of ipsilateral choroid plexus  and draining subependymal vein . **(45-5F)** Coronal T1 C+ MR shows pial angioma  and enlarged choroid plexus . Developmental venous anomaly is seen in the left cerebellar hemisphere .*

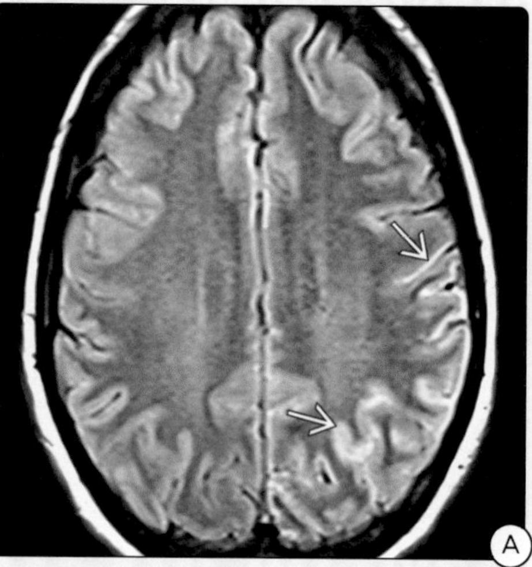

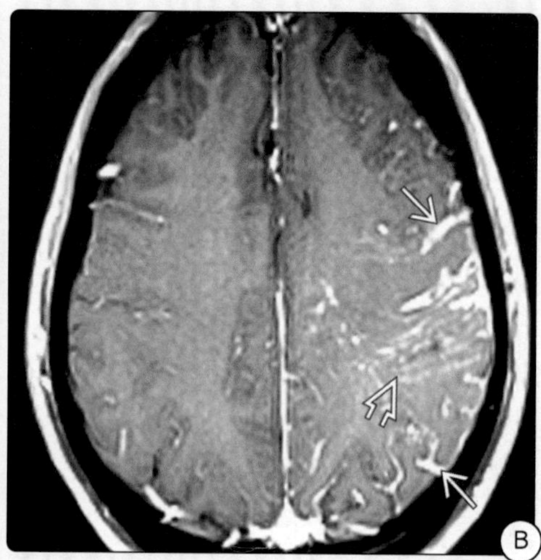

*(45-7A) Axial FLAIR MR in a 25-year-old woman with seizures and SWS shows left parietooccipital sulcal hyperintensity (ivy sign) ➡. (45-7B) T1 C+ FS MR in the same patient shows that the enhancing pial angioma fills the affected sulci ➡. Note the linear enhancing foci caused by enlarged medullary veins ➡ that provide collateral venous drainage into the subependymal veins and galenic system.*

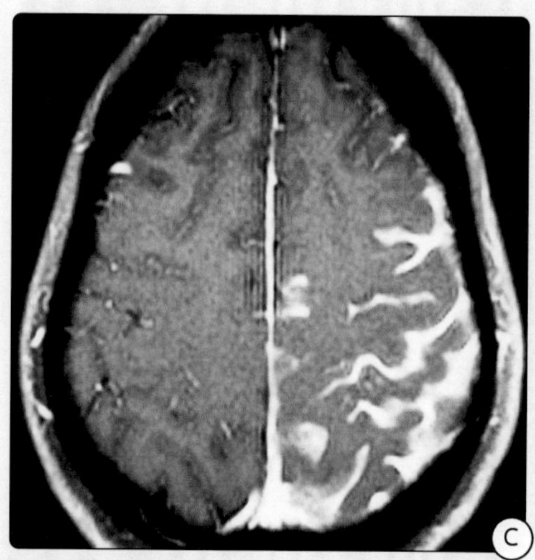

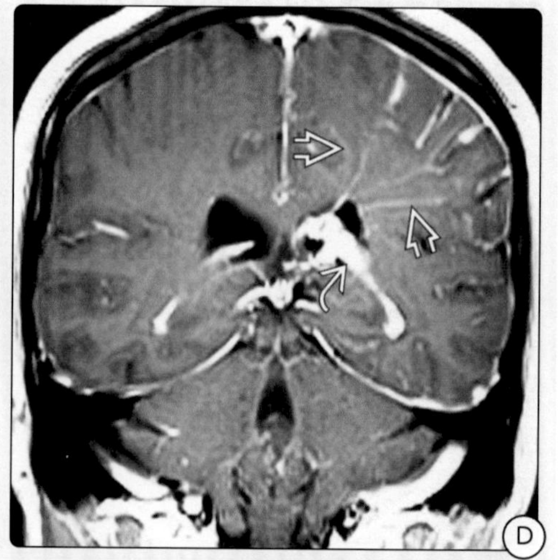

*(45-7C) More cephalad T1 C+ MR in the same patient shows that the sulci and subarachnoid spaces are enlarged, completely filled by the enhancing pial angioma. (45-7D) Coronal T1 C+ MR nicely demonstrates the prominent enhancing medullary veins ➡ as they drain through the hemispheric WM to converge on the subependymal veins that line the lateral ventricles. The ipsilateral choroid plexus ➡ is markedly enlarged.*

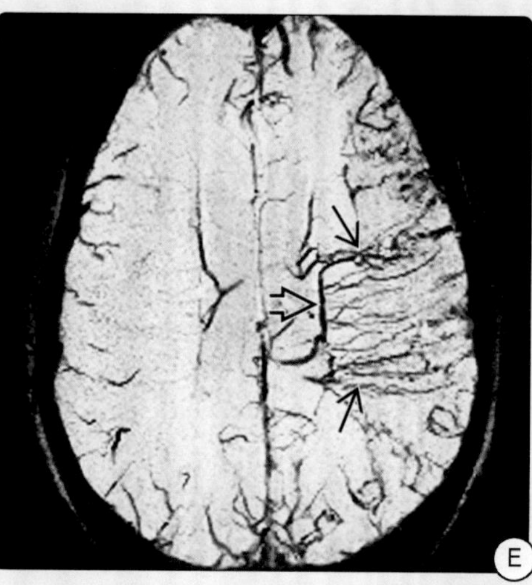

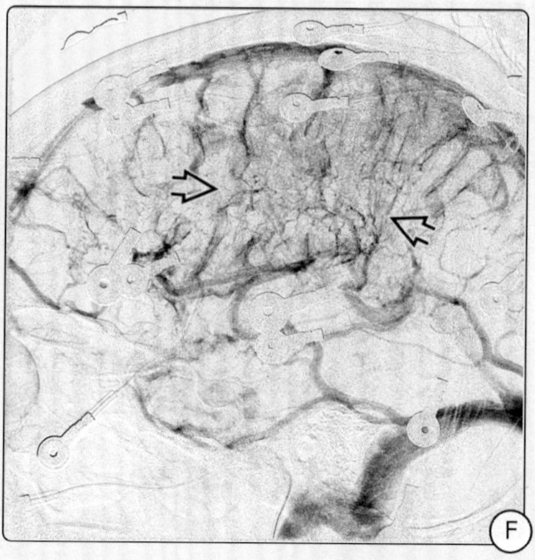

*(45-7E) Axial T2* susceptibility-weighted image (SWI) demonstrates deoxyhemoglobin in the enlarged, tortuous medullary veins ➡ that are slowly draining into enlarged subependymal veins ➡. (45-7F) Venous-phase DSA in the same patient performed as part of a Wada test for language localization shows a paucity of normal cortical veins with a prolonged vascular "blush" caused by contrast stasis in multiple enlarged medullary veins ➡.*

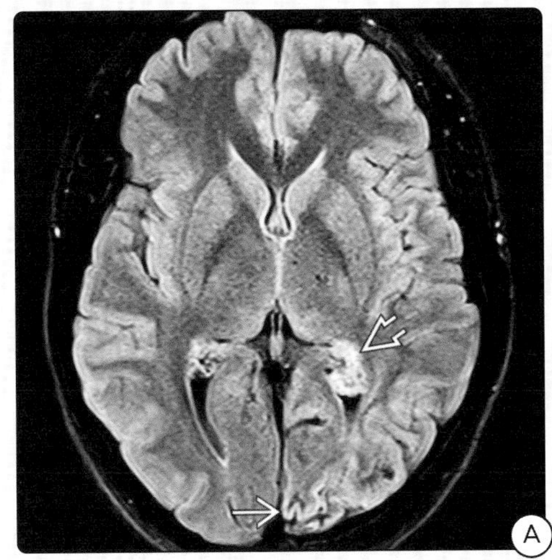
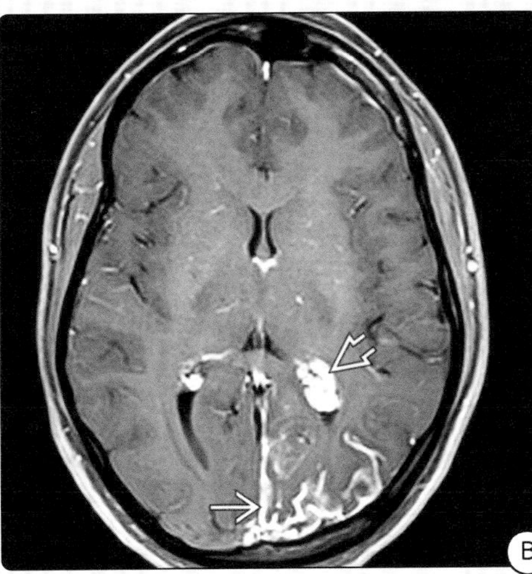

***(45-8A)*** *Axial FLAIR MR in a patient with SWS and left vision loss shows enlarged left choroid plexus glomus ➡ and atrophic, hyperintense occipital gyri with ivy sign ➡.* ***(45-8B)*** *T1 C+ FS MR in the same patient shows enhancing pial angioma ➡ and enlarged ipsilateral choroid plexus ➡.*

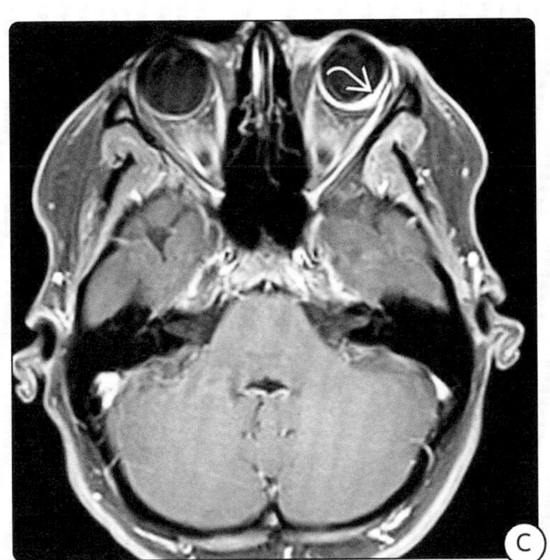
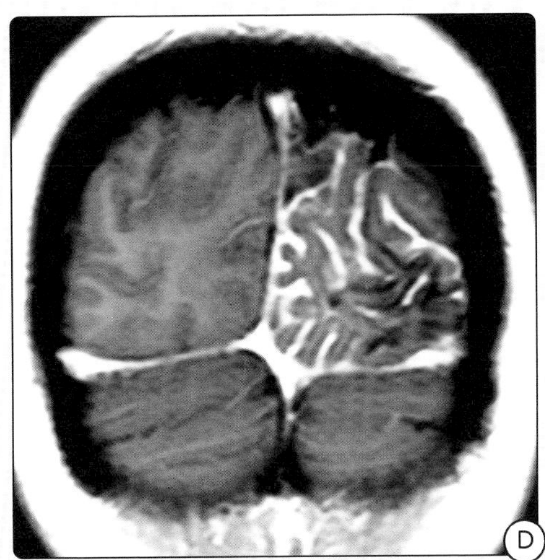

***(45-8C)*** *More inferior T1 C+ FS MR shows enlarged, enhancing diffuse choroidal angioma ➡ in the ipsilateral eye.* ***(45-8D)*** *Coronal T1 C+ MR shows striking volume loss of the left occipital lobe with enhancing pial angioma filling the sulci over the shrunken gyri.*

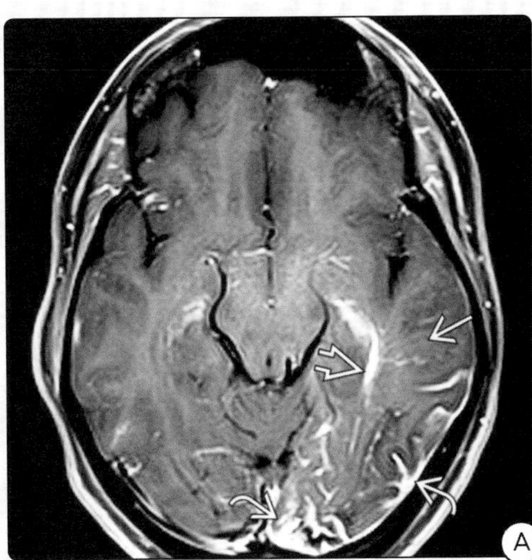
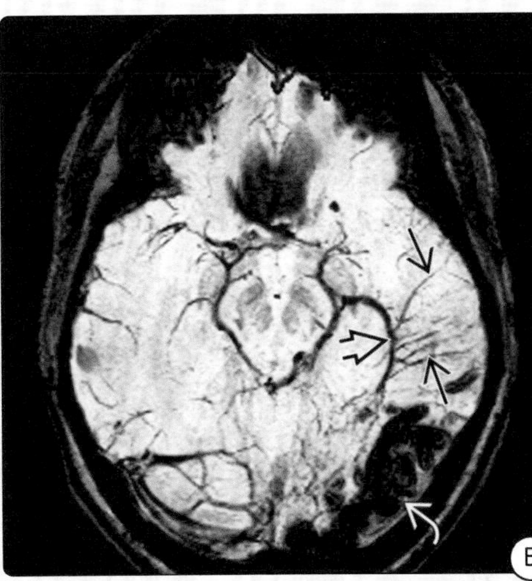

***(45-9A)*** *T1 C+ FS MR in a patient with known SWS shows pial angioma ➡, enlarged, enhancing choroid plexus ➡, and prominent enlarged medullary veins ➡.* ***(45-9B)*** *SWI shows enlarged medullary veins ➡ draining into prominent choroid plexus ➡. Densely calcified dystrophic calcification ➡ in the occipital lobe is present.*

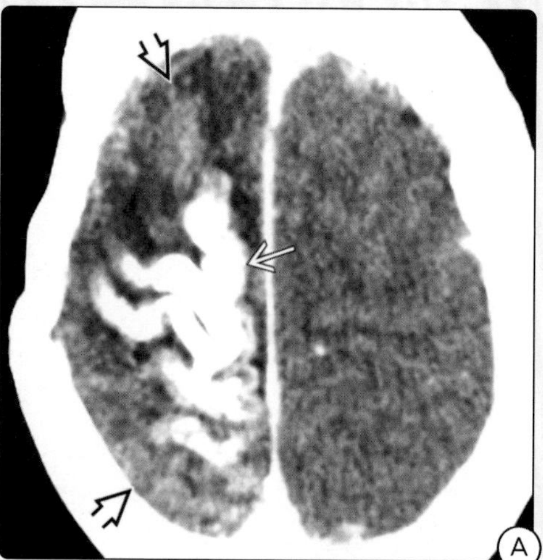

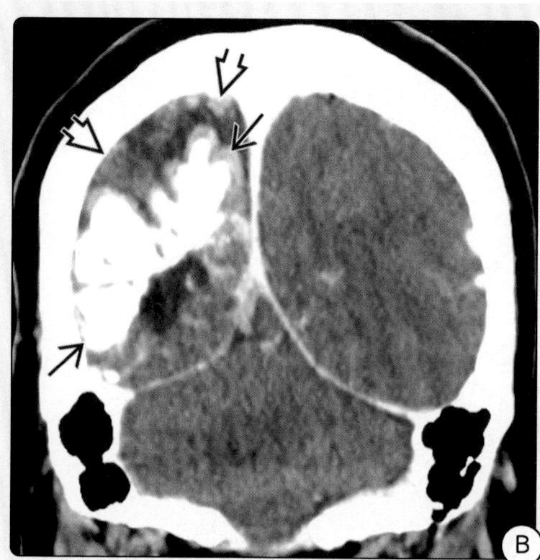

***(45-10A)** CECT in severe SWS shows densely calcified cortex ➡ in severely atrophied right hemisphere. Note diffuse, "hazy" enhancement in the overlying subarachnoid spaces ⇨. **(45-10B)** Coronal CECT shows grossly shrunken, densely calcified brain →. "Hazy" areas of ill-defined enhancement ⇨ are present in the enlarged subarachnoid spaces overlying the atrophic brain.*

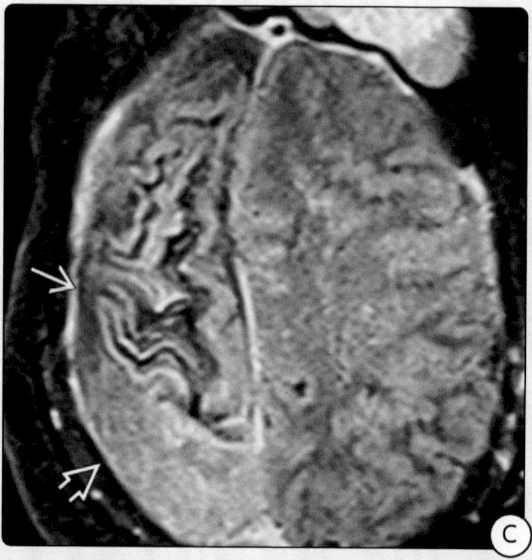

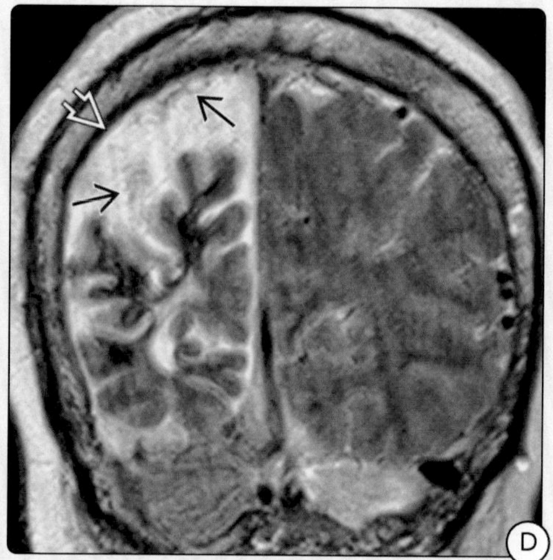

***(45-10C)** Axial FLAIR MR shows the severely atrophic, densely calcified hemisphere with prominent FLAIR ivy sign in the pial angioma ➡. Note "hazy" FLAIR hyperintensity filling the enlarged adjacent subarachnoid space ➡. **(45-10D)** Coronal T2 MR shows enlarged subarachnoid space ➡ overlying the atrophic, shrunken brain that contains linear, web-like, hypointense foci →.*

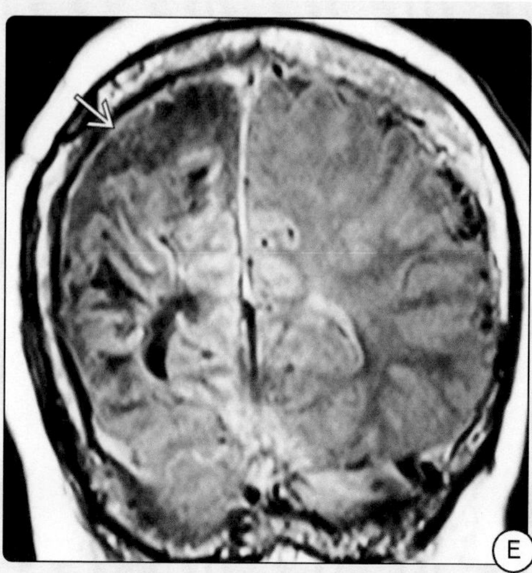

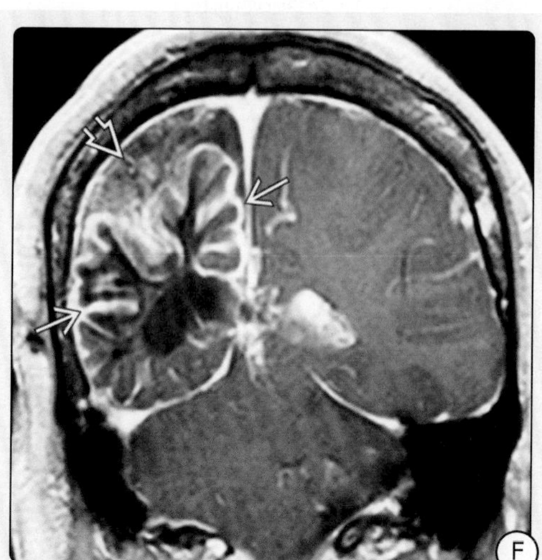

***(45-10E)** Coronal FLAIR MR shows CSF in the enlarged subarachnoid space overlying the atrophic brain does not suppress ➡ and looks "hazy." **(45-10F)** Coronal T1 C+ MR shows classic, strongly enhancing pial angioma ➡ covering the surface of the shrunken, atrophic gyri. Note cloud-like, "hazy" enhancement of enlarged draining veins filling the subarachnoid space ➡. This is severe SWS.*

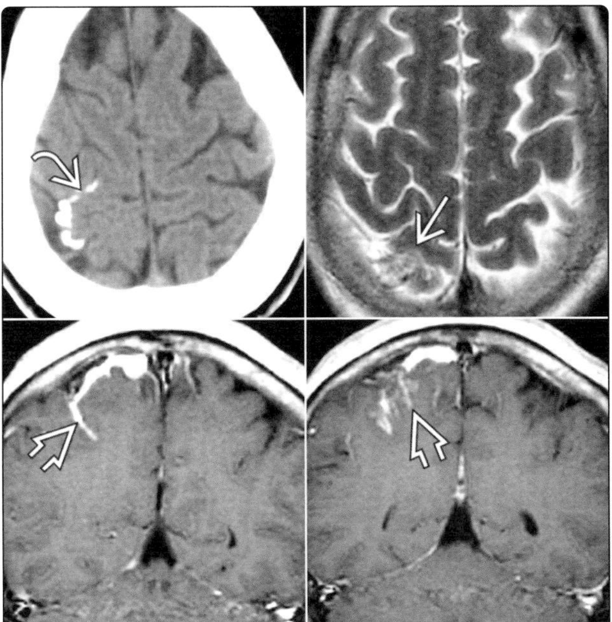

***(45-11) Variant SWS case shows focal calcification ➡, atrophy ➡, and a very localized enhancing pial angioma that fills just a few adjacent sulci ➡.***

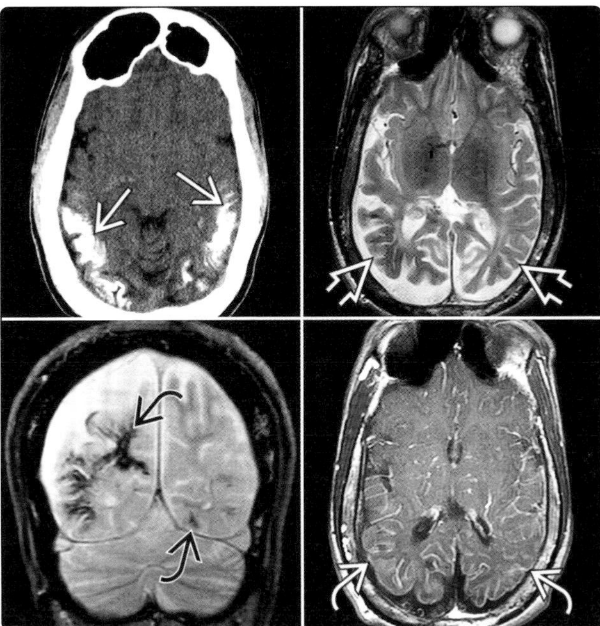

***(45-12) Images from a 17-year-old boy with KTS show bilateral dystrophic parietooccipital parenchymal calcifications ➡ that "bloom" on T2* ➡, parietal occipital atrophy ➡, and extensive bilateral enhancing pial angiomata ➡.***

**CT Findings.** Dystrophic cortical/subcortical calcifications are one of the imaging hallmarks of SWS **(45-5B)**. (Note that the calcifications are in the underlying brain, not the pial angioma). "Tram-track" cortical calcifications along the cerebral sulci under the pial angioma, atrophy, and enlargement of the ipsilateral choroid plexus are typical findings in older children and adults with SWS.

Bone CT shows thickening of the diploë and enlargement with hyperpneumatization of the ipsilateral frontal sinuses.

**MR Findings.** T1 and T2 scans show volume loss in the affected cortex with enlargement of the adjacent subarachnoid spaces **(45-5C)**. Prominent trabeculae and enlarged veins often cross the subarachnoid space, making the CSF appear somewhat grayish or "dirty" **(45-4) (45-10)**.

Dystrophic cortical/subcortical calcifications are seen as linear hypointensities on T2WI that "bloom" on T2* (GRE, SWI) **(45-5D)**. SWI scans often demonstrate linear susceptibility in enlarged medullary veins **(45-7E) (45-9)**. FLAIR scans may demonstrate serpentine hyperintensities in the sulci, the ivy sign **(45-7A) (45-10)**.

T1 C+ shows serpentine enhancement that extends deep into the sulci **(45-11)** and sometimes almost completely fills the subarachnoid space **(45-7C) (45-8D)**. Enlarged medullary veins can sometimes be identified as linear enhancing foci extending deep into the hemispheric white matter **(45-7D)**. The ipsilateral choroid plexus is almost always enlarged and enhances intensely **(45-5E) (45-9)**.

**Angiography.** DSA typically demonstrates a lack of superficial cortical veins with corresponding dilatation of deep medullary and subependymal veins **(45-7F)**. The arterial phase is normal.

### STURGE-WEBER SYNDROME

**Etiology**
- Congenital but sporadic, not inherited
- Postzygotic (i.e., somatic) mutation in *GNAQ*

**Pathology**
- Pial (leptomeningeal) angioma
- Cortical venous ischemia, atrophy
- Parietooccipital > frontal

**Clinical Issues**
- Unilateral facial CM
- Usual cutaneous distribution = CNV1, CNV2 > CNV3
    - Can be bilateral or even absent

**Imaging**
- CT
    - Atrophic cortex
    - Ipsilateral calvarium thick, sinuses enlarged
    - Cortical $Ca^{++}$ (**not** in angioma!) increases with age
- MR
    - Cortical/subcortical hypointensity on T2
    - $Ca^{++}$ "blooms" on T2*
    - Angioma enhances (unilateral 80%, bilateral 20%)
    - Ipsilateral choroid plexus enlarged
    - Enlarged medullary veins

## *PIK3CA*-Related Overgrowth Spectrum

Somatic mutations in the *PIK3CA* gene cause cells to grow and divide abnormally. *PIK3CA* mutations have been identified in patients with a variety of syndromes that are characterized by vascular anomalies and segmental overgrowths. Predominant areas of asymmetric overgrowth include the brain, limbs (including fingers and toes), trunk, and face.

Prior to the identification of PIK3CA as the causative gene, *PIK3CA*-related overgrowth spectrum (PROS) was separated into distinct clinical syndromes. Among many others, these include CLOVES (**c**ongenital **l**ipomatous **o**vergrowth, **v**ascular malformations, **e**pidermal nevi, **s**coliosis/skeletal and spinal syndrome), MCAP (**m**egalencephaly-**ca**pillary **m**alformation), CLAPO syndrome (**c**apillary malformation of the lower lip, **l**ymphatic malformation of the face and neck, **a**symmetry of the face and limbs, **p**artial or generalized **o**vergrowth), and Klippel-Trenaunay syndrome.

The most common malformation in *PIK3CA* mutation syndromes is a fibroadipose vascular anomaly, usually appearing as a venous malformation or mixed lymphatic-venous malformation. The lower extremity muscles are the most common involved site.

**Klippel-Trenaunay syndrome (KTS)**—also called Klippel-Trenaunay-Weber syndrome—is a congenital, sporadic disease characterized by a triad of capillary, lymphatic, and venous malformations with overgrowth of the affected limb. Some KTS cases are linked to somatic activating mutations in *PIK3CA* and are thus classified in PROS disorder.

Capillary malformations are seen in 98% of patients and occur either as cutaneous hemangiomas or port-wine stains. Limb overgrowth, which may include the underlying bones and soft tissues, occurs in 2/3 of KTS patients. Nearly 90% involve the lower limb, and over 2/3 involve a single limb.

Venous varicosities occur in 72% of patients and present as large valveless truncal veins with large varicosities along the lateral aspect of the lower extremities. Lymphatic malformations occur in 11% of KTS patients.

Intracranial neurovascular anomalies occur in 1/3 of cases. Developmental venous anomalies and craniofacial venous malformations are the most common imaging findings **(45-12)**.

### *PIK3CA*-RELATED OVERGROWTH SPECTRUM

**Spectrum of Conditions Includes**

- Klippel-Trenaunay syndrome (KTS)
- CLOVES
- Isolated lymphatic malformation (ILM)
- Megalencephaly-capillary malformation (MCAP/M-CM)
- Hemimegalencephaly (HME)/dysplastic megalencephaly/focal cortical dysplasia type II
- Hemihyperplasia-multiple lipomatosis (HHML)
- Facial infiltrating lipomatosis (FIL)
- Fibroadipose vascular anomaly (FAVA)
- Macrodactyly
- Muscular hemihyperplasia
- Fibroadipose overgrowth (FAO)
- CLAPO
- Epidermal nevus, benign lichenoid keratosis/seborrheic keratosis

## Capillary Malformation-Arteriovenous Malformation

Capillary malformation-arteriovenous malformation (CM-AVM) is a distinct entity that is characterized by a broad phenotypic variability. Multifocal small CMs may occur anywhere in the body, especially in the CNS, spine, and skin. One-third of patients have an arteriovenous fistula (AVF) in muscles, soft tissue, or the CNS.

CM-AVM syndrome is an autosomal dominant syndrome due to mutations in *RASA1* (50% of cases) or *EBHB4* (25%). *RASA1* mutations have been identified in patients with **Parkes-Weber syndrome**. Affected patients present with large CMs, AVFs, and progressive overgrowth of the involved limb.

# Other Neurovascular Syndromes

## Hereditary Hemorrhagic Telangiectasia

### Terminology

Hereditary hemorrhagic telangiectasia (HHT), formerly known as **Osler-Weber-Rendu** or Rendu-Osler-Weber syndrome, is an autosomal dominant monogenetic disorder characterized pathologically by multisystem angiodysplastic lesions. Lesions vary in size from small cutaneous or mucosal telangiectasias to large solid organ arteriovenous malformations (AVMs).

### Etiology

Genetic testing has established several pathogenic gene mutations in HHT. Mutations in two genes (*ENG* and *ACVRL1*/ALK1) cause up to 60-80% of cases (N.B. a negative genetic test does not exclude the diagnosis of HHT). Penetrance increases during lifetime, and in adults over the age of 40 years, it is estimated to exceed 95%.

*ENG* (endoglin) gene mutations cause **type 1 HHT** and are associated with mucocutaneous telangiectases, early onset of epistaxis, pulmonary AVFs, and brain AVMs. *ACVRL1*/ALK1 mutation causes **type 2 HHT**, is associated with milder disease, and presents primarily as GI bleeds and pulmonary arterial hypertension. This mutation causes 35-40% of HHT cases while mutations in a third gene—*SMAD4*—occur in juvenile polyposis/HHT overlap syndrome and account for 2% of cases. Pathogenic mutations in the *HHT3* locus on chromosome 5 and the *HHT4* gene on chromosome 7 result in **HHT type 3** and **HHT type 4**.

### Pathology

Pulmonary AVMs or fistulae develop in ~ 50% of patients with HHT and are most common in HHT type 1 (60-65% compared to 10-20% in HHT type 2). The most common cerebrovascular complication from pulmonary AVMs/AVFs is emboli resulting in brain infarction &/or abscess.

Between 10-20% of patients with a diagnosis of definite HHT have intracranial vascular malformations. Multiple types of cerebral vascular malformations may develop in HHT patients, but two main types are most common: (1) Nidus-type AVMs and (2) capillary vascular malformations. AVFs—common in the lung—are rare in the brain. Nonshunting lesions in HHT include developmental venous anomalies, capillary telangiectasias, and cavernous malformations.

**"Nidal" brain AVMs** account for slightly < 1/2 of all HHT neurovascular manifestations and are found in 10% of all patients. Nearly 60% are solitary, whereas multiple lesions are present in 40%; ~ 80% are supratentorial, whereas 20% are infratentorial. Most brain AVMs in the HHT population are symptomatic, although between 85-90% are Spetzler-Martin grade 2 or less.

**Capillary vascular malformations** account for slightly over 1/2 of all neurovascular manifestations of HHT. They are typically supratentorial (86%), are often peripherally located in the brain, and are almost always < 1 cm.

**Capillary telangiectasias** are distinct from capillary vascular malformations and consist of numerous thin-walled ectatic capillaries interspersed in normal brain parenchyma. Feeding arteries are absent, although sometimes a draining vein can be identified. Brain capillary telangiectasias are relatively rare in HHT (2-4%). They are typically found in the pons or medulla and are **occult on DSA**.

Other manifestations of HHT include pial AVFs and nonshunting lesions, such as **developmental venous anomalies** (12%) and **cavernous malformations** (3-4%). **Pial AVFs** are rare, accounting for just 1% of all HHT-related brain vascular malformations. **Malformations of cortical development**—usually perisylvian polymicrogyria—are found in 12% of HHT cases.

### HEREDITARY HEMORRHAGIC TELANGIECTASIA: ETIOLOGY AND PATHOLOGY

**Etiology**

- Type 1 HHT
  - Endoglin (*ENG*) mutation
  - Mucocutaneous telangiectases, epistaxis, pulmonary AVFs/brain AVMs
- Type 2 HHT
  - *ACVRL1*/ALK1 mutation
  - Milder; predominantly GI bleeds

**Pathology**

- Neurovascular malformations in 10-20%
  - > 50% multiple
  - Most are supratentorial, superficial, < 3 cm
- 2 main types (~ 50:50)
  - "Nidal" brain AVMs
  - Capillary vascular malformations
- Other intracranial vascular malformations
  - Developmental venous anomaly: 12%
  - Cavernous malformations: 2-4%
  - Capillary telangiectases (mucocutaneous common; rare in brain: 1-3%)
  - Pial AVF: < 1%

## Clinical Issues

**Presentation.** The long-established 2000 Curaçao criteria are the mainstay of HHT clinical diagnosis and include (1) epistaxis (spontaneous, recurrent), (2) telangiectasias (multiple at characteristic sites, such as oral cavity, lips,

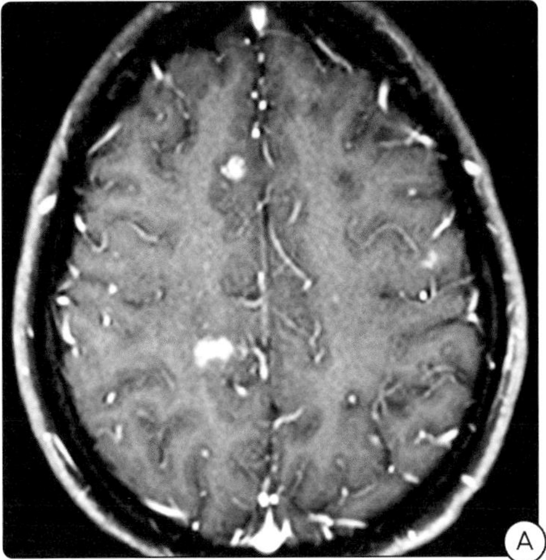


***(45-13A)** T1 C+ FS MR in a 23-year-old woman with HHT shows 2 intensely enhancing lesions in the right hemisphere.*

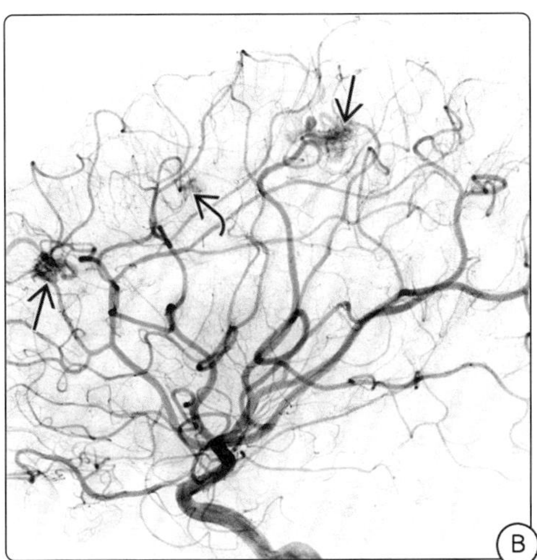


***(45-13B)** DSA of the right ICA shows tangles of vessels ➙ supplied by the anterior cerebral artery (ACA). A 3rd lesion ➙ may be present.*

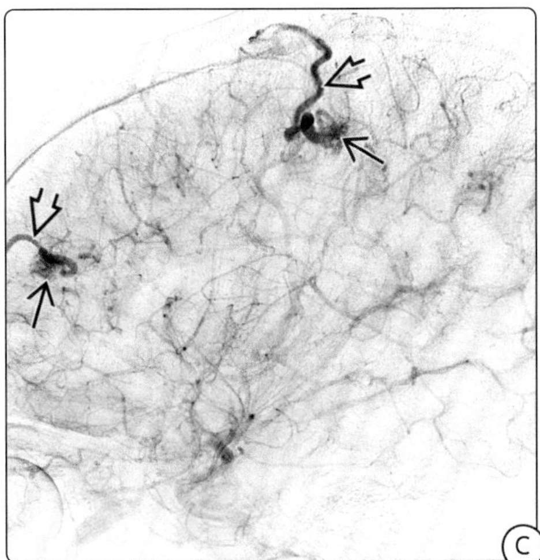


***(45-13C)** Late arterial-phase DSA shows early opacification of cortical veins ➙ draining the lesions ➙. These are "micro" AVMs in HHT.*

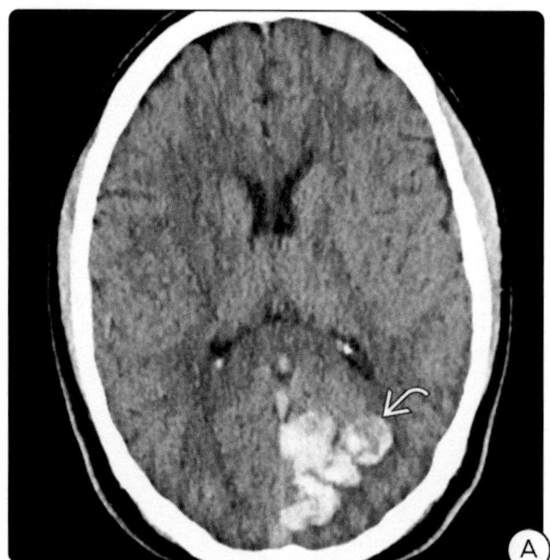

***(45-14A)** NECT in a 24-yo woman with family history of HHT, 3 days of severe headaches shows a left occipital hyperdense hemorrhagic mass ➲.*

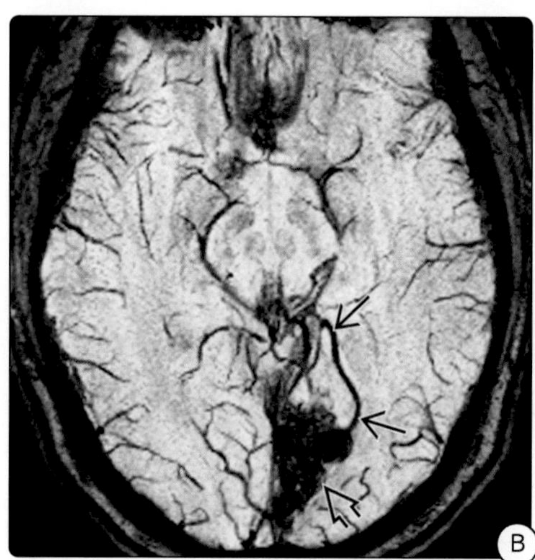

***(45-14B)** MIP SWI shows "blooming" occipital mass ➲, enlarged left posterior cerebral artery (PCA) ➲ supplying the mass.*

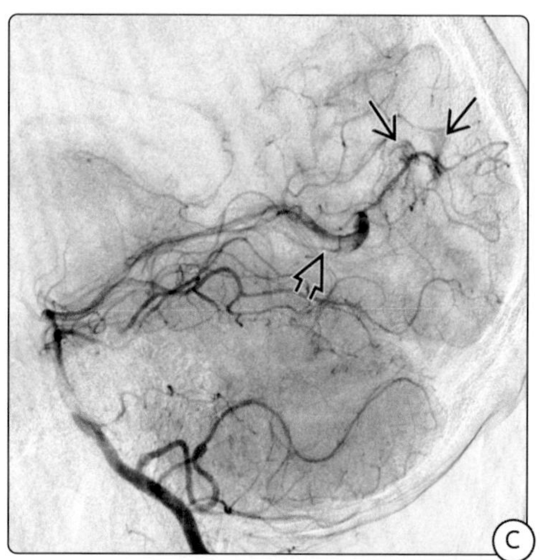

***(45-14C)** DSA shows partially thrombosed PCA ➲ with stagnating flow and vascular blush ➲. This is hemorrhagic, partially thrombosed AVM.*

fingers, and nose), (3) visceral lesions (e.g., pulmonary, hepatic, cerebral or spinal AVMs), and (4) family history (first-degree relative with HHT). Three or more criteria establish the definite diagnosis of HHT. The recent integration of nasal endoscopy in children with suspected HHT has increased the diagnostic sensitivity of the Curaçao criteria.

The most common features of HHT are epistaxis and telangiectases on the lips, hands, tongue, and oral mucosa. Epistaxis typically begins by age 10 while 80-90% have nosebleeds &/or GI bleeding by age 21. The onset of visible telangiectases is generally 5-30 years later than for epistaxis. Almost 95% of affected individuals eventually develop mucocutaneous telangiectases.

HHT patients should be screened for cerebral vascular malformations at least once during their clinical evaluation. Current guidelines also suggest careful attention to all family members (including children) of an index case.

**Natural History.** HHT displays age-related penetrance with increasing manifestations developing over a lifetime; penetrance approaches 100% by age 40. Epistaxis increases in frequency and severity and, in some cases, can require multiple transfusions or even become life threatening.

Although most HHT-associated brain AVMs are small and have a low Spetzler-Martin grade, 20% present with rupture, and nearly 50% are symptomatic. Treatment options include surgical resection, stereotactic radiosurgery, &/or embolization.

Shunting of air, thrombi, and bacteria through pulmonary AVMs can cause TIAs, strokes, and cerebral abscesses. Heritable pulmonary arterial hypertension (HPAH) is a rare but severe complication of HHT.

## Imaging

Brain MR without and with contrast enhancement is the recommended screening procedure for patients diagnosed with HHT and, when possible, should be obtained within the first six months of life. Molecular diagnostics may obviate further imaging. In adults, if no AVMs are detected on initial MR scans, further screening for cerebral AVMs is unnecessary.

Although some HHT-associated **AVMs** are large **(45-14)**, nearly 90% are small (Spetzler-Martin ≤ 2). Large lesions can demonstrate prominent "flow voids" on T2WI; smaller lesions are seen as "speckled" enhancing foci on T1 C+ studies **(45-13)**.

**Capillary vascular malformations** do not show "flow voids" on MR and are defined by a "blush" of abnormal vessels on the late arterial/capillary phase on DSA or an area of fluffy stain-like enhancement on T1 C+ MR. A dilated feeding artery that empties directly into a draining vein is typical of an **AVF**.

**Capillary telangiectasias** are most common in the pons and are angiographically occult without a visible feeding artery or draining vein on DSA. Capillary telangiectasias are usually invisible on T2/FLAIR. A faint brush-like area of enhancement is seen on T1 C+, whereas T2*/SWI sequences show decreased signal intensity.

**HEREDITARY HEMORRHAGIC TELANGIECTASIA: IMAGING**

**Capillary Vascular Malformations**

- < 1 cm in diameter
- Feeding artery, vein often visible on DSA but not enlarged
- No "flow voids" on MR
- "Blush" of fluffy, stain-like enhancement on T1 C+

**Arteriovenous Malformations**

- Most are Spetzler-Martin grades ≤ 2
    - Multiple AVMs: 40%
- Large lesions rare
    - "Flow voids" on T2WI present
- Small lesions show "speckled" enhancement on T1 C+
- Feeding artery, nidus, draining vein on DSA

## PHACE Syndrome

### Terminology

PHACE syndrome is an acronym for **p**osterior fossa malformations, **h**emangioma, **a**rterial cerebrovascular anomalies, **c**oarctation of the aorta and cardiac defects, and **e**ye abnormalities (sometimes called PHACES with the addition of the less common **s**ternal clefting or **s**upraumbilical raphe). PHACE syndrome is sporadic with an unknown pathogenesis.

### Pathology

Hemangiomas are—by definition—found in 100% of PHACE patients. Hemangiomas are true vascular neoplasms and are the most common benign tumor of infancy, occurring in 2-3% of neonates and 10-12% of children under one year of age.

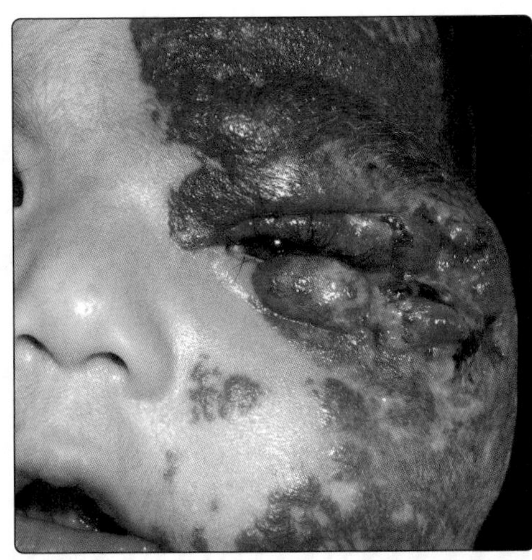

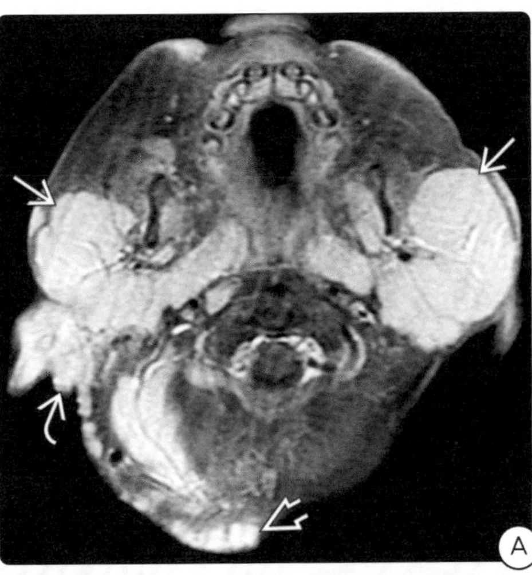

***(45-15)** Clinical photograph of a patient with PHACES shows a typical facial infantile hemangioma. (Courtesy S. Yashar, MD.) **(45-16A)** T1 C+ FS MR in the same case shows intensely enhancing hemangiomas in massively enlarged parotid glands ➡ and the right ear ➡. Hemangioma also infiltrates the scalp ➡ and posterior cervical space.*

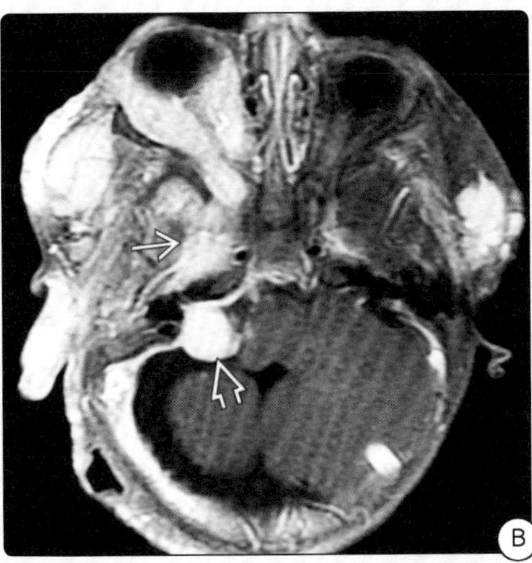

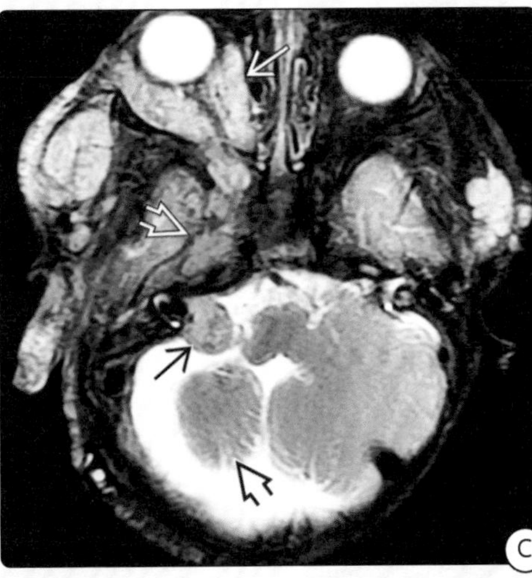

***(45-16B)** T1 C+ FS MR shows intracranial extension of the hemangioma into the cavernous sinus ➡ and cerebellopontine angle (CPA) cistern ➡. **(45-16C)** T2 MR in PHACES shows orbital ➡, cavernous sinus ➡, CPA hemangioma ➡, and ipsilateral cerebellum hypoplasia ➡.*

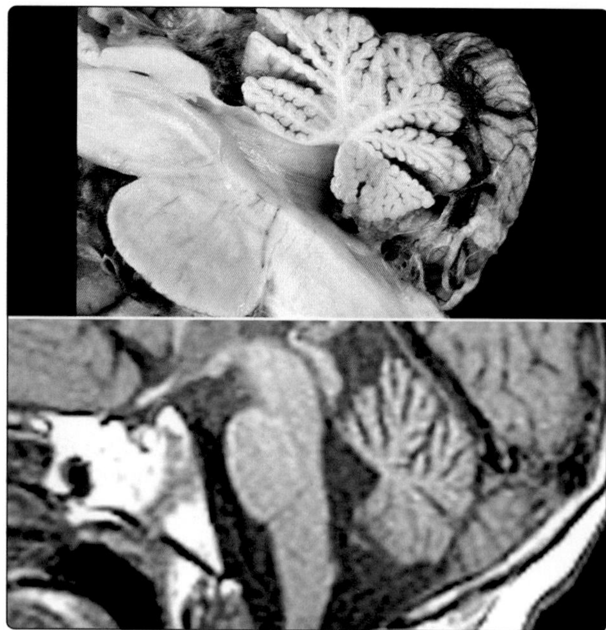

*(45-18) (Top) Sagittal autopsy in ataxia-telangiectasia (A-T) shows severe atrophy of the vermis and cerebellum. (Bottom) Sagittal T1 MR in a 4-yo child with A-T shows striking vermian atrophy. (Courtesy S. Blaser, MD.)*

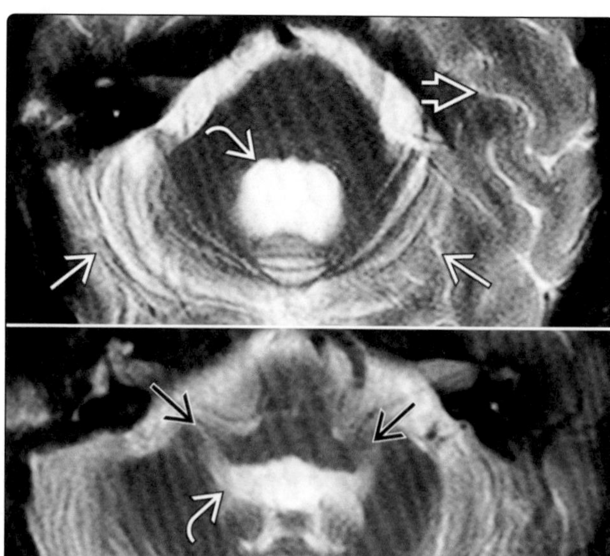

*(45-19) Axial T2 MR images in patient with A-T shows normal supratentorial brain and marked cerebellar atrophy with enlarged 4th ventricle and lateral recesses.*

The majority are sporadic, nonsyndromic lesions; only 20% meet the diagnostic criteria for PHACE.

## Clinical Issues

PHACE is characterized clinically by a large infantile hemangioma (IH) that is associated with multiple developmental defects **(45-15)**. A definitive diagnosis of PHACE is determined when a **craniofacial hemangioma** is present together with one or more characteristic extracutaneous anomalies.

## Imaging

MR is the best technique to evaluate the presence and extent of craniofacial hemangiomas and to delineate coexisting intracranial malformations **(45-16)**. T1 scans depict callosal dysgenesis and cerebellar anomalies. Gray matter heterotopias are best seen on T2WI. Proliferating hemangiomas appear hyperintense on T2WI and may exhibit prominent internal "flow voids." Intense homogeneous enhancement following contrast administration is typical.

## Differential Diagnosis

The major differential diagnosis of PHACE is **Sturge-Weber syndrome** (SWS). The facial hemangioma of PHACE is often mistaken for the port-wine stain of SWS. Patients with SWS lack the noncutaneous systemic manifestations of PHACE. The intracranial hemangioma of PHACE is usually more focal and mass-like, often involving the cerebellopontine angle or cavernous sinus.

### PHACE(S) SYNDROME

**Terminology**
- **P**osterior fossa malformations
- **H**emangioma
- **A**rterial cerebrovascular anomalies
- **C**oarctation of aorta and cardiac defects
- **E**ye abnormalities
- ± **S**ternal clefting or supraumbilical raphe

**Pathology**
- Hemangiomas (vascular neoplasm, not malformation)
- Ipsilateral cerebellar hypoplasia
- Posterior fossa cystic lesions (e.g., Dandy-Walker) common
- Arterial stenoses/occlusions, saccular aneurysms, aberrant vessels

**Clinical Issues**
- Hemangiomas proliferate, then involute

**Imaging**
- T1 C+ FS MR to delineate hemangiomas
- CTA/MRA to evaluate for vascular anomalies

# Ataxia-Telangiectasia

Ataxia-telangiectasia (A-T) syndrome, a.k.a. Louis-Bar syndrome, is a rare neurocutaneous autosomal recessive syndrome caused by *ATM* (ataxia-telangiectasia mutated kinase) mutations. Oculocutaneous telangiectasias, progressive cerebellar degeneration, and infantile onset of Ataxia are characteristic clinical features **(45-18)** **(45-19)**. How *ATM* loss leads to cerebellar degeneration is unknown. Heterozygous, loss-of-function germline variants in *ATM* have been associated with increased lifetime risk of cancers (ATM hereditary cancer syndrome).

## Blue Rubber Bleb Nevus Syndrome

Blue rubber bleb nevus syndrome (BRBNS), also called Bean syndrome, is a rare disorder characterized by multiple venous malformations in the skin, GI, and musculoskeletal system. BRBNS is caused by a sporadic, activating somatic mutation in the receptor tyrosine kinase or *TEK*, the gene encoding TIE2. *TEK* is a controller of endothelial cell assembling and remodeling that organizes the vascular network and recruits the perivascular cells necessary for stabilizing vessel walls. The same mutation also occurs in sporadic multifocal venous malformations. *PIK3CA* mutations have been implicated in some patients with BRBNS.

BRBNS usually affects the skin, oral cavity, and GI tract. Small, raised, bluish, soft, compressible, rubber- or "bleb"/grape-like lesions are the clinical hallmarks of this disorder and tend to occur on the palms, soles, trunk, and perineum **(45-20)**. The most common presentation is iron deficiency anemia caused by intestinal bleeding.

CNS manifestations are rare (10-15% of cases), variable, nonspecific, and tend to occur late in the disease. Reported imaging manifestations include venous thrombosis, multiple brain cavernomas, and noncavernomatous venous malformations **(45-21)**. An extensive network of developmental venous anomalies with or without sinus pericranii **(45-22)** may be present **(45-23)**.

## Wyburn-Mason and Cerebral Arteriovenous Metameric Syndrome

**Wyburn-Mason syndrome** (WMS), a.k.a. racemose angioma or congenital unilateral retinocephalic vascular malformation syndrome, is a rare nonhereditary neurocutaneous syndrome that presents with multiple but unilateral AVMs of the brain, orbit, and face. Craniofacial vascular malformations can involve the eyelids and orbits as well as the retina and optic nerve. Lesions range from barely visible to large tangles of dilated, tortuous vessels in the retina &/or brain. Patients with extensive retinal AVMs are at high risk for visual loss, whereas patients with brain AVMs are at risk for parenchymal hemorrhage.

Vascular malformations can involve the orbits, face, and brain simultaneously. **Cerebral arteriovenous metameric syndrome** (CAMS) causes maxillofacial and intracranial AVMs.

**Cerebrofacial venous metameric syndrome** (CVMS) is a complex disorder in which patients have a constellation of venous vascular malformations affecting soft tissues, bone, dura, eye, and brain. The most commonly recognized form of CVMS is Sturge-Weber syndrome, but a spectrum of slow-flow venous, cavernous, and possibly even hemangiomatous lesions in the face and brain occurs. Lesions are classified into three groups (CVMS 1-3) according to the embryonic metamere affected.

*Selected References: The complete reference list is available on the eBooks+ version included with purchase.*

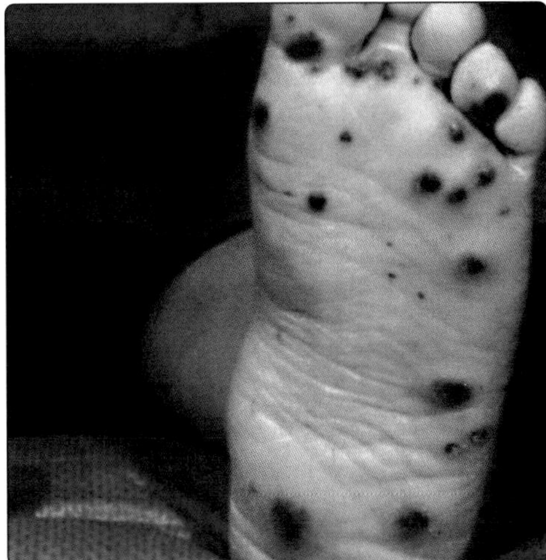

***(45-20)** Clinical photograph of a patient with BRBNS shows multiple elevated and bluish skin "blebs" on the foot. (Courtesy AFIP Archives.)*

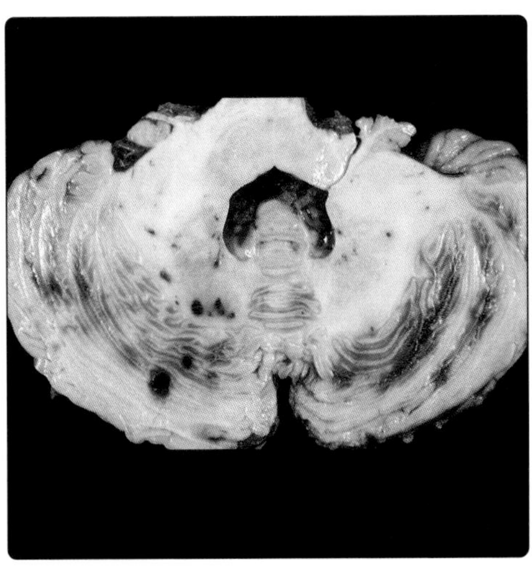

***(45-21)** Axial cut section through the cerebellum shows multiple developmental venous anomalies (DVAs) characteristic of BRBNS. (R. Hewlett, MD.)*

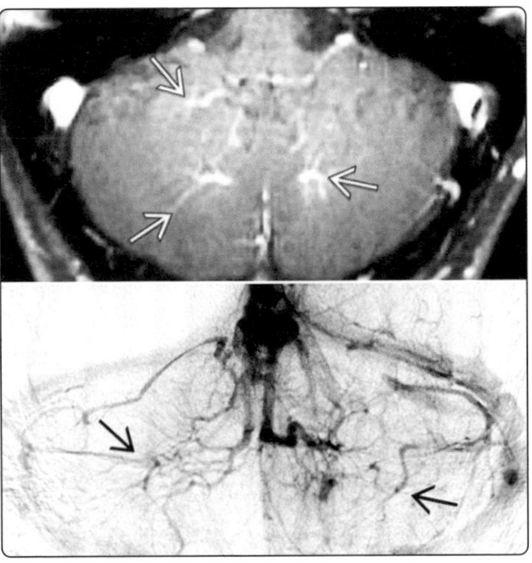

***(45-22)** (Top) T1 C+ FS MR in a patient with probable BRBNS shows bilateral enhancing DVAs ➡. (Bottom) AP DSA shows bilateral DVAs ➡.*

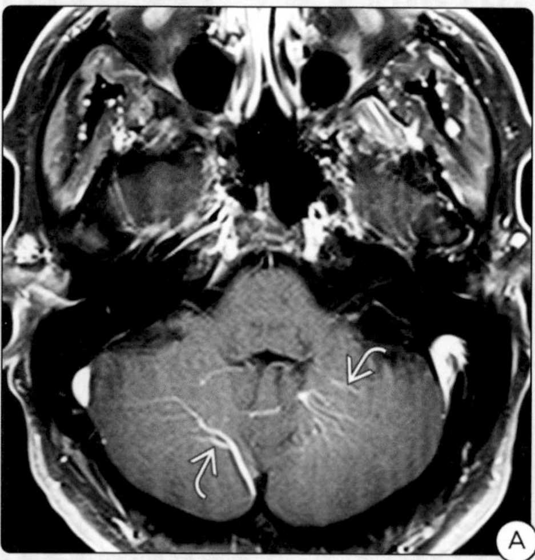

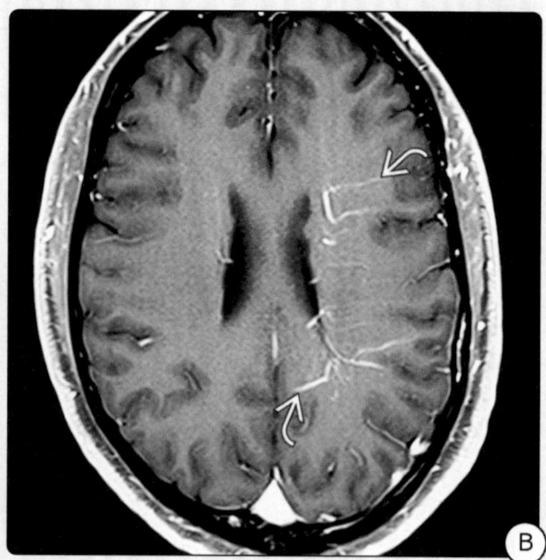

***(45-23A)** T1 C+ FS MR in a patient with BRBNS shows 2 DVAs ➦ in the cerebellar hemispheres. **(45-23B)** More cephalad T1 C+ FS MR shows additional DVAs in the left cerebral hemisphere ➦.*

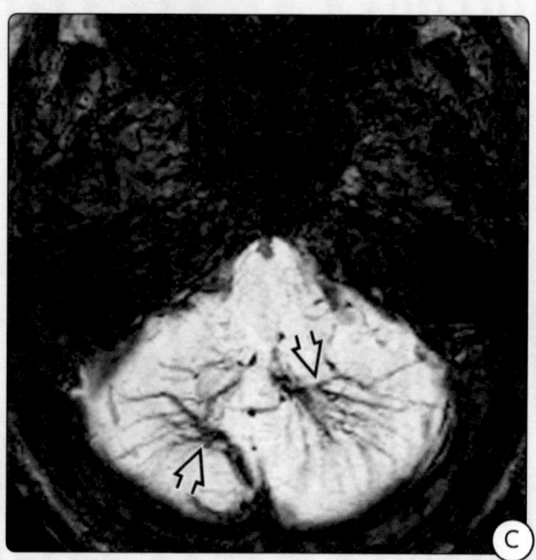

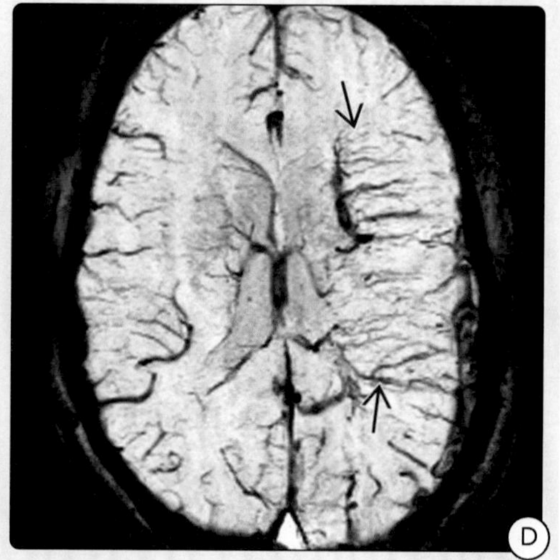

***(45-23C)** Axial MIP of the SWI beautifully delineates deoxyhemoglobin in the enlarged tributaries of both cerebellar DVAs ➩. **(45-23D)** More cephalad MIP SWI shows the markedly enlarged medullary veins ➩ that are prominent tributaries of the huge, nearly holohemispheric DVA.*

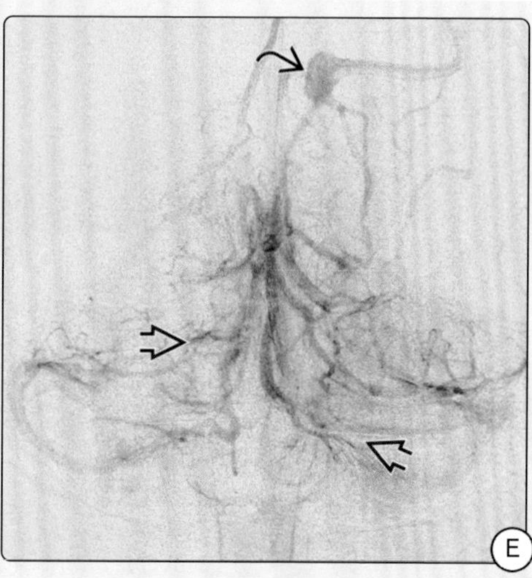

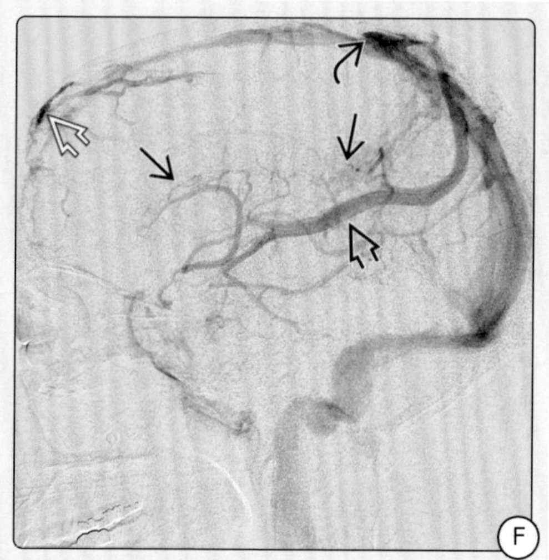

***(45-23E)** AP view of the vertebral angiogram shows 2 large DVAs ➩ in the cerebellar hemispheres. Note presence of a venous varix ➦ draining the DVAs. **(45-23F)** DSA of the left internal carotid angiogram, venous phase, shows a large DVA ➩ draining into an unusually prominent vein of Trolard ➩ that empties into a sinus pericranii ➦. Another, smaller left frontal sinus pericranii is also present ➩.*

# Anomalies of the Skull and Meninges

*Anomalies of the skull and meninges represent maldevelopment of the embryonic mesenchyme. These include cephaloceles, congenital calvarial defects, and other meningeal malformations, including lipomas.*



## Cephaloceles

Cephaloceles are external protrusions of CNS contents through a calvarial defect, usually in the midline. Cephaloceles can occur in the occipital, parietal, frontal, petrous apex, or intrasphenoidal regions.

"Cephaloceles" or "encephaloceles" are generic terms for the protrusion of intracranial contents through a calvarial or skull base defect **(46-1)**. Cephaloceles that contain herniations of brain tissue, meninges, and CSF are called **meningoencephaloceles**. If the meninges and accompanying CSF are herniated *without* brain tissue, the lesion is termed a **meningocele**. **Glioceles** are glial-lined, CSF-containing cysts. **Atretic cephalocele** (APC) is a small defect that contains just dura, fibrous tissue, and degenerated brain tissue.

Cephaloceles can be congenital or acquired and are defined by their contents and location. The most common congenital cephaloceles are occipital, frontoethmoidal, parietal, and skull base cephaloceles.

Cephalocele imaging has four goals: (1) Depict the osseous defect, (2) delineate the sac and define its contents, (3) map the course of adjacent arteries and determine the integrity of the dural venous sinuses, and (4) identify any coexisting anomalies.

### Occipital Cephaloceles

#### Terminology and Classification

Three subtypes of occipital cephalocele (OC) are recognized and identified according to the involved bone(s). From most to least extensive, they are **occipitocervical** (involving the occipital bone, foramen magnum, and neural arches of the upper cervical spine), **low occipital** (involving the occipital bone and foramen magnum) **(46-3)**, and **high occipital** (involving only the occipital bone).

High OCs and low OCs are the most common and are typically located in the midline of the occipital bone between the lambda and foramen magnum. They are sometimes divided into two subtypes: Supra- and infratorcular OCs.

## Clinical Issues

OCs account for 75% of cephaloceles in European and North American White patients but are relatively rare in South and Southeast Asia. There is a 2.4:1 male predominance.

OCs are usually recognized at birth as an occipital or suboccipital soft tissue mass **(46-1)**. Size varies from small to very large. The term "giant" OC is used when the size of the OC is equal to or greater than the size of the head. In such cases, the affected infant is often microcephalic with visible craniofacial disproportion.

Neurodevelopmental outcome in infants with OCs is related to cephalocele size and contents as well as the presence and type of associated abnormalities.

## Imaging

Bone CT with 3D reconstruction delineates the osseous defect well, and multiplanar MR best depicts the sac and its contents. The herniated brain—which can derive from both supra- and infratentorial structures—is always abnormal, appearing dysmorphic, disorganized, and dysplastic. Depending on the size of the cephalocele, severe traction and distortion of the brainstem and supratentorial structures can be present **(46-2)**.

Dura and CSF-filled structures (including the fourth ventricle and sometimes part of the lateral ventricles) are often contained within the sac. In addition to delineating the sac and its contents, identifying the course and integrity of the dural venous sinuses is essential for preoperative planning.

Hydrocephalus occurs in 60-90% of posterior cephaloceles. At least 1/2 of all patients with OCs have associated

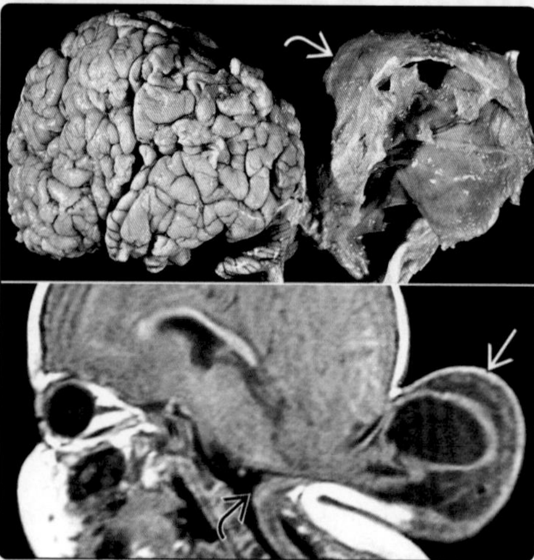

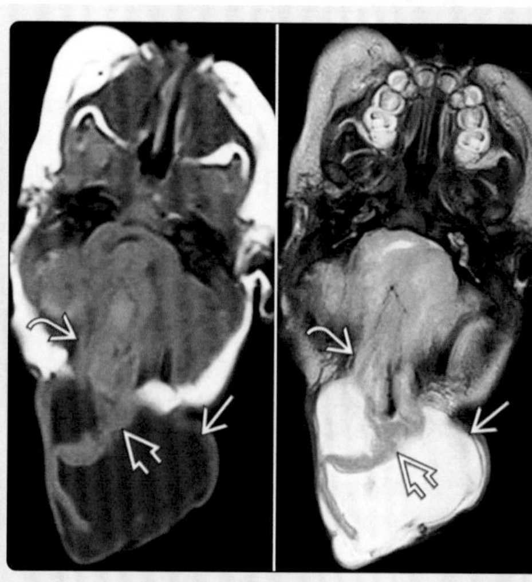

***(46-1)** (Top) Autopsy shows occipital cephalocele ➡, brain with pachy-/polymicrogyria. (Courtesy E. T. Hedley-Whyte, MD.) (Bottom) Sagittal T1WI shows occipitocervical meningoencephalocele ➡ with traction of the cervicomedullary junction ➡. **(46-2)** (L) T1WI, (R) T2WI show occipital cephalocele that contains meninges and CSF ➡ along with dysplastic brain ➡. Note traction and distortion of the cerebellum ➡.*

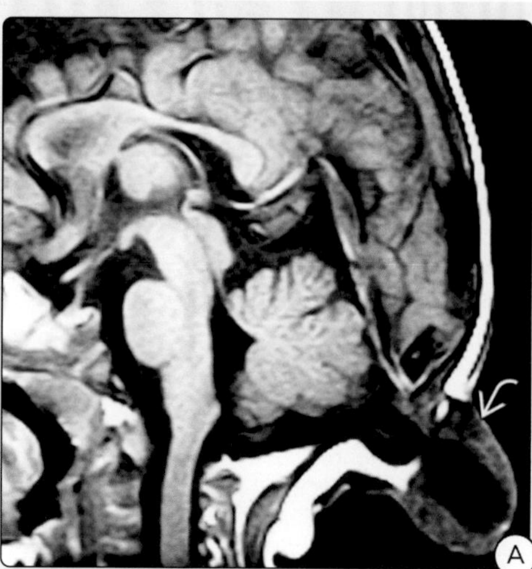

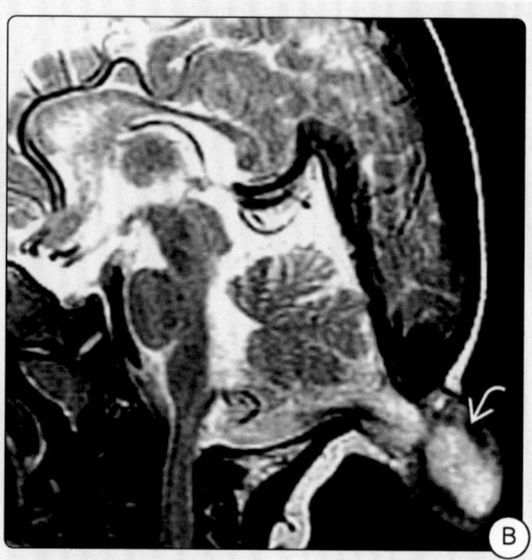

***(46-3A)** Sagittal T1WI shows a low occipital cephalocele ➡ involving the occipital bone and foramen magnum. The defect is below the torcular Herophili and above neural arches of the cervical spine. **(46-3B)** Sagittal T2WI shows the cephalocele ➡ is fluid filled and does not contain visible brain. There is slight traction on the cerebellar vermis, but it is not herniated into the cephalocele.*

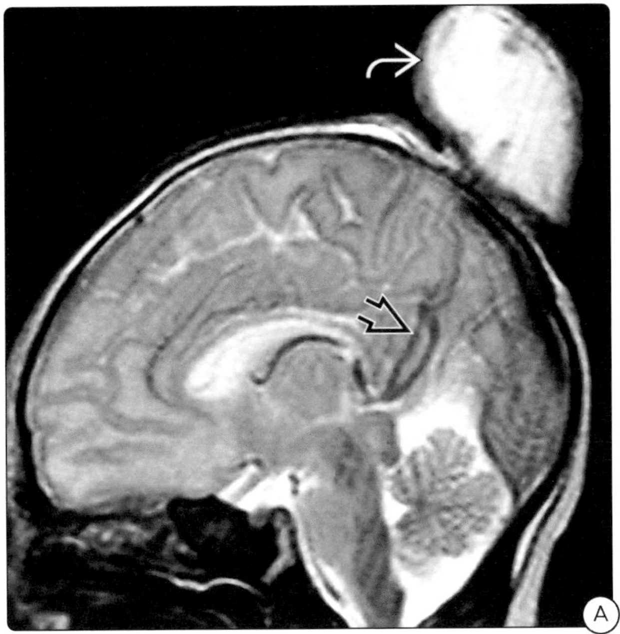

*(46-4A) Sagittal T2WI shows classic parietal cephalocele in the midline over the posterior vertex ➡. The cephalocele is associated with a persistent falcine sinus ⇨.*

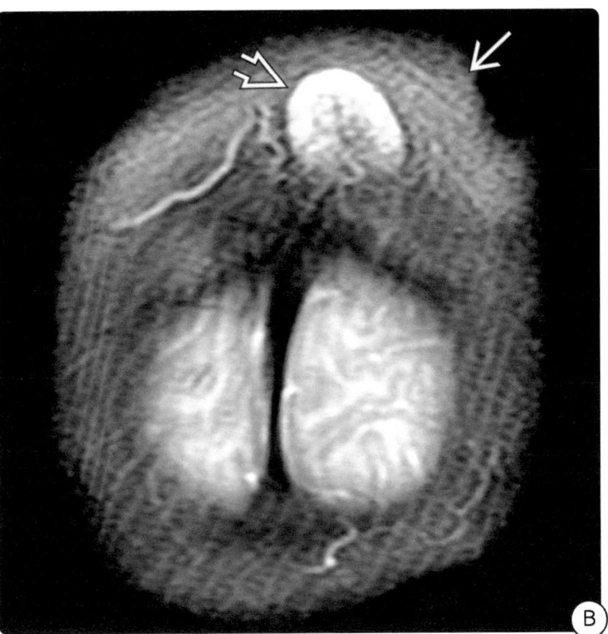

*(46-4B) Coronal T2WI shows a scalp mass ➡ with underlying parietal cephalocele ➡. (Courtesy K. Moore, MD.)*

abnormalities, such as callosal dysgenesis, Chiari 2, Dandy-Walker spectrum disorders, and gray matter heterotopias.

## Parietal Cephaloceles

Parietal cephaloceles compose just 5-10% of all cephaloceles. Most have underlying brain and vascular anomalies, such as a persistent falcine sinus or sinus pericranii **(46-4)**.

MR best delineates cephalocele contents. Defining the position of the superior sagittal sinus and adjacent cortical draining veins with MRV, CTV, or DSA prior to surgery is essential.

## Atretic Cephaloceles

APCs are occult or rudimentary cephaloceles that present clinically as midline scalp masses near the posterior vertex **(46-5)**. APCs are congenital skull defects with herniation of rudimentary intracranial structures through the defect. Most are covered by skin and consist of meninges &/or neuronal or glial cells.

Typical finding is a midline osseus defect within the sagittal suture **(46-6A)**. Venous anomalies are common. A recent review identified fenestration ("splitting") of the superior sagittal sinus in almost 1/2 of all cases **(46-7)**. Other vascular anomalies include a persistent falcine sinus (47%) **(46-6B)**, vertical positioning of the straight sinus (44%), absent straight sinus (40%), and vein of Galen anomalies (27%). Prognosis depends on the coexistent intracranial abnormalities.

## Frontoethmoidal Cephaloceles

Frontoethmoidal cephaloceles are the most common type of cephalocele seen in Southeast Asia. Brain tissue, CSF, and leptomeninges herniate into the midface, typically the forehead or dorsum of the nose **(46-13)**.

**Frontonasal** cephaloceles represent 40-60% of frontoethmoidal cephaloceles. Brain herniates into the forehead between the frontal bones above and the nasal bones below **(46-8)**. In **nasoethmoidal** cephaloceles (30%), the sac herniates through a midline foramen cecum defect into the prenasal space. The cribriform plate is deficient or absent; the crista galli may be absent or bifid. **Naso-orbital** and combined **nasoethmoidal and naso-orbital** are less common location-based subtypes of frontonasal cephaloceles **(46-14)**.

The management of frontoethmoidal cephaloceles is surgical. Careful preoperative, imaging-based planning minimizes the risk of intra- and postoperative complications. NECT scans show a well-demarcated, heterogeneous, mixed-density mass that extends extracranially through a bony defect. MR shows a soft tissue mass in direct contiguity with the intracranial parenchyma.

## Skull Base Cephaloceles

Skull base cephaloceles account for 10% of all cephaloceles **(46-11)**. MR of skull base cephaloceles is essential to delineate the sac contents **(46-10)**. The pituitary gland, optic nerves and chiasm, hypothalamus, and third ventricle can all be displaced inferiorly into the cephalocele **(46-12)**. Associated anomalies, such as corpus callosum dysgenesis and an azygous anterior cerebral artery, are common.

*(46-5)* *Skin-covered atretic parietal cephalocele is associated with a dura-lined sinus tract and a persistent falcine sinus.* *(46-6A)* *3D bone CT in a patient with midline scalp lesions shows a 1-cm, well-demarcated skull defect in the middle of the sagittal suture.*

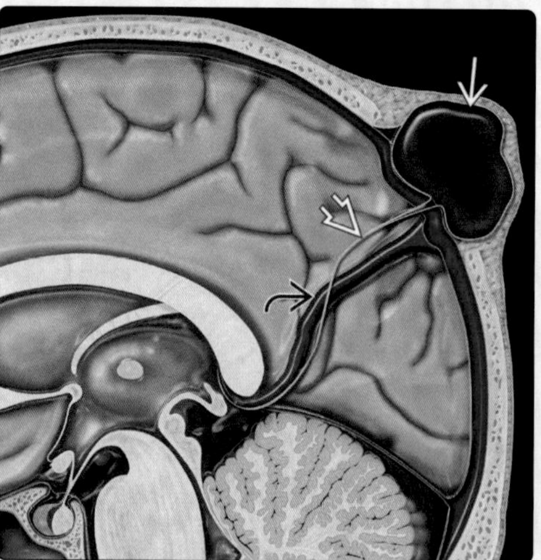

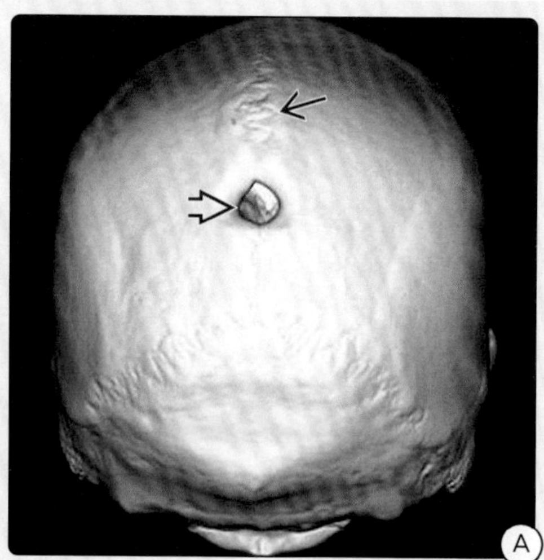


*(46-6B)* *Lateral NECT in the same case shows the midline skull defect, absent straight sinus with a large persistent falcine sinus coursing superiorly towards the defect, and an atretic cephalocele. (Courtesy G. E. Morgan, MD.)* *(46-7A)* *3D-rendered bone CT in a child with an atretic parietal cephalocele demonstrates a small, well-demarcated midline skull defect.*

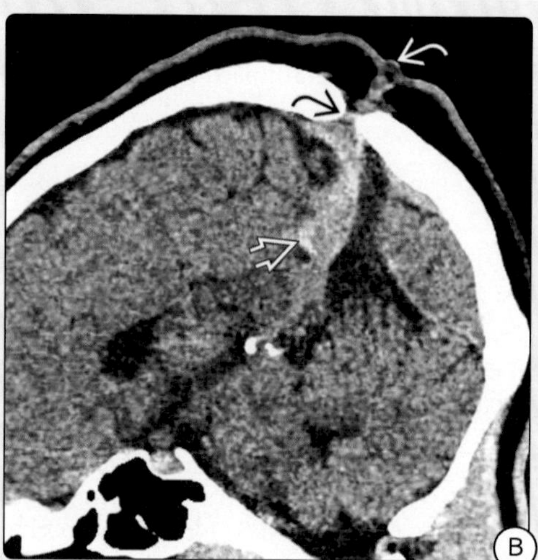


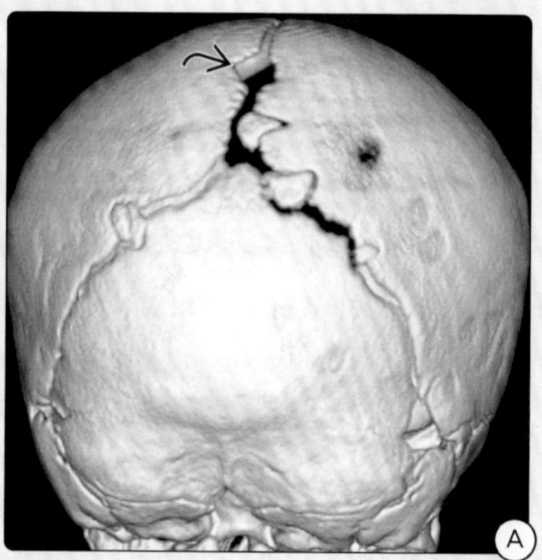


*(46-7B)* *CTA in the same patient demonstrates a persistent falcine sinus and atretic cephalocele passing between the split superior sagittal sinus.* *(46-7C)* *Sagittal T2 FS in the same patient demonstrates the persistent falcine sinus and a tiny atretic cephalocele. (Courtesy K. Moore, MD.)*

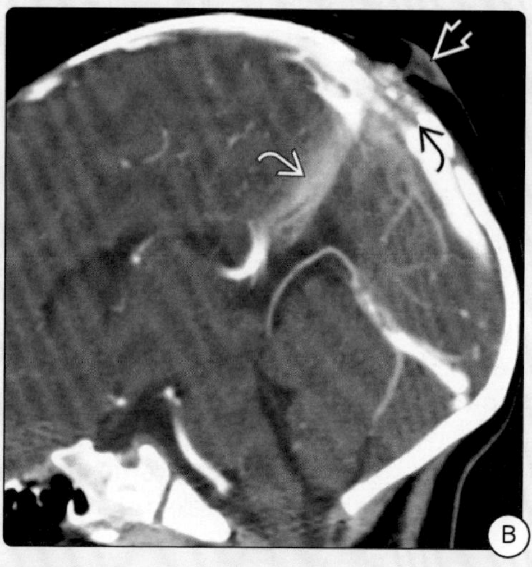


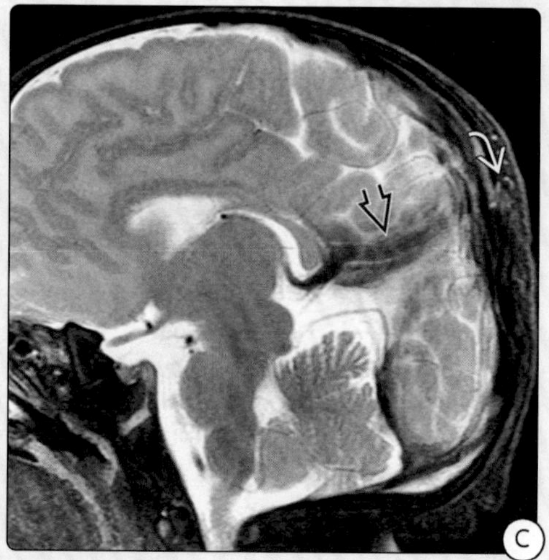

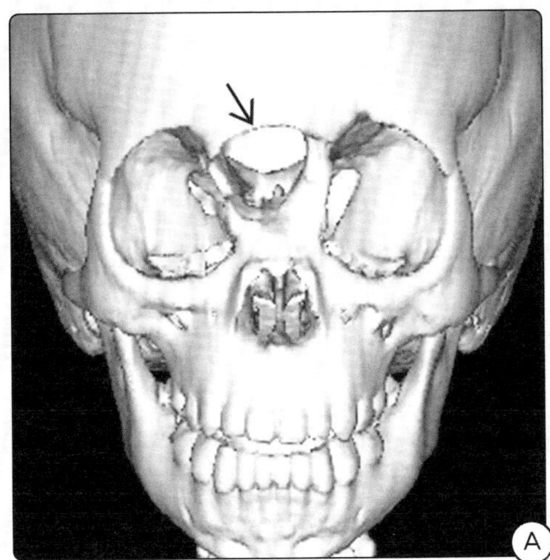

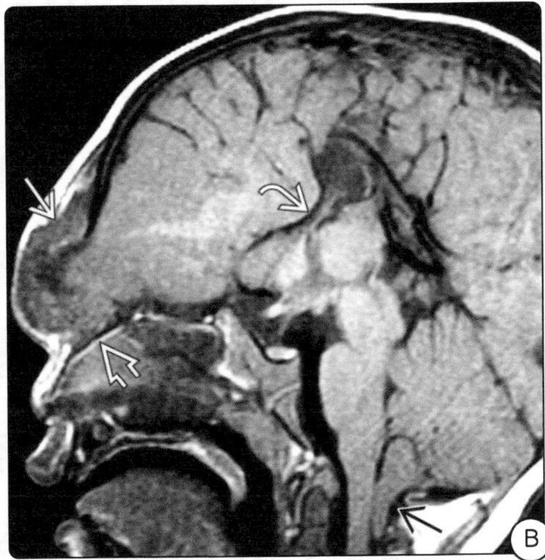

***(46-8A)*** *3D reformatted bone CT shows a well-delineated frontonasal bony defect ⇒ just above the bridge of the nose.* ***(46-8B)*** *Sagittal T1WI shows a soft tissue mass ➡ protruding through a patent fonticulus frontalis ➡. Note absent corpus callosum ➡, Chiari 1 ⇒.*

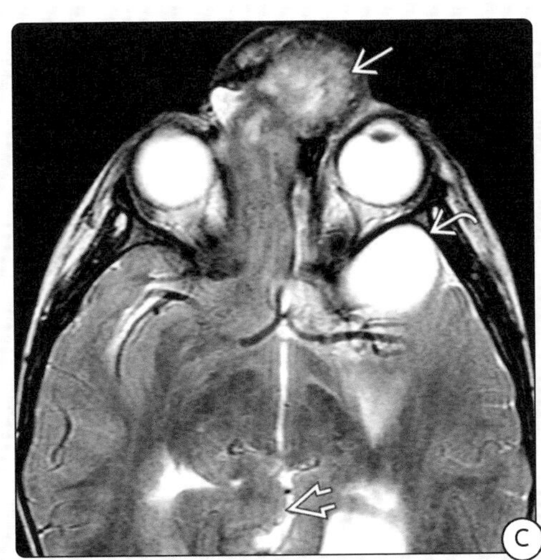

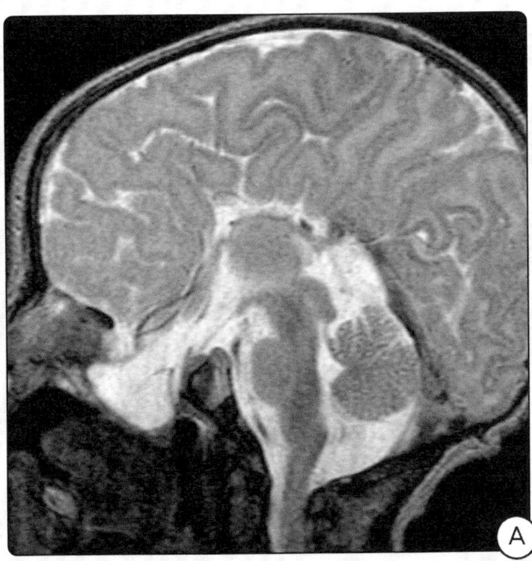

***(46-8C)*** *T2WI shows cephalocele is mostly dysplastic brain ➡. Note arachnoid cyst ➡, polymicrogyria ➡. (Courtesy M. Michel, MD.)* ***(46-9A)*** *Sagittal T2WI shows a sphenoethmoidal cephalocele. Note extreme retraction of the anterior recesses and optic chiasm into the cephalocele. Agenesis of the corpus callosum is present, and the anterior cerebral arteries are retracted into the defect.*

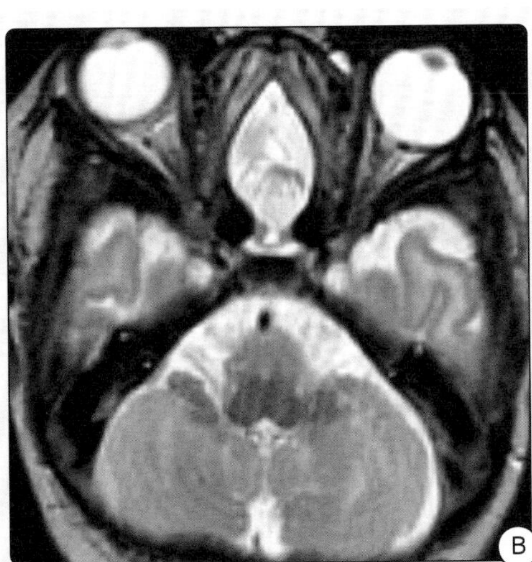

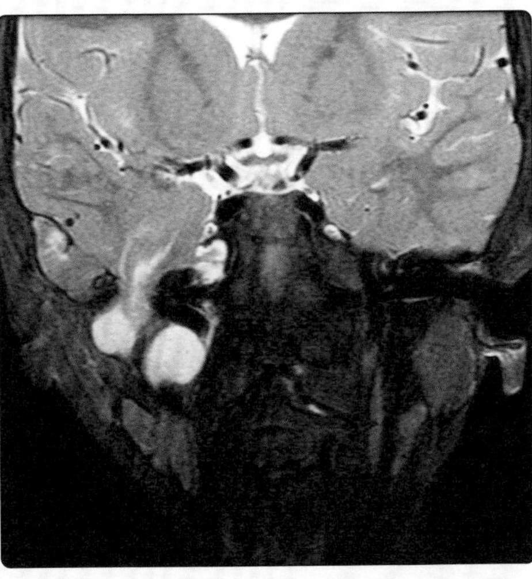

***(46-9B)*** *Axial T2WI shows the sphenoethmoidal cephalocele with retracted optic chiasm.* ***(46-10)*** *Coronal T2WI shows an unusual temporal encephalocele with part of the temporal lobe herniating through a defect in the floor of the sphenoid sinus.*

*(**46-11A**) (L) Autopsy of sphenoethmoidal cephalocele shows central skull base defect ⇨. (R) Basal view of brain shows cephalocele →. (**46-11B**) Sagittal view of brain in the same case shows cephalocele ⇨, pachygyria, corpus callosum dysplasia. (Courtesy E. T. Hedley-Whyte, MD.)*

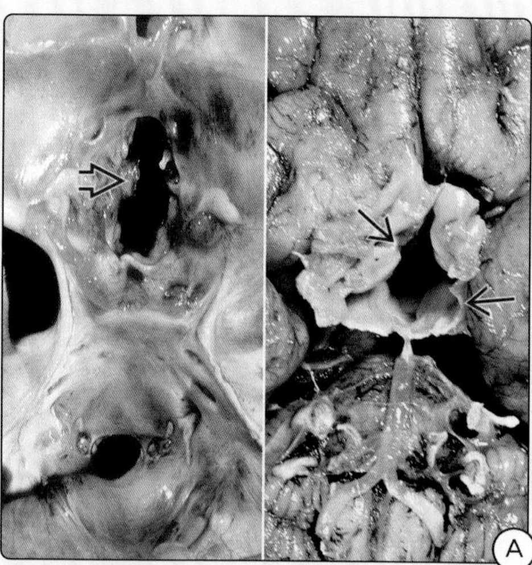


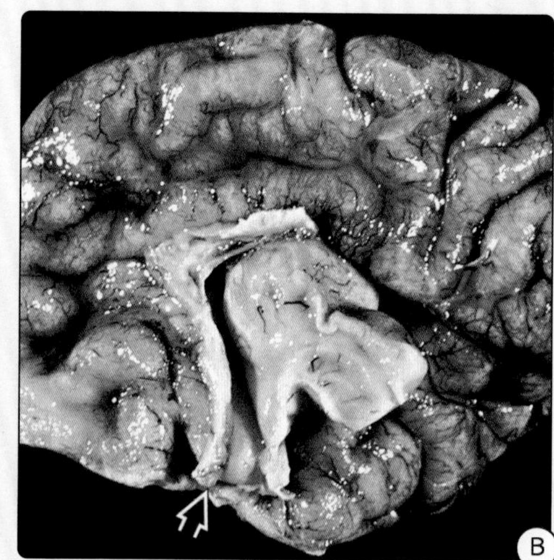


*(**46-12**) Sagittal T1WI shows sphenoethmoidal cephalocele ⇨. Hypothalamus, anterior 3rd ventricle are retracted into the sac. (**46-13**) Clinical photograph of an infant shows a large frontonasal cephalocele.*

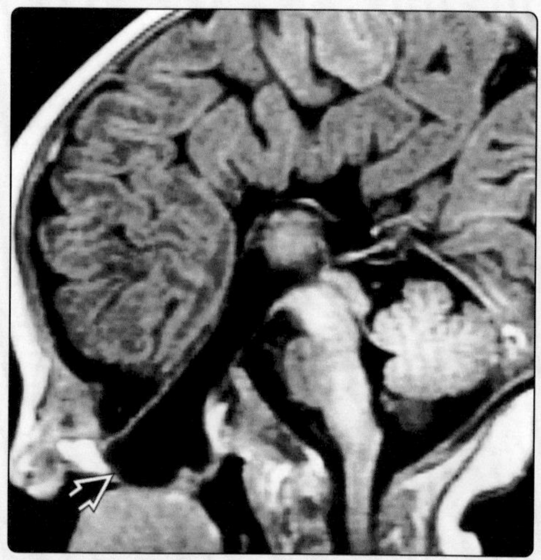

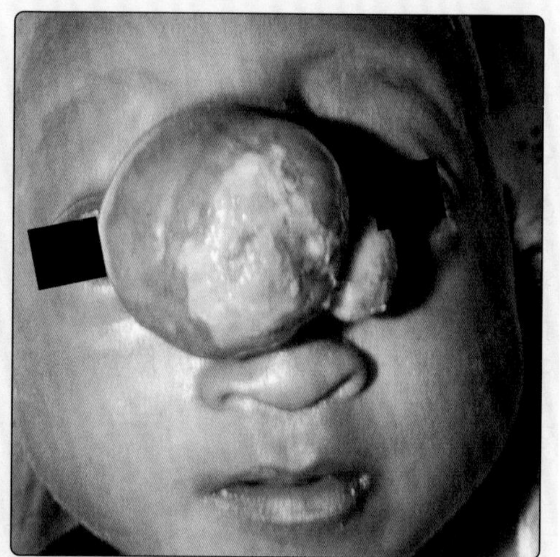

*(**46-14A**) Coronal T2WI in a 13-day-old girl shows a nasoethmoidal cephalocele ⇨ with dysplastic brain ⇨ clearly herniating in front of and below an intact crista galli ↷. (**46-14B**) Sagittal T2WI in the same case shows the nasoethmoidal cephalocele ⇨ contains dysplastic brain with signal intensity resembling gray matter.*

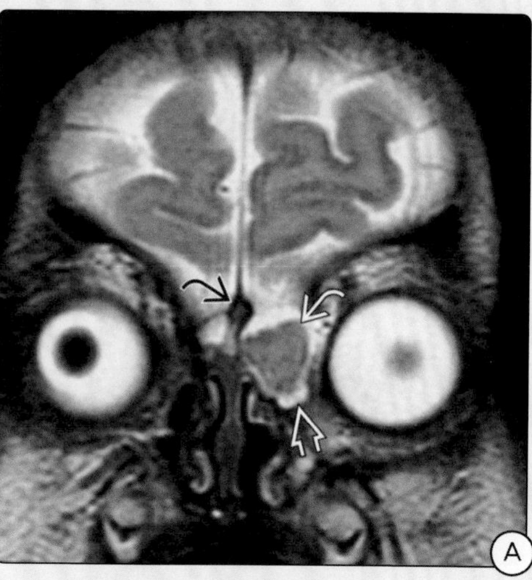


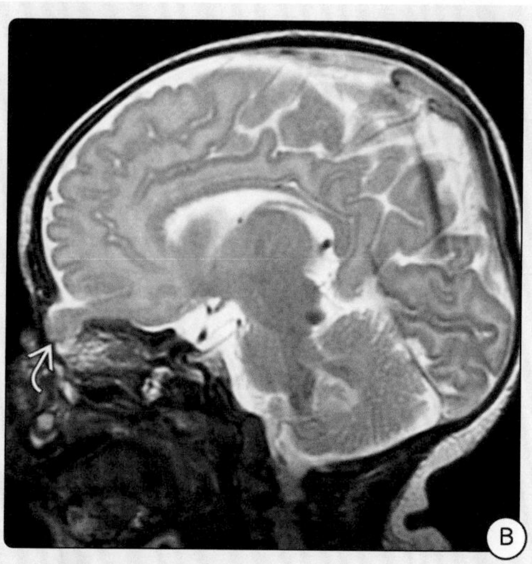

**CEPHALOCELES**

**Occipital Cephaloceles**
- Most common in European/North American White patients
- 75% of cephaloceles
- Typically contains dysplastic brain

**Frontoethmoidal Cephaloceles**
- Southeast Asian predominance
- 10-15% of cephaloceles
- Frontonasal (40-60%) = forehead
- Nasoethmoidal (30%) = nose

**Parietal Cephaloceles**
- 5-10% of cephaloceles
- Most are atretic ± falcine sinus, sinus pericranii

**Skull Base Cephaloceles**
- 10% of cephaloceles
- Brain anomalies common (e.g., callosal dysgenesis)

# Craniosynostoses

## Craniosynostosis Overview

Craniosynostosis (from Greek meaning skull + together + bone interlocking and fastening) refers to early fusion of one or several cranial sutures resulting in craniofacial abnormalities.

The craniosynostoses are a heterogeneous group of disorders characterized by abnormal head shape resulting from premature fusion of the skull sutures. Any of the skull sutures can be prematurely fused. Craniosynostosis can be nonsyndromic (70-75% of cases) or syndromic and may affect a single suture or multiple sutures.

The cranial sutures form relatively late (at around 16 weeks of gestation). As long as the brain grows rapidly, the calvarium expands. As brain growth slows, the sutures close.

The normal order of closure is metopic first, followed by the coronal and then the lambdoid sutures. The sagittal suture normally closes last. Craniosynostosis occurs when osseous obliteration of one or more sutures occurs prematurely. Premature closure means bones with persisting open sutures will develop in a compensatory way, usually without limiting the growth of brain volume.

In 85% of cases, craniosynostosis is a sporadic (i.e., nonsyndromic) abnormality with no clear genetic association. In the other 15%, craniosynostosis occurs as part of an identifiable syndrome (i.e., syndromic craniosynostosis). One or multiple sutures can be affected.

True synostosis must be distinguished from positional deformities. In contrast to craniosynostosis (rare), nonsynostotic head shape problems are benign entities caused by external mechanical forces that mold the infant skull (common). The sutures themselves are normal. This is often referred to as "deformational" or **"positional" plagiocephaly** or **positional brachycephaly** (plagiocephaly—"skewed"—simply refers to an asymmetry of the head). Here, the altered head shape is due to positioning of the head with respect to its surroundings (in utero, at birth, or postnatally) and is **not** caused by sutural stenosis. Treatment is nonsurgical.

## Nonsyndromic Craniosynostosis

Nonsyndromic craniosynostoses (NCSs) occur in the absence of a recognizable syndrome, although a likely pathogenic germline variant has been reported in nearly 10% of children with NCSs.

Craniosynostosis results in restricted growth around the fused suture. Clinically, this growth pattern leads to abnormal bulging or bossing of bone plates that have patent sutures, causing characteristic dysmorphic craniofacial features.

Approximately 60% of all single-suture craniosynostosis cases involve premature fusion of the sagittal suture followed in frequency by those that involve the coronal (22%) and metopic (15%) sutures. Lambdoid craniosynostosis is very rare, causing just 2% of all cases.

Craniosynostosis is generally classified by head shape. There are four major abnormal head shapes: **Scaphocephaly** or **dolichocephaly** (long and narrow, associated with sagittal synostosis), **brachycephaly** (broad and flattened, bicoronal synostosis), **trigonocephaly** (triangular at the front, from metopic synostosis) **(46-15)**, or **plagiocephaly** ("skewed," from unilateral coronal or lambdoid synostosis). Focal synostosis or diffuse bony ridging or "beaking" along the affected suture are typical findings **(46-16)**. Compensatory spreading of the noninvolved sutures is common **(46-17)**.

CT is required to determine whether part or all of the affected suture(s) is fused. Thin-section CT scans with multiplanar reconstruction and 3D shaded surface display (SSD) are invaluable for detailed evaluation and preoperative planning. MR is helpful to rule out coexisting anomalies, such as hydrocephalus, corpus callosum dysgenesis, and gray matter abnormalities.

**CRANIOSYNOSTOSIS**

**Normal Suture Development**
- Late (16-weeks gestation)
- Metopic closes first, sagittal closes last

**Pathology**
- Location
  - Sagittal (60%): Scaphocephaly
  - Coronal (22%): Brachycephaly
  - Metopic (15%): Trigonocephaly
  - Lambdoid (2%)
  - Multiple (5%)
- Gross pathology
  - Suture obliterated by diffuse or focal bony "beaking"
  - Compensatory spreading of noninvolved sutures

*(46-15) Bone CT of trigonocephaly shows triangular anterior pointing of the skull ➡. In the transverse plane, calvarium appears widened.*

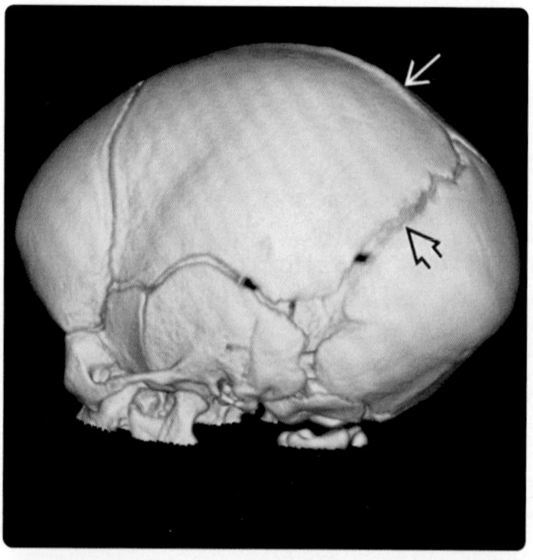

*(46-16) 3D CT of scaphocephaly shows fusion and ridging of sagittal suture ➡ with compensated widened lambdoid suture ⇨.*

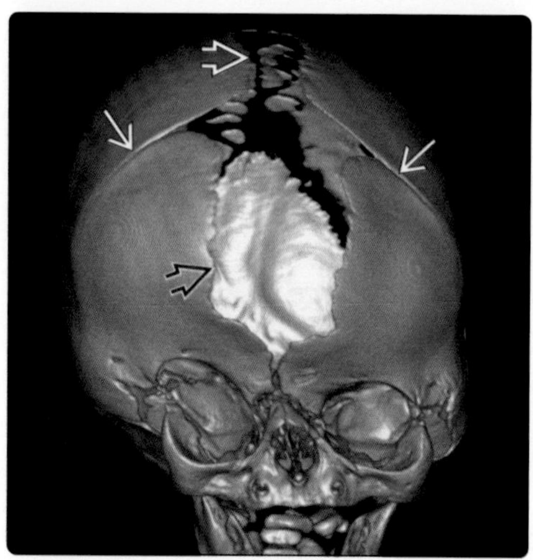

*(46-17) 3D CT in an infant with Apert syndrome shows widened metopic ⇨ and sagittal sutures ➡, bilateral coronal synostosis ➡.*

## Syndromic Craniosynostoses

A minority of craniosynostosis cases are related to craniofacial syndromes, such as Apert or Crouzon syndrome. Syndromic craniosynostoses account for just 25-30% of all cranial stenoses but are much more likely to be associated with additional craniofacial or skeletal anomalies. These include limb abnormalities, dysmorphic facial features, and skull deformity. In addition, brain malformations are common, and developmental delay is more frequent. In contrast to NSCs (in which the sagittal suture is most often affected), bilateral coronal synostosis is the most common pattern in these patients.

Examples of syndromic craniosynostoses include Apert syndrome (a.k.a. **acrocephalosyndactyly type 1**). Bilateral coronal synostosis is the most common calvarial anomaly **(46-17)**. Hypertelorism, midface hypoplasia, and cervical spine anomalies are common.

Of all the syndromic craniosynostoses, patients with Apert syndrome are most severely affected in terms of intellectual disability, developmental delay, CNS malformations, hearing loss, and limb anomalies. Intracranial anomalies occur in > 1/2 of all cases and include hydrocephalus, callosal dysgenesis, and abnormalities of the septi pellucidi (25-30% each).

# Meningeal Anomalies

Anomalies of the cranial meninges commonly accompany other congenital malformations, such as Chiari 2 malformation. **Lipomas** and **arachnoid cysts** are two important intracranial abnormalities with meningeal origin. Arachnoid cysts were considered in detail in Chapter 32. We therefore conclude our discussion of congenital anomalies by focusing on lipomas.

## Lipomas

The 2021 WHO classification of CNS tumors no longer includes mention of intracranial lipomas as potentially neoplastic. Because lipomas do not demonstrate neoplastic behavior, it is more appropriate to consider them on the spectrum of malformative overgrowths that arise during brain development. We include lipomas in this chapter because of their frequent association with other congenital malformations.

Fat—adipose tissue—is not normally found inside the arachnoid. Therefore, any fatty tissue inside the skull or spine is abnormal. Because fat deposits commonly accompany congenital malformations, such as callosal dysgenesis or tethered spinal cord, imaging studies should be closely scrutinized for the presence of additional abnormalities.

### Terminology

So-called ordinary lipoma is the most common of all soft tissue tumors and is composed of mature adipose tissue. "Complex lipomatous lesions" may contain other mesenchymal tissues, such as striated muscle, and have sometimes been referred to as **choristomas**.

### Etiology

Lipomas were once thought to be congenital malformations of the **embryonic meninx primitiva** (the undifferentiated mesenchyme). The primitive meninx normally differentiates into the cranial meninges, invaginating along the choroid fissure of the lateral ventricle. Maldifferentiation and persistence of the meninx was thought to result in

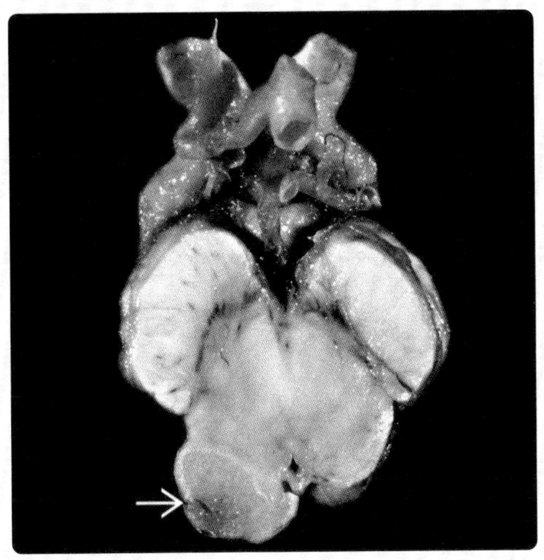

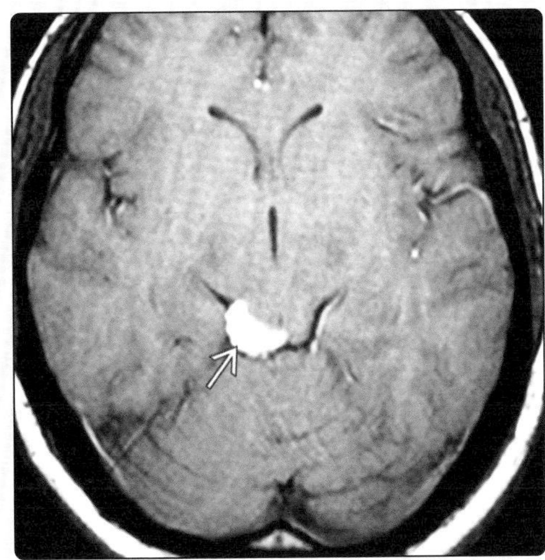

***(46-18)** Autopsy case demonstrates subpial lipoma ➡ attached to quadrigeminal plate. (Courtesy E. T. Hedley-Whyte, MD.) **(46-19)** T1 MR shows hyperintense lipoma ➡ is attached to the quadrigeminal plate without a distinct medial border.*

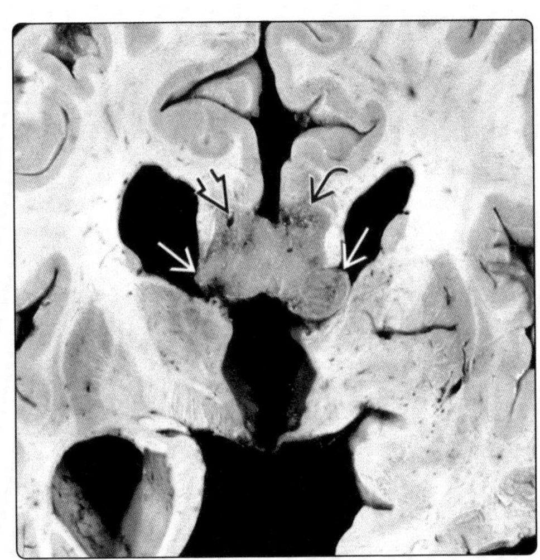

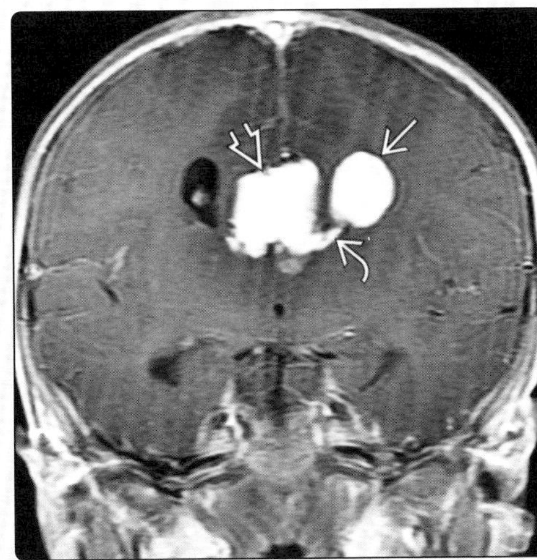

***(46-20)** Autopsy of complete corpus callosum agenesis shows a midline interhemispheric lipoma ➡. Note encased anterior cerebral arteries ➡, lipoma extension through choroidal fissures into lateral ventricles ➡. **(46-21)** Coronal T1 C+ in an 11-month-old shows corpus callosum agenesis with a large, bulky interhemispheric lipoma ➡ that extends through the choroidal fissure ➡ into the left lateral ventricle ➡.*

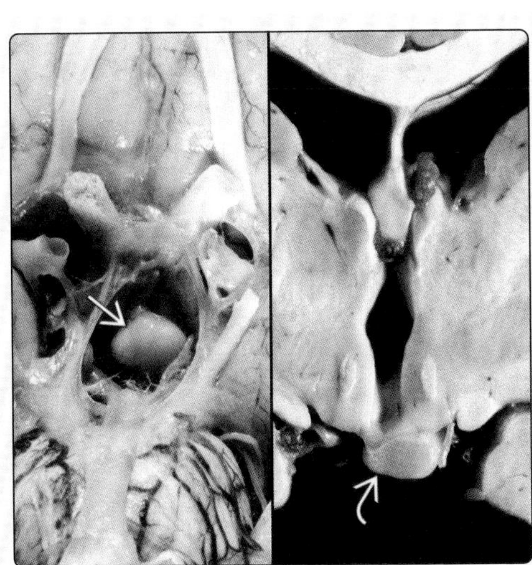

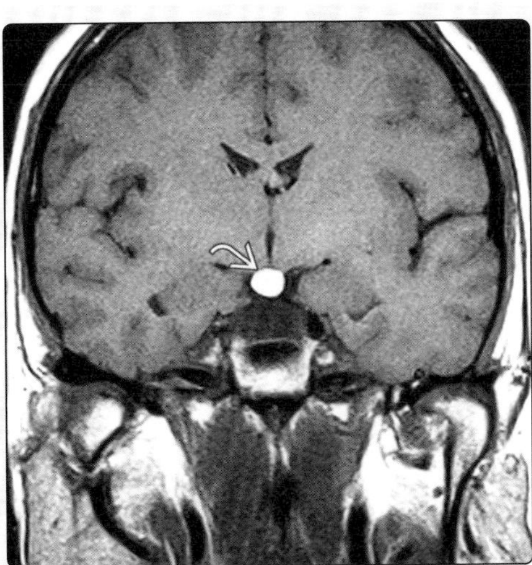

***(46-22)** (L) Basal view of autopsy shows suprasellar lipoma ➡. (R) Coronal section shows lipoma ➡ is attached to hypothalamus. (Courtesy J. Townsend, MD.) **(46-23)** Coronal T1WI shows incidental finding of suprasellar lipoma ➡.*

deposits of mature adipose tissue, i.e., fat, along the subpial surface of the brain and spinal cord and within the lateral ventricles.

Recent fluorescence in situ hybridization (FISH) and comparative genomic hybridization (CGH) studies have identified clonal cytogenetic aberrations in nearly 60% of ordinary systemic lipomas.

## Pathology

**Location.** Nearly 80% of intracranial lipomas are supratentorial, and most occur in or near the midline. The interhemispheric fissure is the most common overall site (40-50%). Lipomas curve over the dorsal corpus callosum, often extending through the choroidal fissures into the lateral ventricles or choroid plexus **(46-20)**.

Between 15-25% are located in the quadrigeminal region, usually attached to the inferior colliculi or superior vermis **(46-18)**. Approximately 15% are suprasellar, attached to the undersurface of the hypothalamus or infundibular stalk **(46-22)** **(46-23)**. About 5% of lipomas are found in the sylvian fissure.

Approximately 20% of lipomas are infratentorial. The cerebellopontine angle cistern is the most common posterior fossa site (10%).

Lipomas are generally solitary lesions that vary from tiny, barely perceptible fatty collections to huge, bulky masses. Most are < 5 cm in diameter.

**Gross Pathology.** Lipomas appear as bright yellow, lobulated soft masses **(46-18)**. They usually adhere to the pia and underlying parenchyma. At least 1/3 encase adjacent vessels &/or cranial nerves. Lipomas are composed of mature, nonneoplastic-appearing adipose tissue with relatively uniform fat cells.

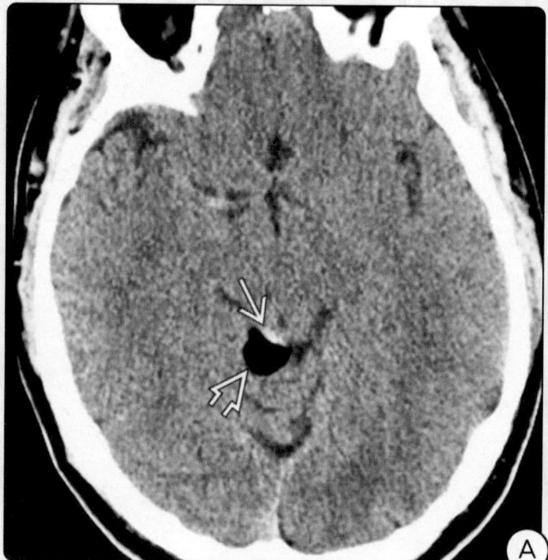


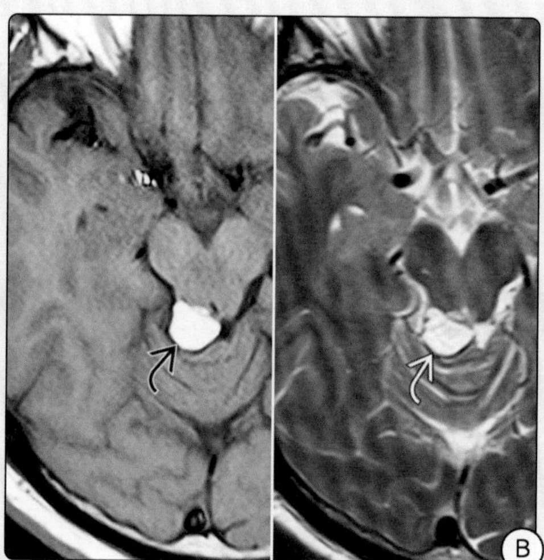


***(46-24A)* NECT in a 46-yo woman imaged for stroke shows a well-delineated hypodense mass ➡ with focal calcification ➡ attached to the dorsal midbrain. *(46-24B)* (L) T1WI shows the mass ➡ is uniformly hyperintense and appears to focally infiltrate the quadrigeminal plate. (R) The mass remains hyperintense on T2 FSE ➡ because of J-coupling.**

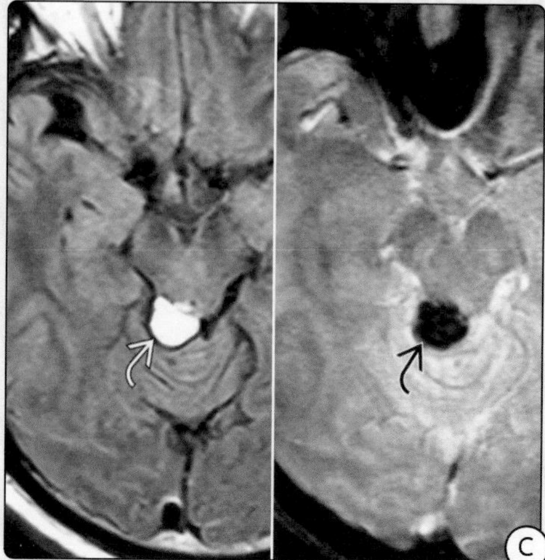


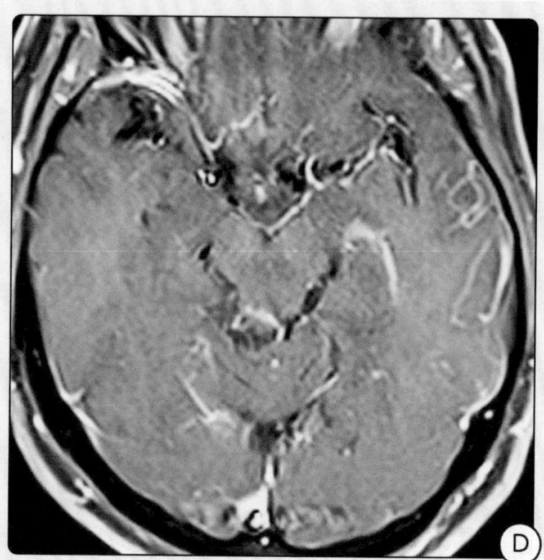


***(46-24C)* (L) The mass is hyperintense on FLAIR ➡ but "blooms" and is very hypointense on T2* GRE ➡ (R). *(46-24D)* The mass suppresses on T1 C+ FS. This is incidental tectal plate lipoma.**

**INTRACRANIAL LIPOMAS: ETIOLOGY AND PATHOLOGY**

**Etiology**
- 2 theories
  - Maldifferentiation of embryonic meninx primitiva
  - Genetic aberration

**Pathology**
- Usually solitary
- Supratentorial (80%)
  - Interhemispheric fissure (40-50%)
  - Quadrigeminal (15-25%)
  - Suprasellar (15%)
- Infratentorial (20%)
- Gross appearance: Lobulated, yellow
- Microscopic: Mature, nonneoplastic adipose tissue

## Clinical Issues

Lipomas are relatively rare, accounting for < 0.5% of intracranial masses. They can be found in patients of all ages.

Lipomas are rarely symptomatic and are usually incidental findings on imaging studies. Headache, seizure, hypothalamic disturbances, and cranial nerve deficits have been reported in a few cases. Lipomas are benign lesions. They may grow during periods of significant body growth early in life or with increases in overall body fat. Some may expand with corticosteroid use.

Lipomas encase vessels and nerves, so they are generally considered "leave me alone" lesions **(46-26)**. Surgery has high associated morbidity and mortality.

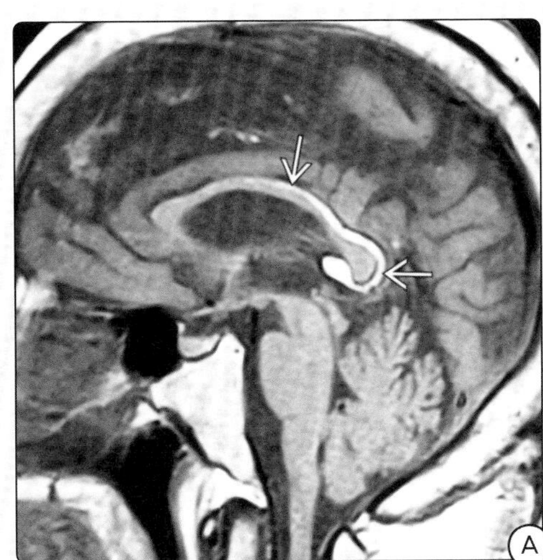


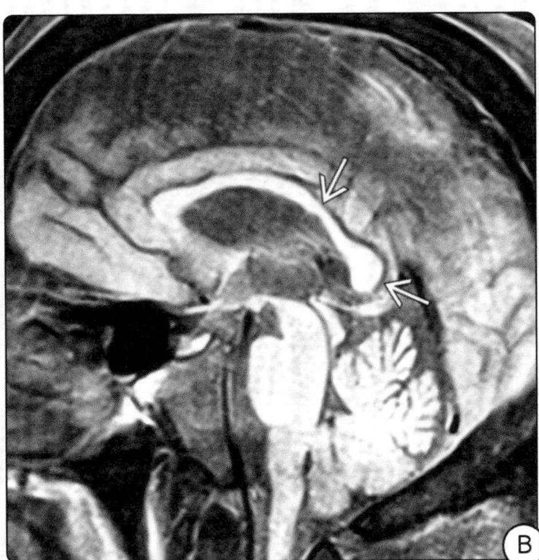


***(46-25A)** Sagittal T1WI in a 47-yo man shows incidental finding of interhemispheric lipoma along the superior surface of the corpus callosum. **(46-25B)** T1 FS in the same case shows the lipoma suppresses completely.*

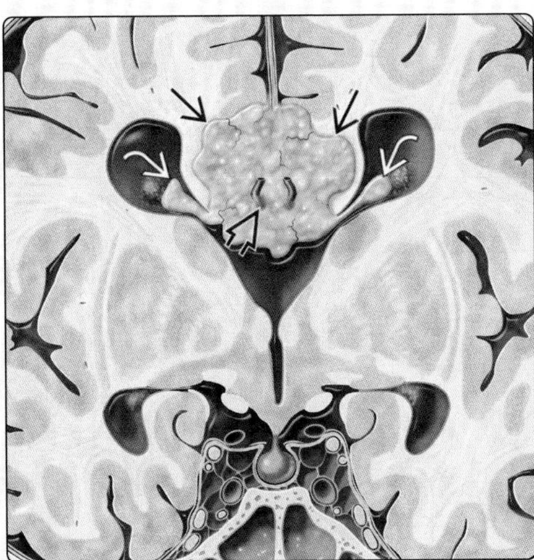

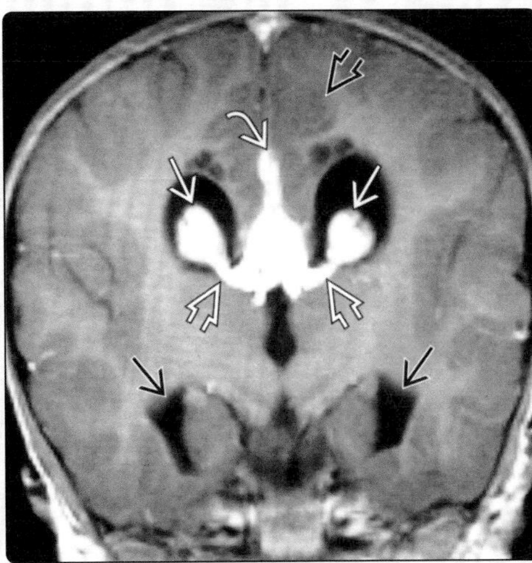

***(46-26)** Graphic shows callosal agenesis with lipoma encasing anterior cerebral arteries. Note lipoma extension through choroidal fissures into lateral ventricles. **(46-27)** Coronal T1WI shows callosal agenesis with large interhemispheric lipoma that extends through choroidal fissures into lateral ventricles. Other visible anomalies include cortical dysplasia, vertically oriented temporal horns.*

## Imaging

**General Features.** Lipomas are seen as well-delineated, somewhat lobulated extraaxial masses that exhibit fat density/signal intensity.

Two morphologic configurations of interhemispheric fissure lipomas are recognized on imaging studies: A **curvilinear** type (a thin, pencil-like mass that curves around the corpus callosum body and splenium) **(46-25A)** and a **tubulonodular** type (a large, bulky interhemispheric fatty mass) **(46-21)**. Dystrophic calcification occurs in both types but is more common in tubulonodular lesions.

**CT Findings.** NECT scans show a hypodense mass that measures -50 to -100 HU **(46-24A)**. Calcification varies from extensive—nearly 2/3 of bulky tubulonodular interhemispheric lipomas are partially calcified **(46-28A)**—to none, generally seen in small lesions in other locations. Lipomas do not enhance on CECT scans.

**MR Findings.** Lipomas follow fat signal on all imaging sequences. They appear homogeneously hyperintense on T1WI **(46-19)** and become hypointense with fat suppression **(46-24D)**. Lipomas exhibit chemical-shift artifact in the frequency-encoding direction.

Signal on T2WI varies. Fat becomes hypointense on standard T2WI but remains moderately hyperintense on fast spin-echo studies because of J-coupling **(46-24B)**. Fat is hypointense on STIR and appears hyperintense on FLAIR **(46-24C)**. No enhancement is seen following contrast administration.

On SWI, lipomas show hyperintensity surrounded by a low signal intensity band along the fat-water interface that is more prominent than seen on T2* GRE sequences **(46-24C)**.

Other CNS malformations are common. The most frequent are corpus callosum anomalies. These range from mild dysgenesis (usually with curvilinear lipomas) to agenesis (with bulky tubulonodular lipomas) **(46-27)** **(46-28)**.

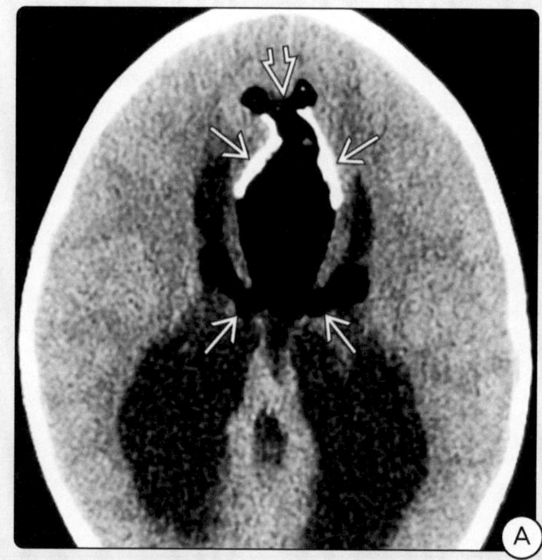


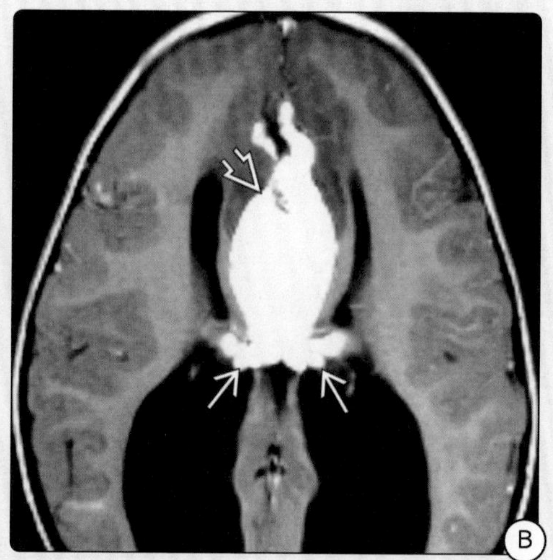


***(46-28A)** NECT shows corpus callosum agenesis with parallel, nonconverging lateral ventricles. Large, partially calcified tubulonodular interhemispheric lipoma ➡ extends into both lateral ventricles through choroidal fissures ➡. **(46-28B)** T1WI shows the hyperintense interhemispheric lipoma ➡ between parallel, nonconverging lateral ventricles. Note extension into lateral ventricles through choroidal fissures ➡.*

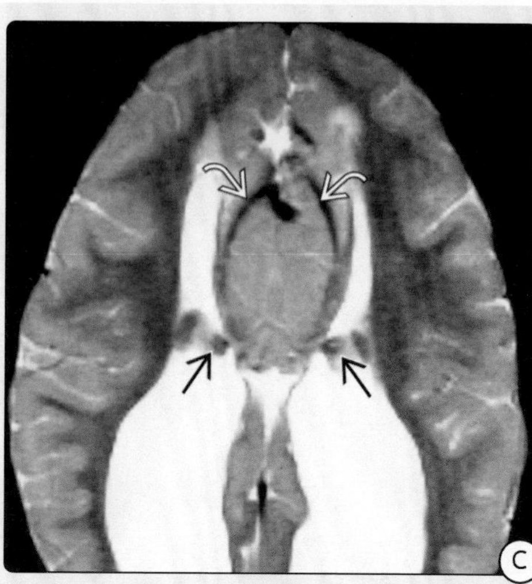


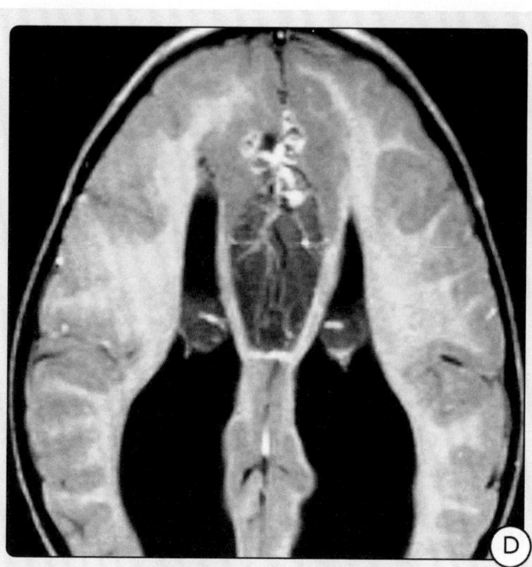


***(46-28C)** Standard non-FSE T2WI shows the lipoma is relatively hypointense compared to its signal on the T1WI. Note extension into lateral ventricles ➡, hypointensity from calcifications ➡. **(46-28D)** The lipoma suppresses on T1 C+ FS.*

## Differential Diagnosis

Although fat does not appear inside the normal CNS, it *can* be found within the dura and cavernous sinus. **Metaplastic falx ossification** is a normal variant that can resemble an interhemispheric lipoma. Dense cortical bone surrounding T1-hyperintense, fatty marrow is the typical finding.

The major differential diagnosis of intracranial lipoma is unruptured **dermoid cyst**. Dermoids generally measure 20-40 HU, often calcify, and demonstrate more heterogeneous signal intensity on MR.

### INTRACRANIAL LIPOMAS

**Clinical Issues**
- < 0.5% of intracranial masses
- Usually found incidentally; "leave me alone" lesions

**Imaging**
- NECT: -50 to -100 HU
    - Calcifications rare, except in tubulonodular lesions
- MR: "Just like fat"
    - Other intracranial malformations common
    - Often surrounds, encases vessels/nerves

**Differential Diagnosis**
- Dermoid cyst
- Falx ossification

*Selected References: The complete reference list is available on the eBooks+ version included with purchase.*

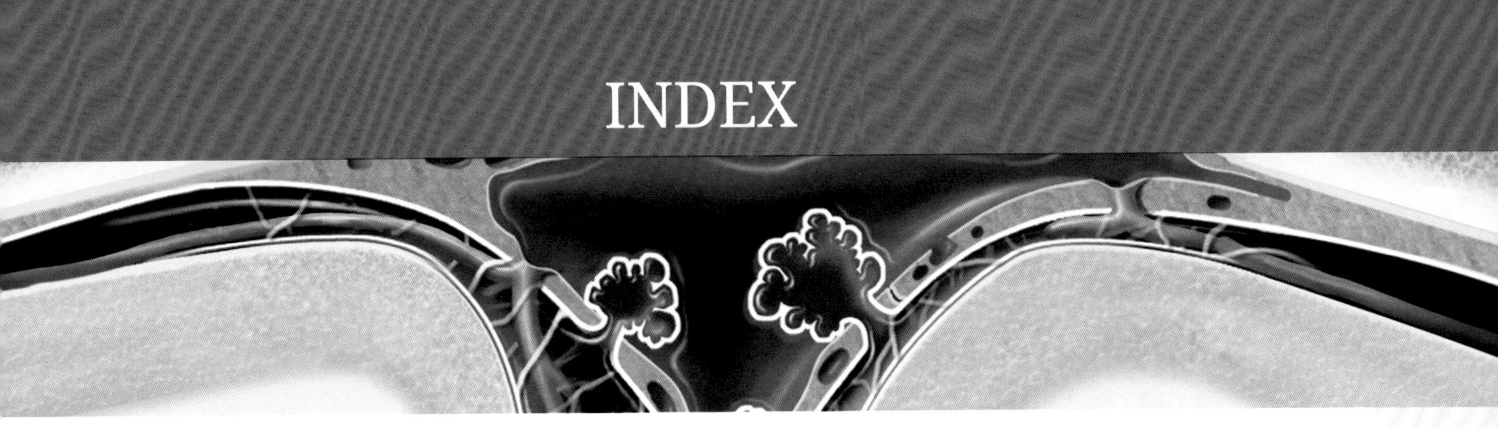

# INDEX

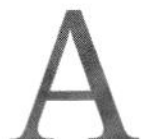

# INDEX

# INDEX

# INDEX

# INDEX



# B

# INDEX

# INDEX

# INDEX

# INDEX

# INDEX

# INDEX

# INDEX

# D

# INDEX



# E

# INDEX

# INDEX

# F

# G

# H

# INDEX

# INDEX

# INDEX



# I

# INDEX

# INDEX



# J



# K



# L

# M

# INDEX

# INDEX



# N

# INDEX

# INDEX

# INDEX



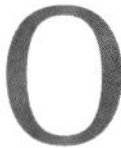

# P

# INDEX

# INDEX

# Q



# R

# S

# INDEX

# INDEX

# INDEX

# INDEX



# U



# V

# INDEX

# W



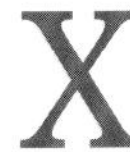

# Y



# Z